P9-CCY-206

WILLARD & SPACKMAN'S
OCCUPATIONAL THERAPY

Tenth Edition

WILLARD & SPACKMAN'S OCCUPATIONAL THERAPY

Elizabeth Blesedell Crepeau, PhD, OTR, FAOTA
Professor
Occupational Therapy Department
School of Health and Human Services
University of New Hampshire
Durham, New Hampshire

Ellen S. Cohn, ScD, OTR, FAOTA
Clinical Associate Professor
Occupational Therapy Department
Sargent College of Health and Rehabilitation Sciences
Boston University
Boston, Massachusetts

Barbara A. Boyt Schell, PhD, OTR, FAOTA
Professor and Chair
Occupational Therapy Department
Brenau University
Gainesville, Georgia

104 Contributors

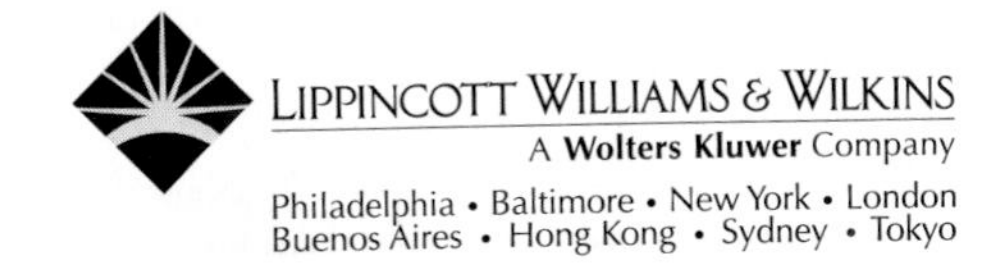

LIPPINCOTT WILLIAMS & WILKINS
A Wolters Kluwer Company
Philadelphia • Baltimore • New York • London
Buenos Aires • Hong Kong • Sydney • Tokyo

Senior Acquisitions Editor: Timothy L. Julet
Managing Editor: David Payne
Marketing Manager: Debby Hartman
Project Editor: Jennifer Ajello
Indexer: Mary Kidd
Designer: Risa Clow
Typesetter: Techbooks
Printer: Quebecor World

530 Walnut Street
Philadelphia, Pennsylvania 19106

351 West Camden Street
Baltimore, Maryland 21201-2436 USA

Printed in the United States of America

Library of Congress Cataloging-in-Publication Data

Willard and Spackman's occupational therapy.—10th ed. / [edited by] Elizabeth Blesedell Crepeau, Ellen S. Cohn, Barbara A. Boyt Schell ; 104 contributors.
p. ; cm.
Includes index.
ISBN 0-7817-2798-7
1. Occupational therapy. I. Title: Occupational therapy. II. Willard, Helen S. III. Crepeau, Elizabeth Blesedell. IV. Cohn, Ellen S., V. Schell, Barbara A. Boyt.
[DNLM: 1. Occupational Therapy. 2. Occupational Therapy—trends. 3. Rehabilitation, Vocational. WB 555 W692 2003]
RM735 .029 2003
615.8'515—dc21 2002031288

To purchase additional copies of this book, call our customer service department at **(800) 638-3030** or fax orders to **(301) 824-7390.** For other book services, including chapter reprints and large quantity sales, ask for the Special Sales department.

For all other calls originating outside of the United States, please call **(301)714-2324.**

***Visit Lippincott Williams & Wilkins on the Internet:* http://www.1ww.com.** Lippincott Williams & Wilkins customer service representatives are available from 8:30 am to 6:00 pm, EST, Monday through Friday, for telephone access.

03 04 05 06 07
1 2 3 4 5 6 7 8 9 10

When citing chapters or sections of chapters from this book, please use the appropriate form. The correct APA format is as follows:

[Chapter author last name, I.] (2003). [Chapter title]. In E. B. Crepeau, E. S. Cohn, & B. A. B. Schell (Eds.), *Willard and Spackman's occupational therapy* (10th ed., pp. x–x). Philadelphia: Lippincott, Williams & Wilkins.

The tools of our minds and the tools of our hands
are of meaningless use without deep and personal reasons of the heart
to set their purpose and guide their use.

PAUL BROCKELMAN

DEDICATION

Maureen Neistadt, ScD, OTR, FAOTA

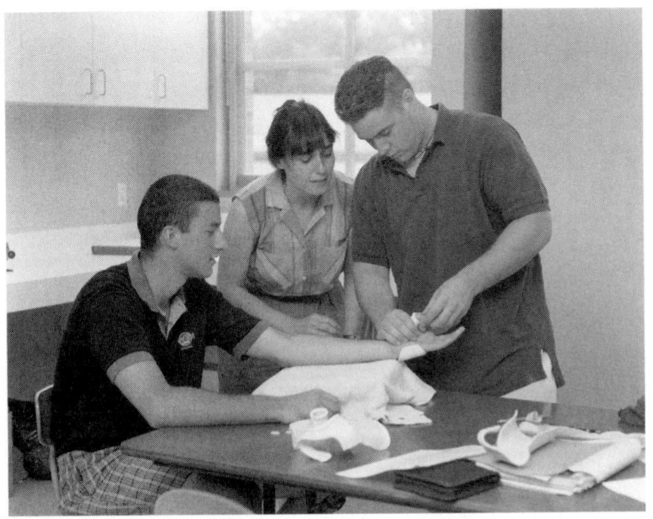
(Courtesy of G. Samson, Photographic Services, University of New Hampshire, Durham, NH.)

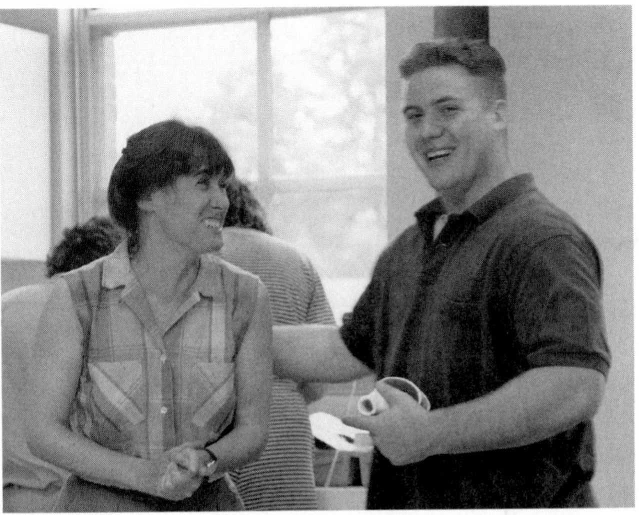
(Courtesy of G. Samson, Photographic Services, University of New Hampshire, Durham, NH.)

Maureen Neistadt was a dedicated teacher, scholar, and generous colleague. She served with Elizabeth Crepeau as co-editor of the ninth edition of *Willard and Spackman* and began the planning for this edition. Her work on *Willard and Spackman* was informed by her commitment to student learning and rigorous scholarship. She was an innovative teacher who enabled students to experience the excitement of inquiry, challenge their assumptions, and push the boundaries of their learning. Students admired her ability to synthesize and clearly explain complex processes. This same clarity was evident in her writing. She made major contributions to the occupational therapy literature on clinical reasoning, the neurobiology of learning for people with cognitive disabilities, and the education of occupational therapy students. Maureen consistently enacted the highest values of the profession. She established and maintained authentic relationships with everyone. Her energy, enthusiasm, and humor were contagious.

Because of these many qualities, we dedicate this book to her memory.

Elizabeth Blesedell Crepeau

Ellen S. Cohn

Barbara A. Boyt Schell

CONTRIBUTORS

Diana M. Bailey, EdD, OTR, FAOTA
Associate Professor
Tufts University—Boston School of Occupational Therapy
Medford, MA

Beverly K. Bain, EdD, OTR, FAOTA
Project Coordinator RSA Technology Grant
New York University
Occupational Therapy Department
New York, NY

Olga Baloueff, ScD, OTR/L, BCP
Associate Professor
Tufts University—Boston School of Occupational Therapy
Medford, MA

Laura Barrett, MS, OTR/L
Associate Director of Rehabilitation
Illinois Department of Human Services
Chicago—Read Mental Health Center
Chicago, IL

Gary M. Bedell, PhD, OT
Postdoctoral Research Fellow
Center for Rehabilitation Effectiveness
Sargent College of Health and Rehabilitation Sciences
Boston University
Boston, MA

David Beer, MA
Associate
Conifer Research
818 Dempster Street
Evanston, IL

Rosmary Bigsby, ScD, OTR/L, FAOTA
Clinical Assistant Professor of Pediatrics
Brown University School of Medicine
Infant Development Unit
Department of Pediatrics
Providence, RI

Cheryl Trautmann Boop, MS, OTR/L
Occupational Therapist
Wee Care Pediatric Rehabilitation/Ty Cobb Healthcare System, Inc.
Royston, GA

Catana Brown, PhD, OTR, FAOTA
Associate Professor
The University of Kansas University Medical Center
Occupational Therapy Education Department
Kansas City, KS

Mary Ellen Buning, PhD, OTR/L, ATP
Assistant Professor
Department of Rehabilitation Science and Technology
School of Health and Rehabilitation Sciences
University of Pittsburgh
Pittsburgh, PA

Ann Burkhardt, MA, OTR/L
Director, Occupational Therapy
NY Presbyterian Hospital
Columbia Presbyterian Center
New York, NY

Florence Clark, PhD, OTR, FAOTA
Professor and Department Chairperson
Department of Occupational Science and Occupational Therapy
University of Southern California
Los Angeles, CA

Barbara Acheson Cooper, PhD
Professor Emeritus
Institute of Applied Health Sciences
School of Rehabilitation Science
McMaster University
Hamilton, ON
Canada

Kathleen Hilko Culler, MS, OTR/L
Research Occupational Therapist
Rehabilitation Institute of Chicago
Chicago, IL

Debora A. Davidson, MS, OTR/L
Assistant Professor
Occupational Therapy Program
Maryville University
St. Louis, MO

Regina Ferraro Doherty, MS, OTR/L
Senior Occupational Therapist
Massachusetts General Hospital
Department of Occupational Therapy
Boston, MA

Cathy Dolhi, MS, OTR/L, FAOTA
Assistant Professor
Occupational Therapy Department
Chatham College
Pittsburgh, PA

Brian J. Dudgeon, PhD, OTR
Assistant Professor
Department of Rehabilitation Medicine
University of Washington
Seattle, WA

Winnie Dunn, PhD, OTR, FAOTA
Professor and Chair
Occupational Therapy Education
University of Kansas University Medical Center
Kansas City, KS

Susan Emerson, MEd, OTR, CHT, CEES
Rehab To Work Medical Consultants
York, ME

Joyce M. Engel, PhD, OTR/L
Associate Professor
Division of Occupational Therapy
Department of Rehabilitation Medicine
University of Washington
Seattle, WA

Cynthia F. Epstein, MA, OTR, FAOTA
Executive Director
Occupational Therapy Consultants, Inc.
Somerset, NJ

Mary Evanofski, OTR/L
Organizational Development Specialist
Dartmouth Hitchcock Medical Center
Lebanon, NH

Mary Evenson, MPH, OTR/L
Academic Fieldwork Coordinator
Tufts University—Boston School of Occupational Therapy
Medford, MA

Mary Feldhaus-Weber
Head Injury Survivor
Jamaica Plain, MA

Sherlyn Fenton, MS, OTR, CWCE
Director of Rehabilitation
OTR Group, Inc.
Holliston, MA

Linda Florey, PhD, OTR, FAOTA
Chief, Rehabilitation Services
University of California at Los Angeles
Neuropsychiatric Institute
Los Angeles, CA

Kirsty Forsyth, PhD, OTR, SROT
Research Specialist
Occupational Therapy Department
University of Illinois at Chicago
Chicago, IL

Patricia Gagnon, OTR/L, CWCE
Operations Manager
The Therapy and Spine Center of Peabody
WorkWELL Occupational Health Services
Peabody, MA

Gordon Muir Giles, PhD, OTR, FAOTA
Associate Professor
Samuel Merritt College
Director of Neurobehavioral Program
Crestwood Behavioral Health, Inc.
Oakland, CA

Clare G. Giuffrida, PhD, OTR/L, FAOTA
Assistant Professor
Occupational Therapy Department
University of Florida
Gainesville, FL

Kathleen Golisz, MA, OTR, BCN
Assistant Professor
Associate Director of Clinical Education
Mercy College
Occupational Therapy Program
Dobbs Ferry, NY

Stephanie Grant, MS, OTR
Bone Works
Gainesville, GA

Lou Ann Sooy Griswold, PhD, OTR/L, FAOTA
Department Chair and Associate Professor
Occupational Therapy Department
School of Health and Human Services
University of New Hampshire
Durham, NH

Ruth Ann Hansen, PhD, FAOTA
Professor and Graduate Coordinator
Occupational Therapy Program
Department of Associated Health Professions
Eastern Michigan University
Ypsilanti, MI

Betty Risteen Hasselkus, PhD, OTR, FAOTA
Emeritus Professor
Occupational Therapy Program
University of Wisconsin at Madison
Madison, WI

Alexis D. Henry, ScD, OTR/L, FAOTA
Assistant Professor
Occupational Therapy Department
Sargent College of Health and Rehabilitation Sciences
Boston University
Boston, MA

Jim Hinojosa, PhD, OT, FAOTA
Professor and Chair
Department of Occupational Therapy
The Steinhardt School of Education
New York University
New York, NY

Margo B. Holm, PhD, OTR/L, FAOTA, ABDA
Professor and Director of Postprofessional Education
Occupational Therapy Department
School of Health and Rehabilitation Sciences
University of Pittsburgh
Pittsburgh, PA

Evelyn G. Jaffe, MPH, OTR, FAOTA
Occupational Therapy Consultant
Maternal and Child Health
Community Mental Health
Tiburon, CA

Anne Birge James, MS, OTR/L
Assistant Professor
Occupational Therapy Department
Division of Health Professions
University of Hartford
West Hartford, CT

Margaret Kaplan, PhD, OTR
Clinical Assistant Professor
Occupational Therapy Program
State University of New York at Downstate
Brooklyn, NY

Gary Kielhofner, DrPH, OTR, FAOTA
Wade/Meyer Chair
Department of Occupational Therapy
University of Illinois at Chicago
Chicago, IL

Kirsten M. Kohlmeyer, MS, OTR/L
Occupational Therapist
Special Education District of Lake Country
Lake Forest, IL

Wendy J. Kraft, OTR/L
Occupational Therapy Department
Healthsouth New England Rehabilitation Hospital
Woburn, MA

Penny Kyler, MA, OTR, FAOTA
Public Health Analyst
Public Health Analyst Genetics Services Branch
Maternal and Child Health Bureau
Rockville, MD

Elizabeth Larson, PhD, OTR
Assistant Professor
Occupational Therapy Program
Department of Kinesiology
University of Wisconsin at Madison
Madison, WI

Mary Law, PhD, OT Reg (C)
Professor and Associate Dean
School of Rehabilitation Science
Institute Applied Health Sciences
McMaster University
Hamilton, ON
Canada

Mary Lawlor, ScD, OTR/L, FAOTA
Associate Professor
Department of Occupational Science and Occupational Therapy
University of Southern California
Los Angeles, CA

Mary Lou Leibold, MS, OTR/L
Assistant Professor
Occupational Therapy Department
Chatham College
Pittsburgh, PA

Lori Letts, MA, OT Reg (Ont)
Assistant Professor
School of Rehabilitation Science
McMaster University
Hamilton, ON
Canada

Kathleen Doyle Lyons, MS, OTR/L
Doctoral Student
Occupational Therapy Department
Sargent College of Health and Rehabilitation Sciences
Boston University
Boston, MA

Elisa Renee Marks, MS, OTR, CHT
Clinical Specialist II—Hand Therapy
Kaiser Permanente—Woodland Hills
Occupational Therapy Department
Wooland Hills, CA

Kimberly D. Marks, MS, OTR/L
Cerebral Palsy Association of Eastern Massachusetts, Inc.
North Shore Infant Toddler Program
Salem, MA

Cheryl Mattingly, PhD
Professor
Department of Occupational Science and Occupational Therapy
Department of Anthropology
University of Southern California
Department of Occupational Therapy
Los Angeles, CA

Linda Haney McClain, PhD, OTR/L, FAOTA
Director of Special Services
Department of Education
Pueblo of Laguna
Division of Early Childhood
Laguna, NM

Susan McDonough, B. App. Sc (OT)
Occupational Therapist
St. Vincent's Mental Health Service
Melbourne, Victoria
Australia

Juli McGruder, PhD, OTR/L
Professor
School of Occupational Therapy and Physical Therapy
University of Puget Sound
Tacoma, WA

Kryss McKenna, PhD, BOccThy (Hons)
Senior Lecturer
Department of Occupational Therapy
University of Queensland
Queensland
Australia

Susan Cook Merrill, MA, OTR/L
Academic Fieldwork Coordinator and Assistant Professor
Occupational Therapy Department
School of Health and Human Services
University of New Hampshire
Durham, NH

Tamara L. Mills, MS, OTR/L
Research Associate
Rehabilitation Science and Technology Department
School of Health and Rehabilitation Sciences
University of Pittsburgh
Pittsburgh, PA

Shelley Mulligan, PhD, OTR/L
Associate Professor
Department of Occupational Therapy
School of Health and Human Services
University of New Hampshire
Durham, NH

Maureen E. Neistadt, ScD, OTR/L, FAOTA
Associate Professor
Occupational Therapy Department
School of Health and Human Services
University of New Hampshire
Durham, New Hampshire

Deborah Pinet O'Mahony, MA, OTR/L
Occupational Therapist
Catholic Medical Center
Manchester, NH

Kenneth Ottenbacher, PhD, OTR, FAOTA
Director
Division of Rehabilitation Sciences
Associate Director
Sealy Center on Aging
University of Texas Medical Branch at Galveston
Galveston, TX

Suzanne M. Peloquin, PhD, OTR, FAOTA
Professor
Department of Occupational Therapy
School of Allied Health Sciences
University of Texas Medical Branch at Galveston
Galveston, TX

Judith M. Perinchief, MS, OTR/L
Assistant Professor
Occupational Therapy Department
Temple University
College of Allied Health Professions
Philadelphia, PA

Greg Pitts, MS, OTR/L CHT
Kentucky Hand and Physical Therapy
Lexington, Kentucky

Michael Pizzi, MS, OTR/L, CHES, FAOTA
Wellness Lifestyle Coach and Consultant
President
Pizzi Wellness and Health Association, Inc.
New York, NY

Janice Miller Polgar, PhD, OT Reg (Ont)
Associate Professor
School of Occupational Therapy
Faculty of Health Sciences
Elborn College
London, ON
Canada

Loree A. Primeau, PhD, OTR, OT (C)
Associate Professor and Chair
Department of Occupational Therapy
School of Allied Health Sciences
University of Texas Medical Branch at Galveston
Galveston, TX

Karen Halliday Pulaski, MS, OTR/L
Occupational Therapist
Moses Cone Memorial Hospital
Greensboro, NC

Patricia J. Rigby, MHSc OT Reg (Ont)
Assistant Professor and Graduate Coordinator
Department of Occupational Therapy
Faculty of Medicine
University of Toronto
Toronto, ON
Canada

Elizabeth A. Rivers, MA, OTR/L, RN
Retired Burn Rehabilitation Specialist
Regions Medical Center
St. Paul, MN

Pamela Roberts, MSHA, OTR
Quality Practice Coordinator
Cedars-Sinai Medical Center
West Los Angeles, CA

Joan C. Rogers, PhD, OTR/L, FAOTA, ABDA
Professor and Chair
Occupational Therapy Department
School of Health and Rehabilitation Sciences
University of Pittsburgh
Pittsburgh, PA

Graham David Rowles, PhD
Professor of Geography and Director
Sanders-Brown Center on Aging
University of Kentucky
Lexington, KY

Mary Sands, MS Ed, OTR, FAOTA
Professor Emeritus
Occupational Therapy Assistant Department
Orange County Community College
Middletown, NY

Janette K. Schkade, PhD, OTR
Dean
School of Occupational Therapy
Texas Woman's University
School of Occupational Therapy
Denton, TX

Mark R. Schmeler, MS, OTR/L, ATP
Director
Center for Assistive Technology
University of Pittsburgh Medical Center Health System
Pittsburgh, PA

Jodi Schreiber, MS, OTR/L
Independent Occupational Therapy Consultant
Pittsburgh, PA

Sally Schultz, PhD, OTR
Professor and Coordinator of Graduate Programs
School of Occupational Therapy
Texas Woman's University
Denton, TX

Kathleen Barker Schwartz, EdD, OTR, FAOTA
Professor
Occupational Therapy Department
San Jose State University
San Jose, CA

Sharan L. Schwartzberg, EdD, OTR, FAOTA
Professor and Chair
Tufts University–Boston School of Occupational Therapy
Medford, MA

Alice C. Seidel, EdD, OTR/L
Associate Professor
Occupational Therapy Department
School of Health and Human Services
University of New Hampshire
Durham, NH

Alice Shafer, MS, OTR/L, FAOTA
Principal Consultant
ASCA Consulting Group
Wayland, MA

Elizabeth R Skidmore, MS, OTR/L
Research Associate
University of Pittsburgh
Occupational Therapist
University of Pittsburgh Medical Center
Pittsburgh, PA

Pat Sue Spear, OTR/L
Occupational Therapist
Richie MacFarland Children's Center
Stratham, NH

Elinor Anne Spencer, MA, OTR/L, FAOTA
Occupational Therapist and Consultant
Calais Regional Hospital
Calais, ME

Jean Cole Spencer, PhD, OTR, FAOTA
Professor
School of Occupational Therapy
Texas Women's University
Houston, TX

Debra Stewart, MSc, OT Reg (Ont)
Assistant Clinical Professor
School of Rehabilitation Science
McMaster University
Hamilton, ON
Canada

Ronald G. Stone, MS, OTR/L
Professor
University of Puget Sound
Occupational Therapy
Tacoma, WA

Susan Strong, MSc OT Reg (Ont)
Assistant Clinical Professor
School of Rehabilitation Science
Institute of Applied Health Sciences
McMaster University
Hamilton, ON
Canada

Barbara Biggs Sussenberger, MS, OTR
Associate Professor
Occupational Therapy Department
School of Health and Human Services
University of New Hampshire
Durham, NH

Yvonne L. Swinth, PhD, OTR/L
Associate Professor
School of Occupational and Physical Therapy
University of Puget Sound
Tacoma, WA

Joan Pascale Toglia, MA, OTR
Associate Professor and Program Director
Occupational Therapy Department
Mercy College
Dobbs Ferry, NY

Robin Underwood, MS, OTR/L
Academic Fieldwork Coordinator and Assistant Professor
Occupational Therapy Department
Brenau University
Gainesville, GA

Judith D. Ward, PhD, OTR/L
Associate Professor
Occupational Therapy Department
School of Health and Human Services
University of New Hampshire
Durham, NH

Janet Waylett-Rendall, OTR, CHT
Rehab Technology Works
San Bernadino, CA

Barbara Prudhomme White, PhD, OTR/L
Assistant Professor
Occupational Therapy Department
School of Health and Human Services
University of New Hampshire
Durham, NH

Ann A. Wilcock, PhD, DipCOT, BAppScOT, GradDipPH
Associate Professor
Occupational Therapy
University of South Australia
Adelaide, South Australia
Australia

Wendy Wood, PhD, OTR/L, FAOTA
Associate Professor
Division of Occupational Science
Department of Allied Health Sciences
Medical School
Chapel Hill, NC

Elizabeth J. Yerxa, EdD, LHD(hon), ScD(hon), OTR, FAOTA
Distinguished Professor Emerita
Department of Occupational Science and Occupational Therapy
University of Southern California
Los Angeles, CA

Mary Jane Youngstrom, MS, OTR, FAOTA
Clinical Instructor
Occupational Therapy Education
University of Kansas Medical Center
Kansas City, KS

PREFACE

Willard and Spackman's Occupational Therapy has a long tradition that extends back to the 1st edition published in 1947. Helen Willard and Clare Spackman, colleagues who taught together at the Occupational Therapy Program at the University of Pennsylvania, co-edited the 1st through 4th editions. They turned the editorial responsibilities over to Helen Hopkins and Helen Smith, faculty members at Temple University and Tufts University, respectively. Hopkins and Smith edited the 5th through the 8th editions. Maureen Neistadt and Elizabeth Crepeau edited the 9th edition.

We have revised and updated the 10th edition to reflect the changes in knowledge in occupational therapy and occupational science in the past 5 years. This edition retains much of the basic organizational structure established in the 9th edition, an approach that focused on questions students want to know about occupational therapy and the people who seek occupational therapy.

Unit I addresses the history of the field, the emerging discipline of occupational science, and occupational therapy practice today and in the future. Unit II is concerned with the people who seek and receive our services—who they are as individuals embedded in cultural, socioeconomic, and family systems. Students want to learn about their occupational therapy colleagues and what they will be doing together.

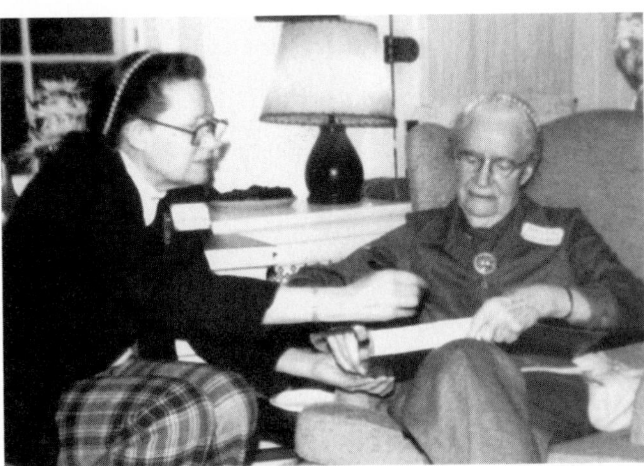

Ms. Clare Spackman and Ms. Helen Willard autographing the 5th edition of Occupational Therapy. (Courtesy of the Archives of the American Occupational Therapy Association, Inc. Bethesda, MD.)

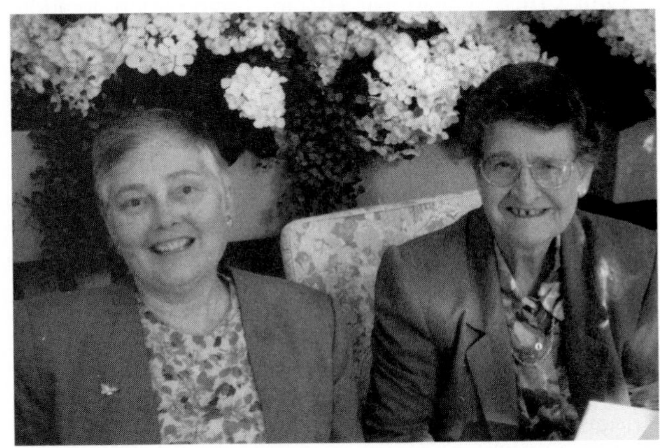

Dr. Helen Hopkins and Ms. Helen Smith, editors of the 5th through 8th editions of Willard and Spackman's Occupational Therapy. (Courtesy of H. Hopkins.)

Unit III begins to answer these questions with a discussion of the roles of occupational therapists and occupational therapy assistants, the clinical reasoning process, and professional development. Units IV and V provide in-depth analyses of therapeutic relationships and occupational and activity analysis, all of which are key to occupational therapy evaluation and intervention. Subsequent units further articulate aspects of the role of occupational therapy practitioners. Unit VI delineates the conceptual bases of practice. Units VII and VIII address occupational therapy evaluation and intervention. Units IX and X describe the specific diagnoses or problems that bring people to occupational therapy. Finally, Units XI and XII discuss issues related to working in various practice arenas, ethics, research, and challenges for the future.

The 10th edition has many new chapters and features. In Unit I, Ann Wilcock argues for an expansion of services to include a public health focus to occupational therapy. Unit II, Persons Seeking Occupational Therapy, includes new chapters on spirituality and the meaning of place. These chapters distill current literature about these important topics that have not been addressed extensively in occupational therapy texts. We are delighted to have 16 color plates of Mary Feldhaus-Weber's paintings and mixed media that chronicle her recovery from a head trauma. Her chapter has been expanded to describe her life since the previous edition of the book; thus it provides a 20-year perspective on the ongoing recovery of a head injury survivor.

Unit III, focusing on occupational therapy practitioners, now includes a chapter on professional development considerations for occupational therapy practitioners. Because of the centrality of occupational behavior perspectives we have more extensive coverage of these in Unit VI, Conceptual Basis for Practice. We have also included the person–environment–occupation frame of reference articulated by Mary Law and her colleagues in Canada. Unit VII, Occupational Therapy Evaluation, now includes chapters that address evaluation of educational activities and communication and interaction skills and socioemotional factors.

Unit VIII, Occupational Therapy Intervention, in addition to the revised content, now addresses childrearing and caregiving, education, and community integration as well as manual wheelchairs, seating, and positioning. Unit X, Diagnostic Considerations in Adult and Older Adult Practice, now includes a chapter on interventions for people with serious mental illness.

All of the evaluation and intervention units have been revised to demonstrate more explicitly how the client's occupational interests and concerns are integrated into the therapy process. In addition, there is an expansion of coverage to address the broad range of settings, including education-based, community-based, and medically-based programs. Unit XI, Issues in Service Provision, includes a chapter that delineates consultation and program development. Another chapter examines the ethical and legal responsibilities of practitioners working with vulnerable populations, a concern that has had little attention in occupational therapy literature. The research chapter in Unit XII has been completely revised. This new chapter describes how to examine research literature critically and the value of evidence-based practice. We feel that mastery of the research competencies delineated in Unit XII form the basis for an introduction to research and the research process.

This edition adopts the new terminology of the International Classification of Function (formerly known as ICIDH-2) and the Occupational Therapy Practice Framework (from the American Occupational Therapy Association). One of the most notable and—from a practical perspective—vexing challenges was this changing terminology. The evolution of the Occupational Therapy Practice Framework through various drafts paralleled our editorial work on *Willard and Spackman*. We struggled to keep pace with these changes as the book evolved.

Because we are aware of the power of language to influence the way we think, we have attempted to be as inclusive as possible in descriptors of individuals. Consequently, to the extent possible we used the term occupational therapy practitioner to represent the certified occupational therapist and certified occupational therapy assistant. We have tried to avoid language that reflects bias and labels people with disabilities. We have used nonmedical model language to the extent that this was appropriate. As in the 9th edition, we have struggled with terminology that refers to the individual who seeks occupational therapy—be that a patient, client, consumer, or student.

Throughout the text are special features that expand and extend the text of the chapter. In addition to case studies and case analyses, the reader will find research, ethics, and historical notes. A new feature, "What's a Practitioner to Do?" presents practice dilemmas for students to consider. Many of these features pose questions for student reflection and discussion. The appendices now include a table describing commonly used assessments and their sources. The appendices also include examples of Web sites useful to occupational therapy practitioners and the people who seek our services.

We are grateful to our many colleagues who have given us feedback about the 9th edition and their hopes for the 10th edition. Our efforts have been to create a book that reflects the best aspects of our field—and that reflects positively on the former editors and contributors. Their contributions to previous editions of *Willard and Spackman*, and to the knowledge base of occupational therapy and occupational science created the foundation upon which this text is based. It is our hope that this edition honors the past and provides a pathway to future generations of occupational therapy practitioners.

ACKNOWLEDGMENTS

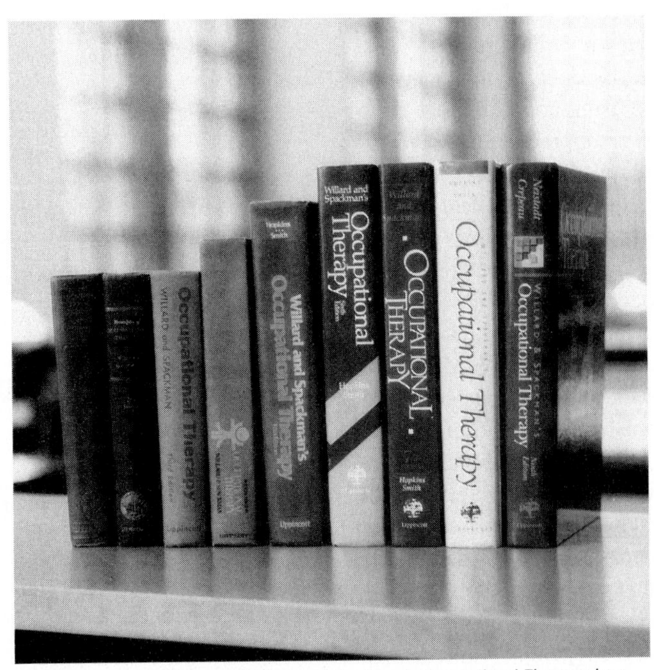

The nine previous editions of Willard and Spackman's Occupational Therapy show the expansion of knowledge in the field. (Courtesy of L. Nugent, Photographic Services, University of New Hampshire, Durham.)

Planning began for the 10th edition of *Willard and Spackman* during the winter of 1998–1999, 1 year after the 9th edition was released.

At that time, Maureen was recovering from a year of multiple surgeries and a round of chemotherapy for ovarian cancer. She and Betty approached the planning of this edition with every hope and expectation that they would edit the book together. Sadly, this did not occur. Maureen's cancer returned in December 1999. Over the next 6 months, it became clear that she would not have the strength to maintain an active editorial role. In June, Betty and Maureen discussed additional editors and recruited Ellen Cohn and Barbara Schell to join the editorial team. Betty, Ellen, and Barb began working during that summer as Maureen continued bravely to fight the cancer that took her life on September 22, 2000. Since that time, Maureen's spirit has infused and supported our work together. It is our hope that this edition reflects her vision and spirit.

One of the more exciting aspects of editing a major text in the field has been to see its transformation over the past 5 years. We have new research advancing our knowledge of occupation and occupational therapy and new terminology to express this knowledge. The field seems to be changing in front of our eyes, and, in fact, the terminology did continue to change through various drafts of the Practice Framework, which we were trying to incorporate into the book. As the chapters came in, these changes virtually marched across our desks. Our weekly conference calls, while sometimes filled with the mundane details associated with a task such as this, were more often dominated by our excitement of seeing the book unfold before us.

We believe we have been involved in what Jonsson, Josephsson, and Kielhofner called an engaging occupation. This is a concept that emerged from their study of the experience of retirement, but we feel that it applies just as well to our occupation of editing *Willard and Spackman*. The editorial role requires great commitment, intensity, and responsibility, much like the engaging occupations Jonsson and his colleagues described. Moreover, the editorial challenges are matched by great enjoyment and pleasure, particularly in the relationships we have developed with the contributors, the personnel at Lippincott, Williams & Wilkins, and everyone else who has worked with us on this book. The rewards of this process and the meaning we derive from it stem largely from these relationships, which Jonsson, Josephsson, and Kielhofner would call an occupational community. We would like to thank the many people in our occupational community for their role in making this book a reality.

Our experience of working together has brought us renewed appreciation for the value of collaborative effort. This work has been characterized by deep commitment to the task before us, a willingness to listen and challenge each other's thinking, and the capacity to appreciate the particular strengths that each of us brings to the process. We have supported each other during our grief, and have learned the value of a common commitment to the healing process. Many times, we have invoked Maureen's spirit to provide her wisdom and great humor. Beyond our "Willie Work," our weekly conference calls invariably included discussions of our families, pets, gardens, and cooking. We discussed movies, books, our perennial flower beds, and magnolias on a regular basis—as well as admonishing each other to take time away from the book to engage in our other valued occupations. It is our hope that this collaborative effort will continue the tradition established by the previous editors of this text and honor their many contributions to the field.

Our families—husbands, children, and grandchildren—put up with our preoccupations. Ellen's children helped us all keep this task in perspective; Maggie repeatedly asked "Are you done?" and Adrienne repeatedly asked to use the computer so she could "IM" her friends. Eve, Barb's dog routinely reminded her when it was time to take an exercise break. Betty's cats, George and Fluffy, continued to interrupt her work, looking for attention and for her assistance in letting them in or out. We are incredibly fortunate to have loving and understanding husbands—Rod, Larry, and John—who supported our work on the book while maintaining the texture of life in our homes, and mostly with good humor about the sheer volume of editing *Willard and Spackman*.

We are especially honored and privileged to have worked closely with 104 contributors who shared their vision of occupation therapy. All are deeply committed to articulating the art and science of occupational therapy. For that, we thank them. We thank the following people who assisted us in the preparation of this book:

PHOTOGRAPHS AND HISTORICAL DOCUMENTS

- John Adams, Gary Samson, Ron Bergeron, and Doug Prince, Lisa Nugent, and Beverly Conway: University of New Hampshire Photographic Services Department, Durham, NH.
- Mary Binderman: Wilma West Library, American Occupational Therapy Foundation, Bethesda, MD.
- Elaine Chu and Karen Jacobs: Occupational Therapy Department, Sargent College, Boston University, Boston, MA.
- Kindra Clineff and the staff and members of Steppingstones, Portsmouth, NH.
- Regina Ferraro Doherty: Massachusetts General Hospital, Boston, MA.
- Cheryl Harmeling and Occupational Therapy Associates: Watertown, MA.
- Lucia Grochowska Littlefield and Deborah Amani: Sargent College GKM Instructional Resource Center, Boston University, Boston, MA.
- Kenneth Ottenbacher University of Texas Medical Branch, Galveston, TX.
- Maggie Paine: *University of New Hampshire Magazine*.
- John Schell: University of Georgia, Athens.

SECRETARIAL AND ADMINISTRATIVE SUPPORT

- Christine Diaz and Alice Vosburg: Occupational Therapy Department, University of New Hampshire, Durham, NH.
- Elly Leary: formerly of the Occupational Therapy Department, Boston University, Boston, MA.
- Donna Rinaldi and Meg Trafton: Dover Secretarial Services, Dover, NH.

PROFESSIONAL COLLEAGUES AND STUDENTS

With gratitude and appreciation, we acknowledge our faculty colleagues at the University of New Hampshire, Boston University, and Brenau University for their assistance, support, insightful feedback, and willingness to listen to endless conversations about *Willard and Spackman*. In particular, we would like to thank the following individuals:

BOSTON UNIVERSITY

- Sue Berger and Nancy Lowenstein and their students.
- Meaghan Callahan and Emily Nielson, class of 2002.
- Wendy Coster, Alexis Henry, Deane McCraith, and Linda Tickle-Degnen.

UNIVERSITY OF NEW HAMPSHIRE

- Becky Alwood and Stacey Lehrer, occupational therapy students.
- Classes of 2002 and 2003.
- Lou Ann Griswold, Douglas Simmons, Susan Merrill, Barbara Prudhomme White, Raelene Shippee-Rice, and Cinthia Gannett.

BRENAU UNIVERSITY

- Jennifer Moody class of 2003.
- Ahlem Selme, Fulbright Scholar, University of Georgia.
- Classes of 2004 and 2005.
- Robin Underwood, Sara Brayman, and John White.
- Helen Ray.

LIPPINCOTT, WILLIAMS & WILKINS

Current and former Lippincott, Williams & Wilkins personnel have provided consistent assistance and support:

- Administrative support: Amy Amico, Natalie Casp, Frank Musick, Erin Seifert.
- Editorial personnel: Margaret Biblis, Tim Julet, Susan Katz , Ulita Lushnycky, David Payne, Nancy Peterson.

REVIEWERS

We are grateful to the reviewers who critiqued the book proposal and new chapters in this edition. They provided us with helpful feedback that has resulted in a stronger book. A number of reviewers wished to remain anonymous and are not listed below.

- Judith E. Bowen, MPA, OTR
  Occupational Therapy Department
  University of Texas—Pan American
  Edinburg, TX
- Linda DiJoseph, MS, OTR, FAOTA, BCN
  Occupational Therapy Department
  Gannon University
  Erie, PA
- Gwendolyn Gray, MA, OTR/L
  Occupational Therapy Program
  Tuskegee University
  Tuskegee, AL
- Cynthia Haynes, MEd, OTR/L
  Occupational Therapy Department
  Philadelphia University
  Philadelphia, PA
- Tracy Jirikowic, PhD
  Special Education/Rehabilitation Medicine
  University of Washington
  Seattle, WA
- Lindsey J. Lawrence, BGS, COTA/L
  Occupational Therapy Assistant Program
  Jefferson Community College
  Louisville, KY
- Sue Leicht, MS, OTR/L, BCN
  Occupational Therapy Department
  Ithaca College
  Ithaca, NY
- Mary A. Matteliano, MS, OTR/L
  Occupational Therapy Department
  University at Buffalo, State University of New York
  Buffalo, NY
- Gail F. Metzger, MS, OTR/L
  Occupational Therapy Department
  Alvernia College
  Reading, PA
- Ann Moscony, MA, OTR/L, CHT
  Pain Relief and Physical Therapy
  Philadelphia University
  Media, PA
- Teresa Norris, PhD, OTR
  Occupational Therapy Department
  University of Tennessee at Chattanooga
  Chattanooga, TN
- S. Maggie Reitz, PhD, OTR/L, FAOTA
  Occupational Therapy & Occupational Sciences
  Towson University
  Towson, MD
- Barbara G. Sarbaugh, MA, OTR/L
  Department of Occupational Therapy
  Xavier University
  Cincinnati, OH
- Patricia Schaber, MA, OTR/L
  Program in Occupational Therapy
  University of Minnesota
  Minneapolis, MN

BRIEF CONTENTS

CONTENTS

RECURRING DISPLAYS

HISTORICAL NOTES

RESEARCH NOTES

WHAT'S A PRACTITIONER TO DO?

ETHICS NOTES

CASE STUDIES

LIFE ISSUES TO CONSIDER IN PRACTICE

BOXES

CASE ANALYSIS

WILLARD & SPACKMAN'S OCCUPATIONAL THERAPY

UNIT *one*

Occupational Therapy and Occupational Science: Past, Present, and Future

Learning Objectives

After completing this unit, readers will be able to:

- Identify the confluence of movements that fostered the founding of occupational therapy and explain how this history provided the moral and philosophical grounding for occupational science.
- Delineate beliefs that have persevered throughout the profession's history concerning the relation of occupation to adaptation.
- Explain how occupational therapy's history has contributed to the opportunities and challenges that practitioners face today.
- Define the academic discipline of occupational science and describe the ways occupational science has fostered change in the practice of occupational therapy.
- Define occupational therapy and its scope of practice today.
- Discuss the future role of occupational therapy in promoting health for all.

Occupational therapy has a rich history that continues to influence the evolution of the field and its related academic discipline, occupational science. These chapters review this history and show how our past continues to challenge and inspire us. The opening chapter reviews our history, most especially major turning points in the focus and philosophy of the field. The second chapter delineates the development of occupational science, its influence on education and practice, and the major findings of its research. The last chapter opens with a brief overview of contemporary occupational therapy practice and identifies major themes addressed throughout this volume. The unit closes with a challenging call to contribute to the development of a public health perspective for occupational therapy that is concerned about the health of all citizens. (*Note:* Words in **bold** type are defined in the Glossary.)

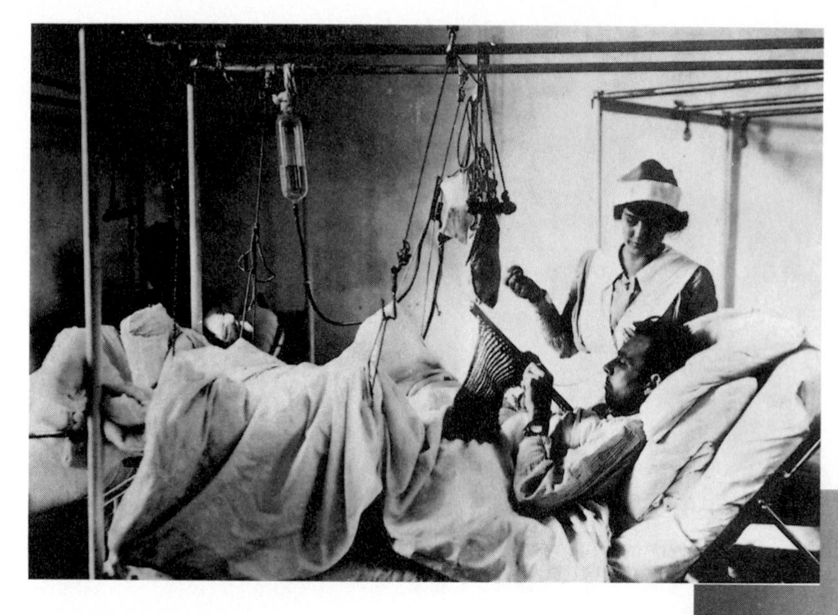

Occupational therapy intervention has evolved in response to changes in health care. (Photos courtesy of the archives of the American Occupational Therapy Association, Inc., Bethesda, MD.) (*top*) Bedside occupational therapy during World War I: Miss Hitchcock; a reconstruction aide; and Corporal Lane, patient—Base Hospital, Charearoux, France. (*middle*) Winifred Conrick Kahmann working with children at the James Whitcomb Riley Hospital for Children. Kahmann, a leader in the field for many years, founded occupational therapy programs at Riley Hospital and the Long Hospital for Adults, the Indiana Occupational Therapy Association in 1936, and the Occupational Therapy and Physical Therapy Programs at the Indiana School of Medicine in 1958. She served as the first occupational therapist to be elected president of the American Occupational Therapy Association in the early 1950s. (*bottom*) Occupational therapy in the 1970s involved the use of facilitation techniques to support movement and assumed that improved performance would naturally follow. Today, there is increased understanding of the importance of embedding such techniques within activities that are directly connected to the occupational interests and motivations of individual clients.

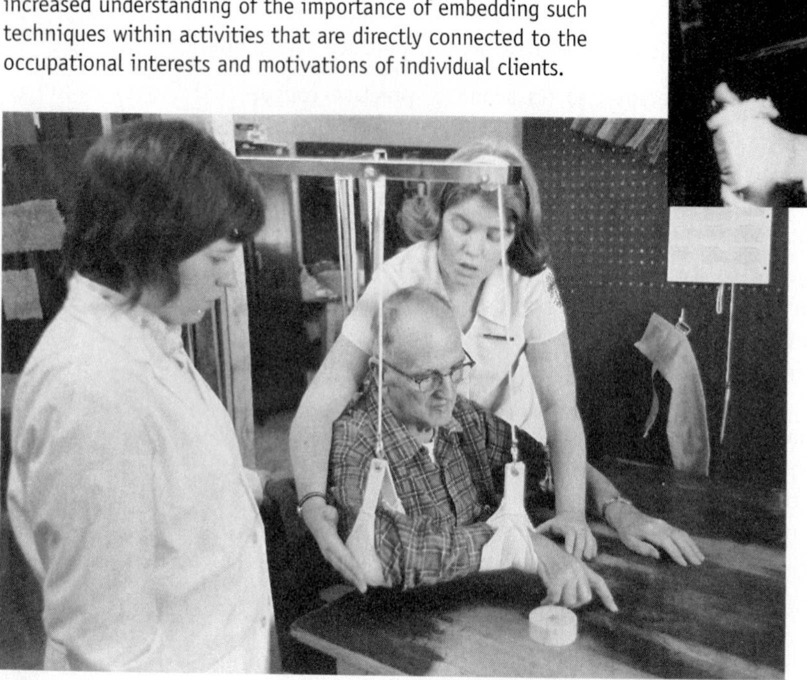

CHAPTER 1

THE HISTORY OF OCCUPATIONAL THERAPY

KATHLEEN BARKER SCHWARTZ

William Rush Dunton (1947) wrote the history of occupational therapy for the first edition of *Willard and Spackman's Occupational Therapy*. As the profession enters the twenty-first century, it is an honor to follow in Dunton's illustrious footsteps. This history describes the evolution of the profession from its inception in 1917 to today and examines the ideals and leadership that have helped shape its development.

THE FOUNDING IDEALS

The Founders

The individuals who gathered together in Clifton Springs, New York, on March 17, 1917, to found the National Society for the Promotion of Occupational Therapy (NSPOT; later renamed the American Occupational Therapy Association, AOTA) were drawn together by a strong belief in the therapeutic value of occupations. Because they came from a variety of professional backgrounds and experiences they created a vision of occupational therapy far richer and more complex than if they had been of the same discipline. The five founders attending the meeting were William Rush Dunton Jr., Eleanor Clarke Slagle, George Edward Barton, Susan Cox Johnson, and Thomas Bessell Kidner. Although Susan E. Tracy and Herbert James Hall did not attend, they have been described as near founders (Peloquin, 1991) because of their leadership in promoting occupations.

Dunton, frequently referred to as the Father of Occupational Therapy, was a leading advocate of occupational therapy through his prolific writing and numerous professional presentations. Dunton was a psychiatrist who initially became convinced of the value of occupation through his work as supervisor of the occupation classes at Sheppard Pratt Hospital in Maryland. He proposed that occupational therapy represented a continuation of the **moral treatment** approach to the mentally ill introduced in the previous

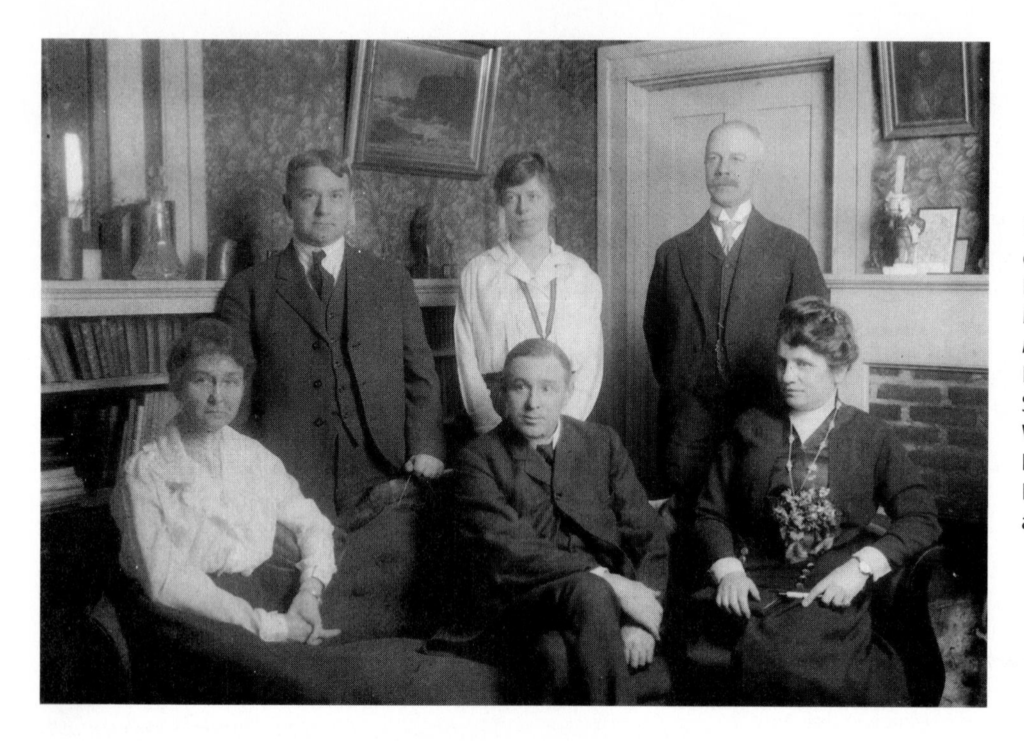

FIGURE 1–1. The founders of occupational therapy at Consolation House, Clifton Springs, New York, March 1917. Front row (*left to right*): Susan Cox Johnson, George Edward Barton, and Eleanor Clarke Slagle. Back row (*left to right*): William Rush Dunton, Isabelle Newton, and Thomas Bessell Kidner. (Photo courtesy of the archives of AOTA, Bethesda, MD.)

century (Dunton, 1917). As Dunton was the profession's father, Slagle was its mother. Slagle was a welfare worker first attracted to the therapeutic value of occupation through her association with Julia Lathrop and Jane Addams of Hull House. Later as director of occupational therapy at Phipps Clinic, she implemented **habit training** as a way to structure engagement in occupations for the seriously mentally ill (Slagle, 1924). Slagle became legendary for the political and administrative expertise she demonstrated as executive secretary of the AOTA, a position she held for 15 years.

Barton, the host of the founding meeting, was an architect who came to understand the value of occupation through his own efforts to cure himself of tuberculosis and paralysis. As an embodiment of his conception of a proper healing environment, Barton created Consolation House—a school, workshop, and vocational bureau—from a small house and barn in Clifton Springs, New York. It was a place where individuals could engage in occupations to strengthen their bodies, clarify their minds, and discover "a new life upon recovery" (Barton, 1920, p. 307). Barton lived only until 1923, but Consolation House remains his legacy to occupational therapy.

Johnson was a former arts and crafts teacher who became director of occupation at Montefiore Hospital in New York and lecturer at Columbia Teachers College. She was a strong advocate for the use of handcrafts in occupational therapy as a way to help individuals regain self-confidence, redirect their thoughts, and strengthen their bodies through the use of graded physical exercise (Johnson, 1920). Kidner was vocational secretary to the Canadian Military Hospitals and a former architect. He was an ardent supporter of the use of occupations in prevocational rehabilitation and proposed the creation of the "preindustrial shop" as a way for convalescent soldiers to return to work or acquire a new vocation (Fig. 1-1) (Kidner, 1925, p. 188).

The Philosophy of Occupational Therapy

Dunton (1917) traced the roots of occupational therapy back to the philosophical movement known as moral treatment, which originated in Europe in the nineteenth century. In France, Philippe Pinel (1809, p. 260) proposed a "*revolution morale*" to replace the view that individuals with mental illness were dangerous, were incurable, and should be locked away with a **humanitarian** approach of kindness and a regimen of daily life that consisted of creative and recreational occupations to restore mental health. Moral treatment hospitals in the United States, such as Friend's Asylum in Pennsylvania and McLean Hospital in Massachusetts, were equipped with craft shops and garden and recreational areas to promote occupational engagement. The treatment programs at Sheppard Pratt Asylum were still influenced by moral treatment when, in 1902, Dunton was appointed assistant physician and supervisor of occupation classes. Dunton clearly saw the connection, and at the founding meeting, he proposed that moral treatment could be described in philosophy and practice as a comprehensive occupational therapy program (Bockoven, 1971).

Adolph Meyer (1922), a professor of psychiatry at Johns Hopkins University and a mentor of Dunton's and Slagle's, took the ideas fundamental to moral treatment and built on them to create his own philosophy of occupation therapy. To the humanitarian approach of moral treatment and its occupational regimen, Meyer added the idea that mental

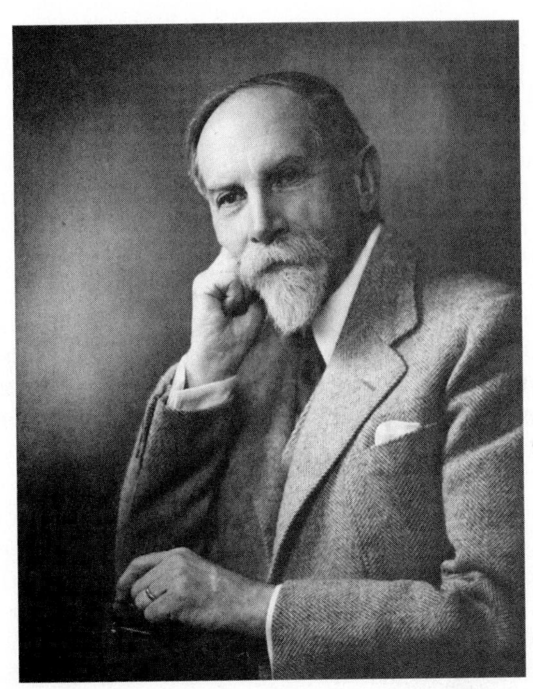

FIGURE 1–2. Adolf Meyer, renowned psychobiologist and author of *The Philosophy of Occupation Therapy* (1922). (Photo courtesy of the archives of AOTA, Bethesda, MD.)

illness was largely a problem of adaptation, habit deterioration, and lack of balance of work and play. The solution he proposed included habit training, as exemplified by the programs run by Slagle, and therapeutic programs designed to provide opportunities for engaging in occupations that were pleasurable, creative, and educational (Fig. 1-2).

The Art of Occupational Therapy

In the early 1900s, creative arts and crafts had become popular as a result of the Arts and Crafts movement that originated in England with William Morris and John Ruskin. The movement sought to ameliorate the negative effects of industrialization by advocating a return to a simpler life in which the body and mind could be engaged in occupations that yielded fine hand-crafted objects (Boris, 1986).

The founders of occupational therapy recognized the therapeutic value of the creative, pleasurable experience that handcrafts provided. The occupation program Tracy (1910, p. 7) created at Adams Nervine Asylum in Boston engaged patients in the weaving of "rugs and finer fabrics, basket work, bookbinding and clay modeling." The occupation classes Dunton supervised at Sheppard Pratt included weaving, art, metalwork, and bookbinding (Fields, 1911). Under the supervision of Slagle at Phipps Clinic, "groups of patients with raffia and basket work, or with various kinds of handiwork and weaving and bookbinding and metal and leather work took the place of the bored wall flowers and mischief-makers" (Meyer, 1922, p. 3). Johnson (1920, p. 69), the former arts and crafts teacher, clearly recognized the creative value handcrafts had in occupational therapy:

> *Handcrafts have a special therapeutic value as they afford occupation that combines the elements of play and recreation with work and accomplishment. They give a concrete return and provide a stimulus to mental activity and muscular exercise at the same time, and afford an opportunity for creation and self-expression.*

The Science of Occupational Therapy

At the time the profession was founded, it was a popular belief that science could be used to reform all of society's ills, including poverty, poor education, corrupt city politics, and inefficient business practices (Taylor, 1911). Indeed scientific discoveries in the twentieth century had resulted in vastly improved medical care compared to the disorganized, unsanitary conditions prevalent in hospitals in the previous century.

The founders recognized the importance of being able to establish the effectiveness of occupational therapy scientifically if the profession was going to be well recognized. Barton (c. 1920) proposed that time and motion studies might provide a model for occupational therapy research. Dunton (1928) led an effort to analyze occupations systematically. He also tried to address two problems that could inhibit research in occupational therapy: funding and methodology. He proposed the creation of a foundation to sponsor research in occupational therapy. "To the present it has not been possible to make any grants for research, and all that has been done has been by the self sacrifice of individuals" (NSPOT, c. 1923, p. 3). Regarding methodology, he recognized that it was not easy to study the therapeutic effects of occupation on individuals, because the medium and process were complex and therefore difficult to reduce to the discreet variables required by the existing research paradigm.

> *[We] are unable to present the results of research because psychologists have not yet given us the formulae for judging the emotional effect of pounding a copper disk into a nut dish. . . . In other words, we lack a quick and snappy means of measuring the emotions (Dunton, 1934, p. 325).*

He advocated that occupational therapists look beyond the current research models.

Summary

The founders' conception of occupational therapy was guided by a **humanistic** philosophy that recognized the full complexity of the individual and the therapeutic process that would enable individuals to adapt to the "problems of living" (Meyer, 1922, p. 4). They also acknowledged the importance of developing a science of occupation to establish the profession's legitimate place within the medical disciplines. The founders defined the use of occupation broadly, to include habit training, handcrafts, graded physical exercise, and the preindustrial shop. Although each founder emphasized a different aspect of the benefits of occupation, they all shared the belief that meaningful engagement in occupation was the key to creating a healthy body and mind.

EXPANSION AND SPECIALIZATION

The World Wars and the Rehabilitation Movement

According to Dunton (1947), World War I provided the impetus for the founding of NSPOT in 1917. NSPOT served as a clearing house for information on reconstruction aides and monitored the emergency training programs that were organized in Boston, New York, and Milwaukee. Ultimately, 1200 reconstruction aides provided bedside occupations to wounded soldiers at hospital bases in Europe. They were praised by the Surgeon General's Office as being "worth their weight in gold" (Quiroga, 1995, p. 164).

After World War I, the development of occupational therapy was relatively slow until the United States entered World War II in 1941. The demand for trained personnel greatly increased, with the military hospitals alone needing more occupational therapists than existed in the entire country (Dunton, 1947). This prompted the development of new educational programs, so that by 1945 there were 21 programs and 3224 occupational therapists (Arestad & Westmoreland, 1946).

Recent scientific discoveries resulted in much higher survival rates for the wounded than were seen during World War I, and the focus in occupational therapy shifted from bedside handcrafts such as basketry and weaving to more functional, job-related occupations such as carpentry (Fig. 1-3). The newly created departments of physical medicine and rehabilitation in Veterans Administration hospitals produced a high demand for occupational therapists who could treat physically impaired soldiers. After the war, the need for rehabilitation services continued to grow, stimulated by the Rehabilitation Act of 1954. Comprehensive rehabilitation centers were built in the private sector using the interdisciplinary model of the Veteran's Administration system. Howard Rusk, head of rehabilitation and physical medicine at New York University, called attention to the shortage of rehabilitation personnel, including occupational therapists, needed to work with the "5,300,000 persons in the nation who suffer from chronic disability" (Lack of Trained Personnel, 1954). The passage of Medicare legislation in 1965 further increased the demand for occupational therapy services to meet the needs of the aged, chronically ill, and disabled.

Specialization

By the 1960s, the profession of occupational therapy had two distinct specialty areas—physical disabilities and psychosocial dysfunction—and one emerging area—pediatrics. Advances in medical rehabilitation required occupational therapists to possess specialized knowledge and technical skills for treating individuals who have physical dysfunction. The occupational therapy schools revised the curriculum to include kinesiology, neurology, prosthetics, activities

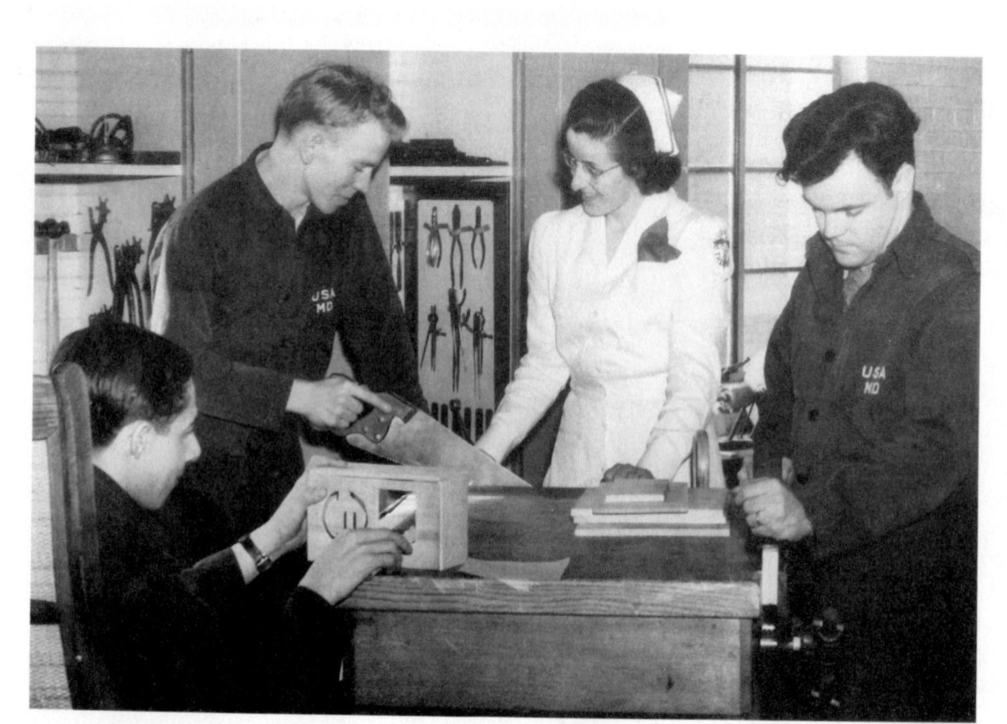

FIGURE 1–3. Wilma L. West, head of orthopedics occupational therapy, Walter Reed General Hospital, Washington, DC, 1943–1944. West was a founder of the American Occupational Therapy Foundation and its president from 1972 to 1982. She was also president of the AOTA from 1961 to 1964 and Eleanor Clarke Slagle lecturer in 1967. (Photo courtesy of the archives of AOTA, Bethesda, MD.)

of daily living, adaptive equipment, work simplification, and prevocational evaluation and to de-emphasize the teaching of arts and crafts (West & McNary, 1956). Specialization was also advocated by those who believed it would increase their status among other health professionals (Higher Status Near, c. 1960). AOTA sought closer ties with the American Medical Association in the hope of increasing the profession's scientific and medical credibility.

To establish a more scientific basis for psychiatric practice, it was proposed that occupational therapy align itself with psychoanalytic theory (Fidler & Fidler, 1954). However, the deinstitutionalization movement of the 1960s and 1970s resulted in the closing of state hospitals, the opening of community mental health centers, and the adoption of a milieu treatment approach. In theory, this should have provided an opportunity for occupational therapists to start up and supervise Consolation Houses throughout the country. In reality, funding was insufficient to provide essential services for the mentally ill who were displaced from the institutions. Occupational therapists failed to create a definitive niche for themselves among the professionals vying for the limited fiscal resources. Woodside (1971), believing that the situation was serious, warned about the possible demise of occupational therapy practice in psychiatry in a paper presented at the Fiftieth Annual Conference of the American Occupational Therapy Association.

> *Psychiatric occupational therapy could cease to exist because other professions are rapidly absorbing our body of knowledge, they appear to the public to be offering the same services that we offer, and they are selling their programs to other professionals and the public more effectively than we are (p. 229).*

At the same time, pediatrics was emerging as a popular specialty. This was partly owing to the passage of PL 94-142 Education of the Handicapped Children Act in 1975, which required that children with handicaps receive the necessary therapy to ensure full participation in the school setting. It was also a result of the growing body of theory and research that had began to emerge in pediatric occupational therapy practice from leaders such as Ayres (1963).

Summary

The world wars and the rehabilitation movement stimulated the growth of the profession and helped increase public awareness of occupational therapy's benefits. These factors, as well as ties between the AOTA and the American Medical Association, fostered a closer link between occupational therapy and medicine. Practice within the medical system increased the pressure on practitioners to narrow their focus through specialization. Although specialization brought with it more recognition and technical expertise, it threatened the generalist approach, which was holistic and occupation centered. The closer bond with medicine and the medical model brought the profession into conflict with some of its founding ideals.

A TIME OF QUESTIONING

Re-Evaluating the Direction of the Profession

The crisis in psychosocial practice and the emphasis on technique and modality in physical dysfunction practice prompted leaders in the profession to question the direction the profession was taking. Reilly (1962) criticized the movement away from occupation, and she challenged the profession to redirect its efforts toward developing a body of knowledge based on a thorough understanding of the nature of occupation. Only then could the profession fulfill the founder's "truly great and magnificent" vision "[t]hat man through the use of his hands as they are energized by mind and will, can influence the state of his own health" (Reilly, 1962, p. 2). Yerxa (1967) reminded therapists that the **reductionistic** view of the medical model that looked at patients only in terms of a specific diagnosis or body part was incompatible with "authentic occupational therapy." She said, "Philosophically we do not see man as a 'thing' but as a being whose choices allow him to discover and determine his own Being" (Yerxa, 1967, p. 8) (Fig. 1-4). Shannon (1977, p. 229) criticized the mechanistic nature of the medical model and occupational therapists' willingness to view the patient as a "mechanistic creature susceptible to manipulation and control via the application of techniques." He urged practitioners to stop the "derailment of occupational therapy" and return to the founding philosophy of moral treatment.

One source of the problem was a conflict between two **paradigms:** The scientific medical paradigm based on a reductionistic, mechanistic view of individuals and the occupation and moral treatment paradigm based on a humanistic and holistic view of the individual (Kielhofner & Burke, 1977). An unanticipated consequence of the expansion of the profession was that the values of the medical model overshadowed those of the founding philosophy of occupational therapy. The views inherent in the medical model represented a shift away from the humanistic approach of moral treatment, which was concerned with an individual's overall well-being, toward a mechanistic and problem-oriented intervention, which was concerned with a particular diagnosis. This tension was not evident to the founders, who encouraged occupational therapy to embrace both medical science and moral treatment. Perhaps that was because in the founding years the medical model had not yet emerged as the dominant perspective.

Theory and Research in Occupational Therapy

The problem for the profession was twofold. First, the perspective of the medical model had eclipsed many of the

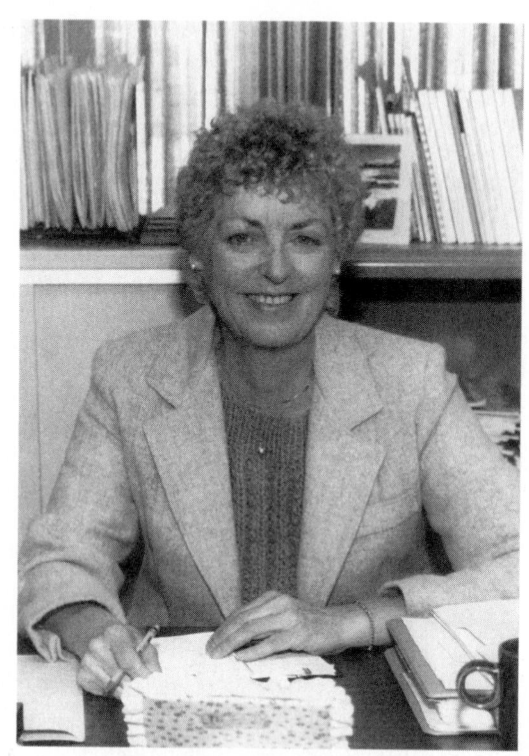

FIGURE 1–4. Dr. Elizabeth J. Yerxa, professor emeritus of the University of Southern California, was chair of the university's occupational therapy department from 1976 to 1988. She has received numerous awards, including the AOTA Award of Merit for her leadership in the profession, and was the Eleanor Clarke Slagle lecturer in 1966. (Photo courtesy of the archives of AOTA, Bethesda, MD.)

ideals inherent in the philosophy of occupation as articulated by the founders (Kielhofner & Burke, 1977). Equally troubling was the fact that the profession did not have a science unique to occupation or much research to justify its practice (Reilly, 1962). Anecdotal evidence and an intuitive belief in the benefits of occupation were not sufficient to persuade the scientific community of the therapy's efficacy. Clearly, the profession needed to develop a body of knowledge that fully described the nature of occupation. In addition, it had to engage in systematic research to demonstrate the effectiveness of occupational therapy. It should be noted that in 1960 other health professions such as nursing, physical therapy, and art and music therapy shared a similar lack of research and theory (Gritzer & Arluke, 1985). Medicine itself was far from having all the answers, but it had set the scientific standard that all health professions had to meet if they were to succeed in the medical community.

Why was there so little research and theory development within the profession up to the 1960s? There were several reasons. First, there were few occupational therapists who had earned doctoral degrees and who could conduct research. Most scholars outside the discipline were not interested in studying the field. Second, there was little pressure within health care to demonstrate the efficacy of treatment until the late 1970s. Beginning in 1980, Medicare and other health insurance third-party payers instituted a policy of reimbursing only for services for which treatment benefits were clearly documented. Third, there was little funding for occupational therapy research. The situation had not changed much since 1923 when Dunton had advocated the establishment of a foundation within the profession to sponsor research. Finally, there was the issue of research methodology. It was difficult to design research that could capture the richness and complexity of the occupational therapy process using the reductionistic scientific paradigm.

Dunton (1934, p. 325) had addressed this problem when he urged therapists to develop new methods of research to avoid reducing the occupational therapy process to "fractions, tangents, and cosines." The scholars who seemed to understand occupational therapy best were from the social sciences rather than from medicine. For example, Gregory Bateson (1956, p. 188), a well-know anthropologist, gave his description of the process of occupational therapy in a presentation at the annual American Occupational Therapy Conference, held in San Francisco:

> *Every act of creation is an act of discovery and the message which [occupational therapy] is trying to communicate is a discovery. . . . The modality is somehow to be the carrier for a message to the patient. A message about himself, his relationship to the human universe and the relationship between himself and you.*

Bateson's words gave eloquent expression to what the founders and succeeding generations of occupational therapists saw as the essence of the therapeutic process. Researchers had to find the methodologies that would enable them to study successfully occupational therapy in all its complexity.

Summary

The 1960s and 1970s were a time of questioning the direction the profession appeared to be taking. Leaders during this period, such as Reilly (1962) and Yerxa (1967), argued that the profession's rapid growth and increased recognition within the medical system brought it into conflict with some of the founding ideals. In particular, they were concerned that the profession was losing its focus on holistic, humanistic, occupation-centered treatment as it sought specialization. As this history has shown, the founders originally intended that both medical science and moral treatment philosophy would inform occupational therapy. The founders did not anticipate that a dichotomy would develop between the two perspectives. The leaders of the 1960s and 1970s recognized and articulated this development. They challenged the profession to bridge the gap between the two perspectives and to practice both the art and science of occupational therapy (Fig. 1-5).

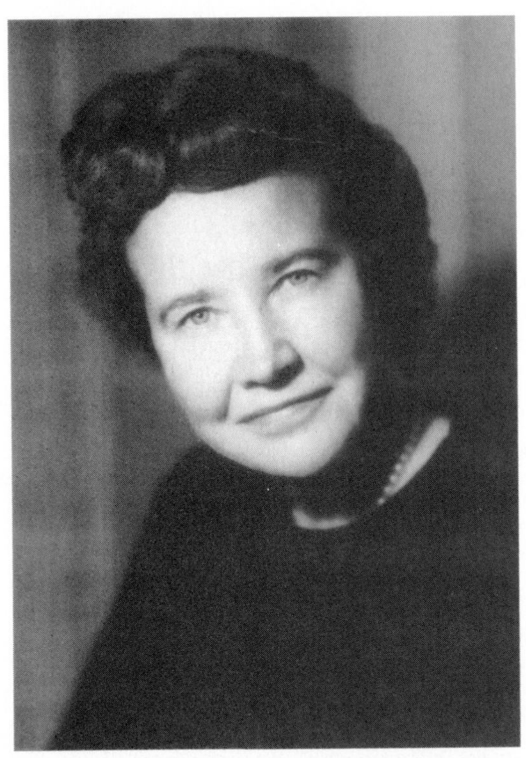

FIGURE 1–5. Dr. Mary Reilly, professor emeritus of the University of Southern California, was director of the university's Graduate Programs from 1962 to 1977. She was named a charter member of the Academy of Research of the American Occupational Therapy Foundation for her exemplary contributions to the development of a paradigm for occupational therapy practice and was the Eleanor Clarke Slagle lecturer in 1961. (Photo courtesy of the archives of AOTA, Bethesda, MD.)

RECLAIMING OCCUPATION: OCCUPATION-CENTERED THEORY, RESEARCH, AND PRACTICE

The profession heeded the warnings of the 1960s and 1970s as it turned its efforts toward promoting occupation-centered theory, research, education, and practice. Reilly (1969) and co-workers proposed occupational behavior as a theoretical construct to explain occupation through its emphasis on occupational roles, human adaptation, competency, and work and play. This work expanded on Meyer's (1922) philosophy of occupation therapy in which he emphasized the importance of occupation, habit training, adaptation, and the balance of work and play. Later, Kielhofner and Burke's Model of Human Occupation, which evolved out of their work with Reilly, added the dimensions of motivation and the influence of the environment on occupational behavior (Kielhofner, 1997). Other occupation-centered theoretical constructs that have been proposed include the ecology of human performance (Dunn, Brown, & McGuigan, 1994) and occupational adaptation (Schkade & Schultz, 1992). Within the practice areas, several theoretical models have been developed, including sensory integration (Ayres, 1972) neurodevelopmental treatment (Bobath, 1980), and cognitive disabilities (Allen, 1985). Thus, since the 1980s, the profession has made substantial progress toward developing theoretical models that can guide occupational therapy intervention. Clark and co-workers (1991) are helping to lead these efforts as they develop occupational science, the academic discipline of occupation.

During this period, led by occupational therapy scholars, the amount of published research surged. The change was most apparent in *The American Journal of Occupational Therapy* (*AJOT*), which from 1947 to 1970 featured articles written by those outside the field, with occupational therapists being listed as second or third authors. Now occupational therapists were the primary contributors. The American Occupational Therapy Foundation (AOTF) was founded in 1965 to provide financial support for occupational therapy research. The foundation created *The Occupational Therapy Journal of Research* to disseminate occupational therapy research and practice. AOTF is currently funding research in evidence-based practice (Tickle-Degnen, 2000). To address the issue of methodology, scholars have adapted research designs from the sciences and social sciences and have used both qualitative and quantitative data to capture the complexity of occupation and the occupational therapy process. The research by Clark and co-workers (1997) is an excellent example of the study of effectiveness of occupational therapy with a group of healthy older adults. The Clinical Reasoning Study, funded by AOTF (Mattingly & Gillette, 1991), illustrates how ethnographic research can inform practice.

Occupational therapy practice has grown dramatically since the 1980s. It has expanded beyond hospitals into private homes, public schools, nursing homes, hospices, community centers, and the workplace. In 2000, the Accreditation Council for Occupational Therapy Education listed 138 accredited professional programs and 176 accredited technical programs. The most recently approved Standards for an Accredited Educational Program for the Occupational Therapist require that students understand the meaning and dynamics of occupation and that they be able to develop occupationally based intervention plans (AOTA, 1999). The recent decision that occupational therapy become a profession that requires a master's degree for entry-level practice means that occupational therapists will be better prepared to lead the profession's future in the creation of practice that is occupation centered and evidence based.

CONCLUSION

This history has shown that a major challenge to occupational therapy has been the development of a theoretical body of knowledge rooted in a science that is consistent with the profession's philosophical assumptions. The founders articulated the philosophy of occupational therapy. They left to succeeding generations the work of building the science of occupation. That work has proved to be a daunting task:

> *Being at the beginning of the development of a profession is both exciting and scary. It means admitting that there is much that we cannot know, and acknowledging that many years of arduous development of research and educational preparation of the professional occupational therapist may be required. . . . [It] is going to take as many years to begin to move toward realizing this potential and generating a knowledge base as it has taken medicine and law (Fidler, cited in Miller, Sieg, Ludwig, Shortridge, & Van Deusen, 1988, p. 24).*

We have yet to fully meet this challenge and must rely on future generations to complete the task. In this work, we are all connected by a common bond: the shared belief in the value of occupation. Practitioners today still hold the assumptions that Dunton (1919, p. 10) expressed in the *Credo for Occupational Therapists:* "That occupation is as necessary to life as food and drink. That every human being should have both physical and mental occupations . . . which they enjoy. . . . That sick minds, sick bodies, sick souls may be healed through occupation." Occupational therapy retains as its fundamental concern the individual's capacity to live a satisfying life through engagement in occupations that bring fulfillment and joy. It is the profession's legacy.

References

Allen, C. (1985). *Occupational therapy for psychiatric disorders: Measurement and management of cognitive disabilities*. Boston: Little Brown.

American Occupational Therapy Association [AOTA]. (1999). Standards for an accredited educational program for the occupational therapist. *American Journal of Occupational Therapy, 53*, 575–582.

Arestad, F. H., & Westmoreland, M. G. (1946). Hospital service in the United States. *Journal of the American Medical Association, 130*, 1085.

Ayres, A. J. (1963). The development of perceptual-motor abilities: A theoretical basis for treatment of dysfunction [Eleanor Clarke Slagle Lecture]. *American Journal of Occupational Therapy, 17*, 221–225.

Ayres, A. J. (1972). *Sensory integration and learning disorders*. Los Angeles: Western Psychological Services.

Barton, G. E. (1920). What occupational therapy may mean to nursing. *The Trained Nurse and Hospital Review, 64*, 304–310.

Barton, G. E. (c. 1920). The movies and the microscope. *Occupational Therapy*, 75–89. [Archives of the Wilma L. West Library, American Occupational Therapy Foundation, Bethesda, MD.]

Bateson, G. (1956). Communication in occupational therapy. *American Journal of Occupational Therapy, 10*, 188.

Bobath, K. (1980). *A neurophysiological basis for the treatment of cerebral palsy*. London: Heinemann Books.

Bockoven, J. S. (1971). Legacy of moral treatment: 1800's to 1910. *American Journal of Occupational Therapy, 25*, 223–225.

Boris, E. (1986). *Art and labor: Ruskin, Morris, and the craftsman ideal in America*. Philadelphia: Temple University.

Clark, F., Azen, S., Zemke, R., Jackson, J., Carlson, M., Mandel, D., Hay, J., Josephson, K., Cherry, B., Hessel, C., Palmer, J., & Lipson, L. (1997). Occupational therapy for independent-living older adults. *Journal of the American Medical Association, 278*, 1298–1326.

Clark, F., Parham, L. D., Carlson, M., Frank, G., Jackson, J., Pierce, D., Wolfe, R., & Zemke, R. (1991). Occupational science: Academic innovation in the service of occupational therapy's future. *American Journal of Occupational Therapy, 49*, 1015–1018.

Dunn, W., Brown, C., & McGuigan, A. (1994). The ecology of human performance: A framework for considering the effect of context. *American Journal of Occupational Therapy, 48*, 595–607.

Dunton, W. R. (1917). History of occupational therapy. *The Modern Hospital, 8*, 380–382.

Dunton, W. R. (1919). *Reconstruction therapy*. Philadelphia: Saunders.

Dunton, W. R. (1928). *Prescribing occupational therapy*. Springfield, IL: Thomas.

Dunton, W. R. (1934). The need for and value of research in occupational therapy. *Occupational Therapy and Rehabilitation, 13*, 325–328.

Dunton, W. R. (1947). History and development of occupational therapy. In H. S. Willard & C. S. Spackman (Eds.). *Principles of occupational therapy* (pp. 1–9). Philadelphia: Lippincott.

Fidler, G., & Fidler, J. (1954). *Introduction to psychiatric occupational therapy*. New York: Macmillan.

Fields, G. E. (1911). The effect of occupation upon the individual. *The American Journal of Insanity, 68*, 103–109.

Gritzer, G., & Arluke, A. (1985). The making of rehabilitation: A political economy of medical specialization, 1890–1980. Berkeley: University of California Press.

Higher status near, doctor tells therapists. (c. 1960). [Archives of the Department of Occupational Therapy, San Jose State University, San Jose, CA.]

Johnson, S. C. (1920). Instruction in handcrafts and design for hospital patients. *The Modern Hospital, 15*, 69–72.

Kidner, T. B. (1925). The hospital pre-industrial shop. *Occupational Therapy and Rehabilitation, 4*, 187–194.

Kielhofner, G. (1997). *Conceptual foundations of occupational therapy*. Philadelphia: Davis.

Kielhofner, G., & Burke, J. (1977). Occupational therapy after 60 years: An account of changing identity and knowledge. *American Journal of Occupational Therapy, 31*, 674–689.

Lack of trained personnel felt in rehabilitation field. (1954, January 25). *New York Times*. [Archives of the Department of Occupational Therapy, San Jose State University, San Jose, CA.]

Mattingly, C., & Gillette, N. (1991). Anthropology, occupational therapy, and action research. *American Journal of Occupational Therapy, 45*, 972–978.

Meyer, A. (1922). The philosophy of occupation therapy. *Archives of Occupational Therapy, 1*, 1–10.

Miller, J. B., Sieg, K. W., Ludwig, F. M., Shortridge, S. D., & Van Deusen, J. (1988). *Six perspectives on theory*. Rockville, MD: Aspen.

National Society for the Promotion of Occupational Therapy [NSPOT]. (c. 1923). *Circular of information*. Sheppard Hospital Press. [Archives of the Wilma L West Library, American Occupational Therapy Foundation, Bethesda, MD.]

Peloquin, S. M. (1991). Occupational therapy service: Individual and collective understandings of the founders, Part 1. *American Journal of Occupational Therapy, 45*, 352–360.

Pinel, P. (1809). *Traite medico-philosophique sur l'alienation mentale* (2nd ed.). Paris: Brosson.

Quiroga, V. (1995). *Occupational therapy: The first 30 years*. Bethesda, MD: American Occupational Therapy Association.

Reilly, M. (1969). The educational process. *American Journal of Occupational Therapy, 23*, 299–307.

Reilly, M. (1962). Occupational therapy can be one of the great ideas of the twentieth century [Eleanor Clarke Slagle Lecture]. *American Journal of Occupational Therapy, 16*, 1–9.

Schkade, J. K., & Schultz, S. (1992). Occupational adaptation: Toward a holistic approach for contemporary practice. *American Journal of Occupational Therapy, 46*, 829–837.

Shannon, P. D. (1977). The derailment of occupational therapy. *American Journal of Occupational Therapy, 31*, 229–234.

Slagle, E. C. (1924). A year's development of occupational therapy in New York State hospitals. *The Modern Hospital, 22,* 98–104.
Taylor, F. (1911). *The principles of scientific management.* New York: Harper.
Tickle-Degnen, L. (2000). Monitoring and documenting evidence during assessment and intervention. *American Journal of Occupational Therapy, 54,* 434–436.
Tracy, S. E. (1910). *Studies in invalid occupation: A manual for nurses and attendants.* Boston: Whitcomb & Barrows.
West, W., & McNary, H. (1956). A study of the present and potential role of occupational therapy in rehabilitation. *American Journal of Occupational Therapy, 10,* 150–156.
Woodside, H. H. (1971). The development of occupational therapy, 1910–1929. *American Journal of Occupational Therapy, 25,* 226–230.
Yerxa, E. J. (1967). Authentic occupational therapy [Eleanor Clarke Slagle Lecture]. *American Journal of Occupational Therapy, 21,* 1–9.

CHAPTER 2

OCCUPATIONAL SCIENCE: BUILDING THE SCIENCE AND PRACTICE OF OCCUPATION THROUGH AN ACADEMIC DISCIPLINE

ELIZABETH LARSON, WENDY WOOD, and FLORENCE CLARK

Occupational science emerged from the early-twentieth-century values and beliefs of occupational therapy practitioners and promises in the new century to nurture the profession of occupational therapy. Although occupational science and occupational therapy both focus on occupation, they differ in that occupational therapy is a profession and occupational science is an **academic discipline.** A profession is a form of paid employment distinguished by its service to the public through schooled application of a specialized knowledge base and skill (Freidson, 1994). In contrast, an academic discipline is a branch of knowledge, learning, and scholarly inquiry legitimized by university communities that often supports the work of professions. As an academic discipline, occupational science falls within the sciences, not the humanities, since its methods of data collection are systematic, disciplined, and subject to public scrutiny (Carlson & Clark, 1991). Occupational science, because it focuses on human behavior, should be thought of as a social science akin to anthropology, sociology, and psychology and not as a single theory, model, perspective, or frame of reference for occupational therapy.

Occupation is both the central focus of occupational therapy practice and the unit of analysis considered in occupational science. Just as numerous definitions of *culture* exist in anthropology (Moore, 1992; Pierce, 2001), so too have many scholars defined *occupation* (Clark, et al., 1991; Fisher, 1998; Gray, 1997; Hocking, 2000; Kielhofner, 1993; Nelson, 1988; Pierce, 2001; Wilcock, 1998; Zemke & Clark, 1996). These papers provide in-depth reviews of current definitional issues; in this chapter, we define occupation simply as the activities that comprise our life experience and can be named in the culture. Since not every kind of doing is occupation, Carlson and Clark (2001) synthesized existing literature to propose the following five criteria to identify whether a particular form of "doing" is an occupation (Christiansen, 1999; Clark et al, 1991; Gray, 1997; Nelson, 1988; Wood, Towers, & Malchow, 2000). Carlson and Clark's goal is not to offer an airtight definition of occupation but to differentiate occupation from other types of doing.

- Occupations are units of action with identifiable start and end points; a person performing an occupation is doing something that he or she began and can stop doing, such as dining.
- Occupations are repeatable, intentional, and consciously executed. Sleepwalking, or sleeping itself, would not qualify as an occupation; it is, however, crucial that occupational therapists consider the place of sleep in a client's daily routine to achieve a balanced and healthy lifestyle.
- Occupations tend to be meaningful within the context of a person's life. They can contribute to identity. People enact their occupations with some sense of purpose. However, occupations do vary in their degree of meaningfulness; some may be "default" occupations that are low in meaning (like watching a "reality" program on television because we cannot think of anything else to do), whereas others reflect our passions (like ministering to the poor or painting as artistic expression). Yet even if meaningful, not all occupations are healthful: consider, for example, the personal and social costs of tagging the neighborhood with graffiti or spending time finding and taking addictive drugs.
- Occupations are intermediate in terms of scope; they comprise units of doing that fall somewhere between microbehaviors such as stroking one's hair or trimming one's cuticles, and such global life concerns as trying to be a humanistic person.
- Members of the culture label occupations. Everyday language easily labels occupations, because they are composed of customary rather than idiosyncratic activities. Activities such as making a speech and going for a walk meet this criterion of being easily labeled, whereas an activity like meticulously checking the alignment of the teacups in a china closet does not. Since words signify things that people in the culture repeatedly do, new words and terms—for instance, *snowboarding* and *surfing the Net*—emerge when new forms of occupation emerge.

Occupational science specifically focuses on the form, function, and meaning of human occupation (Fig. 2-1). The **form of occupation** refers to aspects of occupations that are directly observable. To study occupational forms, occupational scientists could compare the Japanese style of tatami dining with a common Western style of dining. In the former, participants are seated on the floor on tatami mats, use chopsticks, and typically choose sake as the alcoholic beverage. In the latter, participants sit on chairs, use silverware, and might imbibe a good French wine. The **function of occupation** refers to the ways occupation influences development, adaptation, health, and quality of life. Occupational scientists could study how being fed versus being helped to feed oneself to the maximum extent possible affects the physical health and life satisfaction of residents of health-care institutions. Finally, the **meaning of occupation** refers to the subjective experience of engagement in occupations. People imbue occupations with personal significance or value. Furthermore, occupations are symbolically constituted in a culture and interpreted in context of individuals' life stories. For example, a dining episode with a new acquaintance may be seen as pivotal in shaping one's future, resulting in a romance or even marriage.

1
FORM
Directly observable aspects of occupation

2
FUNCTION
Ways in which occupation serves adaptation

3
MEANING
The significance of occupation within the context of real lives and in the culture

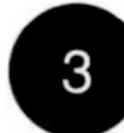

FIGURE 2–1. The three major research orientations of occupational science.

In this chapter we examine the historical events and circumstances that led to the evolution of occupational science in the United States. We describe occupational science as a global movement concerned with providing equitable opportunities to all people in developing their potentials. Next, we review research on the form, function, and meaning of occupation. We conclude by exploring how occupational science has nurtured, and will continue to nurture, occupational therapy.

HISTORICAL NOTE 2–1

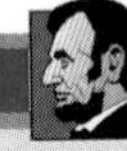

William Dunton's Creed: The Central Role of Occupation

SUZANNE M. PELOQUIN

William Rush Dunton Jr. (1919, p. 17) presented a creed that introduced his book on wartime therapy: "That occupation is as necessary to life as food and drink. That every human being should have both physical and mental occupation. . . . . That sick minds, sick bodies, sick souls, may be healed through occupation." The creed asks therapists to see occupation as a life-giving staple and to engage persons toward the actions that help them build their lives.

Dunton (1955, p. 17) also cited others who had used occupation as part of moral treatment in the nineteenth century, men such as the physician Brush: "Occupation is undoubtedly of very great importance in the treatment of the insane, but the idea of occupation which is satisfied by putting a row of twenty dements to picking hair or making fiber matts is far short of the true aim of occupation."

Comments such as these are cogent reminders that occupation occupies the body, mind, and spirit. Meaningful occupation must drive our inquiry and distinguish our practice. When our therapies fail to engage body, mind, and spirit, our credibility as occupational therapists is at stake.

Dunton, W. R. (1919). *Reconstruction therapy.* Philadelphia: Saunders.

Dunton, W. R. (1955). Today's principles reflected in early literature. *American Journal of Occupational Therapy, 9,* 17–18.

HISTORIC RELATIONSHIP OF OCCUPATIONAL THERAPY TO OCCUPATIONAL SCIENCE

How occupational therapy and occupational science came to be linked historically can be difficult to grasp for an obvious reason: Although occupational therapy emerged in the early twentieth century, occupational science was not formally founded until late in that century. This seeming enigma disappears, however, on investigation of the moral philosophy and body of knowledge on which occupational therapy practice has been based. Tracing the historical foundations of the profession reveals how an academic discipline (occupational science) was both born from and is developing knowledge that guides a pre-existing academic profession (occupational therapy). Four historical turnings or new waves of activity, though overlapping, are especially relevant here:

- The early 1900s, when the core premises of occupational therapy were first formulated.
- The 1920s, when the American Occupational Therapy Association (AOTA) began to make decisions about what comprised an optimal base of knowledge for occupational therapy.
- The 1960s, when critical re-evaluations of the profession's knowledge base occurred and many new theoretical understandings of occupational therapy were generated.
- The late 1980s to 1990s, when occupational science was formally founded and academic curricula explicitly grounded in the science began to be implemented.

The *first turning*, at the start of the twentieth century, is marked by various progressive social and intellectual movements that powerfully informed the new field of occupational therapy: the **settlement-house movement,** the **mental hygiene movement,** the **Arts and Crafts movement** and the philosophy of pragmatism. The settlement-house movement involved progressive social activism to ameliorate the debilitating effects of poverty, industrialization, and cultural alienation suffered by recent immigrants and other disenfranchised persons (Addams, 1910/1990). Proponents of this movement such as Jane Addams, a social worker and eventual Nobel laureate, developed houses in impoverished urban areas as centers of art, music, drama, writing, gardening, crafts, and other creative activities that could help elevate the conditions of those in surrounding neighborhoods, their families, and their cultural communities. The mental hygiene movement similarly endorsed the belief that opportunities for personally meaningful occupations met undeniable human needs. Julia Lathrop, a leader of this movement, along with numerous proponents including Adolf Meyer (1922, 1935/1948), the psychiatrist and pragmatist philosopher who first articulated occupational therapy's philosophical premises, focused on reforming the care of people with mental illness. Mental hygienists promoted public health initiatives to decrease the stigmatization of those with mental illness and to advance their compassionate and enlightened care in institutional and community settings. The Arts and Crafts movement originated in England and spread to the United States out of reaction against the alienating and demoralizing effects of industrialization (Levine, 1986). Its founder, John Ruskin, believed all people were entitled to find happiness in work and thus promoted the idea that acts of creating fine art and crafts could help uplift the human condition on individual and societal levels.

Influential pragmatist philosophers such as William James and John Dewey, among others, lent support to many strong convictions about the potential benefits of everyday occupations promoted by the settlement-house, mental hygiene, and Arts and Crafts movements. Pragmatists viewed human beings as **holistic, agentic,** and teleological (Hooper & Wood, 2002). Being holistic meant that people could not be reduced to dualities—like mind versus body or structure versus function—and that everyday experience could not be understood outside of its environmental context. Being agentic, meant that people were able to develop themselves, their societies, and their cultures through self-directed actions. Human capacities for **agency** were closely tied to the idea of **teleology,** human capacities to foresee and plan the passage of time with a future objective in mind. Converging with the aforementioned social movements, these pragmatist tenets helped create a rich moral and philosophical foundation to occupational therapy—a foundation that today also supports occupational science. Moreover, bolstered by the progressive social movements and philosophy that shaped the field's earliest practices, the founders of occupational therapy conceived of occupation as a sufficiently powerful instrument of health to merit systematic study. In 1917, the National Society for the Promotion of Occupational Therapy (soon to be the AOTA) first called for a science of occupation to advance "occupation as a therapeutic measure," "study . . . the effect–of occupation upon the human being," and to dispense "this knowledge" (AOTA, 1967, p. 4).

The *second turning*, beginning around 1920, marks a time of transition wherein proponents of occupational therapy sought to establish the young field as a legitimate profession. To do so, the earliest practices of occupational therapy and their philosophical and moral premises had to be translated into academic content. Beginning with the field's first formal programs, the field's leaders believed that educational content ought to reflect some balance of basic and applied sciences coupled with practical training (Presseller, 1984). However, which sciences merited inclusion? What was the best balance between basic and applied academic content? How should selected academic content relate to practical skills? Throughout much of the twentieth century, answers to these questions were rendered without benefit of an organized body of knowledge on occupation, for such knowledge did not exist then, nor would it for some time. In addition, occupational therapy's struggle to gain autonomy from medicine affected what students studied at different periods, which consequently influenced occupational therapy practice.

These challenges were evident in the 1920s and 1930s when the AOTA first established and then twice revised educational standards known as *Essentials* (Presseller, 1984). The first educational standards in 1923 deferred largely to medical authorities and sciences to help establish occupational therapy as a viable medical profession. Basic and applied medical content dominated what was then a 1-year program, encompassing the study of anatomy, kinesiology, general medicine and surgery, medical diagnoses and disorders, types of hospitals, and hospital ethics. Less emphasized in the 1923 Essentials were studies in the social sciences of psychology and sociology; the humanities, specifically the historical relationship of arts and crafts to civilization; and the history and theory of occupational therapy. When the Essentials were next revised in 1935 and subsequently approved by the American Medical Association (AMA) for the first time, medical content was expanded to include neurology, physiology, and psychiatry while content in the social sciences remained limited, and content in the liberal arts and humanities was no longer mentioned. These changes reflected the rise of a strict medical model in occupational therapy education. Yet the Essentials were again revised just 3 years later, in 1938, to include sociological content, such as delinquency and crime and also training in clinical techniques appropriate for nonmedical settings: two steps away from a strict medical model.

As this cursory overview suggests, translating occupational therapy's originating practices and premises into a body of knowledge was not easy. While it was first presumed that medical content should properly dominate that knowledge base, ongoing tensions were apparent with respect to how much study of the social sciences and humanities was also needed for occupational therapy's rich philosophical and humanitarian premises to be fully appreciated and clinically applied. As time went on, concern also grew over a growing gap between academic content and theory on the one hand, and the methods and techniques that had come to dominate practice on the other.

In large part due to these mounting issues, a third turning emerged in the 1960s that can be characterized in four ways. First, leaders in occupational therapy increasingly linked their analyses of deficiencies in the field's state of professionalism to its prevailing body of knowledge (e.g., Reilly, 1962a, 1962b; Weimer, 1967; West, 1968). These critiques focused on how the current knowledge base perpetuated a narrow medical approach to education and practice and, hence, the growing schism between theory and practice. Second, the AOTA instituted significant educational reforms by revising its Essentials in 1965, the first revision since 1949 (Presseller, 1984). The 1965 Essentials were ground breaking in several ways: (1) for the first time, a baccalaureate degree was required; (2) for the first time since 1923, content on the humanities was reinserted; and (3) for the first time, an equal emphasis was given to behavioral and social sciences such as psychology, sociology, and human development as was given to medical sciences such as anatomy, physiology, and kinesiology. Crediting a major curriculum study that led to these reforms, Yerxa (1967, p. 2) referred to the early 1960s as a time of an "educational revolution." "It is as if," she wrote, "theory and practice have finally touched hands and found that they respect and need each other" (p. 2). Third, coupled with more critically evaluative stances toward practice and education, occupational therapists generated theories and conceptual frames of reference to help organize the field's knowledge base, unite theory with practice, and promote research (e.g., Ayres, 1963; Llorens, 1970; Mosey, 1968). Influential theoretical advances in the 1960s often addressed humans and their activities from life-span perspectives, signaling a departure from a previously more medically dominated base of knowledge.

Fourth, and perhaps most significant, the work of Mary Reilly and her students at the University of Southern California (USC) directly broke ground for the subsequent founding of occupational science. Reilly (1962a, 1962b, 1974) created a frame of reference known as **occupational behavior** as a guide to practice and education. This frame of reference addressed how childhood exploration and play engendered, in adults, capacities to engage competently in productive work and social relationships. Reilly's students also undertook scholarly analyses of concepts that were central both to occupational behavior and to the philosophical tenets that had first given rise to occupational therapy. For instance, they examined motivational dynamics that affect people's abilities to act as agents (Burke, 1977; Florey, 1969), how environmental context and life history relate to occupational behavior (Moorehead, 1969), and how time use and temporal awareness relate to capacities for adaptation (Kielhofner, 1977).

The *fourth turning* relevant to occupational therapy's historical relationship to occupational science can be dated to 1988 when Elizabeth Yerxa established occupational science as a unique academic discipline sufficient in scope and importance to merit its own doctoral degree at USC (*Proposal for a Doctoral Program*, 1989). Yerxa's genius was in seeing both that the historical evolution of occupational therapy was culminating in the emergence of a new academic discipline and that dedication to that discipline could powerfully advance occupational therapy's time-honored moral and philosophical commitments. Since 1988, incorporation of occupational science in other educational programs has proceeded rapidly on multiple degree levels.

Finally, although this historical analysis has focused on the United States, the ideas and practices that ultimately gave rise to occupational science did not unfold only in this country. Rather, by the late twentieth century, the time was ripe for many occupational therapists around the world, in the context of how occupational therapy had evolved in their societies, to commit themselves to developing a science of occupation. Today, diverse cultural perspectives on the study of occupation are enriching occupational science and are also influencing education and practice around the world.

OCCUPATIONAL SCIENCE AS A GLOBAL SCIENCE AND MOVEMENT

The growth of occupational science on a global scale is evident in conferences and scholarship from the United States, Australia, Canada, Denmark, the United Kingdom, Sweden, Taiwan, Spain, Japan, and New Zealand. As of this writing, for instance, the *Journal of Occupational Science*, founded in Australia, is now in its eighth year of publication; professional journals in the United Kingdom, Scandinavia, and the United States, plus an international journal of occupational therapy, have also published special issues on occupational science (Box 2-1). A total of 13 symposia on occupational science have been held in the United States, 3 in Australia, 3 in Japan, 2 in Sweden, and 1 in Canada. Occupational scientists have presented keynote or invited lectures in South Africa, Korea, Hong Kong, the United Kingdom, Sweden, Australia, Japan, Chile, New Zealand, Denmark, and Taiwan. Consistent with this level of international activity, graduate programs from around the world are founding programs in occupational science. As occupational science has taken root internationally, the traditions and values of the many cultures have shaped its direction and content. U.S. scholars published the earliest papers in occupational science and emphasized the key mission of occupational science as the production of scientific knowledge on occupation (Clark et al., 1991; Yerxa et al., 1990). Reflecting American values of individualism and freedom, these early works presented occupation as largely determined by individual choice and as key in the construction of selfhood, although the relevance of sociocultural systems on both was also recognized. International scholarship has identified the cultural differences in values, beliefs, and sociopolitical structures that have an impact on occupation. For example, in Sweden, workers have much more time for summer vacations than workers in the United States; in South America, more time seems to be devoted to family occupations than in the United States, and in Australia, the presence of the Aborigine people has evoked consideration of occupations that involve being instead of doing (do Rozario, 1994). For these reasons, the question of how and to what extent cultural differences shape the development of occupational science has become particularly important.

BOX 2-1 SPECIAL JOURNAL ISSUES ON OCCUPATIONAL SCIENCE

Clark, F. (Ed.). (2001). [Occupational science: The foundation for new models of practice]. *The Scandinavian Journal of Occupational Therapy, 8* (1).
Johnson, J. A., & Yerxa, E. J. (Eds.). (1990). [Special issue]. *Occupational Therapy in Health Care, 6* (4).
Molineux, M. (Ed.). (2000). Special issue on occupational science. *The British Journal of Occupational Therapy, 65* (5).
Zemke, R. (Ed.). (2000). [Occupational science]. *Occupational Therapy International, 7* (2).

In contrast to the emphasis on individualism by occupational scientists in the United States, Scandinavian occupational scientists emphasize the role of social structures in choices of occupation. Runge (1999, p. 4), a Danish occupational scientist, introduced a social health perspective to point out how a society's prevailing "economical, social, technological, geographical and cultural structures" set the frameworks for how occupation, work, and production are organized. In this view, extremely adverse conditions like starvation, poverty, overconsumption of natural resources, and war are seen both as resulting from human occupation and as causing disease and premature death. Conversely, in altruistic societies where people care for each other and where social occupations are supported by reasonably equitable divisions of resources and power, human occupations potentially have enormously positive results. Occupational scientists influenced by this social health perspective may research topics such as how a nation's economic structure affects the time use and health of its citizens.

Australian occupational therapists' contributions to occupational science have emphasized scholarship, knowledge production, and the promotion of **occupational justice.** In her landmark book *An Occupational Perspective on Health*, Wilcock (1998), developed an elegant theory of the occupational nature of humans from a biological and social perspective; she also mapped out how the perspective of occupational science can contribute to public health worldwide. According to Wilcock, healthy living involves investing time in activities through which participants develop and stretch their capacities at the same time that they respect nature and their ecological surroundings. Wilcock identified three occupational problems that can compromise health. *Occupational imbalance* refers to states in which people are unable to participate in occupations that allow them to exercise their physical, social, and mental capacities. *Occupational deprivation* refers to circumstances in which external forces or situations such as imprisonment or institutionalization prevent people from participating in health-promoting occupations. *Occupational alienation* occurs when people's life activities fail to be in harmony with their natures or environs. Relative to these problems, Wilcock proposed that occupational scientists promote a participatory community model of health in which it is understood that health outcomes are influenced by inequitable distributions of resources and power. In such a model, salient inequalities would be addressed so all people might live in occupationally just societies wherein they "experience satisfaction, purpose, meaning, and ongoing health and well-being through what they do" (Wilcock, 2001, p. 11).

Canadian occupational scientist Townsend (1997) has also focused on issues related to social and occupational justice. Drawing on her ethnographic research, Townsend contended that occupation could both create change in individuals and transform societies. She suggested a new type of occupational therapy practice focused on projects, such as road-side clean up or political activities, or even to helping restructure social values so that the desire for financial security and gain no longer is central in making choices in the Western world about what to do each day. In the Utopian world that she believes occupational therapists can help create, "the ethics of fairness compel us to change the organization of society to create occupational opportunities for everyone" (Townsend, 1997, p. 24).

A strong occupational science movement is emerging in Japan as graduate programs are taking root there. Pronounced differences in Eastern and Western culture and in the structures of the English and Japanese language have rendered meaningful translations of occupational science concepts difficult. The writings of one group of occupational scientists have consequently highlighted the need to identify the ways in which understandings about occupation are not identical across cultural groups and to acknowledge that occupation is, in large part, a culturally saturated phenomenon (Clark, Sato, & Iwama, 2000). Although aspects of occupation that are biologically rooted may lend themselves to universally applicable theories, culturally specific theories may be needed to create a full understanding of occupation and its impact on health throughout the world. Accordingly, both areas of uniqueness associated with local traditions, understandings, and social practices and areas of commonality are likely in new conceptualizations of humans as occupational beings.

The momentum created by the growth of occupational science worldwide has now culminated in the initiation of the International Society of Occupational Scientists (2000). The ISOS aims to promote occupational justice and disseminate occupational science globally to advance world health and to create an international network of occupational scientists that will be engaged in scholarship, debate, and activism.

CURRENT RESEARCH ON OCCUPATION

As occupational science has grown internationally so has a body of knowledge focused sharply on occupation. For the purposes of this review, the research on occupation is organized under the domains of the form, function, and meaning of occupation. These distinctions, however, are made for convenience, because due to the complexity of occupation, researchers often attend to more than one domain for scientific reasons, for instance, to explore how forms of occupation relate to functions or how the meanings of occupations influence their form of expression.

Form of Occupation

To date, studies of the form of occupation have included time diaries to examine time use and subjective occupational experiences, multiple qualitative methodologies to describe engagement in occupation and the orchestration and organization of daily rounds of occupation, and experimental methods to examine the relationship of particular kinds of doing to specific outcomes. In this emerging body of research, particular forms of occupation have constituted a central focus of investigation for advancing several identifiable areas of inquiry.

One such area of inquiry has addressed prevalent therapeutic assumptions regarding performance components, skills, contrived activities, and occupations. In a study of preschoolers receiving occupational therapy, Case-Smith (2000) found that the occupation of play fostered the development of visual and fine-motor skills, suggesting occupation-based interventions altered component skills. Performance of self-care improved only by direct engagement in self-care. These findings suggest that as occupations became more complex, direct links to component skills also became more tenuous. Another study examined how typical toddlers mastered increasingly complex forms of occupation (Bober, Humphry, Carswell, & Core, 2001). Through video analysis, the researchers examined the persistence or on-task time of toddlers performing moderately challenging forms of the occupations of self-feeding and play. Toddlers' persistence in one occupation was only modestly related to persistence in the other. Bober and colleagues explained these findings as related to environmental variations, suggesting that contrived activities enacted in contrived situations may not facilitate independence as well as meaningful occupations enacted in natural contexts. At the other end of the age spectrum, Cooke, Fisher, Mayberry, and Oakley (2000) found that adults with Alzheimer disease could handle and use materials needed to perform daily activities in their familiar home environs, but they had difficulty locating objects, solving problems, using helpful cues, or knowing when to ask for help. Thus though abilities to perform routine occupational forms were retained, day-to-day performance was potentially undermined by difficulties dealing with novelty or solving problems that required higher-level cognitive skills.

Another area of inquiry has examined how people with various disabilities orchestrate a range of occupations and create altered forms of occupation in response to disability. A study of adolescents returning to school following spinal cord injury revealed various physical barriers (e.g., being assigned classroom seating in an awkward place) and attitudinal barriers (e.g., not being challenged by teachers) that curtailed participation in vital dimensions of life (Mulcahey, 1992). A study of women with spinal cord injuries underscored the persistent needs of participants to plan in order to foresee all possible barriers and contingencies involved in traveling outside usual adapted realms (Quigley, 1995). Quigley's findings of rigid structuring of daily schedules suggest a positive relationship with reduced opportunities for spontaneity. Borell, Lilja, Sviden, and Sadlo (2001), in their study of older adults with health challenges, discovered that some participants retreated from their occupations when disability was perceived as too large a barrier to overcome. In contrast, others persisted in engaging in their occupations despite perceived odds against success.

Occupational scientists have also investigated how family and paid caregivers orchestrate daily rounds of occupation for those in their care. In Segal's (1998) study, parents of children with attention deficit and hyperactivity **unfolded** occupations that made up morning and after-school routines to focus on their children's needs and promote successful completion of routines or homework. Instead of cooking while overseeing homework, these mothers found alternatives like purchasing food or having someone else cook so they could help their children with homework. In another study, mothers of children with severe disabilities used sophisticated strategies to prioritize daily routines in ways that promoted or sustained their children's health (Larson, 2000). Once their children's health was stable, these mothers inserted activities to promote independence. In similar fashion, paid caregivers for adults with Alzheimer disease promoted participation in daily activities by anticipating problems, decreasing waiting time between activities, managing the "tone" or calmness of activities, and preventing both physical and emotional harm (Hasselkus, 1992).

Another line of research has examined how various forms of occupation are embedded within daily life and patterned in time. In Blanche's (1998) study, adults often **enfolded** play or enjoyable activities with their work, suggesting that people often do not engage in play and work as discrete occupations in time and space. Similarly, working-class parents used two different strategies to accomplish household work and facilitate play with and by their children (Primeau, 1998). One strategy segregated play from work, creating sequential routines throughout the day that gave parents time to focus on needed tasks; the other strategy interspersed play with work, infusing household work with a playful nature. Farnsworth (1998), in studying juvenile offenders, discovered that study participants engaged in passive leisure 80% of the time, many having dropped out of school lost the daily structure once provided, including opportunities to participate in sports or other hobbies.

Finally, in contrast to the definition of **occupational form** offered in this chapter, Nelson (1988) defined the term as the pre-existing physical elements and social cultural contexts that elicit, guide, or structure human performance. Nelson's conceptualization of occupational form has led to study of a core premise of occupational therapy: that the use of occupation fosters therapeutic ends. Outcomes of engaging with enriched occupational forms—that is, those involving actual performance, more natural physical materials, or added purpose—have been contrasted with outcomes of engaging with less enriched occupational forms such as rote exercise, imagery in the absence of physical doing, or observing someone else do something (see Ferguson & Trombly, 1997; Hartman, Miller, & Nelson, 2000; Wu, Trombly, & Lin, 1994). A meta-analysis of studies of occupational form found that, in contrast to less enriched forms, enriched occupational forms moderately enhanced performance outcomes, especially in the area of movement kinematics (Lin, Wu, Tickle-Degnen, & Coster, 1997).

Function of Occupation

Occupational therapists have historically been concerned with the relationship of occupation to health. Contemporary

RESEARCH NOTE 2–1

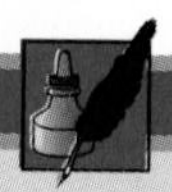

Meta-Analysis: A Tool for Synthesis of Research Findings

KENNETH J. OTTENBACHER

In their practice, occupational therapists must synthesize and translate information derived from research into practical knowledge and skills that can be used in clinical and community practice. Often the results of individual research studies can be confusing or even contradictory. There are many reasons why two or more studies examining the same research question might produce conflicting results, including differences in sample sizes, in the ways in which outcome measures were collected, in the intensity or duration of treatment, or in the types of statistical analyses conducted. These factors can make it difficult for the therapist to interpret and translate results from multiple studies. Fortunately, a method, referred to as meta-analysis, has been developed to help researchers and clinicians to synthesize large numbers of studies.

In a meta-analysis, systematic rules are used to search the literature and gather information from multiple investigations in a standardized manner. The results of multiple studies are converted to a common metric that allows the investigator to combine statistical results across several studies. Baker and Tickle-Degnen (2001) found 25 individual studies that examined the effectiveness of occupational therapy for clients with multiple sclerosis. Using the procedures associated with meta-analysis, they were able to demonstrate that occupational therapy interventions produced positive effects in several areas such as dressing, bathing, and ambulation.

Modern methods of research synthesis, such as meta-analysis, provide a mechanism for synthesizing and interpreting research studies on the effectiveness of interventions used by occupational therapists.

Baker, N. A., Tickle-Degnen, L. (2001). The effectiveness of physical, psychological, and functional interventions in treating clients with multiple sclerosis: A *meta-analysis*. *American Journal of Occupational Therapy*, 55, 324–331.

occupational scientists broadly conceptualize the function of occupation as encompassing considerations not only of health but also of adaptation, life-span development, and quality of life. To date, a variety of research approaches has been employed to investigate these functions, including naturalistic case studies, survey research, experience sampling methods, and randomized clinical trials.

Various theorists have proposed that the power of occupation as an instrument of adaptation—a vital means by which living beings adapt to their environs to support their survival and realize their potential—was honed through the evolutionary process of natural selection (Reilly, 1974; Wilcock, 1998; Yerxa et al., 1990). Models of research based on captive nonhuman primates have been used to investigate the long-standing assumption that occupational engagement is necessary for adaptation. A naturalistic study of sifakas, primitive primates, found that the environment had to support specific qualities of occupational behavior if optimal adaptedness was to be sustained. These qualities include **intentionality,** the quality of being about something; **purposiveness,** the quality of organizing multiple actions in accord with some goal; and agency, the quality of being able to affect other beings or material things (Wood, Towers, & Malchow, 2000). Relative to these behavioral qualities, Wood (2002) studied two groups of zoo chimpanzees to illustrate how differing constellations of social and physical ecological features influence adaptation. The adaptive benefits of particular environments (or their lack) were evident in the occupational behaviors and usual patterns of time use as influenced by the interaction of social and physical ecological features.

The relationship of occupation to adaptation has also been studied with respect to the adaptive living strategies of humans. For example, a 53-year-old woman with cerebral palsy used technology and social supports and set routines of activity to maintain both her independence and others' perceptions of her as mentally competent (McCuaig & Frank, 1991). Conversely, people with postpoliomyelitis syndrome, a condition that imposes new functional losses over time, reportedly altered their patterns of occupation as new functional losses arose while also striving to maintain positive emotions, social relations, and plans for the future (Jönsson, Möller, & Grimby, 1999). Clark and colleagues (1996), who studied older adults living in an urban apartment complex, identified 10 life domains and adaptive strategies used by these elders. For example, in the domain of psychological well-being and happiness elders strove to keep active or maintain positive states of mind; in the domain of activities of daily living they used informal and formal help to support their adaptation to aging and decreased abilities.

Occupational scientists have also focused on critical dimensions of quality of life, such as subjective well-being and life satisfaction. Survey research of a large population of adult Swedes examined how happiness related to satisfaction in life relative to the domains of self-care, leisure, work, and sexual relationships (Bränholm & Fugl-Meyer, 1994; Fugl-Meyer, Bränholm, & Fugl-Meyer, 1991). Factor analysis revealed a significant relationship between preferences for specific activities and occupational roles; in turn, this relationship was found to be related both to life satisfaction in the studied domains and to measures of happiness. Kennedy (2001) used the experience sampling method to ask women with HIV, at random intervals across the day, to describe how their symptoms and pain related to their current occupations and the physical environments in which those occupations were occurring. Participants reported experiencing fewer symptoms and less pain during productive tasks and higher levels of energy during leisure. Lo and Huang's (2000) study of optimistic intentions suggests that these intentions influenced the amount of time people were happy or unhappy during their daily occupations. Participants who tried to enjoy their occupations experienced greater well-being than those who made no such efforts.

Finally, a comprehensive investigation of the functions of occupation involved a randomized controlled clinical trial in which multiple positive outcomes pertaining to health and quality of life were studied as a function of older adults' participation in a program of **lifestyle redesign** (Clark et al., 1997). This program of lifestyle redesign, led by occupational therapists, involved helping people identify and put into practice plans for experiencing healthier, fuller, and more satisfying lives through their occupational endeavors (Jackson, Carlson, Mandel, Zemke, & Clark, 1998). Of 361 culturally diverse older adults who participated in the trial, one third was enrolled in the lifestyle redesign program over a 9-month period; the remaining two thirds were assigned to control groups. Findings indicated that, compared to controls, those in the lifestyle redesign program demonstrated greater gains in life satisfaction, mental health, vitality, quality of social interaction, and physical functioning and an absence of bodily pain and emotional problems. Six months after treatment ended, participants had maintained approximately 90% of these original treatment benefits (Clark et al., 2001).

Meaning of Occupation

To study the meaning of occupation, occupational scientists have addressed such issues as the relationship of meaning to self-expression and identity, the personal and cultural significance of occupations, how meaning influences choices of occupation, and felt experiences of occupation. Because the meanings of occupation are typically invisible and not easily inferred from overt behavioral expression (Hasselkus & Rosa, 1997), qualitative methods have mostly been used to explore how individuals perceive, experience, think, and talk about what they do.

Self-esteem and a sense of personhood are linked to the ability to engage in occupations. For instance, a young man with chronic schizophrenia experienced an increased sense of self-worth and more confidence in his abilities to contribute to others and control his illness after he participated in an occupation-focused community program (Legault & Reberio, 2001). Conversely, men with traumatic brain injuries were described feeling like less than real men after having lost their ability to provide for their families or to compete at sports (Gutman & Napier-Klemic, 1996).

Other studies have examined how occupational meanings relate to what people do and believe. Hasselkus, Dickie, and Gregory (1997) found that occupational therapists experienced either satisfying or dissatisfying responses to "doing" occupational therapy based on their favored treatment methods, beliefs, and past practices. Another study noted that the multiple ways in which lesbian occupational therapists experienced exclusionary work climates—often in the context of occupations like lunch with colleagues—related to how they adjusted their behavior to ensure a sense of safety and collegiality (Jackson, 2000). Humphry and Thigben-Beck (1997) demonstrated that specific beliefs about child development and society influenced how parents of different ethnic backgrounds went about feeding their infants and toddlers. Along a similar vein, Frank and colleagues (1997) found that Orthodox Jewish couples regarded engagement in certain daily occupations as ways of practicing their spiritual beliefs, thereby giving their lives meaning and purpose. The meaning of craftwork by crafters who sell their work in informal venues such as craft fairs was found to be closely linked to being part of a household economy where goods and services were exchanged by family members (Dickie, 1998).

Subjective experiences have also been studied in individuals who are unable to communicate easily in words, due to developmental age or some disabling condition. In one study, parents of typically developing children, children with autism, and children with developmental delays provided home videos that had been made of their children at 9 to 12 months of age (Baranek, 1999). Retrospective analysis of these videos found variations in sensory processing and social responsiveness among groups, thus illuminating salient differences in the children's subjective experiences of doing things and suggesting that early symptoms of autism can be detected. More recently, Baranek, Chin, Greiss, Yankee, Hatton, and Hooper (2001) examined the relationship of occupational performance to sensory processing in children with Fragile X syndrome. Children who avoided self-controlled sensory experiences had low levels of engagement in self-care and play; conversely, those with aversions to external touch demonstrated a trend toward greater independence in self-care.

It is important to stress again that research studies often encompass simultaneous attention to the form, function, and meaning of occupation. For example, the study of mothers of children with severe disabilities cited in the discussion of occupational form demonstrated the close relationship of form to meaning (Larson, 1998). In this work, meaning drove maternal work, sustaining the mothers' hopes for progress despite their children's serious impediments. To achieve development-promoting routines, these mothers continually negotiated obstacles like securing and maintaining desired services, managing unique child-care and medical procedures, and balancing conflicting family needs. In the randomized clinical trial on lifestyle redesign cited in the occupational function section (Clark et al., 1997), the degree to which the program was tailored to the participants' occupational challenges, needs, and wants contributed to positive outcomes, demonstrating the pivotal relationship of occupational meaning to occupational function.

OCCUPATIONAL THERAPY AND OCCUPATIONAL SCIENCE: TODAY AND TOMORROW

The relationship of an academic discipline to a profession can and should be deeply nurturing (Freidson, 1994): an ideal that today epitomizes the relationship of occupational science to occupational therapy. For instance, it is clear that knowledge generated in occupational science has substantiated the soundness and importance of core beliefs about the value of occupation that gave rise to occupational therapy. It is also clear that this body of knowledge is advancing evidence-based practice in occupational therapy, an indispensable requirement of practice today (Tickle-Degnen, 1999). Across a wide spectrum of age and disability categories, research in occupational science offers strong evidence to support highly individualized interventions. These interventions are (1) centered around occupations people find especially meaningful and important; (2) attuned to how cultural, social, and physical contexts influence what people do; and (3) responsive to the full complex of routines and occupational challenges that comprise a person's life. Various studies have also illuminated a plethora of adaptive strategies by which people manage their occupations and daily challenges, as well as specific factors that can undermine individuals' sense of competency, self-identity, and self-esteem.

Advances in occupational science are also bringing about new ways of conceptualizing services in accord with credible evidence. For example, the concept of lifestyle redesign (Clark et al., 1997; Jackson et al., 1998; Mandel, Jackson, Zemke, Nelson, & Clark, 1999; Womack & Farmer, 1999) is now being applied in research or practice to diverse consumer groups, including older adults living in the community (Womack & Farmer, 1999), as well as to individuals with spinal cord injury who have recurrent pressure sores (NIDRR Grant #H133G000062) and for weight loss (USC private practice offers lifestyle redesign weight loss program, 2001). Just as occupational therapists in the early twentieth century developed programs to address public health needs such as tuberculosis and mental illness, occupational therapy practitioners in this century will adapt the concept of lifestyle redesign to confront today's public health challenges such as depression, diabetes, obesity, cancer, and heart disease.

CONCLUSION

Because occupational science is designed to produce a clear and systematic understanding of how occupation influences health and well-being, it is not surprising that it has already paved the way for important advances in occupational therapy. Yet, studying occupation remains enormously challenging precisely because occupation is so complex and ubiquitous on the one hand, yet so seemingly transparent, and hence apt to be taken for granted on the other. Occupational scientists must now develop methodologies to elucidate how everyday occupations and occupational patterns relate to biological, physiological, and subjective measures of health and well-being across the life span; salient ecological dynamics must also be explicated at personal, social, and cultural levels. If achieved, such scientific advances would most assuredly nurture a bright future for occupational therapy.

References

Addams, J. (1910/1990). *Twenty years at Hull House*. Urbana: University of Illinois Press.

American Occupational Therapy Association [AOTA]. (1967). *American Occupational Therapy Association: Then and now: 1917–1967*. Rockville, MD: Author.

Ayres, A. J. (1963). The development of perceptual-motor abilities: A theoretical basis for treatment of dysfunction [Eleanor Clarke Slagle Lecture]. *American Journal of Occupational Therapy, 17*, 221–225.

Baranek, G. T., (1999). Autism during infancy: A retrospective video analysis of sensory-motor and social behaviors at 9–12 months of age. *Journal of Autism and Developmental Disorders, 29*, 213–224.

Baranek, G. T., Chin, Y. H., Greiss, L. M., Yankee, J. G., Hatton, D. D., & Hooper, S. R. (2001). Sensory processing correlates of occupational performance in children with Fragile X syndrome. Manuscript submitted for publication.

Blanche, E. (1998). Play and process: The experience of play in the life of the adult. Ann Arbor, MI: University Microfilms International.

Bober, S. J., Humphry, R., Carswell, H. W., & Core, A. J. (2001). Toddlers' persistence in the emerging occupations of functional play and self-feeding. *American Journal of Occupational Therapy, 55*, 369–376.

Borell, L., Lilja, M., Sviden, G., & Sadlo, G. (2001). Occupation and signs of reduced hope: An exploration study of older adults with functional impairments. *American Journal of Occupational Therapy, 55*, 311–316.

Bränholm, I. B., & Fugl-Meyer, A. R. (1994). On non-work activity preferences: Relationships with occupational roles. *Disability and Rehabilitation, 16*, 205–216.

Burke, J. P. (1977). A clinical perspective on motivation: Pawn versus origin. *American Journal of Occupational Therapy, 31*, 255–258.

Carlson, M., & Clark, F. (1991). The search for useful methodologies in occupational science. *American Journal of Occupational Therapy, 45*, 235–241.

Carlson, M., & Clark, F. (2001, October). *Occupation in relation to the self*. Presented at the Thirteenth Annual Occupational Science Symposium, University of Southern California, Los Angeles.

Case-Smith, J. (2000). Effect of occupational therapy services on fine motor and functional performance in preschool children. *American Journal of Occupational Therapy, 54*, 372–380.

Christiansen, C. (1999). Defining lives: Occupation as identity: An essay on competence, coherence, and the creation of meaning. *The American Journal of Occupational Therapy, 53*, 547–558.

Clark, F., Azen, S. P., Carlson, M., Mandel, D., LaBree, L., Hay, J., Zemke, R., Jackson, J., & Lipson, L. (2001). Embedding health-promoting changes into the daily lives of independent living older adults: Long term follow-up of occupational therapy intervention. *The Journals of Gerontology Series B, Psychological Sciences and Social Sciences, 56*, 60–63.

Clark, F., Azen, S. P., Zemke, R., Jackson, J., Carlson, M., Mandel, D., Hay, J., Josephson, K., Cherry, B., Hessel, C., Palmer, J., & Lipson, L. (1997). Occupational therapy for independent-living older adults: A randomized controlled trial. *Journal of the American Medical Association, 278*, 1321–1326.

Clark, F., Carlson, M., Zemke, R., Frank, G., Patterson, K., Ennevor, B. L., Rankin-Martinez, A., Hobson, L. A., Crandall, J., Mandel, D., & Lipson,

L. (1996). Life domains and adaptive strategies of a group of low-income well older adults. *American Journal of Occupational Therapy*, *50*, 99–108.

Clark, F., Parham, D., Carlson, M. E., Frank, G., Jackson, J., Pierce, D., Wolfe, R. J., & Zemke, R. (1991). Occupational science: Academic innovation in the service of occupational therapy's future. *American Journal of Occupational Therapy*, *45*, 300–310.

Clark, F., Sato, T., & Iwama, M. (2000). Towards the construction of a universally acceptable definition of occupation. *The Japanese Journal of Occupational Therapy*, *34*, 9–14.

Cooke, K., Fisher, A., Mayberry, W., & Oakley, F. (2000). Differences in activities of daily living process skills with and without Alzheimer's disease. *Occupational Therapy Journal of Research*, *20*, 87–105.

Dickie, V. (1998). Households, multiple livelihoods, and the informal economy: A study of American crafters. *Scandinavian Journal of Occupational Therapy*, *5*, 109–118.

do Rozario, L. (1994). Ritual, meaning and transcendence: The role of occupation in modern life. *Journal of Occupational Science: Australia*, *1*, 46–53.

Farnsworth, L. (1998). The time use and subjective experience of occupations of young male and female legal offenders. Ann Arbor, MI: University Microfilms International.

Ferguson, J., & Trombly, C. (1997). The effect of added-purpose and meaningful occupation on motor learning. *American Journal of Occupational Therapy*, *51*, 508–515.

Fisher, A. G. (1998). Uniting practice and theory in an occupational framework. *American Journal of Occupational Therapy*, *52*, 509–521.

Florey, L. L. (1969). Intrinsic motivation: The dynamics of occupational therapy theory. *American Journal of Occupational Therapy*, *23*, 319–322.

Frank, G., Bernardo, C. S., Tropper, S., Noguchi, F., Lipman, C., Maulhart, B., & Weitze, L. (1997). Jewish spirituality through actions in time: Occupations of young orthodox Jewish couples in Los Angeles. *American Journal of Occupational Therapy*, *51*, 199–206.

Freidson, E. (1994), *Professionalism reborn: Theory, prophecy, and policy*. Chicago: University of Chicago Press.

Fugl-Meyer, A., Bränholm, I., & Fugl-Meyer, K. (1991). Happiness and domain-specific life satisfaction in adult northern Swedes. *Clinical Rehabilitation*, *5*, 25–33.

Gray, J. M. (1997). Application of the phenomenological method of conceptualization to the concept of occupation. *Journal of Occupational Science: Australia*, *4*, 5–17.

Gutman, S. & Napier-Klemic, S. (1996). The experience of head injury on the impairment of gender identity and gender role. *American Journal of Occupational Therapy*, *50*, 535–544.

Hartman, B., Miller, B., & Nelson, D. (2000). The effect of hands on occupation versus demonstration on children's recall memory. *American Journal of Occupational Therapy*, *54*, 477–483.

Hasselkus, B. (1992). The meaning of activity: Day care for persons with Alzheimer disease. *American Journal of Occupational Therapy*, *46*, 199–206.

Hasselkus, B., Dickie, V., & Gregory, C. (1997). Geriatric occupational therapy: The uncertain ideology of long term care. *American Journal of Occupational Therapy*, *51*, 132–139.

Hasselkus, B., & Rosa, S. (1997). Meaning and occupation. In C. Christiansen & C. Baum (Eds.), *Occupational therapy: Enabling function and well-being* (pp. 363–377). Thorofare, NJ: Slack.

Hocking, C. (2000). Occupational science: A stock take of accumulated insights. *Journal of Occupational Science*, *7*, 58–67.

Hooper, B., & Wood, W. (2002). Pragmatism and structuralism in occupational therapy: The long conversation. *American Journal of Occupational Therapy*, *56*, 40–50.

Humphry, R., & Thigben-Beck, B. (1997). Caregiver role: Ideas about feeding infants and toddlers. *Occupational Therapy Journal of Research*, *17*, 237–263.

Kennedy, B. (2001). *Effects of context on health: A strategy for occupational redesign*. Paper presented at the American Occupational Therapy Association annual conference, Philadelphia.

Kielhofner, G. (1977). Temporal adaptation: A conceptual framework for occupational therapy. *American Journal of Occupational Therapy*, *31*, 235–242.

Kielhofner, G. (1993). Occupation as the major activity of humans. In H. L. Hopkins & H. D. Smith (Eds.), *Willard & Spackman's Occupational Therapy* (8th ed., pp. 137–144). Philadelphia: Lippincott.

Larson, E. A. (1998). Reframing the meaning of disability to families: The embrace of paradox. *Social Science and Medicine*, *47*, 865–875.

Larson, E. (2000). The orchestration of occupation: the dance of mothers. *American Journal of Occupational Therapy*, *54*, 269–280.

Legault, E., & Reberio, K. (2001). Occupation as means to mental health: A single-case study. *American Journal of Occupational Therapy*, *55*, 90–96.

Levine, R. (1986). Historical research: Ordering the past to chart our future. *Occupational Therapy Journal of Research*, *6*, 32–42.

Lin, K.-C., Wu, C.-Y., Tickle-Degnen, L., & Coster, W. (1997). Enhancing occupational performance through occupationally embedded exercise: A meta-analytic review. *Occupational Therapy Journal of Research*, *17*, 25–47.

Llorens, L. A. (1970). Facilitating growth and development: The promise of occupational therapy [Eleanor Clarke Slagle Lecture]. *American Journal of Occupational Therapy*, *24*, 93–101.

Meyer, M. (1922). The philosophy of occupation therapy. *Archives of Occupational Therapy*, *1*, 1–10.

Meyer, M. (1935/1948). The mental hygiene movement. In A. Lief (Ed.), *The commonsense psychiatry of Dr. Adolf Meyer: Fifty-two selected papers* (pp. 576–589). New York: McGraw-Hill.

Moore, A. (1992). *Cultural anthropology: The field study human beings*. San Diego, CA: Collegiate.

Moorehead, L. (1969). The occupational history. *American Journal of Occupational Therapy*, *23*, 329–334.

Mosey, A. C. (1968). *Occupational therapy: Theory and practice*. Medford, MA: Pothier Brothers.

Mulcahey, M. (1992). Returning to school after a spinal cord injury: Perspectives from four adolescents. *American Journal of Occupational Therapy*, *46*, 305–312.

Nelson, D. L. (1988). Occupation: Form and performance. *American Journal of Occupational Therapy*, *42*, 633–641.

Pierce, D. (2001). Untangling occupation and activity. *American Journal of Occupational Therapy*, *55*, 138–145.

Presseller, S. R. (1984). Occupational therapy education: Yesterday, today, and tomorrow. *Dissertation Abstracts International*, 45(12), 3777B (UHI No. 8504293).

Primeau, L. (1998). Orchestration of work and play within families. *American Journal of Occupational Therapy*, *52*, 188–195.

Proposal for a doctoral program in occupational science. (1989). Unpublished manuscript, University of Southern California, Department of Occupational Therapy, Los Angeles.

Quigley, M. (1995). Impact of spinal cord injury on life roles of women. *American Journal of Occupational Therapy*, *49*, 780–786.

Reilly, M. (1962a). Occupational therapy can be one of the greatest ideas of 20th century medicine [Eleanor Clarke Slagle Lecture]. *American Journal of Occupational Therapy*, *16*, 1–9.

Reilly, M. (1962b). A psychiatric occupational therapy program as a teaching model. *American Journal of Occupational Therapy*, *20*, 61–67.

Reilly, M. (1974). *Play as exploratory learning: Studies of curiosity behavior*. Beverly Hills, CA: Sage.

Runge, U. (1999, September). *Occupational health from a social point of view*. Paper presented at the Nordic Congress, Trondheim.

Tickle-Degnen, L. (1999). Evidence-based practice forum—Organizing, evaluating, and using evidence in occupational therapy practice. *American Journal of Occupational Therapy*, *53*, 537–539.

Townsend, E. (1997). Occupation: Potential for personal and social transformation. *Journal of Occupational Science: Australia*, *4*, 18–26.

USC private practice offers lifestyle redesign weight loss program. (2001). *University of Southern California Department of Occupational Science and Occupational Therapy Newsletter*, *2*, 5.

Weimer, R. W. (1967). From the president: After fifty years, what stature do we hold? *American Journal of Occupational Therapy, 5*, 262–267.

West, W. L. (1968). Professional responsibility in times of change [Eleanor Clarke Slagle Lecture]. *American Journal of Occupational Therapy, 22*, 9–15.

Wilcock, A. (1998). *An occupational perspective on health*. Thorofare, NJ: Slack.

Wilcock, A. A. (2001). Occupational utopias: Back to the future. *Journal of Occupational Science, 8*, 5–12.

Womack, J. & Farmer, P. (1999). Strong roots, flexible branches: Community-based occupational therapy at the Vanderbilt apartments. *OT Practice, 4*, 17–21.

Wood, W. (2002). Ecological synergies in two groups of zoo chimpanzees: Divergent patterns of time-use. *American Journal of Occupational Therapy, 56*, 160–170.

Wood, W., Towers, L., & Malchow, J. (2000). Environment, time-use, and adaptedness in prosimians: Implications for discerning behavior that is occupational in nature. *Journal of Occupational Science, 7*, 14–27.

Wu, C., Trombly, C., & Lin, K.-C. (1994). The relationship between occupational form and performance: A kinematic perspective. *American Journal of Occupational Therapy, 48*, 679–697.

Yerxa, E. J. (1967). Authentic occupational therapy. [Eleanor Clarke Slagle Lecture]. *American Journal of Occupational Therapy, 21*, 1–9.

Yerxa, E., Clark, F., Frank, G., Jackson, J., Parham, D., Pierce, D., Stein, C., & Zemke, R. (1990). An introduction to occupational science: A foundation for occupational therapy in the 21st century. *Occupational Therapy in Health Care, 6*, 1–17.

Zemke, R., & Clark, F. (1996). *Occupational Science: The Evolving Discipline*. Philadelphia: Davis.

CHAPTER 3

OCCUPATIONAL THERAPY PRACTICE

SECTION I: Occupational Therapy Practice Today
SECTION II: Population Interventions Focused on Health for All

SECTION I

Occupational Therapy Practice Today

ELIZABETH BLESEDELL CREPEAU
ELLEN S. COHN
BARBARA BOYT SCHELL

- Linda is a 35-year-old carpenter who accidentally cut the tendons across the back of her right, dominant, hand at work. She lives with her partner, Susan, in a house surrounded by a garden to which they devote considerable time and energy. Robin, an occupational therapist, custom-made a hand splint for Linda that positions and protects her hand while it is healing. Robin also showed her how to manage her wound care as part of her daily self-care routine. Together they discussed what activities Linda could realistically and safely do, both at home and at work. Robin encouraged her to use the two fingers on her injured hand that were not involved as much as possible and suggested that she might want to use the coming weeks to do the computer work needed to get her year-end taxes ready, since Linda owns her own business.
- Jack is a 14-year-old junior high student with developmental disabilities. He has been successfully included in the public school setting, but he, his family, and his educational team must begin planning for his transition from school to life after graduation. At a recent educational-planning meeting Jack stated that he would like to take the local bus with his peers to his weekly after-school sports program rather than driving with his mother each week. Jack has never used public transportation and has little understanding of how to manage money. He is not sure what he would like to do when he grows up but knows he wants to live in his own apartment someday.
- Jack, Pete, and Harry like to attend the Bridges program at the local recreation center. Bridges is a member-directed program for people who sustained brain injuries. This morning, the newspaper group discussed ideas for articles for the next monthly issue. Members selected topics and went to the recreation center's computer room to search the Web for ideas. When they arrived at the computer room, Sally, a certified occupational therapy assistant, helped each member set up a computer with the appropriate adaptations.

- Maplewood Industries is a furniture company whose employees have experienced many work-related repetitive trauma injuries. John, an occupational therapist, has a contract with Maplewood to conduct a work-site assessment to identify how the various workstations could be changed to avoid repetitive trauma injuries. He also has been working with the company health nurse to develop and implement an employee-training program to prevent the onset of these injuries.
- Mrs. Oak is a retired schoolteacher whose husband of 52 years died the past spring. She has just moved into a small apartment in a life-care community. Her daughter, who lives in another state, is concerned that her mother seems depressed and is not adjusting to her new setting, even though there are many activities there for her to enjoy. Pam, the occupational therapist, interviewed Mrs. Oak about her lifelong interests and activities and is helping Mrs. Oak adapt her routines to this setting.

These five scenarios represent the diversity of occupational therapy intervention for occupational therapy clients, be they individuals, groups, or organizations. Linda wants to be able to return to work and her garden. Like most adolescents, Jack wants to be more autonomous from his parents, use public transportation, live in his own apartment someday, and learn job skills to prepare him for life after high school. The members of the Bridges program want to be able to contribute to their group and the broader community and to enjoy time with their friends. The manager at Maplewood Industries wants to be sure that his employees do not develop repetitive trauma injuries because of his concern for them as human beings and for the company's productivity. Mrs. Oaks wants to find a way to live meaningfully in her new life as a widow, and her daughter wants her to be as comfortable as possible. As these scenarios demonstrate, occupational therapy practitioners provide services to a variety of clients in many settings, from hospitals and schools to community programs and businesses. These services include direct intervention with individuals to programming for groups to consultation within organizations. In all cases, occupational therapy practitioners are concerned with enabling people to participate as fully as possible in society and to meet their individual goals. The overarching goal of occupational therapy is to improve the health and quality of life of people through engagement in meaningful and important occupations.

DEFINITION OF OCCUPATIONAL THERAPY

Occupational therapy is the art and science of helping people do the day-to-day activities that are important and meaningful to their health and well-being through engagement in valued occupations. The *occupation* in occupational therapy comes from an older use of the word, meaning how people use or "occupy" their time. As such, occupational therapy refers to all of the activities that occupy people's time and give meaning to their lives. Occupation includes the day-to-day activities that enable people to sustain themselves, to contribute to the life of their family, and to participate in the broader society (American Occupational Therapy Association [AOTA], in press). Occupational engagement is important because it has the capacity to contribute to health and well-being (Clarke et al., 1997; Glass, Mendes de Leon, Marottoli, & Berkman, 1999; Law, Seinwender, & Leclair, 1998). As the scenarios that opened this chapter illustrate, occupational therapy practitioners provide individual intervention as well as consultative services that foster community participation, prevention, and wellness of groups in a wide range of settings.

Contemporary occupational therapy practice draws on the historical roots of the profession, filtered through current occupational therapy, health, and human service research and practice. Meyer (1977/1922), for example, in his oft-quoted address to the National Society for the Promotion of Occupational Therapy asserted, "Our role consists in giving opportunities rather than prescriptions. There must be opportunities to work, opportunities to do, and to plan and create, and to use material (p. 641). Englehardt (1977), and more recently Pörn (1993), asserted that health is measured by an individual's adaptive capacity and engagement in daily activities. In her Eleanor Clark Slagle Lecture, Yerxa (1967) explained that authentic occupational therapy focuses on clients' humanity and their ability to choose and initiate activities that provide the basis for the discovery of meaning. She further argued that authentic occupational therapy requires that the practitioner "in every professional act defines the profession" and, in doing so, enters into a reciprocal relationship characterized by mutual care and that "to care means to be affected just as surely as it means to affect" (p. 8). Later in her address, Yerxa called for practitioner engagement in research to promote the development of the knowledge base of profession. These themes translate into three principles to guide contemporary occupational therapy: client-centered practice, occupation-centered practice, and evidence-based practice.

Client-Centered Practice

At the core of occupational therapy is the commitment to focus on the client as an active agent seeking to accomplish important day-to-day activities. Occupational therapy practitioners often work with people who are disempowered (Townsend, 1996). Clients seek care and professional help to "gain mastery over their affairs" (Rappaport, 1987, p. 122). To be client centered, practitioners must be willing to enter the client's world to create a relationship that encourages the other to enhance his or her life in ways that are most meaningful to that person. Practitioners strive to understand the client as a person embedded in a particular context consisting of family and friends, socioeconomic

ETHICS NOTE 3–1

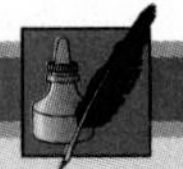

Should Peter Testify?

PENNY KYLER and RUTH ANN HANSEN

Peter is in rehabilitation and is being sought out to testify in a trial about a major oil spill. The accident was alleged to be caused by an error in judgment by the captain of an oil tanker. Peter's therapist is aware that her client has cognitive deficits, and she has questions about whether he can give reliable testimony. However, she is unfamiliar with the legal process of testifying and is not certain what Peter will be asked during his testimony. Her knowledge of the oil spill is based on news media coverage and from hearing Peter talk about it. She is aware that he appears anxious about being asked to testify, since he talks of nothing else during their therapy sessions.

- **What is the therapist's obligation to Peter?**
- **What should she do to determine if Peter is capable of testifying?**
- **What, if any, obligation does she have to the legal system?**

status, culture, etc. In a client-centered model, practitioner and client collaboratively engage in the therapeutic process (Law, 1998). Mattingly (1991) asserted that this process is narrative in nature, which means the practitioner and client create an understanding of the client's past, present, and future story. Mattingly further asserted that the future story is co-constructed and constantly revised in the midst of therapy. Practitioners strive to understand human feelings and intentions as well as the deeper meaning of people's lives through what Clark (1993) called occupational storytelling. In contrast, occupational storymaking occurs in the midst of therapy. It is that imaginative process through which clients create and then enact new occupational identities (Clark, 1993).

Occupation-Centered Practice

Contemporary occupational therapy emphasizes occupational engagement. Clients seek occupational therapy because they need help engaging in their valued occupations. The emphasis on occupational engagement stems from the profession's beliefs, substantiated by emerging research, that people's occupations are central to their identity and that they can reconstruct themselves through their occupations (Jackson, 1998). Occupations are not isolated activities but are connected in a web of daily activities that help people fulfill their basic needs and contribute to their family, friends, and broader community. Occupation-centered practice focuses on meaningful occupations selected by clients and performed in their typical settings (Fischer, 1998; Pierce, 1998). Systematic assessment of clients' occupations and priorities are vital to occupation-centered practice. This information—when coupled with careful analyses of the person's capacities, the task's demands, and the performance context—provides the basis for intervention. Intervention goals are directly connected to the person's occupational concerns, and intervention methods capitalize on the person's occupational interests. In this way, both the means (methods) and the ends (goals) of therapy involve intervention grounded in the occupations of the client (Fisher, 1998; Gray, 1998; Trombly, 1995).

Evidence-Based Practice

One of the important trends in health care is the growing requirement to base intervention decisions on "the conscientious, explicit, and judicious use of current best evidence" (Sackett, Rosenberg, Muir Grany, Haynes, & Richardson, 1996, p. 71). This process, called evidence-based practice, entails being able to integrate research evidence into the clinical-reasoning process to explain the rationale behind interventions and predict probable outcomes—or, as Gray asserted, "doing the right things right" (cited in Holm, 2000, p. 576). Beyond "doing the right things right," evidence-based practice involves being able to explain occupational therapy recommendations to clients in a language clients will understand (Tickle-Degnen, 2000). Furthermore, intervention grounded in the customs of the field no longer meets the ethical requirement to "fully inform the service recipients of the nature, risks, and potential outcomes of any interventions" (American Occupational Therapy Association [AOTA], 1994, p. 1037).

The challenge for occupational therapy practitioners is threefold. First, to practice occupational therapy based on research evidence, practitioners must know how to access, evaluate, and interpret relevant research. Second, practitioners must have the capacity to collect data to support their intervention recommendations. Third, once practitioners understand the possible interventions and related outcomes, they need to communicate the probable outcomes to clients and/or their care providers, so clients can decide whether to participate in occupational therapy intervention. Not only must practitioners be willing to examine intervention practices to see if they are effective but also they must be open to changes in their intervention patterns when the evidence suggests more effective approaches than the ones they typically use.

OCCUPATIONAL THERAPY PRACTITIONERS

Clients are, of course, an essential component of occupational therapy intervention, but occupational therapy practitioners are the other part of the equation. Practitioners use their clinical-reasoning abilities to actualize their knowledge and skills in practice. Just as clients have an occupational history, so do practitioners. They are also embedded in personal, social, and cultural contexts that shape their worldview. These include their preferred theories and intervention techniques, the practical realities of the setting in which they practice, and the team members with whom they work (Schell & Cervero, 1993).

Like clients, practitioners come with particular strengths and limitations that influence their interactions with others. These strengths and limitations influence how practitioners frame client problems and use the intervention context to benefit clients.

CONCLUSION

Occupational therapy is a complex process that involves collaborative interaction between the practitioner and the client embedded in the intervention context. Occupational therapy intervention must be grounded in research and focused on the client as an occupational being. The therapeutic process evolves as the practitioner and client work together to analyze carefully the client's occupations and performance limitations. Because occupational therapy is a "doing with" and not a "doing to" profession, there is an improvisational aspect of intervention that requires the practitioner and client to coordinate their actions to achieve the client's goal. The rest of this book delineates the various aspects of occupational therapy. It emphasizes consistently that best practice involves (1) understanding and respecting clients, (2) collaborating with clients to achieve their occupational goals, and (3) using interventions that are supported by research.

As you start your career, our challenge to you is to strive to achieve the ideals of the profession. First, be aware of the influence of your beliefs and your personal and professional contexts and how these influence your actions. Second, consistently challenge yourself to listen to your clients so that you can facilitate their autonomy and engagement in desired occupations. Third, use the most effective assessment instruments and interventions to support the progress of your clients. Fourth, advocate for your clients so they can obtain the services they need and learn to advocate for themselves. Finally, systematically evaluate your practice to ensure that your interventions enable your clients to engage in those occupations they value most. The people whose scenarios opened this chapter remind us that, in the words of Yerxa et al. (1989), "people are most true to their humanity when engaged in occupation" (p. 7). Our job is ultimately to help people realize their humanity through occupational engagement.

SECTION II

Population Interventions Focused on Health for All

ANN A. WILCOCK

This section considers how occupational therapy practitioners can extend their expertise into the field of population health. It does so from the point of view of a public health approach to preventing illness and disability and promoting positive health and well-being. The World Health Organization (WHO) began advocating that kind of approach over half a century ago; however, funding for public health approaches has been limited. One reason for limited spending on prevention is the need to fund ongoing remedial programs. A second reason for poor funding of preventive programs is the belief that modern medicine can treat illnesses caused by poor lifestyle choices. Although government spending on preventive programs has been limited, a public-health approach continues to make economic sense, because it is generally cheaper to prevent something than it is to manage a problem once it occurs.

In terms of occupational therapy, a public health approach makes more than economic sense. Population health, wellness, and preventive programs introduce people to the idea of entirely different values of life related to understanding the natural world and the place of occupation as a biologically and socially health-maintaining and-promoting entity. This public health approach has the potential to create a different, saner, and healthier world. However, to go that far requires occupational therapy practitioners to be politically persuasive toward occupationally just environments and policies, to seek out opportunities to inform people at large about the relationship between occupation and health, and to develop programs outside the health-care systems. The creation of occupationally just environments would enable everyone, including those with social as well as mental and physical illness, disability, and handicap, to consider afresh the habits of a lifetime. The *Ottawa Charter for Health Promotion*—hereafter referred to as "the Charter" (World Health Organization [WHO], Health and Welfare, Canada, Canadian Public Health Association, 1986)—articulates a public health perspective. The Charter provides the organizing structure for this section. Selected examples of current population research and initiatives are also provided to illustrate possibilities. As the latter tend to be scarce, this section takes a futures perspective rather than an informative, prescriptive one based on current practice.

There have been, and are, many occupational therapy practitioners whose roles extend beyond the amelioration of illness to the promotion of optimal states of health in line with WHO philosophies. They and others, understand that, if "things" were different, practitioners could play an important role in public health as it is currently conceived. However, like many governments the majority of occupational therapy practitioners have largely ignored public health approaches, even when articulated by leaders in the field. There is a tendency to wait for employment in the field to be initiated and provided by others. Although specific jobs for occupational therapy practitioners to address population level needs are rare, there are opportunities that can be developed.

OCCUPATIONAL THERAPY TOWARD PUBLIC HEALTH

Public health involves more than sanitation, epidemics, and the control of infectious diseases. Last (1987), a late-twentieth-century biographer of public health, defined it as

> *the combination of sciences, skills and beliefs that is directed to the maintenance and improvement of the health of all the people.* (p. 3)

From that it can be seen that public health, in addition to the prevention of illness, embraces health promotion which, according to the Charter (WHO, 1986), is the process of enabling people to increase control over, and to improve, their health. The Charter definition continues:

> *To reach a state of complete physical, mental and social well-being, an individual or group must be able to identify and to realize aspirations, to satisfy needs, and to change or cope with the environment. Health is, therefore, seen as a resource for everyday life, not the objective of living. Health is a positive concept emphasizing social and personal resources, as well as physical capacities. Therefore, health promotion is not just the responsibility of the health sector, but goes beyond healthy life-styles to well-being.* (p. 2)

That definition, although not using the word *occupation* itself, clearly is in tune with the concept of occupational therapy's potentially positive role in maintaining and enhancing health. Few occupational therapy practitioners would argue with this statement. Indeed, it is through their occupations that people realize aspirations, satisfy needs, and change or cope with the environment. So theoretically, at least, it appears that occupational therapy and public health are in alignment.

Public health is now viewed as a dynamic discipline in which people from many different, and sometimes surprising, spheres of interest interact. According to Last (1987), it has to be responsive, not only to the historical and cultural context but also to available facts about perceived human need and social values. Public health requires scientific and technical capabilities to intervene effectively within rapidly changing social and biological environments. With that in mind, population intervention by occupational therapy practitioners is a dynamic process in which practitioners work alongside others from diverse fields. This approach should be responsive to historical and cultural occupation for health needs, patterns, and values, ready to intervene appropriately and rapidly in response to occupational changes of a social, biological, or environmental nature. Population intervention should be informed by research and meet the needs of individuals and communities according to the notions of **occupational justice,** which is a justice that recognizes individual differences in equity of opportunity.

To be effective in population intervention, occupational therapy practitioners need to appreciate and show others how their education relates to the scope of public health. While based in large part on medical science, public health also embraces a social model of health, occupational health and safety, and epidemiological research. Although many occupational therapy practitioners may feel appropriately qualified to participate in public health programs, some need additional course work not covered in their entry-level curriculum. In addition, postgraduate course work in relevant subjects may be useful for practitioners.

For public health authorities to accept that occupational therapy practitioners have something useful to offer, it is

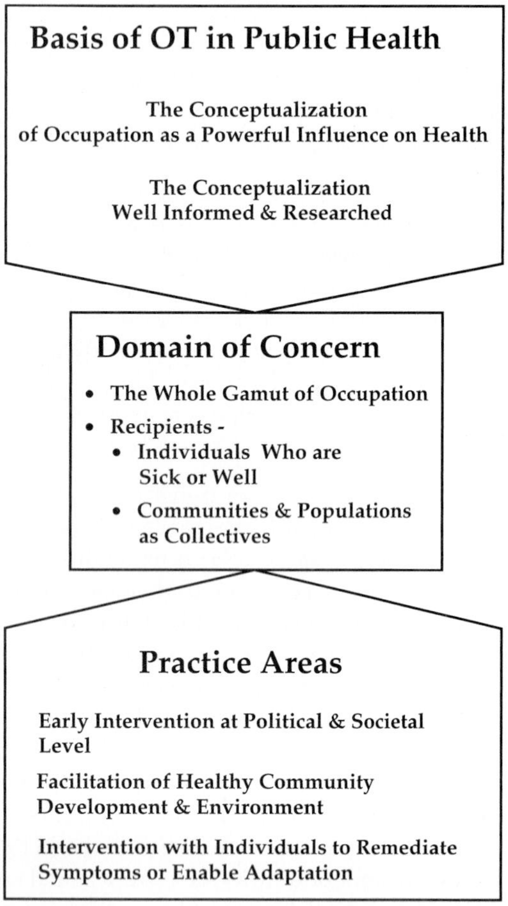

Basis of OT in Public Health

The Conceptualization
of Occupation as a Powerful Influence on Health

The Conceptualization
Well Informed & Researched

Domain of Concern

- The Whole Gamut of Occupation
- Recipients -
  - Individuals Who are Sick or Well
  - Communities & Populations as Collectives

Practice Areas

Early Intervention at Political & Societal Level

Facilitation of Healthy Community Development & Environment

Intervention with Individuals to Remediate Symptoms or Enable Adaptation

FIGURE 3–1. Occupationally focused public health.

necessary to be clear about a direction that an occupationally focused public health could espouse. It requires reacceptance within the profession that occupation is a powerful influence on health and that everyone—individuals who are sick or well, communities, and populations—should be part of the profession's domain of concern (Fig. 3-1). It also requires acceptance that occupationally based intervention at the political and societal levels is as important and as relevant to occupational therapy as treating one patient at a time to remediate symptoms or enable adaptation.

As early as 1934, LeVesconte suggested that occupational therapists take a preventive role in the community. LeVesconte argued that in collaboration with social workers, occupational therapists could establish programs aimed at social and economic reorganization. Now it is argued, similarly, that in collaboration with many diverse disciplines, occupational therapy practitioners could establish programs aimed at social, economic, and health management reorganization through initiatives highlighting people's occupational needs for health and well-being.

Also in the 1930s, Losada (1936) wrote about potential for occupational therapy in the field of preventive medicine, reasoning that it could be an agent for positive health. Very

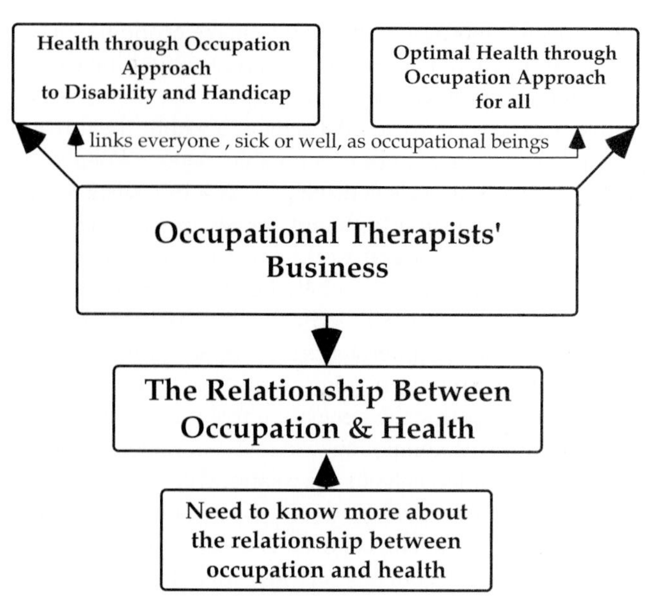

FIGURE 3–2. The basis of the business of occupational therapy.

few, if any, occupational therapists took such a path at that time. It was not until the 1960s and 1970s that a health-promotion and preventive approach that combined notions of occupation with others about health again made a serious debut into occupational therapy literature. People who had either an "occupation" focus to their work or a "public health" focus led this approach. Both arrived at the conclusion that the relationship between occupation and health was paramount, that it was occupational therapists' business, and that they needed to know more about it (Fig. 3-2).

Reilly (1969), and others in her wake, argued that way when she developed her "occupational behavior" perspective toward the treatment of disability and handicap. At about the same time, West (1967), along with a group of leaders in the health and wellness field, encouraged practitioners to focus, through occupation, on "maintaining optimum health rather than . . . intermittent treatment of acute disease and disability" (p. 312). The combination of a health through occupation approach to disability and handicap, as well as an optimal health approach for all, links everyone, sick or well, as occupational beings. Together those approaches suggest that occupational therapy has something to add to the health experience of everyone, if both biomedical and public health philosophies are accepted as the domain of concern. This argument remains true if an occupational perspective of mental, physical, and social health is taken instead of one confined to a biomedical model.

West, in 1968, envisaged that in the future occupational therapists would function as health agents with responsibility toward enabling normal growth and development. In a "new mold" they would consider more fully the socioeconomic, cultural, and biological causes of disease and dysfunction. When considering what appeared to be the growing importance of prevention, she put forward the idea that occupational therapists could offer programs in primary prevention to stop disability or illness from occurring at all and in secondary prevention to effect early detection and retardation of progression to more serious conditions (West, 1969). A year later, at the Fifth International Congress of the World Federation of Occupational Therapists (WFOT), she proposed a health model for occupational therapy practice. This model translated the profession's long-held focus on activities of daily living (ADL) for people with disability to one that centered on a balanced regime of age-appropriate, work-play activities for people before the advent of disease or disability (West, 1970). She called for a client/community-centered practice to enrich development of people's physical, mental, emotional, social, and vocational abilities.

Cromwell (1970), at the same WFOT congress, addressed what she described as a global trend toward preventive as opposed to curative programs and advocated the search for more universal systems of world health care by considering how different nations combated the problems facing them. She saw that the profession's concern about patients' behavior in ordinary environments, where they live, work, and play, was a universal phenomenon of great importance to health and argued for occupational therapists to move into "well care." Similarly, the occupational therapist in prevention programs was the topic of Finn's (1972) Eleanor Clarke Slagle Lecture. Later, she (1977) proposed the development of a model of practice addressing the issue of the significance of occupation to human life. Finn based her argument on the idea that primary prevention is directed toward what keeps people in a state of health rooted on an understanding of the relationship between the basic structural elements of society and of health. It followed, she observed, that practitioners working within primary prevention would make their contribution with a greater understanding of how occupation can keep people in a state of health, according to an understanding of the relationship between health and occupation, which is a basic structural element of society. Those far-sighted occupational therapists were in tune with population health initiatives of the times, for it was in 1978 that WHO, at Alma Ata, made the famous plea: "Health for all by the year 2000." Calling for a new approach to health care that achieved more equitable distribution of resources to close the gap between the haves and have nots, the WHO declaration stressed the importance of the reorientation of health professions toward preventive programs well integrated with curative, rehabilitative, and environmental measures.

Such a plea at a time when economic constraints effectively curbed the development of new trends appears to have been ignored. Prevention did not become, and is still not, a priority in health service offerings. Improved global health was not achieved by the year 2000. Likewise, West's, Cromwell's, and Finn's forecasts were not to come to fruition in any real way. Therefore, occupational therapy practitioners, like other health professionals, did not make that paradigm shift. The majority of health professions remained concentrated on clinical rather than on community programs and on reversing the ill-health states of individuals rather than on taking a proactive stance toward preventing illness and promoting health at population levels.

Public health and world health authorities made another urgent call for action across the globe after the first International Conference on Health Promotion that was held in Ottawa in November 1986 (WHO, 1986). Sponsored by WHO, primarily in response to growing expectations for new public health movements around the world, 212 individuals from 38 countries were invited to participate. Among them were health, lay, and other professional workers from government, voluntary, and community organizations; politics; administration; and academics. The open dialogue of the conference, while recognizing all regions, focused on industrialized countries. At the meeting, the Charter was drawn up, aimed at stimulating action toward achieving the "Health for all by the year 2000" objective of the conference at Alma Ata. It called on other international governments, nongovernment and voluntary organizations, and people in all walks of life to join forces "to advocate the promotion of health in all appropriate forums and to support countries in setting up strategies and programs for health promotion" (p. 5).

TAKING A FUTURES PERSPECTIVE

"Moving into the future" is one of the major headings in the Charter. And this and other messages contained in the Charter are worthy of consideration. The Charter begins with a sentence in which goodness of fit with occupational therapy principles of practice are obvious:

> *Health is created and lived by people within the settings of their everyday life; where they learn, work, play, and love. (p. 8)*

Consider, for example, how well the Charter's vision of health meshes with Neistadt and Crepeau's (1998) description of occupational therapy as "the art and science of helping people to do the day-to-day activities that are important to them despite impairment, disability, or handicap" (p. 5). This is in line with Humphry's (2002) recent articulation of occupation as an interactive process between the person and the environment, resulting in socially expected or freely chosen activities that are "culturally valued, coherent patterns of actions" (p. 172). These would include daily activities; instrumental activities of daily living, work, education, play, leisure, and social participation (American Occupational Therapy Association Commission on Practice [AOTA], in press).

A population approach could extend Neistadt and Crepeau's (1998) description by eliminating the words "despite impairment, disability, or handicap" and inserting, instead, a few more words. It would then read that occupational therapy is the art and science of helping all people to engage in the day-to-day activities that are important to them and to their health and well-being. The holistic nature of the phrase includes those people with disability and handicap but does not single them out as different. That last point is emerging as important in terms of social justice as put forward by numerous support groups for people with special needs.

The Charter continues its "moving into the future" suggestions with other notions that are congruent with occupational therapy ideology. One example is the idea that "health is created by caring for oneself and others" and "by being able to take decisions and have control over one's life circumstances" (p. 5). This idea is germane to my own findings from historical research that when people lived naturally, in a way similar to other species in the wild, nature itself imposed self-health occupational regimes (Wilcock, 1998, 2001). Occupation for self-health in the natural environment is an in-built survival mechanism but one that we need to consider consciously in the artificial environment in which many people now live. This artificial environment no longer provides self-health opportunities of the same kind or to the same extent; but for thousands of years, when life was decidedly more adventurous, unpredictable, and freer of constraints, people engaged in an occupation continuum of activity and rest according to diurnal variation and the seasons. Through these occupations, people kept their physical, mental, and social capacities honed and healthy. To survive, people dealt with many and various challenges to provide for their daily requirements and depended on the social collective of the community in which they lived. People, often in consultation with kin and other community members, would have determined what occupations made them feel better when they were sick, whether their health improved with restful or energetic activity. It is probable that they also made use of their apparent inventive capacities to adapt occupations or tools to enable the carrying out of ADL despite dysfunction. It was not until late in the nineteenth century that trained medical personnel began to replace these lay approaches to health maintenance (Wilcock, 1998, 2001).

It has not been possible to ensure, as the Charter prescribes, "that the society one lives in creates conditions that allow the attainment of health by all its members" (p. 5). Daily, the newspapers, even in the most advanced countries in the world, tell a tale of hopelessness, despair, and illness created by people not being able to cope or to fit into their environment and its demands. Drug and alcohol abuse are rife; depression and youth suicide abound; family discord, poverty, lack of autonomy and power, aggression, and crime are accepted as the norm; and long waiting lists for hospitals and medical care are common for all but the affluent. Many of the reasons for such unhealthy outcomes may be that socioeconomic/political planners have insufficiently considered the occupational needs of people. The environments created by their endeavors are not ones in which occupational justice abounds, so that some people are unable to find meaning, to reach adequately toward their occupational potential or, in some cases, to meet basic sustenance and safety needs through what they do.

One reason for this inattention to occupation is the insufficient evidence about the relationship between occupation and health on which to base decisions. This points to the need for occupational therapy practitioners and occupational scientists to extend their "health" research into population issues around basic occupational determinants or prerequisites of health. For example, a study I conducted with a student group explored a sample of 140 people's self-reported perceptions and experiences of well-being. Participants named specific occupational factors related to their own experience of well-being, such as leisure, achievement, selfless activity, religious practice, and work. When these were grouped together into one "occupation" category, engagement in occupation with particular meaning to them was the most frequent response, ranking above social relationships—the issue that has seemed to receive most mention in other explorations (Wilcock et al., 1998).

Blaxter's (1990) study of 9000 adults in the United Kingdom, revealed that people there describe health variously, such as never being ill or diseased, having energy, and being physically or psychologically fit or functionally able. Some participants were not able to articulate any views. She concluded that views of health are multidimensional and differ over the life course and between genders. Some of Blaxter's results point to an occupational component. Her survey found that *energy*, inclusive of physical and psychosocial vitality, was "the word most frequently used by all women and older men to describe health" (pp. 24–25) and most often was expressed as enthusiasm about work. For younger men, energy came a close second to fitness, a category that "stressed strength, athletic prowess, [and] the ability to play sports" (pp. 24–25). Young people, particularly, associated health with other well-publicized health occupations, like "virtuous" eating patterns, exercise, and not drinking or smoking, citing "the role of 'bad habits' in the causation of disease" (p. 24). Of even more interest from an occupational perspective is the notion of "health as function," which was again most frequently mentioned by older people. This view of health incorporated ideas about being able to perform physically demanding work, to participate in "social, family and community activity," "being fit to work" or to "work despite an advanced age," as well as "being mobile or self-sufficient" (p. 28). Some, including the young, saw health as "being able to do what you want to when you want to" (p. 28).

For those in the middle years, psychosocial well-being was the most frequently cited concept for describing self-health. Often associated with health as energy, as social relationships, or as function, psychosocial well-being was a separate concept that some used to describe "spirituality, mental alertness, happiness, enjoyment, and a relaxed attitude" (p. 29).

Blaxter's findings suggest that a considerable number of people link health with occupation but use terms to describe it in the way media reports discuss health, using words such as *physical fitness*, *exercise*, *energy*, *relationships*, and *mental health*, but not the word *occupation*. The lack of the use of the term occupation is hardly surprising, as it is extremely rare to find articles in the popular media discussing the relationship between occupation and health by occupational therapy practitioners. That probably also points to one of the reasons why occupation-related (used in the generic sense) issues of health are seldom the primary concerns of policy makers. Although occupation is regarded as part of the ordinary fabric of life, it is so pervasive in all aspects of life that it is easy to ignore its relationship with health. The paucity of research to demonstrate the relationship of occupation to health may also contribute to this lack of awareness by policy makers. Consequently, research into the relationship between occupation and health and communication of research findings to inform laypeople and policy makers is a necessary aspect of population-based practice.

The Charter named five directions for health promotion action. The subsequent parts of this section delineate these directions, which are reorienting health services, creating supportive environments, strengthening community action, developing personal skills, and building healthy public policy.

REORIENTING HEALTH SERVICES

> *The role of the health sector must move increasingly in a health promotion direction, beyond its responsibility for providing clinical and curative services.* (WHO, 1986, p. 4)

That statement challenges occupational therapy practitioners, along with other health service providers, to embrace an expanded mandate that supports the needs of individuals and communities for a healthier life. The Charter stresses that "the responsibility for health promotion in health services is shared among individuals, community groups, health professionals, health service institutions and governments" (p. 4) working together. This shared responsibility requires open communication between health service providers and those working across broader segments of the environment. Furthermore, the Charter articulates the importance of changes in professional education and training, attention to health (as distinct from ill-health) research, and focus of health services to the holistic needs of individuals.

Most occupational therapists are likely to feel immediately comfortable about the way the Charter suggests a focus on "the total needs of the individual as a whole person" (p. 4). However, despite the profession's idealistic commitment to holism, it can be argued that many of its members have concentrated on the treatment of, or adaptation to, symptoms rather than the whole range of individual occupational needs necessary for health and well-being. Moreover, there are even some aspects of each individual's meaningful occupations not addressed by occupational therapy practitioners to any extent. Depending on the practice setting, vocational, playful, sexual, and creative needs, for example, may sometimes be given only cursory attention in the drive for fast discharge to which many have felt constrained to conform. Practitioners may need to reconsider such initiatives and directions from their own distinct focus to align themselves with the Charter's proposed reorientation. The profession's long-held, but sometimes invisible, philosophical base could benefit from what appears to be the WHO's championing of similar ideas.

To meet the requirements of the sort of reorientation described by the Charter, serious reflection on the part of occupational therapy practitioners is called for. The WHO challenge addressed all health professionals, and the spirit of holistic health with which it is imbued seems to have goodness of fit with many of the ideas and beliefs that form the foundation of occupational therapy. If the profession ignores the directive or chooses not to meet the challenge, a major opportunity to prove the essential nature and worth of occupational therapy will be lost. However, far more serious, the health of large numbers of the world's population may be affected. Occupational factors in health could remain sidelined, or parts of it considered in isolation. Unfortunately, the latter scenario is close to the situation today. That is not to say that the work carried out at present is not of value and important. It is. However, much more needs to be done from both an occupational and a population perspective.

Challenges for Occupational Therapy

Accepting the mandate to support all individual and community needs for a healthier life requires that occupational therapy practitioners in partnership with those they seek to assist, with involved others, and with governments take a proactive stand toward the attainment of occupationally healthy social, political, and economic systems. To do this several fundamental changes are necessary:

1. Be true to the professions' own mandate. This is an often-difficult thing to do, especially when others on the team are frequently in a position of power and

impose their requirements ahead of those that occupational therapy practitioners espouse.

2. Become part of different teams. While in the past occupational therapy practitioners have been team players with medically oriented health professionals, such as physical and speech therapists, medical social workers, and nurses, population intervention calls for sharing power with a range of others. Most important, these include communities and the population itself. They might also include health promotion, community development, and public health practitioners with a variety of different professional backgrounds, including people from sectors outside the broad health-care arena and those with a focus on parts of occupation who may be seen as potentially threatening to the profession. Developing a working relationship with politicians, social planners, research bodies, and the media will be fundamental.
3. Change the emphasis in parts of professional education and training, including fieldwork. Serving the community and working for change at the population level must be emphasized as much as serving the individual. Only through change at the population level can the profession effect change in the occupational health of everyone.
4. Accept and encourage research about the fundamental relationships between occupation and health and health and well-being. Such research should be in addition to outcome research related to medically determined categories of ill health. Research findings about occupation and health may lead to taking a critical stance toward political beliefs and institutions that have a negative impact on people, their health, and their engagement in occupation.
5. For some practitioners, alter the nature of one's employment and employment setting. Instead of working in hospitals and centers specifically for the sick and disabled, practitioners may seek to work in the private sector at many different tasks that aim for health promotion or in community teams that blur rather than accentuate professional differences. They may work as writers, health consultants, or public health researchers. The occupational therapy profession at the national and international levels should support those engaged in these endeavors and recognize them as occupational therapy practitioners with a population focus.

Barriers to Change

To overcome any unexpected impediments in the shift to a population focus, it is important to consider why earlier calls to support the health of all were unsuccessful. Several occupational therapists reflected on the issue during the 1970s. They identified the following factors:

- The daunting number and nature of the social, economic, and political conditions that interfere with health (Grossman, 1977). This remains the case and can be viewed either as a challenge or as a reason to ignore the WHO call.
- The work itself might hold less appeal than work in more acute health services with individuals, because it appeared less defined, less sophisticated, less measurable, and more isolated.
- Positions not designated for occupational therapy practitioners may appear to limit opportunities or to lack professional incentives. These perceived limitations may make it difficult for practitioners to leave the known harbors of traditional health services to work in community institutions (Laukaran, 1977).
- Practitioners might fear the possibility of competition with other professionals in the health promotion field (Laukaran, 1977). Laukaran perceived that these issues had been compounded by long-held values associated with clinically based medicine, for example, that occupational therapy is concerned with ill (defined medically) rather than all people.
- Occupational therapy models may have limited the scope of practice and resulted in gaps in knowledge and theory (Laukaran, 1977). Similarly, Johnson and Kielhofner (1983) argued for fuller development of the profession's knowledge base "concerning social systems and their impact on individuals" to make a contribution to "preventing disease and dysfunctional processes" (p. 191). They contended that "many of those in need of preventive occupational therapy services will not be referred through medical channels, since they are not diseased but are disengaged from daily life" (p. 191).

The problems of 30 or so years ago remain as deterrents today, and reorientation will require a mammoth effort and a different leadership approach in terms of definitions of practice, education requirements, supported research, and informed and critical comment to the outside world. For practitioners making the transition, it will require the commitment and pioneering spirit of the founders.

CREATING SUPPORTIVE ENVIRONMENTS

In its discussion of supportive environments, the Charter calls for the protection of the natural as well as built environments, proposing that any health promotion strategy must address the conservation of natural resources. Idealistically, it goes further when it recommends that taking care of each other, our communities, and our natural environment should be the overall guiding principle for "the world, nations, regions, and communities alike" (p. 3). This guiding principle recognizes the complexity and interrelatedness of societies so that it became clear:

> *Health cannot be separated from other goals. The inextricable links between people and their environment constitutes the basis for a socio-ecological approach to health.* (p. 3)

Occupational therapy practitioners may think that their professional role is not closely connected to wider ecological issues. However, a futures perspective suggests otherwise. First, most people are aware that the natural environment requires urgent attention if future generations are to have a reasonable chance of an environment that supports a healthy life. People through their occupations, particularly in the last century, have caused the deterioration of the environment. Any population health occupational therapy approach has to consider environmental quality within community initiatives. In doing so, it must be proactive at the policy level to prevent further environmental degradation and must lead the way in proposing occupational alternatives that will provide meaning and a healthful future for individuals. Bellamy (1997) provided some ideas of how meaningful occupation that sustains the ecology for all people around the globe might be achieved.

The Charter, when explaining what is involved in the social environment, focuses on the centrality of changing patterns of work and leisure and their impact on health (Fig. 3-3). On more familiar turf for occupational therapy practitioners, it is heartening to read that the delegates in Ottawa considered that

> *work and leisure should be a source of health for people. The way society organizes work should help create a healthy society. Health promotion generates living and working conditions that are safe, stimulating, satisfying and enjoyable.* (p. 3)

Further, the Charter recommends:

> *systematic assessment of the health impact of a rapidly changing environment particularly in areas of technology, work, energy production and urbanization followed by action towards positive health benefit to the population at large.* (p. 4)

Even within more usual environments for occupational therapy, it is possible to enable increased health and well-being through attention to increasing their supportive nature. In that regard, several recent studies by occupational therapists are worthy of note. Brown et al. (2001), in their study of the context and meaning of work, found that environmental issues enhanced meaning and satisfaction and, presumably, resulted in greater psychological and physical health. These findings led the researchers to recommend the establishment of meaningful work environments, which included

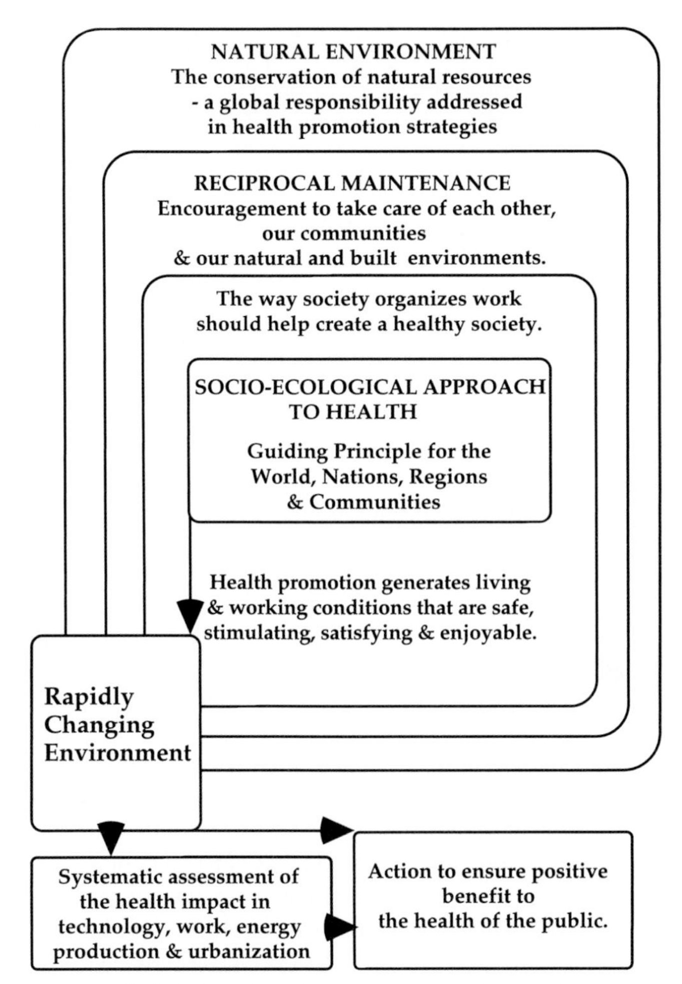

FIGURE 3–3. Creating supportive environments.

> *enhancing personal and professional pride, facilitating self respect for individuals, placing emphasis on the value of learning, providing variety in the workplace and encouraging autonomy and the need for work to include opportunities for creativity, as well as being flexible enough to assist people maintaining significant relationships outside work.* (p. 225)

An interesting study of 22 families carried out by Law, Haight, Milroy, Willms, Stewart, and Rosembaum (1999) explored the constraints that children with physical disability encounter within their environment. It is interesting that Law et al. found that social and institutional environments were greater barriers to occupational engagement than was physical accessibility. Participants suggested that removal of such social and environmental barriers would "enhance their children's ability to participate in occupations of their choice" (p. 108).

In a less familiar example of rehabilitation practice, McDonough describes the challenges of providing a supportive environment within a very different context (What's a Practitioner to Do? 3-1). McDonough's contribution links

WHAT'S A PRACTITIONER TO DO?
Challenging Environments

SUE MCDONOUGH

Wars are the leading injury-related cause of death in Africa (World Health Organization [WHO], 2001). Every 10 min a person, somewhere, is injured or killed by a land mine (Husum, Gilbert, & Wisborg, 2000). More mines are being set than are being cleared. Many of the poorest people of the world have no choice but to enter mine-infested areas to collect wood, grow food, or work for the survival of their families. Survivors of injuries caused by land mines, war, and accidents need rehabilitation: to heal in body and mind, to engage in daily activities, and to participate in their communities. How can this become a reality for people living in some of the poorest and most disadvantaged communities in the world?

In the late 1980s and early 1990s, I was one of several Australian therapists working with an Ethiopian relief agency in Sudan and later in Tigray (in northern Ethiopia). Ethiopia was at that time ravaged by civil wars that had been raging for decades. Its economy, still largely based on small-scale subsistence farming, had been torn apart. Waves of famine, conflict involving both ground troops and aerial bombing, mass movements of people, and murder of educated members of ethnic minority groups all wreaked havoc on the inhabitants. Infant and maternal mortality was high, and life expectancy was low. Many young people, fighting on either side of the conflict, were killed or severely disabled.

In Sudan we found an energetic, organized Tigrayan community based in one main and two smaller care centers on the outskirts of the town Wad Medani. Many people were learning to read and write in their own language for the first time. Some were learning to become tailors or printers. Others fulfilled a range of supporting roles—cooks, drivers, nurses, teachers, administrators. Most were young and disabled. We were struck by the phenomenal industry with which this group approached daily life, which extended to very competitive volleyball and lively Friday-night cultural events. Within this environment, we trained about 20 rehabilitation workers in knowledge and skills to help them care for and rehabilitate the injured.

Within a few years, Tigray came under the control of the popularly supported rebel movement, and it became safe enough for the people based in Wad Medani to return to their homeland. The rehabilitation worker-training program continued at the Central Hospital, a sprawling network of buildings nestled into craggy mountains alongside parched riverbeds. Skillfully camouflaged from the view of fighter jets, the hospital was entirely staffed by Tigrayans. In 1991, the civil war ended. A few years later, after helping to organize some vocational training for disabled fighters, the expatriate therapists were phased out. More than 10 years after that first rehabilitation worker-training program began in Wad Medani, some of rehabilitation workers still work in regional hospitals in Tigray. They are doing so in the absence of the peer support and training that the project had hoped to establish. The rapidly changing political circumstances at the time, made it difficult to pursue the project's broader aim of developing far-reaching services for people with disabilities.

Western-trained therapists have a lot to offer, but how they get involved and what they do are critical. Inevitably, they bring along underlying assumptions about health and life values. It is not easy to be reflective about one's own beliefs, but it is a necessary and ongoing part of the practice of working within another culture (Ingstd & Whyte, 1995). When seeing men who had lost both forearms in explosions being fed by others in preference to using adapted equipment, I was jolted to find how irrelevant the goal of independence can be. Personal independence and meeting family needs are highly valued in some cultures, because doing as much as one can for oneself is critical to survival in situations where there are no formal structures to rely on. However, in the Tigrayan culture, washing or feeding others and eating from a shared plate are everyday means of expressing love among friends and family, able-bodied or disabled. Such a difference illustrates how the meaning attached to the experience of being injured or disabled is culturally determined. We heard some disabled trainees describe their injuries, not as might be expected in terms of loss but more positively as a release from the front line and a lasting outward sign to others of their commitment to their cause. Coping with hunger, war, and death of family members and friends, they explained, was more challenging than losing a leg.

Practitioners who fail to see through their own cultural assumptions risk being ineffective and, worse, doing harm. This is how an experienced Angolan paramedic who trains villagers to provide emergency care for land mine survivors, explains his approach:

> *I begin by finding out how life is there, what the people do to cope, and what they do when different situations arise. I do not need to tell people what I think they need to know, they always ask. (Tromso Mine Victim Resource Center, personal communication, 2000)*

Continues

With basic training and support, health workers and family members can speed healing and reduce the likelihood of lasting disability. For example, caregivers can be made aware of signs of potential problems and shown how to respond. Pressure sores, nerve damage, circulatory problems, poor bone union from inadequate fracture reduction, contractures, and loss of muscle strength are common secondary problems that are avoidable and cause unnecessary suffering. The causes of movement problems, such as pain, joint stiffness, muscle weakness, and spasticity, are often responsive to straightforward treatment that the injured person and his or her family can learn.

Rehabilitation services that address the long- as well as the short-term implications of injury are also important. A study of people with moderate-to-severe physical injuries from land mines in Cambodia and northern Iraq found that the severity of the injury is not a strong indicator of whether or not there will be chronic problems in the future (Husum et al., in press). Despite access to good emergency, surgical, and postoperative care for these people, it was the loss of the means to provide for themselves and their families that was strongly associated with ongoing, and in some cases increasing, pain 1 year after the incident. People with ongoing distress need support, the means to sustain a livelihood, and practical aids like splints and equipment made from low-cost local materials to make moving around and doing everyday activities easier.

Rehabilitation should continue until injured people are home and participating in their local communities. As in Western societies, homes, schools, and workplaces can be adapted to improve access. Those who are unable to continue to do their usual work may need financial and practical help to find alternative work or retraining. In addition, particularly in terms of creating supportive environments, microcredit schemes can make it possible for a disadvantaged family to begin a small income-generating business. More positive community attitudes toward people with disabilities can be nurtured and promoted. Self-help groups are a way of rebuilding hope and lobbying for practical, economic, and political change.

Approaches founded on the strengths of local people are more likely to succeed than those planned and controlled by people outside the community (Werner, 1988). A number of successful models within rehabilitation and related fields offer alternative approaches. Husum et al. (2000) gave a detailed account of how to establish, implement, and evaluate training using the model of a village or jungle university. In Ethiopia, rehabilitation workers were trained to become a part of emerging health services in the region; whereas in Ajoya, Mexico, rehabilitation workers in Project PROJIMO are part of an informal family-like community that serves children with disabilities and their families (Werner, 1988). A program in Thailand improved the lives of disabled people through extensive dialogue with remote communities and by assisting local people to identify and solve their own problems (Hobbs, McDonough, & O'Callaghan, in press).

Listening, learning, and teaching are the basis on which to build sustainable, culturally appropriate services.

Hobbs, L., McDonough, S., & O'Callaghan, A. (in press). *Life after injury*. Penang, Malaysia: Third World Network.

Husum, H., Gilbert, M., & Wisborg, T. (2000). Save lives save limbs. Penang, Malaysia: Third World Network.

Husum, H., Resell, K., Vorren, G. Van Heng, Y., Murad, M., Gilbert, M., & Wisborg, T. (in press). Chronic pain in land mine accident survivors in Cambodia and Kurdistan. *Social Science and Medicine*.

Ingstd, B., & Whyte, S. (1995). *Disability and culture*. Berkeley: University of California Press.

Werner, D. (1988). *Disabled village children*. Palo Alto, CA: Hesperain Foundation.

World Health Organization [WHO]. (2001). World report on violence and health: An update. [On-line]. Available at: www.who.int/violence-injury-prevention. Accessed August 8, 2001.

traditional occupational therapy concerns with very disadvantaged environments and introduces the idea of community action, the strengthening of which is another of the actions proposed as essential in the Charter.

STRENGTHENING COMMUNITY ACTION

To achieve better health for all, the Charter states that communities need to be in "control of their own endeavors and destinies" (p. 4). Occupational therapy practitioners can play a part in this process of strengthening community action. Effective community action is achieved via involvement of community members in all phases of planning, from setting priorities to implementation and evaluation. This direct involvement in the community empowers participants and further strengthens community networks. To develop flexible systems for strengthening public participation and direction of health matters, the Charter recommends that communities require "full and continuous access to information, learning opportunities for health, as well as funding support" (p. 4). Today, although not many practitioners work within community

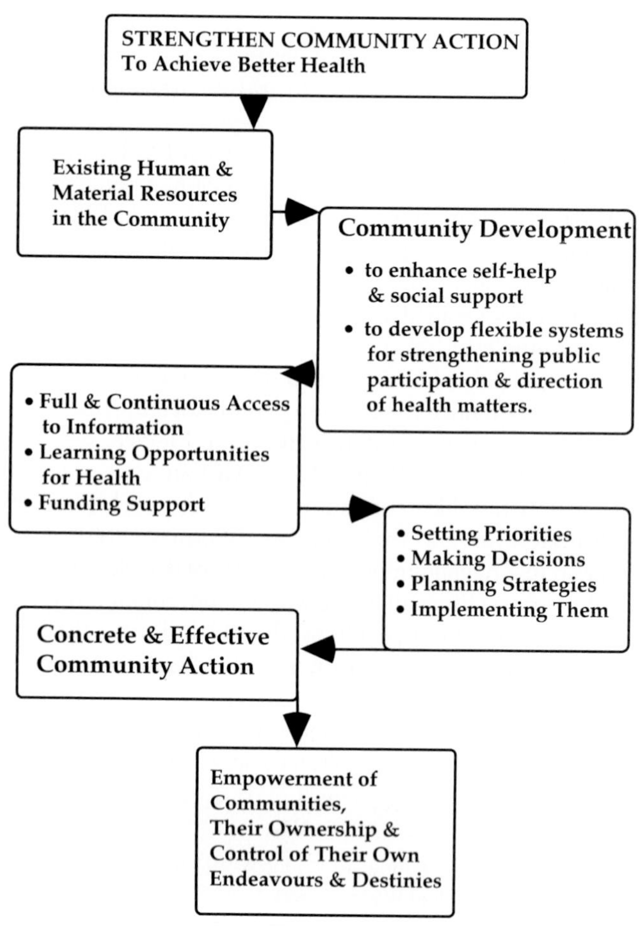

FIGURE 3–4. Strengthening community action.

development in postindustrial societies, quite a number have taken that approach in less-advantaged countries. The establishment of the self-help rehabilitation training described by McDonough is a case in point. It is important for more practitioners to make the transition to community development work, where some of their skills and techniques can enhance social support and facilitate self-help of community members (Fig. 3-4).

In recent decades, community development ideology has influenced occupational therapy practice. For example, a group of clients at a community mental health day treatment center conceived and designed a group learning project to strengthen their community networks as they moved to ex-patient status. Through this project, they sought resources to provide knowledge and practice for themselves and their families to manage the familial and community stressors they anticipated on discharge from the center (Hill, Brittell, & Kotwal, 1989).

Similarly, McColl (1997) described a community-based rehabilitation (CBR) approach as a "strategy within community development for the rehabilitation, equalization of opportunities and social integration of all people with disabilities" (p. 513). This approach, which is consistent with the Charter, involves people with disability and handicap, along with their families and communities in community development. Through this process, communities "learn to listen to disadvantaged and marginalized groups, engage in collective problem solving, and marshal resources which were often previously unknown or underused" (p. 514). The lack of preparation of occupational therapy practitioners and most rehabilitation professionals for work within community development and health promotion can be a barrier (McColl, 1997). However, Twible (1995), another proponent of CBR, found that those therapists who made the transition into the community approach thrived in it, finding it exciting, challenging, and fulfilling.

In taking a population approach within occupational therapy, there would be more to working in community development than the rehabilitation of people with already medically defined disability. It would also include helping the socially and occupationally disadvantaged who are at risk of ill-health in the future. Programs would embrace occupational therapy practitioners as community development workers. These practitioners could enable people to recognize the occupational needs of others as well as their own and to take action to meet such needs more effectively. Thomas (1990), an occupational therapist who worked as a regional training adviser in southeast Asia, described this type of community approach in Pakistan, adjacent to her area of responsibility. There she witnessed the training of local trainers in an integrated rural development project. Extending beyond the sphere of disability, this project embraced socioeconomic needs, including agroforestry, poultry rearing, vocational training, and marketing of local crafts such as carpets, as well as health-care training and health education for school-aged children. Because of the population's low literacy skills, Thomas found that practical training needed to be facilitated by role playing, storytelling, and locally made pictures. This training was slow because many villagers needed to see the results of activities before becoming enthusiastic participants.

DEVELOPING PERSONAL SKILLS

The Charter's fourth strategy for the promotion of population health is the development of personal and social skills. This reflects, in some ways, endorsement of the Wellness Movement, which is primarily an individually focused approach to people making healthy life choices. Some occupational therapy practitioners over the years have espoused wellness models of practice, and literature about it exists in the profession's journals and texts. The Charter recommends that education, practical enhancement of life skills, and information about health be used to help people achieve personal and social development. The approach focuses on

> *increasing the options available to people to exercise more control over their own health, over their environments, and to make choices conducive to health.* (WHO, 1986, p. 4)

Very much in line with traditional occupational therapy ideology, the Charter explains that it is essential to enable "people to learn throughout life, to prepare themselves for all of its stages and to cope with chronic illness and injuries" (p. 4). How it varies from typical occupational therapy procedures is, once again, that the enabling process takes a population approach. Enabling action is facilitated "through educational, professional, commercial and voluntary bodies" within the institutions themselves, in "school, home, work and community settings" (p. 4).

Occupational therapy practitioners who take a population approach have to promulgate, widely and within different types of institutions and organizations, material about their distinctive knowledge—the relationship between occupation and health. Information about occupation and health includes a research-based articulation of concepts relating to occupational satisfaction, meaning, purpose, choice, opportunity, balance, challenges, growth, equity, freedom, creativity, and potential. Practitioners must transmit this information in popular media such as newspapers, magazines, and electronic forums as well as in handouts, promotional material in clinics, and papers in journals. Information should be followed by opportunities for action via workshops, seminars, or individual counseling and, when possible, by client-driven practical skills training. It is perfectly feasible to base even occupational therapy in acute care services on a health and wellness model aimed at the development of personal skills. Follow-up studies could provide essential material to assist with the growth and development of future population public health approaches.

Pols's (2001) study of "best practice" for residents with dementia in low-dependency care is an example of research that combines community and personal development interests. Taking a public health approach within a selected population in South Australia Pols found three best practice principles emerged from in-depth interviews with experts in the field. The first was that residents' needs should drive responses from staff and management, in spite of the progressive decline of the residents' cognitive and functional capacities. The second principle held that an enabling approach is both a feature and a strategy of best practice. Such an approach encourages residents, staff, and management to meet their own needs for autonomy and well-being. The third principle recognized residents, staff, and management as occupational beings in relationship to each other. That principle provided the foundation for the other practices. That is, best practice depends on meeting the occupational needs of all members of the community—residents, staff, and management. Following this research, community initiatives were established to effect change according to these principles.

In similar vein, a study by Baum (1995) of couples in which one of each pair had Alzheimer-type dementia, found that individuals who remain actively engaged in occupation demonstrated fewer disturbing behaviors and required less help with basic self-care. Their caregivers also experienced less stress.

A study by Jonsson, Borell, and Sadlo (2000) focused on retirement as an occupational transition and provided insights into another venue to develop social and personal skills that will maintain and enhance health of older adults. They concluded that preparation for retirement and social policies that encourage social participation of retirees in the community should be explored, for both would provide the structure that many participants felt they lacked in their lives.

This small selection of studies suggests that population initiatives focused on occupationally based community programs are worth developing. In fact, there were two population studies in 1990s even more worthy of mention in that regard. The first was the Well Elderly Study carried out in Los Angeles by a team from the University of Southern California (Clark et al., 1997). The results of that study suggested that the two control groups who engaged in either social activity or no program at all tended to decline over the period of the study. However, significant health, function, and quality-of-life benefits resulted for the occupationally based group. This suggests a preventive capacity for occupational therapy intervention that militates against the health risks of older adults.

The second was another population-based study which examined the association between activities and mortality. Glass et al. (1999) found that

> *social and productive activities (occupations) that involve little or no enhancement of fitness lower the risk of all causes of mortality as much as fitness activities do. This suggests that in addition to increased cardiopulmonary fitness, activity may confer survival benefits through psychosocial pathways. Social and productive activities that require less physical exertion may complement exercise programs and may constitute alternative interventions for frail elderly people.* (p. 478)

These population studies of people without specific disability or illness suggest that occupational needs require close attention, research, and action at the population as well as the individual level. Although the examples provided in this section have been exclusively concerned with the elderly, occupational therapy practitioners could conduct similar research and action with different populations and age groups. Together, these studies support the efficacy of occupational therapy practice and its place in public health as well as acute and rehabilitative medical services. For growth and development in that direction to occur, proactive advocacy in sociopolitical arenas is required. This thought leads to the Charter's last directive for action—that of building healthy public policy.

BUILDING HEALTHY PUBLIC POLICY

A healthy population takes more than a good health-care system with keen, committed, and well-trained health professionals. As the Charter proposes, health has to be "on the agenda of policy makers in all sectors and at all levels" in that they need "to be aware of the health consequences of their decisions and to accept their responsibilities for health" (p. 3). Legislation, fiscal measures, taxation, and organizational change, for example, are not only economically important but also are relevant, in some way, to health policy and outcomes:

> *It is coordinated action that leads to health, income, and social policies that foster greater equity. Joint action contributes to ensuring safer and healthier goods and services, healthier public services and cleaner, more enjoyable environments. (p. 3)*

The Charter's directive is that, in general, the approaches taken should be those of enabler, mediator, or advocate.

- To *enable* all people to achieve their fullest health potential action needs to target equity of opportunities and resources and reduction of the differences in current health status. Targets include creating "supportive environments, access to information, life skills and opportunities for making healthy choices" (p. 2).
- To *mediate* among differing interests in society toward the pursuit of health is a major responsibility of all health-care personnel. Such mediation aims at enabling men and women to take control of political, economic, social, cultural, environmental, behavioral, and biological factors that determine their health.
- To *advocate* for health recognizes that health is a major resource for social and economic development and personal quality of life. Advocacy is aimed at creating favorable conditions and reducing those harmful to health.

Taking a population approach to health means that occupational therapy practitioners need to be able to identify obstacles to the adoption of healthy public policies in non-health and health sectors alike. Identification alone is not enough. Ideas to remove or prevent the obstacles from occurring at all are also required so that policy makers themselves find it easier to frame the healthier choice. In any such advocacy role, occupational therapy practitioners would be addressing their area of specialty, namely, how the legislation or organizational change might affect people's engagement in health-giving occupation.

Such agendas can and should be applied to populations that have been traditionally served by occupational therapy. Gilfoyle, in her 1984 Eleanor Clarke Slagle Lecture, advocated for practitioners:

- To increase their "awareness to include social, economic, and political factors" (p. 576).

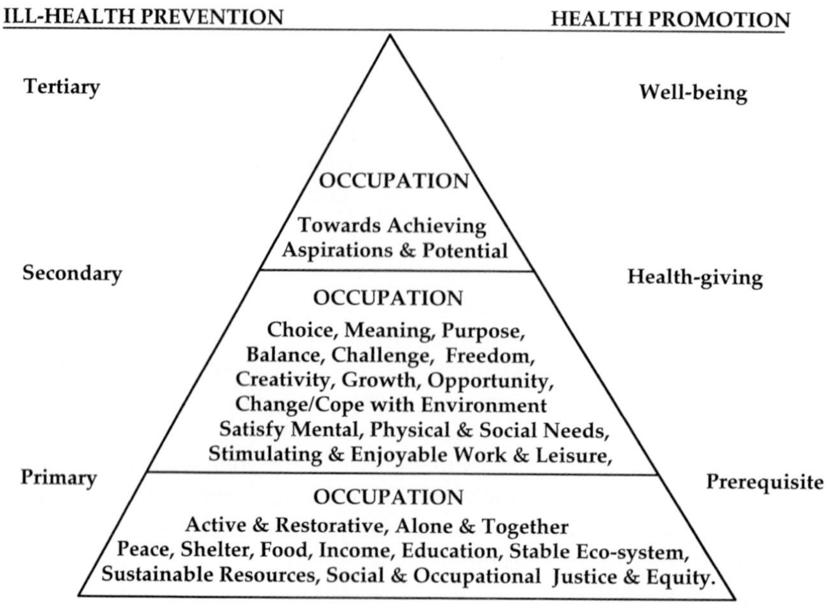

FIGURE 3–5. Daily occupation for health triangle.

- To uncover new understandings of "the value of occupation and the patients' occupational process in promoting their own health" (p. 575).

Other issues need to be pursued to reduce the inequities of opportunities or the obstacles to healthy choices of occupation for many populations of people with handicap or disability of a physical or psychological nature. Taking on the role of advocates or mediators as well as individual enablers for the traditional client group is an obvious step to making policy makers aware of the occupational health needs of the population at large. For example, Pentland, Harvey, and Walker's (1998) study of daily time use of men with spinal cord injuries supported the need to reduce obstacles to healthy occupational opportunities. Their research led to the recommendation that

> *rehabilitation, education, and resources need to go beyond personal care independence such that person's with disabilities can expand their leisure and productivity roles and become better socially and economically integrated into society. (p. 14)*

For appropriate action to take place with this or other populations so that social and economic integration occur equitably across communities or nations instead of case by case, policies may well require change. Even if equal-opportunity legislation is in place, practical intervention at the population level may be necessary to resolve community or environmental access issues.

Addressing the needs of all members of the public, the Charter lists the fundamental conditions and resources that are prerequisite for health. These include peace, shelter, education, food, income, a stable ecosystem, sustainable resources, social justice, and equity. These conditions and resources relate to the basic physiological relationship between occupation and health. They provide the foundation for a visual depiction of occupation for health that may be useful as a population aid in much the same way that the depiction of the daily food triangle is useful (Fig. 3-5).

CONCLUSION

Occupational therapy could make a major contribution to population health by adopting the directions provided in the *Ottawa Charter for Health Promotion*. The major conceptual stumbling block preventing progress in that direction is the dominance of the idea of the "individual" within the profession and the more or less exclusive focus on disability and handicap. While both are important and not to be forsaken in any move toward population intervention, they are so dominant that is difficult to appreciate the occupation for health issues that need attention in the wider social-cultural-political picture. Population-based programs can be as effective as individual ones and are sometimes more so. Such was the case in nineteenth-century Great Britain, when programs to clean up the urban areas and to alter unhealthy work practices were found to effect a far greater improvement in population health than even modern medicine achieved in the twentieth century. Population health programs provide the basic foundation for more effective intervention with individuals.

Occupational therapy practitioners are themselves limited and often frustrated by how little they can achieve because they are hampered by their deference to other biomedically based professions; lack of understanding of their potential contribution; small numbers; and political, social, and economic factors. One way to overcome such professional deprivation and alienation is to bring to public health their concept of the "occupational human" and to be prepared to challenge and analyze population-health research directions and strategies from this perspective.

Taking a futures position is nothing new. Occupational therapy practitioners have always been in the futures business. The nature of their service looks, in practical ways, to the building of capacities in order for their clients to function effectively and well in the future rather than in the here-and-now management of symptoms. That futures focus has marked occupational therapy as different, and capitalizing on this difference will be advantageous in population approaches.

To move effectively into the arena of population intervention focused on health for all requires occupational therapy practitioners to be committed advocates about the relationship between occupation and health and the social-cultural-ecological environments necessary to sustain the occupational prerequisites of health and well-being. Practitioners must put aside their reticence to effect occupational justice across all sectors of the population notwithstanding any political criticism that might incur. Furthermore, they must counteract the economic pressures that maintain imbalanced, unsatisfying, and meaningless occupations; unsupportive and inaccessible occupational environments; and resource depletion. They must also focus attention on public health issues, such as hazards in work, leisure, and domestic environments. Practitioners need to respond to communities that suffer inequities in reaching toward health and well-being as a result of the structure and practices of their societies. Finally, by using community-development principles and practice, practitioners must support and enable all people to keep themselves, their families, their friends, and their societies healthy.

References

American Occupational Therapy Association [AOTA]. (1994). Occupational therapy code of ethics. *American Journal of Occupational Therapy, 48*, 1037–1038.

American Occupational Therapy Association [AOTA]. (in press). Occupational therapy practice framework: Domain and process. *American Journal of Occupational Therapy*.

Baum, C. M. (1995). The contribution of occupation to function in persons with Alzheimer's Disease. *Journal of Occupational Science: Australia, 2(2)*, 59–67.

Bellamy, D. J. (1997). Workaholics anonymous: Putting people back into the equation of livelihood. *Journal of Occupational Science: Australia, 4*(3), 119–125.

Blaxter, M. (1990). *Health and lifestyles*. London: Tavistock/Routledge.

Brown, A., Kitchell, M., O'Neill, T., Lochlier, J., Vosler, A., Kubek D., & Dale, L. (2001). Identifying meaning and perceived level of satisfaction within the context of work. *Work, 16*, 219–226.

Clark, F. (1993). Occupation embedded in a real life: Interweaving occupational science and occupational therapy. [Eleanor Clarke Slagle Lecture]. *American Journal of Occupational Therapy, 47*, 1067–1078.

Clark, F., Azen, S. P., Zemke, R., Jackson, J., Carlson, M., Mandel, D., Hay, J., Josephson, K., Cherry, B., Hessel, C., Palmer, J., & Lipson L. (1997). Occupational therapy for independent-living older adults: A randomized controlled trial. *Journal of the American Medical Association, 278*, 1321–1326.

Cromwell, F. S. (1971). Our challenges in the seventies. In R. Binswanger, Retrout and Spindler, Irerende (Eds.). *Occupational therapy today-tomorrow: Its present position and possibilities of development (pp.232–238). Proceeds of the Fifth International Congress of the World Federation of Occupational Therapists*. Zurich: Basel Karger.

Engelhardt, H. T. (1977). Defining occupational therapy: The meaning of therapy and the virtues of occupation. *American Journal of Occupational Therapy, 31*, 666–672.

Finn, G. L. (1972). The occupational therapist in prevention programs. [Eleanor Clarke Slagle Lecture]. *American Journal of Occupational Therapy, 26*(2), 59–66.

Finn, G. L. (1977). Update of Eleanor Clarke Slagle Lecture: The occupational therapist in prevention programs. *American Journal of Occupational Therapy, 31*(10), 658–659.

Fisher, A. G. (1998). Uniting practice and theory in an occupational framework. *American Journal of Occupational Therapy, 52*, 509–521.

Gilfoyle, E. M. (1984). Transformation of a profession. [Eleanor Clarke Slagle Lecture]. *American Journal of Occupational Therapy, 38*(9), 575–584.

Glass, T. A., Mendes de Leon, C., Marottoli, R. A., & Berkman, L. F. (1999). Population based study of social and productive activities as predictors of survival among elderly Americans. *British Medical Journal, 319*, 478–483.

Gray, J. M. (1998). Putting occupation into practice: Occupation as ends, occupation as means. *American Journal of Occupational Therapy, 52*, 354–364.

Grosman, J. (1977). Preventive health care and community programming. *American Journal of Occupational Therapy, 31*(6), 351–354.

Hill, L., Brittell, T. D., & Kotwal, J. (1989). A community mental health group designed by clients. In J. A. Johnson & E. Jaffe (Eds.). *Health promotive and preventive programs: Models of occupational therapy practice* (pp. 57–66.). New York: Haworth.

Holm, H. B. (2000). Our mandate for a new millennium: Evidence-based practice, 2000, Eleanor Clarke Slagle Lecture. *American Journal of Occupational Therapy, 54*, 575–585.

Humphry, R. (2002). Young children's occupations: Explicating the dynamics of developmental processes. *American Journal of Occupational Therapy, 56*, 171–179.

Jackson, J. (1998). The value of occupation as the core of treatment: Sandy's experience. *American Journal of Occupational Therapy, 52*, 466–473.

Johnson, J., & Kielhofner, G. (1983). Occupational therapy in the health care system of the future. In G. Kielhofner (Ed.). *Health through occupation: Theory and practice in occupational therapy* (pp. 179–195). Philadelphia: Davis.

Jonsson, H., Borell, L., & Sadlo, G. (2000). Retirement: An occupational transition with consequences for temporality, balance and meaning of occupations. *Journal of Occupational Science, 7*(1), 29–37.

Last, J. M. (1987). *Public health and preventive medicine*. Stamford, CT: Appleton & Lange.

Laukaran, V. H. (1977). Toward a model of occupational therapy for community health. *American Journal of Occupational Therapy, 31*, 71–74.

Law, M. (1998). *Client-centered occupational therapy*. Thorofare, NJ: Slack.

Law, M., Haight, M., Milroy, B., Willms, D., Stewart, D., & Rosembaum, P. (1999). Environmental factors affecting the occupations of children with physical disabilities. *Journal of Occupational Science, 6*(3), 102–110.

Law, M., Seinwender, S., & Leclair, L. (1998). Occupation, health, and well-being. *Canadian Journal of Occupational Therapy, 65*, 81–91.

Le Vesconte, H. P. (1934). The place of occupational therapy in social work planning. *Canadian Journal of Occupational Therapy, 2*, 13–16.

Losada, C. A. (1936). Some values in occupational therapy. *Occupational Therapy and Rehabilitation, 15*, 285–289.

Mattingly, C. (1991). The narrative nature of clinical reasoning. *American Journal of Occupational Therapy, 45*, 979–986.

McColl, M. A. (1997). Meeting the challenges of disability. In C. Christiansen & C. Baum (Eds.). *Occupational therapy: Enabling function and well-being* (pp. 508–528). Thorofare, NJ: Slack.

Meyer, A. (1977/1922). The philosophy of occupational therapy. *American Journal of Occupational Therapy, 31*, 639–642.

Neistadt, M. E., & Crepeau, E. B. (1998). Introduction to occupational therapy. In M. E. Neistadt & E. B. Crepeau (Eds.). *Willard and Spackman's occupational therapy* (9th ed., pp. 5–12). Philadelphia: Lippincott.

Pentland, W., Harvey, A. S., & Walker, J. (1998). The relationship between time use and health and well-being in men with spinal cord injury. *Journal of Occupational Science, 5*(1), 14–25.

Pierce, D. (1998). What is the source of occupation's treatment power? *American Journal of Occupational Therapy, 52*, 490–491.

Pols, V. (2001). *Experts views of what is best practice in dementia care for hostel residents*. Unpublished master's thesis, University of South Australia, Adelaide.

Pörn, I. (1993). Health and adaptedness. *Theoretical Medicine, 14*, 295–303.

Rappaport, J. (1987). Terms of empowerment/exemplars of prevention: Toward a theory for community psychology. *American Journal of Community Psychology, 15*(2), 121–145.

Reilly, M. (1969). The educational process. *American Journal of Occupational Therapy, 23*, 299–307.

Sackett, D. L., Rosenberg, W. M. C., Muir Grany, J. A., Haynes, R. B., & Richardson, W. S. (1996). Evidence-based medicine: What it is and what it isn't? *British Medical Journal, 312*, 71–72.

Schell, B. B., & Cervero, R. M. (1993). Clinical reasoning in occupational therapy: An integrative review. *American Journal of Occupational Therapy, 47*, 605–610.

Thomas, K. (1990). A letter from Nepal. In A. A. Wilcock (Ed.). *Health promotion and occupational therapy. Workbook* (pp. 168–169). Melbourne, Australia: World Federation of Occupational Therapists Congress.

Tickle-Degnen, L. (2000). Communicating with clients, family members, and colleagues about research evidence. *American Journal of Occupational Therapy, 54*, 341–343.

Townsend, E. (1996). Institutional ethnography: A method for showing how the context shapes practice. *Occupational Therapy Journal of Research, 16*, 179–199.

Trombly, C. A. (1995). Purposefulness and meaningfulness as therapeutic mechanisms. [Eleanor Clarke Slagle Lecture]. *American Journal of Occupational Therapy, 49*, 960–972.

Twible, R. (1995). Journeying to a new land of hope—A promise for our survival. [Keynote address]. Paper presented at the Australian Association of Occupational Therapists 18th Federal and Inaugural Pacific Rim Conference, Hobart, Australia.

West, W. (1967). The occupational therapists changing responsibilities to the community. *American Journal of Occupational Therapy, 21*, 311–315.

West, W. (1968). Professional responsibility in times of change. [Eleanor Clarke Slagle Lecture]. *American Journal of Occupational Therapy, 22*, 9–15.

West, W. (1969). The growing importance of prevention. *American Journal of Occupational Therapy, 23*, 223–231.

West, W. (1970). The emerging health model of occupational therapy practice. In Binswanger, Retrout and Spindler, Irerende (Eds). *Proceedings of the Fifth International Congress of the World Federation of Occupational Therapists* (pp. 3–7). Zurich: Basel: Karger.

Wilcock, A. A. (1998). *An occupational perspective of health*. Thorofare, NJ: Slack.

Wilcock, A. A. (2001). *Occupation for health: A journey from self health to prescription*. London: College of Occupational Therapists.

Wilcock, A. A., van der Arendt, H., Darling, K., Scholz, J., Siddal, R. Snigg, C., & Stephens, J. (1998) An exploratory study of people's perceptions and experiences of well-being. *British Journal of Occupational Therapy, 61*(2), 75–82.

World Health Organization [WHO]. (1978). *Report of the international conference on primary health care*. Alma Ata, USSR.

World Health Organization [WHO]: Health and Welfare, Canada; & Canadian Public Health Association. (1986). *Ottawa charter for health promotion*. Ottawa, Canada.

Yerxa, E. J. (1967). Authentic occupational therapy. [Eleanor Clarke Slagle Lecture] *American Journal of Occupational Therapy, 21*, 1–9.

Yerxa, E. J., Clark, F., Frank, G., Jackson, J., Parham, D., Pierce, D., Stein, C., & Zemke, R. (1989). An introduction to occupational science: The foundation for occupational therapy in the 21st century. *Occupational Therapy in Health Care, 6(4)*, 1–17.

UNIT *two*

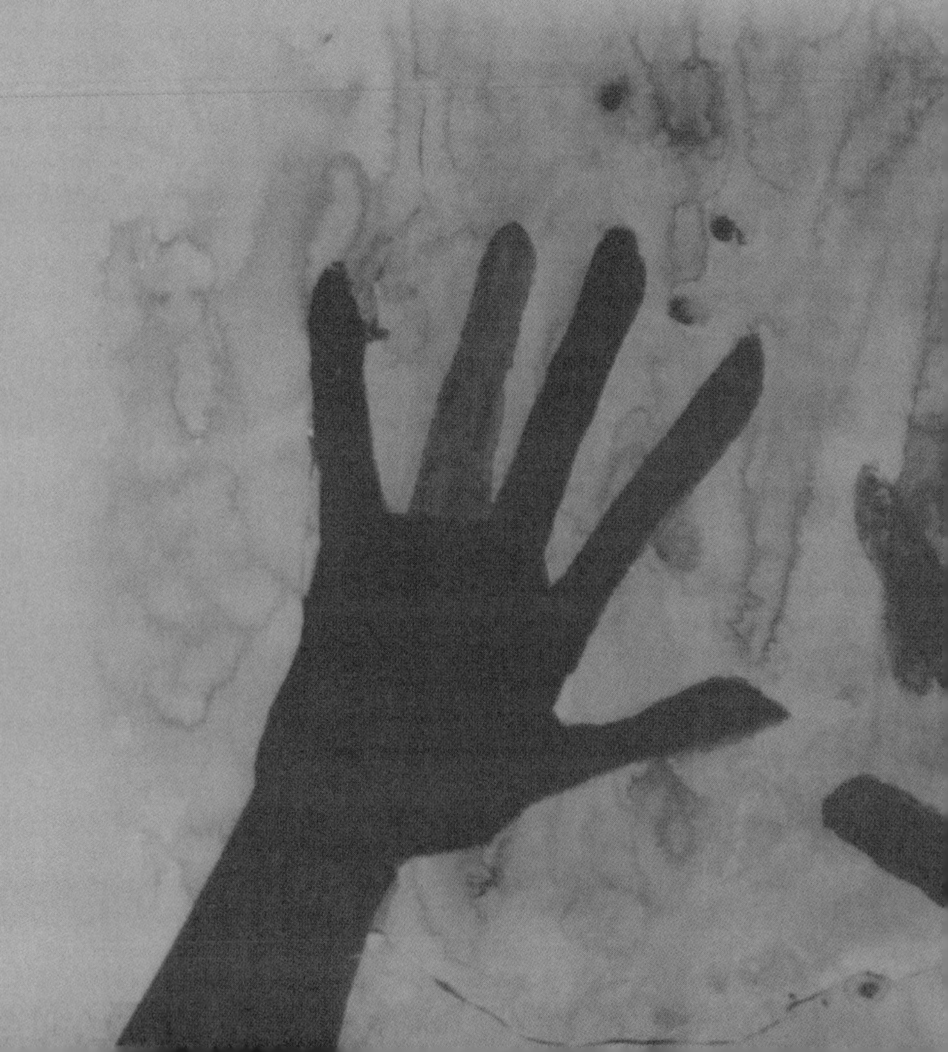

Persons Seeking Occupational Therapy

Learning Objectives

After completing this unit, readers will be able to:

- Begin to explore the experience of brain injury from the perspective of one person.
- Explain and analyze the effect of illness or disability on the family.
- Explain and analyse the effect of illness or disability on occupation.
- Define socioeconomic status and analyze the influence of social inequities on occupation and occupational therapy intervention.
- Define culture and spirituality and analyze their influence on occupation and occupational therapy intervention.
- Discuss the meaning of place and identify how this meaning contributes to an individual's sense of self.

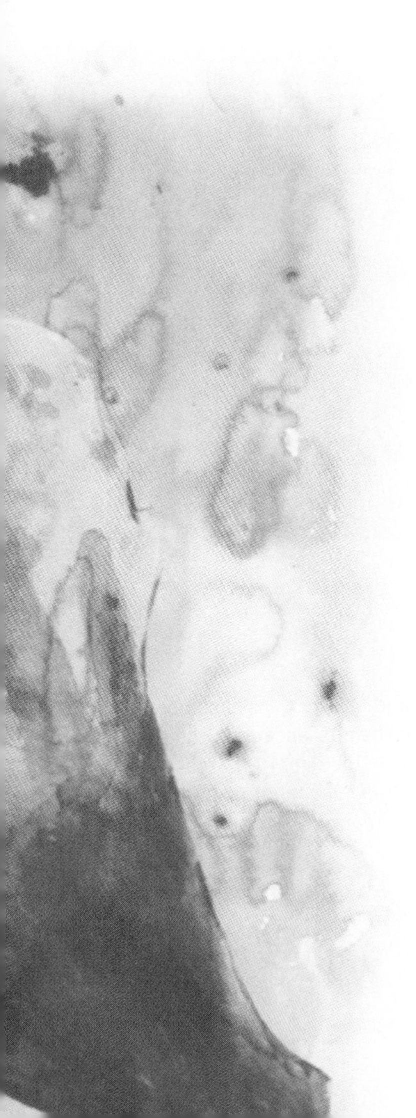

People seek occupational therapy intervention typically because they are unable to carry out tasks and activities that are important to them in their day-to-day lives. The priorities they set in therapy reflect their particular life experiences and circumstances. For example, their family situation, work, socioeconomic status, culture, spiritual beliefs, and sense of place may facilitate or constrain their response to the occupational disruption in their lives. This unit opens with a first-person account of Mary Feldhause-Weber's experience following a traumatic brain injury. It demonstrates that recovery is a transformative process that may continue long after occupational therapy intervention ceases and entails the building of a meaningful existence based in daily occupations and relations with others. The chapters that follow address disability experience from the individual and family perspectives. Subsequent chapters address the influence of culture, socioeconomic status, spirituality, and the meaning of place as contextual aspects of an individual's lived experience. The information in these chapters assist occupational therapy practitioners to understand that each individual brings unique qualities and experiences to the therapy experience, to be sensitive to these differences, and to use each person's unique experiences and strengths to foster his or her recovery. (*Note:* Words in **bold** type are defined in the Glossary.)

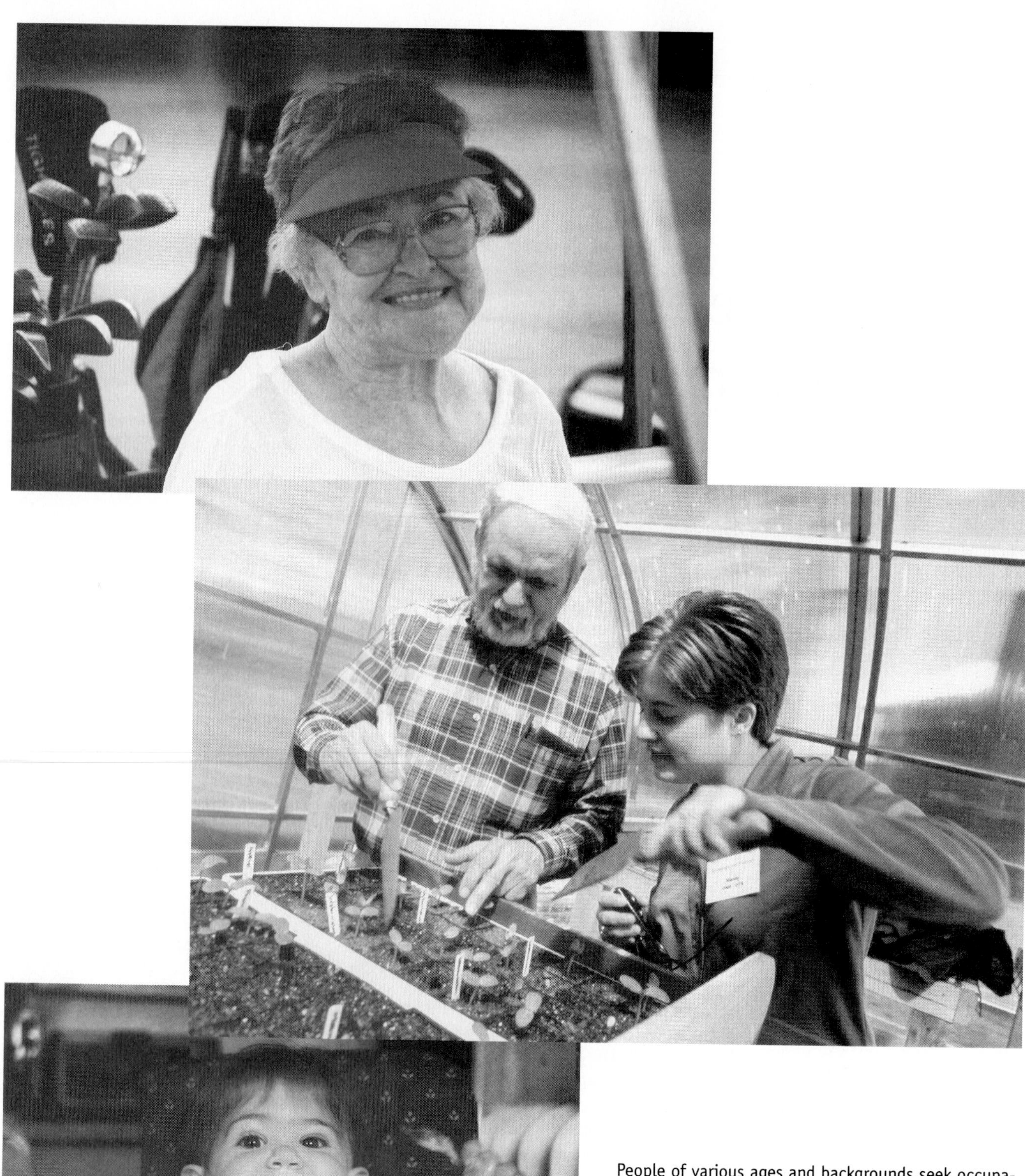

People of various ages and backgrounds seek occupational therapy to enable them to engage in the routines and activities of daily life. (*top*) (Photo courtesy of John Schell) (*middle*) (Photo courtesy of © KINDRA CLINEFF 2001) (*bottom*) (Photo courtesy of Ellen Cohn.)

CHAPTER 4

AN EXCERPT FROM *THE BOOK OF SORROWS, BOOK OF DREAMS*: A FIRST PERSON NARRATIVE

MARY FELDHAUS-WEBER

EDITOR'S PROLOGUE

Mary Feldhaus-Weber was in her 30s, lived in Boston, and was a successful playwright, filmmaker, and television producer. She had produced documentaries for the Public Broadcasting System (PBS). Her plays had been produced off-off-Broadway. She had just finished making *Joan Robinson: One Woman's Story*, an award-winning documentary film about her friend's 3-year struggle with and death from ovarian cancer. In December 1979, 3 weeks before this film was to be telecast on PBS, Mary was the passenger in a car that was struck by a drunk driver. Mary was taken from the demolished car and rushed to a hospital emergency room. Although her head had smashed the car window during the accident, she was released from the hospital that very night. Just 3 days later, Mary began to have seizures. Months later, she was diagnosed as having epilepsy—a seizure disorder—caused by traumatic brain injury. Her brain had been injured when she hit her head during the car accident. She was never hospitalized for this traumatic injury. Her seizures have never been well controlled with medication, and she has not been able to return to work.

What follows is Mary's story of her struggle to live with the effects of her brain injury and seizure disorder—in her own words. This excerpt was taken from her book in progress, *The Book of Sorrows, Book of Dreams*. The first part of the story covers the years 1979 to 1981. Mary dictated this part of her story to friends and occupational therapy students who were working with her. Mary was able to write the final two parts of her story by herself.

Noted throughout the chapter are references to color plates of Mary's paintings.

1979 to 1981

The Accident

Now let me tell you about this. My friend Sally was driving me home at 3 am after working on the "Joan Robinson" film, getting it ready for its national air date. A large American car, going at a high rate of speed, hit the small foreign car we were in, on the passenger side. (I was the passenger.) The car we were in was hit with such intensity that both cars were demolished, totaled (see Color Plate 1: Intersection). My head went through the passenger window sideways. The side of my head above the temple totally shattered the glass, hit with such impact that every piece of glass had been knocked out (see Color Plate 2: The Shattering). People in the emergency room were astonished that I had no facial cuts. I told them my hard Scandinavian head was harder than glass—like stone or a diamond.

I can remember the car lights coming at us. I can remember the sense that we could not get out of the way. I can remember shouting to my friend, "watch out," and then the impact of the car. But strangely, when the car hit, I had the sense that it had not really hit me or the car I was in, that there had been a buffer that was made of time and space. Eternal. Would not break. A shield.

I was also sure that the driver of my car, my friend Sally Schreiber-Cohn, had reached out at the moment of impact and shielded me with her own body. I was absolutely sure this happened. When we got to the hospital, I asked her. She said, "Oh no, I kept both hands on the wheel, of course." If the other car had hit a few inches further back, I probably would have been decapitated. But, it hit where it hit. Sally was bruised and badly shaken up. All the damage has been inside my brain.

One doctor described it as if someone were to have taken Jell-O, the consistency of the brain, and thrown it at a wall as hard as one could. That's how hard the brain hit one side of the skull, and then ricocheted back and hit the other side of the skull, leaving me with right and left side brain injuries. Even though only one side of my head hit the window, both sides of my brain are damaged (see Color Plate 3: Damaged Brain).

Six Months after the Accident

Six months after the accident when I started to have more and more seizures, it became clear that I could no longer live alone and so I had to ask my mother to come from South Dakota to stay with me. I did this with great reluctance because she was 78 and my father wanted her there, taking care of him. When she got here, the thing I remember her saying was that she hadn't realized it had been so bad. Why hadn't I called her sooner? This was the time before the seizures were under any kind of control at all, which is to say, I was very sick.

I sat in the corner day after day, noticing that it was light or dark, noticing that my mother was busy, or sleeping, or crying, noticing that sometimes the phone rang, or that it was the day to see the doctor, noticing that sometimes I had pain in my head. My mother said, "I wonder if a cold wet towel on your head would help?" I think we both remembered that if a horse sprains its leg, you wrap its leg in towels. And so, Mother would get wet towels from the bathroom and wrap them around my head, my brain becoming like a sprained leg, a muscle that wasn't working. Cramped and tense. Convulsing. Filled with fear.

And then because things change and time moves on, the pain would stop, and I would become briefly aware that the couch cover was blue, or that the dog had been rolling in the dust, or that Mother wanted to fix soup for lunch.

And we discovered that after I had a seizure, or as one doctor called them "spells," I didn't have the coordination, or was too confused, to drink soup or hold a spoon. Because Mother liked soup so much, we seemed to try this many times, larger spoons, smaller spoons, bigger cups, smaller cups. It was decided that tomato soup was the easiest. Why, I'm not sure. Finally, I told Mother I did not like soup and had not for years. Therefore, could we try something else?

At this time, I was having constant seizures. There was no time that I was not either having one, getting ready to have one, feeling "spacey," with a strong metallic taste in my mouth, or feeling confused and disoriented after having had one. I felt like the seizures were a powerful force outside of me that suddenly grabbed my brain, me, the essence of me, and with the kind of fury of winds, blizzards, and driving rain, held me under ice (see Color Plate 4: Blue Seizure). While the me that was present could breathe the water under the ice, I knew I was caught, forced to be there. I knew if I struggled even slightly, the pain, the terror, became worse. And for the time the active seizure was roaring on inside me, I had to concentrate on total stillness until the fury dissipated and I was released.

All the drive and the tenacity, the ambition, the creativity, all of the things that had made me who I was did not help in this place. I was terrified, and I was alone. I no longer knew the words to ask or tell anyone what I was living through. I could just sense what hurt, and it hurt less to be absolutely still until the force chose to release me. I had no control of when it seized me or when it chose to release me.

My friend Sally tells me now that looking at me was like watching a candle about to go out. It seemed to her that only 3 percent of me was left.

I felt that I was being annihilated. The me that I had become, lived with, was ceasing to be over and over and over again. It occurred to me that this was what it felt like to die and, for whatever reason, I was dying again and again.

One Year after the Accident

My mother had to return to South Dakota, so I was living alone. One day at the neurologist's office a year after the accident, still confused and in a deep fog. I noticed the doctor's tie. It was a bright, clear yellow Marimeco tie. I stared at the color yellow. It was the first thing to make sense to me since the accident. I understood what I was seeing. The color yellow. The fog lifted for a minute. I understood something, and I had not had to struggle to understand it. I can remember thinking: I am going to be all right.

When I got home that day someone got me a set of poster paints and I painted a small, bright, vivid, yellow daisy (see Color Plate 5: Daisy). And I started painting.

When I began painting I was surprised to find that it didn't turn out so badly, even though I had never painted before.

Painting was one thing I could do all by myself, whether anyone was there or not. It didn't matter if I was spacey or sick. I could just lay down the piece of paper I was working on and continue again after the seizure had come and gone.

Some days I did as many as ten paintings. Looking back, I realize I was desperate to understand my situation. I could hear people talk, but nothing made sense. I looked at their faces. I watched their mouths move, but I could not concentrate on what they were telling me. I can remember thinking: I have to try to explain all this to myself—what is happening to me—because I can't understand anyone else. So I painted. The only time I felt like the person I used to be was when I was painting.

I started finger painting with acrylic paint, wet tissue paper and poster paints. I was drawn to the color and shapes of things. I started to paint brains. I tried to paint the experience of seizures, which I did over and over again (see Color Plate 6: Hemisphere). In a strange kind of way it was like having an artist's model for myself, not a model I could see, but a model which was myself, an internal experience that I then tried to translate into color. The painting gave me something to talk about other than myself. Something to talk about when people came to the house. It was a relief to have something to show someone, to have them look at pieces of paper, not to look at me. It also gave me a way to try to talk about what I was living through. Part of me hoped that the paintings weren't pitiful, because of all the things I did not want to be, to be pitied seemed the very worst.

I was also aware that I had to start from scratch with painting. I had been at the top of my career in film, and now I had to struggle to squeeze the paint tubes. I had to learn to be patient with myself. I was at the very beginning and grateful to be there.

Two Years after the Accident

I still had no real picture of what happened to my brain, to me. I spent a great deal of time thinking about it. Trying to think about it (see Color Plate 7: Dendrites).

I had listened to explanations from doctors, nurses, social workers, and none of them had made sense. All I knew was that I was unable to do the simplest thing, make a bed, tell time, count. Add or subtract. Recognize faces. Tell right from left. Read. Understand what people said to me. Remember things. And perhaps worst of all I did not feel like myself, like "me." I felt like someone, but not like any one I knew. I was a stranger to myself. I was lost (see Color Plate 8: Self-Portrait).

On days that I had constant seizures, I had to ask my friend Sally to come and stay with me. It was at these times we were aware that I was not getting better; in fact, I was barely hanging on.

The everyday litany was long and grim: I fell all the time; I was covered with black and blue marks everywhere. I would come to from a seizure to find that I had bitten the inside of my mouth and was bleeding and had a shard of my broken front tooth sticking out of my bottom lip. Sometimes, I would put my finger in my eyes during a seizure, and the eye would be red and swollen for days. I hit my head. I broke my elbow. It did not seem safe for me to live alone.

I had lost my income when my film company closed after the accident, and I had lost my health insurance with it. Because of these factors, my only option would have been to go on welfare and go into a nursing home. My neurologist felt that if I did that I would likely never come out. I think he had seen too many people become institutionalized. In other words, they had become helpless and had given up.

I still had some small fight left in me; I had been a functional, successful adult. The 3 percent of me that was left was 3 percent of a fighter. We were all counting on the fact that I would keep fighting and I would get better. That somehow I would manage. I also knew I desperately needed someone to help me help myself.

Finally, more than 2 years after the accident, we found someone to help me. Sally had called a therapist friend who said she did know someone who was a gifted occupational therapist and liked dogs. And who was kind. When Sally called the occupational therapist—Anna Deane Scott—she said that she knew very little about head injury. She was a professor at Boston University and the coauthor of a famous occupational therapy textbook and, yes, she did like dogs. She agreed to come to my house to meet me.

When she first met me Anna Deane told me later that I was sitting in the dark on a couch, crying. We talked; she admired my dogs and told me about her own dog. After she left I called her to ask what she thought of the meeting. I was afraid that she might have felt I was beyond help. I asked her how she felt about meeting me. Anna Deane said "I felt sad." She told me the truth. I knew I could trust her.

Every time Anna Deane Scott came over we talked about things in the house that were a problem for me. I was afraid of falling in the shower when I was getting spacey from a seizure, so we got a shower chair and a metal bar on the wall and rubber rugs inside the tub and outside the tub. Each one of these areas we worked on took months to identify the problem and with trial and error find the solutions. But in the case of the shower, finally I was able to take a shower and I was no longer afraid. I was also afraid of burning myself on the flames of my gas stove if I was feeling confused, so we got a large electric hot plate and I could heat something up without being afraid of lighting myself or my clothes on fire.

I had lost the ability to do things; I knew there were steps to take to do any task, but I had no idea which step came first. I later learned that I had lost the ability to sequence, a loss that sometimes occurs when you have had an injury to the frontal lobe of the brain.

Anna Deane and I set out to discover how to teach me to do things again. She said that there was always another way to do something. First we had to find out how I was still able to learn. You will notice when I speak of Anna Deane and myself I always say WE did this, WE decided that. Unlike many other health professionals, Anna Deane felt her role was not to tell me what to do, but to work with me, to empower me. She asked me constantly what was important to me. What did I think of something. What did I want to do. And she LISTENED to me. Extraordinary!

One problem in my life was how to unlock my front door. My house has two doors, an outside door and an inner door, and therefore I have two different keys. If someone would bring me home from the doctor's office, one of the few places that I went, I would often try to get the key in the lock and not be able to. I would try to unlock the door for what felt like hours, over and over again. Desperately trying to get into my own house.

I asked whoever dropped me off to see that I got into the house before they drove off. Often they would have to open the door for me. I felt stupid, unable to do the simplest thing.

Anna Deane watched me try to get into the house and said she understood what the problem was. She said when I couldn't get in the outside door with one key, that I should *try the other key*. It had not occurred to me to try the other key. I would stand endlessly with the wrong key doing it over and over again, but when I had this new strategy, it freed me to get into my own house, and each time I opened the door myself it was such a victory. And I began to feel hope for myself.

Anna Deane and I discovered that while it was impossible for me to just follow or understand verbal directions, if I could also watch someone do a task, listen to the directions, even place my hands on the things at the same time, I could, after a number of tries, do it again myself.

Anna Deane said we could not be sure which parts of my brain were still working, but we had the best chance for success if we used as many senses as possible, hoping we could tap into the areas in my brain that still functioned. When Anna Deane first said this it sounded like the most primitive kind of investigation into unknown territories, all of which were inside me. We were searching for the me that was still there. But she was right. With Anna Deane's help I have learned to do everything [day-to-day self-maintenance activities] over again. Absolutely everything. It is not too strong to say that she gave me my life back.

Another thing that Anna Deane and I worked on was a chart that monitored my daily activities. One of the problems was that I had lost any sense of time. With epilepsy it is important that you take a certain amount of pills, at a certain time every day. It's very simple—if you don't, the seizures come back. You also have to eat and rest regularly in relationship to taking the pills, and before I met Anna Deane, I could not remember if I'd taken a pill, had lunch, let the dogs out; I couldn't tell if it were afternoon or morning, or what day it was.

Gradually, over a period of months and many failures, we worked out a chart on a magnetic blackboard that we divided into morning, afternoon, and evening. We used different colored magnets for different parts of the day, as we discovered that I could understand colors better than words. For every victory, such as the discovery that I still remembered colors, there were dozens of defeats.

Anna Deane said over and over that there was always another way to do something. We just had to find the other way. And every time we failed she learned that much more about my brain, what still worked and how it was working. She said there was no such thing as a "failure." She learned something each time we tried something new.

I, on the other hand, felt the failures very keenly. Because I had been quick and life had come easily to me, I was not used to trying and failing at something simple again and again and again. The things we were trying to do, like a system to get me to remember to take my pills, were both very simple and very important. I was impatient with myself and judged myself by who I had been. For each failure, I shed many tears.

I tried not to cry in front of Anna Deane. My dogs, Desmond and Todd, listened to my crying. I would go to pet them and their fur would be wet. I would be puzzled at first and then remembered I had been crying. And they had been sitting beside me on the couch, wet with my tears.

Anna Deane said that I was doing what I needed to do, grieving over my losses. I had lost a great deal. And that if one didn't grieve and let the past go, it was harder to do new things. That grief could stand in the way of progress (see Color Plate 9: The Color of My Grief). But on the other hand I also needed to look at the balance of things. I needed to find things that still made me happy, gave me pleasure. It became my job each day to do one thing that gave me pleasure (see Color Plate 10: Goblin). This sometimes was as hard to do as the task of grieving. It became obvious to me that the two were connected.

So we refined the magnetic board system further: colored magnets for each time of day, further divided into *take pill; have lunch; feed dogs;* etc. When the activity had been completed, I moved the magnet from the *not-done* category to the *done* category. The chart is large and colorful, and I can look at it from across the room and tell what I've done and what I haven't done yet, and how I'm doing . . . and so, eventually, time and memory seemed somewhat under my control again (see Color Plate 11: Healing Brain).

Anna Deane came to my house every week for an hour and we talked on the phone a number of times between the visits. In the year that I worked with her I could see small changes in my life, and as I got greater control over the details of my life again, the person who I had been started to reemerge. I wasn't making films, but I could change the sheets on my bed. I wasn't writing poetry, but I could dress myself. These may seem like small things, but with each skill I regained I could feel life flowing back into me again.

Another triumph that stands out was the ability to get in and out of buildings. There are many buildings in Boston where you have to buzz the company or office that you are going to, and then they buzz you back and the door opens. I was no more able to decipher this than the Rosetta Stone. It was impossibly complex for me and therefore overwhelming, and therefore tear-producing, and therefore one more thing that I couldn't do.

Anna Deane and I talked about every possible kind of solution and came up with one that worked. The solution was to stand and watch until someone else came along and pushed a button and got in the door; watch how they did it; and either go in with them or do the same thing they did. And it worked.

In large buildings it's still a problem finding the correct office if I haven't been there before, because in the elevator I am not able to understand if 5 is the same as 7 is the same as 9 when the elevator opens. So, I have been lost in the best hospitals in Boston. The people that have taken me went to park their car and against their better judgment let me out, me telling them not to worry about it, that I would meet them at the office. And then, 45 minutes later when I did not show up at the office, and it became clear that there was a problem, various people would be sent to find me. For my part, I would be asking people if this was the fourth floor, etc., etc.

Among the least helpful people to give this kind of simple direction are doctors, nurses, or anyone else from "The Allied Health Professions." Among the most helpful, of course, are the other patients, and all the cleaning and maintenance people. However, Anna Deane and I have not figured a way around this problem, a way to make me independent, to do it all on my own. It is still, sadly, something that makes me cry.

With Anna Deane's help I listened to talking books for reading, and used a calculator to add and subtract, told time with a digital clock, asked people to take me places and not just give me directions, and used the brightly colored arrows that told me which way to turn the thermostat to heat my house and to turn on the water faucets in the shower. In other words, many victories. And more to come.

Sometimes people ask me what kind of fee Anna Deane charged me for this amount of work, and of devotion. The answer is—not one cent. She told me she did not know enough about head injury to charge for her services; it was a learning experience for her too. And, she did not say it, but I knew she knew I did not have a cent to my name.

MAY 1996: SIXTEEN YEARS AFTER THE ACCIDENT

How am I now? I was told that if a function did not come back after a year it would not come back. They were wrong about this in some cases. I have continued to regain things over a period of 16 years. I can discriminate between right and left again, I am much better at recognizing faces—not perfect, but better. I can understand poetry and most abstractions again. I regained my sense of smell. I can read a bit if the print is big. I can write again.

I still can't count. I still can't do multiplication tables or months of the year. I still see double out of one eye. I still have to sit and think a long time about what steps go into a task like putting the laundry in the washing machine and what order those steps should take. I still have balance problems. I still have a lot of seizures—several a day most of the time. I have learned to live with these things—the things that are lost to me and the things that have come back but are different.

I had a battery of [neuropsychological] tests done on me recently, and I still do badly on a number of them. You are reading the writing of someone who now has an IQ still considerably under 100.

I was surprised how many strong feelings I had when I started to answer the simple sounding question—"How are you?" First of all, it is not until I started to get better that I realized how much I had lost. Before that I was too sick or too overwhelmed to notice, to understand the breadth of the loss.

In broad strokes, I lost 10 years of my life where I almost ceased to exist. And I still grieve over that loss; some days it feels like a very big loss, other days it doesn't (see Color Plate 12: Broken Dreams).

So how am I now? I am doing better without having gotten better. In other words, I learned to do a lot of things in new ways just as Anna Deane Scott, the occupational therapist who worked with me, said I would—tell time with a digital clock, read with talking books, write with a large screen, large print computer.

I feel like myself again. I am happy most of the time . . . in fact I seem to be one of the more happy and contented people I know. I have become grateful for things large and small. I am more appreciative of other people. In fact, I think we should all gets stars and bluebirds for getting up in the morning.

The head injury has forced me to look at myself. Look at all the sad, angry parts of me that I did not consider when I was a hotshot television producer. I was too busy working 18-hour days. Being very busy in a high visibility job can be seductive. What you are doing seems so important that you can easily push everything else into a corner. But when you are sitting home, day after day, when the phone isn't ringing off the hook, it is less possible to ignore things.

Being head injured has given me time to look at who I was, how I got there, and to ask myself what I want to do about my life. Counseling also helped me to survive the many assaults to the spirit that can occur when you are forced to endlessly deal with health-care providers. Being a patient can be a grueling life.

I know this will seem strange; it seems strange to me even as I write it down. There is a belief that if you have some sense like sight taken away, your hearing becomes more acute to compensate. In order to understand my own suffering, I have come to better understand the suffering of others.

I also laugh more, am made happy more easily. I am much more at ease with myself. I feel quite literally that I walked and walked and walked through the valley of the shadow of death, stumbling, crying, falling, breaking bones, and finally came out on the other side. When asked about the head injury, I tell people I would not wish it on my worst enemy. Yet strangely, I am also grateful for the journey.

JULY 2001: TWENTY-TWO YEARS AFTER THE ACCIDENT

I continue to live with the physical problems that came from the original injury. And there are still the problems I have because I am who I am. I was on the phone recently with a spit-and-polish person that I don't particularly like. At a point in the conversation, I was not able to understand what she was saying. And then I started perseverating—saying the same word over and over again, which she didn't notice. These signals told me that I was probably about to have a seizure.

I felt frustrated and ashamed. I could do nothing to stop the seizure. Worse still, I thought I might start crying, but I forced myself to be polite. I finally hung up when I began losing the ability to speak. And felt terrible about myself.

I could hear Anne Dean Scott's voice when I used to tell her about this kind of social situation: "Just hang up the phone. And if they don't like it, too bad for them!" A life lesson I have yet to learn. Even after these 22 years I still need to please others at my own expense.

I have had the best help in the world so why don't I learn these lessons? I suppose that is because I am a human being and I still carry the same baggage I had before the accident.

And now I think it is time to tell you about good things.

About 5 years ago a new antiseizure medicine came on the market that has made a large, positive difference in the quality of my life. At long last I have fewer seizures and am more clear headed. I am ME more of the time. It's wonderful.

I have a computer and like it for all the same reasons that everyone else does. Even though I am mostly house bound, I have the world in front of me.

I have always loved animals and now I am active with animal rescue and finding homes for abused, homeless animals (see Color Plate 13: I Stand by While Good Dogs Die). Since a large part of this can be done on the phone or the Internet, I can do this when I am feeling OK.

I have become part of a network of people who care about animals as much as I do. They have no idea that I used to be a filmmaker or even that I was in a terrible accident, although I do tell them about the head injury if there is a reason to. I never have to fear that anyone will feel sorry for me. I am just one more person who is dedicated to helping animals.

I love this part of my life.

In the 22 years since the accident I have gone from not being able to read and write at all or to even turn the pages in a book to be able to write what you are reading right now. I write easily now.

Finally, there is something unexpected that I seldom hear discussed by head-injured survivors or the people who work with them.

The car accident was a crushing, wrenching assault on me. For the first few years after the accident the question that I asked over and over was this: How could God do this to me?

Before the accident, I had been a spiritual person. I believed in a compassionate, wise God who cared about each sparrow that fell and each lily of the field.

After, it seemed like God cared about everything but me.

I was shocked and heart broken that God let this happen. I thought about it constantly and talked to anyone who would listen. I felt twisted and damaged inside and out (see Color Plate 14: When I Think of Dying). And angry. Angry. Angry. You can see this in my paintings (see Color Plate 15: Pain #2).

The years went by and I never came to any understanding. After a time my sorrow blew away like smoke (see Color Plate 16: White Brain).

I understand now that the greatest damage I experienced was the damage no one can see. It left me feeling afraid of things, not trusting in life, not being able to believe in a kind, loving God. I felt alone.

I have had the best occupational therapy and counseling and profited from them. I have learned to do many of the skills of daily living again. I have changed and grown.

And there is more.

My spirit has been the last to heal.

And I am still healing.

POSTSCRIPT: THOUGHTS FOR OCCUPATIONAL THERAPY PRACTITIONERS

One more thought I want to share with you. I've spent a lot of time thinking about what "helps" in the kind of situation I have been in with my head injury. Why could some people get through to me and not others? Why did some people comfort and heal me and other seemingly well-meaning people shame or humiliate me? In other words, What works; What heals? What helps?

I discovered that *power* is at the heart of living with an injury, and *power* is at the heart of getting better. Many of us, particularly women, don't think of ourselves as having power. It is just a word, not something we own or think much about. Yet power is the ability to make things happen.

When I was at my most diminished it felt like everyone was more powerful than I was: from the secretary in the doctor's office who had to take the time to push the right elevator button for me, to the cab driver I had to trust to give back the correct change because I could not count. The people who had to show me to the restroom when I was not capable of finding it. The doctors who filled out the insurance forms so I would get disability payments to buy food and pay the rent. It was a very long list and I was at the bottom. I had to depend on everyone.

Because of the power issues (who has it, who wants it, who needs it, who can share it), I think it is important to check why you are going into the healing professions. Ask yourself tough questions and keep asking them. Questions like, "What do I get out of this work?" "How does this situation make me feel about myself?" "Do I need to have things in black and white or can I bear the uncertainty of all the shades of gray that illness and sorrow present us with?" "Can I trust people, however damaged, to know what is best for themselves?"

So the question I am asking you is this: Can you give over power to another person? Can you honor their own wishes, dreams, abilities? Can you be as interested in their abilities as you are in their disabilities? Can you give them the tools to get their own lives back on track?

And do you listen to people? Do you HEAR what they are telling you? I believe that we are far wiser than we give ourselves or each other credit for.

So, I am telling you that the two most important things you can do as occupational therapy practitioners are to listen and to empower. The people who helped me the most did both of those things. I continue to bless them and to use what they have taught me every day.

You have chosen a profession that helps, restores, teaches, and gives comfort. Some of the finest human beings I have ever met are occupational therapy practitioners.

You speak for us, the people you serve. You are in our corner.

ACKNOWLEDGMENT

Let me tell you about my friend Sally.

Sally Schreiber-Cohn has helped me make this chapter happen, from taking some of the original dictation when I was too sick to do it myself to bringing me art supplies for my painting. Sally and I were friends before the accident and she has stayed my friend through these 22 years. Sally, an artist herself, stuck with me on a day-by-day basis, patient, kind, and worked to see that the artist in me did not die. She has always been in my corner.

Sally is a large part of why I came through all this.

EDITORS' COMMENTS

Mary's story eloquently illustrates concepts we need to think about for all of our clients' stories—the illness experience and the influence of illness, cultural systems, socioeconomic systems, and nonhuman environments on occupation. It also demonstrates that recovery can take many years and that the power of the human spirit and the power of relationships are central to that process. Think about Mary's story as you read the following chapters.

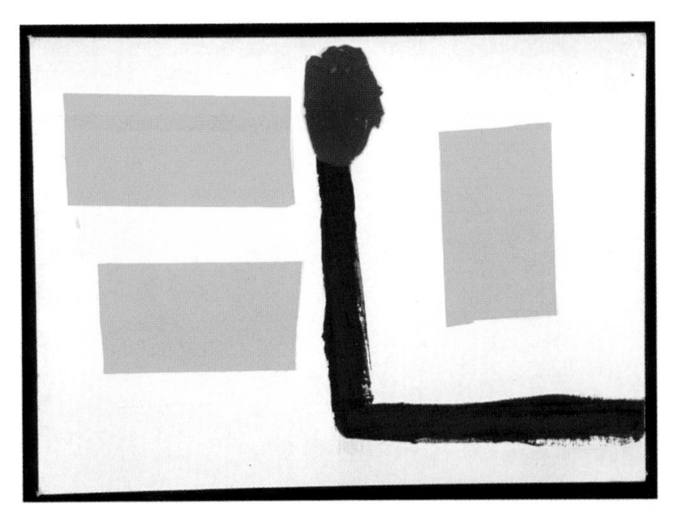

PLATE 1. Intersection: For a long time after the accident my mind played and replayed the car crash. I finally painted it to get the memory outside of myself. Here was the intersection, and here was the car I was in. Then the collision. And then the smashing of the car and of me. (Color plate courtesy of Mary Feldhaus-Weber)

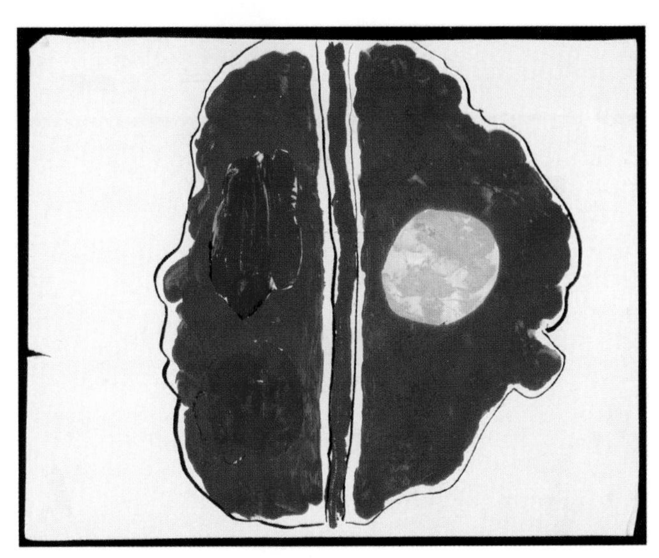

PLATE 3. Damaged Brain: 1981—When I started painting, I painted what I thought my own damaged brain must look like. In this painting I painted a brain that was terribly hurt on both sides—like mine, I thought. Much later, when the doctor ran CAT scans, indeed my brain was damaged on both sides. (Color plate courtesy of Mary Feldhaus-Weber)

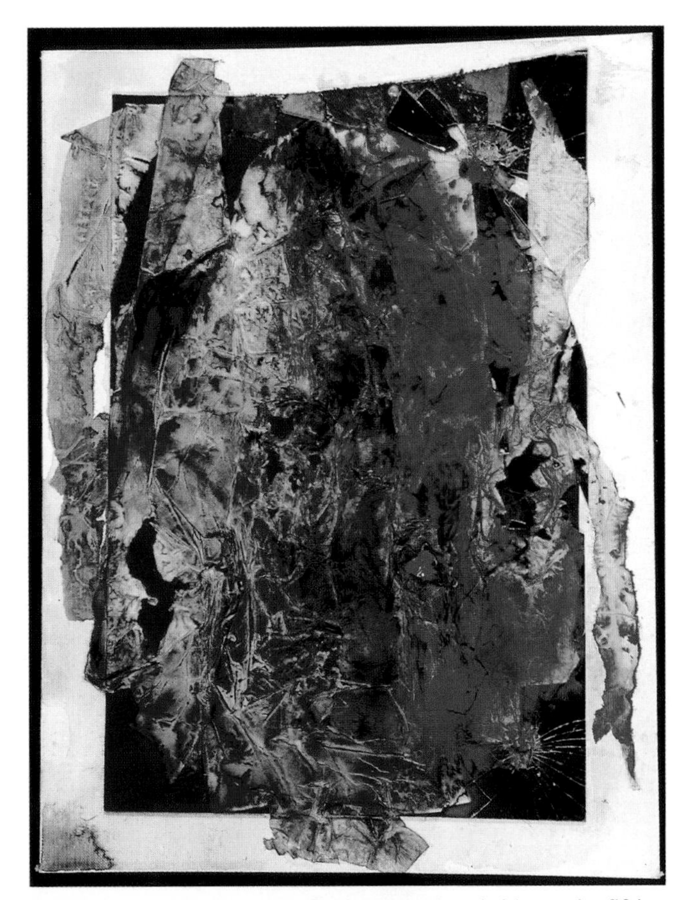

PLATE 2. The Shattering: 11/20/83—I painted this on the fifth anniversary of the accident. I still felt like I was bleeding to death. (Color plate courtesy of Mary Feldhaus-Weber)

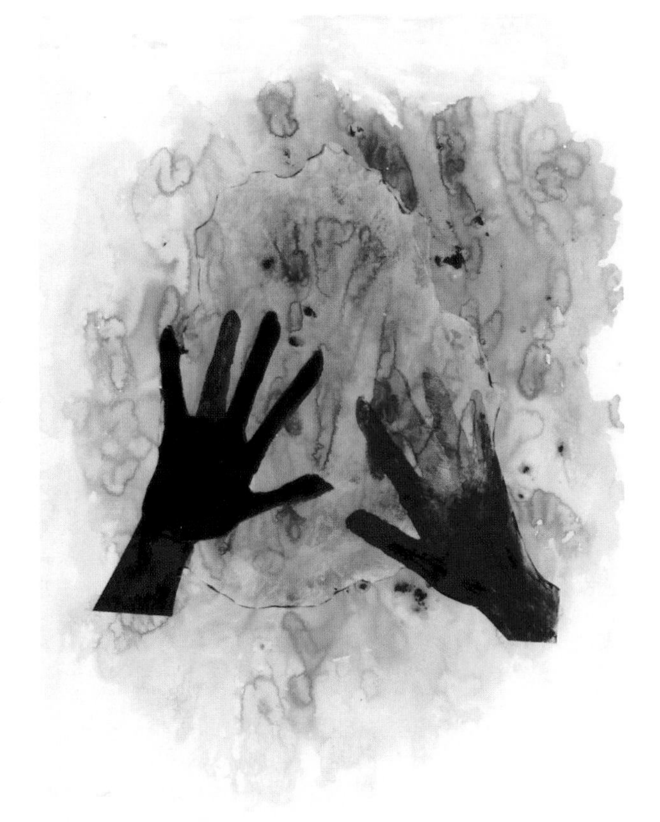

PLATE 4. Blue Seizure: Before we discovered an epilepsy medication that worked I was having constant seizures. This is a picture of what my seizures felt like: a force outside myself (the hands) held my brain under ice. It held me there, terrified, desperate helpless. Until it chose to release me. One of the fingers was red because I sometimes felt pain during the seizures. This picture broke through to a lot of people. My friend Sally said she had witnessed many of my seizures, but never understood how I felt. This painting, she said, was the only thing that helped her "get it". (Color plate courtesy of Mary Feldhaus-Weber)

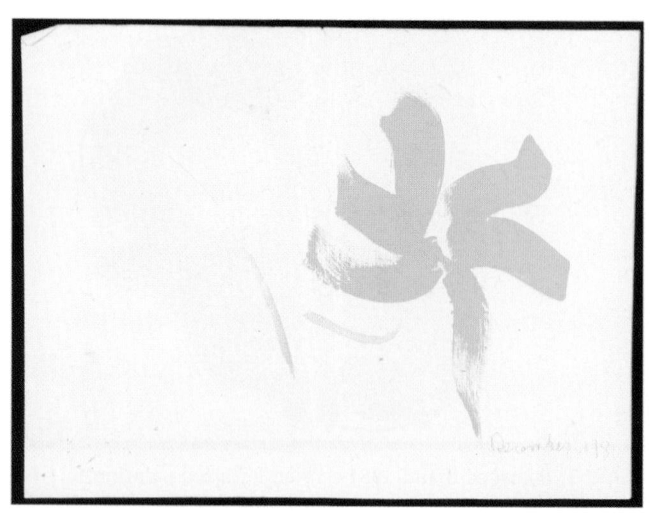

PLATE 5. Daisy: December, 1980—This is the first picture I painted. One year after the accident I painted this modest yellow daisy. I came to this with great desperation. I had never studied painting, but I knew I had to fight to survive or I would be lost. The color of the daisy was the color of my neurologist's tie. (Color plate courtesy of Mary Feldhaus-Weber)

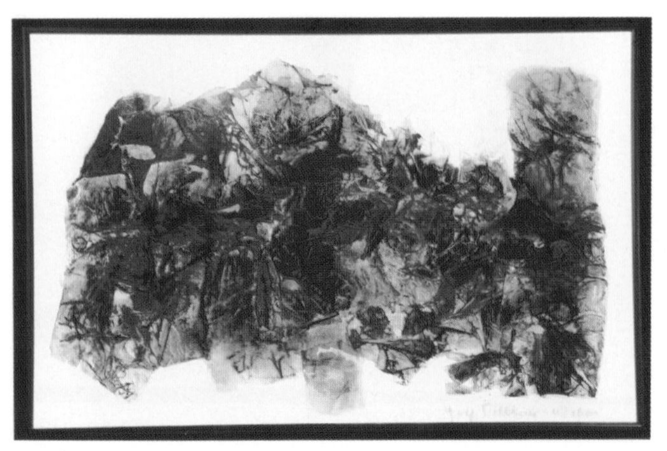

PLATE 7. Dendrites: Painted when I was starting to get better. I began to pick up the jargon of the neurology team I was working with. They explained how parts of the brain communicate. I came home and painted what I thought dendrites might look like. Beautiful and strange. This is one of my favorite paintings. (Color plate courtesy of Susan Mc Ginley)

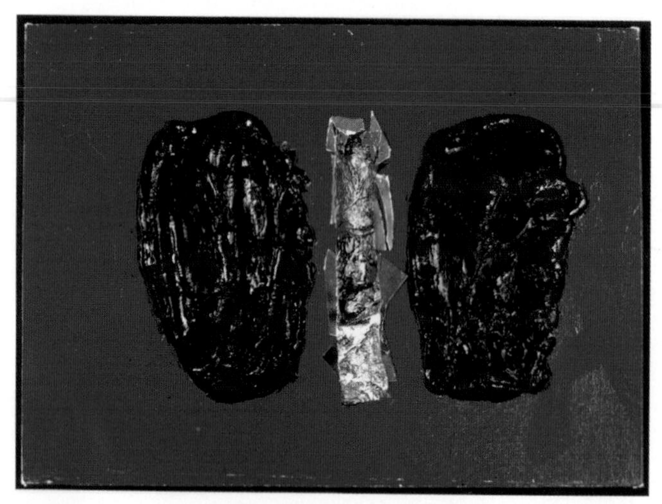

PLATE 6. Hemisphere: Someone told me that for the brain to heal, the two hemispheres of the injured brain had to learn to communicate with each other again—find new pathways that worked. The right side had to take up what the left side used to do. In this picture, I put broken mirrors between the two hemispheres. The idea of my brain ever getting better seemed impossible painful, exhausting. (Color plate courtesy of Mary Feldhaus-Weber)

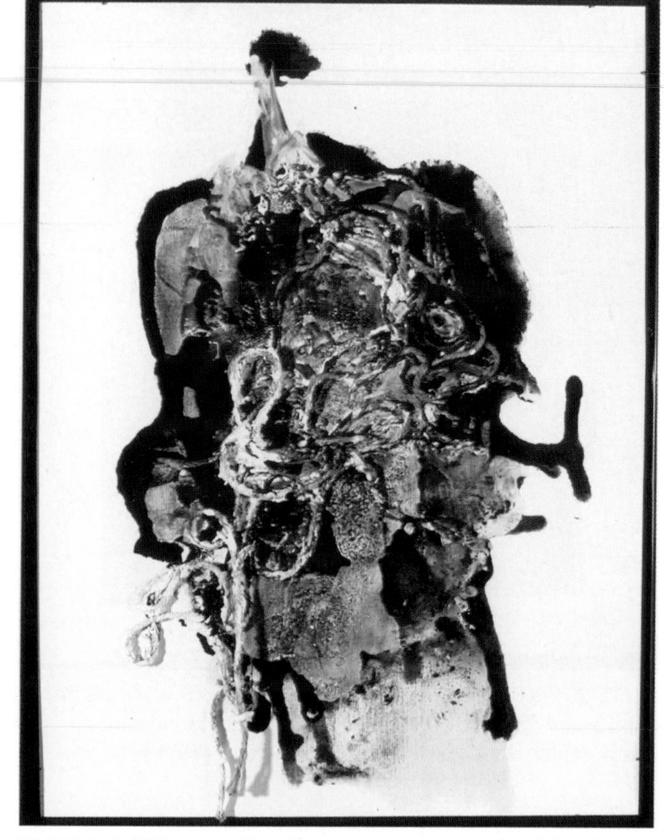

PLATE 8. Self Portrait: The tiny knob was my head. I felt I had ceased to have intelligence. I was just a confused, tattered body. No part of me worked. (Color plate courtesy of Mary Feldhaus-Weber)

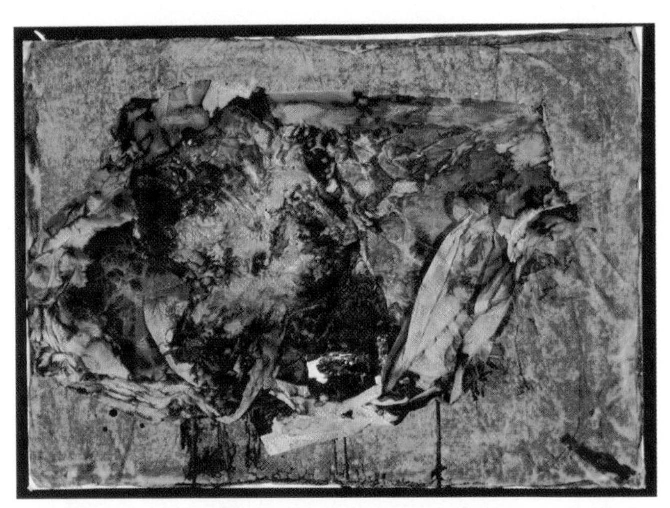

PLATE 9. The Color of My Grief: I connected with a woman in the field of education rehabilitation. With her help I was able to understand the concept of counting again. After several months I was able to count to four. I was thrilled. For some reason I never understood, the agency she was with fired her out of the blue. It was a huge loss to me. Grief upon grief. When you find someone who can help you, they are like gold. I was furious at the people who fired her, and sad beyond words. (Color plate courtesy of Mary Feldhaus-Weber)

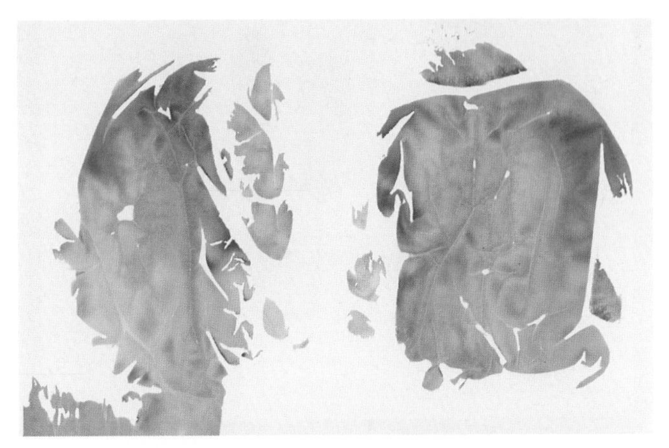

PLATE 11. Healing Brain: Early 1983—This picture shows what I imagined the damaged brain and the healed brain would look like, side by side. (Color plate courtesy of Mary Feldhaus-Weber)

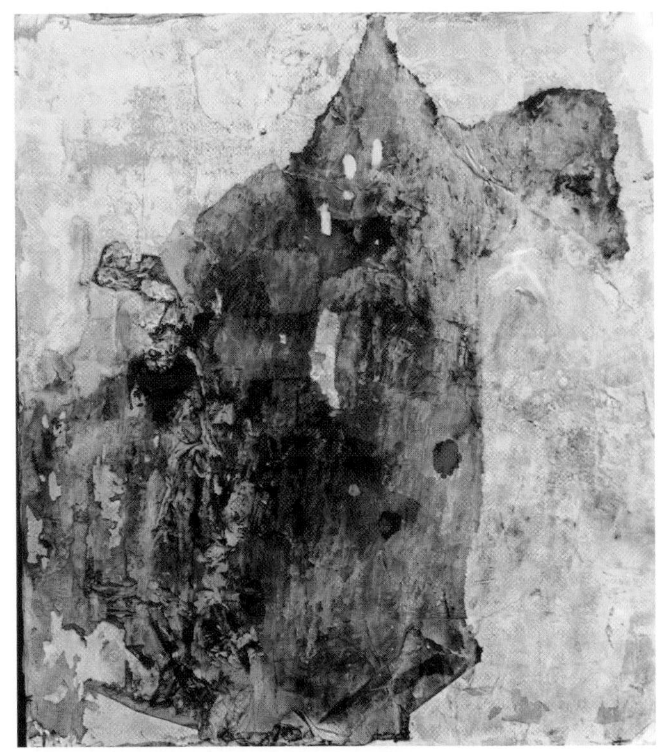

PLATE 10. Goblin: Done for fun. (Color plate courtesy of Mary Feldhaus-Weber)

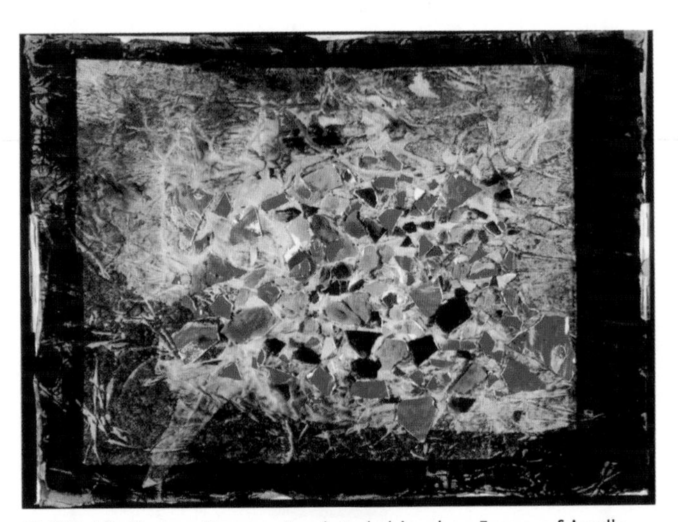

PLATE 12. Broken Dreams: I painted this when I saw a friend's film on TV. I realized that the people I worked with in TV production were moving ahead. I, on the other hand, was sitting at home, having seizures and only able to dial the telephone after many tries. (Color plate courtesy of Mary Feldhaus-Weber)

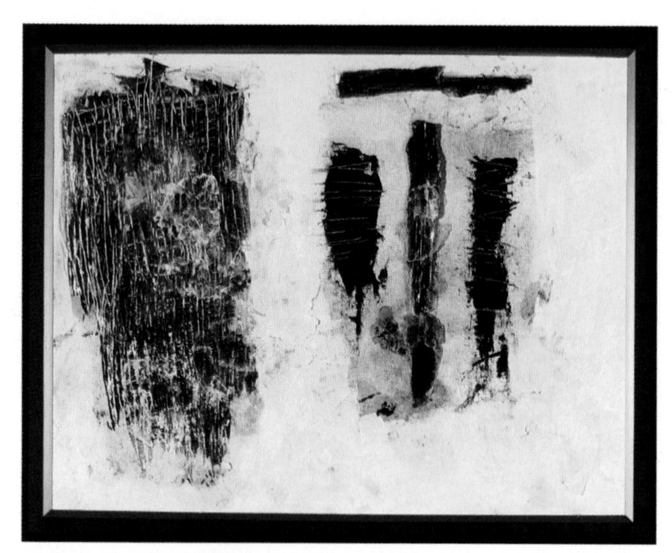

PLATE 13. I Stand By While Good Dogs Die: June, 2001—I have always liked dogs more than anything. I now work as a volunteer with an animal rescue group. I work from home on the telephone when I am able to. Many of the dogs we try to rescue cannot be saved, in spite of our best efforts. There are simply not enough homes to go around. In this picture, I am the figure on the left covered with mica (shiny sheets of mineral), which represents my good intentions. The dogs on the right represent the dogs we can not save. Their spirits are moving upward toward the shining mica, which represents life beyond life. This is my most recent painting. (Color plate courtesy of Mary Feldhaus-Weber)

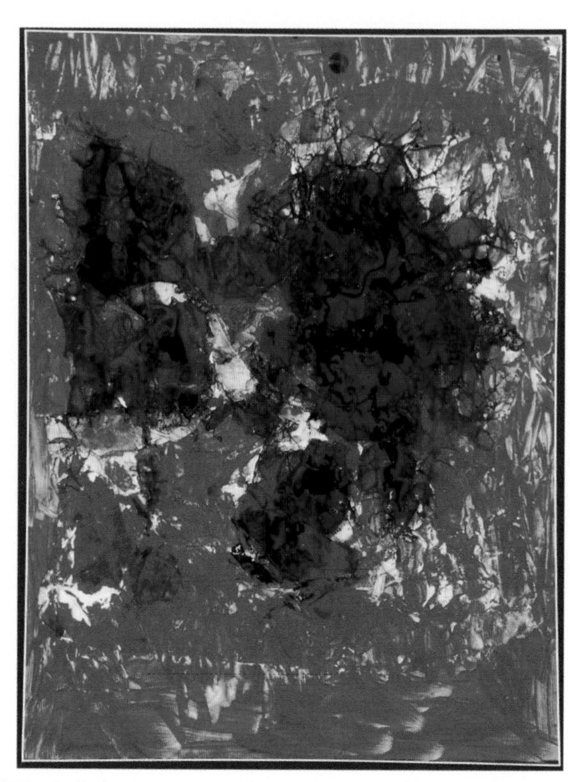

PLATE 15. Pain #2: 1987—More pain, more feeling trapped and desperate. I felt this way a long, long time. My painting was often the only way I had to express it. (Color plate courtesy of Mary Feldhaus-Weber)

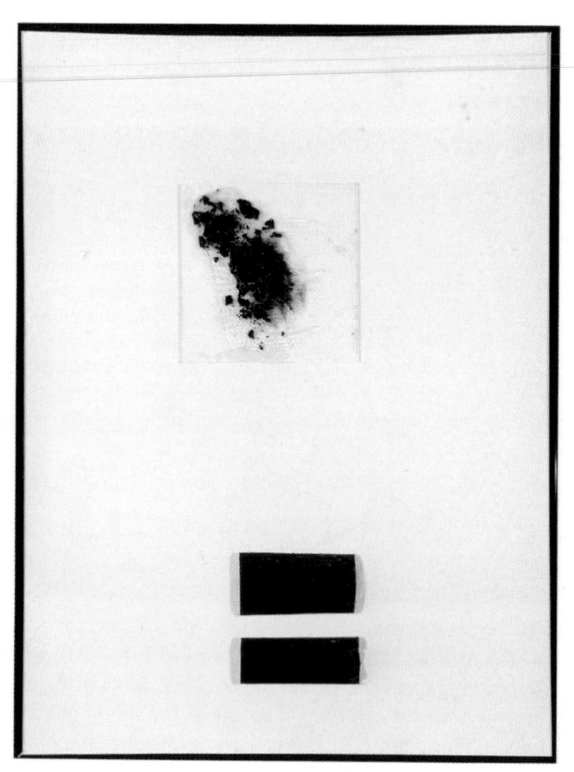

PLATE 14. When I Think of Dying: 10/15/83—As I started to get better, I realized how much I had lost. It was at this time that I thought about suicide. This picture was what I imagined the soul might look like upon leaving the dying body. (Color plate courtesy of Mary Feldhaus-Weber)

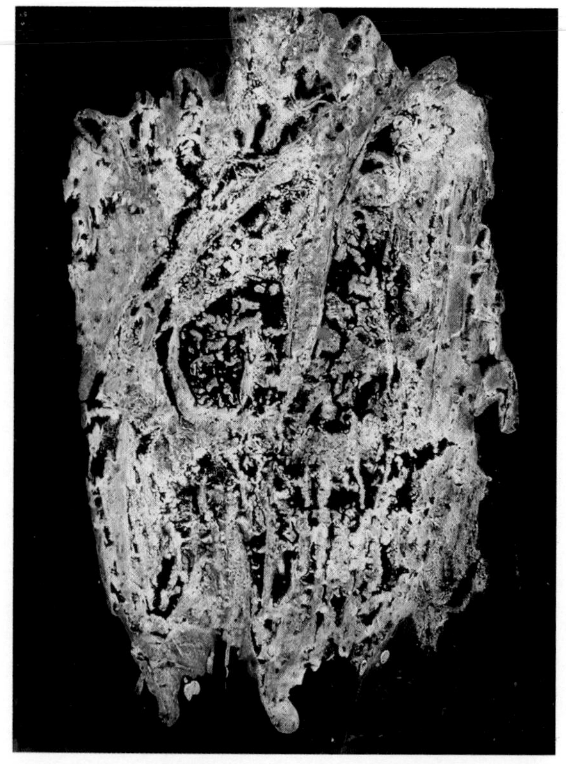

PLATE 16. White Brain: At a certain point I began to make my brain pictures more "decorative", artistic. I was no longer so obsessed with understanding the damage. I was beginning to integrate my feelings about the head injury. (Color plate courtesy of Mary Feldhaus-Weber)

CHAPTER 5

THE ILLNESS AND DISABILITY EXPERIENCE FROM AN INDIVIDUAL PERSPECTIVE

DAVID W. BEER

In this chapter I consider the perspectives of occupational therapy practitioner and client as healer and sufferer, respectively. I am interested in drawing out some of the dimensions of this difference, because as occupational therapy practitioners our understanding of the sufferer's point of view has significant implications for our capacity to engage him or her in meaningful activities. Yet there are characteristics of the roles and experience of practitioners and clients that tend to separate their perspectives. A practitioner has a professional understanding of the body and the person that is based on training that the client, generally, does not have. How many clients, for instance, have actually seen and handled the muscles, tendons, and ligaments of the human arm? Also, many practitioners work in settings that encourage them to restrict their view of clients, reducing them to characteristics directly linked to their afflictions or deficits as exemplars of a disease or syndrome. These settings, and the payment systems that support them, measure client progress (and practitioner effectiveness) against changes in such decontextualized characteristics.

Illness experience, however, is particular to the afflicted person and the world(s) in which he or she lives. An **illness** initially interferes with, and later becomes intertwined with, a particular life, complicating particular relationships, interfering with particular pleasures and activities, requiring particular adaptations, and ultimately, coming to have original significance for a particular person. The generalizing and reducing tendencies of what Frank (1991) called "disease talk" run counter to the development of relationships and understandings, out of which can grow a partnership centered on activities that are meaningful to the client. In approaching this topic, I explore the perspectives of the occupational therapy practitioner and the client through use of constructs that have gained acceptance in anthropological and sociological studies of practitioner and patient or client experiences, including illness and **disease,** sickness, deviance, **liminality,** and **explanatory models.**

ILLNESS AND DISEASE

Since the late 1970s, medical sociology and anthropology have suggested a conceptual distinction between illness and disease, intended to describe the contrast between the perspectives of patients and healing professionals and to place these differing perspectives in their appropriate social and cultural **contexts** (e.g., Frankenberg, 1980; Kleinman, Eisenberg, & Good, 1978). This contrast is a useful one, although potentially problematic (see Hahn, 1984). It reminds us that the perceptions and understandings of this aspect of human experience are positioned—that is, they partly depend on the social and cultural location of the perceiver.

Among other things, this implies that the perceptions of neither client nor healer are completely consistent with reality, meaning with bias- and prejudice-free understandings of the world. Both are influenced by who holds them, why they hold them, what they plan to do with the information, and other concerns. The following conversation, recounted by Kleinman (1988), is useful in illustrating this point. Mrs. Lawler, who has had psoriasis for some time, consults with Dr. Jones, who is reported to be an expert in administering a new treatment for psoriasis:

> *DR. JONES: How long have you had psoriasis?*
> *MRS. LAWLER: Oh, about 15 years.*
> *DR. JONES: Where did it begin?*
> *MRS. LAWLER: I was in college, under lots of pressure from exams, and there is a family history of skin problems. It was winter and I was wearing heavy woolen sweaters that seemed to bother my skin. My diet was . . .*
> *DR. JONES: No, No! I meant where on your skin did you first notice plaques?*
> *MRS. LAWLER: My shoulders and knees. But I had a problem for some time with my scalp that I never . . .*
> *DR. JONES: How has it progressed the past few years?*
> *MRS. LAWLER: These have been difficult years. I mean I have been under great stress at work and in my personal life. I . . .*
> *DR. JONES: I meant, how has your skin problem progressed? (pp. 128–129)*

As shown by this conversation, Mrs. Lawler and Dr. Jones take substantially different views of psoriasis. Mrs. Lawler thinks of psoriasis as she experiences it—as integrated into her ongoing life experience. She locates its beginnings in life events and situations, such as college, examinations, a family history of skin troubles, winter and scratchy sweaters, and diet. She remembers that it was preceded by a scalp problem. She describes its progress in terms of its effect on her life, adding to already significant stress at work and in her personal life.

Dr. Jones thinks of psoriasis as a skin condition that afflicts many people. Psoriasis can be subdivided into different types, each of which has certain causes, follows a certain course, and shares certain characteristics. He wants to know when the first plaques appeared and how far and how rapidly the psoriasis has spread. All of this will help Dr. Jones learn what variety of psoriasis Mrs. Lawler has contracted and whether the new treatment will make a difference.

Mrs. Lawler's understanding of psoriasis is personal. Psoriatic plaques, peeling, itching, and skin disfiguration have become a painful part of the last 15 years of Mrs. Lawler's life, causing her both physical and social suffering. Thinking about psoriasis without thinking about the events and experiences of her life with which it is associated would be impossible. Dr. Jones, on the other hand, must determine whether the psoriasis experienced by Mrs. Lawler is amenable to the new treatment. He must compare certain nonexperiential characteristics of her sickness (e.g., length of time she has suffered, which parts of the body are affected) with those of other patients to know which category of psoriasis she has. Because he is acting as a dermatologist, Dr. Jones ignores much of the personal detail of Mrs. Lawler's story. It is not that he does not care about her; it is that he has a different job to do. He is to attack psoriasis itself, which is located in the body of Mrs. Lawler. Whereas Mrs. Lawler may not easily be able to separate her body, her self, and her life, Dr. Jones does so as a matter of course. For Dr. Jones, Mrs. Lawler's body is not an inseparable part of who she is and how she travels through her world; it is simply the battleground on which he will fight the war against psoriasis.

We construe the terms *disease* and *illness* to refer to the perspectives of the professional healer (in this example, the physician) and the patient, respectively. Which perspective is correct? Should we believe Mrs. Lawler or Dr. Jones? Both accounts can be correct. Mrs. Lawler might very well accept Dr. Jones's entire explanation and likely would approve of the way Dr. Jones uses his account of psoriasis in determining whether and how to treat her. But Mrs. Lawler would never state that Dr. Jones's account explained her experience of psoriasis.

It is important to emphasize just what the patient and professional perspectives are all about. Some accounts suggest that the physician perspective is about reality and the client perspective is about perception, equating the former with hard science and the latter with emotion. A perspective that seems sounder was outlined by Hahn (1984); in this view, some form of suffering or disorder is the common denominator in all therapeutic exchanges, and different parties to the suffering or disorder draw on different sets of ideas and interests, or ideologies, to generate an appropriate explanation for and response to the suffering. In Hahn's conceptualization, illness and disease correspond to the patient and physician views about suffering or disorder.

Occupational therapy practitioners, who often find themselves acting as brokers between physicians and clients, will find in Hahn's conceptualization room for a third point of view concerning the challenges confronted by a given client. Rogers (1982) suggested that much of the difference in viewpoint between medicine and occupational therapy stems from their different understandings of order and disorder. Medicine uses the presence or absence of disease and functional deficit as the basis for perceiving the presence of order or disorder. Occupational therapy, on the other hand, bases its understanding of order and disorder on the occupational performance of the person in question. Occupational performance may be affected by active pathologies, or it may be diminished by capacity changes that are part of normal development. Performance occurs in normal life contexts, not just in clinical settings isolated from regular activity. Performance problems often can be detected only in natural settings; they can seldom be well understood without reference to such settings. A person may have a disease or functional deficit without experiencing disruptions in occupational performance. Likewise, a person may experience a disruption in occupational performance without any disease or functional deficit (Rogers, 1982).

Rogers's (1982) distinction between and among types of order and disorder provides a way to distinguish the practice paradigm of occupational therapy from that of medicine. By itself, however, Roger's distinction does not guarantee that the occupational therapy practitioner will adopt a stance in treatment that includes the client perspective. Occupational therapy practitioners, similar to other therapeutic professionals, are prone to fail to take the client's perspective seriously. This tendency is related to society's view that occupational performance-related disorders are forms of social deviance, and occupational therapy intervention is part of society's effort to control such disorder.

SICKNESS, RECOVERY, LIMINALITY, AND EXPERIENCE

Deviance became an explicit part of formal sociological thought about disease and illness with the work of Parsons (1951). Parsons noted that individuals experiencing illness do not perform their assigned roles in a normal fashion and that, under certain circumstances, there seems to be social acceptance for this deviation from the norm. Parsons termed this situation or condition *sickness*. When people contract disease, they are exempted, temporarily, from their normal social roles. They may stay home from work, miss class, or in other ways avoid normal role behaviors. They are not, however, role free. Instead, sick persons take the sick role, meaning that they are expected to conduct themselves in a way such that they alleviate the conditions that exempt them from normal activity. If one breaks a bone, he or she must have it set and wear a cast. If someone suffers from exhaustion, he or she must rest. In many cases, people must seek the advice of physicians and other health-care professionals, and they must follow that advice. The sick role is temporary; it is obtained under the presumption that the condition that has forced the person out of his or her normal roles will last only a short time. That condition is itself a kind of deviation from the norm (health), and the person is bound by social convention to do whatever is required to alleviate it. In fact, it is the correction of this deviance (sickness) that leads society to permit taking on the sick role, a deviation from the normal performance of social roles. Once the condition has been alleviated, the person, it is assumed, will resume his or her normal roles and activities.

Sickness and the Sick Role

It will be clear to the reader, on reflection, that in our society, the notions of *sickness* and *sick role* are related to the notion of *disease*. I am entitled to take sick leave and receive sick pay covered by sick days, provided either I have something wrong with me that is rooted in a disease or I am pursuing medical advice about a complaint that may, ultimately, turn out to be rooted in a disease. Under some rules, I am permitted to take sick leave to assist with the care of a family member who is suffering from the aforementioned conditions. Nearly always when there is a dispute it is the word of a physician that is considered to be the ultimate authority on whether taking sick days is a legitimate response to what ails me.

Our need to regulate sickness to prescribe a role for those who become ill and to regulate who can and cannot enter into that role suggests a further assumption embedded in the sick role: that sickness is a form of deviance. In this view, participation in activities socially assigned to a particular period of life—school for children, work for adults—constitutes normal activity. Sickness, which excuses one from such activities, is a form of social deviance; hence it must be carefully regulated. Disease, which causes the condition of sickness, is itself a deviation from health. Fighting or working to alleviate disease is the major justification for the sick role.

Occupational therapy practitioners, however, treat many clients who are not going to get better. Because these clients will not, ultimately, be "cured," the sick role and its associated model of social deviance do not really apply. These clients may experience release from social roles to attend to their rehabilitation, but the resumption of these roles, especially for those with severe disability or chronic illness, may remain a question. Whether and, if so, how and when they will resume these roles becomes the object of their rehabilitative process and the focus of much of occupational therapy intervention. This is also the experience of clients recovering from such unpredictable diseases as cancer. Frank (1991) described his permanent membership in what he called the "remission society," a category of people joined by the common knowledge that one telephone call can return them instantly to the tunnel of treatment and uncertainty that the reappearance of cancer cells occasions. One cannot, he suggested, go back to the way things were before one developed cancer. One's life has been

HISTORICAL NOTE 5–1

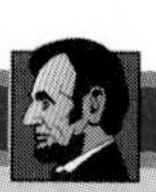

The Power of Persons Seeking Occupational Therapy: The Story of Clifford Beers

SUZANNE M. PELOQUIN

Clifford Beers, a client admitted for depression to three mental institutions between 1900 and 1905, framed an articulate plea for reform. In his book *A Mind That Found Itself,* Beers (1917) used his own experiences to promote change: "For one year no further attention was paid to me than to see that I had three meals a day, the requisite number of baths, and a sufficient amount of exercise" (p. 68). He described his struggle to get simple materials such as a book or paper and pencil, items with which he might occupy himself. After he finally procured these, Beers felt that his reading, writing, and drawing led to his cure. He argued that occupation held healing potential for others. He started the National Committee for Mental Hygiene and through this group advocated many hospital changes, including the use of occupation and recreation.

This story shows us the power of occupation but also shows that persons can shape their destinies and the therapies of their culture. If we stay mindful of the experience of Beers, we might more readily see the strength that dwells in the persons who seek our therapy.

Beers, C. W. (1917). *A mind that found itself.* New York: Longmans, Green.

permanently changed. What is normal for such a person has been transformed.

These considerations suggest that we need to rethink the nature of the experience of disablement. Murphy (1990) suggested that his experience of being physically disabled, "neither sick nor well, neither dead nor fully alive, neither out of society nor wholly in it" (p. 131) is more like a state of permanent liminality than a temporary state of sickness.

Liminality and Disability

The notion of *liminality* is drawn from the writings of anthropologists who study rites of passage—rituals that mark the movement of persons from one status to another (e.g., from child to adult). Such rituals not only mark changes in status but also are considered to be transformative. The Christian ritual of baptism, for instance, not only symbolizes acceptance of certain beliefs but is also felt to cleanse the soul of the baptized person. Anthropologist Turner (1967) observed that such rituals first separate participants from their roles in social life. While participants are separated from their former roles, they undergo transformation through instruction, endowment, surgery, pronouncement, covenant, or magic. Following their transformation, they emerge from their separation and are reintegrated into society, as persons with a new status.

For instance, the bride and groom, before their wedding, separate from the rest of the world by changing clothes, by preparing in isolation from one another, by occupying certain spaces. Then, when it is time for the ceremony, they stand together before a ritual official who is vested with the capacity to make their covenant to live together legally recognized, who evokes promises and intentions from them, and who pronounces them husband and wife. Once this transformation from being unmarried to being married, from being unrelated to being legally bound has occurred, the man and woman become a legally recognized family, meaning, among other things, that their future offspring will be considered the legal heirs of both members of this couple. The new husband and wife emerge from the sacred edifice, home, or courthouse into the world, often to a celebration during which they eat, drink, dance, and engage in other forms of social intercourse with family and friends. Then, finally, they retire together to their home, enacting for the first time, their new status in society as married partners.

During the time when individuals are undergoing change in status, they belong neither to their former nor to their future status. They are liminal because they are betwixt and between social roles. During this time they are, in many rituals, considered dangerous to normal people because of their liminality. But the promise exists that they will be, when all is said and done, reintegrated into society, occupying or enacting a new role, holding a new status, carrying on social life as before. For many disabled people, such reintegration never occurs. They seem dangerous to those nonafflicted persons Goffman (1963) called "normals" precisely because they are physically or psychosocially anomalous. They are not sick, not well, neither dead nor fully alive. They embody disorder. They are never recovered, can never return to the way things used to be.

The disabled person fits into the mold of liminality far better than into the model of social deviance followed by sociologists. Writing about ritual process in primitive societies, Turner (1967) said, "Liminality is frequently likened to death, to being in the womb, to invisibility, to darkness, to bisexuality, to the wilderness, and to an eclipse of the sun or the moon" (p. 59). How well this fits everything we have discussed: the occasional rumor of my death, the social invisibility of the disabled, the attribution of asexuality in the popular mind, the unisex hospital room, and the blurring of roles within the community of the handicapped. The disabled are more than deviants. They are the antiphony of everyday life.

Just as the bodies of the disabled are permanently impaired, so too is their standing as members of society. The lasting indeterminacy of their state of being produces a similar lack of definition of their social roles, which are in any event superseded and obscured by submersion of their identities. Their persons are regarded as contaminated; eyes are averted, and people take care not to approach wheelchairs too closely. (Murphy, 1990)

Disability, Stigma, and Notions of Normality

In addition to painting a more realistic description of the social standing of disabled persons, Murphy's (1990) use of the notion of liminality augments the deviance model of disability and illness in another way. Absent from Parsons' (1951) account of sickness is any careful attention to the variegated and compelling experience of the sick person. The notion of liminality neatly summarizes one vector of the experience of disabled persons living in the contemporary United States, the feeling that one is not quite human, not quite ill, and yet not quite well. This is the feeling to which Murphy, Hockenberry, and other wheelchair users refer when they describe brief encounters with so-called normals. People who do not use wheelchairs act as though the mere presence of a wheelchair gave a normal permission to ignore the person using it, to step on him, or to treat him as an insentient obstacle (Hockenberry, 1995). When such individuals do speak, although the disability is often at the forefront of the minds of both parties of the interaction, both conscientiously avoid mentioning the subject (Murphy, 1990). Such behaviors mark the stigma that is attached to both physical and psychosocial disablement in the contemporary United States. The experience of shame that this stigma engenders in the person with disability is a critical part of the state of being a disabled member of our society.

But the problem with the deviance model goes deeper. Frank (1991) wrote, "Being ill is just another way of living"; it is "nothing special" (p. 3). Suffering, illness, or injury is a part of normal human life; few of us live out our lives without suffering from some form of affliction. As Frank pointed out, by focusing on recovery to the exclusion of the experience of illness, we risk missing completely that part of life. This is even truer for those who suffer from disability or chronic illness. To continue to speak of such conditions in terms of deviance is to deny the degree to which they become integrated with or define the lived world of the afflicted person. Hockenberry—radio and television correspondent, piano student, trainer of developmentally disabled adults, world traveler—never ceases being a "crip." Although he vigorously resists the limitations that normal society attempts to impose on him because of his paraplegia, he does have to deal daily with the personal and social consequences of not having any sensation below the nipples. But for Hockenberry, this is a permanent state; in such circumstances, it makes little sense, and no difference, whether suffering from paraplegia is normal or not. In this case, being "abnormal" has become "normal" (Hockenberry, 1995). There is nothing special to be served by knowing whether Hockenberry's body is normal or not. There is nothing special about knowing the physical details of what is now part of his everyday life, the pathologies, impairments, and functional limitations he suffers, which make him diagnostically similar to some paraplegics but different from others. What is something special is how he lives, experiences, and describes his life.

EXPLANATORY MODELS AND NARRATIVES

Liminality is only one aspect of the experience of disablement. Others we may glean from accounts written by people experiencing disablement: frustration, anger, loss, isolation, guilt, helplessness, personal worthlessness, depression, and pain. All of these feelings are important parts of the experience of disablement. In addition, there are positive feelings: joy, excitement, pride, accomplishment, power, intelligence, fulfillment, and triumph. Such feelings have meaning, ultimately, in the context of a person's life. But how might we best learn of such feelings and the associated events and perspectives that accompany them?

Experience suggests that if we desire to understand our clients, we must invite them to talk about their disabilities or illnesses and listen carefully. Two different (but not mutually exclusive) approaches to conceptualizing this process are explanatory models and illness-disability narratives (IDNs). Explanatory models are personal, often implicit, accounts of illness, held by both practitioners and professionals that describe the nature and origins of the problem and what can be done about it (Kleinman, 1988). IDNs are developing chronicles of key events, situations, personalities, and factors that tell the story of illness. IDNs may also be elicited from both professionals and laypeople (Mattingly, 1994).

Explanatory Models

Kleinman (1988) suggested that explanatory models answer five major questions concerning illness: (1) What is the cause of the affliction? (2) When and how did it begin? (3) What is its pathophysiology or nature? (4) What has been or will be the course of sickness (including degree of severity and type of sick role—acute, chronic, impaired, or other)? (5) What are or should be the available courses of treatment? The notion of explanatory model reminds practitioners that they are not alone in actively seeking to comprehend and give meaning to the problems confronted by their clients. Practitioner explanations of the problem do not encounter a vacuum. The client, the client's family, and other close associates of the client are likely to attempt to make sense of the disruption and discomfort caused by the problem at hand as well. These "theorists" may apply a much wider range of causes and remedies to the problems than do the practitioners.

An example will help clarify the meaning and importance of explanatory models. Donald was born with apparent neurologic sequelae from his mother's heroin abuse

CASE STUDY 5-1

Donald, According to the Occupational Therapist and Mother

[Donald's occupational therapist speaks:] I met this baby first . . . when he was in the neonatal intensive care unit. I'll give you a little bit of statistics [picks up chart to read information from]. He was born full term . . . um . . . on May 29, 1992, and um . . . he was born because of a ruptured membrane. So labor was induced and so it wasn't a . . . a normal birth. . . . He was initially floppy, and they had to give him a bit of oxygen, and he had, um, a seizure about a week later.

Um . . . his mother was also on methadone. She had been doing heroin and then found out she was pregnant, pretty early on in the pregnancy. . . . I'm not sure exactly when, but, um . . . went to a methadone program right away as soon as she found out. And he did show, . . . his name is Donald Peterson, . . . he did show some signs of withdrawal . . . after, um . . . while being in the nursery.

Let's see . . . what else can I tell you about him? Um, he had a little bit of edema—that was shown on the CAT scan, so, so . . . I'm not sure where it was in his brain, but he had some edema somewhere in his brain um . . . I think it was in the temporal area. . . . So we were called in to evaluate him, um, when he was in the intensive care unit. He was reported to be a poor feeder, and they were worried about some tightness in his lower extremities, too.

So I, I saw him . . . once. And um, he was very hard to wake up and to get to an alert stage, even though he was full-term, and he was about a month old when I saw him. And he was tight. His shoulders were tight, his hands were tight, he was irritable . . . and I never did really get him to that full awake stage.

So I saw him one other time and tried to feed him, and um, he, he was a very in-inconsistent sucker. He couldn't coordinate the suck-swallow mechanism. He was just having a hard time. And again, just wasn't alert and just didn't look very good. Um, he was a good-sized baby, he was a big baby, so he wasn't little or frail, um, just had a lot of trouble with state regulation and being tight and just, um, not a calm baby.

Um, and when he left I did meet his mother, an-an, mother and his father and his little brother—her name is Paula—and set up an appointment for her to come as an outpatient. I explained to her what we had seen—that he was a little bit tight, he was irritable and having trouble with feedings—and told her that um, we would like to monitor that to make sure he won't have problems when he gets older. And, um, she was—she seemed to understand and was very agreeable and, um—we scheduled an appointment, and, um, so I've seen him—oh, I think four or five times since then. So, um, and they, she comes consistently and will call if she can't come, and, um, Donald is now going to be 3 months old, I believe, so . . . he's still tiny.

Um, and he's gotten al—his picture has changed since he's—since I've been seeing him. He's now, um, an alert baby. He now tracks visually, which he wasn't doing before. Um, he doesn't cry as much. He can, he calms easier with, um, a pacifier or holding—um, he's still got some, he's got some arching and some tightness in his shoulders and in his back. He tends to keep his hands fisted though that's—the last time I saw him, he looked better with that, with, um, showing some more isolated finger movements and, um, exploring things a little bit with his fingers, fingers on his body or fingers on your hand, um, and I've also worked with the mother a lot, trying to tell her, explain to her what I'm looking at, um, what I'd like to see, what I'd like to see go away, um, like the arching and the tightness, um, and how we can facilitate him in different positions to get him to move and explore optimally without that tightness interfering. . . . And, um, she comes back and she—"Well, I tried putting something behind his head, but—now watch—but he'll lean back anyway and it doesn't really seem to . . ." So we'll try to work together um . . . to problem solve around that.

[Donald's mother speaks:] Donald is a star. Donald is my pride and joy. Donald is my little star. . . . Well [takes deep breath], . . . as as you already know, that Donald has a seizure disorder. Where it's, it's controllable now. When I first had him, he had a real trauma seizure . . . and they put him on medication. You know? And he's supposed to be on his medication until he either grows out of it or 3 years old. But I believe he's gonna go further than that. Cause you can't estimate on a newborn, what's gonna happen in the future. You know? Like we can't see the future. We don't know how Donald's gonna be when he gets older. We don't know if when he make one he might have more seizures, cause he only really had one.

So far his medications been controlling it. Everybody in my house been real careful with him, you know? So, it's been controllable. It's alright now but we don't know how he might look in the future. You know, we don't know tomorrow until tomorrow gets here. But . . . like I said, um . . . it's still considered a disorder because he's taking medication. Dependin' on medication everyday. Takin' phenobarbital everyday. . . .

So . . . he's spoiled. He want you ta hold him. He's a sweet baby. Don't get me wrong. But I knew from the day that he went to intensive care. Like my mother

Continues

says, she knew from that day that I told her that Donald was going to be pinpointed as a special child—special attention—because he had that seizure. So you know everybody really was like watchin' him real close? Now we gettin' a little bit more confidence. Everybody watchin'. Don't get me wrong. They still watchin'. They don't let him cry. He go through like seven arms in my house. He'll be cryin' and somebody pickin' him up. You know? So . . . he, you know? He . . . he be attached to that now. If he whine, he know you gonna pick him up [both laugh]. That's all I have ta do is whhhaaa. "Then somebody will come and pick me up!" So . . . it's not no problem though. Because, like I said, I'm not workin' now so I . . . I don't have nothin' else ta do but enjoy my baby's childhood life. An, you know? Watch 'em grow up.

It's kind of scary because I don't know what the future look like for me as far as him havin' that seizure. We don't know what caused it an' I don't know when one could be triggered. You know? Like when I take him to the doctor to get his um . . . baby shot? They tell me that a . . . a fever can trigger a seizure. An' I be so scared when I get him home that he might have a fever, you know, might catch a fever. But so far, since Donald's been takin' his baby shots? I've been lucky. He hasn't had no temperature. He haven't been real irritable. Been sweet ta be honest with ya. I ain't really had no problems. Not as far as gettin' him a shot.

Like I said, when you got God behind you. I know I did some real devious things, but I been an angel too—don't get me wrong. I think the worst thing in my life that I have done is when I got wrapped up into drugs. You know? But God forgave me. And it's like, he be behind me so . . . I'm okay. An' I got Him . . . you know, He watchin' over Donald. I have so many. I have a lot of people prayin' for him. You know, my grandmother inta church, my uncle inta church. I got an uncle that's a preacher. You know, I have a lot with the church, by me goin' to the church, I have a lot . . . I have a lot of people prayin' for Donald. An' when you have people behind you like that, you know, it makes it better. But that's basically all about Donald.

during the first trimester of her pregnancy with him. Within a week of birth, Donald had a seizure. He showed the signs of problematic neurologic state regulation, alternating between tension and tightness, on the one hand, and floppiness, on the other. Early in his life, it was hard to get Donald aroused to full wakefulness. The occupational therapist that worked with Donald treated him both while he was a patient in the neonatal intensive care unit (NICU) and when he was an outpatient following his discharge from the hospital. The excerpts in Case Study 5-1 were taken from interviews with Donald's therapist and his mother that were conducted by an occupational therapy graduate student during the period when Donald was receiving occupational therapy as an outpatient (Beer, Lawlor, & Mattingly, 1994).

The occupational therapist and the mother had different understandings of Donald's condition and talked about their understandings in very different ways. Thinking of their statements as representing underlying explanatory models, even if we must think of those models as partly formed, is quite useful. Kleinman's (1988) construct gives us a way to organize the comments of each person into a more coherent point of view as well as providing us with some points of contrast.

For instance, we see that the therapist and the mother have defined Donald's problem in different ways, that they used different information to describe the problem, and that their definitions were works in progress that were at different stages of completion. The therapist did not give a name to Donald's condition but instead told us, through use of a variety of specific physiologic details, that Donald suffered from the as yet undetermined and unspecified aftereffects of his mother's heroin abuse. She mentioned edema of the temporal lobe, symptoms of withdrawal, a seizure, poor state regulation, poor coordination of the suck-swallow mechanism, not achieving full alertness, and alternating floppiness and tightness when she saw Donald in the NICU. When she saw Donald as an outpatient, she observed some relaxation of tightness, independent movement of fingers, back arching, more alertness, and improvements in visual tracking. Overall, her statements suggest she noted improvement. In contrast, Donald's mother defined her son's problem more narrowly, as a seizure disorder; she noted that there had only been one seizure thus far and that the seizures were being controlled by medication.

That Donald's occupational therapist and his mother understood his problem differently is not trivial. Each organized her description of Donald and of her activities to assist him around her understanding of Donald's problems. His therapist focused on activities intended to assess and encourage Donald's neurologic development. His mother focused on personal and family efforts intended to prevent a recurrence of the seizure.

Donald's therapist identified the mother's heroin abuse as one of the potential causes of his problems, indicating that he exhibited signs of withdrawal in the NICU. This is consistent with the focus of her description of Donald on signs related to or indicating neurologic functioning. Donald's mother mentioned her drug use, but did not link it directly to Donald's seizure disorder. In fact, she stated her understanding of the problem in a way that supported the family efforts being made to avoid another seizure: "We don't know what caused it an' I don't know when one could be triggered." In related interviews, Donald's mother told us that she received conflicting information about the role of her heroin use in causing Donald's problems. She did, ultimately, identify the use of heroin as a contributor to Donald's problems. At that point, the explanatory models of therapist and mother began to overlap.

Looking toward the future, there is complementarity, but not agreement, between the explanatory models of Donald's therapist and his mother. Donald's therapist did not know what the future would bring for Donald, partly because of her understanding of the workings of the body. It would be hard to tell the extent and permanence of any neurologic damage to Donald's body until it developed further. The seizure a week after birth, the lack of alertness, the variation between floppiness and tightness, and the inconsistent sucking all suggested to Donald's therapist that something neurologic might be wrong. On the other hand, such effects can be (in whole or in part) transient. Donald's increased alertness, his visual tracking, and the reduction of tightness in some parts of his body all suggested that he might grow out of some of the difficulties.

The therapist based her estimations on her observations of and interactions with the child, on the knowledge of neurologic and motor development she obtained from formal education and experience, and on the comments and observations of others whom she consulted about Donald's condition. Her response to her evolving understanding of Donald's condition was threefold. She continued trying to assess his developing capacities and deficiencies. She addressed specific problems, such as fisting of the hands or arching of the back, with specific postures, movements, and activities. And she used activities to support Donald's development to increase his flexibility and strength, to stimulate his perception, and to help him master developmentally appropriate activities and skills.

Donald's mother also did not know what the future would bring for the boy, but her response to not knowing was different from that of Donald's occupational therapist. Donald's mother expressed her immediate concern that Donald would have another seizure. She, with other family members, responded to this concern by making sure Donald took his phenobarbital and by exercising care and watchfulness. Donald's mother credited both strategies with helping him avoid further seizures. Embedded in the family's watchfulness were theories about the kinds of events that might bring on another seizure—fevers induced by inoculations, agitation, and long periods of crying. Family members would not let Donald cry much, and Donald's mother was very careful with inoculations. This line of defense had been successful thus far, as a result of which Donald's family was beginning to feel confident that there might be no more seizures.

If Donald reaches the age of 3 years without incident, he likely will have grown out of seizures and the need to take medication. Donald's mother attributed the fact that Donald had not had another seizure at least partly to having God supporting her. Although she had done some "devious things," the worst of which was her drug abuse, Donald's mother had been "an angel" since that time and felt that God had forgiven her. In addition to her own reformation, Donald's mother pointed to the number of people who were praying for Donald, including a grandmother and an uncle who were "inta church" and an uncle who is a preacher.

Donald's therapist and mother drew on different sets of resources in responding to Donald's condition. Donald's therapist relied primarily on her interactions with Donald, viewing the problem principally as a developmental-neurologic problem, which, while located in Donald's body, could be affected by the appropriate kinds of interaction between Donald and his environment. She extended this idea to Donald's mother and his family when she described ways to adjust the home environment to support Donald in more appropriate postures. Donald's mother drew on substantial social and religious resources in her efforts to prevent future seizures. Family efforts were organized around seeing that Donald took his medication and avoided circumstances that might bring on a seizure. Extended family efforts added the power of God to the efforts of the family, as if to counter the uncertainties of Donald's future well-being.

Explanatory models can be, then, a powerful approach to transforming statements and descriptions into perspectives. Practitioners can elicit material that can be interpreted using the construct of explanatory models through directed, open-ended interview questions, such as the following: "Tell me about your problem." "How did it begin?" "What seems to cause it?" "What can you do about it?" "If you did nothing about it, what would happen?" Statements and ideas that allow the construction of such models can also be collected one statement at a time. Remembering that both clients and practitioners have such models can help practitioners recognize the efforts of clients to understand, interpret, and respond to their ailment, as well as to provide practitioners with one means of understanding the bases of client behaviors that do not seem logical (Beer et al., 1994).

Illness and Disability Narratives

IDNs are developing chronicles of key events, situations, personalities, and factors that tell the story of illness or disability. IDNs share a number of elements with other forms of narrative—actors, setting, plot, desire, dramatic tension, and resolution. IDNs, similar to explanatory models, may be elicited from professionals and laypeople, or they may be constructed from their accounts. They are different from explanatory models, however, in their degree of temporal particularity—their connection to specific events occurring at specific times in particular contexts as well as to specific actors acting at certain times in certain contexts with specific motives. They also differ in the role of temporal ordering and unfolding. In explanatory models, temporality appears, primarily, in the service of causal explanations. In IDNs, temporality is a central structure for organizing plot and tracing the development and resolution of dramatic tension (Mattingly, 1994).

Stories, as the term is used here, should not be confused with chronological accounts of events. Any account that includes actors, provides some sort of setting, and moves in a time-ordered fashion may be considered a chronological account, but a story is different. The actors in a story have concerns, interests, and desires that are either in conflict with one another or with events or circumstances that seem to be out of their control. It is not known if the actors will receive fulfillment of their desires. This question, embedded in the telling of the story, creates an experience of uncertainty for the listener or reader, which may be termed narrative or dramatic *tension*. This tension is what gives a story its life. It animates its plot, its temporal structure of events, and keeps the listener listening or the reader turning the pages. The listener or reader listens for and looks forward to a resolution, some determination as to whether and, if so, how the dramatic tension will be resolved. Often there is a moral or point embedded in the story, which points to how the story is to be made sense of in the context of its telling and which is key to interpreting the story outside the context of its telling.

The term *story* is used here in full knowledge of its common connection to falsehoods and fictions. In fact, stories are constructions, often telescoping years of living and experience into a few hours of talking or even a few paragraphs of transcribed text. But they are not simply made up. Stories about illness or disability are efforts to describe real events and experiences from the perspective of one observer or actor. Although they may not provide accounts that are objectively accurate when mapped onto constant chronological time, stories do provide insight into the lives and perspectives of storytellers. They indicate (by their presence or absence in the story) which events are significant enough to be recounted. They give meaning to those events, shedding further light on the perspective of the storyteller. And they communicate something of the teller's experience of them, as we experience the ebb and flow of dramatic tension and draw analogies to our own experience. Whether a story accurately reflects its teller's original experience at the historical time of the recounted events is a significant issue, but for a practitioner listening to a client, what is important is the client's experience of those events at the time the events are recounted.

In some of our most moving accounts of illness and disability (e.g., Murphy, 1990; Hockenberry, 1995), we know the general outcome before we begin reading. Murphy died in 1990 of respiratory failure, a consequence of increasing pressure from the tumor growing inside his spinal cavity. Hockenberry has become a successful correspondent for NBC News, his third major correspondent position in radio and television reporting. There is, in reading their stories, little tension related to events themselves. These accounts are worth reading for other reasons. Murphy's description of his steadily increasing impairments and functional limitations and of his increasing social isolation, anger, loss, and sense of guilt over the burden he is to his wife, Yolanda, provided an opportunity for him to turn his anthropological gaze on the meaning and experience of disablement in the contemporary United States. As Murphy reflected on his progressing disability, he drew on his knowledge of Mundurucu society, on his Irish Catholic upbringing, and on his experience of alcoholism. He drew on sociologist Erving Goffman's writings about stigma and social interaction; on Oliver Sacks's account of Christina, the "disembodied lady"; and on the reactions of his friends, colleagues, and neighbors to his increasing disablement. He wove these and other materials into his own feelings about his increasing disembodiment and its effect on himself and his family. The resulting IDN is, essentially, a semantic map of Murphy's world.

Hockenberry's account is different. Hockenberry's disablement stemmed from a single accident, an irruption into his biography, and his story was about living in and adjusting to a body that had changed. But it was also about learning what it means to use a wheelchair and figuring out the sorts of uses (e.g., mobility, political activism, social panhandling, personal advantage) for which wheelchairs are appropriate, moral, or healthy. His book makes an interesting contrast with Murphy's. Murphy, an anthropologist, turned his cross-cultural eye inward onto his own life world, defining for his reader the meaning and experience of disability. Hockenberry, with his wheelchair, traveled all over the world, demonstrating in societies from New York to Somalia that it is he, not social or cultural attitudes toward disablement, who defines the limits of his world. His account highlighted the practices and attitudes that variously circumscribe and expand the world of the disabled.

Long narrative works, such as *The Body Silent* and *Moving Violations*, not only show us how actors attribute meaning to disablement and its interface with their lived worlds but also they show us these meanings unfolding across time. One of the critical features of the disablement experience, which the structure of therapy obscures, is its temporal length. Disablement, whether temporary or permanent, is constant and pervasive; and the experience of living it is always more comprehensive than the staccato sequence of therapy appointments. Reading lengthy disablement stories and seeing the meaning of disability unfold in the life of the teller give the reader a sense of the temporal extent of the experience of disability. This is important, because the interest of the disabled client nearly always has more temporal breadth than the interest of the practitioner.

In the accounts of Donald, discussed earlier, the temporal period that is the focus of Donald's mother was nearly 3 years long and implied in her discussion of that period is a concern about the future beyond that initial 3 years. One tension in her account pivoted on the question of whether Donald would have another seizure before his third birthday as well as on whether avoiding a seizure would ensure that Donald would grow into a relatively normal, independent adult. Another tension, not entirely clear in the excerpt printed here, had to do with the extent to which her drug abuse is to blame for Donald's condition. The therapist, in contrast, had a shorter-term interest. For her there were at least two tensions—how would Donald respond to her efforts to reduce the tightness in his fists and the arching of his back and would she be able to help Donald explore the world in a way that would facilitate the rest of his development, despite whatever tightness was present? The temporal span of the narrative tension in the therapist's account was relatively narrow compared to the temporal period that was of interest to the mother.

The purposeful elicitation of stories is an art for experienced interviewers, but the human propensity for storytelling means that almost anyone will tell an IDN, given enough time and a willing listener. Therapeutic settings often provide the rhythm and predictability necessary for a client to feel willing to tell a story, and therapeutic activities may instigate the telling. In addition, a narrative orientation can be used as a frame for combining and interpreting statements made by clients on different occasions over a time period. Either way, a sense of narrative, that actors attribute meaning to their illness or disability by acting and seeing its significance unfold as they live it, makes it possible for practitioners to appreciate the disability experience of the actors. Likewise, the notion that people suffering disability or illness are actively trying to make sense out of what is happening in their lives with explanatory models—by determining what caused the problem, what can be done about it, and what effect doing that will have—suggests to the practitioner that seemingly irrational or meaningless statements or actions by clients may, in fact, make perfect sense from the client perspective. These approaches to understanding the statements of clients constitute a powerful set of tools for understanding the client perspective.

CONCLUSION

Murphy (1990) suggested that the state of being disabled is a kind of permanent liminality. He suggested that, once separated from normal social intercourse, people with disabilities are never fully reintegrated. They are left on the margins of social life, partly integrated and partly not, anomalous for the remainder of their lives. As a conclusion to this reflection on the experience of illness and disablement, I would like to suggest an alternative interpretation of what happens to the person who suffers a disorder that results in disablement.

Were disabled people to be permanently consigned to separation from the rest of society, they would be institutionalized in isolated facilities, never having social interaction with so-called normal persons. Because this is true for only a few such people, to say that they are permanently liminal is to wrest the meaning of liminality. Turner (1967) used the term *liminal* to describe the state of individuals ritually separated from day-to-day social intercourse because they are undergoing social and personal transformation. While they are undergoing this process, they are considered to be dangerous, shifting, anomalous, and even dead. But people who become disabled are more and more often reintegrated into the world. Murphy taught at Columbia University. Hockenberry continues to report for television. Donald lives at home with his family. All were able to leave the hospital, graduate from the rehabilitation clinic, and reside in normal settings. All were able to interact regularly (or are at least were available for interaction) with "normals" who are not wheelchair users, who are not slowly losing control of more and more of their bodies, who are not in danger of seizure at any moment. It seems that all were reintegrated into society, but not as normals.

Being not-normal or other-than-normal has its dangers in this society. For years we have sent anthropologists and other observers off to strange societies to chronicle how other peoples are different from us, as part of a cultural project of comparative self-definition (Fabian, 1983; Wolf, 1982). Part of this process of self-definition is the assumption that others are inferior to us, that otherness is, in fact, prima facie evidence of inferiority. Similar processes of collective self-definition have affected our understanding of the mentally ill, whom we have used to define our sanity and our civility (Foucault, 1972). The construction of minorities—groups of people racially or ethnically or linguistically different from "us" (i.e., white middle-class mainstream American society)—has been a way of justifying unequal distributions of resources and opportunities in our supposedly democratic society.

Now we confront another construction of "other"—the disabled. In our society, people with disabilities culturally define the boundaries of ableness, through existing just across those arbitrary boundaries from able, or normal, people. Their existence as outliers, as others, is critical to maintaining the physical and psychosocial aspects of normalcy. Normals look through them, step on them, bump around them, and obstruct them, because they are positioned just beyond the physical or psychosocial horizon of humanity. When people with disabilities are reintegrated into society they are reintegrated as markers, as personifications of the margins, as not quite human. But they are fully integrated in the sense that the meaning of their existence—in opposition to normalcy—is critical to the maintenance of the notion of normalcy itself. In other words, the transformation that happens in the treatment and rehabilitation process is partly a transformation from normal to abnormal, from able to disabled, from disorder to disordered. Along with this transformation come indications that what has occurred is irreversible and permanent, that there is no road back to what society has defined as normal. However, as Hockenberry demonstrates, the definition of what is normal is also a personal one. Hockenberry incorporates his disability so completely into his daily routine that it is an aspect of himself that he would not change, for to change it would be to deny much of his adult life. This is just the point that people without disabilities miss, that the discomfort they may experience around people with disabilities emanates from themselves and their lack of understanding of the experience of disability.

Fortunately, this is not the end of the story. People with disabilities know that one disability differs from another, that the effect of disability differs from one life to another, and that individuals differ in their capacity to recognize the person who is disabled as more than the disability. Similar to illness, disability is a normal part of life, suffered to some degree by most of us during some part of our lives. Each of us responds to our disability differently. And like illness narratives, disability stories are stories about humanity, about meaning and significance, about challenge and triumph and defeat. Occupational therapy practitioners have opportunities to interact with people with disabilities on a regular basis, and with this comes the opportunity to ask and to listen as such people talk about their experience. Understanding the perspective of people struggling with disabling conditions helps creative practitioners devise treatment that is meaningful to their clients. Knowing how disability affects a person's life, how the person thinks about it, what personal resources a person has for coping all help practitioners understand the way a person responds to treatment. All of this increases the likelihood that treatment will be meaningful.

Moreover, listening to and understanding the perspective of a person with a disability confirms the right of such a person to have a perspective and places a value on it. As participants in the rehabilitation process, practitioners cannot change the response of the world outside rehabilitation to the person with a disability. But they can give these people a sense of their importance; of their humanity; of the legitimacy of their struggles and losses, grief and pain, defeats and triumphs; as well as of their interest to other human beings. Practitioners can counter the tendency in rehabilitation to define people in terms of their disorder, by paying attention to them as whole people, with abilities and disabilities. Practitioners can avoid premature conclusions about their limitations, instead helping them learn to assess and extend their abilities. Practitioners can help clients learn to respond to their social and physical environment creatively, especially in cases in which the environment does not give adequate support. Finally, practitioners can help clients understand that, whatever limitations they may experience, their biography has not yet been written. Ultimately, as Murphy and Hockenberry demonstrated, living is the antidote for the experience of disability.

References

Beer, D. W., Lawlor, M., & Mattingly, C. (1994). *Collaboration, coercion, and compliance in therapeutic relationships*. Paper presented at the American Occupational Therapy Association annual conference, Boston.

Fabian, J. (1983). *Time and the other: How anthropology makes its objects*. New York: Columbia University Press.

Foucault, M. (1972). *Madness and civilization* (A. M. Sheridan Smith, Trans.). New York: Vintage.

Frank, A. (1991). *At the will of the body: Reflections on illness*. Boston: Houghton-Mifflin.

Frankenberg, R. (1980). Medical anthropology and development: A theoretical perspective. *Social Science and Medicine, 14B*, 197–207.

Goffman, E. (1963). *Stigma: Notes on the management of spoiled identity*. Englewood Cliffs, NJ: Prentice-Hall.

Hahn, R. A. (1984). Rethinking "illness" and "disease." In E. V. Daniel & J. F. Pugh (Eds.). *South Asian systems of healing: Contributions to Asian studies* (Vol. 18, pp. 1–23). Leiden: Brill.

Hockenberry, J. (1995). *Moving violations: War zones, wheelchairs, and declarations of independence*. New York: Hyperion.

Kleinman, A. (1988). *The illness narratives: Suffering, healing, and the human condition*. New York: Basic Books.

Kleinman, A., Eisenberg, L., & Good, B. (1978). Culture, illness, and care. *Annals of Internal Medicine, 88*, 251–258.

Mattingly, C. (1994). Therapeutic employment. *Social Science and Medicine, 36*, 811–822.

Murphy, R. (1990). *The body silent*. New York: Norton.

Parsons, T. (1951). *The social system*. New York: Free Press.

Rogers, J. (1982). Order and disorder in medicine and occupational therapy. *American Journal of Occupational Therapy, 36*, 29–35.

Turner, V. (1967). *The forest of symbols: Aspects of Ndembu ritual*. Ithaca, NY: Cornell University Press.

Wolf, E. (1982). *Europe and the people without history*. Berkeley: University of California Press.

CHAPTER 6

DISABILITY EXPERIENCE FROM A FAMILY PERSPECTIVE

CHERYL F. MATTINGLY AND MARY C. LAWLOR

Common sense tells us that most people who come to occupational therapy practitioners live in families of some kind. Even when clients live apart from their families, if they need consistent care, it is very likely that some family members will be instrumental in this care giving. And even in those instances in which no family member is actively involved in care, it is likely that someone from the client's family will be concerned with this care, including the services of the occupational therapy practitioner. Furthermore, the way clients experience disability and how it affects their functioning in the world often depend heavily on the clients' relationships with family members. This is most obvious in pediatric care when the client is a very young child and in geriatric care when spouses and children become involved; but for most people, no matter what the age, ethnicity, socioeconomic status, or geographical location, at times of severe illness or disability, families tend to matter.

Not only do families matter but families shift in response to the issues raised by having a family member with an illness or disability. Roles change. Power relations change. Activities change. The way meals are eaten, vacations are taken, arguments are had, beds are made, money is earned, houses are organized, and myriad other aspects of family life are likely to be affected.

Even though there is nothing startling about any of these statements, families are systematically underconsidered when it comes to health care. Professional training, institutional structures, reimbursement procedures, and reward systems all tend to contribute to the marginalization of families. When occupational therapy practitioners do try to consider the needs of their clients and of family caregivers, they can find themselves addressing a range of issues and facing a number of dilemmas for which they were not prepared. This chapter addresses the place of the family in occupational therapy care and the need to attend to family perspectives in providing services to people with chronic illnesses or disabilities. It highlights some of the interesting problems and opportunities that emerge when practitioners involve families actively in the therapeutic process (Lawlor & Mattingly, 1998). We begin by arguing the need to bring families into the picture and by discussing the recent movement (largely in pediatrics) toward **family-centered care,** raising some questions about what this term might mean in practice. We then look at why families have been so peripheral in the way most health-care professions have defined their practice. The heart of the chapter moves from these more general considerations to an analysis of life issue stories in which practitioners and family members describe their efforts to collaborate in the therapeutic process. In the context of these issues, we highlight some of the intricacies, dilemmas, surprises, and riches of therapeutic work in which families play a central role.

WHY ARE FAMILIES IMPORTANT IN HEALTH CARE?

Public policy efforts related to promoting the health and development of children have been traced to the turn of the twentieth century (Hanft, 1991). The implementation of federal initiatives related to providing services for children with special health-care needs and their families has been documented as early as 1912, with the establishment of the Children's Bureau in Maternal and Child Health (Hanft, 1991) and expanded with the implementation of Title V legislation in 1935 (Colman, 1988). The implementation of **PL 94-142, Part B,** an amendment to the Education for the Handicapped Act (EHA) in 1975, and **PL 99-457, Part H,** an amendment to the EHA in 1986, prompted dramatic changes in the nature of service delivery to children in educational and early childhood settings (Hanft, 1991; Lawlor, 1991). In 1990, EHA was renamed the Individuals with Disabilities Act (IDEA, PL 101-476). Implementation of these services placed new demands on practitioners to reframe traditional medical models of practice to accommodate to the needs of families as well as the child who was referred for services (American Occupational Therapy Association, 1999).

Although the initiative for developing services centered on the needs and values of families began in early childhood programs, many of the principles apply to services for people of all ages. As human service systems moved into the community and people began providing home care, practitioners developed a deeper appreciation of the centrality of families in healing, recovery, and adaptation. Practitioners also recognized that family members often had different perspectives about the needs, priorities, and strengths from those of the professionals. This recognition led to a shift from perceiving family members as people who will carry out the doctors' and practitioners' orders to perceiving family members as people who are most knowledgeable about the client and who are partners in decision making. Family members' perspectives about how the client is doing, what the client needs, what the family needs, and what is most important and meaningful have become part of the clinical dialogue.

The challenge for the occupational therapy practitioner is to collaborate with clients, their families, and other team members in designing a program that builds on a family's strengths and addresses its needs. When done successfully, intervention services are individualized to each family and reflect their unique cultural world. Drawing on the work of Dunst, Trivette, and Deal (1988), we have defined family-centered care as an experience that happens when practitioners effectively and compassionately listen to the concerns, address the needs, and support the hopes of people and their families (Lawlor & Cada, 1993; Lawlor & Mattingly, 1998). Sometimes practitioners can best involve clients and families in the decision-making process by offering multiple options for interventions (Rosen & Granger, 1992). This type of engagement is often described as a means of enabling and empowering families (Deal, Dunst, & Trivette, 1989).

Family-centered care is enacted through the collaborative efforts of family members and practitioners (Edelman, Greenland, & Mills, 1993) and typically is provided through multidisciplinary and interdisciplinary team structures. Partnerships are created based on the establishment of trust and rapport as well as respect for family values, beliefs, and routines (Hanft, 1989). Additional elements of successful collaboration include clarity and honesty in communication, mutual agreement on goals, effective information sharing, accessibility, and absence of blame (McGonigel, Kaufmann, & Johnson, 1991). Successful collaboration occurs when practitioners and family members form relationships that foster a shared understanding of the needs, hopes, expectations, and contributions of all partners (Lawlor & Cada, 1993). Collaboration is much more than being "nice" (Lawlor & Mattingly, 1998; Mattingly, 1998). It involves complex interpretative acts in which the practitioner must understand the meanings of interventions, the meanings of illness or disability in a person and family's life, and the feelings that accompany these experiences.

WHY HAVE FAMILIES BEEN SO MARGINAL AND MISUNDERSTOOD IN HEALTH CARE?

The easiest way to understand why families have not traditionally been better included in decisions about health care is to remember that health-care professionals, including occupational therapy practitioners, are members of professional cultures and work in settings that have institutional cultures. All health-care professions have been powerfully influenced by what anthropologists sometimes call the "culture of Western **biomedicine**" (Good, 1994;

Hahn & Gaines, 1985; Jackson, 2000; Locke & Gordon, 1988; Rhodes, 1991). It is a bit deceptive to speak of one monolithic culture of biomedicine, as though this were some single homogeneous entity. Occupational therapy practitioners, for example, may find they live only partly in the same professional culture as, say, neurosurgeons. And practitioners working within one setting may find that this institutional culture is quite different from another setting in which they have practiced. This can hold true even if both organizations appear outwardly similar—two different rehabilitation hospitals, for instance. But even keeping all these differences and nuances in mind, there are a number of powerful assumptions shared at some level by nearly all health professionals working across a wide variety of settings.

Not only do professionals such as occupational therapy practitioners learn professional skills when they enter the field, they also assimilate a set of values and beliefs that make them members of a professional culture or community of practice (Wenger, 1998). The culture of biomedicine has developed over the past 250 years. (For a detailed reading of this history as a cultural phenomena, see, for example, Foucault, 1973, 1979.) In its development, this culture has provided a powerful view of what it means to be ill and what is expected of the client, the health-care professional, and the client's family or key caregivers. There are some deeply held beliefs about what constitutes an appropriate relationship among professional, client, and family caregivers. These assumptions about the professional–client–caregiver relationship are influenced, in turn, by other basic assumptions about the nature of illness and how it is best treated. Some of these assumptions are especially problematic for rehabilitation professionals such as occupational therapy practitioners who treat clients with chronic illnesses and disabling conditions.

TROUBLESOME ASSUMPTIONS ABOUT DISABILITY, THE ILLNESS EXPERIENCE, AND FAMILIES

Several key assumptions that are particularly potent and particularly tenacious (Gordon, 1988) in the culture of biomedicine, and in occupational therapy, have significantly influenced the way families are drawn into the therapeutic process. We present some life issue examples, written by therapists, that illustrate how these assumptions play out in concrete cases. Case examples are a particularly useful way to look at a professional's assumptions and beliefs, because practitioners often hold these beliefs so unconsciously that they are not even aware they hold them until, in some specific situation, the beliefs are violated. These cases tend to concern surprises as the therapists come to learn something about a client's family that turns out to be extremely important in influencing the meaning and value of therapy and helps the therapist redirect therapeutic interventions in a more efficacious way.

The Disability Belongs to the Individual

One of the most pervasive assumptions in biomedicine is that the professional's task is to treat the individual who has the illness. Sometimes this is narrowly interpreted among health professionals as "treating the pathology," but occupational therapy practitioners are usually sensitive in trying to remember that they are also treating a person who has a disabling condition. The hand therapist is not only treating a hand injury, for example, but also an out-of-work auto mechanic with a wife and three children. And the therapist recognizes that the client whose hand was injured on the job is fearful about his ability to regain his role as family breadwinner.

Put differently, practitioners try to treat what anthropologists speak of as the *illness experience*, rather than simply the disease (Good, 1994; Good & Good, 1994; Kleinman, 1988; Luhrmann, 2000). In the context of occupational therapy, a more accurate term is probably the *disability experience*, for it is certainly possible to have a disability, even one that requires therapy, without being ill. Practitioners try to attend both to the disability as a physiological condition and to the meaning this particular condition carries for the person who has the disability (Mattingly, 1998, 2000; Mattingly & Fleming, 1994). If a practitioner knows a client wants to relearn how to drive, dress independently, eat out at restaurants, or continue to work as an auto mechanic, the practitioner may be able to organize therapeutic tasks that aid the client in carrying out these activities.

However, some goals are far less tangible. This is especially true for goals that concern the client's social world and the connection between functional skills and social relationships. It is artificial to treat only narrowly defined functional skills as though they were unrelated to a client's social world, for a key aspect of the meaning of a condition is how it affects an individual's personal relationships—which is one of the trickier aspects of therapeutic work. By contrast with such goals as learning how to dress oneself and learning wheelchair motility, goals and concerns connected to family relations are much more difficult to define, and they are certainly likely to be hard to measure. Helping a client reclaim his identity as a good father to his 5-year-old daughter even though he has a spinal cord injury, for example, is harder to translate into discrete, skill-based goals than learning how to increase upper body strength or learning how to eat independently. Family-oriented goals are likely to be tied to outcomes that are diffuse, complex, subtle, and difficult to measure, even when they are deeply significant to the client and family. When a client's goals and concerns are tied to shifting family relationships, these may seem out of professional bounds for the occupational therapy practitioner.

Despite the many difficulties in trying to understand a disabling condition as it pertains to a client's role in the family, ignoring this aspect often means being blind to the most significant aspects of the illness (or disability) experience. Ignoring family-oriented goals or the meaning of a disability as it ties to family concerns and family relationships may mean ignoring the person altogether.

The situation given in Life Issues to Consider in Practice 6-1, provided by Mary Black, illustrates the very different identity a client assumes once her family relationships are known. Lily, a woman in her 70s with significant health problems, is almost invisible to the professional staff, except in the psychiatric unit where she resides as an inconvenient collection of medical difficulties. During the course of treatment, the occupational therapist listens to stories Lily tells about her long marriage and family life. Through these stories, Lily is transformed for the therapist into a mother and wife, and her deeper identity, her personhood one might say, is revealed.

Black's case also suggests the difficulty family members may have as they try to interact with health-care professionals in making decisions about the care of their relative. In Black's example, the staff perceived Lily as a burden, because she "misfit" the kinds of psychiatric patients they were accustomed to treating. Her psychiatric diagnosis was vague (and, in Black's view, probably inappropriate), but her medical problems required intense attention. The burden felt by the staff spilled into their relations with the family, so that family members, such that two of Lily's sons, also came to be perceived and treated as burdens, needlessly inconveniencing the staff by coming for a visit at the wrong hours. Although it is easy to understand the staff members' frustration in trying to care for Lily, this case vividly illustrates how family members might feel when they are trying to deal with a difficult family transition and are not supported by many of the health-care professionals. This case also reveals how internal staff issues and other organizational difficulties can cloud the health professionals' recognition of the strengths a family offers, and families, too, can appear as just one more irritation (rather than a resource) in providing services to a client.

The Professional Is the Expert

Traditionally, Western biomedicine has been concerned with curing people. The notion of the professional as healer is important here. The healer is an expert who can both ascertain what is wrong (assess and diagnose) and identify the correct intervention to cure the ailment (treat) (Biesele & Davis-Floyd, 1996; Davis-Floyd, & Sargent, 1997; Good, 1995). The patient's role is a submissive one, offering information as requested, submitting to physical examination, and following the expert's directives for treatment. In this view, health-care professionals make people healthy by curing disease. The concern of the professional is largely with the disease rather than with the person who has the disease (the oncologist fighting the cancer cells with radiation, for instance). The patient's personal history, family situation, and work history are usually of only peripheral importance in the healer's task of diagnosing and treating the pathologic condition that is causing the illness.

Sometimes, this model works. But this is almost never true with occupational therapy clients. Occupational therapy practitioners are well aware that their clients have medical conditions that, by and large, mean living with disabilities. Whereas the hope of medicine has been curing or healing, which implies the ability of the health professional to bring a person from a state of illness to some state of "normalcy" or premorbidity, occupational therapy practitioners are rarely in a position to cure anyone. The people they treat may have rich, full lives, but they are usually living these lives with an impairment that cannot be fixed.

Practices steeped in medical traditions frequently adopt professional–client relationships based on hierarchical models or expert-driven models. The expert model remains prevalent within early childhood practices, despite increasing recognition that elements of this model create barriers to developing collaborative partnerships and understanding family life. The expert model tends to promote dependence within recipients of services, to limit opportunities for families to contribute insights and have their specific concerns and needs addressed, to burden the professional with the unrealistic expectation of always having the expertise to respond to all issues (Cunningham & Davis, 1985), and to organize services in ways that are self-serving to the expert (Howard & Strauss, 1975).

It is not surprising that reliance on expert models fosters relationships between practitioners and family members that incorporate compliance and coercion strategies. This leads to considerable confusion about whether the "story" is one of collaboration, coercion, or compliance (Lawlor & Mattingly, 1998). The issue is not merely a semantics problem. Each approach to working relationships creates distinctly different experiences for all parties. Practitioner judgments that a person is noncompliant, or in the terms used by family members—"bad parent," "bad daughter," and the like—diverts energies away from more reflective analysis or direct attempts to understand alternative perspectives (Trostle, 1988).

The Client Is the Recipient of Care

Another interrelated assumption quite pervasive in biomedicine is that health professionals deliver treatment "to" the person with the disease; they treat a passive patient whose primary task is to receive the cure (e.g., take the medications, undergo the surgery). Although occupational therapy practitioners are well aware that they need "active" clients, rather than passive ones, and that clients must learn to do for themselves, the recipient role reasserts itself in another guise.

LIFE ISSUES TO CONSIDER IN PRACTICE 6-1

Lily and Her Family

MARY BLACK

This story is about a woman I worked with for a short time; no longer than 1 or 2 weeks. I met her about 3 years ago when I was working on a contractual basis on an inpatient psychiatric unit for older adults. I cannot even remember her name or why exactly she was on the psychiatric unit, but I can picture her clearly and remember stories she told me about herself. And I do recall that her declining health and loss of independence resulted in major transitions for herself and her family. Her family made plans for her subsequent living arrangements during her stay in the hospital.

Lily was admitted to the psychiatric unit from the medical floor under confusing circumstances. The feeling conveyed in the morning rounds was that she required more medical management than the psychiatric unit staff could provide, and it was unclear whether she was depressed or disoriented.

Lily had diabetes for many years and came to the unit in a much-weakened state; she needed maximum assistance with self-care and transfers. She had intravenous tubes in her arm and took frequent rests during the day. Most of the time, I saw Lily individually at her bedside; but on a couple of occasions she was able, once in a geri-chair, to attend an afternoon group.

When I first met Lily, she did not strike me as confused or depressed but rather sturdying herself for the inevitable upcoming changes through taking account of her life. Lily was a black woman in her 70s. She told me she was married at 16 to the only man she ever loved. They were married where they grew up, in Mississippi. She wore a "tomato red" dress and had the loan of a car to drive them from the church to the house where they had a party. At the party, the roof or the floor broke (I can't remember which), but she told me, "It was some party." Lily and her husband had 13 children, all now grown. She was very proud that most of them were college educated. This was the first time she had been separated from her husband for so many weeks. She told me they both shared one long pillow. She and her husband, who was also ill, were both going to move into a nursing home together, but it was not yet determined where.

This may sound nostalgic. It was! But through her reminiscing she was able to paint—vividly—highlights and everyday aspects of her life. She had spent her whole life at home, and her family was everything to her. What jolted me then was the reception her children received. Because of the extra care the nursing staff had to provide, they were understandably frustrated. The resentment seemed to be deflected to the family though. Two of Lily's sons came to see her in the morning and were chastised for not being here during visiting hours. They were questioned: "Your brothers and sisters knew, why didn't you?" The family, in turn, did not understand why their mother was on a psychiatric unit and were not given any reasonable answers, because the communication channels between medicine and psychiatry were so ambiguous. They had the feeling their mother was "dumped" there. There were efforts by staff to have her transferred off the floor, but it was unclear as to where. Luckily, the social worker was able to see beyond the internal politics and work with the family on their immediate concern—easing the transition into a nursing home and finding one that would provide care for both their mother and their father.

Together, the social worker and I met with seven or eight of Lily's children to work on this transition. I felt like I was able to confirm to them some of her strengths through my work with her, including interests in working with her hands, efforts in self-care, and brightness of spirit despite her failing health, as well as her quite normal reactions to the losses she felt, of her home and independence, and concern about her husband. Lily had ultimate trust that her family would provide the best they could for her. The social worker was able to provide information and contacts at nursing homes he felt were reputable. We were both able to suggest questions and issues to address when investigating a home. What I remember as well, from the meeting and individually, was just being able to listen to how hard this was for them. It was impossible for any one of them to care for both of their parents, and they were ambivalent about a nursing home. The consolation was that their parents would be together. The family found a home they thought suitable and near enough for most to visit, and Lily was then transferred. I do not know anymore about her after that.

What I found remarkable was the family's closeness, but conversely many of the staff's judgments to the contrary. A "they cannot get it together" and "we want her out of here" attitude prevailed among the staff. I also recognized, coming from a big family myself, that I was easily defensive about these judgments. What I think often happens, as did here, is that territorial issues took precedence over the patient and family concerns. Because of Lily's lovely personality and her family's keen interest and perseverance, the image of her as a burden diminished by her departure, but it was unfortunate her family was not included earlier and that the staff was not more supportive.

Practitioners know that therapy will be successful only if their clients (and often the key family caregivers as well) become motivated to work hard at it. But even as active participants, the clients and family members are often assigned a role as recipients of the instructions offered by occupational therapy practitioners and other rehabilitation experts. While these "active recipients" are sometimes offered a range of choices of goals or preferred activities and practitioners often try to accommodate therapeutic goals into the life of the client or family, practitioners still tend to equate good patients and good families with compliant ones. Thus a quite typical scenario is for the practitioner to assign homework for the client to do between therapy sessions. When family members are involved in therapy, they, too, are assigned roles as facilitators of the home-therapy program. The client and family's primary task is to do their homework faithfully. This family role is regularly underscored by the usual practice of devoting a few minutes of any session to a discussion about how the homework went.

Even though there is nothing necessarily wrong with this kind of collaborative relationship between practitioner and family, it carries some dangers, especially when practitioners are unaware of their power to shift family dynamics and family relationships by pressing family caregivers to become responsible for therapeutic gains. One critical danger is that both practitioners and family members may unconsciously begin to presume that the family's primary role is as a kind of adjunct practitioner. This danger is well illustrated by the case given in Life Issues to Consider in Practice 6-2.

This case story reveals how powerful a practitioner can be in family life, even when she is not present. Practitioners, as we can see, play a role in a family system whether they are aware of it or not. The stronger the partnership between practitioner, client, and family members, the more likely that the practitioner will influence the family outside therapy time in ways he or she had not thought about. In this example—where clearly the therapist (Beth Korby Elenko) and the mother develop an effective partnership—Elenko enters the family world as a kind of absent voice in which she unintentionally reinforces the guilt and sense of inadequacy so prevalent among family caregivers who struggle to care for their family member who has a disability.

Ironically, in her attempts to involve this cooperative and willing family in therapy and to create a partnership with the mother, Elenko may have added pressure to a family already overloaded with responsibility. When the mother begins to voice her weariness of the task, Elenko suddenly recognizes what has happened. Her clever intervention was to suggest that the family take a vacation from therapeutic homework. In her eloquent appeal to the mother to carry out these new instructions, she offers the mother reasons to return family members to being members of a family rather than helpers in a complicated therapeutic home team. The importance of this, and the power of the practitioner to influence family dynamics, is captured in the mother's thank-you the following week. The mother's grateful response also shows how often practitioners may unwittingly be giving family members messages about whether they are good or not based on how faithfully they carry out therapeutic activities. As this mother tells Elenko, she thought if she "didn't do his therapy time religiously every day" she would be a "bad mom."

Illness and Disability Generate Only Negative Experiences

There has been, and continues to be, an assumption that all the effects of illness and disability on a family are negative. This belief also leads to the erroneous conclusion that family reactions to illness and disability are both predictable and shared. In other words, the practitioner might presume to know about the effect of an illness or disability on the family without fully understanding a particular family. These notions get dismissed once one listens to families talk about their experiences. We have been struck by the incredible richness of their stories and the difficulty people have reducing their complex reactions to a few discrete categories such as stress, grief, or acceptance. Some theorists have also attempted to develop theories based on stages of reactions, but the fixedness of these stages has been criticized (Moses, 1983).

Much of the research that has been conducted related to the response of family members to illness or disability has been conducted with parents of children who have special health-care needs. Recently, parents and other family members have offered critiques of this body of research (e.g., Lipsky, 1985), citing the failure of researchers to recognize positive outcomes from these experiences. Researchers have tended to measure such predetermined variables as maternal depression and stress. Critics note that personal reports of other effects, including positive changes in family life, have been discounted. Advocates of the family-centered care movement note the failure of many researchers and practitioners to understand the unique features of family adaptation and coping and assert the need for further research that is grounded in the perspectives of family members. Although it is beyond the scope of this chapter to summarize this body of literature, the assumption that the effects of disability are unilateral and negative must be challenged as both simplistic and inadequate.

Practitioners need to seek understanding of the effects of illness and disability on the families of the people who come to them for assistance. These effects will likely change over time, and the perceptions of the relative stress of families will be shaped by other events in the family and the availability of resources. The presumption that the entirety of a family's experience can be summarized as stressful often leads to misunderstandings and lost opportunities to promote any positive aspects (Lawlor & Mattingly, 1998; Mattingly & Lawlor, 2000). For example, parents who were interviewed in focus groups concerning their experiences with therapists commented on their disappointment that therapists did not tend to celebrate successes with them (Lawlor & Cada, 1993).

LIFE ISSUES TO CONSIDER IN PRACTICE 6-2

My Therapist's Tale

BETH KORBY ELENKO

I recently began treatment of a little boy named Sam. Sam was born with a hemangioma and multiple congenital anomalies. Sam's family includes a mom, a dad, and a 2-year-old sister, Dawn. This family was unusual to me because they came from suburban Chicago, had insurance and regularly attended treatment, which is unique to my work environment. Sam was a child who needed to attend numerous specialists in addition to physical and occupational therapies. His mom never went without her appointment book and never missed an appointment unless she called to reschedule it.

Sam began occupational therapy at 8 months of age after being involved in physical therapy (PT) since 3 months of age. It was the physical therapist who impressed on both the mother and the physician the importance of occupational therapy intervention. My first visit with Sam was a co-treatment transition with PT. During this visit, I spoke to the mother about providing Sam with more normal experiences of sensory-stimulating activities. This mom amazed me; she repeated back everything I told her with those, "So, you're saying, I should . . ." phrases.

On the next appointment, Sam's mom told me all about the new experiences they had had and how she tried everything I told her. I was amazed and excited that this mom would carryover all my treatment goals—this was a therapist's ideal situation.

From then on, Sam's mom would come to therapy reiterating what she had done the previous week and asking what she should work on for the next time. She told me that she set aside an hour each day of "therapy time," during which she carried out the physical therapist's and my instructions. It was always during the evenings so that her husband could occupy Dawn's time. Her husband would also work with Sam an additional hour; and then on weekends when Dawn could spend time at her grandma's house, they would work with Sam together. She told me how difficult it was to live each day running from doctor to doctor to therapists for Sam while trying to maintain a normal family life for Dawn and her husband. If she only knew how much work having a disabled child could be, she would have had Sam first and not had another child.

All of a sudden, I realized that in my excitement of having a mom who would carry out my treatment goals, I forgot to empower this family with just being a family. I then gave Sam's mom "permission" to take a break. A break, which I told her meant time for Sam to be just a baby, just a brother, just a son. A time for Dawn to be just a sister, just a daughter; a time for Mom to be just a mom, just a wife; a time for Dad to be just a dad, just a husband; and a time for all to be just a family, with all the things a family includes. Once I gave that signal that it was okay to be just Sam's mom, I saw the biggest weight lifted off her shoulders, but she looked as if she didn't believe me. I gave her no assignment for the following week, saying that they had lots to work on just learning to be a family. When Sam and his mom returned the following week; the first thing she said was, "Thank you, Beth. I never realized how much we had forgotten how to just be anything but Sam's everything since he was born. I also thought that if I didn't do his therapy time religiously every day that I would be a bad mom and Sam would never develop and catch up. Now I can see that I really need time to enjoy being Sam's as well as Dawn's mom and that Sam needs time just being a baby. We all need a vacation once in a while. Thank you for reminding me that we're all only human, I really appreciated that."

There Is One Family Perspective per Family

Although much of the literature on family-centered care presumes that practitioners come to know all members of the family, we have found that often one member of the family, typically a mother or spouse, serves as the primary contact for the practitioner. It is this individual's perspective that practitioners understand; however, this may be only one of several perspectives held by family members. The case story given in Life Issues to Consider in Practice 6-3 illustrates how misunderstandings about the family can occur.

In many ways, Elizabeth had an extremely difficult job as she tried to negotiate the expectations of the professionals and the views of Jorge held by her husband and his extended family. She was acting as a type of "cultural broker" (Lawlor & Mattingly, 1994, 1998), trying to represent the clinical world to the family and the family world to the clinical staff. The team presumed that Elizabeth's view and the view of her husband and family were highly consistent. Once the team recognized the flaws in their assumptions, they were able to focus on understanding how to ease the burden of being the broker between these two different views, how to promote better communication, and how to better collaborate with the family in identifying intervention priorities and more effective strategies.

LIFE ISSUES TO CONSIDER IN PRACTICE 6-3

The Whole Family

ANONYMOUS

This is a story about Jorge and his family and our attempts as an interdisciplinary team to meet their requests for help in promoting Jorge's development. I was working as an occupational therapist at a regional diagnostic center as a member of a highly cohesive interdisciplinary team. We devoted considerable time toward developing strategies to help families feel more comfortable with the process and prided ourselves in how responsive we were to families. Morning Team (a title based purely on scheduling) was considered to be the "best" team.

We received a referral on a child who was about 18 months old, who was reportedly not progressing well developmentally. His parents were both highly educated and had recently immigrated to the United States from Mexico while the husband, Raul, was completing his doctoral work at a prestigious university. Elizabeth was trained as a teacher but had not gone to work since coming to the United States so that she could devote more time to Jorge and getting the family situated.

When we first met the family, we were surprised with the parents' fluency in English and detected only a slight accent in Raul's speech. The family assured us that they used English primarily, although they continued to speak some Spanish in the home, and would prefer our communication to be in English. They were a striking couple, and I recall our initial conversations and meetings to be unusually comfortable, and there was a sense of immediate rapport that I and several colleagues noted. Jorge was a very "syndromey" looking child. A term that sounds offensive, but reflected our clinical jargon. His somewhat dysmorphic features were particularly apparent because both parents were so striking in their physical attributes. We found Jorge to be developmentally delayed, and I recall my concern that most of his developmental milestones were between 2 and 6 months of age. Jorge was able to propel himself forward on his feet in a manner that simulated walking, but his balance was poor and he would inevitably crash (into walls, furniture, or the floor) because he was unable to control the forward momentum that he would generate. I remember this sense of how active, out of control, and socially disconnected this child appeared and can still visualize him, even though it has been at least 7 years since I last saw the family.

As a group, we were disappointed in our evaluation findings and were somewhat overwhelmed by the sadness of the story, as we found little to be optimistic about for Jorge's future development. We felt that the family was the primary strength but expressed concern that Elizabeth might easily become overburdened with the full-time care of this infant, who seemed to give so little back in terms of social responsiveness. In addition, we decided to focus on safety concerns and identify some other means of mobility while we worked on promoting more age-appropriate development. We continued to see the family for a period of several weeks while we made arrangements for early intervention services in their community.

One morning, I was scheduled for a follow-up visit with Jorge and Elizabeth and the speech and physical therapists. We had not seen them for several weeks because they had canceled an appointment. When they came in, I was shocked to see wounds around Jorge's mouth. Elizabeth was also quite anxious about this and told us that Jorge had bitten into a live electrical wire. She saw this as a violation of her commitment to us to work and keep Jorge safe and clearly was horrified that the accident had happened. We at first assumed that her distress was primarily due to guilt, but we sensed that there was a lot more she had to tell us. We were all standing awkwardly at the entrance of the clinic when she proceeded to tell us what a living hell her life was. Her efforts to follow our direction by keeping Jorge safe and providing more meaningful developmental experiences were viewed by her husband as poor mothering, giving up on his firstborn son, and failing to provide the appropriate home environment. In addition, Raul's extended family called from Mexico regularly to remind her that their firstborn son would carry the family name and needed to be encouraged to his full potential. For example, using the helmet, trying to facilitate more mature walking patterns, and adapting the home to make it safer were viewed as signs of her inadequacies. Our perspective that we were family oriented and working collaboratively with the family was clearly out of focus.

LIFE ISSUES TO CONSIDER IN PRACTICE 6-4

My Father

My father was terminally ill and in a coronary intensive care unit. I caught a flight, as I had done many times over the spring, and joined my gathering siblings. I went directly from the airport to the hospital and met a brother. A friendly and sympathetic nurse approached us and talked about her approach to care. When she described herself as "family centered," I felt both relieved and jarred by her comments, because family-centered care had been the focus of my research and teaching. When I have thought about this encounter, which I have many times, I conjure up the theme from the *Twilight Zone* as a kind of background music.

Shortly after we entered my father's room, the nurse returned and asked us to leave because she had some procedures to do. My sister questioned her a little bit about this, because she had been with our father during the day and evening shifts and had been allowed to stay.

We were troubled about leaving the room, because we had made a promise to my father that he would not die alone. My professional self knew that this was quite presumptuous, given the nature of hospital life and the fact that many hospitals require that you follow visiting hours, particularly in intensive care units. However, as a member of a family that loved this man deeply we just knew that we would need to be there. We left the room and waited in the unit day room. After more than 20 min had gone by, my brother and I returned to check. The nurse was doing an invasive procedure that we had understood would not be done. When we spoke to the nurse, she talked about the fact that she was the one with the nurse's license and we should not be challenging her. She indicated that she did not agree with our decision not to continue procedures. We tried to find out why she did not agree, because we obviously wanted to do the right thing, and I was still very much hoping that someone would come up with something that would turn things for the better. However, our efforts to understand where the nurse was coming from seemed to generate more defensive reactions. I am sure we were also not the easiest people to talk with at the time because of our stress and distress. Needless to say, a difficult and disturbing series of discussions followed.

The next day another nurse who cared for my father came on duty. At one point she came into the room and asked how my sister and I were doing. She then started crying and apologizing profusely for her tears, which she feared were unprofessional. As she tried to explain why she was so upset, she began talking about why she had grown so fond of our father. Many of the characteristics she spoke about were aspects that were also endearing to the family. I was struck by how much this nurse, who was providing the care, cared. She also shared that watching us with our father made her think about her own father and that "She couldn't do it" (presumably referring to our kind of deathbed vigil).

THE OCCUPATIONAL THERAPY PRACTITIONER AS THE AGENT OF FAMILY-CENTERED CARE

One of the greatest challenges for practitioners is understanding how their own lived experience shapes their interactions with family members in the course of providing services for patients and clients. Conceptual models of practice and theory regarding family systems and human development, ethics, and public and institutional policies all contribute to our framework for family-centered interventions. However, practitioners, as the instruments for intervention, bring their own selves and their cultural views of families into clinical interactions.

Occupational therapy practitioners come to their profession with life experiences of being a member of a family. This lived experience of growing up in a family significantly shapes who we are as practitioners, particularly in situations in which practitioners are getting to know a family and seeking to understand their needs, priorities, values, hopes, and resources. These assumptions about family life tend to be quite tacit, and we are often not aware of their influence unless we actively reflect on our actions. Guided reflection through mentorship and supervision, as well as discussions with other team members concerning beliefs about specific families, are essential components of intervention planning and implementation with clients and their families.

The story given in Life Issues to Consider in Practice 6-4 was shared by one of us to illustrate how these multiple perspectives on families intersect in the course of clinical interactions.

The first nurse spoke eloquently about the principles of family-centered care, but the family's experience with her was quite contradictory to her espoused beliefs. The second nurse, who was found to be truly a partner in this ordeal, perceived her caring actions as unprofessional. The members of the family felt much more supported by the second nurse and also felt that they were active participants in making decisions for their father. The first nurse seemed to understand the principles of providing family-centered care, but the family's experiences left them confused, upset, and chastised for interfering with the work of the nurse.

Why did these two experiences feel so different? These two nurses were colleagues and worked under the prevailing philosophy of the unit that included being responsive to the needs of families and developing effective partnerships with family members. Perhaps the difference can be partially explained by the fact that the first nurse seemed to perceive the involvement of family members as interfering with her role as the nurse. The second nurse was confused about her perceptions of how a nurse behaved and her personal response to the situation. She seemed to fear that sharing emotions and getting personally involved would diminish her professionalism. In implementing family-centered care, practitioners must move beyond the rhetoric and develop roles as practitioners that integrate the need for supportive relationships within the context of the work of providing care.

CONCLUSION

In this chapter, we highlighted many of the challenges involved in attempting to respond to the needs of clients and their families. Challenges are coupled with opportunities. As practitioners discover ways of getting to know families and understanding their perspectives, opportunities emerge for practitioners to construct richer, more meaningful experiences. The more meaningful the experience, the more likely treatment will be efficacious.

We have found that discussions of opportunities must be tempered with specific cautions. Approaches to getting to know families must be noninvasive, sensitive, nonjudgmental, and respectful of the parameters for privacy and disclosure that individuals indicate. Understanding a perspective does not presume that, as an occupational therapy practitioner, you are responsible for intervening in every dimension of that perspective. Family-centered care is implemented most effectively in situations in which interdisciplinary efforts are well coordinated and effectively communicated. In situations in which practitioners are working in relative isolation, caution must be exercised to ensure that they are practicing within the bounds of their expertise and appropriately facilitating access to other resources as needed.

We intuitively recognize that such things as our ethnicity, nationality, geographical home, and perhaps even our religion provide us with powerful cultural worlds. These aspects of our background help make us who we are, culturally speaking. We are often not fully aware that our profession and our family also offer cultural worlds that shape some of our deepest assumptions, beliefs, and values. This chapter concerns a kind of cultural intersection between the practitioner (acting as a member of a professional culture) and a client (acting as a member of a family culture). Practitioners, of course, have families, and clients often have professions. However, when practitioners and clients meet during occupational therapy intervention, the practitioner's professional and institutional cultures are particularly significant in shaping how the practitioner defines good intervention and a good professional-client relationship.

ACKNOWLEDGMENTS

This chapter was supported by data obtained through three research projects. One study was supported by grant MCJ-060745 from the Maternal and Child Health Program (Title V, Social Security Act), Health and Services Administration, Department of Health and Human Services. Appreciation is expressed to the American Occupational Therapy Foundation for their support of pilot work related to that study. Research was also supported by grant number R01 HD 38878 from the National Institute of Child Health and Human Development. The contents of this chapter are solely the responsibility of the authors and do not necessarily represent the official views of any of these agencies. We also would like to express our appreciation to the many children, families, therapists, and practitioners who have participated in these research efforts and who have willingly shared their experiences.

References

American Occupational Therapy Association. (1999). *Occupational therapy services for children and youth under the Individuals with Disabilities Education Act* (2nd ed.). Bethesda, MD: Author.

Biesele, M., & Davis-Floyd, R. (1996). Dying as a medical performance: The oncologist as Charon. In C. Laderman & M. Roseman (Eds.). *The performance of healing* (pp. 291–321). New York: Routledge.

Colman, W. (1988). The evolution of occupational therapy in the public schools: The laws mandating practice. *American Journal of Occupational Therapy, 42,* 701–705.

Cunningham, C., & Davis, H. (1985). *Working with parents: Frameworks for collaboration*. Philadelphia: Open University Press.

Davis-Floyd, R., & Sargent, C. (1997). *Childbirth and authoritative knowledge: Cross-cultural perspectives*. Berkeley: University of California Press.

Deal, A., Dunst, C., & Trivette, C. (1989). A flexible and functional approach to developing individualized family support plans. *Infants and Young Children, 1*(4), 32–43.

Dunst, C., Trivette, C., & Deal, A. (1988). *Enabling and empowering families: Principles and guidelines for practice*. Cambridge, MA: Brookline.

Edelman, L., Greenland, B., & Mills, B. (1993). *Building parent professional collaboration: Facilitator's guide*. St. Paul, MN: Pathfinder Resources.

Foucault, M. (1973). *The birth of the clinic: An archaeology of medical perception*. New York: Vintage.

Foucault, M. (1979). *Discipline and punish: The birth of the prison*. New York: Vintage.

Good, B. (1994). *Medicine, rationality, and experience*. Cambridge, UK: Cambridge University Press.

Good, B., & Good, M. J. (1994). In the subjunctive mode: Epilepsy narratives in Turkey. *Social Science in Medicine*, *38*, 835–842.

Good, M. J. (1995). *American medicine: The quest for competence*. Berkeley: University of California Press.

Gordon, D. (1988). Clinical science and clinical experience: Changing boundaries between art and science in medicine. In M. Locke & D. Gordon (Eds.). *Biomedicine examined* (pp. 257–295). Dordrecht: Kluwer Academic.

Hahn, R. A., & Gaines, A. D. (Eds.). (1985). *Physicians of Western medicine*. Norwell, MA: Reidel.

Hanft, B. (1989). *Family-centered care: An early intervention resource manual*. Rockville, MD: American Occupational Therapy Association.

Hanft, B. E. (1991). Impact of public policy on pediatric health and education programs. In W. Dunn (Ed.). *Pediatric occupational therapy: Facilitating effective service provision* (pp. 273–284). Thoroughfare, NJ: Slack.

Howard, J., & Strauss, A. (1975). *Humanizing health care*. New York: Wiley.

Jackson, J. (2000). *Camp pain: Talking with chronic pain patients*. Berkeley: University of California Press.

Kleinman, A. (1988). *The illness narratives: Suffering, healing, and the human condition*. New York: Basic Books.

Lawlor, M. C. (1991). Historical and societal influences on school system practice. In A. Bundy (Ed.). *Making a difference: OTs and PTs in public schools* (pp. 1–15). Chicago: University of Illinois.

Lawlor, M. C., & Cada, E. (1993). Partnerships between therapists, parents, and children. *OSERS News in Print*, *V*(4), 27–30.

Lawlor, M. C., & Mattingly, C. (1994). *Understanding family-centered care*. Unpublished manuscript, concept paper.

Lawlor, M., & Mattingly, C. (1998). The complexities in family-centered care. *American Journal of Occupational Therapy*, *52*, 259–267.

Lipsky, D. K. (1985). A parental perspective in stress and coping. *American Journal of Orthopsychiatry*, *55*, 614–617.

Locke, M., & Gordon, D. (Eds.). (1988). *Biomedicine examined*. Dordrecht: Kluwer Academic.

Luhrmann, T. M. (2000). *Of two minds: The growing disorder of American psychiatry*. New York: Knopf.

Mattingly, C. (1998). *Healing dramas and clinical plots: The narrative structure of experience*. Cambridge, UK: Cambridge University Press.

Mattingly, C. (2000). Emergent narratives. In C. Mattingly & L. C. Garro (Eds.), *Narrative and the cultural construction of healing* (pp. 181–211). Berkeley: University of California Press.

Mattingly, C., & Fleming, M. (1994). *Clinical reasoning: Forms of inquiry in a therapeutic practice*. Philadelphia: Davis.

Mattingly, C., & Lawlor, M. (2000). Learning from stories: Narrative interviewing in cross-cultural research. *The Scandinavian Journal of Occupational Therapy*, *7*, 4–14.

McGonigel, M. J., Kaufmann, R. K., & Johnson, B. H. (Eds.). (1991). *Guidelines and recommended practices for the individualized family service plan*. Bethesda, MD: Association for the Care of Children's Health.

Moses, K. L. (1983). The impact of initial diagnosis: Mobilizing family resources. In J. Mulick & S. Pueschel (Eds.). *Parent-professional partnerships in developmental disability services* (pp. 11–34). Cambridge, MA: Academic Guild.

Rhodes, L. (1991). *Emptying beds: The work of an emergency psychiatric unit*. Berkeley: University of California Press.

Rosen, S., & Granger, M. (1992). Early intervention and school programs. In A. Crocker, H. Cohen, & T. Kastner (Eds.). *HIV infection and developmental disabilities: A resource for service providers* (pp. 75–84). Baltimore: Brookes.

Trostle, J. A. (1988). Medical compliance as an ideology. *Social Sciences in Medicine*, *27*, 1299–1308.

Wenger, E. (1998). *Communities of practice*. Cambridge, UK: Cambridge University Press.

CHAPTER 7

CULTURE, RACE, ETHNICITY, AND OTHER FORMS OF HUMAN DIVERSITY IN OCCUPATIONAL THERAPY

JULI McGRUDER

CULTURE AND OTHER FORMS OF HUMAN DIVERSITY IN OCCUPATIONAL THERAPY

Culture can be defined in many ways. In occupational therapy, culture has been defined as learned, shared experience that provides "the individual and the group with effective mechanisms for interacting both with others and with the surrounding environment" (Krefting & Krefting, 1991, p. 102). Because occupational therapy practitioners aim to discover and support clients' agency in making meaning in everyday actions and activities, they, of necessity, interact with the cultural worlds into which their clients have been socialized (Mattingly & Beer, 1993).

Culture is just one distinguishing human characteristic, however, and should not be used to stand in for other forms of human difference. Dyck (1992) warned occupational therapy practitioners not to confuse culture and other sources of difference when she wrote:

> *A reliance on culture as distinct beliefs, values, and customary practices to explain nonadherence and difficulties in the therapeutic process is misguided. The everyday social and work conditions that shape health experiences and behaviors must also be recognized. These, in turn, are forged within a socio-economic and political environment. (p. 696)*

This specific criticism of the use of the culture concept in occupational therapy is informed by three more general criticisms of conceptualizations of culture: that the concept, misused, has a tendency to essentialize, reify, and mystify human difference. To *essentialize* is to take complex multifaceted phenomena, like the lifeways, ideas, and all that a group of humans has acquired by learning and reduce them to a few basic and inherent "essences" that explain this group in totality. Descriptions that essentialize are often ahistorical, and in that way, they distort. To *reify* is to "thing-ify," to take an abstract and to treat it as a fixed and concrete thing with definable boundaries. Treating culture as a thing can promote stereotyping. Reifying culture ignores the interactive nature of humans as creators of culture situated in environments that change. To *mystify* is to obscure important causes, contributing factors, or results of a phenomenon. For example, when Moynihan (1965) referred to the African-American family as a "tangle of pathology," he obscured the economic and political factors that underlay cultural phenomena he was criticizing. Attempts to define or discuss culture must avoid reproducing these errors and fallacies. With that precaution in mind, let's examine a list of agreed on defining attributes of culture.

WHAT CULTURE IS: AN AGREED ON LIST

Culture Is Real, Learned, Shared, Malleable and Dynamic, and Invisible

While not concrete or tangible, culture is real. When someone falls ill because of a curse, the illness is real. When someone feels peace or joy, because appropriate rituals have appeased supernatural beings, the emotional state is significant and real. We cannot see or touch culture but its effects surround us, rendering it a very real force.

Culture Is Not Inherited: It Is Learned

Beliefs and values are taught to us both explicitly and tacitly in our families and communities and by mass media. Most readers will not have learned much about spirits, curses, or propitiation rituals but will have been taught in thousands of ways that they are each unique individuals with inalienable rights. The idea that we are individuals with a free will and a "natural" right to our own opinions seems a given to Americans today, but it is a cultural idea, quite foreign to others. Observers from other cultures have commented on the ways we entrain this idea of individual self-determination in children. I once counted how many decisions a middle-class European American preschooler was offered in her first waking hour of the day. The decisions—about simple things like what to wear, where to dress, what to eat—numbered around 20. The child was actively being taught about her individuality and her right to choose. Later that evening, as adults were discussing where to go for dinner, this child announced, "Those are your ideas, and I have ideas of my own." She had internalized the dominant cultural ideal of individual independence at age 3.

Culture Is Not Idiosyncratic, But Is Shared in Human Society

Although it may be carried in the minds of individuals, as some have argued, culture's manifestations are social. How do you greet your grandfather? With a kiss on the cheek? A hug? A hello? A kiss on the back of his hand? Or do you shake his hand and then kiss your own and place it over your heart, as a respectful child in coastal East Africa would? Scholars of culture may dispute whether it is the greeting behavior itself or the shared understanding that underlies it that is the locus of culture, but all would agree that culture is shared socially. As such, it is most easily perceived in interactions between and among people.

Cultures Adapt

While culture is real and has incredible staying power, it is not static, fixed, or immutable. Values, attitudes, aesthetics, lifeways, arts, morals, customs, laws, and the many other things that are included in culture can change in response to the forces of history, politics, and economics. Culture is malleable and dynamic. Even a cursory glance at the advertising media of the United States in the twenty-first century would reveal that we think light brown or beige skin, narrow muscular buttocks, large chests, and full lips are aesthetically pleasing in either gender. Was it always so? No. For example, before the Industrial Revolution, when peasants labored outdoors, suntanned skin was not considered aesthetically pleasing, but a mark of low class. The North American and European leisured classes of the preindustrial era took pains to protect the whiteness of their skins, even while enjoying outdoor activities. It was not until workers went indoors to sunless factories that sun tanning became a mark of expendable income and leisure time and thus became culturally valued.

Cultures change as human groups encounter each other. A young child who was a recent immigrant from the Philippines made me chuckle when she asked if I knew the

Filipino dish "spaghetti." But spaghetti is Italian, right? Unless you remember that Marco Polo brought pasta to Italy from Asia. When my neighbor's children in Zanzibar, Tanzania, received toy pistols as gifts and enacted a gun battle while singing Tupac Shakur's hit "California Love," they reminded me of the powerful influence of mass culture exported by the West and the quickening pace of culture change. An African friend, quizzical about the representations she saw in mass media, asked me if African Americans were frequently outlaws. When groups of humans come in contact, they influence each other's cultures by imitation, innovation, and even coercion.

Culture Is Invisible

Culture is invisible, especially to those who participate in it. It is taken for granted. When we meet cultural ways that are different from our own, we perceive the otherness, the strangeness of the other group's ways. Still, it takes repeated experiences with entering other cultural spaces, coupled with introspection, just to make our own cultural assumptions visible to us. In Western culture, we accept without question the unity of consciousness and continuity of personhood as givens, as natural. But the "nature" of human nature is a culturally constructed entity, invisible to us, because we are immersed in it. Many cultures include ideas about the consciousness and personhood that would strike us as unusual.

WHAT CULTURE IS NOT

Ethnic and Racial Diversity

Culture is not the same as **ethnicity** or race. *Culture* is not a polite synonym for the word *race*, although people who are uncomfortable with discussing race and ethnicity sometimes use it that way. Ethnic groups, according to Weber's (1922/1968) classic definition, are groups that "entertain a subjective belief in their common descent because of similarities of physical type or of customs or of both, or because of memories of colonization and migration" (p. 389). Ethnic identity can be self-selected and built from within a group or imposed from outside it. As such, it is dynamic and fluid, changing in response to social change (Cornell & Hartmann, 1998). Race and ethnicity are socially constructed categories; concepts agreed on in public and private discourse that can only be understood in the context of the history of their employment in a particular place.

Moreover, race—although an operative concept in American social life, politics, economics, and entertainment marketing—is not a biological entity. Biologists have shown that there is more variation within than between the so-called races of humans, thus invalidating the categorization on a statistical basis. To say that race is a bogus concept biologically or that it is socially constructed, however, does not mean that race is not psychologically or socially real. Dealing with race relations is a very real part of life for many humans. Humans are killed and are denied or given rights and privileges based on race. Although race and ethnicity are not the same as culture, the historical experience of oppression—or, for that matter, of privilege—based on racial or ethnic group membership can shape culture.

Large groups, like those based on race, language, religion, or national origin, are often more heterogeneous than homogeneous and may not share much overlap in cultural beliefs, attitudes, and practices. For example, though African Americans are grouped in a racial category, cultural practices vary within the group (Llorens, 1971). American citizens of African descent who have voluntarily migrated from Africa or who have come from the Caribbean have cultural beliefs, practices, and habits that are different from those of other African Americans. Racial bias or discriminatory treatment is something that most Americans of African descent have experienced, however, and some commonly held cultural beliefs and practices have been organized in response to this experience. Race, ethnicity, class, religion, language group, sexual orientation, and gender diversity all interact and affect the cultural adaptation of groups of people.

Language Group Diversity

Because occupational therapy practitioners rely on interviews for gathering data relevant to treatment planning, perhaps the diversity that most complicates the treatment process is language diversity. Some practitioners are naive about issues surrounding cross-cultural communication (Wardin, 1996). Wardin surveyed occupational therapists to identify both difficulties in cross lingual communication and examples of successful interaction during the evaluation process. She found that, when family members or professional translators were not available, gestural communication could be relied on. Yet, gestures are not universal, and without an understanding of what gestures mean in different cultural contexts, therapy practitioners risk insulting their clients. In North America when we gesture for someone to come close we flex the index finger, and the more pleading and apologetic we are, the more likely we are to minimize the range and the size of this beckoning gesture. In East Africa, a polite "come here" signal must be made with the whole hand and forearm and to use a digit or minimize the size of the gesture is a serious insult. Signaling okay with thumb and index or with a thumbs-up seems positive and benign to many of us, but in some cultures these gestures are obscene. Even a smile can be misinterpreted. Smiles may be seen as sly indications of the smiler's superiority or that the one smiled at is appearing foolish. One foreign student in the United States noted that he felt he should return to his room to make certain his trousers' fly was closed, because he could think of no other reason for his fellow students to persist in grinning at him so. Clearly, nonverbal communication is an inadequate basis on which to form a therapeutic relationship across cultures.

Many respondents to Wardin's (1996) study worked in systems in which they relied on family members for translation. Problems occur, however, when family members serve as interpreters, frequently because they give help or suggest responses on evaluations. Furthermore, junior family members may experience role strain when required to ask personal questions of, or assertively give directions to, more senior family members. Federal legislation is interpreted to mandate provision of translation services in primary health-care facilities (National Center for Cultural Competence, 2000). Useful guidelines for working with interpreters have been published (e.g., Setness, 1998).

Compared to citizens of other nations, those of the United States are more often monolingual and less aware of cross-cultural communication issues. Wardin's (1996) study showed that practitioners who were functionally bilingual reported more effective practice strategies, even with clients whose languages they did not speak. Thus there is evidence that language study sensitizes practitioners to issues caused by limited English proficiency. Communication is not a simple or straightforward process. When analyzed closely, it can be seen as fraught with so many complications that one is amazed we understand each other at all. Practitioners acknowledge the need for skillful use of interpreters and for active listening to check that the meaning received is the one intended and to attend to both verbal and nonverbal aspects of communication.

MYTHS, STEREOTYPES, XENOPHOBIA, AND GENERALIZATIONS

With regard to multicultural awareness, a **myth** is an unfounded or poorly founded belief that is given uncritical acceptance by members of a group. Myths operate in support of existing or traditional practices and institutions. **Stereotypes** are mental pictures based on myths that lead people to associate a characteristic or set of characteristics with particular groups of people. **Xenophobia** is an unreasonable fear or hatred of those different from ourselves. Is xenophobia just part of human nature, as some have argued, or is it taught and learned, handed down from adults to children, as part and parcel of a social group's culture? The fact that xenophobia can be unlearned and that some humans are consistently attracted to those who are different from themselves argues against a view of humans as naturally suspicious of other humans not of their own group.

The tendencies to generalize, however, and to cluster perceptions in memory do appear to be an inherent part of the human mental apparatus. Piaget (1969) described the development of children's thinking in terms of forming and refining schemata for grouping objects and creatures in the natural world around them. Thinking about such cognitive clustering can provide some insights into how myths and stereotypes about groups of others are formed. It is a way to begin to undo some of the myths and stereotypes we may have incorporated into our own thinking about human diversity.

Let's say that at some point in your youth you heard the phrase *woman driver*. The circumstances under which you heard this language employed allowed you to understand quickly that this was a phrase meant to disparage the abilities of women to operate motor vehicles safely and efficiently. Having heard the phrase used once or twice, you internalized this concept, even if just on a trial basis. With this concept embedded in your mental apparatus, however, you were readily able to incorporate and file away in this conceptual category any and all instances you may have noted personally or heard about in which a female did indeed operate a motor vehicle in an ineffective or unsafe manner. Conversely, there was no handy cognitive schema in which you might mentally record, in a ready-made category, all incidents or reports of males driving badly. Challenged to recall instances of or anecdotes about bad driving by females and by males, you would much more readily retrieve from memory all those precoded instances of bad driving by females. A concept is introduced, and as with a self-fulfilling prophecy, evidence begins to be amassed through experience; experience filtered through previously learned cognitive categories. You might well conclude that women are worse drivers than men. Then you would be confronted with a different reality. Insurance actuarial tables show that, in fact, women are better drivers than men and insurance companies, large and small, honor that truth in the way they structure differential rates for coverage by gender.

Humans cannot turn off the grouping, generalizing, and schemata-building aspects of their minds. However, they can rigorously examine the generalizations they make about other humans and the conclusions they draw. To practice competently and ethically with a diversity of individuals and groups, health-care professionals accept the responsibility to examine their generalizations.

Generalizations about cultural or racial groups are not all negative or destructive. Health-care professionals have sometimes found it useful to generalize from published lists of characterizations of particular ethnic, cultural, or language groups. One such list contrasts beliefs, values, and practices of Native Americans with those of Anglo-European Americans, so all statements included are considered relative comparisons. In contrast to European Americans, Native Americans are characterized as (Joe & Malch, 1992)

- More group than individual oriented.
- Having respect for elders and experts.
- Viewing time and place as permanent and settled.
- Being introverted and avoiding ridicule or criticism of others.
- Being pragmatic and accepting of what is.
- Emphasizing responsibility for family and self more than authority over or responsibility for larger social groups.
- Attending to how others behave more so than to what they say they think or feel, and seeking harmony.

This may be useful information to have as a starting point for observations of and conversations with a particular Native American client or family, but it is important to remain open to the possibility that the individual or various family members may espouse and enact all, some, or none of these beliefs and values. If, for example, the hypothetical client were an urban American Indian Movement activist leader, it would be unlikely that she would concern herself only with self and family or pragmatically accept the status quo. The more information that you have about social history and context of an individual or family group, the better able you will be to discern whether published descriptions of these cultural others apply.

Attempts to generalize from knowledge of another's religion present particular difficulties. While North Americans and Europeans tend to give a religious tradition complete allegiance, excluding the possibility of participating in religious practices springing from other traditions, this is not the rule worldwide. Muslims in North, West, and East Africa, for example, do not experience rituals aimed at recognizing or propitiating capricious and problematic spirits as contradictory to or disrespectful of their Islamic faith. Similarly, spirit possession and animal sacrifice practices by Brazilians practicing candomblé or Cubans practicing santeria, both of which blend elements of Christianity with worship of West African deities, do not see these as interfering with their practice of Roman Catholicism. Conservative orthodox leaders of Sunni Islam or of Roman Catholicism may frown on such practices, but their disapproval is somewhat moot from the perspective of the practitioner–client relationship and attempts at cross-cultural understanding. Medical anthropologists have long observed that, faced with adversity, humans generally try any and all remedies they perceive as useful, even if those remedies do not fit into one systematic worldview or set of beliefs in the supernatural.

It is also wise to consider the forces of assimilation in applying generalizations. As previously mentioned, mass media and interactions with other social group members provide a powerful impetus for cultural or racial minorities to adopt dominant group values, beliefs, and practices. This is seen most readily in generations born to immigrant citizens. A client's personal ethos (worldview and approach to life) may well be a creative blend of cultural elements from the previous society, or older generation's culture, and the new society and culture he or she has entered.

Finally, it is also important to realize that the process of generalizing about culturally different others is multidirectional. As you interact with those different from you and test hypotheses based on your learned generalizations, others will be doing the same in regard to you. Myths and stereotypes about all cultural and racial groups, including European Americans, abound. Books such as Henry Louis Gates's *Colored People* (1994), Anne Fadiman's *The Spirit Catches You and You Fall Down* (1997), and Anna Deavere Smith's *Twilight, Los Angeles, 1992* (1994) and *Fires in the Mirror* (1993) provide priceless insights into cultural and racial myth making and stereotyping in America. See What's a Practitioner to Do? 7-1 to identify generalizations and assumptions about culture beliefs and practices.

CULTURE AND OTHER FORMS OF DIVERSITY IN OCCUPATIONAL THERAPY THEORY AND PRACTICE

Mattingly and Beer (1993) offered two reasons for occupational therapy practitioners to strive for an accurate understanding of their clients' cultural backgrounds: to allow for collaboration in goal setting and treatment planning and to individualize therapy. I would add two others: to ensure accurate assessment and to increase the likelihood of equitable treatment. Underlying all of these goals of culturally sensitive treatment is the imperative that we establish accurate empathy for our clients.

More than 90% of occupational therapy practitioners are European Americans (American Occupational Therapy Association, 1991). Only 76% of the U.S. population is European American. African Americans, Hispanic and Latino Americans, and Native Americans are underrepresented in our profession. While race and ethnicity are not the same as culture, they are attributes that, like culture, are marked as differences in North American society. As such, they can create challenges to interpersonal understanding between individuals coming from different groups, just as class and culture do. The American Occupational Therapy Association (AOTA) does not keep statistics on the class backgrounds of practitioners, but it seems safe to hypothesize that occupational therapy practitioners come from a narrower range of class backgrounds than do their clients. Furthermore, all practitioners share the socializing influence of higher education. A recent study showed strong agreement among occupational therapists of different races on a list of beliefs and values, whereas these same respondents ascribed different sets of values to ethnic groups other than their own (Pineda, 1996). Respondents in two surveys described a struggle between therapists and families over helping and caring for an ill or recently disabled person (Pineda, 1996; Wardin, 1996). This clash of values centered on the idea of personal independence. A family's desire to do things for an ill or disabled loved one should not be demeaned nor devalued by practitioners, simply because the occupational therapy profession (and European American culture) value independence over interdependence.

Still, practitioners may feel trapped between the families' wishes and the demands of third-party payers, whose reimbursement for services is contingent on attainment of the productivity and independence that the dominant culture values. To solve this conundrum practitioners need a clear understanding of their own cultures as well as those of

WHAT'S A PRACTITIONER TO DO? 7-1
Examining Generalizations and Assumptions

This is a true story with some identifying details altered to protect confidentiality.

SaMol, a 50-year-old Cambodian, and his wife are war refugees who sought asylum in the United States 12 years ago. After their escape from Cambodia and while they were in refugee camps in Thailand they were separated from their six children. The entire family suffered terribly during this period. In particular, one of their daughters, Bonnie (who has Americanized the spelling of her name) almost died during her escape from the Khmer Rouge. Eventually, the children emigrated to France, Thailand, and the United States. Once in the United States, SaMol, desperate to find his children, wrote letters to Thai authorities for assistance in locating them. Finally, after sending many letters and a few sums of money, SaMol located all of his children and reunited his family in the Pacific Northwest.

Once the family was reunited, SaMol agreed to an arranged marriage between Bonnie and Ry, another war refugee from Thailand. Ry had come to the United States several years earlier and can speak both English and Khmer. Ignoring tradition, Bonnie and Ry met once before the Buddhist ceremony that blessed their union. Soon after his daughter's marriage, SaMol fell ill.

SaMol began complaining of mild headaches and tiredness, a general malaise, some nausea, and weakness. Ry, his new son-in-law, accompanied him to the doctor's office. SaMol had suffered many worse things, and so he did not complain of these symptoms forcefully to Ry. And in translating, Ry followed his father-in-law and perhaps minimized the degree of discomfort these symptoms caused SaMol. The doctor asked a few questions about the daily occurrence of SaMol's symptoms and diagnosed depression. The physician knew from published reports that Southeast Asians frequently somatize negative emotions—that is, instead of complaining directly about feeling down or being depressed, they describe physical symptoms. The physician prescribed antidepressants.

Several trips to the doctor ensued when the antidepressants brought no relief. At no point did the physician elicit the family history and discover that the recent developments in SaMol's life would be cause for joy and not depression. The physician ordered a brain scan only when SaMol developed lower extremity partial paralysis. The scan showed a tumor in the brainstem. By then it was almost inoperable; but given the alternative of certain death, the doctor recommended trying to remove it. After surgery, SaMol never regained consciousness.

SaMol was moved to the long-term care wing where he was expected to regain consciousness. Betsy, SaMol's occupational therapist, began a program of sensory stimulation, range of motion, and positioning. Betsy gradually learned of the dramatic saga of this family and came to feel very close to Ry and Bonnie. She learned that Ry worked as a teacher's assistant in the same school one of her sons attended. She came to understand that since his father-in-law's illness, Ry had assumed the role of head of the family, over his mother-in-law; his wife, Bonnie; and her siblings. Therefore, he took the lead in interacting with health professionals in his father-in-law's interest. It is his traditional role, based on age and gender, facilitated by his mastery of English. Communicating through Ry, Betsy discovered that the family wanted SaMol at home. Consequently, the focus of the occupational therapy program shifted to training the family in SaMol's care.

Late one Saturday morning, Betsy received a call from Ry who told her that SaMol had died and that a funeral was to be held in the family home. He asked her if she would come over that day. Betsy agreed to attend, although she was surprised by the request and surprised at how quickly a funeral had been planned since SaMol had just died. After she hung up, she realized she did not know how to dress. She put on the dressiest, darkest suit in her closet and carefully selected matching pumps. She called a friend to take care of her two sons, aged 7 and 9.

Once she arrived at SaMol's home, however, she noticed that others were casually dressed, children were playing, men were drinking, and women were cooking. Everyone was chatting. Some were smoking. The small house was packed with people. She wondered how Ry had pulled so many together so quickly. "Where are your boys?" Ry asked her, having seen their photos on Betsy's desk and knowing one from the school where he worked. Betsy explained that she had sent them to her friend's house. Ry seemed puzzled. Soon the food was ready, and Betsy joined in eating with the others. As she took a seat in the front room, she noted a small shrine with a picture of SaMol; fruit and flowers were arranged in front of it.

When all were finished eating, Ry asked Betsy if she would come with the family to the hospital where SaMol's body lay. Betsy went along, out of respect for the family's grief and because she felt they might need her help to feel comfortable on her turf, the hospital. A contingent of 20 people went to the hospital to view SaMol's body. Many wept. Then Ry explained to Betsy that they

Continues

had come to the hospital not only to sit with SaMol's body but to use the chapel. "Could you lead us in some Christian prayers there?" he asked. Betsy was astounded and panicked for a moment. Unbeknownst to Ry, Betsy was no longer a practicing Christian. Still, Betsy did not want to offend, so she accompanied Ry and his community of 20, one of whom was videotaping, to a nondenominational chapel.

In the chapel, there was a Bible, a Jewish prayer book, a Koran, some pews, and a single kneeler up front. Betsy went up front and knelt to pray with her back to the others, since that was consistent with religious customs familiar to her. Some community members seemed nonplused, but all followed suit, kneeling and facing the front of the chapel. Betsy quickly composed a prayer asking God to give the widow and her children strength and to keep the recently reunited family together. Then she said the Lord's Prayer. Ry and other members of the group thanked her.

The group returned to the family home, for at 6:00 P.M. Buddhist monks were coming to chant prayers for SaMol. Betsy returned to the house. She then asked Ry when this next part might end, so that she could make a graceful exit. "This chanting is now three days," Ry replied. Betsy listened for a short time and then made apologies and left.

Several months later, she saw Ry and Bonnie at a grocery store. Ry was happy to announce that, at Bonnie's mother's urging, they had conceived a child. He explained it was necessary to do so as soon as possible, so that SaMol's essence would be able to return to their family instead of finding its way into another. In this way, the family would again be reunited. Certainly, Betsy's prayer for family unity had helped, Ry said. If the child was a girl, Bonnie wanted to name her Betsy.

For another glimpse into the experiences of refugees coming from Southeast Asia to the United States, view the award-winning documentary film *Becoming American* (Levine & Levine, 1981).

QUESTIONS AND EXERCISES

1. How many assumptions and generalizations about unfamiliar others can you identify in this tale?
2. How did the assumptions of all of the people—particularly of SaMol, Ry, the doctor, and Betsy—affect what happened in the story?
3. Many people assume that Southeast Asian immigrants to the United States have come here merely for economic opportunity. How does the story call that assumption into question?

their clients, so that they may negotiate therapy goals that meet clients' needs. The process of negotiation begins with the recognition that personal independence is not a value-neutral concept. Rather, it is a cherished cultural ideal of the dominant culture in North America, and it is not held in such high regard by people of many other cultural groups.

Cultural differences enter into the process of assessment not only at the level of achieving understanding and empathy for the client but also at the level of choosing evaluation instruments and strategies and interpreting results. By their very nature, standardized norm-referenced assessment tools make assumptions about normalcy that may be culture bound. Most testing instruments assume characteristics of modal individuals, often based on middle-class European or European American lifeways and experiences. For example, Law (1993) found that current activities of daily living (ADL) and instrumental activities of daily living (IADL) reflected North American dominant cultural values regarding independence and individual rights. Table 7-1 summarizes other occupational therapy literature that supports the need to tailor evaluation strategies with care given cultural, racial, ethnic, and class diversity.

Racial minorities, particularly African Americans, have less access to health care than do European Americans and suffer higher mortality and morbidity rates from a host of common disease processes (Advisory Board of the President's Initiative on Race, 1998; American Medical Association Council on Ethical and Judicial Affairs, 1990; Evans, 1992). Limited access to health-care services seems especially evident for high-tech interventions, costly surgical procedures, and lengthy rehabilitation services. Yet, even relatively low cost rehabilitative interventions may not be equitably distributed across racial groups. A retrospective review of rehabilitation services provided to clients with hip fractures discovered that factors unrelated to clinical presentation in part determined whether clients were referred for occupational therapy and physical therapy. Race appeared to be the factor that determined the frequency of therapy sessions; African Americans were more likely than other groups to receive a lower frequency of post–hip fracture treatment (Hoenig, Rubenstein, & Kahn, 1996). Once an accurate understanding of the client is achieved and valid assessment strategies selected, the practitioner's role is as an advocate for the client to receive needed services. Evans (1992) recommended that European Americans carefully reexamine their assumptions any time they perceive a client of color as unlikely to benefit from rehabilitation services and to be certain that myths, stereotypes, or generalizations do not cloud their vision.

Humphry (1995) described how chronic poverty, an experience unequally shared across cultural and racial groups in the United States, depersonalizes and erodes the sense of self, alters children's developmental progression, and

TABLE 7–1. **OCCUPATIONAL THERAPY LITERATURE ON CULTURALLY SENSITIVE ASSESSMENT**

Reference	Description of Work	Effects of Diversity on Test Scores
Bowman & Wallace (1990)	Quasi-experimental study; n = 22 white preschoolers of low SES compared to 22 higher SES preschoolers (matched for age, race, sex, hand dominance, height, and weight) on a battery of 12 assessments	Lower SES subjects scored as functioning at significantly lower developmental levels in hand strength, visuomotor integration, and praxis. Therapist should consider the effects of social class when interpreting results of tests of hand strength, the Beery Test of Visual-Motor Integration, and the Praxis on Verbal Command subtest of the SIPT. Vestibular functioning and other SIPT measures of praxis did not differ significantly between the groups.
Janelle (1992)	Quasi-experimental study; n = 13 nondisabled and 8 congenitally physically disabled adolescents (matched for IQ, age, race and SES) compared for locus of control as measured by the Nowicki-Strickland Locus of Control Scale	Unanticipated finding that disability status did not correlate with locus of control; rather race was the only variable significantly correlated with locus of control scores. African American subjects in both groups scored more external than European-American subjects; but given small number of African American subjects, the author viewed this result with caution, considered that SES might have been a hidden factor in difference by race and recommended further research.
Myers (1992)	Description and discussion based on clinical observation of Hmong children and their families in an early intervention program	No standardized test of development, motor functioning, or sensory integration has included the Hmong population in norming. Approach to interpretation of standardized testing should be one of item analysis, description of patterns of behavior, and augmentation of test results via extended or multiple observations in the child's home environment. Some oft-tested skills may be absent or delayed secondary, not to developmental delay, but to lack of family expectation, exposure, and practice.
Miller (1992)	Description and discussion of observations based on experience of trying to administer standardized tests, such as the Peabody Test of Motor Development, to orphans in Cambodia	Children had such limited experience with toys and with one-on-one mental play stimulation with an adult that author quickly abandoned this assessment strategy. Author devised an observation checklist and used knowledge of development and neurodevelopmental treatment to make judgments about children's areas of competence.
Fudge (1992)	Description and discussion of observations based on the experience of administering the Peabody Test of Motor Development to children with kwashiorkor and other forms of malnutrition in Guatemala	Author concluded that children's limited exposure to test materials made it impossible to interpret test results as indicators of motor function. As children responded to novel play tasks, Peabody Test of Motor Development format allowed observations about early cognitive functioning and imitative learning.
Packir (1994)	Quasi-experimental study; compared 15 Sri Lankan mother-child dyads to U.S. established norms for the Nursing Child Assessment Satellite Training scales	Sri Lankan dyads scored significantly below norms on cognitive and social emotional growth-fostering subscales. Norms are unlikely to apply to this population; cultural differences in parenting, differential valuing of various temperaments of infants and children, and different social norms of parent-child interaction (e.g., frequency of sustained direct eye contact) limit cross-cultural application of this instrument.
Cermack, Katz, McGuire, Greenbaum, Peralta, and Maser-Flanagan (1995)	Quasi-experimental study; n = 25 North Americans and 56 Israelis who had suffered a cerebrovascular accident; subjects compared via the Loewstein Occupational Therapy Cognitive Assessment	Only one subtest—the Orientation to Time Test—revealed a significant difference between American and Israeli groups for subjects with either left or right cerebrovascular accident. Authors unsure whether age differences between the two groups or cultural differences underlay better performance by Israeli group with lower mean age. Authors also consider differences between performance of subjects with left vs. right cerebrovascular accident.

TABLE 7-1. **OCCUPATIONAL THERAPY LITERATURE ON CULTURALLY SENSITIVE ASSESSMENT**

Reference	Description of Work	Effects of Diversity on Test Scores
Colonius (1995)	Quasi-experimental study; n = 27 Native American (Tlingit and Haida) and 7 non-Native American children from the same preschools in Alaska; compared with norms for the FirstSTEP developmental screening test	Native American children scored significantly higher than norms in the motor domain and significantly lower than norms in the cognitive and language domains. Non-Native peers of a similar SES (based on inclusion in Head Start preschool) scored at or above normative means. Given norms and performance of the small sample of non-Native children, differences in performance across groups seem more related to culture than to SES. Author recommends caution in application of FirstSTEP norms to Native American children in Alaska.

SES, socioeconomic status; *SIPT,* Sensory Integration and Praxis Tests.

causes potential conflicts between practitioners and clients or their caregivers around the five universal problems of time orientation, activity, human relationships, human nature, and control of natural forces. These values conflicts have implications, not only for testing that purports to measure locus of control and human motivation but also for how we represent humans and human occupation in occupational therapy theory. Occupational therapy theoreticians continually build and refine models for practice. The profession values this scholarly activity. Refinement takes place as scholars open their work for criticism and debate among their peers. Rigorously examining the culture-based assumptions of a practice model is one way to test it.

From its inception, occupational science has embraced narrative, or story making, as the best means to understand clients' experiences of their illness or disability (Clark, 1993). The emphasis in occupational science on emic (insiders') perspectives gives it the potential to cross cultural barriers. Concern with the client's own account of his or her life is part of the occupational therapy tradition (Frank, 1996). In the application of narrative methods of assessment across cultures, however, it is important to recognize that what is a satisfying narrative to Western minds has a particular linear structure. That structure has been discussed (and prescribed) in Western culture since Aristotle's time. Proponents of narrative methods of evaluation admit that the "story" arrived at by the client (and family) and practitioner is the result of a negotiation between the client's telling and the practitioner's reconstruction of the story (Frank, 1996). When occupational therapy practitioners interview clients to discover their activity goals or the meanings that activities hold for them sometimes elicit stories that make no sense to them. The task for ethical practitioners is to push themselves outside the comfortable but invisible confines of their own culture and class to attempt an accurate understanding of their clients' worldviews and life situations. Doing so is a necessary step in collaborative goal setting, accurate assessment, individualized treatment planning, and equitable treatment provision. See Life Issues to Consider in Practice 7-1 for one example of the process of cross-cultural negotiation across several kinds of diversity.

ACHIEVING MULTICULTURAL COMPETENCE AS AN OCCUPATIONAL THERAPY PRACTITIONER

Approaches to multicultural competence education are sometimes dichotomized as culture-specific versus culture-universal or culture-general models (Bandy, 1994; Bennet, 1986; Freeman, 1993). Culture-specific models endeavor to inform learners about expected differences between groups, usually in a didactic way. Others are described by way of lists of traits, beliefs, or customary practices. These models are aimed at increasing cultural sensitivity, defined as an openness to the cultural values of others (Dillard, Andonian, Flores, MacRae, & Shakir, 1992). In contrast, culture-general models emphasize that all humans have culture and thereby attempt to avoid reifying differences between self and other. The approach to understanding others is via self-awareness. The assumption is made that those who better understand themselves will better understand their own culture and thus will be able to understand that of others. This component of multicultural competence training has been called *cultural awareness* (Dillard et al., 1992). After reviewing multicultural competence education literature, Bandy (1994) concluded that activities aimed at increasing both cultural awareness and cultural sensitivity are important and that, used together, they have the potential to offset deficiencies inherent in using only one or the other.

Programs aimed at increasing awareness of one's own culture often begin with examination of dominant North American cultural values, making those values less invisible

LIFE ISSUES TO CONSIDER IN PRACTICE 7-1

Negotiating across Multiple Layers of Diversity

Material for this case story is based in part on interview transcripts from a study conducted by Crenshaw (1996). Some names and circumstances have been altered to protect informant anonymity and provide closure for the case study.

John Banks is a 41-year-old African-American father of nine children, the youngest of whom, Tyler, has multiple disabilities and medical conditions related to a chromosomal anomaly. Joanne, John's wife, works full time as a secretary and has health-care benefits through a health maintenance organization (HMO). John chooses to work only part time so that the family will not be disqualified for Medicaid assistance. The family's income, at the poverty level, places them among our country's many working poor. John and Joanne agree that the specialty children's hospital, to which they have access via their Medicaid coverage, provides better, more complete, and more sophisticated therapy services than does the HMO. John, Joanne, and the other eight children in the family are able bodied and generally healthy. John is involved in the care of his son Tyler, who is now 3 years old and functions at approximately the 6-month level. John is Tyler's primary caregiver during the day and attends all parent-professional case conferences related to Tyler's ongoing early intervention program.

John has attended parent support-group meetings and 2 years earlier joined a state-level policy-planning council for early intervention services, as a parent member. Through these experiences, John has become knowledgeable about the services available in the state but is frustrated with state-level agencies' perceived slowness and lack of responsiveness to the needs of families with disabled children.

Currently John Banks and Rita Connor, a 26-year-old European American who is Tyler's occupational therapist, are involved in a conflict about the elements of programming in Tyler's treatment plan. The occupational therapist has recommended play therapy and is standing firm behind that suggestion. John is seeking expensive exercise equipment and a powered wheelchair for Tyler and is refusing the play therapy. Rita does not agree that Tyler needs the exercise equipment or is ready for power mobility. She has the authority to block John's request for these items by not providing the state with the necessary therapeutic rationale for their procurement. She reports that she sees John as unrealistic and in denial. John is angry about the therapist's interference with his getting for his child what he believes the child needs.

Bettina Crenshaw, an African-American occupational therapist-consultant, intervened by meeting with John and giving him uninterrupted time to talk about his son, his perceptions of therapy, and his feelings. During the interview John revealed the following:

- His perception that the range of services available is not made clear to the African-American community, asking, "Why would they have these services and then hide the fact that they provide these services?"
- His perception that as an African-American male he is often disrespected and challenged by European American care providers to prove that he is not "trying to get something for nothing." African-American parents, said John, often see the health-care system as adversarial and exclusive. He related this to the dominant culture myth that many African-Americans are welfare frauds.
- His perception that the family had received services that were "human and sincere" from some European American care providers and thus that race differences could be breached and cooperation forged. He related several stories about a caring European American female pediatrician once employed by the children's hospital.
- His spiritual beliefs and the deep intangible connection he shares with his nonverbal child. John commented that "the spirituality that is in African American culture is not one that is understood in the European American culture." John described how from the first instant that he saw an early ultrasound image of his son, before any problems were even diagnosed, he had a spiritual connection to the child: "The spirit spoke out to me and I cried. . . . I sat on the edge of the bed, picked up the picture and cried. I knew immediately something was wrong." He went on to say that he and Joanne never considered abortion as an option, but decided to let their son's spirit determine his fate. John sees his son as having a strong spirit and will to live.
- His idea that play therapy would be frivolous and that Tyler needs to work hard, with the most intense therapy possible during the early intervention period, as this will determine his course later on. "We don't have time to waste with play; we need to work."

The following elements of cross-cultural conflict are apparent in the case:

Continues

- A class and race conflict based on the historical denial and present barriers to equal access to health care for African Americans that makes it difficult for John to trust that the therapist has his or Tyler's best interests at heart. This is intensified by the current struggle over health-care reform and John's fear that he will lose access to the children's hospital.
- A cultural conflict involving values related to work. John may be misperceived as having a weak work ethic because of his rational choice to limit his income earning so as not to lose Medicaid benefits and because of myths and stereotypes that exist in the dominant culture about both African Americans and welfare recipients.
- A potential cultural conflict between John and the therapist over the relative values of spirituality and science and technology, given John's assertion that European Americans don't understand his spirituality and occupational therapy's position as an allied medical service in the children's hospital.
- A potential gender-based cultural conflict with John favoring strength, exercise, technology, and motor skills (male ideal) and the occupational therapist valuing (or is perceived as valuing) social-emotional, cognitive, and interaction skills (female ideal) to be developed through play.

At the same time, by carefully listening to John, many bases for agreement and keys to cooperation are revealed:

- John and Joanne have enjoyed good relations with specific European American care providers in the past so the trust barrier can be overcome. They have a history of good relations with a European American female who was perceived as "human and sincere."
- John's remarks about work being more necessary and more serious than play actually reveal a strong valuing of work, a work ethic perhaps stronger than the therapist's.
- John's desire for high-tech exercise equipment and power mobility devices belie a faith in science and technology that is typically considered a mainstream dominant culture value. He likely does not experience his spiritual beliefs as being in conflict with this faith in technology as an aid to human progress.
- John's belief in the existence and strength of Tyler's spirit opens a door to an understanding of play as a means to develop that spirit.
- John has clearly internalized the importance of early intervention and has learned to be an advocate for his child within a complex system.

Bettina suggested several avenues for rebuilding a cooperative working relationship between Rita and John so Tyler could benefit from the good intentions of both. As a professional service provider, Rita has the responsibility to begin the process of resolving the conflict.

- *Accord John respect.* Rita should use his title and surname when addressing him (i.e., Mr. Banks). He is her senior and, in accordance with norms of African American culture, should be addressed formally until he explicitly gives permission for her to call him John (Evans, 1992; Willis, 1992).
- *Assume that John earnestly seeks what is best for his child.* Convey this assumption to him and, for that matter, to all parents (Crenshaw, 1996). Make it clear that Tyler has a right to the best combination of services possible, and work diligently toward that end. Elicit and respect John and Joanne's opinions of Tyler's care.
- *Rigorously avoid conversing with co-workers about personal matters* while providing care to Tyler and do not indulge in idle chitchat during sessions. Such behavior is read as a lack of concern and as not having one's mind on one's work. Adopt a serious, but warm, attitude (Willis, 1992).
- *Rigorously avoid conveying agreement with any stereotypes* of African Americans or welfare recipients as somehow not worthy of the best services available. Similarly, if Rita disagrees with or disproves of the family's decisions about the pregnancy, the size of their family, or work schedules she must keep these entirely out of the conversation. Her role is to help the family not to judge it. Poverty is not, in and of itself, a dysfunction (Humphry, 1995; Willis, 1992).
- *Open a discussion with John* about his spiritual connection with Tyler and seek to understand and appreciate it. It is an asset to Tyler's development.
- *Elicit from John his aims and goals* as regards the desired exercise equipment and power mobility devices. Remain open and use active listening.
- *Once these views are understood, build from them,* negotiating a view of the problem and its treatment that both the practitioner and the client's parents can agree on (Kleinman, 1988). For example, present the occupational therapy belief that play is the antecedent of work. Present play therapy as a way to exercise Tyler's spirit through awakening his understanding of cause and effect and the way that the physical world works. Given John's interest in high technology and Tyler's limited motor control, plan to incorporate in play therapy some work with microswitches or computer keyboards to activate toys or games. Explain the

Continues

skills of understanding cause and effect and operating switches as prerequisites to learning to use power mobility equipment and augmentative communication devices. Offer hope that Tyler will one day be able to profit from these high-tech assistive devices. Develop a series of goals to work toward skilled use of joystick controls and other kinds of switches, with a timeline for consideration of powered mobility for Tyler.

QUESTIONS AND EXERCISES

1. What actions could Rita have taken to avoid the conflict that developed between her and the Banks family?
2. Brainstorm a list of other scenarios in which collaborative goal setting may be a challenge given cultural, racial, ethnic, language, or social-class differences between a hypothetical practitioner and a hypothetical client or family.
3. Organize a debate, assigning teams in your class to support or refute the following assertion: It is more important for occupational therapy interventions to meet clients' or clients' families' perceived needs than to alter clients' perceptions so that they take a more biomedical view of health problems.
4. Access and view the videotape *Equal Partners: African American Fathers and Systems of Health Care* (National Fathers' Network, 1996) to hear fathers of children with disabilities talk about the challenges they face.

Crenshaw, B. (1996). *Parent satisfaction with family-centered services in African American families: A pilot study.* Unpublished master's thesis, University of Puget Sound, Tacoma, WA.

Evans, J. (1992). Nationally speaking—What occupational therapists can do to eliminate racial barriers to health care access. *American Journal of Occupational Therapy, 46,* 679–683.

Humphry, R. (1995). Families who live in chronic poverty: Meeting the challenge of family-centered services. *American Journal of Occupational Therapy, 49,* 687–693.

Kleinman, A. (1988). *The illness narratives: Suffering, healing and the human condition.* New York: Basic Books

National Fathers' Network (Producer). (1996). *Equal partners: African American fathers and systems of health care.* [Videotape]. (Available from Kindering Center, Bellevue, WA.)

Willis, W. (1992). Families with African American roots. In E. W. Lynch & M. J. Hanson (Eds.). *Developing cross-cultural competence: A guide for working with young children and their families.* Baltimore, MD: Brooks.

to those who have assimilated them. Table 7-2 lists are some areas in which the values orientation of the dominant culture and that of the occupational therapy profession come together to create a strong bias that we must be aware of—and be willing to give up—when working with others whose values may be different (Humphry, 1995; Pineda, 1996; Sanchez, 1964).

For European American practitioners, learning to establish accurate empathy begins with acknowledgment of the privileges and advantages inherent in membership in the

BOX 7–1 ACKNOWLEDGING PRIVILEGE INHERENT IN DOMINANT GROUP MEMBERSHIP

- If I wish, I can arrange to be in the company of people of my race most of the time.
- I can avoid spending time with people whom I was trained to mistrust and who have learned to mistrust my kind or me.
- If I should need to move, I can be pretty sure of renting or purchasing housing in an area that can afford and in which I would want to live.
- I can be pretty sure that my neighbors in such a location will be neutral or pleasant to me.
- I can go shopping alone most of the time, pretty well assured that I will not be followed or harassed. Whether I use checks, credit cards, or cash, I can count on my skin color not to work against the appearance of financial reliability.
- I can turn on the television or open to the front page of the paper and see people of my race widely represented.
- When I am told about our national heritage or about "civilization," I am shown that people of my color made it what it is. . . . I can be sure that my children will be given curricular materials that testify to the existence of their race.
- I can arrange to protect my children most of the time from people who might not like them.
- I do not have to educate my children to be aware of systemic racism for their own daily physical protection.
- I can be pretty sure that my children's teachers and employers will tolerate them if they fit school and workplace norms; my chief worries about them do not concern others' attitudes toward their race.
- I am never asked to speak for all the people of my racial group.
- I can remain oblivious of the language and customs of persons of color who constitute the world's majority without feeling in my culture any penalty for such oblivion

(Adapted from McIntosh, P. (1997). White privilege and male privilege: A personal account of coming to see correspondences through work in women's studies. In R. Delgado & J. Stefancic (Eds.). *Critical white studies: Looking behind the mirror* (pp. 291–299). Philadelphia: Temple University Press.)

TABLE 7-2. **VALUES ORIENTATIONS**[a]

European American Culture and Practitioners[b]	Examples of Evidence
Value the future over the present and value long-range planning and delaying gratification	Writing plans with long-term goals Undergoing discomfort now with the idea that a better result will occur later (wearing burn garments) Emphasizing saving (the grasshopper and ant morality tale)
Value individuality and place the good of one individual over that of the rest of the social group	Feeling parents should orient the family's emotional and/or financial resources toward the developmental needs of a child with a disability
See the locus of identity as the individual and define the social unit primarily as the nuclear family	Feeling that hierarchical authority relationships in families are undesirable Expecting clients to have individuals goals for their well-being without consultation with socially significant others, or if others are involved in goal setting, often select one (spouse, parent, or offspring)
Value independence over interdependence and group members doing for themselves over being served by others	Assuming that clients will want to perform their own hygiene, grooming, toileting, and other ADL and that independence in these activities is superior to reliance on another Assuming that it is unfair to expect others to care for patient, the concept of "caregiver burden"
Desire and value control and do not readily acquiesce to situations others may see as fate	Assuming everything has a cause and relentlessly seeking a natural cause to explain the incidence of disease Having a book on the best-seller list that tries to solve the conundrum of why bad things happen to good people Seeing a belief in personal causation and an internal locus of control as marks of normalcy
See science and technology as a source of control over the natural world, including humans	Noting the elaboration of technological assistive devices, weather prediction and measurement equipment, nuclear weapons, and genetic engineering Believing the adage The Lord helps those who help themselves
Value physicality and doing over introspection and being	Seeing expenditures on sporting and gaming equipment outpace expenditures on books Realizing that mass media images of activity far outnumber depictions of thinking, conversing, reading, or other less-active pursuits
Believe that humans are nearly perfectible and value discipline and learning as a means toward that end	Noting the proliferation of self-help books, infant learning protocols, and flash cards. Believing in the adage Spare the rod and spoil the child

[a]Summarized from Humphry (1995), Pineda (1996), and Sanchez (1994).
[b]Orientations shared by the dominant European-American culture and the occupational therapy profession on which many clients will differ.

dominant group (Evans, 1992; Matala, 1993). This is not an easy step, but it is a necessary one. Dominant cultural group members may have been raised with the myths that one may pull himself up by his boot straps and that hard work always pays off. Moreover, they may have worked very hard for their achievements. Thus they come to see their status as a just reward and wonder why others have not achieved similarly. The privileges, small and large, that accompany dominant group membership status may be invisible to them. Box 7-1 shows a sampling of such privileges, taken from a longer list by McIntosh (1997).

Cultural sensitivity follows when learners are aware of their own value orientations and are ready to explore those of others nonjudgmentally. Contact with empowered persons whose cultural, racial, ethnic, class, gender, or sexual orientation is different from one's own is the most highly valued sort of activity for increasing cultural sensitivity (Bandy, 1994). The learner must be willing to be uncomfortable by entering environments in which he or she will have the experience of being the numerical minority. While face-to-face contact and immersion in culturally distinct environments is extremely useful, much can also be learned from reading autobiographies and novels written by those different from oneself. Sometimes a well-written novel does more to pull the reader into the protagonist's perspective and help him or her develop empathy than hours of lectures on the same cultural group could accomplish. Didactic works that take a positive approach in employing cross-cultural generalizations with necessary caution include Wells and Black's *Cultural Competency for Health Professionals* (2000) and Lynch and Hanson's *Developing Cross Cultural Competence* (1992); The former was written specifically for occupational therapy practitioners.

CONCLUSION

Developing multicultural competence is a challenge, but the learning that occurs along the way can be a joy. Nothing is more interesting than the varieties of ways humans use to solve the problems of daily living. Looking for culture through careful observation of and interaction with others coupled with introspection of self enables the establishment of accurate empathy between practitioner and client. Cultural difference then becomes a basis for understanding and working together and not a barrier to therapeutic gains.

References

Advisory Board of the President's Initiative on Race. (1998). One America in the 21st century: Forging a new future. Available at: www.whitehouse.gov/Initiatives/OneAmerica/cevent.html. Accessed January 15, 2001.

American Medical Association Council on Ethical and Judicial Affairs. (1990). *Black-white disparities in health care. Journal of the American Medical Association*, *263*, 2344–2346.

American Occupational Therapy Association. (1991). *1990 Member data survey: Summary report*. Rockville, MD: Author.

Bandy, N. (1994). *Educating occupational therapists for multicultural competence*. Unpublished master's thesis, University of Puget Sound, Tacoma, WA.

Bennet, J. (1986). Modes of cross-cultural training: conceptualizing cross-cultural training as education. *International Journal of Cultural Relations*, 10, 179–196.

Bowman, O. J., & Wallace, B. A. (1990). The effects of socioeconomic status on hand size and strength, vestibular function, visuomotor integration and praxis in preschool children. *American Journal of Occupational Therapy*, *44*, 610–622.

Cermack, S. A., Katz, N., McGuire E., Greenbaum, S., Peralta, C., & Maser-Flanagan, V. (1995). Performance of Americans and Israelis with cerebrovascular accident on the Loewenstein Occupational Therapy Cognitive Assessment (LOTCA). *American Journal of Occupational Therapy*, *49*, 500–506.

Clark, F. (1993). Occupation embedded in a real life: Interweaving occupational science and occupational therapy. *American Journal of Occupational Therapy*, *47*, 1067–1078.

Colonius, G. (1995). *Measurement accuracy of the FirstSTEP: A comparison between Alaska native children and the FirstSTEP norms*. Unpublished master's thesis, University of Puget Sound, Tacoma, WA.

Cornell, S., & Hartmann, D. (1998). *Ethnicity and race: Making identities in a changing world*. Thousand Oaks, CA: Pine Forge.

Dillard, M., Andonian, L., Flores, O., MacRae, A., & Shakir, M. (1992) Culturally competent occupational therapy in a diversely populated mental health setting. *American Journal of Occupational Therapy*, *46*, 721–726.

Dyck, I. (1992). Managing chronic illness: An immigrant woman's acquisition and use of health care knowledge. *American Journal of Occupational Therapy*, *46*, 696–705

Evans, J. (1992). Nationally Speaking—What occupational therapists can do to eliminate racial barriers to health care access. *American Journal of Occupational Therapy*, *46*, 679–683.

Fadiman, A. (1997) *The spirit catches you and you fall down: A Hmong child, her American doctors and the collision of two cultures*. New York: Farrar, Straus & Giroux.

Frank, G. (1996). Life histories in occupational therapy clinical practice. *American Journal of Occupational Therapy*, *50*, 251–264.

Freeman, S. (1993). Client-centered therapy: The universal within the specific. *Journal of Multicultural Counseling and Development*, *18*, 173–179.

Fudge, S. (1992). A perspective on consulting in Guatemala. *Occupational Therapy in Health Care*, *8*, 15–37.

Gates, H. L. (1994). *Colored people: A memoir*. New York: Knopf.

Hoenig, H., Rubenstein, L., & Kahn, K. (1996). Rehabilitation after hip fracture—Equal opportunity for all? *Archives of Physical Medicine and Rehabilitation*, *77*, 58–63

Humphry, R. (1995). Families who live in chronic poverty: Meeting the challenge of family-centered services. *American Journal of Occupational Therapy*, *49*, 687–693.

Janelle, S. (1992). Locus of control in nondisabled versus congenitally physically disabled adolescents. *American Journal of Occupational Therapy*, *46*, 334–342.

Joe, J. R., & Malach, R. S. (1992). Families with Native American roots. In E. W. Lynch & M. J. Hanson (Eds.). *Developing cross-cultural competence: A guide for working with young children and their families* (pp. 127–164). Baltimore, MD: Brookes.

Kleinman, A. (1988). *The illness narratives: Suffering, healing and the human condition*. New York: Basic Books

Krefting L., & Krefting, D. (1991). Cultural influences on performance. In C. Christiansen and C. Baum (Eds.). *Occupational therapy: Overcoming human performance deficits* (pp. 101–124). Thorofare, NJ: Slack.

Law, M. (1993). Evaluating activities of daily living: Directions for the future. *American Journal of Occupational Therapy*, *47*, 233–237.

Levine, K., & Levine, I. W. (Producers). (1981). *Becoming American*. [Film]. In association with WNET 13, Iris Film and Video. (Available from New Day Films, Franklin Lakes, NJ.)

Llorens, L. (1971). Black culture and child development. *American Journal of Occupational Therapy*, *25*, 144–148.

Lynch, E. W., & Hanson, M. J. (Eds.). (1992). *Developing cross-cultural competence: A guide for working with young children and their families*. Baltimore, MD: Brookes.

Matala, M. R. (1993). Race relations at work: a challenge to occupational therapy. *British Journal of Occupational Therapy*, *56*, 434–436.

Mattingly, C., & Beer, D. (1993). Interpreting culture in a therapeutic context. In H. Hopkins & H. D. Smith (Eds.). *Willard and Spackman's occupational therapy* (8th ed., pp. 154–161). Philadelphia: Lippincott.

McIntosh, P. (1997). White privilege and male privilege: A personal account of coming to see correspondences through work in women's studies. In R. Delgado & J. Stefancic (Eds.). *Critical white studies: Looking behind the mirror* (pp. 291–299). Philadelphia: Temple.

Miller, L. (1992). Evaluating the developmental skills of Cambodian orphans. *Occupational Therapy in Health Care*, *8*, 73–87.

Moynihan, D. P. (1965, March). *The Negro Family: The case for national action*. [The Moynihan Report]. Washington, DC: U.S. Department of Labor, Office of Planning and Research.

Myers, C. (1992). Hmong children and their families: Consideration of cultural influences in assessment. *American Journal of Occupational Therapy*, *46*, 737–744.

National Center for Cultural Competence (2000, winter). Linguistic competence in Primary Health Care Delivery Systems, Implications for Policy Makers. Policy Brief 2. Available at: http://gucdc.georgetown.edu/nccc/ncccpolicy2.html. Accessed September 17, 2001.

Packir, R. (1994). *Comparison of Sri Lankan and American mother-child dyads on the NCAST.* Unpublished master's thesis, University of Puget Sound, Tacoma, WA.

Piaget, J. (1969). *Science of education and the psychology of the child* (D. Coltman, Trans.). New York: Viking.

Pineda, L. (1996). *Occupational therapists' multicultural competence and attitudes toward ethnically and culturally different clients*. Unpublished master's thesis, University of Puget Sound, Tacoma, WA.

Sanchez, V. (1964). Relevance of cultural values for occupational therapy programs. *American Journal of Occupational Therapy*, *18*, 1–5.

Setness, P. (1998). Culturally competent health care. *Postgraduate Medicine*, *103*, 13–16.

Smith, A. D. (1993). *Fires in the mirror: Crown heights, Brooklyn and other identities*. New York: Dramatists Play Service, Inc.

Smith, A. D. (1994). *Twilight Los Angeles, 1992: On the road: A search for American character*. New York: Double day.

Wardin, K. (1996). A comparison of verbal assessment of clients with limited English proficiency and English speaking clients in physical rehabilitation settings. *American Journal of Occupational Therapy, 50*, 816–825.

Weber, M. (1968). *Economy and society: An interpretive sociology* (E. Fischoff, Trans., G. Roth & C. Wittich, Eds.). New York: Bedminster. (Original work published 1922.)

Wells, S. A., & Black, R. M. (2000). *Cultural competency for health professionals*. Bethesda, MD: American Occupational Therapy Association.

CHAPTER 8

SOCIOECONOMIC FACTORS AND THEIR INFLUENCE ON OCCUPATIONAL PERFORMANCE

BARBARA SUSSENBERGER

The focus of this chapter is the influence of socioeconomic factors on people seeking occupational therapy. How do social and economic factors influence individual occupation in health and illness? Why and how do we need to take this into account as occupational therapy practitioners? Essentially I am talking about the importance of recognizing that there are supports and constraints on the options available to individuals in their occupational performance; it means that the kinds of choices and chances people have open to them in their education, jobs, leisure interests, living arrangements, self-care, and well-being are significantly affected by socioeconomic factors. When working at its best, occupational therapy services can assist clients to examine and expand their choices and resources.

Each of us occupies a "social position" that is individually and socially defined and constructed. Social positions are defined and constructed by the differences and inequalities among people or groups of people "that are consequential for the lives they lead, most particularly for the rights or opportunities they exercise and the rewards or privileges they enjoy" (Grabb, 1997, pp. 1–2). Social and material inequities refer to such resources as education, jobs, housing, and health care. At the individual level, our social position shapes our values, beliefs, and view of the world. As you can imagine, all of these are directly related to our interactions with clients and the effectiveness of any of our occupational therapy interventions and outcomes. The values, beliefs, and material resources of our clients have a high degree of variation and may be quite different from our own. We have to ensure that our services are directed to clients' needs and values and that client–practitioner communications are mutually understood. This means that the occupational therapy practitioner has to develop the ability to look at the world in the way the individual client sees it. Issues such as these need discussion and study in the educational preparation and day-to-day practice of occupational therapy practitioners.

DEFINING AND CONTEXTUALIZING SOCIOECONOMIC FACTORS

What Do We Mean by the Terms *Socioeconomic Status, Class, Stratification,* and *Social Inequalities*?

On the surface, it may seem as if the meaning of *socioeconomic status* (SES) were self-evident, but there are several terms that are used to indicate a recognition of social inequalities, and each has a slightly different meaning. SES is used to refer to occupational, educational, and income achievements by individuals or groups. Each of these categories has a level of social prestige or power. Through measurements of these achievements, the relative status of an individual or group can be compared to another (Johnson, 2000).

You may be more familiar with the term *class* to indicate differences. We frequently hear such differences through use of the terms *lower class*, *working class*, *middle class*, and *upper class*. Class is often used interchangeably with SES; however, while SES refers to differences among individuals, class is used as a way to indicate differences among groups (Gilbert & Kahl, 1993). To varying degrees, all societies are stratified by classes or class divisions; in some societies, classes are rigid and legally defined, whereas others (such as the United States) have "open" class systems, meaning that the differences are not legally enforced and that there is room for potential mobility between classes. Sociologist use the term *stratification* to refer to "studies of structured social inequality" (Marshall, 1994, p. 512). The United States, which is an industrialized, free-market society, is stratified largely according to economic rewards; and as Scase (1992) observes, such a social system is divided into "patterns of opportunity" (p. 42). *Social inequality* is used to refer to the unequal rewards and opportunities for different individuals or subgroups within a group or for groups within a society (Marshall, 1994).

Changing one's social or economic position in the social system, even within an open system, is not a straightforward matter of individual desire or ambition. Inequalities or the "patterns of opportunity" are persistent social problems, denoting that the United States offers less economic mobility than other rich countries (Economic Policy Institute, 2001). At the same time, there is the persistent American Dream, with its ideal of achievement and upward mobility.

Generational upward mobility can be observed at the individual SES level when a member of the younger generation has achieved more years of education, followed by employment in a prestigious profession, compared to the background of his or her parents. Upward mobility can be observed during the course of an individual's life span, often through what we sometimes call "career ladders" (Gilbert & Kahl, 1993). It is also possible for a person to experience downward mobility through such life events as illness, job loss, or unanticipated family difficulties. In our work settings, occupational therapy practitioners are often in a position to see people at a time in their personal history when they are struggling with losing their social, economic, and physical well-being. Illness and many other difficult life events can easily destabilize and shift the life course of a person. These are some of the factors we have to consider when we approach a new client.

In this chapter, the term *socioeconomic factors* is used to focus and stress the need to recognize that there are inequities of material resources and opportunities between and among individuals and groups of people in our society, all of which have multiple implications for the many facets of a person's occupational performance. A large share of our clients are struggling, not only with the health-related issues that brought them into contact with occupational therapy but also with meeting their personal and financial responsibilities day by day or week to week. In addition, as health-care professionals, we must remember that there are many people who do not even have access to health care because of their economic status. One of the roles of occupational therapy practitioners is a concern for the health and well-being of all members of our society. The individual practitioner may act on this level of social concern through social or political advocacy activities in our state and national associations.

The Intersections of Class, Gender, Race, Ethnicity, Age, and Disability

The notion of status, class differences, or inequalities in the United States is not an appealing one (Fig. 8-1). Americans typically avoid talking about this problem (Fussell, 1983; hooks, 2000). The idea that we all have equal chances and equal opportunities is one that we want to believe is true, that we can all go to the schools of our choice, enter any

STAHLER
HOW IS THE WORLD DIVIDED?
RACE, GENDER, CLASS & RELIGION

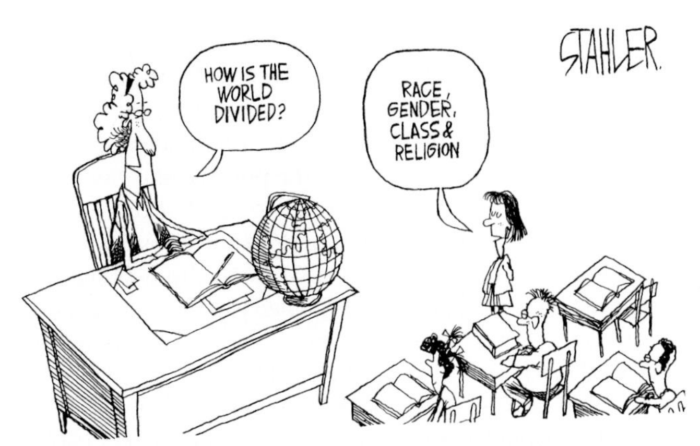

FIGURE 8–1. Divisions in our society are frequently unstated; however, they are implicitly understood through personal observations and experiences. (Jeff Stahler, reprinted by permission of Newspaper Enterprise Association, Inc.)

occupation we desire, and be free to participate in any leisure activity that appeals to us is the idealized version of our social system. On the other hand, we know from our individual experiences that this ideal is not so easily realized. Most of us have had to change or modify our plans or hopes and desires because we did not have the necessary resources to obtain what we wanted. The word *resource* is used broadly to include both material and social factors. The ability to meet our needs or achieve what we want out of life depends on a variety of factors; quite often, it is financial, but not entirely. Our individual support system may help us get through a difficult period more successfully than having substantial financial assets. There are multiple socioeconomic barriers confronting individuals and groups of people as they attempt to actively achieve their hopes and ambitions.

Inequalities are socially and materially enacted through the dynamic and changing interrelationships of such variables as class, gender, race, ethnicity, age, and disability. There are moments when these variables may intersect and we discover that one may take primacy over another. An example is obtaining a membership in a country club. Membership fees at an exclusive country club may be expensive, costing thousands of dollars. But in addition to the cost factor, there may also be an unstated criterion about membership that prevents the entry of an individual; it may be race, ethnicity, marital status, or occupation. Although an individual may have the financial resources for membership, another dynamic of our stratified social system could intersect and act as a barrier to joining the club.

Having the necessary financial resources or educational preparation is not all that affects entry into certain occupations. Other forms of social inequities can block the road to one's ambitions. Women have found it particularly difficult to enter some professions and jobs and to participate in some activities because of gender bias. Although opportunities have been rapidly changing and expanding, there are still fields that are hostile terrains for women. And there continue to be roles that are predominately perceived to be women's work (Apter, 1993; Hesse-Biber & Carter, 2000).

Race and ethnicity are two significant variables that affect the chances and choices of individuals. Educational opportunities and career paths are not equally open or accessible, and levels of health status are affected. The Children's Defense Fund (2001) reports that in 1999, approximately 12.1 million children were considered poor. Minority children are disproportionately poor: 33.1% of African American children and 30.3% of Hispanic American children compared to 13.5% of white children and 11.8% of Asian and Pacific Island children. Many of the health-related issues of minority groups are due to inadequate or unavailable medical care. However, people who are poor do not form a homogenous group, and we cannot equate race and ethnicity with being poor; indeed, to do so is a form of racism. On the other hand, we need to recognize that members of minority groups are at a greater risk of living in poverty because of racism. Some of the discussions of economic inequality that follow in this chapter refer to the experiences of members of minority groups because the issues of racism and poverty are so closely interrelated.

Age is another variable that shapes opportunity. Bee (2000) refers to Riley's term *age strata* to describe how all societies have some sorts of shared expectations and demands of its members based on age. *Ageism* is used to identify and describe discrimination based on age, but not all cultures perceive aging in a negative way (Bee, 2000). Aging is not perceived positively in the United States. Despite substantial research to the contrary, people in the age category we might call young-older adulthood are often seen as over the hill and too old to perform certain educational or vocational tasks. Although it is against the law to discriminate when hiring people, the 60-year-old man or woman who wants to (or needs to) make a career or even a job change does not find many open doors, regardless of his or her experience, skills, or educational background. Perhaps we will see a real decrease in ageism in this country along with the aging of the large Baby Boomer generation. Attitudes and social practice about age may soon change as members of the older generation in the United States forge new models and lifestyles of aging that will force all of us to develop other ways of looking at life-span development and occupational performance in the later years of adulthood.

People with disabilities have found educational, employment, and leisure opportunities blocked, regardless of their individual skills and abilities or financial resources. Accessible recreational resources are only recently being expanded or developed for persons with disabilities. Medical and technological advances have enabled people to be independent in the community, but that independence cannot be fully realized without access to education, jobs, or recreational resources. The social and political actions at the basis of the Americans with Disabilities Act and earlier legislation aimed at equal opportunities for people with disabilities reflect the efforts and outcomes to influence the inequities of the legal and social structures (Trattner, 1994). It is as important to alter the popular misperceptions of disability as it is to pass legislation, and occupational therapy practitioners are in a unique position to help make these changes (Bowman, 1992).

Despite the legislation intended to eliminate or reduce the social and economic inequalities that exist, and regardless of our professed beliefs in equal opportunity, life's choices and chances are not equal. This means that the occupational performance of an individual is mediated by many social and economic variables. The foregoing discussion is intended to point out variables that dynamically intersect. Sometimes the constraint on the individual is primarily because of economic disadvantages, but other times it might be gender, race-ethnicity, age, or disability that intervenes and blocks the individual's choices. The intersections of race, ethnicity, gender, age, disability, and sometimes geographic region are dynamic and specific—they change with the situation, and they change across time.

How Is Poverty Defined?

Poverty refers to the lack of material resources that are necessary for subsistence. At the social policy level, to help people acquire the necessary material resources and to determine who qualifies for assistance, poverty has to be defined in a way that it can be measured, this is what is commonly called the poverty line. This line, also referred to as the poverty threshold, is defined by the U.S. Census Bureau (2001a) as:

> *a set of money income thresholds that vary by family size and composition to determine who is poor. If a family's total income is less than that family's threshold, then that family, and every individual in it, is considered poor. The poverty thresholds do not vary geographically, but they are updated annually using the Consumer Price Index.* (p. 1)

In 1999, the poverty threshold for a single person was $8,501, and for a two-parent family with three children, it was $13,423 (U.S. Census Bureau, 2001b).

This definition of poverty lends itself to a great deal of debate since it does not account for geographical differences, relative standards of living, or the quality of life or well-being. Over time, some adjustments for minimum standards have been made at local levels based on such assumptions as considering that a minimum standard of living includes having electricity or a full bath. There are misconceptions and debates about how many people are poor, who are the poor, and who is at risk of being poor. Most researchers and human service agencies begin to examine those questions by using statistics collected by the U.S. Census Bureau, with the poverty threshold as a measure. But critics claim that the poverty line is pegged too low and thus serves as a way to lower the total number of people in poverty (Albelda, Folbre, & The Center for Popular Economics, 1996; Brouwer, 1998; Miringoff & Miringoff, 1999).

Living on the poverty line has a number of implications for the occupational performance of an individual or members of a family budget at or near the poverty line would impose severe constraints on the smallest kind of recreational outings like ball games, movies, or any kind of family excursion. Eating out would be impossible. Baby-sitters or summer camp would be too costly. Books, video games, toys, or music lessons could not be considered, neither would gifts or parties or special kinds of food for birthdays. Holidays would have to be planned and saved for across the whole year, and even then, they would have to be kept to a minimum (Sidel, 1996).

Who Is Poor? Who Is at Risk of Being Poor?

Certain categories of people are more at risk than others to living in poverty. Here are some examples (Dalaker & Proctor, 2000):

- Of all age groups, it is children (people under 18 years of age) who are most likely to be poor. Although the figures were down from preceding years, in 1999, the child poverty rate was 16.9%.
- The most vulnerable are related children under 6. The rate for this category in 1999 was 18.0%.
- The poverty rate for African Americans was 23.6% in 1999—about three times higher than for white non-Hispanics.
- Female-householder families represented the highest category of families in poverty, at 53%.

These figures give us some ideas about the extent of poverty and the categories of the population that are most vulnerable to the problem. But statistics can be, and often are, used in ways that mislead us into constructing stereotypes of who the poor are. In many ways, poverty is everywhere. Much of the stigma about poverty is directed toward those who are at risk. The tendency in our social system is to look at individuals or groups as "the problem" rather than looking at the social structural constraints that produce the problems (Scase, 1992).

Statistics used to record the number of people in poverty represent complexities embedded in our social system; the composition of the census categories shift and change with time as the political economy and the demographics change. The terms *working poor* and *the new poor* are used to identify what some of those complexities are and how some of those changes happen to individuals.

Working poor refers to a growing number of people who are working full time but whose wages do not raise them or their families above the poverty line. The new poor is a term used to describe a group of people who have fallen into poverty because of certain circumstances. For example, the economic consequences of a serious illness, divorce, unemployment, layoff, or other unplanned life change can start a downward spiral into poverty (Sidel, 1996).

One of the changes since the 1980s is the growing polarization between the rich and the poor, leaving what is called the "shrinking middle class." We are seeing a growth in the group of working poor and a downward slide for many who were once in the middle-income bracket. In the early 1990s, almost half the distribution of household income was in the top 20% while the bottom 20% of U.S. households received only 3.6% (Sidel, 1996). In that decade, it was the highest wage earners who experienced the greatest growth in salaries, they earned more than 95% of all workers, a 62.7% gain for chief executive officers (CEOs; Economic Policy Institute, 2001).

THESE PEOPLE USED TO IRRITATE ME...
UNTIL I WAS LAID OFF
STAHLER

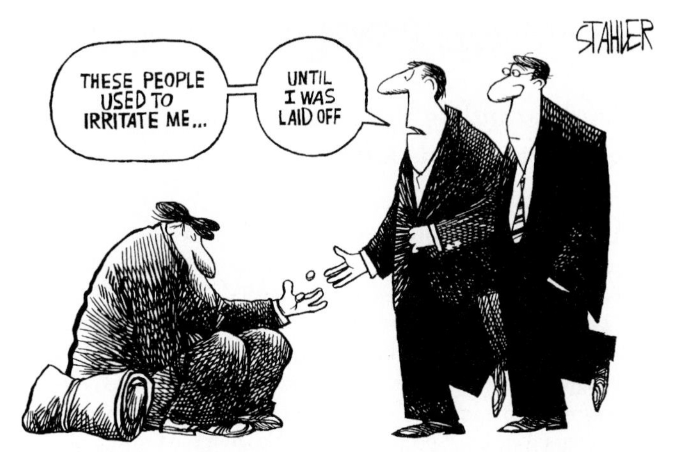

FIGURE 8–2. Our ability to empathize with people is often limited by the view from our own social position. (Jeff Stahler, reprinted by permission of Newspaper Enterprise Association, Inc.)

THE EFFECTS OF SOCIOECONOMIC FACTORS ON OCCUPATIONAL PERFORMANCE

Much of the social science research indicates that degrees of stratification are both internally and externally imposed. It is easy to see how this happens at the individual level; we develop our view of the world through the world in which we live. We want to join clubs and live in neighborhoods where we know people and where we feel comfortable (Gilbert & Kahl, 1993). This helps explain the tendency of the stratified social system to reproduce itself. But Gilbert and Kahl (1993) remind us that changes in society are continuous and that they transform lives, expectations, and possibilities. Shifts in the economy change job opportunities, and technological developments cause some fields to become obsolete while creating entirely new occupations. Mass media show us varieties of lifestyles that influence our ideas and ambitions. There is a constant tension between change and continuity in the social system, and the individual experience is a part of that dichotomy (Fig. 8-2).

Education

Starting off in poverty places children on a precarious educational trajectory.

> *Poor youths tend to score lower on national tests of reading, math, and vocabulary. They are twice as likely to repeat a grade. They have more behavior problems and are three times more likely to be expelled from school. The high school dropout rate of low-income 16 to 24 year olds is twice that of middle-income youths and 11 times that of wealthy children. The chances of earning a bachelor's degree are only half as good for poor high school sophomores as for the non-poor. (Sherman, 1997)*

The extent and quality of education are critical factors in the life course of an individual and are essential for survival, because employment opportunities are tied to educational attainment (Miringoff & Miringoff, 1999). Access to public education is a fundamental part of realizing the American Dream of being able to advance. The institution of the public school system played a "major role in establishing the democratic values of the nation" (Peterson, 1994, p. 234). But neither educational opportunities nor the quality of educational experiences is equitably distributed in our social system (Sennet & Cobb, 1972). School systems are a reflection of the beliefs, values, and structural inequality of the broader social system. Some who are concerned with issues of educational inequality claim the schools promote "an officially sanctioned system of privilege for the few, the powerful, and the able" (Books, 1998, p. xi).

Studies show that there is a positive correlation between school quality and the rate of future earnings (Albelda et al., 1996). School districts are based on residential patterns, and the schools in neighborhoods where the poverty rates are high tend to be overcrowded, understaffed, and undersupplied; their maintenance and repair are neglected, the nonhuman environment is unsafe, and the human environment is often violent (Kozol, 1991, 1995; Mooney, Knox, & Schact, 2000). It is not hard to imagine, given school environments such as these, that students get the message that they are not considered valuable resources for the future of society. A 15-year-old girl described her perceptions to Kozol (1995):

> *It's more like being 'hidden.' It's as if you have been put in a garage where, if they don't have room for something but aren't sure if they should throw it out, they put it where they don't need to think of it again. (pp. 37–38)*

It is also easy to understand the views of the world that children develop in settings such as these can differ substantially from those of children in well-financed school systems.

The foundation of life goals is the vision that people have for their future. This vision is based on a sense of capability and competence that is difficult to develop when schools are neglected and deprived of even the most basic of resources.

RESEARCH NOTE 8–1

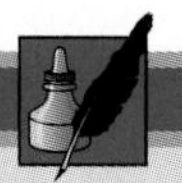

Understanding the Influence of Culture and Socioeconomic Influences on Occupational Choice

ELIZABETH CREPEAU

Understanding the lived experience of people seeking occupational therapy requires understanding their particular opportunities, expectations, and challenges. Farnsworth's (2000) study of time use and occupational engagement of Australian adolescent offenders over a 7-day period offers insights into their daily lives. Farnsworth used the experience sampling method which involved the participating adolescents wearing a beeper that was programmed to signal them at random intervals. She found that this group of adolescents were in productive occupations only 10% of the time they were beeped and were engaged in 30% more passive leisure than typical Australian adolescents. Because the adolescent offenders were likely to be out of school, they did not have opportunities to learn and to engage in sports and other extracurricular activities. They were further limited by a lack of financial resources and opportunities. Studies such as this one demonstrate the dynamics between social structures, financial resources, and opportunities and how they may enhance or constrict engagement in occupation and ultimately well-being. This study also suggests the importance of remaining in school as a way of sustaining occupations that foster development. Understanding the time use of young offenders can assist occupational therapy practitioners when designing interventions to foster engagement in occupations that offer the challenge, structure, and organization to support skill development and intrinsic motivation.

Farnsworth, L. (2000). Time use and leisure occupations of young offenders. *American Journal of Occupational Therapy, 54*, 315–325.

Kozol (1995) relates an illustration of a dream limited by opportunity that was told to him by a teacher in the South Bronx:

> *Many of the ambitions of the children . . . are locked in at a level suburban kids would scorn. It's as if the very possibilities of life have been scaled back. Boys who are doing well in school will tell me, 'I would like to be a sanitation man.' . . . In this neighborhood, a sanitation job is something to be longed for.* (p. 125)

One of the outcomes of more education is that it provides more opportunity structures for individuals to advance in jobs (Scase, 1992). The connections among education and work and upward mobility are clear, but again there is a tendency for the reproduction of social inequalities. Educational institutions in some high poverty areas may provide programs to fill only certain kinds of job markets, which are low in status, low in salary, and offer no security or advancement possibilities (Gilbert & Kahl, 1993). Students in these schools are channeled into such jobs without having other kinds of options available (Kozol, 1995).

Economic and social science research showed a growing disparity in the 1990s between those who can attend college and those who find the economic barriers too great for them or their children. Reasons for this are identified as largely due to increased tuition rates combined with decreased availability of tuition assistance. This means that families in the higher income brackets can be more readily assured that their children will have the opportunities for the professional careers that a college education provides (Peterson, 1994). Because education is such a critical element in the ability to lessen the risk of being poor or to achieve upward mobility, the effect of access to a college education has enormous consequences for the future of the children who are now in poverty.

Work

In the occupational therapy process, as we collaborate with clients to develop their long-term goals and objectives, education and paid work are often central concerns. Our direct services focus on the clients' abilities and functional skills in relation to their short- and long-term goals, but we do not always consider the goals in the broader context of the trends and issues of the economy. When a client is ready to return to work, it can be an indicator of success of our interventions, but can we describe the labor market to the client and assist in developing alternative strategies if certain kinds of jobs become scarce or if the client's skills become less marketable?

The upward mobility of an individual or the reduction of the risk of falling into poverty depends on the availability of educational opportunities and access to particular forms of work. Mobility is also inspired by the desire or hope to enter a particular profession or job. From the examples cited earlier, we know that in the absence of support and material resources individual aspirations are reduced or scaled back. Research consistently shows that parents' SES influences their children's level of educational attainment and career (Bee, 2000). Children growing up in areas of high unemployment and poor jobs have fewer chances and choices about work, and they perceive their choices as limited. Children also have fewer models of worker roles if their parents or other family members are unemployed or underemployed;

the environment and its limitations promote the tendency to the reproduction of stratification.

The job market varies with international, national, and regional economies at any given time, and thus employment opportunities are far from static. The late 1990s had a low overall unemployment rate, but looking behind that kind of statement reveals that there were different experiences for different groups. It is not surprising that the unemployment rate is higher in areas where the poverty rate is high, especially for young African Americans and Hispanics in poor urban neighborhoods (Economic Policy Institute, 2000). There are fewer job possibilities in these neighborhoods, and the quality of the schools is generally poor. The result is that young people with poor educational backgrounds have less competitive job market skills. Furthermore, the kinds of jobs that are available in neighborhoods with high poverty rates rarely offer benefits such as health care, nor do they open up chances for security or advancement (Albelda et al., 1996). Entry into work is ideally an active process of matching available opportunities with a person's skills and interests. Skill development depends not only on the person's innate abilities and aspirations but also on the quality of his or her educational preparation and the opportunities that are accessible.

In addition to problems of unemployment, are those associated with the working poor. We often think of low wage earners as teenagers in summer jobs, but estimates show that up to 43% of the minimum wage earners were full time in 1994, and 64% of them were women (Albelda et al., 1996). Many workers try to increase their incomes by taking on a second, third, and sometimes even a fourth job. But for those who are on the lower end of the scale, this strategy has limited success—in fact it tends to reproduce the problems of lower paying jobs. Hesse-Biber and Carter (2000) described this dilemma: "Due to lack of education or low socioeconomic status, these women supplement one poor job with another equally poor job" (p. 149). These difficulties or barriers to getting out of poverty caused by low-wage jobs are often further complicated by the demands of parenting, which can conflict with demands at work. Resources such as available childcare and transportation are difficult to obtain for the working poor (Henly, 1999).

Handler (1995) asked this question: "If the problem is poverty, and the vast majority of the poor are working and not on welfare, then what is the problem with work?" (p. 39). Trends in the labor market have implications for our future and for our clients who need to return to work. Over the years, there has been an overall decline in real wages, a decrease in the availability of jobs in the manufacturing sector, an increase in part-time work, and an increase in jobs without benefits; furthermore, the better jobs have increasingly higher education and skill requirements (Brouwer, 1998; Handler, 1995). The loss of manufacturing jobs in the United States since the 1980s, owing to a shift in the global economy, is significant because those jobs typically offered better paying opportunities for people with low educational backgrounds and minimum skills (Peterson, 1994).

Since the 1980s, developments in technology and international trade arrangements make it possible for corporations to relocate their production and other aspects of their operations to areas with the cheapest labor. Corporate downsizing and mergers have become commonplace since the 1980s. These transactions are usually accompanied by large layoffs, which have sometimes put entire communities out of work. Corporate executives and people working in middle management have not escaped the effects.

For example, a well-to-do corporate executive was given 9 months' notice that the division he headed was being closed by the company. During those 9 months, he searched, but could not find an equivalent job. He and his family were forced to move from their comfortable suburban home into a modest apartment. The social life of the entire family changed because they no longer had the same financial resources; as they lost contact with their old friends, tensions built up in the family, which heightened the feelings of instability and anxiety (Newman, 1988). This story is not about the experience of living at the poverty line; but instead, it illustrates that downward mobility can happen at any income level and that it reverberates through every activity of the whole family system.

Women's work and career patterns have differed from men's largely because they have taken time out for child rearing or other caretaker roles. This interrupted pattern of employment increases women's economic vulnerability, because career achievement and economic success are associated with working continuously (Bee, 2000). Divorce also increases women's liability to poverty. Sidel (1996) told about one woman who, after 23 years of marriage, was divorced by her husband. He subsequently left the state and provided no financial support for her or their children. In a few months, she found that her annual income went from $70,000 to $7,000. Her job as a home health aide was not enough to keep her out of poverty. Although she and the children went without heating oil for a winter and sold some household appliances, such as the dishwasher, she was unable to keep up payments on their home. The bank foreclosed on the mortgage, and she and her children found themselves homeless. Although she was able to obtain work, she had a relatively limited educational background and her prior work experience did not allow her to compete for jobs that would pay an adequate salary. This vulnerability continues into older adulthood for women retirees; their employment pattern of being in and out of the labor force also affects whether or not they have been able to accrue adequate retirement benefits (Bee, 2000).

Play and Leisure

Children learn and develop through their play activities. Not only does play help them learn about themselves as individuals but it is how they acquire their fundamental socialization skills. For adults, play and leisure occupations have similar roles of providing the experiences through which one learns about oneself, about others, and about the world. The neighborhoods described by Kozol (1991, 1995) are in areas overrun by poverty, crime, neglect, and abuse, in the form of polluting industries and incinerators. In some instances, parents are afraid to let their children play outdoors because of the high rate of crime and violence in the neighborhood. As noted earlier, the financial constraints required when living at the poverty line provide little room for toys, games, or such luxuries as music and sports lessons.

"Leisure, like work is stratified" (Kelly & Godbey, 1992, p. 120). You can see socioeconomic gradations in travel advertisements in your Sunday papers directed at specialized groups for "luxury class" or "budget" accommodations. You can see parents who take their children to a fast-food outlet, because it is too costly to go to a restaurant with three children. Some of the leisure research indicates that there are class differences not just with the economic differences of recreational choices but also with the type of activities in which people participate. Many of these patterns are linked to family and educational backgrounds that tend to be repeated by the children as they grow into adulthood (Gilbert & Kahl, 1993).

There is concern that leisure time is decreasing for people in the United States (Schor, 1992). The Economic Policy Institute (2001) reported the following about families' loss of leisure time:

> *Middle-class, married couple family's income grew 9.2% from 1989 to 1998, however a substantial part of this growth reflected a growth in family work hours, up 182 hours to 3,600 total or about 4.5 extra full-time weeks a year since 1989. (p. 7)*

And minorities feel the squeeze even more: "An average middle-income African American family with children needed over 12 more weeks of work than the average white family in order to reach the middle-income ranks" (p. 8).

The reasons given for the loss of available hours to enjoy leisure occupations are generally related to problems about trends in the job market. As companies cut back on the number of employees, the people who are kept on have more work to do and are afraid of losing their jobs; they feel they cannot refuse when asked to work overtime (Schor, 1992). Some employees invest more and more hours in their work to stay competitive in the job market in case their company merges or downsizes. Others are simply working more than one job, sometimes as many hours as they can to avoid or escape poverty. In situations such as these, leisure becomes even more important to a person's health and well-being, but time for leisure is problematic. Schor (1992) noted:

> *People report their leisure time has declined by as much as one third since the 1970s. Predictably, they are spending less time on the basics like sleeping and eating. Parents are devoting less time to their children. Stress is on the rise, partly owing to the 'balancing act' of reconciling the demands of work and family life. (p. 5)*

The juggling act of time and work for women is typically complicated by their additional hours of responsibilities in nonwaged household chores. Hesse-Biber and Carter's (2000) review of several studies that examined the number of hours invested in household chores by men and women showed that women consistently spend more hours than men on housework. This is often referred to as *women's double day*.

Health and Illness

Studies of socioeconomic differences in health and illness consistently illustrate patterns of relationships. The increase in chronic health conditions and limitations in daily activities present greater problems for the poor and working poor (Bee, 2000). One of the explanations for this relationship is reduced access to medical care for people in the lower income levels. Another explanation is the connection between poverty or low income and poor housing and the quality of the environment.

The higher poverty rates associated with race and ethnic groups are also reflected in studies of their health status (Berger, 1994).

> *African Americans also have shorter life expectancies than whites, and have higher rates of specific diseases; Hispanics have significantly lower rates of heart disease but suffer from other diseases at higher rates; some of these differences appear to be linked to variations in health habits and social class. (Bee, 2000, p. 126)*

Some of the large-scale, longitudinal research undertaken to examine the relations between class and health status have shown that even if specific causes of death are eliminated, there are still class differences in health status (Marmot et al., 1994). This means the focus of the solution cannot be disease specific. Higher income is associated with better health; however, we have seen that one of the trends in the economy is a widening wage gap between the rich and the poor. As the wage gap widens, there is a corresponding overall decline in the health of the population (Institute for the Future, 2000). Poverty, and its corresponding problems with nutrition, housing, and safety, places young children at risk for years of developmental problems and reduced life chances (Miringoff & Miringoff, 1999). The importance of the availability of resources for mothers and infants is a crucial factor in addressing the problems of poverty for those who are at highest risk.

The health of an individual is not largely determined by the health system. Individual health has more to do with other factors, identified earlier. For example, the quality of our environments, our educational experiences, the kind of job we have, the availability and quality of our social support system, and our self-perception all affect our health status. (Kelly & Godbey, 1992). Everyday activities and routines can make the difference in our health status, but given the descriptions of the daily problems people encounter, a healthy lifestyle is not that simple to establish or sustain. Some of the differences in social-class-related health habits are smoking, diet, and exercise. Poorer health habits are associated with lower education and lower income (Rice, 1994). Good nutrition—a central component of health—is a challenge for people below the poverty line, even for the most informed and creative cook. Furthermore, there is a strong connection between good health habits and a sense of personal control (Bee, 2000). But personal control or autonomy is difficult to feel when one is employed in a low paying job, is vulnerable to layoffs, or experiences other major stressors.

THE POLITICAL ECONOMY OF THE HEALTH-CARE SYSTEM

The health-care system in the United States has been described as unique (Shi & Singh, 1998); it reflects the cultural beliefs and values of this particular free-market system. It is a highly dynamic, complex, fragmented, and stratified system of competition, regulation, and reimbursement (Fig. 8-3). The United States is the only industrialized country in the world that does not have some form of national health insurance, which would ensure access to health care for all of its citizens. Embedded in the system is a tension between market justice and social justice. Corporate competition and individual responsibility tend to prevail. People who are on the lower end of the economic scale have two health-care concerns: access to care and quality of care when there is access.

Health care is not accessible to a significant and increasing number of people; 40–42 million people are estimated to have no health insurance, and another 52 million people are thought to have insufficient coverage (Brouwer, 1998; Institute for the Future, 2000; Shi & Singh, 1998). Those who are uninsured and in the poorest health have to postpone seeking medical help or have difficulty getting the care they need (Shi & Singh, 1998). It is not surprising that these groups experience higher death rates (Albelda et al., 1996).

Quality of care is also an issue. Kozol (1991) noted reports about the quality of health care in New York hospitals intended to serve the poor where there is "no working microscope to study sputum samples, no gauze or syringes" and where personnel were "running out of sutures in the operating room" (p. 116). Many times people choose not to seek health care in places such as this because they knew the system was dangerous to their health (Abraham, 1993).

The shifts in the economy since the 1980s and the mix of jobs and industries in it have added to the numbers of uninsured, because so much of our ability to obtain health coverage is linked to our job. In fact, it is the low-paying, low-skill jobs that are least likely to offer health insurance (Shi & Singh, 1998), and many of the new jobs that have been created in the 1990s are part time and offer no health benefits (Lee, Soffel, & Luft, 1994). Allen (1995) illustrated the links among employment, health insurance, and poverty with the following example. A 46-year-old single mother of two boys, who had worked for 26 years in a billing department of a hospital became seriously ill and was hospitalized for 2 weeks. Her illness caused her to lose more time at work, and eventually she used up all her vacation and sick time. As the bills accumulated, her older son's tuition at school had to be put on hold; she turned off her telephone and stopped the cable television services. She eliminated all the expenses she could, but the family still faced eviction and homelessness because she was behind in rent.

Elements of publicly financed health-care benefits such as Medicare and Medicaid are present and supported. Medicaid was intended to assist the poor who have no health coverage, however, many are not covered because of eligibility requirements and other regulations that create obstacles to care (Abraham, 1993). Furthermore, the range and scope of these programs are often the object of political debate. Despite the recognition that millions of people are uninsured or underinsured for their health needs, the arguments about reforming the system show little tendency to coming to agreement

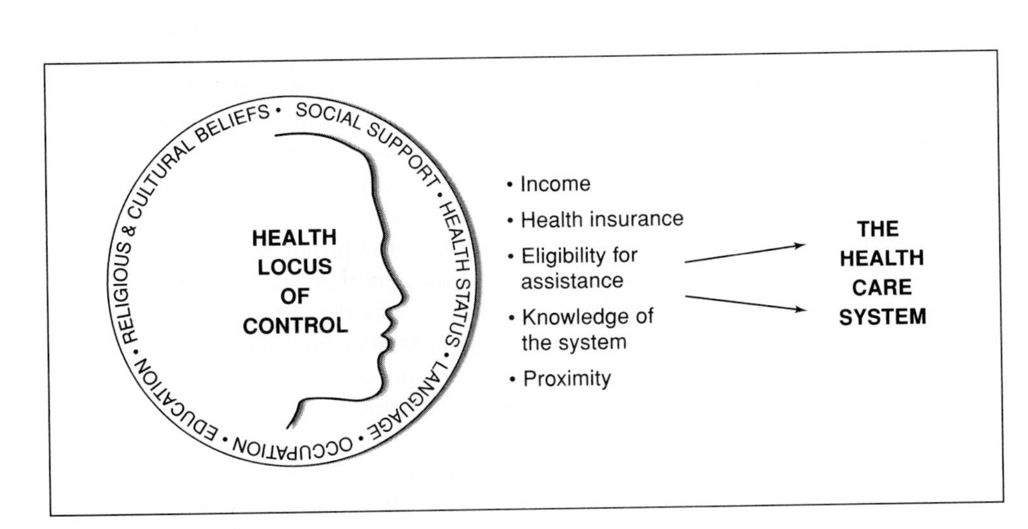

FIGURE 8–3. Individual decisions made when seeking and using services in the health-care system are based on the influence and interaction of many internal and external factors.

about how to "fix" it. Until such agreement is achieved, people living in poverty will continue to have difficulty gaining access to adequate health care.

OCCUPATIONAL THERAPY SERVICES—ARE THEY EQUITABLE? WHOM DO WE SERVE?

The preceding discussion on socioeconomic factors focused on domains of concern for occupational therapy practitioners: education, work, play and leisure, and health and illness. I have examined and discussed issues of social and economic inequities of a stratified social system. The ways in which health care is organized and delivered is a reflection of the larger system. Peloquin (1993) noted that one of the constructs that compromise the caring expressions of health practitioners is the "health care provision system that is driven by business, efficiency, and profit" (p. 936). We need to recognize that occupational therapy is a part of the health-care system and that our patterns of practice may reflect aspects of the inequities discussed in this chapter.

One of the occupational hazards of a health-care professional is a tendency to begin to think of clients in categories; patients, clients, consumers, or students: We have a caseload, we have a really interesting traumatic brain injury, or we have required numbers of treatment units per day. All of these terms are abstractions of what we really intend to offer in the occupational therapy process. As occupational therapy practitioners, we like to argue that one of the strengths of the profession is that we gear our approach to the whole person, but do we? Or how do we? That phrase does not simply mean that we address the physical and psychosocial domains in our outcome goals for a consumer with carpal tunnel syndrome. It means we have to learn about the consumer as "Ms. Smith" in the terms of her world, her perceptions, her experiences, and her realities of it. We have to develop "multicultural competencies" (Pope-Davis, 1993) and understand the cultural complexities we encounter in our practice through the kind of active-reflective process discussed in the preceding chapter. And we have to learn and understand the socioeconomic supports and constraints of Ms. Smith's world and integrate that knowledge into our work with her. We have to do this to be effective in our services to each person with whom we work. Without this, the follow-through or carryover of our services is unlikely. This is getting harder to do in today's health-care system, in which we may see Ms. Smith only two to five times, and those limited times are highly structured around specific outcome goals. For our interventions to be truly effective and ethical, they have to be geared to the contextual realities of each of our clients.

The first principle of the *Occupational Therapy Code of Ethics* states that occupational therapy personnel are responsible for providing services "in a fair and equitable manner"; included in this principle is that we need to "recognize and appreciate the cultural components of economics, geography, race, ethnicity, religious and political factors, marital status, sexual orientation, and disability" (American Occupational Therapy Association, 2000, pp. 614–615). But sometimes our services are discriminatory. In addition to our individual personalities and experiences, which affect our relationships with clients, all the attributes that make us professionals may be factors that contribute to a distancing between ourselves and our clients. Purtilo and Haddad (1996) use several examples to point out the difficulties that may emerge between a practitioner and a client because of SES differences. These differences can influence how we feel and what we do about our therapeutic interventions with clients in such dimensions as our capacity to empathize or our ability to understand daily routines and priorities that differ from our own (Purtilo & Haddad, 1996). As Olson (2001) observed "most occupational therapists in the United States are members of the dominant white middle-class culture; the privilege that they have experienced based upon race and socioeconomic standing must be acknowledged" (p. 184). We may not be consciously aware of how our client interactions are affected by these factors, but we may act it out in subtle ways. In addition to concern about individual clients, occupational therapy practitioners also have to recognize the inequities of the broader social system and must "move beyond seeing success as due to one's personal effort" (p. 184).

Many of our assessment tools contain categories of occupational performance skills and habits. Because we have to objectify our documentation, the categories of occupational performance become abstract and we tend to lose sight of the complexities. This problem is clearly illustrated in Chapter 7. Although the effect of socioeconomic factors on occupational performance are not directly addressed, Dunn, Brown, and McGuigan (1994) referred to the need for us to consider the effect of "context" and question if "standardized functional assessments are valid for capturing what is actually known about the person's performance in the natural context" (p. 605). On-site home and job site visits are examples of how the practitioner can come in direct contact and observation of the client in his or her own environment. Knowledge and understanding of the client's home and work environments greatly increase the effectiveness of our interventions. However, the context of these visits may also bring the practitioner into conflict with values, priorities, and resources available for self-care, diet, or other occupational performance components. Practitioners find themselves overwhelmed and intimidated at times by the social and economic barriers that challenge their clients. Home or job site visits are not always possible to undertake, but we can become more familiar with the neighborhoods in which our clients live and work as a matter of our own orientation to our work settings.

As occupational therapy practitioners, we often feel compromised by what services we can offer our clients compared to what we want to offer. Our services are constrained by the particulars of reimbursement, and that system in health care does take such things as the socioeconomic status of our clients into account through the inequities of the private or public health insurance programs. So how do we give the maximum to each and every client and stay within the constraints of the system? We want to keep our focus on the ideals of what services we could offer. One practitioner made a decision always to include a note or a list of occupational therapy services recommended as the ideal for her clients with the documentation for services that were allowed for reimbursement. This kind of daily documentation practice keeps the gaps between the ideal and the real in the forefront. It helps maintain a focus on ethical practice, and it communicates the gaps to third-party payers. There are active and proactive approaches we can take individually or through organizations to promote and support change in the system, but our focus on ethical ideals of occupational therapy have to become a part of our day-to-day work, otherwise we become a part of the problem, not a part of the solution.

The majority of health and human service professionals would say that they learned their most important lessons from their clients. These stories are usually about how the professional lacked an understanding of the situation and the client set her straight about how things really were. This means we have to listen, and in order to listen we have to ask the right questions and give the time and space for the answers. Some studies have shown that physicians interrupt their patients after 18 sec of their attempts to describe or explain their symptoms or problems (Frishman, 1996). We do not know how long occupational therapy practitioners wait and listen to clients' responses before trying to categorize them or attempting to resolve a problem based on personal ideas and assumptions about what would be best. Fortunately, there are some instructive lessons in the occupational therapy literature in the form of qualitative research contributions that show us the benefits of asking and listening (Peloquin, 1993, 1995; Wood, 1996).

Clark et al. (1996) identified "adaptive strategies" of a group of low-income, older, well adults as a way to describe how and what they did to successfully maintain their engagement in occupations that were of personal and individual significance. They recognized that the environment required particular kinds of adaptation. Issues such as safety in the neighborhood had to be taken into account, as did the financial resources available for recreation or for activities of daily living. This study placed personal importance as a first consideration and put it in the context of the older adults' living environment and financial constraints. The authors enabled us to see the potential for preventive services that are informed by the values and beliefs of individuals as well as by socioeconomic constraints.

Fidler's (1996) lifestyle performance model also offers a construct that would take the individual and environmental context into account. The model "stresses an initial focus on individual interests, capacities, and customary patterns of daily living as the basis for defining and prioritizing any intervention" (p. 141). Whatever assessment tools we choose to use, we need to put the emphasis on the individual's priorities, resources, and constraints. This means that we have to integrate knowledge and consideration of socioeconomic factors. A large part of the occupational therapy process is enabling our clients' problem solving; we need to know how to assist in realizing goals, which means we have to know how clients can obtain necessary resources. If we can do this, we can help people break through some of the barriers to their goals.

INCORPORATING KNOWLEDGE OF SOCIOECONOMIC FACTORS INTO OUR PRACTICE

At the beginning of the chapter, I described occupational therapy services as being most effective when they assist clients to expand the choices and resources that are available to them. To accomplish this promise of occupational therapy requires knowledge of the communities in which we work and the networks of social, medical, educational, voluntary public, and private organizations that make up potential resources. It requires knowledge of the policy definitions of eligibility for various forms of assistance. And it involves having experience in the community, knowing its politics and its economy, and asking questions.

- Where are the jobs and what kind are they?
- What is the unemployment rate?
- What are the schools like?
- What are the characteristics of the community and the population served by the agencies where we work?

A lot of this kind of knowledge and experience we learn firsthand, and we learn from others—professionals, volunteers, and especially our clients. Very often, the issues themselves can shape the focus of group sessions with some of our clients in which all members contribute to each others' knowledge base. For example, job readiness groups, money management groups, and cooking (for three on a poverty-line budget) groups that draw on knowledge and direct experience of the clients' environments are excellent vehicles for clients to learn new strategies and identify new resources.

LESSONS FROM CLIENTS

The following vignettes describe four lessons learned from clients to illustrate some of the points discussed throughout the chapter about the effect of socioeconomic factors on occupational performance.

Work

An occupational therapy group at a day treatment center was intended to enable its members to build job readiness skills in eight sessions. Two sessions of this group were devoted to how to write résumés. However, the jobs that the clients were hoping to get did not require résumés. The kinds of jobs people were looking for included waitress, hardware store clerk, janitor, and counter help in a fast-food chain; jobs such as these require being able to fill out forms, and, most important, being able to interact and communicate effectively in a short interview. The notion of a résumé being such an important tool in the clients' job searches came from the occupational therapy practitioner's own experience as a health-care professional. The two sessions of the group that were devoted to this topic were lost time that could have been spent role playing the kind of interviews the clients might encounter.

Play and Leisure

A client at a mental health center gave me an effective lesson in choices. I asked the client to complete an interest inventory of leisure activities, a commonly used assessment tool. He was asked to check those activities that he enjoyed doing and those he did not enjoy. A third column asked him to check any of the activities that he would like to learn to do. His response was to check the third column for the entire list. When I asked him to discuss his responses, he explained that he had never had the opportunity to learn to do any of the activities on the list. His background information confirmed his explanation; his childhood was spent moving from one foster home to another, and he had few memories of play or toys. Some of the activities on the list required special equipment or instruction; in other words, they required resources that were unavailable to him. Later, he was able to make up his own list of leisure interests based on his experiences that were not on the "official" occupational therapy list he was given to complete.

One Monday morning a client told me about taking her children on a trip over the weekend. As she described the trip, it became clear that her experiences and mine were very different. She finally got up the courage to take the public bus to a city park, where she and her children had a picnic lunch and a paddleboat tour around the pond in the center of the park. The bus trip was < 5 miles, but she and her children had never been in that section of the city before, because, as she explained, she had never thought about being able to leave the housing project or the neighborhood where she lived. Furthermore, neither she nor her two school-age children had ever been on a picnic. Her weekend activity with her children was an adventure that took a lot of courage to try out some new skills and ideas that were inspired by the encouragement and coaching of other group members in the program.

Self-Care

An occupational therapy colleague once told me about a client she worked with on transfer skills for bathing and toileting. More by chance than by design, the practitioner did a follow-up home visit a few weeks after discharge. To the practitioner's surprise, the client's home had no indoor plumbing. The occasional showers that were accessible to the former client were at the home of a friend a few miles away. The client had been too self-conscious to tell the practitioner at the rehabilitation center that the resources that were available at home for personal hygiene were different from the practitioner's assumptions. The skills the client needed at home were not the same as those that were worked on during the therapy sessions at the rehabilitation center; but they could have been, if the practitioner had known more about the client.

CONCLUSION

The foregoing examples all indicate that despite the best intentions, it is quite possible for a practitioner to implement an intervention strategy without adequate or accurate client information. Within the client–practitioner relationship there is a power dynamic that is often intimidating for clients because of the professional–patient roles. Even when we feel as if our planning with a client were a collaborative effort, we may have imposed our ideas and values in such a way that the client feels compelled to comply. This may be especially true for clients who are less educated than their health professionals. The socioeconomic factors discussed throughout this chapter come into play in our relationships with clients and their families.

While listening and learning from individual clients are paramount to effective occupational therapy interventions, we also have to remember that this approach individualizes the underlying problems of the social structural constraints. The social system has a tendency to produce and reproduce problems of stratification (Scase, 1992). On the one hand, we have to work with and understand each client individually with knowledge of the particulars of their resources, but this can obscure the larger issues resulting from the kind of social and material inequities I have discussed. As the profession of occupational therapy advocates for practice models that are truly client centered and that move away from the institutionalized medical model to community settings and health promotion, it is even more incumbent on us to incorporate and apply knowledge of social, economic, and political factors that affect the health and well-being of people. We have to be able to work at both levels—the individual level and the social policy level—to offer occupational therapy services that are ethical, effective, and equitable.

References

Abraham, L. (1993). *Mama might be better off dead: The failure of health care in urban America*. Chicago: University of Chicago Press.

Albelda, R., Folbre, N., & The Centre for Popular Economics. (1996). *The war on the poor: A defense manual*. New York: New Press.

Allen, L. (1995, December 31). Family's careful balance collapses during illness. *The New York Times*, section A p. 27.

American Occupational Therapy Association. (2000). Occupational therapy code of ethics. *The American Journal of Occupational Therapy, 54*, 614–616.

Apter, T. (1993). *Working women don't have wives: Professional success in the 1990s*. New York: St. Martin's.

Bee, H. L. (2000). *The journey of adulthood* (4th ed.). Upper Saddle River, NJ: Prentice-Hall.

Berger, K. (1994). *The developing person through the life span*. New York: Worth.

Books, S. (Ed.). (1998). Invisible children in the society and its schools. Mahwah, NJ: Erlbaum.

Bowman, O. J. (1992). Americans have a shared vision: Occupational therapists can help create the future reality. *American Journal of Occupational Therapy, 46*, 391–396.

Brouwer, S. (1998). *Sharing the pie: A citizen's guide to wealth and power in America*. New York: Holt.

Children's Defense Fund. (2001). Frequently asked questions about child poverty. Available at: www.childrensdefense.org. Accessed on April 18, 2001.

Clark, F., Carlson, M., Zemke, R., Frank, G., Patterson, K., Ennevor, B., Rankin-Martinez, A., Hobson, L., Crandall, J., Mandel, D., & Lipson, L. (1996). Life domains and adaptive strategies of a group of low-income, well older adults. *American Journal of Occupational Therapy, 50*, 99–108.

Dalaker, J., & Proctor, B. (2000). Poverty in the United States: 1999. [U. S. Census Bureau, Current Population Reports, Series P60-210]. Available at: www.census.gov/hhes/www/poverty.html. Accessed on: March 27, 2001.

Dunn, W., Brown, C., & McGuigan, A. (1994). The ecology of human performance: A framework for considering the effect of context. *American Journal of Occupational Therapy, 48*, 595–607.

Economic Policy Institute. (2000). The state of working America 2000–01. Introduction available at: www.epinet.org/books/swa2000/swa2000 intro.html. Accessed on: May 2, 2001.

Economic Policy Institute. (2001). Issue Guide. Minimum wage: Frequently asked questions. Available at: www.epinet.org/Issueguides/ minwagefaq.html. Accessed on: May 2, 2001.

Fidler, G. (1996). Life-style performance: From profile to conceptual model. *The American Journal of Occupational Therapy, 50*, 139–147.

Frishman, R. (1996, August). Quality of care: Don't be a wimp in the doctor's office. *Harvard Health Letter, 21*, 1–2.

Fussell, P. (1983). *Class: A guide through the American status system*. New York: Touchstone.

Gilbert, D., & Kahl, J. (1993). *The American class structure: A new synthesis* (4th ed.). Belmont, CA: Wadsworth.

Grabb, E. G. (1997). *Theories of social inequality: Classical and contemporary perspectives* (3rd ed.). New York: Harcout Brace.

Handler, J. (1995). *The poverty of welfare reform*. New Haven, CT: Yale University Press.

Henly, J. (1999). Barriers to finding and maintaining jobs: The perspectives of workers and employers in the low-wage labor market. In J. Handler. & L. White (Eds.). *Hard labor: Women and work in the post-welfare era* (pp. 48–75). Armonk, NY: Sharpe.

Hesse-Biber, S., & Carter, G. (2000). *Working women in America: Split dreams*. New York: Oxford University Press.

hooks, b. (2000). *Where we stand: Class matters*. New York: Routledge.

Institute for the Future. (2000). *Health and health care 2010: The forecast, the challenge*. San Francisco: Jossey-Bass.

Johnson, A. (2000). *The Blackwell dictionary of sociology: A user's guide to sociological language* (2nd ed.). Malden, MA: Blackwell.

Kelly, J., & Godbey, G. (1992). *The sociology of leisure*. State College, PA: Venture Publishing.

Kozol, J. (1991). *Savage inequalities: Children in America's schools*. New York: HarperCollins.

Kozol, J. (1995). *Amazing grace*. New York: Crown.

Lee, P., Soffel, D., & Luft, H. (1994). Costs and coverage: Pressures toward health care reform. In P. Lee, P. & C. Estes (Eds.). *The nation's health* (4th ed, pp. 204–213). Boston: Jones & Bartlett.

Marshall, G. (Ed.). (1994). *The concise Oxford dictionary of sociology*. Oxford, UK: Oxford University Press.

Marmot, M., Smith, G., Stansfeld, S., Patel, C., North, F., Head, J., White, L., Brunner, E., & Feeney, A. (1994). Health inequalities and social class. In P. Lee & C. Estes (Eds.). *The nation's health* (4th ed., pp. 34–40). Boston: Jones & Bartlett.

Miringoff, M., & Miringoff, M. (1999). *The social health of the nation: How America is really doing*. New York: Oxford University Press.

Mooney, L, Knox, D., & Schacht, C. (2000). *Understanding social problems* (2nd ed.). Belmont, CA: Wadsworth/Thomson Learning.

Newman, K. S. (1988). *Falling from grace: The experience of downward mobility in the American middle-class*. New York: Vintage Books.

Olson, L. (2001). Child psychiatry in the USA. In L. Lougher (Ed.). *Occupational therapy for child and adolescent mental health* (pp. 173–191). New York: Churchill Livingstone.

Peloquin, S. M. (1993). The patient-therapist relationship: Beliefs that shape care. *The American Journal of Occupational Therapy, 47*, 935–942.

Peloquin, S. M. (1995). The fullness of empathy: Reflections and illustrations. *The American Journal of Occupational Therapy, 49*, 24–31.

Peterson, W. C. (1994). *Silent depression: The fate of the American dream*. New York: Norton.

Pope-Davis, D. B. (1993). Exploring multicultural competencies of occupational therapists: Implications for education and training. *The American Journal of Occupational Therapy, 47*, 838–844.

Purtilo, R., & Haddad, A. (1996). *Health professional and patient interaction* (5th ed.). Philadelphia: Saunders.

Rice, D. (1994). Health status and national health priorities. In P. Lee & C. Estes (Eds.). *The nation's health* (4th ed., pp. 45–58). Boston: Jones & Bartlett.

Scase, R. (1992). *Class*. Minneapolis: University of Minnesota Press.

Schor, J. (1992). *The overworked American: The unexpected decline of leisure*. New York: Basic.

Sennett, R., & Cobb, J. (1972). *The hidden injuries of class*. New York: Norton.

Sherman, A. (1997). Poverty matters: The cost of child poverty in America. [Washington, DC: The Children's Defense Fund]. Available at: www.childrensdefense.org. Accessed on: April 18, 2001.

Shi, L., & Singh, D. (1998). *Delivering health care in America: A systems approach*. Gaithersburg, MD: Aspen.

Sidel, R. (1996). *Keeping women and children last: America's war on the poor*. New York: Penguin.

Trattner, W. (1994). *From poor law to welfare state: A history of social welfare in America* (5th ed.). New York: Free Press.

U.S. Census Bureau. (2001a). How the Census Bureau calculates poverty. Available at: www.census.gov/hhes/poverty/povdef.html. Accessed on: March 27, 2001.

U.S. Census Bureau. (2001b). Poverty thresholds in 1999. Available at: www.census.gov/hhes/poverty/threshld99.html Accessed on: May 10, 2001.

Wood, W. (1996). Delivering occupational therapy's fullest promise: Clinical interpretations of "Life domains and adaptive strategies of a group of low-income, well older adults." *American Journal of Occupational Therapy, 50*, 109–112.

CHAPTER 9

THE MEANING OF PLACE AS A COMPONENT OF SELF

GRAHAM D. ROWLES

THE PERSON–ENVIRONMENT RELATIONSHIP IN OCCUPATIONAL THERAPY

Place in Human Experience

Increased recognition of the role of the environment in conditioning human experience began to permeate occupational therapy during the 1980s (Barris, 1986; Barris, Kielhofner, Levine, & Neville, 1985; Kiernat, 1982, 1987). It is now widely accepted that full understanding of a person cannot be achieved independently of an appreciation of environmental context—the place in which he or she dwells. Occupational therapists have proposed several recent theories of the person–environment relationship that emphasize this interdependence (Christiansen & Baum, 1997; Dunn, Brown, & McGuigan, 1994; Kielhofner, 1995; Law et al., 1996; Schkade & Schultz, 1992). These transactional theories are moving away from simple sequential stimulus–response conceptualizations of the individual as influenced by the environment and the environment as modified by human action and toward directly acknowledging the degree to which the relationship involves the blending of person and place in human experience (Chapter 18). There is growing realization that the self is in and of rather than separate from the individual's environment and that lives are intimately and inextricably immersed in place.

There is also increasing recognition that each person's relationship with environment cannot be considered independently of an historical context and the accumulation of experiences of place over time (Settersten, 1999; Wheeler, 1995). Each person is born in a particular location, into a particular family configuration, into a particular culture, and into a specific birth cohort. Over the course of life, each individual is molded by experience—a melding of physiological capability, individual agency, and circumstance—in a manner that profoundly influences the person he or she becomes.

Phenomenological Perspective

Effective occupational therapy practice requires more than cursory inspection of a person's physical setting and compilation of a brief personal history. Probing deeper, it is important to understand each person from the perspective of an experienced context—the life world within which he or she conducts daily activities, defines the self, and receives occupational therapy intervention. From such a phenomenological perspective, how does the person experience his or her world? To what extent has he or she created the physical setting of home, with its familiar furniture, memorabilia, and photographs, as an expression of self, perhaps over the course of decades? To what extent is he or she continuing to manipulate the setting in accommodating to changing needs and abilities in ways that facilitate maintaining a sense of self, agency, and a meaningful life? Alternatively, in what ways is he or she a prisoner of space, constrained by the configuration and accoutrements of the setting and trapped in a place that is increasingly confining and restrictive? In essence, what is the meaning of dwelling in a particular place and what are the implications of this meaning for the practice of occupational therapy? To answer such questions, it is important to understand complex dimensions of meaning that characterize the phenomenon of *dwelling* and that nurture a therapeutically desirable sense of *being in place* (Rowles, 1991, 2000).

Relevance to Occupational Therapy

Developing a sense of each person's environmental, life course, and phenomenological contexts is of paramount importance to practitioners because occupational therapy interventions are invariably framed against the backdrop of a person's unique sense of self and of being in place. Interventions that take an individual out of place—for example, those that occur in a hospital, clinic, or rehabilitation environment—are invariably compromised because the agenda of the person is necessarily expanded to cope with accommodation to an unfamiliar setting. In some cases, treatment in a hospital or clinical setting is inevitable because of the availability of specialized equipment and personnel. This does not obviate the need for understanding the dimensions of a person's being in place. Rather, it makes such understanding even more important when designing treatment settings that create a level of environmental comfort conducive to effective occupational therapy practice.

DIMENSIONS OF BEING IN PLACE

A person's sense of being in place is a complex and dynamic phenomenon (Rowles, 1978; Rubinstein & Parmalee, 1992; Tuan, 1977). Several underlying themes or dimensions can be identified (Box 9-1).

BOX 9–1 DIMENSIONS OF BEING IN PLACE

USE OF SPACE

Immediate physical activity: Range of motion and functional capability-related movement in the proximal environment.

Everyday activity: Routine and often repeated daily trips along familiar pathways involved in the conduct of daily life.

Occasional trips: Vacations and long-distance trips, generally involving overnight stays.

ORIENTATION IN SPACE

Personal schema: Physiologically based axial orientation that enables the individual to maintain balance and distinguish left from right, front from back, and up from down.

Specific schemata: Cognitive linear maps of regularly traveled pathways, including an awareness of environmental cues that facilitate successfully traversing space.

General schema: An implicit cognitive map of the world as known, which can be evoked and mentally constituted at diverse scales and in diverse manifestations that vary according to the circumstances in which it is invoked.

EMOTIONAL AFFILIATIONS WITH PLACE

Personal: Emotions evoked by personal experiences within particular locations that imbue settings with meaning and significance for the individual may be positive or negative.

Shared: Mutually developed emotions for place refined through interaction over time among residents of a shared environment.

VICARIOUS PARTICIPATION IN SPATIALLY AND/OR TEMPORALLY DISPLACED ENVIRONMENTS

Reflective: Involvement in places of one's past (either the current environment as it was in the past or previously experienced places located elsewhere).

Projective: Vicarious projection into contemporary places that are geographically displaced from the individual's current location.

Using Space

At its most fundamental and easily observable level, being in place involves patterns of occupation, of activity in using space. Space is used on multiple levels. First is the domain of immediate physical activity or range of motion. This involves activities of daily living; for example, the functional ability to reach for a high shelf or to crouch without difficulty to pin up a skirt. Use of space on this level becomes a primary focus of occupational therapy when activity becomes limited through illness or accident.

On a larger scale, we traverse the physical environment and trace regular pathways of everyday activity that over

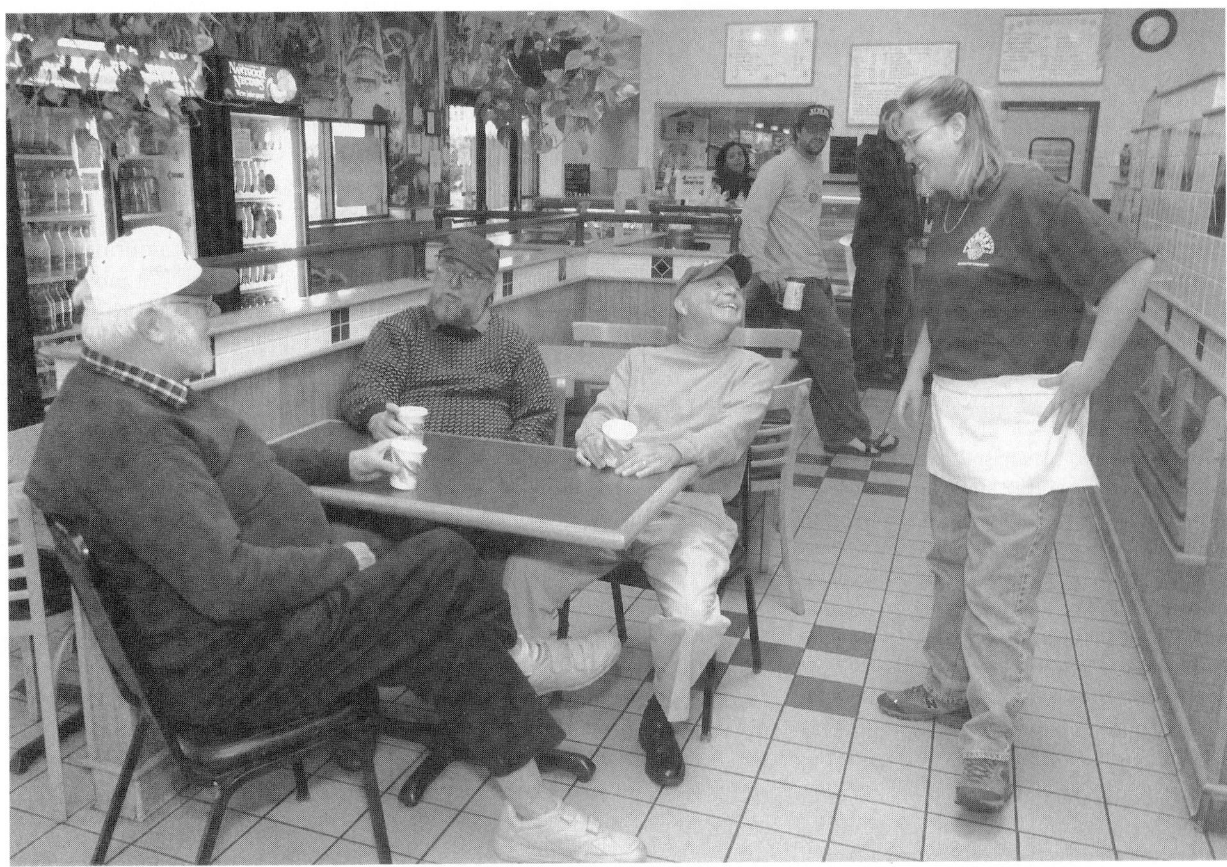

FIGURE 9–1. The everyday habit of breakfast at a local eatery forms important relationships. (Photo courtesy of D, Prince, University of New Hampshire Photographic Services Durham, NH.)

time may become habitual (Rowles, 1978, 2000; Seamon, 1980). Each weekday morning, we walk to the corner of our street to catch the bus to work. On Sundays, we drive a familiar route to church. Over time, we tend to develop a regular time–space rhythm and routine in use of the physical environment that becomes taken for granted and subconscious as our body adapts to the setting (Fig. 9-1). Recent occupational therapy research suggests that deeper understanding of habits and habituation may hold the key to important therapeutic interventions (American Occupational Therapy Foundation, 2000).

The regular routine of everyday behaviors is enriched or disrupted by occasional trips that take us beyond our daily round. We vacation in a distant state or make an annual visit to stay with a relative. After a motor accident, we may spend a period recuperating in a rehabilitation hospital some way from our home.

Over the life course, patterns of using space gradually evolve in concert with changing capabilities and resources. The infant is restricted to a crib or playpen. The child, under a parent or sibling's watchful eye, may be permitted to play in the garden or in the neighborhood. Access to a first automobile significantly increases spatial range and in adulthood may lead to a propensity to travel far and wide. With advancing years, the space within which we physically reside and travel may become limited once again as we become environmentally vulnerable.

Patterns of using space are closely intertwined with the manner in which we cognitively orient ourselves in the environment. This involves a physiological orientation within the axial system of the human body that provides the ability to discriminate up from down, left from right, and front from back. This personal schema is taken for granted. Its critical role may be fully recognized only when we become *dis*oriented through a health condition such as Ménière disease that affects balance, the secondary effects of medication, or excessive consumption of alcohol.

Physiologic orientation is a necessary but not sufficient condition for moving around in the environment. It is also necessary to develop mental images, cognitive maps of the configuration of the environment that guide us as we traverse space (Downs & Stea, 1973). Over time, we develop detailed cognitive awareness of paths we trace each day. This awareness may involve an array of environmental cues, comprising specific schemata that mark each route we take: The more familiar the journey, the more implicit the schemata. The first time we walk an unfamiliar route, we are acutely aware of directions, the environmental cues that

ETHICS NOTE 9–1

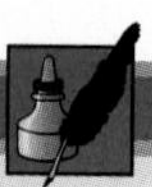

The Question of Driving Safety

PENNY KYLER and RUTH HANSEN

Louise is a 71-year-old widow who has traveled widely and been an active and lively participant in the cultural scene of her small town. In addition, she has driven from the East Coast to New Mexico several times in the last few years to attend an opera festival. Six months ago, Louise experienced a moderate cerebral vascular accident with resultant left hemiparesis and left side neglect. She is currently at home living alone. She has grown tired of having to depend on friends and neighbors for rides to various places. For the past 2 weeks, Louise has been driving by herself on the streets of her small community. She mentioned just at her last therapy session that she plans to make her trip westward for the opera season.

QUESTIONS AND EXERCISES

1. **As her home health therapist, what are your legal and ethical responsibilities? To Louise, to the members of her community, and to the public at large?**
2. **What, if any, are Louise's obligations to her community?**
3. **How should the therapist handle the information regarding Louise's driving, if she has not gotten the information directly from Louise?**

friends have related mark the places to turn or to cross the street. But as we repeatedly pass along this way, the need to use these cues recedes into the subconscious.

Cognitive awareness of regular pathways is embedded within a general schema. This implicit cognitive map of the world as we know it is characteristically centered on our home. It involves detailed awareness of zones of immediately adjacent space; for example, the surveillance zone—the area within the visual field in which we may develop strong visual or mutually supportive relationships with neighbors characterized by a high level of everyday reciprocity (Rowles, 1981) (Fig. 9-2). We may also be familiar with space beyond the visual field, which becomes identified as our neighborhood. Moving farther away from home, cognitive awareness of space becomes progressively sketchier. There may be limited cognitive knowledge of the configuration of spaces beyond our own community, city, or town. The exception is a limited number of "beyond spaces." These are places we have visited on occasional trips, settings in which we lived in the past, or familiar places where relatives reside. We may retain detailed images of the configuration of such places.

Life-course transitions in the use of space are paralleled by evolution in the manner in which we orient in space. In childhood, the experienced environment may be limited to our home and surroundings in the immediate vicinity. As experience increases and we become more geographically liberated, our cognitive world becomes more extensive. A cosmopolitan mobile pattern of life in adulthood may lead to familiarity with environments throughout the world and an acute sense of their configuration and spatial relationship to one another. If we lead a life focused on a single urban neighborhood or rural community, our orientation may be equally rich and detailed but more locally focused. Finally, as we grow older, the tricks of memory and the sheer volume of accumulated place experiences may result in complex overlapping cognitive images within which specific locations may be known simultaneously as they were during a series of different times in their existence. Our awareness of a less frequently visited location may be a residual memory of its past rather than an accurate image of its current configuration. Indeed, when we return to such a setting we may no longer recognize it and may become disoriented.

Meaning in Place

Patterns of use and cognitive orientation to place parallel the development and reinforcement of distinctive place-related emotions (Altman & Low, 1992; Seamon, 1984). Some of these are individual and highly personal. They may express a sense of affinity with places where key life events transpired—where we met our future spouse, made love for the first time, or experienced a traumatic event. Mere presence in such places may evoke memories, the resurrection in consciousness of key incidents in our lives, and strong visceral emotions. As life experiences accumulate, frequently inhabited places where multiple events occurred over an extended period of time become suffused with an array of emotions, reflecting a place biography of self and setting.

Other place-related emotions are shared. They arise from common habitation of a space—for example, an inner-city neighborhood—by a cohort of residents who, through their interaction and shared experiences, gradually come to imbue the place with its own personality, identity, and meaning as a social space (Rowles, 1978; Suttles, 1969). Long-time residents of changing neighborhoods may share complex emotional identification with a collage of the many different places it has been over the course of their lives, ranging from vibrant new development to rundown and largely abandoned slum.

Recognition of the critical role of time in human experience allows us to understand being in place as far more than the physical occupation of a space, the use of orientation skills, and the development of emotional affiliation with particular locales. Through the uniquely human capacity to remember, to imagine, and to project ourselves mentally into spaces beyond our immediate visual field, we can vicariously participate in spaces displaced in space and time. We can return in our minds to the places of our childhood (Chaudhury, 1999). We can project ourselves into the contemporary

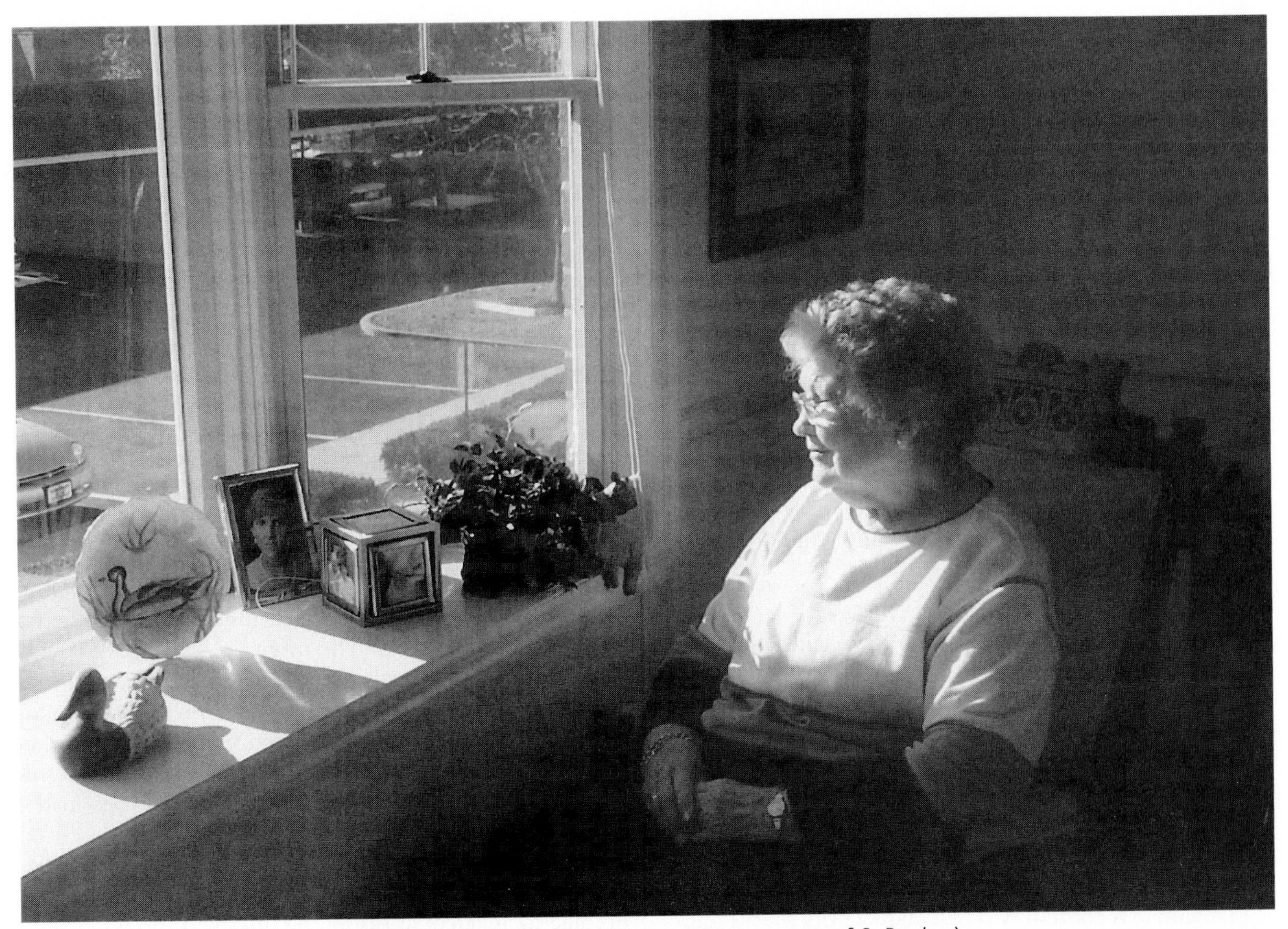

FIGURE 9–2. The surveillance zone. (Photo courtesy of G. Rowles.)

environments of family members and imagine what they might be doing half a continent away as we watch a televised national weather forecast that informs us it is raining where they live (Rowles, 1978).

The ability to traverse space and time in our mind and inhabit an experiential world much larger than the immediate and contemporary physical setting is nurtured and reinforced by the artifacts with which we surround ourselves. Particular items of furniture, treasured personal possessions, scrapbooks, and photographs all serve as cues to the resurrection or stimulation of place experience in consciousness (Belk, 1992; Boschetti, 1995; Csikszentmuhalyi & Rochberg-Halton, 1981). Such items convey a sense of identity; capture essential elements of our autobiography; and in so doing, help us define and maintain a sense of self. We become the places of our lives—where we live and what we own.

To summarize, the *spaces* of our life become transformed into the *places* of our life through a variety of physical, cognitive, emotional, and imaginative processes of habitation that imbue existence with meaning and personal significance. Contemporary physical presence is only a small part of being in place. It is merely the overtly observable and most readily apparent aspect of a complex self that has gradually evolved over the life course, with the accumulation and integration of a plethora of life-shaping and person-forming experiences in the different places we have occupied from birth until the present.

Meaning of Home

The most intense expression of being in place characteristically involves our relationship with home—usually, although not invariably, the dwelling where we reside. In this location we find the most sophisticated expressions of human relationship with the environment with respect to all levels of being in place—use, cognitive orientation, emotional affiliation, and vicarious involvement (Marcus, 1995; Rubinstein, 1989; Sixsmith, 1986; Zingmark, Norberg, & Sandman, 1995). Indeed, being in place entails being "at home." Home is territory—a place of possession and ownership that may be fiercely defended. Home is a place of safety and security. Often, home is the spatial fulcrum of our life, a place of centering that may become the core of our being and a location from which we venture forth into a potentially hostile world outside and beyond and to which we return for shelter. Home is a place of freedom, a location where we can let go and be ourselves. Home is a repository of the items we have accumulated that catalog our history and define who we are. Beyond the personal significances with which such items can be imbued, home often also becomes a locus of expression as we present ourselves to visitors, neighbors, and those who pass by, through the way in which we maintain and decorate the property and care for our yard. Because of the complex interweaving of these themes over an extended period of residence, home may come to be viewed as a sacred place and the seat of a person's very being and identity (Eliade, 1959). Little wonder that, for many people, to abandon one's home is, in a quite real sense, to contemplate a severance from self.

MAKING SPACES INTO PLACES OVER THE LIFE COURSE

Being in place and its relationship to self is a dynamic phenomenon. Throughout the life course, as we move from location to location, we are constantly creating and re-creating place as a component of personal identity. With every move, we slough off elements of our past. With every move, we carry selected elements of this past with us and meld them with new experiences and the influence of new environments as we create a contemporary lifestyle and sense of being in place in the present. This selective process of transference allows us to maintain a continuity of self and identity that is reinforced by an evolving relationship with the places of our life (Twigger-Ross & Uzzell, 1996).

Transitions and Disruptions of Being in Place

A variety of circumstances result in changes in an individual's relationship with place that have important consequences for sense of self and well-being. Among the most profound are changes in personal capability. During the first portion of life, such changes are generally liberating. As we progress from infancy through childhood and into adolescence, the geographical world tends to expand as physical and mental capabilities develop and access is gained to an ever-wider array of resources (education, income, transportation). Competence tends to increase within an increasingly diverse array of environments. At the other end of the life course, as we grow old, physical and sensory decrements may become restrictive and confining, at least with respect to our physical use of space. It may become more difficult to venture abroad, to maintain our home, even to climb the stairs to an upstairs bedroom.

Lives are also lived within the context of constantly changing environments. New roadways disruptively slice through neighborhoods, the physical landscape changes with the addition of new buildings or the deterioration and demolition of old ones, new populations migrate into formerly stable residential enclaves, and both natural and human-made disasters transform the landscapes of our life. In youth, such change may be a source of stimulation and new opportunity; but as we grow older, we may become less resilient in accommodating to such external environmental changes. Regardless of its source, change in people's relationship with the environment, whether in situ change or relocation, has become a predominant motif of life in contemporary Western societies.

Creating and Re-Creating Place

A fundamental human tension exists between the need for familiarity, security, and a sense of continuity and an urge to explore and to venture forth into the unknown (Balint, 1955; Buttimer, 1980). This tension is expressed in sequential habitation of the environments of our life through processes whereby we constantly create and re-create place as an expression of an evolving self (Rowles & Watkins, In press). Most people exhibit residential inertia and reluctance to move. The intensity of this inertia may vary over the life course and among different generations with many young people exhibiting greater enthusiasm for relocation and many elders expressing a desire to age in place (Callahan, 1992; Tilson, 1990). However, when relocation does occur, there are certain constancies in the manner in which people accommodate to change.

People with a history of frequent relocation often become experienced place makers. With every relocation they become more adept at sustaining links with places of their past even as they accommodate to opportunities provided by new settings. The process involves several overlapping elements: Each serves to preserve a continuity of self. First, there is a tendency for holding on manifest in routine ways of accommodating to the stress of separation from environments of our past. Contact with previous settings may be maintained through periodic return visits, telephone calls to former neighbors, or maintaining ongoing correspondence. Maintaining links with the places and the self of the past may also involve transferring treasured artifacts, including photographs and memorabilia that serve as cues to key events and locations in personal history (Boschetti, 1995; Paton & Cram, 1992).

A second element of creating and re-creating place is a recurring process of moving on; personal growth through active investment in each new setting. Often this involves lifestyle change because of accommodation to illness, disability, or other changed circumstances. The process may involve the use of learned strategies for making new friends and becoming involved in the local social milieu, such as making conscious efforts to visit new neighbors or co-residents (Reed & Payton, 1996). It may entail efforts, sometimes subconscious, to re-create elements of the familiar in each new setting. For example, some people re-create place and facilitate the maintenance of a comfortable routine in the use of space by arranging their furniture in a configuration similar to that which existed in their previous residence (Hartwigsen, 1987; Toyama, 1988). The re-creation of place may also involve the selective transfer of artifacts and possessions and their arrangement within a new space in ways that serve to define and reinforce an evolving sense of self (Belk, 1992; Boschetti, 1995).

Creation and re-creation of place are lifelong processes. During the first part of life, acts of accumulation tend to be dominant motifs within this process. Thus, as a student apartment gives way to the condominium of the young professional, the first single-family home, and a series of progressively larger dwellings in parallel with changing needs as we find a partner and establish a family, we tend to accumulate more and more possessions—possessions that may come to define our persona. There is preliminary evidence that as we grow older and, in many cases, are obliged to move from spacious dwellings to residences with progressively less space, this process may gradually give way to a process of divestiture that involves a carefully reasoned but emotionally taxing reduction of inventory and placing priority on retaining items of particular personal and self-defining significance (Morris, 1992). For elders, a continuing sense of being in place may be closely related to the ability to accomplish this process in a manner that facilitates the retention of ongoing identity.

THE PLACE OF PLACE IN OCCUPATIONAL THERAPY

This chapter suggests that understanding a person's sense of self and well-being is intimately linked to a phenomenological life-course-based understanding of an evolving person–environment relationship. Within this rubric, definition of *person* is expanded to emphasize the role of autobiography in defining the self. The concept of *environment* is elaborated and recast as the experiential notion of place. This reconfiguration is more than semantic novelty. Rather, it provides the basis for deeper understanding of aspects of the experienced world of the client that have important implications for practice.

At the most fundamental level there is a need for occupational therapy practitioners to become more intimately attuned and sensitive to the complexity of each client's being in place. It is not enough solely to observe a person's contemporary architectural setting and identify the physical barriers that interfere with the performance of daily occupational tasks. Admittedly, it is important for practitioners to become advocates for client-centered environmental design that enhances occupational performance through design modification and the use of assistive devices. But while this may be necessary as a first step in seeking interventions to improve functional performance, it is not sufficient if the goal is to enable the client to realize his or her full potential for attaining the highest possible quality of life. To accomplish this more sophisticated objective, it is necessary to embrace a broader understanding of place as a component of therapy—to develop place therapy (Scheidt & Norris-Baker, 1999).

What would an occupational place therapy look like? More than a rigid set of prescribed procedures, such a therapy would focus primarily on attitude and the practitioner's manner of relating to each client. It would focus on identifying customary patterns in the use of space, the role of habit and routine in these behaviors, and ways in which interventions can minimize disruption of habits and routines or create new ones consonant with a client's personal history. It would focus on identifying the manner in which clients cognitively orient their daily behaviors in relation to the places of their lives and normatively use such constructions in accommodating to personal or environmental change. Such information would enable the practitioner to provide appropriate support and re-orientation in response to changed circumstances. It would explicitly focus on the implications of disrupting longstanding emotional attachments to specific environments and to the artifacts contained in those environments and seek ways of compensating for such disruptions; for example, facilitating the transfer of key personal possessions when relocation is necessary (Wapner, Demick, & Redondo, 1990). And it would focus on framing interventions within the constraints and opportunities provided by the myriad environments that clients vicariously inhabit in their minds—environments displaced in space and/or time—that often are key elements in their definition of self. In this domain, key occupational therapy intervention might include reminiscence therapy or other types of activity that serve to maintain the connection of clients with the places of their lives that constitute their experiential world (Burnside & Haight, 1994; Chaudhury, 1999).

Translating such lofty aspirations into practical terms in the context of home and relocation, possibilities for facilitating adjustment to either reduced physical capability in situ or a needed relocation include preparation strategies, ranging from anticipatory modeling of change (Hunt & Pastalan, 1987) through processes of "constructing familiarity" (Reed & Payton, 1996) to psychotherapy based on "ecoanalysis of the home" (Peled & Schwartz, 1999). Such strategies are designed to prepare clients to deal with the consequences of separation from familiar place and routine and to facilitate the re-creation of place in a manner consistent with changed circumstances.

It is important to add words of caution at this point. First, for some people, expressions of self and of being in the world derive from dimensions of life other than place and home. It can be argued that such "placeless" persons may be alienated from their environment and perhaps, by extension, from self. Nonetheless, it is important to avoid the dangers of romanticism and to avoid a stereotypical view of the role of place in people's lives. Second, occupational place therapy may be more appropriate for some clients than for others. For example, persons with lengthy histories and multiple experiences of accommodating to change both within their indigenous environment and through experience in place-making gained from frequent relocations may be adept at accommodating to lifestyle and behavioral changes necessitated by a needed occupational therapy intervention. But what of those who have been more residentially stable and who have been accustomed to lifelong routines of using a single space and relating to only a few places? Such individuals may experience great difficulty in abandoning familiar routines; adjusting the nature of their being in place in a familiar residence; or, should relocation be necessary, transforming a new space into a place. For these individuals change may be particularly traumatic.

CONCLUSION

There is a tendency in contemporary society to assume that individuals achieve successful rehabilitation merely by returning to former levels of physical functioning and behavioral competence. Such a view is myopic and demeaning with respect to the richness of human experience. When a practitioner advocates removal of a potentially hazardous throw rug from a client's hallway, offers assistance in rearranging the client's space to accommodate a disability, or provides training in the use of the latest occupational therapy gadget, he or she may be effectively enhancing the safety of the home and the physical competence of the client while diminishing the client's sense of control and autonomy. The interventions may mean discarding a rug inherited from a favorite grandmother and transported from home to home over a lifetime—an artifact that is an enduring symbol of family history and continuity. Rearranging the space may move important family photographs beyond the visual field of a favorite chair that, itself, was formerly by the window but has been moved to a safer location that no longer affords a view of activities in the surveillance zone outside. The gadget that the therapist finds so innovative and helpful may achieve its overt purpose but reinforce a sense of inadequacy and incompetence in an individual who might be even better served by accommodating to a disability through a less overtly intrusive strategy.

Historically, the past few decades may come to be known as an era in which our technology exceeded our humanity as humankind lapsed into hedonistic obsession with material and technological ingenuity. By reinvesting in meaning through place, it may be that occupational therapy can help us rediscover our humanity. By seeking new ways to enable individuals to maintain an enduring sense of being in place as a component of the self, the practice of occupational therapy can become elevated to a higher plane.

References

Altman, I., & Low, S. M. (Eds.). (1992). *Place attachment*. New York: Plenum.

American Occupational Therapy Foundation. (2000). 1999 Habits conference supplemental issue. *Occupational Therapy Journal of Research, 20*(Suppl. 1), 2S–143S.

Balint, M. (1955). Friendly expanses—Horrid empty spaces. *International Journal of Psychoanalysis, 36*(4/5), 225–241.

Barris, R. (1986). Activity: The interface between person and environment. *Physical and Occupational Therapy in Geriatrics, 5*, 39–49.

Barris, R., Kielhofner, G., Levine, R. E., & Neville, A. M. (1985). Occupation as interaction with environment. In G. Kielhofner (Ed.). *A model of human occupation: Theory and application* (pp. 42–62). Baltimore: Williams & Wilkins

Belk, R. W. (1992). Attachment to possessions. In I. Altman & S. M. Low (Eds.). *Place attachment* (pp. 37–62). New York: Plenum.

Boschetti, M. A. (1995). Attachment to personal possessions: An interpretive study of the older person's experiences. *Journal of Interior Design, 21*(1), 1–12.

Burnside, I., & Haight, B. (1994). Reminiscence and life review: Therapeutic interventions for older people. *Nurse Practitioner, 19*(4), 55–61.

Buttimer, A. (1980). Home, reach and the sense of place. In A. Buttimer & D. Seamon (Eds.). *The human experience of space and place* (pp. 166–187). New York: St. Martin's.

Callahan, J. J. (1992). Aging in place. *Generations, 16*, 5–6.

Chaudhury, H. (1999). Self and reminiscence of place: A conceptual study. *Journal of Aging and Identity, 4*(4), 231–253.

Christiansen, C., & Baum, C. (1997). Person-environment-occupational performance: A conceptual model for practice. In C. Christiansen & C. Baum (Eds.). *Occupational therapy: Enabling function and well-being* (pp. 46–70). Thorofare, NJ: Slack.

Csikszentmuhalyi, M., & Rochberg-Halton, E. (1981). *The meaning of things: Domestic symbols and the self*. New York: Cambridge University Press.

Downs, R. M., & Stea, D. (Eds.). (1973). *Image and environment: Cognitive mapping and spatial behavior*. Chicago: Aldine.

Dunn, W., Brown, C., & McGuigan, A. (1994). The ecology of human performance: A framework for considering the effect of context. *American Journal of Occupational Therapy, 48*(7), 595–607.

Eliade, M. (1959). *The sacred and the profane*. New York: Harcourt, Brace & World.

Hartwigsen, G. (1987). Older widows and the transference of home. *International Journal of Aging and Human Development, 25*(3), 195–207.

Hunt, M. E., & Pastalan, L. A. (1987). Easing relocation: An environmental learning process. In V. Regnier & J. Pynoos (Eds.). *Housing the aged: Design directives and policy considerations* (pp. 421–440). New York: Elsevier.

Kielhofner, G. (1995). *A model of human occupation: Theory and application* (2nd ed.) Baltimore: Williams & Wilkins.

Kiernat, J. M. (1982). Environment: The hidden modality. *Physical and Occupational Therapy in Geriatrics, 2*, 3–12.

Kiernat, J. M. (1987). Promoting independence and autonomy through environmental approaches. *Topics in Geriatric Rehabilitation, 3*, 1–6.

Law, M., Cooper, B., Strong, S., Steward, D., Rigby, P., & Letts, L. (1996). The person-environment occupation model: A transactive approach to occupational performance. *Canadian Journal of Occupational Therapy, 63*, 9–23.

Marcus, C. C. (1995). *House as a mirror of self: Exploring the deeper meaning of home*. Berkeley, CA: Conari.

Morris, B. R. (1992). Reducing inventory: Divestiture of personal possessions. *Journal of Women and Aging, 4*(2), 79–92.

Paton, H., & Cram, F. (1992). Personal possessions and environmental control: The experiences of elderly women in three residential settings. *Journal of Women and Aging, 4*(2), 61–78.

Peled, A., & Schwartz, H. (1999). Exploring the ideal home in psychotherapy: Two case studies. *Journal of Environmental Psychology, 19*, 87–94.

Reed, J., & Payton, V. R. (1996). Constructing familiarity and managing the self: Ways of adapting to life in nursing and residential homes for older people. *Ageing and Society, 16*, 543–560.

Rowles, G. D. (1978). *Prisoners of space? Exploring the geographical experience of older people*. Boulder, CO: Westview.

Rowles, G. D. (1981). The surveillance zone as meaningful space for the aged. *The Gerontologist, 21*(3), 304–311.

Rowles, G. D. (1991). Beyond performance: Being in place as a component of occupational therapy. *American Journal of Occupational Therapy, 45*(3), 265–271.

Rowles, G. D. (2000). Habituation and being in place. *Occupational Therapy Journal of Research, 20* (Suppl. 1), 52S–67S.

Rowles, G. D., & Watkins, J. F. (In press). History, habit, heart and hearth: On making spaces into places. In K. W. Schaie, H.-W. Wahl, H. Mollenkopf & F. Oswald (Eds.). *Aging in the community: Living environments and mobility*. New York: Springer.

Rubinstein, R. (1989). The home environments of older people: A description of the psychosocial processes linking person to place. *Journals of Gerontology, 44*, S45–S53.

Rubinstein, R., & Parmalee, P. A. (1992). Attachment to place and the representation of the life course by the elderly. In I Altman & S. M. Low (Eds.). *Place attachment* (pp. 139–163). New York: Plenum.

Scheidt, R. J., & Norris-Baker, C. (1999). Place therapies for older adults: Conceptual and interventive approaches. *International Journal of Aging and Human Development, 48*(1), 1–15.

Schkade, J. K., & Schultz, S. (1992). Occupational adaptation: Toward a holistic approach for contemporary practice, part 1. *American Journal of Occupational Therapy, 46*, 829–837.

Seamon, D. (1980). Body subject, time-space routines, and place ballets. In A. Buttimer & D. Seamon (Eds.). *The human experience of space and place* (pp. 148–165). London: Croom Helm.

Seamon, D. (1984). Emotional experience of the environment. *American Behavioral Scientist, 27*(6), 757–770.

Settersten, R. A. (1999). Lives in time and place: The problems and promises of developmental science. Amityville, NY: Baywood.

Sixsmith, J. (1986). The meaning of home: An exploratory study of environmental experience. *Journal of Environmental Psychology, 6*, 281–298.

Suttles, G. D. (1969). *The social order of the slum*. Chicago: University of Chicago Press.

Tilson, D. (Ed.). (1990). *Aging in place: Supporting the frail elderly in residential environments*. Glenview, IL: Scott, Foresman.

Toyama, T. (1988). *Identity and milieu: A study of relocation focusing on reciprocal changes in elderly people and their environment*. Stockholm: Department for Building Function Analysis, the Royal Institute of Technology.

Tuan, Y. F. (1977). *Space and place: The perspective of experience*. Minneapolis: University of Minnesota Press.

Twigger-Ross, C., & Uzzell, D. L. (1996). Place and identity processes. *Journal of Environmental Psychology, 16*, 205–220.

Wapner, S., Demick, J., & Redondo, J. P. (1990). Cherished possessions and adaptation of older people to nursing homes. *International Journal of Aging and Human Development, 31*(3), 219–235.

Wheeler, W. M. (1995). *Elderly residential experience: The evolution of places as residence*. New York: Garland.

Zingmark, A., Norberg, K., & Sandman, P.-O. (1995). The experience of being at home throughout the lifespan: Investigation of persons 2 to 102. *International Journal of Aging and Human Development, 41*(1), 47–62.

CHAPTER 10

SPIRITUALITY: MEANINGS RELATED TO OCCUPATIONAL THERAPY

SUZANNE M. PELOQUIN

Within this discussion of the person seeking therapy some thought must turn to **spirituality** for reasons psychologist Maslow (1970) argued well:

> *I want to demonstrate that spiritual values have naturalistic meaning, that they are not the exclusive possession of organized churches, that they do not need supernatural concepts to validate them, that they are well within the jurisdiction of a suitably enlarged science, and that, therefore, they are the general responsibility of all mankind.* (p. 33)

Personality, according to most humanistic psychologists, includes a spiritual dimension, whether one names it *spiritual* or not. To understand people means to consider that dimension.

This is a thumbnail discussion of (1) the meaning of spirituality as it relates to occupational therapy; (2) the profession's position on spirituality; and (3) the relevance of spirituality to three professional concerns: person, context, and occupation. Often the discussion turns to the language we use because, as Becvar (1997) suggested, "Language is the means by which individuals come to know their world and in their knowing simultaneously construct it" (p. 4).

SPIRITUALITY: MEANINGS RELATED TO OCCUPATIONAL THERAPY

Meanings from Everyday Language

> *Spirit: an animating or vital principle.*
> *Spiritual: relating to, consisting of, or affecting the spirit.*
> *Spirituality: the quality or state of being spiritual.*
> *Religion: a personal set or institutionalized system of religions attitudes, beliefs, and practices.* (Mish et al., 1995)

Individuals turn to dictionary definitions of terms to access social agreement on their meanings. Although the distinctions between the terms *spirituality* and *religion* are noteworthy in the listing above, they are further elaborated in everyday usage. For example, as individuals occupy themselves with daily living, much spontaneous conversation reflects their awareness of spirituality in the naturalistic sense that Maslow (1970) described. An audience judges a dance routine spirited. A teacher sees hostile play and calls it mean spirited. Those regrouping after a flood are said to show strength of spirit. One senses a kindred spirit when befriending a stranger. Impressed by creative acts, one asks what inspired them. This sampling of colloquialisms shows that we understand the human spirit as a blend of liveliness, moral presence, psychic energy, emotional courage, social connection, and creative action. Our language reveals an implied knowledge of the spiritual nature of individuals, a nature that can also express itself through religion. Each of these manifestations of spirit can be seen in occupational therapy practice.

Meanings from the Professional Literature

The literature on spirituality is wide ranging, with the meanings of spirituality and religion discussed more directly. Theologians; psychologists, historians, and, with increasing frequency since the 1980s, health-care practitioners have explored the construct and offered definitions. Attempts at reconciling diverse definitions have led most to see spirituality as multifaceted. Elkins, Hedstrom, Hughes, Leaf, and Saunders (1988) are but one group of scholars who synthesized the construct's many elements:

- Belief in a transcendent dimension to life.
- Belief in some meaning and purpose to life.
- Belief in a sense of personal mission.
- Belief that life is infused with sacredness.
- Belief that material values are of themselves insufficient.
- Altruism.
- Idealism.
- Awareness of the tragic realities of human existence.
- Awareness that having a spiritual sense bears fruit.

These elements are spiritual values that do not imply religiosity. They do, however, imply convictions about how to occupy a life. By comparison, religion is understood to be a more organized and culturally shaped avenue for spiritual expression (Rosenfeld, 2000). In so far as they constitute or reflect personal values held by those seeking occupational therapy, elements of spirituality and religious practice matter.

Meanings from Occupational Therapy's History

In occupational therapy, discussion of spirituality is not just a recent event. Early in the profession's history, prominent individuals involved in its development described occupation's connections with the human spirit. Barton (1920) believed that through occupation, a person's spirit could triumph over despair and disability. He thus chose a phoenix rising from flames as emblem for Consolation House, a school and workshop he opened for convalescents (Barton, 1968).

Dunton (1919), another of the profession's founders, saw the roots of occupational therapy in moral treatment, the nineteenth-century practice of using occupations in supportive environments for individuals with mental illness. His creed conveyed belief in the healing power of occupation:

> *That occupation is as necessary to life as food and drink. That every human being should have both physical and mental occupations. That all should have occupations which they enjoy. . . . . That sick minds, sick bodies, sick souls, may be healed through occupation. (p. 17)*

In an address to graduating students, Kidner (1929) shared this spiritual legacy with the next generation:

> *May you realize in increasing measure the value of certain spiritual things which are the real making of life, but which we call by many common names. Kindness, humanity, decency, honor, good faith—to give these up under any circumstances whatever would be a loss greater than death itself. (p. 385)*

In more recent years, many practitioners have addressed spirituality more tacitly, and often within the discussion of other constructs, such as the meaning and purpose of occupation (American Occupational Therapy Association [AOTA], 1994, 1995), the core values of the profession (AOTA, 1993; Peloquin, 1995), the reflective and caring nature of practitioners (Parham, 1987; Yerxa, 1980), the art of practice (Mosey, 1981; Peloquin, 1989), wellness (Johnson, 1986; White, 1986), and the quality of patients' lives (do Rozario, 1994). The absence of an explicit naming of spirituality may relate in part to Kroeker's (1997) observation that such integration has been difficult in modern times during which therapy has been narrowly understood as technical expertise that targets objective problems.

Toward the end of the twentieth century, however, Canadian occupational therapy practitioners revisited spirituality explicitly, identifying it as a central component in client-centered practice (Department of National Health and Welfare [DNWH] & Canadian Association of Occupational Therapists [CAOT], 1983; CAOT, 1991). They later placed spirituality at the core of the Canadian model of occupational performance (CAOT, 1997). Other practitioners soon addressed the topic directly: Yerxa (1991) discussed human experience as filled with spiritual meaning, Egan and Delaat (1994) named spirit the essence of individuals, and Urbanowski and Vargo (1994) characterized spirituality as the meaning found in life. In 1997, both the *American Journal of Occupational Therapy* and the *Canadian Journal of Occupational Therapy* published special issues in which authors discussed spirituality, religion, and occupational therapy from perspectives as diverse as philosophy, theory, practice, ethics, and research.

The spiritual natures of those seeking occupational therapy have concerned occupational therapy practitioners since the profession's founding, sometimes being very much in the foreground of therapeutic efforts and other times being more in the background. Concern with the human spirit seems linked in vital ways with concern for the ways in which individuals occupy their lives.

RELEVANCE TO THE PROFESSION'S CORE CONCERNS

So far this discussion has grounded the relevance of spirituality to occupational therapy in the meanings that are associated with spiritual themes found in everyday language, literature, and the profession's history. The discussion will now turn to additional links among spirituality, persons and their contexts, and human occupation.

Persons as Central to Practice

Maslow's (1970) argument, remember, was that because people are spiritual, spirituality is the responsibility of everyone. Occupational therapy practitioners have echoed that argument as part of holistic and client-centered practice. Urbanowski and Vargo (1994) saw spirituality as an integral part of a person's makeup; Egan and Delaat (1997) said that spirituality is the individual. Christiansen (1997) argued that denial of a spiritual dimension fragments an understanding of people. The logic of these assertions leads to this conclusion: If occupational therapy practitioners profess that the perspectives, values, needs, and strengths of individuals will direct their interventions, they must address the spiritual dimensions of those perspectives and values, needs and strengths.

Psychologist Wink (1999) reminded those in helping roles that spiritual perspectives and values may vary according to social and cultural factors, including historical cohort, ethnicity, and gender. The spiritual quest of Luke Skywalker, he said, might have more appeal to Baby Boomers than to older Americans. Those with an Eastern spirituality may favor contemplative expressions. Women, he thought, may seek the sacred in interpersonal relations and men, in heroic myths. If practitioners can see spirituality as another form of diversity, their need to attend to it seems clear (Westbrooks, 1998).

Needs and strengths uncovered by occupational therapy practitioners may also be spiritual. Physician Rousseau (2000) noted that "spiritual suffering often manifests as physical or psychologic problems and shares many features with depression, including feelings of hopelessness and worthlessness as well as a sense of meaninglessness" (p. 2000). Strengths that practitioners identify, such as motivation, social connection, and courage, can also be seen as spiritual.

Contexts as Awakening to Spirituality

We know that individuals function within contexts that change over time; these shape their perspectives and values, needs and strengths. Since the 1980s, Western culture has seen a surge of interest in spirituality. Books such as Moore's (1992) *Care of the Soul* and Moyers's (1993) *Healing and the Mind* were best-sellers; the covers of *Life*, *Newsweek*, and *Time* have promoted feature articles on the subject.

Perhaps in response to such interest, alternative medicine now includes natural and more transcendent modes of healing, such as herbal therapy, aromatherapy, massage, t'ai chi, and yoga. An increasing number of scientific studies examine the influences of spirituality and religion on physical and mental health (Koenig, 1999; Levin, 1994). Current health promotion efforts endorse a holistic focus on mind, body, and spirit (Bowen, 1999). Institutional care holds a similar focus, with the construction of gardens, butterfly rooms, and other spiritual havens. Johnson (1998) noted that the standards for the Joint Commission for the Accreditation of Health Care Organizations now formalize a patient's right to care that honors spiritual values. A new field called neurotheology posits that the human brain is hardwired to experience transcendence (Begley, 2001). Many name this surge of interest an awakening to spirituality. Given occupational therapy's history, it seems a *re*awakening.

Occupations as the Making of Lives and Worlds

It is easy to move from an understanding of the human spirit found in casual conversation to a reframing of occupational therapy as engaged with spirituality. One construct that prompts most to see a spiritual dimension in occupation is that of *making*, as described in this poem by Petersen (1976):

> *There is a shouting SPIRIT deep inside me:*
> *TAKE CLAY, it cries,*
> *TAKE PEN AND INK,*
> *TAKE FLOUR AND WATER,*
> *TAKE A SCRUB BRUSH,*
> *TAKE A YELLOW CRAYON,*
> *TAKE ANOTHER'S HAND—*
> *AND WITH ALL THESE SAY YOU,*
> *SAY LOVING,*
> *So much of who I am*
> *Is subtly spoken in my making. (p. 61)*

I have elsewhere shared my grasp of this passage—that meaningful occupation animates and extends the human spirit (Peloquin, 1996, 1997). When practitioners take part in this process, they enact the profession's tacit philosophy—that people are the makers of their lives and worlds. Most philosophers, such as Scarry (1985), also see the world-making function of persons:

As one maneuvers each day through the realm of tablecloths, dishes, potted plants, ideological structures, automobiles, newspapers, ideas about families, streetlights, language, city parks, one does not at each moment actively perceive the objects as humanly made; but if for any reason one stops and thinks about their origins, one can with varying degrees of ease recover the fact that they all have human makers. (p. 312)

The image of someone in the act of making is one in which human being (its character, heart, or spirit) flows into human doing. To see occupation as the making of lives and worlds is a spiritual perspective.

The language of making is important to occupational therapy practitioners because colloquialisms rename many tasks as acts of making. We name hair care/grooming, for example, but we also hear it described as an act of making oneself presentable or likeable. What we call cooking, we also call the making of a meal within a much larger making of home or tradition. We may call the occupational performance work, but we can see it more deeply as making a living or making a family or community. What we call cognition, we can also see as making sense, choice, or inquiry. When we take this perspective, we can see the spirit in occupation. Other professionals see merit in this perspective. For example, Westbrooks (1998), a social worker, said, "It is intriguing to note the mystical overtone given to constructs associated with spirituality, as if spirituality does not and could not exist in the concrete activities of daily living" (p. 78).

Unruh (1997) explored the writings of individuals who loved to garden; there she found a spiritual dimension valued by many. Smith (1991), for example, said: "There is nothing more spiritually satisfying than an early morning spent crawling around on my hands and knees, sinking my fingers into the soil" (p. 143). For those inspired by gardening, a reclamation of that capacity is a deep restoration in which practitioners share. Restorative occupations are as varied as the individuals who cherish them; they may include gourmet cooking, dance, Bible class, and river rafting. Individuals inspired by occupations built around religious rituals warrant the same regard that we accord to those who love gardening. When we help others engage in occupations with meaning, we engage their spirits whether we name the action spiritual or not.

PRACTICAL APPLICATIONS

Suggestions for the manner in which spirituality can be integrated into occupational therapy are important to consider. Discussing such suggestions, Low (1997) noted that we ought not perceive the mandate to attend to spirituality as one of becoming spiritual counselors.

Many practitioners already attend to the human spirit in ways that are embedded in what they do (Egan & Delaat, 1994), often as part of an underground practice that is less discussed or documented (Christiansen, 1997; Mattingly & Fleming, 1994). The change suggested here is one of openly acknowledging the depth of our engagement so that we can recognize the importance of spiritual values—ours and those of clients—as they are enacted in practice.

Urbanowski and Vargo (1994) noted that accessing the meaning of daily activities from individuals is central to occupational therapy. They suggested interview questions that might help:

- *How will your life be different?*
- *What is the one thing that you never want to lose?*
- *Who are the most important people in your life?*
- *What won't you be able to do? What might you do instead? (p. 91)*

None of these questions is radically new, and variations appear in existing protocols. The suggestion is that we be mindful that such questions move discussion to matters of the spirit and that we ought to listen to these matters well and without judgment.

Kirsh (1996) and Collins (1998) said that such questions structure a narrative approach, in which individuals reflect about their occupations. The invitation to tell one's story—of everyday occupations or an imagined future—can also nest in therapy sessions. Swarbrick and Burkhardt (2000) suggested that the use of media with transcendent potential, such as art, music, or nature activities, can prompt and support communication on a spiritual level.

After an assessment of needs and strengths, collaborative goal setting will include aims related to spiritual expression when these are important to the individual. A Jewish woman wanting to keep a kosher home might say of her rituals, "Those are the rules I live by. Just like everybody lives by the rules of gravity" (Frank et al., 1997, p. 205). Her practitioner must respond to the importance of such beliefs. Spencer, Davidson, and White (1997) saw the goal attainment scaling used by Lloyd (1986) as an apt tool in such a circumstance. The tool permits what is called *hope work* in the setting of goals, work such as imagining possibilities and evaluating future choices. Goals with real meaning to the client must take high priority in planning interventions.

Interventions that flow from clients' goals help them engage or reengage in meaningful occupations or, as Christiansen (1997) called them, "activities of the spirit." If an individual's preferred occupation is unfamiliar to the practitioner, such as keeping a kosher home might be, members of the clergy or spiritual advisers might be accessed (Swarbrick & Burkhardt, 2000). Competence in activity analysis, however, means that, as with any novel occupation, a practitioner will invite the individual, friends, or family members to fully describe the task.

During the intervention process, the therapeutic use of self has been noted as a primary mode of reaching and inspiring others (Collins, 1998; Egan & Delaat, 1994; Mosey, 1981; Peloquin, 1989; Urbanowski & Vargo, 1994). Many practitioners thus recognize suggestions to integrate spirituality as enactments of the use of self. To open oneself to the values of another is an outcome of having empathy, and empathy touches the spirit: "Empathy in health care practice is the enactment of the conviction that, empowered by someone's willingness to understand, the patient will gather the requisite measure of courage" (Peloquin, 1995, p. 26).

CONCLUSION

When it comes to discerning a spiritual dimension in occupational therapy, it helps to consider the kinds of seeing that cause three-dimensional pictures to emerge from designs called *stereograms*. Stereograms are bright patterns, their overall effect much like gift wrapping. Experts give this cue for finding the third dimension: Gaze through the pattern to some point beyond it (Baccei, 1994). This broad way of seeing, freed from a fix on details but still led by them, yields a vibrant picture. The discovery is awesome.

The dimensionality of the stereogram can go unnoticed. The deep dimension emerges only when a viewer knows how to look. The patterns of human occupation and occupational therapy seem much like stereograms. Two dimensions of practice—those relating to the body and to the mind—are readily seen. The spiritual dimension takes a more discerning eye. Gazing past the details of practice—the handles on rakes, the covers on jars—to the point beyond them, we can see a spiritual aim. The lesson of this chapter is that we must.

Occupation, the core of our therapy, animates and extends the human spirit. We participate in that animation. This discovery is a reawakening that clarifies our responsibility. We must explicitly attend to the spiritual dimension of human occupation and affirm the spiritual values that transform a person's engagement in occupations into the making of lives and worlds.

ACKNOWLEDGMENT

Portions of this chapter were revised from "Nationally Speaking: The Spiritual Depth of Occupation: Making Worlds and Making Lives," by S. M. Peloquin. Copyright 1997 by the American Occupational Therapy Association, Inc. Reprinted with permission.

References

Mish, F. C., et al. (1995). Merriam Webster's Collegiate Dictionary. Springfield, MA: Merriam Webster.

American Occupational Therapy Association [AOTA]. (1993). Core values and attitudes of occupational therapy practice. *American Journal of Occupational Therapy, 47*, 1085–1086.

American Occupational Therapy Association [AOTA]. (1994). Position paper: Purposeful activity. *American Journal of Occupational Therapy, 48*, 467–468.

American Occupational Therapy Association [AOTA]. (1995). Position paper: Occupation. *American Journal of Occupational Therapy, 49*, 1015–1018.

Baccei, T. (1994). *In Disney's magic eye—A new bag of tricks*. Kansas City, MO: Andrews & McNeel.

Barton, G. E. (1920). What occupational therapy many mean to nursing. *Trained Nurse and Hospital Review, 64*, 304–310.

Barton, I. G. (1968). Consolation house, fifty years ago. *American Journal of Occupational Therapy, 22*, 340–345.

Becvar, D. S (1997). *Soul healing: A spiritual orientation in counseling and therapy*. New York: Basic Books.

Begley, S. (2001, January 29). Searching for the God within. *Newsweek*, 59.

Bowen, J. R. (1999, December 20). Health promotion in the new millennium. *OT Practice, 12*, 14–18.

Canadian Association of Occupational Therapists [CAOT]. (1991). *Occupational therapy guidelines for client-centered practice*. Toronto: Author.

Canadian Association of Occupational Therapists [CAOT]. (1997). Enabling occupation: An occupational perspective. Ottawa: Author.

Christiansen, C. (1997). Acknowledging a spiritual dimension in occupational therapy practice. *American Journal of Occupational Therapy, 3*, 169–172.

Collins, M. (1998). Occupational therapy and spirituality: Reflecting on quality and experience in therapeutic interventions. *British Journal of Occupational Therapy, 61*, 280–284.

Department of National Health and Welfare & Canadian Association of Occupational Therapists. (1983). *Guidelines for the client-centered practice of occupational therapy* (Cat. H39-33/1983/E). Ottawa: Author.

do Rozario, L. (1994). Ritual, meaning, and transcendence: The role of occupation in modern life. *Journal of Occupational Science, 1*, 46–53.

Dunton, W. R. (1919). *Reconstruction therapy*. Philadelphia: Saunders.

Egan, M., & Delaat, M. D. (1994). Considering spirituality in occupational therapy practice. *Canadian Journal of Occupational Therapy, 61*, 95–101.

Egan, M., & Delaat, M. D. (1997). The implicit spirituality of occupational therapy practice. *Canadian Journal of Occupational Therapy, 64*, 115–121.

Elkins, D. N., Hedstrom, L. J., Hughes, L. L., Leaf, J. A., & Saunders, C. S. (1988). Toward a humanistic-phenomenological spirituality. *Journal of Humanistic Psychology, 28*(4), 5–18.

Frank, G, Bernardo, C. S., Tropper, S., Noguchi, F., Lipman, C., Maulhardt, B., & Weitze, L. (1997). Jewish spirituality through actions in time: Daily occupations of Orthodox Jewish couples in Los Angeles. *American Journal of Occupational Therapy, 51*, 199–206.

Johnson, E. (1998). Integrating health care and spirituality: Considerations for ethical and cultural sensitivity. *Maryland Nurse, 17*, 5.

Johnson, J. (1986). Wellness and occupational therapy. *American Journal of Occupational Therapy, 40*, 735–758.

Kidner, T. B. (1929). Address to graduates. *Occupational Therapy and Rehabilitation, 8*, 379–385.

Kirsh, B. (1996). A narrative approach to addressing spirituality in occupational therapy: Exploring personal meaning and purpose. *Canadian Journal of Occupational Therapy, 63*, 55–61.

Koenig, H. (1999). Exploring links between religion/spirituality and health. *Scientific Review of Alternative Medicine, 3*, 52–52.

Kroeker, P. T. (1997). Spirituality and occupational therapy in a secular culture. *Canadian Journal of Occupational Therapy, 64*, 122–126.

Levin, J. S. (1994). *Religion in aging and health*. Thousand Oaks, CA: Sage.

Lloyd, C. (1986). The process of goal setting using goal attainment scaling in a therapeutic community. *Occupational Therapy in Mental Health, 6*, 19–30.

Low, J. F. (1997). Religious orientation and pain management. *American Journal of Occupational Therapy, 51*, 215–219.

Maslow, A. H. (1970). *Religions, values and peak experiences*. New York: Viking.

Mattingly, C., & Fleming, M. (1994). *Clinical reasoning: Forms of inquiry in a therapeutic practice*. Philadelphia: Davis.

Moore, T. (1992). *Care of the soul: A guide for cultivating depth and sacredness in everyday life*. New York: HarperCollins.

Mosey, A. C. (1981). *Occupational therapy: Configuration of a profession*. New York: Raven.

Moyers, B. (1993). *Healing and the mind*. New York: Doubleday.

Parham, D. (1987). Nationally speaking: Toward professionalism: The reflective therapist. *American Journal of Occupational Therapy, 41*, 555–561.

Peloquin, S. M. (1989). Sustaining the art of practice in occupational therapy. *American Journal of Occupational Therapy, 43*, 219–226.

Peloquin, S. M. (1995). The fullness of empathy: Reflections and illustrations. *American Journal of Occupational Therapy, 49*, 24–31.

Peloquin, S. M. (1996). Using the arts to enhance confluent learning. *American Journal of Occupational Therapy, 50*, 148–151.

Peloquin, S. M. (1997). Nationally speaking: The spiritual depth of occupation: Making worlds and making lives. *American Journal of Occupational Therapy, 3*, 167–168.

Petersen, J. (1976). *A book of yes*. Niles, IL: Argus.

Rosenfeld, M. S. (2000, January 17). Spiritual agent modalities for occupational therapy practice. *OT Practice 1*, 17–21.

Rousseau, P. (2000). Spirituality and the dying patient. *Journal of Clinical Oncology, 18*, 2000–2002.

Scarry, E. (1985). *The body in pain: The making and unmaking of the world*. New York: Oxford University Press.

Smith, M. (1991). *Beds I have known: Confessions of a passionate amateur gardener*. New York: Fireside.

Spencer, J., Davidson, H., & White, V. (1997). Helping clients develop hopes for the future. *American Journal of Occupational Therapy, 51*, 191–198.

Swarbrick, P., & Burkhardt, A. (2000). Spiritual health: Implications for the occupational therapy process. *Mental Health Special Interest Quarterly, 23*, 1–3.

Unruh, A. M. (1997). Spirituality and occupation: Garden musings and the Himalayan blue poppy. *Canadian Journal of Occupational Therapy, 64*, 156–160.

Urbanowski, R., & Vargo, J. (1994). Spirituality, daily practice, and the occupational performance model. *Canadian Journal of Occupational Therapy, 61*, 88–94.

Westbrooks, K. L. (1998). Spirituality as a form of functional diversity: Activating unconventional family strengths. *Journal of Family Social Work, 4*, 77–87.

White, V. (1986). Promoting health and wellness: A theme for the eighties. *American Journal of Occupational Therapy, 41*, 743–747.

Wink, P. (1999, Spring). Addressing end-of-life issues: Spirituality and inner life. *Generations*, 75–80.

Yerxa, E. J. (1980). Occupational therapy's role in creating a future climate of caring. *American Journal of Occupational Therapy, 34*, 529–534.

Yerxa, E. J. (1991). Seeking a relevant, ethical, and realistic way of knowing for occupational therapy. *American Journal of Occupational Therapy, 45*, 199–204.

UNIT *three*

Occupational Therapy Practitioners: The Occupational Therapist and the Occupational Therapy Assistant

Learning Objectives

After completing this unit, readers will be able to:

- Define clinical reasoning and explain important cognitive processes required for effective clinical reasoning.
- Describe four different facets of clinical reasoning and explain their importance.
- Identify the different facets of clinical reasoning based on personal reflection, practitioner's descriptions, and case studies.
- Describe the common stages of expertise development and the roles of experience and reflection in that developmental process.
- Describe and explain the necessary components of the occupational therapist–occupational therapy assistant partnership, including the supervisory relationship.
- Explain the process of establishing service competency.
- Describe credentialing for both entry-level practice and post-entry-level specialization.
- Summarize key aspects of the occupational therapy roles of practitioner, educator, manager, entrepreneur, advocate, and research/scholar.

The clinical reasoning process is the focus of the first chapter of this unit. This multifaceted approach, described by Schell, involves scientific, narrative, pragmatic, and ethical reasoning. In the second chapter in this unit, Schell, Crepeau, and

Cohn describe the evolution of professional competence from entry level through a variety of roles that experienced practitioners assume. Finally, Mary Sand describes the collaborative relationship between occupational therapists and occupational therapy assistants. This relationship is based on their preparation to enter the field and their interdependent roles. (Note: Words in bold type are defined in the Glossary.)

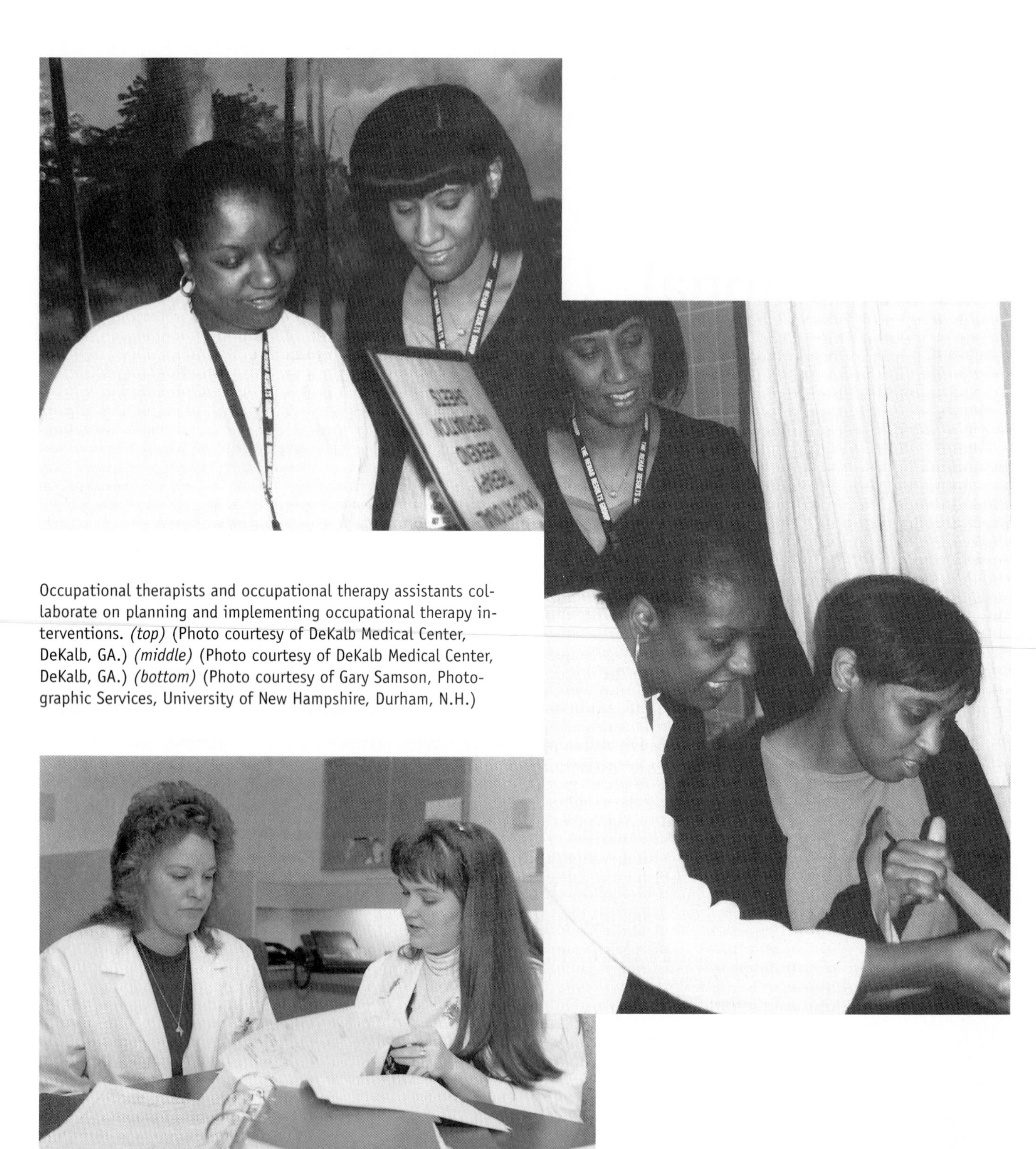

Occupational therapists and occupational therapy assistants collaborate on planning and implementing occupational therapy interventions. *(top)* (Photo courtesy of DeKalb Medical Center, DeKalb, GA.) *(middle)* (Photo courtesy of DeKalb Medical Center, DeKalb, GA.) *(bottom)* (Photo courtesy of Gary Samson, Photographic Services, University of New Hampshire, Durham, N.H.)

CHAPTER 11

CLINICAL REASONING: THE BASIS OF PRACTICE

BARBARA A. BOYT SCHELL

Clinical reasoning is the process used by practitioners to plan, direct, perform, and reflect on client care. It is a complex and multifaceted process. To consider clinical reasoning requires engaging in a **metacognitive** analysis. In simple terms, that means thinking about thinking. This is important, because newcomers to the field may incorrectly understand clinical reasoning as something that practitioners choose to do or consider it a form of occupational therapy intervention theory. It is neither of those things. Whenever you are thinking about or doing occupational therapy for an identified individual or group, you are engaged in clinical reasoning. It is not a question of whether you are doing it, only a question of how well. Furthermore, there are many practice theories discussed throughout this text that will inform your clinical reasoning. However, the theories about clinical reasoning discussed in this chapter are theories about occupational therapy practitioners and their reasoning processes, not about clients. Keep in mind these important distinctions as you become mindful of your own clinical reasoning processes.

This chapter examines clinical reasoning from several perspectives. The case study presented in What's a Practitioner to Do? 11-1—adapted, with name changes, from a situation I actually observed—provides an example of an encounter between an occupational therapist, Terry, and her client, Mrs. Munro. Read this case study before continuing with the text, paying special attention to the different kinds of issues and problems that the occupational therapy practitioner has to address.

CLINICAL REASONING: A WHOLE BODY PROCESS

With the case study in mind, let's explore the nature of clinical reasoning. Perhaps one of the first things to note is that clinical reasoning is a whole body process. That is one reason it is a different experience to read a case study than to be the practitioner in the situation. Some clinical reasoning involves straightforward thinking processes that the practitioner can easily describe. Examples include assessing occupational performance, such as daily living skills and work behaviors. Occupational therapy practitioners use their observations and theoretical knowledge to identify

WHAT'S A PRACTITIONER TO DO? 11-1
Determining Appropriate Recommendations

Terry, an occupational therapist, goes up to a client's room in the neurology unit of a regional medical center. Along the way, she shares her thoughts with Barb, a researcher who is observing her practice. Terry fills Barb in on the client they are about to see. The client, Mrs. Munro, is a widow who lives alone in a house in town. A couple of days earlier, she suffered a stroke—a right cerebrovascular accident (CVA)—and was brought by a neighbor to the hospital. Mrs. Munro has made a rapid recovery and demonstrates good return of her motor skills. She still has some left-sided weakness and incoordination, along with some cognitive problems. She is a delightfully pleasant older woman and is anxious to return home.

Terry is seeing this client for the third time, and her primary concern is to assess whether Mrs. Munro has any cognitive residual effects from her stroke that would put her at serious risk if she returned home alone. Terry plans to do some more in-depth activities of daily living (ADL) with her to see how well Mrs. Munro demonstrates safety awareness. Terry thinks she will probably have Mrs. Munro get out of bed, obtain her clothing and hygiene supplies, perform her morning hygiene routines at the sink, and then get dressed. Terry wants to see the degree to which Mrs. Munro is spontaneously able to manage these tasks as well has how good her judgment appears to be. Terry's thought is that if she can engage Mrs. Munro in several multistep activities that also require her to perform in different positions Terry should be able to detect any cognitive and motor problems that pose a serious safety threat.

When Terry arrives at the room, she greets Mrs. Munro who says, "I am so excited. The doctor says I can go home tomorrow."

Terry turns to Barb and raises her eyebrows, as if to say, "I told you so." On the way to the room, Terry had told Barb that she was worried that the physician managing Mrs. Munro's case tended to think that as soon as clients can physically get up, they can go home. Terry went on to defend the physician by saying that in today's cost-conscious environment, doctors were under a lot of pressure to not keep clients in the hospital.

As Terry converses with Mrs. Munro about generalities, she notices that Mrs. Munro is already dressed in her housecoat. When she talks to Mrs. Munro about doing some self-care activities, it becomes apparent that the client has already completed her bathing and dressing routines, with help from nursing. When Terry suggests that she perhaps brush her teeth and comb her hair, Mrs. Munro is happy to get up out of bed, but notes that her neighbor never did bring in her dentures. Mrs. Munro sits on the edge of the bed, and after a reminder from Terry, puts on her slippers. She then stands and walks to the nearby sink, finds her comb, and combs her hair. While she is doing this Terry looks around for some other ideas about what to do, since Mrs. Munro has already completed the self-care tasks Terry had planned to do with her.

Terry's eyes light on some wilted flowers by the bed. She suggests to Mrs. Munro that she might want to dispose of the flowers and clean the vase so it will be ready to pack when it comes time to go home. Mrs. Munro agrees and proceeds to walk somewhat unsteadily over to the vase. Picking it up, she carries it to the sink, where she pulls out the dead flowers. Terry follows her, staying slightly behind and within reach of Mrs. Munro. When Mrs. Munro stops after removing the flowers, Terry suggests she rinse out the vase, which she does. She then dries it and returns the vase to the bedside table. Terry reminds her to throw out the dead flowers. While Mrs. Munro does this, they begin to talk some more about her plans to return home.

Mrs. Munro tells Terry that she has lived in her home for 40 years, and even though her husband died over 10 years ago, she still feels his presence there. He used to love her cooking, and she still cooks three meals a day for herself. She starts to cry when they talk about cooking, but then cheers up. Terry tells her that it might be safer if she had someone around the house for a few weeks, until she recovers a bit more from her stroke. Mrs. Munro thinks she can get some help from her neighbor. Terry says she is also going to suggest some home-care therapy, just to make sure she is safe in the kitchen, bathroom, and so on, noting, "We sure don't want to see you have a bad fall just when you are doing so well after your stroke."

After reviewing some coordination exercises for Mrs. Munro's left hand, Terry says good-bye. Terry and Barb leave the room. Terry stops at the nurses' station to note in the chart that Mrs. Munro demonstrated good safety awareness in familiar tasks at her bedside but did require cuing to complete multistep tasks. Terry also notes some motor instability in task performance during ambulation. Terry recommends a referral to a home health occupational therapy practitioner "to assess safety and equipment needs during bathroom activities, meal preparation, and routine homemaking tasks." Terry comments to Barb, as they walk off the unit, that she thinks Mrs. Munro did pretty well, but Terry remains concerned about the risks once Mrs. Munro goes home and particularly when she is tired. Terry wants someone to monitor

Continues

Mrs. Munro in a familiar setting to see if she handles her daily routines adequately. Terry would really like to see Mrs. Munro go to a rehab center, but the client has no insurance funding to support that. Terry believes that she might at least be able to get some home care, because there are a few programs around that provide some services to indigent elderly. Staying in her own home seems to be Mrs. Munro's major goal, and Terry is going to do what she can to try to help her attain that goal. Terry will catch up with the social worker later to discuss the need for Mrs. Munro to have good support from any neighbors, friends, or relatives.

QUESTIONS AND EXERCISES

1. How did Terry develop her concerns about Mrs. Munro?
2. How did Terry know what to do when her initial plans didn't work out?
3. What factors seem to guide Terry's recommendations at the end?

relevant client factors that contribute to occupational performance problems. Practitioners also attend to the contextual factors affecting performance. For instance, Terry was able to describe her concerns about Mrs. Munro's safety in returning home. In particular, Terry was addressing self-care and homemaking activities. She had analyzed relevant contextual factors about the home setting and Mrs. Munro's social and financial situation. Terry had identified some impairments in cognition and motor control that were affecting her client's occupational performance skills. This was all information that Terry could readily share with Barb. However, there was more knowledge from the therapy session that Terry either did not or could not put into words.

Part of Terry's clinical reasoning involved body-based knowledge that she gained from her senses. For instance, Terry used her sense of touch to feel the muscle tension (or lack of tension) in Mrs. Munro's affected arm when she was doing an activity or home exercise program. During her evaluation, Terry did some quick stretches to Mrs. Munro's elbow and wrist to see if she could feel evidence of spasticity, an abnormal reflex response commonly found in individuals recovering from a stroke. When Mrs. Munro stood up, Terry carefully gauged the distance she stood from Mrs. Munro, because Mrs. Munro was at some risk of falling. Terry was careful to stand not so close that she crowded or overprotected Mrs. Munro but close enough to protect her should she lose her balance. While close to Mrs. Munro, Terry could smell her, gaining a quick sense of possible hygiene or continence problems. Terry used her voice quality to display encouragement and support. Terry watched and listened carefully for clues about the nature of Mrs. Munro's emotional state. In particular she watched facial expressions and listened for evidence of fear or insecurity during Mrs. Munro's performance of activities. All of these sensations contributed to an image of Mrs. Munro that influenced Terry's practice.

There are other aspects of the clinical reasoning process that are even harder to describe. Fleming (1994a) described this as "knowing more than we can tell" (p. 24). She explained that much of the profession's knowledge is practical knowledge, which is "seldom discussed and rarely described" (p. 25). This tacit knowledge, combined with the rich sensory aspects of actual practice, help explain why reading about therapy and doing therapy are such different experiences.

THEORY AND PRACTICE

There has been a long-standing discussion in many professions about the role of theory in professional practice (Kessels & Korthagen, 1996). Theories help practitioners make decisions, although Cohn (1989) noted that the problems of practice rarely present themselves in the straightforward manner described in textbook theories. Clinical reasoning involves the naming and framing of problems based on a personal understanding of the client's situation (Schön, 1983). In problem identification and problem solution, practitioners blend theories with their own practice experiences to guide their actions. Theoretical knowledge aids the practitioner to avoid unjustified assumptions or the use of ineffective therapy techniques and to reflect on how the clinical experience is similar to or different from theoretical understandings (Parham, 1987). This issue is discussed further in Chapters 12 and 17.

COGNITIVE PROCESSES UNDERLYING CLINICAL REASONING

In the case study, Terry had to remember, obtain, and manage a great deal of information quickly to provide effective and efficient intervention. How did she do it? Research findings from the field of cognitive psychology help explain how practitioners think and how experience combined with reflection fosters increasing expertise. Individuals receive, store, and organize information in **schemata,** or chunks, which are complex representations of phenomena (Bruning, Schraw, & Ronning, 1999). For example, in school, Terry probably learned many of the common problems associated with someone who has had a stroke. She also has seen perhaps 100 people with strokes over the past several years. She has built up a general representation in her mind of what to expect when she receives a referral for someone who has had a stroke. She anticipates that many of these individuals will have thick medical charts, because they almost always have prior medical problems, such as diabetes and high blood pressure. She won't be surprised if the person is overweight. She expects to see impairments in cognition that often affect the person's ability to do everyday tasks, such as dressing, cooking, and driving. As part of her **schema,** Terry has built-in mental rules that help her categorize and detect differences. For instance, although she knows that many people who have strokes have movement impairments, she knows that not all do. Furthermore, when movement is impaired, she expects individuals with a left cerebrovascular accident (CVA) to have right-sided weakness and those with a right CVA to have left-sided weakness. She knows a person's social support systems are critical for promoting an adaptive response to disability. She may use certain cues, such as the presence or absence of frequent family visits, to prompt her to categorize a family as supportive or nonsupportive.

In addition to "chunking" information into schemata, Terry also creates and uses scripts or procedural rules that guide her thinking (Bruning et al., 1999). Just as her schemata help her organize and retrieve her knowledge about common aspects of stroke, scripts help her organize common occurrences or events. For instance, she understands that her role involves responding to the referral by seeing the client, writing her findings on the correct form, providing interventions, communicating verbally with the other team members, and developing discharge plans. Terry likely has scripts about the implications for clients with supportive families and those without. In her experience, a supportive family cares for its family member at home, regardless of the family's financial resources. Alternatively, clients with little family support are more likely to face institutional care. Again, these scripts are formed by Terry's observations and experiences over time and serve the purpose of helping her anticipate likely events.

Schemata and scripts support effective processing of information by providing efficient mental frameworks for handling complex information. Each person individually constructs them. It is no surprise that students and new practitioners often struggle to retain and effectively use their therapy knowledge. It takes time and repetition of experiences to develop effective schemata and scripts. Important aspects of the process are as follows (Bruning et al. 1999; Robertson, 1996; Roberts, 1996):

- *Cue acquisition:* Searching for the helpful and targeted information through observation and questioning.
- *Pattern recognition:* Noticing similarities and differences among situations
- *Limiting the problem space:* Using patterns to help focus cue acquisition and knowledge application to the most fruitful areas.
- *Problem formulation:* Developing an explanation of what is going on, why it is going on, and what a better situation or outcome might be.
- *Problem solution:* Identifying courses of action based on the problem formulation.

These cognitive processes are interactive and rarely occur in a linear fashion. Rather, the mind jumps around between the information at hand and that which has been stored up from prior learning while attempting to make sense of the situation.

ASPECTS OF CLINICAL REASONING

Although there appear to be common processes underlying clinical reasoning, the focus of that mental activity appears to vary with the demands of the problems to be addressed. Fleming (1991) was the first within occupational therapy to describe how occupational therapists seemed to use different thinking approaches, depending on the nature of the clinical problem they were addressing. She referred to this process as the "therapist with the three-track mind" (p. 1007). Since that time others have examined the different aspects of occupational therapy clinical reasoning. The vast majority of this research has been done with occupational therapists, although recent explorations (Lyons & Crepeau, 2001) suggest there is some application for occupational therapy assistants as well. These aspects of clinical reasoning are scientific, narrative, pragmatic, and ethical reasoning. Table 11-1 lists some of the typical questions of the different aspects of clinical reasoning.

Scientific Reasoning

Scientific reasoning is used to understand the condition that is affecting an individual and to decide on interventions that are in the best interest of the client. It is a logical process that parallels scientific inquiry. Two forms of scientific reasoning described in occupational therapy are diagnostic reasoning (Rogers & Holm, 1991) and procedural reasoning (Fleming, 1991, 1994b). Scientific reasoning may also be referred to as treatment planning (Pelland, 1987), in which the therapist uses selected theories both to identify problems and to guide decision making.

Diagnostic reasoning is concerned with clinical problem sensing and problem definition. The process starts in advance of seeing a client. Occupational therapy practitioners, because of their mind-set, primarily look for occupational performance problems. Furthermore, the nature of the problems they expect to find are influenced by the

TABLE 11–1. **ASPECTS AND EXAMPLES OF THE CLINICAL REASONING PROCESS**

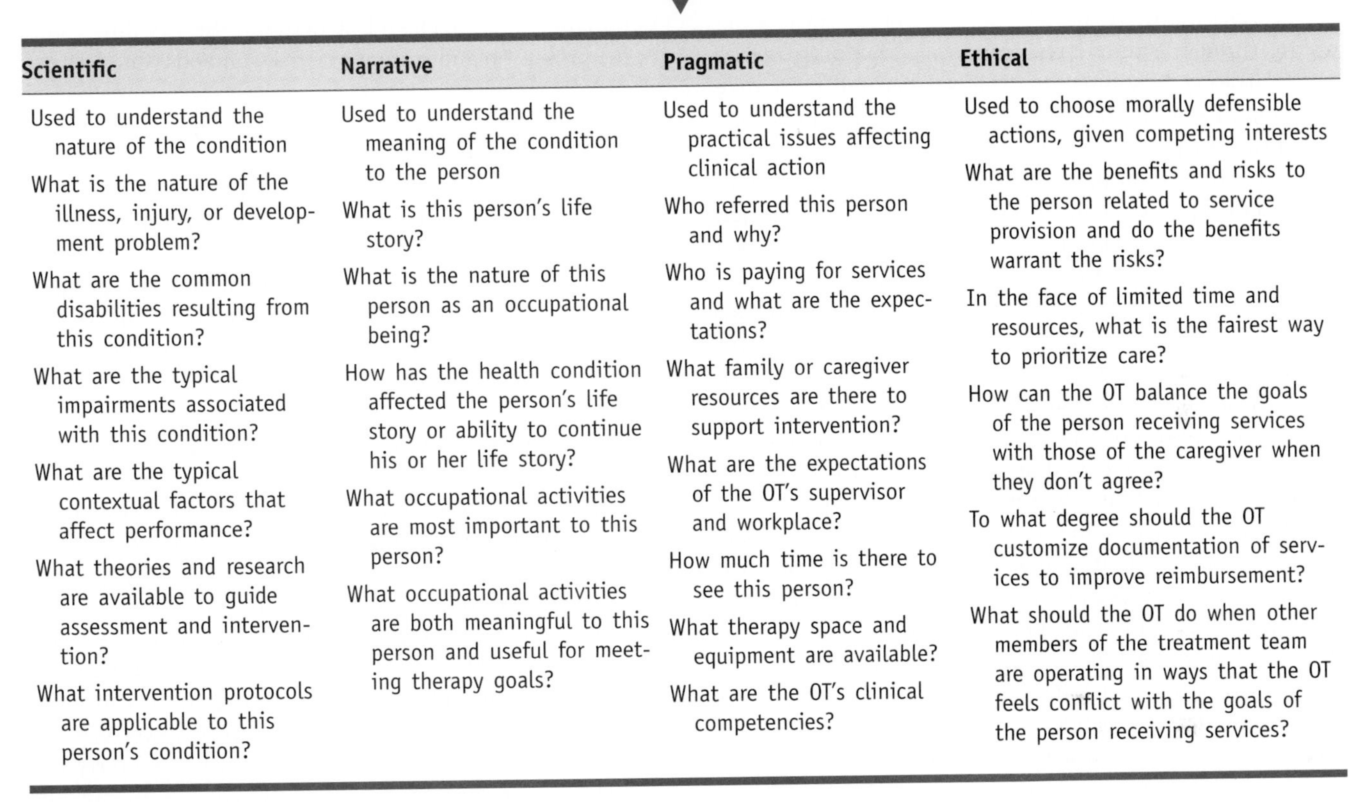

Primary Clinical Reasoning Concerns
What are the person's occupational performance concerns?
What is the person's occupational performance status and potential?
What will be done to improve occupational performance?
How are effective are interventions?
When and how should interventions stop?

Scientific	Narrative	Pragmatic	Ethical
Used to understand the nature of the condition	Used to understand the meaning of the condition to the person	Used to understand the practical issues affecting clinical action	Used to choose morally defensible actions, given competing interests
What is the nature of the illness, injury, or development problem?	What is this person's life story?	Who referred this person and why?	What are the benefits and risks to the person related to service provision and do the benefits warrant the risks?
What are the common disabilities resulting from this condition?	What is the nature of this person as an occupational being?	Who is paying for services and what are the expectations?	In the face of limited time and resources, what is the fairest way to prioritize care?
What are the typical impairments associated with this condition?	How has the health condition affected the person's life story or ability to continue his or her life story?	What family or caregiver resources are there to support intervention?	How can the OT balance the goals of the person receiving services with those of the caregiver when they don't agree?
What are the typical contextual factors that affect performance?	What occupational activities are most important to this person?	What are the expectations of the OT's supervisor and workplace?	To what degree should the OT customize documentation of services to improve reimbursement?
What theories and research are available to guide assessment and intervention?	What occupational activities are both meaningful to this person and useful for meeting therapy goals?	How much time is there to see this person?	What should the OT do when other members of the treatment team are operating in ways that the OT feels conflict with the goals of the person receiving services?
What intervention protocols are applicable to this person's condition?		What therapy space and equipment are available?	
		What are the OT's clinical competencies?	

OT, occupational therapist.

information in the requests for services. Some of Terry's diagnostic reasoning, described earlier, included information about the typical impairments associated with having a stroke.

Procedural reasoning occurs when practitioners are "thinking about the disease or disability and deciding which treatment activities (procedures) they might employ to remediate the person's functional performance problems" (Fleming, 1991, p. 1008). This may involve an interview, an observation of the person engaged in a task, or formal evaluations using standardized tools. In the case study, Terry used a combination of interview and observation, both of which were guided by her working hypothesis that Mrs. Munro had cognitive problems that might affect her safe performance at home. As intervention begins, more data are collected and the occupational therapy practitioner gains a sharper clinical image. This clinical image is the result of the interplay between what the occupational therapy practitioner expects to see (such as the usual course of the disease or disability) and the actual performance of the client. In the case study, there was congruence between Mrs. Munro's abilities and problems in performing activities of daily living and Terry's expectations of someone making a good recovery from a stroke.

Mattingly (1994a) made the point that occupational therapists have a "two-body practice" (p. 37). By that she meant that occupational therapy practitioners view a person in two ways: the body as a machine, in which parts may be broken, and the person as a life, filled with personal meanings and hopes. Much of the procedural reasoning in occupational therapy addresses issues related to the body as machine. The next form of clinical reasoning, narrative reasoning, provides the occupational therapy practitioner with a way to understand a person's illness experience.

Narrative Reasoning

Understanding the meaning that a disease, illness, or disability has to an individual is a task that goes beyond the scientific understanding of disease processes and organ systems. Rather, it requires that practitioners find a way to understand the meaning of this experience from the client's perspective. Mattingly (1994b) suggested that practitioners do this through a form of reasoning called narrative reasoning. Narrative reasoning is so named because it involves thinking in story form. It is not uncommon for an occupational therapy practitioner who is preparing to substitute for another with a client to ask, "So what is her story?" As Kielhofner (1997) noted, narrative reasoning "becomes particularly important for considering how the person's disrupted life story can be constituted or reconstituted" (p. 316).

In the case study, part of Terry's clinical reasoning was concerned with making decisions in light of what was important to Mrs. Munro. This process of collaboration and empathy has been described as "building a communal horizon of understanding" (Clark, Ennevor, & Richardson, 1996, p. 376). Terry gained understanding by listening attentively to Mrs. Munro's stories about her husband and how he loved her cooking. It is apparent from this session that Mrs. Munro's home is more than just a house. It is the place in which she lived with her husband, where he died, and where she still felt his presence. Part of Mrs. Munro's story is that going home is going back to her husband. Should this stroke prevent that, Mrs. Munro would lose more than her independence; she would lose symbolic connections to her husband. Although a logical case might be made that Mrs. Munro should start considering a more supportive living environment, Terry understands that for Mrs. Munro this would not be an acceptable ending. Consequently, Terry worked hard to obtain the support systems that would be necessary for Mrs. Munro to function in her chosen environment, where she will continue her life story.

Often, occupational therapy practitioners work with individuals whose life stories are so severely disrupted that they cannot imagine what their future will look like. Mattingly (1994b) believes that in these situations, skillful practitioners help their clients invent new life stories. To some degree, these stories become visible as the occupational therapy practitioner and the client develop goals together. The use of life stories is also apparent when activities are selected both for their healing potential and their particular significance to the person. To do this, one must first solicit occupational stories from the individual (Clark et al., 1996). With an understanding of clients' past occupational stories, practitioners can help individuals create new stories and new futures for themselves. If Mrs. Munro were more significantly disabled, and in a more extended therapy process, Terry might explore her interest in cooking as an activity that Mrs. Munro liked and that offers many therapeutic opportunities. Further, Mrs. Munro might find that she could express her pleasure in cooking for others by making special treats, first for other clients and then perhaps for neighbors in exchange for their help with chores. During this process, Mrs. Munro would not only be regaining coordination and dexterity, she would be regaining her sense of self as a productive person. This narrative aspect of clinical reasoning, which ultimately focuses on the person as an occupational being, provides a link between the founding values of the profession and current practice demands (Gray, 1998).

Pragmatic Reasoning

Pragmatic reasoning is yet another strand of clinical reasoning that goes beyond the practitioner-client relationship and addresses the world in which therapy occurs (Schell & Cervero, 1993). This world is considered from two perspectives: the practice context and the personal context. Because clinical reasoning is a practical activity, there are a number of everyday issues that have been identified over the years that affect the therapy process. These include treatment resources, organizational culture, power relations among team members, reimbursement issues, and practice trends in the profession (Barris, 1987; Howard, 1991; Neuhaus, 1988; Rogers & Holm, 1991). Studies examining clinical reasoning confirm that occupational therapy practitioners both actively consider and are influenced by their practice contexts (Creighton, Dijkers, Bennett, & Brown, 1995; Schell, 1994; Strong, Gilbert, Cassidy, & Bennett, 1995). An example of pragmatic reasoning in the case study was Terry's use of immediate resources (the flower vase) in Mrs. Munro's room as a therapy tool. Although Terry had thought of appropriate activities related to self-care, she had to identify practical alternatives quickly when it turned out that Mrs. Munro was already dressed. Practical constraints for Terry included (1) the time it would take to move Mrs. Munro to the clinic, where there might be more resources; (2) the need to get the required information on that day, since Mrs. Munro was going home; and (3) the physical constraints of what was available within the room. Terry's invention of a feasible alternative was a product of both her therapeutic imagination and the cues provided within her practice setting.

Terry's attention to the influence of team members demonstrates pragmatic reasoning directed to interpersonal and group issues. She knew the physician had the power to make discharge decisions. She was aware of the pressures on the physician by third-party payers to discharge clients as quickly as possible. Practice requires that practitioners reason about negotiating their clients' interests within the practice culture.

Similar to the practice context, the practitioner's personal situation also is part of the pragmatic reasoning process. A person's clinical competencies, preferences, commitment to the profession, and life role demands outside of work all affect the therapy choices considered and thus enter into the clinical reasoning process. For instance, if a practitioner does not feel safe helping a client stand or transfer to a bed, he or she is more likely to use tabletop activities, which can be done from a wheelchair. Or another occupational therapy practitioner may feel uncomfortable dealing with individuals who have depression and, therefore, may be quick to suggest that such clients are not motivated for therapy. Furthermore, if a practitioner has a young family to go home to, he or she may opt not to schedule clients late in the day, so as to get home as soon as possible. These simple personal issues result in clinical decisions that affect the scope and timing of therapy services. Hooper (1997) suggested that fundamental issues, such as a practitioner's values and general worldview, strongly affect the way an individual constructs his or her clinical reasoning. Such worldviews play an important role in the next kind of reasoning, ethical reasoning.

Ethical Reasoning

All of the forms of reasoning described so far help the practitioner respond to the following questions: What is this person's current occupational situation? What can be done to enhance the person's situation? Ethical reasoning goes one step further and asks the question, What should be done? Rogers (1983) framed these three questions (here paraphrased) in her Eleanor Clark Slagle Lecture and went on to state: "The clinical reasoning process terminates in an ethical decision, rather than a scientific one, and the ethical nature of the goal of clinical reasoning projects itself over the entire sequence" (p. 602). In the case study, Terry's ethical dilemma is to understand Mrs. Munro's personal wishes and to honor them when developing a therapy plan that realistically addresses her limitations. This can be particularly challenging when the pressures of financial realities (such as Mrs. Munro's lack of insurance) affect available options. A number of occupational therapy authors have addressed the ethical aspect of clinical reasoning (Fondiller, Rosage, & Neuhaus; 1990; Howard, 1991; Neuhaus, 1988; Peloquin, 1993), and Chapter 52 of this text is devoted to the issue of the ethics of the profession. The purpose here is to introduce ethical reasoning as yet another of the components of clinical reasoning in occupational therapy.

ETHICS NOTE 11–1

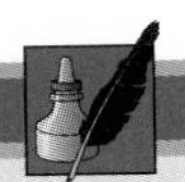

What Are the Ethical Obligations of Robert's Therapist?

PENNY KYLER and RUTH ANN HANSEN

Robert is 25 years old and has sickle cell (SC) anemia. He volunteers at a local SC community program, delivering bottled water to other people who have SC. Medicaid provides coverage for his health care. He has been in the hospital 11 times in the past year with severe abdominal pain and joint pain. During each hospitalization, he receives occupational therapy instructions in energy conservation and joint protection. Today, the occupational therapist walks into the clinic and sees Robert waiting. She turns and walks out mumbling to herself, "It's a waste of my time to treat him. He doesn't follow through on any of my suggestions."

QUESTIONS AND EXERCISES

1. **What are some of the possible reasons that the practitioner is reluctant to treat Robert? Can you justify any of them either ethically or legally?**
2. **Are Robert's goals important? Should his priorities make a difference in setting treatment goals?**
3. **What are possible reasons for Robert's lack of compliance?**

CLINICAL REASONING: A PROCESS OF SYNTHESIS

The preceding section described the aspects of clinical reasoning separately to illustrate the different parts of the process. However, these facets of clinical reasoning are not separate or parallel processes; rather, the opposite appears to be the case. Virtually all the research about clinical reasoning suggests that these different forms interact with each other.

Interactive Process

Scientific, narrative, pragmatic, and ethical reasoning processes are intertwined throughout the therapy process. Indeed, each perspective informs the other. In the case study, Terry's understanding of medical science helped her know what might be potential impairments and performance problems, but her narrative reasoning helped her understand the importance for Mrs. Munro of returning home. Put together, these two forms of reasoning help Terry to an unsaid understanding that there would be a high risk for depression (which could worsen her client's medical condition) if Mrs. Munro did not return to her home, which means so much to her. Furthermore, the practical constraints associated with the setting and Mrs. Munro's reimbursement prompted Terry to reason about the ethics of referring Mrs. Munro to a rehabilitation center (which she couldn't afford), to home alone (where she might not be safe), and finally to home with the support of home health care and neighbors.

Underlying the view of clinical reasoning as an interactive process is the communicative nature of occupational therapy practice. This is because occupational therapy involves "doing with" as opposed to "doing to" clients (Mattingly & Fleming, 1994, p. 178). Practitioners must gain the trust of their client and those persons important in the client's world. They do this by entering the life world of the client (Crepeau, 1991). Once they are in that life world, occupational therapy practitioners can better understand how to help the individual resolve performance problems.

Conditional Process

Not only must practitioners blend different aspects of clinical reasoning in order to interact effectively with their clients but also they must flexibly modify interventions in response to changing conditions. Terry showed her flexibility by inventing an activity with the flower vase when her plan to work with Mrs. Munro on bathing and dressing did not pan out. Creighton et al. (1995) noticed that occupational therapy practitioners preplanned treatments in a hierarchical manner. They observed that practitioners typically brought several sets of supplies to a treatment session. One set would be directed to the expected level of performance, the others to a stage higher and lower than the expected performance. As an example, one practitioner, in preparation for a writing activity with a client who had a spinal cord injury, brought a short writing splint and unlined paper. This practitioner also brought a longer splint to provide wrist support (in case the client's hand control was worse than expected) and lined paper, which required more precision (in case the hand control was better than expected). This practitioner blended scientific and pragmatic concerns in a way that anticipated several possible situations that might occur.

On a larger scale, Fleming (1994c) described the ability of skilled occupational therapy practitioners to "form an image of future life possibilities for the person" (p. 234). The ability to form these images (or schemata, using cognitive terms) seems to require a blend of all the forms of clinical reasoning, along with sufficient clinical experience to have seen a variety of different outcomes with former clients. These images help practitioners select therapeutic activities on a day-to-day basis. For instance, the writing activity for the client who had a spinal cord injury not only is a good activity for increasing coordination but also presages occupations that will enable him to regain control of his life through writing his own checks, signing his name on legal documents, and using various forms of technology for work and play. If this client was an accountant, these would be powerful images. Conversely, if the client was a professional athlete, the occupational therapy practitioner might have to create different activities to allow the client to develop a vision of himself as a future coach or teacher. The activities used in occupational therapy can help meet specific short-term goals and shape long-term expectations. It is in this way that practitioners help individuals reengage in their lives through the use of meaningful occupations.

CONCLUSION

Clinical reasoning is the process used by practitioners to plan, direct, perform, and reflect on client care. It is a whole-body and multisensory process that requires complex cognitive activity. Practitioners develop schemata and scripts as they gain experience, forming the basis of professional knowledge and action. Clinical reasoning is multifaceted and enables practitioners to understand client issues from different perspectives. Practitioners use the logical processes associated with scientific reasoning to understand the client's impairments, disabilities, and performance contexts and to predict the impact these have on occupational performance. Narrative reasoning helps practitioners appreciate the meaning of occupational performance limitations to the client, thus supporting client-centered care. Practitioners use pragmatic reasoning when they address the practical realities associated with service delivery. All of these forms of reasoning lead to an ethical reasoning process by which practitioners select the best therapy action to respond to the client's occupational performance needs.

References

Barris, R. (1987). Clinical reasoning in psychosocial occupational therapy: The evaluation process. *Occupational Therapy Journal of Research, 7,* 147–162

Bruning, R. H., Schraw, G. J., & Ronning, R. R. (1999). *Cognitive psychology and instruction* (3rd ed.). Upper Saddle River, NJ: Merrill.

Clark, F., Ennevor, B. L., & Richardson, P. L. (1996). A grounded theory of techniques for occupational storytelling and occupational story making. In R. Zemke & F. Clark (Eds.). *Occupational science: The evolving discipline* (pp. 373–392). Philadelphia: Davis.

Cohn, E. S. (1989). Fieldwork education: Shaping a foundation for clinical reasoning. *American Journal of Occupational Therapy, 43,* 240–244.

Creighton, C., Dijkers, M., Bennett, N., & Brown, K. (1995). Reasoning and the art of therapy for spinal cord injury. *American Journal of Occupational Therapy, 49,* 311–317.

Crepeau, E. B. (1991). Achieving intersubjective understanding: Examples from an occupational therapy treatment session. *American Journal of Occupational Therapy, 44,* 1016–1024.

Fleming, M. H. (1991). The therapist with the three-track mind. *American Journal of Occupational Therapy, 45,* 1007–1014.

Fleming, M. H. (1994a). The search for tacit knowledge. In C. Mattingly & M. H. Fleming (Eds.). *Clinical reasoning: Forms of inquiry in a therapeutic practice* (pp. 22–33). Philadelphia: Davis.

Fleming, M. H. (1994b). Procedural reasoning: Addressing functional limitations. In C. Mattingly & M. H. Fleming (Eds.). *Clinical reasoning: Forms of inquiry in a therapeutic practice* (pp. 137–177). Philadelphia: Davis.

Fleming, M. H. (1994c). Conditional reasoning: Creating meaningful experiences. In C. Mattingly & M. H. Fleming (Eds.). *Clinical reasoning-forms of inquiry in a therapeutic practice* (pp. 197–235). Philadelphia: Davis.

Fondiller, E. D., Rosage, L. J., & Neuhaus, B. E. (1990). Values influencing clinical reasoning in occupational therapy: An exploratory study. *Occupational Therapy Journal of Research, 10,* 41–55.

Gray, J. M. (1998). Putting occupation in practice: Occupation as ends, occupation as means. *American Journal of Occupational Therapy, 52*, 354–364.

Hooper, B. (1997). The relationship between pretheoretical assumptions and clinical reasoning. *American Journal of Occupational Therapy, 51*, 328–338.

Howard, B. S. (1991). How high do we jump? The effect of reimbursement on occupational therapy. *American Journal of Occupational Therapy, 45*, 875–881.

Kessels, J. P. A. M., & Korthagen, F. A. (1996). The relationship between theory and practice: Back to the classics. *Educational Researcher, 25*(32), 17–22.

Kielhofner, G. (1997). *Conceptual foundations of occupational therapy* (2nd ed.). Philadelphia: Davis.

Lyons, K. D., & Crepeau, E. B. (report—clinical). Case report—The clinical reasoning of a certified occupational therapy assistant. *American Journal of Occupational Therapy, 55*, 577–581.

Mattingly, C. (1994a). Occupational therapy as a two body practice: Body as machine. In C. Mattingly & M. H. Fleming (Eds.). *Clinical reasoning: Forms of inquiry in a therapeutic practice* (pp. 37–63). Philadelphia: Davis.

Mattingly, C. (1994b). The narrative nature of clinical reasoning. In C. Mattingly & M. H. Fleming (Eds.). *Clinical reasoning: Forms of inquiry in a therapeutic practice* (pp. 239–269). Philadelphia: Davis.

Mattingly, C., & Fleming, M. H. (1994). Interactive reasoning: Collaborating with the person. In C. Mattingly & M. H. Fleming (Eds.). *Clinical reasoning: Forms of inquiry in a therapeutic practice* (pp. 178–196). Philadelphia: Davis.

Neuhaus, B. E. (1988). Ethical considerations in clinical reasoning: The impact of technology and cost containment. *American Journal of Occupational Therapy, 42*, 288–294.

Parham, D. (1987). Nationally speaking—toward professionalism: The reflective occupational therapy practitioner. *American Journal of Occupational Therapy, 41*, 555–561.

Pelland, M. J. (1987). A conceptual model for the instruction and supervision of treatment planning. *American Journal of Occupational Therapy, 41*, 351–359.

Peloquin, S. M. (1993). The depersonalization of patients: A profile gleaned from narratives. *American Journal of Occupational Therapy, 49*, 830–837.

Roberts, A. E. (1996). Clinical reasoning in occupational therapy: Idiosyncrasies in content and process. *British Journal of Occupational Therapy, 59*, 372–376.

Robertson, L. J. (1996). Clinical reasoning, part 2: Novice/expert differences. *British Journal of Occupational Therapy, 59*, 212–216.

Rogers, J. C. (1983). Clinical reasoning: The ethics, science, and art. *American Journal of Occupational Therapy, 37*, 601–616.

Rogers, J. C., & Holm, M. B. (1991). Occupational therapy diagnostic reasoning: A component of clinical reasoning. *American Journal of Occupational Therapy, 45*, 1045–1053.

Schell, B. A. B. (1994). The effect of practice context on occupational therapy practitioner's clinical reasoning (Doctoral dissertation, University of Georgia, 1994). *Dissertation Abstracts International*, AAT 9507243.

Schell, B. A., & Cervero, R. M. (1993). Clinical reasoning in occupational therapy: An integrative review. *The American Journal of Occupational Therapy, 47*, 605–610.

Schön, D. A. (1983). *The reflective practitioner: How professionals think in action*. New York: Basic.

Strong, J., Gilbert, J., Cassidy, S., & Bennett, S. (1995). Expert clinicians and student view on clinical reasoning in occupational therapy. *British Journal of Occupational Therapy*, 58, 119–123.

CHAPTER 12

PROFESSIONAL DEVELOPMENT

BARBARA A. BOYT SCHELL, ELIZABETH BLESEDELL CREPEAU, and ELLEN S. COHN

The previous chapter on clinical reasoning provided insight into the cognitive processes of practitioners. In this chapter we look at how practitioners gain expertise and how their roles in practice can change and diversify over the course of a career. These roles include those of educator, manager, entrepreneur, advocate, and researcher–scholar. Since the entry point into the field occurs at the practitioner level, let's start by taking a closer look at some key expectations of practitioners.

PRACTITIONER ROLE

The practitioner role is primarily concerned with client evaluation and related interventions (Crist, 1996). Occupational therapists perform all aspects of the practitioner role. Occupational therapy assistants, working under the supervision of an occupational therapist, provide interventions appropriate to their knowledge and skills. In this book, the term practitioner is used to refer to both the occupational therapist and the occupational therapy assistant. The term therapist is used when discussing information relevant only to the occupational therapist.

Evaluation and Intervention

Using observations, interviews, and standardized assessments, occupational therapists analyze clients' occupational concerns. To understand the client's performance, therapists focus their attention on the nature and influence of specific client factors (such as physical, social, and cognitive skills) as well as outside factors that influence the client (such as physical and social contexts). Intervention approaches may involve provision of services directly to the client (such as skill training) or consultative approaches (such as providing advice on how to modify a worksite or design of a community playground). Both intrinsic and extrinsic factors are addressed strategically to improve occupational performance within the necessary performance contexts. During interventions,

TABLE 12-1. **COMMON PROFESSIONAL CREDENTIALS USED IN THE UNITED STATES**

Credentials		Granting Organization
Entry-Level Credentialing		
ACOTE Accredited	Refers to the status of an occupational therapy educational program that is fully accredited	ACOTE
OTR	Occupational therapist, registered (professional level)	NBCOT
COTA	Certified occupational therapy assistant (technical level)	NBCOT
Advanced Practice and Specialty Certifications		
AP	Advanced Practitioner (for occupational therapy assistants)	AOTA-SCB
BCP	Board Certified in Pediatrics (for occupational therapists)	AOTA-SCB
BCN	Board Certified in Neurorehabilitation (for occupational therapists)	AOTA-SCB
BCG	Board Certified in Geriatrics (for occupational therapists)	AOTA-SCB
ATP	Assistive Technology Practitioner	RESNA
CCM	Certified Case Manager	CCMC
CDRS	Certified Driving Rehabilitation Practitioner	ADED
CHT	Certified Hand Therapist	ASHT
CPE	Certified Professional Ergonomist	BCPE
CVE	Certified Vocational Evaluation Specialist	CCWAVES
NDT	Trained in Neuro-Developmental Therapy	NDTA
SIPT	Certified to administer the Sensory Integration and Praxis Tests	WSP/USC; SII

ACOTE, Accreditation Council for Occupational Therapy Education; *ADED,* Association for Driver Rehabilitation Specialists; *AOTA-SCB,* American Occupational Therapy Association—Specialty Certification Board; *ASHT,* American Society of Hand Therapists, *BCPE,* Board of Certification in Professional Ergonomics; *CCMC,* Commission for Case Manager Certification; *CCWAVES,* Commission on Certification of Work Adjustment and Vocational Evaluation Specialists; *NBCOT,* National Board for Certification of Occupational Therapy; *NDTA,* Neuro-Developmental Training Association; *RESNA,* Rehabilitation Engineering and Assistive Technology Society of North America; *SII,* Sensory Integration International; *WSP/USC,* Western Psychological Service/University of Southern California.

the practitioner maintains an evaluative stance, so that intervention strategies are frequently modified and customized to the emerging needs of the client.

Professional Communication

Communication about occupational therapy services to a wide range of interested parties is an integral part of practice. Some communication may be relatively informal, such as verbally sharing with family members and team members the nature of services provided. More formal presentations may be required to educate payers, employers, or policy makers. In addition, written communication is routinely required to summarize evaluations, intervention progress, and other aspects of service provision. Whatever the form, practitioners are expected to communicate clearly, concisely, and with integrity.

Credentialing and Ongoing Professional Development

Credentialing refers to the methods by which the public can be assured that members of the profession have the necessary knowledge and skills to practice competently. Requirements are delineated by different professional organizations and governmental agencies. For example, in the United States, individuals must complete an educational program approved by the Accreditation Council for Occupational Therapy Education (ACOTE), which includes specified fieldwork requirements, and then pass the certification examination administered by the National Board for Certification of Occupational Therapy (NBCOT). In addition, most of the U.S. state governments regulate practice through licensure or other laws that regulate the delivery of services. Once in the field, practitioners are expected to maintain competence and continually develop expertise (Hinojosa & Blount, 1998). In some cases, specialty credentials may be obtained to reflect increased knowledge and skill in an advanced area. Table 12-1 provides a sampling of major groups that play a role in credentialing practitioners.

DEVELOPING EXPERTISE

Although the nature of clinical reasoning in occupational therapy is becoming better understood, there is still little empirical research that directly examines its development

TABLE 12-2. **CLINICAL REASONING DEVELOPMENTAL STAGES AND CHARACTERISTICS**[a]

Stage	Years of Reflective Practice	Characteristics
Novice	0	• No experience in situation of practice; depends on theory to guide practice • Uses rule-based procedural reasoning to guide actions, but does not recognize contextual cues; not skillful in adapting rules to fit situation • Narrative reasoning used to establish social relationships, but does not significantly inform practice • Pragmatic reasoning stressed in terms of job survival skills • Recognizes overt ethical issues
Advanced beginner	<1	• Begins to incorporate contextual information into rule-based thinking • Recognizes differences between theoretical expectations and presenting problems • Limited experience impedes recognition of patterns and identification of salient cues; does not prioritize well • Gaining skill in pragmatic and narrative reasoning • Begins to recognize more subtle ethical issues
Competent	3	• Automatically performs more therapeutic skills and attends to more issues • Able to develop communal horizon with persons receiving service • Able to sorts relevant data and prioritize intervention goals related to desired outcomes • Planning is deliberate, efficient and responsive to contextual issues • Uses conditional reasoning to modify intervention, but lacks flexibility of more advanced practitioners • Recognizes ethical dilemmas posed by practice setting, but may be less sensitive to justifiably different ethical responses
Proficient	5	• Perceives situations as wholes • Reflects on expanded range of experiences, permitting more focused evaluation and more flexibility in intervention • Creatively combines different diagnostic and procedural approaches • More attentive to occupational stories and relevance for intervention • More skillful in negotiating resources to meet patient/client needs • Increased sophistication in recognizing situational nature of ethical reasoning
Expert	10	• Clinical reasoning becomes a quick intuitive process—which is deeply internalized and embedded, in an extensive range of case experiences—permitting practice with less routine analysis, except when confronted with situations in which approach is not working • Highly skillful use of occupational story making during intervention to promote long-term occupational performance satisfaction

[a]Modified from Dreyfus and Dreyfus (1986) to include information from Benner (1984); Clark, Ennevor, and Richardson (1996); Creighton, Dijkers, Bennett, and Brown (1995); Mattingly and Fleming (1994); Slater and Cohn (1991); and Strong, Gilbert, Cassidy, and Bennett (1995).

beyond entry level into the profession. There is, however, a large body of research on the development of expertise in a variety of other fields (Boshuizen & Schmidt, 2000). Dreyfus and Dreyfus's (1986) conceptualization of professional expertise has been applied to occupational therapy (Slater & Cohn, 1991). This conceptualization, summarized in Table 12-2, describes changes in the reasoning of occupational therapists as they develop expertise. An underlying assumption of this process is that both experience and reflection about that experience are necessary for expertise to develop. Although the changes listed in Table 12-2 are presented as a hierarchy tied to years of experience, it is important to recognize that development is dynamic and influenced by many factors beyond just the years of experience. Both professional and personal experiences, along with active reflection about those experiences are critical to becoming an expert (Benner, 1984; Gambrill, 1990; Slater & Cohn, 1991).

Practice Experience

The development and advancement of clinical reasoning skills require experience. To some degree, these are issues of attention and memory. Because therapy is a complex process, newcomers to the field have difficulty concentrating on everything at once. It is not until some skills become more automatic that practitioners can concentrate on other parts of the process. As discussed in the Chapter 11, experience is necessary for the development of mental models. These models organize complex information into patterns for rapid recall and use (Boshuizen & Schmidt, 2000; Bruning, Schraw, & Ronning, 1991).

In addition to the development of more automatic skills, experience also allows the practitioner to gain firsthand knowledge of the usual course of events associated with familiar situations. These scripts, sometimes in the form of stories, serve to inform practice over time. The understanding of possible futures, along with ease in performing a variety of technical skills, permits the use of conditional reasoning to guide intervention (Boshuizen & Schmidt, 2000; Mattingly & Fleming, 1994).

An important aspect of experience is that it may not reliably generalize to situations different from the ones in which practitioners have gained some expertise. This observation led Benner (1984) to suggest that expert professionals are expert relative only to particular situations. An expert in an unfamiliar situation may not be expert at all. The context-specific nature of expertise suggests that sustained experience in a particular practice situation may be more effective in developing clinical reasoning than a variety of more superficial experiences in many situations (Cohn, 1989).

Personal Experience

Personal experience can enrich the clinical reasoning process by serving as the basis for empathetic understanding. This, in turn, helps the practitioner enter the life world of another supporting narrative reasoning. For instance, a practitioner who is also a parent may be more realistic about the feasibility of home programs. Conversely, powerful personal experiences may also impede the clinical reasoning process, particularly when practitioners assume another's experience will be just like their own. In spite of these risks, practitioners do find that skillful therapeutic use of self requires a reservoir of personal stories useful in creating therapeutic alliances (Mattingly & Fleming, 1994).

Reflection on Experience

Although necessary, experience alone is not sufficient to ensure advancement in clinical reasoning skills. Schön (1983) proffered the term *reflective practitioner* to describe how experts think critically about their own experience. Reflection happens in two ways. First, practitioners "reflect-in-action" (p. 49). This involves the ability of the practitioner to think in the midst of action and adapt to meet the demands of the situation. Reflection in action most often occurs when the usual approaches aren't working. "Reflection-on-action" (p. 61) is the term Schön uses for critical thinking that occurs after the fact. Reflection about practice, identifying what worked and what didn't, and being open to alternative conceptions are necessary to support the learning associated with advancing expertise. The use of research evidence to support practice and the application of formal theories, along with systematic observation and data collection, can be invaluable aides to the reflection process (Gambrill, 1990; Tickle-Degnen, 2000).

Education

Education is an additional way of developing expertise. This need to continue the development and refinement of clinical reasoning skills is well accepted in most professions, including occupational therapy (Youngstrom, 1998). The value of education is twofold. First, it provides an arena for the development of new knowledge and skills. Second, it supports systematic reflection about past and current practices. This education can take the form of self-directed inquiry, continuing education, and formal education. Self-directed inquiry includes reading or viewing relevant resources as well as networking with others through meetings, study groups, and electronic means. Continuing education involves the completion of short courses of study, such as inservices, workshops, and seminars. Formal education requires enrollment at degree-granting institutions and typically leads to a postprofessional degree in occupational therapy or a related field. Each form of education can support the development of clinical reasoning as well as of specific practice skills, management and consultative expertise, and/or research competence.

CHANGING ROLES AND CAREER OPTIONS

Once individuals gain experience in the practitioner role, it is common for them to seek additional responsibilities and roles. These may build on the practitioner role, as when an individual becomes expert in a particular practice arena and provides mentoring and education to others. Alternatively, as in the case of management and education, new roles may require the addition of knowledge and skills gained from outside occupational therapy, which are then blended with existing professional understandings. The possibilities for career development and expansion for occupational therapy practitioners are practically endless and include the roles of educator, manager, entrepreneur, advocate, and research–scholar (American Occupational Therapy Association, 1993; Yerxa, 1994).

Educator

The processes of teaching and learning are embedded in much of occupational therapy practice. It is not surprising, therefore, that practitioners assume various educational roles, sometimes quite early in their careers. For instance, someone may become a fieldwork educator and provide supervision to occupational therapy students in the practice setting. Practitioners are also frequently asked to provide education to client groups, such as teaching people with arthritis about prevention approaches or parents of children with disabilities about how to select toys. As practitioners gain experience and skills in teaching, they may provide continuing education to others by speaking at conferences and workshops or by developing online educational programs. Finally, individuals may become faculty members at colleges and universities. Each of these roles requires that practitioners learn additional skills related to education (Crepeau, Thibodaux, & Parham, 1999; Crist, 1999). For instance, there is an extensive literature about how learning occurs in children and adults. Understanding learning theory is important for making teaching decisions about the content to be taught, the methods used, the learning environment, and the means of assessing learning. Furthermore, being an effective educator also typically requires that individuals maintain necessary practice skills and engage in scholarship relevant to the education being provided.

Manager

Many practice settings need supervisors, administrators, and program consultants. Some aspects of supervision are already part of the occupational therapist's role, such as the need to provide oversight for occupational therapy assistants and aides. In addition, some aspects of administration, such as the process of ordering and maintaining supplies, are in practitioner expectations. Broader roles can be assumed for coordinating multidisciplinary care as a **case manager** or as a **program manager.** With added education and experience, practitioners can be promoted into positions of authority as supervisors, managers, and administrators. As this occurs, expanded knowledge related to personnel management, organizational theory, and fiscal control are typically required (Schell & Slater, 1998).

Entrepreneur

A significant number of occupational therapists in the United States are self-employed and thus engaged in entrepreneurial roles that may require them to develop new practice opportunities, market these services, negotiate contractual agreements, and manage the relationships necessary for ongoing success (Foto, 1998). Some practitioners may find these skills becoming a greater part of their job expectations or may choose to engage in entrepreneurial activities in addition to their work as an employee. This can be particularly true in regions where occupational therapy services are less well known or in new practice venues where the application of occupational therapy are just being explored.

Advocate

People with disabilities may be excluded from participation in society because of prejudice, lack of understanding, or failure to comply with laws. Yerxa (1994) argued that occupation therapy practitioners should ally themselves with people or groups to advocate for change in society's attitudes. Advocacy is defined as pleading for a cause or proposal. To be effective advocates, practitioners need to understand the effects of current trends in health care and education, laws, political dynamics, social values, economic factors, and cultural issues on access to services and overall well-being. Practitioners may function as advocates by helping clients gain an understanding of their rights and communicating their rights and needs to others so that they may fully participate in society. Practitioners may also advocate on behalf of clients, which may entail representing the client's need to receive support services in a particular setting or to help a client obtain subsidies from a governing agency.

In addition to advocacy related to specific clients, practitioners may advocate for groups via lobbying, public-interest litigation, or public-relations campaigns. For example, practitioners may advocate to a city council to make all public buildings accessible to people with disabilities. Sometimes practitioners must advocate for the profession by representing its concerns to policymakers, legislators, granting agencies, insurance companies, or other payers of services. Such advocacy includes providing testimony about the need for appropriate licensure laws or rules and to support inclusion of occupational therapy services in state or federal legislation.

Researcher–Scholar

Scholars are individuals who seek to develop, evaluate, and synthesize knowledge and to understand critically the implications of knowledge for practice and society (Abreu, Peloquin, & Ottenbacher, 1998). The researcher–scholar role is becoming more important because practitioners are now expected to substantiate their practice by research evidence. As Abreau et al. pointed out, there is a range of knowledge and skills associated with scholarship. Among these are the ability to understand scientific processes; obtain financial and intellectual support; and communicate findings through professional presentations, reports, and journal articles.

CONCLUSION

In the practitioner role, as in all the additional roles described in this chapter, there is a blending of experience, education, and mentorship that is required to progress to higher levels of expertise and broader scopes of responsibility. Peer, employer, and professional associations support this process to some degree. However, the key component in professional development is the personal value that each practitioner puts on the need to continually improve his or her practice.

References

Abreu, B. C., Peloquin, S. M., & Ottenbacher, K. (1998). Competence in scientific inquiry and research. *American Journal of Occupational Therapy, 53,* 751–759.

American Occupational Therapy Association. (1993). Occupational therapy roles. *American Journal of Occupational Therapy, 47,* 1087–1099.

Benner, P. (1984). *From novice to expert.* Menlo Park, CA: Addison-Wesley.

Boshuizen, H. P. A., & Schmidt, H. G. (2000). The development of clinical reasoning expertise. In J. Higgs & M. Jones (Eds.). *Clinical reasoning in the health professions* (2nd ed., pp. 15–22). Boston: Butterworth Heinemann.

Bruning, R. H., Schraw, G. J., & Ronning, R. R. (1991). *Cognitive psychology and instruction* (3rd ed.). Upper Saddle River, NJ: Merrill.

Clark, F., Ennevor, B. L., & Richardson, P. L. (1996). A grounded theory of techniques for occupational storytelling and occupational story making. In R. Zemke & F. Clark (Eds.). *Occupational science: The evolving discipline* (pp. 373–392). Philadelphia: Davis.

Cohn, E. S. (1989). Fieldwork education: Shaping a foundation for clinical reasoning. *American Journal of Occupational Therapy, 43,* 240–244.

Creighton, C., Dijkers, M., Bennett, N., & Brown, K. (1995). Reasoning and the art of therapy for spinal cord injury. *American Journal of Occupational Therapy, 49,* 311–317.

Crepeau, E. B., Thibodaux, L., & Parham, D. (1999). Academic juggling act: Beginning and sustaining an academic career. *American Journal of Occupational Therapy, 53,* 25–30.

Crist, P. (1996). Roles, relationships, and career development. In American Occupational Therapy Association (Eds.). *The occupational therapy manager* (rev. ed., pp. 327–348). Bethesda, MD: Editor.

Crist, P. (1999). Career transition from clinician to academician: Responsibilities and reflections. *American Journal of Occupational Therapy, 53,* 14–19.

Dreyfus, H. L., & Dreyfus, S. E. (1986). *Mind over machine: The power of human intuition and expertise in the era of the computer.* New York: Free Press.

Foto, M. (1998). Competence and the occupational therapy entrepreneur. *American Journal of Occupational Therapy, 52,* 765–769.

Gambrill, E. (1990). *Critical thinking in clinical practice: Improving the accuracy of judgments and decisions about clients.* San Francisco: Jossey-Bass.

Hinojosa, J. & Blount, M.-L. (1998). Nationally speaking: Professional competence. *American Journal of Occupational Therapy, 52,* 699–701.

Mattingly, C., & Fleming, M. H. (1994). *Clinical reasoning: Forms of inquiry in a therapeutic practice.* Philadelphia: Davis.

Schell, B. A. B., & Slater, D. Y. (1998). Management competencies required of administrative and clinical practitioners in the new millennium. *American Journal of Occupational Therapy, 52,* 744–750.

Schön, D. A. (1983). *The reflective practitioner: How professionals think in action.* New York: Basic Books.

Slater, D. Y., & Cohn, E. S. (1991). Staff development through analysis of practice. *American Journal of Occupational Therapy, 45,* 1038–1044.

Strong, J., Gilbert, J., Cassidy, S., & Bennett, S. (1995). Expert clinicians and student view on clinical reasoning in occupational therapy. *British Journal of Occupational Therapy, 58,* 119–123.

Tickle-Degnen, L. (2000). Evidence-based practice forum—Gathering current research evidence to enhance clinical reasoning. *American Journal of Occupational Therapy, 54,* 102–105.

Yerxa, E. J. (1994). Dreams, dilemmas, and decisions for occupational therapy practice in a new millennium: An American perspective. *American Journal of Occupational Therapy, 48,* 586–589.

Youngstrom, M. J. (1998). Evolving competence in the practitioner role. *American Journal of Occupational Therapy, 52,* 716–720.

CHAPTER 13

THE OCCUPATIONAL THERAPIST AND OCCUPATIONAL THERAPY ASSISTANT PARTNERSHIP

MARY SANDS

FRAMEWORK FOR THE OCCUPATIONAL THERAPIST–OCCUPATIONAL THERAPY ASSISTANT PARTNERSHIP

Service delivery in occupational therapy has been and will continue to be influenced by increased demands for productivity, increased access to occupational therapy services, reduced intervention time frames, and increased complexity of problems experienced by occupational therapy clients. These demands increase the importance of teamwork between occupational therapists and occupational therapy assistants to sustain occupational therapy's commitment to client-centered services. The key components of this occupational therapy service provider partnership are supervision, service competency, and collaboration. This chapter explores the critical components of the occupational therapist and occupational therapy assistant partnership with input from occupational therapists and occupational therapy assistants, who provide their perspectives of the therapy team process.

Preparing for Entry to the Field: Understanding the Knowledge Base of Practitioners

Occupational therapy practice involves two levels of preparation: professional and technical. Occupational therapists are certified at the professional level of practice, whereas occupational therapy assistants are certified at the technical level. An occupational therapist has earned either a baccalaureate or a master's degree in occupational therapy from a program accredited by the Accreditation Council for Occupational Therapy Education (ACOTE), has completed a minimum of 6 months of fieldwork, and has passed the national certification examination administered by the National Board for Certification in Occupational Therapy (NBCOT) (American Occupational Therapy Association [AOTA], 1999c). In contrast, an occupational therapy assistant has earned an associate degree from an occupational therapy assistant program accredited by the ACOTE, has completed a minimum of 3 months of fieldwork, and has passed the NBCOT examination for occupational therapy assistants (AOTA, 1999d). Although the occupational therapy component of both levels of education focuses on the common content areas, such as the structure and function of the human body, human development across the life span, and the occupational therapy process, the preparation of the occupational therapist has a greater emphasis on theory, screening and evaluation, management, and research (AOTA, 1999c, 1999d).

Because of the commonalities in their education, occupational therapists and occupational therapy assistants share beliefs and values of occupational therapy; they also share a common language and stock of knowledge. However, because occupational therapists' education focuses more heavily on theory, evaluation, management, and research, they have the legal and ethical responsibility to ensure that occupational therapy services provided by themselves and by any occupational therapy assistants they are supervising meet the highest standards of care. This quality of care is achieved most readily if occupational therapy practitioners respect and honor their common beliefs and different contributions to their mutual work. The supervisory process is a critical component of achieving this ideal.

HISTORICAL NOTE 13–1

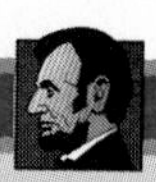

The Scrubwomen of World War I: The Challenge of Practice

SUZANNE M. PELOQUIN

Many see World War I reconstruction aides as the forebears of occupational therapists. Most are less familiar with the circumstances of the aides' recruitment. Dr. Frankwood Williams hoped to have occupational workers on his staff for Base Hospital 117. Although he had gathered several women who wanted to serve, he could not get Washington officials to appoint them. He read about openings for civilian aides, who would serve as scrubwomen with no official connection to the army. Williams suggested that he get his recruits overseas by calling them scrubwomen, and all agreed (Myers, 1948).

These early scrubwomen were Mrs. Clyde Myers, a graduate of Columbia University; Eleanor Johnson, a psychologist; Amy Drevenstedt, a history teacher at Hunter College; Corrine Dezeller, another Columbia graduate; and Laura LaForce, a graduate nurse. They were "divided into squads to clean the quarters assigned" (p. 209) on Ellis Island and moved on from there to reconstruction work overseas.

If we choose to see these women as individuals whose passion for a cause carried them past the hurdles that blocked their way to practice, we might muster a similar passion in the face of circumstances that challenge us today.

Myers, C. M. (1948). Pioneer occupational therapists in World War I. *American Journal of Occupational Therapy*, 2, 208–215.

Supervision

In the occupational therapist–occupational therapy assistant partnership, the occupational therapist supervises the occupational therapy assistant at a level appropriate to two factors: the skill and experience demonstrated by the occupational therapy assistant, and the skill and knowledge required for specific intervention procedures. Supervision should cultivate and promote learning for both the supervisor and the supervisee.

> *Supervision is a mutual undertaking between the supervisor and the supervisee that fosters growth and development; assures appropriate utilization of training and potential; encourages creativity and innovation; and provides guidance, education, support, encouragement, and respect while working toward a goal.* (AOTA, 1999b, p. 592)

Entry-level practitioners have completed their educational programs and have passed the appropriate certification examinations. They have less than 1 year's experience and are prepared to practice in a generalist setting (AOTA, 1999a). The responsibilities of entry-level occupational therapists include managing, negotiating, and advocating occupational therapy services and client care. The responsibilities of entry-level occupational therapy assistants are more client related and involve direct service delivery. The success of the occupational therapy team is based on an understanding of the roles of the two practitioners. A major role difference is the responsibility for development and implementation of the occupational therapy treatment program. Occupational therapists have this responsibility. A therapist may (1) select appropriate assessment and intervention techniques and carry them out unassisted, (2) delegate specific procedures to an occupational therapy assistant based on previously established service competencies, or (3) delegate most of the intervention to a certified occupational therapy assistant with the required service competencies. When using either of the last two options, occupational therapists and occupational therapy assistants need to rely on effective supervision and communication.

Various levels of supervision are required and depend on the level of acuity and complexity of the client population, the interventions being used, and the expertise of the occupational therapy assistant. Supervision may be close and involve daily contact with assistants who have little experience or who are working with clients who have highly complex problems. However, less supervision is required when practitioners gain more experience and establish service competency (AOTA, 1999b).

Service Competency

A primary consideration in determining an appropriate level of supervision is the confirmation of service competency by the supervising occupational therapist of the occupational therapy assistant's performance of specific treatment activities and techniques.

> *Service competency is the process by which the occupational therapist determines that the occupational therapy assistant can perform tasks in the same way that the occupational therapist would and achieve the same results. If a high degree of competence cannot be assured in this process, the occupational therapist must question the appropriateness of delegating the task. (AOTA, 1999b, p. 593)*

The concept of service competency implies that the occupational therapist delegates a specific task or tasks to the occupational therapy assistant based on the level of competence demonstrated by the assistant in performing the task or tasks in other situations. Because the occupational therapist is responsible for all aspects of occupational therapy service delivery, service competency is critical to the collaborative process and sets the framework for effective supervision. Service competency should be established in areas appropriate to the types of services offered in specific work environments. Establishing service competency is a team effort. The occupational therapy assistant must develop and demonstrate the knowledge and skill required, and the occupational therapist must verify the appropriate use of the knowledge and skill in the process of providing service intervention.

Initial steps in developing service competency should center on the occupational therapist's expectations for quality intervention and a plan and structure for how the occupational therapy assistant will establish service competency. Several avenues for establishing service competency have been successfully used by occupational therapist–occupational therapy assistant treatment teams. Some examples are co-treating; periodic observation of the occupational therapy assistant engaged in service delivery; and the delegated regular review of goals, plans, and documentation for specific client care to the occupational therapy assistant. In the following narrative, Pat (an occupational therapy assistant) and Katherine (an occupational therapist), who work as a team, discuss one way of establishing service competency that fosters communication, develops skills, and ultimately leads to better supervision.

> PAT: *Being able to co-treat is helpful. As an occupational therapy assistant, I am constantly learning by observing my supervisor. When we co-treat, I observe the different things she does with the child and I pick up on it and use it later on.*
>
> KATHERINE: *With co-treatments, I get to have a hands-on approach in treatment implementation. I look at the progress the person has made and I see how the short term and long-term goals are being reached. I get a feeling for what is being done when I'm not there, what is working or not working.*

Collaboration

The key to teamwork is collaboration. Meaningful collaboration occurs when each team member has mastered two requirements: a clear understanding of each role and a respect for the differences and similarities of each role. Furthermore, both the assistant and the therapist must share an appreciation for their unique contributions to their mutual work endeavors (Holmes, 1993). Successful collaboration also depends on effective communication, clarity of expectations, and agreement about mutual responsibilities (Swedberg, 1993).

CLINICAL REASONING IN THE OCCUPATIONAL THERAPIST–OCCUPATIONAL THERAPY ASSISTANT SUPERVISION RELATIONSHIP

Clinical reasoning is the process of considering multiple possibilities when judging specific client situations (Fowler, 1997) and is discussed in greater length in Chapter 11. Research in the clinical reasoning of occupational therapists has identified variable facets of this process. Similar research on the clinical reasoning of occupational therapy assistants is limited to a single case study of an experienced occupational therapy assistant (Lyons & Crepeau, 2001). The findings of this case study suggest that the assistant attended to the same general aspects of care, using similar processes as those identified in empirical studies of the clinical reasoning of occupational therapists. It is reasonable to assume that other assistants would also engage in similar reasoning processes and that the particulars of this reasoning would depend on the assistant's experience. Occupational therapists as managers of therapy programs must delegate tasks appropriately to occupational therapy assistants. In deciding how much structure and supervision an individual occupational therapy assistant will need for a given case, the occupational therapist should consider a variety of factors, including experience and service competency.

Supervision is complicated by the tacit nature of clinical reasoning. Mattlingly and Fleming (1994), drawing on work by Polyani, described tacit knowledge as the ability to act effectively rather than the ability to explain those actions. Tacit knowledge is associated with high levels of expertise in which actions proceed without conscious thought; experienced practitioners become so skilled, their actions are automatic. However, the supervisory process relies on sharing experiences and thoughts—in essence, making the tacit explicit. Consequently, "by the very nature of their role, occupational therapy assistants cannot allow their reasoning to remain tacit" (Lyons & Crepeau, 2000). Therefore, both the supervising occupational therapist and the occupational therapy assistant must take the time to uncover the assistant's tacit knowledge about the client's response to intervention.

Supervising Entry-Level Versus Experienced Occupational Therapy Assistants

Supervision of entry-level occupational therapy assistants differs from supervision of those with more than 1 year's experience. Verifying basic knowledge, as well as new knowledge and skills as they are developed, is a required function of the occupational therapist–occupational therapy assistant collaborative process. Service competency can be established at different levels, and the level of service competency an occupational therapy assistant has accomplished is an important consideration in the clinical reasoning process. An occupational therapy assistant at the entry level may achieve service competency in certain assessment procedures, such as assessing the safety in dressing for a person who has had a total hip replacement or observing the classroom behavior of a child with attention deficit hyperactivity disorder. Assistants with more experience and expertise in a practice setting might develop service competency in more complex assessment procedures, such as assessing the abilities of a client with early-stage Alzheimer disease to plan and carry out meal preparation for a small family gathering. In both instances, service competency is limited to the ability to follow the assessment protocol and to achieve the same results as the occupational therapist, but it does not extend to the application of the assessment results to the therapeutic program.

An entry-level occupational therapy assistant may demonstrate skill in performing a specific therapy technique, such as supervising meal preparation to ensure energy conservation and joint protection or performing child care with a mother who is wheelchair dependent. In contrast, an experienced occupational therapy assistant may have achieved service competency in more complex intervention strategies. Work experience within the setting, concentrated exposure to the use of intervention procedures by supervising occupational therapists, and knowledge acquired from in-service training and continuing education activities all contribute to the occupational therapy assistant's level of competency. To think about these issues read What's a Practitioner to Do? 13-1 and respond to the questions at the end of the scenario.

Though extremely important, the establishment of service competencies is only one aspect of the partnership between the occupational therapist and occupational therapy assistant. Experienced assistants require less supervision in their work with clients. This level of supervision may be routine, occurring every 2 weeks at the work site with the opportunity for additional supervision in the intervening time (AOTA, 1999b). Depending on the expertise of the occupational therapy assistant and the setting, this supervision may even be general, which is direct monthly supervision with the opportunity for supervisory contact in the intervening time (AOTA, 1999b). Experienced assistants also provide much needed support by managing the department inventory, finding and obtaining durable equipment, and assisting with the gathering of data for outcome studies. In addition, their experience with activities and occupations make them excellent at adapting and implementing specific activities to meet a client's occupational goals. For example, designing an adapted grip for a fishing pole so that a man with arthritis can continue to pursue his favorite hobby.

Katie (the occupational therapist) and Celeste (the occupational therapy assistant) demonstrate the kind of relationship that develops between two highly skilled occupational therapy practitioners. It is clear from the following short dialogue that Celeste has achieved service competencies in aspects of assessment and intervention; that Katie trusts Celeste's judgment; and that they have an open relationship, which involves trust, mutuality, and availability, even on days when Katie is not working in the same building.

> KATIE: *I feel comfortable handing Celeste an evaluation, because I know she can interpret the technical language and understand what it means relative to what needs be done. I wouldn't feel comfortable doing this if I didn't know her skills. I trust that if Celeste has to make a decision about treatment, it will be a good decision, it will work out, and it won't be a problem. I also know that she's aware of when a decision has to be made by me. An example is a recent Committee on Special Education meeting that Celeste attended in my absence. There were requests made for major changes in a child's treatment program, and Celeste informed the people at the meeting that the requested changes would have to be considered and approved by the occupational therapist.*

WHAT'S A PRACTITIONER TO DO? 13-1
Supervision Decisions

June is a senior occupational therapist in a small outpatient adult rehabilitation section of a community hospital. She has worked on the rehab unit for 4 years, taking the position as a new graduate. June is the only occupational therapist on the unit. Her responsibilities include supervising two occupational therapy assistants, Pearl and Rhonda. Pearl has worked on the rehab unit for 8 years. Rhonda passed the certification examination 9 months ago and worked in a community mental health setting for 6 months before taking this position on the rehab unit. She has worked on the unit for only 3 months. Before Rhonda was hired, June and Pearl worked collaboratively on 90% of the clients referred to the unit for occupational therapy services. An increase in referrals prompted the decision to hire another occupational therapy assistant. Orthopedic conditions are the primary diagnoses of people admitted to the unit.

June recently received a referral for Ann, a 48-year-old elementary-school teacher and mother of three with a diagnosis of rheumatoid arthritis of 2 years' duration. The development and rapid increase of pain and discomfort in her hands and wrists experienced over a 3-month-period led to Ann's diagnosis. Ann lives with her husband and youngest daughter. A regiment of anti-inflammatory drugs controlled Ann's symptoms for about 1 year; however, since that time, the symptoms have increased significantly. Ann's referral to the outpatient rehab clinic came when she complained to her doctor that the drug she was using to control the pain and inflammation in her hands and wrists was no longer effective. In addition to changing her prescription, her doctor referred her to OT for assessment and treatment. Her health insurance approved therapy services twice weekly for 3 weeks.

On Ann's first therapy visit, she is greeted by June, Pearl, and Rhonda. June explains that the first visit involves an assessment of Ann's condition and that Pearl will assist in the initial interview and will be providing services to Ann. June introduces Rhonda and explains that she is observing the assessment as part of her ongoing training and orientation to the rehab unit. During the first 30 min, Pearl and June talk to Ann about her daily activities and what she hopes to achieve in the therapy program. Ann responds that her major concerns are the pain, discomfort, and fatigue she experiences daily. These concerns are heightened by her desire to continue teaching, especially when her daughter enters college in September, and Ann's income will be needed to help with tuition and other college expenses. Ann is encouraging her daughter to live on campus, even through the family lives only 25 miles from the college. Because of Ann's illness, her husband and daughter have assumed a good measure of the responsibility for day-to-day household tasks, such as shopping, doing laundry, and doing regular cleaning. She continues to assume the major responsibility for cooking family meals. The family does not have sufficient income to hire outside help for these daily activities. Ann does not want her illness to interfere with her daughter's chance to experience, what she identifies as "the full value of a college education." For this reason, her main goal for therapy is to develop and learn ways to manage the household responsibilities effectively with less pain. After Pearl leaves, June completes a full motor assessment of Ann's upper extremities and inquires about pain, swelling, and stiffness in other joints.

QUESTIONS AND EXERCISES

If you were June, the supervising occupational therapist:

1. What things would you consider in making the decision to delegate the major responsibility for the treatment program to Pearl?
2. How would you structure your supervision of Pearl for Ann's therapy program?
3. Given Pearl's expertise, what would you expect her to contribute to Ann's intervention?
4. How would you expect Pearl to contribute to the supervisory process?
5. What kind of clinical reasoning would you need to do?
6. How would your answers to these questions differ if Rhonda were the occupational therapy assistant you were to work with? What would be different about how you would supervise and collaborate with Rhonda?

If you were Pearl, the occupational therapy assistant:

1. What would you know about Ann that would assist you in working with June to develop her therapy program. What information would you depend on June to supply?
2. When participating in the supervisory process, what type of information about Ann and the therapy program would you need to share with June?
3. How would sharing this information assist you in your work with Ann?
4. What type of reasoning would you need to do?
5. How would your answers to these questions differ if you were Rhonda? What would be different about how you would collaborate with June?

CELESTE: *I gained my confidence through observing Katie, being trusted with certain responsibilities in the treatment process, and being allowed to share in decision making. Working together, we take up each other's slack. There is a lot of trust; we can rely on each other. I know that Katie's evaluation is a true representation of a child's abilities and deficits. When I am treating and I have a question, I know I can go to Katie and get the answer. Even on days when I am treating alone, I'm comfortable knowing she is only a phone call away.*

PRACTITIONER PERSPECTIVES: A PARTNERSHIP BASED ON MUTUAL TRUST AND RESPECT FOR DIFFERENT INTERESTS AND KNOWLEDGE

Like the dialogue between Katie and Celeste demonstrates, trust is the cornerstone of all successful relationships. Mutual trust sets the framework for effective supervision and communication (Swedberg, 1993, p. 4). When mutual trust and respect exists, occupational therapy assistants can comfortably report what is going on in the treatment process, ask for assistance and/or support when needed, and make and share honest assessments of their skill and knowledge levels. Occupational therapists can delegate tasks based on informed decisions that reflect a clear understanding of the contributions that each will make. The following conversation demonstrates how trust and respect is central to Celeste and Katie's collaborative relationship.

CELESTE: *We give teachers information on home programs and relate them to the types of things the teacher can do in the classroom and pass on to parents. Over the years, we have earned the respect of the teachers by being consistent in what we say and by talking with them when miscommunication has occurred. That has been an important part of our relationship with them.*

The child's environment and culture play big parts in the results we get. It's difficult when there is no carryover at home. We write notes to parents or call them, but even then things are not always carried through. Some parents will bring problems to our attention, like trouble tying shoes, and this is a good indication that the parent will follow through on our suggestions.

KATIE: *Being consistent is important. We will discuss and debate the pros and cons of taking a particular stance about a child's treatment program. We come to a conclusion, and if we really feel strongly about it, we go with it even though others may challenge our position. We may ask for input on legal issues and then consider what we feel is right. The Committee on Special Education may not accept our recommendations, but we stick with what we believe. The decision may be to do the opposite of what we recommend and we say that's fine, this is our report and this is how we stand on this issue.*

CONCLUSION

True collaboration is accomplished when the members of a partnership understand and respect the contributions each one makes. This reciprocity involves a full commitment to working together by listening, accepting, and valuing each other's strengths and mutual engagement in common goals. Well-developed partnerships between occupational therapists and occupational therapy assistants are important to providers of service, receivers of service, and to the viability of the profession.

ACKNOWLEDGMENTS

I wish to thank Kathleen Wilson, OTR; Celeste McAteer, COTA; Katherine Ferrara, OTR; and Patricia Schneider, COTA, for their candid and enthusiastic participation in conversations about their partnerships.

References

American Occupational Therapy Association [AOTA]. (1999a). Glossary: Standards for an accredited educational program for the occupational therapist and the occupational therapy assistant. *American Journal of Occupational Therapy, 53*, 590–591.

American Occupational Therapy Association [AOTA]. (1999b). Guide for supervision of occupational therapy personnel in the delivery of occupational therapy services. *American Journal of Occupational Therapy, 53*, 592–594.

American Occupational Therapy Association [AOTA]. (1999c). Standards for an accredited educational program for the occupational therapist. *American Journal of Occupational Therapy, 53*, 575–582.

American Occupational Therapy Association [AOTA]. (1999d). Standards for an accredited educational program for the occupational therapy assistant. *American Journal of Occupational Therapy, 53*, 583–589.

Fowler, L. P. (1997). Clinical reasoning strategies used during care planning. *Clinical Nursing Research* [On-line serial], 6(4). Retrieve from: www.infotrac.galegroup.com.

Holmes, C. (1993). Challenging old paradigms. *Administration and Management Special Interest Section Newsletter, 9*, 3–4.

Lyons, K. D., & Crepeau, E. B. (2000). The issue is: Clinical reasoning and the challenge of tacit knowledge. Manuscript submitted for publication.

Lyons, K.D., & Crepeau, E.B. (2001). The clinical reasoning of an occupational therapy assistant. *American Journal of Occupational Therapy, 55*, 577–581.

Mattingly, C., & Fleming, M. H. (1994). *Clinical reasoning: Forms of inquiry in a therapeutic practice*. Philadelphia: Davis.

Swedberg, L. (1993). Supervising the advanced certified occupational therapy assistant in a private practice setting. *Administration and Management Special Interest Section Newsletter, 9*, 4–5.

UNIT *four*

Establishing the Therapeutic Alliance

Learning Objectives

After completing this unit, readers will be able to:

- Describe the manner in which occupational therapy practitioners form alliances that honor dignity and convey caring.
- Identify group process mechanisms in large group systems and in small task groups that integrate perspectives of the occupation, the individual, the interpersonal, and the environment.
- Describe methods that establish therapeutic alliances between facilitator and member(s) as well as between member(s) and member(s) and relate the interactive, conditional, and procedural reasoning processes for facilitating a small task group in occupational therapy.

The challenge of occupational therapy practice is to engage people to strive toward their own recovery, growth, development, and well-being. Although society expects people to be motivated to achieve well-being, this motivation is not always the case. Discouragement, depression, and other factors may interfere with full engagement in the therapeutic process. By establishing a therapeutic alliance with those who seek our care, occupational therapy practitioners provide the catalyst to help people engage fully in the process of occupational therapy and achieve their goals. The chapters in this unit provide a vision of what matters most in our therapeutic relationships—making connections, evoking responses, and finding shared meanings. (Note: Words in **bold** type are defined in the Glossary.)

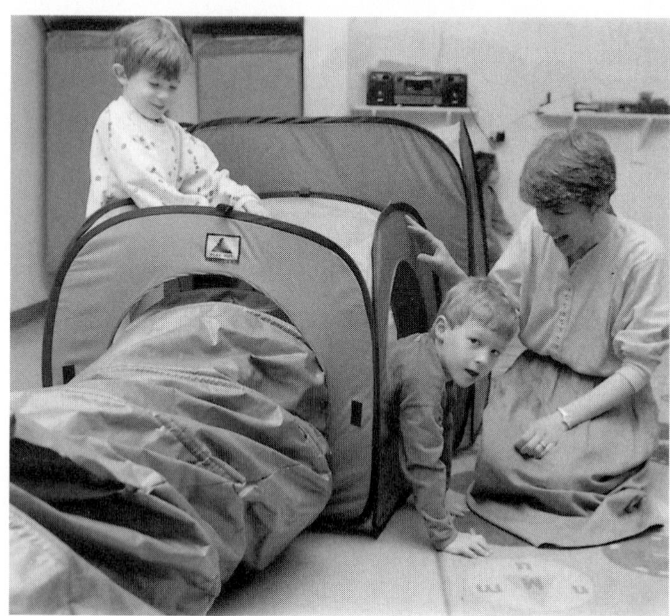

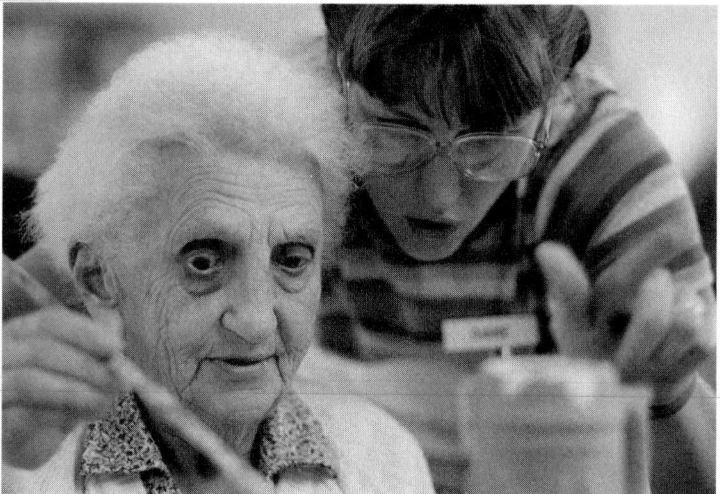

These occupational therapy practitioners are collaborating with clients to address their interests and goals, essential aspects of the therapeutic alliance. *(top)* Therapist with two children crawling in gym. (Photo courtesy of Ron Bergeron, Instructional Services, Dimond Library, University of New Hampshire, Durham, NH). *(middle)* Woman with brush, therapist in background. (Photo courtesy of Gary Samson, Instructional Services, Dimond library, University of New Hampshire, Durham, NH). *(bottom)* Therapist helping older woman. (Photo courtesy of DeKalb Medical Center, DeKalb, GA).

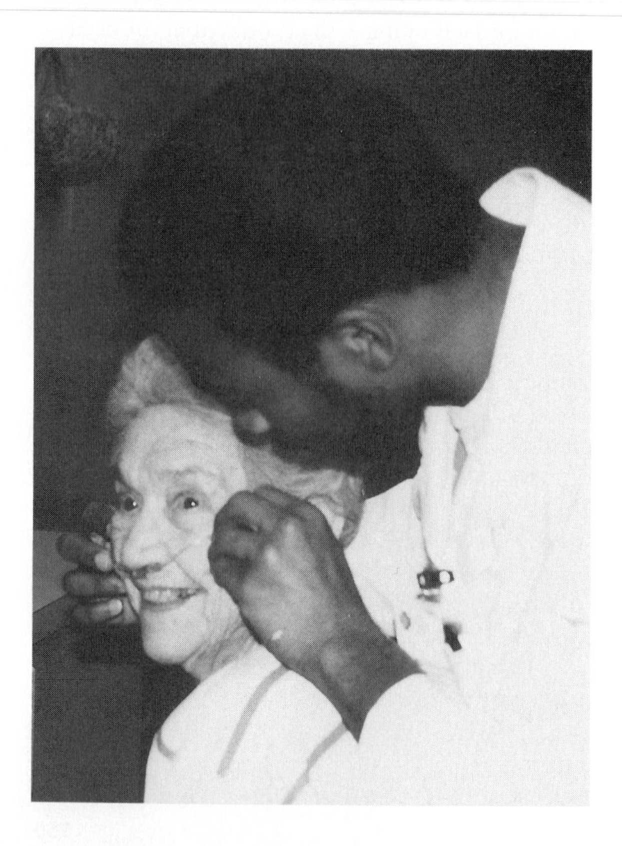

CHAPTER 14

THE THERAPEUTIC RELATIONSHIP: MANIFESTATIONS AND CHALLENGES IN OCCUPATIONAL THERAPY

SUZANNE M. PELOQUIN

THE CHARACTER OF THE RELATIONSHIP

The therapeutic relationship in occupational therapy has been characterized as a manifestation of its artistry and as a process of reaching for the hearts and hands of others. Each of these characterizations is important to consider from the perspectives of practitioners and individuals seeking occupational therapy (Fig. 14-1).

The Relationship as a Manifestation of Artistry

Occupational therapy practice has been described as "the art and science of directing man's participation in selected tasks" (American Occupational Therapy Association Council on Standards, 1972, p. 204). There is an artistry to most professional practices, even those seen as scientific and especially those known as therapy. In her discussion of the art of practice, Mosey (1981) first noted that the art is neither (1) a desire to help others, (2) the skilled application of scientific knowledge, nor (3) the act of being a systematic or sympathetic listener. She wrote, "The capacity to establish rapport, to empathize, and to guide others to know and make use of their potential as participants in a community of others illustrates the art of occupational therapy" (p. 4). The art of the profession's practice, like most art, is a process of making connections, evoking responses, and finding shared meaning.

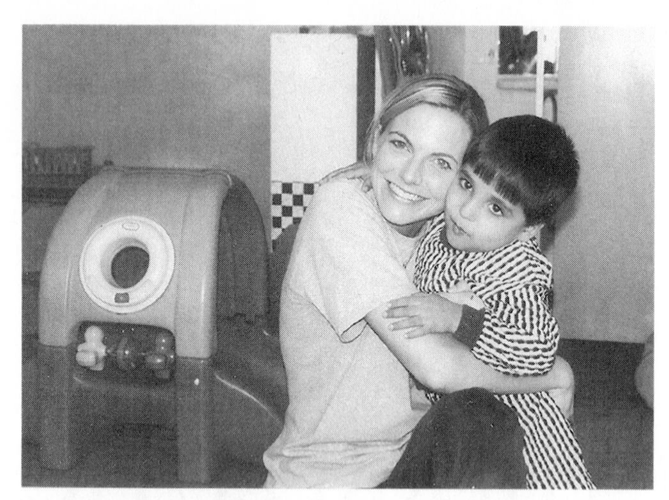

FIGURE 14–1. Reaching for the heart and hands of others. (Photo courtesy of Sharon Cermak.)

Without its art, Mosey claimed, occupational therapy would be an application of knowledge in a sterile vacuum.

One who masters the art of practice perceives and responds to the individual seeking therapy as a whole person, indivisible into parts or subsystems (Mosey, 1981). Although practitioners often reduce the complexity of human problems to understand them more clearly, those who use artistry, Mosey said, reintegrate parts of the problem and clearly see the person. Seeing a person lets a practitioner empathize with feelings and appreciate the personal values that guide occupational performance.

The Core Value: Personal Dignity

A decade after these reflections on the art of practice were made, the American Occupational Therapy Association (1993) identified seven core values that characterize the profession and clarify expectations for the therapeutic relationship: altruism, equality, freedom, justice, dignity, truth, and prudence. These values derive from guiding documents, such as the profession's philosophy statement and code of ethics. For practitioners who work among divergent populations, in varied settings, and with distinct frames of reference, this affirmation of shared professional values gives clear direction about how occupational therapists should be in practice.

Within the American Occupational Therapy Association's (1993) elaboration of core values, personal dignity is key; a sound grasp of dignity helps one enact the other values. A practitioner who honors dignity, the core document reads, has an "attitude of empathy" (p. 1086). The term **empathy** is familiar, but its meaning must be clear. What does empathy look like? More pointedly, what does it mean to be empathic in a practice that holds occupation at its center?

The Requisite Attitude: Empathy

Some individuals dismiss discussions of empathy, thinking, "Oh, another rehash of how to decode body language and paraphrase what the client says." Any such dismissal would be hasty, because empathy is much more than these good skills. Katz (1963) described the challenge: "To be a man means to be a fellow man. The human personality becomes human through its association with others" (p. 189). Those who hope for therapeutic associations must see them as forms of fellowship and chances to use their humanity.

How can practitioners establish fellowship with those who seek therapy? Thomas (1983) explained that fellowship rests first on a willingness to *be there*. The disposition to be there is also central to Buber's (1965) concept of dialogue, in which one person turns toward the other, "of course with the body, but also in requisite measure with the soul" (p. 10). The turning within Buber's dialogue is an empathic action that transcends any procedures; it asks for more of who one is than of what one does. Likening it to love, Hackney (1978) saw empathy as a qualitative response to people, a potential for understanding others that is possessed by most.

Adler (1931) believed that if practitioners tapped this potential, they would find "the common sense of all mankind" (p. 254). Empathy as a common sense allows individuals to see their likeness to others, recognizing surprise in eyes that widen, stress in brows that furrow, anger in hands that clench. But empathy also prompts a respect for differences. At its deepest level, Egan (1986) explained, empathy is a way of seeing with the eyes of others to appreciate *their* views of the world. To be present to others empathically is to take a stand from which one shares their experiences. Such a stance is aptly named an understanding.

Perhaps the most cited description of empathy is that of psychologist Rogers (1975):

> *It means entering the private world of the other and becoming thoroughly at home in it. It involves being sensitive, moment to moment, to the changing felt meanings which flow in this other person, to the fear or rage or tenderness or confusion or whatever, that he/she is experiencing. It means temporarily living in his/her life, moving about in it delicately without making judgments. . . . In some sense it means that you lay aside your self and this can only be done by a person who is secure enough in himself that he knows he will not get lost in what may turn out to be the strange and bizarre world of the other.* (p. 3)

In his early writings, Rogers (1957) underscored the as-if thinking of empathy; one thinks and feels and moves as if one were in the other's world. This imaginative work lets caregivers distinguish their clients' experiences from their own. This is the hallmark of empathy: "In order to help people who are sick, we must know what it is like to be in their shoes but, at the same time, also know very well that we are not in their shoes" (Reiser & Schroder, 1980, p. 46).

Practitioners sometimes seem ambivalent about the intimacy of empathy. They worry that "they may not be able to extricate themselves from the net of feeling" (Katz, 1963, p. 25).

When overwhelmed with the feelings of others, it is not empathy that individuals enact, but sympathy. Olinick (1984) judged sympathy "an immature, imperfect empathy" (p. 139). Sympathetic helpers grasp the feelings of others but focus more on the pain that they take from that encounter than the comfort they give through their presence. A true empathizer, said Katz (1963), abandons his or her self-consciousness in the encounter. Even when a helper engages in a profound act of empathy, the "power to recover" (p. 139) remains.

Such recovery is possible because empathy does not exact a fusion with the pain of another but a connection with the person of another. This connection implies a recognition of pain but not without a simultaneous grasp of the dignity and courage that are also there. Empathy, in health-care practice, is the enactment of the conviction that, empowered by someone's willingness to understand, a person will gather courage. The empathic way of being conveys a fierce faith in personal dignity. It is central to the art of therapy.

The Relationship as a Reaching for Hands and Heart

Because the manner of "being with" in occupational therapy is a unique enactment of "doing with," it is important to consider portrayals of that relationship. One aspiring to be an empathic helper must know what such a practitioner looks like. A vibrant image emerges in the book *The Healing Heart* (Carlova & Ruggles, 1946). This biography of Ora Ruggles, reconstruction aide, chronicles an early story of occupational therapy from World War I through the 1940s. Because it deals openly with the values that Ruggles held and the relationships that she shared, the story serves well as a lesson in the therapeutic relationship.

The title of the book comes from a comment made twice by Ruggles, once at the start of her story and again at the end. On the first occasion, Ruggles walked into the barracks at Fort McPherson after a day's work and was strangely quiet. When pressed by others to share her thoughts, Ruggles said, "It is not enough to give a patient something to do with his hands. It's the heart that really does the healing" (Carlova & Ruggles, 1946, p. 69). Later, when she retired, she was asked about the most important part of her work. She echoed her early discovery: Reach for the patient's heart. Reaching for hearts and hands thus becomes an apt characterization of the therapeutic relationship in occupational therapy.

In *The Healing Heart*, Ruggles exemplified an empathic attitude. At Fort McPherson, she worked among soldiers with war injuries. Her two enormous wards were the scenes of horseplay among those who could move about and stone-faced staring from those who could not. A tall and attractive redhead, Ruggles drew much attention on the day she first walked the wards. One patient named Hap, who had no legs and only one arm, made Ruggles laugh with his flirtatious comments and impish grin. When she said that she would keep the men occupied with basket weaving, Hap quipped that he'd rather keep her occupied. Another patient, named Kilgore, called Hap a legless clown, not man enough to keep anyone occupied. The men grew silent. Ruggles moved to Hap's side and put her hand on his shoulder, saying "Don't mind him, Hap! Man is far more than an arm or leg" (Carlova & Ruggles, 1946, p. 57). Her words went deep. Within minutes, more than 20 men clamored into her class.

Because of his disability, Hap could only pass reeds to the other men; Ruggles saw his silence grow as his incapacity became clear. She spent much time thinking about what Hap could do. She went to the artificial limb shop, where limb making was still rather crude. She described and sketched what she wanted: a leather device from which metal braces and a clamp would protrude. Later she approached Hap, cautioning him against too much hope as she slipped the device over his stump and secured a brush in its clamp. As Hap painted tentative lines of color onto the rim of a basket, he whooped with joy. He practiced secretly for days before showing his skill. The men responded with delight; even Kilgore was impressed. Overwhelmed, Ruggles began a practice that she kept for years. She slipped away into a closet and let the tears flow. That closet was the first of Ruggles's many "crying corners" (Carlova & Ruggles, 1946, p. 63) from which she emerged ready to resume her care.

Kilgore's behavior troubled Ruggles. During one class, a soldier said that Kilgore would not try basket weaving because he knew he would fail. Challenged, Kilgore sat for an hour, weaving furiously. When another soldier judged the result "not bad," Kilgore drove his fist down to destroy the basket. Ruggles asked a physician about Kilgore's past. The physician told her that the man had once been a cowboy and that he now hated his wartime actions. Ruggles consulted the foreman of the blacksmith shop and then found Kilgore, who told her he would make no more baskets. Ruggles showed him a design for spurs and asked if he would help her start a metalworking class. Within the hour he was in the shop, where he mastered the work quickly. His drinking, gambling, and outbursts stopped; and after discharge, he started an ironwork plant that grew to be the largest in the Southwest. Kilgore wrote to Ruggles, years later:

> *I've been doing a lot of thinking lately, Ruggie. It started out last week when some of the boys around town asked me to run for mayor. It makes me realize, again, how much I owe you. I wonder what the boys who asked me to run for mayor would think if they knew an army doctor once scribbled on my medical record, "This man is a menace to society." (Carlova & Ruggles, 1946, p. 91)*

Ruggles's interactions with Hap and Kilgore depict a practitioner whose relationship with others reflects the best of empathy. Ruggles reached for the hearts as well the hands of her patients. By creating fellowship, she practiced artistry as she engaged them in occupations.

The Enactment of Empathy: Poignant Illustrations

Scenes in *The Healing Heart* show more of Ruggles's artistry and other aspects of empathy. Beyond its communication of fellowship, empathy has been said to consist of (1) a turning of the soul, (2) a recognition of likeness and uniqueness in another, (3) an entry into the other's experience, (4) a connection with the other's feelings, and (5) a power to recover from that connection and feel a personal enrichment. Each of these aspects of empathy assumes a unique character in occupational therapy, an interpersonal encounter within which a practitioner brings not just the self but the objects and tools of everyday life.

Turning of the Soul

Empathy requires a turning to another that is a turning of the soul. One example of Ruggles's turning, not just to solve a problem but to capture its deeper meaning, was her interaction with a child named Ruby. When Ruggles first met Ruby, she saw an unattractive 12-year-old who retaliated against the taunts of other children by ruining their work. Hoping to learn the child's interests, Ruggles asked Ruby if she might like sewing. The child responded, "Why? So I can grow up and be an old maid and sit at home with my sewing? Is that what you do?" (Carlova & Ruggles, 1946, p. 215) Although Ruggles's initial urge was to "wallop" Ruby, she checked her temper and thought, "This girls dislikes people because she can see they dislike her. I must alter my attitude. . . . I must show Ruby that I love her" (p. 215). This turning of soul prompted Ruggles to ask what Ruby aimed to be when she grew up. In a tiny voice, Ruby said she hoped to work in a beauty parlor. Ruggles softened as she saw this child in light of her yearning for beauty. She taught Ruby how to shampoo and set her own hair, and she arranged for her to spend time in a beauty shop. Over time, Ruggles noticed a change; as Ruby worked so closely with others, her inner beauty emerged. Ruggles's turning of the soul prompted a similar turning in Ruby.

Recognition of Likeness

Another aspect of empathy is a recognition of likeness in another, a grasp of the commonality of personal problems. Ruggles's work with an 11-year-old boy named Ramon showed her capacity to see his need for belonging and to structure occupations to meet that need. Ramon had little muscular control, and he twitched and jerked constantly. Painfully shy, he hid himself in dark corners so he would not be noticed. One day, when the rest of Ruggles's charges complained that their clay was so lumpy that they were wasting time pressing it though a screen, Ruggles thought of Ramon. She walked him from a corner into the center of the workroom. As soon as he saw the others making clay figures, he reproached Ruggles for suggesting that he join the group. Ruggles countered by showing him how to press clay through the screen. Here, his uncontrolled movements worked to his advantage, and the other children patted him on the back and thanked him for producing clay with such fine texture. Ramon felt useful and appreciated and after a short period was no longer shy. The task gave him a chance to connect with others in a venture that highlighted fellowship more than differences.

Recognition of Uniqueness

Empathy also requires a recognition of uniqueness in the other, and Ruggles's practice in a "mental ward" at Fort McPherson introduced her to some dramatic examples of the unique behaviors of schizophrenia during an era before psychotropic medications. One day a patient announced that he was General Pershing and that Ruggles ought to salute him. She did. Another patient whispered as they were working that he was a German spy. He and Ruggles agreed on a set of signals they used for communicating. Ruggles knew that another patient was a bird lover who stood for hours by the barred windows. One day while hallucinating, he asked what the birds were doing in Ruggles's hair. Without skipping a beat, Ruggles said, "Oh those. Their nest was blown away and I'm sort of helping them out until I find another one" (Carlova & Ruggles, 1946, p. 100). Calmed, he praised the quality of her nest. She learned to salute, pass secret signals, and live with imagined birds as she worked with the men. Her matter-of-fact acceptance of their uniqueness permitted their engagement with her and with the work that calmed them.

Entering into the Experience of the Other

Central to empathy is the act of entering into the experience of another to understand what it must be like. Ruggles's interaction with a man named Leo showed her sensitive participation in the lives of her patients. Poverty troubled many of the patients in another setting, the Olive View sanatorium, especially those with families. Ruggles ran a shop in the hospital where patients could sell their crafts to defray expenses. After Leo arrived he was sent to bed with a high fever. He was restless and troubled; he had a wife and four children to support, and his small farm was mortgaged. His family needed $15.25 a month to keep the farm. The physician thought Leo's temperature too high and work with Ruggles too risky. Although Ruggles accepted that decision at first, as Leo's condition worsened she reopened the question. Ruggles thought that Leo's deterioration was more mental than physical. She proposed to work with him at bedside but to stop if his temperature rose. The physician agreed.

Ruggles told Leo that he could make $20 a month selling leatherwork. Although his first efforts were crude, before long he was producing fine items. His first earnings amounted to $22.65. The physician pronounced him well enough to work outside the ward. Leo became Ruggles's assistant, helping other patients as soon as he secured his $15.25. Ruggles's work was credited with saving Leo's farm, his pride, and his life. Her willingness to enter into his life experience had engaged him.

Connection with Feelings

Ruggles's work among people in pain offered many occasions for her to connect with their feelings. While she was on the ward one day, a young soldier shot with shrapnel in 65 places caught her eye as he frantically scanned the room. Kilgore warned her that the young man was about to explode his feelings, and that she'd better go. Ruggles told Kilgore that she would stay. The soldier spoke of screams in the trench where he fell with his wounded friends. An artillery blast blew him free, and he woke to find parts of bodies, torn and bloody, scattered all over. "I was the only man alive," he said, "and I wished I was dead" (Carlova & Ruggles, 1946, p. 88). Ruggles sat near the boy for a long time, feeling sick and weak. Kilgore whispered that now she too had been through the war and that she ought not listen next time. "No," Ruggles said, "if I can help, I'll stay" (p. 88). Ruggles's patients often needed to speak of their anguish and share their pain. Her staying power in the face of their feelings confirmed her empathy.

Power to Recover from the Connection

Ruggles's power to recover from connecting with the deep feelings of others, another of the actions that earmarks empathy, stayed strong. She saw dignity and courage alongside the pain. She turned to friends who would listen. She changed jobs to work with different populations. She saw the results of her efforts. She applied to herself the principles of therapy, finding strength in occupations. Always, Ruggles saw her practice as one from which she drew the personal growth that is the promise of empathy. Through occupational therapy, patients found their courage. And Ruggles knew that in "helping others, she helped herself" (Carlova & Ruggles, 1946, p. 191). As the years passed, she felt the growing presence of a supreme spirit and "felt more than rich" (p. 192).

Empathy assumes a unique character in occupational therapy, a practice in which occupation is central. The story of Ora Ruggles portrays a caring and competent practitioner whose vision of the therapeutic relationship was to reach for hearts and hands.

Professional Visions of the Therapeutic Relationship

The American Occupational Therapy Association's (1993) late-twentieth-century elaboration of the core values that shape the therapeutic alliance might be called the profession's vision for the new millennium. In the absence of this formal document, practitioners had previously turned to other sources, such as the story of Ruggles, for cues about how they should be in practice. Perhaps no source better illustrates the evolution of the profession's vision of the therapeutic relationship during the twentieth century than *Willard and Spackman's Occupational Therapy*. From the first edition to the present, this text has offered contributions from individuals working in a variety of practice arenas. The book has served as a primary tool in educating students, often introducing them to a vision of the therapeutic relationship. This embedded vision has changed over the years.

The Vision of the 1940s: An Emphasis on Competence

We saw a vision of the therapeutic relationship depicted in the work of Ruggles. By the 1940s, that vision had changed. Contributors to Willard and Spackman's 1947 edition of *Occupational Therapy* proposed skill-oriented and impersonal relationships. Although they mentioned caring intentions, they emphasized professional competence.

Wade (1947) viewed a good relationship as one in which a skilled therapist earned respect, admiration, and confidence. She saw the successful therapist as one who had mastered two skills to "support patient equilibrium." The first was tact, in which "adjustment is always made to the patient" because "these patients are hypersensitive to implications expressed in words, by tone of voice, mannerism or facial expression" (p. 84). The second skill was "complete self-control in order to prevent untimely expression of a spontaneous emotional reaction" (p. 84). A therapist's tact and control were essential to a patient's equanimity; spontaneity and personal expression were discouraged.

Reaching out was thought important if done with objectivity. The therapist had to see the patient's situation but keep an objective attitude: "The technic [*sic*] of doing this is similar to that used by the adult in correlating his thoughts with those of a child" (Wade, 1947, p. 84). If the therapist had to be a good listener, it was because "it is frequently necessary to play this role" (p. 84). The "good approach" needed to be "within normal limits" (p. 85), which meant restricted to impersonal matters. The bottom line for professional behavior was that one be "impersonal in relationships" (p. 84).

This press for impersonality was not limited to mental health practice. Fay and March (1947) discussed the therapeutic relationship in general hospitals and listed several directives, a few of which follow:

> *Do's*
> *Be encouraging and hopeful and foster a desire in the patient to get well.*
> *Be understandingly sympathetic.*
> *Be friendly and sincere.*
> *Be impersonally personal.*
> *Don't's [sic]*
> *Don't show alarm, horror or sorrow.*
> *Don't argue. Be a good listener.*
> *Don't talk of depressing or distressing subjects.*
> *Don't show racial, religious or political prejudices.*
> *(pp. 125–126).*

The vision of the patient–therapist relationship in the 1947 edition of Willard and Spackman's *Occupational Therapy* reflects a striving for behaviors that objectified and formalized the encounter to make it more professional. Warm traits and spontaneous expressions were discouraged. Perhaps the closest any single contributor in the 1947 edition came to the idea of caring was Gleave (1947), who wrote in her chapter on pediatric services:

> *Ability to talk with children rather than to or at them is an asset. Every effort should be made to bring out the child's ideas, to get him to express himself freely and naturally. . . . She must make the child feel that she is his friend while holding his respect and maintaining discipline when problems arise. (p. 148)*

Gleave mentioned friendship as acceptable within the context of working with children, for whom, perhaps, the need for impersonality was less crucial. The vision of the 1940s differs from the more personal practices of Ruggles. The approach was impersonal because a "professional" approach was thought best.

The Vision of the 1980s: An Emphasis on Caring

Contributors to later editions of *Willard and Spackman's Occupational Therapy* again focused on the personal character of the relationship, with an emphasis on the caring seen in the profession's early years. By the 1983 edition, the term *therapeutic relationship* had taken hold, and a therapist's caring attitude and capacity to be personal assumed much significance (Hopkins & Smith, 1983). A knowledge of self was deemed "most important," and Frank's (1958) work on the therapeutic use of self (the use of one's personal abilities and strengths as a tool in therapy), was endorsed. As if in recognition of a prior emphasis on the objectivity of professionalism, Hopkins and Tiffany (1983) cited a new image: Purtilo's integrated characterization of "the personal-professional self" (p. 95). Purtilo (1978), a physical therapist, had proposed a blend of traits, hoping to minimize conflicts for those who struggled with whether to be personal or professional in their relationships:

> *[The personal-professional self] incorporates actions that communicate caring into the patient health professional interaction; he recognizes efficiency as a trait which can express caring when it does not impose rigid limits on the interaction. (p. 148)*

Hopkins and Tiffany (1983) elaborated on the precise meaning of a therapeutic relationship:

> *The therapist's own self-confidence, the therapist's ability to be honest and open in the relationship and the extent to which the therapist is able to communicate "unconditional positive regard" and empathy for the client will affect the client's ability to invest in the relationship. (pp. 94–95)*

Here we see a reaffirmation of values held by Ruggles.

Tiffany (1983) similarly underscored the practitioner's being "attuned to the principle of facilitating the client's own personal search for purpose, meaning, and self-actualization" (p. 291). Open and personal communication was vital to understanding a client's search for purpose. Within that open relationship, activities were seen as "facilitators for transactions between people" (Hopkins & Tiffany, 1983, p. 95). The vision of the 1980s is clear: Personal relationships held much respect.

When one studies the vision of the therapeutic relationship in occupational therapy over time, one sees that it has always been a blend of competent and caring features. If practitioners enact the alliance in many different ways today, some of those differences may relate to this changing vision. In spite of this varying emphasis on professional competence and personal caring, however, the commitment to collaborate with clients has been long-standing.

Collaboration: A Fundamental Action

A practitioner who collaborates with a client in planning and completing interventions does so when the alliance is considered a partnership. Assumptions that support a collaborative approach are well represented in the occupational therapy literature of the 1940s, even at a time when the relationship was kept impersonal and the term *collaborate* was not used. These assumptions can be summarized: The patient is rational and able to make choices. The patient is free to choose or reject therapeutic services. The therapist is but a teacher and a motivator in the process of therapy; real agency lies with the patient.

Excerpts from Willard and Spackman's (1947) *Occupational Therapy* highlight various aspects of the profession's commitment to collaborate. McNary (1947), for example, wrote: "An activity entered into without a purpose is not occupational therapy" (p. 10). The corollary view was that the practitioner shared the purpose of any activity. Edgerton (1947) said that "the ability to relate an activity to the need of the individual is one of the characteristics that distinguishes the occupational therapist from . . . the crafts instructor" (p. 42). Here is strong support for sharing the merits of any plan: Clients can understand. Given a statement of purpose, clients can choose.

Personal choice was vital, even in the 1940s. Wade (1947) said that "if the patient is unable to participate actively in the plan, its existence should be kept in his consciousness as a justification for the task" (p. 90). If collaboration in planning seemed impossible, she suggested that the therapist should at least explain the reasons for the task. If the person seeking therapy was cognitively impaired, for example, it may have seemed easier to abandon such explanations, but Wade advised that therapists explain at whatever level of understanding is possible. Even if brief or simple, information invites participation.

Literature on collaboration from the 1980s builds on beliefs of the 1940s. Reed and Sanderson (1983) asked practitioners to see a "valuable, worthwhile person, even if the client does not respond readily to the program" (p. 153). The client's right to challenge services, they said, increases a practitioner's responsibility to give helpful information "in a manner that is comprehensive and at a rate that can be absorbed" (p. 154). The mandate of the 1980s built on such rights. Choice had to be given, because individuals could self-direct.

Years before the press for client-centered practice was as strong as it is today, the occupational therapy literature encouraged practitioners to collaborate with those seeking therapy. The profession's long-standing commitment to *working with* clients *rather than doing to* them is foundational to the client-directed collaboration endorsed today (American Occupational Therapy Association [AOTA], 1995b).

Images of Practitioners: The Other Side of the Relationship

After discussion of the therapeutic relationship from the perspective of the practitioner, it seems important to consider that relationship from the perspective of the client. The stories that clients tell about their experiences with occupational therapy practitioners show their views of the alliance quite colorfully. The following fictional story says much about one therapist:

> *Brunhilde, the misplaced Viking Lady, comes tapping on my door every afternoon in an effort to intimidate me into going to Occupational Therapy. She marches around the seventh floor telling all the patients that their doctor has "ordered" Occupational Therapy, and they must come IMMEDIATELY. She herds them out in the hall and they mill around until she lines them up in two columns and goosesteps them out the door. (Rebeta-Burditt, 1977, p. 114)*

A full reading of this novel shows that the patient, Cassie, saw some professionals as compassionate. Her satirical barbs targeted only those whose demands for control threatened her autonomy. Because Brunhilde seems uncaring, this image of the practitioner is disturbing.

It makes sense that clients will gather an impression of practitioners' behaviors and that often those behaviors are compressed into vivid images. In the story of Brunhilde, Cassie was frustrated by a controlling therapist; she formulated the image of a fearsome Viking. Regrettably, a number of other stories portray occupational therapy practitioners as uncaring. It seems important to understand, evaluate, and learn from these.

The Practitioner Seen as Technician, Parent, or Covenanter

To frame an understanding of clients' stories, it may help to turn to the writings of May (1983), a physician who thought about health-care relationships in terms of images. May found images helpful, both in clarifying the functions of individuals and in setting standards for their performance. He argued that "the image tells a kind of compressed story" (p. 17) that introduces not only the basic actor but also the person with whom the actor relates. An image quickly describes the alliance. The image of a physician as a priest, for example, introduces the physician as having mystical power; the patient, as responding in awe. The image of an occupational therapist as a Viking Lady introduces a practitioner called to battle; a client, cowering in fear. The image is far removed from that of Ruggles's reaching for heart and hands.

From among the several images of physicians described by May (1983), three—technician, parent, and covenanter—also emerge from stories about occupational therapists. Essentially, technical practitioners are most concerned with technique, parental practitioners with help or control, and covenanting practitioners with partnerships. Each of these images reflects a markedly different enactment of a practitioner's understanding of how to be both competent and caring in practice.

The Practitioner as Technician

The occupational therapy practitioner who functions as a technician commits foremost to good technique, valuing most the competence reflected in effective procedures (May, 1983). A therapist whose main focus is on methodology, return of function, or the task at hand is often seen as a technician. Although the image may seem cold, the technical practitioner sees excellent performance and procedures as the best way to show care. Stories of technicians in action can be instructive, however.

In *No Laughing Matter* (Heller & Vogel, 1986), Heller described his ordeal with Guillain-Barré syndrome and the time he spent with an occupational therapist who might "be surprised or contrite to find out now of the very considerable anguish" he experienced so often in his sessions with her (p. 166). Methodology and gain were most important to this therapist:

> *In occupational therapy, as soon as I could sand a block of wood (with a need to rest both arms, it was written, after seven repetitions), a change was made to a coarser grade of sandpaper, increasing the amount of force required, and it was just as punishing and demoralizing for me to have to execute them as it had been in the beginning. (pp. 166–167)*

Heller's impression was that therapy meant to keep him "always at a standstill" (p. 166). His personal need was clear—to make some gain and feel it. The therapist, oblivious to his need, used a well-known method of increasing the challenge. Goals for improvement came from a standard protocol, not from collaboration with Heller. Heller thus felt anguish.

Another story, told in verse, also portrays a technician. The opening lines note the patient's dilemma: "Preserve me from the occupational therapist, God/She means well, but I'm too busy to make baskets" (McClay, 1977, p. 106). This well-intended therapist made no attempt to hear her patient or to discuss meaningful occupations; the exchange fell short of a relationship.

Oh, here she comes, the therapist, with
scissors and paste,
Would I like to try decoupage?
"No," I say, "I haven't got time."
"Nonsense," she says, "You're going to
live a long, long time."
That's not what I mean,
I mean that all my life I've been
doing things
for people, with people. I have to
catch up
on my thinking and feeling. (p. 107)

One can claim that occupational therapy is a process that uses meaningful occupation only if practitioners pursue meaning from their clients' perspectives. The therapist in this poem offered techniques; she used age, diagnosis, and disability to determine her choice of activity. She never inquired about the woman's need, which was to reflect. Activities chosen either because a protocol or provider deem them important may have purpose, but they are questionable therapy when they lack meaning. This therapist might have offered occupations that invited reflection, but she did not. So it is in many stories. An overzealous commitment to the technical competence seen in effective procedures leaves clients wondering if practitioners care.

The Practitioner as Parent

The image of a parent seems more personal than that of a technician. But the parental image can be either positive or negative, depending on the manner in which control is provided or help is given (May, 1983). The practitioner who supports another person, while trying to meet some need, conveys the image of a good parent. An excess of either help or control can squelch the relationship. When helpers become overly controlling or paternalistic, clients can rebel. When practitioners become too nurturing, clients can feel disempowered.

Brunhilde, the fictional Viking Lady, was a negative parental figure who used control for the patient's own good. Rule-bound and paternalistic, she ignored her patients' autonomy. By contrast, Hanlan (1979) praised the parental helpers she thought were good:

I was . . . impressed with the equanimity of occupational and physical therapists as they worked all day with severely handicapped people, some with terminal illnesses . . . just "hanging in there," which is really the most essential ingredient. (p. 28)

The steadfast support of practitioners who help with basic activities shapes the image of a good parent.

The fictional story about an activities therapist named Meg shows a valid concern with control (Gibson, 1979). Meg asked patients in a private psychiatric hospital to design and make living room drapes. She got them to accept the idea, and they were enthusiastic about the project. The psychiatrist later commended her skilled handling of the situation. She acknowledged that it was a handling, a manipulation with questionable appropriateness. Her psychiatrist friend answered:

I don't think you did any—violence to their being; the idea was in them or you couldn't have wooed it out. And dealing with patients always takes some handling, the question is only is it for their benefit or yours. (p. 51)

This psychiatrist's rationale is common; paternalistic control is justified if used for the person's own good. The parental practitioner assumes that control and help, choice and decision making should come from the practitioner who has greater knowledge and wisdom about the client's good. The image that a client draws from such behavior is that of a parent. This view differs from the image of reaching for a person's heart to facilitate the search for personal meaning and self-actualization.

The Practitioner as Covenanter

The image of a covenanter, drawn from biblical stories, is more like partnership or friendship (May, 1983). A covenanter acknowledges that any relationship is a gift and works toward reciprocity in the exchange. When acting out of a spirit of covenant, the practitioner sees professional knowledge and skills as resources that are no more important than a client's experiences, perspectives, and strengths. Therapy occurs in a trusting relationship within which both parties draw and give some good. Acknowledging that power and knowledge may not always be balanced, the covenanting practitioner uses personal strengths and professional skills to encourage the other (May, 1983).

Some stories portray occupational therapy practitioners as friends and partners who work to support the goals of others. Benziger (1969), for example, described her hospitalization for depression, remembering the occupational therapist as her "new friend" (p. 48). She shared her first impression of the therapist:

A few days later the first person I had met there who made any real sense came into my room. She was the occupational therapist—a term I've always hated. She was kind, interested, enthusiastic, full of ideas, and intelligent. (p. 47)

This therapist trusted Benziger, followed through on promises made, and supported her will to get well. She valued Benziger's dignity and pressed her to see her own strengths. Crafts served as prompts for their discussions of life:

"You know, you go at your work too hard, too fast, too desperately—and too frenetically."

> *"I guess I do, but that's the way I feel . . ."*
> *She said, "You are an intelligent person, and you will help yourself to get well quickly."*
> *"You know," I answered, "you're the first person who has mentioned intelligence versus non intelligence, instead of sanity. You make me feel like a human being . . ." I was grateful. I should not forget her.* (p. 49)

Another image of practitioner as friend appeared in Donaldson's (1976) account of his unwarranted 15-year confinement in mental institutions:

> *While I waited, I found OT fun. Young, overweight Baldylocks had about five of us . . . showing compassion and understanding to all of us. He let me spend afternoons learning the touch system of typing. . . . Baldylocks started taking the OT men and a half dozen from upstairs for a two-hour walk on the grounds each Wednesday.* (pp. 245–246)

Donaldson exercised, cooked, and learned lathe work from Baldylocks—all satisfying activities that he helped choose. In this oppressive environment, he saw and valued his therapist's commitment to caring ways and competent work.

Clients' stories suggest that the behaviors of practitioners can evoke images of technicians, parents, or covenanted friends—portrayals that show different enactments of competence and caring. Such stories can help us understand how clients perceive us when we choose to emphasize either competence or caring.

Variable Emphases on Competence and Caring

Each image of occupational therapy practitioners—technician, parent, and covenanter—shows a clients' experience of how competence and caring are enacted. It seems important to note that positive images reflect the actions of practitioners who are competent and caring in ways that match a client's needs. Practitioners must consider, in sometimes brief exchanges, what each person needs from the relationship. This challenge is a real one. Often, an individual's words, manner, and personal style will give cues about how to respond. Although some individuals prefer that practitioners relate to them as technicians or parents, most seek a person who equalizes competence and caring to become a partnering friend.

THE CONTEXT AND ITS INFLUENCE ON RELATIONSHIP

The therapeutic relationship in occupational therapy has been shaped by the profession's visions, but no less so than by influential contexts that have been temporal, social, and physical. Any alliance is embedded within and affected by some context, a fact well illustrated by markedly different descriptions of professional alliances in occupational therapy during the 1940s and the 1980s. As times and places and players in health care change, so do interpersonal behaviors. To see a therapeutic alliance only in terms of the dynamics between a therapist and client would be an oversimplistic view. Individuals who partner in any venture find both opportunity and constraint from the locale, group, or culture within which the alliance occurs. And so it is with therapy.

Societal Beliefs That Shape Care

Prevalent societal beliefs shape the contexts within which practice occurs. Such beliefs have affected occupational therapy since its inception, when as Yerxa (1980) said, "it began in a climate of caring" (p. 532). One notable change in the last quarter of the twentieth century was the sense that the climate of health-care practice had become less caring. It is not surprising that the profession's affirmation of personal relationships in the 1980s emerged in response to uncaring practices. Patients at that time were describing experiences with practitioners as difficult, sharing their grasp of the problem with the words dehumanizing or depersonalizing. These abstractions have continued into present times to become a shorthand expression for careless behaviors.

If practitioners are to avoid behaviors felt as uncaring, they must know what these are. Woven through a large number of clients' stories is a profile of impersonal attitudes and actions that clients say strip them of courage when they need it most. Clients say that helpers depersonalize practice by (1) failing to see the personal consequences of illness and disability; (2) denying the feelings of those whom they treat; (3) dismissing clients and their concerns; (4) failing to show, in even small ways, that they themselves feel and can appreciate a clients' pain; (5) engaging in distancing behaviors; (6) withholding vital information; (7) being silent or aloof; (8) acting brusquely; and (9) misusing their power. The personal hurts in their stories are clear.

If practitioners can envision and enact both competence and caring, as clients' stories indicate that they can, what beliefs cause them to act impersonally? Three contextual beliefs compromise social behaviors and inhibit caring environments: that the rational fixing of problems is best; that methods and protocols are the primary agents in therapy; and that delivery systems should be driven by business, efficiency, and profit. These beliefs can prompt caregivers to act as cold technicians or controlling parents, rather than as covenanted partners who cherish personal relationships.

The Emphasis on Rational Fixing

One societal force that compromises caring actions is the belief that illness and disability are diagnosable problems that should be solved. When Hodgins wrote in 1964, after experiencing a stroke, he described the patient and the caregiver as perceiving illness differently:

> *In stroke two basic sets of assumptions could govern treatment. One set proceeds from what the patient*

perceives or thinks he perceives; the other comes from what the doctor knows or thinks he knows. The two are very different sets of things. (p. 842)

Hodgins argued that health-care professionals often disregard a patient's perception of what ought to be done. Some helpers do not see that human understanding is as important as a solution to the problem.

Van Eys (1988), a physician, regretted such limited insight. He discussed the hemisected worldview in which "diseases become problems, and patients become dissected into such problems" (p. 21). Clients resent this narrowness of view. It feels impersonal when caregivers see their disease and the mechanisms of their bodies but not their experience of illness and unease, not its meaning to them, and surely not their feelings.

Disregard for parts of people disturbed Murphy (1987), an anthropologist who wrote of his disabling illness: "The full subjective states of the patient are of little concern in the medical model of disability, which holds that the problem arises wholly from some atomic or physiological disorder and is correctable by standard modes of therapy—drugs, surgery, radiation, or whatever" (p. 88). The question for practitioners becomes, What is the problem with treating bodies when they need fixing? Most clients answer that when they appear "as a physiological mechanism, the doctor may neglect personal communication in favor of the immediate scientific task at hand" (Leder, 1984, p. 36). The press to fix problems in rational and formulaic ways makes it easier for one to neglect feelings and easier to justify being silent, curt, or aloof.

The consequence of a too-strong commitment to rationale fixing—of the disease, the body, or the occupational problem—is a disregard that feels care-less. Are occupational therapy practitioners among those who commit to rational fixing? Mattingly (1991) gave most practitioners cause for concern when she said, "Therapists can come to reduce their practice to a manipulation of the physical body, forgetting how much their interventions are directed to a person's life" (p. 986).

The Reliance on Methods and Protocol

A second societal belief that compromises caring is an overvaluation of the techniques, procedures, and modalities that solve the problem. When they are ill, people seek concern as well as solutions, but they often find technique. Hodgins (1964) loathed the discovery: "As so-called science more and more enters medicine, the heedless or routine physician will be accordingly tempted to withdraw his humanity and wait for specifics" (p. 843). Hodgins considered the treatments needed for cure and the humanity needed for care as different but inseparable parts of care. When a drug or a procedure works well on a problem, however, a practitioner may think less about the need to make personal connections. Sacks (1983) rejected the argument that helpers must use only treatments or protocols. When facing surgery, he wondered:

What sort of man would Swan be? I know he was a good surgeon, but it was not the surgeon but the person that I would stand in relation to, or, rather, the man in whom, I hoped, the surgeon and the person would be wholly fused. (p. 92)

Cassell (1985), a physician, shared this belief: "Doctors who lack developed personal powers are inadequately trained. . . . Doctors are themselves instruments of patient care" (p. 1).

When methods and protocols are effective, however, they can take the upper hand. Helpers side with what works, so that a challenge to the procedure also threatens them. Lear (1980) remembered the upshot of such an identification when her husband, Hal, a urologist, requested a milder painkiller: "The resident got angry. He said, 'There is a medication ordered for pain for you. If you want it, you can have it. If not, you'll get nothing.' And he walked out" (p. 41).

Helpers can wrap themselves in their procedural authority, binding themselves so tightly in their concern for the right method that it is no wonder they seem constrained. They will never be seen as personal if they offer knowledge or skills instead of themselves. Hodgins (1964) thought that personal encounters are often what patients need most: The patient "will draw courage as he perceives human understanding underlying the professional techniques of those into whose care he has been given" (p. 841). Unhappily, concern for personal issues seems to matter little in the formulaic belief that correct procedures give best results.

Occupational therapy practitioners admit that techniques can preempt caring. Yerxa (1980) argued that "technique, once employed in the service of human needs, is rapidly moving us toward a society of total technology in which our ways of thinking and being themselves become so technical that we lose sight of other ways of thinking and being" (p. 530). Parham (1987) discussed the case of Longmore, a former faculty member at the University of Southern California Program in Disability and Society:

He was subjected to long hours of occupational therapy training for self-care skills although he had no intention of performing these time-consuming tasks independently at home. He planned to hire an attendant who would expedite the process, freeing him to use his time and energy to pursue more stimulating and productive activities. (p. 556)

Situations such as this one led King (1980) to conclude that "therapists have ignored their instinct for caring" (p. 525).

Delivery Systems Driven by Business, Efficiency, and Profit

The third societal belief that compromises caring is that delivery systems must, above all else, be efficient and profitable. This belief preceded the advent of managed care by several years. Peabody (1930) stated the upshot of this problem well when he argued that "hospitals, like other institutions, founded with the highest human ideals, are apt to deteriorate into dehumanized machines" (p. 33).

The Business of Delivery Systems

Any business that offers service to large numbers of people—whether a hospital, prison, or community agency—may suffer from clients' complaints about being ignored. As Sarason (1985) wrote, "The clinician becomes a rationer of time, and that obviously sets drastic limits on the degree to which the ever-present client need for caring and compassion can be met" (p. 170). Such rationing affected a young man with AIDS in a busy clinic: "I just feel like they don't care" (Peabody, 1986, p. 172).

Because of their lifesaving functions, hospitals can compromise caring. Hodgins (1964) discussed the estrangement that occurs: "The stroke victim is most likely to encounter, as his first medical ministrant, a physician to whom he is a total stranger. Since speedy hospitalization is usually a first goal in stroke, treatment by strangers is likely to continue" (p. 839).

Peabody (1930) explained one consequence to the patient of a lifesaving business conducted among strangers:

> *He loses his personal identity. He is generally referred to, not as Henry Jones, but as "that case of mitral stenosis in the second bed on the left." . . . It leads, more or less directly, to the patient being treated as a case of mitral stenosis, and not a sick man. (p. 31).*

The problem is a matter of focus; the institutional eye sees the relevance of saving Henry's life but does not capture the wider clinical picture—that although "Henry happens to have heart disease, he is not disturbed so much by dyspnea as he is by anxiety for the future" (p. 34).

The Efficiency of Delivery Systems

If the business of delivery systems is problematic, so is their efficiency. Murphy (1987) discussed the structure and control of institutions, describing them as systems of schedules and shifts: "The hospital has all the features of a bureaucracy, and, like bureaucracies everywhere, it both breeds and feeds on impersonality" (p. 21). The impersonality is well illustrated in Saxton's (1987) account:

> *The scariest part of the hospitalization for me was not the surgery but the doctor rounds. On the mornings when these rituals were scheduled, the nurses and aides awakened us much earlier than usual. . . . Then they would come, the surgeons, the residents, and the interns. . . . They entered our ward, about fifteen adults. . . . Strange long words were uttered; bandages were opened and quickly closed. (p. 53)*

Gebolys (1990) recalled that only on the fourth day of her hospital stay did a nurse's aide wash her hair, bloody and dirty from an automobile accident. The aide did so after her shift was over because the highly regulated day precluded this helping task. Sacks (1983) concluded that "the hospital, in short, is a singular mixture, where freedom and bondage, warmth and coldness, human and mechanical, life and death, are locked together in perpetual combat" (p. 24).

The battle sometimes seems insane. Brice (1987) recalled a nurse in the recovery room whom she asked for a blanket. The nurse "barked, 'I just brought you one; I'm not going to bring you another' and disappeared" (p. 31). People can bring caring to delivery systems; there will be no fellowship if they bring only efficiency.

The Profit of Service Provision

A profit-driven focus in health care has also received much criticism. Within a profit ethos, knowledge has coin value, cure is a high-priced commodity, and ill people are buyers. Success and solvency turn into treatment goals, and efficiency the means to achieve them. In this scheme, more status accrues from procedures that cure than from manners that care.

Practitioners face a major quandary when the client's need for time and compassion competes with the institution's need to prosper. When high regard falls to those who accumulate the most billable units of time, it becomes harder to justify moments spent noticing, listening, or communicating. One physician explained: "Whose agent I was became a pressing, daily, moral problem. I know what it is to have divided loyalties, to want to give up the fight, to rationalize away the internalized conflict" (Sarason, 1985, pp. 170–171). Although few helpers buy the idea that clients are mere customers, many budget their caring actions. Individuals feel the cuts as hurtful. Lear (1980) hated that he had not attended to his patients' experiences. He thought: "Damn it, doctors should know. They should care. Say how're they are treating you? How's the food? Accommodations comfortable? Staff courteous. . . . He himself would never even have thought to ask. Didn't that make him negligent too? Ah. Bingo!" (p. 43).

Occupational therapy practitioners speak openly about their frustrations with a profit ethos. Howard (1991) noted that growing caseloads are a real concern since productivity and efficiency have become top-priority goals (Howard, 1991). She also argued that technological approaches seem valued more than the holistic use of a variety of methods. The climate seems one of cost containment rather than caring. Burke and Cassidy (1991) named the dilemma a "disparity between reimbursement driven practices and the humanistic values of occupational therapy" (p. 173). The enormity of the challenge pressed Grady (1992) to ask: "Is there still enjoyment in occupational therapy, or have we become so controlled with the realities of productivity, reimbursement, and modalities that we are failing to see the process as part of the outcome" (p. 1063)?

During the twentieth century, growing distress over the impersonality of technical or parental care led to measures that defend personal rights: quality of care requirements, the Patient's Bill of Rights, and informed consent laws. These measures protect clients against systems that demand financial solvency and technical competence but dismiss caring. Laws push uncaring helpers to at least honor human rights. But a commitment to caring cannot be legislated; it must be inspired by a vision of the therapeutic relationship that keeps caring central.

The Profession's Affirmation of a Climate of Caring

Several leading occupational therapy practitioners reaffirmed the need for a climate of caring in the 1980s because they saw dangers fomenting in delivery systems "not oriented to the human being" (Baum, 1980, p. 514). In an effort to renew the profession's commitment to caring, Baum made this point: "Occupational therapy harnesses will and gives the individual control through activity. That is human, that is care" (p. 515). Technical skills, other leaders argued, serve practitioners well if they "promote movement and flexibility within therapeutic relationships" (Gilfoyle, 1980, p. 520). Therapy, they said, needs to be grounded in commitment to a person. Gilfoyle wrote:

> *The caring therapist directly knows a client as a unique individual, as someone in his or her own right, not as an average, a generality, or number on the Gaussian curve . . . [it] is the art of "being with the person"; it is something you feel. (p. 520)*

"The caring," said Gilfoyle, "is not the taking-care-of the person, but helping the person to learn to take care of himself/herself" (p. 519). Yerxa (1980) saw deliberations on caring as measures of the profession's success. She said that "our practice in the future should be evaluated not only on the basis of measurable scientific outcomes, but also by what it contributes to individual human dignity" (p. 534). She identified the challenge of the future as that of embracing and preserving a climate of caring.

Preserving the Relationship

In the last two decades, we have been mindful of Yerxa's (1980) challenge. The profession has affirmed the value of caring, the art of practice, and the therapeutic relationship. We have taken a public stand regarding the core values that will guide practice, naming human dignity essential (AOTA, 1993). We support client-centered care (AOTA, 1995a; Neidstadt, 1995). We promote occupations with meaning to those who seek our services (AOTA, 1994, 1995b). We use interactive and narrative reasoning to learn a person's concerns (Clark, Carlson, & Polkinghorne, 1997; Fleming, 1991; Mattingly, 1998). We support collaboration with those who seek our help (AOTA, 1995b; Ponte-Allan & Giles, 1999). We examine uncaring practices (Jackson, 2000). We support caring behaviors as part of professional development (Fidler, 1996; Sands, 1995). We publish inquiries into the art of practice (Spencer, Davidson, & White, 1997; Weinstein, 1998) and the effects of the therapeutic relationship (Dunkerley, Tickle-Degnen, & Coster, 1997; Neuhaus, 1997; Yuen, 1996).

Alongside these efforts, however, we continue to see trends to dismiss the art of practice and caring, many of these from profit-driven managed care systems. These systems sharpen a focus on accountability, efficiency, and profit and call into question the merits of empathy and artistry. The commitment made to a climate of caring in the 1980s needs reaffirmation today. The challenge, as always, is for practitioners to meet clients' needs and sustain the profession's artistry.

ETHICS NOTE 14–1

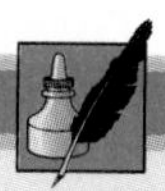

How Can a Practitioner Balance Conflicting Ethical Obligations?

PENNY KYLER and RUTH ANN HANSEN

Jamie, a 14-year-old, has an attention deficit disorder and juvenile-onset diabetes. Some of the kids in his neighborhood know that Jamie has needles for insulin injections. They have forced him to give them some of the needles. Then they sell them to substance abusers. Jamie has confided to his occupational therapy practitioner that he is afraid to tell his parents about this and is afraid of what the kids will do to him if he does tell.

QUESTIONS AND EXERCISES

1. **The occupational therapy practitioner has obligations and duties to several individuals and groups. Identify them. Which group or individual should receive the highest priority?**
2. **What conflicts are present between the role of being a caring professional and that of preventing harm?**
3. **Discuss the concepts of personal autonomy, the right to privacy, the right to confidentiality, and the obligations to do good and avoid doing harm as they relate to this situation.**

CONCLUSION

In his reflections about education, Davies (1991) offered an opinion that may help place the current challenge in perspective and close this discussion. From his position on a state governing board, he saw that the essential function of board members was to inspire education. A question that he thought they must ask is this: "Are we helping to create an environment in which teaching and learning are honored and can flourish?" (p. 58). He said that the making of such an environment is a call to engender a restlessness throughout the system, disturb complacency, and insist that rules be broken when there is good and sufficient reason.

Occupational therapy practitioners must see their rational, technical, and managerial functions—marks of their competence—as a vital part of good practice. But they must also make a climate of caring by creating environments in which personal relationships can flourish. To do so in some practice settings may mean engendering a restlessness, disturbing complacency, and insisting that rules be broken.

Calls from our forbears to reach for hearts as well as hands have real meaning today. We can inspire health-care systems. We can touch hearts—if we choose to reach for them. We can make care happen—if we are empathic in all of our doing. We can practice our art—if we establish fellowship. The challenge to create therapeutic relationships in occupational therapy can be framed with a simple question that we each must ask: As I engage others in occupation, am I also caring?

ACKNOWLEDGMENTS

The American Occupational Therapy Association granted the author permission to revise and combine her original works from the *American Journal of Occupational Therapy*: Linking purpose to procedure during interactions with patients. (1988). *42*(12), 775–781; Sustaining the art of practice. (1989). *43*(4), 219–226; The patient-therapist relationship in occupational therapy: Understanding visions and images. (1990). *44*(1), 13–21; The depersonalization of patients: A profile gleaned from narratives. (1993). *47*(9), 830–837; The patient-therapist relationship: Beliefs that shape care. (1993). *47*(10), 935–942; The fullness of empathy: Reflections and illustrations. (1995). *49*(1), 24–31.

References

Adler, A. (1931). *What life should mean to you*. Boston: Little, Brown.

American Occupational Therapy Association [AOTA]. (1993). Core values and attitudes of occupational therapy practice. *American Journal of Occupational Therapy, 47*, 1085–1086.

American Occupational Therapy Association [AOTA]. (1994). Position paper: Purposeful activity. *American Journal of Occupational Therapy, 48*, 467–468.

American Occupational Therapy Association [AOTA]. (1995a). Concept paper: Service delivery in occupational therapy. *American Journal of Occupational Therapy, 49*, 1029–1031.

American Occupational Therapy Association [AOTA]. (1995b). Position paper: Occupation. *American Journal of Occupational Therapy, 49*, 1015–1018.

American Occupational Therapy Association Council on Standards. (1972). Occupational therapy: Its definition and functions. *American Journal of Occupational Therapy, 26*, 204–205.

Baum, C. M. (1980). Occupational therapists put care in the health system. [Eleanor Clarke Slagle Lecture]. *American Journal of Occupational Therapy, 34*, 505–516.

Benziger, B. (1969). *The prison of my mind*. New York: Walker.

Brice, J. (1987). Empathy lost. *Harvard Medical Letter, 60*, 28–32.

Buber, M. (1965). *Between man and man*. New York: Macmillan.

Burke, J. P., & Cassidy, J. C. (1991). Disparity between reimbursement-driven practice and humanistic values of occupational therapy. *American Journal of Occupational Therapy, 45*, 173–176.

Carlova, J., & Ruggles, O. (1946). *The healing heart*. New York: Messner.

Cassell, E. J. (1985). *Talking with patients. Volume 1: The theory of doctor-patient communication*. Cambridge, MA: MIT Press.

Clark, F., Carlson, M., & Polkinghorne, D. (1997). Legitimacy of life history and narrative approaches in the story of occupation. *American Journal of Occupational Therapy 51*, 313–317.

Davies, G. K. (1991). Teaching and learning: What are the questions? *Teaching Education, 4*, 57–61.

Donaldson, K. (1976). *Insanity inside out*. New York: Crown.

Dunkerley, E. Tickle-Degnen, L., & Coster, W. J. (1997). Therapist-child interactions in the middle minutes of sensory integration treatment. *American Journal of Occupational Therapy, 51*, 799–805.

Edgerton, W. B. (1947). Activities in occupational therapy. In H. S. Willard & C. S. Spackman (Eds.). *Principles of occupational therapy* (pp. 40–59). Philadelphia: Lippincott.

Egan, G. (1986). *The skilled helper: A systematic approach to effective helping*. Monterey: Brooks/Cole.

Fay, E. V., & March, I. (1947). Occupational therapy in general and special hospitals. In H. S. Willard & C. S. Spackman (Eds). *Principles of occupational therapy* (1st ed., pp. 118–137). Philadelphia: Lippincott.

Fidler, G. S. (1996). Developing a repertoire of professional behaviors. *American Journal of Occupational Therapy, 50*, 583–587.

Fleming, M. H. (1991). The therapist with the three-track mind. *American Journal of Occupational Therapy, 45*, 1007–1014.

Frank, J. (1958). The therapeutic use of self. *American Journal of Occupational Therapy, 12*, 215.

Gebolys, E. (1990). Inadequacies, inequities and inanities in modern medicine—A personal experience. *Occupational Therapy Forum, 12*, 6–7, 13–18.

Gibson, W. (1979). *The cobweb*. New York: Atheneum Press.

Gilfoyle, E. (1980). Caring: A philosophy of practice. *American Journal of Occupational Therapy, 34*, 517–521.

Gleave, G. M. (1947). Occupational therapy in children's hospitals and pediatric services. In H. S. Willard & C. S. Spackman (Eds.). *Principles of occupational therapy* (pp. 141–174). Philadelphia: Lippincott.

Grady, A. P. (1992). Nationally speaking-Occupation as vision. *American Journal of Occupational Therapy, 46*, 1062–1065.

Hackney, H. (1978). The evolution of empathy. *Personnel and Guidance Journal, 56*, 35–38.

Hanlan, M. (1979, November). Living with a dying husband. *Pennsylvania Gazette*, 25–28.

Heller, J., & Vogel, S. (1986). *No laughing matter*. New York: Avon.

Hodgins, E. (1964). Whatever became of the healing art? *Annals of the New York Academy of Sciences, 164*, 838–846.

Hopkins, H. L. & Smith, H. D. (Eds.). (1983). *Willard and Spackman's occupational therapy* (6th ed.). Philadelphia: Lippincott.

Hopkins, H. L., & Tiffany, E. G. (1983). Occupational therapy: A problem solving process. In H. L. Hopkins & H. D. Smith (Eds.). *Willard & Spackman's occupational therapy* (6th ed., pp. 89–100). Philadelphia: Lippincott.

Howard, B. S. (1991). How high do we jump? The effect of reimbursement on occupational therapy. *American Journal of Occupational Therapy, 45*, 875–881.

Jackson, J. (2000). Understanding the experience of noninclusive occupational therapy clinics: Lesbians' perspectives. *American Journal of Occupational Therapy, 54*(1), 26–35.

Katz, R. L. (1963). *Empathy: Its nature and uses*. London: Free Press of Glencoe.

Kidner, T. B. (1929). Address to graduates. *Occupational Therapy and Rehabilitation, 8*, 379–385.

King, L. J. (1980). Creative caring. *American Journal of Occupational Therapy, 34*, 522–528.

Lear, M. (1980). *Heartsounds*. New York: Simon & Schuster.

Leder, D. (1984). Medicine and paradigms of embodiment. *Journal of Medicine and Philosophy, 9*(1), 29–43.

Mattingly, C. (1991). The narrative nature of clinical reasoning. *American Journal of Occupational Therapy, 45*, 998–1005.

Mattingly, C. (1998). *Healing dramas and clinical plots. The narrative structure of experience*. New York: Cambridge University Press.

May, W. (1983). *The physician's covenant: Images of the healer in medical ethics*. Philadelphia: Westminster.

McClay, E. (1977). *Green winter: Celebrations of old age*. New York: Reader's Digest.

McNary, H. (1947). The scope of occupational therapy. In H. Willard & C. Spackman (Eds.). *Principles of occupational therapy* (pp. 10–22). Philadelphia: Lippincott.

Mosey, A. C. (1981). *Occupational therapy: Configuration of a profession*. New York: Raven.

Murphy, R. F. (1987). *The body silent*. New York: Henry Holt.

Neidstadt, M. E. (1995). Methods of assessing clients' priorities: A survey of adult physical dysfunction settings. *American Journal of Occupational Therapy, 49*, 428–436.

Neuhaus, B. E. (1997). Including hope in occupational therapy practice: A pilot study. *American Journal of Occupational Therapy, 51*, 228–234.

Olinick, S. L. (1984). Empathy and sympathy. In J. Lichtenberg, M. Bornstein & D. Silver (Eds.). *Empathy I* (pp. 25–166). New York: Analytic.

Parham, D. (1987). Nationally speaking-Toward professionalism: The reflective therapist. *American Journal of Occupational Therapy, 41*, 555–561.

Peabody, B. (1986). *The screaming room: A mother's journal of her son's struggle with AIDS*. New York: Macmillan.

Peabody, F. W. (1930). *Doctor and patient papers on the relationship of the physician to men and institutions*. New York: Macmillan.

Ponte-Allan, M. & Giles, G. M. (1999). Goal setting and functional outcomes in rehabilitation. *American Journal of Occupational Therapy, 53*, 646–649.

Purtilo, R. (1978). *Health professional/patient interaction*. Philadelphia: Saunders.

Rebeta-Burditt, J. (1977). *The cracker factory*. New York: Macmillan.

Reed, K. L., & Sanderson, S. R. (1983). *Concepts of occupational therapy*. Baltimore: Williams & Wilkins.

Reiser, D., & Schroder, A. K. (1980). *Patient interviewing: The human dimension*. Baltimore: Williams & Wilkins.

Rogers, C. R. (1975). Empathic: An unappreciated way of being. *Counseling Psychologist, 5*(2), 2–10.

Rogers, C. R. (1957). The necessary and sufficient conditions of therapeutic personality change. *Journal of Consulting Psychology, 21*, 95–103.

Sacks, O. (1983). *Awakenings*. New York: Dutton.

Sands, M. (1995). Readying occupational therapy assistant students for level II fieldwork: Beyond academic to personal behaviors and attitudes. *American Journal of Occupational Therapy, 49*, 150–152.

Sarason, S. B. (1985). *Caring and compassion in clinical practice*. San Francisco: Jossey-Bass.

Saxton, M. (1987). The something that happened before I was born. In M. Saxton & F. Howe (Eds.). *With wings: An anthology of literature by and about women with disabilities* (pp. 51–57). New York: Feminist Press.

Spencer, J., Davidson, H., & White, V. (1997). Helping clients develop hope for the future. *American Journal of Occupational Therapy, 51*, 191–198.

Thomas, L. (1983). *The youngest science: Notes of medicine-watcher*. New York: Viking.

Tiffany, E. G. (1983). Psychiatry and mental health. In H. L. Hopkins & H. D. Smith (Eds.). *Willard and Spackman's occupational therapy* (6th ed., pp. 267–229). Philadelphia: Lippincott.

Van Eys, J. & McGovern, J. P., (Eds.). (1988). *The doctor as a person*. Springfield, IL: Thomas.

Wade, B. D. (1947). Occupational therapy for patients with mental disease. In H. Willard & C. Spackman (Eds.). *Principles of occupational therapy* (pp. 81–117). Philadelphia: Lippincott.

Weinstein, E. (1998). Elements of art of practice in mental health. *American Journal of Occupational Therapy, 52*, 563–569.

Willard, H. S., & Spackman, C. S. (Eds.). (1947). *Principles of occupational therapy*. Philadelphia: Lippincott.

Yerxa, E. J. (1980). Occupational therapy's role in creating a future climate of caring. *American Journal of Occupational Therapy, 34*, 529–534.

Yuen, H. K. (1996). Case report: Management of avoidance behaviors using direct and indirect psychological methods. *American Journal of Occupational Therapy, 50*, 578–582.

CHAPTER 15

GROUP PROCESS

SHARAN L. SCHWARTZBERG

GROUP PROCESS: LARGE GROUP SYSTEMS AND SMALL TASK GROUPS

Occupational therapists work within large group systems such as schools and hospitals and in small task groups for therapeutic aims, peer support, organizational goals, and evaluation purposes. For example, in a hospital setting the practitioner may lead a dressing group for a couple of patients with hip fractures and in the community facilitate a peer support group for 10 individuals who have experienced head injury. Other settings, as illustration, that require **group process** skills are being a consultant to a large school board to evaluate accessibility of community facilities and assisting a family and other caretakers to learn feeding techniques for a child who has difficulty feeding himself or herself.

ECOLOGICAL SYSTEMS ANALYSIS

To appreciate group process fully, it is helpful to understand **ecological systems analysis,** an integrative perspective of the individual, interpersonal relationships, and the environment. Use of the ecological systems model in occupational therapy (Howe & Briggs, 1982) draws on Bronfenbrenner's (1979) work in human development and on general systems theory. Howe and Briggs call attention to understanding behavior as an interaction between the individual with an inherent biopsychosocial makeup and a given environmental system.

LARGE GROUPS

The ecological notion of relationship between person and environment is instrumental to understanding an integrative perspective of large groups, such as the community or institutional setting, as context for individual and interpersonal relationships. As Dunn, Brown, and McGuigan (1994) explained, human behavior and performance cannot be understood outside of context (physical, temporal, social, and cultural features).

Community

Understanding a community as a large group can tell practitioners about the various sociocultural perspectives of individuals and subgroups. An analysis may include concerns such as racial and ethnic background, religious affiliations, educational backgrounds, occupational roles, and sexual orientation as well as community resources for vocational, cultural, leisure, and educational pursuits. Of equal importance, but not as easy to identify, are the various values, beliefs, and attitudes of a community.

Institutional Settings

Traditional institutions—such as hospitals, clinics, and schools—remain standard to the environmental diet of a therapist. Each has its own mission and philosophy, values, and hierarchy that influence the leader and individuals, be they patient, client, student, staff, or administrative personnel. As in the community setting, institutional norms may be covert or made explicit. With rapid change in health-service delivery systems, one can expect frustration because of clashes in values and unclear boundaries. To illustrate, practitioners and consumers accustomed to unlimited care may question the ethics of managed care. When angry and disillusioned, they appear resistant in group meetings.

SMALL TASK GROUPS

There are many types of small task groups in occupational therapy. They can be broadly classified for purposes of therapy, peer support, the focus process, and consultation and supervision.

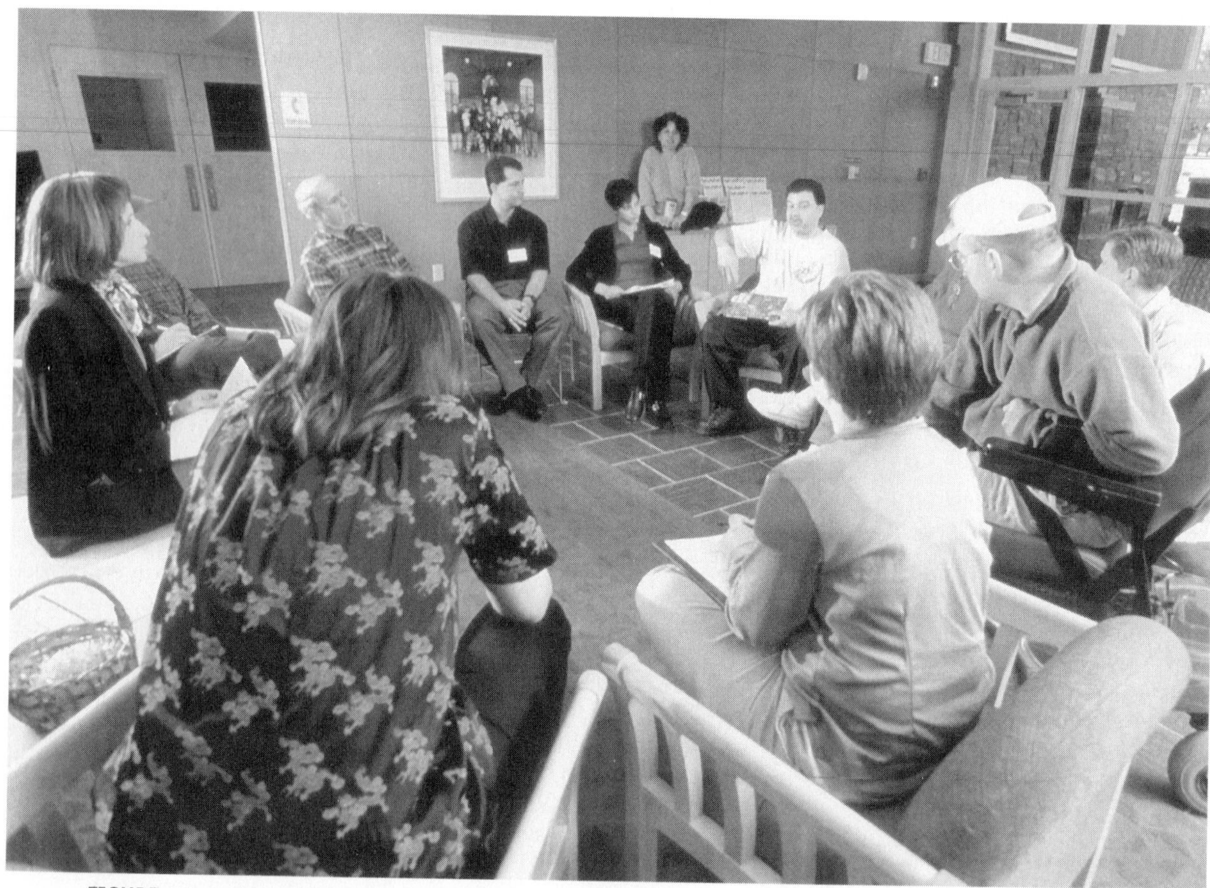

FIGURE 15–1. Occupational therapy often occurs within a group format. (Photo courtesy of Kindra Clinetf.)

Therapeutic Groups

Most task groups in the category of therapeutic groups have individual change as a primary aim. The therapeutic tasks are designed for the purposes of restoration or development of functioning in client factors and areas of occupational performance; they may also serve aims of prevention and may offer support of existing strengths. Group membership is usually small, ordinarily from 6 to 10 patients (Fig. 15-1).

Peer Support Groups

Peer support groups are designed to provide support for individuals, their families, caretakers, and partners who have in common a medically related problem, diagnosis, or disability. The degree to which professionals are involved varies a great deal from active involvement as teacher and leader to a consultative role as facilitator. These task groups can be quite large or small, depending on the format. If the material is didactic, rather than process oriented, a larger group can be accommodated. According to Howe and Schwartzberg (2001), occupational therapists also play a role in naturally occurring support groups, such as those found in wellness programs, religious organizations, and the workplace. They characterized these groups as functional groups. It is predicted that the occupational therapist's professional role in such community-based programs will expand in the near future.

Focus Groups

Focus groups are small groups used for the purpose of tapping opinions. These task groups are increasingly popular for studying a theme to generate research hypotheses or to organize discussion around material on a restricted topic. We can expect focus groups to gain popularity in occupational therapy with the increased need for qualitative research related to functioning and time-limited intervention regimes.

Consultation and Supervision Groups

As practitioners work more independently, there will be an increased need for peer support, supervision, and consultation. Group supervision, both disciplinary and interdisciplinary, is a viable option. One can expect a trend in this direction, as large occupational therapy departments with supervisory staff diminish and more practitioners work in private and community-based practices in isolation of others with similar training. Occupational therapists will also increasingly be called on to supervise occupational therapy assistants, aides, and other caretakers. The group format should serve this need both educationally and economically.

HISTORICAL NOTE 15–1

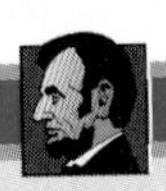

The Story of the Healing Heart: Doing with Persons as a Unique Alliance

SUZANNE M. PELOQUIN

The biography of Ora Ruggles chronicles the kind of service that reconstruction aides rendered during World War I. A schoolteacher who had graduated from San Diego Normal School and taken courses in the manual arts, Ruggles quickly engaged each of her patients. Her competence, warmth, and concern inspired awe and gratitude in many of them. The title of her biography, *The Healing Heart*, derives from a comment Ruggles made to her peers. As she walked into the army barracks at Fort McPherson one evening, her friends asked about her unusual silence. Ruggles explained that she had made a great discovery, simple yet so effective. When pressed to share, she offered this fine keepsake: "It is not enough to give a patient something to do with his hands. You must reach for the heart as well as the hands. It's the heart that really does the healing" (Carlova & Ruggles, 1946, p. 69). The comment still has meaning five decades later. Ruggles described an interactive form of doing with others that transforms the use of occupation into an alliance named "occupational therapy." Within a health-care system that presses so many to do things to their clients, this alliance is remarkable.

Carlova, J., & Ruggles, O. (1946). *The healing heart*. New York: Messner.

PAST AND PRESENT TRENDS IN THERAPEUTIC GROUPS

Occupational therapy group intervention is the combination of structured, adapted group process and tasks or a set of activities aimed at fostering change and adaptation in people with acute or chronic illness, impairments, or disability. The occupational therapist's use of group process requires knowledge of group process theories and **group dynamics,** understanding of conceptual models that describe group principles and parallel therapeutic techniques, and knowledge of empirical research on variables related to the small task-oriented group (both nonclinical and therapeutic). Group therapists must be able to use this information, along with their knowledge of pathology, wellness, and the use of meaningful occupation, to reason about the individual in the group context.

Historical Overview

A contemporary occupational therapy group consists of more than simply two or three people doing solitary activities in the same room. Nevertheless, it was not uncommon to find such parallel interaction constituting group treatment in the profession's early years (Howe & Schwartzberg, 1986).

TABLE 15-1. **COMPARISON OF THERAPEUTIC USES OF GROUP PROPERTIES**

Group Properties	Occupational Therapy	Verbal Psychotherapy	Peer Support
Leader involvement	Very central	Not central	Not central
Purposeful activity	Very central	Not central	Not central
Structure and format	Very central	Not central	Somewhat central
Practice	Very central	Somewhat central	Not central
Teaching and learning	Very central	Somewhat central	Very central
Socialization and outside action	Somewhat central	Not central	Very central
There and then	Not central	Very central	Somewhat central
Here and now	Very central	Very central	Very central

Today, it is incongruous to have occupational therapy conducted in groups without therapist consideration of the unique properties of the group format. When occupational therapy groups are compared to verbal psychotherapy and peer support groups, the group properties receive different emphasis (Table 15-1). Occupational therapy's unique perspective of the group as a format for service delivery is further understood through descriptions of past and current practices. Separate historical periods have been identified (Howe & Schwartzberg, 1986, 1995), and the focus of group involvement during each of these eras is outlined in Table 15-2.

Current Status

The use of group treatment in occupational therapy is often mistaken as primarily restricted to practice in mental health or to the treatment of children or the elderly. Duncombe and Howe (1985) established that "60% of occupational therapists in all areas of practice lead groups in treatment" (p. 163); 10 years later they found a slight decrease to 52% (Duncombe & Howe, 1995). This negligible difference, they surmised, is due to a decrease in the number of occupational therapists working in large medical and psychiatric hospitals. Predictably, a shift toward community- and school-based practice and cost-containment measures, including managed care, will increase the use of group treatment in the near future. The role of group leader as educator and consultant should grow as occupational therapists form partnerships with consumers in peer support groups and family care, as well as with other care extenders and health professionals in group practice plans.

Reports also specifically document the value of group occupational therapy for patients with physical problems, such as Parkinson disease (Gauthier, Dalziel, & Gauthier, 1987), head injuries (Lundgren & Persechino, 1986), and rheumatoid arthritis (Van Deusen & Harlowe, 1987). Individual treatment is fast becoming viewed as a luxury as practitioners move toward interdisciplinary group treatment models that are more cost-efficient and capitalize on the therapeutic properties of groups (Marmer, 1995; Morris, Andreassi, & Lichtenberg, 1994). Projects like Trahey's (1991) study of services to individuals who underwent a total hip replacement demonstrate not only the therapeutic value but also the cost effectiveness of occupational therapy group treatment compared to individual treatment as the primary format for care in rehabilitation settings.

TABLE 15-2. **ERAS OF GROUP WORK IN OCCUPATIONAL THERAPY**[a]

Era	Focus of Group Involvement
Project (1922–1936)	Project completion
Socialization (1937–1953)	Social activity
Group dynamics–process (1954–1961)	Interpersonal dynamics
Ego building–psychodynamic (1962–1961)	Ego reconstitution
Adaptation (1970–1990s)	Social adaptation
Wellness (1990s–present)	Engagement in occupations

[a]Historical analysis from Howe and Schwartzberg (2001).

DEFINITIONS AND TYPES OF OCCUPATIONAL THERAPY GROUPS

Duncombe and Howe (1985) identified 10 types of groups commonly used in occupational therapy: exercise, cooking, tasks, activities of daily living, arts and crafts, self-expression, feelings-oriented discussion, reality-oriented discussion, sensorimotor or sensory integration group, and educational. Occupational therapy groups remain for the most part activity groups that are small sized (<10 members, usually about 6) and popularly focus on therapeutic goals such as task skills,

TABLE 15–3. **OCCUPATIONAL THERAPY GROUP VARIABLES**

Setting
Therapeutic factors
Goals: short term and long term
Duration of group
Composition of group
Time frame and format
Population
Group size
Frame of reference
Open versus time limited, closed membership
Member selection and preparation
Contraindications

communication and socialization skills, and physical abilities (Duncombe & Howe, 1995).

At least 12 group variables describe an occupational therapy group (Table 15-3). Each variable needs to be considered in the formation and design of a therapeutic group. One of the most important of these variables, the group setting (inpatient or outpatient) has an impact on the group goals and techniques used. The relationship between group orientation or format and therapeutic focus is given in Table 15-4.

MODELS IN OCCUPATIONAL THERAPY: ROLES OF LEADER, GROUP MEMBER, AND ACTIVITY

Several different group approaches are used in occupational therapy and to varying degrees; each has its own articulated theoretical perspective. Selected occupational therapy group approaches are identified in Table 15-5. The roles of the leader, group member, and activity vary among the models. Differences in the models deserve attention when applied to practice. The reader is referred to the original works for details about each approach.

The functional group model (Howe & Schwartzberg, 1986, 1988, 1995, 2001; Kielhofner, 1992) is considered a generic group model in occupational therapy. It incorporates four key concepts: purposeful activity, self-initiated action, spontaneous action, and group-centered action. Howe and Schwartzberg (1988) explained how to enhance group process through group structure:

> *To accomplish this result within the functional group model, the following factors should be considered in planning, running, and reviewing the group: (1) maximum involvement through group-centered action, (2) a maximum sense of individual and group identity, (3) a "flow" experience, (4) spontaneous involvement of members, and (5) member support and feedback. These five major categories should be reviewed individually in terms of the parameters to be considered by the leader or co-leaders. It is suggested that the Group Session Plan Protocol be used to organize and formulate the clinical reasoning process for group interventions.* (p. 3)

Leader techniques and procedures for conducting a group are described later in this chapter.

COMPARISON TO GROUP FORMATS OF OTHER PROFESSIONS

As shown in Table 15-1, the occupational therapy group format is significantly different from verbal psychotherapy groups conducted by other professionals, such as psychiatrists, psychologists, nurses, and social workers. In verbal group psychotherapy, for example, the emphasis is often on talking, insight, and understanding. In a psychodynamic or interpersonal model of group treatment, the **there-and-then experience,** or past experience, which is often familial, is used as a means to understand present-day conflicts. The **here-and-now**

TABLE 15–4. **OCCUPATIONAL THERAPY GROUP SETTINGS, GOALS, AND TECHNIQUES**

	Goals and Techniques	
Group Orientation or Format[a]	**Inpatient**	**Outpatient**
Interpersonal and dynamic	Support, containment	Social change, insight
Behavioral and educational	New skills and attitudes, structure	Here-and-now experiences
Support	Acceptance	Legitimization, information, decreased isolation
Maintenance and rehabilitation	Safety, reevaluation, discharge planning	Adaptation, resources, minimize stress

[a]Categories adapted from Vinogradov and Yalom's (1989) classification of outpatient groups.

TABLE 15-5. **SELECTED OCCUPATIONAL THERAPY GROUP APPROACHES AND THEORETICAL CONSIDERATIONS**

Group Approach	References
Task-oriented group	Fidler (1969)
Functional group model	Howe and Schwartzberg (1986, 1995, 2001)
Directive group therapy	Kaplan (1988)
Activity group	Borg and Bruce (1991), Mosey (1973a, 1973b)
Developmental group	Mosey (1970)
Psychoeducational group	Lillie and Armstrong (1982)
Structured five-stage integrative group therapy	Ross (1991)
Peer support group	Schwartzberg (1994, 1999), Lowenstein and Schwartzberg (1999)
Theoretical Considerations	
Theoretical base	
Function–dysfunction continuum	
Behaviors indicating function or dysfunction	
Postulates of change	

experience, or immediate experience, in the group is examined as a projection of the patient's past and provides members with an opportunity to test new and more adaptive interpersonal styles. These groups require members to have a fair degree of abstract capability and self-control over their behavior.

In contrast, as a general rule, occupational therapy groups focus as much as possible on shared doing and adjusted experience within the here-and-now experience. Groups are structured and graded so that members with modest to more advanced social and cognitive skills may participate. Mosey's (1973a) classification of group interaction skills is often used to designate the type and level of interaction required in an activity group. These levels are parallel group, project group, egocentric-cooperative group, cooperative group, and mature group. They range from the parallel level, with maximal leader support and structure and little expectation for interaction around a task, to the mature level, with minimal leader intervention with a high degree of interaction required for task completion and social-emotional satisfaction.

A nonprogressing but multilevel scheme is the hierarchical task analysis developed by Allen (1985). This task analysis is used to group patients according to their cognitive capabilities. Group tasks of varying complexity are chosen accordingly.

GROUP PROCESS AND SMALL TASK GROUPS

The practice of group work in occupational therapy involves observation and interaction as well as the procedures of assessment, designing, planning, evaluating, analyzing, responding, and documenting. Authentic use of group process in occupational therapy is an interactive occupation-based perspective. In reasoning and practice, the practitioner must always consider the group dynamics relationships among person, occupation, and environment. The following discussion is an examination of intervention with small groups rather than with large institutional groups, in which other techniques are applied.

Observation

The leader looks for information about the group's process in several areas. All aspects of the group are considered dynamic and, therefore, are constantly changing, which makes observation difficult and challenging.

Group as System: Group Process, Phase, and Dynamics

Groups progress through stages of development when therapeutic conditions have been achieved, such as clear, mutual goals and trust. **Group phases,** indicating the stages of group development in terms of leader, group member, and activity roles, are identified in Table 15-6. When observing the group's development, leaders look at the group's phase in relation to decision-making patterns; membership and leadership roles; and the level and type of participation patterns, such as who initiates communication, who talks to whom, and the tone of voice members and leaders use.

Individual Member in System

In addition to the group as a whole, the leader observes the group member in relation to other members, the leader, and

TABLE 15-6. **SAMPLE ROLES AND PHASES OF GROUP DEVELOPMENT**

Roles	Formation	Development	Termination
Leader	Set climate, provide structure, offer support	Grade actions, facilitate	Aid separation, reinforce gains
Member	Identify purpose	Collaborate, initiate	Evaluate, express reactions
Activity	Form goals, establish trust	Purposeful action	Review

the group task. These observations of group dynamics may be informal or structured around a task designed to demonstrate certain skills and behaviors such as cooperativeness, mobility, attention span, memory, concentration, and assertiveness. The observation task may also include functional activities, such as collaborative work, cooking, or other activities of daily living. Depending on the setting and length of treatment, and when possible, the therapist may also conduct pregroup interviews as a means to observe, establish rapport, and gain information about a potential group member.

Leader and Co-Leader Self-Awareness

An equally important area of observation is the leader's own behavior and internal reactions. It is good practice for group leaders to write group process notes after each group meeting. In these notes, practitioners describe their personal reactions, thoughts, and the critical events in the group. It is beneficial to share observations of the group and of each other with a co-leader. These observations are helpful in clinical supervision and in analysis of countertransference. The leaders' insights into their own family patterns and dynamics, including parental or sibling relationships, are a rich source of information for the therapist. Such exploration can inform therapists about areas of their own misperceptions as well as maladaptive responses of group members.

Group, Member, and Leader Observations

The observation of group process is conducted at the following levels: the group, the individual members in relation to the group and subgroups, the individual members and the group in relation to the leader or co-leaders, and all in relation to a task or activity. In addition, for the purposes of feedback, the practitioner may look for opportunities to observe the group member in functional contexts outside the group, such as in the community, school, work, and family environments.

Interaction: Establishing a Therapeutic Alliance Through Group Process

Therapeutic factors unique to occupational therapy groups have been isolated in preliminary studies. They include creativity and self-esteem, relaxation and diversion, enjoyment, increased skills, and concentration (Finn, 1989; Webster, 1988; Webster & Schwartzberg, 1992). Given the extensive research on therapeutic factors in verbal psychotherapy groups, the factors found in common with occupational therapy groups deserve emphasis. The therapeutic factors identified by Yalom (1985) found in both occupational therapy and psychotherapy groups are group cohesiveness, interpersonal learning/output, and instillation of hope (Falk-Kessler, Momich, & Perel, 1991; Finn, 1989; Howe & Schwartzberg, 1986; Webster & Schwartzberg, 1992). These factors are focal points for selecting leadership strategies that promote therapeutic alliances through the group process.

Leader to Members

An important aspect of group therapy practice, as well as individual therapy practice, is the therapist's use of self in the group. Leaders serve particular roles and use techniques, which they are continually attempting to perfect to achieve therapeutic goals. The primary roles of the leader include observer, group designer, role model, and climate setter (supporting and substituting actions as needed in the group). A skilled leader always weighs individual and group needs and chooses the strategies and techniques he or she will use by considering past responses and immediate as well as long-term therapeutic goals (Fig. 15-2).

The leadership strategies commonly used include genuineness and empathy, modeling behavior, reality testing, communicating, and planning the group activity through activity analysis and adaptation (Howe & Schwartzberg, 1986, 1995). Particular use of these strategies and related techniques depends on the group's goals and conceptual framework, the group's phase of development, and the practitioner's relationship with the group members.

Group Members to Group Members

The practitioner and members of a group have work to accomplish goals in a group. Nevertheless, some problems commonly surface in group work, including difficulty establishing trust with the leader and other group members, dependency on the leader, difficulty setting goals, misdirected anger, competition among group members, subgrouping, withdrawal from the group or task, lack of skill, absenteeism, members leaving the group meeting and premature termination from the group, external

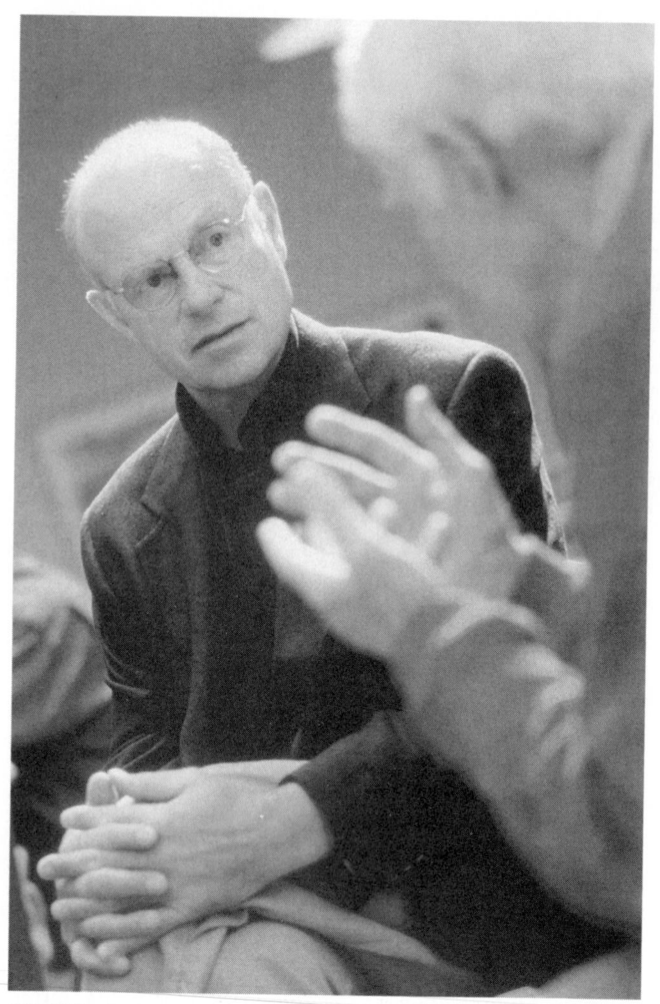

FIGURE 15–2. A peer leader listens carefully to a group member. (Photo courtesy of Kindra Clinetf.)

conflicts and pressure (e.g., from family), and interference from outside the group (e.g., interruptions from other services, such as the laboratory). When one of these problems arises, it must be examined separately and interpreted differently, depending on the practitioner's theoretical framework.

Co-Leaders

In working together, co-leaders assist in the physical and emotional management of the group. This is particularly important when the group is large or when members require considerable individual attention because of cognitive, physical, or social-emotional limitations. As in any professional interaction, ethical dilemmas are bound to arise. In group interventions, such concerns typically involve issues related to confidentiality and cost-benefit issues. Co-leaders can assist each other in sorting out an appropriate course of action. In addition, co-leaders are model participants in the group, demonstrating healthy interaction and ways of resolving conflict with others.

It is useful to have supervision with both leaders present. These sessions help the leaders work out differences of opinion, conflicts, and rivalry that inevitably exist when co-leading a group. When possible, a more experienced therapist co-leads with a beginning practitioner. The experienced practitioner serves as a model and can provide supervision. Often the co-leaders' relationship draws attention from the group. For example, members may be competitive with a novice therapist in fear of losing the more senior leader's attention. Through an accepting relationship with both leaders members can alter their perceptions. They may react differently when expected to share in the future. As model participants in groups, the co-leaders provide members an opportunity to observe a working, productive, teaching–learning relationship.

Reasoning Processes

Group leadership in occupational therapy requires time in designing the overall group plan and individual session plans. The leader also evaluates individual sessions and member progress and the overall group progress. In community settings in which the practitioner is working with a well or natural group, an assessment of population-based needs and resources is conducted. Protocols for assessing community resources, program development, design, and evaluation require strategies focused on promoting services relevant to the group as a whole. The latter emphasis is concerned with a population of people rather than with an individual member, as in the following discussion.

Assessing Individual Members and the Group

Assessment is an ongoing process that usually begins with meeting the group member before the first session. The practitioner may have a formal referral or may see a group member as part of a larger program. Groups may also be used for the sole purpose of evaluation. This is common in inpatient settings, in which patients are discharged rapidly and the main goal of hospitalization is evaluation and discharge planning.

It is through interactive reasoning that the leader comes to know members' perceived experience of their disabilities (Fleming, 1991) and to understand how they affect their functioning. Interactive reasoning enables the therapist to be truly empathic and for trust to develop within the group. In coming to know the members, the leader conveys and models warmth, support, and acceptance. In the group setting, interactive reasoning occurs not only between the practitioner and the client but also among other group members and the group as a whole. The degree to which this is successful influences the proportion to which therapeutic factors of cohesiveness, interpersonal learning, and instillation of hope are achieved.

In some settings, the registered occupational therapist evaluates patients and develops a plan, and the certified occupational therapy assistant actually conducts the group.

The registered therapist provides supervision as well. Service delivery arrangements and use of staff resources vary from setting to setting.

Designing

The group's design has several components. The design is usually written in the form a group protocol that includes group and, if possible, individual members' short- and long-term goals; selection criteria for membership; group size and composition; group methods, techniques, and activity modalities; time and location of the group meeting and group leaders' names; and referral procedures. Protocols aid therapists in communicating with other professionals and prospective group members.

Planning and Evaluating

Evaluation is continuous throughout the group's existence and, when possible, involves the group members. After evaluating each session, the leaders create detailed individual group session plans with categories similar to the overall, more generalized plan. When there is a major shift in client population, the leader may also modify the general group plan. In time-limited groups (MacKenzie, 1995) sessions are highly focused, and circumscribed goals are made explicit to members. The therapist must be highly active in promoting a therapeutic climate conductive to goal achievement.

Analyzing and Responding

Each group situation is analyzed separately and continuously if the group is ongoing. To respond, the therapist uses the group's history as well as individual members' histories of strategies that were successful or unsuccessful. In an open group with changing membership, the leader's experience with similar situations becomes particularly useful. In a closed or time-limited group, the membership remains consistent from session to session. In these cases, the therapist can use prior experience for analyzing and responding, and the group can become its own control.

FOCUS ON THERAPEUTIC FACTORS

To illustrate the reasoning involved in analyzing and responding to group process, the three therapeutic factors—group cohesiveness, interpersonal learning, and instillation of hope—will be used as a focus for three case situations, presented in What's a Practitioner to Do? boxes. Although presented separately here, a leadership strategy may promote more than one factor and outcome. The strategies detailed (Andrews, 1995; Howe & Schwartzberg, 1995; Mattingly & Fleming, 1994) are those commonly applicable to occupational therapy, however, it is not an exhaustive list.

- *Group cohesiveness:* "Cohesiveness refers to the attraction that members have for their group and for the other members. The members of a cohesive group are accepting of one another, supportive, and inclined to form meaningful relationships in the group. Cohesiveness seems to be a significant factor in successful group therapy outcome" (Yalom, 1985, p. 69).
- *Interpersonal learning—output:* "Interpersonal learning is the group therapy equivalent of such individual therapy factors as self-understanding or insight, working through the transference, and the corrective emotional experience. Interpersonal learning involves the identification, the elucidation, and the modification of maladaptive interpersonal relationships. . . . Three basic assumptions upon it rests: 1. interpersonal theory, 2. the group as a social microcosm, and 3. the here-and-now" (Yalom, 1983, p. 45). This therapeutic factor involves improving skills for getting along with others. (Yalom, 1985).
- *Instillation of hope*: "Group members are at different points along a collapse/coping continuum and can gain hope from observing others, especially others with similar problems, who have profited from therapy" (Yalom, 1983, p. 41).

DOCUMENTING

Clinicians must consult their individual facilities, third-party payers, federal privacy laws, and state requirements for specific information concerning appropriate documentation and billing for group evaluation and treatment. Practitioners usually document each member's progress separately after group sessions as well as ideally keep records of the group's progress as a whole for the purposes of analysis and supervision. As mentioned earlier, group protocols, session plans, and process notes are other forms of documentation commonly used in group practice.

RESEARCH

Problems and Strengths

Much remains to be understand about the use of group process in occupational therapy and about the best methods for teaching students and therapists how to use this important tool. A strength is the apparent value of the group to its members and to health-care delivery as a cost-effective treatment.

The practice of documenting group process and content is diminishing as therapists are under increasing pressures to be efficient and cost effective. In fact, Duncombe and Howe (1995) found that 55% of 75 therapists in their study reported no difference in the rate charged for individual versus group treatment. Furthermore, they reported that 94% of the 219 respondents kept individual documentation rather than for the group as a whole or both. There is a danger that economic incentives will undermine the relationship between the individual and the group as a whole, exactly the inherent therapeutic value of group treatment.

Current Research

Studies strongly suggest differences in outcomes when activity groups are compared with psychotherapy groups (DeCarlo & Mann, 1985; Eklund, 1999; Klyczek & Mann, 1986; McDermott, 1988; Mumford, 1974; Schwartzberg, Howe, & McDermott; 1982). Eklund (1999) compared psychiatric outpatients receiving group-based occupational therapy with a matched group of patients receiving the usual treatment of verbal therapy. Supporting an occupation-based approach, her results indicated that the occupational therapy group was helpful for some psychiatric patients on a variety of outcome variables relating to occupational performance, global mental health, and psychiatric symptoms.

In addition, there are studies that provide evidence to the effectiveness of the functional group model—an interactive occupational model of group work—as an intervention format with the well elderly (Clark et al., 1997; Jackson, Carlson, Mandel, Zemke, & Clark, 1998; Mandel, Jackson, Zemke, Nelson, & Clark, 1999) and other populations that is also cost-efficient (Howe & Schwartzberg, 2001). The findings of the well-elderly studies are particularly significant given the strong evidence, from a long-term large population-based study, that social engagement and interaction are highly related to longevity (Glass, Mendes de Leon, Marottoli, & Berkman, 1999).

WHAT'S A PRACTITIONER TO DO? 15-1
Group Cohesiveness

Mrs. Clark was looking forward to a vacation in Florida, although somewhat apprehensive about her husband's upcoming retirement. He had worked hard as a loyal employee of a men's clothing store; however, he had no other interests or involvement in his home. The latter was "wife business." The store was about to go into bankruptcy and now, at age 68, Mr. Clark was forced to retire. Pleased with an opportunity to go to her niece's wedding, Mrs. Clark put on her best new high-heeled shoes for an evening of dancing. Hours later, she was rushed to a local emergency room and 4 days later, a rehabilitation hospital. Mrs. Clark slipped while dancing and broke her hip and several bones in the wrist of her dominant hand. The recovery seemed to go well until she got home. Mr. Clark was of no help and was in an agitated depression since his retirement. Once the visiting nurses association stopped home services, Mrs. Clark went for outpatient occupational therapy at the rehabilitation center. She was feeling angry, unsupported, and frustrated with her limited mobility and loss of homemaker roles.

In attending one of the occupational therapy groups for patients with hip replacements, Mrs. Clark found relief. Many of the other patients were older than Mrs. Clark, and she had an opportunity to help them and at the same time be nurtured. Many stories were told about husbands retiring and acting "helpless," about children not visiting, and the like.

LEADERSHIP STRATEGIES

- Design activities that have "maximal involvement of members through group-centered action" (Howe & Schwartzberg, 1995).
- Maintain a "maximal sense of individual and group identity" (Howe & Schwartzberg, 1995).
- Provide and invite member support.
- Demonstrate genuineness and empathy.
- Self-disclose one's own feelings and reactions in an authentic and prudent fashion.
- Be active in listening and responding.
- Consider judiciously "doing for patients" (Mattingly & Fleming, 1994).
- Look for ways to encourage joint problem solving.
- Demonstrate acceptance and affirmation.
- Contemplate reframing problems in a more positive manner (Andrews, 1995).

QUESTIONS AND EXERCISES

From the perspective of group cohesiveness, which calls attention to member support, acceptance, and individual identity, be alert to the following questions:

1. How can the leader structure range-of-motion and functional activities to promote maximal sharing and joint problem solving?
2. What role can the leader play in helping the members reframe their problems in a more positive way?

WHAT'S A PRACTITIONER TO DO? 15-2
Interpersonal Learning—Output

A support group for people who have experienced head injury is assembling for its usual weekly meeting. The group is now in its second year of meeting at the founding member's home (Facilitator A). An occupational therapist is present as co-facilitator (Facilitator B).

FACILITATOR B: I'd like to have the older members introduce themselves and tell their stories and have other people have a chance to tell their stories. [This is a group ritual for starting meetings.]
MEMBER A: I'm not going first.
FACILITATOR A: Should we get labels?
FACILITATOR B: Yes, that helps.
FACILITATOR A: I will go and get labels for everybody because that helps a lot.
MEMBER A: I really don't like that.
FACILITATOR B: Why's that?
MEMBER A: Because it really bothers me.
FACILITATOR B: What bothers you?
MEMBER A: Labels.
FACILITATOR B: You mean name tags? Why?
MEMBER B: Because it's distracting?
MEMBER A: Because it's insulting.
MEMBER B: Why?
MEMBER C: For brain-injured people?
MEMBER D: For anyone.
MEMBER C: My ability before my brain injury was to remember everything about a person. Now I forget their names. But I remember everything about them. I guess . . .
MEMBER B: Member A was saying that she objected, Facilitator A, to name tags.
FACILITATOR A: But why?
FACILITATOR B: I think that we just starting out talking . . .
MEMBER A: That was a very noncompassionate thing for me to say, because I strengthen my memory by not having things like name tags so I can really work on remembering names. I have to be compassionate that there are people who have strength in other things that I have more trouble with, and that name tags are necessary.
MEMBER D: Since we're not together every day. If we were, we might remember.
MEMBER B: So Member A said she didn't want to be the first one to tell her story.
FACILITATOR B: Facilitator A?
FACILITATOR A: I had a car accident four and a half years ago . . .

LEADERSHIP STRATEGIES

- Invite spontaneous involvement.
- Invite member feedback.
- Model desired behaviors.
- Clarify, explain, understand, and interpret what is happening in the group as a framework for change.
- Reality test.
- Encourage feedback and consensual validation.
- Be concrete and bridge group experiences to situations outside of the group.
- Invite gentle confrontation.
- Look for ways to create choices (Mattingly & Fleming, 1994).
- Encourage members to compare experiences and impressions.
- Encourage members to identify problems in group that are familiar and similar to difficulties in outside functioning.

QUESTIONS AND EXERCISES

From the perspective of interpersonal learning, which calls attention to understanding and interpreting what is happening in the group, concreteness, and comparing experiences, be mindful of the following questions:

1. In what ways can the facilitator use the group process so that Member A feels accepted and understood rather than encouraged to further castigate herself for lacking compassion and, at the same time, get feedback from other members about their impressions?
2. How might the facilitator create new choices by relating this exchange to outside experiences? Typically, individuals with a head injury may be unaware of or attempt to conceal problems in functioning to avoid being viewed as disabled and in doing so may sabotage assistance offered.

In contrast, although differences have been noted (Finn, 1989; Webster, 1988), similarities have also been found between members' perceptions of the therapeutic value of occupational therapy groups and the perspectives of members of psychotherapy groups (Eklund, 1997; Falk-Kessler, Momich, & Perel, 1991; Webster & Schwartzberg, 1992). In addition, there appear to exist unique roles and helping factors when peer-led groups are compared with professional-led groups in occupational therapy (Sacenti, 1988; Schwartzberg, 1994). Furthermore, Howe and

WHAT'S A PRACTITIONER TO DO? 15-3
Installation of Hope

Maria, a teen mother, entered the hospital after slashing her wrists and threatening to throw her baby out the window. John, a teenaged young man, entered the hospital after repeated attempts to beat his father. He was smoking pot at school, often truant, and when at home he spent most of his days locked in his room not eating or sleeping. Terry, an anorexic woman, entered the hospital after she returned from a college semester abroad. Her parents found that she had not eaten in a week. Receiving a B-average grade report apparently precipitated the event.

The group was making holiday greeting cards using stencils, stamps, silk screens, and a word processor. Options ranged from placing stickers on preworded cards to creating designs for silk screening on the computer. While doing the activity, members talked about their family disappointments, hopes, accomplishments, and losses of confidence. The therapist structured the activity so that everyone succeeded in making an attractive product.

LEADERSHIP STRATEGIES

- Design group so that there is a "flow experience" (Howe & Schwartzberg, 1995).
- Structure success into activities and process.
- Encourage exchange of "personal stories" (Mattingly & Fleming, 1994).
- Comment on member successes as they happen (Andrews, 1995).
- Highlight positive themes in the group (Andrews, 1995).

QUESTIONS AND EXERCISES

From the perspective of instillation of hope, which calls attention to structuring success experiences, exchange of personal stories, and supporting positive themes in the group, be alert to the following questions:

1. How can the activity be graded from simple to fairly complex so that members' decrease in perceptual, cognitive, and social functioning is not apparent and the developmental needs of adolescents and the 3- to 5-day hospital length of stay is taken into consideration?
2. It is recognized that parallel task groups intrinsically create conditions that promote interaction between patients (Schwartzberg, Howe, & McDermott, 1982). How can the leader gently invite members to share feelings of hope, being sensitive to members' feelings of disappointment, and at the same time not contaminate the natural flow of communication?

RESEARCH NOTE 15–1

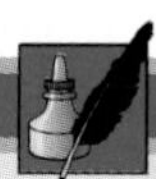

Group Process

KENNETH J. OTTENBACHER

Clinical research is a collaborative and communal process. When describing the communal nature of research, Thomas (1974) observed that research

> *sometimes looks like a lonely activity, but it is as much the opposite of lonely as human behavior can be. There is nothing so social, so communal, so interdependent. An active field of science is like an immense intellectual anthill; the individual almost vanishes into the mass of minds tumbling over each other, carrying information from place to place, passing it around at the speed of light. (p. 101)*

The cooperative and communal nature of occupational therapy research is reflected in the use of therapeutic groups. An example of the effectiveness of therapeutic groups in occupational therapy practice was reported by Scott (1999). Occupational therapy students led community-based wellness groups involving older adults, homeless persons, women in a shelter, and people with mental illness. The groups established wellness awareness learning contracts and individual wellness and health promotion goals. After 4–6 weeks of community-based group intervention, the individual goals were objectively examined using the method of goal attainment scaling. Improvements were noted in individual wellness and health promotion goals for both the students and the community-based clients.

Scott, A. H. (1999). Wellness works: Community service health promotion groups led by occupational therapy students. *American Journal of Occupational Therapy, 53*, 566–574.

Thomas, L. (1974). *The lives of a cell. Notes of a biology watcher*. New York: Viking.

Schwartzberg (1995) "demonstrate that group format has an effect on the quality and quantity of interaction, meaning assigned to the group action, and members' functional status" (p. 221).

Future research in all settings in which occupational therapists use group treatment should address both outcomes related to function and client perceptions of group treatment. Regardless of group format, it would be of interest to know, for example, if patient perceptions of therapeutic factors are related to functional outcomes, or vice versa. Further studies in activity group analysis and the meaning of restricted variables would also support the endeavor to explain the therapeutic use of group process in occupational therapy (Adelstein & Nelson, 1985; Henry, Nelson, & Duncombe, 1984; Kremer, Nelson, & Duncombe, 1984; Nelson, Peterson, Smith, Boughton, & Whalen, 1988; Steffan & Nelson, 1987; Steffan, 1990). Finally, in this era of managed and rationed care it would be of interest to study (1) individual and group treatment outcomes in relation to amount of treatment time required and staff resources; (2) treatment time required with various occupational therapy group modalities and strategies in relationship to diagnosis, functional problems, resources, and severity of illness; and (3) therapeutic factors in occupational therapy groups compared to verbally oriented, interdisciplinary, and peer formats.

CONCLUSION

The past and present trends in group process as a tool of occupational therapy were introduced. Models of group treatment in occupational therapy were described, and the procedural aspects of this practice highlighted. Some recent research on the use of group treatment was summarized; and, as examples, a few principles in need of verification were identified.

References

Adelstein, L. A., & Nelson, D. L. (1985). Effects of sharing versus nonsharing on affective meaning in collage activities. *Occupational Therapy in Mental Health: A Journal of Psychosocial Practice and Research, 5*(2), 29–45.

Allen, C. K. (1985). *Occupational therapy for psychiatric diseases: Measurement and management of cognitive disabilities*. Boston: Little, Brown.

Andrews, H. B. (1995). *Group design and leadership: Strategies for creating successful common theme groups*. Boston: Allyn & Bacon.

Borg, B., & Bruce, M. A. (1991). *The group system: The therapeutic activity group in occupational therapy*. Thorofare, NJ: Slack.

Bronfenbrenner, U. (1979). *The ecology of human development: Experiments by nature and design*. Cambridge, MA: Harvard University Press.

Clark, F., Azen, S. P., Zemke, R., Jackson, J., Carlson, M., Mandel, D., Hay, J., Josephson, K., Cherry, B., Hessel, C., Palmer, J., & Lipson, L. (1997). Occupational therapy for independent-living older adults: A randomized controlled trial. *Journal of the American Medical Association, 278*, 1321–1326.

DeCarlo, J. J., & Mann, W. C. (1985). The effectiveness of verbal versus activity groups in improving self-perceptions of interpersonal communication skills. *American Journal of Occupational Therapy, 39*(1), 20–27.

Duncombe, L. W., & Howe, M. C. (1985). Group work in occupational therapy: A survey of practice. *American Journal of Occupational Therapy, 39*(3), 163–170.

Duncombe, L. W., & Howe, M. C. (1995). Group treatment: Goals, tasks, and economic implications. *American Journal of Occupational Therapy, 49*(3), 199–205.

Dunn, W., Brown, C., & McGuigan, A. (1994). The ecology of human performance: A framework for considering the effect of context. *American Journal of Occupational Therapy, 48*(7), 595–607.

Eklund, M. (1997). Therapeutic factors in occupational group therapy identified by patients discharged from a psychiatric day centre and their significant others. *Occupational Therapy International, 4*(3), 198–212.

Eklund, M. (1999). Outcome of occupational therapy in a psychiatric day care unit for long-term mentally ill patients. *Occupational Therapy in Mental Health, 14*(4), 21–45.

Falk-Kessler, J., Momich, C., & Perel, S. (1991). Therapeutic factors in occupational therapy groups. *American Journal of Occupational Therapy, 45*(1), 59–66.

Fidler, G. S. (1969). The task-oriented group as a context for treatment. *American Journal of Occupational Therapy, 23*(1), 43–48.

Finn, M. (1989). *Patients' perceptions of occupational therapy groups: Interview generated factors*. Unpublished master's thesis, Tufts University, Boston School of Occupational Therapy, Medford, MA.

Fleming, M. H. (1991). The therapist with the three-track mind. *American Journal of Occupational Therapy, 45*(11), 1007–1014.

Gauthier, L., Dalziel, S., & Gauthier, S. (1987). The benefits of group occupational therapy for patients with Parkinson's disease. *American Journal of Occupational Therapy, 41*(6), 360–365.

Glass, T. A., Mendes de Leon, C., Marottoli, R. A. & Berkman, L. F. (1999). Population based study of social and productive activities as predictors of survival among elderly Americans. *British Medical Journal, 319*, 478–483.

Henry, A. D., Nelson, D. L., & Duncombe, L. W. (1984). Choice making in group and individual activity. *American Journal of Occupational Therapy, 38*(4), 245–251.

Howe, M. C., & Briggs, A. K. (1982). Ecological systems model for occupational therapy. *American Journal of Occupational Therapy, 36*(5), 322–327.

Howe, M. C., & Schwartzberg, S. L. (1986). *A functional approach to group work in occupational therapy*. Philadelphia: Lippincott.

Howe, M. C., & Schwartzberg, S. L. (1988). Structure and process in designing a functional group. *Occupational Therapy in Mental Health: A Journal of Psychosocial Practice and Research, 8*(3), 1–8.

Howe, M. C., & Schwartzberg, S. L. (1995). *A functional approach to group work in occupational therapy* (2nd ed.). Philadelphia: Lippincott.

Howe, M. C., & Schwartzberg, S. L. (2001). *A functional approach to group work in occupational therapy* (3rd ed.). Philadelphia: Lippincott, Williams & Wilkins.

Jackson, J., Carlson, M., Mandel, D., Zemke, R., & Clark, F. (1998). Occupation in lifestyle redesign: The well elderly study occupational therapy program. *American Journal of Occupational Therapy, 52*(5), 326–336.

Kaplan, K. L. (1988). *Directive group therapy: Innovative mental health treatment*. Thorofare, NJ: Slack.

Kielhofner, G. (1992). *Conceptual foundations in occupational therapy*. Philadelphia: Davis.

Klyczek, J. P., & Mann, W. C. (1986). Therapeutic modality comparisons in day treatment. *American Journal of Occupational Therapy, 40*(9), 606–611.

Kremer, E. R. H., Nelson, D. L., & Duncombe, L. W. (1984). Effects of selected activities on affective meaning in psychiatric patients. *American Journal of Occupational Therapy, 38*(8), 522–528.

Lillie, M., & Armstrong, H. (1982). Contributions to the development of psychoeducational approaches to mental health service. *American Journal of Occupational Therapy, 36*(7), 438–443.

Lowenstein, A., & Schwartzberg, S. L. (1999). A support group for head injured individuals: Stories from the peer leader and facilitator. In S. Ryan and E. McKay (Eds.). *Thinking and reasoning in therapy: Narratives from practice* (pp. 94–106). Cheltenham, UK: Thornes.

Lundgren, C. C., & Persechino, E. L. (1986). Cognitive group: A treatment program for head injured adults. *American Journal of Occupational Therapy, 40*(6), 397–401.

MacKenzie, K. R. (1995). Rationale for group psychotherapy in managed care. In K. R. MacKenzie (Ed.). *Effective use of group therapy in managed care* (pp. 1–25). Washington, DC: American Psychiatric Press.

Mandel, D. R., Jackson, J. M., Zemke, R., Nelson, L., & Clark, F. A. (1999). *Lifestyle redesign: Implementing the well elderly program*. Bethesda, MD: American Occupational Therapy Association.

Marmer, L. (1995, October 2). Group treatment works well in stroke recovery. *Advance for Occupational Therapists,* 13.

Mattingly, C., & Fleming, M. H. (1994). Interactive reasoning Collaborating with the person. In C. Mattingly & M. H. Fleming (Eds.). *Clinical reasoning: Forms of inquiry in a therapeutic practice* (pp. 178–196). Philadelphia: F. A. Davis.

McDermott, A. A. (1988). The effect of three group formats on group interaction patterns. *Occupational Therapy in Mental Health: A Journal of Psychosocial Practice and Research, 8*(3), 69–89.

Morris, P. A., Andreassi, E., & Lichtenberg, P. (1994, August 25). Preparing for community living. *OT Week,* 20–21.

Mosey, A. C. (1970). The concept and use of developmental groups. *American Journal of Occupational Therapy, 24*(4), 272–275.

Mosey, A. C. (1973a). *Activities therapy*. New York: Raven.

Mosey, A. C. (1973b). Meeting health needs. *American Journal of Occupational Therapy, 27*(1), 14–17.

Mumford, M. S. (1974). A comparison of interpersonal skills in verbal and activity groups. *American Journal of Occupational Therapy, 28*(5), 281–283.

Nelson, D. L., Peterson, C., Smith, D. A., Boughton, J. A., & Whalen, G. M. (1988). Effects of project versus parallel groups on social interaction and affective responses in senior citizens. *American Journal of Occupational Therapy, 42*(1), 23–29.

Ross, M. (1991). *Integrative group therapy: The structured five-stage approach* (2nd ed.). Thorofare, NJ: Slack.

Sacenti, L. (1988). *Mastery and levels of participation in members of two groups for chronic pain: Self-help and professionally led*. Unpublished master's thesis, Tufts University, Boston School of Occupational Therapy, Medford, MA.

Schwartzberg, S. L. (1994). Helping factors in a peer-developed support group for persons with head injury. Part 1: Participant observer perspective. *American Journal of Occupational Therapy, 48*(4), 297–304.

Schwartzberg, S. L. (1999). The use of groups in the rehabilitation of persons with head injury: Reasoning skills employed by the group facilitator. In C. Unsworth (Ed.). *Cognitive and perceptual dysfunction: A clinical reasoning approach to evaluation and intervention* (pp. 455–471). Philadelphia: F. A. Davis.

Schwartzberg, S. L., Howe, M. C., & McDermott, A. (1982). A comparison of three treatment group formats for facilitating social interaction. *Occupational Therapy in Mental Health: A Journal of Psychosocial Practice and Research, 2*(4), 1–16.

Steffan, J. A. (1990). Productive occupation in small task groups of adults: Synthesis and annotations of the social psychology literature. In A. C. Bundy, N. D. Prendergast, J. A. Steffan, & D. Thorn (Eds.). *Review of selected literature on occupation and health* (pp. 175–281). Rockville, MD: American Occupational Therapy Association.

Steffan, J. A., & Nelson, D. L. (1987). The effects of tool scarcity on group climate and affective meaning within the context of a stenciling activity. *American Journal of Occupational Therapy, 41*(7), 449–453.

Trahey, P. J. (1991). A comparison of the cost-effectiveness of two types of occupational therapy services. *American Journal of Occupational Therapy, 45*(5), 397–400.

Van Deusen, J., & Harlowe, D. (1987). The efficacy of the ROM dance program for adults with rheumatoid arthritis. *American Journal of Occupational Therapy, 41*(2), 90–95.

Vinogradov, S., & Yalom, I. D. (1989). *A concise guide to group psychotherapy*. Washington, DC: American Psychiatric Press.

Webster, D. (1988). *Patients' perceptions of therapeutic factors in occupational therapy groups*. Unpublished master's thesis, Tufts University, Boston School of Occupational Therapy, Medford, MA.

Webster, D., & Schwartzberg, S. L. (1992). Patients' perception of curative factors in occupational therapy groups. *Occupational Therapy in Mental Health: A Journal of Psychosocial Practice and Research 12*(1), 3–24.

Yalom, I. D. (1983). *Inpatient group psychotherapy*. New York: Basic Books.

Yalom, I. D. (1985). *The theory and practice of group psychotherapy* (3rd ed.). New York: Basic Books.

Suggested Reading

Bruce, M. A. (1988). Occupational therapy in group treatment. In D. W. Scott & N. Katz (Eds.). *Occupational therapy in mental health Principles in practice* (pp. 116–132). Philadelphia: Taylor & Francis.

Cole, M. B. (1998). *Group dynamics in occupational therapy: The theoretical basis and practice application of group treatment* (2nd ed.). Thorofare, NJ: Slack.

Fazio, L. S. (2001). *Developing occupation—centered programs for the community: A workbook for students and professionals*. Upper Saddle River, NJ: Prentice-Hall.

Kaplan, K. (1986). The directive group: Short-term treatment for psychiatric patients with a minimal level of functioning. *American Journal of Occupational Therapy, 40*(7), 474–481.

Posthuma, B. W. (1996). *Small groups in counseling and therapy: Process and leadership* (2nd ed.). Needham Heights, MA: Allyn & Bacon.

Ross, M. (1987). *Group process: Using therapeutic activities in chronic care*. Thorofare, NJ: Slack.

UNIT *five*

Analyzing Occupation and Activity

Learning Objectives

After completing this unit, readers will be able to:

- Define and explain activity analysis, theory-focused activity analysis, and occupation-based activity analysis.
- Analyze activities and occupation-based activities for contextual demands and performance skills.
- Grade and adapt activities and occupations to meet the needs of clients.

Occupational therapy practitioners analyze activities and occupations to understand their component parts, their possible meanings to clients, and their therapeutic potential. Occupational therapy intervention is based in engaging clients in meaningful occupations to enable or improve their ability to meet their goals and participate in daily life. Consequently, the analytic processes practitioners bring to their work is at the core of occupational therapy practice. This unit describes these processes and links them to clinical reasoning, evaluation, and intervention. (*Note:* Words in **bold** type are defined in the Glossary.)

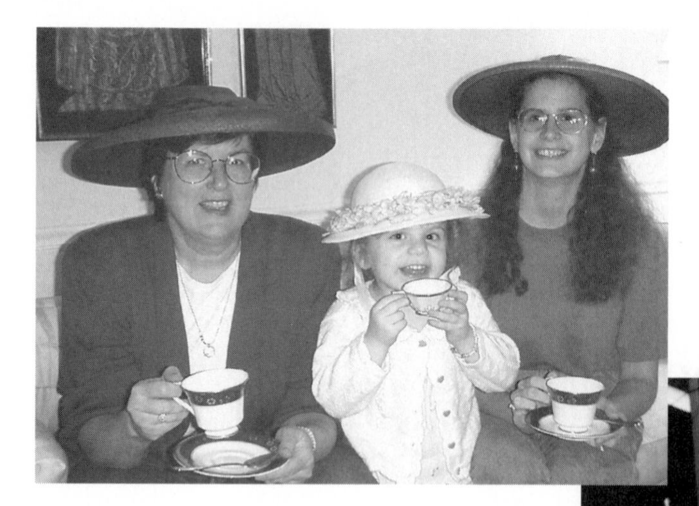

(top) Sipping tea with a grandchild models important aspects of a culture. (Courtesy of John Schell.) *(middle)* The context and meaning of sewing shoes are different from those of sewing to make clothing for the family. (Courtesy of Dennis Abbott.) *(bottom)* New leisure pursuits are offered to this man in an adult day program. (Courtesy of John Adams, Photographic Services, University of New Hampshire, Durham.)

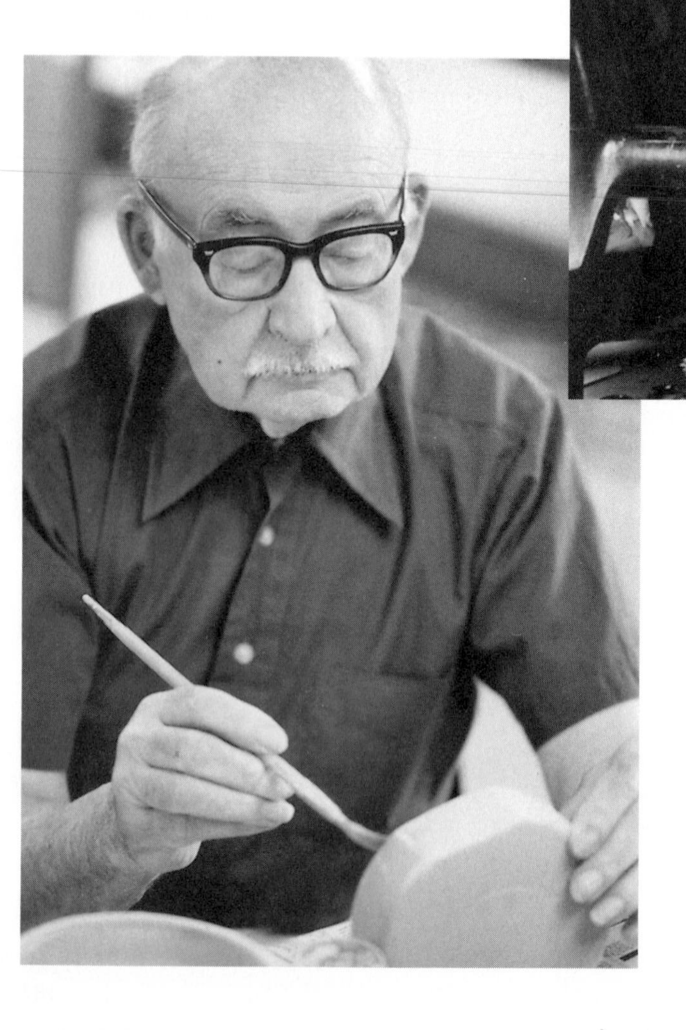

CHAPTER 16

ANALYZING OCCUPATION AND ACTIVITY: A WAY OF THINKING ABOUT OCCUPATIONAL PERFORMANCE

ELIZABETH BLESEDELL CREPEAU

This chapter describes three central components of occupational therapy practice: activity analysis, theory-focused activity analysis, and occupation-based activity analysis. These analytic processes are ways of thinking used by occupational therapy practitioners to understand activities and occupations, their demands and therapeutic potential, the skills required to do them, and the potential meanings ascribed to them. These thought processes contribute to the clinical reasoning of practitioners during occupational therapy evaluation and intervention.

Recent discussion in the field has attempted to make the distinction among activity, task, and occupation (Gray, 1998; Nelson, 1988; Pierce, 2001; Trombly, 1995a). One approach is to create a hierarchy in which tasks and activities are nested within the broader category of occupation (Law et al., 1996; Trombly, 1995a). Another is to differentiate between task and activity by asserting that activity is context free whereas task refers to a person's actual performance in context (Hagendorn, 1995, 1997; Watson, 1997). Pierce (2001) argued that activities are abstract concepts that describe general human experience and are shared within the culture. These activities are made concrete when people engage in them. From Pierce's perspective, engagement in an activity transforms it to an occupation when a particular person or persons act in a specific context. For example, swimming is an activity that many people would identify as an occupation. However, the person who swims for a team in an Olympic pool has a different occupational experience from someone who swims on a private beach at the family's lakeside cottage and from an inner-city child who swims at the public pool. Pedretti and Early (cited in American Occupational Therapy Association [AOTA], in press) used the term *occupation-based activity* to describe clients' engagement in occupations. For the purpose of this chapter, I will adopt these terms, as they provide a way of differentiating

TABLE 16-1. **CONTEXT(S)[a]: Context refers to a variety of interrelated conditions within and surrounding the client that influence performance.**

Area	Definitions	Examples
Cultural	"Customs, beliefs, activity patterns, behavior standards, and expectations accepted by the society of which the individual is a member. Includes political aspects, such as laws that affect access to resources and affirm personal rights. Also includes opportunities for education, employment, and economic support" (AOTA, 1994, p. 1054)	Ethnicity, family, attitude, beliefs, values
Physical	"Nonhuman aspects of contexts. Includes the accessibility to and performance within environments having natural terrain, plants, animals, buildings, furniture, objects, tools, or devices" (AOTA, 1994, p. 1054)	Objects, built environment, natural environment, geographic terrain, sensory qualities of environment
Social	"Availability and expectations of significant individuals, such as spouse, friends, and caregivers. Also includes larger social groups which are influential in establishing norms, role expectations, and social routines" (AOTA, 1994, p. 1054)	Relationships with individuals, groups, or organizations; relationships with systems (political, economic, institutional)
Personal	"Features of the individual that are not part of a health condition or health status" (World Health Organization, 2001, p. 15); personal context includes age, gender, socioeconomic status, and educational status	Twenty-five-year old unemployed man with a high school diploma
Spiritual	The fundamental orientation of a person's life; that which inspires and motivates that individual	Essence of the person, greater or higher purpose, meaning, substance
Temporal	"Location of occupational performance in time" (Neistadt & Crepeau, 1998, p. 292)	Stages of life, time of day, time of year, and duration
Virtual	Environment in which communication occurs by means of airways or computers and computers and an absence of physical contact	Realistic simulation of an environment, chat rooms, radio transmissions

[a](AOTA, in press). Copyright (in press) by the American Occupational Therapy Association, Inc. Reprinted with permission.

activity analysis (the thought processes practitioners use when thinking about activities in general) from occupation-based activity analysis (analysis of a person's actual occupational engagement within a specific context).

Context includes the external physical, social, and cultural environments in which people function, as well as the internal or personal aspects, such as age, gender, motivation, and stage in the life cycle (AOTA, in press). Table 16-1 lists the AOTA *Practice Framework* definitions for terms related to context. Lave (1988), an anthropologist, makes a distinction between the potential uses of contexts and the ways people actually interact with them. She used the term *arena* to describe the places in which an activity occurs, such as a library, school, or hospital. In contrast, she used the word *setting* to describe those aspects of the arena that the person attends to. For example, two different individuals going to a library are likely to use the library in different ways and to construct different meanings from their experiences. The man entering the library with his young child will most likely go to the children's section to look at colorful picture or chapter books. He is likely to sit on a small chair or a pillow while reading to his child. Later, he may help the child select books to take home. In contrast, a scholar is more likely to go to her library carrel to work on her current research project. The carrel is likely to be arranged in a particular way and to contain books and papers specific to the study being pursued. Thus, while the library as an arena remains the same, the library as a setting differs from person to person. The distinction Lave makes between arena and setting is similar to the distinction Pierce makes between activity and occupation. Arena and activity provide the external context and demands for people to engage in occupations within individually constructed settings.

Because occupational therapy practitioners are concerned about their clients as occupational beings, they need to have a broad understanding of both activities as culturally defined concepts and how people transform those activities into personally enacted and meaningful occupations. Adopting this distinction means that activity analysis enables the identification of the potential ways in which the activity may be enacted, the range of places in which it might occur, and the potential cultural and personal meanings that could be ascribed to it. In contrast, occupation-based activity analysis is centered in a person's occupational choices and experience embedded in his or her uniquely interpreted context. These occupations provide meaning and purpose to the person's life (Clark et al., 1991; Gray, 1998; Nelson, 1997; Pierce, 2001). Meaning is individually interpreted.

Using the library example, it is likely if you talked to the father about the meaning of going to the library with his child that he might mention the pleasure he derives from instilling in his child the value and enjoyment of reading and the quiet time they share together. He might recall his

RESEARCH NOTE 16–1

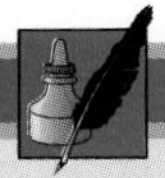

The Benefits of Occupational Engagement

KENNETH J. OTTENBACHER

In a previous edition of this text, Hopkins and Smith (1983) wrote:

> *It is through our activities that we are connected with life and with other human beings. Through the activities in which we engage, we learn about the world, test our knowledge, practice skills, express our feelings, experience pleasure, take care of our needs for survival, develop competence, and achieve mastery over our destinies. (p. 296)*

The day-to-day practice of occupational therapy reflects the fact that our activities, our behaviors, and the products of our occupations combine to give us a sense of who we are and help define us as social beings. This relationship between daily occupations and social roles is illustrated by a recent investigation by Eakman and Nelson (2001). In this study, individuals with traumatic brain injury who prepared a simple meal were significantly more likely to recall the steps and procedures used to complete the meal-preparation tasks than a comparable group of subjects who were given only written and verbal instructions regarding meal preparation. The amount of time and attention devoted to both groups was the same. The difference between the two groups was that one group engaged in the occupation of meal preparation and the other group only read or heard about the task. The authors demonstrated that the act of participating in an occupation (preparing a meal) by people with brain injury was important in retaining and understanding the steps necessary to complete the task.

Eakman, E. M., & Nelson, D. L. (2001). The effect of hands-on occupation on recall memory in man with traumatic brain injuries. *The Occupational Therapy Journal of Research, 21,* 109–114.

Hopkins, H. L., & Smith, H. D. (1983). *Willard and Spackman's occupational therapy.* Philadelphia: Lippincott.

childhood and the times he went to the library with one of his parents. Alternatively, he might explain that he never had the opportunity to go to the library with his father because his father had abandoned the family. The latter experience would create an entirely different meaning and motivational structure for this father–child occupation. As this example illustrates, the different experiences, values, and beliefs of clients make the interpretation of meaning a particularly complex aspect of practice. This difficulty is exacerbated by differences in socioeconomic status and culture between practitioners and their clients (Kielhofner & Barrett, 1998; see also Unit III). It is the practitioner's responsibility to develop the therapeutic relationships that foster an understanding of clients and their world (Crepeau, 1991; Peloquin, 1995; see also Chapter 14).

ACTIVITY ANALYSIS AND CLINICAL REASONING

Occupational therapy practitioners draw on their education, knowledge of activities, and clinical experience when analyzing activities (Neistadt, McAuley, Zecha, & Shannon, 1993). This analysis is so automatic that it is often ignored or unappreciated, becoming another aspect of the tacit nature of clinical reasoning (Mattingly & Fleming, 1994; Schell & Cervero, 1993). Practitioners analyze activities from the perspective of practice theories to understand problems in performance and intervention strategies appropriate from that theoretical perspective. Their analysis is also based on access to particular activities and the degree to which they are willing to engage in trial and error or experimentation to understand activities more fully.

Studies that have attempted to make activity analysis an objective process have demonstrated that the number of variables is so great that the goal of objectivity would be exceedingly difficult to achieve (Llorens, 1986; Neistadt et al., 1993; Trombly, 1995a). Adopting the distinction between activity analysis and occupation-based activity analysis renders this concern moot. If the outcome of activity analysis is to understand the potential demands of an activity, objectivity is not the goal. Rather, identifying the multiple demands, skills, and potential meanings of the activity enables practitioners to have a deeper understanding of this activity in general.

In contrast, occupation-based activity analysis is a highly individualized process because it is embedded in the particular perspective of the person, the person's occupational performance problems, and the performance context. This analysis occurs within top-down evaluation models that first attempt to understand the person as an occupational being before identifying occupational performance and barriers to effective performance (Coster, 1998; Fisher, 2001; Hocking, 2001; Polatajko, Mandich, & Martini, 2000; Trombly, 1995b). These client-centered evaluation models address the ability of a person to engage in a valued occupation and the interplay between actual performance, activity demands, and context (Law, 1998).

This chapter focuses on three levels of analysis: activity analysis, theory-focused activity analysis, and occupation-based activity analysis. Activity analysis is the exploration of the typical contexts, demands, and potential meanings that could be ascribed to an activity. Theory-focused activity analysis examines the properties of an activity from the perspective of a particular practice theory to understand the activity's therapeutic potential. Used in this way, both activity analysis and theory-focused activity analysis are abstract, because they involve exploring and understanding the activity for its potential in relation to occupational therapy evaluation and intervention. In contrast, occupation-based activity analysis focuses on individuals engaging in occupations within their unique physical, cultural, and social environments. By blending these analytic models, practitioners can gain an understanding of the particular ways in which clients relate to their occupations and can then use their knowledge of activity and practice theories to harness those occupational activities for therapeutic purposes. This understanding is achieved through all three forms of analysis.

ACTIVITY ANALYSIS

Activity analysis is a way of thinking about activities. Practitioners must perform quick analyses while working with clients. In addition, occupational therapy practitioners may also think about activities for their therapeutic potential, for instance by sizing up new games, cooking gadgets, and other objects or activities. Activity analysis addresses the typical demands of an activity, the range of skills involved in its performance, and the various cultural meanings that might be ascribed to it. The goal of activity analysis is to understand as much as possible about an activity, including the particular skills required to do it competently and its relation to participation in the world at large (Cynkin, 1995). It is this knowledge of activities, their properties, and their potential cultural meanings that sensitizes practitioners to the occupations of their clients and helps practitioners know which particular activities to suggest to them.

Activity Analysis Format

The activity analysis format is based on the organization of the *Occupational Therapy Practice Framework* (AOTA, in press). The *Occupational Therapy Practice Framework* is designed to reflect the current practice of occupational therapy and its concern for supporting occupational engagement and social participation of individuals in our society. Activity analysis focuses on the identification of activity demands and performance skills. Activity demands include aspects of the activity such as the objects typically used, the space and social demands of the activity, and the skills required to carry it out (AOTA, in press). Performance skills are subdivided into motor skills, process skills, and communication/interaction skills. Table 16–2 presents the activity analysis format, Table 16-3 provides a description of performance skills, and Table 16-4 contains an abbreviated list of body functions.

THEORY-FOCUSED ACTIVITY ANALYSIS

Theory-focused activity analysis has a different perspective. Rather than examining the properties of an activity to understand its demands in general, theory-focused activity analysis examines these properties from a theoretical perspective. By using the principles of a particular practice theory, occupational therapy practitioners analyze activities as they think about performance problems addressed by this theory. The potential therapeutic intervention should be consistent with the theory and will likely entail the grading and adaptation of the occupations chosen by the client.

Each theory articulates a view of function, dysfunction, and the use of occupations to enable clients to improve their performance. This understanding directs practitioners to the particular evaluation and intervention strategies of that theory. For example, problems in motor performance may impede the ability of clients to cook, an occupation for many people. If the poor motor performance is caused by an inability to hold and lift objects due to poor strength, a biomechanical approach would be appropriate. This approach improves motor performance by increasing strength through added resistance to or increased repetitions of motions embedded in an occupation, in this case, cooking (Fisher, 1998). If the client's abil-

HISTORICAL NOTE 16–1

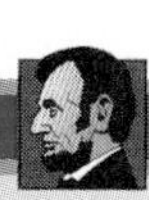

The Long-Standing Need for Activity Analysis: George Barton's Beliefs

SUZANNE M. PELOQUIN

George Edward Barton, originator of the idea of founding a society to promote occupation as therapy, grasped the concept of activity analysis. He often used medical analogies to explain the therapeutic effects of occupation. He suggested that when Adam was cast from the Garden of Eden, he was given this divine prescription: "Work by the sweat of the brow" (Barton, 1915a). More specifically, Barton thought that any medicine listed as a therapeutic agent in the *Materia Medica* had an occupational parallel. He explained that if a doctor might prescribe leukotoxin benzol to a patient with leukemia, the occupational therapist could lead that same person to work at a canning factory where the fumes of hot benzine would have a similar effect (Barton, 1915b).

The particulars of Barton's analysis now seem quaint. The fact remains, however, that if an occupation is to be deemed therapeutic, it must withstand a rigorous analysis of its possible benefits. If the facts are outdated, the concept endures.

Barton, G. E. (1915a). Occupational nursing. *Trained Nurse and Hospital Review*, 54, 138–140.

Barton, G. E. (1915b). Occupational therapy. *Trained Nurse and Hospital Review*, 54, 335–338.

TABLE 16-2. **ACTIVITY ANALYSIS FORMAT**[a]

Activity	• Describe the activity in one to two sentences.
Objects used and their properties	• Describe the tools, materials, and equipment used in the process of carrying out the activity. • Consider the potential symbolism/meaning of the objects and their properties; describe them.
Space demands	• Describe the physical context in which the activity is being analyzed, using the categories listed below; be specific. Describe the arrangement of furniture. Describe the placement of equipment. Describe the lighting. Describe the level of noise and other distractions that may be present. Is this the typical context for this activity? If not, what other contexts might be appropriate? Briefly describe them.
Social demands	• Describe the social and cultural demands or the range of demands that may be required by this activity or elicited by engagement in this activity, using the categories listed below. Describe other people involved in the activity. What is their relationship to each other? What do they expect from each other? Describe the typical rules, norms, and expectations involved in doing this activity. Describe the cultural and symbolic meanings typically ascribed to this activity. Speculate about other social contexts in which the activity might be performed. How might the rules, expectations, and meanings vary from this setting?
Sequence and timing	• List the sequential steps (no more than 15) of the activity as it is being analyzed. Include any timing requirements, such as waiting for glue to dry, bread to rise, etc. • How much flexibility exists in the sequence and timing of the steps of this activity? • Does this activity typically occur at a specific time of day (e.g., bathing and dressing typically occur in the morning)?
Required actions	• For each category below, select the five most important performance skills that would be required to carry out the activity. List and briefly describe them (Table 16-3 describes these skills). Motor skills. Process skills. Communication/interaction skills. • How much flexibility exists for people with skill deficits, e.g., what is the potential for grading and adaptation?
Required body structures and functions	• Briefly list the body structures (parts of the body) used to perform this activity. • Briefly list the essential body functions necessary to engage in this activity (Table 16-5 lists these functions).
Safety hazards	• List potential safety hazards for this activity. Think especially of children, people with cognitive and judgment problems, etc.

[a]AOTA (in press). Copyright (in press) by the American Occupational Therapy Association, Inc. Adapted with permission.

ity to cook is hampered by poor motor performance caused by the inability to complete complex movement patterns, a biomechanical approach is not appropriate. Rather, the multicontext theoretical perspective analyzes cooking from its simple to complex movement patterns, an entirely different way of understanding the performance skills required to cook. For examples of theory-focused activity analysis, see the tables in Chapter 30, Section 5. Table 16-5 presents the format of theory-focused activity analysis.

OCCUPATION-BASED ACTIVITY ANALYSIS

In contrast to activity analysis and theory-focused activity analysis, occupation-based activity analysis places the person in the foreground. It takes into account the particular person's interests, goals, abilities, and contexts, as well as the demands of the activity itself. These considerations shape the practitioner's efforts to help the person reach his or her goals through carefully designed evaluation and intervention. Top-down evaluation models, such as those described by Coster (1998), Fisher (2001), Hocking (2001), Polatajko et al. (2000), and Trombly (1995b), embed occupation-based activity analysis within the evaluation process, though their terminology in describing this process differs. Within the evaluation process, all models identify the person's ability to perform valued occupations and to understand the strengths and weaknesses of his or her performance before detailed assessment of the underlying capacities that support that performance. The selection and design of the particular therapeutic occupations are derived from the practitioner's

TABLE 16-3. **PERFORMANCE SKILLS**[a]

PERFORMANCE SKILLS

Features of what one does, not what one has, related to observable elements of action that have implicit functional purposes (adapted from Fisher & Kielhofner, 1995, p. 113).

MOTOR SKILLS: skills in moving and interacting with task, objects, and environment (A. Fisher, personal communication, July 9, 2001).

POSTURE relates to the stabilizing and aligning of one's body while moving in relation to task objects with which one must deal.
- **Stabilizes:** maintains trunk control and balance while interacting with task objects such that there is no evidence of transient (i.e., quickly passing) propping or loss of balance that affects task performance.
- **Aligns:** maintains an upright sitting or standing position, without evidence of a need to persistently prop during the task performance.
- **Positions:** positions body, arms, or wheelchair in relation to task objects and in a manner that promotes the use of efficient arm movements during task performance.

MOBILITY relates to moving the entire body or a body part in space as necessary when interacting with task objects.
- **Walks:** ambulates on level surfaces and changes direction while walking without shuffling the feet, lurching, instability, or using external supports or assistive devices (e.g., cane, walker, wheelchair) during the task performance.
- **Reaches:** extends, moves the arm (and when appropriate, the trunk) to effectively grasp or place task objects that are out of reach, including skillfully using a reacher to obtain task objects.
- **Bends:** actively flexes, rotates, or twists the trunk in a manner and direction appropriate to the task.

COORDINATION relates to using more than one body part to interact with task objects in a manner that supports task performance.
- **Coordinates:** uses two or more body parts together to stabilize and manipulate task objects during bilateral motor tasks.
- **Manipulates:** uses dexterous grasp-and-release patterns, isolated finger movements, and coordinated in-hand manipulation patterns when interacting with task objects.
- **Flows:** uses smooth and fluid arm and hand movements when interacting with task objects.

STRENGTH AND EFFORT pertains to skills that require generation of muscle force appropriate for effective interaction with task objects.
- **Moves:** pushes, pulls, or drags task objects along a supporting surface.
- **Transports:** carries task objects from one place to another while walking, seated in a wheelchair, or using a walker.
- **Lifts:** raises or hoists task objects, including lifting an object from one place to another, but without ambulating or moving from one place to another.
- **Calibrates:** regulates or grades the force, speed, and extent of movement when interacting with task objects (e.g., not too much or too little).
- **Grips:** pinches or grasps task objects with no "grip slips."

ENERGY refers to sustained effort over the course of task performance.
- **Endures:** persists and completes the task without obvious evidence of physical fatigue, pausing to rest, or stopping to "catch one's breath."
- **Paces:** maintains a consistent and effective rate or tempo of performance throughout the steps of the entire task.

PROCESS SKILLS: "skills . . . used in managing and modifying actions en route to the completion of daily life tasks" (Fisher & Kielhofner, 1995, p. 120).

ENERGY refers to sustained effort over the course of task performance.
- **Paces:** maintains a consistent and effective rate or tempo of performance throughout the steps of the entire task.
- **Attends:** maintains focused attention throughout the task such that the client is not distracted away from the task by extraneous auditory or visual stimuli.

KNOWLEDGE refers to the ability to seek and use task-related knowledge.
- **Chooses:** selects appropriate and necessary tools and materials for the task, including choosing the tools and materials that were specified for use prior to the initiation of the task.
- **Uses:** uses tools and materials according to their intended purposes and in a reasonable or hygienic fashion, given their intrinsic properties and the availability (or lack of availability) of other objects.
- **Handles:** supports, stabilizes, and holds tools and materials in an appropriate manner and that protects them from damage, falling, or dropping.
- **Heeds:** uses goal-directed task actions that are focused toward the completion of the specified task (i.e., the outcome originally agreed on or specified by another) without behavior that is driven or guided by environmental cues (i.e., "environmentally cued" behavior).
- **Inquires:** (a) seeks needed verbal or written information by asking questions or reading directions or labels (b) asks no unnecessary information questions (e.g., questions related to where materials are located or how a familiar task is performed).

TEMPORAL ORGANIZATION pertains to the beginning, logical ordering, continuation, and completion of the steps and action sequences of a task.
- **Initiates:** starts or begins the next action or step without hesitation.
- **Continues:** performs actions or action sequences of steps without unnecessary interruption such that once an action sequence is initiated, the individual continues on until the step is completed.
- **Sequences:** performs steps in an effective or logical order for efficient use of time and energy and with an absence of (a) randomness in the ordering and/or (b) inappropriate repetition ("reordering") of steps.

TABLE 16–3. *(continued)*

- **Terminates:** brings to completion single actions or single steps without perseveration, inappropriate persistence, or premature cessation.

ORGANIZING SPACE AND OBJECTS pertains to skills for organizing task spaces and task objects.

- **Searches/Locates:** looks for and locates tools and materials in a logical manner, including looking beyond the immediate environment (e.g., looking in, behind, on top of).
- **Gathers:** collects together needed or misplaced tools and materials, including (a) collecting located supplies into the workspace and (b) collecting and replacing materials that have spilled, fallen, or been misplaced.
- **Organizes:** logically positions or spatially arranges tools and materials in an orderly fashion (a) within a single workspace and (b) among multiple appropriate workspaces in order to facilitate ease of task performance.
- **Restores:** (a) puts away tools and materials in appropriate places, (b) restores immediate workspace to original condition (e.g., wiping surfaces clean), (c) closes and seals containers and coverings when indicated, and (d) twists or folds any plastic bags to seal.
- **Navigates:** modifies the movement pattern of the arm, body, or wheelchair to maneuver around obstacles that are encountered in the course of moving through space such that undesirable contact with obstacles (e.g., knocking over, bumping into) is avoided (includes maneuvering objects held in the hand around obstacles).

ADAPTATION relates to the ability to anticipate, correct for, and benefit by learning from the consequences of errors that arise in the course of task performance.

- **Notices/Responds:** responds appropriately to (a) nonverbal environmental/perceptual cues (i.e., movement, sound, smell, heat, moisture, texture, shape, consistency) that provide feedback with respect to task progression and (b) the spatial arrangement of objects to one another (e.g., aligning objects during stacking). Notices and, when indicated, makes an effective and efficient response.
- **Accommodates:** modifies his or her actions or the location of objects within the workspace, in anticipation of or in response to problems that might arise. The client anticipates or responds to problems effectively by (a) changing the method with which he or she is performing an action sequence, (b) changing the manner in which he or she interacts with or handles tools and materials already in the workspace, and (c) asking for assistance when appropriate or needed.
- **Adjusts:** changes working environments in anticipation of or in response to problems that might arise. The client anticipates or responds to problems effectively by making some change (a) between working environments by moving to a new workspace or bringing in or removing tools and materials from the present workspace or (b) in an environmental condition (e.g., turning on or off the tap, turning up or down the temperature).
- **Benefits:** anticipates and prevents undesirable circumstances or problems from recurring or persisting.

COMMUNICATION/INTERACTION SKILLS: refer to conveying intentions and needs and coordinating social behavior to act together with people (Forsyth & Kielhofner, 1999; Forsyth, Salamy, Simon, and Kielhofner, 1997; and Kielhofner, 2002).

PHYSICALITY pertains to using the physical body when communicating within an occupation.

- **Contacts:** makes physical contact with others.
- **Gazes:** uses eyes to communicate and interact with others.
- **Gestures:** uses movements of the body to indicate, demonstrate, or add emphasis.
- **Maneuvers:** moves one's body in relation to others.
- **Orients:** directs one's body in relation to others and/or occupational forms.
- **Postures:** Assumes physical positions.

INFORMATION EXCHANGE refers to giving and receiving information within an occupation.

- **Articulates:** produces clear, understandable speech.
- **Asserts:** directly expresses desires, refusals, and requests.
- **Asks:** requests factual or personal information.
- **Engages:** initiates interactions.
- **Expresses:** displays affect/attitude.
- **Modulates:** uses volume and inflection in speech.
- **Shares:** gives out factual or personal information.
- **Speaks:** makes oneself understood through use of words, phrases, and sentences.
- **Sustains:** keeps up speech for appropriate duration.

RELATIONS relates to maintaining appropriate relationships within an occupation.

- **Collaborates:** coordinates action with others toward a common end goal.
- **Conforms:** follows implicit and explicit social norms.
- **Focuses:** directs conversation and behavior to ongoing social action.
- **Relates:** assumes a manner of acting that tries to establish a rapport with others.
- **Respects:** accommodates to other people's reactions and requests.

TABLE 16–4. **LIST OF BODY FUNCTIONS**[a]

Function	Examples
Mental	Consciousness, orientation, intellect, global psychosocial, temperament and personality, energy and drive, attention, memory, psychomotor, emotional, perceptual, thought, higher-level cognitive, language, calculation
Sensory	Seeing, hearing, vestibular, taste, smell, proprioceptive, touch
Voice and speech	Voice, articulation, fluency
Cardiovascular and respiratory systems	Exercise tolerance
Neuromusculoskeletal and movement related	Joint mobility, muscle power, muscle tone, muscle endurance

[a]Adapted from World Health Organization (2001).

TABLE 16–5. **THEORY-FOCUSED ACTIVITY ANALYSIS**

- Briefly describe the activity.
- Name the practice theory.
- How does this theory define
  - Function?
  - Dysfunction?
  - Change?
- Analyze an activity and then respond to these questions::
  - Using the principles of this theoretical perspective, how can the activity be graded to improve skills?
  - Using the principles of this theoretical perspective, how can the activity be adapted to improve performance?

TABLE 16–6. **OCCUPATION-BASED ACTIVITY ANALYSIS FORMAT**

Factor	Activity
Who is this person?	• List this person's goals. • What occupational activities are most important to this person? • How have these goals and occupational activities been influenced by performance problems?
Select an occupational activity to analyze	• Briefly describe one of the person's occupational activities and why this is important to him or her.
Objects used and their properties	• Describe the tools, materials, and equipment used to carry out this occupation. • Consider the potential symbolism/meaning of the objects and their properties to this individual; describe them.
Space demands	• Describe the physical context in which the occupational activity is being analyzed using the categories listed below. Be specific. • Describe the arrangement of furniture. • Describe the placement of equipment. • Describe the lighting. • Describe the level of noise and other distractions that may be present. • Is this the typical context for the person to engage in this occupational activity? If not, briefly describe how it is different.
Social demands	• Describe the specific social and cultural context of this occupational activity using the categories listed below. • Describe the other people involved. What are their relationships to each other? What do they expect from each other? • Describe the typical rules, norms, and expectations involved. • What are the cultural and symbolic meanings the person assigns to this occupational activity?
Sequence and timing	• List the sequential steps (no more than 15) of the activity as it is being analyzed. Include any timing requirements, such as waiting for glue to dry, bread to rise, etc. • How much flexibility exists in the sequence and timing of the steps of this occupational activity? • Does the client perform this occupational activity at a specific time of day? • How does this occupational activity relate to the person's habits and routines?
Required actions	• For each category list and describe the individual's strengths and deficits in occupational performance. Motor skills. Process skills. Communication/interaction skills.
Required body structures and functions	• Describe any assets and deficits in body structures and function that influenced the person's occupational performance. Should these be evaluated further?
Safety hazards	• Are there potential safety hazards when this person engages in this occupational activity?

ETHICS NOTE 16–1

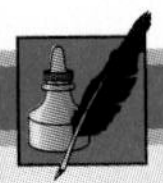

Using Analysis to Meet a Client's Goals

PENNY KYLER and RUTH A. HANSEN

Karla is receiving home-health occupational therapy because of a cerebral vascular accident. She has a flaccid left arm and is left-handed. She is also a new mother, who wants to be able to diaper her infant. Because she is concerned about the environment she does not believe in disposable diapers and wants to use cloth diapers and diaper pins. Karla has shared this desire with her therapist. The therapist has never seen or used cloth diapers and, in fact, has never diapered a child. The therapist does not want to seem incompetent. She develops a treatment plan that focuses on balance. The therapist has Karla dusting to improve her balance so she can reach her goal of diapering her child.

QUESTIONS AND EXERCISES

1. **How should the therapist proceed with developing a treatment plan?**
2. **Does the therapist have any obligation to discuss with the patient her lack of experience in this area?**
3. **What ethical concerns could be raised relative to the mother's environmental concerns versus the concerns for what is best for the newborn?**

understanding of the client and his or her goals, the barriers to performance, and the therapeutic interventions the practitioner deems appropriate to pursue. See Table 16-6 for a format to guide occupation-based activity analysis.

GRADING AND ADAPTATION

Intervention strategies typically involve the use of grading and adaptation. Grading and adaptation facilitate therapeutic change and support engagement in occupation. While these processes typically occur during intervention, understanding the potential for grading and adaptation of a wide variety of activities and from various theoretical perspectives is a useful skill for occupational therapy practitioners.

Practitioners grade occupations to improve the client's underlying capacities and skills (Fisher, 2001). The grading of an occupation-based activity involves sequentially increasing its demands to stimulate improvement in the person's function. Depending on the nature of the client's performance problems and the practice theory or theories selected by the practitioner to address these problems, the particular way of grading will vary. For example, a practitioner working with a child who wants to ride a two-wheeled bicycle but who is unsuccessful at balancing sufficiently may grade the activity from a sensory integrative theory perspective by encouraging the child to participate in a variety of balance-enhancing activities. Activity choices may include play on air mattresses, suspension bridges, and large inflated balls. The activities are less challenging than the bicycle but are anticipated to enhance overall postural adjustment and balance skills, eventually leading up to improved bicycle-riding performance (with or without training wheels to start). In contrast, a motor learning perspective might have the same child practicing posture and balance skills on a stationary bicycle, carefully removing supports to allow for greater balance demands, until the child was ready to ride a bicycle with training wheels. Practitioners monitor clients and adjust their grading to be sure that the level of demand is at the appropriate level to stimulate therapeutic change but not so difficult as to frustrate the person, that is, to create the "just right challenge."

The goal of adaptation is to allow the person continued involvement in a valued occupation that can no longer be pursued. Rather than striving to improve the functional capacity of the individual, adaptation focuses on changing the demands of the activity so they are within the person's ability level. These adaptations may involve the modification of the occupation itself by reducing its demands, the use of assistive devices, or changes in the physical or social environment (Fisher, 2001). Changing the demands of the occupation may involve making it simpler cognitively or reducing the physical skills required to do it. Adaptive equipment, such as reachers or holders, may be used to enable dressing. Voice-recognition software may be used for someone who can no longer use a keyboard. Adaptation may also involve changing the social world through the provision of assistance by another person, such as a personal-care attendant or family member, to help with bathing and dressing each morning and evening. With degenerative conditions, these adaptations may need to be made repeatedly as the individual's skills diminish. AIDS, cancer, arthritis, and other chronic illnesses might require daily adaptation because of the fluctuating levels of function typical of these conditions.

CONCLUSION

This chapter describes three types of analyses: activity analysis, theory-focused activity analysis, and occupation-based activity analysis. Use of these strategies requires practitioners to understand the following:

- The general properties and demands of activities as they are customarily performed in given settings and cultures.
- How to select activities that are occupationally relevant to clients.
- How to select and grade activities based on theoretical knowledge to bring about therapeutic change or to improve performance.

- How to use occupations valued by clients to achieve their goals as occupational beings

These core skills are critical for effective occupational therapy evaluation and intervention. All three processes ultimately center on occupation and its capacity to motivate people to act and to create meaning in their lives. Brockelman (1980), a philosopher, recognized the importance of occupation in the following statement: "The tools of our minds and the tools of our hands are of meaningless use without deep and personal reasons of the heart to set their purpose and guide their use" (p. 24). It is through practitioners' deep understanding of people as occupational beings that effective occupational therapy intervention occurs.

References

American Occupational Therapy Association [AOTA]. (1994). Uniform terminology for occupational Therapy—Third edition. *American Journal of Occupational Therapy, 48*, 1047–1054.

American Occupational Therapy Association. (In press). Occupational therapy practice framework: Domain and process. *American Journal of Occupational Therapy.*

Brockelman, P. T. (1980). *Existential phenomenology and the world of ordinary experience: An introduction.* Lanham, MD: University of America Press.

Clarke, F., Parham, D., Carlson, M., Frank, G., Jackson, J., Pierce, D., Wolfe, R. J., & Zemke, R. (1991). Occupational science: Academic innovation in the service of occupational therapy's future. *American Journal of Occupational Therapy, 45*, 300–310.

Coster, W. (1998). Occupation-centered assessment of children. *American Journal of Occupational Therapy, 52*, 337–344.

Crepeau, E. B. (1991). Achieving intersubjective understanding: Examples from an occupational therapy treatment session. *American Journal of Occupational Therapy, 44*, 311–317.

Cynkin, S. (1995). Activities. In C. B. Royeen (Ed.). *The practice of the future: Putting occupation back into therapy: AOTA self-study series* (Module 7; pp. 1–52). Rockville, MD: American Occupational Therapy Association.

Fisher, A. G. (1998). Uniting practice and theory in an occupational framework. [Eleanor Clarke Slagle Lecture]. *American Journal of Occupational Therapy, 52*, 509–521.

Fisher, A. G. (2001). *Assessment of motor and process skills: Vol. 1. Development, standardization, and administration manual* (4th ed.). Fort Collins, CO: Three Stars Press.

Fisher, A., & Kielhofner, G. (1995). Skill in occupational performance. In G. Kielhofner (Ed.), *A model of human occupation: Theory and application* (2nd ed., pp. 113–128). Baltimore: Williams & Wilkins.

Forsyth, K., & Kielhofner G. (1999). Validity of the assessment of communication of interaction skills. *British Journal of Occupational Therapy, 62*, 69–74.

Forsyth, K., Salamy, M., Simon, S., & Kielhofner. G. (1997). *Assessment of communication and interaction skills.* Chicago: University of Illinois, Model of Human Occupation Clearing House.

Gray, J. M. (1998). Putting occupation into practice: Occupation as ends, occupation as means. *American Journal of Occupational Therapy, 52*, 354–364.

Hagendorn, R. (1995). *Occupational therapy: Perspectives and processes.* Edinburgh, UK: Churchill Livingstone.

Hagendorn, R. (1997). *Foundations for practice in occupational therapy* (2nd ed.). New York: Churchill Livingstone.

Hocking, C. (2001). Implementing occupation-based assessment. *American Journal of Occupational Therapy, 55*, 463–469.

Kielhofner, G., & Barrett, L. (1998). Meaning and misunderstanding in occupational forms: A study of therapeutic goal setting. *American Journal of Occupational Therapy, 52*, 345–353.

Kielhofner, G. (2002). Dimensions of doing. In G. Kielhofner (Ed.), *A model of human occupation: Theory and application* (3rd ed., pp. 114–123). Baltimore: Lippincott Williams & Wilkins.

Lave, J. (1988). *Cognition in practice: Mind, mathematics and culture in everyday life.* Cambridge, UK: Cambridge University Press.

Law, M. (Ed.). (1998). *Client-centered occupational therapy.* Thorofare, NJ: Slack.

Law, M., Cooper, B. A., Strong, S., Stewart, D., Rigby, P., & Letts, L. (1996). The person-environment-occupation model: A transactive approach to occupational performance. *Canadian Journal of Occupational Therapy, 63*, 9–23.

Llorens, L. A. (1986). Activity analysis: Agreement among factors in a sensory processing model. *American Journal of Occupational Therapy, 40*, 103–110.

Mattingly, C., & Fleming, M. H. (1994). *Clinical reasoning: Forms of inquiry in a therapeutic practice.* Philadelphia: Davis.

Neistadt, M. E., & Crepeau, E. B. (Eds.). (1998). *Willard and Spackman's occupational therapy* (9th ed.). Philadelphia: Lippincott-Raven.

Neistadt, M. E., McAuley, D., Zecha, D., & Shannon, R. (1993). An analysis of a board game as a treatment activity. *American Journal of Occupational Therapy, 47*, 154–160.

Nelson, D. L. (1988). Occupation: Form and function. *American Journal of Occupational Therapy, 42*, 633–642.

Nelson, D. L. (1997). Why the profession of occupational therapy will flourish in the 21st century. *American Journal of Occupational Therapy, 51*, 11–24.

Peloquin, S. M. (1995). The fullness of empathy: Reflections and illustrations. *American Journal of Occupational Therapy, 49*, 24–31.

Pierce, D. (2001). Untangling occupation and activity. *American Journal of Occupational Therapy, 55*, 138–146.

Polatajko, H. J., Mandich, A., & Martini, R. (2000). Dynamic performance analysis: A framework for understanding occupational performance. *American Journal of Occupational Therapy, 54*, 65–72.

Schell, B. A., & Cervero, R. M. (1993). Clinical reasoning in occupational therapy: An integrative review. *American Journal of Occupational Therapy, 47*, 605–610.

Trombly, C. A. (1995a). Occupation, purposefulness and meaningfulness as therapeutic mechanisms. [Eleanor Clarke Slagle Lecture]. *American Journal of Occupational Therapy, 49*, 960–972.

Trombly, C. A. (1995b). *Occupational therapy for physical dysfunction* (4th ed.). Baltimore: Williams & Wilkins.

Watson, D. E. (1997). *Task analysis: An occupational performance approach.* Bethesda, MD: American Occupational Therapy Association.

World Health Organization (WHO). (2001). *International classification of functioning, disability, and health (ICF).* Geneva: Author. (Available at: www.who.int/icidh/)

UNIT *six*

Conceptual Basis for Practice

Learning Objectives

After completing this unit, readers will be able to:

- Identify the relationship between theory and practice.
- Explain the importance of theory to the development of professional knowledge.
- Explain the historical heritage of occupation-based perspectives, rehabilitation perspectives, developmental and neurological perspectives, and learning perspectives.
- Define and explain the assumptions, strengths, and limitations of these perspectives.
- Compare and contrast these perspectives and their utility for occupational therapy practice.

Occupational therapy practice is guided by various theories and frames of reference. These are evolving as research further articulates their effectiveness in occupational therapy evaluation intervention. This unit opens with occupation-based perspectives, which provide the baseline for occupational therapy evaluation and intervention. These perspectives help us understand the individual as an occupational being embedded in a social and environmental context. For example, from an occupational perspective we could say that Mary Weber (see Chapter 4) has difficulty engaging in activities of daily living, work, leisure, and social participation primarily because she has difficulty sequencing and organizing tasks. Because her ability to sequence and organize tasks is so impaired, she can no longer work in her profession, manage her finances, prepare meals, shop, drive, or use public transportation without assistance. This is where theory helps. Occupation-based perspectives allow us to identify those occupations that are most important to Mary, her strengths and weaknesses, and the supports within her physical and social worlds. With this information, we can identify specific goals to assist her to do those things that she identified as most important. Because the source of most of Mary's problems is in sequencing and organizing tasks, we could use an evaluation and intervention approach developed for these types of problems. Joan Toglia's multicontext approach, for instance, is a practice approach grounded in learning theory that provides practitioners with specific ideas about how to proceed with Mary's evaluation and intervention. In contrast, if Mary's problems were primarily physical, then practice theories derived from rehabilitation perspectives would be helpful. This unit presents an overview of the different conceptual bases of practice most frequently used by occupational therapy practitioners. (*Note:* Words in **bold** type are defined in the Glossary.)

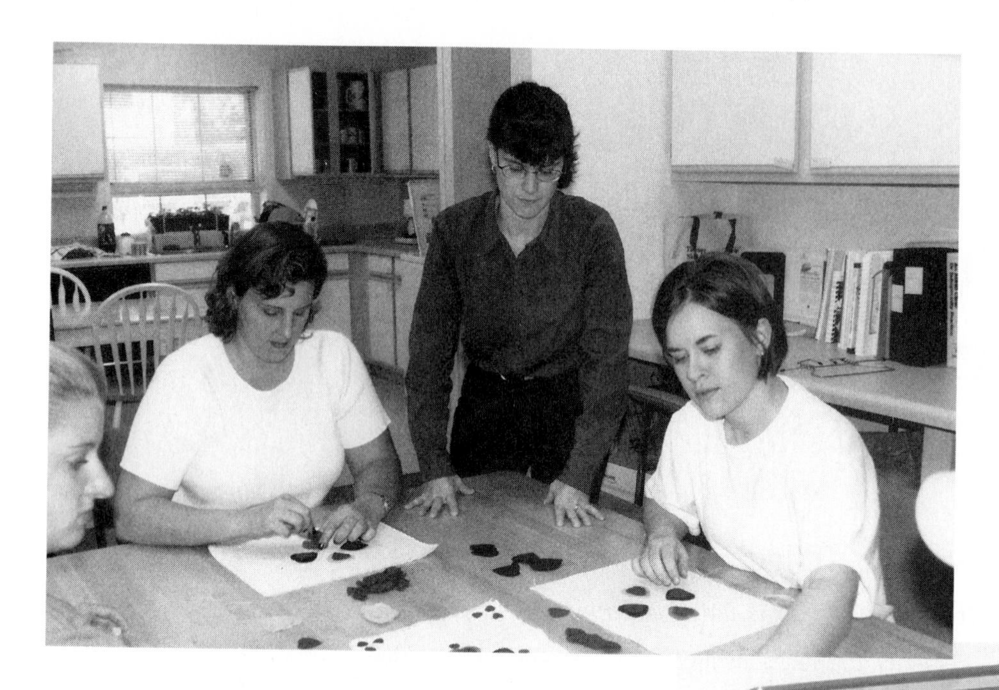

The developmental, rehabilitative, and learning approaches to occupational therapy evaluation and intervention. *(top)* (Courtesy of Barbara Schell.) *(middle)* (Courtesy of KINDRA CLINEFF, Copyright 2001.) *(bottom)* (Courtesy of Ron Bergeron, Photographic Services, University of New Hampshire, Durham.)

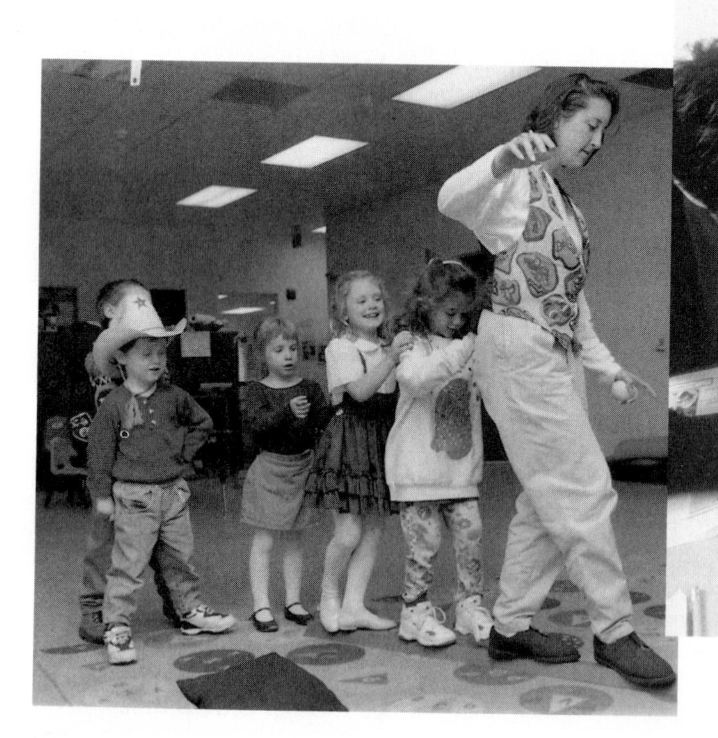

CHAPTER 17

THEORY AND PRACTICE IN OCCUPATIONAL THERAPY

ELIZABETH BLESEDELL CREPEAU and
BARBARA A. BOYT SCHELL

Becoming an occupational therapy practitioner involves learning the knowledge, skills, and values of the field. An important part of this process is the ability to understand and use theoretical knowledge (Parham, 1987). Theoretical knowledge or ideas, when combined with the practitioners' personal and professional experiences, form the basis for professional action. The combination of all these factors results in the development of individual professional paradigms, or mental models, that practitioners use to guide their actions (Cervero, 1988; Griswold, 1995; Törnebohm, 1991). An individual's professional paradigm involves an integration of the following elements:

- The practitioner's underlying beliefs, values, and commitments (Hooper; 1997; Törnebohm, 1991).
- The practitioner's occupational therapy knowledge, abilities, and skills, including theories, evaluation, and intervention strategies (Griswold, 1995; Törnebohm, 1991).
- The practitioner's professional values as expressed in a commitment to the field and to people who seek his or her care (Törnebohm, 1991).

Practitioners draw on their professional paradigms as they work to enhance their clients' abilities to engage in valued occupations. Through experience, professional paradigms become highly developed and provide a great resource for practitioners to reflect about their practice and the problems encountered by their clients (Griswold, 1995; Schön, 1983; Törnebohm, 1991). See Chapters 11 and 12 to learn more about these clinical reasoning processes and how they are developed. Of particular interest for Unit VI is the exploration of theoretical knowledge and why it is important for effective occupational therapy practice.

WHAT IS THEORY?

In the broadest sense, a theory is a set of ideas or concepts that people use to guide their actions (Morse, 1997). A theory reflects an image or explanation of why or how a phenomenon occurs. When fully developed, a theory defines concepts and states relationships among them (Morse, 1997), giving people the tools to understand, explain, or predict phenomena (McColl, Law, & Stewart, 1993). Types of theories range from **personal theories,** which are private understandings about the issue of concern, to **formal theories,** which are publicly articulated, published, and validated to varying degrees by scientific study. For example, one occupational therapy student indicated that she had learned to suspect a violent or abusive cause whenever a woman came to the clinic with tendon and nerve injuries from lacerations to the palms of her hands. The student had noticed, while working as an aide, that such women described using their hands to protect their faces when attacked by abusers using knives and hence would get knife wounds on the palms of their hands. This is an example of a personal theory, because the student had never really even talked about her observations, much less researched or published her impressions. However, her personal theory did serve to guide her thinking to some degree. Alternately, another student might find that she was able to use information from both cognitive and occupational behavior theories to understand why a client in a nursing home did not seem motivated to dress herself or to take her medications. In this case, the student is using one or more formal theories to support her clinical reasoning. Practitioners have access to an increasing number of formal theories that they can use to guide their practice.

Readers may also come across other terms related to theories, such as practice models and frames of reference. Generally, such terms are used to describe the level of development or complexity of a theory or as a way to differentiate practice guidelines from more formal theory (Mosey, 1992). For purposes of this chapter, these distinctions are not so important. More critical is the ability to understand the differing purposes or scopes of major theories used in the profession, the components of these theories, and how well these theories have been validated by research and found useful in practice. Table 17-1 provides

TABLE 17–1. **DEFINITIONS OF COMMONLY USED TERMS**[a]

Term	Definition	Function	Examples
Paradigm	Provides a conceptual structure for understanding the world; within a profession, provides an accepted orienting structure for the profession, its values, beliefs, and knowledge	Supports a field's identity by providing a common focus	Through engagement in occupations, people find meaning, health, and well-being
Professional model	Delineates and defines the scope or area of concern for a profession; articulates the overall beliefs and knowledge of the profession; is derived from the profession's paradigm	Defines the scope of practice	*Occupational Therapy Practice Framework*
Theory	Describes an image or provides an explanation of why or how a phenomenon occurs and how that phenomenon can be controlled	Organizes observations and understandings for easier use	See both formal and personal theories for examples
Formal theory	Explains observable events or relationships by stating a series of abstract propositions or principles; based on systematic research with carefully defined concepts and explanations of relationships among these concepts	Systematically explains predicts, or describes phenomena	Model of Human Occupation; Ecology of Human Performance; Occupational Adaptation; Person–Environment Occupation Model
Personal theory	Private understandings based on experience	Helps individuals articulate their experience	A practitioner's theory that her female clients' hand wounds are the result of protecting themselves from physical abuse
Frame of reference	Guides practice by delineating the beliefs, assumptions, definitions, and concepts within a specific area of practice; drawn from a theoretical base and has a particular view of the function–dysfunction continuum; delineates evaluation processes and intervention strategies that are consistent with the theoretical base	Guides a specific area of practice	Sensory integration; self-advocacy; rehabilitation; *American Occupational Therapy Association Practice Guidelines*

[a]Reprinted from Kielhofner (1997), McColl et al. (1993), Morse (1997), Mosey (1992), and Turner (1986).

definitions of theoretical terms commonly used in occupational therapy literature.

SCOPE OF PRACTICE

Broadly accepted professional knowledge about occupational therapy is often articulated in major documents approved and published by professional organizations, such as the American Occupational Therapy Association and the Canadian Occupational Therapy Association. These documents, such as the *Guide to Occupational Therapy Practice* (Moyers, 1999), *Occupational Therapy Practice Framework* (American Occupational Therapy Association [AOTA], in press), and the Canadian model of occupational performance (Townsend, 1997) serve as general guides to the profession and define its **scope of practice.** They provide frameworks that delimit the profession's range of interest and focus attention on those aspects of human functioning that are of greatest concern to occupational therapy practitioners (Moyers, 1999). Such documents often attempt to distill the assumptions, knowledge, values, and beliefs commonly accepted throughout the profession (Mosey, 1981) and evolve to reflect the changing nature of professional practice. The knowledge base is derived from research in occupational therapy, occupational science, and disciplines beyond the field.

Although such documents are useful in helping frame the general concerns of the profession and as such serve as good starting points for students, they rarely reflect the detailed information provided by various formal theories. Formal theories explain observable events or relationships by stating a series of abstract propositions or principles. These theories are based on systematic research and carefully defined concepts and explanations of the relationships among those concepts (Turner, 1986). Formal theories are publicly shared through presentations at professional meetings and publications in research journals and texts. This public sharing promotes critical analysis of theoretical assumptions, which in turn serves to gradually refine theories in response to continued analysis and research.

WHY IS THEORY IMPORTANT?

One of the most perplexing issues for occupational therapy students as they go into the field is the frequency with which they find practitioners who cannot immediately tell them the specific theory being used in a given intervention session. Such experiences can lead students to wonder why learning theory is important. It is helpful to think about how practitioners use theory and why theory is important. First, theory is important because it is part of the knowledge base of the field and an essential aspect of each practitioner's professional paradigm (Argyris & Schön, 1974). However, practitioners do not necessarily retain the sources of the knowledge that form their professional paradigm. For instance, practitioners are generally ethical in their practice, but few would be able to list all the specific terms associated with their ethical knowledge. With increased experience, practitioners tend to integrate knowledge in such a way that it becomes automatic (Argyris & Schön, 1974; Schön, 1983, 1987). Think about how infrequently experienced drivers pay attention to the mechanics of operating a car. In the same way, practitioners' use of theoretical knowledge becomes automatic, and they "just do" therapy. So, although theoretical knowledge may be embedded in the professional paradigm, it is part of the data practitioners bring to the

RESEARCH NOTE 17–1

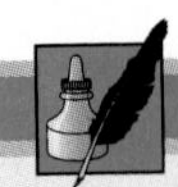

Theories Provide Conceptual Scaffolding and Show Relationships among Variables

KENNETH J. OTTENBACHER

Theories have multiple functions in practicing professions such as occupational therapy. Theories provide a conceptual scaffolding for the interpretation of observations and are used to explain practice by showing how variables and events are related. For instance, a theory of motor learning might explain the relationship between feedback and feedforward mechanisms in the learning, performance, and retention of a sensorimotor skill such as buttoning a shirt. Theories also help summarize existing knowledge and point out directions for new research.

A theory is most useful when it helps a therapist predict what will occur in treatment. A theory of motivation and compliance might assist a therapist in predicting which clients are most likely to engage in specific intervention activities and which clients are likely to resist those same activities. One important goal of research is to confirm the predictions derived from theories. Ideas and clinical hunches that are systematically examined by research may lead to theory (induction), or research may be used to test existing theory (deduction). This circular process of integrating research and theory helps provide a dynamic clinical environment in which theories improve practice and practice advances theory. Many opportunities exist for occupational therapy researchers to advance existing theory and improve practice. For example, research on psychosocial theories of depression has shown that depression can be averted when people are given an opportunity to gain personal meaning from everyday occupations and when they believe that there is choice and control in their lives (Kapci, 1998). These are activities inherent in many occupational therapy intervention programs.

Kapci, E. G. (1998). Test of the hopelessness theory of depression: Drawing negative inferences from negative life events. *Psychological Reports*, 82, 355–363.

TABLE 17-2. **EVALUATING THEORETICAL KNOWLEDGE FOR ACTION**

General Question	Specific Questions
What theory or theories are embedded in your practice?	• What theoretical knowledge do you use? • Which theories are personal and which are public?
What is the theory's focus?	• Who developed the theory? • What is it trying to explain? • What kind of clients or settings was it intended for? • How well does it match your therapy needs?
How do you know?	• On what data is this knowledge based? • What literature relates to this knowledge? • How relevant is the literature to your needs?
How well do you know?	• How was the knowledge developed? • How were the data collected? • How were data analyzed and interpreted? • What were the research circumstances?
How will your understanding shape your practice decisions?	• How does the theory enhance your understanding? • What are its strengths and limitations? • How does this information affirm your current approaches? • How does it contradict your current approaches? • What different approaches will you use based on your understanding?
What additional information do you need?	• What further questions do you have? • What sources can help answer those questions? • How will you access this information?

Adapted from Watson (2000)

therapeutic encounter (Rogers, 1983, 1986). It helps practitioners name and frame the problems they encounter (Parham, 1987, Schön, 1983, 1987).

Theory may be particularly important for new practitioners, who have little experience to draw on. It can be seen as borrowed experience, a thinking frame (Neistadt, 1998), or a metaphor (Parham, 1987) to assist new practitioners in their clinical reasoning. For experienced practitioners, theory helps their reflective processes as they work to articulate reasons for their actions and evaluate the effectiveness of those actions in light of existing theory and the responses of their clients. The current emphasis on evidence-based practice in health care is an attempt to have all practitioners be more systematic in understanding the sources and validity of knowledge they use in practice. For practice to improve, it is practitioners' ethical responsibility, routinely and systematically, to check their professional paradigms against emerging theory and research.

EVALUATING KNOWLEDGE AND REFLECTIVE INQUIRY

It is essential to view theory as evolving knowledge. It is not a fixed, objective truth. Because theory involves the evolution of knowledge—whether it is formal theory or personal theory derived from professional experience and reflective inquiry—it needs constant examination and testing. This can involve continued research about the theory, critical examination of the research supporting the theory, or the reflective inquiry described by Schön (1983) and summarized in Chapter 12. Table 17-2 lists six questions that practitioners can use to guide the process of examining theoretical knowledge. These questions can be used to promote examination of published research and theories as well as to guide practitioner reflections on specific practice situations.

CONCLUSION

It is essential for a profession to have a base of knowledge grounded in well-articulated and specified theories that, in turn, provide scientific support for practice and test the effectiveness of occupational therapy interventions. The remaining chapters in this unit summarize many of the current theories and frames of reference in occupational therapy. These form the knowledge base of the profession and are an important aspect of practitioners' professional paradigm. These theories address occupational behavior, rehabilitation, development, and learning; all areas central to knowledge development and practice in occupational therapy. One of the challenges of professional practice is the need to bridge the gap between current theoretical knowledge and practitioners' use of such knowledge within their professional paradigm. Taking a reflective stance toward practice assists practitioners in understanding their clinical reasoning and in exploring the theoretical underpinnings of that process.

References

American Occupational Therapy Association, [AOTA]. (In press). Occupational therapy practice framework: Domain and process. *American Journal of Occupational Therapy*.

Argyris, C., & Schön, D. A. (1974). *Theory in practice: Increasing professional effectiveness*. San Francisco: Jossey-Bass.

Cervero, R. M. (1988). *Effective continuing education for professionals*. San Francisco: Jossey

Griswold, L. A. (1995). *Professionalization of occupational therapists: A study of emergent identities*. Unpublished doctoral dissertation, University of New Hampshire, Durham.

Hooper, B. (1997). The relationship between pretheoretical assumptions and clinical reasoning. *American Journal of Occupational Therapy, 51*, 328–338.

Kielhofner, G. (1997). *Conceptual foundations of occupational therapy* (2nd ed.). Philadelphia: Davis.

McColl, M. A., Law, M., & Stewart, D. (1993). *Theoretical basis of occupational therapy: An annotated bibliography of applied theory in the professional literature*. Thorofare, NJ: Slack.

Morse, J. M. (1997). Considering theory derived from qualitative research. In J. M. Morse (Ed.). *Completing a qualitative project: Details and dialogue* (pp. 163–188). Thousand Oaks, CA: Sage.

Mosey, A. C. (1981). *Occupational therapy: Configuration of a profession*. New York: Raven.

Mosey, A. C. (1992). *Applied scientific inquiry in the health professions: An epistemological orientation*. Rockville, MD: American Occupational Therapy Association.

Moyers, P. A. (1999). Guide to occupational therapy practice. *American Journal of Occupational Therapy, 53*, 247–322.

Neistadt, M. E. (1998). Teaching clinical reasoning as a thinking frame. *American Journal of Occupational Therapy, 52*, 221–229.

Parham, D. (1987). Toward professionalism: The reflective therapist. *American Journal of Occupational Therapy, 41*, 555–561.

Rogers, J. C. (1983). Clinical reasoning: The ethics, science, and art. *American Journal of Occupational Therapy, 37*, 601–616.

Rogers, J. C. (1986). Clinical judgment: The bridge between theory and practice. In American Occupational Therapy Association (Ed.). *Target 2000: Occupational therapy education* [Proceedings]. Rockville, MD: Editor.

Schön, D. A. (1983). *The reflective practitioner: How professionals think in action*. New York: Basic Books.

Schön, D. A. (1987). *Educating the reflective practitioner*. San Francisco: Jossey-Bass.

Törnebohm, H. (1991). What is worth knowing in occupational therapy. *American Journal of Occupational Therapy, 45*, 451–454.

Townsend, E. (Ed.). (1997). *Enabling occupation: An occupational therapy perspective*. Ottawa, Ont.: Canadian Occupational Therapy Association.

Turner, J. H. (1986). *The structure of sociological theory* (4th ed.). Belmont, CA: Wadsworth.

Watson, G. H. (2000). Oh no! Its theory O! *Quality Progress, 33*(10), 16.

CHAPTER 18

THEORIES DERIVED FROM OCCUPATIONAL BEHAVIOR PERSPECTIVES

SECTION I

An Overview of Occupational Behavior

LAURA BARRETT
GARY KIELHOFNER

During the 1960s and 1970s, Mary Reilly, with her colleagues and graduate students, developed a theoretical tradition at the University of Southern California that has had a broad and lasting influence on the field of occupational therapy. As Reilly (1969) argued, the purpose of occupational behavior was to articulate a general theory of occupational therapy "that would explain why occupation was the media and method of the field" (p. 303). In what remains the most central paper of this tradition, Reilly (1962) stated its central premise: "that man, through the use of his hands as they are energized by his mind and will, can influence the state of his own health" (p. 2).

HISTORICAL CONTEXT OF OCCUPATIONAL BEHAVIOR

Reilly's effort to develop occupational behavior came at a time when the field had built a strong alliance with medicine (Kielhofner & Burke, 1977; Shannon, 1972). Reilly challenged the field to consider that medicine's influence had resulted in occupational therapy losing sight of its original purpose and mission. In particular, she argued that occupational therapy had failed to achieve the promise of the vision of its founders concerning the potential of occupation as a force in the health of humans. Following medicine's lead, occupational therapy defined the impact of patient engagement in activity in narrow terms based on biomedical and psychoanalytic knowledge. Reilly (1969) argued that it was important to distinguish occupational therapy from medicine, noting: "It is the task of medicine to prevent and reduce illness; while the task of occupational therapy is to prevent and reduce the incapacities resulting from illness" (p. 300). Based on the recognition that occupational therapy had a different purpose from medicine, Reilly stressed building a base of knowledge about occupation and its impact on human welfare from the point of view of the social sciences. Hence the concepts of occupational behavior are mainly based on ideas from philosophy, psychology, social psychology, sociology, and anthropology.

DEFINITION AND THEMES OF OCCUPATIONAL BEHAVIOR

Occupational Behavior Defined

Occupational behavior consists of those activities that occupy a person's time, involve achievement, and address the economic realities of life (Reilly, 1962, 1966). Occupational behavior is longitudinal in the sense that it constitutes the complete developmental continuum from childhood play to adult work (Black, 1976; Moorhead, 1969; Reilly, 1962; Shannon, 1972). Occupational behavior involves the daily routine of work, play, and rest within a physical, temporal, and social environment (Matsutsuyu, 1971; Shannon, 1972). Moreover, occupational behavior involves interaction with the complex, interrelated environments in which people function (Dunning, 1972; Gray, 1972; Parent, 1978; Reilly, 1966).

Occupational Behavior Themes

Work and Play Adaptation

The concepts of occupation and adaptation are closely linked. To begin with, occupation is the landscape on which the person adapts. From birth on, the human being is challenged to deal with the necessary tasks of everyday living. This process begins with the infant's struggle to overcome gravity, proceeds through learning the necessary tasks of self-care and cultural competency, and culminates in the challenge of taking on adult responsibility for productivity (Black, 1976; Matsutsuyu, 1971; Reilly, 1962).

Adaptation in occupation requires that individuals have and exercise basic occupational skills, including motor, social decision-making, time use, self-care, and specific work and play abilities (Black, 1976; Kielhofner, 1977; Shannon, 1972). When these occupational skills are intact, the person is able to adapt; when illness or disability compromise these skills, adaptation is threatened. Hence, occupational behavior calls attention to how disease and disability affect occupational skills and to how these skills can be optimized in the face of chronic impairments.

People cope and adapt in their lives through engagement in occupations. This idea is contained in a range of writing emphasizing that human adaptation through occupation involves the ability to fill time, to find meaning, and to contribute productively to society (Florey, 1969; Kielhofner, 1977; Matsutsuyu, 1971; Reilly, 1962). Occupation is also a means of generating the capacity for adaptation. For example, in play the child learns and integrates the rules and skills that will be required in later life (Robinson, 1977). Through play, children experience, explore, and test the world and learn about their own capacities, how the world responds to their efforts, and what expectations others have for their behavior (Hurff, 1980; Michelman, 1971; Robinson, 1977). Finally, people adapt through occupation because they respond to the expectations of society and validate themselves as social members (Matsutsuyu, 1971).

The Motivation for Occupation

The human need to exercise capacity and to achieve a degree of personal mastery over self and the environment is central to Reilly's (1962) argument. Much thinking at the time was dominated by the psychoanalytic and behavioral tradition that emphasized sexual and physiological needs; consequently, Reilly's assertion of the need for mastery and filling life with occupation was an important turning point for the field.

Occupation is intrinsically motivating; as a result, people engage in occupation for its own sake—that is, for the rewards of learning, control, and mastery that occur in the midst of performance (Florey, 1969). The intrinsic motive of occupation changes over the life span, beginning with the early motive of curiosity, which fuels exploration; proceeding to a competency motive for learning, and ultimately to the adult motive for achievement (Florey, 1969; Reilly, 1966, 1974).

Experiencing oneself as an agent able to achieve desired outcomes is the product of healthy occupation; it also is the foundation for being motivated to engage in occupation (Burke, 1977). When occupation is prevented or disturbed, this sense of competence is threatened. Interest as expressed in occupational engagement provides an outlet for personal needs and expression of capacity. Knowing a person's interests is the key to knowing how he or she is individually motivated (Borys, 1974).

Overall, the focus on motivation within the occupational behavior tradition is important for underscoring two points. The first is recognizing that humans have a psychological need for occupation and that when they lack occupation they suffer. The second is attending to the subjective, experiential aspect of occupation along with the objective, functional dimension.

Temporal Adaptation

Occupation is the main way that people occupy time, and this perspective spawned interest in the theme of temporality. This theme of temporality can be traced back to the founders of the field, who emphasized that health could be measured by how effectively people filled time with activity (Kielhofner, 1977; Shannon, 1972). Two ideas to emerge from this interest in temporality were balance and habits.

Achieving an appropriate balance between the demanding activities of work and the restorative activities of play and rest were seen as essential to health (Kielhofner, 1977; Shannon, 1972). Health is realized in the rhythm of alternating forms of activity and rest and the quality of those behaviors that fill time. A lack of balance can, of itself, constitute a failure in healthy living. Therefore, when impairment disrupts the balance of occupational life, it is important to restore that balance.

Habits are the basic structures that give order to daily behavior in time (Kielhofner, 1977). Habits account for behaviors that become automatic when repeated over time. Furthermore, habits integrate skills into routines of action organized to meet the daily demands of life. Hence it is not sufficient just to have basic occupational skills; rather, those skills have to be organized into behavioral patterns that fulfill environmental expectations and achieve balance.

HISTORICAL NOTE 18–1

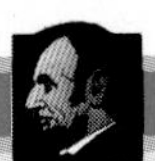

Slagle's Use of Habit Training: Practice Based on Reason

SUZANNE M. PELOQUIN

Eleanor Clarke Slagle, one of the founders of the Society for the Promotion of Occupational Therapy, taught habit training to patients with mental illness. Believing that occupations could be useful and even curative when done habitually, she selected patients who were regressed and chronically ill.

Each patient in habit training was encouraged to get into a routine and to then assume responsibility for it. Excerpts from one patient's case convey a sense of the practice:

> ***May 3, 1926—Admitted to habit training. Will not dress or undress self. Clothing untidy and unbuttoned. Wets and soils the bed. Eats excessively. Masturbation frequent.***
> ***June 1 to June 30—Washes and dresses self. Wets and soils less frequently. Polishes floor when continuously supervised. Does low-grade occupation.***
> ***July 10 to September 22, 1926—Speaks occasionally. Told superintendent that he was "slightly improved." Works on braid-weave rug. Helps attendant with cleaning and clears dishes from table at meals. Appetite more normal. (Wilson, 1929, pp. 196–197)***

The belief that treatment needed to be directed by reason and purpose predated more current discussions of theory and frames of reference. Since the profession's inception, hypotheses about the nature of a patient's problems and the effects of a therapist's actions have helped guide treatment.

Wilson, S. C. (1929). Habit training for mental cases. *Occupational Therapy and Rehabilitation*, 8, 189–197.

Occupational Roles

The concept of **roles** provides a way of thinking about human interaction with the task-oriented environment (Moorhead, 1969). Roles mediate between the requirements of the social environment and the contributions of the individual. They are behavioral expectations that accompany a person's occupied position or status in a social system and serve as the primary means through which individuals express occupational behavior (Heard, 1977). Occupational roles begin with the play of the child; proceed through the familial, friendship, and student roles; continue in the adult work role; and culminate in the role of retiree. This sequence of occupational roles is referred to as the occupational career (Black, 1976; Heard, 1977; Kielhofner, 1977; Matsutsuyu, 1971; Moorhead, 1969; Reilly, 1966).

Two role-related concepts are (1) socialization, the series of environmentally based learning experiences (e.g., role modeling, experiences with chores) by which individuals come to acquire necessary role attitudes and behaviors, and (2) the process of occupational choice, through which people select and commit themselves to occupational roles (Matsutsuyu, 1971; Moorhead, 1969).

THE IMPACT OF OCCUPATIONAL BEHAVIOR ON THE FIELD

Occupational behavior was designed to be a theory that informed occupational therapy practice. Because the concepts of occupational behavior were deemed complex and multifaceted, case method was the primary means of exploring the applicability of occupational behavior concepts (Line, 1969; Reilly, 1969). Many occupational behavior articles attempted to illustrate the relevance of concepts to practice through case presentations. These efforts not withstanding, the occupational behavior tradition was criticized as being difficult to apply in practice. One example of such criticism was Mosey's (1986) observation that the occupational behavior tradition contained no less than 28 different papers that met her criteria for frames of reference. Given such diversity, she wondered whether the body of knowledge was too disparate to be effectively applied.

The impact of occupational behavior on occupational therapy is probably not best measured by its direct application in practice. Rather, its importance lies in its overall influence on the directions of the field and its richness in generating new traditions. Three effects are probably most notable:

- Occupational behavior has been successful in calling occupational therapy's attention to the need to emancipate itself from medicine and define its practice around the construct of occupation. Since the late twentieth century, this process has been described as building a paradigm for the field (Kielhofner, 1997). From this point of view, occupational behavior can be said to have been responsible for generating the field's present paradigm.
- The occupational behavior tradition is the basis for the occupational science movement currently centered at the University of Southern California. Proponents of occupational science are attempting to build a scientific discipline around the study of occupation.
- The occupational behavior tradition is the foundation out of which the model of human occupation (Kielhofner, 2002) and other occupation-based frames of reference developed. The remaining sections of this chapter delineate some of these models.

Largely, the aim of these models has been to synthesize many of the themes of occupational behavior into a framework suitable to guide practice.

CONCLUSION

In the end, occupational behavior is probably best appreciated on two accounts. First, as this chapter illustrates, the literature of occupational behavior is still a rich source of now-classical arguments and papers in the field. Second, occupational behavior is historically important for having shaped the identity and direction of occupational therapy and for having provided the foundations for modern scholarship and practice.

SECTION II

The Model of Human Occupation

GARY KIELHOFNER
KIRSTY FORSYTH
LAURA BARRETT

INTELLECTUAL HERITAGE

The Model of Human Occupation (MOHO) grew out efforts to articulate a theory to guide practice that reflected a focus on occupation. It was first introduced in the 1980s (Kielhofner & Burke, 1980) and was discussed in texts that reflect the cumulative refinements of the theory and its application (Kielhofner, 1985, 1995, 2002). Today, MOHO includes contributions from researchers and practitioners throughout the world. It provides a way of thinking about people's occupational adaptation and about the process of therapy. Its concepts address motivation for occupation, the routine patterning of occupations, the nature of skilled performance, and the influence of environment on occupation (Fig. 18-1). The model provides a broad framework for gathering data about a client's circumstances, for generating an understanding of the client's occupational strengths and limitations, and for selecting and implementing a course of occupational therapy.

ASSUMPTIONS OF MOHO

MOHO incorporates a systems view of the human being that emphasizes two main points. The first point is that

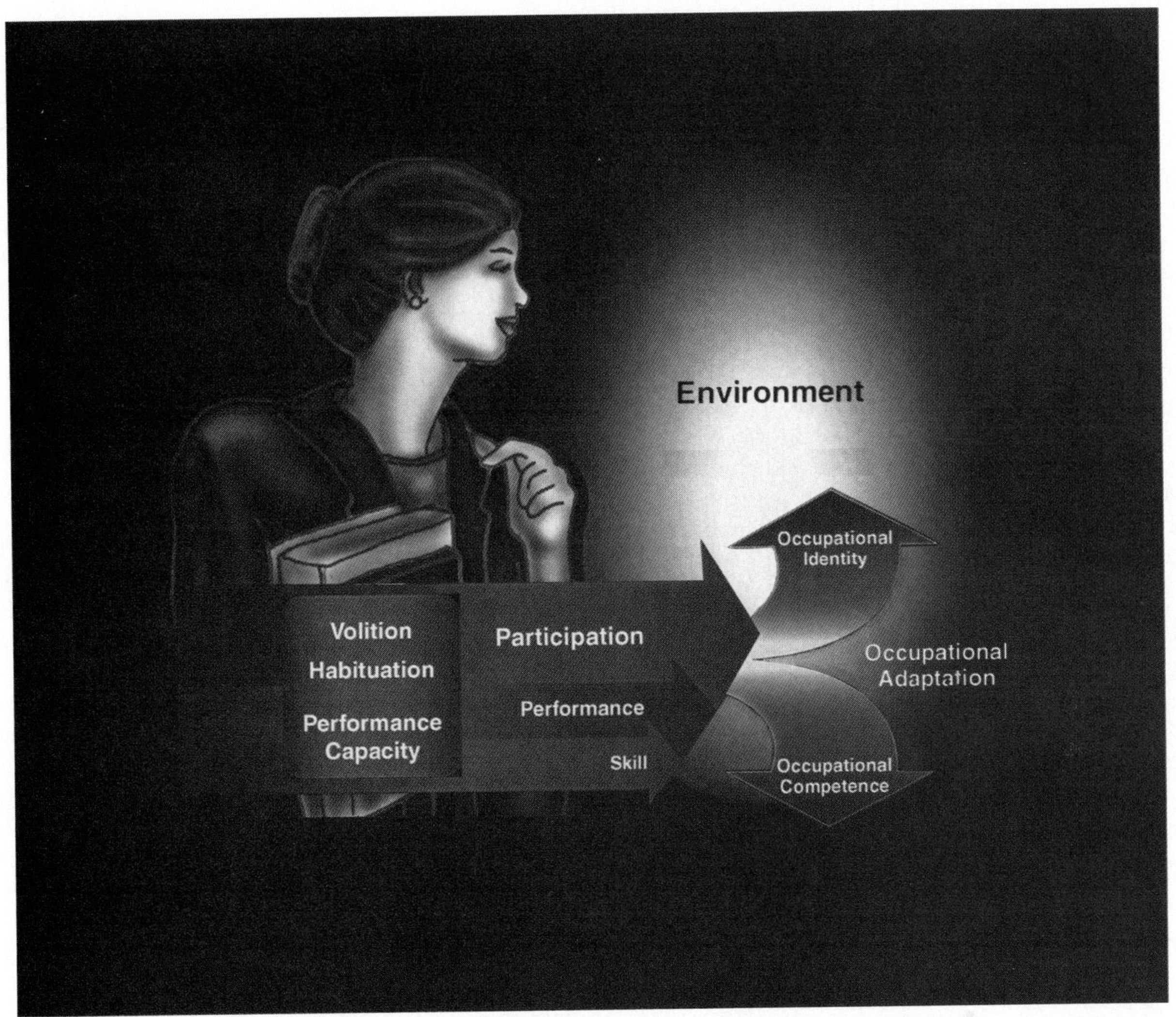

FIGURE 18–1. The process of occupational adaptation. (Reprinted with permission from Kielhofner, 2002.)

behavior is dynamic and context dependent. That is, a person's inner characteristics interact with the environment to create a network of conditions that influence a person's motivation, actions, and performance. The second point is that occupation is essential to self-organization. That is, by doing things, people maintain or alter their capacities and generate ongoing experiences that affirm or reshape their motivation. Therefore, people's characteristics reflect what they have done in the past. Consistent with this principle, the model views therapy as a process by which people are helped to do things in order to shape their abilities, self-concepts, and identities. MOHO envisions occupational therapy as engaging people in occupation, which helps maintain, restore, or reorganize their occupational lives.

The following statements characterize this model's implicit assumptions:

- Occupational adaptation is dynamic and context dependent; therefore, what a person does in work, play, and self-care is a function of the interaction among person, characteristics of motivation, life patterns, and performance capacity with the environment. All clients have the potential for change and to become more occupationally adaptive through occupational therapy.
- Occupation is essential to self-organization; therefore, the central mechanisms of change in therapy are what the client does and what the client thinks and feels about his or her doing.
- Client occupational problems tend to be complex and deserve the careful attention of a comprehensive theoretical approach and well-developed tools of intervention.
- Practitioners must actively use theory as a way to understand clients and decide the course of occupational therapy.
- MOHO-based intervention is client centered; the unique characteristics of the client should inform

intervention and should be based on a collaborative approach with the client.

BASIC MOHO CONCEPTS

To explain how occupations are chosen, patterned, and performed, MOHO conceptualizes the human as composed of three elements: volition, habituation, and performance capacity. *Volition* refers to the process by which persons are motivated toward and choose what they do. *Habituation* refers to a process whereby people organize their actions into patterns and routines. *Performance capacity* refers both to people's underlying objective mental and physical abilities and to their lived experience that shapes performance. These concepts are discussed in greater detail in the following subsections.

Volition

At the core of volition are thoughts and feelings about doing things, such as enjoying, valuing, and feeling competent. The thoughts and feelings people have about doing things ultimately concern the issues of mastery, enjoyment, and valuation of what they have done. Consequently, volitional thoughts and feelings pertain to:

- A person's effectiveness in acting on the world.
- What the person holds as important.
- What the person finds enjoyable and satisfying.

These three areas are referred to as personal causation, values, and interests, respectively.

Personal Causation

Personal causation refers to people's capacities and effectiveness. People all observe themselves through the commonsense lens of their culture, building up a store of knowledge about what kinds of capacities they have in relationship to their environmental demands and expectations. As people do things, they generate thoughts, along with feelings of confidence or insecurity, about their physical, mental, and social abilities. They reflect on how effective they are in using their capacities to achieve their desired outcome. Consequently, people also develop thoughts and feelings about their effectiveness in using their capacities and the compliance or resistance of their environment to their efforts.

Values

Choices for occupations are also influenced by values. Values are composed of beliefs and commitments that define what is good, right, and important (Grossack & Gardner, 1970; Kalish & Collier, 1981; Klavins, 1972; Lee, 1971; Smith, 1969). They influence people's views of what is worth doing and the proper way to act. Values are felt as obligations, and people cannot behave contrary to their values without feeling guilty or inadequate. Conversely, people experience a sense of belonging and correctness when they enact their values.

Values specify what is worth doing, how to perform, and what goals or aspirations deserve commitment. Because values belong to a commonsense, cultural view of life, they are usually associated with strong emotions (e.g., feelings of security, worthiness, belonging, or accomplishment) (Bruner, 1990).

Interests

The experience of pleasure and satisfaction in occupation generates interests. Interests begin with natural dispositions (e.g., the tendency to enjoy physical or intellectual activity). They further develop through the acquisition of tastes generated from the experience of pleasure and satisfaction derived from occupational engagement (Matsutsuyu, 1969). Therefore, the development of interests depends on available opportunities to engage in occupations.

Being interested in an occupation means feeling attraction based on anticipation of positive experience. This attraction may come from positive feelings associated with such factors as the exercise of capacity, intellectual or physical challenge, fellowship with others, or aesthetic stimulation. People are more likely to enjoy what they can perform with some level of proficiency. Each person has a unique preference for certain occupations or for particular ways of performing.

Volitional Processes

Together, personal causation, values, and interests contribute to a pattern of thoughts and feelings embedded in a cycle of anticipation, choice, involvement, and subsequent interpretation. Volition predisposes people to attend to the world and anticipate possibilities for action in particular ways. That is, their attraction to occupations, beliefs about capacity, and convictions about performance primarily influence what they notice and search out in the world. People make both activity and occupational choices. The former are everyday choices for action, and the latter are choices concerning occupations that will become an extended or permanent part of their lives.

Habituation

Habituation organizes behavior into recurrent patterns that are integrated into the rhythms and customs of the physical, social, and temporal world. Repeated action within specific contexts establishes habituated patterns of doing. By virtue of developing a way of doing something likely to be repeated, habituation evokes the very actions that sustain it. Habituated patterns of action are governed by habits and roles. Together, they weave the patterns in which people typically traverse their days, weeks, and seasons; their homes, neighborhoods, and cities; and their families, work organizations, and communities.

Habits

Habits involve learned ways of doing things that unfold automatically. Through repeated experience, people acquire a kind of map for appreciating and behaving in familiar environments. Habits operate in cooperation with context, using and incorporating the environment as a resource for routine doing (Dewey, 1922). Because of habits, people intuitively know when it is time to leave for work, what turns to take when driving there, and what step comes next when performing a familiar work task. Habits locate people in the unfolding events and places of everyday life and steer their behavior in the right direction. Habits influence how people perform routine activities, use time, and behave.

Roles

Internalized roles give people an identity and a sense of the obligations that go with that identity. People see themselves as students, workers, and parents and recognize that they should behave in certain ways to fulfill those roles. Much of what people do is done *as* a spouse, parent, worker, student, and so on. The expectations that others hold for a role and the nature of the social system in which each role is located serve as guides for learning how to behave within most roles. Thus, through interaction with others, people internalize an identity, an outlook, and a way of behaving that belongs to the role (Sarbin & Scheibe, 1983). Once internalized, this role serves as a kind of framework for looking out on the world and for acting. Roles shape behavior. Therefore, when people engage in an occupation within a given role, that role may be reflected in their style of dress, their demeanor, and their actions. Roles place expectations on people for task performance and for time use, thereby providing structure and regularity to life and channeling people's actions into necessary patterns and tasks. Because of roles and habits, most routines of daily life unfold automatically and predictably. Habituation allows people to appreciate and cooperate with their physical, temporal, and sociocultural ecologies to do routine behavior efficiently and automatically.

Performance Capacity

The capacity for performance is affected by the status of musculoskeletal, neurological, cardiopulmonary, and other bodily systems that are called on when doing things. Performance also calls on mental, or cognitive, abilities such as memory and planning. Occupational therapy models have addressed the problem of performance capacity from an objective point of view, focusing on physical and mental capacities as phenomena that can be observed, measured, and modified (Ayres, 1972, 1979, 1986; Trombly, 1989).

A new perspective within MOHO (Kielhofner, Baz, Hutson, & Tham, 2002) offers a different but complimentary way of addressing performance capacity. This view of performance focuses on subjective experience and its role in human performance. The approach brings the concepts of mind and body together, demonstrating how they are dual aspects of the same thing. It also offers a way of going beyond current concepts of body and mind to understand how the body is mindful and the mind, embodied. These concepts emphasize how the body has an intelligence of its own, especially as it pertains to everyday performance, and that the foundations of abstract mental processes are found in bodily experience (Husserl, 1962; Merleau-Ponty, 1962).

Contribution of the Environment to Occupational Adaptation

Just as components of the person are interrelated and interdependent, people and their environments are also inseparable. MOHO conceptualizes the environment as consisting of both a social and a physical dimension. These offer opportunities, resources, demands, and constraints that have a potential impact on the person. The physical environment consists of the natural and human-made spaces and the objects within them. The social environment consists of groups of individuals and the occupational forms that members of those groups perform (Nelson, 1988). Groups provide and assign roles to their members and constitute social space in which those roles are enacted, according to group ambiance, norms, and climate. Thus groups allow and prescribe the kinds of things their members can do. Occupational forms are rule-bound sequences of action that are oriented to a purpose, sustained in collective knowledge, culturally recognizable, and named. Said simply, occupational forms are the things that are available to do in any social context (Nelson, 1988).

Any performance setting consists of spaces, objects, occupational forms, and/or social groups. Typical settings for occupational forms are the home, neighborhood, school, or workplace. Whether and how the characteristics of the physical and social environment of a setting influence people depends on their values, interests, personal causation, roles, habits, and performance capacities. Because each individual is unique in regard to these aspects of the self, any environment will have somewhat different effects on those within it.

Interactions of Volition, Habituation, Performance Capacity, and the Environment

The things people do and how they think and feel about them reflect a complex interplay of motives, habits and roles, abilities, and the environment. Volition, habituation, and performance capacity always operate in concert with each other and the environment, making simultaneous contributions to participation. Occupational adaptation cannot be fully understood without reference to these contributing factors. Every moment is potentially infused with influences from and interactions with volition, habituation, and performance capacity. These parts of the person and the environment resonate together, creating conditions out of which thoughts, feelings, and doing emerge. Examples of such resonance are the anxiety from a lack of belief in skill that interferes with performance and is exacerbated by environmental demands, old habits reinforced by the environment's interference with new volitional choices, and the pull of values that maintain motivation despite pain caused by engagement in a valued activity. In these and other circumstances, values, interests, personal causation, roles, habits, performance capacity, and the environment are always tethered into a dynamic whole. What people do, think, and feel come out of that dynamic whole.

Skills

Within occupational performance, we carry out discrete purposeful actions. For example, making coffee is a culturally recognizable occupational form in many Western cultures. To do so, one engages in such purposeful actions as *gathering* together coffee, coffee maker, and cup; *handling* these materials and objects; and sequencing the steps necessary to brew and pour the coffee. The actions that make up occupational performance are referred to as skills. Skills are goal-directed actions that a person uses while performing (Fisher, 1998; Fisher & Kielhofner, 1995; Forsyth, Salamy, Simon, & Kielhofner, 1998).

In contrast to performance capacity, which refers to underlying ability, skill refers to discrete functional actions. There are three types of skills: motor skills, process skills, and communication and interaction skills. Detailed taxonomies of the functional actions that make up each of the three types of skills have been developed as part of the process of creating assessments of skill. Fisher (1998) and colleagues (Bernspang & Fisher, 1995; Doble, 1991) have developed the taxonomies of motor and process skills that make up the Assessment of Motor and Process Skills (AMPS). Forsyth, Lai, and Kielhofner (1999) and Forsyth, Salamy, Simon, and Kielhofner (1998) developed a taxonomy of communication and interaction skills that make up the Assessment of Communication/Interaction Skills (ACIS).

Occupational Identity and Competence

Over time, what people do creates their occupational identity. This identity, generated from experience, is the cumulative sense of who people are and wish to become as occupational beings. The degree to which people are able to sustain a pattern of doing that enacts their occupational identity is referred to as occupational competence. The two essential elements of occupational adaptation entail the creation of an occupational identity and the ability to enact this identity in a variety of circumstances.

APPLYING THE MODEL IN PRACTICE

Problems encountered in volition, habituation, performance capacity, and the environment may all contribute to an individual becoming disengaged from his or her occupations. When this is the case, the occupational therapy practitioner uses MOHO as a framework for understanding the interrelated factors that contribute to occupational dysfunction. The therapist evaluating a particular client will discover the unique way in which these factors are involved in that person's occupational adaptation and dysfunction. In assessment, therapists collect information to answer questions they generate from this theoretical perspective.

Table 18-1 lists examples of clinical questions derived from MOHO. These questions and observations can be used if the therapist is using a fairly situated method of gathering data. Table 18-2 shows the standardized assessment tools that have been developed from this conceptual model of practice and how they relate to the theory's constructs. These tools provide relatively structured and standardized ways of collecting MOHO-based information, if it is required. MOHO identifies what volitional, habit, and performance changes can be anticipated from engaging clients in occupational forms (Kielhofner, 2002). It also identifies the kinds of therapeutic strategies that will support these client changes (Kielhofner, 2002).

RESEARCH

More than 80 studies on MOHO have been completed and published since the 1980s. A full reference list may be found on line (www.uic.edu/hsc/acad/cahp/OT/MOHOC). The amount of research on this model is steadily increasing. Moreover, studies of MOHO are becoming more methodologically sophisticated, since a tradition of research has been established. This research includes studies that tested MOHO concepts and led to refinement of the theory. It also includes research that examined how MOHO-based assessments work in practice, how its concepts influence therapeutic reasoning, what happens in therapy, and the outcomes achieved from therapy based on MOHO. MOHO has been studied with a wide range of quantitative and qualitative research methods. Much of the research has taken place across national and cultural boundaries, which has provided evidence for cross-cultural relevance of the model. Future priorities for MOHO research are to determine more accurately the mechanism of change that underlies MOHO-based

TABLE 18–1. **CLINICAL QUESTIONS RELATED TO MOHO CONSTRUCTS**

MOHO Construct	Clinical Question
Person	
Personal causation	• What is this person's view of personal capacity and effectiveness and how does it affect the choice, experience, interpretation, and anticipation of doing things? • What abilities or limitations stand out in this person's view of self? • Is the sense of capacity accurate? • Is this person aware of abilities and limitations?
Values	• What is the organizing theme in this person's sense of values? • What things are most important to this person to do? • What standards or other criteria does this person use to judge his or her own performance?
Interests	• Can this person identify personal interests? • What occupations does this person enjoy doing? • What are the aspects of doing that this person enjoys most (e.g., physical challenge, intellectual stimulation, social contact, and aesthetic experience)?
Roles	• What is the overall pattern of role involvement of this person? • Does this person have roles that positively affect his or her identity, use of time, and involvement in social groups? • Is the person overinvolved or underinvolved in roles? • How important is each role to the person?
Habits	• Does this person have well-established habits? • What kind of routine does this person have and is it effective?
Performance capacity	• How do experiences (e.g., pain, fatigue, dizziness, confusion, or altered bodily perceptions) influence this person's occupational performance?
Environment	
Physical and social	• Do the spaces in which this person performs his or her occupations represent physical barriers or supports that impact performance? • Do the objects this person uses support performance? • Do interactions with others support or inhibit this person's performance? • Do the social groups of which this person is a member support the assumption of meaningful roles?
Skill	
Motor	• Does this person have adequate bending, reaching, coordinating, grasping skill to complete occupational forms?
Process	• Does this person have adequate sequencing, terminating, adjusting skill to complete occupational forms?
Communication and interaction	• Does this person have adequate posture, articulation, modulation, assertion skill to complete occupational forms?

therapy, to map out more clearly the dynamics of change and the factors that support change, and to study outcomes of MOHO-based occupational therapy.

CONCLUSION

The model of human occupation has been in development for 25 years. A substantial literature exists including the most recent edition of the text (Kielhofner, 2002) which is a comprehensive and current compendium of theory, application and research. Additionally a website (*www.uic.edu/hsc/acad/cahp/*OT/MOHOC) is a source of contemporary resources and information. For example, more information on the assessments noted in Table 18-2 can be found on this website. Some of the assessments can be downloaded and information on obtaining the others is contained in the website. The website maintains an updated bibliography on MOHO and opportunity to join a listserv of therapists interested in the model.

TABLE 18–2. **MOHO-BASED ASSESSMENTS, THE CONCEPTS ON WHICH THEY PROVIDE DATA, THE METHODS THEY USE, AND THE POPULATION FOR WHICH THEY ARE DESIGNED.**

	Occupational Adaptation		*Volition*			*Habituation*		*Skills*		
Concepts Addressed by the Assessment	**Identity**	**Competence**	**Personal Causation**	**Values**	**Interests**	**Roles**	**Habits**	**Motor**	**Process**	**Communication/ Interaction**
Assessment of Communication and Interaction Skills										■
Assessment of Motor and Process Skills								■	■	
Assessment of Occupational Functioning			■	■	■	■	■	■	■	■
Child Occupational Self-Assessment		■	■	■	■	■	■	■	■	■
Interest Checklist					■					
MOHO Screening Tool			■	■	■	■	■	■	■	■
NIH Activity Record			■	■	■	■	■			
Occupational Circumstances Assessment: Interview and Rating Scale			■	■	■	■	■	■	■	■
Occupational Performance History: Interview 2	■	■	■	■	■	■	■			
Occupational Questionnaire			■	■	■	■	■			
Occupational Self-Assessment		■	■	■	■	■	■	■	■	■
Occupational Therapy Psychosocial Assessment of Learning			■	■	■	■	■			
Pediatric Interest Profile			■		■	■				
Pediatric Volitional Questionnaire			■	■	■					
Role Checklist				■		■				
School Setting Interview										
Volitional Questionnaire			■	■	■					
Worker Role Interview			■	■	■	■	■			
Work Environment Impact Scale										

NIH, National Institutes of Health.

		Environment		*Method of Data Collection*			*Population*			
Performance	**Participation**	**Physical**	**Social**	**Observation**	**Self-Report**	**Interview**	**Children**	**Adolescents**	**Adults**	**Elderly**

SECTION III

Occupational Adaptation

SALLY SCHULTZ
JANETTE K. SCHKADE

INTELLECTUAL HERITAGE

Occupational adaptation (OA) is a theory that describes the integration of two concepts long present in occupational therapy thinking: occupation and adaptation. The intellectual heritage dates back to the writings of Adolph Meyer (1922) and continues through several key contemporary theorists (Gilfoyle, Grady, & Moore, 1981; King, 1978; Llorens, 1970; Selye, 1956). Occupational Adaptation offers a description of an internal adaptation process that occurs through occupation and for occupation. Two initial theoretical articles describing occupational adaptation appeared in 1992 (Schkade & Schultz, 1992; Schultz & Schkade, 1992). Interventions with specific populations were first published in 1993 (Schkade & Schultz, 1993) and a model outlining home-health interventions appeared in 1994 (Schultz & Schkade, 1994). Numerous practice models and population-specific applications have appeared over the years (Crist, Royeen, & Schkade, 2000; Garrett & Schkade, 1995; Pasek & Schkade, 1996; Ross, 1994; Schkade, 1999; Schkade & McClung, 2001; Schultz, 1997; Werner, 2000).

The theory of OA originated as part of the process in which a Ph.D. program in occupational therapy was instituted at Texas Woman's University (TWU) in 1994. This theory is the research focus for the doctoral program. In 1998, the entry-level master's curriculum at TWU was reframed to emphasize the theory of Occupational Adaptation.

GUIDING ASSUMPTIONS

The theory of OA makes six assumptions about human adaptation that address the significance of the adaptive process in normal human growth and development. These assumptions apply to everyone, whether they are clients or not.

- Competence in occupation is a life-long process of adaptation to internal and external demands to perform.
- Demands to perform occur naturally as part of the person's occupational roles and the context (person–occupational–environment interactions) in which they occur.
- Dysfunction occurs because the person's ability to adapt has been challenged to the point that the demands for performance are not satisfactorily met.
- At any stage of life, the person's adaptive capacity can be overwhelmed by impairment, physical or emotional disability, and stressful life events.
- The greater the level of dysfunction, the greater the demand for changes in the person's adaptive processes.
- Success in occupational performance is a direct result of the person's ability to adapt with sufficient mastery to satisfy the self and others.

CONSTRUCTS IN THE THEORY OF OCCUPATIONAL ADAPTATION

The constructs of OA are consistent with the guiding assumptions. Figure 18-2, the OA process diagram, demonstrates a systematic explanation of how people adapt to perform their everyday occupations. The diagram organizes the interplay of the constructs into a sequence that reflects a typical flow between the constructs. In other words, the OA process diagram shows a snapshot view of an individual's adaptive processes at a single point in time. The diagram depicts the interaction between the person and the environment through occupation and the process of adaptation when challenges occur in occupational roles. It is this representation of the process of OA that provides the practitioner with the means, methods, and goals of intervention.

ANALYSIS OF THE OA PROCESS DIAGRAM

At first glance, the OA process diagram (Fig. 18-2) appears complex; however, it can be divided into three parts, with each part representing the three aspects of mastery.

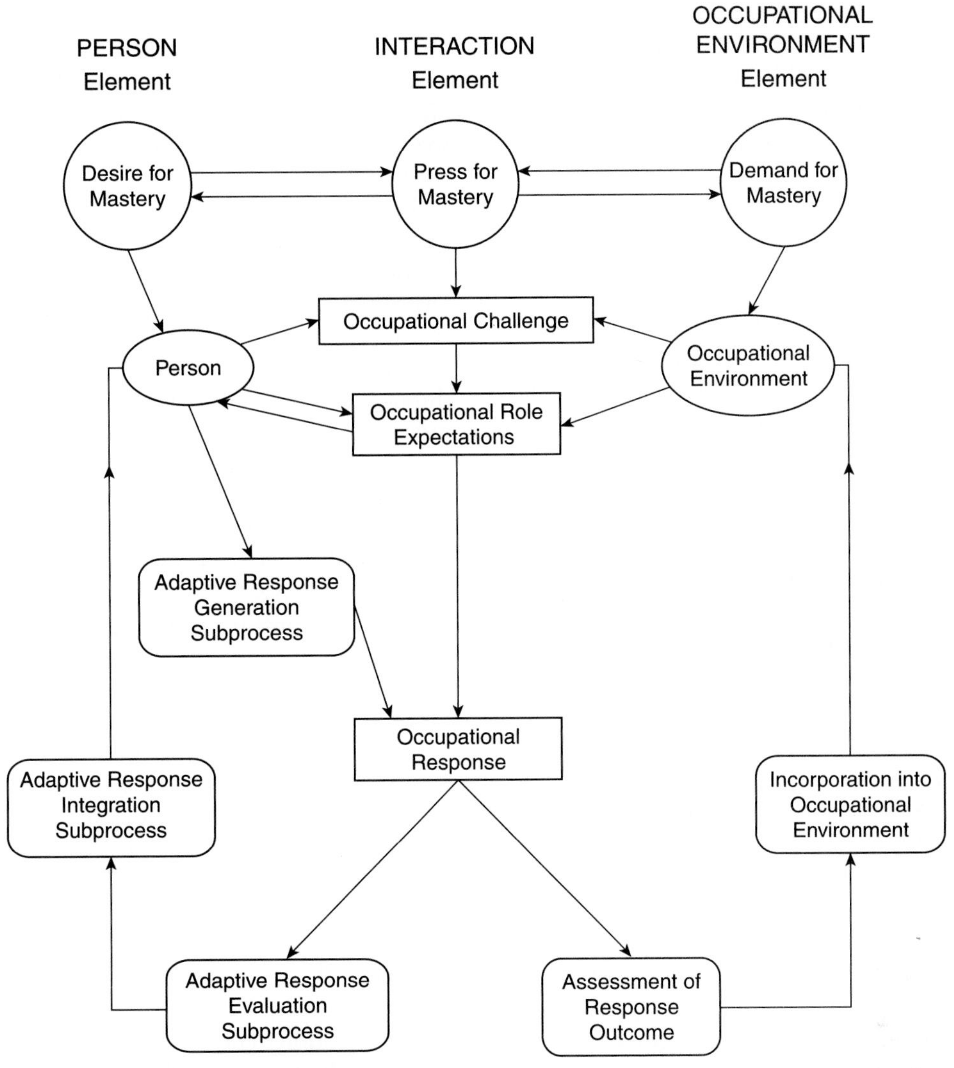

FIGURE 18–2. Occupational adaptation process showing the relationships among occupational adaptation constructs. (Reprinted with permission from Schkade and Schultz, 1992.)

The left side of the diagram shows the processes related to the person–person systems, adaptive response generation, evaluation, and integration. These processes are activated by the *desire for mastery*.

The right side of the diagram shows the processes related to the environmental–occupational environment, assessment by the occupational environment, and integration into the occupational environment. These processes are activated by the *demand for mastery*.

The middle of the diagram shows the interaction between the person and the environmental–occupational challenge, occupational roles, and occupational response. These processes result from the *press for mastery*.

Occupational adaptation is not about mastery per se. Rather, it is the constant presence of the desire, demand, and press for mastery in occupational contexts that provide the impetus for adaptation. In other words, these constants reflect pervasive and ongoing influences. The person seeking to respond masterfully in occupational situations will engage in the adaptive processes.

KEY DEFINITIONS AND CONSTRUCTS IN THE THEORY

OA presents the adaptation process as emerging from an interaction between the person (consisting of idiosyncratic sensorimotor, cognitive, and psychosocial systems) and occupational environment (consisting of work, play, and leisure and self-maintenance functions) in response to occupational challenges. Person systems are what they are because of genetic, environmental, and experiential subsystems that feed into them to create the idiosyncratic nature of individuals. Likewise, in the occupational environments, physical, social, and cultural subsystems feed into and create the nature of specific occupational environments, or contexts in which occupation occurs. Occupational challenges occur within the context of performing occupational roles. Performance expectations from the occupational environment and from the person's own internal expectations influence the challenge experience.

Adaptation Subprocesses

An individual uses three adaptation subprocesses when facing an occupational challenge: the adaptive response generation subprocess, the adaptive response evaluation subprocess, and the adaptive response integration subprocess. These subprocesses plan the occupational response, evaluate it, and integrate its outcome into the person as adaptation.

The adaptive response generation subprocess is the anticipatory portion of the adaptation process. It consists of two components: the adaptive response mechanism and the adaptation Gestalt. The adaptive response mechanism creates a plan of action for the occupational response. The plan calls for the individual to program the three person systems (the Gestalt) to execute the plan of action. The occupational response is the outcome of the interplay between the mechanism and the Gestalt. It is assumed that the individual attempts to generate responses that result in some degree of **relative mastery.**

In the adaptive response evaluation subprocess, the individual assesses his or her experience of mastery. As this is a personal assessment, the evaluation is relative to the individual (hence, the term relative mastery). To evaluate relative mastery, individuals assess the following:

- Personal experience of efficiency (use of time, energy, and resources).
- Effectiveness (extent to which their desired goal was achieved).
- Satisfaction to self and society (the extent to which they are personally satisfied with the response and the extent to which they believe their social system assesses the response to be satisfactory for its expec-tations).

If the evaluation subprocess indicates that the individual needs to change his or her interaction with the environment in similar circumstances, the necessary adaptation occurs because of action of the adaptive response integration subprocess. The **occupational environment** also evaluates the outcome of the occupational response. Consequently, the potential for change in the occupational environment is also present.

EVALUATION, INTERVENTION, CLIENT—PRACTITIONER INTERACTIONS

The theory of OA is not a collection of techniques but a way of thinking that guides and organizes the intervention process. The essential task of the practitioner is to acknowledge and facilitate the client as the agent of therapeutic change. The practitioner sets the stage for the client to progressively assume the agency role. This is critical in influencing the client's internal adaptation process. To reiterate, the internal adaptation process is the focus for intervention with the theory of occupational adaptation.

In all phases of intervention, collaboration between the client and the practitioner is essential. The goal of intervention is to facilitate the client's ability to make his or her own adaptations for engaging in occupational activities that are personally meaningful. This is accomplished by enhancing the function of the client's internal adaptation process through using a client-selected occupational role to guide intervention. The therapist evaluates the client's ability to carry out activities within that role and determines what is helping or hindering the client's experience of relative mastery in those activities. A plan is then developed to enhance the capabilities and minimize the negative effect of disabling conditions.

The plan consists of two types of intervention: occupational readiness and occupational activity. Occupational readiness addresses deficits in motor, process, and communication/interaction performance skills to prepare clients for occupational activity. Occupational readiness might include a splint to support the hand in a more functional position, exercise to strengthen weak muscles, training in social skills, or other interventions. Occupational activity engages the client in tasks that are a part of the occupational role selected by the client. An important intervention principle is that all three person systems are always present in every occupational response. This principle requires that practitioners always think holistically when planning and carrying out interventions. For example, using an OA approach, Ford (1995) facilitated an elderly client's own adaptive processes in her role as homemaker. Because of this intervention, the client took more responsibility for upgrading her goals and initiating her own adaptations, such as placing a coffee maker where she could reach it from her wheelchair.

STRENGTHS AND LIMITATIONS

The strengths of this particular theoretical perspective lie in its holistic orientation and its adherence to ideas of occupation and adaptation inherent in the profession's history and philosophy (Schultz & Schkade, 1997). It provides an organized way to think and communicate about occupational therapy intervention that is occupation based, process oriented, and client focused. Other strengths are OA's compatibility with new terminology coming from the World Health Organization (2001) and its concern with the ability of individuals and groups of individuals to participate fully in society. From an OA standpoint, occupation plays a significant role as a facilitator in social participation. Likewise, we believe that dysfunction in occupation becomes a significant participation restriction. Limitations have yet to be identified, as this theory is quite new; however, they will surface as practitioners report their experience using this theory and in research designed to test its principles in intervention.

RESEARCH

Research on the effectiveness of OA intervention has included a variety of methods. Clinical research on groups of clients has involved comparison of standard facility approaches with an OA approach. A sample of research findings to date includes advances in functional independence for clients who have suffered a cerebrovascular accident (CVA) (Gibson & Schkade, 1997) and for patients who have had a hip fracture (Jackson & Schkade, 2001). Buddenberg and Schkade (1998) reported that post–hip fracture patients who underwent OA intervention performed better at discharge on tasks they had not been previously trained on than a group that was treated with standard facility protocols. In a 6-week study in which clients served as their own control group, CVA patients stood longer when engaged in personally meaningful occupation than when engaged in standard facility protocol activities (Dolecheck & Schkade, 1999). Using a case study research method, three CVA clients who had been discharged from therapy as having reached a plateau in mobility, showed significant gains in mobility when treated in their homes using OA principles (Johnson & Schkade, 2001). These studies represent only a portion of the research efforts to determine the effectiveness of OA theory in applications.

CONCLUSION

Occupational Adaptation is one way for practitioners to think about, describe, and plan, occupation-based intervention designed to promote participation in a wellness context and remediate participation restriction in a dysfunctional context.

SECTION IV

The Ecology of Human Performance

WINNIE DUNN
LINDA HANEY McCLAIN
CATANA BROWN
MARY JANE YOUNGSTROM

The purpose of this section is to introduce the Ecology of Human Performance (EHP) framework as a model for considering context in occupational therapy practice. The fundamental theoretical postulate of the EHP framework is that **ecology,** or the interaction between a person and the context, affects human behavior and task performance. Human performance is a transactional process through which the person, the context, and the task performance affect each other. Each transaction influences a person's future performance range and options, because the person, the context, or the available performance range may be modified by the context or a particular person variable. Frequently, the person–context match is the most apparent performance issue. **Therapeutic intervention** from an EHP perspective occurs as collaboration among the person, the family and the occupational therapy practitioner. It is designed to facilitate occupational performance. Occupational therapy intervention expands the person's performance range by changing the following variables: the person, the context, the task, or the transactions among them.

INTELLECTUAL HERITAGE

Scholars from many disciplines have explored the interaction between organisms and their environments. Environmental psychologists have emphasized the relationships between people and their physical environments (e.g. Holahan, 1986; Wicker, 1979). Hart (1979) considered the environment as a medium for social interactions and pointed out that the environment could support social competence; Bronfenbrenner (1979) also discussed the social aspects of context as part of an ecological model for human development. Auerswald (1971) argued that a holistic ecological perspective enabled the practitioner to be concerned with the performance environment as well as the performance demands the person must face.

Occupational therapy theory has long been concerned with the construct of context (i.e., environment, in much of the occupational therapy literature). Earlier perspectives focused on manipulation or selection of contexts as part of the intervention process supporting change or adaptation. Llorens (1970) employed the construct of context by explaining occupational therapy intervention as a process of providing environments that assist people when their developmental evolution has been disrupted. Fidler and Fidler (1978) conceived of context as important as clients develop mastery through their interactions with aspects of the environment. King (1978) characterized interventions as the use of the environment to elicit an adaptive response.

Other occupational therapy theories conceptualized the person and context relationship within general systems theory in which the person and environment are interdependent as they interact in the system of input, throughput, and output. The Model of Human Occupation (Kielhofner & Burke, 1980), occupational science (Clark et al., 1991), and Nelson's (1988) description of the dynamics of occupational form (i.e. context) and occupational performance draw on general systems theory.

Several recent occupational therapy theories provide different models for considering person, environment, and occupation relationships with an appreciation for the importance of context. Occupational Adaptation (Schkade & Schultz, 1992) gives equal weight to person and environment features and sees occupation as the means by which people adapt. In the Person–Environment–Occupation Model (Law et al., 1996), occupational performance is viewed as the dynamic experience that occurs when a person engages in purposeful activities within an environment. The Person–Environment Occupational Performance Model (Christiansen & Baum, 1997) sees occupational performance as influenced by intrinsic factors (psychological and biological) as well as extrinsic factors (social and cultural).

The Ecology of Human Performance perspective describes context as the lens through which a person views task performance opportunities (Dunn, Brown, & McGuigan, 1994). The EHP model elucidates five intervention options that differ in terms of the intervention target (person, task, context) and the intervention goal (resolve or prevent a problem, enhance performance). An intention of EHP is to provide a framework that encourages interaction and collaboration among disciplines. The framework is not intended for occupational therapy application exclusively but can be, and has been, used by other disciplines to analyze and design assessments and interventions for particular person, task, and context interactions.

ASSUMPTIONS UNDERLYING THE ECOLOGY OF HUMAN PERFORMANCE

People and their contexts are unique and dynamic. It is impossible to understand the person without also understanding the person's context. Individuals influence contexts and contexts influence individuals. A person's performance range is determined by the transaction between the person and the context. It is through engagement in tasks that persons and contexts transact.

Contrived contexts are different from natural contexts. When compared to natural environments, contrived contexts may either facilitate or inhibit performance. Assessment and intervention best approximate the person's true performance when enacted in natural environments.

Occupational therapy practice involves promoting self-determination and inclusion of persons with disabilities in all contexts. The occupational therapy process begins when the person served and/or the family of the person served identifies what the person wants or needs. Occupational therapy practice includes making changes in systems so that people with disabilities receive the full rights and privileges they are due.

Independence includes using contextual supports to meet the person's wants and needs. The use of assistive devices or other people does not mean the client is dependent. Intervention strategies that adapt or alter the environment are not reserved for use only when restorative interventions have failed.

DEFINITIONS

Person

A *person* is an individual with his or her own configuration of abilities; experiences; and sensorimotor, cognitive, and psychosocial needs. Persons are unique and complex; therefore, precise predictability about their performance is impossible. The meaning a person attaches to task and contextual variables strongly influences performance (Dunn, Brown, McClain, & Westman, 1994).

Task

A *task* may be considered an objective set of behaviors necessary to accomplish a goal. An infinite variety of tasks exists for every person. Roles shape a person's tasks. Tasks take on meaning only in the transactional relationship of the person, task, and context. It is through this process that tasks become occupations.

Performance

Performance is composed of both the process and the result of the person interacting with context to engage in tasks. The transaction between the person and the context determines the performance range. A person's skills, abilities, and experiences, along with contextual facilitators and barriers, determine whether a particular task falls within the performance range. The performance range is fluid, changing across time as person and context features change.

Context

Context has two aspects: temporal and environmental. Although temporal aspects are determined by the person, temporal features become contextual because of the social and cultural meaning attached to them.

Temporal Aspects

- *Chronological:* Individual's age.
- *Developmental:* Stage or phase of maturation.
- *Life cycle:* Place in important life phases, such as career cycle, parenting cycle, or educational process.
- *Disability status:* Place in continuum of disability, or terminal nature of illness (American Occupational Therapy Association [AOTA], 1994).
- *Period:* Measurable span of time during which a task exists or continues; includes the steps of a task, when it takes place, and how long and how often it occurs.

Environment

- *Physical:* Nonhuman aspects of contexts; includes accessibility to and performance within environments having natural terrain, plants, animals, buildings, furniture, objects, tools, or devices.
- *Social:* Availability and expectations of significant individuals, such as spouse, friends, and caregivers; includes larger social groups that are influential in establishing norms, role expectations, and social routines as well as organizations, institutions, and political and economic systems.
- *Cultural:* Customs, beliefs, activity patterns, behavior standards, and expectations accepted by the society of which the individual is a member; includes political aspects (e.g., laws that affect access to resources and affirm personal rights) and opportunities for education, employment, and economic support (AOTA, 1994).

Person–Context–Task Transaction

The person–context transaction in task performance is the major variable that ultimately governs the performance range. Ecology, or the transaction between a person and the context, affects task performance; task performance, in turn, affects the person, the context, and the person–context transaction.

Therapeutic Intervention

Therapeutic intervention is a collaboration among the person, the family, and the occupational practitioner (Fig. 18-3). It is directed at meeting performance needs using the strategies discussed next.

- *Establish or restore a person's abilities to perform in context.* One intervention option is to establish or restore a person's skills or abilities. The establish intervention leads to the attainment of a new skill or ability. The restore option leads to the reestablishment of a lost skill or ability. **Establish and restore interventions** target the person; the outcome is a new or renewed skill or ability. The skills acquired in an establish/restore intervention include sensorimotor, cognitive, and psychosocial skills. Furthermore, establish/restore interventions encompass education in the tasks themselves (e.g., money management, parenting, leisure activities, job tasks). From an EHP perspective, establish/restore interventions should not occur in isolation but in relation to tasks that are needed or wanted by the person.
- *Alter actual context or task in which people perform.* Therapeutic interventions can alter the context or task within which the person performs. This intervention emphasizes selecting a context or task that enables the person to perform with current skills and abilities. This includes placing the person in a different setting or task that more closely matches current skills and abilities, rather than changing the present setting or task to accommodate needs. In the **alter intervention,** nothing is changed about the person, the context, or the task, but a better match is made. For example, a one-story house would be a better match for someone who has motoric problems that make stair climbing difficult. In an alter intervention addressing the cultural context, a religious institution that is harmonious with the person's beliefs and values may be identified to meet wants and needs.
- *Modify (adapt) contextual features and task demands so they support performance in context.* When employing **modify (adapt) intervention** strategies, the occupational therapy practitioner finds ways to revise the current context or task demands to support performance in the natural setting. Modify (adapt) approaches encompass compensatory techniques. Features of the context or task are changed so that the task becomes available to the person. Most of the time, occupational therapy practitioners focus on modifications to the physical environment; however, all types of contextual features are amenable to change. For example social networks can be modified to provide the needed supports, norms and belief systems can be changed within systems, and temporal modifications (e.g., duration or sequence in which a person engages in a task) can be changed.

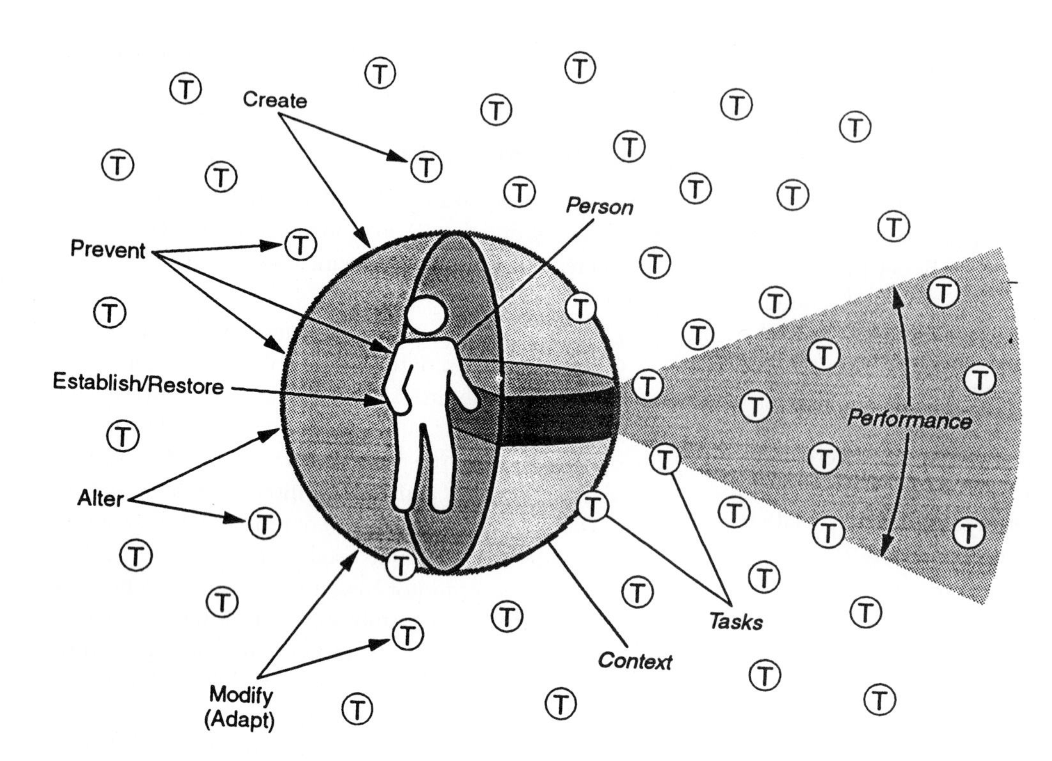

FIGURE 18–3. The interventions available within the ecology of human performance framework. *Arrows,* the focus of each intervention approach.

- *Prevent the occurrence or evolution of performance problems in context.* Therapeutic interventions can **prevent** the occurrence or evolution of barriers to performance in context. Sometimes practitioners can predict that without intervention certain negative outcomes are likely to occur. Practitioners can design interventions to change the course of events. These interventions may address person, context, task, or a combination of these variables to change the course, thereby sustaining functional performance. Therefore, prevent strategies may look like establish/restore, adapt, or alter interventions. The difference is prevent strategies occur before the problem develops.
- *Create circumstances that promote more adaptable or complex performance in context.* Providers can also **create interventions** that promote performance in context. The create intervention does not assume a disability is present or that any factors would interfere with performance. The create intervention focuses on providing enriched contextual and task experiences that will enhance performance for all persons in the natural contexts of life (Dunn, Brown, McClain, & Westman, 1994; Dunn, Brown, & McGuigan, 1994).

APPLICATION TO PRACTICE

Occupational therapy practitioners intervene when people have difficulty with the tasks that make up their occupations. The ecology of human performance framework not only considers performance but also consistently considers the unique nature of performance in context. The primary theoretical postulate fundamental to the EHP framework is that ecology, or the transaction between the person and the context, affects human behavior and task performance and that performance can be understood only in context. Likewise, task performance affects the person, the context, and the person–context transaction. Therefore, occupational therapy evaluation and intervention options are not restricted to the person variables that affect human performance but also consider the effects of the context and the person–context match and the effect of the tasks themselves on human performance.

STRENGTHS AND LIMITATIONS

The EHP framework has several strengths. First, it provides an explicit link among the person, tasks, and contexts for performance in daily life. By linking these concepts together, professionals are more likely to include all aspects of performance in assessment and planning. Second, the EHP framework offers an expansive concept of intervention by illustrating different ways to consider the performance challenge (i.e., the five approaches to intervention). Third, the EHP provides a communication vehicle among disciplines. The model employs common language, thereby providing professionals from several disciplines a common conceptual model for collaborating model in practice and research.

The limitations of the EHP framework relate to the need for additional work to verify the nature of the proposed relationships. For example, we do not know the effectiveness of the various interventions in practice or when and how to select them for optimal outcomes. In addition, we made assumptions as we developed this framework, and these assumptions must be verified as work in this area proceeds.

RESEARCH

We have conducted studies with colleagues from other disciplines to evaluate the use of EHP. Researchers designed a measure of rehabilitation context based on the EHP (Teel, Dunn, Jackson, & Duncan, 1997, 2001). They found that context is best characterized as a holistic concept and that the caregiver's belief that participation is critical to positive rehabilitation outcomes is an important feature of context. With another team, we used EHP to support both adult education programs and college teaching (Bulgren et al., 1997). This study linked the most common interferences to learning and used the EHP interventions to design a system of interventions for more inclusive teaching. Another team used EHP to design a test of grocery shopping and an effective intervention to teach grocery shopping to persons with severe and persistent mental illness who live in the community (Brown, Rempfer, & Hamera, 2002). Finally, the EHP constructs underlie the design and validation of the sensory profile measures for infants, toddlers, children and adults (Brown, Tolefson, Dunn, Cromwell, & Filion, 2001; Dunn, 1999; 2001). These studies indicate that people with and without disabilities have distinct patterns of performance in relation to their sensory contexts and that knowing these patterns provides guidance for selecting EHP interventions.

CONCLUSION

The EHP framework provides a way to understand the transactional nature of person, task, performance, and context. Using this framework, practitioners can collaborate with the person and family members to identify performance needs and develop strategies to enhance performance.

SECTION V

The Person–Environment–Occupation Model

DEBRA STEWART
LORI LETTS
MARY LAW
BARBARA ACHESON COOPER
SUSAN STRONG
PATRICIA J. RIGBY

INTELLECTUAL HERITAGE

The Person–Environment–Occupation (PEO) model was developed to facilitate occupational therapists' understanding of the dynamic nature of occupational performance. A simple Venn diagram (Fig. 18-4) depicts the PEO model as three interrelated elements of person, environment, and occupation. Occupational performance emerges from the overlap of the three circles and represents the fit or congruence among the three elements. The PEO model describes occupational performance as the outcome of a **transactional relationship** (Saegert & Winkel, 1990) that exists among people; their occupations; and the environments in which they live, work, and play (Law et al., 1996). This relationship is dynamic in nature, as the three elements are always changing and influencing each other. Thus occupational performance is changing constantly over a lifetime (Fig. 18-5).

A group of six occupational therapists at McMaster University (Hamilton, ON) reviewed the literature in diverse fields of study and applied relevant findings to current occupational therapy practice (Law et al., 1994, 1997). These fields of study include environment–behavior studies (EBSs), psychology, and occupational therapy. EBSs include research from disciplines of environmental psychology, social science, anthropology, human geography, and architecture. All of these disciplines have contributed to the

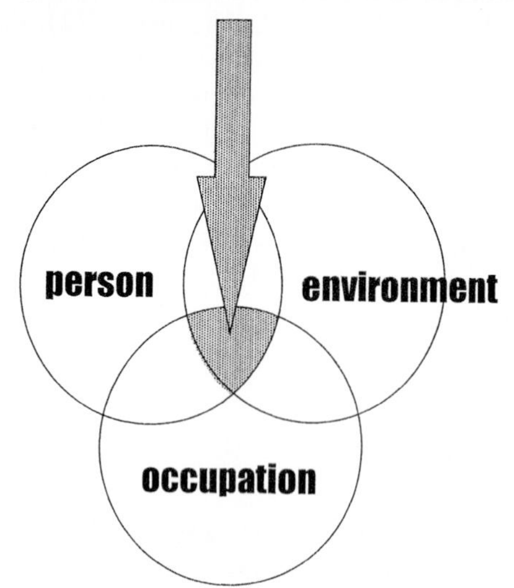

FIGURE 18–4. Person–environment–occupation relationship. (Adapted with permission from Law et al., 1996.)

understanding about the relationship between the behavior of persons and their environments. The concepts and assumptions of several EBS theorists are particularly relevant to occupational therapy beliefs and values. For example, Bronfenbrenner's (1977) ecological systems model emphasizes the social nature of individuals who interact with all levels of the environment to develop and bring meaning to their lives. Lawton and Nahemow's (1973) ecological theory of aging describes the interactive relationship between an individual and the environment as it affects the degree of adaptation that the individual is able to achieve. This theory of adaptation is similar to the views of Csikszentmihalyi and Csikszentmihalyi (1988) in the field of psychology. They describe the relationship between the challenges of an activity and individual skills in their theory of flow. The work of these theorists offers relevant ideas for occupational therapists when considering both person and environmental issues in practice, and these ideas allow sufficient flexibility to include the concept of occupational performance as a critical variable.

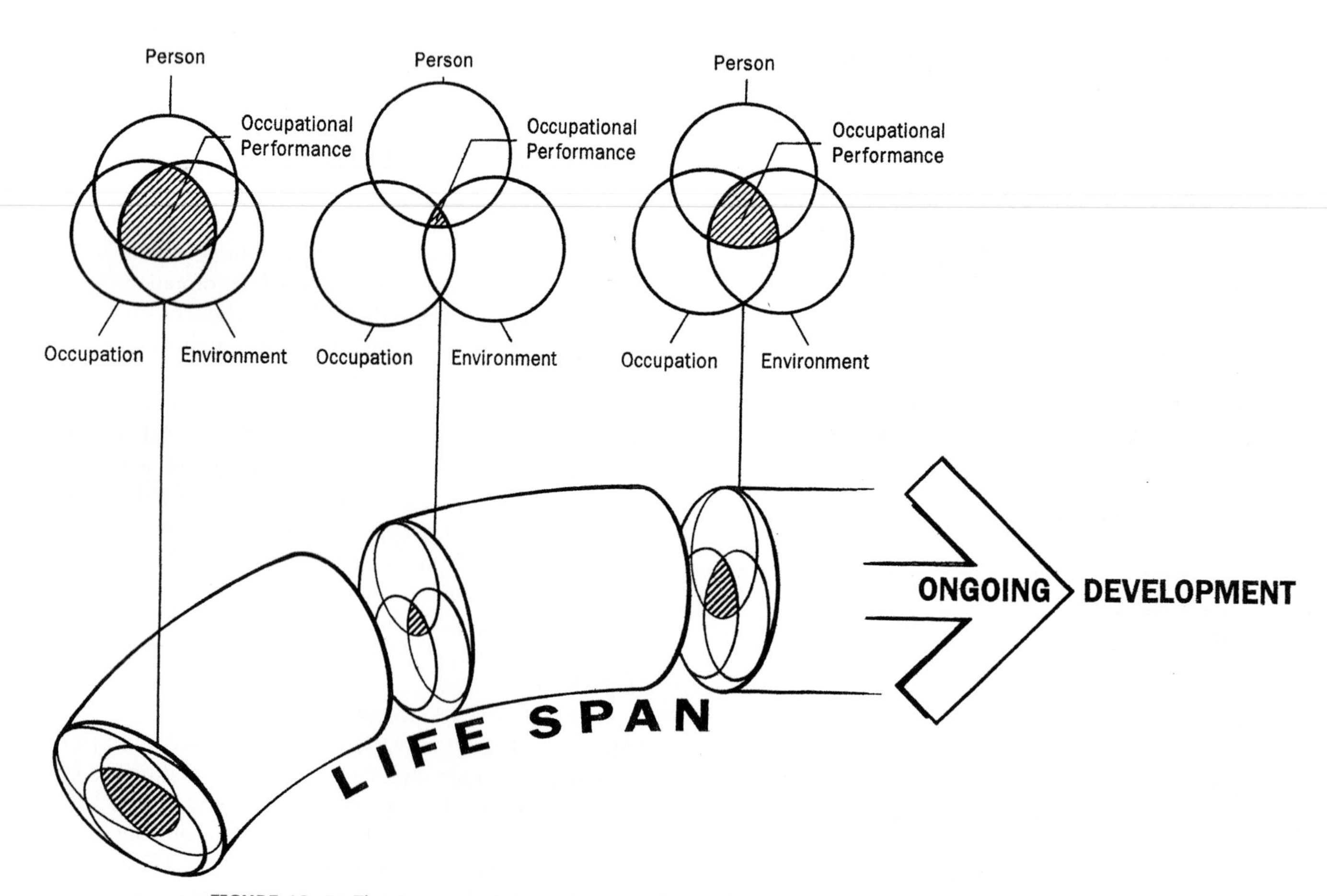

FIGURE 18–5. The person-environment-occupation model of occupational performance across the life span, illustrating hypothetical changes in occupational performance at three different points in time. (Reprinted with permission from Law et al., 1996.)

The PEO model integrates these theories with current Canadian guidelines for client-centered practice (Canadian Association of Occupational Therapists [CAOT], 1997). Furthermore, the model is congruent with current global models of health, such as the revised International Classification of Functioning, Disability, and Health (ICF) (World Health Organization, 2001), which also acknowledges the interactions of person and environment in the process of health and well-being. Thus the PEO model is a synthesis of multidisciplinary approaches to person–environment relations and the unique perspective of occupational therapy.

DEFINITIONS

The PEO model is purposefully flexible, which is similar to many environment–behavior approaches. The elements of the model are broadly defined to allow adaptation and expansion for specific practice situations.

Person

The *person* (or group of people) is considered to be a unique being who assumes a variety of ever-changing and simultaneous roles. These roles vary across time and context in their importance, duration, and meaning. The person is viewed holistically as a composite of mind, body, and spirit. These qualities include physical, cognitive, and affective attributes (skills and functions) and life experiences. Each person calls on these components, as well as a set of learned and innate skills, to facilitate occupational performance.

Environment

A broad definition of *environment* gives equal importance to cultural, social, physical, and institutional/organizational elements. The environment is viewed as the context in which behavior takes place, and it provides cues to an individual (or group of people) about what to do or what is expected. For example, a community hall can be used as a classroom, a party room, a temporary church, or a public meeting room. A person relates to the environmental cues and behaves accordingly. In addition, elements in the environment can be viewed as barriers or supports to occupational performance. This emphasizes the need to understand a person's perception of his or her environment, as well as the barriers and supports present, when addressing the environment with this model.

Occupation

The term *occupation* embraces all self-care, productive, and leisure pursuits. The concepts of activities, tasks, and occupations are viewed as nested within each other. Activities are considered to be the basic units of tasks; tasks are sets of purposeful, related activities; and occupations are groups of self-directed, functional tasks and activities in which a person engages over a life span. To illustrate this, the activities of using a computer keyboard and a word-processing program are nested in the task of writing an academic paper, which is part of the occupation of completing the coursework required in a first-year occupational therapy program. The PEO model recognizes that occupations vary across the life span and bring meaning to a person's life.

Occupational Performance

Occupational performance is the outcome of the transaction of the person, the environment, and the occupation. In the model shown in Figure 18-5, the degree of fit or congruence among the three elements is indicated by the amount of overlap of the three circles, which represents occupational performance. Occupational performance is a dynamic, ever-changing experience of a person engaged in purposeful activities, tasks, and occupations within an environment.

ASSUMPTIONS

The assumptions of this model focus on the three elements and their relationships.

- The person is a dynamic, motivated, and ever-developing being, who is always interacting with the environment. Behavior cannot be separated from environmental influences, temporal factors, and physical and psychological characteristics.
- Environments are constantly changing, and as they change, the behavior necessary to accomplish a goal changes.
- Environments can have enabling or constraining effects on occupational performance.
- The environment is often more amenable to change than the person.
- Occupations are complex, pluralistic, and necessary for quality of life and well-being. They meet a person's intrinsic needs for self-maintenance, expression, and fulfillment within the context of his or her personal roles and environment.
- The relationship among the three elements of person, environment, and occupation is transactional, meaning that it is mutually interwoven and difficult to separate. The outcome of this transactional relationship is called occupational performance. The key assumption of the PEO model is that person, environment, and occupation interact continually across time and space in ways that increase or decrease their congruence: The

closer the fit, the greater the overlap or occupational performance.

- Occupational performance changes over a lifetime as individuals constantly renegotiate their view of self and their roles as they ascribe meaning to occupations and the environments around them.

EFFECTS ON EVALUATION, INTERVENTION, AND CLIENT–PRACTITIONER INTERACTION

The PEO model supports a collaborative partnership among clients, occupational therapy practitioners, and the people in the clients' environments. Client-centered practice is a theoretical underpinning of the PEO model, as the occupational therapy practitioner is expected to address occupational performance issues that have been identified by the client. Concepts from environment–behavior studies acknowledge that a person's perceptions and beliefs about his or her environments and occupations influence subsequent occupational performance.

The PEO model provides a useful framework for the identification and assessment of occupational performance. It supports a temporal approach to evaluation, focusing on the changing nature of occupational performance and the relationships among person, environment, and occupation. An occupational therapy evaluation begins with identification of occupational performance strengths and challenges, using a client-centered measure, such as the Canadian Occupational Performance Measure (Law et al., 1998). The PEO model then guides the practitioner to identify barriers and supports to occupational performance through an analysis of the three major elements of person, environment, and occupation as they relate to the identified occupational performance issues. Furthermore, the relationships between person and environment, person and occupation, and environment and occupation assist the practitioner to understand fully the enabling and constraining influences on occupational performance. This encourages occupational therapy practitioners to use evaluation methods that take place continuously throughout the occupational therapy process, rather than in a time-limited, linear approach.

The profession of occupational therapy has developed numerous measures to evaluate the person in areas of physical, social, cultural, and affective components. The profession's uniqueness is closely tied with our skills in the analysis of occupations, tasks, and activities. Evaluation of the environment has not received as much attention from occupational therapy practitioners, although this is slowly changing. The authors of the PEO model reviewed a wide repertoire of well-validated measures to assess the environment, which were developed in occupational therapy and other disciplines (Cooper, Letts, Rigby, Stewart, & Strong, 2001; Letts et al., 1994). Use of these measures is encouraged for the profession to gain a better understanding of the environmental influences on a person's life.

The PEO model also encourages practitioners to expand intervention approaches by considering the multidimensional concepts and relationships that influence occupational performance. There are multiple avenues for facilitating change in person, environment, and/or occupation that result in improved occupational performance. Personal change may be addressed in individuals, families, groups, communities, and/or organizations. Strategies to change the environment can be directed at the micro and/or macro level. Some examples of environmental strategies are

- Improving physical access in indoor and outdoor environments.
- Establishing a social network of support for an individual.
- Influencing change in the cultural beliefs of a community toward people with disabilities through education and information.
- Advocating for accommodations within an organization to promote inclusion and participation of all persons.

Occupation is the third element of the model and represents one of the unique perspectives that occupational therapy practitioners bring to intervention. Through adaptation or modification of activities, tasks, and occupations, we enable occupational performance. The PEO model emphasizes the need to consider the transactional relationships of occupations with people and the environments in which they are performing these occupations to address clients' occupational performance issues and goals. The model also guides practitioners to recognize the temporal nature of these relationships, because people, environments, and occupations are constantly changing. Thus the resources or intervention strategies needed at one point in time may be quite different later on.

LIMITATIONS AND STRENGTHS OF THE MODEL

The PEO model is a conceptual model and as such requires occupational therapy practitioners to apply it to their specific practice setting. The simplicity of the model may be a limitation in some situations, because it does not answer the questions practitioners have about specific evaluation methods and/or intervention techniques. On the other hand, its simplicity can be a strength, as the model can be used in all settings, with all ages of people, and with all types of client populations to guide the thinking and clinical decision making of occupational therapy practitioners. Its flexibility allows practitioners to expand on specific evaluation and intervention methods to suit their situation.

A limitation of the PEO model relates to the fact that it is a relatively new model of practice and has not received extensive testing. This is changing rapidly, however, as practitioners become more familiar with the model and begin to apply it to numerous practice settings and situations involving individuals (or groups) who are experiencing problems in occupational performance.

RESEARCH

We and our students (Strong et al., 1999) have conducted numerous research studies since the mid-1990s to determine the validity of the PEO model. Results support the transactional nature of the relationship among person, environment, and occupation. Studies have included the relationship between older persons and the physical environment (Cooper & Stewart, 1997), persons with mental health problems and the work environment (Strong, 1998), successful work (re)entry for persons with disabilities (Westmorland, Williams, & Strong, 2000), environmental factors influencing children's participation in occupations (Law et al., 1999), the temporal nature of occupational performance for young people with disabilities in transition to adulthood (Stewart, Law, Rosenbaum, & Williams, 2001), and the cultural sensitivity of the PEO model (McKye, Shin, & Letts, 1998).

As occupational therapy practitioners and researchers become more familiar with the PEO model, the number of clinical research studies is increasing. One study used the PEO model as a conceptual framework to explain the effect of environmental sensitivity on occupational performance (Peachy-Hill & Law, 2000). A study about the meaning of occupation as a quality-of-life factor for a group of older persons in a nursing home was guided by the PEO model (Green & Cooper, 2000). The qualitative data were organized and analyzed using the PEO model, contributing to the validation of the model.

Future research is planned in a continuing effort to validate the PEO model and to apply it to daily occupational therapy practice. A current study is exploring successful occupational therapy experiences from client and practitioner perspectives. This may lead to the development and testing of new intervention strategies that focus on person–environment–occupation relations.

CONCLUSION

The PEO model guides occupational therapy practitioners to consider the dynamic, transactional relationships that comprise occupational performance. Research to date supports the validity of the PEO model, and further study is underway. The model's flexibility and simplicity facilitate its use in all occupational therapy practice settings.

References

American Occupational Therapy Association [AOTA]. (1994). Uniform terminology for occupational therapy—Third edition. *American Journal of Occupational Therapy, 48,* 1047–1054.

Auerswald, E. H. (1971). Families, change, and the ecological perspective. *Family Process, 10,* 263–280.

Ayres, A. J. (1972). *Sensory integration and learning disorders.* Los Angeles: Western Psychological Services.

Ayres, A. J. (1979). *Sensory integration and the child.* Los Angeles: Western Psychological Services.

Ayres, A. J. (1986). *Developmental dyspraxia and adult onset apraxia.* Torrance, CA: Sensory Integration International.

Bernspang, B., & Fisher, A. (1995). Differences between persons with a right or left cerebral vascular accident on the assessment of motor and process skills. *Archives of Physical Medicine and Rehabilitation, 75,* 1144–1151.

Black, M. M. (1976). The occupational career. *American Journal of Occupational Therapy, 30,* 225–228.

Borys, S. S. (1974). Implications of interest theory. *American Journal of Occupational Therapy, 28,* 35–38.

Bronfenbrenner, U. (1977). Toward an experimental ecology of human development. *American Psychologist, 32,* 513–531.

Bronfenbrenner, U. (1979). *The ecology of human development.* Cambridge, MA: Harvard University Press.

Brown, C., Rempfer, M., & Hamera, E. (2002). Teaching grocery shopping skills to people with schizophrenia. *Occupational Therapy Journal of Research, 22, Suppl (1),* 90s–91s.

Brown, C., Tolefson, N., Dunn, W., Cromwell, R., & Filion, D. (2001). The adult sensory profile: Measuring patterns of sensory processing. *American Journal of Occupational Therapy, 55,* 75–82.

Bruner, J. (1990). Act of Meaning. Cambridge, MA: Harvard.

Buddenberg, L. A., & Schkade, J. K. (1998). A comparison of occupational therapy intervention approaches for older patients after hip fracture. *Topics in Geriatric Rehabilitation, 13*(4), 52–68.

Bulgren, J. A., Gilbert, M. P., Hall, J., Horton, B., Mellard, D., & Parker, K. (1997). *Accommodating adults with disabilities in adult education programs: National field test.* Lawrence, KS: University of Kansas Institute for Adult Studies.

Burke, J. P. (1977). A clinical perspective on motivation: Pawn versus origin. *American Journal of Occupational Therapy, 31,* 254–258.

Canadian Association of Occupational Therapists [CAOT] (1997). *Enabling occupation. An occupational therapy perspective.* Ottawa, ON: Author.

Christiansen, C., & Baum, C. (1997). Person-environment-occupation performance: A conceptual model for practice. In C. Christiansen & C. Baum (Eds.). *Occupational therapy: Enabling function and well-being* (2nd ed., pp. 46–70). Thorofare, NJ: Slack.

Clark, F. A., Parham, D., Carison, H. E., Frank, G., Jackson, J., Pierce, D., Wolfe, R. J., & Zemke, R. (1991). Occupational Science: Academic innovation in the service of occupational therapy's future. *American Journal of Occupational Therapy, 45,* 300–310.

Cooper, B., Letts, L., Rigby, P., Stewart, D., & Strong, S. (2001). Measuring environmental factors. In M. Law, C. Baum & W. Dunn (Eds.). *Measuring occupational performance: Supporting best practice in occupational therapy* (pp. 229–256). Thorofare, NJ: Slack.

Cooper, B., & Stewart, D. (1997). The effect of a transfer device in the homes of elderly women. *Physical and Occupational Therapy in Geriatrics, 15,* 61–77.

Crist, P. A., Royeen, C. B., & Schkade, J. K. (2000). *Infusing occupation into practice* (2nd ed.). Bethesda, MD: American Occupational Therapy Association.

Csikszentmihalyi, M., & Csikszentmihalyi, I. S. (1988). *Optimal experience: Psychological studies in flow in consciousness.* Cambridge, UK: Cambridge University Press.

Dewey, J. (1922). *Human nature and conduct.* New York: Holt.

Doble, S. (1991). Test-retest and interrater reliability of a process skills assessment. *Occupational Therapy Journal of Research, 11,* 8–23.

Dolecheck, J. R., & Schkade, J. K. (1999). Effects on dynamic standing endurance when persons with CVA perform personally meaningful activities rather than non-meaningful tasks. *Occupational Therapy Journal of Research. 19*(1), 40–53.

Dunn, W. (1999). *The sensory profile manual.* San Antonio: Psychological Corp.

Dunn, W. (2001). *Infant toddler sensory profile manual.* Unpublished manuscript.

Dunn, W., Brown, C., McClain, L., & Westman, K. (1994). The ecology of human performance: A contextual perspective on human occupation. In C. B. Royeen (Ed.). *AOTA self-study series: The practice of the future: Putting occupation back into therapy* (Module 1). Rockville, MD: American Occupational Therapy Association.

Dunn, W., Brown, C., & McGuigan, A. (1994). The ecology of human performance: A framework for considering the effect of context. *American Journal of Occupational Therapy, 48,* 595–607.

Dunning, H. (1972). Environmental occupational therapy. *American Journal of Occupational Therapy, 26,* 292–298.

Fidler, G. S., & Fidler, F. W. (1978). Doing and becoming: Purposeful action and self-actualization. *American Journal of Occupational Therapy, 32,* 305–310.

Fisher, A. (1998). Uniting practice and theory in an occupational framework. *American Journal of Occupational Therapy, 52,* 509–520.

Fisher, A., & Kielhofner, G. (1995). Skill in occupational performance. In G. Kielhofner (Ed.). *A model of human occupation: Theory and application* (2nd ed., pp. 113–117). Baltimore: Williams & Wilkins.

Florey, L. L. (1969). Intrinsic motivation: The dynamics of occupational therapy theory. *American Journal of Occupational Therapy, 23,* 319–322.

Ford, K. (1995). Occupational adaptation in home health: A therapist's viewpoint. *Home Health and Community Special Interest Section Newsletter, 2*(1), 2–4.

Forsyth, K., Lai, J., & Kielhofner, G. (1999). The assessment of communication and interaction skills (ACIS): Measurement properties. *British Journal of Occupational Therapy, 62*(2), 69–74.

Forsyth, K., Salamy, M., Simon, S., & Kielhofner, G. (1998). *A users guide to the assessment of communication and interaction skills (ACIS).* Bethesda, MD: American Occupational Therapy Association.

Garrett, S., & Schkade, J. K. (1995). The occupational adaptation model of professional development as applied to level II fieldwork in occupational therapy. *American Journal of Occupational Therapy, 49,* 119–126.

Gibson, J., & Schkade, J. K. (1997). Effects of occupational adaptation treatment with CVA. *American Journal of Occupational Therapy, 51,* 523–529.

Gilfoyle, E., Grady, A., & Moore, J. (1981). *Children adapt.* Thorofare, NJ: Slack.

Gray, M. (1972). Effects of hospitalization on work-play behavior. *American Journal of Occupational Therapy, 26,* 180–185.

Green, S., & Cooper, B. A. (2000). Occupation as a quality of life constituent: A nursing home perspective. *British Journal of Occupational Therapy, 63,* 17–24.

Grossack, M., & Gardner, H. (1970). *Man and men: Social psychology as social science.* Scranton, PA: International Textbook.

Hart, R. (1979). *Children's experience of place.* New York: Irvington.

Heard, C. (1977). Occupational role acquisition: A perspective on the chronically disabled. *American Journal of Occupational Therapy, 31,* 243–247.

Holahan, C. J. (1986). Environmental psychology. *Annual Review of Psychology, 37,* 381–307.

Hurff, J. (1980). A play skills inventory: A competency monitoring tool for the 10-year old. *American Journal of Occupational Therapy, 34,* 651–656.

Husserl, E. (1962). *Ideas: General introduction to pure phenomenology* (W. R. B. Gibson, Trans.). London: Collier Books.

Jackson, J. P., & Schkade, J. K. (2001). Occupational adaptation model vs. biomechanical/rehabilitation models in the treatment of patients with hip fractures. *American Journal of Occupational Therapy, 55,* 531–537.

Johnson, J., & Schkade, J. K. (2001). Effects of occupation-based intervention on mobility problems following a cerebral vascular accident. *Journal of Applied Gerontology, 20*(1), 91–110.

Kalish, R. A., & Collier, K. W. (1981). *Exploring human values.* Monterey, CA: Brooks/Cole.

Kielhofner, G. (1977). Temporal adaptation: A conceptual framework for occupational therapy. *American Journal of Occupational Therapy, 31,* 235–242.

Kielhofner, G. (1985). *A model of human occupation: Theory and application.* Baltimore: Williams & Wilkins.

Kielhofner, G. (1995). *A model of human occupation: Theory and application* (2nd ed.). Baltimore: Williams & Wilkins.

Kielhofner, G. (1997). *Conceptual foundations of occupational therapy* (2nd ed.). Philadelphia: Davis.

Kielhofner, G. (2002). *A model of human occupation: Theory and application* (3rd ed.). Baltimore: Williams & Wilkins.

Kielhofner, G., & Burke, J. P. (1977). Occupational therapy after 60 years: An account of changing identity and knowledge. *American Journal of Occupational Therapy, 31,* 675–689.

Kielhofner, G., Baz, T., Hutson, H., & Tham, K. (2002). Performance capacity and the lived body. In G. Kiehofner (Ed.). *The model of human occupation: Theory and application* (3rd ed., pp. 81–98). Baltimore: Williams & Wilkins.

Kielhofner, G., & Burke, J. P. (1980). A model of human occupation, part one. Conceptual framework and content. *American Journal of Occupational Therapy, 34,* 572–581.

King, L. J. (1978). Toward a science of adaptive responses. *American Journal of Occupational Therapy, 32,* 429–437.

Klavins, R. (1972). Work-play behavior: Cultural influences. *American Journal of Occupational Therapy, 26,* 176–179.

Law, M., Baptiste, S., Carswell, A., McColl, M. A., Polatajko, H., & Pollock, N. (1998). *Canadian Occupational Performance Measure* (3rd ed.). Ottawa, ON: CAOT Publications.

Law, M., Cooper, B., Stewart, D., Letts, L., Rigby, P., & Strong, S. (1994). Person-environment relations. *Work, 4,* 228–238.

Law, M., Cooper, B., Strong, S., Stewart, D., Rigby, P., & Letts, L. (1996). The person-environment-occupation model: A transactive approach to occupational performance. *Canadian Journal of Occupational Therapy, 63,* 9–23.

Law, M., Cooper, B., Strong, S., Stewart, D., Rigby, P., & Letts, L. (1997). Theoretical contexts for the practice of occupational therapy. In C. Christiansen & C. Baum (Eds.). *Enabling function and well-being* (2nd ed., pp. 72–102). Thorofare, NJ: Slack.

Law, M., Haight, M., Milroy, B., Willms, D., Stewart, D., & Rosenbaum, P. (1999). Environmental factors affecting the occupations of children with physical disabilities. *Journal of Occupational Science, 6*(3), 102–110.

Lawton, M. P., & Nahemow, L. (1973). Toward an ecological theory of adaptation and aging. In W. Preiser (Ed.). *Environmental design research* (pp. 24–32). Stroudsburg, PA: Dowden, Hutchison & Ross.

Letts, L., Law, M., Rigby, P., Cooper, B., Stewart, D., & Strong, S. (1994). Person-environment assessments in occupational therapy. *American Journal of Occupational Therapy, 48,* 608–618.

Line, J. (1969). Case method as a scientific form of clinical thinking. *American Journal of Occupational Therapy, 23,* 308–313.

Llorens, L. A. (1970). Facilitating growth and development: The promise of occupational therapy. *American Journal of Occupational Therapy, 24,* 93–101.

Matsutsuyu, J. S. (1969). The interest check list. *American Journal of Occupational Therapy, 23,* 323–328.

Matsutsuyu, J. (1971). Occupational behavior: A perspective on work and play. *American Journal of Occupational Therapy, 25,* 291–294.

McKye, A., Shin, J., & Letts, L. (1998). Cultural sensitivity of the person-environment-occupation (PEO) model. *Book of abstracts.* Number A142. Montreal, CA: World federation of occupational therapists.

Merleau-Ponty, M. (1962). *Phenomenology of perception* (C. Smith, Trans.). London: Routledge & Kegan Paul.

Meyer, A. (1922). The philosophy of occupational therapy. *Archives of Occupational Therapy, 1,* 1–10.

Michelman, S. S. (1971). The importance of creative play. *American Journal of Occupational Therapy, 25,* 285–290.

Moorhead, L. (1969). The occupational history. *American Journal of Occupational Therapy, 23,* 329–334.

Mosey, A. C. (1986). *Psychosocial components of occupational therapy.* New York: Raven.

Nelson, D (1988). Occupation: Form and performance. *American Journal of Occupational Therapy, 42,* 633–641.

Parent, L. H. (1978). Effects of a low-stimulus environment on behavior. *American Journal of Occupational Therapy, 32,* 19–25.

Pasek, P. B., & Schkade, J. K. (1996). Effects of a skiing experience on adolescents with limb deficiencies: An occupational adaptation perspective. *American Journal of Occupational Therapy, 50,* 24–31.

Peachy-Hill, C., & Law, M. (2000). Impact of environmental sensitivity on occupational performance. *Canadian Journal of Occupational Therapy, 67,* 304–313.

Reilly, M. (1962). Occupational therapy can be one of the great ideas of 20th century medicine. *American Journal of Occupational Therapy, 16,* 1–9.

Reilly, M. (1966). A psychiatric occupational program as a teaching model. *American Journal of Occupational Therapy, 20,* 61–67.

Reilly, M. (1969). The educational process. *American Journal of Occupational Therapy, 23,* 299–307.

Reilly, M. (Ed.). (1974). *Play as exploratory learning: Studies of curiosity behavior.* Beverly Hills, CA: Sage.

Robinson, A. L. (1977). The arena for acquisition of rules for competent behavior. *American Journal of Occupational Therapy, 31,* 248–253.

Ross, M. M. (1994, August 11). Applying theory to practice. *OT Week,* 16–17.

Saegert, S., & Winkel, G. H. (1990). Environmental psychology. *Annual Review of Psychology, 41,* 441–477.

Sarbin, T. R., & Scheibe, K. E. (1983). A model of social identity. In T. R. Sarbin & K. E. Scheibe (Eds.). *Studies in social identity* (pp. 5–28). New York: Praeger.

Schkade, J. K. (1999). Student to practitioner: The adaptive transition. *Innovations in Occupational Therapy Education, 1,* 147–156.

Schkade, J. K., & McClung, M. (2001). *Occupational adaptation in practice: Concepts and cases.* Thorofare, NJ: Slack.

Schkade, J. K., & Schultz, S. (1992). Occupational adaptation: Toward a holistic approach to contemporary practice, Part 1. *American Journal of Occupational Therapy, 46,* 829–837.

Schkade, J. K., & Schultz, S. (1993). Occupational adaptation: An integrative frame of reference. In H. Hopkins & H. Smith, (Eds.). *Willard and Spackman's occupational therapy* (8th ed., pp. 87–91). Philadelphia: Lippincott.

Schultz, S. (1997). *Treating students with behavior disorders: An institute.* Paper presented at the American Occupational Therapy Conference, Orlando, FL.

Schultz, S. & Schkade, J. K. (1997). Adaptation. In C. Christiansen & C. Baum (Eds.). *Occupational therapy: Enabling function and well being* (2nd ed., pp. 458–481). Thorofare, NJ: Slack.

Schultz, S., & Schkade, J. K. (1992). Occupational adaptation: Toward a holistic approach to contemporary practice, Part 2. *American Journal of Occupational Therapy, 46,* 917–926.

Schultz, S., & Schkade, J. K. (1994, September). Home health care: a window of opportunity to synthesize practice. *Home & Community Health, AOTA Special Interest Section Newsletter, 1*(3), 1–4.

Selye, H. (1956). *The Stress of Life.* New York: McGraw-Hill.

Shannon, P. (1972). Work-play theory and the occupational therapy process. *American Journal of Occupational Therapy, 26,* 169–172.

Smith, M. B. (1969). *Social psychology and human values.* Chicago: Aldine.

Stewart, D., Law, M., Rosenbaum, P., & Williams, D. (2001). A qualitative study of the transition to adulthood for youth with physical disabilities. *Physical and Occupational Therapy in Pediatrics, 21,* 3–21.

Strong, S. (1998). Meaningful work in supportive environments: Experiences with the recovery process. *American Journal of Occupational Therapy, 52,* 31–38.

Strong, S., Rigby, P., Stewart, D., Law, M., Letts, L., & Cooper, B. (1999). Application of the person-environment-occupation model: A practical tool. *Canadian Journal of Occupational Therapy,* 66, 122–133.

Teel, C., Dunn, W., Jackson, S., & Duncan, P. (1997). The role of the environment in fostering independence: conceptual and methodological issues in developing an instrument. *Topics in Stroke Rehabilitation,* 4(1), 28–40.

Teel, C., Dunn, W., Jackson, S., & Duncan, P. (2001). *Development of the Environmental Independence Interaction Scale (EIIS).* Unpublished manuscript.

Trombly, C. A. (1989). *Occupational therapy for physical dysfunction.* Baltimore: Williams & Wilkins.

Werner, E. (2000). *Families, children with autism and everyday occupations.* Unpublished doctoral dissertation. Nova Southeastern University, Fort Lauderdale, FL.

Westmorland, M., Williams, R., & Strong, S. (2000). *Workplace perspectives: Successful work (re)entry for persons with disabilities* [Research report]. Hamilton, ON: McMaster University, School of Rehabilitation Science, Work Function Unit.

Wicker, A. W. (1979). *An introduction to ecological psychology.* Cambridge, UK: Cambridge University Press.

World Health Organization. (2001). *International classification of function, disability, and health* (ICF). Geneva: Author. Retrieved March 1, 2002, from www.who.int/icf/icftemplate.cfm

CHAPTER 19

THEORIES DERIVED FROM REHABILITATION PERSPECTIVES

SECTION I: Rehabilitation Perspectives
SECTION II: Rehabilitative Frame of Reference
SECTION III: Biomechanical Frame of Reference

SECTION I

Rehabilitation Perspectives

ALICE C. SEIDEL

DEFINING REHABILITATION

Rehabilitation is the process of restoring an individual's capacity to participate in functional activities when this capacity has been altered or limited by a physical or mental impairment. The rehabilitation process is "the combined and coordinated use of medical, social, educational and vocational measures for training and retraining the individual to the highest levels of functional ability" (Hagedorn, 1997, p. 42). Rehabilitation activities include "adaptive or compensatory occupations in which assistive devices, alternative or compensatory strategies or modifications of physical or social environments" (Fisher, 1998, p. 513) are provided to enable clients' participation in daily living activities. Rehabilitation does not cure the illness or replace lost organ function, but it does enable performance of self-care, work, and leisure activities (Dutton, 1995; Gullickson & Licht, 1968; Mattingly & Fleming, 1993).

The World Health Organization's (2001) International Classification of Functioning, Disability, and Health defines terminology associated with rehabilitation: impairment, activity limitation, and participation restriction. Impairment is a "problem in body function or structure such as a significant deviation or loss" (p. 8). For example, a person with an amputation of his or her right forearm has an impairment of the right upper extremity. When impairment limits an individual's performance of a task, he or she has an activity limitation. An activity limitation is "difficulty in executing activities" (p. 8). The person with an impaired right upper extremity is unable to tie his or her shoes; therefore, he or she has an activity limitation. When a person with a persistent disability is unable to complete activities that fulfill the essential responsibilities and duties of a social role, he or she experiences participation restriction. Participation restriction entails the inability to work or to participate in the community by going to church, joining community organizations, etc. The World Health Organization (WHO) model includes physical, social, and attitudinal environmental factors that influence individuals' performance in daily living activities and participation in society. These definitions provide a framework for describing levels of function among clients who participate in rehabilitation.

HISTORICAL ROOTS OF REHABILITATION

Before the early nineteenth century, family members cared for persons with disabilities in their homes. Outside of the immediate family unit, few people knew about the needs of individuals with physical or mental disabilities. Individuals with disabilities were isolated and sheltered from societal attitudes about disabilities. In an effort to educate others about the needs of their impaired members, caregiving families formed groups. These groups, based on families' experiences, became the first formal organizations that advocated for the needs of persons with impairments. They represented the earliest efforts to shift the issues of disability from the family to society. Contemporary consumer advocacy groups and government programs that fund rehabilitation programs and services continue this long tradition of societal participation in meeting the needs of persons with disabilities (Groce, 1992; Gullickson & Licht, 1968).

The shift of care from the family unit to the community led to the development of rehabilitation institutions and programs. The education and advocacy efforts of family organizations led to the creation of rehabilitation facilities. As women, the primary caregivers, entered the workforce, the idea of placing a family member with a disability in a residential rehabilitation center gained social acceptance. Early facilities did not attempt to teach residents how to achieve independence or functional competence to care for themselves; instead, they provided shelter and basic care (Groce, 1992). This concept of rehabilitation as caregiving remained unchanged until World War II (WWII). After WWII, rehabilitation facilities started teaching residents how to function as independently as possible when performing their activities of daily living (ADL), when in their homes and conducting instrumental activities of daily living (IADL), and when participating in society through work and community activities.

WWII veterans who returned from the battlefields with disabilities were the catalysts of this change in the philosophy of rehabilitation. Medical advances in the treatment of war injuries enabled large numbers of soldiers to survive, despite permanent physical impairments. These disabled veterans returned to their hometowns and wanted to resume their former social, family, and worker roles. Society could not ignore the needs of men and women who had lost their ability to function while serving their country (Groce, 1992; Gullickson & Licht, 1968).

To meet the needs of these soldiers, veterans' hospitals, built in the United States during WWI to provide residential care for veterans, expanded to include restorative services. Funded by the government, veterans' hospitals became national leaders in advancing the philosophy of rehabilitation. They provided the most up-to-date medical, social, and vocational services to return veterans to their social roles. Federal funding provided financial support to train occupational therapists, physical therapists, and vocational counselors to meet the needs of these veterans. The post-WWII era marked the beginning of long-term government funding of rehabilitation programs, facilities, and personnel (Groce, 1992).

Rehabilitation became a medical specialty in the years after WWII. Medical advances enabled people to survive acute and chronic illnesses and traumatic injuries. However, these survivors often had disabilities that prevented them from participating fully in society. These changes in health and illness patterns led to the development of a medical specialty called rehabilitation medicine, or physical medicine. Specialists in rehabilitation medicine, called physiatrists, serve the medical needs of individuals with physical impairments. Initial efforts to organize rehabilitation medicine as a specialty occurred in veterans' hospitals, which provided a service-delivery model for the development of civilian rehabilitation centers (Gullickson & Licht, 1968).

Rehabilitation medicine highlighted the importance of enabling people with chronic illness and impairments to live productive lives. It also introduced the concept of a treatment team composed of professionals trained in the area of rehabilitation. The rehabilitation team usually includes a physiatrist, physical therapist, occupational therapy practitioner, vocational counselor, and a rehabilitation nurse. Additional members may include a prosthetist, orthotist, speech and language pathologist, therapeutic recreation specialist, and psychologist.

Much of the early writing about rehabilitation as a medical specialty suggests that the restoration of physical function dominated the philosophy and goals of programs and professionals. In contrast, rehabilitation services for persons with mental illness garnered minimal attention and, when mentioned, focused on community reentry (Fidler, 1993).

EFFECT OF LEGISLATION ON REHABILITATION

Federal legislation that funded rehabilitation programs, facilities, services, and training for personnel helped advance rehabilitation in the United States. Vocational rehabilitation received its initial funding in 1918 and 1920 from legislation enacted to support rehabilitation services for individuals with physical impairments. The 1943 amendments to the earlier vocational rehabilitation legislation funded medical and psychiatric rehabilitation services. The 1943 amendments strengthened the ability of rehabilitation programs to serve the vocational needs of persons with mental impairments. Subsequent amendments in 1954 and 1963 expanded the concept of rehabilitation from a biorehabilitation to a social rehabilitation model. The shift to a social rehabilitation model emphasized the restoration of individuals to their fullest potential as participants and contributors in family and community groups (Reed, 1984). The concept of social rehabilitation resulted in federal funds for research and the training of rehabilitation personnel, such as occupational therapy practitioners, to provide services that enabled persons with disabilities to function in social, family, and community activities (Reed, 1984).

The social movements of civil rights and deinstitutionalization of persons with chronic mental impairments influenced American rehabilitation services and programs during the 1960s and 1970s. The philosophical underpinnings of these movements stimulated the independent living movement that advocated for community reintegration of persons with physical impairments. The independent living movement, funded by vocational rehabilitation amendments, created community-based programs, such as wheelchair repair shops and transportation services, for people confined to wheelchairs. These services enabled people with disabilities to live in group homes or assisted-living apartments. Most important, the movement advocated persistently and loudly for the inclusion of persons with disabilities in the mainstream of community life. Rehabilitation professionals and consumers involved in the independent living movement laid the foundation that would eventually become the American Disabilities Act (ADA) of 1993—landmark legislation that ensures the rights of people with disabilities to participate fully in society. Further evidence of societal changes about the place and role of persons with disabilities is evident in the revisions of WHO's (2001) classification of functioning, disability, and health, which now includes social participation as a primary criterion for determining individuals' engagement in daily activities and roles.

OCCUPATIONAL THERAPY AND THE REHABILITATION MOVEMENT

Concern for the preservation and restoration of an individual's functional abilities made occupational therapy practitioners early advocates for rehabilitation services. During WWI, "reconstruction aides" provided restorative services at battlefield sites to soldiers suffering from battle fatigue and mental trauma. Reconstruction aides, who later would become trainers of future generations of occupational therapy practitioners, used vocational-based crafts, such as woodworking, to teach soldiers trades they could use in civilian work roles. Reconstruction aides returned from the battlefields to continue their restorative work with soldiers in veterans' hospitals. They would eventually establish similar programs in civilian hospitals and train nurses and social workers in the use of activity to rehabilitate individuals institutionalized with mental impairments.

The growth of rehabilitation services after WWII led to an increased demand for trained occupational therapy practitioners. Because of the large number of soldiers returning from WWII with permanent physical injuries, occupational therapy practitioners began to specialize in the rehabilitation of individuals with physical impairments. The specialty of "physical disabilities" gained popularity among therapists. The areas of prosthetics, orthotics, and the application of assistive devices expanded to become integral parts of the rehabilitation process.

When rehabilitation moved toward a community model, occupational therapy practitioners often spearheaded the development and implementation of programs that occurred in independent-living centers or transitional housing settings. Because these settings are in the community, occupational therapy practitioners facilitate the development of social participation skills in their clients.

CONCLUSION

The historical roots of rehabilitation reflect societal and legislative initiatives so that the needs and the desires of persons with chronic illnesses and impairments are met and they can live productive lives. Occupational therapy practitioners, through their focus on occupation, have contributed significantly to the development of rehabilitation as a team oriented, medical specialty. The remaining sections of this chapter describe two practice theories or frames of reference (FORs) derived from rehabilitation principles: the rehabilitation and biomechanical frames of reference.

SECTION II

Rehabilitative Frame of Reference

ALICE C. SEIDEL

PHILOSOPHY

The rehabilitative frame of reference embraces the philosophy of rehabilitation: to enable a person with physical or mental disability or chronic illness to achieve maximum function in the performance of his or her daily activities. When medical or surgical remediation of impairment is not possible or successful, rehabilitation is the next intervention strategy (Hagedorn, 1997; Trombly, 1995a). Rehabilitation emphasizes an individual's abilities; therefore, the rehabilitative FOR focuses on compensatory methods, assistive devices, and environmental modifications the individual needs to function in spite of his or her impairment.

INTELLECTUAL HERITAGE

Knowledge bases that contribute to the rehabilitative frame of reference include the medical sciences and the physical and social sciences. The medical sciences help practitioners understand the influence of pathological processes on an individual's abilities to function in ADL and IADL. Physical sciences help practitioners understand the biomechanics of human movement, design or select assistive devices that promote function, and modify an environment to help an individual with a disability function more effectively. The social sciences contribute important knowledge about how individuals and societies respond to chronic illness and disability.

DEFINITIONS AND ASSUMPTIONS

Rehabilitation is the processes of helping a person with a disability perform competently in his or her social roles and daily activities. The rehabilitation FOR emphasizes the teaching of compensatory techniques: the use of adaptive and assistive equipment and the modification of social and physical features of environments that inhibit function. Dutton (1995) identified five assumptions of the rehabilitative frame of reference:

- With compensation strategies and techniques, an individual can restore independence when the underlying impairment cannot be remediated.
- A person's level of motivation affects the extent to which an individual regains independence.
- Environments in which a person performs influence his or her motivation for independence.
- Rehabilitation involves the teaching–learning process; therefore, the person needs sufficient cognitive skills to learn and to apply compensatory methods. Motivation enables the individual to participate fully in the teaching–learning process.
- Clinical reasoning, used by the practitioner, begins with the individual's goals and functional capabilities, moves to the environments in which the person will function, and then to the types of compensatory strategies the person needs to use his or her capabilities.

EFFECTS ON EVALUATION

In the rehabilitative FOR, evaluation identifies a client's goals and function in self-care and social participation, such as work and leisure activities. The results of this evaluation provide a picture of the person's capabilities and competencies in daily activities. The occupational therapist uses several types of assessment methods: observations of client performance in selected activities, interviews about a client's daily living priorities, and client self-reports about his or her level of competency in daily activities (Dutton, 1995). Most commonly, the therapist uses all three assessment methods to evaluate a client's function in daily activities.

Throughout an evaluation, the occupational therapist pays attention to several factors associated with an individual's functional status, including

- Characteristics of physical and social environments in which the client functions.
- Equipment and economic resources used by the client.
- Levels of supervision and assistance available to the client.
- Developmental expectations for the client's performance.
- Motor, process, and social interaction skills that are absent or are limiting a client's function.

The practitioner's analysis of evaluation data provides a picture of the client's capabilities and areas that need intervention (Dutton, 1995; Trombly, 1995a).

MECHANISMS FOR CHANGE

Occupational therapy practitioners using the rehabilitative frame of reference assume that the client's impairment is stabilized and cannot be altered by therapeutic interventions. The client's capacity to function in daily activities, however, can be changed through the use of compensatory methods and adaptive equipment. Therefore, the teaching–learning process is a major part of occupational therapy intervention. The practitioner teaches the client compensatory methods to perform ADL, IADL, and ways to apply these new techniques to his or her daily activities and participation in life situations (Trombly, 1995a; WHO, 2001).

Change in a client's functional abilities depends on several client-centered factors. The plan of intervention must be based on goals established in collaboration with the client (Law & Mills, 1998). The client must be motivated to participate in the teaching–learning process and to use new compensation methods or assistive devices. The client's processing skills influence his or her ability to learn and apply new compensatory methods. The environment in which therapy occurs is essential to a client's learning. This environment needs to include the necessary equipment, objects, support, and feedback systems that contribute to the client's commitment to change and that match his or her learning style (Fisher, 1998; Trombly, 1995a).

Practitioner–client collaboration is important in the rehabilitative FOR (Dutton, 1995; Trombly, 1995a). The rehabilitative frame of reference uses daily living, work, and leisure activities as the purposeful activities of occupational therapy intervention. Treatment programs occur in the environment that is natural for the performance of the daily activities (Fisher, 1998). For example, a practitioner would teach a client compensatory methods for bathing in a fully equipped bathroom that contains the assistive devices and equipment the client needs to achieve competent performance. Opportunities to practice and apply the newly learned compensatory methods are important elements of the intervention process. The client is expected to cooperate in learning and to practice new compensatory strategies (Hagedorn, 1997). By participating in the problem-solving process of treatment, clients learn skills they will use outside the therapeutic milieu. Practitioners use reinforcement and demonstration to create environments that support learning. An important factor in the therapeutic relationship is the occupational therapy practitioner's creativity in devising compensatory methods, adaptive equipment, and learning environments that fit with the client's goals, capabilities, and limitations (Trombly, 1995a).

STRENGTHS AND LIMITATIONS

The rehabilitative frame of reference has enjoyed a long and successful history in occupational therapy because it includes the core values of occupational therapy. It focuses on client-centered capabilities and daily activities (Hagedorn, 1997). The therapeutic relationship focuses on the client and requires collaboration to problem solve and create compensatory methods for the client's performance of everyday activities. The evaluation process addresses a client's interests, roles, resources, environments, and support systems, thereby providing the occupational therapy practitioner a holistic perspective of a client's function in daily activities.

There are limitations to the rehabilitative FOR, which cannot be overlooked. Some ADL and IADL instruments lack reliability and validity data and are designed specifically and exclusively for a particular setting (Dutton, 1995). This absence of reliability and validity data limits the use of these evaluations in outcomes research.

Successful outcomes in the rehabilitative frame of reference depend heavily on client commitment and participation in the teaching–learning process. When compensatory methods do not work or a client is unable to learn new approaches, this frame of reference provides no alternatives. The rehabilitative FOR is linked closely to the medical model and, particularly, to physical rehabilitation, which emphasizes the individual with a physical impairment. Therefore, the rehabilitative frame of reference is most closely associated with the physical disabilities area of occupational therapy practice. The rehabilitative frame of reference is seldom presented as a model for designing occupational therapy programs for clients with mental impairments.

FUTURE RESEARCH

An important area for research in the rehabilitative frame of reference is the establishment of reliability and validity for ADL and IADL evaluation instruments so therapists can use these assessment tools to conduct functional outcome studies of the rehabilitative frame of reference. Another area of research is the use of the rehabilitative FOR in occupational therapy programs for individuals with mental impairments. Because client commitment is a requisite for successful outcomes under this model, the application of a client-centered approach to goal setting within a rehabilitative frame of reference is also an appropriate area for occupational therapy research.

CONCLUSION

Linked closely to physical medicine, the rehabilitation FOR emphasizes clients' use of assistive equipment, adaptive compensatory methods, and environmental modifications to restore their function in daily activities. The evaluation process assesses clients' level of competency in performing daily self-care, leisure, and work activities and their goals for improving function in these areas. Change in clients' function results from occupational therapy practitioners use of the teaching-learning process in which adaptive strategies are learned and practiced by clients. Successful outcomes in the rehabilitation FOR depend upon clients' motivation and commitment to improve their functional competence in daily occupations.

SECTION III

Biomechanical Frame of Reference

ANNE BIRGE JAMES

The **biomechanical** frame of reference is used to treat individuals with activity limitations due to **impairments** in biomechanical body structures and functions, including structural instability, decreased strength, limited range of motion (ROM), and poor endurance. The main tenet of the biomechanical approach is that occupational performance can be regained through addressing underlying impairments that limit performance of activities (Hagedorn, 1997; Trombly, 1995a).

Treatment within the biomechanical FOR focuses on preventing or decreasing impairments through the use of activity and exercise, which may be purposeful or rote (Kielhofner, 1997). The treatment modalities may not be inherently meaningful to the client, but meaning is thought to be created through the ultimate goal of restoring the client's capability to engage in occupation.

INTELLECTUAL HERITAGE

The biomechanical FOR derives its foundation from the biomedical sciences, which are reductionistic—that is, they focus on correcting the underlying problem to restore health (Yerxa, 2001). An understanding of pathology, wound healing, precautions, and prognosis for disorders that have an impact on the musculoskeletal system is crucial for setting safe and realistic goals. Knowledge of the cardiopulmonary system is also necessary for managing clients with endurance deficits (Kielhofner, 1997).

Applied physical sciences also contribute to the biomechanical FOR, including kinesiology and exercise physiology. Kinesiology helps practitioners understand the biomechanics of human movement (Zemke, 1995). Exercise physiologists have published extensively on optimal programs to increase strength, flexibility, and endurance. Occupational therapy practitioners using a biomechanical FOR can apply this knowledge to a treatment program that restores occupational performance.

DOMAIN OF PRACTICE AND UNDERLYING ASSUMPTIONS

The domains of concern addressed through a biomechanical FOR are structural stability, strength, ROM, edema, and endurance, including both cardiopulmonary and muscle endurance (Kielhofner, 1997; Pedretti & Early, 2001). Assumptions of the biomechanical FOR include

- Most activities have a biomechanical dimension (Kielhofner, 1997).
- People with biomechanical impairments may have difficulty with occupational performance (Kielhofner, 1997).
- Biomechanical impairments can be corrected through varied treatment methods, including adjunctive modalities, which prepare the client for occupational performance (e.g., passive stretching), and enabling activities, which are not purposeful but allow practice of component skills needed for occupational performance (e.g., pegboards) (Pedretti & Early, 2001).
- The underlying pathology must be considered so that realistic and appropriate goals can be set, i.e., the prognosis for improvement of the biomechanical deficit is good, and treatment will enhance body structures without harming them.
- While some spontaneous improvement in activities of daily living may occur as biomechanical body functions and structures improve, transitional activities ensure that gains in biomechanical function are transferred into the client's occupational performance (Perr & Bell, 2000).

EFFECTS ON EVALUATION, INTERVENTION, AND CLIENT–PRACTITIONER INTERACTIONS

Evaluation begins with a careful review the client's medical record so that the pathology, precautions, and prognosis are clear to the therapist. The occupational therapist should assess the client's compliance with the precautions within the context of daily activities.

A top-down approach is recommended to ensure that the relationship between specific biomechanical impairments and occupational performance is clear (Trombly, 1995a). Assessment of the biomechanical impairments should then focus on those impairments that appear to be influencing occupational performance and can be expected to improve with direct treatment (Trombly, 1995a). Typical assessments of biomechanical impairments used by occupational therapists are described in Chapter 25, Section 1.

Treatment is aimed at reducing biomechanical impairments; however, goals must reflect expected improvements in occupational performance (Trombly, 1995b). Treatment goals written at the impairment level must be linked to related activities; for example, the client will increase right elbow flexion to 130° to facilitate fastening cardigan garments. Writing goals that target the impairment often makes it easier to document interim progress.

Activity analysis focused on the biomechanical aspects of the task is necessary to determine how much remediation of impairment is needed to reach activity goals (Pedretti, 2001). Treatment goals need not aim for normal strength to enable performance of the activity goals.

Many treatment techniques are commonly used within the biomechanical FOR. Static orthotics increase joint stability or position a joint to prevent deformity (Coppard & Lynn, 2001). Dynamic orthotics can increase ROM at a joint (Coppard & Lynn, 2001). A variety of stretching exercises are used to maintain or increase passive ROM (Zemke, 1995). Reducing edema that interferes with movement can be done through elevation, compressive wraps, active exercise, or specialized massage (Kasch & Nickerson, 2001). Strength can be improved through a wide array of exercises or activities that elicit a maximum contraction from the weak muscles. Exercises for weak muscles may include assistance to help the client move, whereas stronger muscles must work against resistance to enhance strength (Kasch & Nickerson, 2001; Zemke, 1995). Muscle endurance is crucial for activities that are repetitive or lengthy and can be improved through activities that work the muscles at submaximal contractions for relatively long periods of time (Zemke, 1995). Cardiovascular endurance can be addressed through graded activities aimed at gradually increasing the client's tolerance to physical activity (Atchison, 1995; Matthews, 2001; Zemke, 1995).

Occupational therapy practitioners are trained to see the connection between biomechanical impairments and occupational performance deficits; however, this connection is often not clear to clients. When using a biomechanical FOR, the practitioner must explain the purpose of the treatment activities in relationship to the occupational performance goals.

STRENGTHS AND LIMITATIONS

The main advantage of the biomechanical FOR is that it directly addresses the impairments that limit occupational performance. Addressing underlying impairments restores activity performance more efficiently than using compensatory strategies, because the client can generalize gains made in underlying impairments to many activities, whereas compensatory strategies are often task specific (Sabari, 2000; Trombly, 1995a).

The biomechanical FOR fits well into occupational therapy practice *if* the link between occupational performance and biomechanical deficits remains in the forefront of treatment planning and implementation. If the focus shifts exclusively to the biomechanical impairments, the practitioner slips out of an occupational therapy framework altogether, raising significant ethical issues regarding scope of practice.

The biomechanical FOR is reductionistic and does not take into account important parameters, such as clients' interests and motivation for treatment. This limitation can be overcome by combining the biomechanical FOR with other frames of reference that are more client centered, such as the occupational behavior frames of reference (see Chapter 18).

The biomechanical FOR has a narrowly focused domain. Clients with biomechanical impairments may also have neurosensorimotor deficits that are not addressed through this approach, for example, problems with muscle timing, decreased coordination, impaired balance, hyposensory or hypersensory deficits, and acute or chronic pain. The integration of the biomechanical FOR with other approaches can be used successfully to overcome the narrow focus.

Clients may have biomechanical impairments that cannot be restored through therapy. The rehabilitation FOR can be used to enable a client to compensate for permanent biomechanical impairments, while a biomechanical FOR can be used to address impairments that will respond to direct treatment (Kielhofner, 1997; Trombly, 1995a). The rehabilitation FOR can also be used for temporary compensation to increase performance in the short term, as gains in biomechanical body structures or functions frequently take weeks or months.

FUTURE RESEARCH

The biomechanical requirements of specific activities are not well described in the literature (Kielhofner, 1997).

Studies that examine the minimum biomechanical requirements for common ADL may facilitate the activity analysis used to link biomechanical deficits to limitations in activity performance and may facilitate appropriate goal setting.

Treatment using a biomechanical FOR often incorporates rote exercise, although the treatment principles can be applied to purposeful activities as well. Many studies have looked at the impact of purposeful activity on client participation in treatment and found that participation is typically improved when purposeful, rather than rote, activity is used (Dolecheck & Schkade, 1999; Melchert-McKearnan, Deitz, Engel, & White, 2000; Thomas, 1996). These studies suggest that treatment with purposeful activity could be more effective, which has implications for therapists who frequently use rote tasks. Few studies, however, have examined the effect of purposeful activity on body function or activity-based outcomes. Further research is needed in this area.

EDITORS' CONCLUSION

The rehabilitation and biomechanical frames of reference focus on clients' physical impairments and the impact of these impairments on their engagement in daily occupations. Practitioners using the rehabilitation FOR teach clients to compensate for their physical impairments, whereas practitioners using the biomechanical FOR focus on remediation of specific client impairments. A practitioner may use both frames of reference simultaneously with any given client, teaching adaptation for those impairments that are not likely to improve and offering remedial intervention for impairments that have the potential to improve. Before using either approach, practitioners need to consider its strengths and weaknesses relative to each client's particular situation and priorities. These approaches are most effective when combined with other frames of reference, because that way they provide a holistic approach to care that is consistent with the foundations of occupational therapy practice.

References

Atchison, B. (1995). Cardiopulmonary diseases. In C. A. Trombly (Ed.). *Occupational therapy for physical dysfunction* (4th ed., pp. 875–892). Baltimore: Williams & Wilkins.

Coppard, B. M., & Lynn, P. (2001). Introduction to splinting. In B. M. Coppard & H. Lohman (Eds.). *Introduction to splinting: A clinical-reasoning and problem-solving approach* (pp. 1–33). St. Louis: Mosby.

Dolecheck, J. R., & Schkade, J. K. (1999). The extent of dynamic standing endurance is effected when CVA subjects perform personally meaningful activities rather than nonmeaningful tasks. *Occupational Therapy Journal of Research, 19*, 40–54.

Dutton, R. (1995). *Clinical reasoning in physical disabilities*. Baltimore: Williams & Wilkins.

Fidler, G. S. (1993). The challenge of change to occupational therapy practice. In R. P. F. Cotrell (Ed.). *Psychosocial occupational therapy* (pp. 15–19). Bethesda, MD: American Occupational Therapy Association.

Fisher, A. G. (1998). Uniting practice and theory in an occupational framework. *American Journal of Occupational Therapy. 52*, 509–521.

Groce, N. (1992). *The U. S. Role in international disability activities: A history and look towards the future*. [Grant G0087C2013]. Oakland, CA: World Institute on Disability.

Gullickson, G., & Licht, S. (1968). Definition and philosophy of rehabilitation medicine. In S. Licht (Ed.). *Rehabilitation and medicine* (pp. 1–13). Baltimore: Waverly.

Hagedorn, R. (1997). *Foundations for practice in occupational therapy* (2nd ed.). New York: Churchill Livingstone.

Kasch, M. C., & Nickerson, E. (2001). Hand and upper extremity injuries. In L. W. Pedretti & M. B. Early (Eds.). *Occupational therapy: Practice skills for physical dysfunction* (5th ed., pp. 833–866). St. Louis: Mosby.

Kielhofner, G. (1997). *Conceptual foundations of occupational therapy* (2nd ed.). Philadelphia: Davis.

Law, M., & Mills, J. (1998). Client-centered occupational therapy. In M. Law (Ed.). *Client-centered occupational therapy* (pp. 1–18). Thorofare, NJ: Slack.

Matthews, M. M. (2001). Cardiac and pulmonary diseases. In L. W. Pedretti & M. B. Early (Eds.). *Occupational therapy: Practice skills for physical dysfunction* (5th ed., pp. 966–980). St. Louis: Mosby.

Mattingly, C., & Fleming, M. H. (1993). *Clinical reasoning: Forms of inquiry in a therapeutic process*. Philadelphia: Davis.

Melchert-McKearnan, K., Deitz, J., Engel, J. M., & White, O. (2000). Children with burn injuries: Purposeful activity versus rote exercise. *American Journal of Occupational Therapy, 54*, 381–390.

Pedretti, L. W. (2001). Joint range of motion. In L. W. Pedretti & M. B. Early (Eds.). *Occupational therapy: Practice skills for physical dysfunction* (5th ed., pp. 285–315). St. Louis: Mosby.

Pedretti, L. W., & Early, M. B. (2001). Occupational performance and models of practice for physical dysfunction. In L. W. Pedretti & M. B. Early (Eds.). *Occupational therapy: Practice skills for physical dysfunction* (5th ed., pp. 3–12). St. Louis: Mosby.

Perr, A., & Bell, P. F. (2000). Moving from simulation to real life. In J. Hinohosa & M.-L. Blount (Eds.). *The texture of life: Purposeful activities in occupational therapy* (pp. 234–257). Bethesda, MD: American Occupational Therapy Association.

Reed, K. L. (1984). *Models of practice in occupational therapy*. Baltimore: Williams & Wilkins.

Sabari, J. S. (2000). Using activities as challenges to facilitate development of functional skills. In J. Hinojosa & M.-L. Blount (Eds.). *The texture of life: Purposeful activities in occupational therapy* (pp. 215–233). Bethesda: American Occupational Therapy Association.

Thomas, J. J. (1996). Materials-based, imagery-based, and rote exercise occupational form: Effect on repetitions, heart rate, duration of performance, and self-perceived rest period in well elderly women. *American Journal of Occupational Therapy, 50*, 783–789.

Trombly, C. A. (1995a). Theoretical foundations for practice. In C. A. Trombly (Ed.). *Occupational therapy for physical dysfunction* (4th ed., pp. 15–27). Baltimore: Williams & Wilkins.

Trombly, C. A. (1995b). Planning, guiding, and documenting therapy. In C. A. Trombly (Ed.). *Occupational therapy for physical dysfunction* (4th ed., pp. 29–40). Baltimore: Williams & Wilkins.

World Health Organization [WHO]. (2001). *International classification of impairments, disabilities and handicaps*. Geneva: Author. Available at: www.who.int/icidh. Accessed January 10, 2002.

Yerxa, E. J. (2001). The social and psychological experience of having a disability. In L. W. Pedretti & M. B. Early (Eds.). *Occupational therapy: Practice skills for physical dysfunction* (5th ed., pp. 470–492). St. Louis: Mosby.

Zemke, R. (1995). Remediating biomechanical and physiological impairments in motor performance. In C. A. Trombly (Ed.). *Occupational therapy for physical dysfunction* (4th ed., pp. 405–422). Baltimore: Williams & Wilkins.

CHAPTER 20

DEVELOPMENTAL AND NEUROLOGICAL PERSPECTIVES

SECTION I

Overview of Infant and Child Developmental Models

ROSEMARIE BIGSBY

HISTORICAL PERSPECTIVE ON DEVELOPMENTAL MODELS

The scientific view on human development as a process changed dramatically during the twentieth century. Until the 1980s, developmental theorists viewed development as a predictable, stepwise sequence that depended on maturation of the central nervous system (CNS). Now they see development as a variable process that depends on a complex interaction between a child's biological endowment, the immediate caregiving environment, the community, and the society or culture within which the child is being raised (Freel, 1996; Wachs, 1992).

THE HIERARCHICAL MODEL: CONTINUITY AND PREDICTABILITY IN NORMAL DEVELOPMENT

Early views on development were dominated by observational studies of motor and cognitive development (Gesell, 1928; Piaget, 1952) that presumed a **hierarchical model**—that is, one in which normal development occurs in a predictable sequence of steps. Scholars proposed that the process underlying this linear developmental progression was biologically pre-determined and directly related to hierarchical changes in CNS development. Although increasingly complex functions are known to emerge as the CNS develops, brain–behavior relationships are not necessarily as direct as was previously thought, and early notions of the interdependence of fine and gross motor performance are being challenged (Simons, Mandich, Ritchie, & Mullett, 2000). What the hierarchical model leaves unexplained are the variability and flexibility seen in motor and cognitive behavior among both typically and atypically developing children as well as the profound influence of CNS plasticity and the environment on development.

CONTEXTUAL MODELS: THE IMPACT OF EXPERIENCE AND FEATURES OF THE ENVIRONMENT

Periods of variability in performance were recognized by early theorists, who described them as a time of "interweaving" of new unrefined behaviors with old established ones (Gesell, 1928), an adaptation sequence involving assimilation of new with previous experiences, accommodation to changing circumstances, and eventual progression to a new, higher level of functioning (Piaget, 1952). This theory of adaptation held a dominant role in occupational therapy, because it incorporates adjustment to disruption or change as well as the roles of purposeful activity, self-direction, and motivation in coping with stress and challenge (Gilfoyle, Grady, & Moore, 1981; King, 1978; Llorens, 1969). Still, this model failed to address the periods in normal development—often just before a shift to a higher level of performance—when infants and young children not only exhibit variability in their behavior but also actually appear to lose previously acquired skills. Using motor development as an example, McGraw's longitudinal study during the 1930s was one of the first to suggest that such periods of disorganization may, in fact, perform a function: to fuel development (Dalton, 1996). Decades later, theorists returned their attention to these processes, recognizing that motor development is dynamic and variable, "a product of not only the central nervous system but also of the biomechanical and energetic properties of the body, the environmental support, and the specific (and sometimes changing) demands of the particular task" (Thelen, 1995, p. 81).

Dynamical explanations for development of motor control were first put forth by Bernstein (1967), who questioned the feasibility of a motor system that relies on a centrally programmed one-to-one relationship between CNS connections and action. Bernstein proposed that movements are the product of coordinated action by groups of muscles and are subject to the biomechanical constraints imposed by the weight and size of the limbs, as well as the demands and opportunities for flexibility inherent in the environment. **Dynamical theory** posits that the disequilibrium seen before a change in development is the response of a stable system to perturbations imposed by one or several of the foregoing influences. A characteristic of the coordinative structures that support movement is that they are self-regulating (i.e., they are "attracted" to their previous stable state after a perturbation, such as the introduction of a new task or challenge). However, in a dynamic system, a temporary loss of stability provides the opportunity for change to a new movement strategy. As development proceeds, changes in the body and new task-related challenges within the environment combine to disrupt an otherwise stable pattern of movement, permitting flexibility of response and eventual change. If there is sufficient flexibility within postural components, new movement strategies will be attempted under varying conditions and constraints and then reinforced through use (Sporns & Edelman, 1993). The broader the range of "affordances" (i.e., facilitators for action) available within the environment, the greater the possibilities for change (Gibson, 1979). Thus action, in and of itself, provides an influence on perceptual and motor experience that is unique to the individual (van der Meer & van der Weel, 1999).

Dynamical theory does not specifically address the various degrees of purposefulness and motivation inherent in a task, although the potential influence of such psychosocial factors on development is significant (Thelen, 1995). Sameroff and Fiese (2000) emphasize the need to focus beyond biological risk and genetic endowment to examine not only environment but also, more specifically, the combined contributions of child and caregiver to early development. Thus the child, the caregiver, and the social and physical environment each may contribute substantially and interdependently to developmental outcome. This transactional model acknowledges potential effects of socioeconomic status, social support, infant–caregiver reciprocity, and individual behavioral characteristics of infants and caregivers on development. Rather than focusing on single factors, such as medical risk, practitioners who wish to assist families in optimizing child outcomes are now encouraged to consider the family within its environment as a contextual unit and to involve family members when assessing needs and identifying priorities for intervention. This approach to service provision, termed *family-centered care* (Dunst, Johanson, Trivette, & Hamby, 1991) brings health-care professionals closer to understanding the complex interplay of factors that influence a growing child's health and development.

BROADENING FRAMES OF REFERENCE FOR INTERVENTION TO INCORPORATE CHANGING VIEWS

Occupational therapy practitioners need to draw from various developmental models to construct principles for effective pediatric intervention. As research continues to identify factors that influence development to a greater or lesser extent, developmental models, and the treatment principles based on them, need to be continually modified. In the interim, it may be useful to approach developmental intervention from two broad perspectives: elements of developmental risk and protection (Werner, 2000) and goodness of fit (Lester et al., 1994). Occupational therapy practitioners might ask. What are the elements of risk and of protection inherent in this child–family system that can influence development? How can occupational therapy intervention be used to reduce risk and strengthen protective factors within the child, the family, and the environment. In this approach, the individual needs of the child and caregivers (elements of risk) and the capacities of each (elements of protection) are assessed within the context of the environment. The focus of interventions is to achieve a fit between the needs and capacities of the child and those of each member of the family system, while considering environmental affordances and influences.

CONCLUSION

The following sections of this chapter discuss two occupational therapy frames of reference that were derived from hierarchical theory. In light of more current theories, each frame of reference has undergone its own developmental process, emerging in a modified form that takes into account some of the converging influences on development. Successful occupational therapy practitioners avoid basing their interventions on a single frame of reference, which could be grounded in out-dated theory, and remain conscious of the need to continue to assess the validity of the theories that underlie their approaches to developmental intervention.

SECTION II

Neurodevelopmental Theory

BARBARA PRUDHOMME WHITE

Origins of the Intervention Approach
Evolving Perspectives in NDT
The NDT Approach Currently Defined
Summary of Research Literature
Conclusion

ORIGINS OF THE INTERVENTION APPROACH

Neurodevelopmental treatment (NDT) was developed in England during the 1940s by the Bobaths, a husband–wife team who dedicated much of their lives to improving the well-being of individuals with **cerebral palsy** (CP) (Bly, 1991, 2001; Breslin, 1996; Girolami & Campbell, 1994; Law, Missiuna, Pollock, & Stewart, 2001; Valvano & Long, 1991). Karel, a physician, and Berta, a physical therapist, developed the approach together in the hope of improving motor behavior in individuals with cerebral palsy while decreasing the secondary deformities, such as contractures, associated with the disorder. The Bobaths applied neuroscience theories available at the time to their clinical observations of motor behavior in people with cerebral palsy. Some of their greatest contributions included identifying the importance of intervening early with children who have CP and proposing that clients with CP should be treated with strategies that address the neurological and developmental components of the condition.

The Bobaths drew on early understanding of human neuroplasticity and theorized that treatment should target a reorganization of brain areas that support motor behavior. They suggested two primary ways for carrying this out: by positioning individuals so that their abnormal movements and motor tone are reduced or eliminated and by facilitating individuals in new, more typical movement patterns. The Bobaths theorized that if individuals with CP experienced typical movement patterns, their brains would accommodate new motor memories that could support normal purposeful movement (Ottenbacher, Biocca, & De Gremer, 1986; Royeen & DeGangi, 1992; Valvano & Long, 1991). Thus NDT began, and continues to be defined, as a remediative approach that focuses on changing aspects of the physical factors that support the individual's ability to move.

EVOLVING PERSPECTIVES IN NDT

The Bobaths considered their theory to be a living concept (Bly, 1991, 2001), an intervention approach that could adapt over time as new knowledge and handling techniques emerged. Indeed, NDT was modified by both the Bobaths and other practitioners so much since its inception that current NDT intervention is defined and presented quite differently from its earlier forms.

Initially, NDT techniques were developed to inhibit abnormal **muscle tone** and reflexes and to encourage normal movement primarily through the practitioner's handling and positioning of individuals with CP. Sessions were focused on physical handling by the practitioner to reduce increased tone and abnormal movement patterns influenced by reflexes, followed by **facilitation** of both passive and active movement once tone and abnormal posturing seemed to be reduced. Key areas for controlling movement were identified as the neck, shoulders, hips, and pelvic area. Intervention targeted postural control in these proximal locations through supported positions, so that movement of the extremities and head could be facilitated (Bly, 1991, 2001; Brelin, 1996; Ottenbacher et al., 1986; Valvano & Long, 1991).

Current NDT incorporates many of the original aspects of the approach, including postural alignment of the key areas of motor control, inhibitory or facilitory techniques to influence muscle tone temporarily, and facilitation of normal movement patterns (Bly, 2001). However, a number of aspects have been changed or added. For example, current NDT incorporates the vestibular and somatosensory systems' influence on movement. Moreover, active involvement of the individual in meaningful motor acts has replaced passive movement controlled by the practitioner. An individual's active problem solving, motivation in coordinating movement for a purpose, and repetition of the movement all draw on knowledge gained from motor control theory, which is now embedded into NDT (Barry, 1996; Bly, 2001; Breslin, 1996; DeGangi & Royeen, 1994; Royeen & DeGangi, 1992; Valvano & Long, 1991). Furthermore, the influence of distal– proximal control of movement, in addition to proximal–distal control, is now considered a relevant aspect of understanding and treating motor barriers and facilitating movement potentials in clients with cerebral palsy (Bly 2001; Breslin, 1996; DeGangi, 1994).

THE NDT APPROACH CURRENTLY DEFINED

NDT's initial concepts were based on the available knowledge and theories about human movement. The Bobaths expected that their approach would evolve as new knowledge emerged. However, in the process of adapting to both theoretical concepts and intervention strategies, NDT has become more difficult to define as a unique intervention framework. Increasingly, practitioners use NDT techniques as a part of an integrated approach that blends handling, positioning, skill practice, sensory cues, verbal feedback, function, and purpose within an occupational therapy framework (Breslin, 1996; DeGangi & Royeen, 1994; Law et al., 2001).

There are at least two ways to view the current state of NDT. The initial view still considers NDT to be a unique intervention approach because of the practitioner handling and positioning to promote more typical movement patterns. The inclusion of additional intervention strategies (e.g., sensory stimulation and cues, practice, functional activity) could be interpreted as adaptations to NDT theory and practice based on current knowledge, further enhancing its potential effectiveness. Another view is that NDT has become less of a unique approach and more of a set of strategies that are blended into best-practice guidelines or other frames of reference for both occupational and physical therapy practitioners. This is the more common approach currently observed in pediatric therapy (DeGangi & Royeen, 1994; Law et al., 2001).

NDT practitioners who view their intervention as a unique approach tend to specialize within the CP population, focusing primarily on motor function (Adams, Chandler, & Schulman, 2000; Barry, 1996; Bly, 2001; Breslin, 1996; Girolami & Campbell, 1994; Kluzik, Fetters, & Coryell, 1990; Valvano & Long, 1991). Since individuals with CP lack normal muscle tone and movement patterns that stabilize the body during motion, various compensations are frequently observed, specifically in the proximal joints (e.g., shoulders, hips, and pelvic area). These compensations are referred to as active *blocking* or *fixing*, both NDT terms that describe the tensing of muscles for stabilization of the body against gravity. Prolonged use of these abnormal motor patterns by people with CP is believed to result in shortened muscles and restricted movement. In addition, NDT practitioners hypothesize that continued use of these motor blocks and abnormal movement patterns leads to increased deformity, further restriction of movement, and neural motor memories that perpetuate the abnormal motor patterns (Barry, 1996; Bly, 2001; Girolami & Campbell, 1994; Royeen & DeGangi, 1992; Valvano & Long, 1991). Intervention is focused on reducing the use of motor blocks, strengthening little-used muscles, and elongating foreshortened muscles for less restricted movement.

Although other aspects of individual functioning may be considered, arguably the primary targets of intervention in a more purely NDT approach are factors or components associated with motor proficiency. This approach, however, seems to be less common in pediatric therapy, and most practitioners subscribe to integrated and blended approaches to intervention (DeGangi & Royeen, 1994). This second view proposes that many of the strategies that began as pure NDT intervention for clients with cerebral palsy—such as modification of motor tone and abnormal posturing, postural alignment, and facilitation of movement through key points of control—are currently blended with strategies from other theoretical intervention perspectives, at least for practitioners using NDT, within an occupational therapy framework.

A blended approach includes aspects of sensory integration intervention (somatosensory and vestibular influences on movement), the use of sensory cues and feedback in adapting movement, the practice of motor skills in functional contexts (motor learning), functional occupation-focused intervention, and consideration of cognitive–emotional–social aspects of motivation and meaning making (Bly, 2001; Breslin, 1996; DeGangi & Royeen, 1994). Thus the targets of intervention from this second perspective include facilitation of specific motor competencies but are arguably just as focused on broad aspects of functional performance in age-appropriate and desired occupations as well as psychosocial needs, essentially creating a systems perspective.

Although the clinical application of NDT would likely look similar, the two perspectives reflect differences in practitioners' theoretical perspectives and concentrations. Moreover, the clinician's perspective of how NDT is used in practice has implications for the design and interpretation of efficacy research.

SUMMARY OF RESEARCH LITERATURE

Research support for the effectiveness of NDT as a unique intervention approach has not been particularly supportive of the method in achieving improved motor function in individuals with CP. Still, the authors of one current study (Adams, Chandler, & Schulman, 2000) reported that a 6-week intervention using NDT facilitated improved gait characteristics in children with cerebral palsy. Butler and Darrah (2000), reporting for the American Academy of Cerebral Palsy and Developmental Medicine (AACPDM), summarized efficacy research from 1956 through 2000 that studied NDT interventions for individuals with cerebral palsy. It is the most comprehensive **meta-evaluation** of NDT research to date. Of 58 possible studies, 16 met the criteria determined acceptable for both population (CP) and research methods. The findings of this report suggest that while NDT may be helpful in increasing active range of motion during treatment, no evidence supports long-term changes that produce more normal movement patterns or increased functional activity in individuals with cerebral palsy who have undergone NDT interventions. The authors noted that there were gaps in the body of evidence available and suggested future directions for research.

Research is lacking, for example, regarding the long-term effects of compensatory movement patterns in individuals with cerebral palsy, regarding differences in outcome between early and late NDT intervention, and regarding how or whether spasticity or increased tone is affected during intervention. Moreover, NDT research is hampered by inadequate outcome measures, lack of consistency in intervention techniques, and the length of time used to study the interventions. Finally, the differences in motor impairment among the participants in group design studies makes it difficult to interpret individual changes as a result of NDT intervention. Consistent evidence from these efficacy studies of increased active movement in individuals with cerebral palsy during treatment may offer opportunities for future research focused on the potential influence of NDT techniques on tone reduction as well as possible increased comfort and cooperation during therapy (Butler & Darrah, 2000).

CONCLUSION

Further research is needed to investigate whether NDT, as a unique frame of reference for treatment, is an effective intervention for individuals with cerebral palsy. To date, there is little supportive evidence to suggest that NDT approaches alone are effective for long-term changes in motor function. On the other hand, many practitioners use NDT strategies as part of an integrated intervention approach, influenced by an occupational performance framework (Breslin, 1996; DeGangi, 1994; DeGangi & Royeen, 1994; Ottenbacher et al., 1986; Royeen & DeGangi, 1992). It is likely that in the context of being "packaged" with other approaches, NDT may be most effective. Thus future research using NDT techniques may be more productive if it is focused on investigating the efficacy of the overall intervention package (i.e., occupational therapy or physical therapy) of which NDT techniques play a part, rather than on a specific component in the delivery of services.

SECTION III

Sensory Integration

OLGA BALOUEFF

DEFINITION

Sensory integration (SI) refers to both a neurophysiological process and a theory of the relationship between the neural organization of sensory processing and behavior (Ayres,

1972a, 1972b, 1989; Lane, Miller, & Hanft, 2000). Ayres (1989), the occupational therapist who developed this theory, defined SI as:

> *[T]he neurological process that organizes sensation from one's own body and from the environment and makes it possible to use the body effectively within the environment. The spatial and temporal aspects of inputs from different sensory modalities are interpreted, associated, and unified. Sensory integration is information processing. (p. 11)*

INTELLECTUAL HERITAGE OF THE FRAME OF REFERENCE

Jean Ayres (1920–1988), an accomplished therapist, teacher, and scholar, began developing the theory of sensory integration in the 1960s and continued to redefine it until her death in 1988. Ayres's early work was influenced by Rood and the Bobaths, who addressed the relationship of sensory stimuli to motor responses in the treatment of neuromuscular dysfunction, and by Piaget, who stressed the early sensorimotor experiences as the foundation for cognitive development. Ayres's clinical work with adults and children with neurological and learning problems led her to the study and assessment of neurobehavioral functioning, including the perceptual and motor contributions to learning.

ASSUMPTIONS AND NEUROBEHAVIORAL CONCEPTS

Several assumptions are central to SI theoretical construction (Ayres 1972a, 1979; Fisher & Murray, 1991; Kimball, 1999; Parham & Mailloux, 2001).

- *Sensory nourishment:* Sensory input is critical for brain function; to promote optimal neural integration, the individual must actively organize and use sensory input to interact with the environment.
- *Adaptive response:* When people experience a challenging but not overwhelming level of sensory stimulation to their CNS (i.e., just the right amount of challenge) and successfully respond to it, an adaptive response takes place, which contributes to the development of sensory integration.
- *Plasticity within the CNS:* Through adaptive responses to environmental demands (i.e., purposeful activities), changes occur at the neuronal synaptic level.
- *Developmental sequence:* Sensory integrative processes occur in a developmental sequence as the CNS organizes adaptive responses to sensory information with increasing levels of complexity.
- *CNS organization:* The brain functions both as an integrated whole and as hierarchically organized interactive systems; cortical centers depend on the functioning of the brainstem and thalamus for the organization and interpretation of incoming sensory information.
- *Sensory modalities convergence:* Convergence (integration) of sensory input from all sensory modalities occurs in the reticular formation (brainstem and thalamus), which has a widespread influence over the rest of the brain.
- *Inner drive:* People have an inner impetus to develop sensory integration through their participation in sensorimotor activities and activity preference; the more inner directed the activities, the greater the potential for improving neural organization.

EVALUATION OF SI DYSFUNCTION

Evaluation of sensory integrative functioning is a multifaceted process based on assessment data from a number of sources (Mulligan, 2000). It requires an understanding of the presenting problems in relation to children's daily occupations and life participation in the context of their families, school, and other significant environments (Cohn & Cermak, 1998; Coster, 1998; Parham & Mailloux, 2001). Cohn and Cermak (1998) proposed that the assessment process should begin with an exploration of the significant occupations of the children and the family, focusing on parental concerns, priorities, and aspirations for their children's engagement in age-appropriate activities.

Assessment tools for determining SI dysfunction include interviews and questionnaires, sensory reactivity checklists, standardized tests, and clinical observations. Contextual considerations are always taken into account.

Interviews and Questionnaires

Interviews and questionnaires are given to gather pertinent information, such as referral background; reason for referral; developmental milestones; sensory reactivity; and sensitivity to auditory, tactile, proprioceptive, visual, and vestibular input during daily activities. Teachers' and parents' perceptions of the children's temperament, coping styles, performance in ADL, feeding, play, school work, and social participation are explored as well. The interviewer should also include the children's own perception of their problems, their strengths, reason for referral, and personal goals. Exploration of parental hopes for the outcomes of occupational therapy is at the center of the evaluation process (Cohn & Cermak, 1998; Cohn, Miller, & Tickle-Degnen, 2000).

Clinical Observations

Informal and formal observations of clients' occupational performance are part of the evaluation process. Informal and unstructured observations of children in their natural settings may include, but are not limited to, the sitting posture, handling of writing tools, and frustration tolerance with the complexity of a task. On the playground, children's level of participation in games and enjoyment with the activity are also observed. Formal clinical observations of muscle tone and cocontraction, reflex integration, symmetry, oculomotor, and postural reactions supplement the Sensory Integration and Praxis Tests (SIPT).

Standardized Testing

The primary instrument for identification of sensory integration dysfunction is the SIPT (Ayres, 1989). The SIPT evolved from earlier test batteries developed by Ayres (1972b, 1975, 1980): the Southern California Sensory Integration Test (SCSIT) and the Southern California Postrotary Nystagmus Test (SCPNT). The SIPT is composed of 17 subtests measuring four SI domains: tactile, vestibular, and proprioceptive processing; form and space perception and visual-motor coordination; praxis; and bilateral integration and sequencing (Ayres, 1989). Testing is administered individually and takes about 2 hours. The SIPT is appropriate for clients aged 4 years through 8 years, 11 months. Administration and interpretation of the SIPT requires specialized training (SIPT certification).

As needed, additional testing of specific performance areas or components is administered, such as play, activities of daily living, school function, psychosocial, sensorimotor, and cognitive skills. Neuropsychological testing may also be part of a comprehensive evaluation.

SENSORY INTEGRATION PATTERNS OF DYSFUNCTION

Dysfunction in sensory integration (DSI) refers to the "inability to modulate, discriminate, coordinate, or organize sensation adaptively" (Lane et al., 2000, p. 2). DSI is an heterogeneous group of disorders characterized by problems in CNS processing of sensory input (Parham & Mailloux, 2001). Over the years, different systems of categorization for disorders of sensory integration have been generated (Ayres, 1989; Lane et al., 2000; Mulligan, 2000; Parham & Mailloux, 2001). Four major categories of DSI are seen as recurring themes addressed by practitioners and scholars: **sensory modulation dysfunction** (SMD), **developmental dyspraxia, bilateral integration and sequencing dysfunction,** and **sensory discrimination dysfunction** (Kimball, 1999; Lane et al., 2000; Parham & Mailloux, 2001).

Sensory modulation dysfunction is a problem "in the capacity to regulate and organize the degree, intensity, and nature of response to sensory input in a graded and adaptive manner" (Lane et al., 2000, p. 2). Three response patterns reflect this inability to react appropriately to sensory input from the body or environment (Hanft, Miller, & Lane, 2000; Lane et al., 2000):

- *Overresponsivity to incoming sensory input (sensory defensiveness)*: Manifested by a constellation of behaviors (e.g., avoidance, anxiety, overreaction, aggression) in the carrying out of some daily life routines; tactile defensiveness and gravitational insecurity are examples of hyperresponsivity to ordinary tactile and vestibular sensations, respectively.
- *Underresponsivity to incoming sensations*: Reflected for some individuals in intense and exaggerated sensation-seeking behaviors to counterbalance a hyporesponsivity to certain sensory input (e.g., vestibular and proprioceptive); for others, it is manifested in a failure to attend or register relevant sensory stimuli, raising safety concerns in carrying out daily tasks.
- *Fluctuating responsivity*: Characterized by fluctuations and rapid shifts from greater to lesser sensory modulation; it renders people inefficient in their interaction with the environment.

Developmental dyspraxia is a difficulty with the planning and execution of movement patterns of a skilled or nonhabitual nature and originates in childhood. It refers to a "disruption in sensory processing and motor planning" (Lane et al., 2000, p. 2). Some children with praxis problems experience difficulty with the processing of tactile and proprioceptive input (somatodyspraxia). Others have problems with the cognitive element or ideation of organizing their activities in novel and unstructured situations (Parham & Mailloux, 2001).

Bilateral integration and sequencing dysfunction is thought to reflect problems in central vestibular processing. Deficits in coordinating the two sides of the body, poor equilibrium reactions, low muscle tone, difficulties in communication, poor right–left discrimination, and a lack of clearly defined hand dominance are common manifestations of this type of disorder. Sensory discrimination dysfunction involves problems in the organization and interpretation of the temporal and spatial characteristics of sensory stimuli.

CLIENT–PRACTITIONER INTERACTION AND EXPECTED OUTCOMES OF SI INTERVENTION

Although the specific objectives of SI intervention may vary according to each client's individual characteristics and type of dysfunction, several general outcomes of therapy are expected, based on SI theory and practice (Ayres, 1972a, 1979; Cohn & Cermak, 1998; Cohn et al., 2000; Koomar & Bundy, 1991; Parham & Mailloux, 2001):

- Development of increasingly more organized behavioral responses to environmental demands.
- Increase in the duration and frequency of adaptive responses.
- Improvement in gross and fine motor skills.
- Improvement in cognitive, language, and academic performance.
- Increase in perceived competence, self-confidence, and self-esteem.
- Enhancement of occupational engagement, self-regulation, and social participation.
- Enhancement of child and family quality of life.

Ayres (1972b, 1979) referred to therapy as an art. The role of the therapist is to provide a therapeutic situation that elicits the person's "inner urge for action and growth and drives him toward a response that furthers maturation and integration" (Ayres, 1972a, p. 256). Koomar and Bundy (1991) further identified SI therapy as an "art and a science." To provide SI intervention, occupational therapists need proficiency in clinical reasoning skills, education in SI theory, and training in the art and science of SI therapy. Several characteristics are proper to the SI therapeutic milieu (Ayres, 1972a, 1979; Kimball, 1999; Koomar & Bundy, 1991; Parham & Mailloux, 2001). Treatment is individualized, reflecting the client's unique characteristics, and promotes participation by encouraging self-direction and active involvement in tasks. Activities are chosen to tap the person's motivation and inner drive to respond through adaptive responses. There is also a "just right" balance between structure and freedom. The therapist uses clinical reasoning skills to assess when to step back, when to allow the client to choose the activity, when to step in and modify or discontinue the activity, and when to introduce a specific type of sensory input.

APPLICATION OF SI THEORY TO OCCUPATIONAL THERAPY PRACTICE

Over the years, the sensory integrative frame of reference has led to several innovative approaches designed to address children's sensory-processing issues and development of functional skills within the contexts of their daily lives (DeGangi, 2000; Dunn, 1997, 1999; Wilbarger, 1995; Wilbarger & Wilbarger, 1991; Williams & Shellenberger, 1994). Assessment tools have been developed to capture children's responses to various sensations, including the range of behavioral and emotional responses generated by sensory experiences in the course of their daily routines (DeGangi & Poisson, 2000; Dunn, 1999). These tests—judgment-based questionnaires given to the child's caregivers—are instrumental in identifying which types of sensory input are more likely to "be contributing to or creating barriers to functional performance" (Dunn, 1999, p. 2). They also provide direction for planning and developing family-centered interventions.

Addressing problems of self-regulation in children within the context of their daily lives is a prevalent area of practice for occupational therapists with a SI perspective. Williams and Shellenberger (1994) developed the Alert Program to help school-aged children learn to monitor, maintain, and change their level of arousal so that it is appropriate for a given task or situation. This program, widely used by occupational therapists working in schools, offers specific strategies that incorporate SI techniques with cognitive approaches.

DeGangi's (2000) clinical research with infants and toddlers addresses early regulatory disorders as manifested in problems of affect, behavior, and sensory reactivity. Principles from SI theory are used to address the child's constitutional problems and to help parents adapt their care-giving approaches to promote their child's well-being.

Recognizing the importance of integrating sensory experiences into daily routines, Wilbarger (1995) coined the term *sensory diet*. A sensory diet is analogous to a daily nutritional diet or meal plan, in that the right combination of sensory-related activities is vital to keep a person functioning at his or her optimal level of arousal and performance throughout the day (Wilbarger & Wilbarger, 1991). This concept is used to educate people about their sensory needs and in developing family-centered therapeutic interventions.

EVIDENCE-BASED PRACTICE OF SI INTERVENTIONS

Despite the wide use of sensory integration interventions (Case-Smith & Miller, 1999; Cohn et al., 2000), conflicting reports exist regarding its effectiveness (Cermak & Henderson, 1990; Hoehn & Baumeister, 1994; Holm, 2000; Vargas & Camilli, 1999; William, 1999). At present, the claim that SI intervention is effective has not been substantiated by empirical studies (Holm, 2000; William, 1999). Vargas and Camilli (1999) conducted a meta-analysis of the results of 22 sensory integration efficacy research studies published from 1972 to 1997. They reached three principal conclusions. First, in studies comparing SI treatment to no treatment, sensory integration approaches were found to be more effective in the earlier studies (1972–1982), but this effect was not seen in more recent studies. Second, the largest gains were found in the areas of psychoeducational and motor performance, not in the sensory-perceptual areas (a major goal of SI therapy). Third, SI methods were found to be as effective as various alternative treatment practices. As Holm (2000) stated, "The results of the study provide us with a stark reminder of the difference between preferred practice and evidence-based practice" (p. 577).

Future research should concentrate on developing new models to examine the effects of SI methods in a variety of domains (Cermak & Henderson, 1990; Holm, 2000). Promising research is currently being developed in the area of sensory modulation disorders. Miller and McIntosh (1998) are systematically studying sensory modulation disorders in regard to its behavioral manifestations and the use of SI intervention to remediate and improve the lives of clients with this type of syndrome. Family perspectives regarding the goals of SI therapy for children with sensory modulation disorders and measures to evaluate them have been proposed by Cohn and Cermak (1998) and Cohn et al. (2000). Understanding the perceptions of parents and children receiving SI therapy is an essential part of occupational therapy services. Likewise, including parents' hopes and goals for therapy is at the core of family-centered care and a major quality control factor (Cohn & Cermack, 1998).

CONCLUSION

In summary, critical analysis of SI theory and practice should remain an ongoing process as interventions are being used in a variety of contexts and with various populations. Gathering evidence about the efficacy of sensory integration is a mandate for all of those who espouse its approaches in treatment.

References

Adams, M. A., Chandler, L. S., & Schulman, K. (2000). Gait changes in children with cerebral palsy following neurodevelopmental treatment course. *Pediatric Physical Therapy, 12*(3), 114–120.

Ayres, A. J. (1972a). *Sensory integration and learning disorders*. Los Angeles: Western Psychological Services.

Ayres, A. J. (1972b). *Southern California sensory integration tests*. Los Angeles: Western Psychological Services.

Ayres, A. J. (1975). *Southern California postrotary nystagmus test manual*. Los Angeles: Western Psychological Services.

Ayres, A. J. (1979). Sensory integration and the child. Los Angeles: Western Psychological Services.

Ayres, A. J. (1980). *Southern California sensory integration tests*. Los Angeles: Western Psychological Services.

Ayres, A. J. (1989). *Sensory integration and praxis tests*. Los Angeles: Western Psychological Services.

Barry, M. J. (1996). Physical therapy interventions for patients with movement disorders due to cerebral palsy. *Journal of Child Neurology, 11*(1), S51–S60.

Bernstein, N. (1967). *The coordination and regulation of movements*. London: Pergamon.

Bly, L. (1991). A historical and current view of the basis of NDT. *Pediatric Physical Therapy, 3*, 131–135.

Bly, L. (2001). Historical and current view of the basis of NDT. Available at: www.ndta.org/aboutNDTA/historical.html. Accessed February 11, 2001.

Breslin, D. M. (1996). Motor-learning theory and the neurodevelopmental treatment approach: A comparative analysis. *Occupational Therapy in Health Care, 10*(1), 25–40.

Butler, C., & Darrah, J. (2000). American Academy for Cerebral Palsy and Developmental Medicine (AACPDM) evidence report: Effects of neurodevelopmental treatment (NDT) for cerebral palsy. Available at: www.aacpdm.org/home_basic.html. Accessed December 10, 2000.

Case-Smith, J., & Miller, H. (1999). Occupational therapy with children with pervasive developmental disorders. *American Journal of Occupational Therapy, 53*(5), 506–513.

Cermak, S. A., & Henderson, A. (1990). The efficacy of sensory integration procedures, Part II. *Sensory Integration Quarterly, 28*(1), 1–5.

Cohn, E. S., & Cermak, S. A. (1998). Including the family perspective in sensory integration outcomes research. *American Journal of Occupational Therapy, 52*(7), 540–546.

Cohn, E., Miller, L. J., & Tickle-Degnen, L. (2000). Parental hopes for therapy outcomes: Children with sensory modulation disorders. *American Journal of Occupational Therapy, 54*(1), 36–43.

Coster, W. (1998). Occupation-centered assessment of children. *American Journal of Occupational Therapy, 52*(5), 337–344.

Dalton, T. C. (1996, Winter). Reconstructing John Dewey's unusual collaboration with Myrtle McGraw in the 1930s. *Newsletter of the Society for Research in Child Development*, 1–3, 8–10.

DeGangi, G. (2000). *Pediatric disorders of regulation in affect and behavior: A therapist's guide to assessment and treatment*. San Diego: Academic Press.

DeGangi, G. A. (1994). Examining the efficacy of short-term NDT intervention using a case study design: Part 2. *Physical and Occupational Therapy in Pediatrics, 14*(2), 21–61.

DeGangi, G., & Poisson, S. (2000). Infant-toddler symptom checklist: Long version. In G. DeGangi (Ed.), *Pediatric disorders of regulation in affect and behavior: A therapist's guide to assessment and treatment* (pp. 335–340). San Diego: Academic.

DeGangi, G. A., & Royeen, C. B. (1994). Current practice among neurodevelopmental treatment association members. *American Journal of Occupational Therapy, 48*(9), 803–809.

Dunn, W. (1997). The impact of sensory processing abilities on the daily lives of young children and their families. A conceptual model. *Infants and Young Children, 9*(4), 23–35.

Dunn, W. (1999). *Sensory profile: User's manual*. San Antonio, TX: Psychological Corp.

Dunst, C. J., Johanson, C., Trivette, C. M., & Hamby, D. W. (1991). Family-oriented early intervention policies and practices: Family-centered or not? *Exceptional Children, 58*, 115–126.

Fisher, A. G., & Murray, E. A. (1991). Introduction to sensory integration theory. In A. G. Fisher, E. A. Murray, & A. C. Bundy (Eds.). *Sensory integration theory and practice* (pp. 3–26). Philadelphia: Davis.

Freel, K. S. (1996). Finding complexities and balancing perspectives: Using an ethnographic viewpoint to understand children and their families. *Zero to Three, 16*, 1–7.

Gesell, A. (1928). *Infancy and human growth*. New York: Macmillan.

Gibson, J. J. (1979). *The ecological approach to visual perception*. Boston: Houghton Mifflin.

Gilfoyle, E. M., Grady, A. P., & Moore, J. C. (1981). *Children adapt*. Thorofare, NJ: Slack.

Girolami, G. L., & Campbell, S. K. (1994). Efficacy of a neuro-developmental treatment program to improve motor control in infants born prematurely. *Pediatric Physical Therapy, 6*, 175–184.

Hanft, B. E., Miller, L. J., & Lane, S. J. (2000). Toward a consensus in terminology in sensory integration and practice: Part 3: Observable behaviors: Sensory integration dysfunction. *Sensory Integration Special Interest Section Quarterly, 23*(3), 1–4.

Hoehn, T. P., & Baumeister, A. A. (1994). A critique of the application of sensory integration therapy to children with learning disabilities. *Journal of Learning Disabilities, 27*(6), 338–350.

Holm, M. B. (2000). Our mandate for the new millennium: Evidence-based practice. [Eleanor Clarke Slagle Lecture]. *American Journal of Occupational Therapy, 54*(6), 575–585.

Kimball, J. C. (1999). Sensory integrative frame of reference. In P. Kramer & J. Hinojosa (Eds.), *Frames of reference for pediatric occupational therapy* (pp. 119–204). Baltimore: Williams & Wilkins.

King, L. J. (1978). Toward a science of adaptive responses. *American Journal of Occupational Therapy, 32*, 429–437.

Kluzik, J., Fetters, L., & Coryell, J. (1990). Quantification of control: A preliminary study of neurodevelopmental treatment on reaching in children with spastic cerebral palsy. *Physical Therapy, 70*, 65–78.

Koomar, J. A., & Bundy, A. C. (1991). The art and science of creating direct intervention from theory. In A. G. Fisher, E. A. Murray, & A. C. Bundy (Eds.). *Sensory integration theory and practice* (pp. 234–250). Philadelphia: Davis.

Lane, S. J., Miller, L. J., & Hanft, B. E. (2000). Toward a consensus in terminology in sensory integration theory and practice: Part 2. *Special Interest Section Quarterly, 23*(2), 1–3.

Law, M., Missiuna, C., Pollock, N., & Stewart, D. (2001). Foundations for occupational therapy practice with children. In J. Case-Smith (Ed.). *Occupational therapy for children* (4th ed., pp. 39–70). St. Louis: Mosby.

Lester, B. M., McGrath, M. M., Garcia-Coll, C. T., Brem, F. S., Sullivan, M. C., & Mattis, S. B. (1994). Relationship between risk and protective factors, developmental outcome and the home environment at 4-years-of-age in term and preterm infants. In H. Fitzgerald, B. M. Lester, & B. Zuckerman (Eds.). *Children in poverty: Research, health care, and policy issues* (pp. 197–227). New York: Garland.

Llorens, L. (1969). Facilitating growth and development: The promise of occupational therapy. *American Journal of Occupational Therapy, 24*, 93–101.

Miller, L. J., & McIntosh, D. N. (1998). The diagnosis, treatment, and etiology of sensory modulation disorder. *Sensory Integration Special Interest Section Newsletter, 21*(1), 1–4.

Mulligan, S. (2000). Cluster analysis of scores of children on the sensory integration and praxis tests. *Occupational Therapy Journal of Research, 20*(4), 256–270.

Ottenbacher, K. J., Biocca, Z., & De Gremer, G. (1986). Quantitative analysis of the effectiveness of pediatric therapy: Emphasis on the neurodevelopmental treatment approach. *Physical Therapy, 66*, 1096–1101.

Parham, D. L., & Mailloux, Z. (2001). Sensory integration. In J. Case-Smith, (Eds.). *Occupational therapy for children* (4th ed., pp. 329–379). St. Louis: Mosby.

Piaget, J. (1952). *The origins of intelligence in children*. New York: International Universities Press.

Royeen, C. B., & DeGangi, G. A. (1992). Use of neurodevelopmental treatment as an intervention: Annotated listing of studies. *Perceptual and Motor Skills, 75*(1), 175–194.

Sameroff, A. J., & Fiese, B. H. (2000). Transactional regulation: The developmental ecology of early intervention. In J. P. Shonkoff & S. J. Meisels (Eds.). *Handbook of early childhood intervention* (pp. 135–157). New York: Cambridge University Press.

Simons, C. J., Mandich, M., Ritchie, S. K., & Mullett, M. D. (2000). Assessment of motor development in very low birth weight infants. *Journal of Perinatology, 20*(3), 172–175.

Sporns, O., & Edelman, G. M. (1993). Solving Bernstein's problem: A proposal for the development of coordinated movement by selection. *Child Development, 64*, 960–981.

Thelen, E. (1995). Motor development: A new synthesis. *American Psychologist, 50*, 79–95.

Valvano, J. & Long, T. (1991). Neurodevelopmental treatment: A review of the writings of the Bobath's. *Pediatric Physical Therapy, 3*, 125–129.

Van der Meer, A. L., & van der Weel, F. R. (1999). Development of perception in action in healthy and at-risk children. *Acta Paediatrica Supplement, 88*(429), 29–36.

Vargas, S., & Camilli, G. (1999). A meta-analysis of research on sensory integration treatment. *American Journal of Occupational Therapy, 53*(2), 189–198.

Wachs, T. D. (1992). *The nature of nurture*. Newbury Park, CA: Sage.

Werner, E. E. (2000). Protective factors and individual resilience. In J. P. Shonkoff & S. J. Meisels (Eds.). *Handbook of early childhood intervention* (pp. 115–132). New York: Cambridge University Press.

Wilbarger, P. (1995). The sensory diet: Activity programs based on sensory processing theory. *Sensory Integration Special Interest Section Newsletter, 18*(2), 1–4.

Wilbarger, P., & Wilbarger, J. L. (1991). *Sensory defensiveness in children aged 2–12*. Denver: Avanti Educational.

William, R. A. (1999). Controversial practices: The need for a reacculturation of early intervention fields. *Topics in Early Childhood Special Education, 19*(3), 177–188.

Williams, M. S., & Shellenberger, S. (1994). *How does your engine run? A leader's guide to the Alert program for self-regulation*. Albuquerque: Therapy Works.

CHAPTER 21

LEARNING PERSPECTIVES

SECTION I

Overview of Learning Theory

CLARE G. GIUFFRIDA
MAUREEN E. NEISTADT

Occupational therapy clients spend most of their intervention time **learning** different strategies to become more independent. Consequently, occupational therapy practitioners need to know something about learning and learning theory. Learning can be defined as "a relatively permanent change in the capacity for responding, resulting from practice and experience, persists with time, resists environmental changes, and can be generalized in response to new tasks and situations" (Schmidt & Lee, 1999, p. 264). Furthermore, "Such changes cannot be attributed to temporary body states induced by illness, fatigue, or drugs" (Hergenhahn, 1976, p. 9). Learning is one process that allows the person to cope with the changing demands of the environment and along with memory is the most important mechanism in humans by which the environment influences behavior (Kandel, Kupfermann, & Iversen, 2000). When we learn, we acquire knowledge about the world that results in changed behavior. Memory, an important component in learning, involves the processes by which the knowledge acquired is encoded, stored, and later retrieved.

Philosophers since Plato (427–347 B.C.E.) and Aristotle (384–322 B.C.E.) have debated over whether the nature of knowledge is primarily determined by the mind (rationalism) or by sensory experience (empiricism). Beginning in the mid-nineteenth century, this debate about the nature of learning evolved into a psychology debate about the best way to explain learning. Some theorists, such as Pavlov (1849–1936), Watson (1878–1958), and Skinner (1904–1990), felt that learning was best explained by observing and describing relationships between behaviors and observable events (associationism, behaviorism). Others, such as the Gestalt psychologists (late nineteenth to mid-twentieth century) and Piaget (1896–1980), felt that learning was best explained by making inferences about the mental activities underlying observed behaviors (cognitive theorists). Since the late 1950s, the dominant perspective in learning theory focuses on **information processing.** Information processing addresses mental representations and cognitive processing and delineates the structure and processing of information from sensory input through response output by the person. In these approaches, it is hypothesized that each person acts on information by using various mental operations. Information is actively transformed, stored, and retrieved as the person acts adaptively in the environment.

Information processing accounts of learning and cognition are, however, in contrast to ecological approaches, such as those proposed by Gibson in the late 1960s. Gibson viewed people and animals as embedded in their environment. Thus perception and behavior can be understood only by understanding the environment and the information that it makes available (Neisser, 1992). Although both the information processing and the ecological approaches consider the role of information in the environment, their views of learning and cognition differ significantly. Information processing accounts of learning model the structure and processing of information by the person. Ecologically valid accounts of learning, however, reflect that there is no need to process or represent information, since information is always in the environment. Effective action is possible because the individual can perceive the environment and what possibilities for action it affords. Since about 1950, alternative models of learning were developed to accompany these significant changes in orientation to learning (Hergenhahn, 1976; Hintzman, 1978; Ormrod, 1990). These models represent different assumptions about human learning, how it occurs, and what is important to the learning process.

Along with these shifts in explaining learning, ongoing developments in the neurosciences, such as noninvasive structural and functional brain imaging techniques, are increasingly being used to further our understanding of the brain processes involved in learning and memory. Biomedical and behavioral techniques used to study the brain have contributed to a more detailed knowledge of the forms of learning and memory that influence human performance. These different kinds of learning and memory follow different rules, involve different brain sites, and require different neurochemical events (Rosenzweig, 1998). Both behavioral and biomedical investigators examine human learning and memory with experimental designs that now include multiple measures on the same participants across different types of tasks.

Occupational therapy practitioners influenced by changes in the field of human learning and the neurosciences use behavioral, cognitive behavioral, and dynamic interactive information processing accounts of learning in their everyday practice. The ecological approach to direct perception and action has not specifically influenced occupational therapy learning approaches, although its influence is evident in the occupational literature that is focused on the effects of the environment on performance. Specific behavioral and cognitive behavioral approaches to learning in occupational therapy are discussed in Sections 2 and 3. Sections 4, 5, and 6 discuss three intervention theories derived from an information processing perspective on learning. This section provides an overview of the information processing perspective, showing how it can be applied to occupational therapy evaluation and intervention.

LEARNING AS INFORMATION PROCESSING

The information processing perspective suggests that learning is a process mediated by the brain; the brain interprets and relates external sensory impressions and internally stored concepts with each other, much as a computer relates keyboard inputs with internally stored programs (Kantowitz & Roediger, 1980). This information processing system works best when the information or task to be learned is meaningful to the learner and the learner is actively involved in the learning activity (Jarus, 1994; Mathiowetz & Haugen, 1994). This approach relies heavily on computer metaphors and simulation and modeling of expert learning systems (Baddeley, 1990). It does not take into account learning that is socially situated or mediated through interaction and context.

From an information processing perspective learning requires effective sensory reception, brain processing, and motor behavior for either movement or communication. Errors in this information processing system can lead to errors in occupational performance. For example, people who have difficulty with visual acuity may frequently spill things in the kitchen because they cannot see objects clearly. Individuals with slowed brain processing may have difficulty driving on high-speed, heavily trafficked roads because they cannot process the multiple, rapid inputs fast enough to make safe driving decisions. People with impaired motor responses may have difficulty carrying out a wide range of functional activities or knowing how to perform simple functional activities, such as opening a door. Research has indicated that the brain processing part of this information system operates at different levels of capacity over time and yields different types of learning.

Levels of Information Processing and Learning

In therapy, clients can learn new ways to function independently or with assistance. This can involve learning specific procedures, such as learning how to transfer from a bed to a chair or learning how to navigate a wheelchair to move around a nursing home environment. This learning can be

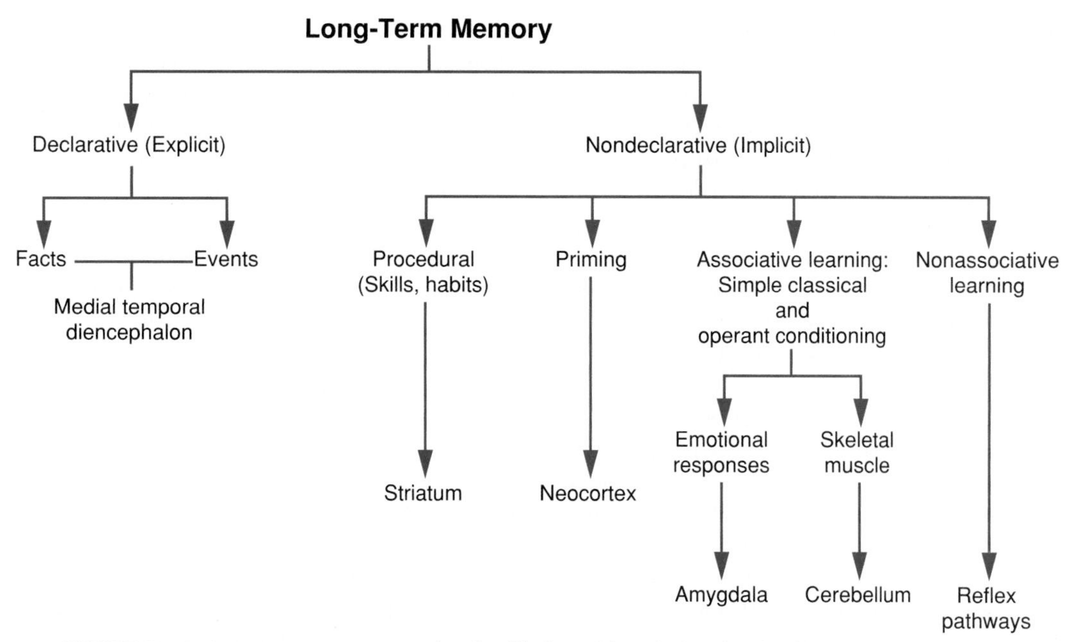

FIGURE 21–1. Long-term memory can be classified as either declarative (explicit) or nondeclarative (implicit). Declarative memory involves the factual knowledge of people, places, events, and things and what those facts mean. Long-term storage of explicit memory involves the temporal lobe system. Nondeclarative memory includes information about how to perform something, a memory that is recalled unconsciously. It is typically involved in training, reflexive motor, or perceptual acts. Different forms of implicit memory are acquired through different forms of learning and involve different brain regions. (Data from Kandel et al., 2000; Squire, 1992; Squire & Zola Morgan, 1991.

both conscious and explicit and not conscious and implicit, depending on what is learned and remembered. Likewise, memory can differ according to whether the items or procedures learned were learned consciously or not. One kind of memory forms the basis for conscious recollections of facts and events (Fig. 21-1). This is termed **declarative memory** to signify that an image or proposition can be brought to mind or declared by a person recognizing or recalling what was learned. Declarative memory can be contrasted with a collection of nonconscious memory abilities, which is termed **nondeclarative memory.**

Nondeclarative memory includes information that is acquired during skill learning (motor skills, perceptual skills, and cognitive skills). It also includes habit formation, simple classical conditioning, priming, and other knowledge expressed through performance. Nondeclarative memory refers to a mixed group of abilities whereby experience alters behavior nonconsciously, without providing access to any memory content. Occupational therapy approaches that help clients learn focus on different aspects of the explicit and implicit learning and memory process.

Regardless of the type of learning or the learning demands, all healthy adults have the capacity to engage in three types of learning that require differing degrees of information processing: **association, representational,** and **abstract learning** (Goldstein & Oakley, 1985). Association learning, which happens when an individual makes an association between two events, is mediated by subcortical or, in some cases, cerebellar structures in the brain. A cigarette smoker who learns to associate smoking with drinking a cup of coffee at the end of a meal in a restaurant illustrates this type of learning. For that person, the arrival of the coffee triggers an automatic response to light up a cigarette. Associative learning has its origins in the stimulus–response models of conditioned learning introduced by behavioral psychology. Learning that is based on forming associations between events is used in behavioral approaches to learning.

Representational learning involves the "formation of durable internal (including linguistic) representations or images of events, and the creation of a spatio-temporal framework into which events are organized and from which they are retrieved" (Goldstein & Oakley, 1985, p. 14). This type of learning is mediated by the hippocampus and neocortex. It takes into account the role of imagery, schemes, and scripts used to guide learning. Representational learning is illustrated by becoming familiar with cooking a new recipe. Initially, a person might follow the recipe step by step. However, with practice, he or she will begin to rely less and less on the cookbook and more and more on the memory of the recipe and the action sequences needed to complete it. That is, the person will have developed an internal image of how to make this particular dish and this representation and script for cooking will guide the person's cooking performance.

Abstract learning is the "acquisition and storage of rules, knowledge and facts abstracted from events, independently of spatio-temporal context" (Goldstein & Oakley, 1985, p. 14).

This type of learning is mediated by the neocortex and includes principled learning. Abstract learning is illustrated by a client with a stroke who derives the principle of always starting with the affected extremity from one session of upper extremity dressing training and then applies that principle to lower extremity dressing without being cued to do so.

Abstract learning requires more complex information processing than representational and association learning, and representational learning requires more complex information processing than association learning. The neurological capacity for abstract learning develops gradually throughout childhood and adolescence. Children may rely more heavily on association and representation learning than on abstract learning, because they have not yet fully developed the ability to think abstractly. Healthy adolescents and adults have access to all three types of learning, but those with brain dysfunction may not. Adolescents and adults with severe brain dysfunction may rely exclusively on association learning, whereas those with lesser dysfunction may still have access to representational or even abstract learning.

Transfer of Learning

Association, representational, and abstract learners all have different capacities for transferring learning from one activity to another. Within the multicontext treatment approach Toglia (1998) identified degrees of transfer along a continuum from transfer to very similar to transfer to very different activities. Spontaneous transfer of learning across very different activities is also known as generalization.

People relying on association learning can, at best, accomplish near transfer of learning—tasks different in one or two characteristics (Toglia, 1998). These individuals have difficulty transferring learning across different situations, with different sets of stimuli. For instance, a teenager with congenital brain dysfunction who was using association learning might be able to learn to make a cup of instant coffee if the necessary supplies (mug, instant coffee, etc.) were set out on the kitchen counter in exactly the same way with the same cues given by the same person each time that task was practiced. If any aspect of the activity presentation changed, the association learner might not be able to make the cup of coffee. An association learner would be able to transfer this learning only to very similar situations (e.g., to a setup in the same kitchen where the mug or the brand of instant coffee had been changed). The best learning environment for association learners, then, is the home setting where they will be doing self-care and home management activities.

People engaged in representational learning are able to tolerate changes in activity setup, because they have an internal image of activity performance against which to compare the immediate environmental stimuli. For instance, representational learners know to look for missing ingredients in the setup for an instant coffee preparation activity. They are likely able to show near and intermediate—tasks different in three to six characteristics (Toglia, 1998)—transfer of learning. That is, after learning to make instant coffee with a given set of supplies in a given kitchen, this learner might be able to make a cup of instant coffee in a different kitchen with different supplies (different mug, kettle, brand of coffee, and such). These learners might be able to transfer some task strategies learned in therapy clinics to their home settings.

The conceptual framework of representational learners, however, is limited and is insufficient to deal with major changes in activity presentation. Therefore, home settings are the better learning environments for these learners also. Representational learners, for example, are not able to problem solve past a broken stove while making a cup of instant coffee because they would be working with only one image of how the activity can be done. Abstract learners, by contrast, are able to create alternative images for activity completion based on past experiences. When faced with a broken stove, the abstract learner looks for an alternative way to heat the water, based on the abstract knowledge that to heat water, one has to apply some form of energy to it (e.g., microwaves). Abstract learners are able to show far and very far transfer of learning—tasks conceptually similar but different in all but one or two characteristics (Toglia, 1998). For example, after learning to make instant coffee in a kitchen, abstract learners are able to figure out how to make a cup of instant coffee at a campsite, with supplies that are totally different in appearance from the ones used during training. Abstract learners, then, are able to transfer activity strategies learned in hospital or outpatient settings to their homes.

EVALUATION OF CLIENTS' LEARNING CAPACITIES

Because learning capacities (association, representational, abstract) are associated with specific abilities to transfer learning, occupational therapists can evaluate clients' learning capabilities by assessing their abilities to transfer learning across different activities. To evaluate transfer of learning, a therapist can change a functional task from one session to the next and see how the client responds. For example, a bathing activity using a basin on the bedside table could be done with soap and toiletries laid out in a line on the table next to the basin one day and with soap and toiletries laid out in a cluster the next. The client who is unable to perform the activity with this change may not be capable of new learning at all. A client who is confused by this change in task presentation is showing difficulty with near transfer (one characteristic changed) and may be using primarily association learning. A client who can bathe even with changes in position (sitting in a bedside chair instead of lying in bed with the head of the bed raised), arrangement of toiletries, and environment (television or radio on instead of off or washing in the bathroom rather than at bedside) is showing capacity for intermediate transfer (three to six characteristics changed) and is demonstrating a capacity for representational learning. A client who can bath successfully in the shower, with soap and toiletries jumbled together in a plastic basket, is showing both far transfer from the bed bath situation and a capacity for abstract learning.

Clients' abilities to transfer learning can change through the course of intervention owing to spontaneous neurological recovery from medical conditions, such as stroke and head injury, and the neurobiological effects of learning (Bach-y-Rita, 1981; Kertesz, 1985; Neistadt, 1994). Clients' transfer of learning capacities, then, should not be considered a static characteristic and must be reevaluated on an ongoing basis.

INTERVENTION RECOMMENDATIONS RELATED TO LEARNING CAPACITIES

General guidelines for intervention can be recommended based on clients' assessed learning capabilities. When clients show no learning capacity on evaluation, the therapist needs to recommend adapting the environment and providing clients with whatever assistance they need to perform their daily activities safely.

Clients who show association learning need a focus on functional activity training, with consistent task setups and intervention schedules. Once an association learner had mastered a particular functional activity with consistent task setups, then it is appropriate to vary the activity setup by one characteristic (e.g., changing from pullover to button down shirt for dressing). Association learners need tremendous amounts of repetition to learn, so behaviors like activities of daily living (ADL) must be practiced at least five times a week.

For clients who show representational learning, the occupational therapy practitioner can vary three to six characteristics from one intervention session to the next (e.g., changing the style and texture of clothing and moving from bedside to bathroom for dressing). These clients may need less repetition for learning and so may need only three or four intervention sessions per week for ADL training. Abstract learners can be taught the principles behind adapted functional activity performance during an initial intervention session and may need only a few sessions of practice with the practitioner after that. For example, abstract learners with total hip replacement (THR) may need only a few sessions to learn the proper precautions and the techniques for using long-handled equipment for dressing. Once abstract learners understand the principles of long-handled equipment use, they might be able to practice on their own and become proficient with the devices.

CONCLUSION

Application of learning theory perspectives to practice can help practitioners continually think of more effective ways to teach clients skills and activity adaptations. The remaining sections of this chapter provide background on other approaches to practice derived from learning theory.

SECTION II

Behaviorism

GORDON MUIR GILES

For the behaviorist, observable behavior is itself the fundamental subject of study (Catania & Harnad, 1988). Rather than a single school, behaviorism is best viewed as a general orientation to experimental and clinical work (Giles & Clark-Wilson, 1999). The term *learning theory* is often used to describe the philosophical foundations of behaviorism (Kazdin, 1994). Various terms are used to refer to behavioral intervention approaches, including behavior therapy, behavior modification, and applied behavioral analysis (Kazdin, 1994). This section provides an overview of some of the basic concepts of learning theory and how occupational therapy practitioners may apply these concepts.

INTELLECTUAL HERITAGE

Watson (1913) has been called the father of American behaviorism. Watson thought that the only legitimate subject of scientific study was observable behavior, and he viewed speculation about consciousness as irrelevant to the study of behavior. During the 1950s, principles derived from learning theory began to be applied to the treatment of mental health problems (Thompson, 1988). Wolpe (1958) developed the principles of systematic desensitization and Eysenck and

Rachman (1965), in England, began to define behavioral treatment of psychological problems. Under the theoretical influence of Skinner, behavioral principles were applied in mental hospitals to ameliorate some of the more handicapping behaviors exhibited by individuals with severe and chronic mental illness (Thompson, 1988). In addition to the pharmacological treatments that became available at the time, behavioral methods were central to the wave of deinstitutionalization that occurred in the 1960s. Beginning in the late 1960s, cognitive therapies developed as a separate approach, but behavior therapy has remained a dynamic subspecialty in psychological theory and has continued to develop new methods to help individuals with behavioral health problems (Epstein, 1992; Kaplan, 1990).

ASSUMPTIONS

It is commonly assumed that individuals consciously determine a course of action and then act on their decision (Hefferline, Keenan, & Hartford, 1958; Nisbett & Wilson, 1977; Svartdal, 1991). There is, however, considerable evidence that people have little insight into the true determinants of their own behavior (Bargh & Chartrand, 1999; Nisbett & Wilson, 1977; Park, 1999). Learning theory provides an alternative account of the "voluntary" behavior traditionally attributed to a freely acting individual.

- The frequency of occurrence of a behavior depends on its reinforcement contingencies (i.e., it is selected by its consequences) (Skinner, 1938).
- Environmental cues, habits, and the person's reinforcement history influence behavior in ways that are unavailable to introspection (Bargh & Chartrand, 1999; Nisbett & Wilson, 1977; Wegner & Wheatley, 1999).
- The therapy practitioner's role is to organize factors that influence the person's behavior (otherwise left to chance) to assist in the learning and maintenance of adaptive behavior (Giles & Clark-Wilson, 1999).

THEORETICAL PRINCIPLES OF BEHAVIORISM

Fundamental to the behaviorists' understanding of behavior is the law of effect, first established by Thorndike (1898). The law of effect states that if an organism's response to a given stimulus is followed by a pleasant event, the association formed between the stimulus and the response is strengthened; if the response is followed by an aversive event, the association is weakened.

In learning theory, classes of behavior are identified by reference to how they originate. Three types of learning can be identified that correspond to different classes of behavior: **classical conditioning, operant conditioning,** and **vicarious learning.** In classical (Pavlovian) conditioning, responses originate with the stimuli that elicit them and are called respondents. This class of responses is illustrated by the stimulus– response (S–R) relationship of reflexes. Through classical conditioning, species-specific responses developed through natural selection (unconditioned response; UCR) can come under the influence of new stimuli (conditioned stimuli; CS), leading to a new response (conditioned response; CR). Classical conditioning may be best considered a mechanism by which organisms map important regularities in their environment (Rescorla, 1988). Classical conditioning underlies important human phenomena, such as anxiety and anger, and is implicated in physiological mechanisms (e.g., psychoneuroimmunology) (Ader & Cohen, 1993).

In operant conditioning, behaviors are considered to develop as a result of the effect they have on the environment. Operants are said to be emitted because they do not require an eliciting stimulus (as is necessary in classical conditioning). The consequences of operants may either raise or lower the rate at which they subsequently occur (are emitted). Events that follow an operant and that raise the frequency of responding are called reinforcers, and events that lower the frequency of responding are called punishers. Mapping the relationships between responses and their consequences establishes the contingencies of **reinforcement** or punishment. Altering the antecedents (social or physical circumstances or events that precede a behavior) can change the likelihood that a behavior will occur (e.g., the presence or absence of a red light alters the likelihood that a driver will stop at an intersection). Antecedent control provides techniques for altering the behavior of persons with profound cognitive impairments, such as those with dementia or those in acute recovery from brain injury for whom learning may be problematic (Giles & Clark-Wilson, 1999).

The third type of learning is observational, or vicarious, learning (Bandura, 1977). Vicarious learning occurs when an individual observes another person engaging in a behavior. The individual need not engage in the behavior (or be reinforced) to later emit the behavior; however, whether and how often the behavior is emitted may depend on its consequences. Modeling, a form of vicarious learning, is often used in behavior therapy to reduce anxiety and build skills and may play a significant role in the beneficial effects of group skills training.

APPLICATION OF BEHAVIORAL PRINCIPLES WITH CLINICAL POPULATIONS

The theoretical principles described in this section—and further described in basic texts on behavior therapy such as that of Kazdin (1994)—are often directly applicable to occupational therapy interventions with clients. Accurate assessment is essential to behavior therapy and attempts to identify the factors that helped establish and maintain maladaptive behaviors. Behavior is observed objectively and accurately and without value judgments. A detailed description of a problematic behavior includes an analysis of antecedents (what comes before the event), the behavior itself, and the consequences of the behavior for the individual. These are called antecedent-behavior-consequence (ABC) records. Positive consequences for an individual may include direct rewards (getting what he or she wants) or avoiding situations that are experienced as aversive (Giles & Clark-Wilson, 1999). Behavioral interventions involve changing the contingencies of reinforcement to support the development of more adaptive behaviors. In addition, assessment may reveal that the client has limited coping skills or strategies. Interventions may help the client develop skills to replace the maladaptive strategies previously used in an attempt to control the environment (Giles & Clark-Wilson, 1999).

When practitioners add a reinforcer, they are attempting to alter the contingencies of reinforcement that accrue to a particular behavior and to increase the likelihood of its occurrence. Reinforcement may be of two types: primary or secondary. Primary reinforcers are often social (e.g., praise or social attention) or tangible (e.g., food items or access to preferred activities). Secondary reinforcers are symbols that stand for primary reinforcers and include things such as tokens or points that can be traded for primary reinforcers (money is an example of a powerful secondary reinforcer). The use of secondary reinforcers provides flexibility in the organization of reinforcement programs (Giles & Clark-Wilson, 1993, 1999).

Behavioral interventions used by occupational therapy practitioners can be divided into behavioral-management interventions and skill-building interventions. Behavioral-management interventions are intended to increase prosocial and health-promoting behaviors and decrease antisocial and health-threatening behaviors. Skill-building programs are intended to help individuals with inadequate functional or coping skills acquire needed skills (e.g., meal preparation in a population of individuals with mental retardation or social skills in a group of adolescents with schizophrenia).

Behavioral programs often involve formal and clearly articulated contracts. An example of a formal contract used for therapeutic purposes is a point reward system for appropriate behavior used in a treatment setting for adolescents with conduct disorder. Behavioral principles may also guide the occupational therapy practitioner in the absence of a formal behavioral program. For example, in working with patients with chronic pain, the practitioner may encourage independence in functional behaviors and limit attention from staff and family members for chronic pain behaviors (Romano, Jensen, Turner, Good, & Hops, 2000).

RESEARCH REGARDING BEHAVIORAL INTERVENTIONS IN OCCUPATIONAL THERAPY

Behavior therapy has been shown to be a highly effective form of intervention for individuals with various types of health problems (McEachin, Smith, & Lovaas, 1993; Romano et al., 2000; Speed, 1996). Research contrasting behavior therapy with more standard forms of therapy either shows no difference or favors the behavioral skills-building approach (Basmajian et al., 1987; Liberman, Wallace, Blackwell, Kopelowicz, & Vaccaro, 1998). Research published in the occupational therapy literature is more limited but is generally favorable (e.g., Giles, Ridley, Dill, & Frye, 1997; O'Neill, Gwinn, & Adler, 1997).

SECTION III

Cognitive Therapy

GORDON MUIR GILES

In the 1960s and 1970s, Beck (1963; 1967), Beck, Rush, Shaw, and Emery (1979), Ellis (1962; 1973), Meichenbaum (1977), and Dobson (1988) developed cognitive therapy (CT). Also called cognitive behavior therapy this approach has been used as a frame of reference in occupational therapy (Duncombe, 1998). For the cognitive therapist, the clients' cognitions about the self, the world, and the future are of central importance. Like behavior therapy, CT is best considered a family of approaches, which includes cognitive therapy, problem-solving training, coping skills training, and other approaches (Dobson, 1988). However the cognitive therapy of Beck et al. (1979) has been particularly influential and is the primary focus of this section.

INTELLECTUAL HERITAGE

CT was developed partly because behavior therapy, owing to its lack of cognitive explanations, could not address many important mental health problems (N. B. Allen, 1998; Beck, 1993; Dobson, 1988). Despite the differences between CT and behavioral approaches there remain many similarities, including a strong emphasis on the analysis of specific problems (detailed analysis of actual events), practice of skills outside treatment (homework), short-term intervention, the use of measurable behavioral and affective changes as the criteria for success, and emphasis on empirical validation (Beck, 1993; Dobson, 1988). Other important influences on CT are the emergence of cognitive psychology, particularly information processing theory, and the development of methods to analyze cognitive events (Beck, 1993; Dobson, 1988).

ASSUMPTIONS

Central to the distinction between behavior therapy and CT is that the cognitive therapist recognizes the importance of the client's appraisal of events in the development and continuation of mental disorders (McMullin, 2000). The following assumptions undergird CT approaches:

- Appraisal processes influence affect and behavior.
- Altering cognitions may alter affect and behavior.
- **Thinking errors** contribute to the development and maintenance of irrational beliefs and maladaptive behavior; therapists help clients learn to dispute or counter irrational thoughts and ways of perceiving the world (McMullin, 2000).

A wide variety of techniques have been developed by cognitive therapists to assist clients counter irrational beliefs. CT has received considerable empirical support (King & Ollendick, 1998) and has been demonstrated to be effective in the treatment of many mental health disorders (Beck, 1993; Dobson, 1989; Nauta, Hospers, Kok, & Jansen, 2000; Scott, 1997).

BASIC PRINCIPLES OF CT

Unlike many forms of psychotherapy, in CT, the therapist is active and directive (McMullin, 2000). The cognitive therapist is interested in the patient's habitual ways of thinking about the self, the world, and the future (the cognitive triad). A central idea in CT is that it is the person's thoughts about events and not the events themselves that lead to distress. The cognitive therapist uses a process of guided discovery to assist clients to uncover the irrational beliefs that cause distress or maladaptive patterns of behavior. A formulation approach is used in which the therapist tries to grasp the client's core beliefs and ways of understanding the world. Clients are believed to have automatic thoughts—things that they tell themselves—that are so habitual that clients may have no awareness of them. The automatic thoughts may be highly abbreviated forms of subvocal speech, such as single words or simple phrases, with which clients assign meaning to ongoing events. Automatic thoughts reflect habitual and often erroneous forms of thinking. For example, believing that it is possible to know what another person is thinking (usually inferring a negative evaluation of the self).

Core schemas, built up over many years, describe the fundamental ways a person thinks about the self, others, and the world. They affect the person's perceptions of the environment and influence the person's actions. Core schemas cannot be accessed directly and are inferred from the client's automatic thoughts and behavior. The schemas can be presented as a series of if/then statements about the self, people, and the world. For example, "If I am open about my feelings, then people will ridicule and despise me." Schemas (through which the client's experiences are processed) can stand in the way of awareness of events that are inconsistent with expectations (Beck et al., 1979). Core schemas cannot be modified directly but may be changed by helping the client change his or her thoughts (McMullin, 2000).

CT uses an array of intervention techniques to help clients make consistent changes in their behavior and thought so as to influence their mood and other aspects of their mental health (McMullin, 2000). The intervention approach is fundamentally collaborative. Intervention is focused and usually short term; it addresses specific goals, often defined early in intervention by the development of a problem list on which the client and therapist agree. By asking questions about the client's beliefs, the therapist assists him or her to uncover the underlying irrational beliefs or cognitive distortions that lead to distress or maladaptive behavior.

It should be emphasized, however, that CT is not about replacing negative self-talk with positive self-talk (happy talk) but rather aims to replace negative thoughts with more realistic appraisals to reduce the impact of distorted thinking styles. Clients are encouraged to examine the advantages and disadvantages of certain beliefs, to challenge their ideas logically, talk back to their thoughts, and subject their beliefs to experimental challenge. Specific disorders have been found to have specific types of maladaptive beliefs associated with them. For example, individuals with alcohol abuse may continue to drink because of permissive beliefs such as "One drink won't hurt me" or "I cannot have fun, relax, or make friends unless I drink" (Beck, Wright, Newman, & Liese, 1993).

RELEVANCE OF COGNITIVE APPROACHES TO OCCUPATIONAL THERAPY

The emphasis of CT on cognitive appraisal fits the biopsychosocial model recognized as appropriate for occupational therapy. The combination of CT and occupational therapy allows therapists the opportunity to examine meaning associated with functional activities (Giles, 1985). The focus on each client's cognition appraisal process leads to the individualization of each client's intervention plan and the development of specific objectives. Within the CT framework, the occupational therapy practitioner establishes a collaborative relationship, acts as an educator and coach, models a scientific attitude, questions irrational beliefs, and uses meaningful activities to access and change cognitions and appraisals that are detrimental to the client's competencies.

Assessment frequently includes a client interview, questions about cognitions during practical activities, the use of formal assessments, and the use of self-assessments and ratings (Duncombe, 1998: Giles, 1985). Cognitive therapy is used by occupational therapy practitioners to help clients with schizophrenia (Goldman & Quinn, 1988; Greenberg et al., 1988; Stein & Nikolic, 1989), depressive illness (Lichtenberg, Kimbarow, MacKinnon, Morris, & Bush, 1995), eating disorders (Giles, 1985; Nauta et al., 2000; Telch, Agras, & Linehan, 2000), substance-abuse problems (Beck et al., 1993; Marlatt, 1978;), anger-control problems (Grogan, 1991a, 1991b; Steffen, 2000), and stress management (Mitchel, 2000; Stein & Smith, 1989). CT is also used in occupational therapy for wellness and health promotion (Mitchell, 2000; Steffen, 2000; Stein & Nikoloc, 1989; Stein & Smith, 1989).

RESEARCH REGARDING THE USE OF CT IN OCCUPATIONAL THERAPY

Cognitive therapy has been shown to be a highly effective form of intervention for individuals with various types of mental health problems (Beck, 1993; Dobson, 1988; McMullin, 2000). Research published in the occupational therapy literature is more limited but is generally favorable (e.g., Mitchell, 2000; Stein & Nikolic, 1989; Stein & Smith, 1989).

SECTION IV

Cognitive Disability Frame of Reference

STEPHANIE GRANT

INTELLECTUAL HERITAGE

Allen developed the cognitive disability model based on observations she made when treating clients with psychiatric illnesses. Initially, Allen predicated the model on Piagetian principles, developing her six cognitive levels after Piaget's six substages of cognitive growth (Allen, 1982; Sweetingham, 1996). Later, Allen (1987) introduced concepts from Soviet psychology to the model, arguing this is "the only branch of the social sciences that has used the concept of activity as the central focus of study" (p. 564). In conjunction with these ideas, she infused the model with more contemporary neuroscience concepts, specifically the information processing approach to understanding cognition and function (Allen, 1987; Allen, Earhart, & Blue, 1992; Katz & Heinmann, 1990; Sweetingham, 1996). More recently, Allen (1999) returned to an emphasis on the Piagetian influence of structuralism and now refers to the model as the functional information processing model.

ASSUMPTIONS

An overarching framework for this model is the pattern of assumptions about what a client can do, will do, and may do (Allen, Earhart, & Blue, 1995). What a client can do is based on biological factors and is the aspect of the client's function that is measured by Allen cognitive levels. What a client will do is influenced by psychological factors, such as motivation, fears, or meaningfulness of the activity being performed. What a client may due is a reflection of how much support he or she receives from his or her social systems, including family, friends, and caregivers.

- The severity of a mental disorder can be judged by the consequences it has on a person's capacity to think, do, and learn.
- Mild mental disorders can be compensated for by learning psychological substitutes for normal mental processes.
- Severe mental disorders can be associated with limited mental abilities that cannot be corrected by what the person says or does.
- Severe mental disorders can be compensated for by providing environmental substitutes for normal mental processes and identifying normal processes that can still be used.
- The remaining mental abilities can be engaged to do realistic activities that are meaningful to the client, practical for caregivers, and sustainable over time.
- When people are unable to learn to use psychological compensations effectively, environmental compensations can improve the quality of life for them and their long-term caregivers (C. K. Allen, 1998).

Similar mental structures predict similar performance (Allen, 1999). The practitioner identifies the underlying mental structures of a given activity to predict similar performance in other activities. Allen defined underlying mental structures as "the mental components used to organize thinking and learning processes" (p. 2). She indicated that successful performance of an activity occurs when these mental structures are available to the person and match the demands of the activity.

DEFINITIONS

- *Cognitive disability:* An impairment in task behavior relative to cognitive skill; measured via Allen cognitive levels.
- *Allen cognitive levels:* Ordinal hierarchical scale, ranging from 0.8 to 6.0, used to describe the status of cognitive ability (Table 21-1).
- *Cognitive performance modes:* Describe the progression of cognitive ability within each cognitive level.
- *Underlying mental structures:* "The mental components used to organize thinking and learning processes" (Allen, 1999, p. 2) include: attention, memory, speed, perception, orientation to time and social rules, cause and effect, and verbal communication.
- *Allen Cognitive Level Screen (ACLS):* Leather lacing activity designed to determine the cognitive level of clients functioning between levels 3.0 and 6.0. Clients are assessed on how they perform three leather stitches of increasing complexity.
- *Large Allen Cognitive Level Screen (LACLS):* Leather lacing activity that it is larger than the ACLS and enables clients with low-vision to engage in the screening.

TABLE 21-1. **ALLEN COGNITIVE LEVELS**[a]

Title	Cognitive Level	Description
Planned activities	6.0	Able to think about actions before performing them; considers the needs of others; attends to abstract cues, the potential outcome of an action, safety hazards, and social expectations
Independent learning	5.0	Able to explore new actions and make fine motor adjustments; attends to surface properties, spatial properties, feelings; remembers the effects of previous actions to learn new activities
Goal-directed learning	4.0	Able to complete a goal, perform self-care independently, and comply with directions; attends to eye-catching visual cues, familiar actions that accomplish a goal, possessions, and errors
Manual actions	3.0	Able to handle objects, follows one-step cues within the context of familiar activity, and repeat/learn movement patterns; attends to gross hand use and size, shape, and function of familiar objects
Postural actions	2.0	Able to move body for sitting, standing, walking, and balance; attends to barriers in environment and large objects
Automatic actions	1.0	Able to use protective responses (withdrawing from noxious stimuli); attends to all five senses with focus on survival
Coma	0.0–0.8	Unconscious, no response to stimuli or only reflexive responses (flexion–extension, eyes, hands, and mouth open and close spontaneously)

[a]Adapted from Allen (1997).

- *Routine Task Inventory (RTI):* Assessment of ADL that examines client, caregiver, and occupational therapy practitioner observations of function and assigns cognitive levels to each activity assessed.
- *Allen Diagnostic Module (ADM):* Series of standardized craft activities designed to verify the score obtained the ACLS and to predict functional outcomes.
- *Sensory stimulation kits:* Two kits (I and II) that stimulate all five senses and are designed to assess cognitive levels 0.8 through 3.2.
- *Allen battery:* Describes all the cognitive disability assessments.

EFFECTS ON EVALUATION, INTERVENTION, AND CLIENT–PRACTITIONER INTERACTIONS

When using the cognitive disability model, the occupational therapy practitioner begins an evaluation by conducting an interview to establish a rapport with the client before administering the ACLS. The practitioner uses the leather lacing screening to assess the client's cognitive level. If a score of ≥3.0 is obtained, the practitioner can choose to use the ADM or the RTI-2 to verify the score. When the practitioner is confident of the score obtained, he or she may use of the handbook *Understanding Cognitive Performance Modes* (Allen et al., 1995) as a starting place for predicting the client's best ability to function relative to his or her cognitive level. The handbook, a nearly essential guide for using the ACLS, lists abilities and a level-specific safety checklist, which can help guide intervention. If the score cannot be determined from the ACLS, a sensory stimulation kit can be used to determine cognitive levels <3.2.

Arguably, the most effective use of the cognitive levels is in determining what type of environmental and/or social support is indicated to facilitate a client's best ability to function (Allen et al., 1992). The occupational therapy practitioner determines if intervention to affect occupational performance improvement should be focused directly on the client, his or her caregivers, or both. The emphasis of intervention for clients with higher cognitive levels is to teach the client. For clients with lower cognitive levels, the practitioner focuses on caregivers; and for clients at the middle range of the cognitive levels, teaching is aimed at both the client and the caregivers.

STRENGTHS AND LIMITATIONS

Use of the cognitive disability model is an effective method for quickly identifying a disturbance in cognition as it relates to everyday function. This model is effective at identifying the potential function of a client relative to underlying mental structures. The cognitive disability model has been considered a departure from a core occupational therapy belief, which contends that activity improves physical and mental well-being (Kielhofner, 1997; Sweetingham, 1996). If change in the underlying mental structures is desired, this model can measure that change (or even track a decline), but it does not seek to effect that change. The concepts related to the higher cognitive levels within this model are not well articulated and may seem confusing, especially to the occupational therapy practitioner who is new to the model. Examples for facilitating clients with higher cognitive disability are needed. Although the model has a lot of use, the therapist must undergo a long learning curve to understand all the aspects of the model fully and to make the link to clinical practice.

ETHICS NOTE 21–1

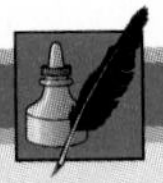

What Are the Ethical Uses of Evaluations?

PENNY KYLER and RUTH HANSEN

An occupational therapist, Justine, takes a job as a contract therapist in a nursing home. The other therapist who works there has told Justine that her responsibility is to do initial and follow-up evaluations with all residents and that she needs to use the Allen cognitive level evaluation method. The results of the evaluations will be used for placement and level of care considerations in the facility. A new person is admitted to the hospital with a diagnosis of amyotrophic lateral sclerosis (ALS). Justine does not feel that the ACL is an appropriate assessment for this person. She knows that it is supposed to be used as a screening tool.

QUESTIONS AND EXERCISES

1. **What, if anything, should Justine do in this situation?**
2. **What is her obligation to the resident with ALS?**
3. **What is her obligation to the other nursing home residents?**

RESEARCH

Studies of the cognitive disability model have focused largely on reliability and validity of the ACLS (including the ACL-E, ACL-PS, and ACL-90) and the RTI (and RTI-2). Several studies have established that the ACLS has interrater reliability (Keller & Hayes, 1998; Penny, Mueser, & North, 1995; Henry, Moore, Quinlivan, & Triggs, 1998). Allen et al. (1992) determined that the ACLS has test-retest reliability.

There is research to support that the ACLS has concurrent (congruent) and construct validity as well. Mayer (1988) established that the ACLS has congruent validity with the Wechsler Adult Intelligence Scale-Revised (WAIS-R) (a measure of fluid intelligence) and thus is useful as an indicator of learning potential. Velligan, True, Lefton, Moore, and Flores (1995) studied the concurrent validity of the ACLS with the Functional Needs Assessment and found that the ACLS "is a valid measure of concurrent level of adaptive functioning" (p. 107). Keller and Hayes's (1998) study provided preliminary support for the construct validity of the ACLS (ACL-90) and concluded that the ACL may be a direct measure of adaptive functioning.

The ACLS has also been found to be a measure of cognitive dysfunction associated with organicity and a predictor of community functioning (David & Riley, 1990; Henry et al., 1998). Studies done on the RTI have revealed its value as an occupational therapy assessment tool and that daily living skills on the RTI are related to cognitive level (Heinmann, Allen, & Yerxa, 1989; McAnanama, Rogosin-Rose, Scott, Jaffe, & Kelner, 1999).

CONCLUSION

The cognitive disability model is effective in the evaluation and treatment of a person's adaptive functioning relative to cognitive ability. The model is useful in multiple settings and assists the therapist to establish a quick and accurate understanding of a person's present cognitive functioning as it relates to daily activity.

SECTION V

Multicontext Treatment Approach

JOAN PASCALE TOGLIA

COMPONENTS OF THE MULTICONTEXT APPROACH

The multicontext treatment approach addresses the issue of generalization in cognitive rehabilitation. Although it was designed for clients with brain injury, it has also been applied to clients with psychiatric disabilities (Josman, 1998). The multicontext approach is based on the dynamic interactional model of cognition (Toglia, 1992, 1998). It was influenced by clinical practice with persons with brain injury and cognitive and educational psychology literature on learning and generalization (Bransford, 1979; Brown, 1983, 1988).

The multicontext treatment approach views learning as an interaction between internal (person) and external (activity demands and context) variables. Internal variables include the following:

- Characteristics of the learner, such as previous experiences, knowledge, values, personality, coping style, motivation, and emotions.
- Structural capacity or inherent, fixed abilities.
- Self-awareness or knowledge and beliefs regarding one's abilities as well as monitoring and regulating performance.
- Processing strategies, or small units of behavior that contribute to the effectiveness and efficiency of performance.

External variables include activity parameters, such as the number of items and steps, arrangement, familiarity, predictability, and movement requirements, as well as contextual factors, such as the physical, social, and cultural context.

Problems in processing information and learning are understood by analyzing the dynamic interaction between the person, the activity, and the context (Toglia, 1998). When the activity demands or context changes, the type of cognitive strategies and self-monitoring skills required for efficient performance change as well. Dynamic assessment is used to identify external conditions that increase and decrease cognitive symptoms.

In the multicontext approach, separate cognitive perceptual skills are not addressed. Intervention focuses on increasing efficiency and effectiveness of processing strategies and self-monitoring techniques within purposeful and occupation-based activities. Activity parameters and the context are systematically varied, while the same strategies and self-monitoring techniques are practiced across different situations to facilitate learning and generalization (Toglia, 1991). The components of the multicontext approach are summarized in Table 21-2 and described in the following sections.

TABLE 21–2. **COMPONENTS OF THE MULTICONTEXT TREATMENT APPROACH**

Intervention Components	Description
1. Specify a Processing Strategy for Transfer *The behavior that should be observed in a variety of different tasks*	**Strategies: 2 types** **Internal—**Strategy uses self-cues, self-reminders, self-instructions, self-questions, mental rehearsal, or visualization; client is taught to simplify activities by attending to one step or part at a time, mentally rehearsing performance before actual performance, and verbalizing instructions during performance. **External—**Strategy uses aids or interactions with environmental stimuli, such as checklists, anchor for scanning, highlighting critical points, finger pointing during scanning, and memory notebook. Strategies may also be characterized by their range of application; some are effective only in selected tasks and environments, whereas others are nonspecific and effective in a wide variety of contexts.
2. Analyze Activity and Establish Criteria for Transfer *Transfer of learning can occur at different levels*	Gradually vary the physical or surface features of the activity while keeping the underlying strategy consistent. **Near transfer (Very Similar)—**Alternate form of the same task; only one to two activity parameters are changed; activity is easily recognizable. **Intermediate Transfer (Somewhat Similar)—**Three to six activity parameters are changed; activity shares some physical features with the original task but similarities are less obvious. **Far Transfer (Different)—**All activity parameters are changed except for one or two; activity is conceptually the same but physically different. **Very Far Transfer (Very Different)—**Transfer of what has been learned in intervention to everyday functioning.
3. Practice Application of the Strategy in Multiple Activities and Contexts	• Transfer increases with the number of examples and situations provided • Include practice in identifying situations in which the strategy does not apply • Difficulty level is not increased until evidence of far transfer is observed
4. Train Awareness (Metacognitive Training) *Self-monitoring and self-regulatory skills are needed to move the client beyond the cued condition*	**Self-Awareness Skills include the ability to:** • Evaluate task difficulty in relationship to one's own abilities • Predict or anticipate consequences • Recognize errors or obstacles during task performance • Monitor and adjust responses according to feedback from the task
5. Consider Learner Characteristics *Information is better learned and retained when the client can relate it to previously learned material*	**Motivation and Active Participation are Enhanced when:** • Intervention activities are individualized and tailored to the client's personality, interests, occupations, and experiences • The goals are defined concretely (e.g., measurable scores, charts, graphs of self-ratings for each task) • Each new intervention activity is connected with previous intervention activities and experiences • The Clients are assisted in gaining a sense of control over their symptoms

From: Toglia J (1996). A multicontext approach to cognitive rehabilitation. Supplemental manual to workshop conducted at New York Hospital-Cornell Medical Center, New York, N.Y.

Specifying a Processing Strategy for Transfer

A dynamic approach to evaluation examines the extent to which performance changes with cues, activity modification, or practitioner mediation (see Chapter 25, Section 2). Responsiveness to cues or mediation indicates learning potential. In intervention, behaviors that are targeted for change are those that interfere with performance of a wide range of activities and are responsive to cues or mediation. In addition, minimal awareness of performance limitations is necessary. Table 21-3 presents examples of inefficient processing strategies or behaviors that may be addressed in intervention by teaching the client to use more efficient strategies. The behavior(s) that are targeted for change in the multicontext approach may not be the client's most obvious cognitive symptoms but rather are behavior(s) that are easily modifiable, as determined through dynamic assessment. Once the behavior(s) targeted for change are identified, the client is taught to use a processing strategy that enhances performance in a variety of different situations.

TABLE 21-3. **SAMPLE PROCESSING STRATEGIES**

Inefficient Strategies (behaviors targeted for change)	**Efficient Strategies** (behaviors emphasized in intervention)
Omits details or steps	Highlights, circles, underlines relevant details
Overfocuses on pieces	Attends to the whole context before attending to details
Haphazard approach	Prioritizes, preplans, groups materials together, arranges items in order of use before activity
Responds impulsively	Paces and modulates speed of action
Sidetracked with irrelevant information	Covers, reduces, or removes information

Activity Analysis, Establishment of Criteria for Transfer, and Practice in Multiple Activities and Contexts

Transfer of learning is not all or none. Different levels of transfer are viewed on a continuum that represents activities or learning situations that gradually differ in physical similarity. The more two situations or activities are physically similar, the easier it is to transfer strategies learned in one situation to the other (Davidson & Sternberg, 1998; Toglia, 1991). In intervention, the client practices the same processing strategy in activities and contexts that gradually differ. Activity parameters are analyzed and manipulated to place increasing demands on the ability to transfer learning within a "just right" challenge level. A just right challenge level is indicated by occasional cues (<25%) for successful performance. Key activity parameters are adapted and remain constant to match a just right challenge level while other activity parameters are varied. For example, the number of items, choices, steps, or rules may remain the same across all activities, while the type of activity and activity context are varied.

Intervention progresses in a horizontal manner and emphasizes sideways learning. An example of intervention activities presented along the transfer continuum is shown in Table 21-4. The targeted strategy (e.g., use of a checklist) is practiced in activities that require approximately equivalent skills and abilities but vary in physical appearance. Transfer of learning demands are increased along the transfer continuum, while activity demands remain at the same level and are not increased until spontaneous strategy use along the entire transfer continuum is observed.

The transfer continuum represents a guideline for progression of intervention activities, not absolute levels. If clients have difficulty in transferring use of a strategy, the physical similarity of intervention activities and contexts is changed very slowly; for other clients, intervention progresses quickly along the continuum and the focus is on practicing strategies in activities that vary widely in appearance (far transfer).

Training in Self-Awareness: Metacognitive Training

Training in self-awareness is embedded throughout intervention (see Chapter 30, Section 5). To function across different activities and contexts, clients needs to be able to monitor their performance and know when a particular strategy should be applied. Several authors have found that training in self-monitoring increases the probability of transfer of cognitive skills (Belmont, Butterfield & Ferretti, 1982; Borkowski & Burke, 1996; Brown, 1988; Cornoldi, 1998; Ford, Weissbein, Smith, & Gully, 1998; Roberts & Erdos, 1993).

Learner Characteristics

The client needs to be an active participant in intervention. Table 21-2 lists some ways to enhance client motivation and active participation. In addition, the use of structured subgoaling and journaling methods that help clients focus on here-and-now performance, self-monitor their progress, and reflect on their activity experiences can enhance motivation and participation (see Chapter 30, Section 5) (Toglia, 1998).

TABLE 21-4. **THE TRANSFER CONTINUUM**

Strategy emphasized in all activities: Use checklist to gather and keep track of items while:							
Making vegetable salad (6–8 items)	Making fruit salad (6–8 items)	Setting table for dinner	Packing 6–8 items in lunch box	Packing 6–8 items in bag for an overnight stay	Putting 6–8 appointments in calendar	Completing 6–8 party invitations	Completing 6 errands
Very Similar			**Somewhat Similar**		**Different**		**Very Different**

STRENGTHS, LIMITATIONS, AND RESEARCH

The multicontext approach aims to change the person's use of strategies and self-monitoring skills within a just right challenge level. It combines adaptation of the activity and context with a focus on changing the person's processing strategies and self-awareness skills across a wide range of situations. Some clients are not responsive to cues and do not have any awareness of their cognitive limitations. Other clients may be responsive to cues only at a very low level of performance, so that small changes will not make a meaningful impact on occupational performance within the intervention time frame. In these cases, approaches that do not require learning or generalization are preferred. The multicontext approach is best suited for individuals who show responsiveness to cues or practitioner mediation and display at least vague acknowledgment of limitations.

The use of the multicontext approach has been illustrated through case reports (Golisz, 1998; Landa-Gonzalez, 2001; Toglia, 1998). Although there is no research comparing the use of the multicontext approach with other intervention strategies, there is increasing evidence to support the critical components of the approach, such as strategy training (Cicerone et al., 2000; Fasotti, Kovacs, Eling, & Brouwer, 2000; Nelson & Lenhart, 1996; Niemeier, 1998; Trexler, Webb, & Zappala, 1994), awareness (metacognitive) training (Cicerone & Giacino, 1992; Fertherlin, 1989; Schlund, 1999; Tham, Ginsburg, Fisher, & Tegner, 2001), and the use of a wide range of activities and situations in intervention (Cicerone et al., 2000; Levine et al., 2000; Llyod & Curvo, 1994; Niemeier, Cifu, & Kishore, 2001; Sohlberg & Raskin, 1996).

CONCLUSION

The multicontext treatment approach challenges practitioners to identify behaviors that show potential for change rather than focusing on specific cognitive impairments. It provides practitioners with guidelines for selecting, grading, and progressing treatment activities using a "sideways method" to facilitate learning and transfer of strategies. Research is needed that examines the characteristics of clients who are best able to benefit from this approach.

SECTION VI

Motor Learning: An Emerging Frame of Reference for Occupational Performance

CLARE G. GIUFFRIDA

Motor **learning** theory can be thought of as a collection or set of ideas from the movement sciences that is used to explain the acquisition and modification of movements. There is no one motor learning theory but several different concepts, theories, and research evidence proposed to explain both the learning and the control of movement (Shumway-Cook & Woollacott, 2001). The act of motor learning includes more than simple motor processes, because it can involve learning new strategies for sensing and perceiving as well as moving. One ecological view suggests that motor learning emerges from the interaction of perception–cognition and action. Newel (1991) described it as the search for task solutions involving new strategies for perceiving and acting. These strategies emerge from the interaction of the individual with the task and the environment. Since the 1990s, studies of movement learning in both typical people and individuals with disabilities have significantly influenced the occupational therapy practitioner's knowledge and approach to clients who are learning and relearning skilled movements after injury.

INTELLECTUAL HERITAGE

Since the 1990s, several occupational therapists (Jarus, 1994, 1995; Haugen & Mathiowitz, 1995; Mathiowitz & Haugen, 1994; Poole, 1991; Sabari, 1991) have introduced movement science concepts, principles, and research from the field of motor behavior into occupational therapy. For many years, the motor behavior field primarily focused on investigating the nature, cause, acquisition, and modification of movements. From this research, theories, models, and principles to explain motor learning and control have emerged (Schmidt & Lee, 1998). These different theories, models, and principles reflect the changing focus of the motor behavior field as it has developed.

Starting in the late 1970s, the motor behavior field shifted from a strict behavioral, stimulus–response orientation to a cognitively based information processing framework. During this period, there was a focus on studying the mental and neural events hypothesized to support and produce movement. Researchers in neurophysiology and motor behavior attempted to find an association between motor behavior and neurological processes to understand the control of movement (Adams, 1987). As interest in the neural mechanisms of motor control increased, interest in motor learning and information processing gradually declined. Concurrently, there was also a shift from examining how the nervous system controlled movements to studying the mechanics and dynamics of movement control. However, counterintuitive information processing explanations about the beneficial effects of difficult learning contexts (Shea & Morgan, 1979) and the advantages of less feedback during practice (Salmoni, Schmidt, & Walter, 1984) provoked renewed interest in the study of both the neural mechanisms and the mental processes underlying movement learning. This interest was supported with advances in the cognitive sciences and ongoing exploration of brain and motor behavior relationships particularly in the 1990s, the decade of the brain.

COMMONALITIES BETWEEN MOTOR LEARNING AND OCCUPATIONAL THERAPY

Motor behavior scientists have traditionally focused on motor learning investigations with "normal" individuals, whereas occupational therapy has focused on restoring or rehabilitating occupational performance in clients (Schmidt & Lee, 1998). However, many neurorehabilitation intervention approaches within occupational therapy are based on implicit and explicit assumptions about motor control and learning in the normal individual (Mathiowitz & Haugen, 1994). Since the 1980s, those assumptions have been challenged by motor control and learning research across several fields. This research has led to moving away from using reflexive and hierarchical models of motor learning toward using less prescriptive and more distributed models of motor learning, programming, and control (Schmidt & Lee, 1998). This shift in knowledge has implications for how occupational therapy practitioners teach clients new movement sequences, such as how to get out of bed after a stroke or how to use a long-handled reacher.

MOTOR LEARNING

Schmidt and Lee (1998) described motor learning as a set of processes associated with practice and experience leading to permanent changes in the capacity for responding and producing skilled action. This definition highlights four aspects essential to learning:

- Motor learning is the process of acquiring the capability for skilled action.
- Motor learning results from experience or practice.
- Motor learning is inferred, based on behavior, and not measured directly.
- Motor learning produces permanent changes in behavior.

Learning is distinguished from temporary improvements in performance and is highlighted by relatively permanent changes in behavior. Learning is assessed by testing the knowledge after clients have completed practice. If the behavior is learned, it is evident on a retention test, which is a test after practice. Learners' posttraining performance and their ability to generalize their skill, therefore, become ways to assess the effectiveness of the training or rehabilitation program. The most effective practice conditions become those leading to the most accurate performance by the person on a novel version of the task or on the task practiced under novel conditions. For the occupational therapy practitioner planning intervention sessions, this means incorporating more task novelty into sessions to test the client's learning after practicing functional skills.

The goals of practice, training, and therapy become long-term retention, generalizability, and task learning that is resistant to altered contexts. These goals are highly congruent with occupational therapy's emphasis on function and intervention to restore or enhance independence in functional tasks necessary to fulfill occupational roles.

INFORMATION VARIABLES AS FEEDBACK

Feedback is information that the learner receives about performance while learning a skill or a new occupational performance. This information is frequently under the control of the teacher or therapist. Feedback informs learn- ers about the proficiency of their response while or after making the response and appears critical for learning. For example, in occupational therapy, as individuals practice putting on items of clothing, they receive feedback from their sensory receptors, environment, and therapist concerning their success with that activity. This feedback can be further divided into **intrinsic feedback** and **extrinsic feedback.**

Intrinsic Feedback

Intrinsic feedback includes information that is gathered through the individual's available sensory avenues, such as proprioception and vision. This form of information feedback occurs as the person is performing the movement skill. Feedback is then compared to a learned reference of correct movement. If there is no reference of correctness, the learner is unable to use feedback to detect errors and correct the movement. Feedback may be used in early learning to generate or modify each successive movement pattern. Later in the learning process, feedback helps the learner compare the movement executed with the reference of correctness that was developed (Poole, 1991). Clients who have sensory impairments or diminished sensory acuity have difficulty getting the feel of a movement or its correctness based on limited feedback from the intrinsic sensory mechanisms.

Extrinsic Feedback

Extrinsic feedback is provided verbally to the learner about task success and performance. This feedback from an external source supplements intrinsic feedback (Schmidt & Lee, 1998). It can be given concurrently with the task and/or at the end of the task. Extrinsic feedback can be provided as **knowledge of results** and as **knowledge of performance.**

Knowledge of Results

Knowledge of results (KR) is verbal, terminal, postaction information feedback about the movement outcome in terms of the environmental goal (Schmidt & Lee, 1998). Knowledge of results provides information about errors, thus giving the learner information about whether to modify the movement on the next attempt. For example, the occupational therapist could say, "You reached for the plate, not the cup" or "Your shirt is on backward."

Knowledge of Performance

Knowledge of performance (KP) is verbal postaction information feedback about the correctness of the movement pattern that the learner makes (Schmidt & Lee, 1998). It is directed toward improving the movement pattern rather than just the outcome of the movement in the environment. For example, the occupational therapist could say, "You need to lean forward in your chair to reach for the cup" or "You need to push with both arms to make the scooter go faster." Motor learning theorists suggest that more research is needed on KP and KR, as therapists seem to provide both in intervention sessions (Winstein & Schmidt, 1990).

Salmoni et al. (1984), in a review of the effects of KR on performance, described KR as providing an energizing, guiding, and informational function for the learner. Knowledge of results seems to guide the learner away from error toward the correct response. It tells the learner what went wrong and indicates how to correct it on the next trial. For example, if the therapist tells the client that he or she has reached for the plate and not the cup, then the next time the client will reach for the cup. Thus KR has a prescriptive role and provides guidance for the learner. Knowledge of results can also keep the learner alert and motivated, particularly for mundane tasks or long practice periods. This is important in therapy, because KR can make extended, difficult intervention sessions more interesting and keep the client engaged.

Knowledge of results, however, can also detract from the learning process. Research has shown that frequent feedback compared to reduced schedules of feedback may be detrimental to the learning process (Winstein & Schmidt, 1990; Wulf, Shea, & Rice, 1996). This finding runs counter to the traditional viewpoint that less frequent feedback degrades learning (Adams, 1971; Thorndike, 1927). Motor learning research indicates that too much KR can be counterproductive to individuals' learning, if it interferes with their processing of intrinsic information about the movement skill or interferes with their developing error detection capability. How patients use feedback effectively in therapy and how and when therapists provide feedback are important questions for future motor learning research in occupational therapy.

INFORMATION VARIABLES AS PRACTICE CONDITIONS

Practice, like feedback, is important to learning and to motor learning in therapy sessions. Typically, the more a person practices, the more he or she learns and remembers. Therefore, in therapy, it is advisable to practice, practice, practice—because the amount of practice is considered to be the strongest influence on motor learning (Nicholson, 1996). However, it is also helpful to know what practice conditions support and optimize learning, so that therapy sessions can be structured to maximize the patient's learning.

Massed and Distributed Practice

Massed practice is defined as continuous practice with no rest periods or as practice sessions in which the practice time is longer than the rest period between practices. In massed practice, for example, if a client practices transfers, the practice time for the transfer is greater than the time period between the first and second practice of the transfer. On the other hand, **distributed practice** is defined as practice interspersed with more time spent resting between practice sessions. For example, the time spent resting equals or is greater than the time the client spends practicing the transfer. Distributed practice enhances performance and learning more than massed practice, but this seems to be specific to the learning of continuous tasks, such as driving. For discrete tasks, which have a specific beginning and end, such as picking up a cup, research evidence is not as clear as to the effects of massed versus distributed practice (Schmidt & Lee, 1998). Further research in this area might guide the therapist's scheduling of effective practice sessions for clients.

Whole- and Part-Task Practice

Whole and part practice involve practicing the entire activity or just its component parts. Using a work simulator, such as a Baltimore Therapeutic Equipment (BTE), is an example of **part practice;** and practicing a complete transfer, such as bed to chair, is an example of **whole practice** (Poole, 1991). Several studies indicate that unless the component parts are subskills of each other or natural components of the task, part practice is not as beneficial as whole practice (Winstein, Gardner, McNeal, Barto, & Nicholason, 1989).

In a recent motion analysis study of part- and whole-task performance of a signature task. Ma and Trombly (2001) found a difference in handwriting performance across practice conditions in a group of elderly persons. Elderly participants in the whole-task practice condition demonstrated a more forceful and smoother movement for picking up a pen and writing their name than the participants in the part-task practice condition. This research, although limited, suggests that practicing this task in its entirety leads to a smoother and more natural movement pattern being used by participants. This research finding is important to therapists, because part practice is often used by therapists who are taught to break activities into component parts for ease of teaching and learning.

Mental Practice

Mental practice involves performing or running through the activity in one's mind without accompanying physical practice. Research indicates that mental practice cannot replace physical practice, but it can produce effects on tasks requiring accuracy in performance rather than on tasks tapping strength or endurance. It is hypothesized that mental practice triggers neural circuits underlying previously learned physical movement sequences (Leonard, 1998). For clients temporarily unable to practice physically, mental practice or rehearsal of occupational performance tasks may provide a reasonable alternative and supplement to intervention (Shumway-Cook & Woollacott, 2001).

Constant Versus Variable Practice

Constant practice involves practicing the same movement task in the same way for every trial. In constant practice, there are no variations in task conditions. Practicing buttoning the same size button, donning the same blouse, and using the same size spoon at all meals are examples of constant practice. **Varying practice** involves altering the conditions of the task across practice trials. Practicing buttoning different size buttons, putting on different types of blouses, and using different sizes of spoons are examples of variable practice. Variable practice appears to be more effective than constant practice, although research in this area indicates that this practice condition is constrained by a variety of person, task, and environmental factors (Lai, Shea, Wulf, & Wright, 2000; Van Rossum, 1990).

Schedule of Practice

Schedule of practice takes into account how different tasks practiced together are grouped or ordered in a practice session. In therapy, this involves multitask practice. Blocked or rote practice is repetitive practice of one task before the next task is introduced, for example, practicing sit to stand several times before practicing another therapeutic skill. Random practice is alternating, nonsystematic, but repetitive practice of each task in a set of tasks, for example, one trial practicing sit to stand, one trial practicing using a reacher, one trial practicing stand to sit, and then repeating this set of trials in any order.

Contextual Interference

The **contextual interference** effect refers to the specific finding that practice of multiple tasks in a random or nonsystematic but repetitive way results in depressed performance but greater retention and transfer for the learner. This is as compared to practicing multiple tasks in a repetitive, blocked, or systematic manner. In blocked practice, the learner performs more proficiently during the practice session but later demonstrates less retention and memory for the skill as compared to random practice.

There are several cognitive explanations for this difference in performance from practice schedules. Most researchers suggest that in random practice the learner uses more controlled and strategic cognitive processing (Shea & Morgan, 1979), has more opportunities for reconstructing the action plan (Lee & Magill, 1983), and/or has less task interference than in blocked practice (Shewokis, Del Rey, & Simpson, 1998). This difference in processing or interference during practice, therefore, causes the learner in random practice to perform poorly during practice. However, because of the increased cognitive efforts encountered in random practice, learners remember and generalize the movement skill better than from blocked practice.

The implications of this phenomenon on client intervention are significant. It suggests that methods of practice such as drill or rote practice are not necessarily the most effective for learning. On the contrary, practicing a variety of tasks in a nonsystematic way is more successful for learning. Therefore, the therapist may not need to make task practice simple or easy but, perhaps, should make it more demanding and effortful for the client. By varying the order of tasks practiced, the client becomes cognitively engaged, and more effective learning can occur.

Brady's (1998) review of this effect in applied settings supported the potency of random versus blocked effects. What remain elusive, however, are the specific boundary conditions for this effect across person, task, and environmental conditions. In occupational therapy, there is limited research examining this effect with different tasks and patient populations (Hanlon, 1996).

Guidance

In the practice condition of guidance, the learner is physically guided through the movement task to be learned. Generally, research in this area indicates that physically **guiding** a learner through the task is no more effective than allowing the client to engage in unguided practice (Shumway-Cook & Woollacott, 2001). However, guidance may be useful for acquainting the client with the requirements of the task.

MOTOR LEARNING THEORIES

Theories of motor learning are groups of distinct ideas about the nature and cause of the acquisition or modification of movement. Different theories include Adams's (1971) closed-loop theory of learning, Schmidt's (1975) schema theory, information processing–based theories (Glass & Holyoak, 1986), and Newell's (1991) systems and ecological–based motor control theory of learning as exploration.

In addition, there are several stage theories of motor learning that look at the process of motor learning over time and how the person, task, and environment act to constrain the learning process. For example, Gentile (1992) proposed a two-stage theory of motor skill acquisition that reflects the goal of the learner in each stage. In the first stage, the goal is to understand the task dynamics. In this stage, the learner gets the idea of the movement, develops strategies relevant to the goal, and recognizes and understands the features of the environment critical to the organization of the movement. In the second stage, the learner refines the movement. Other stage models of motor learning also emphasize how the learner goes from the novice to the expert stage and the processes involved (Fitts & Posner, 1967).

Each of these motor learning theories provides different explanations of the processes and factors significant in motor learning. They all, however, stress that the learner is actively involved in the process and that there is an interaction between the learner and the environment. A detailed exploration of these theories is beyond the scope of this book, and the reader is referred to the original articles on these theories.

MOTOR LEARNING POSTULATES FOR OCCUPATIONAL THERAPY EVALUATION AND INTERVENTION

Information variables, practice conditions, and theories derived from motor learning provide a framework for assessing and treating clients in occupational therapy. The following principles can guide occupational therapy:

- Motor learning is the individual's active process of acquiring the capability for skilled action through practice and experience and results in permanent changes in behavior.
- Learning occurs when performers are encouraged to develop their own movement solutions; however, training occurs when performers are provided with solutions to problems (Nicholson, 1996).
- Learning is best assessed by performance after, not during, practice.
- Practice and feedback are the two most important variables affecting motor learning.
- Creating practice conditions that are difficult (e.g., providing reduced knowledge of results and varying the practice schedule) creates an optimal motor learning environment for the client, as intense cognitive effort has to occur.

Contemporaneous motor learning theories are based on a systems model of the individual, the task, and the environment and on a distributed model of motor control. In the motor learning theories proposed by Schmidt and Lee (1999), practice produces a cumulative change in behavior and with practice a more appropriate representation of action is developed. However, perception action theorists, such as Newell (1991), stress that motor learning is a process of increased coordination between perception and action that is consistent with the task and the environment. Practice, therefore, becomes a search for the most effective strategies to solve the task, given the learning and environmental constraints.

THE IMPACT OF MOTOR LEARNING PRINCIPLES ON OCCUPATIONAL THERAPY EVALUATION AND INTERVENTION

Motor learning principles provide a guide for assessing and treating the client. These principles encourage active involvement of the learner in the process. However, this also means providing or altering the practice context so that the client receives reduced knowledge of results and performance and encounters difficulty in the practice context. Providing therapy in this way may be difficult for therapists wanting to encourage and support the client while also simplifying task demands.

STRENGTHS AND WEAKNESSES OF THE FRAMEWORK

The motor learning approach is based on research evidence mostly from normal motor learning, although evidence for this approach is increasing from patient populations. However, it does seem reasonable to assume that the evidence from typical motor learning applies to clients engaged in normal motor learning or relearning of activities; it remains to be supported by more robust motor learning research on atypical populations. Equally, the theory needs to be systematically explored with clients who have different learning needs and different movement problems. It may not be the approach to use with clients who have difficulty learning.

CONCLUSION

In order to function more effectively in their daily lives, clients often learn new movement strategies in occupational therapy. This section reviewed the primary concepts, principles, and theories derived from motor learning research that are influencing the delivery of occupational therapy services for clients with functional movement problems. Practitioners need to be aware of this ongoing research and how contemporaneous interpretations of the process of motor learning continue to impact occupational therapy.

References

Adams, J. A. (1971). A closed-loop theory of motor learning. *Journal of Motor Behavior, 3*, 111–150.

Adams, J. A. (1987). Historical review and appraisal of research on the learning, retention, and transfer of human motor skills. *Psychology Bulletin, 101*, 41–74.

Ader, R., & Cohen, N. (1993). Psychoneuroimmunology: Conditioning and stress. *Annual Review of Psychology, 44*, 53–85.

Allen, C. K. (1982). Independence through activity: The practice of occupational therapy (psychiatry). *American Journal of Occupational Therapy, 36*, 731–739

Allen, C. K. (1987). Activity, occupational therapy's treatment method. [Eleanor Clarke Slagle Lecture.] *American Journal of Occupational Therapy, 41*, 563–575.

Allen, C. K. (1997). *Use of Allen's Cognitive Levels in rehab, psych, geriatrics and physical disabilities*. Ormand Beach, FL: Allen Conferences.

Allen, C. K. (1998). Cognitive disability frame of reference. In M. E. Neistadt & E. B. Crepeau (Eds.). *Willard and Spackman's occupational therapy* (9th ed., pp. 555–557). Philadelphia: Lippincott.

Allen, C. K. (1999). *Structures of the cognitive performance modes*. Ormand Beach, FL: Allen Conferences.

Allen, C. K., Earhart, C. A., & Blue, T (1992). *Occupational therapy treatment goals for the physically and cognitively disabled*. Rockville, MD: American Occupational Therapy Association.

Allen, C. K., Earhart, C. A., & Blue, T. (1995). *Understanding cognitive performance modes*. Ormand Beach, FL: Allen Conferences.

Allen, N. B. (1998). Cognitive psychotherapy. In S. Bloch (Ed.). *An introduction to the psychotherapies* (pp. 167–191). Oxford, UK: Oxford Medical.

Bach-y-Rita, P. (1981). Brain plasticity as a basis of the development of rehabilitation procedures for hemiplegia. *Scandinavian Journal of Rehabilitation Medicine, 13*, 73–83.

Baddeley, A. (1990). When practice makes perfect. In A. Baddeley (Ed.). *Human memory* (pp. 143–175). Boston: Allyn & Bacon.

Bandura, A. (1977). *Social learning theory*. Englewood Cliffs, NJ: Prentice-Hall.

Bargh, J. A., & Chartrand, T. L. (1999). The unbearable automaticity of being. *American Psychologist, 54*, 462–479.

Basmajian, J. V., Gowland, C. A., Finlayson, M. A. J., Hall, A. J., Swanson, L. R., Stratford, P. W., Trotter, J. E., & Brandstater, M. E. (1987). Stroke treatment: Comparison of integrated behavioral-physical therapy vs. traditional physical therapy programs. *Archives of Physical Medicine and Rehabilitation, 68*, 267–272.

Beck, A. T. (1963). Thinking and depression. I. Idiosyncratic content and cognitive distortions. *Archives of General Psychiatry, 9*, 36–46.

Beck, A. T. (1967). *Depression: Clinical, experimental, and theoretical aspects*. New York: Harper and Row.

Beck, A. T. (1993) Cognitive therapy: Past, present and future. *Journal of Consulting and Clinical Psychology, 61*, 194–198.

Beck, A. T., Rush, A. J., Shaw, B. F., & Emery, G. (1979). *Cognitive therapy of depression*. New York: Guildford.

Beck, A. T., Wright, F. D., Newman, C. F., & Liese, B. S. (1993). *Cognitive therapy of substance abuse*. New York: Guildford.

Belmont, J. M., Butterfield, E. C., & Ferretti, R. P. (1982). To secure transfer of learning: Instruct self management skills. In D. K. Detterman & R. J. Sternberg (Eds.). *How and how much can intelligence be increased* (pp. 147–154). Norwood, NJ: Ablex.

Borkowski, J. G., & Burke, J. E. (1996). Theories, models, and measurements of executive functioning: An information processing perspective. In G. R. Lyon & N. A. Krasnegor (Eds.). *Attention, memory and executive function* (pp. 235–262). Baltimore: Brookes.

Brady, F. (1998). A theoretical and empirical review of the contextual interference effect and the learning of motor skills. *Quest, 50*(3), 266–293,

Bransford, J. (1979). Human cognition: Learning, understanding and remembering. Belmont, CA: Wadsworth.

Brown, A. (1983). Learning, remembering and understanding. In J. Flavell & E. Markman (Eds.). *Handbook of child psychology* (vol. 3, pp. 77–158). New York: Wiley.

Brown, A. (1988). Motivation to learn and understand: On taking charge of one's own learning. *Cognition and Instruction, 5*, 311–321.

Catania, A. C., & Harnad, S. (Eds.). (1988). *The selection of behavior*. Cambridge, UK: Cambridge University Press.

Cicerone, K. D., Dahlberg, C., Kalmar, K., Langenbahn, D. M., Malec, J. F., Bergquist, T. F. et al. (2000). Evidence-based cognitive rehabilitation:

Recommendations for clinical practice. *Archives of Physical Medicine and Rehabilitation, 81*, 1596–1615.

Cicerone, K. D., & Giacino, T. J. (1992). Remediation of executive function deficits after traumatic brain injury. *NeuroRehabilitation, 2*, 12–22.

Cornoldi, C. (1998). The impact of metacognitive reflection on cognitive control. In G. Mazzoni & T. O. Nelson (Eds.). *Metacognition and cognitive neuropsychology* (pp. 139–159). Mahwah, NJ: Erlbaum.

David, S. K., & Riley, W. T. (1990). The relationship of the Allen Cognitive Level Test to cognitive abilities and psychopathology. *American Journal of Occupational Therapy, 44*, 493–497.

Davidson, J. E., & Sternberg, R. J. (1998). Smart problem solving: How metacognition helps. In D. J. Hacker, J. Dunlosky, & A. G. Graesser (Eds.). *Metacognition in educational theory and practice* (pp. 47–68). Mahwah, NJ: Erlbaum.

Dobson, K. S. (1988). *Handbook of cognitive-behavioral therapies*. New York: Guildford.

Dobson, K. S. (1989). A meta-analysis of the efficacy of cognitive therapy for depression. *Journal of Consulting and Clinical Psychology, 57*, 414–419.

Duncombe, L. (1998). The cognitive behavioral model in mental health. In N. Katz (Ed.). *Cognition and occupation in rehabilitation* (pp. 165–191). Bethesda, MD: American Occupational Therapy Association.

Ellis, A. (1962). *Reason and emotion in psychotherapy*. New York: Stuart.

Ellis, A. (1973). *Humanistic psychotherapy: The rational-emotive approach*. New York: Julian.

Epstein, L. H. (1992). Role of behavior theory in behavioral medicine. *Journal of Consulting and Clinical Psychology, 60*, 493–498.

Eysenck, H. J., & Rachman, S. (1965). *The causes and cures of neurosis*. San Diego, CA: Knapp.

Fasotti, L., Kovacs, F., Eling P., & Brouwer, W. H. (2000). Time pressure management as a compensatory strategy training after closed head injury. *Neuropsychological Rehabilitation, 10*, 47–65.

Fertherlin, J. M. (1989). Self-instruction: A compensatory strategy to increase functional independence with brain injured adults. *Occupational Therapy Practice, 1*(1), 75–78.

Fitts, P. M., & Posner, M. I. (1967). *Human performance*. Belmont, CA: Brooks/Cole.

Ford, J. K., Weissbein, D. A., Smith, E. M., & Gully, S. M. (1998). Relationship of goal orientation, metacognitive ability and practice strategies with learning outcomes and transfer. *Journal of Applied Psychology, 83*, 218–233.

Gentile, A. (1992). The nature of skill acquisition: Therapeutic implications for children with movement disorders. In H. Forssberg & H. Hirschfield (Eds.). *Movement disorders in children* (pp. 31–40). Basel: Karger.

Giles, G. M. (1985). Anorexia nervosa and bulimia: An activity oriented approach. *American Journal of Occupational Therapy, 39*, 510–517.

Giles, G. M., & Clark-Wilson, J. (1993). *Brain injury rehabilitation: A neurofunctional approach*. San Diego, CA: Singular.

Giles, G. M., & Clark-Wilson, J. (1999). *Rehabilitation of the severely brain injured adult: A practical approach*. Cheltenham, UK: Thornes.

Giles, G. M., Ridley, J. E., Dill, A., & Frye, S. (1997). A consecutive series of adults with brain injury treated with a dressing retraining program. *American Journal of Occupational Therapy, 51*, 256–266.

Glass A. J., & Holyoak, K. J. (1986). *Cognition*. New York: Random House.

Goldman, C. R., & Quinn, F. L. (1988). Effects of a patient education program in the treatment of schizophrenia. *Hospital and Community Psychiatry, 39*, 282–286.

Goldstein, L. H., & Oakley, D. A. (1985). Expected and actual behavioural capacity after diffuse reduction in cerebral cortex: A review and suggestions for rehabilitative techniques with the mentally handicapped and head injured. *British Journal of Clinical Psychology, 24*, 13–24.

Golisz, K. M. (1998). Dynamic assessment and multicontext treatment of unilateral neglect. *Topics in Stroke Rehabilitation, 5*, 11–28.

Greenberg, L., Fine, S. B., Cohen, C., Larson, K., Michaelson-Baily, A., Rubinton, P., & Glick, I.D. (1988). An interdisiciplinary psychoeducational program for schizophrenic patients and their families in an acute care setting. *Hospital and Community Psychiatry, 39*, 277–281.

Grogan, G. (1991a). Anger management: A perspective for occupational therapy (Part 1). *Occupational Therapy in Mental Health, 11*(2/3), 135–148.

Grogan, G. (1991b). Anger management: Clinical implications for occupational therapy. *Occupational Therapy in Mental Health, 11*(2/3), 149–171.

Hanlon, R .E. (1996). Motor learning following unilateral stroke. *Archives of Physical Medicine and Rehabilitation, 77*, 811– 815.

Haugen, J., & Mathiowetz, V. (1995). Contemporary task-oriented approach. In C. Trombly (Ed.). *Occupational Therapy for Physical Dysfunction* (3rd ed., pp. 510–529). Baltimore: Williams & Wilkins.

Hefferline, R. F., Keenan, B., & Hartford, R. A. (1958). Escape and avoidance conditioning in human subjects without their observation of the response. *Science, 130*, 1338–1339.

Heinmann, N. E., Allen, C. K., & Yerxa, E. J. (1989). The routine task inventory: A tool for describing the functional behavior of the cognitively disabled. *Occupational Therapy Practice, 1*, 67–74.

Henry, A. D., Moore, K., Quinlivan, M., & Triggs, M. (1998). The relationship of the Allen Cognitive Level Test to demographics, diagnosis and disposition among psychiatric inpatients. *American Journal of Occupational Therapy, 52*, 638–643.

Hergenhahn, B. R. (1976). *An introduction to theories of learning*. Englewood Cliffs, NJ: Prentice-Hall.

Hintzman, D. L. (1978). *The psychology of learning and memory*. San Francisco: Freeman.

Jarus, T. (1994). Motor learning and occupational therapy: The organization of practice. *American Journal of Occupational Therapy 48*, 810–816.

Jarus, T. (1995). Is more always better? Optimal amounts of feedback in learning to calibrate sensory awareness. *Occupational Therapy Journal of Research, 15*, 181–197.

Josman, N. (1998). The dynamic interactional model in schizophrenia. In N. Katz (Ed.). *Cognition and occupation in rehabilitation* (pp. 151–164). Bethesda, MD: American Occupational Therapy Association.

Kandel, E. R., Kupfermann, I., & Iversen, S. (2000). Learning and memory. In E. R. Kandel, J. H. Schwartz, & T. M. Jessell (Eds.). *Principles of neural science* (pp. 1227–1245). New York: McGraw Hill.

Kantowitz, B. H., & Roediger, H. L. III (1980). Memory and information processing. In G. M. Gazda & R. J. Corsini (Eds.). *Theories of learning* (pp. 332–69). Itasca, IL: Peacock.

Kaplan, R. M. (1990). Behavior as a central outcome in health care. *American Psychologist, 45*, 1211–1220.

Katz, N., & Heinmann, N. (1990). Review of research conducted in Israel in cognitive disability instrumentation. *Occupational Therapy in Mental Health, 10*, 1–15.

Kazdin, A. (1994). *Behavior modification in applied settings* (5th ed.). Pacific Grove, CA: Brook/Cole.

Keller, S., & Hayes, R. (1998). The relationship between the Allen Cognitive Level Test and the Life Skills Profile. *American Journal of Occupational Therapy, 52*, 851–856.

Kertesz, A. (1985). Recovery and treatment. In K. M. Heilman & E Valenstein (Eds.). *Clinical Neuropsychology* (2nd ed., pp. 481–505). New York: Oxford University Press.

Kielhofner, G. (1997). *Conceptual foundations of occupational therapy*. Philadelphia: Davis.

King, N. J., & Ollendick, T. H. (1998). Empirically validated treatments in clinical psychology. *Australian Psychologist, 33*, 89–95.

Lai, Q., Shea, C. H., Wulf, G., & Wright, D. L. (2000). Optimizing generalized motor program and parameter learning. *Research Quarterly for Exercise and Sport, 71*, 10–24.

Landa-Gonzalez, B. (2001). Multicontextual occupational therapy intervention: A case study of traumatic brain injury. *Occupational Therapy International, 8*, 49–62.

Lee, T. D., & Magill, R. A. (1983). The focus of contextual interference in motor-skill acquisition. *Journal of Experimental Psychology, 9*, 730–746

Leonard, C. (1998). The neuroscience of motor learning, In C. T. Leonard (Ed.). *The neuroscience of human movement* (pp. 203–229). St. Louis: Mosby Year Book.

Levine, B., Robertson, I. H., Clare, L., Carter, G., Hong, J., Wilson, B. A., Duncan, J., & Stuss, D. T. et al. (2000). Rehabilitation of executive functioning: An experimental-clinical validation of goal management training. *Journal of International Neuropsychological Society, 6,* 299–312.

Liberman, R. P., Wallace, C. J., Blackwell, G., Kopelowicz, A., & Vaccaro, J. V. (1998). Skills training versus psychosocial occupational therapy for persistent schizophrenia. *American Journal of Psychiatry, 155,* 1087–1091.

Lichtenberg, P. A., Kimbarow, M. L., MacKinnon, D., Morris, P. A., & Bush, J. V. (1995). An interdisciplinary behavioral treatment program for depressed geriatric rehabilitation inpatients. *Gerontologist, 35,* 688–690.

Llyod, L., & Curvo, A. (1994). Maintenance and generalization of behaviors after treatment of persons with traumatic brain injury. *Brain Injury, 8,* 529–540.

Ma, H., & Trombly, C. (2001). The comparison of motor performance between part and whole tasks in elderly persons. *American Journal of Occupational Therapy, 55,* 62–67.

Marlatt, G. A. (1978). Craving for alcohol, loss of control and relapse: A cognitive-behavioral analysis. In P. E. Nathan & G. A. Marlatt (Eds.). *Experimental and behavioral approaches to alcoholism* (pp. 271–314). New York: Plenum.

Mathiowetz, V., & Haugen, J. (1994). Motor behavior research: Implications for therapeutic approaches to central nervous system dysfunction. *American Journal of Occupational Therapy, 48,* 733–745.

Mayer, M. A. (1988). Analysis of information processing and cognitive disability theory. *American Journal of Occupational Therapy, 42,* 176–183.

McAnanama, E. P., Rogosin-Rose, M. L., Scott, E. A., Jaffe, R. T., & Kelner, M. (1999). Discharge planning in mental health: The relevance of cognition to community living. *American Journal of Occupational Therapy, 53*(2), 129–135.

McEachin, J. J., Smith, T., & Lovaas, O. I. (1993). Long-term outcome for children with autism who received early intensive behavioral treatment. *American Journal of Mental Retardation, 97,* 359–372.

McMullin, R. E. (2000). *The new handbook of cognitive therapy techniques.* New York: Norton.

Meichenbaum, D. (1977). *Cognitive-behavior modification: An integrative approach.* New York: Plenum.

Mitchell, E. (2000). Managing career stress: An evaluation of a stress management programme for carers of people with dementia. *British Journal of Occupational Therapy, 63,* 179–184.

Nauta, H., Hospers, H., Kok, G., & Jansen, A. (2000). A comparison between a cognitive and a behavioral treatment for obese binge eaters and obese non-binge eaters. *Behavior Therapy, 31,* 441–461.

Neisser, U. (1992). Two themes in the study of cognition. In H. L. Pick, P. Van Den Broek, & D. C. Knill (Eds.). *Cognition* (pp. 333–340). Washington, DC : American Psychological Association.

Neistadt, M. E. (1994). The neurobiology of learning: Implications for treatment of adults with brain injury. *American Journal of Occupational Therapy, 48,* 421–430.

Nelson, D. L., & Lenhart, D. A. (1996). Resumption of outpatient occupational therapy for a young woman five years after traumatic brain injury. *American Journal of Occupational Therapy, 50,* 223–228.

Newell, K. M. (1991). Motor skill acquisition. *Annual Review of Psychology, 42,* 213–237.

Nicholson, D. (1996). Motor learning, In C. M. Fredericks and L. K Saladin (Eds.). *Pathophysiology of the motor system* (pp. 238–251). Philadelphia: Davis.

Niemeier, J. P. (1998). The lighthouse strategy: Use of a visual imagery technique to treat visual inattention in stroke patients. *Brain Injury, 12*(5), 399–406.

Niemeier, J. P., Cifu, D. X., & Kishore, R. (2001). The lighthouse strategy: Improving the functional status of patients with unilateral neglect after stroke and brain injury using a visual imagery intervention. *Topics in Stroke Rehabilitation, 8*(2), 10–18.

Nisbett, R. E., & Wilson, T. D. (1977). Telling more than we can know: Verbal reports on mental processes. *Psychology Review, 84,* 231–259.

O'Neill, M. E., Gwinn, K. A., & Adler, C. H. (1997). Biofeedback for writer's cramp. *American Journal of Occupational Therapy, 51,* 605–607.

Ormrod, J. E. (1990). *Human learning: Principles, theories, and educational applications.* New York: Macmillan.

Park, D. C. (1999). Acts of will? *American Psychologist, 54,* 461.

Penny, N. H., Musser, K. T., & North, C. T. (1995). The Allen Cognitive Level Test and social competence in adult psychiatric patients. *American Journal of Occupational Therapy, 49,* 420–427

Poole, J. (1991). Application of motor learning principles in occupational therapy. *American Journal of Occupational Therapy, 45,* 531–537.

Rescorla, R. A. (1988). Pavlovian conditioning: It's not what you think it is. *American Psychologist, 43,* 151–160.

Roberts, M. J., & Erdos, G. (1993). Strategy selection and metacognition. *Educational Psychology, 13,* 259–266.

Romano, J. M., Jensen, M. P., Turner, J. A., Good, J. A., & Hops, H. (2000). Chronic pain patient-partner interactions: Further support for a behavioral model of chronic pain. *Behavior Therapy, 31,* 415–440.

Rosenzweig, M. R. (1998). Historical perspectives on the development of the biology of learning and memory. In J. Martinez & Kesner, R. (Eds.). *Neurobiology of learning and memory* (pp. 1–53). San Diego, CA: Academic.

Sabari, J. S. (1991). Motor learning concepts applied to activity based intervention with adults with hemiplegia. *American Journal of Occupational Therapy, 45,* 523–536.

Salmoni, A. W., Schmidt, R. A., & Walter, C. B. (1984). Knowledge of results and motor learning: A review of critical appraisal. *Psychological Bulletin, 95,* 355–386.

Schlund, M. W. (1999). Self awareness: Effects of feedback and review on verbal self reports and remembering following brain injury. *Brain Injury, 13*(5), 375–380.

Schmidt, R. A. (1975). A schema theory of discrete motor skill learning. *Psychological Review, 82,* 225–260.

Schmidt, R. A., & Lee, T. (1999). *Motor control and learning.* Champaign, IL: Human Kinetics.

Scott, J. (1997). Advances in cognitive therapy. *Current Opinion in Psychiatry, 10,* 256–260.

Shea, J., & Morgan, R. (1979). Contextual interference effects on the acquisition, retention and transfer of a motor skill. *Journal of Experimental Psychology, 5,* 179–187.

Shewokis, P., Del Rey, P., & Simpson, K. (1998). A test of retroactive inhibition as an explanation of contextual interference. *Research Quarterly Exercise and Sport, 69,* 70–74.

Shumway-Cook, M., & Woollacott, M. (2001). *Motor control: Theory and practical applications.* Baltimore: Williams & Wilkins.

Skinner, B. F. (1938). *The behavior of organisms.* New York: Appelton-Century-Crofts.

Sohlberg, M. M., & Raskin, S. A. (1996). Principles of generalization applied to attention and memory interventions. *Journal of Head Trauma Rehabilitation, 11*(2), 65–78.

Speed, J. (1996) Behavioral management of conversion disorder: Retrospective study. *Archives of Physical Medicine and Rehabilitation, 77,* 147–154.

Squire, L. R. (1992). Memory and the hippocampus: A synthesis from findings with rats, monkeys, and humans. *Psychological Review, 99,* 195–231.

Squire, L. R., Zola-Margan, S. (1991). The medial temporal lobe memory system. *Science, 253* (5026), 1380–1386.

Steffen, A. M. (2000). Anger management for dementia caregivers: A preliminary study using video and telephone interventions. *Behavior Therapy, 31,* 281–299.

Stein, F., & Nikolic, S. (1989). Teaching stress management techniques to a schizophrenic patient. *American Journal of Occupational Therapy, 43,* 162–169.

Stein, F., & Smith, J. (1989). Short-term stress management programme with acutely depressed in-patients. *Canadian Journal of Occupational Therapy, 56,* 185–191.

Svartdal, F. (1991). Operant modulation of low level attributes of rule governed behavior by nonverbal contingencies. *Learning and Motivation, 22,* 406–420.

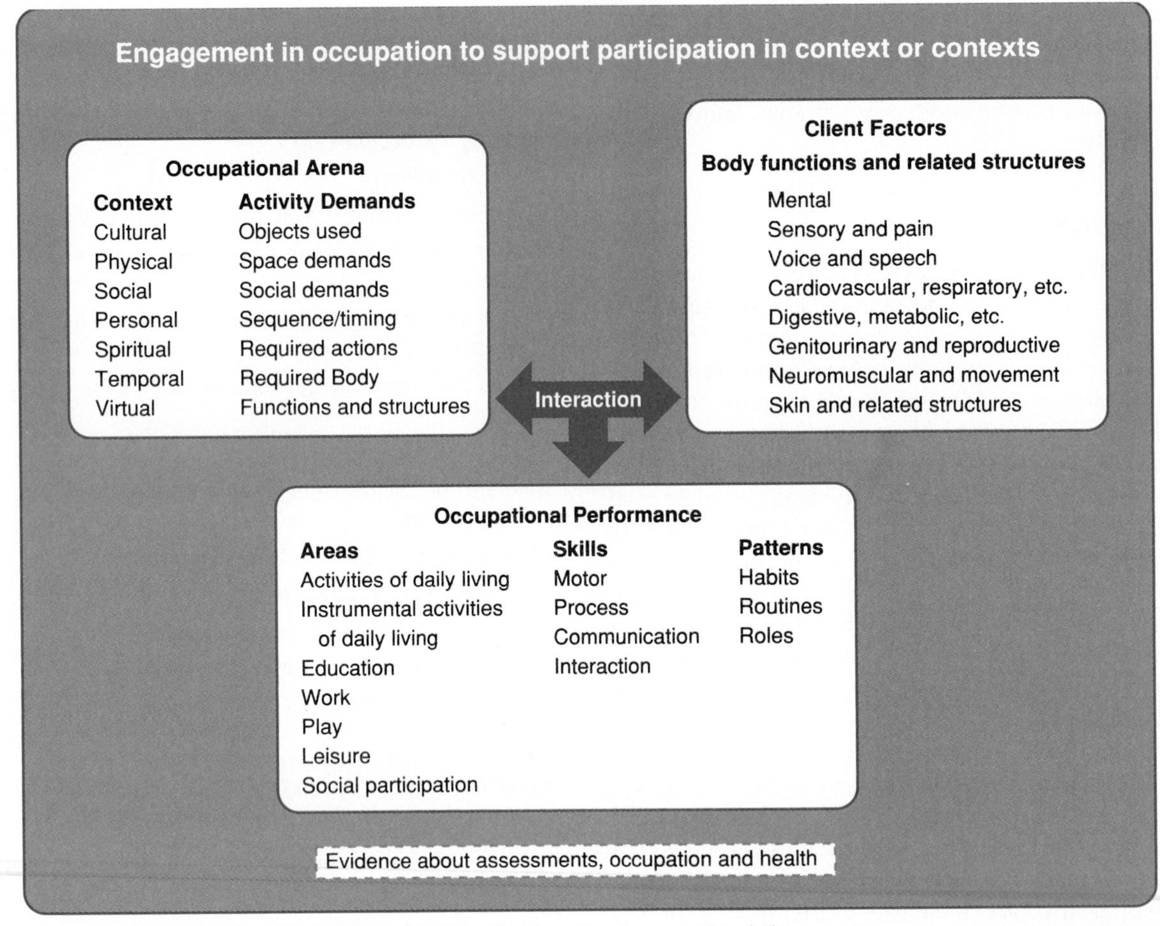

FIGURE 22–1. The domain of occupational therapy.

10. Develop goals for intervention that are consistent with the client's priorities and are feasible in light of evaluation findings (AOTA, in press).

Together these steps result in a thorough and effective evaluation necessary for intervention planning. The evaluation process is described more fully in the following section.

Review Preliminary Information

Clients come to occupational therapy with a past history, a living present, and a desire for the future. Most likely, clients seek the services of occupational therapy because of some difficulty with daily activities or occupations. Practitioners need to understand the client's history and specific reasons for seeking services; whether other practitioners are also providing intervention; and, if available, the medical, educational, or social history of the client. Referral information may be in the form of a phone call from the client or caregiver, a written report from another professional, or standard protocol in a particular setting where all clients are evaluated by occupational therapists. Formal records or reports often help practitioners develop initial images or understanding of the clients they are about to meet. These initial images are provisional until practitioner and client actually meet. Formal diagnoses of clients' health conditions may be available and may provide practitioners with initial cues about potential occupational performance problems. However, the diagnoses cannot tell practitioners how clients are experiencing their problems and the effect of the conditions on their occupations. Practitioners must remain open to understanding the uniqueness of each client they evaluate.

Interview Client

When meeting a client for the first time, practitioners should introduce themselves and explain the purpose of the visit. It is important to understand, from the client's perspective, what brought the client (which may be the person with the problem or the caregiver) to occupational therapy. The response can reveal the client's most immediate concerns. Many clients are anxious about the evaluation, about the problems that have brought them to occupational therapy, and about the disruptions those problems have caused in their lives. It is the practitioner's job to

make clients feel comfortable and safe through respectful and empathetic interactions. This interaction starts during the interview. Section 2 of this chapter provides specific guidelines about how to conduct interviews, and Unit IV addresses the therapeutic alliance.

Guiding Questions

Trombly (1995) urged therapists to use a top-down approach to evaluation. To use a top-down approach, therapists first focus on clients' occupational performance rather than beginning the evaluation with an emphasis on potential underlying performance component limitations. Hocking (2001) advised therapists to begin with interviews focused on the meaning of occupation for the client. This requires an understanding of significance of the major occupational themes in the person's life—past, present, and projected. For example, a therapist hired by a public health department to assist families living in urban poverty might begin the occupational therapy evaluation by asking clients to describe their day and then follow-up with probing questions to understand how those daily activities connect to the clients' life purpose.

The second focus for data gathering is to gain understanding of the functions of occupation for clients. This aspect addresses the relative importance of different occupational areas and the contribution that each of these makes to the person's development and lifestyle. Understanding the form of occupation involves establishing the quality of the client's occupational performance by observing the client actually engage in desired occupations in relevant contexts, while keeping the expectations of the context in mind. Table 22-1 lists questions that can be useful in understanding a client's occupational concerns.

TABLE 22-1. **GUIDING QUESTIONS THAT ADDRESS MEANING, FUNCTION, AND FORM OF OCCUPATIONS**

Meaning of Occupation
Who is the client?
How does this client describe himself or herself?
How does the client's occupations relate to his or her identity?
What is the meaning to the client's of his or her occupations?
How do the client's occupations connect to his or her life purpose?
Why is the client seeking service?
What are the client's current concerns about engaging in daily life activities?
What meaning or identity does the client wish to achieve?
In what areas of occupation is the client successful?
What areas of occupation are problematic?
What is the client's occupational history?
What are the client's occupational priorities and desired outcomes?
Function of Occupation
What is the client unable to do?
How does the current occupational situation affect ongoing development?
Who is affected by the client's challenges?
How do the occupations of key persons or groups support the client?
How do the occupations of key persons or groups hinder the client?
How might key persons or groups provide better support to the client?
Form of Occupation
What actions are required to complete the occupation successfully?
Where can the occupation be observed?
When and how often can it be observed?
What is the quality of client's occupational performance?
What performance standards apply to important occupations?
What occupational performance areas meet quality expectations?
What occupational performance areas do not meet quality expectations?
What will happen as a result of performing the occupation?
What contexts support engagement in desired occupations?
What contexts are inhibiting engagement?
What are the client's strengths?
What are the client's vulnerabilities?

Adapted from Hocking (2001).

Synthesize Information from Interview

Based on the information shared in the interview, the practitioner and client collaboratively name and frame the areas of occupation most important to the client (Schon, 1983). The practitioner and client identify the most relevant and meaningful occupations to further evaluate. Synthesis requires practitioners to listen carefully to client and caregiver concerns and focus on the most salient issues. Often, assessments such as the Canadian Occupational Performance Measure (Law, Baptiste, McColl, Opzoomer, Polatajko, & Pollock, 1990) and the School Function Assessment (Coster, Deeney, Haltiwanger, & Haley, 1998), help both the therapist and the client prioritize key areas.

Observe Occupational Performance and Identify Factors Influencing Performance

Once priorities are established, therapists observe clients performing the activities important to the occupation.

Therapists note the quality of performance, performance patterns, and activity demands. Therapists may use standardized assessments of performance skills for this part of the evaluation. Chapter 23 discusses the relative merits of formal and informal assessments and helps practitioners select the types of assessments most appropriate for a variety of evaluation needs. Chapters 24, 25, and 26 offer detailed descriptions of various areas of occupation, performance skill, client factors, and contextual evaluations.

During observations of clients' occupational performance, practitioners begin to hypothesize about what factors might be contributing to performance. To generate hypotheses about performance, therapists analyze the interaction between clients and the demands of the occupation or activity in relevant contexts and identify the facilitators and barriers to engagement in desired occupations.

To be successful in occupational performance, clients need to be proficient in the skills necessary for activity performance and to be able to orchestrate those skills into the desired or necessary occupational form. For example, to interact with peers during a kick-ball game on the playground during recess, 10-year-old Jeremy needs to interpret the social cues of his peers, know how to join the group, have the motor and language skills to play kick ball, understand the rules of the game, wait his turn, and cope with frustration if someone catches his fly ball and causes his team to have an out. If the occupational therapist observes difficulties with kicking, running, and balance, he or she would specifically assess Jeremy's motor skills. If Jeremy engages in ritualistic hand flapping while waiting his turn, a more through evaluation of dominating habits may be indicated. Perhaps Jeremy has just moved to the school from a different country and is observed standing at the edge of the field with a bewildered look on his face. In this case, the therapist may want to further explore Jeremy's prior cultural experiences.

Interpret Assessment Data to Identify Facilitators and Barriers to Performance

The goal of occupational therapy is to support clients' occupational performance in everyday life activities. Thus occupational therapists analyze transactions between clients and their performance contexts as enacted through occupation. Careful analysis of all factors results in identification of facilitators and barriers to performance. Facilitators and barriers may be found in many areas. For example, the stigma associated with mental illness may serve as a barrier to Sara, a mother with a serious mental illness parenting her 4-year-old son, Mike. Because society continues to have certain views about mental illness, Sara may be reluctant to seek support because she fears loss of custody of Mike. In this situation, societal attitudes are barriers to the Sara's performance as a parent. The activity demands may also create barriers to performance, as would be the case when a young child was unable to join a mixed age group of children playing a very complex game with multiple steps and constantly changing rules. Conversely, facilitators can support occupational performance. Proper positioning and lifting techniques may assist shipping clerks perform their job. The facilitators and barriers may be internal to clients, such as a strong desire to succeed, or external, as when adaptive devices are used to support performance.

Develop and Refine Hypotheses

Once therapists understand the quality of clients' occupational performance in context and possible factors influencing performance, they need to check out their hypotheses about performance problems systematically. For instance, consider a client named Peter who was having trouble putting his T-shirt on. The therapist might believe the problem was shoulder range of motion or muscle strength. The therapist would then assess the joint flexibility and strength of the affected arm. If Peter can move his shoulder through its full range of motion, the therapist eliminates joint flexibility from the hypothesis list and assesses functional muscle strength to see if that is a contributing factor. If the shoulder muscles are weak, the therapist identifies shoulder weakness as one contributing factor. Of course, in most cases, there will be a blend of several physical, social, or emotional factors that contribute to performance.

Collaboratively Create Goals with Clients

Once the occupational therapy evaluation is complete and the client's occupational performance is understood, the therapist must reexplore the client's stated priorities and life situation. The first step is to review the occupational therapy evaluation with clients and any important caregivers. Feasible intervention goals and activities are described at that time. For therapy to be most effective, clients and the significant people in their lives must own the plan. To do this, they must both understand and value the intervention goals and recommendations. Therapists must actively seek their clients' perspective and listen carefully to design effective interventions.

FACTORS AFFECTING EVALUATION

Client evaluation, like all of occupational therapy, is shaped by the practice arena or setting in which it occurs. In some settings, such as an early intervention program, therapists may perform numerous assessments to provide a comprehensive summary for long-term intervention. Alternatively, therapists in an acute care psychiatric setting may be able to screen only areas of primary concern and use that information to recommend continued evaluation and

RESEARCH NOTE 22–1

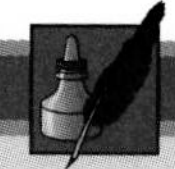

The Practice Claims of the Profession Must Be Verified by Research

KENNETH J. OTTENBACHER

One of the complex challenges facing the field of occupational therapy is to integrate the methods of evidence-based health care into occupational therapy practice and education to establish evidence-based occupational therapy. Evidence-based health care, sometimes referred to as evidence-based practice (EBP), was defined by Sackett, Richardson, Rosenberg, and Haynes (1997) as "the conscientious and judicious use of current best evidence from clinical care research in the management of individual patients." A total of 12 evidence-based practice centers have been established in the United States, with funding from the Agency for Health Research and Quality (formerly the Agency for Health Care Policy Research) in the Department of Health and Human Services. These centers are responsible for collecting evidence and developing guidelines for evidence-based practice for specific medical conditions and disorders, including heart disease, breast cancer, and stroke.

In her Eleanor Clarke Slagle lecture, Holm (2000) raised the challenge of creating evidence-based occupational therapy to clinicians, educators, and researchers. To achieve this goal, we must first ask some basic questions. Where do the data for evidence-based occupational therapy come from? And who is responsible for generating, collecting, and interpreting these data? Systematic evaluation and goal setting involving the client, family members, and other professionals are the first steps in establishing evidence-based occupational therapy.

Holm, M. B. (2000). Our mandate for the new millennium: Evidence-based practice. [Eleanor Clarke Slagle Lecture]. *American Journal of Occupational Therapy, 54,* 575–585.

Sackett, D. L., Richardson, W. S., Rosenberg, W., & Haynes, R. B. (Eds.). (1997). *Evidence-based medicine: How to practice and teach EBM.* New York: Churchill Livingstone.

intervention in another setting. Furthermore, the client's ability to communicate occupational concerns may improve as the therapeutic relationship is developed. For instance, someone with an acute hand injury may be mostly concerned with pain relief and protection of the hand. Once those short-term concerns are addressed, the client may be able to attend to the larger occupational implications of the hand injury. Finally, when services are provided to populations, therapists must use assessments that are likely to achieve the greatest yield across a variety of individuals. In all cases, the client's concerns and priorities serve to frame the therapist's decisions in the evaluation process.

ONGOING EVALUATIONS

In some settings, ongoing evaluations are conducted formally at set intervals determined by the policies of the setting and the requirements of payers. In other settings, ongoing evaluations are done informally as part of the intervention. Practitioners document occupational performance throughout intervention, modifying intervention as appropriate. The purposes of an ongoing evaluation are to (1) assess the client's progress since the last evaluation, (2) reassess the client's priorities for intervention, (3) update the client's potential postintervention situation, (4) revise the statements of about potential performance problems or capacities, and (5) revise intervention goals to reflect the client's priorities given any changes since the last evaluation.

OUTCOME EVALUATIONS

Outcome evaluations are generally conducted shortly before a client is ready to complete occupational therapy and are used to determine the client's ability to perform desired occupations. The steps of the outcome evaluation are the same as those for the initial evaluation, except that the preliminary information includes the record of the client's progress in occupational therapy. The purposes of an occupational therapy outcome evaluation are to (1) assess client progress since the initial evaluation, (2) document the status of the client's occupational performance and the factors supporting and inhibiting performance, (3) document recommendations for facilitating occupational performance, (4) document recommendations for any needed continued services, and (5) document effectiveness of occupational therapy to address the client's ability to engage in meaningful occupation.

CONCLUSION

Although the occupational therapy evaluation process was presented in a linear manner in this chapter, in practice,

the process is recursive and dynamic. The practitioner and client are continuously modifying and revising initial hypotheses. The ultimate purpose of the evaluation is to understand the client as an occupational being, thus supporting the design and implementation of successful intervention.

SECTION II

The Interview Process in Occupational Therapy

ALEXIS D. HENRY

After reviewing the preliminary information about a client, interviewing is the first step in conducting a client-centered evaluation and developing an occupational profile (AOTA, in press). Interviewing is an essential skill for one of the most common assessment procedures used by occupational therapy practitioners. The goals of interviewing are both product and process. Beyond gathering information (product), interviews are useful because they help develop a therapeutic alliance with the client (process).

WHAT IS INTERVIEWING?

Interviewing has been defined as a shared verbal experience, jointly constructed by the interviewer and the interviewee, organized around the asking and answering of questions (Mishler, 1986). Although your job as the interviewer is primarily to ask the questions and the client's job as the interviewee is primarily to answer, effective interviewing does not proceed in a stilted, stimulus–response manner. Rather, you and the client are attempting to achieve some shared understanding of a particular reality. That reality is the client's story.

When you first meet a client, the information that you are most likely to have is a label that identifies the client as having a particular type of problem. Most often, this label takes the form of a diagnosis; for example, the client may have a diagnosis of schizophrenia, arthritis, or a learning disability. The diagnosis is likely to lead you to make certain assumptions about the occupational performance problems the client might have, based on either your past experience with other individuals with that same diagnosis or your textbook knowledge of the diagnostic condition. In reality, information such as a client's diagnosis has limited usefulness in influencing the course of intervention. To develop a meaningful intervention plan, you must know the particulars of the client's situation—and you need to know them from the client's perspective. In other words, you need to understand the client's story (Fig. 22-2).

When a practitioner considers how the client's present situation fits into the client's larger life story, the practitioner is thinking narratively about the client (Clark, 1993: Frank, 1996; Helfrich & Kielhofner, 1994; Mattingly, 1991; Mattingly & Fleming, 1994). A narrative or life story approach involves considering the particular set of circumstances that describe the clients' life before they came for intervention, how clients view their life now, and where clients see their life going after intervention. When thinking narratively, the practitioner strives to understand clients' values and motives to make interventions meaningful.

Interviews are strategies that can help you think about clients in narrative terms. The client's story, goals,

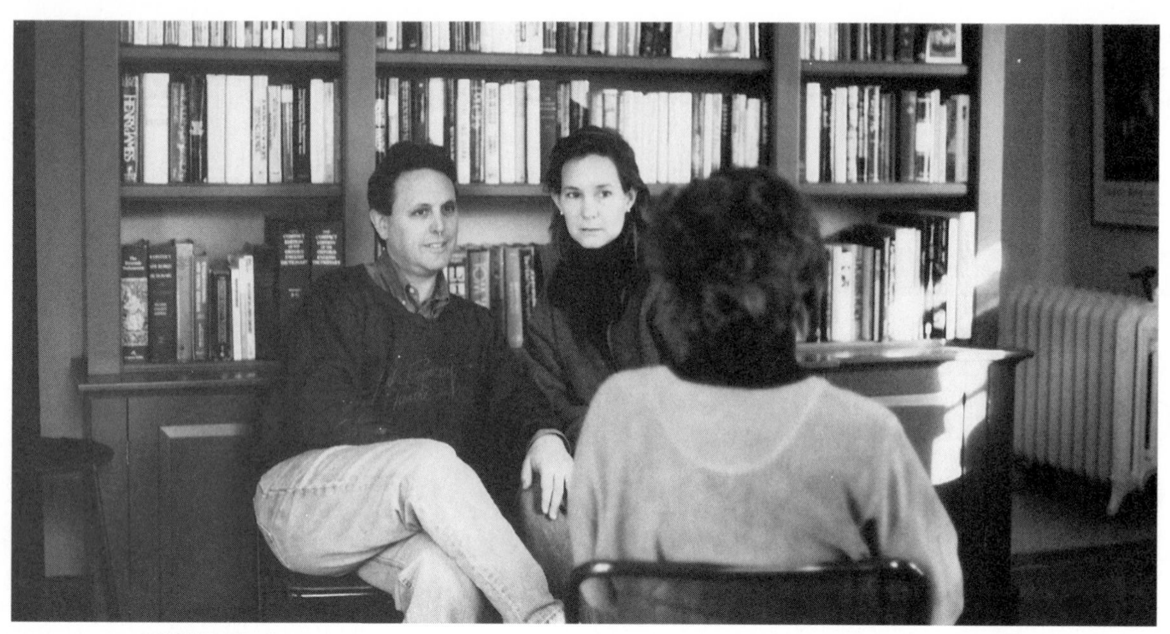

FIGURE 22–2. An occupational therapist interviewing parents about their 4-year-old child.

concerns, and aspirations are essential for determining the course of intervention. When there is a mismatch between your perception and the client's perception of what is needed, intervention is likely to become stalled (Mattingly, 1991). A shared perception of what is needed can best be achieved through a dialogue between you and the client.

Interviews are structured strategies for engaging the client in a dialogue, although interviews function best when they proceed as a normal conversation, rather than as a formal question-and-answer session. The interview should always take place at the beginning of the intervention process and has the important goal of gathering specific information about the client. In this way, an interview is one of many of procedures that might be used in a comprehensive evaluation of a client. However, because it is an interaction between you and the client, an interview is also an intervention that can have therapeutic value in its own right. In the context of an interview, you and the client together can begin to construct a new life story for the client (Mattingly & Fleming, 1994).

WHEN AND WHOM TO INTERVIEW

The Initial Interview: Interview as Assessment

Because interviewing is an integral part of a comprehensive evaluation of a client's occupational functioning, it most frequently occurs at the beginning of your work with a client. In my own practice, an interview is almost always my first significant interaction with a new client. Before administering any other assessment, I sit down with a client to talk. During that initial interaction, I have two primary goals. The first is to begin to understand the client's story. Who is this person? What brought him or her here? Where does the client hope to go after intervention? The answers to these questions shape the suggestions that I make for the work we can do together in the time we have. The second, but not unrelated, goal is to begin to form a collaborative relationship with the client. These and other goals of interviewing are discussed later in this section.

During the Course of Therapy: Interview as Intervention

Although interviewing is virtually always done at the beginning of an intervention process, the beginning is not the only time an interview may be appropriate. An interview that occurs after your work with a client has begun can be both a form of reevaluation and an intervention. Such interviews are usually less structured than the data-gathering process used during the formal initial evaluation phase. This more informal kind of interaction can involve you and the client reviewing what has happened thus far and anticipating and planning for the future. This discussion can help the client construct an image of a future self who is able to do more than he or she can do now. Such images are important in making the intervention something the client can commit to and invest in (Helfrich & Kielhofner, 1994; Polkinghorne, 1996). In addition, reviewing you work together can be a useful strategy when you seem to be at a stuck point, when it seems that the intervention is not progressing. Together, you and the client can ask, "Why is this not working?" and "What can we do to make things better?" In these ways, interviewing is a collaborative tool that is used repeatedly throughout the intervention process.

Interviewing Older Adolescents and Adults

Most older adolescents and adults that you encounter in practice are appropriate candidates for interviewing. The techniques for interviewing that are discussed later in this section apply, for the most part, to interviewing individuals of these ages. However, some clients are not appropriate candidates for interviews or should be interviewed only in highly structured situations. For example, individuals with severe depression may have difficulty concentrating on and responding to interview questions; people with mania may be too distracted by external stimuli to attend to an interview. Clients with psychosis may have such disorganized thinking that their answers to questions are difficult to understand. People with expressive or receptive language deficits (e.g., aphasia) either may not comprehend questions or may not be able to respond even if they understand. If an interview is approached as a conversation, a time when you and the client are going to talk, rather than as a formal evaluation of the client, then either continuing or discontinuing the interview (if that seems necessary) can be done without making the client feel as if he or she had failed the evaluation.

Interviewing Children and Younger Adolescents

Although pediatrics is one of the largest practice areas in occupational therapy, until recently there were virtually no interview procedures developed to gather data on children's occupational behavior directly from children, and there was only one interview developed for use with adolescents (Black, 1976). Some advances have been made in developing interview and other self-report procedures for use with children; some of these procedures are discussed later in this chapter.

Children pose a unique challenge for the interviewer. The ability of children to describe their experiences and their feelings depends on their acquisition of the requisite cognitive, linguistic, and social skills (Stone & Lemanek, 1990). Before the age of 7 or 8, most children describe themselves only in terms of observable characteristics and behaviors and make differentiations between themselves and others on the basis of these observable traits, rather than on internal states. For example, a young child may be able to describe herself in terms of physical attributes (e.g., "I have blue eyes"), possessions (e.g., "I have a cat"), or preferred activities (e.g., "I like to ride my bike"). However, these notions about the self are not integrated into a global self-concept (Stone & Lemanek, 1990). In addition, young children may have difficulty labeling or verbally communicating their subjective emotional state (LaGreca, 1990). Young children also have difficulty relating events in a temporal order, especially if the events happened in the (relatively) distant past.

At around age 8, children acquire a more global sense of the self. After this age, children are better able to report on their thoughts and feelings and to provide more accurate information on diverse experiences and situations. During adolescence, the capacity for self-reflection increases further. Adolescents have the capacity to describe themselves in abstract psychological and interpersonal terms, rather than the concrete, physical terms used by younger children. In addition, adolescents begin to evaluate their own thoughts and behaviors critically and to analyze others' reactions to their behavior (Stone & Lemanek, 1990). Thus as self-awareness increases, older children and younger adolescents are able to respond to interview questions with increasing sophistication. However, the increased use of social comparisons and greater psychological awareness that come as children age may contribute to a tendency to respond to interview questions in a socially desirable manner (Stone & Lemanek, 1990).

Other factors may influence the way in which children and adolescents respond during interview situations. One of the most important to consider is the inherent power imbalance in the relationship between a child and an adult interviewer (Cohn, 1994). Adults, generally, have greater social power than children; children are, for the most part, socialized to respond to adults in ways they think adults want to hear. Because of the power imbalance, whether real or merely perceived, children may unintentionally fabricate answers to questions to please an adult interviewer (Cohn, 1994).

Establishing rapport and a sense of trust are critical to the successful interview. Engaging a child in a play activity or a discussion about a favorite book or movie before the interview can help establish rapport. Honest communication with adolescents about the reasons for the interview and the confidential nature of the interview can help instill trust. Age-appropriate communication is another key to a successful interview. With young children, the use of simple vocabulary, short sentences, and concrete, direct questions (e.g., "What do you do during school?") are recommended (Cohn, 1994). Adolescents can usually answer more open-ended questions (e.g., "Tell me about how school has been going for you.").

Finally, the process of gathering information concerning children's occupations should involve other people in the child's environment, including parents and teachers (LaGreca, 1990). Because children are under the social control of others, their behavior in one environment may not be the same as their behavior in another environment. Thus it is important to gather information from the multiple contexts within which the child functions. Moreover, because others refer children for intervention, usually a parent, it is important to understand and respect the perspective of those who may be distressed by the child's behavior (LaGreca, 1990).

HISTORICAL NOTE 22–1

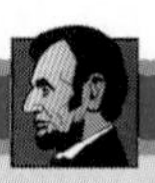

Ruggles's Work with People as Part of the Evaluation

SUZANNE M. PELOQUIN

Ora Ruggles, reconstruction aide, helped many individuals through the use of occupation. One difficult patient at Fort McPherson initially worried her, so she consulted his doctor for more information. She learned that Kilgore was a cowboy whose wartime experience had fueled an anger he suppressed.

Ruggles approached the foreman of the blacksmith shop. She then found Kilgore, showed him a design for spurs, and asked him if he would help her start a metal-working class. Within the hour, Kilgore was busily working in the shop. Years later, he wrote Ruggles about his personal reconstruction, made possible through her having correctly grasped his problems and strengths:

> *I've been doing a lot of thinking lately, Ruggie. It started out last week when some of the boys around town asked me to run for mayor. . . . It makes me realize again, Ruggie, how much I owe you. I wonder what the boys who asked me to run for mayor would think if they knew an army doctor once scribbled on my medical record, "This man is a menace to society." (Carolva & Ruggles, 1946, p. 91)*

Kilgore's gratitude is clear; it speaks to his having been seen not as the personification of a problem but as a person with real strengths. Such an evaluation can spark in many clients the courage that they need for change.

Carlova, J. & Ruggles, O. (1946). *The healing heart.* New York: Messner.

WHY INTERVIEW

Understanding the Client's Story

The single most important reason to interview the client is so that you can better understand how the client sees things. As I discussed, the interview is an opportunity for clients to tell you their story. Mattingly (1991) noted, "a disability is something that interrupts and irreversibly changes a person's life story . . . therapy can be seen as a short story within the patient's longer life story" (p. 1000). During the course of the interview, you are trying to uncover the plot of the client's story. Before the interview, you might have some general information about the client; and through the interview, you try to fill in' the particulars of the story. Thus the main questions should be similar to the following:

- What happened?
- How did this person come to you?
- What was a typical day like before the client came to you?
- What was and is important to this person?
- Where does the client hope to go after he or she leaves you?

Asking and valuing the answers to these questions is what it means to be "client centered" (Law, 1998). The answers individualize and prioritize your intervention with that particular client.

Building the Therapeutic Alliance

Because an interview is an interaction between two persons, a relationship begins to develop during the course of the interview. Through the interview, you want to establish a relationship with the client that will help you together set and attain the goals of intervention. The manner in which you conduct the interview either fosters or inhibits the development of that relationship. As you talk with clients, your ability to communicate a sense of concern and respect for the individual and the information being shared and your ability to be real and genuine in the interaction go a long way to establishing this relationship.

The client has come to you for help. For the client to feel that you are someone who can be of help, a sense of safety, trust, and collaboration must develop between the two (Okun, 1997). An interview can enhance a sense of collaboration between you and the client, because it gives you an opportunity to communicate that you care about what is important to the client. To the extent that you have a collaborative relationship with the client, you will be much more likely to achieve intervention goals (Neistadt, 1995; Tickle-Degnen, 1995).

Gathering Information and Developing the Occupational Profile

Occupational therapy interviews are used to gather information about the client's functioning in occupations. Most interviews consider the client's current or recent functioning; some also take a historical perspective and seek to understand the client's functioning over time. Although the specific questions vary across different interviews, in general, interviews solicit information about clients' daily use of time; past and current role involvement (e.g., worker, student, homemaker, parent); play and leisure participation; and values, goals, and sense of competence relative to occupations. Some interviews include questions about the client's current environment (human and nonhuman), so you can evaluate whether the environment supports or constrains the person's functioning. This information forms the occupational profile (AOTA, in press).

It is important to gather information about the client's past functioning, because it is often one of the best predictors of future functioning. The disability, limitations, and restrictions associated with a particular health condition may predict a client's future to some extent (World Health Organization [WHO], 2001). But the successes a person has had in the past, particularly the recent past, are often resources on which the client can draw. Clients' goals and sense of competence indicate their desire and motivation to return to their prior life.

Observing Behavior

During the course of an interview, you have an opportunity to observe the client's behavior. The client's ability to participate in an interview can reveal much about his or her current functioning. You can make observations about the client's energy level, stamina, affect, comprehension, memory, concentration, thought organization, physical appearance, and interpersonal behavior.

- Is the client able to engage actively through a 45-min interview without fatiguing?
- Does the client appear depressed or elated?
- Does the client's memory seem intact? For example, is the client able to remember the dates of her last five jobs and relate them to you in chronological order?
- Does the person comprehend the questions being asked?
- Is the client able to convey his history in a manner that you can understand and follow?
- Is the person's thinking organized and goal directed or is the client tangential (i.e., does the client seem to get off track)?
- Is the person appropriately dressed and groomed for the situation or does the client appear unkempt?
- Is the person friendly and forthcoming with information or does the client seem angry, hostile, or resistant to being interviewed?

The extent to which the client engages with you during an interview may indicate the extent to which the client will engage in interventions. Of course, if clients appear to be defensive or resistant during the interview, it is important for you to ask yourself if there is something that you are doing to make the client feel defensive.

In my own practice, I make the kinds of behavioral observations described in the foregoing as I interview a client. In doing so, the initial interview serves as a kind of screening procedure that indicates other performance-based assessments that might be appropriate to administer.

Identifying Client Strengths and Potential Problem Areas

As the interview progresses and you begin to achieve a deeper understanding of the person's story and observe the client's behavior, you should begin to formulate an initial sense of the client's strengths or assets as well as problems that might be addressed by occupational therapy interventions. All clients, regardless of disability, bring certain strengths (current competencies, past experiences, and environmental supports and resources) to their work with you. It is important to identify these early on, as the client will be able to draw on these assets over the course of the intervention.

A set of problems will also begin to take shape from the things the client tells you and the things you observe. It is important to remember, however, that this initial idea about the problems is tentative and subject to revision as you and the client begin to work together. Moreover, your perspective of the problems the client faces may not be the same as the client's perspective. You must share your initial impression with the client to confirm the extent to which you are seeing things in the same way. This involves restating what you have perceived as the client's major concerns and sharing your impressions and observations during the interview regarding the client's strengths and potential problems. By engaging in mutual problem setting, you set the groundwork for a client-centered, collaborative relationship. Toward the end of the interview, you might say to the client, "Well, from what you've told me, it sounds like you are concerned about . . ., and it seems to me that you are also having some difficulty with . . ." The goal is for both of you to arrive at an agreement about the problems the client faces.

Clarifying Your Role in the Setting

You can also use the end of an interview to elaborate on and clarify your role in the setting and the work you and the client may do together. Do not be surprised if the client does not know what occupational therapists do. At this point, you can explain what services occupational therapy offers, what options might be available to the client, whether you and other providers (e.g., physical therapist, nurse, or social worker) might be working with the client together or whether the client might be referred to another provider for a service not offered by occupational therapy. This is the time to make initial recommendations about the possible interventions.

Establishing Priorities for Intervention

Once you and the client agree on the work to be done, you have explained your role and the services that occupational therapy can offer, and have made some initial recommendations for intervention, then you and the client can work collaboratively to establish intervention priorities. Being client centered means that the client's priorities should be your priorities; however, it is important to recognize other factors that can influence the recommendations you make. For example, you might be influenced by the services most easily provided in your setting, your own interests and competencies, or funding and reimbursement. The client's goals and priorities are central in determining the course of intervention. Engaging the client in goal setting and prioritizing is a good way to finish up an interview.

HOW TO INTERVIEW

It may seem that interviewing should come naturally; after all, you talk to people every day. But, in fact, much of our day-to-day communication with other people is quite superficial. When you conduct an interview with a client, you are engaging in a dialogue with the express purpose of trying to understand that person so that you can be helpful (Okun, 1997). Thus *therapeutic communication* differs from day-to-day conversation in fundamental ways. Developing communication skills needed to become an effective interviewer takes time and experience. The skills of effective interviewing and ways to structure a therapeutic interview are discussed below.

The Skills of Effective Interviewing

Preparing

Preparing for the interview is an important first step. Before conducting an interview, you should prepare yourself, the client, and the environment. In preparing yourself, you should have some notion of the questions you want to ask. Several occupational therapy interview procedures have been published in recent years (discussed below). I strongly recommend using one of the existing interview procedures, rather than developing your own, because these methods have generally been examined in terms of reliability and validity.

If you are a novice interviewer, you should practice before interviewing your first client. Observing experienced interviewers and noting how they structure the interview, asking questions, and responding to information the client shares are good ways to begin to develop a sense of how an interview flows. You might also practice administering the interview to a colleague or supervisor and ask that person to give you feedback. Videotaping and critiquing your practice interviews is another useful way to hone your interviewing skills.

Before conducting an interview with a client, you should read the available preliminary information on the client. This information may give you some initial ideas about areas to focus on during the interview. Moreover, information about the client's diagnosis or presenting problem will give you an idea of how actively the client can participate in the interview—whether he or she might tolerate only a short interview or might not be ready for an interview at this time. Nursing staff or others in close contact with the client might have useful information how the client is doing that day.

In addition to preparing yourself, you should prepare the client for the interview. I rarely approach a person whom I have never met before and ask if I can interview him or her on the spot. Rather, I approach a client, introduce myself, and briefly explain my role in the setting. Then I will ask permission to do the interview, telling him or her briefly about the content and purpose of the interview, and schedule an appointment. Scheduling an appointment (even if just for later that same day) gives the client a degree of control; the client has some choice about when he or she will see you. Some times of the day are better than others for many persons. For example, many people with depression feel worse in the morning and experience improvements in their mood and energy level as the day progresses. By allowing clients to have some degree of control in a situation in which they may feel out of control, you help set the tone for a collaborative relationship.

Finally, you need to pay some attention to the environment in which you will conduct the interview. Obviously, a private space is the most desirable. Some of the questions you will be asking are highly personal, and a private space will make you both feel more comfortable. You should not make assumptions about which questions are personal for a particular client. It is common to see a client display an emotional response to a particular question that the therapist thought was neutral. Chairs should be an appropriate distance apart (3 or 4 feet). The room should be at a temperature that is comfortable for both of you and should be well lighted. Have tissues and water available. If it is not possible to have a private space, then create some sense of privacy in a more open space by arranging the chairs in a corner of the room. If possible, I prefer not to interview a client when he or she is in bed.

Questioning

Interviewing involves the asking of questions. The way you pose those questions influences the quality and amount of information you can obtain and thus the level of understanding of the client's story you can achieve. How you ask questions also influences how you are perceived by the client and affects the development of your relationship with the client. In general, open-ended questions encourage clients to tell their story and are more likely to yield meaningful information than are closed questions that require only yes or no answers or very brief responses. For example, the question "Do you like your job?" can be answered yes or no. However, the statement "Tell me what you liked about your job" will likely result in a more elaborated response by the client. In addition, the use of probes and follow-up questions (e.g., "Tell me more about that") encourages the client to relate his or her story. During the course of an interview, it is likely that you will ask two types of questions: Those that are factual or descriptive (e.g., "What do you do for work?") and those that are intended to elicit more narrative data. Narrative questions yield data on events in the client's life and his or her perceptions and motives concerning those events (e.g., "Tell me about a time when work was going very well for you."). Kielhofner and Mallinson (1995) suggested that effective interviewing involves a weaving of these two ways of questioning. There may be certain clients for whom a more structured, factual approach to questioning is appropriate. For example, a client whose thinking is disorganized may have difficulty answering more open-ended or narrative questions in a coherent manner but may be able to respond to a more structured question, such as "Where do you live?" It will usually be apparent when you need to use a more structured approach to the interview.

During the interview, you want to be conscious of whether the questions you are asking are making the client anxious or uncomfortable. Your intention is to put the client at ease. To do this, it is best if your questions are open, clear, singular (i.e., you ask only one question at a time) nonjudgmental, and encourage the client to tell his or her story. You want to avoid putting the client on the defensive. Sometimes, questions that begin with the word *why* (e.g., "Why did you do that?") have the unintended effect of making clients feel that they owe you an explanation about their feelings or behavior (Okun, 1997). Particularly during the initial interview, it is more useful to assume a neutral, nonjudgmental stance (Bradburn, 1992).

Responding

An interview needs to be more than a series of questions on your part, interspersed with answers from the client. You must respond to the information that the client is sharing with you. There are many ways of doing this. Often, because of a desire to help, the therapist's impulse is to respond with advice or suggestions. However, particularly during an initial interview, you want to resist this impulse, at least until you have come to the end of the interview. Before that, it is doubtful that you will have sufficient information on which to base advice. But, even though you want to resist giving advice until you have achieved some understanding of the client's story, you still need to respond.

During the course of the interview, your responses should primarily be attempts to paraphrase what the client has just said. **Paraphrasing** is more than just repeating what the client has said. It involves trying to capture the essence of what the client said and restating it in your own words to communicate your desire to understand (Denton, 1987). Paraphrasing helps you communicate to clients that you have listened to, heard, understood, and valued the information being shared with you. Paraphrasing also allows you to confirm that you have, in fact, clearly understood the client.

There are two general types of responses that you can use during an interview: **content responses** and **affective responses.** Content responses are used when you want to clarify the facts or communicate that you have understood what the client means. A content response might begin like this: "So, you're saying that . . ." Content responses clarify information and meaning. Affective responses are used when you want to reflect the underlying effect or feeling tone that the client is communicating. An affective response might begin like this: "It seems like you're feeling . . ." or "In that situation, I might have felt . . ." An affective response should be phrased somewhat tentatively until you have confirmed that the client actually feels that way. Affective responses communicate that you are trying to understand and are concerned about how the client feels.

Attending and Observing

Attending involves the use of both nonverbal and verbal behaviors that help communicate your interest in the client and can facilitate the development of therapeutic rapport. Nonverbal behaviors include positions and movements of the face and body as well as qualities of the voice, such as tone, intensity, and speed (Tickle-Degnen, 1995). Having your chair and the client's chair either facing each other or slightly angled, about 3 feet apart, allows you to see the client fully and the client to see you. You can communicate your interest in the client by making frequent eye contact. Other nonverbal behaviors that communicate interest include head nodding, smiling, and leaning forward.

Verbal behaviors, such as saying "uh-huh," "humm," "yes," and "go on," let the client know that you are listening and encourage the client to continue with his or her story. Tickle-Degnen (1995) noted that tone of voice is an important attribute to attend to. A cheerful tone of voice is not always the most appropriate to use. Rather, a tone of voice that is genuine and conveys concern about the client may be more effective. Effective interviewers often accommodate their bodies, movements, and tone of voice to be in sync with the client's (Bradburn, 1992; Tickle-Degnen, 1995).

Attending also involves observing how the client seems to be feeling as the interview progresses. Does the client seem to be fatiguing? Does the interview content seem to be emotionally difficult for the client? If you sense that the client is finding the interview difficult, you should verify this. For example, questions such as "How are you doing?" and "Are you getting tired?" communicate that you are concerned about the client. A common side effect of psychiatric medications is dry mouth; offering a glass of water is another way of showing that you are attending. Observing also involves noting the client's behavior as the interview progresses.

Listening

Finally, although it seems obvious to say so, throughout the interview, you need to listen to the client. Listening effectively allows you to respond effectively. Paying close attention to both the content and the underlying feeling or affect takes energy. Listening is more difficult than it sounds, because there are many distractions to effective listening. There can be external distractions, such as activity in the environment, or internal distractions, such as your thoughts about a meeting you just came from or your next client. Even when your attention is focused on the client, there can be distractions. Denton (1987) identified blocks to effective listening: thinking about the person, thinking for the person, and thinking ahead of the person.

Thinking about the person involves making judgments about the client's lifestyle, morals, and motives; such judgments can create distance between you and the client and interfere with your being able to understand the client's perspective. When you think for the client, you prematurely think about solutions to his or her problems. Because one aim of the interview is to facilitate a collaborative relationship with the client, prematurely offering solutions diminishes the client's role in the relationship and can reinforce the client's sense of helplessness. Thinking ahead of the person involves rushing the client through his or her story just to get the facts. This can happen when you feel you already know the story, when the client is relating too many or seemingly irrelevant details, or when you feel pressed for time (Denton, 1987). The reality is that you never already know the story; each person's story is unique. However, if the client is giving you more detail than you need at the moment and you begin to run out of time, you can respectfully redirect the client by saying something like, "I can hear that this topic is very important to you. Perhaps we should set another time to really talk about this. Right now, I need to ask you some questions about something else."

Finally, particularly if you are a novice interviewer, you can be distracted from listening because you are thinking about what you should say next. If you are thinking about what you should say next then you are not listening to the client. "Effective listening occurs only when you are paying attention to your patient instead of yourself" (Denton, 1987, p. 13). One way to improve your listening skills is to learn to use silence effectively. Most of us feel uncomfortable with silence and feel a need to fill a silent space as soon as it occurs. However, if you can feel comfortable taking a brief silent pause to think about what the client has just said and about what you might say next, then you will not need to prepare your next question while the client is talking. You can even say to the client, "I'm just taking a moment to think about what you've said." Rarely will you need more than 10 sec to do this.

Structuring the Interview

Regardless of the type of interview you use, there are three phases to an interview: the opening, the body , and the closure (Denton, 1987).

Opening

At the opening of the interview, you let the client know the purpose of the interview. Even though you probably did so when you made the appointment for the interview, you might want to reintroduce yourself, to say again that you are an occupational therapist, and to describe briefly your role in the setting. You should then explain the purpose of the interview and the types of questions that you will be asking.

Body

The body is the exploration and development phase of the interview, the time when you and the client are actively constructing the client's story. Although specific interview procedures often provide a recommended sequence of questions, it is good idea to enter into this phase of the interview with relatively general and neutral questions that allow you to begin to sketch the background of the story. Because I am interested in clients' occupations, I often begin by asking clients to tell me how they spend their time on a typical day. Such a broad question tends to be nonthreatening but allows me to begin to develop a picture of the clients' roles. Subsequent questions serve to fill in the details. Some clients are forthcoming and are able to relate their stories easily; others need much support and structure. It is during this phase that you will call on your skills in listening, attending, responding, and questioning.

Closure

Toward the end of the interview, you will need to begin to put closure on the session. It is important not to end the interview abruptly. Make sure that you allow sufficient time to summarize information, identify important themes in the client's story, and address how you and the client will work together. This will often be the time that you and the client mutually begin to set goals for intervention. As the interview comes to an end, you should let the client know what the next steps will be and when you will see him or her again. You might set a time for your next appointment. You should also thank the client for sharing his or her story with you.

OCCUPATIONAL THERAPY INTERVIEWS

Since the 1980s, a variety of interview procedures have been developed for use with both children and adults. The interview procedures reviewed next provide methods of collecting information directly from the intended service recipient or client. There are also interview procedures that allow you to collect data from other informants, usually caregivers or parents. For example, the Play History collects information on a child's participation in play from a parent (Behnke & Fetkovich, 1984; Parks, Oakley, & Fonseca, 1998). Interviews that collect data from informants other than the intended service recipient are not described here, but are reviewed elsewhere in this book. All of the interviews reviewed in this chapter can assist you in developing an occupational profile of clients, and all have demonstrated at least preliminary evidence of reliability and validity.

Interviews for Use with Children and Adolescents

The School Setting Interview

The School Setting Interview (SSI) is a collaborative interview that allows children and adolescents with disabilities (including physical, developmental, and emotional/behavioral) to describe the impact of the environment on their functioning in multiple school settings (e.g., classroom, playground, gymnasium, corridors) and to identify any needs for accommodations (Hoffman, Hemmingsson, & Kielhofner, 2000). Appropriate for students from about age 9 through high school, the SSI requires about 40 min to administer. The SSI was originally developed in Sweden and has been translated into English. Initial studies indicate that the SSI has good test–retest reliability, is useful for identifying students' unmet needs for school environment accommodations, and can be used to examine student–environment fit in school settings (Hemmingsson & Borrell, 1996, 2000).

Adolescent Role Assessment

The Adolescent Role Assessment (ARA) is the only occupational therapy interview specifically targeted for adolescents (Black, 1976). The ARA is a semistructured interview procedure that gathers information on the adolescent's occupational role involvement over time and across domains. The 21 questions of the ARA cover six areas: childhood play, socialization within the family, school functioning, socialization with peers, occupational choice, and anticipated adult work. The ARA has been found to have acceptable test–retest reliability, and scores on the ARA are able to discriminate between psychiatrically hospitalized adolescents and nonhospitalized adolescents (Black, 1982). The general content of the ARA appears to yield useful information on an adolescent's functioning in occupations; however, some questions may be dated. Given the paucity of interview procedures specifically targeted for adolescents, further development and refinement of the ARA and similar interviews should be a priority.

Interviews for Use with Adolescents and Adults

The Occupational Circumstances Assessment—Interview Rating Scale

The new version of the Occupational Circumstances Assessment—Interview Rating Scale (OCAIRS), by Haglund, Henriksson, Crisp, Fredhiem, and Kielhofner (2001), represents a revision of the original OCAIRS developed by Kaplan and Kielhofner (1989). The OCAIRS provides a method for gathering data on a client's occupational adaptation. It includes a semistructured interview and a 21-item rating scale. The items cover the client's personal causation, values and goals, interests, roles, habits, skills, previous experiences, physical and social environments, and overall occupational participation and adaptation. The OCAIRS can be used with adolescent and adult clients who have a variety of disabilities; it takes about 1 hour to administer and rate.

Much of the work on the revised version of the OCAIRS has been done in Sweden, and there is a translated version. Studies have shown the revised OCIARS to have acceptable internal consistency and excellent interrater reliability (Haglund, Thorell, & Walinder, 1998a; Lai, Haglund, & Kielhofner, 1999). OCAIRS scores are able to discriminate between clients who need occupational therapy intervention and those who do not and between those with different severities of psychiatric disorders (Haglund et al., 1998a, 1998b).

The Occupational Performance History Interview—Second Version

The Occupational Performance History Interview—Second Version (OPHI-II) is a historical interview that gathers information about a client's occupational adaptation over time and can be used with adolescents and adults in a variety of settings (Kielhofner et al., 1997). The OPHI-II is a recent revision of the original OPHI (Kielhofner, Henry, & Walens, 1989). It consists of three parts: a semistructured interview concerning the client's occupational life history, three rating scales, and a life history narrative. The flexible interview format is designed to gather information in five thematic areas (activity/occupational choices, critical life events, daily routines, occupational roles, and occupational behavior settings). The three ratings scales provide a measure of the client's interests, values, and confidence; the client's ability to sustain satisfying occupational participation; and the impact of the environment on the client's occupational life. The life history narrative provides a qualitative description of the client's history. The OPHI-II can be administered in about 1 hour.

The validity of the original OPHI was examined in studies of individuals with physical and psychiatric disabilities (Henry, 1994; Lynch & Bridle, 1993; Mauras-Nelson & Oakley, 1996). A recent international study of the OPHI-II (using six different language versions) provided evidence of the internal consistency and construct validity of its three rating scales (Kielhofner, Mallinson, Forsyth, & Lai, 2001).

The Worker Role Interview

The Worker Role Interview (WRI) is a semistructured interview that gathers data on psychosocial and environmental factors related to work. It is appropriate to use with any individual whose disability has had an impact on his or her participation in work (Handelsman, 1994; Velozo, Kielhofner, & Fisher, 1998). The WRI is composed of a set of 28 recommended questions and an accompanying 17-item rating scale; it was developed to be compatible with the Model of Human Occupation. The items form six subscales that reflect the worker's sense of personal causation, values, interests, roles, and habits related to work as well as the influence of the environment. Studies indicate that the WRI has good inter-rater and test–retest reliability and demonstrates evidence of internal consistency and construct validity (Biernacki, 1993; Velozo et al., 1999).

The Work Environment Impact Scale

The Work Environment Impact Scale (WEIS) is a semi-structured interview and rating scale designed to examine how individuals with disabilities experience the work environment (Corner, Kielhofner, & Olson, 1998). The WEIS is intended for use with individuals who are currently working or are actively anticipating returning to a specific job or type of work. The WEIS asks questions regarding work environment factors such as space, social supports, temporal demands, objects used, and job functions. The scale items reflect the extent to which environmental factors affect performance; satisfaction; and the physical, social, and emotional well-being of the worker. Studies of the WEIS provide evidence of its construct validity and internal consistency (Corner, Kielhofner, & Lin, 1997; Kielhofner, Lai, Olson, Haglund, Ekbadh, & Edlund, 1999).

The Canadian Occupational Performance Measure

The Canadian Occupational Performance Measure (COPM) is a client-centered semistructured interview procedure designed to measure clients' perceptions of their occupational performance over time (Law, Baptiste, McColl, Opzoomer, Polatajko, & Pollock, 1998). During the initial evaluation, the therapist interviews clients about their functioning in the areas of self-care, productivity, and leisure. Clients are asked to identify any activities that are difficult for them to do in each area and to indicate how important it is for them to be able to do those activities. Finally, clients are asked to identify their five most important problems and to rate their performance and level of satisfaction in those activities. The importance of the activity to the client, the quality of the client's performance, and the client's level of satisfaction are all rated by the client using similar 10-point scales. The specific focus of the COPM on client-identified problems is intended to facilitate collaborative goal setting between the therapist and client. The COPM can also be used for reevaluation and to detect changes in the client's perceptions over time; thus it has utility as an outcome measure.

Across multiple studies, the COPM has been shown to have good test–retest reliability (Law et al., 1998). Other studies have provided evidence of concurrent and construct validity of the COPM (Carpenter, Baker, & Tyldesley, 2001; McColl, Paterson, Davies, Doubt, & Law, 2000). Studies using the COPM as an outcome measure indicate that it is sensitive to change following rehabilitation interventions (Bodiam, 1999; Carpenter et al., 2001).

ADJUNCTS TO INTERVIEWS: PAPER-AND-PENCIL SELF-REPORT MEASURES

In addition to interviewing, paper-and-pencil self-report measures can be useful for obtaining information from clients. Self-report measures include surveys, forms, and checklists that the client completes. Sometimes, the client can complete a form or checklist on his or her own, making this a convenient way to obtain information. More often, however, you should be present when the client completes the measure to ensure that he or she comprehends what is being asked and is responding appropriately. Just as with interviews, self-report measures may not be appropriate for all clients.

In practice, self-report measures should not be used as substitutes for face-to-face interviews with the client. They can be a helpful adjunct, however, because they tend to gather detailed information on a specific topic, such as time use or interest patterns. They are most useful when administered in conjunction with an interview. Once a client has completed a self-report measure, he or she and the therapist should review the form together. Self-report measures help focus the discussion around a particular topic or issue.

Self-Report Measures for Children and Adolescents

The Pediatric Interest Profiles

The Pediatric Interest Profiles (PIPs) are paper-and-pencil surveys of play and leisure interests designed to be used with children and adolescents (Henry, 2000). The three versions of include the Kid Play Profile (KPP), for children aged 6 to 9; the Preteen Play Profile (PPP), for children aged 9 to 12; and the Adolescent Leisure Interest Profile (ALIP), for adolescents aged 12 to 21. Each version asks the youth to report his or her interest and/or participation in a variety of age-appropriate leisure activities and to indicate his or her feelings of enjoyment and competence in the activities. The PIPs also ask whether the youth does the activities alone or with others. The kid and preteen versions use pictorial representations of play activities.

Total scores for the three versions of the PIPs have acceptable test–retest reliability (Henry, 2000). In addition, scores on the ALIP have been found to discriminate between adolescents with and without disabilities (Henry, 1998).

Children's Assessment of Participation and Enjoyment and the Preferences for Activities of Children

The Children's Assessment of Participation and Enjoyment (CAPE) is a two-part self-report measure that gathers information on children's participation in everyday activities outside of mandated school activities (King, Law, King, et al., 2001). The CAPE is intended for children aged 6 and up. In phase 1, the child (or child and parent) indicates how often he or she has done a variety of activities in the previous 4 months. In phase 2, a practitioner interviews the child about the activities in which the child participates, focusing on enjoyment in the activities and where and with whom the activities are done. Like the PIPs, activity items are represented pictorially. A preliminary study indicates that the CAPE has good test–retest reliability.

The Preferences for Activities of Children (PAC) examines a child's preferences for activities (CanChild Centre for Childhood Disability Research [CanChild], 2001). The child sorts 50 activity cards, indicating whether he or she would "really," "sort of," or "not" like to do each activity.

The PAC and the CAPE can be used together or separately. Examination of the reliability and validity of the CAPE is underway. Both measures are undergoing addition development.

Self-Report Measures for Adults

Interest Checklists

Interest checklists are among the most commonly used self-report measures. Interest checklists are used to tap a client's level of interest in a range of activities, most often leisure activities. Age-targeted measures of interest in activities are likely to yield more relevant data than a general measure, because leisure interests vary widely across the age span. Interest checklists are useful for identifying problems related to leisure and for identifying potential activities to use in treatment.

One of the oldest checklists is the Neuro Psychiatric Institute (NPI) interest checklist (Matsutsuyu, 1969). The NPI interest checklist contains 80 activity items, grouped into five categories: activities of daily living, manual skills, cultural and educational activities, physical sports, and social and recreational activities. When completing the checklist, the client indicates strong, casual, or no interest in the activity (Rogers, 1988). The original NPI interest checklist was found to have acceptable test–retest reliability (Weinstein, 1979) and to show evidence of construct and predictive validity (Barris, Kielhofner, Burch, Gelinas, Klement, & Schultz, 1986; Ebb, Coster, & Duncombe, 1989; Henry, 1994). Kielhofner and Neville (1983) modified the NPI interest checklist to include questions concerning changes in activity preferences over time and the desire to participate in interests in the future.

Gregory (1983) described two self-report measures of activity involvement specifically designed for older adults. Total scores on both the Activity Index (which taps activity interest and participation) and the Meaningfulness of Activity Scale (which taps feelings of enjoyment, autonomy, and competence relative to activities) demonstrated good test–retest reliability with small pilot samples. Scores on both measures were also correlated positively with a measure of life satisfaction.

The Role Checklist

The Role Checklist (RC) is a two-part, paper-and-pencil inventory of 10 occupational roles, including worker, student, family member, homemaker, caregiver, volunteer, and hobbyist (Oakley, Kielhofner, Barris, & Reichler, 1986). The first part of the RC examines the client's past, present, and future intentions related to performance of each role. The second part examines the value the client assigns to each role. Studies indicate that the RC has good test–retest reliability (Barris, Oakley, & Kielhofner, 1988), is sensitive to role changes (Hallett, Zasler, Maurer, & Cash, 1994), and discriminates between adults without disabilities and those with psychiatric or physical disabilities (Dickerson, 1999).

Occupational Self-Assessment

The Occupational Self-Assessment (OSA) is a self-report measure designed to gather data on clients' perceptions of their occupational competence (21 items) and the impact of the environment on their functioning (8 items) (Baron, Kielhofner, Iyenger, Goldhammer, & Wolenski, 2001). The OSA also asks clients to indicate the importance of specific areas of functioning and to identify priorities for change, making it particularly useful in conjunction with an interview. The OSA can be used as an initial assessment and as a follow-up or outcome measure that captures client-reported change in functioning. Preliminary international studies indicate that the OSA has acceptable internal consistency and is relevant across different cultures (Iyenger, 2001; Kielhofner & Forsyth, in press).

The Occupational Questionnaire

The Occupational Questionnaire (OQ) is a paper-and-pencil measure that gathers data on time-use patterns and feelings about time use (Smith, Kielhofner, & Watts, 1986). When completing the OQ, clients indicate their main activity during each half hour of a typical day and classify each activity as either school, work, ADL, recreation, or rest. Clients then rate each activity, indicating how well they do the activity, how important the activity is, and how enjoyable the activity is. Studies indicate that the OQ has acceptable test–retest reliability and shows evidence of concurrent and construct validity (Kielhofner & Brinson, 1989; Smith et al., 1986; Smynteck, Barris, & Kielhofner, 1985).

CONCLUSION

In addition to providing information about a client's functioning in specific occupations, interviews are among the most useful strategies available to practitioners both to understand better the client's perspective of his or her situation and to enhance the working relationship with the client. Each of the interviews and self-report measures discussed in this section has its unique characteristics. Practitioners should choose the combination of interview and other assessments that best fits the needs of their clients and setting.

References

American Occupational Therapy Association (In press). Occupational therapy practice framework: Domain and process. *American Journal of Occupational Therapy*.

Barris, R., Kielhofner, G., Burch, R. M., Gelinas, I., Klement, M., & Schultz, B. (1986). Occupational function and dysfunction in three groups of adolescents. *Occupational Therapy Journal of Research, 6*, 301–317.

Barris, R., Oakley, F., & Kielhofner, G. (1988). The Role Checklist. In B. Hemphill (Ed.). *Mental health assessment in occupational therapy. An integrative approach to the evaluation process* (pp. 73–91). Thorofare, NJ: Slack.

Behnke, C. J., & Fetkovich, M. M. (1984). Examining the reliability and validity of the Play History. *American Journal of Occupational Therapy, 38*, 94–100.

Biernacki, S. D. (1993). Reliability of the Worker Role Interview. *American Journal of Occupational Therapy, 47*, 797–803.

Black, M. M. (1976). Adolescent Role Assessment. *American Journal of Occupational Therapy, 30*, 73–79.

Black, M. M. (1982). Adolescent Role Assessment. In B. Hemphill (Ed.). *The evaluative process in psychiatric occupational therapy* (pp. 49–53). Thorofare, NJ: Slack.

Bodiam, C. (1999). The use of the Canadian Occupational Performance Measure for the assessment of outcome on a neurorehabilitation unit. *British Journal of Occupational Therapy, 62*, 123–126.

Bradburn, S. L. (1992). *Psychiatric occupational therapists' strategies for engaging patients in treatment during the initial interview*. Unpublished masters thesis, Tufts University, Medford, MA.

CanChild Centre for Childhood Disability Research [CanChild]. (2001). PAC: Preferences for Activities of Children. Hamilton, ON, Canada: McMaster University: Author.

Carpenter, L., Baker, G. A. & Tyldesley, B. (2001). The use of the Canadian Occupational Performance Measure as an outcome of a pain management program. *Canadian Journal of Occupational Therapy, 68*, 16–22.

Clark, F. (1993). Occupation embedded in real life: Interweaving occupation science and occupational therapy. [Eleanor Clarke Slagle Lecture]. *American Journal of Occupational Therapy, 47*, 1067–1078.

Cohn, E. (1994). *Interviewing children*. Unpublished manuscript, Boston University.

Corner, R. A., Kielhofner, G., & Lin, F.-L. (1997). Construct validity of a work environment impact scale. *Work: A Journal of Prevention, Assessment and Rehabilitation, 9*, 21–34.

Corner, R., Kielhofner, G. & Olson, L. (1998). *Work Environment Impact Scale (WEIS)* (Version 2.0). Chicago: Model of Human Occupation Clearinghouse, Department of Occupational Therapy, University of Illinois.

Coster, W., Deeney, T., Haltiwanger, J., & Haley, S. (1998). *School function assessment*. San Antonio, TX: Psychological Corp.

Denton, P. L. (1987). *Psychiatric occupational therapy: A workbook of practical skills*. Boston: Little, Brown.

Dickerson, A. E. (1999). The Role Checklist. In B. J. Hemphill-Pearson (Ed.). *Assessments in occupational therapy in mental health: An integrative approach* (pp. 175–191). Thorofare, NJ: Slack.

Ebb, E. W., Coster, W., & Duncombe, L. (1989). Comparison of normal and psychosocially dysfunctional male adolescents. *Occupational Therapy in Mental Health, 9*(2), 53–74.

Frank, G. (1996). Life histories in occupational therapy clinical practice. *American Journal of Occupational Therapy, 50*, 251–264.

Gregory, M. (1983). Occupational behavior and life satisfaction among retirees. *American Journal of Occupational Therapy, 37*, 548–552.

Haglund, L., Henriksson, C., Crisp, M., Friedheim L., Kielhofner, G. (2001). *The Occupational Circumstances Assessment—Interview and Rating Scale (OCAIRS)* (Version 2.0). Chicago: Model of Human Occupation Clearinghouse, Department of Occupational Therapy, University of Illinois.

Haglund, L., Thorell, L., & Walinder, J. (1998a). Assessment of occupational functioning for screening of patients to occupational therapy in general psychiatric care. *Occupational Therapy Journal of Research, 4*, 193–206.

Haglund, L., Thorell, L., & Walinder, J. (1998b). Occupational functioning in relation to psychiatric diagnoses: Schizophrenia and mood disorders. *Nordisk Journal of Psychiatry, 52*(3), 223–229.

Hallett, J. D., Zasler, N. D., Maurer, P., & Cash, S. (1994). Role change after traumatic brain injury. *American Journal of Occupational Therapy, 48*, 241–246.

Handelsman, D. (1994). *The construct validity of the Worker Role Interview for the chronic mentally ill*. Unpublished master's thesis, University of Illinois at Chicago.

Helfrich, C., & Kielhofner, G. (1994). Volitional narratives and the meaning of therapy. *American Journal of Occupational Therapy, 48*, 319–326.

Hemmingsson, H., & Borell, L. (1996). The development of an assessment of adjustment needs in the school setting for use with physically disabled students. *Scandinavian Journal of Occupational Therapy, 3*, 156–162.

Hemmingsson, H., & Borell, L. (2000). Accommodation needs and student-environment fit in upper secondary school for students with severe physical disabilities. *Canadian Journal of Occupational Therapy, 67*, 162–173.

Henry, A. D. (1994). *Predicting psychosocial functioning and symptomatic recovery of adolescents and young adults with a first psychotic episode: A six-month follow-up study*. Unpublished doctoral dissertation, Boston University.

Henry, A. D. (1998). Development of a measure of adolescent leisure interests. *American Journal of Occupational Therapy, 52*, 531–539.

Henry, A. D. (2000). *The Pediatric Interest Profiles: Surveys of play for children and adolescents*. San Antonio, TX: Therapy Skill Builders.

Hocking, C. (2001). Implementing occupation-based assessment. *American Journal of Occupational Therapy, 55*, 463–469.

Hoffman, O. R., Hemmingsson, H., & Kielhofner, G. (2000). *A user's manual for the School Setting Interview (SSI)* (Version 1.0). Chicago: Model of Human Occupation Clearinghouse, Department of Occupational Therapy, University of Illinois.

Iyenger, A. (2001). *A study of the psychometric properties of the OSA*. Unpublished master's thesis, University of Illinois at Chicago.

Kaplan, K., & Kielhofner, G. (1989). *Occupational case analysis interview and rating scale*. Thorofare, NJ: Slack.

Kielhofner, G., & Brinson, M. (1989). Development and evaluation of an aftercare program for young and chronic psychiatrically disabled adults. *Occupational Therapy in Mental Health, 9*(2), 1–25.

Kielhofner, G., Forsyth, K. (In press). Measurement properties of a client self report for treatment planning and documenting therapy outcomes. *Scandinavian Journal of Occupational Therapy*.

Kielhofner, G., Henry A. D., & Walens, D. (1989). *A user's guide to the Occupational Performance History Interview*. Rockville, MD: American Occupational Therapy Association.

Kielhofner, G., Lai, J. S., Olson, L., Haglund, L., Ekbadh, E., & Edlund, M. (1999). Psychometric properties of the work environment impact scale: A cross-cultural study. *Work: A Journal of Prevention, Assessment and Rehabilitation, 12*, 17–77.

Kielhofner, G., & Mallinson, T. (1995). Gathering narrative data through interviews: Empirical observations and suggested guidelines. *Scandinavian Journal of Occupational Therapy, 2*, 63–68.

Kielhofner, G., & Neville, A. (1983). *The modified interest checklist*. Unpublished manuscript, University of Illinois at Chicago.

Kielhofner, G., Mallinson, T., Crawford, C., Nowak, M., Rigby, M., Henry, A., Walens, D. (1997). *A user's guide to the Occupational Performance History Interview–II (OPHI-II)* (Version 2.0). Chicago: Model of Human Occupation Clearinghouse, Department of Occupational Therapy, University of Illinois.

Kielhofner, G., Mallinson, T., Forsyth, K., & Lai, J.-S. (2001). Psychometric properties of the second version of the Occupational Performance History Interview. *American Journal of Occupational Therapy, 55*, 260–267.

King, G., Law, M., Hurley, P., Hanna, S., King, S., Rosenbaum, P., Kertoy, M., & Young, N. (2001). *A preliminary test-retest reliability study of the CAPE*. Unpublished manuscript, Canada: CanChild Centre for Childhood Disability Research, McMaster University, Hamilton, ON, Canada.

King, G., Law, M., King, S., Harms, S., Kertoy, M., Rosenbaum, P., Young, N. (2001). CAPE: Children's Assessment of Participation and Enjoyment. Hamilton, ON, Canada: CanChild Centre for Childhood Disability Research, McMaster University.

LaGreca, A. M. (Ed.). (1990). *Through the eyes of the child. Obtaining self-reports from children and adolescents*. Boston: Allyn & Bacon.

Lai, J.-S., Haglund, L., & Kielhofner, G. (1999). The Occupational Case Analysis Interview and Rating Scale: Construct validity and directions for future development. *Scandinavian Journal of Caring Sciences, 13*, 267–273.

Law, M. (Ed). (1998). *Client-centered occupational therapy*. Thorofare, NJ: Slack.

Law, M., Baptiste, S., Carswell, A., McColl, M. A., Polatajko, H., & Pollock, N. (1998). *Canadian occupational performance measure* (3rd ed.). Toronto: Canadian Association of Occupational Therapists.

Law, M., Baptiste, S., McColl, M., Opzoomer, A., Polatajko, H., & Pollock, N. (1990). The Canadian Occupational Performance Measure: An outcome measure for occupational therapy. *Canadian Journal of Occupational Therapy, 57*, 82–87.

Law, M., Cooper, B., Strong, S., Stewart, D., Rigby, P., & Letts, L. (1996). The Person-Environment-Occupation Model: A transactive approach to occupational performance. *Canadian Journal of Occupational Therapy, 63*, 9–23.

Lynch, K. B., & Bridle, M. J. (1993). Construct validity of the occupational performance history interview. *Occupational Therapy Journal of Research, 13*, 231–240.

Matsutsuyu, J. (1969). The interest checklist. *American Journal of Occupational Therapy, 23*, 323–328.

Mattingly, C. (1991). The narrative nature of clinical reasoning. *American Journal of Occupational Therapy, 45*, 998–1005.

Mattingly, C., & Fleming, M. H. (1994). *Clinical reasoning. Forms of inquiry in a therapeutic practice*. Philadelphia: Davis.

Mauras-Nelson, E., & Oakley, F. (1996, April). *Bone marrow transplantation: Implications on function*. Poster presentation at the American Occupational Therapy Association's annual conference, Chicago.

McColl, M. A., Paterson, M., Davies, D., Doubt, L., & Law, M. (2000). Validity and community utility of the Canadian Occupational Performance Measure. *Canadian Journal of Occupational Therapy, 67*, 22–30.

Mishler, E. G. (1986). *Research interviewing: Context and narrative*. Cambridge, MA: Harvard University Press.

Neistadt, M. E. (1995). Methods of assessing clients' priorities: A survey of adult physical dysfunction settings. *American Journal of Occupational Therapy, 49*, 428–436.

Oakley, F., Kielhofner, G., Barris, R., & Reichler, R. (1986). The Role Checklist: Development and empirical assessment of reliability. *Occupational Therapy Journal of Research, 6*, 157–170.

Okun, B. F. (1997). *Effective helping. Interviewing and counseling techniques*. Pacific Grove, CA: Brooks/Cole.

Parks, R. A., Oakley, F., & Fonseca, M. (1998). Play development in children with HIV infection: A pilot study. *American Journal of Occupational Therapy, 52*, 672–675.

Polkinghorne, D. E. (1996). Transformative narratives: From victimic to agentic life plots. *American Journal of Occupational Therapy, 50*, 299–305.

Rogers, J. C. (1988). The NPI interest checklist. In B. J. Hemphill (Ed.). *Mental health assessment in occupational therapy. An integrative approach to the evaluation process*. Thorofare, NJ: Slack.

Rogers, J. C., & Holm, M. B. (1991). Occupational therapy diagnostic reasoning: A component of clinical reasoning. *American Journal of Occupational Therapy, 45*, 1045–1053.

Schon, D. A. (1983). *The reflective practitioner: How professionals think in action*. New York: Basic Books.

Smith, N. R., Kielhofner, G., & Watts, J. H. (1986). The relationship between volition, activity pattern and life satisfaction in the elderly. *American Journal of Occupational Therapy, 40*, 278–283.

Smyntek, L., Barris, R., & Kielhofner, G. (1985). The model of human occupation applied to psychosocially functional and dysfunctional adolescents. *Occupational Therapy in Mental Health*, 5(1), 21–40.

Stone, W. L., & Lemanek, K. L. (1990). Developmental issues in children's self-reports. In A. M. LaGreca (Ed.). *Through the eyes of the child. Obtaining self-reports from children and adolescents* (pp. 18–55). Boston: Allyn & Bacon.

Tickle-Degnen, L. (1995). Therapeutic rapport. In C. A. Trombly (Ed.). *Occupational therapy for physical dysfunction* (4th ed., pp. 277–285). Baltimore: Williams & Wilkins.

Trombly, C. (1995). Occupation: Purposefulness and meaningfulness as therapeutic mechanisms. 1995 Eleanor Clarke Slagle Lecture. *American Journal of Occupational Therapy, 49*, 960–972.

Velozo, C., Kielhofner, G., & Fisher, G. (1998). *A user's guide to the Worker Role Interview (WRI)* (Version 9.0). Chicago: Model of Human Occupation Clearinghouse, Department of Occupational Therapy, University of Illinois.

Velozo, C., Kielhofner, G., Gern, A., Lin, F., Azhar, F., Lai, J., & Fisher, G. (1999). Worker Role Interview: Toward validation of a psychosocial work-related measure. *Journal of Occupational Rehabilitation*, 9(3), 153–168.

Weinstein, J. (1979). *The generation of profiles of adolescent interests*. Unpublished master's thesis, University of Southern California at Los Angeles.

World Health Organization (WHO). (2001). *ICIDH-2: International classification of functioning, disability and health* (final draft, full version). Geneva: Author.

CHAPTER 23

CRITIQUING ASSESSMENTS

JANICE MILLER POLGAR

Evaluation has two main purposes in the practice of occupational therapy: as part of the therapy process to help determine occupational performance issues (Townsend et al., 1997) and to provide support for the evidence base of the profession (Hamer & Collinson, 1999; Sackett, Straus, Richardson, Rosenberg, & Haynes, 2000). When a **standardized assessment** is used, it is crucial that the occupational therapist has critiqued the instrument to determine its appropriateness for the individual or group to be evaluated as well as the purpose of the evaluation. The occupational therapist must ensure that the method of test development, standardization, development of norms, and psychometric properties meet acceptable standards when determining the test's clinical utility. This chapter explains why it is important to appraise these instruments critically and discusses each component of a thorough instrument critique.

The primary purpose of this chapter is to present sufficient information to enable an adequate critique of assessments used in occupational therapy. It is not meant to provide the reader with a detailed discussion of the various statistical analyses involved in test development or establishment of psychometric properties. I review issues of test development and standardization, reliability and validity, and the influence of culture and disabilities on test use. Sources for more detailed information are identified in the references. In the literature, several labels are used to identify a measurement tool, including *test*, *instrument*" *evaluation*, *measurement*, and *assessment*. I use the labels *assessment*, *instrument*, and *test* in this chapter.

MEASUREMENT

Measurement is the process of assigning numbers to represent quantities of a trait, attribute, or characteristic or to classify objects (Nunnally & Bernstein, 1995). It enables therapists to understand aspects of clients' performances, abilities, or personal characteristics. An important distinction here is that measurement enables therapists to quantify aspects of individuals but not the individuals themselves. It provides a means to define behaviors operationally and, by quantifying these behaviors, to make comparisons between individuals or to compare the same person at two different times (Law, 1987).

Some fundamental assumptions of measurement are critical to an understanding of the properties of psychometrically sound instruments (Barclay, 1991). The definition of measurement presented above assumes that psychological, sociological, and biological functions are observable and thus measurable. A second assumption is that what is observable and quantifiable corresponds to aspects of human behavior. For example, the Rotter (1966) internal–external (I-E) scale yields a numerical score that is inferred to measure the individual's level of personal causation; the pattern of responses on the test items is considered to represent the multifaceted construct of personal causation. Third, it is assumed that these measures have a normal distribution in the population (this concept is discussed later), and finally, it is assumed that some traits are relatively stable across time whereas others are expected to change. Measurements are used in different ways, depending on the purpose of a given evaluation.

PURPOSES OF EVALUATION IN OCCUPATIONAL THERAPY

Three main purposes have been identified for evaluation (Kirshner & Guyatt, 1985). The first purpose is descriptive. When the practitioner's intent is to describe individuals within a group or to describe differences among members of a group, an instrument should be chosen that measures the desired attribute comprehensively (Law, 1987). For example, if an occupational therapist is interested in describing a child's ability to operate a powered wheelchair, the instrument should measure all components considered necessary for this task.

The second purpose is to predict either future function or function in a related area (Kirshner & Guyatt, 1985). The practitioner may be interested in understanding the relation between performance on a measure of motor skills in infancy and subsequent performance on a test of fine motor skills at the age of 5. Alternatively, the therapist might be interested in determining the relation between achievement of a certain score on a vocational test and function on the job site.

Finally, practitioners use measurement to evaluate outcomes of therapeutic intervention (Kirshner & Guyatt, 1985). In this instance, it is important to use an instrument that will detect change that has occurred (Gowland et al., 1991; Law, 1987). This last purpose provides evidence to support our practice.

Whether an instrument is employed to describe an individual or group, to predict function, or evaluate outcome, the results of testing are used to make decisions. From this testing, therapists determine the suitability of clients to return to work or to their community, whether clients are suitable candidates for therapeutic intervention, and the types of intervention that are likely to be most effective. Therapists also make decisions about the efficacy of their practice. These decisions have important implications to the practitioner's practice and to the lives of their clients. Because of the importance of these decisions, it is crucial that occupational therapists critique instruments relative to test construction, reliability and validity, and applicability to the client group under consideration.

CRITIQUING ASSESSMENTS

Box 23-1 provides an outline to guide the critique of an instrument. Each of the major technical considerations is discussed below.

BOX 23–1. FORMAT FOR CRITIQUING ASSESSMENTS

I. General Information
   A. Title
   B. Author
   C. Publisher
   D. Time required to administer
   E. Materials required
   F. Cost
II. Description of Purpose of Assessment
   A. Type/purpose of assessment (description, prediction, evaluation)
   B. Target population
   C. Item description (response format, content)
   D. Traits or aptitudes evaluated (total score and subscales)
III. Practical Evaluation
   A. Ease of administration
   B. Clarity of directions
   C. Scoring procedures
   D. Examiner qualifications and training
IV. Technical Considerations
   A. Norms
      1. Type (percentiles, standard scores, etc.)
      2. Standardization sample
      3. Standardization procedures
   B. Reliability
      1. Test–retest
      2. Alternate form
      3. Internal consistency
      4. Split-half
      5. Cronbach's alpha
      6. Kuder-Richardson
   C. Validity (evidence to support the construct)
      1. Content
      2. Internal structure
      3. Response processes
      4. Relationship to external variables
V. External Reviewers' Comments (information from published evaluations of the assessment)
VI. Summary of Strengths and Weaknesses of the Assessment

Test Construction

The test manual should explicate the manner in which the test has been constructed. It should give sufficient information so the individual evaluating the test is able to determine that it was developed in a logical, systematic, and stringent fashion. The following sections present information about how tests should be constructed and what should be considered when critiquing an unfamiliar test.

Defining the Construct

The current *Standards for Psychological and Educational Measurement* (American Educational Research Association, American Psychological Association, & National Council on Measurement in Education [AERA], 1999) suggests broadening the understanding of a construct from something that is abstract and cannot be directly measured to the concept, characteristic, behavior, etc. that a test is designed to measure. It further suggests that there are many means of expressing these characteristics and of interpreting scores derived from such tests. Thus it must be made clear how the test developers conceptualize the construct and the manner in which it can be measured.

The first step in test construction is to define, explicitly, the construct or concept of interest and to generate hypotheses about how this construct will manifest itself (Zeidner & Most, 1992). Definition of the construct requires that the test developers articulate their understanding of the construct and its content domain. The definition of the construct comes from a sound understanding of the relevant literature (Benson & Clark, 1982; DePoy & Gitlin, 1998). From clinical experience and support from the literature, an operational definition of the construct is developed, and the significant factors contributing to it are identified and defined. An operational definition is one that states under which conditions a behavior will be labeled as the desired construct (Pedhazur & Schmelkin, 1991). For example, on the McCarthy Scales of Children's Abilities, the construct of arm coordination is operationally defined as the ability to bounce a ball and to catch a beanbag and throw it through a target (McCarthy, 1972). The information concerning conceptualization and definition of the construct and related variables should be included in the test manual.

Potential users must go through a similar procedure when evaluating the suitability of the test. If the users are not familiar with the area, they too should review the pertinent literature (Zeidner & Most, 1992). Users must explicitly articulate their conceptualization of the construct and its dimensions and compare their understanding of the construct with that stated in the test manual. If this comparison yields a match between conceptualizations, support is gained for the clinical usefulness of the instrument. Furthermore, users must compare their purpose and use of the test with that stated by the test developers.

Item Development

Development of the test items is an involved process, and detailed discussion is beyond the scope of this chapter. In terms of test critique, however, it is important to review test items for the following features:

- Congruence of the items with the conceptualization of the construct found in the test manual or related literature.
- Representativeness of the dimensions of the construct.
- Clarity of items to avoid ambiguity.
- Possibility of bias for certain clients (Murphy & Davidshofer, 1991).

Scales of Measurement

It is important to determine the type of measurement scale that is used. There are four scales of measurement: nominal, ordinal, interval, and ratio (Pedhazur & Schmelkin, 1991; Portney & Watkins, 2000). The nominal scale involves mutually exclusive categories (e.g., female versus male; geographic location). Often these categories are given numbers (e.g., male = 1; female = 2), but these numbers are not meaningful in a quantitative way. This scale simply identifies differences with no attempt to quantify or order those differences.

The second level is the ordinal scale. This scale involves rank ordering of scores. The order indicates greater (or better) than, but no inference can be made about the magnitude of the difference between scores.

Interval scales are the third level. This type of scale is the most common in measures found in occupational therapy. The intervals between scores are equal, so comparisons can be made between individuals (Pedhazur & Schmelkin, 1991). However, zero is not an absolute point on these scales. Because zero is arbitrary, ratio comparisons between scores cannot be made (Pedhazur & Schmelkin, 1991; Portney & Watkins, 2000). For example, if person A scores 20 on a test of self-esteem and person B scores 40 on the same test, it is not meaningful to say that person B has twice as much self-esteem as person A. To make such a comparison meaningful, zero must be a fixed point.

On ratio scales, zero does have a fixed point and ratio comparisons can be made (Pedhazur & Schmelkin, 1991). To use these scales, absence of the attribute being measured must be meaningful. When measuring liquid volume, for example, a score of zero indicates the absence of liquid. In occupational therapy, range of motion can be understood on a ratio scale because there can be absence of measurable movement around a joint, and it is meaningful to indicate that a person gained twice as much movement from one measurement to the next.

Development of Norms

Many of the tests used by occupational therapists are norm referenced (Anastasi & Urbina, 1997; Murphy &

Davidshofer, 1991). Norms are statistics that are generated from a well-defined group that has been evaluated using the test in a standardized manner (Wiersma & Jurs, 1990). Usually, but not necessarily, norms are measures of the average performance of this reference group. These statistics are used to make comparisons between the individual tested and the reference group (i.e., the norms provide a point of reference for comparing the individual's score).

It is crucial to understand that the norms provided in the manual are not definitive norms (Murphy & Davidshofer, 1991). Instead, they represent the performance of the individuals who were tested for the development of the norms. The usefulness of the norms for making a meaningful interpretation of an individual's score depends on the information given about the characteristics of the sample used to create the norms, the method of recruiting the sample, and the degree to which the sample represents the test's target population.

At some point in the development of the test, a target population is identified (Murphy & Davidshofer, 1991; Wiersma & Jurs, 1990). The population defines the group for which the test is intended. The test manual should clearly state the intended target population. Before using a test, the therapist must determine that it is intended to evaluate people with characteristics similar to those of the client.

Wiersma and Jurs (1990) list three criteria for evaluating the usefulness of the norms, related to the target population: They should be representative, relevant, and recent. The sample represents the target population when the distribution of characteristics of the population is reflected in the sample. A test that is targeted for national (or international) use must demonstrate that the norms were developed in a way that represents the distribution of region, urban, and rural living; gender; ethnicity; and any other relevant characteristics of the national or international population (Murphy & Davidshofer, 1991; Wiersma & Jurs, 1990). A test that is intended to provide information about performance at different ages must use a sample that is made up of individuals of each age. For example, researchers developing a test that provides norms for children at 6-month intervals should ensure that children at each of the targeted ages were included in the norming sample.

The test manual should include clear information about the selection of the norming sample. Random sampling procedures should be used. These involve selection based on the distribution of the characteristics of the population identified, not on convenience (Wiersma & Jurs, 1990). The sample size should be sufficient to minimize measurement errors and to maximize the confidence the test user has in the norms provided. The procedures for administering the test to the sample subjects and the time of administration should also be identified in the test manual.

The norming sample should be relevant to the target population (Wiersma & Jurs, 1990). It should have characteristics similar to the population. Norms that have been developed from the motor performance of adults are of little use in providing a meaningful interpretation of the motor performance of preschoolers.

Finally, norms should be recent (Wiersma & Jurs, 1990). Test material can become dated. For example, tests developed before the mid-1970s that require knowledge of linear measurement will not reliably test this knowledge in Canadian children today. Before the mid-1970s measurement was expressed in imperial units. At that time, the metric system was introduced, and Canadian children were no longer taught imperial units of measurement. Today, questions involving knowledge of imperial units are not meaningful to young Canadians. Furthermore, over time, performance or attributes may change in the population.

Standardized Scores

Raw scores are usually converted into another form to facilitate comparison and meaningful interpretation. These forms include percentiles, stanines, standard scores, and age- or grade-equivalent scores (Murphy & Davidshofer, 1991; Wiersma & Jurs, 1990). These forms will be discussed presently, but first I review some basic statistical concepts related to test scores.

There are three measures of central tendency: mean, median, and mode. The mean is the arithmetic average of the cumulative measures (Murphy & Davidshofer, 1991; Portney & Watkins, 2000). The median is the point in the distribution of scores that divides the scores in half (i.e., 50% of the scores are above the median and 50% are below it). The mode is the most frequently occurring score. It is important to know which of these measures of central tendency is being reported.

For a given population, scores are considered to be distributed normally. In the normal distribution, the bulk of the scores are at the center of the range, with fewer scores found at the extremes (Portney & Watkins, 2000). The range of the distribution is the span between the lowest and highest score. The variance indicates the dispersion of the scores. The standard deviation (SD) is the square root of the variance and is the most common method of dividing the normal distribution. It represents the spread of the scores in the same units as the test score (Wiersma & Jurs, 1990). Approximately 68% of the scores fall within -1.0 and $+1.0$ SD, 95% fall within -2.0 and $+2.0$ SD, and 99% fall within -3.0 and $+3.0$ SD (Portney & Watkins, 2000).

The percentile rank is expressed as a whole number between 1 and 99. The number represents the percentage of people who scored at or below a given score (Portney & Watkins, 2000; Wiersma & Jurs, 1990). An individual whose score is at the 75th percentile performed equal to or better than 75% of those tested. Percentile rank is an ordinal scale, so the intervals between the ranks are not equal (Wiersma & Jurs, 1990). It is considered to have a normal distribution, and the majority of the scores fall around the 50th percentile (Portney & Watkins, 2000).

Stanine is the abbreviation for standard-nine (Wiersma & Jurs, 1990). This method of standardizing scores divides the normal distribution into nine components, each making up one half of a standard deviation to provide equal units of measure. It minimizes the tendency to overinterpret small differences in scores, but it may not be sufficiently sensitive to detect small changes (Wiersma & Jurs, 1990).

Standard scores use the standard deviation to obtain a scale with equal intervals. These scores have been termed *z*-scores (Witt, Elliott, Gresham, & Kramer, 1988). The *z*-scores express an individual's score in terms of standard deviation above or below the mean, providing ease of interpretation (Wiersma & Jurs, 1990).

Age- or grade-equivalent scores relate the individual's performance on the test to that of the typical individual of a particular age or grade (Murphy & Davidshofer, 1991). It is crucial that the sample used to create the norms has sufficient representation of the comparison grades or ages.

In summary, the norms of the test provide the comparison group needed to make a meaningful interpretation of the obtained score. The group used to create the norms should represent and be relevant to the test's target population and should be current. The methods used for establishing the norms and the type of standardized score used should be clearly identified in the test manual.

Test Standardization

As stated earlier, tests are used to describe people, make comparisons, or evaluate performance. Because of the effect that decisions from test scores have on the lives of people, it is important that as many extraneous factors as possible are eliminated from the method of administering, scoring, and interpreting the scores (Murphy & Davidshofer, 1991). Test standardization procedures are used to ensure the maximum level of consistency in testing situations.

The test manual should clearly describe the arrangement of the testing environment, the presentation of materials, standardized instructions, and time limits (AERA, 1999). When the test developers have made modifications to any of these areas to accommodate individuals with different abilities, these modifications should be clearly indicated so they can be replicated in appropriate situations. Moreover, the manual should include clear guidelines for scoring the test and interpreting the scores.

It is not possible to standardize all aspects of test administration. Some aspects of the environment, such as noise or the examinee's mood at the time of testing, are not controllable. Because of these uncontrollable factors, which can affect the reliability of the test, it is important to follow the standardized instructions of the test exactly. Failure to do so will affect the reliability of the test scores (AERA, 1999). It is also important to ensure that the test user is adequately trained or prepared to administer the test. Some tests indicate the type of training necessary for administration. Indeed, some tests are not available except to those who hold the necessary qualifications.

Reliability

Definition

A standardized test used to evaluate the performance of an individual or to measure the existence of a specified trait yields a score. It is important to demonstrate that the score resulting from the use of a test is consistent and repeatable. Consistency and repeatability are aspects of **reliability,** defined as "the consistency of . . . measurements when the testing procedure is repeated on a population of individuals or groups" (AERA, 1999, p. 25). Reliability is based on the correlation coefficient and referred to as a reliability coefficient. The reliability coefficient can range from 0 to +1, with 0 indicating no consistency and +1 indicating perfect consistency. Reliability approaching +1 is desirable.

An instrument is considered to be reliable when a similar score is achieved on repeated administration. It is important to distinguish that a similar score, not an identical one, is the aim in reliability (Siegel, 1989). When an instrument is reliable, it is expected that on subsequent testing an individual will achieve scores that are consistent with, but not necessarily identical to, previously achieved scores. To understand why identical scores are not expected, an explanation of some of the assumptions of reliability, or classical test theory, is important. A test score is considered to consist of three components:

- The obtained score.
- The true score, considered to be a hypothetical, unobservable quantity of the specific attribute under consideration (Carmines & Zeller, 1979).
- Measurement error.

The relation between these components is expressed by Equation 23-1:

$$\text{obtained score} = \text{true score} + \text{measurement error} \qquad (23\text{-}1)$$

In other words, every obtained score is made up of two components: a portion of the score that reflects the "true" quantity of an attribute and random errors that contribute to inconsistency in the measurement (Murphy & Davidshofer, 1991). It is assumed that no relation exists between true scores and the error component. Reliability is high when the proportion of the obtained score owing to measurement error is low. Below, I discuss the sources of measurement error further.

Factors That Contribute to Error in Testing

There are several factors that contribute to error in testing. These factors can be classed as factors related to the test itself, those related to the situation of testing, those related to the individual being tested, and those related to the examiner. Factors related to the test include how stringently the test was constructed, the adequacy of the directions for administering and scoring the test, test length, homogeneity of test content, effect of bias, and the construction of the items (Isaac & Michael, 1971; Murphy & Davidshofer, 1991).

Various environmental or situational factors may contribute to error. The environment might be distracting, time limits may induce undue stress, or the length of the assessment may contribute to fatigue (Isaac & Michael, 1971).

Many factors related to the individual can contribute to variance in the obtained score. Some factors are relatively stable, such as level of ability, knowledge or skills, personality, or the level of comfort with a particular response mode (e.g., multiple choice) (Murphy & Davidshofer, 1991). Other factors are more inconsistent, such as motivation, practice with test items, fatigue, anxiety, or other emotional states (Murphy & Davidshofer). Factors related to the examiner include familiarity and training for the specific test and assessment process, adherence to standardized instructions, and the ability to establish an effective evaluation atmosphere (Isaac & Michael, 1971). These factors occur on a random basis and are not easily quantifiable. Therefore, therapists must estimate their potential influence on an individual's obtained test score.

Types of Reliability

Test–Retest Reliability

Test-retest reliability is a measure of the consistency of an assessment over time. It has also been termed *stability*, because it estimates the stability of the measurement over time (Jensen, 1980). This form of reliability is determined by administering an evaluation on two occasions, separated by a time interval. Nunnally and Bernstein (1995) suggested that a desirable separation is 2 weeks. With a shorter time period, the examinee may remember the test items; with a longer time period, actual changes might occur. Test–retest reliability is estimated by determining the correlation or association between scores obtained on two testing occasions. A correlation approaching +1.0 suggests that a test is stable across time.

Test–retest reliability is meaningful only when the trait being measured is expected to be stable over the testing interval (AERA, 1999). An evaluation of mood, for example, is not expected to yield consistent results over a period of weeks, for mood is considered to fluctuate. Alternatively, a trait such as adult height is stable and should yield little variability in the obtained scores over repeated measurements. Many attributes measured in occupational therapy are not as clearly consistent or inconsistent as the examples just given. In each case, practitioners considering the test must compare their understanding of the construct or attribute being measured with that explicated in the test manual to assess whether that attribute is stable and thus whether an indication of stability is essential.

An estimate of the test's stability is necessary when the measurement is used as an outcome measure (Jensen, 1980). Test stability should not be affected by maturation unless such is accounted for in the scoring procedures (Murphy & Davidshofer, 1991).

Evaluation of a test's stability can be confounded by several factors. There may be changes in the individual on the trait being measured between the test administrations (Jensen, 1980). Sometimes, simple exposure to a test may cause the individual to reflect on the trait or attribute, resulting in a change in subsequent test performance. Carmines and Zeller (1979) termed this phenomenon *reactivity*. A historical event may occur between administrations that could influence the score (Kerlinger, 1973). The individual may remember the test items or practice with the materials, which would result in inflation of the estimate of stability (Carmines & Zeller, 1979).

Alternate Form Reliability

The establishment of reliability using alternative forms has some similarities to test–retest reliability because it is estimated by testing the same group of people on two separate occasions (Carmines & Zeller, 1979). However, it differs from test–retest reliability estimation because of its use of two distinct, but parallel, forms of a test. When estimating alternative form reliability, the test administration should occur about 2 weeks apart to account for day-to-day fluctuations in performance (Nunnally & Bernstein, 1995).

Occasionally, in occupational therapy treatment, clients' performance in a specific area must be evaluated repeatedly. Repeated administrations of the same instrument causes problems, because the clients may remember test items or practice them. Thus repeated exposure to the same test may artificially inflate the obtained score. The use of parallel forms minimizes the influence that memory or practice can have on inflating the estimated reliability. These two forms should not differ in "any systematic way" (Carmines & Zeller, 1979, p. 40). Computation of the reliability coefficient between these forms establishes their equivalence.

Internal Consistency

Both the alternative form and test–retest reliabilities require two separate test administrations to determine reliability. As discussed, this separation of administrations of the test may make it difficult to determine whether the difference between the scores is due to test unreliability or to other sources of error, such as the individual's memory, actual changes in the trait, or a historical event (Carmines & Zeller, 1979; Jensen, 1980; Kerlinger, 1973). One means of eliminating the influence of time separation is to estimate reliability from a single test administration. These methods determine the internal consistency of the test (Carmines & Zeller, 1979; Nunnally & Bernstein, 1995; Pedhazur & Schmelkin, 1991).

The simplest and crudest type of internal consistency is split-half reliability (Nunnally & Bernstein, 1995; Pedhazur & Schmelkin, 1991). In this method, dividing the test items in half and obtaining the correlation between the two halves determine reliability. Commonly, performance is compared between even- and odd-numbered items or the first half of the items and the second half.

This method calculates the correlation between the two halves so, unless a correction is made, the resulting reliability coefficient will underestimate the reliability of the whole test (Carmines & Zeller, 1979). Use of the Spearman-Brown formula makes a statistical correction so that the estimated reliability reflects the total test and not the compared halves (Carmines & Zeller, 1979).

The limitation of the split-half method of estimating reliability is that the variety of ways of dividing the items can result in different reliability coefficients (Carmines & Zeller, 1979). More sophisticated methods of estimating internal consistency take into account the variety of ways of grouping the test items (Carmines & Zeller, 1979; Nunnally & Bernstein, 1995; Pedhazur & Schmelkin, 1991). These analyses give an indication of the consistency of the "responses across the various items of the test" (Zeidner & Most, 1992, p. 59). Internal consistency takes into account the correlation of each item with every other item as well as with the total score. These inter-item and item-total correlations provide an estimate of how consistent the items are with each other.

High internal consistency suggests that the test items measure a homogeneous construct. When low internal consistency exists, the representation of a single construct in a test must be questioned. The items that do not correlate highly with other items or with the total test may measure a different construct. A test that is intended to measure a narrowly defined construct should have high internal consistency (Zeidner & Most, 1992).

The most common ways to estimate the internal consistency are through the use of Cronbach's (1951) alpha or the Kuder and Richardson (1937) formula. These methods provide the "theoretical average of all possible split-half correlations" (Green, 1991, p. 29). In other words, the formulas used to calculate internal consistency generate a matrix of the inter-item and item-total correlations in the calculation of reliability. Cronbach's alpha is computed when the items are scored in a nondichotomous manner. When the scoring is dichotomous, the Kuder-Richardson formula is used. For further information on the theory and calculations of internal consistency, see the reference list.

Standard Error of Measurement

Procedures used to establish reliability involve testing groups of individuals (Zeidner & Most, 1992). Reliability estimation gives the potential test user an indication of the test's consistency. In instances when the therapist would like to understand how close the obtained score is to the true score for an individual, the estimates from group data can be used to calculate the standard error of measurement (SEM). The SEM indicates how much variability in the test scores can be attributed to error (Murphy & Davidshofer, 1991). As can be seen from Equation 23-2, as reliability increases, the SEM decreases:

$$\text{SEM} = \text{SD}\sqrt{1-r_{xx}} \qquad (23\text{-}2)$$

where SD refers to the standard deviation of the group from which the reliability (r) is calculated. It can be seen that the SEM is always less than the SD, except in the unlikely occurrence that the reliability equals zero. In this extreme case, the SEM would equal the standard deviation.

Once the SEM has been calculated, a confidence interval can be constructed around the obtained score. A confidence interval is defined as the range in which it can be stated that a certain score will fall, with a specified degree of confidence (Portney & Watkins, 2000). The degree of confidence is determined from the properties of the normal distribution. Previously, the approximate distribution of scores within the normal distribution was identified for ease of understanding. To calculate a confidence interval, the precise SD that corresponds to 95% of the distribution, for example, must be used. Thus from the normal distribution, 95% of the scores fall within −1.96 and +1.96 SD from the mean and 99% fall within −2.54 to +2.54 SD from the mean (Anastasi & Urbina, 1997). To construct a 95% confidence interval, the SEM is multiplied by 1.96 (Murphy & Davidshofer, 1991). Thus the true score is known, with 95% confidence, to fall between the obtained score −1.96(SEM) and the obtained score + 1.96(SEM). Similarly a 99% confidence interval is constructed by multiplying the SEM by 2.54.

Suppose a 5½-year-old child achieves a score of 55 on the McCarthy Scales of Children's Abilities (McCarthy, 1972). From the test manual, it is known that the SD equals 7.3 and the reliability is 0.75. From the foregoing formula, the SEM is calculated at 3.65. To construct a 95% confidence interval, 3.65 (the SEM) is multiplied by 1.96 (the SD), resulting in 7.15, which is rounded to 7. The confidence interval is then 55 ± 7, or 48 to 62. Thus it can be said with a 95% level of confidence that the child's true score falls within the range of 48 to 62. It can be seen from this example how the standard error of measurement can be used to provide an estimate of the range in which the child's true score would fall, providing a more meaningful interpretation of performance.

How Reliable Should a Test Be?

The question of how reliable a test should be does not have a ready answer. The purpose of the test should be considered when deciding whether the reliability reported is acceptable (Salvia & Ysseldyke, 1985). Tests that are used to make decisions about a person, such as determining whether he or she is capable of returning to work, should have a higher level of reliability than tests that are intended to serve as screening or descriptive instruments (King-Thomas & Hacker, 1987; Salvia & Ysseldyke, 1985; Murphy & Davidshofer, 1991). Similarly, those instruments that attempt to categorize individuals, such as a test that is used to assign cognitive levels, should have a high degree of reliability (Murphy & Davidshofer, 1991).

The following minimal levels of reliability should be considered as guidelines. It is also useful to remember that the reliability coefficient estimates the proportion of the score making up the true score. A reliability coefficient of 0.80 indicates that 80% of the variance in the score is true variance and 20% of the variance of the score is due to errors of measurement. Thus when a reliability coefficient of 0.50 is reported, the amount of the score that can be attributed to the true score is equivalent to that attributed to error. Generally, a reliability coefficient of 0.90 is considered to be high, 0.80 moderate, 0.70 low, and 0.60 generally unacceptable for clinical use (Murphy & Davidshofer, 1991).

It is recommended that when a test score is to be used to make significant decisions about an individual, such as placement decisions, a minimum level of reliability of 0.90 should be reported (King-Thomas & Hacker, 1987; Nunnally & Bernstein, 1995; Salvia & Ysseldyke, 1985). When a test is to be used for screening, a minimum level of reliability of 0.80 is considered appropriate (King-Thomas & Hacker, 1987; Salvia & Ysseldyke, 1985). Wiersma and Jurs (1990) suggest that, because attitudes are more difficult to quantify, reliability coefficients are likely to be lower and that a minimum level of reliability of 0.70 is acceptable for attitude tests. If the test has been administered to a group and the data are reported for the group as a whole, a minimum level of 0.60 has been suggested (Salvia & Ysseldyke, 1985).

It is important to remember that the reliability reported reflects the specific situation and the sample used to collect the data. The method used to collect the data to establish reliability should be clearly stated in the test manual. The potential test users must ensure that they understand the type of reliability that has been reported, the appropriate means of establishing that specific reliability, and its applicability for the purpose of the test. Table 23-1 summarizes this information. With this information and the reported reliability coefficient, the potential test users can make an informed decision about the usefulness of the test for their purposes.

Validity

Definition

Contemporary understanding of **validity** is that it is a unitary concept and that the establishment of validity is the process of accumulating evidence to support the underlying construct that an evaluation is considered to measure (Cronbach, 1988; Messick, 1988, 1989, 1995). This notion is relevant not only to the interpretation of the test score but to the social consequences of that interpretation. The current edition of *Standards for Educational and Psychological Testing* defines validity as "the degree to which evidence and theory support the interpretations of test scores entailed by proposed uses of tests" (AERA, 1999, p. 9). Messick (1989) added that validity is the "adequacy and appropriateness of inferences and actions based on test scores" (p. 13). Furthermore, evidence for validity is concerned with the relevance and utility of scores for particular individuals or groups and the significance of the value attributed to the score or underlying construct as they related to the social consequences for the individual or group (Messick, 1995).

What can we draw from these defining statements? First, let's consider the ideas of appropriateness, meaningfulness, and usefulness, which are relevant to how the evaluation is used and the consequences of the inferences made from interpretation of the scores. Appropriateness refers to the question of whether the construct and elements of the evaluation are suitable for the population of persons to be evaluated and the context and purpose of the evaluation. Meaningfulness is associated with the articulation of the underlying construct and how it explains or describes the trait being measured. Finally, usefulness is concerned with the utility of the evaluation in terms of the information that is

TABLE 23-1. **RELIABILITY COEFFICIENTS, TYPE OF RELIABILITY, AND SOURCES OF VARIABILITY**

Reliability Coefficient	Type of Reliability	Sources of Variability
Test–retest	Stability	Length of time between testing; stability of trait measured; memory of test items; actual change in trait measured
Alternate form	Equivalence of parallel forms (equivalence and stability if forms are administered at two times)	Ability to generate parallel forms
Split-half	Internal consistency	Method of splitting items; length of test; consistency of test content
Cronbach's alpha; Kuder-Richardson 20 and 21	Internal consistency	Consistency of test content

gained from the test results in consideration of the effort required to undertake the evaluation. Evidence of validity, as it provides support for the underlying construct, is necessary to justify a particular evaluation with a specific population in a given context.

These statements are very clear that it is not the test that has validity. Rather, validity relates to the interpretations and actions derived from the resulting scores (Messick, 1988, 1989, 1995). There are implications here for both test developers and test users. Both empirical and theoretical evidence of validity are required to provide support for these interpretations and actions. Thus an assessment must be based on a well-founded or articulated theoretical construct, and there should be empirical evidence to support the hypotheses derived from the theory. Otherwise, the inferences made from the test scores are without meaning and are not justifiable.

In addition, these definitions suggest a variety of uses of the test results. Consequently, evidence of validity must be provided for each of the intended uses. When first using an evaluation, the occupational therapist must be clear on its intended use. How will the test score be interpreted and how will that interpretation affect the client's life? Is the therapist's intended use of the evaluation congruent with that articulated by the test developers? The answers to these questions influence the appropriateness, meaningfulness, and usefulness of inferences made from the test scores.

Before I discuss sources of validity evidence, I will describe two threats to validity: construct underrepresentation and construct irrelevance (AERA, 1999, Messick, 1989, 1995). Construct underrepresentation refers to an inadequate sampling of the construct domain in the test items—that is, content is missing. The resulting interpretation of the score is not comprehensive, because the test did not tap some content, underlying processes, or response that is important to the understanding of the construct. Examples of construct underrepresentation are given in subsequent sections.

Construct-irrelevant variance is present when test scores are influenced by processes or abilities that are not pertinent to the construct (AERA, 1999; Messick, 1988, 1995). Here, the person evaluated must have a certain level of ability, skill, or knowledge extraneous to the construct being measured to make a response or to achieve satisfactory score. A valid interpretation of a low score cannot be made because it cannot be determined whether the score reflects performance on the construct or some other ability. An example of this type of variance is a test of arithmetic ability that requires reading comprehension to complete the problems satisfactorily.

The following discussion presents different sources of evidence to support construct validity. These sources include evidence from examination of content, response processes, structure of the test, and relationship to external variables (AERA, 1999; Messick, 1989; Moss, 1995). Together this evidence enables the test developer or user to construct an argument for the validity relating to appropriateness, meaningfulness, and relevance of inferences and actions based on test scores.

Evidence of Validity Derived from Content

The current *Standards for Educational and Psychological Testing* refers to content as themes, wording, item format, response method, and guidelines for procedures for administration and scoring. In other words, not only is the actual content of the test items important evidence but so too are the processes that underlie the respondent's interpretation of the items and the response format. Construct representativeness is interpreted here as how well the content of the evaluation represents the hypothesized content domain and structure. Construct relevancy considers how relevant the content, means of interpretation, and response format are to the construct. For example, if a test of visual perception required language to signify a response, language skills could be a source of construct irrelevant variance.

Validation of the content of a test begins at the test development stage. As noted, the initial stages of test construction begin with a clear articulation of the theory underlying the construct. Theoretical ideas have three purposes: operationally define the construct—that is, what behaviors are considered to indicate the construct (Pedhazur & Schmelkin, 1991); state hypotheses of the structure and elements of the construct; and describe the relationship among these elements (Messick, 1988; 1989). From there, a blueprint is developed to guide the content, item difficulty, and proportion of the test that focuses on particular dimensions of the theoretical construct to be represented.

Validation of the content is derived from consideration of the sampling of the construct domain—that all aspects of the domain are adequately covered, that the content is relevant to the construct, and that the underlying processes necessary for satisfactory interpretation of test items and response are also relevant (AERA, 1999; Messick, 1988, 1989). One means of gathering this evidence is through the examination of the content by a panel of experts to determine relevance and representativeness. For example, consider an instrument designed to measure performance in activities of daily living (ADL). The test developers articulate their understanding of the construct of ADL, create items considered to measure ADL performance, and assemble these on an evaluation. Evidence of the representativeness and relevance of the content is provided by a review of the evaluation by occupational therapists who are considered to be experts and who determine that the construct, as defined, is adequately represented by the items and that these items and the response means are relevant to ADL.

When a test is used with a population different from that for which it was originally intended or for a different purpose, the test user must examine the content to determine that it is appropriate for that population or purpose. In particular here, issues of relevance are important. The test user must determine whether any aspects of test administration, item interpretation, or response format are a source of bias for the intended purpose or population (AERA, 1999; Messick, 1988, 1989, 1995).

Inferences of low scores that are based on content can suggest only that the respondent was not competent in taking the test. It cannot be interpreted that the individual is incompetent on the underlying skill, has inadequate knowledge, or has less of a specific trait. Other sources of variance may contribute to this low score (Messick, 1989). Again, it is important to review the test content in light of the construct definition and domain to identify any sources of bias that may disadvantage or give unfair advantage to any particular group or individual.

Evidence from Test Structure

To compile evidence from the structure of the test, it is necessary to examine the relationship of the hypothesized structure of the construct to the structure of the evaluation (AERA, 1999; Messick, 1989). This examination is completed through empirical analysis of the relationship between the items (inter-item) and to the total score (AERA, 1999). If the conceptual framework suggests that the underlying construct is unidimensional, then analysis of the relationship between the items should reveal a single dimension. Alternately, if a multidimensional structure is hypothesized, then analysis should support this structure with multiple dimensions of content that are distinct from each other and congruent with the structure hypothesized from the theory. More simply put, if the construct is hypothesized to have three dimensions, factor analysis should confirm that number. Items that load on those factors should have content congruent to articulation of the construct. In addition, the scoring structure should reflect the theorized dimensionality of the construct (Messick, 1989).

Evidence from Response Processes

Part of the hypotheses of the construct includes the underlying processes that are necessary for a correct response (AERA, 1999). Examination of how respondents arrive at a response provides evidence for this element of the validity argument. For example, a professional certification examination may be hypothesized to require clinical reasoning to achieve a correct response. It is only through examination of an individual's approach to answering questions on this examination that evidence is provided to support or refute this hypothesis. In situations such as this example, directly questioning the respondents on their approach to gaining an answer is appropriate.

The issue of construct irrelevance is important here. As indicated previously, evidence must be provided that the means of deriving an answer and indicating a response are relevant to the construct. This evidence is important during test construction; but, more important for occupational therapists, it is necessary when considering a test that was not developed for the population or purpose for which the therapist intends. Evidence must be provided that these elements of validity are not a source of bias for the clients.

Evidence from the Relationship to External Variables

When examining the relationship to other variables, therapists are considering the "extent to which the test's relationship with other tests and non-test behavior reflects the expected high, low, and interactive relations implied in the theory of the construct being assessed" (Messick, 1989, p. 45). Here the user is looking for convergent evidence (i.e., the test is highly related to other tests or nontest behavior that is theoretically related to the construct) or divergent evidence (i.e., the test is not related to other tests or nontest behavior that is theoretically not related to the construct). Both convergent and divergent evidence provide necessary information for understanding the theoretical construct and the therapist's ability to measure it. This evidence is derived from empirical studies.

Historically, there are two types of studies that are important here (AERA, 1999): predictor and concurrent studies. Predictor studies provide evidence that performance on the test predicts performance on a criterion later in time. Clinically, such evidence is useful for guiding decisions on who will benefit from a given intervention. Concurrent studies provide evidence of the relationship between the test and a given criterion at the same point in time. Such studies are useful when examining different methods for measuring the same construct or when analyzing a client's behavior or abilities (AERA, 1999).

When a measure is used for evaluative purposes, evidence of responsiveness is important (Gowland et al., 1991; Guyatt, Walter, & Norman, 1987; Kirshner & Guyatt, 1985; Law, 1987). Test responsiveness is defined as "the capability of an instrument to detect clinically meaningful change in an attribute, characteristic, or function" (Guyatt et al., 1987, cited in Gowland et al., 1991, p. 7). For example, suppose an occupational therapist wanted to determine whether the participants in a task group developed improved self-esteem as a result of involvement in the group. The therapist could measure the participants' self-esteem before they begin the group and again on the group's termination and then determine whether a significant difference exists between the two measures. To make a meaningful interpretation of the results, the therapist must be confident that the instrument was capable of detecting any change that had occurred.

Examination of the relationship to other variables provides information about group differences. It may support predicted differences between groups with different characteristics, suggesting that the meaning of the score is different for members of different groups (AERA, 1999). It is important to provide evidence that the differences are congruent

TABLE 23-2. **VALIDITY EVIDENCE: PURPOSE AND METHOD OF DETERMINATION**

Evidence	Information	Method of Determination
Content	Content adequately samples the domains of the construct and reflects its hypothesized structure	Support for content is found in the literature and expert opinion
Response processes	The means of deriving and indicating a response is congruent with construct hypotheses	Examination of how respondent forms and indicates a response
Test structure	Structure of the test, e.g., dimensions or scores congruent with that of underlying construct	Examination of relationship of items to each other and with total test
Relationship to external variables	Test scores relate to other measures or nontest behaviors as predicted by theoretical construct	Empirical studies of hypothesized relationships

with hypotheses derived from the construct and not the result of some source of construct irrelevance.

Social Consequences

There is some debate as to whether consideration of the social consequences of inferences and actions based on a test score are relevant to the validity argument (Lees-Haley, 1996; Messick, 1988, 1989, 1995; Zimiles, 1996). However, both Messick and the current *Standards for Educational and Psychological Testing* make a compelling argument that these consequences need to be considered in the evaluation process, although they do not, in and of themselves, provide evidence for the validity argument. Social consequences refer to the implications that inferences made and actions taken from the test score have on the life of the individual tested. High-stakes testing involves evaluation in which the results carry significant implications for the life of the individual, such as access to education, treatment, or a career; the value associated with a labeling derived from the score; and costs that result from actions based on the score (Haertel, 1999). How are these important for occupational therapists?

When therapists assess a client, they do so from a particular theoretical framework, tacit or otherwise. This framework guides what they measure, the meaning they give to a score, and the way they interpret that score. Furthermore, it influences the label that results, for example, performance on certain measures of motor performance could result in a child being labeled as having developmental coordination disorder. It is important to recognize the value associated with a label and whether the value attributes positive or negative connotations in the lives of clients.

The results of practitioners' assessments guide who will receive intervention, and the theoretical ideas of change resulting from therapy help indicate when therapy should cease. There are implications here for costs—both actual and in time and effort—for the therapist and the client. Given the economic state of many health-care systems, the evidence that supports decisions related to where therapy efforts will be directed, in what manner, and for how long is crucial.

Constructing the Validity Argument

The preceding discussion of various sources of evidence concerning the validity of inferences and actions based on test scores suggests a dynamic and continuing process. An initial argument to support the use and interpretation of test scores is constructed from the available evidence. However, subsequent studies may provide information that weakens the initial argument when hypothesized relationships are not supported or new sources of construct irrelevance are uncovered. This fluidity underscores the importance for occupational therapists to examine evidence to determine that the proposed use of the test is appropriate and that the interpretation of the scores can be made with some degree of confidence (Table 23-2).

FAIR TESTING PRACTICES

It is the responsibility of the test user to take whatever measures are possible to minimize bias in testing for particular groups. Because the outcome of occupational therapy evaluation has implications not only for the lives of clients but also for the distribution of scarce health-care dollars, therapists must seriously consider whether an evaluation is fair for their clients and what extraneous variables might influence their scores. The *Standards for Educational and Psychological Testing* describes four aspects of **fair testing,** reflecting the idea that testing does not need to be identical for all groups, but evidence should exist that interpretation of the score is valid, without undue influence of construct underrepresentation or irrelevance (AERA, 1999). Sources of bias should be identified and eliminated, when feasible, so they do not alter the meaning of scores obtained by clients. When bias cannot be removed, satisfactorily, then the evaluation should not be used.

All clients should be treated in an equitable manner with respect to the context and purpose of the test and the way in which the test scores are used; they should all have a reasonable opportunity or means to demonstrate their competence on the construct measured. Differences in outcomes across groups do not necessarily mean that one group is disadvantaged relative to another. However, such differences need to be examined to determine whether such a situation is present. Finally, all groups should have a similar opportunity to learn or practice knowledge or behaviors measured by the test (AERA, 1999). For the purposes of this chapter, two specific instances of fair testing practices will be considered: considerations related to culture and to persons with disabilities.

Culture-Fair Evaluation

In many countries, cultural diversity is increasing. Occupational therapists may be required to assess an individual whose first language is not the official language of the country. The literature reviewed for this section focused on tests developed in English and the effect of their use for individuals whose first language is not English. There are two main issues here: the influence of a native language, other than English, on interpretation of and response to test items and the influence of cultural expectations, behaviors, values, etc. on test performance (AERA, 1999; Jensen, 1980; Lam, 1991).

Even within North America and among people whose first language is English, there is a disparity of culture (Jensen, 1980). The life experience of people living in remote areas of the Arctic is vastly different from that of individuals living in urban areas, and both are vastly different from the experience of many people of color. So it is evident that the issue of cultural fairness in assessment is not a simple one to resolve. This section discusses these issues and presents some of the recommendations that have been made to minimize the influence of cultural diversity in the assessment situation.

Language can significantly confound the results obtained on an assessment. When the assessment requires a verbal response or when the test items contain a substantial verbal component, the test may measure language ability more than the underlying construct (AERA, 1999). Language ability affects the reliability of the test by increasing the error component. It is crucial to ascertain the intelligibility of the test items and instructions for individuals whose first language is not English (Jensen, 1980).

One seemingly obvious means to minimize the language issue is to translate the test directly. However, this approach is not as useful as it appears, because language is dynamic, filled with cultural and historical context. Many words or phrases do not have the same meaning when translated from one language to another. For example, *poser un lapin à quelqu'un* is idiomatic French, meaning "to stand someone up." This phrase literally translates to English as "lay a rabbit on someone," which creates quite a different visual image from the French meaning. Direct translation does not account for the dynamic and contextual nature of language.

Test content is another area affected by cultural and language diversity (Lam, 1991). The naming of common objects differs, even among English-speaking cultures. For example, in the United Kingdom, the words *nappy*, *petrol*, and *bonnet* refer to a diaper, gasoline, and the hood of a car. British children who are asked to point to a diaper do not share the North American label for the item and may not be able to identify the target object. Similarly, concepts may differ between cultures. To return to an earlier example, the Woodcock-Johnson Psychoeducational Test Battery (Woodcock, 1978), asks examinees to perform arithmetic calculations using imperial measures. Since Canadian children learn the metric system of measurement, they cannot correctly perform the calculations.

Behavioral expectations vary from one culture to another (AERA, 1999). Children in one culture may be discouraged from responding directly to an adult or from engaging in a detailed conversation. Such behavior is considered rude. On an assessment for which children are expected to express their ideas, children of this culture would perform poorly, not because their ideas are ill-formed but because their cultural expectations preclude them from engaging in a long conversation, thus altering the meaning of their obtained score.

The perception of time and the speed of completion of tasks may vary among cultures. People from cultures in which speed is not emphasized, as it is in North America, will not perform as well on a timed test. Again, scores achieved by these individuals may not reflect their actual ability.

The actual test situation may be unfamiliar for people from some cultures (Lam, 1991). The very act of placing people into a testing situation may put them at a disadvantage. Similarly, some individuals may not be familiar with the completion of computer-marked response cards or may have limited experience using a paper and pencil or a computer. The means of indicating a response in these situations requires skills or exposure to media that are not universal.

The foregoing discussion illustrates the complexity of the issue of performing assessments with individuals of a culture different from the one for which the instrument was standardized. The *Standards for Educational and Psychological Testing* presents several standards to minimize the potential disadvantage to individuals of a diverse culture. These standards, and the recommendations from other writers, which follow, recognize that it is not generally feasible to create a test that may be considered free of cultural bias. It is the ethical responsibility of the examiner to ensure that measures have been taken to minimize the cultural bias (AERA, 1999, Jensen, 1980).

The *Standards for Educational and Psychological Testing* recommends that tests and their use for non-English speakers and those who speak certain English dialects "should be designed to reduce threats to the reliability and validity of test score inferences that may arise from language differences" (AERA, 1999, p. 97). The ability of non-English speakers to understand the test items and instructions should be ascertained, perhaps through the administration of practice items (Jensen, 1980). Test items should be reviewed, during the development phase, by representatives of minority groups to eliminate or modify items with a cultural bias (Jensen, 1980). When language modifications have been made to tests originally developed in English, information should be provided in the test manual to document those modifications and their influence on the psychometric properties of the test.

Therapists must be cognizant of the threats to the validity of the interpretation and inferences of obtained scores when the client is not a native English speaker and/or has a different cultural background. Practitioners have a responsibility to make or use modifications to the evaluation that minimize this threat while realizing that these will affect psychometric properties. If adequate evidence is not available, then the resulting scores cannot be interpreted in a meaningful way—that is, the therapist can have no confidence that the score represents performance on the underlying construct or is the result of construct-irrelevant variance of language or cultural aspects.

ISSUES IN THE EVALUATION OF PEOPLE WITH DISABILITIES

Because of the nature of the occupational therapy profession, the clients whom therapists assess have some form of disability. It is important to recognize the various ways in which a disability will limit performance on a test and, equally, to understand how tests can be misused with this group of individuals. As with the use of tests for people of diverse cultures, the issues here are complex, and the solutions are often incomplete.

The influence of language proficiency on test score interpretation was described earlier. Individuals with language impairments are disadvantaged on a test with a significant language component in the content or administrative process. Individuals who lost their ability to hear at a prelinguistic stage have particular difficulty with language skills (Baker, 1991), as the auditory deficit limits their ability to interact with the aural environment.

Perception of the presentation of the test items raises difficulties for people with a variety of disabilities. Auditory information is perceived with difficulty by those with a hearing impairment (Baker, 1991). Clients with a visual impairment may not perceive information presented visually (Taylor, Sternberg, & Richards, 1995). A learning disability may interfere with the ability to process the information presented.

Individuals whose disability affects motor skills may have difficulty indicating a response when a movement is required (Hacker & Porter, 1987). These clients may have difficulty interacting with the test stimuli or maintaining a proper sitting position during the test; they may not have sufficient endurance to complete the assessment (Hacker & Porter, 1987).

Satisfactory performance on a test depends, in part, on the ability to engage in the testing situation. Individuals with behavioral or emotional problems, cognitive impairment, or learning disability may have difficulty with engagement (Taylor et al., 1995). These individuals may need assistance interacting with the examiner and the test materials and remaining engaged in the testing situation for the required time. A cognitive impairment may limit the person's ability to comprehend verbal or written instructions (Salvia & Ysseldyke, 1985; Taylor et al., 1995). Similarly, a person with aphasia may have difficulty understanding instructions or providing a verbal response (Taylor et al., 1995).

A distinction is made in some sources concerning accommodation versus modification of assessments (Education Accountability Act, 2000, Individuals with Disabilities Education Act Amendments [IDEA], 1997). Accommodations are considered to be changes that enable a person to participate in an assessment but do not alter content (breadth and depth, performance requirements, response method, reliability, or validity) (Ministry of Education, 2000). Modifications, on the other hand, are more significant changes to the assessment and do have implications for reliability, validity, and subsequent inferences made from obtained scores.

As with modification of tests to minimize the influence of cultural diversity, there are no simple solutions to establishing a test that is fair for individuals with disabilities. The *Standards for Educational and Psychological Testing* (AERA, 1999) recommends that practitioners who modify any test for use with an individual with a disability do so with the assistance of an expert in psychometrics. Furthermore, the test user should have knowledge about the manner in which the disability might affect the reliability and validity of the inferences of the test score. Test developers should report any modifications that they have made to the test for its use with persons with disabilities and report the effect of these modifications on the psychometric properties.

When conducting evaluations with children with disabilities in the school system, occupational therapists must know the regulations that govern such assessment. I will describe two examples of these regulations: the U.S. IDEA Amendment of 1997 and the Education Accountability Act of the province of Ontario, Canada. Both pieces of legislation require that students with disabilities be afforded the opportunity to participate in state or provincial standardized testing. Evaluation must be conducted in such a way that the score can be meaningfully interpreted to reflect the child's performance on the underlying construct and not be biased by some extraneous variable (i.e., irrelevant to the construct), such as language or motor ability (Education Accountability Act, 2000; IDEA, 1997).

Both IDEA and the Education Accountability Act indicate that modifications or accommodations are to be used, as appropriate, providing there is evidence of reliability and validity with the specific modifications. These modifications are to be similar to those identified in the students' individual education plans as needed for their engagement in academic activities. Specific modifications include changes to time requirements, format of administration or response, language, setting, and individual or group administration. Specific accommodations include alteration of test administration (large print, Braille translation, interpreter for the hearing impaired, multiple sessions), response method (oral response, use of computer access devices), and setting (segregated area) (Assistance to States for the Education of Children with Disabilities and Early Intervention Program for Infants and Toddlers with Disabilities, 1999; Ministry of Education, 2000).

IDEA (1997; Assistance to States for the Education of Children with Disabilities and Early Intervention Program for Infants and Toddlers with Disabilities, 1999) further requires the following provisions: Evaluations should be

- Free of racial and or cultural bias.
- Available and administered in the student's native language or by some other mode of communication.
- Examined for evidence of validity for the specified purpose.
- Administered (and interpreted) by trained and knowledgeable personnel.
- Administered according to the standards of the test developer.

This discussion of the challenges of evaluating clients with disabilities in a fair manner underlines the responsibility of the therapist for an appropriate, meaningful, and relevant interpretation of the obtained score. Satisfactory validity evidence must be present to support the intended purpose of the test and the interpretation of the scores and the actions that arise from that interpretation. Particularly when the outcome of the evaluation has the potential to influence education, employment, or living situation, the therapist must be able to demonstrate the validity of the inferences made from the score. This responsibility is not one to be taken lightly.

CONCLUSION

This chapter provided an overview of issues with which an occupational therapist must be familiar to critique an assessment. A number of sources are available that provide reviews of published tests. The *Mental Measurements Yearbook* (e.g., Conoley, 1995) provide reviews of most of the commercially available tests. Each successive edition reviews tests published since the last edition and updates reviews of the major tests. *Tests in Print* (e.g., Murphy, Impara, & Plake, 1999) provides descriptive information and bibliographies. There are several journals that publish reviews of a wide variety of tests, along with their reliability and validity, and theoretical discussions of these properties. Some of the more useful ones are *Educational and Psychological Measurement*, *Journal of Applied Psychology*, *Journal of Chronic Diseases* (now *Journal of Clinical Epidemiology*), and *Psychological Assessment*.

This chapter is meant to be an overview of the critical concerns in the critique of evaluations. It is not intended to include a detailed discussion of all aspects, formulas, and calculations of test construction, item analysis, reliability, and validity. More detailed information and reviews of commonly used assessments in occupational therapy are available in the literature.

ACKNOWLEDGMENTS

Jennifer Landry, School of Occupational Therapy, Dalhousie University, and Linda Miller, School of Occupational Therapy, The University of Western Ontario, provided valuable feedback on an earlier draft of this chapter. Joseph Hansen, Detroit Country Day School, provided French language consultation. Jackie Klee, School of Occupational Therapy, The University of Western Ontario, helped edit the current draft. Ernest Skakun, Division of Studies in Medical Education, University of Alberta, provided many lively discussions of psychometrics that helped frame some of the ideas in this chapter.

References

American Educational Research Association, American Psychological Association, & National Council on Measurement in Education [AERA]. (1999). *Standards for educational and psychological testing*. Washington, DC: American Psychological Association.*

Anastasi, A., & Urbina, S. (1997). *Psychological testing* (7th ed.). Upper Saddle River, NJ: Prentice Hall.*

Assistance to States for the Education of Children with Disabilities and Early Intervention Program for Infants and Toddlers with Disabilities: Final Regulations, 64 Fed. Reg. 12406 (1999). (to be codified at 34 C.F.R. §§ 300, 303).

Baker, R. M. (1991). Evaluation of hearing-impaired children. In K. E. Green (Ed.). *Educational testing: Issues and applications* (pp. 77–107). New York: Garland.

Barclay, J. R. (1991). *Psychological assessment: A theory and systems approach*. Malabar, FL: Krieger.

Bensen, J., & Clark, F. (1982). A guide for instrument development and validation. *American Journal of Occupational Therapy, 36*(12), 789–800.

Carmines, E. G., & Zeller, R. A. (1979). *Reliability and validity assessment*. Newbury Park, CA: Sage.*

Conoley, J. C. (Ed.). (1995). Mental measurement yearbook. New York: Buros Institute.

Cronbach, L. J. (1951). Coefficient alpha and the internal structure of tests. *Psychometrika, 16*, 297–334.

Cronbach, L. J. (1988). Five perspectives on validity. In H. Wainer & H. Braun (Eds.). *Test validity* (pp. 3–17). Hillsdale, NJ: Erlbaum.

DePoy E., & Gitlin, L. N. (1998). *Introduction to research: Understanding and applying multiple strategies* (2nd ed.). St. Louis, MO: Mosby.*

Education Accountability Act (2000). Toronto, ON: Queen's Printer for Ontario.

Gowland, C., King, G., King, S., Law, M., Letts, L., MacKinnon, E., Rosenbaum, P., & Russell, D. (1991). *Review of selected measures in neurodevelopmental rehabilitation* (Neurodevelopmental Clinical Research Unit Rep. No. 91-2). Hamilton, ON, Canada: Neurodevelopmental Clinical Research Unit.

Green, K. E. (1991). Reliability, validity, and test score interpretation. In K. E. Green (Ed.). *Educational testing: Issues and applications* (pp. 27–38). New York: Garland.

Guyatt, G., Walter, S., & Norman, G. (1987). Measuring change over time: Assessing the usefulness of evaluative instruments. *Journal of Chronic Diseases*, 40(2), 171–178.

Hacker, B. J., & Porter, P. B. (1987). Use of standardized tests with the physically handicapped. In L. King-Thomas & B. J. Hacker (Eds.). *A therapist's guide to pediatric assessment* (pp. 35–40). Boston: Little, Brown.

Haertel, E. (1999). Validity arguments for high-stakes testing: In search of evidence. *Educational Measurement, 18*(4), 5–9.

Hamer, S., & Collinson, G. (1999). *Achieving evidence-based practice: A handbook for practitioners*. Edinburgh: Tindall.

Individuals with Disabilities Education Act Amendments [IDEA], U.S.C.A. § 600 et seq. (1977).

Isaac, S., & Michael, W. B. (1971). *Handbook in research and evaluation*. San Diego, CA: EdITS.

Jensen, A. R. (1980). *Bias in mental testing*. New York: Free Press.

Kerlinger, F. A. (1973). *Foundations in behavioral research*. New York: Holt, Rinehart & Winston.

King-Thomas, L., & Hacker, B. J. (Eds.). (1987). *A therapist's guide to pediatric assessment*. Boston: Little, Brown.

Kirshner, B., & Guyatt, B. (1985). A methodological framework for assessing health indices. *Journal of Chronic Diseases, 38*(1), 27–36.

Kuder, G. F., & Richardson, M. (1937). The theory of the estimation test reliability. *Psychometrika, 2*, 151–160.

Lam, T. C. M. (1991). Testing of limited English proficient children. In K. E. Green (Ed.). *Educational testing: Issues and applications* (pp. 125–167). New York: Garland.

Law, M. (1987). Measurement in occupational therapy: Scientific criteria for evaluation. *Canadian Journal of Occupational Therapy*, 54(3), 133–138.

Lees-Haley, P. R. (1996). Alice in validityland, or the dangerous consequences of consequential validity. *American Psychologist, 51*, 981–983.

McCarthy, D. (1972). *McCarthy scales of children's abilities*. San Antonio, TX: Psychological Corp.

Messick, S. (1988). The once and future issues of validity: Assessing the meaning and consequences of measurement. In H. Wainer & H. Braun (Eds.). *Test validity* (pp. 33–45). Hillsdale, NJ: Erlbaum.

Messick, S. (1989). Validity. In R. L. Linn (Ed.). *Educational measurement* (pp. 13–103). New York: Macmillan.

Messick, S. (1995). Validity of psychological assessment: Validation inferences from person's responses and performances as scientific inquiry into score meaning. *American Psychologist*, 50(9), 741–749.

Ministry of Education. (2000). *Individual education plans: Standards for development, program planning, and implementation*. Toronto: Author.

Moss, P. A. (1995). Themes and variations in validity theory. *Educational Measurement, 14*, 5–13.

Murphy, K. R., & Davidshofer, C. O. (1991). Psychological testing: principles and applications (2nd ed.). Englewood Cliffs, NJ: Prentice-Hall.

Murphy, L. L., Impara, J. C., & Plake, B. S. (Eds.). (1999). *Tests in print V: An index to tests, test reviews and the literature on specific tests*. Lincoln: University of Nebraska Press.

Nunnally, J. C., & Bernstein, I. H. (1995). *Psychometric theory* (3rd ed.). Toronto: McGraw-Hill.*

Pedhazur, E. J., & Schmelkin, L. P. (1991). *Measurement, design and analysis: An integrated approach*. Hillsdale, NJ: Erlbaum.*

Portney, L. G., & Watkins, M. P. (2000) *Foundations of clinical research: Applications to practice* (2nd ed.). Upper Saddle River, NJ: Prentice Hall.*

Rotter, J. (1966). Generalized expectancies for internal versus external control of reinforcement. *Psychological Monographs*, *80*, 1–28.

Sackett, D. L., Straus, S. E., Richardson, W. S., Rosenberg, W., & Haynes, R. B. (2000). *Evidence-based medicine: How to practice and teach EBM* (2nd ed.). Edinburgh, UK: Churchill Livingstone.

Salvia, J., & Ysseldyke, J. E. (1985). *Assessment in special and remedial education* (3rd ed.). Boston: Houghton Mifflin.

Siegel, L. S. (1989). A reconceptualization of prediction from infant test scores. In M. bornstein & N. A. Krasnegor (Eds.). Stability and continuity in mental development (pp. 89–103). Hillsdale, NJ: Erlbaum.

Taylor, R. L., Sternberg, L., & Richards, S. B. (1995). *Exceptional children: Integrating research and teaching* (2nd ed.). San Diego, CA: Singular.

Townsend, E., Stanton, S., Law, M., Polatajko, H., Baptiste, S., Thompson-Franson, T., Kramer, C., Swedlove, F., Brintnell, S., & Campanile, L. (1997). *Enabling occupation: An occupational therapy perspective*. Ottawa, ON, Canada: CAOT.

Wiersma, W., & Jurs, S. G. (1990). *Educational measurement and testing* (2nd ed.). Needham Heights, MA: Allyn & Bacon.

Witt, J. C., Elliott, S. N., Gresham, F. M., & Kramer, J. J. (1988). *Assessment of special children*. Glenview, IL: Scott, Foresman.

Woodcock, R. (1978). *Woodcock-Johnson psycho-educational battery*. Hingham, MA: Teaching Resources.

Zeidner, M., & Most, R. (1992). *Psychological testing: An inside view*. Palo Alto, CA: Consulting Psychologists.

Zimiles, H. (1996). Rethinking the validity of psychological assessment. *American Psychologist*. *51*, 980–981.

*This source provides more detailed information and/or is a review of assessments commonly used in occupational therapy.

CHAPTER 24

EVALUATION OF AREAS OF OCCUPATION

SECTION I: Activities of Daily Living and Instrumental Activities of Daily Living
SECTION II: Therapeutic Driving and Community Mobility
SECTION III: Work Activities
SECTION IV: Educational Activities
SECTION V: Play and Leisure

SECTION I

Activities of Daily Living and Instrumental Activities of Daily Living

JOAN C. ROGERS
MARGO B. HOLM

This section focuses on the evaluation of areas of occupation classified as activities of daily living (ADL) and instrumental activities of daily living (IADL) in the occupational therapy practice framework (American Occupational Therapy Association [AOTA], in press). Dysfunctions in ADL and IADL, formerly labeled disability in the classification system of the World Health Organization (1980), are termed *activity limitations* in the International Classification of Functioning, Disability, and Health (ICF, 2001) framework. Evaluation is a key aspect of the occupational therapy process because it establishes the direction for therapeutic actions. Core questions to be addressed concerning the evaluation of ADL and IADL are the following:

- What use is to be made of the evaluation data?
- What activities are to be evaluated?
- What parameters of activity performance are to be evaluated?
- How are activities to be evaluated?
- How are evaluation data to be integrated for clinical decision making?
- What instruments are available to aid data gathering?

These questions provide the organizational scheme for this section and each question is addressed in sequence.

PURPOSE OF EVALUATION OF ADL AND IADL

ADL and IADL may be evaluated for different purposes. At the level of individual client care, evaluation may be done to (1) screen for activity limitations, (2) assess activity limitations to plan occupational therapy intervention, or (3) facilitate decision making concerning actions such as discharge disposition or legal competence for independent living. At the programmatic level, evaluation may be done to document the need for program expansion or development and to appraise outcomes. Before starting an evaluation, the practitioner must determine how the information will be used so that appropriate and sufficient data are obtained.

Screening

Screening involves a cursory evaluation to determine if a more intensive evaluation is needed. It is a case-finding procedure intended to separate individuals who have or are at risk for developing activity limitations from those who do not have or are not at risk for developing activity limitations. Because screening procedures are often applied to large groups of individuals, such as all applicants for an independent living program or all new clients in an outpatient clinic, they should be brief, easy to administer, and inexpensive. At the same time, they must have sufficient sensitivity to detect activity limitations, so that individuals who have such limitations are not incorrectly classified as not having them and, therefore, not needing further evaluation and help. Screening procedures do not need to be done by occupational therapy practitioners. They form the basis of any referral to occupational therapy and may be conducted by health-care, social services, and educational personnel; potential clients; and family members of potential clients.

Evaluation

Evaluation of ADL and IADL is more comprehensive and detailed than screening and must be conducted by an occupational therapy practitioner. Its purpose is to identify the ADL and IADL for which limitations are present or may be developing. Evaluation data may be used to plan and monitor occupational therapy interventions or to assist in decision making relative to disposition, competency, conservatorship, and/or involuntary commitment. The extent of data gathering depends on the specific purpose for which the evaluation is being conducted.

Plan and Monitor Occupational Therapy Interventions

Before practitioners intervene to improve performance of ADL or IADL, they must evaluate clients' baseline performance. When an evaluation is conducted to plan occupational therapy intervention, four types of data are needed (Rogers, Holm, & Stone, 1997). First, activities in which performance is deficient need to be identified. To target intervention appropriately, the identification of deficits needs to be precise. Knowing that clients have a limitation in oral hygiene is insufficient for planning intervention. The evaluation needs to inform practitioners about the specific components of oral hygiene (e.g., removing dentures, preparing denture solution) that clients can and cannot perform. Occupational therapy intervention can then be targeted to develop or compensate for the components that are dysfunctional, while simultaneously maintaining and enhancing those that are functional.

Second, data are needed about the cause or causes of the activity limitation. For example, a limitation in cooking might be caused by low vision, a wheelchair–inaccessible kitchen, a lack of proficiency in cooking, or poor motivation to cook. Occupational therapy intervention for a limitation in cooking is different for each of these causes. Problems caused by low vision might be alleviated through assistive technology, such as a high-intensity light. Elimination of architectural barriers might remedy the inaccessible kitchen. Training might be initiated to improve cooking skills, and apathy may be approached through a structured program of activities meeting a client's interests and abilities. As these examples illustrate, to understand the etiology of an activity limitation, data about occupational areas (ADL, IADL) need to be supplemented with data about activity demands (visual acuity) and contexts (physical structures).

Third, the occupational therapy evaluation should provide data about clients' capacities for modifying their activity performance. These data also assist in establishing an overall approach to occupational therapy intervention. Interventions involving skill acquisition are feasible for clients who demonstrate the ability to learn, whereas environmental modifications are appropriate for those lacking this ability.

Fourth, the evaluation should yield data about the kinds of occupational therapy interventions that are most likely to develop or improve performance. When an evaluation is conducted with the intent of providing intervention, it must go beyond describing activity limitations to providing data that enable practitioners to create a therapeutic situation that will likely move clients along the continuum of dysfunction to function. The practice of occupational therapy incorporates a broad array of restorative, compensatory, and preventive interventions that can be brought to bear on activity limitations and their precursors. An essential yield of the evaluation process is a narrowing down of this array so that occupational therapy practitioners can select those interventions that are most likely to elicit positive outcomes within the projected time constraints for therapy.

The first two types of evaluation data—identifying activity limitations and their causes—are diagnostic in nature. The last two types of evaluation data—determining clients' modifiability and ascertaining potential interventions—are therapeutically oriented. All four types of data are needed to devise adequate intervention plans. Once an intervention is implemented, its effects on performance need to be monitored. Hence, re-evaluations need to be undertaken periodically to ascertain if the intervention is alleviating the activity limitations; if not, a change of approach is needed.

Facilitate Decision Making

Clients may be also referred for evaluation of ADL and IADL to facilitate decision making about eligibility or disposition. The ability to care for oneself and one's home lies at the interface between independent and supported or assisted living. Supported living represents a continuum of options that includes in-home services (e.g., chore services), personal care homes, assisted living centers, foster homes, group homes, independent living centers, supervised apartments, and transitional apartments. Within each setting, a range of supports is offered to maintain or enhance daily living skills. At the extreme dependency end of this continuum is institutionalization (e.g., long-term care facility) where all ADL and IADL needs can be met.

Each point on this continuum, as well as each service or facility, has ADL and IADL requirements that must be met for eligibility or admission. For example, depending on the site, residents may or may not need to manage their own medications or keep their rooms clean and tidy. When ADL and IADL are evaluated to serve these types of eligibility or disposition decisions, the evaluation may be less comprehensive and detailed than when it is done to plan individual interventions. The primary question to be answered through the evaluation is, Does the client meet the functional criteria? This question can generally be answered by identifying activities in which limitations are present.

A somewhat similar evaluation objective occurs when occupational therapy practitioners are asked to make recommendations regarding legal competence for independent living. This usually involves competence in caring for oneself or competence in managing one's property. Difficulties with the first type of competence lead to legal proceedings called guardianship, whereas difficulties with the second type of competence involve conservatorship. Evaluation may also be requested in conjunction with involuntary commitments to psychiatric facilities to appraise the influence of psychiatric status on daily living. Individuals are usually not competent or incompetent; rather competence is exhibited in some activities but not in others. When competence is used in the legal sense, the capacity to make judicious or responsible decisions usually takes precedence over the capacity to perform activities. Individuals who have the ability to procure services and supervise caregivers in managing their personal care and living situation are viewed as competent, even though they may not be able to perform these activities themselves. Thus occupational therapy evaluations conducted with guardianship, conservatorship, or involuntary commitment in mind must take into account the decisional capacities and supervisory skills needed by clients.

Programmatic Uses

Although this section emphasizes evaluation for individual client care, it is important to recognize that data gathered about clients may be aggregated for programmatic purposes. For example, data about the ADL and IADL characteristics of clients served in an occupational therapy clinic may be used to document the extent of particular activity limitations and to support the development of new or expanded programs to manage them. In the current health-care climate of cost effectiveness and cost containment, group data are increasingly being used to evaluate the outcomes of occupational therapy programs, occupational therapy interventions, and even the productivity of individual occupational therapy practitioners (DeJong & Sutton, 1995).

CONTENT OF ADL AND IADL EVALUATION

One of the first decisions occupational therapy practitioners must make when approaching an ADL or IADL evaluation concerns the specific activities to be evaluated. In making this decision, multiple conceptual and practical issues need to be taken into account. Terms (i.e., concepts) used in reference to ADL and IADL need to be understood. The application of these concepts in practice through their operationalization, including activity analysis, needs to be critically appraised. Most important, clients' needs must be recognized and the implications of terminology and its operationalization for clients' care must be carefully considered.

Differences in Terminology

Conceptually, ADL could apply to all activities that individuals perform routinely. The term *activities of daily living* was coined by Deaver to refer to a wide range of behavior patterns considered necessary for meeting the demands of daily living (United States Department of Education, 1982). In the Occupational Therapy Practice Framework (OTPF: AOTA, in press), ADL are divided into 11 activity categories: bathing/ showering, bowel and bladder management, dressing, eating, feeding, functional mobility, personal device care, personal hygiene and grooming, sexual activity, sleep/rest, and toilet hygiene. IADL also make up 11 activity categories: care of others, care of pets, child rearing, communication device use, community mobility, financial management, health and maintenance, home establishment and management, meal preparation and clean up, safety procedures and emergency responses, and shopping.

The OTPF (AOTA, in press) provides a nomenclature and organizational scheme for occupational therapy practitioners. Other health-care and social services practitioners may be unfamiliar with this terminology and may use other terms to refer to these same ADL and IADL concepts or may use the same terms but define them differently. For example, the term *ADL* is generally restricted to activities involving functional mobility and personal care. Ambulation and wheelchair mobility, transfers, feeding, hygiene, toileting, bathing, and dressing are typically covered under ADL. Synonyms for ADL are *basic ADL*, *physical ADL*, *basic self-maintenance*, *physical self-maintenance*, and *personal self-maintenance* (Fillenbaum, 1988; Lawton, 1972; Lawton & Brody, 1969). Similarly, the term *IADL* is generally applied to activities required for independent living and includes telephone use, shopping, food preparation, housekeeping, medication management, financial management, and getting around one's community. Laundering and leisure may also be considered under IADL. Synonyms for IADL are *independent living skills*, *advanced ADL*, and *extended ADL* (Lawton & Brody, 1969; Nouri & Lincoln, 1987). More recently, the acronym AADL—for advanced activities of daily living—has come into use to capture activities that are more physically strenuous than IADL (Reuben, Laliberte, Hiris, & Mor, 1990). AADL include participating in active sports that may cause the individual to become winded or to work up a sweat, walking 1 mile or more without resting, walking ¼ mile or more without resting, entertaining at home, visiting the homes of others, going out to eat with others, working at a hobby, and traveling out of town. In the OTPF (AOTA, in press), these activities are classified as play, leisure, or social participation.

Occupational therapy practitioners need to be aware of the differences in terminology and use when communicating with other professionals and when selecting evaluation instruments. Practitioners must know how to respond appropriately to a referral for an IADL evaluation. Table 24-1 lists specific activities commonly found on ADL and IADL measures related to functional mobility, personal care, and home management.

Operationalization of Concepts

Before functional mobility, personal care, and home management activities can be evaluated, they must be operationally defined—that is, the occupational therapy practitioner must know the precise meaning of each term. An operational definition is one that provides guidelines for measurement (Rothstein, 1985). It is an instructional tool that informs practitioners about the activities that are to be evaluated and the components of those activities (Eakin, 1989). For example, because feeding is an abstract concept, it cannot be observed. Feeding takes on concreteness and precision when it is operationalized as "moving solid and liquid food from dinnerware to the mouth." The movement of solid and liquid food from dinnerware to the mouth is observable and measurable.

A single concept may be operationalized in different ways, as is illustrated by the following definitions of feeding independence, which are on three widely used functional assessments:

On the Barthel Index (Barthel) independence in feeding is defined as:

> *The patient can feed himself from a tray or table when someone puts the food within his reach. He must put on an assistive device if this is needed, cut up food, use salt and pepper, spread butter etc. He must accomplish this in a reasonable time. (Mahoney & Barthel, 1965, p. 62)*

On the Katz Index of ADL (Index of ADL), independence in feeding is defined as:

> *Gets food from plate or its equivalent into mouth; (precutting of meal and preparation of food, as buttering bread, are excluded from evaluation). (Katz, Ford, Moskowitz, Jackson, & Jaffe, 1963, p. 915)*

On the Functional Independence Measure (FIM™), independence in feeding is defined as:

> *All of the tasks described as making up the activity are typically performed safely, without modification, assistive devices, or aids, within a reasonable amount of time. (Uniform Data System for Medical Rehabilitation [UDSMR], 1993, p. III-4)*

> *Subject eats from a dish, while managing all consistencies of food, and drinks from a cup or glass with the meal presented in the customary manner on a table or tray. The subject uses a spoon or fork to bring food to the mouth; food is chewed and swallowed. Performs safely. (p. III-6)*

Thus Mr. Miles, a client who can perform hand-to-mouth actions but cannot cut his food, is dependent in feeding

TABLE 24–1. **FUNCTIONAL MOBILITY, PERSONAL CARE, AND HOME MANAGEMENT ACTIVITIES INCLUDED IN EVALUATION TOOLS**

Functional Mobility

Move in bed
- Shift position
- Turn
- Sit

Transfer
- Bed
- Chair
- Bathtub
- Shower
- Car

Sit in chair

Stand

Walk
- Level surface
- Environmental terrain
- Ramps
- Curbs
- Stairs

Community mobility
- Get in or out of residence
- Cross street
- Around neighborhood
- To bus stop

Work-related
- Bending, kneeling, stooping
- Lifting and carrying
- Reaching
- Pushing and pulling
- Manipulating

Personal Care

Feeding/eating
- Feed from dish
- Drink from cup, glass, straw
- Use utensils
- Cut food
- Manage finger food
- Bite and chew
- Swallow

Hygiene
- Clean teeth/dentures
- Brush, comb hair
- Shave
- Apply makeup
- Groom nails

Bathe
- Upper body
  - Face
  - Hands
  - Arms
  - Trunk
- Lower Body
  - Groin
  - Buttocks
  - Upper legs
  - Lower legs/feet

Dress
- Upper body
  - Front opening garments
  - Pull over garments
  - Brassiere
  - Corset/brace
  - Hearing aid/eye glasses
- Lower body
  - Underclothing
  - Slacks/skirt
  - Socks, stockings
  - Shoes
  - Brace, prosthesis
  - Fasteners

Toileting
- Handle clothing
- Wipe
- Flush
- Control bladder
- Control bowels

Communicate
- Comprehend spoken language
- Comprehend written language
- Comprehend symbols
- Express basic needs
  - Speech
  - Writing
  - Sign/gesture

Home Management

Meal preparation
- Prepare cold food
- Prepare hot food
  - Use appliances/utensils
  - Use oven
  - Use stovetop

Housecleaning
- Light housecleaning
  - Dust
  - Tidy up
  - Wash and dry dishes
- Heavy housecleaning
  - Vacuum
  - Wash windows
  - Clean bathtub, refrigerator, stove

Finances
- Manage cash exchanges
- Write checks
- Balance checkbook
- Keep financial records
- Assemble tax records

Shopping
- For food
- For clothing
- For household necessities

Telephoning
- Locate number
- Dial telephone
- Give messages
- Receive messages

Medication management
- Manage containers
- Take as directed
- Refill prescription

Laundry
- Wash clothes
- Manage drying clothes
- Put clothes away properly

Time management
- Plan, organize, follow through
- Keep track of appointments

Transportation
- Drive car
- Public transportation

on the Barthel but independent on the Index of ADL. Furthermore, because he needs to use feeding utensils with enlarged handles, he cannot be rated as fully independent on the FIM™. His rating on the FIM™ would also be reduced because he tends to choke when swallowing liquids, a component of feeding that is not included on the Barthel or Index of ADL.

As might be expected because of their increased complexity, the operational definitions of IADL are more varied than those for ADL. The domain of meal preparation illustrates this point well. On the Instrumental Activities of Daily Living Scale (IADL Scale), which is generally considered to be the prototype instrument for IADL, the highest level of competence is described as "plans, prepares, and serves adequate meals independently" (Lawton, 1972, p. 133). Comparable items on the Nottingham Extended ADL Index inquire about the ability to make a hot drink and hot snack alone and easily (Nouri & Lincoln, 1987). Thus, a rating of independence in cooking achieved on the Nottingham Extended ADL Index implies less competence than a rating of independence on the IADL Scale.

Concepts are operationalized so that occupational therapy practitioners know what to look for when conducting an evaluation. The operationalization of concepts is similar to the process of activity analysis, by which activities are broken down into the functional subactivities needed to complete them. In Table 24-2, we analyzed the content of the Barthel, Index of ADL, and FIM™ definitions of independent feeding and added the activity analysis from the Klein-Bell ADL Scale (Klein & Bell, 1979). Given the data previously presented about Mr. Miles's feeding abilities, his feeding performance is rated on the four instruments, using able and unable as the measurement scale. By reviewing the subactivities, the nature of Mr. Miles's eating limitations and abilities can be described explicitly.

The Barthel identified limitations in cutting food and spreading butter, the FIM™ identified a swallowing dysfunction, and the Klein-Bell ADL Scale noted problems in cutting food and swallowing liquid without choking. However, only the scoring system of the Klein-Bell ADL Scale, which allows subactivities to be rated individually, yields evaluation data that enable occupational therapy interventions to be targeted precisely to the dysfunctional activity components. The Barthel, Index of ADL, and FIM™ do not yield retrievable data about subactivity performance, because they are global scales. On global scales, activity domains (e.g., feeding, dressing) are rated as a unit rather than by the subactivities making up these domains. Although subactivities are taken into account in the operational definition of an activity, these details become lost (Settle & Holm, 1993). On the Barthel, for example, because of Mr. Miles's inability to cut food and spread butter, he is rated as dependent in feeding; however, the instrument records only his overall dependency in feeding and not where this dependency occurs.

TABLE 24-2. **ACTIVITY ANALYSIS OF MR. MILES'S FEEDING BY INSTRUMENT**

	Mr. Miles's Performance	
Instrument	**Able**	**Unable**
The Barthel (Mahoney & Barthel, 1965)		
Put on assistive device	X	
Feed self	X	
Cut food		X
Use salt and pepper	X	
Spread butter		X
Index of ADL		
Get food from plate (or its equivalent) into mouth	X	
FIM™ (Uniform Data System for Medical Rehabilitation, 1993)		
Eats all food consistencies from a dish	X	
Drinks from a cup/glass	X	
Uses a spoon or fork to bring food to mouth	X (with device)	
Chews food	X	
Swallows food		X (unsafe)
Klein-Bell ADL Scale (Klein & Bell, 1979)		
Eat Solid food		
Grasp fork/spoon	X	
Cut food		X
Spear food portion with fork	X	
Place portion inside mouth	X	
Chew	X	
Swallow	X	
Eat Semisolid food		
Scoop food portion onto utensil	X	
Place food inside mouth	X	
Eat Liquid food		
Scoop food portion from bowl	X	
Place food portion inside mouth	X	
Drink		
Grasp container	X	
Bring container to mouth	X	
Intake liquid without spilling	X	
Swallow liquid without choking		X

Practice Guidelines: Content

Client-centered care requires that the occupational therapy evaluation responds to the unique needs and living situations of individuals. Practitioners can expect the activities of concern for a 29-year-old homemaker who is caring for three young children to be different from those of concern for a 49-year-old business executive; and the evaluations of these clients need to be tailored to take their lifestyle differences into account. Occupational therapy practitioners need to give careful attention to the way in which they operationalize ADL and IADL, whether this operationalization occurs through the instruments they select to administer or the informal procedures they implement.

Our review of several definitions of feeding and meal preparation made it apparent that clients may be made more or less independent or dependent in an activity, depending on how it is defined and measured by the practitioner. Because of the loss of descriptive data, global scales are less useful for planning occupational therapy interventions than are scales that employ detailed activity analyses. Global scales may be more useful when screening for activity limitations than when evaluating with the intent to intervene. Because global scales are less sensitive to change, they are also less useful for documenting progress resulting from rehabilitation.

PARAMETERS OF ADL AND IADL EVALUATION

The activities classified as ADL and IADL define the content of the occupational therapy evaluation for these areas. When planning an evaluation, decisions must be made about the parameters of activity performance to evaluate as well as the content of the evaluation. What is it about activity performance that practitioners want to know? Do they want to learn where an activity is performed, when it is performed, or how it is performed? The parameters of activity performance direct attention to the dimensions of ADL and IADL that are to be evaluated. Parameters of activity performance are a part of the operational definition of an activity (Eakin, 1989; Rothstein, 1985). In our review of the operational definitions of feeding on the Barthel, Index of ADL, and FIM™ scales, we considered not just feeding but independence in feeding. Independence was the parameter used to evaluate feeding. In general, ADL and IADL evaluation provides data about those activities that clients can do safely, independently, efficiently, and adequately and those activities for which supervision, assistance, or modification is required because of deficits in safety, independence, efficiency, or adequacy.

Evaluative Approaches

The parameters of activity performance may be evaluated through qualitative or quantitative approaches. In the qualitative approach, activity performance is described. In the quantitative approach, it is measured. Both approaches incorporate clinical reasoning to integrate evaluative data and ascertain its meaning.

Qualitative Approach

In the qualitative approach to evaluation, the salient characteristics of clients' activity performance are described. These descriptions are used to formulate inferences about clients' performance on the evaluation parameters of interest. A practitioner might note, for instance, that a client, Mr. Brand, could not sufficiently bend (flex) at the waist to reach his feet with his hands and could not sufficiently bend (hip external rotation; knee flexion) his lower extremities to move his feet closer to his hands. From these observations, the practitioner might infer that the client is unable to don socks and other lower extremity garments and thus rates Mr. Brand as dependent in lower extremity dressing. Both the data and the conclusions drawn from the data are managed qualitatively.

Quantitative Approach

In the quantitative approach to evaluation, the evaluation parameters of interest are quantified through the assignment of numbers (Wade, 1992). Numbers can aid in determining the severity of dysfunction and the extent of improvement or deterioration. However, they can also lead to misinterpretations and erroneous conclusions, which is why it is important to understand the numbers that are generated by various measures and the mathematical procedures that can be appropriately applied to them. Each of the four levels of measurement—nominal, ordinal, interval, and ratio—is applicable to ADL and IADL evaluation.

Nominal measurement involves the use of discrete categories. For example, dressing limitations might be diagnosed as 1 = related to physical impairment, 2 = related to cognitive impairment, and 3 = related to emotional impairment. The numbers *1*, *2*, and *3* merely indicate different types of dressing limitations. There is no implication that a limitation of emotional etiology, which is assigned a 3, is better or worse or more or less than a limitation having a cognitive or physical basis, which are given a 2 and 1, respectively. Nominal measurement is essentially a process of grouping similar data and naming or labeling it (Fox, 1969; Wade, 1992). Nominal data cannot be added and subtracted, because these manipulations have no numeric meaning.

Ordinal measurement entails a rank ordering of scores. A dressing limitation, for example, may be rated as: 1 = requires minimal assistance, 2 = requires moderate assistance, and 3 = requires maximal assistance. In this case, a 1 signifies less limitation than a 3. However, the difference between requiring minimal and moderate assistance and between requiring moderate and maximal assistance—that is, between a 1 and 2 or a 2 and 3—are unknown. Hence, it cannot be stated that a client who receives a 2 has twice as much dressing limitation as the one receiving a 1. To make such a comparative statement, the unit of measurement (e.g., amount of assistance) must have the same quantitative meaning at each point on the scale. Thus, for example, caregivers must expend twice as much energy assisting clients scoring 2 than they do assisting clients scoring 1.

Ordinal measurement may also be devised using an activity-descriptive approach. In this approach, each point on a scale is defined in terms of specific activity behaviors. Dressing performance might be scaled as follows: 3 = locates, selects, and dons appropriate clothing; 2 = dons but cannot locate or select appropriate clothing; and 1 = cannot locate, select, or don appropriate clothing. In this example, dressing is scaled based on features that are inherent to, as well as essential to, activity performance.

In interval measurement, the unit of measurement has the same quantitative meaning at any point on the scale. A 5-lb weight loss represents the same amount whether the weight loss occurs from 105 to 100 lb or from 350 to 345 lb. Because of this quality, comparative statements can be made, as the difference between any two scores is equal. At this level of measurement, scores can be added and subtracted, but not multiplied or divided. Unfortunately, it is difficult to create equal-interval scales in regard to ADL and IADL because it is difficult to determine the weight to attach to individual activities.

Ratio measurement is distinguished by having a definite or fixed zero point as well as an equal-interval scale. An example of ratio measurement would be measuring the time a client takes to complete dressing. Timing would begin when the first piece of clothing is picked up and would terminate when the last piece of clothing was donned. The time elapsed from start to finish would be the client's score. All arithmetic operations can be applied to ratio data.

Parameters of Activity Performance for Description and Measurement

The parameters of activity performance that occupational therapists are most interested in evaluating are value, independence, safety, and quality (i.e., efficiency, adequacy, and acceptability). Figure 24-1 provides an overview of the parameters discussed.

Value

When evaluating the meaning of activity performance and activity performance dysfunctions to clients, data about the **value** that they place on different activities is essential. Value reflects the importance or significance of an activity to the client. As an evaluation parameter, value is usually used in reference to the independent performance of activities. Chiou and Burnett (1985), for example, ascertained that of 15 ADL, the ability to move indoors independently was most valued by clients with stroke. Similarly, Atwood, Holm, and James (1994) determined that nursing home residents reported higher capability in personal care activities for which independence was most valued. Because our actions as humans are influenced by our values, ascertaining the relative value that different activities have for clients is useful for establishing intervention priorities and for negotiating target intervention outcomes with them.

Independence

The most common parameter used to measure activity performance is the level of **independence** clients exhibit when performing an activity. A rating of independence or able means that clients are able to perform an activity by themselves. Conversely, a rating of **dependence** or unable means that clients are unable to perform an activity by themselves, in other words, that help is required. When activity performance is not totally independent, a more refined measurement scale may be used to quantify the extent of independence. For example, activity performance may be rated as 75% independent, 50% independent, or 25% independent. Alternately, the reference point used to measure limitations may be the effort exerted by caregivers, rather than clients. For example, caregivers may provide no, minimal, moderate, or maximal assistance of one or more persons to the client.

When assistance is required to complete an activity, the type of help needed may be added to the rating scale. Three general types of assistance are recognized and are rank ordered from least to most assistive as follows: assistive technology, nonphysical assistance, and physical assistance. Assistive technology—which is also referred to as assistive devices, adaptive equipment, technical aids, and self-help aids—qualifies as the least assistive type of help when it enables activity performance to be adaptive but independent. Clients who can feed themselves using utensils with enlarged or elongated handles fit this definition. The use of assistive technology is treated differently on different functional assessments. On some instruments, assistive technology is included in the definition of independent performance; whereas on others, it receives a lower rating—for example, the FIM™ (UDSMR, 1997) and the Health Assessment Questionnaire (Fries, Spitz, Kraines, & Holman, 1980). Hence, even though assistive technology may enable clients to perform activities by themselves, on some instruments those clients cannot receive the highest independence rating. Nonetheless, they would still be rated higher than clients requiring other kinds of assistance. The rationale behind using a lower score is that by using assistive technology, activity performance is not done in a normative manner—that is, in the manner in which it is usually done by adults in the client's culture.

In terms of independence, a client who requires nonphysical help is considered to be less dependent than one who needs physical, hands-on help. Nonphysical help takes into account an array of techniques, including activity setup,

VALUE

Independence is important	Independence is not important

INDEPENDENCE

Independence	Dependent
Able	Unable
100% Independent	0% Independent
No assistance	Maximal assistance • from 1 person • from 2 persons

No assistance	Assistive technology	Non-physical assistance • Setup • Supervision • Standby assist • Verbal assist • Nonverbal assist • Encouragement • Instruction	Physical assistance • Physical guidance • Physical assistance

I believe I can	I believe I cannot

SAFETY

Safe	Unsafe
No risk • Client performance • Environment	At risk • Client performance • Environment

ADEQUACY
Efficiency of Action

No difficulty	Severe difficulty
Without difficulty	Unable to do
No pain	Severe pain
Pain does not interfere with performance	Pain prevents performance
Seconds/minutes	Hours
Fatigue does not interfere with performance	Fatigue prevents performance

Acceptability of Outcome

Meets normative standards	Does not meet normative standards
Satisfied	Dissatisfied
Satisfied 100% of the time	Satisfied 0% of the time
Previous experience	No previous experience
Recent experience	Infrequent experience
Frequent experience	Infrequent experience
Resources adequate to meet needs	Resources inadequate to meet needs
Absence of aberrant activity behaviors	Presence of aberrant activity behaviors

FIGURE 24–1. Parameters used to evaluate ADL and IADL performance.

supervision, standby assistance, and verbal and nonverbal encouragement and guidance. Activity setup, also known as stimulus control, involves preparing the materials and environment for activity performance. Examples of activity setup are opening milk cartons and sugar packets. Supervision means that the caregiver is available to monitor activity performance and to intervene if problems arise. Standby assistance is similar to supervision, except that the caregiver must be physically present and in close proximity to the client at all times. A caregiver who is reviewing checks for accuracy after they have been written is an example of supervision, whereas walking alongside a client who is using a walker is an example of standby assistance.

Verbal guidance means using words, either spoken or written, to instruct clients about activity performance or to prompt them to initiate or continue it. Examples are reminding clients to brush their teeth or telling them how to do a bathtub transfer. Nonverbal guidance involves the use of demonstration, which is also called modeling, or gestures to instruct clients about activity performance or prompt them to initiate or continue it. Examples include demonstrating a bathtub transfer or tapping on a client's foot to draw attention to the need to put socks on. Encouragement differs from guidance in that the intent is to motivate clients rather than to teach them. "You are doing a great job" is an example of a motivational statement.

Although there is substantive consensus that the need for nonphysical help only implies greater independence than does the need for physical help, there is less consensus about the rank order of the techniques grouped under nonphysical help. For instance, is activity setup less assistive than giving verbal cues or demonstrating how an activity is to be done? Because of this lack of consensus, these techniques are arranged differently on different scales.

Physical assistance includes physically guiding clients to do an activity or part of an activity as well as doing it for them; both of these techniques require direct, hands-on contact with clients. When physical guidance is used, the expectation is that clients will participate in the action once they understand what is to be done; whereas when physical assistance is used, the expectation for clients is that they cooperate with caregiving. Examples of physical guidance are inserting a client's hand into the armhole of a garment and positioning a client's hands on a walker. If the practitioner puts a shirt on a client or lifts a client from a chair, he or she is giving physical assistance.

Perceived self-efficacy is another facet of independent activity performance. Perceived self-efficacy refers to clients' beliefs about their ability to perform activities independently. If the distance between the bed and a wheelchair looks like the Grand Canyon to clients and they believe that they cannot execute the transfer successfully, it is likely that they will not perform the transfer. Self-perceptions of performance capability influence activity performance as significantly as actual capabilities (Gage, Noh, Polatajko, & Kaspar, 1994). Perceived self-efficacy is activity specific. Hence it is measured only in relation to specific activities. For example, clients may rate the extent to which they believe they can perform a bed-to-wheelchair transfer independently.

Safety

Safety refers to the extent to which clients are at risk when engaged in activities. As used here, safety is applied to the way in which clients interact with objects and their environments to perform activities. Safety is not a quality of the environment per se, but rather of the person-activity-context transaction. Although a bathtub safety rail is a safety feature, its presence in the bathroom will not improve clients' safety unless it is actually used, and used correctly, when bathtub transfers are executed. Unsafe features of a home, on the other hand, may indicate unsafe activity performance or increased risk. A can of bacon grease on the stove or an electrical cord traversing a sink suggests that the client, or someone else in the home, has unsafe daily living habits.

On some functional assessment instruments (e.g., FIM™), safety is included in the judgment of independence. In other words, to be rated as independent, clients must perform an activity safely. However, because clients may be able to execute activities by themselves and yet do so unsafely, it is advantageous to rate safety separately from independence. This situation often occurs as the ability to do ADL and IADL begins to decline due to the progression of disease, such as dementia. Clients will continue to prepare meals, for example, but burn themselves or the food more often than previously. Safety and independence are related but distinct evaluation parameters.

Safety may also include risks associated with poor judgment and decisions as well as those related to physical actions. Clients who take too much or too little medication may be acting in a manner that will lead to health risks. Those who leave the door unlocked at night or flash $20 bills around while standing at the bus stop may also be acting unsafely. The risk to personal safety is the core factor being evaluated under this parameter.

Although safety has always been recognized as a critical evaluation parameter in occupational therapy, researchers are only beginning to devise scales to measure it separately from independence in activity performance (Letts & Marshall, 1995). When working with clients, it is often difficult to decide where the line between safe and unsafe performance should be drawn and to determine when activity performance is sufficiently unsafe that independence should be restricted. As occupational therapy practice moves more into clients' homes; interfaces more with the legal system for the purposes of guardianship, conservatorship, and involuntary commitment, and becomes more oriented toward prevention and health promotion, safety will increasingly shift to the forefront of evaluation technology.

Adequacy

Adequacy of activity performance is a complex evaluation parameter that refers to the efficiency of the action or process used to execute activities as well as the acceptability of the outcome or product of that action. When dressing, for example, movement may be efficient or inefficient. When dressing is completed, the individual may look neat or disheveled. Similarly, when paying bills, clients may take each bill in turn or shuffle them like a deck of cards. The checks written in payment for the bills may or may not correspond with the amount due or to the correct bill. The distinction between action/process and outcome/product may be blurred on assessments. Parameters emphasizing the efficiency of action or process usually come under the following headings: difficulty, pain, fatigue and dyspnea, and duration. Those emphasizing the acceptability of the outcome or product of action are generally categorized under these headings: normative standards, satisfaction, experience, and aberrant activity behaviors.

Difficulty

Difficulty refers to the perceived ease with which an activity is accomplished. Rehabilitation theorist Verbrugge (1990) argued that difficulty is the most appropriate way to measure activity limitations because ratings of difficulty come from clients, whereas ratings of the amount of assistance required to complete activities come from clients' caregivers. Caregiver ratings of assistance may be more reflective of the assistance given than of the assistance that is actually needed. The Functional Status Index (FSI), an activity limitation measure designed for use with adults with arthritis, uses a four-point scale of no, mild, moderate, and severe difficulty (Jette, 1980). The Health Assessment Questionnaire (HAQ), another activity instrument designed for clients with arthritis, also employs a four-point scale. The HAQ scale considers without any difficulty, with some difficulty, with much difficulty, and unable to do (Fries et al., 1980).

The level of difficulty experienced during activity performance is increasingly being viewed as a marker of preclinical disability—that is, as a symptom that indicates that the individual is at risk for decline in function even though the precise nature of that decline is not yet apparent (Fried, Herdman, Kuhn, Rubin, & Turano, 1991). Unless the onset of pathology is sudden, such as that arising from a car accident or stroke, it is likely that clients will find it harder to perform activities before they are unable to perform them at all. Along similar lines, an increase in perceived difficulty or the spread of difficulty from more difficult (e.g., heavy housework) to easier (e.g., oral hygiene) activities may signal the progression of occult disability.

Pain

Pain is the discomfort or sensation of hurting that is experienced during activity performance and may continue after performance has stopped (Jette, 1980). In relation to activity performance, the component of pain that is of most concern is the extent to which it interferes with performance. Interference may be ascertained in relation to specific activities, such as walking or dressing. Alternately, interference may be gauged more globally in reference to clients' general activity level (McDowell & Newell, 1996). Because of pain, activities may be modified, done at a slower pace, done less often or adequately, or eliminated from one's daily routine. In addition to interference with activities, it may be useful to note the presence or absence of pain, the location and distribution of pain, the intensity of pain (none, mild, moderate, severe), and/or the character of the pain experienced (shooting, burning, dull).

Fatigue and Dyspnea

Fatigue is the discomfort or sensation of tiredness, weariness, or exhaustion that is experienced during or after activity performance (Hart & Freel, 1982; Tack, 1991). When fatigued, clients describe themselves as tired and needing to rest (Freal, Kraft, & Coryell, 1984). Fatigue and dyspnea often occur together. Dyspnea is a sensation of difficult or labored breathing (Gift, 1987). Clients describe their symptoms of dyspnea as feeling short of breathe, not getting enough air, chest tightness, and finding it hard to move air (Janson-Bjerklie, Carrieri, & Hudes, 1986). Fatigue and dyspnea may interfere with the ability to do activities and may be exacerbated by activity performance. Similar to pain, they may lead to modifications in the manner in which activities are done, a slower pace, decreases in participation in activities, and the transfer of responsibility to others. An interesting aspect of fatigue and dyspnea is that they can result from too much (e.g., strenuous housework) as well as too little (e.g., sedentary lifestyle) physical activity (Gift & Pugh, 1993). They may be a component of both physical (e.g., chronic lung disease) and mental (e.g., anxiety) illness. As with pain, the fatigue/dyspnea–activity limitation relationship is generally approached by ascertaining the extent of interference with specific activities and usual activity level. Scales may also record the presence or absence, the amount (none, a lot), and the severity (mild, severe) of the fatigue or dyspnea (McDowell & Newell, 1996).

Duration

The **duration** of activity performance—that is, the time needed to complete an activity—is often used as a measure of efficiency. Less time is interpreted as meaning increased efficiency. In essence, time gives a measure of the speed of performance. Some functional assessment instruments include a time criterion in the definition of independence. The FIM™ specifies, for example, that activities must be completed in "reasonable time" (UDSMR, 1997). Practitioners often comment on activities being completed "within normal limits." It is interesting that neither the average length of time adults take nor the minimum time they need to perform various ADL and IADL has been calculated.

Although time to activity completion provides a ratio scale for measuring activity performance, it is cumbersome data to collect in the clinical situation, because it requires the use of a stopwatch and the designation of precise beginning and ending points for each activity. Furthermore, the time needed to complete activities depends on the reason for engaging in the activity. Dressing to do housecleaning is likely to take less time than dressing to go out to work. Time is also a poor marker of efficiency for clients who are impulsive or manic, because they may rush through activities with little consideration for safety or adequacy. Although such individuals may prepare a meal in record time, for example, the food may be unappetizing and the kitchen cluttered with pots and cooking utensils when they are finished.

Societal Standards

In moving from looking at the efficiency of action or process to the acceptability of the outcome or product of that action, the question of adequacy or acceptability to whom must be addressed. One approach to evaluating the quality of activity outcomes or products is to evaluate those results against the normative expectations of society. Accordingly, for example, humans are expected to maintain personal cleanliness and not to overdraw their checking accounts. Although there may be a wide, rather than a narrow, line between what is acceptable and unacceptable, activity performance that consistently goes outside the line will be labeled unacceptable, inappropriate, or inadequate according to **societal standards.** In applying normative standards, practitioners must be careful to make allowance for cultural diversity.

Satisfaction

A second parameter of acceptability of task outcomes or products is **satisfaction.** Satisfaction refers to the experience of pleasure and contentment with one's performance (Yerxa, Burnett-Beaulieu, Stocking, & Azen, 1988). As a parameter of performance, it is likely that satisfaction interacts with an individual's willingness to engage in an activity. If clients fail to derive satisfaction from their activity performance, they may restrict their participation. In relating satisfaction to activity performance, a dichotomous scale may be used consisting of satisfied or dissatisfied, or satisfaction may be rated according to the proportion of time over a defined interval that clients experienced satisfaction (e.g., 100%, 75%, and so on) or the degree of satisfaction may be rated on a likert scale (e.g., not satisfied at all to extremely satisfied) (Law et al., 1998; Yerxa et al., 1988; Pincus, Summey, Soraci, Wallston, & Hummon, 1983). Caregivers of clients may also be asked to rate the extent to which they are satisfied with the care recipient's activity performance. This procedure has the potential for providing practitioners with information about the normative expectations for activity performance within the family unit.

Experience

Experience refers to the direct participation in an activity that an individual has accumulated. The assumption is that experience provides practice, which perfects performance and outcomes. All humans generally learn activities classified as functional mobility or personal care over the course of childhood and adolescence. As activities basic to and essential for daily living, they are practiced regularly over adulthood. Possible exceptions to this norm include hair care that is done by beauticians, fingernail care that is done by manicurists, and toenail care that is done by podiatrists. Nonetheless, the societal expectation is that all adults have a wide range of experience with these activities and perform them adequately. However, a similar expectation does not hold for IADL, for which humans have more options. Clients, therefore, may not have developed proficiency in all IADL activities. Some may have no experience in preparing meals, doing the laundry, or managing finances. Clients' activity performance history is essential for understanding their current performance level. An activity limitation is interpreted differently for a client who has had no or little prior experience performing the activity than for one who had been doing it immediately premorbidly.

In addition to past experience, recent or current experience must also be evaluated. When activities are not performed regularly, the proficiency needed to do them can fall into disuse or become obsolete with technological advances. Inquiries about recency and frequency of activity experience are generally approached by ascertaining clients' skills and habits in ADL and IADL (Rogers & Holm, 1991a). Skill refers to the capability to do an activity, whereas habit refers to usual or routine activity performance. In their activity repertoires, all humans have activities that they usually do not perform but that they can perform if situations arise when they have to do them or want to do them. For example, you may know how to cook but prefer to let your spouse do this on a daily basis. However, if your spouse goes away on a business trip, you are able to cook dinner for yourself. Inquiries about activity skills are generally phrased in this manner: "Can you [name the activity]?" Inquiries about habits are generally phrased this way: "Do you [name the activity]?"

Resources

When an evaluation is conducted to assist in discharge decisions, the resources available to clients must be taken into account as well as the clients' skills. Consider, for example, Ms. Cross and Ms. Lum, who are unable to use the range and oven safely to prepare hot food. Ms. Cross has a niece who lives on the same city block as she does and is willing to assist her in preparing hot meals. Ms. Lum lives in a rural community, which does not have a Meals-on-Wheels program, and her neighbors are elderly themselves and unable to assist her. Although the meal preparation skills of both of these clients are the same, Ms. Lum is at greater risk for adverse outcomes than Ms. Cross because

TABLE 24-3. **ABERRANT ACTIVITY BEHAVIORS OBSERVED DURING ACTIVITY PERFORMANCE EVALUATIONS**

Functional Mobility	Personal Care	Home Management
Moving in bed • Drops onto bed • Rocks to gain enough momentum to get up from bed Transferring • Drops during standing pivot • Grabs onto clothing of caregiver Sitting in chair • Drops down Standing • Falls deliberately Walking • Refuses to walk • Staggers • Weaves • Paces • Wanders Moving around the community • Gets lost Walking around work • Does not adhere to safety guidelines during mobility	Feeding/eating • Refuses to eat • Drools • Coughs, chokes, gags • Has delayed swallow; does not swallow • Has disturbing tongue movements • Eats too fast or too slowly or only certain foods • Spits food out of mouth • Stuffs food in mouth • Takes another person's food • Eats spoiled food Performing hygiene • Bites nails • Spits nails on floor Bathing • Refuses to bathe • Fear of water, hair washing • Neglects to wash some body parts • Fails to rinse soap Dressing • Resists dressing • Sleeps in street clothes • Dons clothes inside out/backward • Dons clothes on wrong body part • Dons underclothes on top of street clothes • Layers clothes inappropriately • Takes clothes off at inappropriate times or places • Wears the same clothes every day • Dons another person's clothes • Dons nonclothing items • Ignores weather conditions Toileting • Urinates in inappropriate places • Defecates in inappropriate places Communicating • Makes sexual gestures/advances • Is verbally aggressive • Is physically aggressive	Preparing meals • Burns food • Cooks food inadequately • Uses too much spice • Forgets to turn off stove/oven Housecleaning • Dusts inadequately • Leaves dirt on floor • Forgets to remove garbage • Cleans inadequately (bathtub, stove) • Keeps spoiled food Managing finances • Forgets to pay bills • Makes errors in calculating costs • Throws out bills or money • Gives money away Shopping • Goes on a spending sprees • Can't remember what to buy Telephoning • Calls a person repeatedly, thus being annoying • Calls police inappropriately • Neglects to give a message Managing medications • Takes too much or too little • Stops taking • Takes at the wrong time Managing laundry • Stores soiled clothes Managing time • Forgets appointments • Comes for appointments at wrong time Using transportation • Forgets where car is parked • Gets lost • Gets on wrong bus • Confused about destination

she has less supportive living resources available to her. Thus when discharge decisions are at stake, the evaluation of ADL and IADL becomes meaningful only when deficits are linked to resources (Williams, et al., 1991).

Aberrant Activity Behaviors

The activity analyses used on ADL and IADL instruments are based on the way in which activities are normally performed—that is, the way in which they are usually performed by individuals without disabilities. However, individuals with cognitive impairments, such as those associated with dementia, traumatic brain injury, schizophrenia, and mental retardation, may exhibit behaviors that are aberrant or abnormal. For example, they may pocket food in their cheeks or spit food out. In contrast to the subactivities derived from activity analyses, which are to be encouraged during intervention, aberrant behaviors are to be extinguished or reduced in frequency. Table 24-3 lists some common aberrant activity-related behaviors. These behaviors are not well represented on available ADL and IADL instruments, with the exception of the Routine Task Inventory, an instrument specifically devised for use with a psychiatric population (Allen, 1985).

Evaluation Parameters and Measurement Instruments

This discussion of evaluation parameters has emphasized individual items and the scores assigned to them. Item scores are often summed to obtain a total score. The total score provides a summary index of the client's overall status on the concept that is being evaluated (e.g., ADL, IADL). Several scoring systems may be used on these measures. Most common, item scores are simply added, thus giving equal weight to all items on the scale. In this type of system, bathing and grooming, for example, make an equal contribution to the total score. On some instruments, items are differentially weighted to take into account the value or consequences that they have for activity limitations or overall occupational status. Bathing, for example, might be given double the weight of grooming, because it contributes twice as much to disablement. Item weights may be assigned through expert opinion or statistical methods. Intrinsic to each scoring system are assumptions about the relative value of each activity item to the total score. Occupational therapy practitioners need to be aware of these scoring systems so that they can correctly interpret their clients' scores.

Most instruments used in professional fields, such as occupational therapy, medicine, rehabilitation, and education, do not have the precision required to qualify as interval measures. They are ordinal measures. Nonetheless, even though they do not meet the criteria for interval measures, they are often commonly treated and interpreted in that way (Eakin, 1989; Merbitz, Morris, & Grip, 1989; Wade, 1992). In other words, the unit of measurement is treated as equal from point to point (e.g., minimal, moderate, maximal assistance) when it is not. Item ratings are added to obtain total scores; and statistical operations, such as means and standard deviations, are calculated. Occupational therapy practitioners need to be cautious about assuming that scales that appear to have equal measurement intervals are in fact interval scales. Rasch analysis has the capability of converting ordinal scales to interval ones (Wright & Linacre, 1989), thereby resolving the dilemma associated with nonequal interval scales. Rasch analysis has been applied to the FIM™ (UDSMR, 1997) and the Assessment of Motor and Process Skills (AMPS; Fisher, 1999).

Practice Guidelines: Parameters

The parameters for describing or measuring ADL and IADL performance are independence, safety, and adequacy. Although there are options in the ways in which these parameters may be operationalized, practitioners should evaluate them regardless of the specific activity or activities being evaluated. They are essential to competent activity performance. Activity performance that is not independent indicates a need for assistance from technology or humans. Activity performance that is independent but unsafe places clients at risk. Activity performance that is independent but marginal or inadequate restricts clients' role participation and may also place them at risk. Deficits in activity independence, safety, and adequacy indicate a need for occupational therapy interventions or for supportive services for ADL or IADL.

In view of the number of activities involved in ADL and IADL, practitioners need to devise rules of thumb, or conceptual shortcuts, for deciding which activities to include in the evaluation and the order in which they should be evaluated. Activity hierarchies provide a basis for devising these conceptual shortcuts. Activity hierarchies arrange activities according to their level of difficulty. They enable practitioners to assume that clients passing items at an intermediate level would pass all easier items but would likely fail more difficult ones. Thus, by using background information about clients, practitioners hypothesize about their functional level, start the evaluation with an activity at a reasonable point on the hierarchy, and stop the evaluation after two or three items have been failed.

The development of the Index of ADL was based on a Guttman scaling-type approach; the Index ranks ADL, in order of increasing difficulty, as feeding, continence, transfers, toileting, dressing, and bathing (Katz et al., 1963). Guttman scaling of the IADL Scale ranks the performance of older adults from least to most difficult as follows: uses telephone; takes care of all shopping needs; plans, prepares, and serves adequate meals independently; maintains light housework independently; does all laundry; travels by car or public transportation; takes medications with correct dosage at right time; and manages all financial tasks, except major purchases or banking (Lawton & Brody, 1969). Rasch analysis has provided a substantive boost to the delineation of activity hierarchies, and practitioners can anticipate considerable advances in this regard in the future (Bray, Fisher, & Duran, 2001; Fisher, 1993; Velozo, Magalhaes, Pan, & Leiter, 1995).

By combining information from the different evaluation parameters, practitioners can obtain information valuable for targeting intervention outcomes. Take for example, Mrs. Morris, a client with low vision, who indicates that independence in financial management is most important to her and, furthermore, that this is the activity for which she requires the most assistance. The practitioner would probably want to negotiate with her to intervene, at least initially, on an easier task—one in which she is also dependent but for which less assistance is required, such as cooking. The reason for selecting an easier task is that the disparity between Mrs. Morris's current and desired performance is less, and the practitioner gauges her rehabilitation potential in cooking to be better than that of financial management. Client-centered practice is not violated when practitioners assist their clients in establishing feasible goals.

The occupational therapy evaluation yields data about clients' activity abilities and limitations. Although the occupational therapy process focuses on preventing, remediating, or compensating for dysfunctions in activity performance, practitioners need to document activities that clients can perform as well as those that they cannot perform. Clients' abilities are as significant as their limitations for their adjustment to living with a activity limitations.

ADL AND IADL EVALUATION METHODS

Practitioners may use a combination of data-gathering methods to assess clients' ADL and IADL. The fundamental or basic methods are asking questioning, observing, and testing. The specific procedures used to gather data within each of these methods range from unstructured to structured. When questions or observations about activity performance are sufficiently structured, and when the questions or observations yield numerical scores, these methods are transformed into testing. Other methods of learning about clients' performance, such as client care conferences or record review (e.g., medical, school, work), rely on these three basic methods.

Each data-gathering method has advantages and disadvantages. The questioning method of data gathering is more subjective than observation, and this subjectivity may reduce reliability. Questioning is also less expensive and less labor intensive. Interviews and questionnaires can be administered by less costly personnel rather than by observational instruments, because they require less skilled judgment on the part of the assessor. Moreover, clients are not placed at physical risk for injury when they talk about their activity performance, as they may be when they actually perform activities. Hence, there is little need for skilled personnel to monitor risk.

When observation is structured, it has the potential for increasing the reliability of evaluation results compared to questioning, because the meaning of items is clear. Item ambiguity is reduced because the items must be operationalized to be performed. In turn, increased reliability increases the ability to detect change, a critical factor for practitioners who seek to improve activity performance through intervention. As we alluded to previously, the disadvantages of observation over questioning are that it is more time consuming and more costly in terms of space, equipment, and personnel.

Although no data-gathering method is intrinsically superior to the others, one method may be better for some evaluation purposes than others or for some clinical situations than others. A practitioner's selection of a particular method or a combination of methods is largely determined by the overall purpose for conducting the evaluation in conjunction with practicalities, such as the time allowed for the evaluation and the equipment available (Holm & Rogers, 1989). However, practitioners need to be aware that the methods are not necessarily equivalent and do not always yield the same data about clients' performance of ADL and IADL (Sager, et al., 1992).

Asking Questions

In the questioning method of data gathering, questions are posed about ADL and IADL. The questioning method may be implemented in an oral or a written format, using interviews or questionnaires, respectively. Neither format requires face-to-face contact. Interviews may be conducted over the telephone. Questionnaires may be completed while waiting for an appointment or mailed out in advance of a session. The degree of structure imposed on the interview or the questionnaire may vary considerably.

Table 24-4 provides data about the bathing performance of two clients that were obtained through questioning. The evaluation of bathing consisted of five questions. The first question, "Can you bathe yourself?" was the most general and allowed clients the most leeway in interpreting the meaning of "bathe yourself." Questions 2 through 5 asked about specific components of bathing. These questions used activity analysis to breakdown "bathe yourself" into four components—transferring in and out of the bathtub, lowering the body to the bottom of the bathtub, washing the body, and washing specific body parts. As these case data illustrate, the conclusion about a limitation in bathing depends on the questions asked by the practitioner. If only the most general question about bathing (question 1) had been asked, neither client would have been identified as having a bathing limitation. By applying the activity analysis approach, both clients were identified as having a limitation in bathing, but the site of the dysfunction was different. Furthermore, questioning of Ms. Beech about how she bathed, elicited the information that she showered in the bathtub. This information led the practitioner to reverse the conclusion about a bathing limitation because showering eliminates the need to sit in the bathtub. When Ms. Bern was questioned about how she washed her feet and back, she indicated that she soaked them while in the bathtub because she was unable to reach them. She also indicated that she felt that she bathed inadequately because her toes and back were constantly itchy and her back had a rash. Thus the decision of bathing limitation was retained for Ms. Bern.

It is preferable to have clients respond to questions about their activity performance because they are the most knowledgeable about it. They have the opportunity for daily self-observation. However, if they have not performed activities in a while, they may report their abilities inaccurately, because

TABLE 24-4. **DATA OBTAINED ABOUT BATHING PERFORMANCE FROM ASKING QUESTIONS, OBSERVING, AND TESTING**

	Data from Asking Questions	
Question	**Ms Bern**	**Ms Beech**
1. Can you bathe yourself?	yes	yes
2. Can you get in and out of the bathtub by yourself?	yes	yes
3. Can you lower yourself to the bottom of the bathtub?	yes	no
4. Can you wash yourself?	yes	yes
5. Can you wash your entire body including your feet and back?	no	yes

	Data from Observing	
Bathing Step	**Mr. Kline**	**Mr. Market**
1. Move into tub	I (instability when lifting foot to step into tub)	I (knelt on floor, crawled into tub)
2. Lower to tub bottom	Dependent—moderate physical assistance, S	(Crawling precluded this step)
3. Fill tub with water	I, S, A	I (filled tub with cool water; emptied hot water tank)
4. Wash upper body	I, S, A	Dependent—verbal and manual guidance, S, A
5. Wash lower body	I, S, A	Dependent—verbal and manual guidance, S, A
6. Rise from tub bottom	Dependent—moderate physical assistance, S	I, S (had difficulty getting feet under body; poor motor planning)
7. Move out of tub	I, S, A	I, S, A
8. Dry upper body	I, S, A	Dependent—instruction not effective, S, neglected back
9. Dry lower body	I, S, A	I, S, A

	Data from Testing	
	Score	
Test	**Mr. Kline**	**Mr. Market**
FIM™		
• Bathing	7	5
• Transfer	3	7

I, independence; *S*, safety; *A*, adequacy.

they believe they can perform activities that they actually can no longer perform.

There are also numerous situations in which clients are unable to respond on their own behalf. For example, they may be too physically ill or too depressed to participate in questioning. They may lack insight into their problems or be unable to respond reliably, as might occur with cognitive impairment, or they may refuse to respond, as might be the case with personality disorders or when clients fear that negative decisions may follow from giving the information (e.g., institutionalization). In these situations, caregivers or other proxies may be asked to respond on behalf of clients. To a great extent, the usefulness of the information obtained from caregivers or proxies depends on their familiarity with the ADL and IADL of the client. For example, if the caregiver or proxy has not actually observed a client bathing, or has not done this for some time, the information given about bathing may be based more on opinion than data.

In addition, there are known biases in the reporting tendencies of caregivers and proxies. Family proxies are prone to perceive clients as more disabled than clients perceive themselves, and they perceive clients as more disabled than do professional caregivers (e.g., nurses). Furthermore, spouses tend to be more negative in their evaluations of activity performance than other family members (Rubenstein, Schairer, Wieland, & Kane, 1984). It is likely that the responses of caregivers are influenced by their own coping styles, which may lead them to minimize or magnify performance dysfunctions.

Evaluation parameters such as independence, safety, and aberrant activity behaviors can be readily observed by caregivers and proxies. For some evaluation parameters, however, clients are the only appropriate respondents. Inquiries, for instance, about values, perceived self-efficacy, satisfaction with performance, and activity-related pain are subjective, and indices of these parameters are difficult for others to observe.

The questioning method is particularly useful for screening for activity limitations, because a large number of activities can be queried in a short amount of time. However, it is less useful when evaluating limitations for the purposes of intervention, because clients may not be able to describe their limitations in sufficient detail to target the components of activities that are problematic. Furthermore, clients do not have the medical, rehabilitation, and occupational therapy knowledge to isolate the factors that may be causing limitations. Nonetheless, questioning is usually the data-gathering method of choice when information is needed about daily living habits—that is, about what clients usually do on a daily basis. Although it is theoretically possible to assess ADL and IADL habits through observation, it is generally not practical to do so because this would require a series of observations, preferably in the natural setting (e.g., home, nursing home, group home) and at the time of day that the activities usually occur. Consequently, habits are generally evaluated through questioning. Similarly, questioning is a primary mode of learning about clients' ADL and IADL experience. The only other way to retrieve information about past performance is to examine existing records (medical, school, work, or other).

Observing

In the observation method, practitioners obtain data by watching clients as they perform activities. Practitioners may observe activity performance under natural or laboratory conditions. Under natural conditions, performance is observed within the context that it usually takes place or is expected to take place. This includes the location (home) and objects (bathtub, soap) usually used for activities and, if possible, the routine time that activities take place. These conditions can often be met in long term-care settings and home care. For example, practitioners may observe clients bathe, groom, dress, and feed themselves as they perform their morning care routines. When clients are seen in the hospital or outpatient clinics, observation of activity performance takes places under laboratory conditions. The laboratory may be the occupational therapy clinic or the temporary space occupied by clients (e.g., the hospital room).

Table 24-4 provides data, obtained through observation, about the bathing performance of two clients. An advantage that the observation method has over the questioning method is the descriptive detail that it provides about performance. When activity performance is at risk for limitations or when limitations are already present, the characteristics of performance exhibited by clients play an essential role in planning intervention. Mr. Kline's bathing performance, for example, is characteristic of motor impairment, whereas Mr. Market's is characteristic of cognitive impairment. Interventions can be planned with these impairments in mind. The descriptive detail gleaned through observation is extremely difficult to elicit in an interview or through a questionnaire.

When clients engage in an activity, they apply their abilities to accomplish it with available human and material resources—that is, within a specific context. The significance of context to activity performance may be illustrated by thinking about the dysfunction that you would encounter if you prepared dinner this evening in your neighbor's house rather than in your own. You would need to spend time locating food, cooking utensils, and pots and pans. You might be afraid of cutting yourself while paring carrots because the knife is not sharp. You may burn the chicken because you are accustomed to a gas rather than an electric range. You may forget to rotate the potatoes in the microwave because your appliance has a revolving tray. You may have difficulty expanding your recipes to provide for eight individuals as opposed to the four in your family. As this scenario illustrates, the physical and social context in which activity performance takes place has a strong influence on the quality of performance outcomes.

Regardless of where an evaluation is done, the influence of context on activity performance must be taken into account so that valid conclusions about performance can be drawn. Occupational therapy clinics are designed to promote function and have numerous adaptive features to compensate for impairments. These features may make it easier for clients to perform activities in the clinic than in their own homes. Conversely, however, performance may be more difficult because clients are unfamiliar with the clinic. When an evaluation is done in the home, clients have the advantage of using their own activity objects in the confines of existing architecture. The social context is changed, however, because to conduct an evaluation, practitioners oversee activity performance, and their mere presence may affect the manner and the adequacy of the activities performed.

As an objective data-gathering method, observation has the advantage of minimizing the subjective, distorting aspects associated with self-reports and proxy reports. However, the generalizability of clients' performance in laboratory settings to real-world situations is problematic. Research has suggested that evaluation results obtained in the laboratory differ from those obtained in clients' homes (Haworth &

Hollings, 1979). Similar to proxy reports, observation is appropriate only for evaluation parameters that are observable. In contrast to both self-reports and proxy reports, however, observation provides practitioners with the opportunity to analyze impairments that may be interfering with activity performance.

Testing

When questions and observations are systematically structured and when a numerical score or a category system is used to describe activity performance, the questions or observations constitute a test (Cronbach, 1970). The traditional approach to testing has been norm referenced. The purpose of norm-referenced testing is to compare a client's performance on a test to that of others on the same test (Popham, 1990). Norm-referenced tests are useful for answering questions like this: How do the home management skills of Mrs. Zone, who is 65 years old and has arthritis and cardiopulmonary disease, compare with others her age who are living independently in the community? Norm-referenced testing requires evaluation under standardized conditions. Hence, the materials used in the test are specified, the instructions given to clients are detailed, the procedures for administering the test are outlined, and the manner of scoring clients' responses is designated. Standardization is needed to ensure the reliability and validity of test results. As Christiansen (1991) noted, standardization "creates formidable difficulties if one is concerned with getting an accurate picture of the characteristic level of functional performance under everyday circumstances, which vary from one person to the next" (p. 377).

An alternate model of testing is provided by the criterion-referenced approach. The purpose of criterion-referenced testing is to compare a client's performance on a test to a performance standard (Popham, 1990). Criterion-referenced tests stress activity mastery and address questions such as this: Can Mrs. Zone perform all activities, or procure the services, needed to live in the community by herself? Criterion-referenced tests often incorporate activity analyses, and the degree of structure imposed on testing is often more flexible than for norm-referenced testing.

Data obtained on the FIM™ for Mr. Kline and Mr. Market are recorded in Table 24-4. A score of 7 on the FIM™, a criterion-referenced instrument, denotes complete independence, a score of 5 signifies the need for supervision or setup, and a score of 3 indicates the need for moderate assistance from a helper. Because Mr. Market's bathing dysfunction is likely due to cognitive impairment, the FIM™ may not be the most appropriate instrument to use, according to the instrument guidelines, for it is heavily oriented toward medical diagnoses.

Norm-referenced and criterion-referenced testing employ a static evaluation strategy. Clients' activity performance is tested once to determine their performance status at that point in time. A newer testing strategy, called dynamic, interactive, or process assessment, evaluates clients' performance, while interactively providing interventions to determine their potential for improving performance (Haywood & Tzuriel, 1992; Missiuna, 1987). The outcomes of dynamic assessment are the identification and diagnosis of activity limitations, the determination of effective intervention strategies for developing or restoring activity performance or for compensating for deficits, and the determination of the potential for rehabilitation (Rogers et al., 1997). It provides answers to questions such as these: What types of technological or human assistance does Mrs. Zone require to perform everyday tasks independently, safely, and adequately? Does Mrs. Zone have the potential for improving her performance? Dynamic assessment focuses on measuring changes in activity performance and identifying interventions used during the evaluation that effected those changes, so that they can be used during intervention. Hence, standardization is not necessary, and practitioners can tailor the evaluation to the clients' needs. Dynamic assessment manages the formidable difficulties presented by standardization mentioned by Christiansen (1991).

Practice Guidelines: Method

In conducting the occupational therapy evaluation, practitioners have a choice of data-gathering methods and options within each method. Perhaps the best data-gathering strategy is to use a combination of methods and sources, relying on the convergence of data for the best profile of clients' activity abilities and limitations. Discrepancies in the evaluation data need to be clarified and reconciled. For example, when questioned about grocery shopping, clients may indicate independence, whereas caregivers state dependence. However, the two responses are not necessarily at variance, because clients may be responding in terms of their capacities (e.g., "I could do it if I had to.") and caregivers may be responding in reference to their habits (e.g., "She does not go shopping."). Similarly, a practitioner may ascertain through performance testing that clients can execute bed to wheelchair transfers. Yet clients may insist that they cannot. The inconsistency may arise because, although clients perform the transfer when the practitioner is present, they feel insecure about their abilities when they have to execute transfers on their own. In both of these examples, the use of different data sources identified a performance discrepancy between skill and habit that would not have been apparent through the use of one source alone (see Chapter 27, Section 1).

An effective strategy for combining data-gathering methods is to begin the evaluation with a questioning procedure. The primary purposes of the questioning procedure are to provide an overall profile of clients abilities and limitations, to understand clients' priorities for learning how to manage their limitations, and to target activities requiring in-depth evaluation. Questioning is then followed by an observational procedure. The purposes of the observational procedure are to identify the deficit components of activities already identified as dysfunctional or at risk for dysfunction through questioning; to hypothesize about the underlying cause of the performance deficit; to identify the most likely interventions for managing the deficit, which may be remedial, compensatory, or preventive; and to ascertain the clients' potential for improving their performance. The evaluation is then complete because the practitioner has the data needed to intervene. If the observational procedure raises questions about the clients' activity performance abilities previously delineated through questioning, these activities can also be subject to observational procedures.

ADL and IADL are evaluated on entry to occupational therapy to provide a measure of clients' baseline performance status. An intervention to improve activity performance may then be initiated. The intervention may be short term and limited in scope, such as the prescription of a walker and training in using it correctly and safely, or it may be more long term and intensive, such as homemaker training. Regardless of the extent and length of the intervention, reevaluation of ADL and IADL performance is needed to ascertain whether the intervention is resulting in improvement, whether the intervention should be continued or changed, or whether maximal benefit from occupational therapy has been achieved and activity performance has reached a plateau. The best strategy for reevaluation is to re-administer the evaluations done at baseline. This involves using the same ADL and IADL content, the same measurement parameters, and the same data-gathering methods. By keeping all three factors constant at baseline and at any subsequent reevaluations, the possibility of detecting change—attributable to intervention—in clients' performance is increased. If the evaluation content, parameters, or methods vary from one point in time to another, the same evaluative data are not available for comparison, and the potential for detecting change is reduced. For example, if activity performance is evaluated in the occupational therapy clinic by using observation immediately before discharge and by using a telephone survey sometime after discharge, it is not possible to determine if an alteration in activity performance is the result of a client's deterioration or improvement or is the result of the change in data-gathering method (observation versus questioning).

INTEGRATING EVALUATION DATA

The evaluation data obtained through questioning, observing, and testing methods must be analyzed, synthesized, and interpreted. Practitioners function as data processors and managers in grouping data that are similar into categories, resolving discrepancies, and, finally, putting forth an occupational therapy diagnosis that integrates the findings into a cohesive problem statement that is simultaneously capable of functioning as the end point of the evaluation and the beginning point of intervention. This integration of data is accomplished through diagnostic reasoning, which is a component of clinical reasoning (Rogers, 1983; Rogers & Holm, 1991b).

The clinical reasoning of practitioners resembles a dialectical process in which practitioners argue with themselves about the interpretation of the data. Evidence supporting one interpretation is weighed against evidence rejecting that interpretation. The pros and cons for each interpretation are summed, so to speak, and the interpretation is selected that has the most supporting or compelling evidence. If the evidence fails to support sufficiently one interpretation over another, more evaluative data are collected in an attempt to break the tie and make one interpretation more cogent than the other(s). Through this process, the practitioner arrives at a cohesive understanding of the ADL and IADL performance of the client and of an appropriate therapeutic action (i.e., direct intervention or recommendation). This understanding is presented to clients or their proxies for verification and collaborative decision making concerning the therapeutic action to be implemented.

OCCUPATIONAL THERAPY AND REHABILITATION MEDICINE FUNCTIONAL ASSESSMENTS

Our presentation of occupational therapy and rehabilitation medicine instruments is highly selective. It includes the ADL and IADL sections of instruments that are mandated or recommended by the Centers for Medicare and Medicaid Services (CMS; formerly the Health Care Financing Administration [HCFA]), the FIM™ and WeeFIM™, the Minimum Data Set for Long Term Care (MDS), the Outcome and Assessment Information Set (OASIS), the Inpatient Rehabilitation Facility Patient Assessment Instrument (IRFPAI), and occupational therapy–specific instruments. Key words to use when searching for ADL and IADL instruments are the following: functional assessment, disability evaluation, functional disability, health status, ADL scales, IADL scales, physical function, and quality of life. In selecting instruments for use in clinical practice, psychometric quality and practical considerations must be taken into account. Matching the content, parameters, and data-gathering methods of the instrument to the practitioner's informational needs is an essential practical consideration.

Table 24-5 provides information for the instruments selected for review, including title, purpose for which the

TABLE 24–5. **SUMMARY OF SELECTED ADL AND IADL INSTRUMENTS**

Title	Purpose	Population	Description	Method/Rating	*Psychometric Properties*	
					Reliability	**Validity**
Assessment of Living Skills and Resources (ALSAR)[a]	Assess IADL, identify needs, assign risk, prioritize intervention	Adults	11 IADL skills and related resources for managing deficits (telephoning, reading, leisure, medication management, money management, transportation, shopping, meal preparation, laundering, housekeeping, home maintenance)	Interview with guiding questions; uses a three-point ordinal scale (0 = high, 1 = moderate, 2 = low); a risk score (*R* score) is created by combining skill and resource scores	*Internal:* Cronbach's alpha = 0.91 *Interrater:* skills = average agreement = 86% (72–94%); resources = 95% (78–100%)	*Content:* based on expert judgment of geriatric practitioners *Criterion related:* significant correlation between *R* score and Barthel Index ($r = -0.58$); *R* score predicts changes over 6 months in living situation, hospitalization, or death *Construct:* significant correlations between *R* score and mental status score ($r = -0.26$) suggests adequate sensitivity as a performance measure but not as self-report measure[b]
Assessment of Motor and Process Skills (AMPS)[c]	Examine the relationship between motor and process skills and activity performance to establish current competence and predict IADL performance	Children and adults with impairment	56 calibrated IADL activities (e.g., sweep, repot a plant)[d]	Interview to suggest the familiar activities (two to three) for performance testing; activities observed by a trained, calibrated examiner; activities rated on 16 motor skills (e.g., reaches, lifts) and 20 process skills (e.g., initiates, searches), taking into account physical effort, efficiency, independence, and safety; uses a four-point ordinal scale (1 = unacceptable or deficit; 4 = competent)	*Interrater:* 95% of trained raters ($n = 300$), achieved Rasch goodness-of-fit statistics[e] *Test–retest:* motor, $r = 0.88$; process, $r = 0.86$[f]	*Construct:* validity across age, gender, ethnic, culture, and diagnostic groups and settings (medical and psychiatric)[g]; significant relationships between process scores and mental status (Cambridge Examination for Mental Status in the Elderly, Mini-Mental State Examination) and FIM™ social/cognitive; and the motor scores and FIM™ physical[h]
Canadian Occupational Performance Measure (COPM)[i]	Measure client's perceived change in occupational performance	Children and adults	Activities classified into three areas: self-care (personal care, functional mobility, community management, transportation, shopping, finances), productive (household management, paid/unpaid work), and leisure	Self-report using a semistructured interview; in each occupational area, problems rated for importance from 1 to 10; the five most important problems (regardless of occupational area) then rated for performance and satisfaction (1 = not	*Internal:* for performance, Cronbach's alpha = 0.41–0.56; for satisfaction, 0.71[j] *Test–retest:* intraclass correlation coefficients for	*Content:* Based on a review of instruments *Criterion:* 53% of respondents named spontaneously at least one problem also named on the COPM[k]

				able/not at all satisfied; 10 = do extremely well/extremely satisfied)	performance = 0.80 and for satisfaction = 0.89[j]	
Functional Independence Measure (FIM™)[l]	Measure severity of disability related to physical impairment	Adults with physical impairment	18 activities, 13 with a motor emphasis related to self-care (e.g., feeding, grooming, bathing, dressing upper body, dressing lower body, toileting), sphincter control (e.g., bladder and bowel), mobility (e.g., bed, chair, wheelchair, toilet, tub or shower transfers), and locomotion (e.g., walk or move wheelchair, use stairs); 5 with a cognitive emphasis involving communication (e.g., comprehensive, expression) and social cognition (e.g., social interaction, problem solving, memory)	Observation by a trained observer; uses a seven-point or four-point ordinal scale, grading amount of assistance needed by clients to complete activity; highest score = greatest independence; total score ranges from 18 to 126[m]	*Internal:* using the seven levels, total FIM™ intraclass correlation coefficient = 0.96; motor = 0.96; cognitive 0.91; FIM™ item kappa range from memory (0.53) to stair climbing (0.66)[n]; stable structure of motor and cognitive scales at admission and discharge[o]	*Criterion related:* FIM admission scores predict discharge status and length of stay in rehabilitation; motor function is stronger predictor than cognitive function[p]; high concordance between FIM and Barthel scores[q]
Inpatient Rehabilitation Facility Patient Assessment Instrument (IRFPAI)[E,l,q]	Evaluate baseline functional status and changes in status after medical rehabilitation	Adult clients of inpatient medical rehabilitation	Includes FIM™ items and distance walked or traveled in a wheelchair in feet[F]	Observation by a trained observer; uses a seven-point or four-point ordinal scale grading amount of assistance needed by clients to complete an activity; highest score equals greatest independence; (same scale as FIM™)	Reliability is reported to be higher than that of the MDS	
Klein-Bell Activities of Daily Living Scale[r]	Measure ADL independence to determine current status, change in status, and subactivities to focus on rehabilitation	Children and adults	170 subactivities in six domains (dressing, mobility, elimination, bathing and hygiene, eating, and emergency communication)	Observation; uses a three-point ordinal scale (able to perform, unable to perform, not applicable); expert panel weighted subactivities for importance to health, performance time, performance difficulty, and caregiving burden; weights are used in calculating total score (range = 0–313) (higher scores = greater dependence)	*Interrater:* percent agreement across all items = 92% *Test–retest:* intraclass correlation = 0.98[s]	*Predictive:* correlations between Klein-Bell scores and hours clients required assistance per week for a 5- to 10- month period after discharge[r] *Construct:* Distinguished between children who did and did not have cerebral palsy[s]

Continues

TABLE 24-5. **SUMMARY OF SELECTED ADL AND IADL INSTRUMENTS** *(Continued)*

Title	Purpose	Population	Description	Method/Rating	Psychometric Properties	
					Reliability	**Validity**
Kohlman Evaluation of Living Skills (KELS)[t]	Evaluate ability to live independently and safely in community	Adults with psychiatric diagnoses; clients with mental retardation, brain injury, other cognitive impairments, and older adults	17 activities grouped into five categories: (self-care, safety and health, money management, transportation and telephone, work and leisure); tends to emphasize knowledge component of activities	Combination of interview and performance; uses a three-point scale (0 = independent, 1 or 1/2 = needs assistance)	*Interrater:* percent agreement = 74–94%[u] and 84–94%[v]	*Construct:* residents of sheltered-living situations scored higher than those living independently in community[v] *Criterion related:* significant correlations between KELS and Bay Area Functional Performance Evaluation ($r = -0.84$) and the Global Assessment Scale ($r = 0.78–0.89$)[w]
Minimum Data Set—Section G. Physical Functioning and Structural Problems Scale (MDS)[x]	To describe baseline ADL and track changes in ADL	Residents in long-term care; clients in home care[y]	10 activities (bed mobility, transfer, walk in room, walk in corridor, locomotion on unit, locomotion off unit, dressing, eating, toilet use, personal hygiene, and bathing)	Performance, ascertained from multiple sources, over all shifts during past 7 days; activities rated for self-performance; uses a five-point scale (0 = independent; 4 = total dependence) and support provided using a four-point scale (0 = no; 3 = 2+ person physical assist)[z]	*Interrater:* Spearman Brown average for ADL self-performance = 0.92, for ADL - support = 0.87[A]; weighted kappa = 0.86–0.94 for nursing home residents, 0.84–0.94 for home-care clients[y]	*Construct:* dependence in home-care sample was greater in early-loss ADL (bathing, dressing) than in late-loss ADL (bed mobility, eating)[y]
Milwaukee Evaluation of Daily Living Skills (MEDLS)[B]	Establish baseline behaviors to develop treatment objectives related to daily living skills	Adults with chronic mental health problems	20 subtests (communication, personal care, clothing care, home and community safety, money management, personal health care, medication management, telephone use, transportation usage, time awareness); subtests can be used individually or in combination	Screening, based on information from clients, clients' families, health-care team, and medical record to determine items to be examined; in examination, activities are performed (e.g., dressing), simulated (e.g., bathing) or described (e.g., transportation); each subtest is scored based on number of items completed for that subtest; there is no summary score	*Interrater:* range = 0.57–1.00; most subtests, $r \geq 0.80$	*Content:* based on review of literature and other similar instruments

Outcome and Assessment Information Set B-1 M0640–M0800 (OASIS)[C]	Measure the ability to perform ADL and IADL	Clients in home care	Eight ADL (dress upper body, dress lower body, bathing, toileting, transferring, ambulation/locomotion, feeding or eating, grooming); eight IADL (planning and preparing light meals, transportation, laundry, housekeeping, ability to use telephone, management of oral, inhalant/mist, and injectable medications)	Data may be obtained through various methods; ratings differentiated by task characteristics; scale varies from item to item; zero always equals highest independence level	Deemed stable for home-care field based on its successful applications[D]	*Face:* items are commonly included in ADL and IADL assessments
Performance Assessment of Self-Care Skills (PASS)[G]	Evaluate independent living skills at baseline, after intervention, or for monitoring functional status; provides information for planning intervention or to support service needs	Adults with impairments	26 activities, covering functional mobility (5 items), personal care (3 items), and home management (18 items); there are two protocols, one for use in the client's home and one for use in an occupational therapy clinic; the protocols are identical in terms of activities and performance criteria; however, in the home, clients use their own materials	Performance-based observational tool, yields summary scores of activity independence, safety, and adequacy; uses a four-point ordinal scale (0 = dysfunction; 3 = highest function)	*Decision* (agreement based on mutual observation): total score, independence = 96%, safety = 96%, adequacy = 88%[H]	*Content:* based on interview instruments *Construct:* in independence and adequacy, clients with osteoarthritis, depression, cardiopulmonary disease, macular degeneration, and dementia scored lower than nondisabled older adults; in safety, clients with dementia scored lower than clients with osteoarthritis, depression, cardiopulmonary disease, macular degeneration, and nondisabled older adults
Routine Task Inventory (RT1-2)[I]	Establish level of functional status and document change in status based on Allen Cognitive Levels (ACLs)[J]	Clients with psychiatric diagnoses, including those with cognitive impairments	32 items, covering disability in self-awareness (e.g., grooming, dressing, bathing), situational awareness (e.g., housekeeping, spending money, shopping), occupational role (e.g., planning/doing major role activities, pacing and timing actions), social role (e.g., communicating meaning, following instructions)	Observation or questioning of client (not recommended for Allen cognitive levels 1–4) or proxies; rater matches observations or descriptions of performance to operational definitions for each level of functioning, using a three- to six-point scale, with lower scores indicating lower ability	*Internal:* $r = 0.94$[K] *Interrater:* $r = 0.98$[K] *Test–retest:* $r = 0.91$[K]	*Criterion related:* correlations supported the relationship between functional decline and cognitive impairment on the Mini-Mental State Examination ($r_s = 0.61$)[L] and ACLs ($r_s = 0.54–0.56$)[M]

Continues

TABLE 24-5. **SUMMARY OF SELECTED ADL AND IADL INSTRUMENTS** *(Continued)*

Title	Purpose	Population	Description	Method/Rating	Psychometric Properties	
					Reliability	Validity
WeeFIM™[N]	Measure disability severity related to physical impairment, across health, development, educational, and community settings	Children from 6 months to 7 years	Uses same items as FIM™	Observation, interview or both; uses same rating system as FIM™; scores range from 18 (total dependence) to 126 (complete independence)	*Internal:* adequate consistency across raters and time for children with and without disabilities[O] *Test–retest:* intraclass correlation coefficient, for motor = 0.98, for cognitive = 0.96[O]	*Content:* expert judgment *Construct:* increase of WeeFIM scores with ages 2–5[P]

[a]Williams et al. (1991).
[b]Hilton, Fricke, & Unsworth (2001).
[c]Fisher (1995, 1997, 1999) & www.colostate.edu/programs/AMPS.
[d]See Bray, Fisher, & Duran et al. (2001) regarding the addition of 20 new activities.
[e]Doble, Fisk, Fisher, Ritvo, & Murray (1994).
[f]Doble, Fisk, Lewis, & Rockwood (1999).
[g]For references, see Bray et al. (2001) & Stauffer, Fisher, & Duran (2000).
[h]Robinson & Fisher (1966).
[i]Law (1998).
[j]Bosch (1995).
[k]McColl, Paterson, Davies, Doubt, & Law (2000).
[l]UDSMR (1997) & www.udsmr.org.
[m]A telephone version is available (Jaworski, Kult, & Boynton, 1994).
[n]Hamilton, Laughlin, Fiedler, & Granger (1994).
[o]Linacre, Heinemann, Wright, Granger, & Hamilton (1994).
[p]Heinemann, Linacre, Wright, Hamilton, & Granger (1994).
[q]Gosman-Hedström & Svensson (2000).
[r]Klein & Bell (1979, 1982).
[s]Law & Usher (1988).
[t]McGourty (1979, 1999).
[u]Ilika & Hoffman (1981a).
[v]Tateichi as cited in McGourty (1999).
[w]Ilika & Hoffman (1981b) & Kaufman (1982).
[x]Health Care Financing Administration (1988).
[y]Morris et al. (1997).
[z]Bathing self-performance is rated on a different scale, because bathing is not necessarily performed daily.
[A]Hawes, Morris, Phillips, Mor, Fries, & Nonemaker (1995).
[B]Leonardelli (1988) & Haertlein (1999), which contains a discussion of a potential revised edition.
[C]Center for Health Services & Poilicy Research (1998).
[D]Shaughnessy, Crisler, Schlenker, & Hittle (1999).
[E]cms.hhs.gov/medicare.
[F]Because the FIM™ rates tub & shower transfers and walk and wheelchair in a single item, the PAI also includes these as separately rated items.
[G]Rogers & Holm (1989, 1994, 1999).
[H]Decision consistency was used because the PASS is a criterion-referenced instrument (Rogers, Holm, Beach, Schulz, & Starz, 2001).
[I]Allen, Earhart, & Blue (1992).
[J]Allen (1985, 1990).
[K]Established on original version.
[L]Allen, Kehrberg, & Burn (1992).
[M]Heimann, Allen, & Yerxa (1989).
[N]UDSMR (2000) & www.udsmr.org.
[O]Ottenbacher, Msall, Lyons, Duffy, Granger, & Braun (1997) and Ottenbacher et al. (1996).
[P]Msall, DiGaudio, Duffy, LaForest, Braun, & Granger (1994).

TABLE 24-6. **RESOURCES FOR ADL AND IADL INSTRUMENTS**

Asher, I. A. (1996). *An annotated index of occupational therapy evaluation tools.* Rockville, MD: American Occupational Therapy Association.

Basmajian, J. (Ed.). (1994). *Physical rehabilitation outcome measures.* Toronto, ON: Canadian Physiotherapy Association.

Dittmar, S. S., & Gresham, G. E. (1997). *Functional assessment and outcome measures for the rehabilitation health professional.* Gaithersburg, MD: Aspen.

Ernst, M., & Ernst, N. S. (1984). Functional capacity. In D. J. Mangen and W. A. Peterson (Eds.). *Health, program evaluation, and demography* (Vol. 3, pp. 9–84). Minneapolis: University of Minnesota.

Gallo, J. J., Fulmer, T., Paveza, G. J., & Reichel, W. (2000). *Handbook of geriatric assessment* (3rd ed.). Gaithersburg, MD: Aspen.

Hemphill-Pearson, B. J. (Ed.). (1999). Assessments in occupational therapy mental health: An integrative approach. Thorofare, NJ: Slack.

Herndon, R. M. (Ed.). (1997). *Handbook of neurologic rating scales.* New York: Demos Vermande.

Kane, R. L., & Kane, R. A. (Eds.). (2000). *Assessing older persons: Measures, meaning, and practical applications.* Oxford: Oxford University Press.

Kidd, T., & Yoshida, K. (1995). Critical review of disability measures: Conceptual developments. *Physiotherapy Canada, 47,* 108–119.

Law, M., Baum, C., & Dunn, W. (Eds.). (2001). *Measuring occupational performance: Supporting best practice in occupational therapy.* Thorofare, NJ: Slack.

Lichtenberg, P. A. (Ed.). (1999). *Handbook of assessment in clinical gerontology.* New York: Wiley.

McDowell, I., & Newell, C. (1996). *Measuring health: A guide to rating scales and questionnaires* (2nd ed.). New York: Oxford University Press.

Osterweil, D., Brummel-Smith, K., & Beck, J. C. (2000). *Comprehensive geriatric assessment.* New York: McGraw-Hill.

Spiker, B. (1990). *Quality of life assessment in clinical trials.* New York: Raven.

ter Steeg, A. M., & Lankhorst, G. J. (1994). Screening instruments for disability. *Critical Reviews in Physical and Rehabilitation Medicine, 6,* 101–112.

Wade, D. T. (1992). *Measurement in neurological rehabilitation.* Oxford, UK: Oxford University Press.

instrument was developed or used, target population, description of the content, date-gathering method, scheme for rating activity limitations, and psychometric properties in terms of reliability and validity. Table 24-6 provides resources for ADL and IADL instruments.

CONCLUSION

When planning an occupation-based evaluation, practitioners make decisions about the extent of evaluation required (e.g., screening, evaluation), the activities appropriate for evaluation (e.g., personal care, home management), the method or methods to be used to learn about the patient's activity performance (e.g., asking questions, observing) and the instrument or instruments (e.g., FIM™, PASS) that will structure the data gathering process. Evaluation findings are then discussed with clients and/or their caregivers, and lead to mutually agreed upon intervention goals (e.g., referral, direct treatment) based on the client's needs and preferences. Hence, this decision-making process enables practitioners to plan occupation-based interventions that facilitate clients becoming competent in activities that they wish to do, are required to do, and are expected to do.

SECTION II

Therapeutic Driving and Community Mobility

SHERLYN FENTON
WENDY KRAFT
ELISA MARKS

The ability to move around in the community is critical to engaging in many valued occupations. For some people, the only **community mobility** required may be the ability to safely cross streets and walk to nearby stores. Alternatively, the need to go longer distances requires vehicular transportation. For many people in the United States and other large countries, this means driving. In 1995, 62% of all driver educators were occupational therapy practitioners; the primary health professionals who assist people to regain community mobility (French & Hansen, 1999).

This section describes how occupational therapists assess client community mobility and complete a **therapeutic driving evaluation.** Physicians, individuals with disabilities and their family members, rehabilitation counselors, and insurance case managers are among the many who refer clients to occupational therapy for this service (French & Hansen, 1999). A therapeutic driving evaluation consists of a **predriving assessment,** an **on-the-road practicum,** and an **evaluation report.** The report documents the individual's performance on both predriving and road tests, includes suggestions for equipment resources, and provides therapeutic recommendations regarding the client's driving skills. The ultimate objective of a driving evaluation is to provide the client with a viable plan for community mobility that accommodates the individual's highest level of function while maintaining public safety.

PREDRIVING ASSESSMENT

Occupational therapists begin therapeutic driving evaluations by interviewing clients about their previous driving experience, future requirements as driver and passenger, driving frequency, road conditions, and access to a vehicle. Pertinent medical history and records are reviewed, focusing on neuromuscular, sensory, and mental capacities related to driving skills and whether any limitations are stable or progressive. The neuromuscular examination includes active range of motion, tone, strength, coordination, and sensation. Static and dynamic sitting balance, general endurance, and clients' ability to transfer to and from the vehicle are also assessed. Clients are then asked to display simulated driving skills, such as manipulation of a steering wheel (including possible modifications) and the use of a brake. The therapist observes these simulations for driving feasibility, such as a brake reaction time of less than one second.

It is important to assess clients' abilities to meet their respective state visual regulations. A comprehensive visual evaluation tests clients' **useful field of view** (UFOV), which includes visual acuity for distance, visual fields, convergence, peripheral vision, saccades, color discrimination, and scanning. The use of technology to evaluate UFOV is recommended to ensure validity and reliability (Owsley et al., 1998).

Assessment of mental functions is crucial in the predriving phase, as results help indicate how feasible compensatory strategies will be (French & Hanson, 1999). Perceptual skills that are tested include depth perception, figure ground, form constancy, spatial relations, and unilateral neglect. Cognitive areas that are assessed include attention, insight into disability, visual memory, sequencing, scanning, problem solving, judgment, and cognitive processing time. The therapist also identifies other psychological factors, such as impulse control, frustration tolerance, and anxiety. In addition, clients need to exhibit a full understanding of driving laws. At the conclusion of the predriving assessment, the occupational therapist determines whether clients are ready to pursue the on-the-road practicum.

ON-THE-ROAD PRACTICUM

Clients are evaluated for safe-driving skills within the functional environment of an on-the-road practicum. Client assistive aids and vehicle equipment modifications are evaluated and incorporated at this time. For the road practicum, a rehabilitation program has the choice of using a local commercial driving school instructor in conjunction with a specialized occupational therapist or of providing the service in house with facility-owned equipment and an occupational therapist who has completed the Association for Driver Rehabilitation Specialists (ADED) program to become a **certified driver rehabilitation specialist** (CDRS).

In either case, the first consideration is to establish a predetermined driving route that encompasses the following driving environments: parking lot, quiet residential streets, busy roadways, city congestion, and highway traffic (Galski, Ehle, & Williams, 1998). A driving test route should give opportunities for drivers to demonstrate their ability to search for immediate and potential hazards. Decision-making ability can be determined by appropriate direction and speed control in relation to traffic flow and environmental

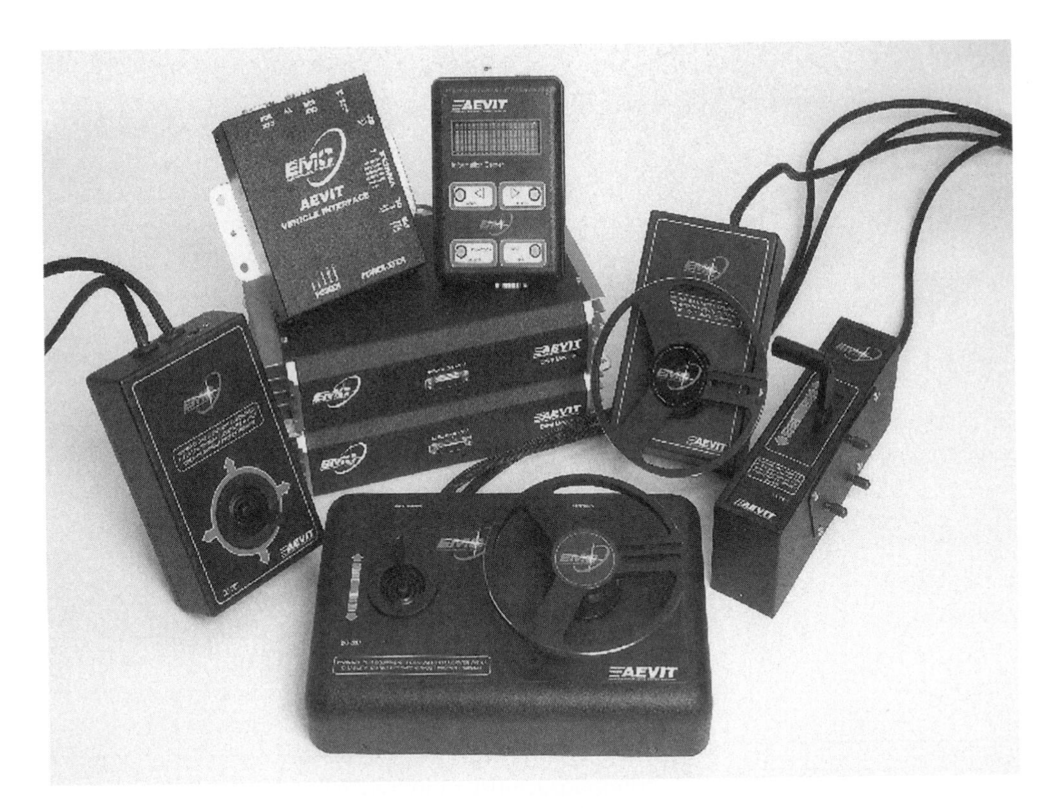

FIGURE 24–2. Electronic mobility controls provide assistive technology to augment driving skills.

situations. Ultimately, the final test route must allow for quick and safe instructor modification options during the actual practicum to ensure client and community safety.

During the road practicum, the evaluator observes the client's ability to operate and practice the systems of the vehicle. When a client requires a primary or secondary driving control, the modification systems should be available at the time of the assessment (Gross, 2001) (Figs. 24-2 and 24-3).

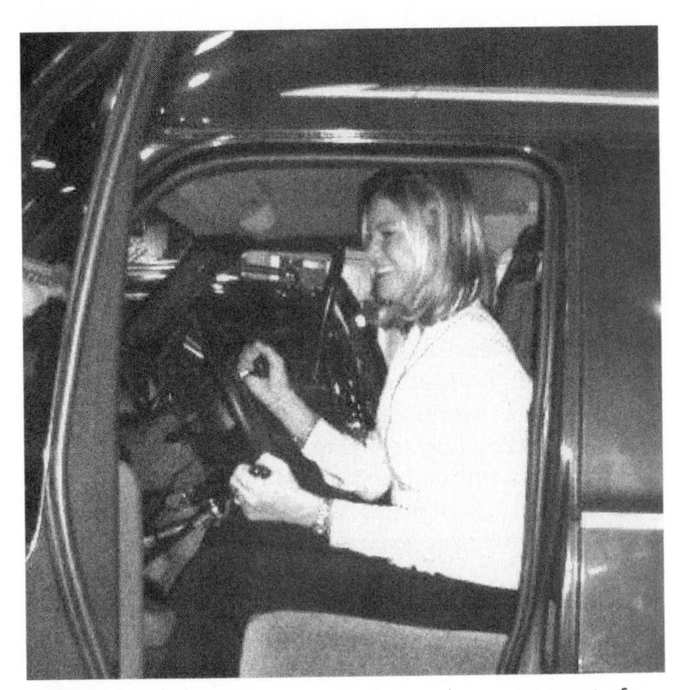

FIGURE 24–3. The driver uses hand controls to compensate for lower extremity paralysis.

EVALUATION INTERPRETATION AND DRIVING REPORT

It is crucial that therapists remain pragmatic in their interpretations following the predriving assessment and road practicum evaluations to maintain objective, client-specific recommendations (Huelskamp, 1997). The most restrictive scenario is that the therapist identifies areas of dysfunction that exclude clients from driving. In this situation, other community mobility resources should be investigated, determined, and implemented to meet clients' needs. When clients display potential yet lack readiness, the therapist recommends that they refrain from current driving and continue with therapy to strengthen deficient areas. When all goes well throughout the clinical assessment and road practicum, the therapist recommends that clients complete their state's registry of motor vehicles criteria and reenter the community as a skilled driver.

CONCLUSION

Historically, programs have focused on experienced drivers with acquired disabilities. However, Wheatley (2001) illustrated the significance of teaching individuals with developmental disabilities how to drive as a newly acquired functional skill. This may be a new area of practice for occupational therapists.

SECTION III

Work Activities

SHERLYN FENTON
PATRICIA GAGNON

"Work can offer a sense of mastery over the environment, as well as a sense of accomplishment and competence leading to an improved quality of life" (Siporin, 1999, p. 23). Occupational therapy practitioners use work-related assessments and interventions for individuals whose abilities to function in competitive work environments have been impaired by developmental disability, physical or emotional illness, or injury (AOTA, 1993).

HISTORICAL OVERVIEW

Occupational therapists have used work tasks to evaluate and rehabilitate persons with mental and physical impairments since the 1920s. In a 1985 *American Journal of Occupational Therapy* special issue on work evaluation, Marshall (1985) described changes in occupational therapy's role relative to work assessment. She noted that "industrial therapy" (p. 287) and treatment programs involving work activities, such as printing and construction, were common in the 1930s and 1940s. At that time, work evaluations consisted of client interviews, job analyses to define duties and requirements, and organization of tasks in a hierarchy of levels. In the 1950s, occupational therapy turned to a more medical model of practice, and attention to work–related evaluations by occupational therapists declined (Harvey-Krefting, 1985). Occupational therapists opting to continue administering work evaluations joined vocational evaluators and work adjusters within the vocational rehabilitation realm.

In the 1970s, occupational therapy theorists began to readdress the importance of work within the larger constructs of occupation (Marshall, 1985), and by the 1980s, medical rehabilitation programs reflected a renewed interest in work and work assessments.

Americans with Disabilities Act

The Rehabilitation Act of 1973 was the only legislation that addressed the civil and working rights of persons with disabilities in the United States before the passing of the **Americans with Disabilities Act** (ADA) on July 29, 1990. The advent of the ADA guaranteed Americans with disabilities access to employment, local and state services, transportation, telecommunications, and public accommodations equal to that of Americans without disabilities (Bowman, 1992).

"*Title 1: Employment* of the ADA was written to prevent employers from discrimination practices against applicants and employees with disabilities. An organization cannot discriminate against an individual with a disability who can perform the **essential functions** of a job with or without **reasonable accommodations.** The essential functions of a job are the job duties a person must be able to perform unaided or with reasonable accommodations. Reasonable accommodations are modifications or adjustments that enable persons with disabilities to perform a job they are otherwise qualified to perform" (Rybski, 1992, p. 412). "In order to ensure that modifications and adaptations fit the individual needs of the worker, it is important to know the objective abilities and limitations of the worker" (Clawson & Noiseux, 2000, p. 32).

Occupational therapists who have attained competency in work environment practices have an expanded role in assessing workers and the work environment within the employment provision of the ADA (Fontana, 1999).

PRACTICE SETTINGS

Occupational therapists and certified occupational therapy assistants treat individuals in work programs in outpatient clinics, hospitals, work sites, sheltered workshops, schools, correctional institutions, long-term care facilities, community-based health centers, private practice, and other environments in which people require skilled assistance to regain vocational function. The ultimate goal is to place the client in the work environment most suitable to his or her level of functioning. This may include volunteer placement and part-time work in addition to full-time, gainful employment (AOTA, 2001b).

Although occupational therapy services can help individuals with many kinds of conditions, such as developmental disabilities and persistent mental illness, in this section, we focus on programs primarily for injured workers, because they are among the most prevalent. Two broad categories of programs for injured workers are industrial rehabilitation programs and ergonomic/work-site consulting. Many occupational therapy practices provide services for both categories. When amenable by the organization, on-site intervention programs provide the therapist with the advantage of observing the jobs directly, which facilitates understanding of the essential functions and demands of the job (Ellexson, 1997).

INDUSTRIAL REHABILITATION EVALUATIONS

Work-based rehabilitation programs focus on the clients' functional abilities as they relate to occupation. Occupational therapists are primary professionals working with clients to assess and determine the appropriate matching of clients, their abilities, job demands, and work environments. Being able to maximize an individual's function by integrating the right performance components and contexts enables the worker to feel productive while providing a sense of connectedness. Therapists have developed assessments and tools to evaluate performance components in the areas of work and productivity.

The **functional capacity evaluation** (FCE) is a comprehensive battery of tests that yields objective measures regarding clients' current levels of function and their abilities to perform work-related tasks. FCE tests often include, but are not limited to, a **physical capacity evaluation** (PCE) and functional standardized and nonstandardized assessments, such as job task simulations and relevant ADL. The data collected and interpreted from these test results are used to evaluate clients' work capacities. The administration procedures for these evaluations must meet five criteria established by the National Institute of Occupational Safety and Health (NIOSH; 1981): safety of administration, reliability, job relatedness, practicality, and productiveness (Iserhagen, 1990).

Intake Interview

The intake interview is the first client contact. The interview focuses on the client's report of past work history, present medical condition, vocational status, and general ethic. Information on previous or reoccurring injuries, results of diagnostic procedures, and medical interventions are considered to determine whether special testing methods are indicated.

During this initial interview, clients complete a functional job description to identify the physical, functional, and psychological demands of their work. The daily vocational tasks are defined in terms of frequency, duration, and methods of work. Lifting, carrying, pushing, pulling, walking, climbing, sitting, standing, driving, and key stroking are a few of the performance components considered and described. The practitioner compares the workers' self-reported job description with the following (Isernhagen & Brown, 1999):

- A functional job description (FJD) as submitted by each client's employer.
- The *Dictionary of Occupational Titles*, the U.S. Department of Labor's (1986) former method.
- O*Net Occupational Information Network, the U.S. Department of Labor's proposed new job categorization method.

This cross-reference provides a comprehensive view of the job's demands and highlights any discrepancies in expectations.

The initial intake interview also addresses clients' subjective perceptions of their ability to participate in the occupational performance areas of bathing, dressing, homemaking, sleeping, and driving. Performance area limitations may be the result of medical restrictions and clients' experiences of pain. Therefore, self-reporting methods are used to determine clients' perceptions of pain. Some commonly used pain scales are the Ransford Pain Drawing (Ransford, Cairns, & Mooney, 1979), the Borg Numerical Pain Scale (Borg, 1982), the McGill Pain Questionnaire (Melzack, 1983, 1987), and the Oswestry (Fairbanks, Davies, & O'Brien, 1980). (See Chapter 30, Section 7 for additional information about pain evaluations.) Comparison of similar scales can support a clinical diagnosis or demonstrate inconsistencies that may indicate abnormal illness behavior. A thorough intake interview is essential in the clinical reasoning phase, while establishing intervention and determining discharge planning.

Physical Capacity Evaluation

The physical capacity evaluation is a significant portion of the FCE. This group of evaluations is often administered by physical therapists and assesses the physical and biomechanical aspects of clients' level of function. The musculoskeletal portion of the assessment involves objective measurements of clients' active range of motion, muscle strength, posture, and gait. Functional hand postures, volumetric measurements, sensation, and cardiopulmonary status are included in the PCE as indicated.

Additional examination techniques may be incorporated for clients with lower back pain to identify nonorganic physical signs. To determine these signs, a group of nine physical tests was developed by Waddell, McCulloch, Kummel, and Venner (1980). Referred to as Waddell signs, these are assessments designed to detect abnormal illness behavior or symptoms not consistent with typical anatomy and physiology.

The results of the PCE, along with documentation received from the client's physician and other medical professionals, provide a baseline of the client's current physical capacity and any performance discrepancies. This information helps the therapist determine if it is appropriate for the client to continue with the FCE. Demonstration of the reliability and validity of physical evaluation results are imperative for third-party payers to support a rehabilitation plan. This is done by selecting valid assessments and by systematically checking to see that the client is demonstrating good faith efforts to complete the assessments. Performing maximum voluntary effort (MVE) tests in a serial fashion allows the therapist to determine the client's intratask consistency (Hildreth, Breidenbach, Lister, & Hodges, 1989; Niemeyer, Matheson, & Carlton, 1989)

The Jamar dynamometer is a tool frequently used to test MVE. Individuals are instructed to apply maximal gross strength for each trial. For the Jamar Dynamometer Endurance Test, clients complete three trials in each of the five dynamometer handle positions. Stokes (1983) recommended that therapists observe the client's grasping patterns and displayed effort. Noted contraction of muscle groups in the forearm, neck, or jaw and visible tightening of tendons typically indicate strong effort, whereas co-contraction of the hand and forearm muscles causing tremors is often observed in individuals who are not putting forth MVE.

In addition to these instruments and tests, several tool activity sorts are used to provide further information on perceived ability and effort. The West Tool Sort, Loma Linda Activity Sort, and Spinal Functions Sort are all means by which the evaluator can compare the client's responses to demonstrated functioning during clinical testing. For example, clients who rate themselves as disabled from lifting a 20-lb bag of groceries on the Spinal Function Sort can be evaluated during a lifting evaluation for intratask consistency. Although these assessment can be useful, isolated use of effort testing can result in inaccurate assessments and documentation (Jacobs, 1991; Niemeyer et al., 1989). Fear of injury, anticipation of pain or anxiety, and lack of clear test procedure instructions all may produce test results that, erroneously, illustrate submaximal effort. Therefore, therapists must document actual test results, objectively report patterns of behavior, and ultimately interpret all data to formulate outcome recommendations.

Functional Capacity Evaluation

A functional capacity evaluation goes beyond measuring a client's biomechanical capacities and is often customized to meet the client's particular situation. Both standardized and nonstandardized assessments are chosen, based on the client's diagnosis, job description, and discharge plan. Commonly used standardized tests include the following:

- Bennett Hand Tool Dexterity Test.
- Minnesota Rate of Manipulation.
- Purdue Peg Board.
- Nine Hole Peg Test.
- O'Connor Finger Dexterity Test.
- Jebsen Hand Function Test.

These all provide information about the client's capabilities and physical tolerances for fine and gross motor skills. Therapists can compare the client's performance with standards derived from tests of relevant populations.

Nonstandardized assessments allow the therapist to assess the client during performance of relevant occupational tasks related to both work and ADL. The therapist's ability to attain a baseline of a client's capability to perform job-simulated tasks is facilitated by several commercially developed work samples. The Valpar Component Work Samples numbers 1–19 and 202–205, the Skills Assessment Module (SAM), the Baltimore Therapeutic Equipment Box, and the West 2A, 3, 4A, and 7 all are used in work evaluations. These tests provide systematic methods of simulating work activities while adhering to NIOSH standards.

An example of the application of a work sample is to evaluate a parcel-delivery worker's ability to complete essential job functions after a low back injury. The Valpar Work Sample number 19 requires the client to read invoices, fill, lift, and move various weighted trays from a variety of heights. The therapist's choosing the most appropriate work samples for the client's job demands is the key to attaining beneficial information for future vocational recommendations.

There are numerous tests available to evaluate clients' capabilities for material handling. Maximal and repetitive lift tests are performed to evaluate strength and knowledge of proper body mechanics and to determine clients' current physical demand level, as categorized by the U.S. Department of Labor. Free-weighted tests and high-technology evaluating equipment both have advantages and drawbacks when used to attempt to assess clients' strength and job skills. Free-weighted tests include the Maximum Isoinertial Effort Test, West 2 Lifting Protocol, and the Progressive Isoinertial Lifting Evaluation (PILE) (Mayer et al., 1988).

The use of highly technological versions of work capacity evaluation devices has paralleled the growth of functional capacity evaluations. The devices simulate and evaluate a wide variety of physical demands, such as lifting, pushing, pulling, and gripping. The Baltimore Therapeutic Equipment (BTE) Work Simulator, the BTE Dynamic Lift, the Lido Work Set, and ERGOS are all examples of commonly used devices. Although these tools provide excellent methods of evaluation, one study has shown that the BTE work simulator tends to overestimate real lifting endurance performance in healthy men (Ting, Wessel, Brintnell, Maikala, & Bhambhani, 2000, p. 184). Experienced therapists soon learn to discern between hard test results and the interpreted abilities of their clients.

Evaluation Interpretation and Documentation

Once the FCE is complete and the results have been interpreted, the therapeutic recommendations are communicated to the individuals authorized to receive the report. Examples of typical recommendations include immediate return to work with or with out limitation, a functional restoration/work hardening program to address limitations in current physical demand levels, vocational counseling, and/or ergonomic analysis.

ERGONOMIC ANALYSIS AND ON-SITE SERVICES

Industries are searching for effective means of preventing injuries at work, and they are turning to occupational therapists as consultants to implement company programs. Industries are looking at their bottom line and are seeing the value of ergonomically based injury-prevention programs and industrial rehabilitation. Therapists who provide such services must be proficient in the areas of **anthropometrics** and **ergonomics.** Anthropometrics describes the physical dimensions and properties of the body, in terms of functional arm, leg, and body movements, made by a worker performing a task. Ergonomics is the science of fitting the task to the worker and not the worker to the task. By improving the interaction of the worker with the equipment, work process, and workstation design, therapists can contribute to workers' well-being.

Ergonomic evaluations include work tolerance screenings, **job site analysis** (JSA), functional job description assessment, job hazard identification, job modification assignment, worker performance evaluations, and reasonable accommodation determination. Other work environment–related services include proper body mechanics training, monitoring safe and effective use of assistive/adaptive therapeutic device technology, and ergonomic principles education.

A successful ergonomic program is reflected in decreased workers' compensation costs, increased productivity and efficiency, and improved morale. Ergonomic programs should involve everyone from the front-line employees to the executive officers. Employers who care about the safety and well-being of their employees take the initiative to implement prevention programs. These organizations reap the benefits of a healthier bottom line. Although ergonomic reform has become a governmental, partisan issue, the previous legislative changes brought on by the ADA, Occupational Safety Health Administration (OSHA), and Workers' Compensation System continue to create a demand for occupational therapy involvement in ergonomic consultation, training, and programming.

Job Site Analysis

Occupational therapy consultants complete a job site analysis as the first step in familiarizing themselves with a work environment or task. The tools most often used in a JSA are a stopwatch, tape measure, counter, video camera, tripod, yardstick, and a variety of force gauges. These tools provide objective methods of assessing physical heights, distances, and work cycles to consider the requirements of force, repetition, and awkward postures.

A review of job descriptions and worker and employer interviews provide information concerning job practices, duration of jobs, and the specific equipment and materials used in jobs. Observation during different work phases, shifts, and seasons (if appropriate or possible) is also essential in realizing both the physical and the psychological demands of the work environment. Work practices and safety procedures need to be considered and adhered to, by therapists (e.g., safety shoes, glasses, and hearing protection) while at the site.

The choice of JSA methods depends on the goal of the analysis or the type of task being evaluated. A manual material handling (MMH) task, such as stocking shelves in a grocery store, may be approached in four ways: psychophysics, static biomechanical models, the NIOSH revised lifting guidelines, and the dynamic biomechanical model.

Psychophysics Model

The psychophysics approach depicts maximum acceptable values for lifting, carrying, pushing, and pulling that are perceived as tolerable by percentages of the working population (Snook & Ciriello, 1991).

Static Biomechanical Model

Under the static biomechanical model, computer software is used to estimate spinal compression force based on posture information. The therapist uses this information to assess the stress and risk of injury involved in handling materials. In 1991, NIOSH revised its lifting guidelines. The appeal of this method is the ease with which the required data can be collected, extrapolated, and interpreted to determine safe lifting practices.

The results of material handling tests are related to the client's job description and extrapolated into a physical demand level of work (PDL) as described by the U.S. Department of Labor (1986) in its *Dictionary of Occupational Titles*. The numeric values achieved from the individual tests are translated into work classifications according to the force (sedentary, light, medium, heavy, and very heavy), frequency, and duration (occasional, frequent, and constant) of lifts achieved during testing (Table 24-7).

Dynamic Biomechanical Model

The dynamic biomechanical model suggests that torsion forces combined with compressive forces increases the risk factors of occupational low back injuries (Buttle, 1995). Occupational therapists observe job motions for examples of torsion and compression (e.g., lifting a heavy load while twisting with feet planted). When the worker's capabilities do not meet the physical demands, as defined by the essential functions of the job, recommendations may include a full FCE

TABLE 24–7. **THE PHYSICAL DEMAND LEVELS OF WORK**[a]

Physical Demand Level	Occasional (0–33% of time; lb)[b]	Frequent (34–66% of time; lb)[b]	Constant (67–100% of time; lb)[b]
Sedentary	10	Negligible	Negligible
Light	20	10	Negligible
Medium	50	20	10
Medium-heavy	75	35	15
Heavy	100	50	20
Very heavy	100+	50+	20+

[a]U.S. Department of Labor (1986).

[b]Defined by the U.S. Department of Labor (1986) as the frequency of "exerting a force," including lifting, carrying, pushing, pulling, or any other physical activity.

with a functional restoration program, a change in jobs, or a reasonable accommodation. Reasonable accommodations include modifying a work schedule, job reassignment, restructuring the workstation, and/or providing more appropriate tools.

Employers must provide reasonable accommodations to qualified persons with a disability unless they can substantiate that the modifications cause undue hardship or a significant safety risk to other workers. Accommodations that strain the financial resources of employers or fundamentally alter the nature of the job are considered undue hardship. An organization's entire resources, such as productivity and quality, are evaluated when determining if a reasonable accommodation qualifies as undue hardship. Most reasonable accommodations, however, can be implemented inexpensively, allowing workers to return to their original duties.

The completed JSA should yield information that will allow the employer to determine the essential functions of the job. Once the functions are determined, a functional job description that accurately depicts the requirements can be written. This job description is the mechanism by which the employer can either reinstate an injured worker with reasonable accommodation or determine if there is the need for screening new employees.

Work Tolerance Screenings

According to the ADA, screenings can be performed after a conditional offer of employment has been made (but before the offer has been finalized) and must test the job's essential functions to be consistent with business necessity. Essential functions that should be included in the preplacement, testing protocol are tasks involving high risk.

OSHA has identified three factors as significant contributors to risk: force, distance (awkward posture), and frequency. Jobs with a history of previously recorded injuries may also be included in the protocol. In the screening evaluation, it is the outcome of the task, not the manner in which the task is performed that matters. Therapists administering work tolerance screenings offer reasonable accommodation options to applicants and workers to assess their ability to meet essential job functions. Although work tolerance screenings can assess the fit between worker and work, they cannot predict future injuries or worker productivity. This is why a full ergonomic program is recommended.

Ergonomics consultation examines the relationship between task demands and worker capabilities in the work environment. The process of referral, evaluation, problem identification, goal establishment, intervention, reevaluation, discharge, and follow-up is necessary when providing both traditional occupational therapy and ergonomics consulting services (Hoelscher & Taylor, 2000).

CONCLUSION

Occupational therapy can play an important and unique role in linking work evaluations to worker's mental, emotional, and physical capacities and to the physical and social environment in the work setting. The profession is well positioned to formulate comprehensive theoretical models of work that should improve and refine present evaluations (Velozo, 1993). As professionals with a sound understanding of occupation and its relevance to injured workers, therapists can be instrumental in future research and development relative to worker assessment and rehabilitation. Using this knowledge, occupational therapists have the opportunity to expand services beyond the injured worker to injury-prevention programs and the development of work programs for individuals with other challenges, such as developmental disabilities, head injuries, and persistent mental illness.

SECTION IV

Educational Activities

YVONNE L. SWINTH

OCCUPATIONAL THERAPY IN EDUCATIONAL SETTINGS

Occupational therapy practitioners work in a variety of educational settings. These include public schools, charter schools, private schools, alternative schools, vocational schools, and university settings (Case-Smith, Rogers, Johnson, 2001). Within these settings, practitioners work with students ranging from infancy through college. Public schools are the most common work setting for occupational therapy practitioners, with almost 25% of all practitioners identifying a public school as their primary work setting (AOTA, 2001a). Therefore, the primary focus of this section is on evaluation of occupational performance within public schools. However, many of the principles discussed can be generalized to any educational setting.

Practice within the schools is guided by federal legislation, with focus on the occupation of education. Occupational therapists began working in the schools after 1935, when federal grants to the states created Crippled Children's Services under a special section of the Social Securities Act (1935). Initially, these services were provided in segregated settings or special schools and primarily to children with orthopedic and neurological impairments (Hanft & Place, 1996). In 1975, the Education of All Handicapped Children Act (EHA) was enacted. This act required states to provide special education and related services, including occupational therapy, to all eligible children ages 6 through 21. Amendments to the EHA in 1986 added services for preschoolers aged 3–5 years and provided incentives for states to develop statewide systems for providing early intervention services to infants, toddlers, and their families.

TABLE 24-8. **KEY CHANGES IN THE IDEA OF 1997**[a]

- Participation of children and youth with disabilities in statewide and districtwide assessment programs
- Expanded participation by parents in any decisions made about their child
- Addition of transition planning starting at age 14, younger if needed
- Supporting professional development to ensure that all school personnel have the needed knowledge and skills to educate children with disabilities
- Increased specificity about eligibility evaluation and reevaluation requirements
- Increased emphasis on student performance and outcomes

[a]Modified from National Information Center for Children and Youth with Disabilities (1998).

In 1990, the EHA was renamed the Individuals with Disabilities Education Act (IDEA), and additional services were added. These include assistive technology devices and services, transition services and increased focus, and funds and programs for children with emotional disturbances. Further amendments were made to the IDEA (PL 105–17) in 1997, which mostly fine-tune the original intent of the law (AOTA, 1999) and include increased emphasis on access to the general education curriculum for students with disabilities (Table 24-8).

Since 1975, the key goals of the IDEA have remained the same (Table 24-9), with an increasing shift from the old paradigm of "if we cannot fix them, we exclude them" to the new paradigm of "disability as a natural and normal part of the human experience" (Silverstein, 2000 p. 1761). Thus the role of occupational therapy under the IDEA has shifted to a focus on contextual factors, such as access to the environment so individuals with disabilities can participate in their environments, rather than on fixing the disability. The IDEA has four parts (A–D); however, in this section I will address only Parts B and C (Part A deals with the general provisions of the IDEA and part D focuses on research and training).

TABLE 24-9. **KEY ASSUMPTIONS OF THE IDEA**[a]

- Equality of opportunity for all individuals
- Full participation (empowerment)
- Independent living
- Economic self-sufficiency

[a]Modified from Silverstein (2000).

TABLE 24-10. **COMMON TERMS IN THE IDEA**[a]

Term	Comments
Free appropriate public education (FAPE)	Special education and related services provided at public expense that meets the standards of the state education agency (SEA)
Individualized education program (IEP)	A commitment of services that ensures that an appropriate program is developed that meets the requirements of the child's unique educational needs
Least restrictive environment (LRE)	The environment that provides maximum interaction with nondisabled peers and is consistent with the needs of the child or student
Related services	Transportation and such developmental, corrective, and other supportive services (including speech/language, audiology, psychological, and physical and occupational therapy services) needed to help the child benefit from special education
Special education	Specially designed instruction at no cost to parents to meet the unique needs of a child with a disability

[a]Modified from National Council on Disabilities (2000).

Under Part C of the IDEA, occupational therapy can be a primary service for infants and toddlers from birth through 2 years of age who are eligible for early intervention services (AOTA, 1999). Part B of the IDEA stipulates occupational therapy, as a related service, for children ages 3–21 for whom the team determines the service is necessary for them to benefit from their special education program. Two key concepts of Part B of the IDEA are a free and appropriate public education (FAPE) in the least restrictive environment (LRE). (Table 24-10 defines key terms found within the IDEA.) The IDEA allows each state and local education agency some latitude in how the federal legislation is implemented as long as the FAPE and LRE provisions are not compromised. Thus there are differences across states and local programs regarding the specifics of how services are provided under the IDEA.

One primary role of the occupational therapy practitioner in the school setting is to contribute to the evaluation process. The practitioner's contribution may be to help the educational team determine eligibility for special education or related services and/or to determine the need for occupational therapy. Several key assumptions underlie the evaluation process in schools under the IDEA that occupational therapy practitioners do not have to address in other settings. These assumptions are briefly discussed below.

UNDERLYING ASSUMPTIONS OF THE EVALUATION PROCESS IN THE SCHOOLS

As with other occupational therapy practice areas, the evaluation process in the schools is dynamic and ongoing and often continues during intervention (Stewart, 2001). According to the IDEA, the evaluation determines whether a child has a disability and the nature and extent of the special education and related services that the child needs. The IDEA does not require use of a specific type of assessment method or tool. Rather, the act requires use of a variety of tools and strategies to gather relevant "functional and developmental information" related to enabling the child to "be involved in and progress in the general education curriculum (Section 300. 532(b))." In addition, the evaluation should help determine children's educational needs and how their disability affects their participation in school activities. Children do not "qualify" for occupational therapy on the basis of testing under the IDEA. Instead, occupational therapy services should be recommended and provided for children if it is necessary for them to "benefit from their special education program" (Section 300. 24) (Fig. 24-4). Even though the evaluation process in the schools is guided by the IDEA, occupation remains core to the occupational therapy practitioners theoretical perspective. Within the educational setting, practitioners draw on the appropriate frames of reference to guide the evaluation process.

A team of qualified individuals—which may include an occupational therapist, school psychologist, special education and general education teachers, physical therapist, and speech and language pathologist—is responsible for conducting the evaluation. The purpose of the evaluation process is to determine the student's needs not only to have access to the educational environment to the maximum extent possible but also to perform within the school setting. In addition, the IDEA requires that the evaluation help determine services that will support a student's ability to demonstrate outcomes with a focus on the general education curriculum. Therefore, the evaluation process is driven by contextual factors (the school environment) and student (client) needs (Dunn, Brown, & McGuigan, 1994).

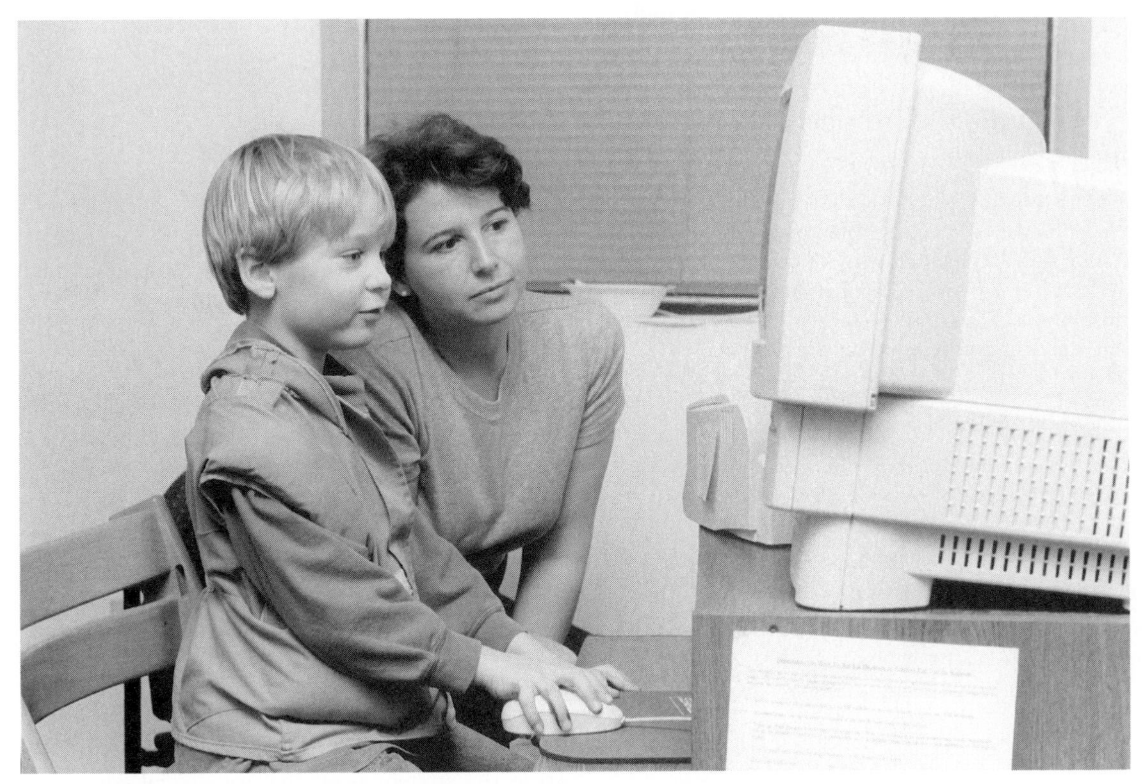

FIGURE 24–4. In the school setting, the occupational therapist focuses on the child's performance related to educational needs. (Courtesy of C. Harmeling and Occupational Therapy Associates Watertown.)

The evaluation process should be individualized (student centered) and should use a top-down approach (Coster, 1998). This means that the occupational therapy evaluation should start by looking at student performance versus evaluating specific performance components out of context. As with any occupational therapy evaluation, a broad view of the student (client) is key and must be considered. Thus the emphasis is on the educational context, including physical, temporal, social, and cultural considerations. Within the educational setting, the focus of special education and related services is on student outcomes. If the educational staff and/or parents require services (e.g., specialized training) to help the student reach his or her outcomes, then the practitioner must address those needs (Primeau & Ferguson, 1999) as well as broader systems issues (e.g., curriculum, environmental adaptations) that may require occupational therapy input and support. Under the IDEA, occupational therapy services are supportive in nature to help the child succeed in school and after-school activities (Giangreco, 2001). Thus, in addition to being provided to the student, services can be provided "on behalf of" the child and "to the parents, teachers and other staff" (Section 300. 347(a)(3)) so that they can better support the child's learning (Table 24-11).

TABLE 24–11. **CLIENTS TO CONSIDER DURING THE OCCUPATIONAL THERAPY EVALUATION PROCESS**

Client	Evaluation Consideration(s)
Student	Gather data regarding the occupational profile and occupational performance
Parent or educational staff	Based on student's occupational profile and occupational performance, determine if there is any need for specific training, support, and/or dissemination of information
System	Based on student's occupational profile and occupational performance, determine if there are any system supports (e.g., environmental modifications, curriculum development) that are needed

ETHICS NOTE 24–1

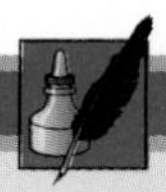

Use of Standardized Assessments

PENNY KYLER and RUTH A. HANSEN

Alane was recently hired by the local elementary school. The school administrator asked Alane to complete sensory screenings of all the children in kindergarten. Alane is expected to use the Sensory Profile (Dunn, 1999) as part of this process. She is unfamiliar with this particular assessment and does not have a complete test manual readily available.

QUESTIONS AND EXERCISES

1. **What is Alane's ethical responsibility to know and understand the levels of reliability and validity when using a standardized test?**
2. **Identify the ethical issues surrounding a therapist's use of standardized assessment procedures.**
3. **Identify the department's area of responsibility for using standardized assessments.**

EVALUATION PROCESS

Occupational therapists in the school setting focus their evaluation on what is needed for the student to engage in meaningful and purposeful school occupations. The occupational therapy assessment addresses the student's strengths and concerns in the occupational performance areas of ADL, education/work, play/leisure, and social participation. In each of these areas, occupational therapists address the performance skills and the physical, sensory, neurological, and cognitive/mental functions of students. First, an occupational profile is developed in collaboration with the team, including the family and student, as appropriate. This profile is followed by an analysis of the student's occupational performance within the educational setting.

Below, I briefly describe the occupational therapy evaluation process. The specific role of the occupational therapist during the evaluation process for any given student depends on the expertise and skills of all the team members as well as the referral concerns. As in all other settings in which occupational therapy practitioners work, the occupational therapist is responsible for the administration of the evaluation methods and measures, the interpretation and documentation of results, and the communication of evaluation results with other team members. However, if an occupational therapy assistant is part of the team, he or she may contribute to any part of the process under the direct supervision of the occupational therapist.

Referral

Generally, the process of referral within the school setting is different from that in a clinical setting. As with any procedure within special education, specific steps can vary from state to state or setting to setting. However, in most situations, if there is a concern about student performance, a team of professionals discusses and implements different strategies within the general education classroom before referring the student for special education. If these strategies are not successful, then the student is referred for a special education evaluation to determine his or her eligibility for services. Occupational therapy may or may not be involved in this step of the process. If the occupational therapist is not involved in the initial evaluation process, then the team may request an occupational therapy evaluation at any time after determining the student is eligible for special education. If the occupational therapist is working in a state where the occupational therapy practice act requires a physician referral for services, then such a referral may be necessary before the implementation of services. If a physician refers a student for an occupational therapy evaluation, the referral does not guarantee services in a school setting. The occupational therapist in the school must first ensure that the student is eligible for special education and then determine if services are necessary for the student to benefit from his or her education program.

Occupational Profile

The occupational profile is developed by gathering data from the student, family, and educational staff (AOTA, in press). Occupational therapy assistants, community providers, and others who know the student also may contribute to the evaluation. The development of the occupational profile occurs over time. Several assessments and procedures have been developed for use in the educational setting that can support the development of the occupational profile. (Table 24-12 summarizes some of these assessments.) Most of these assessments are process oriented and must be completed with input from all team members, including the student and family. Many of the assessments have a problem-solving focus that addresses the student's strengths and concerns as well as contextual factors that may affect student performance and outcomes. Many also help the occupational therapy practitioner identify performance patterns and activity demands. By completing one or more of these process-oriented assessments, the occupational therapy practitioner will have addressed most of the questions outlined within the occupational therapy practice framework (Table 24-13). Box 24-1 summarizes an occupational profile for Kristi, a junior high school student with cerebral palsy.

Analysis of Occupational Performance

Once the occupational profile has been developed, the occupational therapist works with the team to determine if

TABLE 24-12. COMMON EVALUATION METHODS AND TOOLS USED WITHIN EDUCATIONAL SETTINGS

	Participation		Areas of Occupation					Performance Skills	Client Factors
	Characteristics	Contextual Factors	Activity			Experience			
Assessment[a]			Activity Interests	Activity Choices	Subjective Experience	Personal Meaning	Satisfaction		
Process-oriented assessment tools (support gathering data for the occupational profile and analysis of occupational performance)									
Choosing Outcomes and Accommodations for Children(COACH)	■	■	■	■	■	■	■	■	■
Making Action Plan (MAPS)	■	■	■	■	■	■	■	■	■
Planning Alternative Tomorrows with Hope (PATH)	■	■	■	■	■	■	■	■	■
Interview with the student, educational staff, parents, and others	■	■	■	■	■	■	■	■	■
School Function Assessment (SFA)	■	■		■				■	■
Observation	■	■	■	■	■	■	■	■	■
Vermont Interdependent Services Team Approach (VISTA)	■	■	■	■	■	■	■	■	■
Skill-oriented assessment tools (support analysis of occupational performance with specific performance skills, patterns, and tasks)									
Beery Developmental Test of Visual Motor Skills								■	■
Bruininks-Oseretsky Test of Motor Proficiency								■	■
Children's Handwriting Evaluation Scale (CHES)								■	■
Coping Inventory	■				■			■	■
DeGangi-Berk Test of Sensory Integration								■	■
Developmental Test of Visual Perception (DVPT)								■	■
Evaluation Tool of Children's Handwriting (ETCH)								■	■
Gross Motor Function Measure (GMFM)	■							■	■
Knox Preschool Play Scale				■				■	
Interest checklist			■						
Leisure Diagnostic Battery		■	■		■	■		■	
Minnesota Handwriting Assessment								■	■
Motor Free Visual Perception Test (MVPT)								■	■
Peabody Developmental Motor Scales (PDMS)								■	■
Pediatric Evaluation of Disability Inventory (PEDI)	■	■						■	■
Sensory Integration and Praxis Test (SIPT)								■	■
Sensory Profile	■							■	■
Test of handwriting skills								■	■
Test of Visual Perceptual Skills (TVPS)								■	■
Test of Visual Motor Skills (TVMS)								■	■

[a]See Appendix A for further resource information about assessments.

Assessment Process for Kristi

Background

Kristi is a 13-year old student with tetraplegia cerebral palsy. She has received occupational therapy, in the past, in both clinical and school-based settings. Kristi and her family recently moved and the education team in her new school district completed an evaluation to determine her educational needs.

Developing the Occupational Profile

The occupational therapist gathered data for the occupational profile by talking to Kristi and her family and reviewing Kristi's past records. Through this process, the therapist began to develop a summary of Kristi's occupational history and strengths and concerns in the areas of occupation related to Krisiti's educational program. The therapist then observed Kristi in her educational environment. This included academic courses, PE, lunch, and transitional periods (e.g., on and off the bus, between classes). The team also met with Kristi and her parents to complete a McGill Action Planning System (MAPs).

Analysis of Occupational Performance

Based on the data gathered the occupational therapist summarized Kristi's occupational performance (strengths and concerns) related to Kristi's physical, sensory, neurological, and/or mental functions. Since Kristi had some difficulty with handwriting, the therapist also completed a Test of Visual Perceptual Skills and a Test of Visual Motor Skills to assess potential underlying visual perceptual issues affecting Kristi's handwriting performance. The therapist also completed a manual muscle test to determine strength and range of motion.

The occupational therapist summarized the following findings and recommendations to the education team.

Activities of daily living (basic and instrumental)	Kristi is able to take care of her basic self-care needs within her school environment at this time. However, she has difficulty with some dressing activities that may affect her ability to participate in PE activities when she moves to the Jr. High School. Kristi and her mom also want Kristi to take a cooking class as soon as possible to determine Kristi's need for adaptive equipment for cooking.
	Kristi uses a school bus with a lift to get to and from school. She is able to communicate with her peers and teachers without any difficulty.
Education	Kristi is able to participate and complete assignments in her general education classes with accommodations/adaptations. She does require additional time to complete written assignments and utilizes a computer for longer papers. She needs to develop the self-determination skills necessary to independently problem-solve and implement accommodations/adaptations.
Work	Kristi states that she would like to be a lawyer or special education teacher. At age 14, the team will collaborate with Kristi and her parents to begin to develop her transition plan. This plan will support the assessment and address her needs for future environments.
Play/leisure	Kristi rides horses, swims at the YMCA and enjoys playing computer games and watching TV.
Social Participation	Kristi tends to be a loner at school. Her mother states that she is very social when at home with her family, but that she has minimum interaction with other students her age. Kristi reports that she enjoys sports and even though she cannot play, she would like to be involved by keeping scores or helping in some other way.

FIGURE 24–5. Summary of the Assessment Process for Kristi.

more specific assessments are required to help further determine a student's needs. Within the educational setting, the occupational therapist addresses performance in all occupational areas as it relates to the child's educational needs (Table 24-14). As a result, further formal assessment may not be needed. However, this is not always the case. When additional information about occupational performance related to physical, sensory, neurological, and/or mental functions of the student is required, the occupational therapist may use different client factor–oriented tools that are either

TABLE 24–13. **OCCUPATIONAL PROFILE QUESTIONS FROM THE OCCUPATIONAL THERAPY PRACTICE FRAMEWORK**[a,b]

- Who is the student?
- Why was the student referred to special education and/or for an occupational therapy evaluation in the schools?
- What areas of educational occupation (ADL, education, work, play/leisure, and/or social participation) are successful and what are causing problems or risks?
- What contexts support engagement in desired educational occupations, and what contexts are inhibiting engagement?
- What is the student's occupational history?
- What are the student's, family's, and educational staff's priorities and desired target outcomes?

[a]Modified from AOTA (in press).

[b]Adapted for the educational setting.

TABLE 24–14. **OCCUPATIONAL PERFORMANCE AREAS ADDRESSED FROM THE OCCUPATIONAL THERAPY PRACTICE FRAMEWORK**[a,b]

Occupational Performance Area	How Addressed in the Educational Setting
ADL (basic and instrumental)	Cares for basic self needs in school (e.g., eating, toileting, managing shoes and coats; dressing for physical education); uses transportation system and communication devices to interact with others
Education	Participates and performs in the educational environment, including academic (e.g., math, reading, writing), nonacademic (e.g., lunch, recess, after-school activities), prevocational, and vocational activities.
Work	Develops interests, aptitudes, and skills necessary for engaging in work or volunteer activities for transition to community life after graduation from school
Play/leisure	Identifies and engages in age-appropriate toys, games, and leisure experiences; participates in art, music, sports, and after-school activities
Social participation	Interacts with peers, teachers, and other educational personnel during academic and nonacademic educational activities, including extracurricular and preparation for work activities

[a]Modified from Swinth, et al. (in press).

[b]Adapted for the educational setting.

standardized or nonstandardized (Table 24-12). These tools can help determine specific information about occupational performance but should not be used without one or more of the process–oriented methods or tools. In addition, the occupational therapist may use a variety of methods, such as observation, parent or teacher interview, and file review, to support the analysis of a student's performance.

OCCUPATIONAL THERAPY EVALUATION IN OTHER EDUCATIONAL SETTINGS

Even though public schools are the primary educational setting in which occupational therapy practitioners work, therapists also work in other educational settings. These settings may include community colleges, universities, and continuing education settings. Occupational therapy evaluations within these settings are not dictated by the IDEA. Rather, legislation such as the ADA or the Rehabilitation Act (1973) support the evaluation process. However, the basic assumptions outlined in this section (e.g., referral, occupational profile, analysis of occupational performance) are the same.

CONCLUSION

The evaluation process within public schools is guided by federal legislation and occurs within the context of the team. Occupational therapy practitioners contribute their unique training and expertise in the area of occupation to this team process. Using a student- or client-centered and top-down approach, with an emphasis on performance and participation within the educational setting, occupational therapy is able to help support student performance and outcomes within the educational environment. When occupational therapists evaluate occupational performance in other educational settings, the process is similar, but the specific procedures are not guided by the IDEA.

ACKNOWLEDGMENTS

I would like to acknowledge Leslie Jackson, MS, OT; Mary Muhlenhaupt, OT; and Jan Galvin, MPT, for their support in the completion of this chapter.

SECTION V

Play and Leisure

LOREE A. PRIMEAU

WHAT ARE PLAY AND LEISURE?

Although many definitions of *play* and *leisure* have been proposed in the literature, consensus has not been reached on how to define these terms. Lack of definitional clarity for these terms, however, should not prevent occupational therapy practitioners' evaluation of these areas of occupation in their practice with clients. From a pragmatic point of view, play and leisure are powerful tools for practice, and single, precise, and all-purpose definitions that are responsive to the needs of an entire profession may not be required or desired, even if they were possible (Parham & Primeau, 1997). Nevertheless, definitions of play and leisure in the literature tend to converge into four major categories: play and leisure as discretionary time, play and leisure as context, play and leisure as observable behavior or activity, and play and leisure as disposition or experience (Gunter & Stanley, 1985; Rubin, Fein, & Vandenberg, 1983).

Play and Leisure as Time

The category of play and leisure as discretionary time views them as leftover or residual time after obligatory activities, such as paid or unpaid work and self-maintenance tasks, are completed (Gunter & Stanley, 1985; Tinsley & Tinsley, 1982). Play and leisure are defined by what they are not: They are not work or school activities; they are not ADL or IADL. By definition, play and leisure are quantified as the time that is spent by the individual engaged in them. This view of play and leisure lends itself easily to measurement and is often the focus of evaluation in occupational therapy through the use of activity configurations as an assessment tool (Suto, 1998). Although practitioners need to know about their clients' use of time and its relationship to their health and well-being, equally important for evaluation of play and leisure are the contexts in which they occur, the clients' activities, and their experience of those activities.

Play and Leisure as Context

The category of play and leisure as context identifies and describes them in terms of the conditions under which they occur. Environments that are friendly, safe, and comfortable with a variety of materials, objects, people, and activities and that also denote cultural sanctions for play and leisure are more likely to elicit them. Freedom of choice to engage or not to engage in play and leisure and freedom from hunger, fatigue, illness, or other stressors are also identified as conditions conducive to play and leisure (Rubin et al., 1983). Beliefs held by people in a specific culture will determine what is and is not considered to be play and leisure and the conditions under which they occur. Practitioners often draw from this category when they evaluate supports and barriers in their clients' environments that facilitate or hinder their engagement in play and leisure.

One problem with the view of play and leisure as context is that although the conditions described above are necessary for play and leisure, they are not sufficient, meaning that producing such a context does not ensure that play and leisure will emerge in it (Rubin et al., 1983). Because play and leisure are transactions between clients and their environments (Bundy, 2001), clients' play and leisure activities and their experience of them must also be considered.

Play and Leisure as Activity

The category of play and leisure as activity views them as behaviors or activities that can be observed and named.

Taxonomies are used to identify and describe types of play and leisure activities. For example, Primeau and Ferguson (1999) named children's play using the following taxonomy: sensorimotor play, object play, social play, motor play, imaginative play, and game play. Such taxonomies are useful because they provide descriptive criteria for observation and evaluation of clients' play and leisure behaviors, including their interests (Primeau, 1996; Rubin et al., 1983). This view of play and leisure as activity is also easily quantified and measurable. It is familiar to practitioners in the form of many assessments, including checklists used to identify interests as well as strengths and problem areas in performance of play and leisure activities (Suto, 1998). A drawback to the view of play and leisure as activity is lack of consideration of the experience of the activities themselves (Primeau, 1996; Suto, 1998).

Play and Leisure as Experience

The category of play and leisure as experience views them as the overall experience of a client's engagement in play and leisure. Disposition, attitude, and state of mind while participating in play and leisure are of primary importance (Iso-Ahola, 1979; Tinsley & Tinsley, 1982). Personal meanings of play and leisure arise from these subjective experiences (Primeau, 1996). Several qualities of play and leisure as experience have been identified in the literature, including freedom from obligation or constraint, freedom of choice, enjoyment, fun, intrinsic motivation, low work-relation, flow, self-expression, active engagement, aesthetic appreciation, relaxation, internal locus of control, and suspension of reality (Bundy, 1997; Csikszentmihalyi, 1975; Iso-Ahola, 1979; Rubin et al., 1983; Samdahl, 1988; Shaw, 1985; Tinsley, Hinson, Tinsley, & Holt, 1993). Of all these qualities, freedom from constraint and freedom of choice are most often identified as defining characteristics of play and leisure as experience (Henderson, Bialeschki, Shaw, & Freysinger, 1996). Practitioners recognize the importance of evaluating play and leisure as experience by gathering data on clients' points of view through interviews, participant observations, and specific formal assessments.

The view of play and leisure as experience holds the most promise for occupational therapy practice (Bundy, 1993; Primeau, 1996; Suto, 1998). Although evaluation of play and leisure as time, context, and activity are necessary, they are not sufficient to understand clients' participation in play and leisure. Best practice dictates that evaluation of play and leisure as experience must also be conducted to obtain the clearest picture of clients' engagement in them.

GUIDELINES FOR EVALUATION OF PLAY AND LEISURE

Evaluation of play and leisure should be client-centered and should follow a top-down approach. Client-centered evaluation is a collaborative process that combines the perspectives, expertise, and experiences of clients and practitioners to determine what is evaluated, how it is evaluated, and what the focus of intervention is to be. To be truly client-centered, evaluation of play and leisure should occur in clients' natural settings (home, school, work, and community) whenever possible (Townsend, 1997). For practitioners working with children, clients can "include the child, parents, siblings, other family members, peers, teachers, and other adults who are responsible for the child" (Primeau & Ferguson, 1999, p. 470). As the practitioner considers the child in each setting, a new group of individuals may become central to the collaborative process.

A top-down approach to evaluation begins by focusing on clients' participation in play and leisure in home, school, work, and community settings (Trombly, 1993). Clients and practitioners collaboratively identify what the clients want to do, need to do, or are expected to do (Law, Baptiste, McColl, Opzoomer, Polatajko, & Pollock, 1990) and the extent to which they are able to engage in play and leisure in these settings (Coster, 1998). Evaluation of areas of occupation follows to find out how clients' participation in play and leisure is enhanced or limited by the types of activities in which they engage and the manner in which they experience them. Finally, performance skills and client factors are evaluated to determine how limitations or impairments in these areas affect clients' abilities to engage in play and leisure activities.

PARAMETERS FOR EVALUATION OF PLAY AND LEISURE

Client-centered and top-down approaches to evaluation guide practitioners in the process of evaluation, or how to evaluate play and leisure. The client's overall pattern of participation in play and leisure across home, school, work, and community settings is the content, or what needs to be evaluated. I propose that the four definitions of play and leisure described above provide parameters for evaluation that occurs at different levels. Play and leisure as time and as context align with the level of participation, whereas play and leisure as activity and as experience are addressed at the level of areas of occupation. Parameters for evaluation of performance skills and client factors related to play and leisure are drawn from general occupational therapy assessments used to evaluate clients in these areas and are not necessarily specific to play and leisure assessments. Table 24-15 lists assessments that evaluate play and leisure at the levels of participation, areas of occupation, performance skills, and client factors, according to the parameters of time, context, activity, and experience that they address.

Play and Leisure Participation

Play and leisure participation is defined as the client's engagement in play and leisure occupations typically

TABLE 24-15. **ASSESSMENTS OF PLAY AND LEISURE**

Assessment[a]	*Participation*		*Areas of Occupation*					*Performance Skills*	*Client Factors*
	Characteristics	*Contextual Factors*	*Activity*			*Experience*			
			Activity Interests	Activity Choices	Subjective Experience	Personal Meaning	Satisfaction		
Activity Index and Meaningfulness of Activity Scale			■	■	■				
Adult Playfulness Scale					■				
Assessment of Ludic Behaviors (ALB)			■	■	■			■	■
Child Behaviors Inventory of Playfulness					■				
Interest checklist			■						
Knox Preschool Play Scale				■				■	
Leisure Boredom Scale					■		■		
Leisure Competence Measure	■		■		■			■	
Leisure Diagnostic Battery		■	■		■	■		■	
Leisure Interest Profile for Adults			■	■	■				
Leisure Interest Profile for Seniors			■	■	■				
Leisure Satisfaction Scale					■	■	■		
Pediatric Interest Profiles			■	■	■				
Playform		■		■	■			■	
Play History	■	■		■				■	
Qualitative methods (interview, observation)[b]	■	■	■	■	■	■	■	■	■
Self-Directed Search—The Leisure Activities Finder			■						
Test of Environmental Supportiveness (TOES)		■							
Test of Playfulness (ToP)					■				
The Experience of Leisure Scale (TELS)					■				

[a]See Appendix A for author, source, and descriptions of assessments.

[b]See Bundy (1993), Burke and Scaaf (1997), and Florey and Greene (1997) for sample interviews and observation guidelines.

expected of and available to a person of the same age and culture in home, school, work, and community settings (Coster, 1998; Primeau & Ferguson, 1999). Evaluation at the level of participation determines the client's characteristics of play and leisure participation (nature, quality, frequency, and duration) in these settings and the contextual factors that facilitate or hinder his or her participation.

Evaluation of Characteristics of Play and Leisure Participation

Play and leisure participation may be restricted in nature, quality, frequency, or duration. Restrictions are relative to typical participation in each setting. Practitioners compare their clients' participation to that of individuals without participation restrictions to determine clients' degree of participation or participation restriction (World Health Organization, 2001). Practitioners draw from their knowledge base about play and leisure as it occurs naturally in home, school, work, and community settings and from their observations of a typical person engaged in play and leisure in a particular setting to understand the play and leisure of people without restrictions in that setting (Dunn, 1998). Then they may interview their clients and/or observe them to gather data on their participation in play and leisure, including their personal preferences. Finally, practitioners compare this information to that of a person without participation restrictions.

The focus of evaluation is on the nature, quality, frequency, and duration of the client's play and leisure participation. The nature and quality of participation can be addressed by answering the following questions (Coster, 1998): Is the client's participation in play and leisure positive? Does it support the client's physical, cognitive, and psychosocial growth? Is it personally satisfying? Does the client have access to the same opportunities for play and leisure as others of the same age and culture do? Is the client's participation in play and leisure acceptable to others in their settings?

Frequency and duration of participation are related to definitions of play and leisure as time. Does the client participate in play and leisure to the same extent as others in that setting? One study that asked this question found that boys with developmental dyspraxia participated in games on school playgrounds less often and for shorter time periods than boys without developmental dyspraxia (Primeau, 1989), indicating a gap in participation. When gaps in nature, quality, frequency, or duration of participation are found, practitioners must examine contextual factors to identify ways to bridge these gaps (Dunn, 1998).

Evaluation of Contextual Factors

Contextual factors are related to definitions of play and leisure as context. These factors may be physical (built and natural environments), social (groups, networks, social climate), cultural (attitudes and expectations related to ethnicity, behavioral norms, traditions), attitudinal (expectations and willingness of others to accommodate people who are atypical), or organizational (rules, policies, laws) (Cooper, Rigby, & Letts, 1995). Practitioners identify contextual factors in their clients' settings of interest and then determine whether these factors facilitate or hinder participation in play and leisure in those settings. Gathering objective data on contextual factors is not sufficient; practitioners must assess the impact of these factors on their clients' engagement in play and leisure (Dunn, 1998). Interviewing and observing clients in natural settings are optimal methods for doing this. For example, physical accessibility to a restaurant does not ensure that a client living with severe physical disabilities will dine out with friends. Social and attitudinal factors may affect the client's comfort level in that setting, thereby restricting his or her participation. The practitioner would need to ask questions to discover the source of this client's restriction.

Areas of Occupation: Play and Leisure Performance

Definitions of play and leisure as activity and as experience are central to evaluation at the level of areas of occupation. Evaluation focuses on clients' play and leisure performance (what they actually do and their experience while doing it). Practitioners assess clients' play and leisure activities and their experience while engaged in these activities to identify performance limitations and to determine how to enhance performance. Evaluation of **play and leisure activity** considers **activity interests** and **activity choices,** whereas evaluation of play and leisure experience explores subjective experience, personal meaning, and satisfaction with experience.

Evaluation of Play and Leisure Activity

Activity Interests

Interests are defined as "dispositions to find pleasure and satisfaction in occupations and the self-knowledge of enjoyment of occupations" (Kielhofner, Borell, Burke, Helfrich, & Nygard, 1995, p. 47). This definition addresses clients' affective responses to play and leisure activities (often expressed as preferences or as likes, dislikes, and indifferences) and their perceptions and awareness of themselves and their environments (Matsutsuyu, 1969). Assessments of play and leisure activity interests provide information in two areas: preferences and self-knowledge related to interests. Clients are asked to identify their preferences for a variety of play and leisure activities. Based on their responses, practitioners can determine the extent and quality of clients' self-knowledge and awareness of interests. For example, a client living in a cold, land-locked area who identifies scuba diving, surfing, and snorkeling as leisure interests displays limited preferences (only three are identified) and a lack of awareness of the leisure activities that the local environment offers, indicating that this client will most likely encounter limitations in his or her performance of leisure activities.

Activity Choices

Activity choices consist of the activities in which clients engage during play and leisure. Assessments in this area examine what clients do, with whom, and how often. Play and leisure activities are characterized as general categories (object play, games, hobbies, sports) or specific activities (play with blocks, board games, woodworking, soccer). Other areas to explore include whether the activity is done alone or with others (friends, family, or co-workers) and how often a particular play and leisure activity is performed. This indicator of frequency differs from that evaluated at the level of participation, because here practitioners are concerned with clients' individual performance of a specific play and leisure activity, regardless of the setting in which it occurs, to assess clients' history and familiarity with that activity. Returning to the example of the boys with developmental dyspraxia, evaluation of their activity choices would focus on their history and familiarity with games (whether they had played games before and, if so, what types, with whom, and how often) rather than on their overall participation in play on the school playground.

Evaluation of Play and Leisure Experience

Subjective Experience

Subjective experience refers to two aspects of engagement in play and leisure activities: the state of mind with which these activities are approached and the affective experience of engagement in them. State of mind, often termed playfulness, is characterized by freedom from constraint, freedom of choice, intrinsic motivation, internal control, active engagement, and freedom to suspend reality (Bundy, 1997; Henderson et al., 1996). The affective experience of engagement in play and leisure is a positive one, marked by feelings of fun, enjoyment, happiness, satisfaction, and pleasure (Csikzentmihalyi, 1988). Assessments of subjective experience explore these two areas: playfulness and affective experience. Practitioners must remember that the subjective experience of play and leisure transcends cultural definitions of play, leisure, work, and ADL (Primeau, 1996). For example, a mother who described her experience of playing with her children while doing housework as "play-work" stated, "It's like work with an attitude. It's my way to get things done in a fun way. . . . No, [it] isn't exactly what I want to do right now, . . . but I'm getting it done and we're all enjoying it at the same time" (Primeau, 1995, p. 252). Although this woman recognizes that she is restricted in her choice of activity, her use of the words *attitude* and *fun way* demonstrate a playful approach; and her statement *we're all enjoying it* refers to a positive affective experience, suggesting that her subjective experience is one of play and leisure.

Personal Meaning

Personal meaning derives from the subjective experience of play and leisure performance. Satisfaction of conscious or unconscious needs and benefits attributed to this experience create personal meanings, which often become motivation for clients' future engagement in play and leisure activities. Personal meanings can be categorized as physiological (physical fitness, stress reduction and recovery), educational/cognitive (learning, intellectual stimulation), social (social interaction, companionship), psychological (self-identity, self-expression), aesthetic (appreciation of beauty, arts, and symbolic systems of meaning), and spiritual (heightened awareness, transcendent experiences) (Beard & Ragheb, 1980; Driver, Brown, & Peterson, 1991). Evaluation of personal meaning becomes particularly important when practitioners want to increase their clients' repertoire of play and leisure activities (Bundy, 2001) or substitute a new activity for a no longer viable activity (Bundy, 1993). Clients' identified personal meanings can be matched with play and leisure activities that provide those meanings in the form of benefits derived from them, offering new play and leisure options. For example, a study found that bingo, bowling, ceramics, dancing, and volunteer activities were all rated as providing high levels of the benefit of companionship by elderly adults living in the community (Driver, Tinsley, & Manfredo, 1991). Practitioners could suggest these activities, or others that provide a similar benefit for their elderly clients who have expressed a desire for companionship.

Satisfaction with Experience

Satisfaction with experience refers to clients' overall feelings and perceptions related to their play and leisure experiences. Feelings and perceptions can be positive (contentment and satisfaction) (Beard & Ragheb, 1980) or negative (boredom and dissatisfaction) (Iso-Ahola & Weissinger, 1990). Satisfaction with play and leisure experience is thought to have powerful consequences for clients' physical health, mental health, life satisfaction, and personal growth (Driver, Tinsley, & Manfredo, 1991). Evaluation must capture clients' range of feelings and perceptions about their play and leisure satisfaction across all activities and settings in which they participate. For example, in one study, elderly clients' decreased participation in and access to leisure activities did not translate into dissatisfaction with their leisure experience, suggesting that, although their range of activity choices was restricted, even infrequent participation in valued activities added meaning and satisfaction to their lives (Griffin & McKenna, 1998).

Performance Skills and Client Factors

Practitioners can choose from many general occupational therapy assessments and some specific play and leisure assessments designed to assess performance skills and client factors. They can also make informal observations during clients' engagement in play and leisure activities. Specific assessments and observations ensure that practitioners are examining performance skills and body functions and structures actually used by clients in play and leisure activities (Bundy, 2001), thereby increasing the likelihood that the intervention will be focused on outcomes related to clients' participation in play and leisure. For example, practitioners often observe children at play with their peers to assess how their motor, process, and social interaction skills, as well as their physical, cognitive, and psychosocial abilities, affect their play with others.

CONCLUSION

Evaluation of play and leisure is guided by client-centered and top-down approaches and is focused on clients' overall patterns of participation in play and leisure across home, school, work, and community settings. Play and leisure as time (characteristics of participation) and as context (contextual factors) are addressed at the level of participation. Evaluation at the level of areas of occupation considers play and leisure as activity (activity interests, activity choices) and as experience (subjective experience, personal meaning, satisfaction with experience). Evaluation at the levels of performance skills and client factors is conducted using general occupational therapy assessments, specific play and leisure assessments, and observation. Practitioners who use this conceptual framework to evaluate play and leisure are able to design and implement interventions that are directly related to their clients' participation in play and leisure in home, school, work, and community settings.

References

Allen, C. K. (1985). *Occupational therapy for psychiatric diseases: Measurement and management of cognitive disabilities*. Boston: Little, Brown.

Allen, C. K. (1990). *Allen Cognitive Level test manual*. Colchester, CT: Worldwide.

Allen, C. K., Earhart, C. A., & Blue, T. (Eds.), (1992). *Occupational therapy treatment goals for the physically and cognitively challenged*. Rockville, MD: American Occupational Therapy Association.

Allen, C. K., Kehrberg, K., & Burns, T. (1992). Evaluation instruments. In C. K. Allen, C. A. Earhert, & T. Blue (Eds.). *Occupational therapy treatment goals for the physically and cognitively challenged* (pp. 31–68). Rockville, MD: American Occupational Therapy Association.

American Occupational Therapy Association. (1999). *Occupational therapy services for children and youth under the Individuals with Disabilities Education Act* (2nd ed). Bethesda, MD: Author.

American Occupational Therapy Association. (2001a). *American Occupational Therapy Association 2002 AOTA member compensation survey*. Bethesda, MD: Author

American Occupational Therapy Association. (1993). *Occupational therapy: Returning the injured worker to work*. Bethesda, MD: Author.

American Occupational Therapy Association (In press). Occupational therapy practice framework: Domain and process. *American Journal of Occupational Therapy*.

Americans with Disability Act of 1990, Public Law 101–336, 104 Stat. 327–378 (1990).

Atwood, S., Holm, M. B., & James, A. (1994). ADL capabilities and values of long-term care facility residents. *American Journal of Occupational Therapy, 48*, 710–716.

Beard, J. G., & Ragheb, M. G. (1980). Measuring leisure satisfaction. *Journal of Leisure Research, 12*, 20–33.

Borg, G. (1982). Psychophysical bases of perceived exertion. *Medicine and Science in Sports and Exercise, 14*, 377–381.

Bosch, J. (1995). *The reliability and validity of the COPM*. Unpublished master's thesis, McMaster University, Hamilton, ON, Canada.

Bowman, J. (1992). Americans have a shared vision: Occupational therapists can help to create the future reality. *American Journal of Occupational Therapy, 46*, 409–418.

Bray, K., Fisher, A. G., & Duran, L. (2001). The validity of adding new tasks to the Assessment of Motor and Process Skills. *American Journal of Occupational Therapy, 55*, 409–415.

Bundy, A. C. (1993). Assessment of play and leisure: Delineation of the problem. *American Journal of Occupational Therapy, 47*, 217–222.

Bundy, A. C. (1997). Play and playfulness: What to look for. In L. D. Parham & L. S. Fazio (Eds.). *Play in occupational therapy for children* (pp. 52–66). St. Louis: Mosby-Year Book.

Bundy, A. C. (2001). Measuring play performance. In M. Law, C. Baum, & W. Dunn (Eds.). *Measuring occupational performance: Supporting best practice in occupational therapy* (pp. 89–102). Thorofare, NJ: Slack.

Burke, J. P., & Schaaf, R. C. (1997). Family narratives and play assessment. In L. D. Parham & L. S. Fazio (Eds.). *Play in occupational therapy for children* (pp. 67–84). St. Louis: Mosby-Year Book.

Buttle, C. (1995). Ergonomic job analysis. *Rehab Management, 8*, 63–66.

Case-Smith, J., Rogers, J., & Johnson, J. H. (2001). School-based occupational therapy. In J. Case-Smith (Ed.). *Occupational therapy for children* (4th ed., pp. 757–779). Philadelphia: Mosby.

Center for Health Services and Policy Research (1998). *Outcome and Assessment Information Set (OASIS-BI)*. Denver: Author.

Center for Medicare & Medicaid Services. Available: www.udsmr.org Accessed 9/12/02

Chiou, I. L., & Burnett, C. N. (1985). Values of activities of daily living: A survey of stroke patients and their home therapists. *Physical Therapy, 65*, 901–906.

Christiansen, C. (1991). Occupational performance assessment. In C. Christiansen & C. Baum (Eds.). *Occupational therapy: Overcoming human performance deficits* (pp. 375–424). Thorofare, NJ: Slack.

Clawson, C. & Noiseux, J. (2000). A blueprint for accommodation. *Rehabilitation Management, 13*(8), 32–92.

Cooper, B., Rigby, P., & Letts, L. (1995). Evaluation of access to home, community, and workplace. In C. A. Trombly (Ed.). *Occupational therapy for physical dysfunction* (4th ed., pp. 55–72). Baltimore: Williams & Wilkins.

Coster, W. (1998). Occupation-centered assessment of children. *American Journal of Occupational Therapy, 52*(5), 337–344.

Cronbach, L. J. (1970). *Essentials of psychological testing* (3rd ed.). New York: Harper & Row.

Csikszentmihalyi, M. (1975). *Beyond boredom and anxiety*. San Francisco: Jossey-Bass.

Csikszentmihalyi, M. (1988). The flow experience and its significance for human psychology. In M. Csikszentmihalyi & I. S. Csikszentmihalyi (Eds.). *Optimal experience: Psychological studies of flow in consciousness* (pp. 15–35). New York: Cambridge University Press.

DeJong, G., & Sutton, J. P. (1995). Rehab 2000: The evolution of medical rehabilitation in American health care. In P. K. Landrum, N. D. Schmidt, & A. McLean (Eds.). *Outcome-oriented rehabilitation* (pp. 3–42). Gaithersburg, MD: Aspen.

Doble, S. E., Fisk, J. D., Fisher, A. G., Ritvo, P. G., & Murray, T. J. (1994). Functional competence of community-dwelling persons with multiple sclerosis using the Assessment of Motor and Process Skills. *Archives of Physical Medicine and Rehabilitation, 75*, 843–851.

Doble, S. E., Fisk, J. D., Lewis, N., & Rockwood, K. (1999). Test-retest reliability of the Assessment of Motor and Process Skills in elderly adults. *Occupational Therapy Journal of Research, 19*, 203–215.

Driver, B. L., Brown, P. J., & Peterson, G. L. (Eds.). (1991). *Benefits of leisure*. State College, PA: Venture.

Driver, B. L., Tinsley, H. E. A., & Manfredo, M. J. (1991). The Paragraphs about Leisure and Recreation Experience Preference Scales: Results from two inventories designed to assess the breadth of the perceived psychological benefits of leisure. In Driver, B. L., Brown, P. J., & Peterson, G. L. (Eds.), *Benefits of leisure* (pp. 263–286). State College, PA: Venture.

Dunn, W. (1998). Person-centered and contextually relevant evaluation. In J. Hinojosa & P. Kramer (Eds.), *Evaluation: Obtaining and interpreting data* (pp. 47–76). Bethesda, MD: American Occupational Therapy Association.

Dunn, W., Brown, C., & McGuigan, M. (1994). The ecology of human performance: A framework for considering the effect of context. *American Journal of Occupational Therapy, 48*, 595–607.

Eakin, P. (1989). Problems with assessments of activities of daily living. *British Journal of Occupational Therapy, 52*, 50–54.

Education for All Handicapped Children Act of 1975, Pub. L. 94-142, 20 U.S.C. § 1401, Part H, § 677 (1975).

Education for All Handicapped Children Act Amendments of 1986, Pub. L. 99-457, 20.

Ellexson, M. (1997). Work site rehabilitation programs: The future for industrial rehabilitation? *Work Programs Special Interest Section Quarterly, 11*, 1–3.

Fairbanks, J., Davies, J., & O'Brien, J. (1980). The Oswestry low back pain disability questionnaire. *Physiotherapy, 66*, 271–273.

Fillenbaum, G. G. (1988). *Multidimensional functional assessment of older adults: The Duke Older Americans Resources and Services procedures*. Hillsdale, NJ: Erlbaum.

Fisher, A. G. (1993). The assessment of IADL motor skills: An application of many-faced Rasch analysis. *American Journal of Occupational Therapy, 47*, 319–329.

Fisher, A. G. (1995). *Assessment of motor and process skills*. Fort Collins, CO: Three Star Press.

Fisher, A. G. (1997). *Assessment of motor and process skills* (2nd ed.). Fort Collins, CO: Three Star Press.

Fisher, A. G. (1999). *Assessment of motor and process skills* (3rd ed.). Fort Collins, CO: Three Star Press.

Florey, L. L., & Greene, S. (1997). Play in middle childhood: A focus on children with behavior and emotional disorders. In L. D. Parham & L. S. Fazio (Eds.). *Play in occupational therapy for children* (pp. 126–143). St. Louis: Mosby-Year Book.

Fontana, P. (1999). Pushing the envelope: Entering the industrial arena. *OT Practice, 4*, 20–22.

Fox, D. J. (1969). *The research process in education*. New York: Holt, Rinehart & Winston.

Freal, J., Kraft, G., & Coryell, J. (1984). Symptomatic fatigue in multiple sclerosis. *Archives of Physical Medicine and Rehabilitation, 65*, 135–138.

French, D., & Hanson, C. (1999). Survey of driver rehabilitation programs. *American Journal of Occupational Therapy, 53*, 394–397.

Fried, L. P., Herdman, S. J., Kuhn, K. E., Rubin, G., & Turano, K. (1991). Preclinical disability: Hypotheses about the bottom of the iceberg. *Journal of Aging and Health, 3*, 285–300.

Fries, J. F., Spitz, P., Kraines, R. G., & Holman, H. R. (1980). Measurement of patient outcomes in arthritis. *Arthritis and Rheumatism, 23*, 146–152.

Gage, M., Noh, S., Polatajko, H. J., & Kaspar, V. (1994). Measuring perceived self- efficacy in occupational therapy. *American Journal of Occupational Therapy, 48*, 783–790.

Galski, T., Ehle, H., & Williams, J. (1998). Estimates of driving abilities and skills in different conditions. *American Journal of Occupational Therapy, 52*, 268–274.

Giangreco, M. F. (2001). *Guidelines for making choices about IEP services*. Montpelier: Vermont Department of Education. Available: www.uvm.edu/~uapvt/ iepservicess/. Accessed: 7/8/01.

Gift, A. G. (1987). Dyspnea: A clinical perspective. *Scholarly Inquiry in Nursing Practice, 1*, 73–85.

Gift, A. G., & Pugh, L. C. (1993). Dyspnea and fatigue. *Nursing Clinics of North American, 28*, 373–384.

Gosman-Hedström G., & Svensson, E. (2000). Parallel reliability of the Functional Independence Measure and the Barthel ADL Index. *Disability and Rehabilitation, 22*, 702–715.

Griffin, J., & McKenna, K. (1998). Influences on leisure and life satisfaction of elderly people. *Physical and Occupational Therapy in Geriatrics, 15*(4), 1–16.

Gross, M. (2001). Navigating the expanse of driving aids. *Long-Term Rehabilitation Management, 13*, 54–58.

Gunter, B. G., & Stanley, J. (1985). Theoretical issues in leisure study. In B. G. Gunter, J. Stanley, & R. St. Clair (Eds.). *Transitions to leisure: Conceptual and human issues* (pp. 35–51). Lanham, MD: University Press of America.

Haertlein, C. L. (1999). The Milwaukee Evaluation of Daily Living Skills. In B. J. Hemphill-Pearson (Ed.). *Assessments in occupational therapy mental health: An integrative approach* (pp. 245–257). Thorofare, NJ: Slack.

Hamilton, B. B., Laughlin, J. A., Fiedler, R. C., & Granger, C. V. (1994). Interrater reliability of the 7-level Functional Independence Measure (FIM). *Scandinavian Journal of Rehabilitation Medicine, 26*, 115–119.

Hanft, B. E., & Place, P. A. (1996). *The consulting therapist: A Guide for OTs and PTs in schools*. San Antonio, TX: Therapy Skill Builders.

Hart, L., & Freel, M. (1982). Fatigue. In C. Norris (Ed.). *Concept clarification in nursing* (pp. 251–262). Rockville, MD: Aspen.

Harvey-Krefting, L. (1985). The concept of work in occupational therapy: A historical review. *American Journal of Occupational Therapy, 39*, 301–307.

Hawes, C., Morris, J. N., Phillips, C. D., Mor, V., Fries, B. E., & Nonemaker, S. (1995). Reliability estimates for the Minimum Data Set for nursing home resident assessment and care screening (MDS). *Gerontologist, 35*, 172–178.

Haworth, R. J., & Hollings, E. M. (1979). Are hospital assessments of daily living activities valid? *International Rehabilitation Medicine, 1*, 59–62.

Haywood, H. C., & Tzuriel, D. (Eds.) (1992). *Interactive assessment*. New York: Springer-Verlag.

Health Care Financing Administration [HCFA] (1998). *Minimum Data Set, 2.0*. Washington, DC: U.S. Government Printing Office.

Heimann, N. E., Allen, C. K., & Yerxa, E. J. (1989). The Routine Task Inventory: A tool for describing the functional behavior of the cognitively disabled. *Occupational Therapy Practice, 1*, 67–74.

Heinemann, A. W., Linacre, J. M., Wright, B. D., Hamilton, B. B., & Granger, C. (1994). Prediction of rehabilitation outcomes with disability measures. *Archives of Physical Medicine and Rehabilitation, 75*, 133–143.

Henderson, K. A., Bialeschki, M. D., Shaw, S. M., & Freysinger, V. J. (1996). *Both gains and gaps: Feminist perspectives on women's leisure*. State College, PA: Venture.

Hildreth, D., Breidenbach, W., Lister, G., & Hodges, A. (1989). Detection of submaximal effort by use of rapid exchange grip. *Journal of Hand Surgery [Am], 14*, 742–745.

Hilton, K., Fricke, J., & Unsworth, C. (2001). A comparison of self-report versus observation of performance using the Assessment of Living Skills and Resources (ALSAR) with an older population. *British Journal of Occupational Therapy, 64*, 135–143.

Hoelscher, D. & Taylor, S. (2000). Ergonomics consultation: An opportunity for occupational therapists. *OT Practice, 5*, 16–19.

Holm, M. B., & Rogers, J. C. (1999). Performance assessment of self-care skills. In B. J. Hemphill-Pearson (Ed.). *Assessments in occupational therapy mental health: An integrative approach* (pp. 117–124). Thorofare, NJ: Slack.

Holm, M. B., & Rogers, J. C. (1989). The therapist's thinking behind functional assessment, II. In C. Royeen (Ed.). *Assessment of function: An action guide* (pp. 1–36). Rockville, MD: American Occupational Therapy Association.

Huelskamp, S. (1997, August). The road to safety, assessing adaptive driving. *Advance for Directors in Rehabilitation*, 22–28.

Ilika, J., & Hoffman, N. G. (1981a). *Reliability study on the Kohlman Evaluation of Living Skills*. Unpublished manuscript.

Ilika, J., & Hoffman, N. G. (1981b). *Concurrent validity study on the Kohlman Evaluation of Living Skills and the Global Assessment Scale*. Unpublished manuscript.

Individuals with Disabilities Education Act Amendments of 1990. Pub. L. 101-47a6, 20 U.S.C. § 1400–1485 (1990).

Isernhagen, S. (1990). Pre-work screening. *Industrial Rehabilitation Quarterly, 3*(1), 7–47.

Isernhagen, S. & Brown, J. (1999, Winter). Disability evaluations (FCE's) and job analysis methods. *The Isernhagen Work Report*, 4.

Iso-Ahola, S. E. (1979). Basic dimensions of definitions of leisure. *Journal of Leisure Research, 11*, 28–39.

Iso-Ahola, S. E., & Weissinger, E. (1990). Perceptions of boredom in leisure: Conceptualization, reliability, and validity of the Leisure Boredom Scale. *Journal of Leisure Research, 22*, 1–17.

Jacobs, K. (1991). *Occupational therapy work related programs and assessments*. Boston, MA: Little, Brown.

Janson-Bjerklie, S., Carrieri, V. K., & Hudes, M. (1986). The sensations of pulmonary dyspnea. *Nursing Research, 35*, 154–159.

Jaworski, D. M., Kult, T., & Boynton, P. R. (1994). The Functional Independence Measure: A pilot study comparison of observed and reported ratings. *Rehabilitation Nursing Research, 3*(4), 141–147.

Jette, A. M. (1980). Functional Status Index: Reliability of a chronic disease evaluation instrument. *Archives of Physical Medicine and Rehabilitation, 61*, 395–401.

Katz, S., Ford, A. B., Moskowitz, R. W., Jackson, B. A., & Jaffe, M. A. (1963). Studies of illness in the aged: The Index of ADL. *Journal of the American Medical Association, 185*, 914–919.

Kaufman, L. (1982). *Concurrent validity study on the Kohlman Evaluation of Living Skills and the Bay Area Functional Performance Evaluation*. Unpublished master's thesis, University of Florida, Gainesville.

Kielhofner, G., Borell, L., Burke, J., Helfrich, C., & Nygard, L. (1995). Volition subsystem. In G. Kielhofner (Ed.). *A model of human occupation: Theory and application* (2nd ed., pp. 39–62). Baltimore, MD: Williams & Wilkins.

Klein, R. M., & Bell, B. (1979). *The Klein-Bell ADL Scale manual*. Seattle: Educational Resources. University of Washington.

Klein, R. M., & Bell, B. (1982). Self-care skills: Behavioral measurement with Klein- Bell ADL Scale. *Archives of Physical Medicine and Rehabilitation, 63*, 335–338.

Law, M. C., Baptiste, S., Carswell, A., McColl, M. A., Polatajko, H., & Pollock, N. (1998). *The Canadian Occupational Performance Measure* (3rd ed.). Toronto, ON: CAOT Publications.

Law, M., Baptiste, S., McColl, M., Opzoomer, A., Polatajko, H., & Pollock, N. (1990). The Canadian Occupational Performance Measure: An outcome measure for occupational therapy. *Canadian Journal of Occupational Therapy, 57*, 82–87.

Law, M., & Usher, P. (1988). Validation of the Klein-Bell activities of daily living scale for children. *Canadian Journal of Occupational Therapy, 55*, 63–68.

Lawton, M. P. (1972). Assessing the competence of older people. In D. P. Kent, R. Kastenbaum, & S. Sherwood (Eds.). *Research planning and action for the elderly: The power and potential of social science* (pp. 122–143). New York: Behavioral Publications.

Lawton, M. P., & Brody, E. M. (1969). Assessment of older people: Self maintaining and instrumental activities of daily living. *Gerontologist, 9*, 179–186.

Leonardelli, C. A. (1988). *The Milwaukee Evaluation of Daily Living Skills*. Thorofare, NJ: Slack.

Letts, L., & Marshall, L. (1995). Evaluating the validity and consistency of the SAFER tool. *Physical and Occupational Therapy in Geriatrics, 13*, 49–66.

Linacre, J. M., Heinemann, A. W., Wright, B. D., Granger, C. V., & Hamilton, B. B. (1994). The structure and stability of the Functional Independence Measure. *Archives of Physical Medicine and Rehabilitation, 75*, 127–132.

Mahoney, F. I., & Barthel, D. W. (1965). Functional evaluation: The Barthel Index. *Maryland State Medical Journal, 14*, 61–65.

Marshall, E. (1985). Looking back. *American Journal of Occupational Therapy, 39*, 297–299.

Matsutsuyu, J. S. (1969). The interest check list. *American Journal of Occupational Therapy, 23*, 323–328.

Mayer, T., Barnes, D., Kishiro, N., Nichols, G., Gatchel, R., Mayer, H., & Mooney, V. (1988). Progressive isoinertial lifting evaluation: A standardized protocol and normative database. *Spine, 13*, 933–997.

McColl, M. A., Paterson, M., Davies, D., & Law, D. L. (2000). Validity and community utility of the Canadian Occupational Performance Measure. *Canadian Journal of Occupational Therapy, 67*, 22–30.

McDowell, I., & Newell, C. (1996). *Measuring health: A guide to rating scales and questionnaires* (2nd ed.). New York: Oxford University Press.

McGourty, L. K. (1979). *Kohlman Evaluation of Living Skills*. Seattle: Kels Research.

McGourty, L. K. (1999). Kohlman Evaluation of Living Skills. In B. J. Hemphill-Pearson (Ed.). *Assessments in occupational therapy mental health: An integrative approach* (pp. 231–242). Thorofare, NJ: Slack.

Melzak, J. (1983). The McGill pain questionnaire: Major properties and scoring methods. *Pain, 1*, 227–229.

Melzak, J. (1987). Short form McGill pain questionnaire. *Pain, 30*, 191–197.

Merbitz, C., Morris, J., & Grip, J. C. (1989). Ordinal scales and foundations of misinference. *Archives of Physical Medicine and Rehabilitation, 70*, 308–312.

Missiuna, C. (1987). Dynamic assessment: A model for broadening assessment in occupational therapy. *Canadian Journal of Occupational Therapy, 54*, 17–21.

Morris, J. N., Fries, B., Steel, K., Ikegami, N., Bernabei, R., Carpenter, G. I., Gilgen, R., Hirdes, J., & Topinková, E. (1997). Comprehensive clinical assessment in community setting: Applicability of the MDS-HC. *Journal of the American Geriatrics Society, 45*, 1017–1024.

Msall, M. E., DiGaudio, K., Duffy, L. C., LaForest, S., Braun, S., & Granger, C. V. (1994). WeeFIM: Normative sample of an instrument for training functional independence in children. *Clinical Pediatrics, 33*, 431–438.

National Council on Disabilities. (2000). *Back to school on civil rights: Advancing the federal commitment to leave no child behind*. Washington, DC: National Council on Disabilities.

National Information Center for Children and Youth with Disabilities. (1998). The IDEA amendments of 1997. *NICHY New Digest, 26*, 1–40.

National Institute for Occupational Safety and Health. (1981). *Work practice guide for manual lifting* [Technical Report 81-122]. Cincinnati, OH: Author, Division of Biomedical and Behavioral Science.

Niemeyer, L., Matheson, L., & Carlton, R. (1989). Testing consistency of effort: BTE work simulator. *Industrial Rehabilitation Quarterly, 2*, 5–32.

Nouri, F. M., & Lincoln, N. B. (1987). An extended activities of daily living scale for stroke patients. *Clinical Rehabilitation, 1*, 301–305.

Ottenbacher, K. J., Msall, M., Lyons, N. R., Duffy, L. C., Granger, C. V., & Braun, S. (1997). Interrater agreement and stability of the Functional Independence Measure for Children (WeeFIM): Use in children with developmental disabilities. *Archives of Physical Medicine and Rehabilitation, 78*, 1309–1315.

Ottenbacher, K. J., Taylor, E. T., Msall, M. M., Braun, S., Lane, S. J., Granger, C. V., Lyons, N., & Duffy, L. C. (1996). The stability and equivalence reliability of the Functional Independence Measure for Children (WeeFIM). *Developmental Medicine and Child Neurology, 38*, 907–916.

Owsley, C., Ball, K., McGwin, G., Sloane, M., Roenker, D., White, M., & Overley, T. (1998). Visual processing impairment and risk of motor vehicle crash among older adults. *Journal of the American Medical Association, 279*, 1083–1088.

Parham, L. D., & Primeau, L. A. (1997). Play and occupational therapy. In L. D. Parham & L. S. Fazio (Eds.). *Play in occupational therapy for children* (pp. 2–21). St. Louis: Mosby-Year Book.

Pierce, S. (1993). Legal considerations for a driver rehabilitation program. *Physical Disabilities Special Interest Section Newsletter, 16*(1), 1–3.

Pincus, T., Summey, J. A., Soraci, S. A., Wallston, K. A., & Hummon, N. P. (1983). Assessment of patient satisfaction in activities of daily living using a modified Stanford Health Assessment Questionnaire. *Arthritis and Rheumatism, 26*, 1346–1353.

Popham, W. J. (1990). *Modern educational measurement: A practitioner's perspective* (2nd ed.). Englewood Cliffs, NJ: Prentice Hall.

Primeau, L. A. (1989). *A description and comparison of game playing behavior of preadolescent boys 9 to 11 years of age with and without developmental dyspraxia*. Unpublished master's thesis, University of Southern California at Los Angeles.

Primeau, L. A. (1995). *Orchestration of work and play within families*. Unpublished doctoral dissertation, University of Southern California at Los Angeles.

Primeau, L. A. (1996). Work and leisure: Transcending the dichotomy. *American Journal of Occupational Therapy, 50,* 569–577.

Primeau, L. A., & Ferguson, J. F. (1999). Occupational frame of reference. In. P. Kramer & J. Hinojosa (Eds.). *Frames of reference for pediatric occupational therapy* (2nd ed., pp. 469–516). Philadelphia: Lippincott, Williams & Wilkins.

Ransford, A., Cairns, D., & Mooney, V. (1979). The pain drawing as an aid to the psychological evaluation of patients with low back pain. *Spine, 1,* 127–134.

Reauthorization of the Individuals with Disabilities Education Act of 1990, Pub. L. 105-17, 20 U.S.C. (1997).

Rehabilitation Act of 1973, 29 U.S.C. 8504 (1973).

Reuben, D. B., Laliberte, L., Hiris, J., & Mor, V. (1990). A hierarchical exercise scale to measure function at the advanced activities of daily living (AADL) level. *Journal of the American Geriatrics Society, 38,* 855–861.

Robinson, S. E., & Fisher, A. G. (1996). A study to examine the relationship of the Assessment of Motor and Process Skills (AMPS) to other tests of cognition and function. *British Journal of Occupational Therapy, 59,* 260–263.

Rogers, J. C. (1983). Clinical reasoning: The ethics, science, and art. [Eleanor Clarke Slagle Lecture]. *American Journal of Occupational Therapy, 37,* 601–616.

Rogers, J. C., & Holm, M. B. (1989). *Performance Assessment of Self-Care Skills-Revised (PASS-R).* Unpublished manuscript, University of Pittsburgh at Pittsburgh.

Rogers, J. C., & Holm, M. B. (1991a). Older persons with depression: Educational issues. *Topics in Geriatric Rehabilitation, 6,* 27–44.

Rogers, J. C., & Holm, M. B. (1991b). Occupational therapy diagnostic reasoning: A component of clinical reasoning. *American Journal of Occupational Therapy, 45,* 1045–1053

Rogers, J. C., & Holm, M. B. (1994). *Performance Assessment of Self-Care Skills (PASS)* (Version 3.1). Unpublished manuscript, University of Pittsburgh at Pittsburgh.

Rogers, J. C., Holm, M. B., Beach, S., Schulz, R., & Starz, T. W. (2001). *Arthritis Care & Research, 45,* 410–418.

Rogers, J. C., Holm, M. B., & Stone, R. G. (1997). Assessment of daily living activities: The home care advantage. *American Journal of Occupational Therapy, 51,* 410–422.

Rothstein, J. M. (1985). Measurement and clinical practice: Theory and application. In J. M. Rothstein (Ed.). *Measurement in physical therapy* (pp. 1–46). New York: Churchill Livingstone.

Rubenstein, L. A., Schairer, C., Wieland, G. D., & Kane, R. (1984). Systematic biases in functional status assessment of elderly adults. *Journal of Gerontology, 39,* 686–691.

Rubin, K. H., Fein, G. G., & Vandenberg, B. (1983). Play. In E. M. Hetherington (Ed.). *Handbook of child psychology: Vol. 4. Socialization, personality, and social development* (4th ed., pp. 693–774). New York: Wiley.

Rybski, D. (1992). A quality implementation of Title I of the Americans with Disabilities Act of 1990. *American Journal of Occupational Therapy, 46,* pp. 409–418.

Sager, M. A., Dunham, N. C., Schwantes, A., Mecum, L., Halverson, K., & Harlowe, D. (1992). Measurement of activities of daily living in hospitalized elderly: A comparison of self-report and performance-based methods. *Journal of the American Geriatric Society, 40,* 457–462.

Samdahl, D. M. (1988). A symbolic interactionist model of leisure: Theory and empirical support. *Leisure Sciences, 10,* 27–39.

Settle, C., & Holm, M. B. (1993). Program planning: The clinical utility of three activities of daily living assessment tools. *American Journal of Occupational Therapy, 47,* 911–918.

Shaughnessy, P. W., Crisler, K. S., Schlenker, R. E., & Hittle, D. (1998). OASIS. The next 10 years. *Caring, 17*(6), 32–34, 36, 38.

Shaw, S. M. (1985). The meaning of leisure in everyday life. *Leisure Sciences, 7,* 1–24.

Silverstein, R. (2000). An overview of the emerging disability policy framework: A guidepost for analyzing public policy. *Iowa Law Review, 85,* 1757–1802.

Siporin, S. (1999). Help wanted: Supporting workers with developmental disabilities. *OT Practice, 4,* 19–24.

Snook, S., & Ciriello, V. (1991). The design of material handling tasks: Revised tables of maximum acceptable weights and forces. *Ergonomics, 34,* 1197–1213.

Social Security Act of 1935, HR 7260(1935).

Stauffer, L. M., Fisher, A. G., & Duran, L. (2000). ADL performance of black Americans and white Americans on the Assessment of Motor and Process Skills. *American Journal of Occupational Therapy, 54,* 607–613.

Stewart, K. B. (2001). *Purposes, processes, and methods of evaluation. Occupational Therapy for Children* (4th ed., pp. 757–779). Philadelphia: Mosby.

Stokes, H. (1983). The seriously uninjured hand-weakness of grip. *Journal of Occupational Medicine, 25,* 683–684.

Suto, M. (1998). Leisure in occupational therapy. *Canadian Journal of Occupational Therapy, 65,* 271–278.

Swinth, Y. L., Chandler, B., Hanft, B., Jackson, L., & Sheperd, J. (in press). Personel issues in school-based occupational therapy: Supply & demand, preparation, and certification & licensure. Center on Personal Studies in Special Education, Univ. of FL.

Tack, B. B. (1991). *Dimensions and correlates of fatigue in older adults with rheumatoid arthritis.* Unpublished doctoral dissertation, University of California at San Francisco.

Ting, W., Wessel, J., Brintnell, S., Maikala, R., & Bhambhani, Y. (2000). Validity of the Baltimore Therapeutic Work Simulator in the measurement of lifting endurance in healthy men. *American Journal of Occupational Therapy, 55,* 184–190.

Tinsley, H. E., Hinson, J. A., Tinsley, D. J., & Holt, M. S. (1993). Attributes of leisure and work experiences. *Journal of Counseling Psychology, 40,* 447–455.

Tinsley, H. E. A., & Tinsley, D. J. (1982). A holistic model of leisure counseling. *Journal of Leisure Research, 14,* 100–116.

Townsend, E. (1997). *Client-centred occupational assessment.* Unpublished manuscript, Dalhousie University, School of Occupational Therapy, Halifax, NS, Canada.

Trombly, C. (1993). Anticipating the future: Assessment of occupational function. *American Journal of Occupational Therapy, 47,* 253–257.

Uniform Data System for Medical Rehabilitation [UDSMR]. (1993). *Guide for the uniform data set for medical rehabilitation (adult FIM)* (Version 4.0). Buffalo, NY: UB Foundation Activities.

Uniform Data System for Medical Rehabilitation [UDSMR]. (1997). *Guide for the Uniform Data Set for Medical Rehabilitation (including the FIM instrument* (Version 5.1). Buffalo: State University of New York.

Uniform Data System for Medical Rehabilitation [UDSMR]. (2000). *Guide for the Uniform Data Set for Medical Rehabilitation for Children (WeeFIM).* Buffalo: State University of New York.

United States Department of Education (1982). *Annual report of the National Council on the Handicapped.* Washington, DC: US Government Printing Office.

United States Department of Labor. (1986). *Dictionary of occupational titles—Supplement* (4th ed., Appendix C). Washington, DC: US Government Printing Office.

Velozo, C. (1993). Work evaluations: Critique of the state of the art of functional assessment of work. *American Journal of Occupational Therapy, 47,* 203–209.

Velozo, C. A., Magalhaes, L. C., Pan, A., & Leiter, P. (1995). Functional scale discrimination at admission and discharge: Rasch analysis of the Level of Rehabilitation Scale-III. *Archives of Physical Medicine and Rehabilitation, 76,* 705–712.

Verbrugge, L. M. (1990). The iceberg of disability. In S. M. Stahl (Eds.). *The legacy of longevity: Health and health care in later life* (pp. 55–75). Newbury Park, CA: Sage.

Waddell, G. McCulloch, J., Kummel, E., & Venner, R. (1980). Nonorganic physical signs of low pain. *Spine, 5,* 117–125.

Wade, D. T. (1992). *Measurement in neurological rehabilitation.* Oxford, UK: Oxford University Press.

Wheatley, C. (2001). Shifting into drive; evaluating potential drivers with disabilities. *OT Practice,* 12–15.

Williams, J. H., Drinka, T. J. K., Greenberg, J. R., Farrel-Holtan, J., Euhardy, R., & Schram, M. (1991). Development and testing of the Assessment of Living Skills and Resources (ALSAR) in elderly community-dwelling veterans. *Gerontologist*, *31*, 84–91.

World Health Organization. (1980). *International classification of impairments, disabilities, and handicaps: A manual of classification relating to the consequences of disease*. Geneva: Author.

World Health Organization. (2001). *ICF: International Classification of Functioning, Disability, and Health*. Geneva: Author. Available: www.who.int/icidh. Accessed: 9/12/02.

Wright, B., & Linacre, J. M. (1989). Observations are always ordinal; measurements, however, must be interval. *Archives of Physical Medicine and Rehabilitation*, *70*, 857–860.

Yerxa, E. J., Burnett-Beaulieu, S., Stocking, S., & Azen, S. P. (1988). Development of the Satisfaction with Scaled Performance Questionnaire (SPSQ). *American Journal of Occupational Therapy*, *42*, 215–222.

CHAPTER 25

EVALUATION OF PERFORMANCE SKILLS AND CLIENT FACTORS

SECTION I

Sensory and Neuromuscular Function

KIRSTEN KOHLMEYER

Recording and Interpreting Results
Conclusion

Evaluation is a process of gathering data, formulating hypotheses, and making decisions to guide action. Evaluation is necessary to do the following:

- Establish intervention goals and plans.
- Demonstrate efficacy of therapeutic interventions.
- Determine independent-living status.
- Document need for a specific program.
- Facilitate educational or vocational placement.
- Substantiate insurance claims.
- Support litigation.

Evaluation is an ongoing process of collecting and interpreting the data necessary for intervention planning, intervention modification, and discharge planning (Hinojosa & Kramer, 1998). **Assessment** refers to specific tools or instruments used in the evaluation process (American Occupational Therapy Association [AOTA], 1995).

The primary objective of evaluation is to select that combination of data collection approaches that provides the clearest and most complete picture of the individual's level of function, with the least expenditure of time, energy, and cost. Effective evaluation requires a blend of several different kinds of knowledge and skills. A therapist must be

- Effective in obtaining information about their client's occupation performance patterns and concerns (as discussed in earlier chapters).
- Knowledgeable about the health conditions affecting performance, including causes, anticipated course, and prognosis.
- Familiar with a variety of assessment methods, their uses, and their proper administration.
- Able to select assessment methods that are suitable to the client.

The evaluation process includes collecting data from the client and family members, institutional sources such as medical and educational records, and other professionals. The process continues with administration of assessment tools, and it concludes with an analysis and summary of results, specifically how performance deficits affect function (Neistadt, 2000).

When choosing an assessment instrument or strategy, the therapist should be well informed and discriminative. Many types of assessments are available: informal, formal, standardized, nonstandardized, nonreferenced, and criterion-referenced (see Chapter 23 for a discussion of these issues). This section focuses on assessments of sensory, neuromuscular, and neuromotor factors that can affect performance. It provides a general overview; the references cited refer to other sources that give more specific information.

The medical or educational diagnosis may guide a therapist toward specific assessment tools and may provide tentative expectations about the nature of performance deficits. However, diagnosis alone is not an accurate predictor of the factors most influencing occupational performance. Clinical observation of how client factors affect occupational performance is key. Evaluation and intervention need to be prioritized based on the factors that most affect the functional performance areas that are of priority to the client. For example, an individual cannot raise his arm and wants to be able to brush his hair. Is it because he lacks passive range of motion (PROM)? Or lacks the strength? Does he lose his balance with only one or no upper extremity support? Does he know where his arm is in space? Is it a motor-planning problem? The therapist observes other areas of self-care and determines that the client has limited shoulder flexion and external rotation. Given those observations, the clinician (1) checks the medical record for previous injury (e.g., rotator cuff tear); (2) interviews the client for any recent trauma to the area; and (3) initially evaluates PROM, muscle tone, muscle strength, glenohumeral and scapular soft tissue integrity, scapular mobility, and scapulohumeral rhythm. No significant time is spent on sensory examination (the client can feel and manipulate items safely); specific muscle tests of C6, C7, or C8 myotomes (the client's upper extremity strength appears normal distal to the elbow); evaluation of sitting balance; or coordination tests. This is but one example of how the therapist uses information from the client and from observation to identify what client factors should be addressed. The following sections describe assessments commonly used with clients who have sensory and neuromuscular impairments.

SENSORY TESTING

Sensation supplies our nervous system with information that allows us to develop accurate and reliable maps of the environment and ourselves. Problems with the peripheral nervous system diminish transmissions to the brain. Damage to the brain interferes with perception, interpretation, or integration of sensory information. Occupational therapists use sensory testing to detect impairments that may interfere with safety, motor control, motor retraining, speed of performance and, most important, function. Evaluation of sensation is appropriate to consider for clients with peripheral or central nervous system disorders. Typical diagnoses include burn injury, peripheral nerve injury, spinal cord injury, cerebrovascular accident (CVA), brain injury, and complex upper extremity fracture. Results of the sensory evaluation determine the need for teaching precautions against injury, compensatory techniques (personal and environmental), or sensory reeducation. They can also document neural recovery, as in a peripheral nerve injury (Bentzel, 2002; Iyer & Pedretti, 2001; VanDeusen & Foss, 1997).

Professional Roles

Occupational therapists' roles in sensory testing vary slightly, depending on the facility where they work. Areas typically evaluated by therapists include the primary and discriminative somatic systems, which convey sensory information from skin, joints, and skeletal muscles. Other areas that may be evaluated by an occupational therapist or other professionals include the following:

- **Vision:** Light perception, conjugate movement, visual field, visual activity, visual range of motion, and saccade; professionals involved are occupational therapist, optometrist, ophthalmologist, neurologist, neurophthalmologist, or some combination thereof.
- **Hearing:** Responsiveness to auditory stimulation, recognition of auditory stimulation, localization to auditory stimulation, and acuity; professionals involved are audiologist; speech and language pathologist; and ear, nose, and throat (ENT) physician.
- **Olfaction:** Ability to detect and identify various odors and make bilateral comparisons; professionals involved are occupational therapist, speech and language pathologist, and ENT physician.
- **Gustation:** As it relates to taste, salivation trigger, and swallowing; professionals are occupational therapist, speech and language pathologist, and ENT physician.

By having knowledge of data collected by other professionals and the relation of these data to occupational therapy data, therapists can create cohesive intervention strategies (Dunn, 1991). Table 25-1 summarizes sensory components of tests frequently used by occupational therapists and other professionals.

Somatic Sensation Testing

General Methodology Principles

The following principles apply to all somatic sensation testing (Bentzel, 2002; Van Deusen & Foss, 1997):

- Explain the procedure to the client; ask for feedback or questions.
- Give instructions when the client's eyes are not occluded; demonstrate on noninvolved extremity if there is one.
- Test a nonaffected area to:
  Determine client's understanding.
  Establish what is normal for that individual.
- Occlude the client's vision (e.g., with a manila folder, screen, eyes closed); have client open eyes in between tests to avoid dizziness or disorientation.
- Apply stimuli:
  Proximal to distal.
  Randomly interspersed with nonpresentation trials.
  On dorsal and ventral surfaces.
- If client cannot respond verbally, he or she can point to a duplicate stimulus or picture or replicate movement if appropriate.
- Enter results on form; date and sign it.
- Scoring, definitions, and recording methods should be consistent.

The environment should be conducive to testing. The client should understand the general purpose and specific procedure and be able to actively participate and communicate responses. Specific testing procedures for primary and discriminative somatic sensation are delineated below.

Primary Somatic System

Light Touch

One test is to determine the client's ability to feel light touch.

- *Stimulus:* A light touch on a small area of the client's skin with a cotton swab, eraser tip, or therapist's fingertip.
- *Response:* Client gives an indication when the stimulus is felt by saying "now" or "yes," describing the feeling, or pointing to the location (Bentzel, 2002; Dunn, 1991; Iyer & Pedretti, 2001).

Fine gradations of light touch can be evaluated using the Semmes-Weinstein Calibrated Monofilament Test. This test controls the amount of force applied to the client's hand by a calibrated, hand-held instrument. This type of evaluation is particularly important for clients with peripheral nerve involvement. The Semmes-Weinstein test has intrainstrument, interinstrument, intrarater, and interrater reliability as well as administration and interpretation guidelines (Bentzel, 2002; Fess, 1995).

Pain

Other tests determine the client's ability to feel pain.

- *Stimulus:* A safety pin with one sharp and one blunt end; the therapist applies mixed sharp and dull stimuli randomly and using the same degree of pressure.
- *Response:* The client indicates when and which stimulus is felt by answering "sharp" or "dull."
- *Note:* The pin should be cleaned with an alcohol swab before and after testing (Bentzel, 2002; Iyer & Pedretti, 2001).

Temperature

Therapists test the client's ability to distinguish variations in temperature.

- *Stimulus:* Capped test tubes (metal conducts heat better than glass)—one filled with ice water and the other with hot tap water (tolerable to normal touch); the

TABLE 25-1. **SUMMARY OF SENSORY COMPONENTS OF TESTS USED BY OCCUPATIONAL THERAPISTS**[a]

Test Name	Sensory/Perceptual Subtest	*Sensory Areas Addressed*				
		O	**G**	**A**	**Vis**	**S**
Balcones Sensory Integration Screening	Finger to nose					
	Standing balance				■	
	Visual motor forms Arm postures				■	
	Stereognosis					
	Tactile graphics					■
Beery Developmental Test of Visual Motor Integration					■	■
DeGangi-Berk Test of Sensory Integration	Postural control items					
Miller Assessment for Preschoolers	Foundations Index				■	■
	Coordination Index				■	
	Complex Task Index					■
	Behaviors and Observations					
Motor Free Visual Perception Test	All subtests				■	
Sensory Integration and Praxis Tests	Visual subtests				■	
	Somatosensory subtests					
Quick Neurological Screening Test	Figure recognition and production				■	■
	Palm form recognition			■		
	Sound patterns					■
	Double simultaneous stimuli					
	Arm and leg extension			■	■	■
	Stand on one leg					
	Behavior irregularities					
Sensory Integration Praxis Tests	Visual subtests				■	
	Somatosensory subtests					■
Test of Visual Motor Skills					■	
Test of Visual Perceptual Skills (nonmotor)	All subtests				■	

[a]Data from Ayres (1989), Compton (1984), Keyser and Sweetland (1984), King-Thomas and Hacker (1987), Mitchell (1985), Sattler (1982), and Sweetland and Keyser (1986). Reprinted with permission from Dunn (1991).

O, olfactory; *G,* gustatory; *A,* auditory; *Vis,* visual; *S,* somatosensory; *Ves,* vestibular; *P,* proprioceptive; *LD,* learning disabled.

See Appendix A for author, source, and description of assessments.

therapist randomly uses each stimulus, keeping it on the client's body surface long enough to allow a temperature change to occur on the skin (approximately 1 sec).

- *Response:* The client indicates which stimulus is felt by answering "hot" or "cold" (Bentzel, 2002; Dunn, 1991; Iyer & Pedretti, 2001).

Discriminative Somatic System

Tactile Localization

The occupational therapist may also test the client's ability to localize touch.

- *Stimulus:* The therapist touches the client's skin with an eraser tip, cotton swab, or fingertip; the intensity

Ves	P	Age Group	Diagnosis	Validity	Reliability	Norms
		Primary grades	Learning; neurological behavior			130 children 6–9 years
		2–15 years	Developmental; neurological LD	Construct	Interrater	1039 normal
		3–5 years	Developmental delays	Construct	Test–retest	101 normal; 38 delayed
		2 years, 9 months–5 years	Developmental at-risk	Criterion-relation	Test–retest	1200 normal
		4–8 years	All types	Construct	Test–retest	881 normal; 22 states
		4–9 years	Learning and behavior problems	Construct; criterion; content	Test–retest; interrater	1997 children
		5+ years	Neurological	Interrater	Test–retest	1231 normal; 1008 LD
		4–8 years, 11 months for sensory tests	Learning problems		Test–retest	Somato 935; normal visual 240; normal
		4–12 years, 11 months	Learning problems	Content; criterion	Internal consistency	1000+ normal
		4–12 years, 11 months	Learning problems	Content; criterion	Internal consistency	962 normal

and duration of the stimulus significantly influence accuracy of response.

- *Response:* After each stimulus, the client opens his or her eyes and places a finger on or describes the area touched (Bentzel, 2002; Iyer & Pedretti, 2001).

Two-Point Discrimination

Clients are tested for their ability to perceive two distinct stimuli when touched with two stimuli simultaneously.

- *Stimulus:* An aesthesiometer (Fig. 25-1), Boley gauge, or paper clip is used; the therapist applies two points simultaneously along the longitudinal axis in the center of the zone to be tested, with equal light pressure to the palmar surface of the forearm, hand, and fingers; the therapist adjusts the distance between the double stimuli during testing to identify the amount of distance needed between the two stimuli before the client perceives them both; one-point application trials are interspersed with test trials.

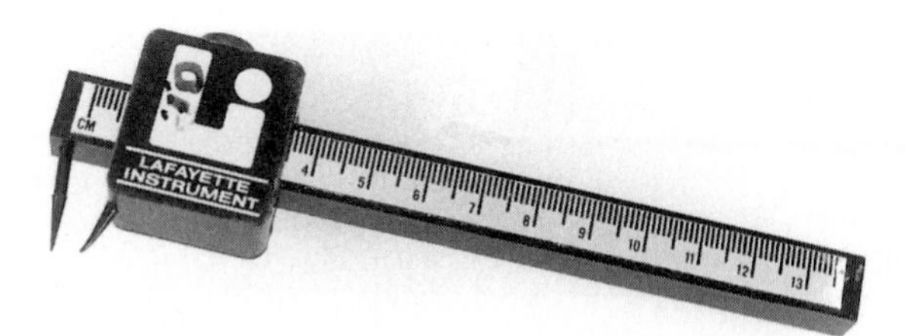

FIGURE 25–1. An aesthesiometer. (Courtesy of the Rehabilitation Institute of Chicago.)

- *Response:* The client identifies the stimulus by saying "one point" or "two points"; a score is recorded for each skin area examined; several normative values exist for the distance between the felt double stimuli (Bentzel, 2002; Dunn, 1991)

Stereognosis

Stereognosis is the ability to identify objects tactually.

- *Stimulus:* The therapist puts a common object in the client's hand (e.g., pen, key, quarter, cotton ball); the client is asked to manipulate and identify the object.
- *Response:* The client names the object as it is identified, describes the properties if unable to name object, or points to a choice from a photograph or display of identical objects (Bentzel, 2002; Dunn, 1991; Wheatley, 2001).
- *Note:* This test is not appropriate for clients who are unable to manipulate objects on their own.

Proprioception

Proprioception is the ability to identify limb position in space without vision.

- *Stimulus:* The therapist holds the body part being tested laterally to avoid cutaneous input and slowly, passively positions the joint being tested; joints are tested singly and in combination.
- *Response:* The client is asked to reproduce the position with the opposite extremity. If unable to copy the limb position, a verbal response may be given such as "up" or "down," or the client may use a gesture or point to directional arrows (Bentzel, 2002; Iyer & Pedretti, 2001).

Kinesthesia

Kinesthesia is movement sense.

- *Stimulus:* The therapist holds the body part being tested laterally to reduce tactile input and moves the joint up or down; the level of detection of kinesthesia is influenced by velocity (it is easier to detect brisk movement).
- *Response:* After each stimulus, the client indicates in which direction the body part was moved (Iyer & Pedretti, 2001).

Recording Results

Recorded results should be specific enough to enable future comparison of progress and to communicate useful information to others. Sensibility tests can show variability both within and between evaluators, depending on how the tests are performed (Mielke, Novak, Mac Kinnon & Feely, 1996). Sensation can be recorded as intact, impaired, or absent. Recording options include graphic methods (Fig. 25-2), diagrams, peripheral nerve distribution, dermatome distribu-

Two Point Discrimination
N: .3-.6 cm
P: .6-1.2 cm
S: 1.2....cm

Pain/Temp L		Pain/Temp R		Proprioception L		Proprioception R				
	C4				Shoulder					
	C5				Elbow					
	C6				Wrist			L		R
	C7				Hand				C6	
	C8								C7	
	T1								C8	

Note. N=no apparent deficit; P=partial deficit; S=severe deficit; NE=not examined. Recordings made in unshaded areas.

FIGURE 25–2. Sensory record for pain-temperature and two-point discrimination by dermatome and for proprioception by joint. (Reprinted with permission from the Rehabilitation Institute of Chicago.)

tion (Fig. 25-3), the number correct, and the number of trials (such as stereognosis).

Interpreting Results

Therapists must be alert to the influence of cognitive, perceptual, psychosocial, and motor deficits on sensory performance. Some clients may not be able to attend to or appreciate the abstract nature of tests used to evaluate sensation. They may have difficulty comprehending instructions, may guess at responses, or may find the procedure irrelevant and so not fully participate. It is important to ask clients to describe (if able) what they feel. Observe clients during functional activities. Do they use proper force when grasping an object? Do they acknowledge or feel uncomfortable when touched? Are they aware of the position of their extremities when getting dressed? Do they drop items when not looking directly at the item? If sensation appears to be a contributing source to performance problems, accurately identify which deficits contribute to the problems. Educate the client, team members, and caregivers to the deficits and potential functional ramifications, such as safety issues, compensatory techniques, and environmental adaptations to facilitate sensory awareness and processing (Dunn, 1991; Okkema, 1993a).

RANGE OF MOTION

Range of motion (ROM) is the arc of motion through which a joint passes. **PROM** is the arc of motion through which the joint passes when moved by an outside force. **Active range of motion (AROM)** is the arc of motion through which the joint passes when moved by muscles acting on the joint. Joint structure and the integrity of

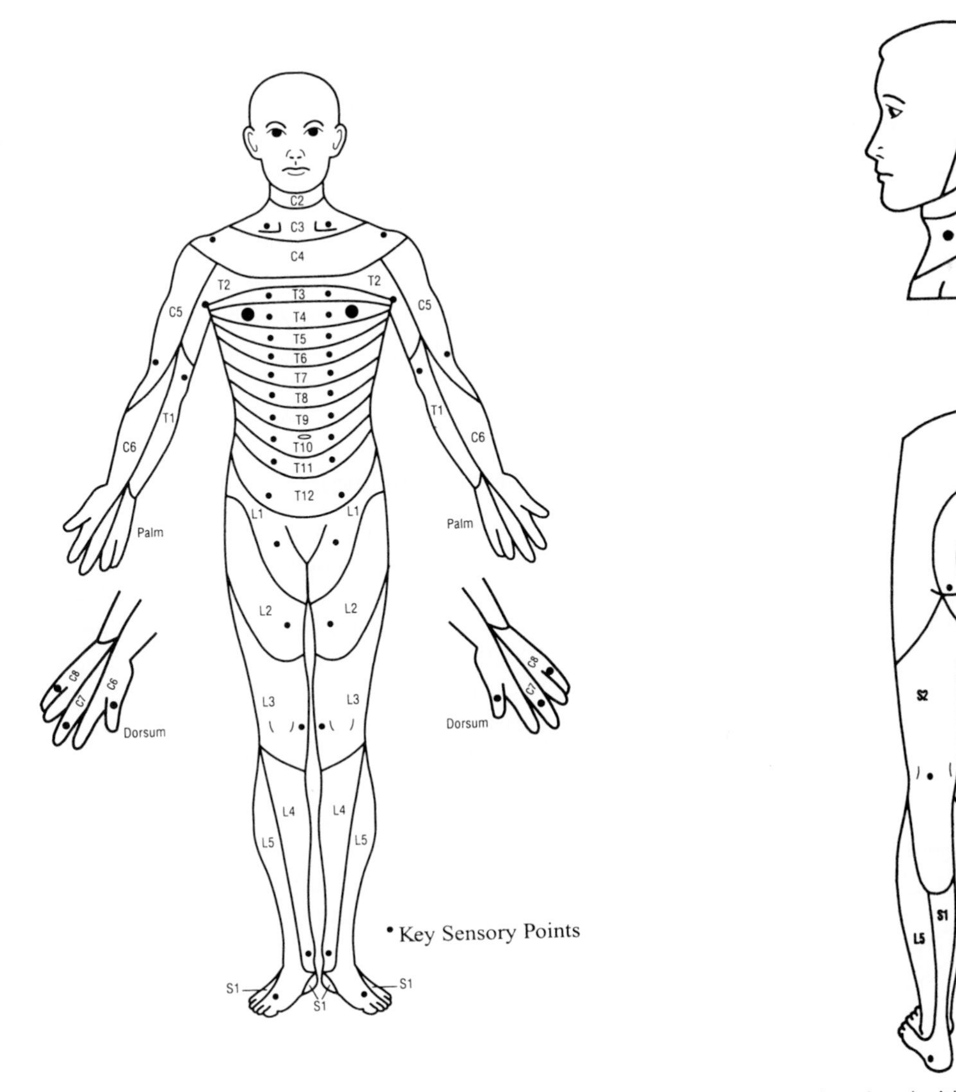

FIGURE 25–3. Dermatome chart for recording results of sensory testing. (Reprinted with permission from the American Spinal Injury Association, 2000.)

surrounding tissues determine the directions and limits of motion for any given joint (Gillam & Barstow, 1997; Pedretti, 2001a; Trombly & Podolski 2002).

The occupational therapist evaluates ROM to:

- Determine limitations that affect function.
- Determine limitations that may produce deformity.
- Determine additional range needed for function.
- Keep a record of progression or regression.
- Determine appropriate intervention goals.
- Determine the need for splints, assistive devices, or both.
- Select appropriate intervention modalities, positioning techniques, and other strategies to decrease limitations.

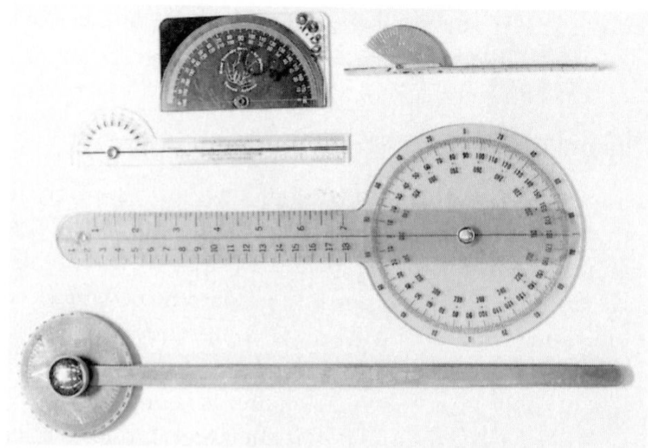

FIGURE 25–5. Goniometers. (Courtesy of the Rehabilitation Institute of Chicago.)

Goniometric Measurement Tools

A **goniometer** is the instrument used to measure joint ROM. Goniometers can be metal or plastic, come in several sizes, and are available from medical and rehabilitation equipment companies (Figs. 25-4 and 25-5).

Goniometer Parts and Functions

- *Protractor:* A half-circle attached to the stationary bar that contains a scale of degrees from 0 to 180 in each direction; permits measurement of motion in opposite directions (e.g., flexion and extension).
- *Stationary bar:* Attached to the axis.
- *Movable bar:* Attached to the axis.
- *Axis:* Where the two bars are riveted together; acts as the fulcrum; must move freely, yet be tight enough to remain where set when the goniometer is removed from the body segment after joint measurement.

A neutral zero method for measuring and recording is recommended by the Committee on Joint Motion of the American Academy of Orthopedic Surgeons. Most clinics use this 180° system, in which the following standards are used (Gillam & Barstow, 1997; Pedretti, 2001a; Trombly & Podolski, 2002):

- 0° is the starting position for all joint motions.
- Anatomic position is the starting position.
- 180° is superimposed as a semicircle on the body in the plane in which the motion will occur.
- The axis of the joint is the axis of the semicircle or arc of motion.
- All joint motions begin at 0° and increase toward 180°.

Other measurement systems used include the 360° system, in which 180° is the starting position and motion goes toward 0° (Gillam & Barstow, 1997; Pedretti, 2001a; Trombly & Podolski, 2002).

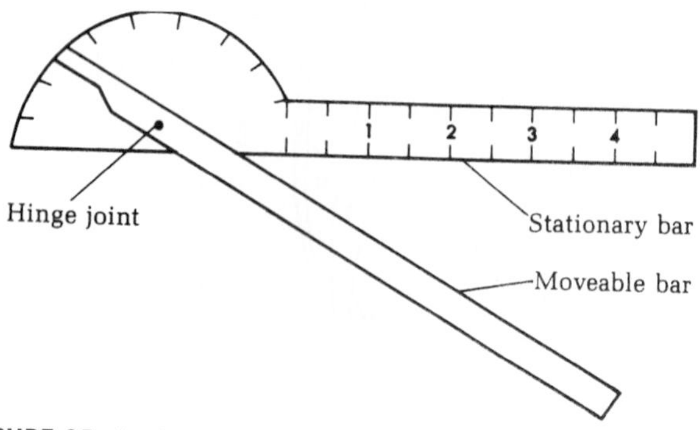

FIGURE 25–4. A goniometer.

General Principles

Formal joint measurement is not necessary with every client, especially when limited ROM is not anticipated. Typical diagnoses that may necessitate closer attention include arthritis, fractures, CVA, and spinal cord injury. AROM can be visually observed during activities of daily living (ADL) or by having the client move through various positions (Killingsworth & Pedretti, 2001). All joints can be put briefly through PROM.

Normal ROM varies from one person to the next. Ranges are listed in the literature and on most recording forms. The therapist could also measure the client's uninvolved extremity as a normal comparison. A medical history should be noted for any previous joint injury or secondary diagnosis affecting ROM. The ROM can be limited by pain. Joints should not be forced beyond the point of resistance during PROM (Pedretti, 2001a).

When evaluating ROM, the therapist may need to provide outside support or stability so the individual is free to concentrate and attempt the desired movement, as opposed to "fixing" to even sit upright (Pedretti, 2001a). The therapist should also evaluate scapular mobility, thoracic spinal extension, and head and neck positioning before proceeding with shoulder joint measurements, as these all affect glenohumeral joint motion.

Finally, before conducting an actual evaluation, therapists need to know the average normal ROM, how the joint moves, and how to position themselves, the clients, and the joints for measurement. Therapists should think about comfort as well as body mechanics to protect themselves and clients while placing the goniometer and providing support to the joint being tested.

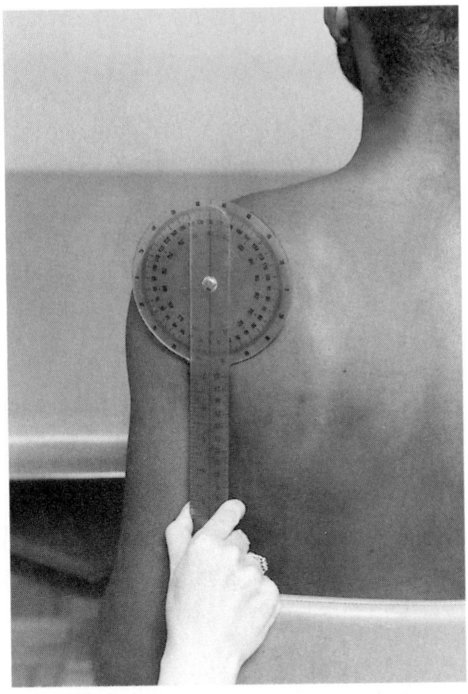

FIGURE 25–6. Goniometric measurement of shoulder abduction—starting position. (Courtesy of the Rehabilitation Institute of Chicago.)

ROM Evaluation Procedure

1. Position the client comfortably.
2. Explain and demonstrate to the client what is being done and why.
3. Stabilize joint proximal to joint being measured.
4. Observe available movement by having the client move the joint or by moving the joint passively to get a sense of joint mobility.
5. Place the goniometer axis over the joint axis in the starting position (the stationary bar goes over the stationary bone proximal to the joint and parallel to the longitudinal axis of the bone; the movable bar goes over movable bone distal to the joint and parallel to the longitudinal axis of the bone). Face the top of goniometer's protractor away from the direction of movement so the goniometer dial (end of the movable bar) does not go off the measurement scale.
6. Record the number of degrees at the starting position.
7. Hold the body part securely above and below the joint being measured; gently move the joint through the available PROM. Do not use excessive force. Note any crepitus. Stop at any point of pain or at the end of the range. (The axis of motion for some joints coincides with bony landmarks; other joint axes are found by observing the movement of the joint to determine the point around which the motion occurs.)
8. Return the limb to the resting position.
9. Record the number of degrees at the final position. Note in which position the joint measurement was taken when more than one position can be used (e.g., shoulder internal or external rotation).
10. Date and sign the form.

Figures 25-6 through 25-11 show examples of goniometric measurements for shoulder abduction, elbow flexion, and wrist extension. Factors that influence the accuracy and reliability of goniometer measurement include the type of support given to the body part, the body part being measured, bulking clothing, the environment (e.g., temperature), the time of day, client fatigue, the client's reaction to pain, and the examiner's experience (Flowers,

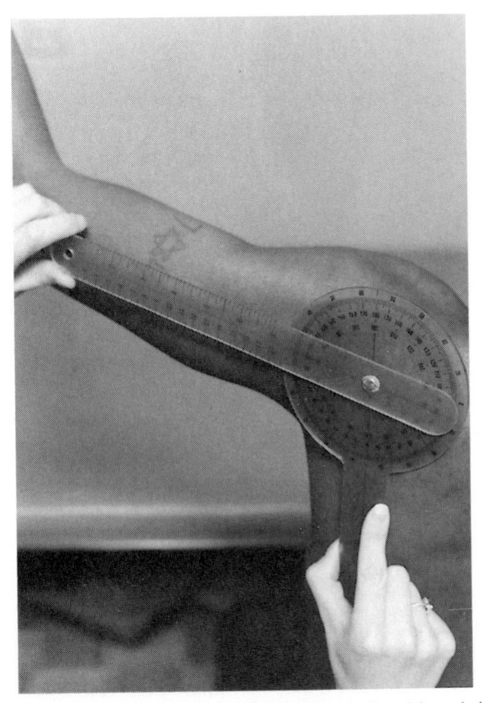

FIGURE 25–7. Goniometric measurement of shoulder abduction. (Courtesy of the Rehabilitation Institute of Chicago.)

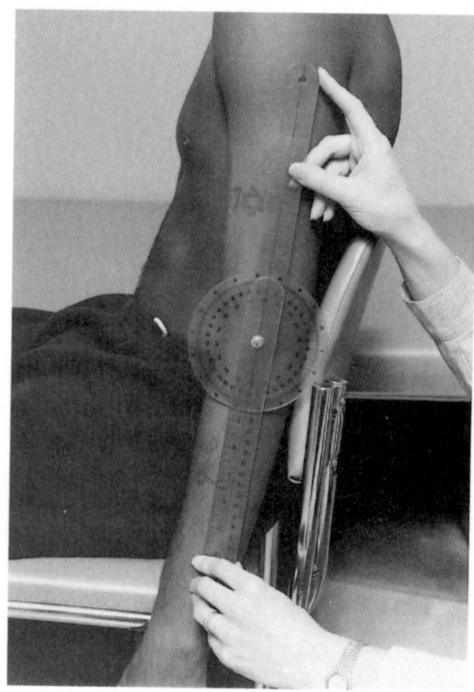

FIGURE 25–8. Goniometric measurement of elbow flexion—starting position. (Courtesy of the Rehabilitation Institute of Chicago.)

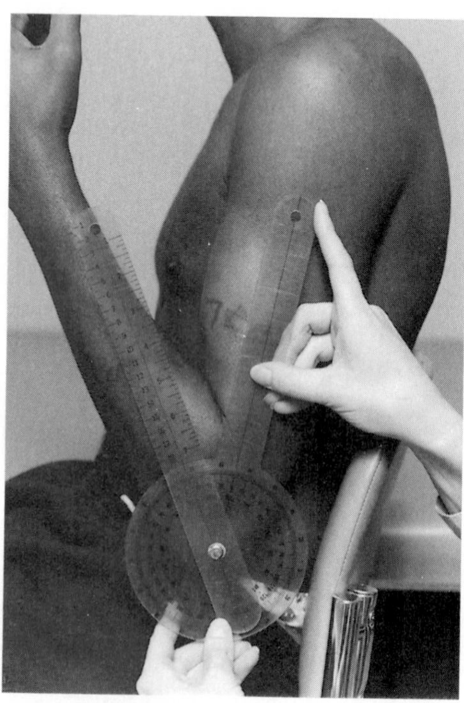

FIGURE 25–9. Goniometric measurement of elbow flexion. (Courtesy of the Rehabilitation Institute of Chicago.)

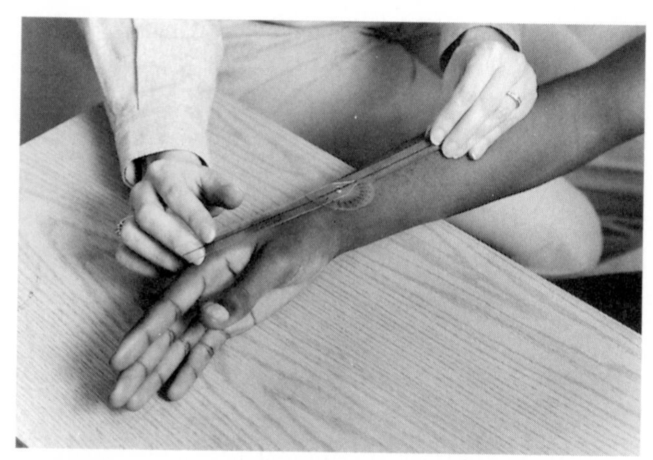

FIGURE 25–10. Goniometric measurement of wrist extension—starting position. (Courtesy of the Rehabilitation Institute of Chicago.)

Stephens-Chisar, LaStayo, & Grakante 2001; LaStays & Wheeler, 1994; Pedretti, 2001a; Riddle, 1992; Wei, McQuade, & Smidt, 1993).

Recording Results

When using the 180° system, the evaluator should record the number of degrees at the starting position and the number of degrees at the final position after the joint has passed through the maximal possible arc of motion. Normal ROM starts at 0° and increases toward 180° (Pedretti, 2001a). A limitation can be indicated at either end of the scale; for example, at the elbow joint, the measurements could be as follows:

0–140°	normal
20–140°	limited extension
0–100°	limited flexion

A sample form for recording ROM measurements is shown in Figure 25-12.

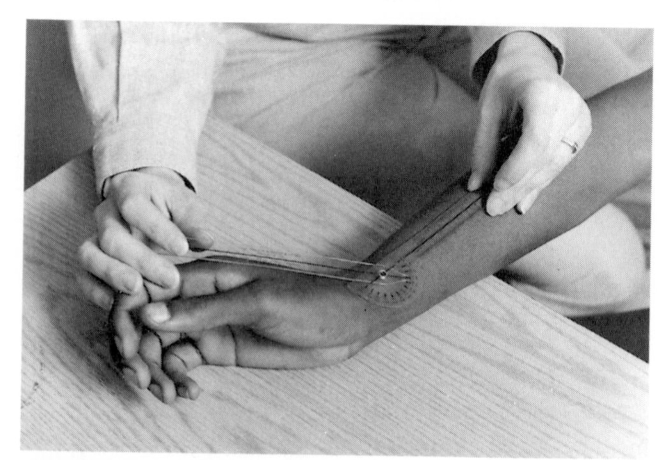

FIGURE 25–11. Goniometric measurement of wrist extension. (Courtesy of the Rehabilitation Institute of Chicago.)

Name:

RIC #:

Physician:

JOINT RANGE MEASUREMENTS

AROM	AROM	PROM	PROM				PROM	PROM	AROM	AROM
Date	Date	Date	Date				Date	Date	Date	Date
				< - Left	Right - >					
				Flexion	0-180	Shoulder				
				Extension	0-60	Shoulder				
				Abduction	0-180	Shoulder				
				External Rotation	0-90	Shoulder				
				Internal Rotation	0-70	Shoulder				
				Horiz. Abduction	0-90	Shoulder				
				Horiz. Adduction	0-45	Shoulder				
				Flexion	0-150	Elbow				
				Supination	0-80	Elbow				
				Pronation	0-80	Elbow				
				Flexion	0-80	Wrist				
				Extension	0-70	Wrist				
				Ulnar Dev.	0-30	Wrist				
				Radial Dev.	0-20	Wrist				
				M.P. Flexion	0-50	Thumb				
				I. P. Flexion	0-80	Thumb				
				Abduction	0-70	Thumb				
				M. P. Flexion	0-90	Index F.				
				M. P. Extension	0-45	Index F.				
				P. I. P. Flexion	0-100	Index F.				
				D. I. P. Flexion	0-80	Index F.				
				M. P. Flexion	0-90	Long F.				
				M. P. Extension	0-45	Long F.				
				P. I. P. Flexion	0-100	Long F.				
				D. I. P. Flexion	0-90	Long F.				
				M. P. Flexion	0-90	Ring F.				
				M. P. Extension	0-45	Ring F.				
				P. I. P. Flexion	0-100	Ring F.				
				D. I. P. Flexion	0-90	Ring F.				
				M. P. Flexion	0-90	Little F.				
				M. P. Extension	0-45	Little F.				
				P. I. P. Flexion	0-100	Little F.				
				D. I. P. Flexion	0-90	Little F.				

FIGURE 25–12. Form for recording ROM measurements. (Reprinted with permission from the Rehabilitation Institute of Chicago.)

Interpreting Results

A therapist should focus on ranges that fall below functional limits—that is, the amount of joint range necessary to perform ADL and other desired occupations without the use of special equipment. The therapist should evaluate what is causing the decreased range. Is it pain, edema, muscle weakness, skin adhesions, spasticity, bony obstruction or destruction, or soft tissue contracture? Is the cause changeable? Is it possible to increase the active range or prevent further loss by stretching, strengthening, orthotic management, casting, or modalities? Intervention goals should reflect the identified problem. If the available range is not expected to change, the practitioner should focus on adaptive techniques or the use of adaptive equipment to perform the desired task (Pedretti, 2001a; Trombly & Podolski, 2002).

MUSCLE TONE

Definitions

Muscle tone can be defined in several ways. Barrows (1980) defined it as resistance offered by a muscle to a stretch when a joint is passively moved. Brooks (1986) defined muscle tone as resistance to stretch that is generated by lower motor neuron activity, viscoelastic properties of muscles and joints, and sensory feedback. Chusid and DeGroot (1988) stated that tone is a continuous mild contraction of the muscle tissue in its resting state. Preston (2001) added that muscle tone depends on the integrity of the peripheral and central nervous system mechanisms as well as muscle contractility, elasticity, and extensibility.

Normal muscle tone varies from person to person and can depend on age, gender, and occupation. Normal tone can be characterized by the ability to move against gravity, shift between stability and mobility, use muscles in groups or selectively, and balance between agonist and antagonists (Preston, 2001). The level of tone in a muscle can be increased or decreased by damage to the nervous system (Fig. 25-13).

Hypotonia

Hypotonia is characterized by decreased muscle tone resulting from hyporesponsiveness to sensory stimulation and efferent commands. Clinically, muscles appear soft, flabby, and lax. This, in addition to weak co-contraction around the proximal joints, may result in a wider range for PROM. Deep tendon reflexes are diminished or absent. Hypotonia occurs in primary muscle diseases, cerebellar lesions, lower motor neuron disorders, and the initial phases of CVA and spinal cord injury (Mathiowetz & Bass-Haugen, 2002; Preston, 2001; Trombly & Podolski, 2002).

Spasticity

Spasticity is a motor disorder characterized by a velocity-dependent increase in tonic stretch reflexes, with exaggerated tendon jerks, resulting from hyperexcitability of the stretch reflex as one component of the upper motor neuron syndrome (Katz, Rovai, Brait, & Rymer, 1992; Katz & Rymer, 1989). The selective nature of spasticity results in a disruption of synergistic movement caused by an imbalance between muscle groups. Clinically, characteristics of spasticity include hypertonic muscles, hyperactive deep tendon reflexes, clonus, abnormal spinal reflexes, increased resistance to passive movement, and decreased motor coordination. Spasticity occurs in upper motor neuron disorders such as multiple sclerosis, cerebral palsy, spinal cord injury, CVA, and traumatic brain injury (Preston, 2001; Sabari, 1997; Trombly, 2002; Warren, 1991).

Spasticity is influenced by postural reflex mechanisms as well as by extrinsic factors such as contracture, anxiety, temperature extremes, and emotional or physical pain. It can be characterized as mild, moderate, or severe (Table 25-2).

Rigidity

Rigidity is the simultaneous increase of muscle tone in agonistic and antagonistic muscles that results in increased resistance to passive movement in any direction throughout the ROM. "Lead pipe" rigidity is characterized by a feeling of constant stiffness throughout the available ROM. Cogwheel rigidity is characterized by a tremor superimposed on the rigidity, causing alternate contraction and relaxation throughout the ROM. Rigidity occurs in extrapyramidal system lesions such as Parkinson disease, encephalitis, and tumors. Rigidity and spasticity may both be present in a muscle group (Cooperman, Forwell, & Hugos, 2002; Preston, 2001).

Hypotonia (Floppy; Flaccid)	Normal Muscle Tissue	Hypertonia (Spasticity; Rigidity)
LESS ◄- - - -	- - - - - - - - - - - - - - -	- - - -► MORE

FIGURE 25–13. Muscle tone changes that may occur with damage to the central nervous system.

TABLE 25-2. **CATEGORIES OF SPASTICITY**[a]

Mild Spasticity	Moderate Spasticity	Severe Spasticity
Stretch reflex occurs in last quarter of range	Stretch reflex occurs in midrange	Stretch reflex occurs in initial quarter of range
Slight imbalance in tone between agonist and antagonist	Marked imbalance of tone between agonist and antagonist	Severe imbalance of tone between agonist and antagonist
Mild increased resistance to passive stretch	Considerable resistance to passive stretch; able to move through full PROM	Marked resistance to passive movement unable to complete full PROM
May exhibit slight decreased mobility and ability to perform fine, selective movements	May exhibit slow gross movements that require increased effort; may show decreased coordination	Significant decreased or lack of active movement; may exhibit joint contractures

[a]Modified from Mathiowetz and Bass Haugen (1995).

Muscle Tone Assessment

The occupational therapist assesses muscle tone to:

- Establish a baseline.
- Plan intervention and select intervention methods.
- Train the client in special methods or use of assistive devices to accomplish functional tasks.
- Structure environmental factors to minimize negative effects of abnormal tone.

To date, it has been difficult to achieve both reliability and validity when measuring muscle tone. There is no standardized procedure. The available electromyographic, biomechanical, and myotonometric methods have varying degrees of success. Often, evaluation equipment is expensive and more suited to research than to clinical applications (Preston, 2001; Worley, Bennett, Miller, Miller, Walker, & Harmon, 1991).

Numerous clinical methods for assessing muscle tone exist. The most common method is to grasp the body part gently and firmly and to move it briskly through the desired movement pattern. The Ashworth (1964) scale grades tone from 0 (no increase in tone) to 4 (limb is rigid in flexion or extension). Bohannon and Smith (1987) modified Ashworth's scale by adding an additional level, incorporating the angle at which resistance appears, and controlling the speed of passive movement with a 1-sec count (Table 25-3). A tone assessment scale has been developed in an attempt to address the relationship between abnormal tone and posture and associated reactions (Gregson, Leathley, Moore, Sharma, Smith, & Watkins, 1999).

Brennan (1959) measured the ROM that is possible before resistance to movement is felt. King (1987) established a five-point rating scale for each of four functions: presence of tone, AROM, alternating movement, and resistance to passive movement. Bobath (1978) described a method of evaluating the combined effects of tone and primitive reflexes. Clients' limbs are moved in normal patterns of use, and the adaptation of the different muscle groups to changes in position is noted. Fugl-Meyer, Jaasko, Leyman, Olson, and Steglind (1975) established an objective method for measuring function and movement in hemiparetic clients (Table 25-4).

TABLE 25-3. **MODIFIED ASHWORTH SCALE**[a]

Grade	Description
0	No increase in muscle tone
1	Slight increase in tone, manifested by a catch and release or by minimal resistance at the end of ROM when affected part is moved in flexion or extension
+1	Slight increase in muscle tone, manifested by a catch, followed by minimal resistance throughout remainder (less than half) of ROM
2	More marked increase in muscle tone through most of ROM, but affected part easily moved
3	Considerable increase in muscle tone; passive movement difficult
4	Affected part rigid in flexion or extension

[a]Reprinted with permission from Bohannon and Smith (1987).

TABLE 25-4. **FUGL-MEYER SCALE OF FUNCTIONAL RETURN AFTER HEMIPLEGIA**[a]

Grade	Movement of Shoulder, Elbow, Forearm, and Lower Extremity
I	Muscle stretch reflexes can be elicited
II	Volitional movements can be performed within dynamic flexor-extensor synergies
III	Volitional motion is performed by mixing dynamic flexor-extensor synergies
IV	Volitional movements are performed with little or no synergy dependence
V	Normal muscle stretch reflexes

[a]Data from Fugl-Meyer, Jaasko, Leyman, Olson, and Steglind (1975).

Various electrophysiologic quantifications of spasticity exist but may or may not be clinically useful (Sehgal & McGuire, 1998).

Recording Results

When recording results, the therapist should note the position in which testing was done, the presence of abnormal reflexes, as well as any external factors that may influence results. This may include environmental temperature, time of day, and medications. The therapist should note the presence, degree, distribution, and type of abnormal tone, as well as its effect on the client's ability to perform ADL. This can be done graphically, with a table, or in narrative form.

Interpreting Results

For clients who have abnormal tone, therapists should ask the following types of questions:

- Does it affect function?
- What influences the tone?
- Is it the position of the head, hips, or trunk?
- Does a combination of muscle tones exist?
- Do medications have an effect on tone and related function?
- Do facilitation or inhibitory techniques have any short- or long-term effect?

If low tone is present, a muscle test can determine the degree of weakness. If recovery from low tone is expected, graded exercise and therapeutic activity are appropriate. Adaptive equipment may be necessary on a short- or long-term basis. Positioning should protect weak muscles from overstretching.

High muscle tone makes it impossible to conduct accurate muscle testing and necessitates techniques to maintain ROM, perform ADL, and position in patterns opposite the spastic patterns. Inhibitory techniques depend on the nature and severity of the disability, abnormal tone distribution, and other concomitant problems (Preston, 2001; Mathiowetz & Bass-Haugen, 2002; Warren, 1991).

MUSCLE STRENGTH

Definition and Purpose

Muscle strength can be defined as "the ability to demonstrate a degree of power of a muscle when movement is resisted, as with objects or gravity" (Jacobs, 1999, p. 142). Clinical assessment of muscle strength examines the maximal contraction of a muscle or muscle group when apparent weakness or difficulties with function exist. Muscle weakness is typically seen in lower motor neuron disorders, primary muscle diseases, and neurological diseases. Disabilities that cause disuse or immobilization, such as burns, arthritis, and amputation, can also cause weakness (Pedretti, 2001b; Trombly & Podolski, 2002).

Assessment of muscle strength can

- Facilitate diagnosis in some neuromuscular conditions (e.g., spinal cord injury, peripheral nerve lesion).
- Establish a baseline and ongoing measure to assess intervention effectiveness.
- Determine if weakness is limiting performance.
- Determine the need for compensatory measures or assistive devices on a temporary or long-term basis, depending on the nature of the disability.
- Identify muscle imbalances that may require strengthening, if possible, or orthotic intervention to prevent deformity.

Muscle strength can be measured by spring scales, tensiometers, dynamometers, weights, or manual resistance. The evaluation of muscle strength does not measure endurance, coordination, or performance capabilities (Pedretti, 2001b; Simmonds, 1997; Trombly & Podolski, 2002)

General Principles

Gross muscle testing evaluates the strength of groups of muscles that perform specific movements at each joint (e.g., elbow flexors). Manual muscle testing evaluates individual muscles (e.g., biceps, brachialis, brachioradialis). A therapist might first observe functional performance and then decide to focus on a certain muscle group based on the outcome of the observation. Specific muscle testing may be necessary for people with certain diagnoses, such as spinal cord injury, Guillain-Barré syndrome, and peripheral nerve injury, to determine preventative and restorative approaches to support performance. Clients with other diagnoses, such as generalized weakness, lower extremity amputation, or hip replacement, may require only gross muscle testing as a screen for determining limitations affecting performance.

To perform muscle testing, a therapist needs to know the muscles and their functions, the anatomic position and direction of muscle fibers, and the angle of pull on the joints. Substitution patterns (i.e., when a muscle or muscle group attempts to compensate for lack of function in a weak or paralyzed muscle) should be expected and targeted (e.g., shoulder external rotation and eccentric lengthening of biceps versus triceps elbow extension in gravity-eliminated position).

Muscle testing cannot be accurately used with clients who have upper motor neuron disorders. In these clients, hypertonic muscle tone and movement tend to occur in gross synergistic patterns and may be influenced by primitive reflexes (Pedretti, 2001b). Note that in people with spinal cord injury (an upper motor neuron disorder), the

TABLE 25-5. **MUSCLE TESTING GRADES**[a]

Number Garde	Word or Letter Grade	Definition
0	Zero (0)	No muscle contraction can be seen or felt.
1	Trace (T)	Contraction can be felt, but there is no motion.
1−	Poor minus (P−)	Part moves through an incomplete ROM with gravity eliminated.
2	Poor (P)	Part moves through a complete ROM with gravity eliminated.
2+	Poor plus (P+)	Part moves through incomplete ROM (< 50%) against gravity or through complete ROM with gravity eliminated against slight resistance.
3−	Fair minus (F−)	Part moves through an incomplete ROM (> 50%) against gravity.
3	Fair (F)	Part moves through complete ROM against gravity.
3+	Fair plus (F+)	Part moves through a complete ROM against gravity and slight resistance.
4	Good (G)	Part moves through a complete ROM against gravity and moderate assistance.
5	Normal (N)	Part moves through complete ROM against gravity and full resistance.

[a]Reprinted with permission from Pedretti (2001b).

muscles being tested are those innervated by spinal cord segments above the level of the injury.

Gravity influences muscle function. Gravity-eliminated positions are used with O to P+ (or 0 to 2+) grades. Movements against gravity are used with F to N (or 3 to 5) grades. Definitions for muscle grades are relatively standard (Table 25-5). Assignment of muscle grades depends on clinical judgment, knowledge, and examiner experience. The amount of resistance given (e.g., slight, moderate, or full) is determined by the client's age, gender, body type, and occupation and varies from one muscle group to the next. The therapist must consider the size and relative muscle power and leverage used when giving resistance. That is, the practitioner would not apply the same force to finger flexors as to shoulder flexors (Hilsop, Montgomery, Connelly, & Daniels, 1995; Kendall, McCreary, & Provance, 1993; Pedretti, 2001b; Simmonds, 1997; Trombly & Podolski, 2002).

In individual cases, positioning for muscle testing in the correct plane may not be possible due to medical precautions, immobilization devices, trunk instability, or weakness. Modifications in positioning and grading are cited for individual tests in muscle testing manuals (Hilsop et al., 1995; Kendall et al., 1993). Lamb (1985) discussed various aspects of manual muscle testing, including variables of testing procedures, reliability, and validity issues. Differences in methods (e.g., force application, stabilization, and positioning) and strength determination during controlled studies are discussed by Smidt and Roger (1982).

Procedure for Muscle Testing

Whether performing gross or manual muscle testing, certain general procedures apply (Pedretti, 2001b).

1. Determine the available PROM of the joint associated with the muscles being examined.
2. Position and stabilize the body part proximal to the part being tested.
3. Demonstrate or describe the test motion.
4. Ask the client to perform the movement.
5. Palpate by placing fingerpads firmly and gently over the muscle tendon or belly.
6. Observe the client's movement.
7. Ask the client to hold the position.
8. For grades above fair (or 3), resist
   In the opposite direction of test movement.
   At the end of available ROM.
   On the distal end of the moving bone.
   As close to a perpendicular direction as possible.

Table 25-6 suggests a sequence of upper extremity muscle testing that streamlines the clinical evaluation process. Figures 25-14 through 25-19 illustrate specific muscle testing techniques in both gravity-eliminated and against-gravity positions. Techniques for testing for shoulder abduction (middle deltoid), elbow flexion (biceps), and wrist extension (extensor carpi radialis longus) are shown.

Comparison of Two Philosophies

There are primarily two dominant philosophies and methods for clinical evaluation of muscle strength; one proposed by Kendall et al. (1993) and the other by Daniels and Worthingham (1986). Each philosophy defines muscle grades slightly differently.

The Kendall philosophy uses isometric hold, or break, tests. The muscle strength required to hold the test position, with few exceptions, is considered equivalent to the muscle strength required to complete the test movement. It also recommends using assistive movements into antigravity

TABLE 25–6. **SUGGESTED SEQUENCE FOR UPPER EXTREMITY MUSCLE TESTING**[a,b]

Back lying (supine)	
Grades N to F	
Scapula abduction and upward rotation	
Shoulder horizontal abduction	
All tests for forearm, wrist, and fingers can be given in the back-lying position if necessary	
Grades P to 0	
Shoulder abduction	Hip external rotation
Elbow flexion	Hip internal rotation
Elbow extension	Foot inversion
Hip abduction	Foot eversion
Hip adduction	
Face lying (prone)	
Grades N to F	
Scapula depression	Shoulder horizontal abduction
Scapula adduction	Elbow extension
Scapula adduction and downward rotation	Hip extension
Shoulder extension	Knee flexion
Shoulder external rotation	Ankle plantar flexion
Shoulder internal rotation	
Grades P to 0	
Scapula elevation	Scapula adduction
Scapula depression	
Side lying	
Grades N to F	
Hip abduction	Foot inversion
Hip adduction	Foot eversion
Grades P to 0	
Shoulder flexion	Knee flexion
Shoulder extension	Knee extension
Hip flexion	Ankle plantar flexion
Hip extension	Ankle dorsiflexion
Sitting	
Grades N to F	
Scapula elevation	Hip flexion
Shoulder flexion	Hip external rotation
Shoulder abduction	Hip internal rotation
Elbow flexion	Knee extension
All forearm, wrist, finger, and thumb movements	Ankle dorsiflexion with inversion
Grades P to 0	
All forearm, wrist, finger, and thumb movements	
Ankle dorsiflexion with inversion	

[a]Reprinted with permission from Pedretti (2001b).

[b]See Table 25-5 for more detailed information.

N, normal; *F*, fair; *P*, poor; *0*, zero.

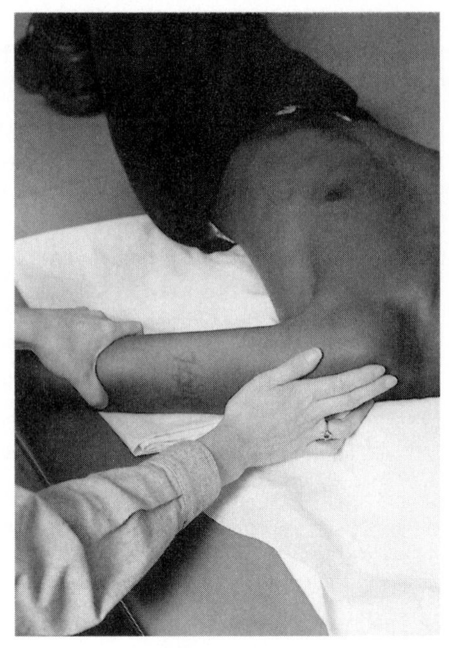

FIGURE 25–14. Muscle testing for shoulder abduction (middle deltoid) in the gravity-eliminated position. (Courtesy of the Rehabilitation Institute of Chicago.)

positions, rather than frequent position changes, and uses percentage values. Table 25-7 shows the Kendall muscle grades and their definitions.

Alternatively, the Daniels and Worthingham grading is based on the following three factors (Table 25-8):

- Amount of resistance that can be given manually to a contracting muscle.
- Ability of the muscle to move a part through the complete ROM.
- Evidence of the presence or absence of contraction.

The two methods are compared in Tables 25-9 and 25-10.

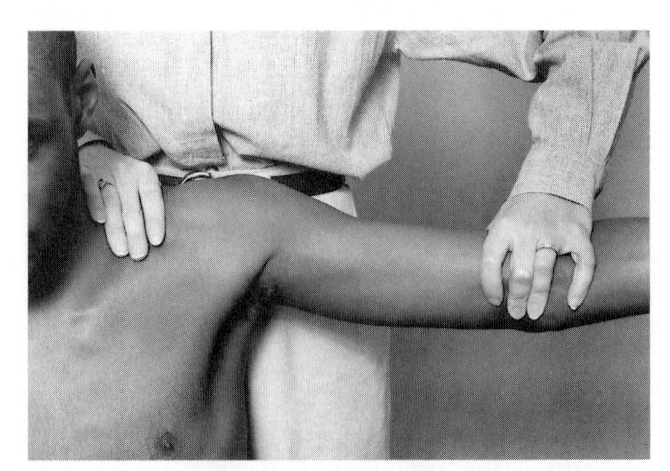

FIGURE 25–15. Muscle testing for shoulder abduction (middle deltoid) in the against-gravity position. (Courtesy of the Rehabilitation Institute of Chicago.)

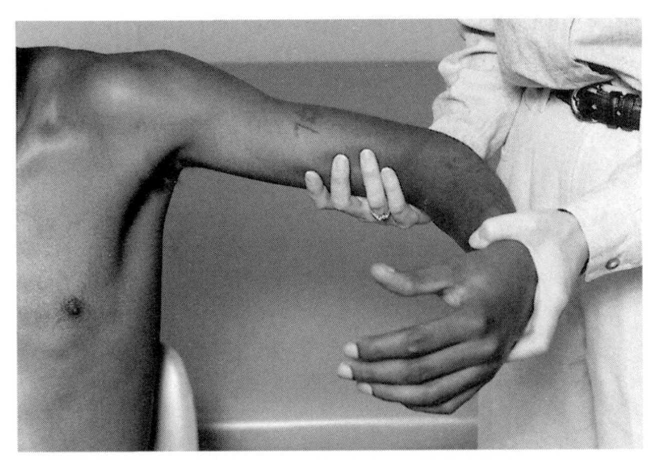

FIGURE 25–16. Muscle testing for elbow flexion (biceps) in the gravity-eliminated position. (Courtesy of the Rehabilitation Institute of Chicago.)

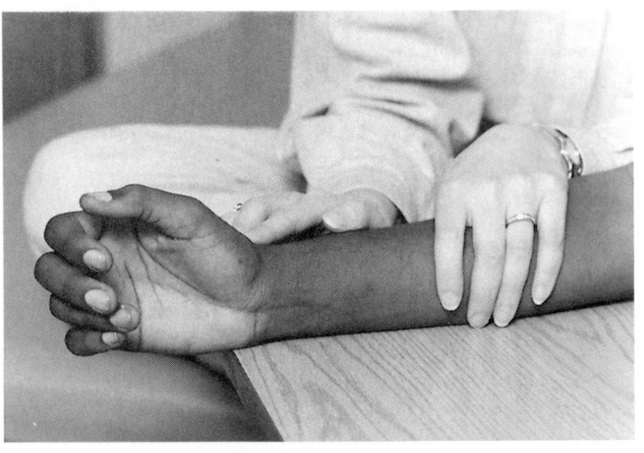

FIGURE 25–18. Muscle testing for wrist extension (extensor carpi radialis longus) in the gravity-eliminated position. (Courtesy of the Rehabilitation Institute of Chicago.)

Hand Strength

For evaluation of hand strength, the American Society of Hand Therapists (1981) recommends standard methods of measurement on which norms are based. Standardized positioning and instructions are also recommended by Mathiowetz, Volland, Kashman, and Weber (1985). Elbow position, forearm position, the type of dynamometer, and the handle position of the dynamometer can influence results and, therefore, must remain consistent (Bellace, Healy, Besser, Byron, & Hohman, 2000; Hamilton, Balnare, & Adams 1994; Oxford, 2000; Richards, Olson, & Palmiter-Thomas, 1996). Grip strength is measured by a standard adjustable-handle dynamometer (Fig. 25-20). The client is seated with shoulder adducted, elbow flexed at 90°, and forearm in the neutral position. The average of three successive forceful grips is taken (Pedretti, 2001b; Trombly, & Podolski, 2002).

Pinch strength is tested on a standard pinch dynamometer in three ways (Figs. 25-21 and 25-22:

- *Palmar pinch:* Thumb tip to index finger
- *Lateral pinch:* Thumb pulp to lateral aspect of middle phalanx of index finger
- *Three-point pinch:* Thumb tip to tips of index and long fingers

The average of three successive trials is taken (Pedretti, 2001; Trombly & Podolski, 2002).

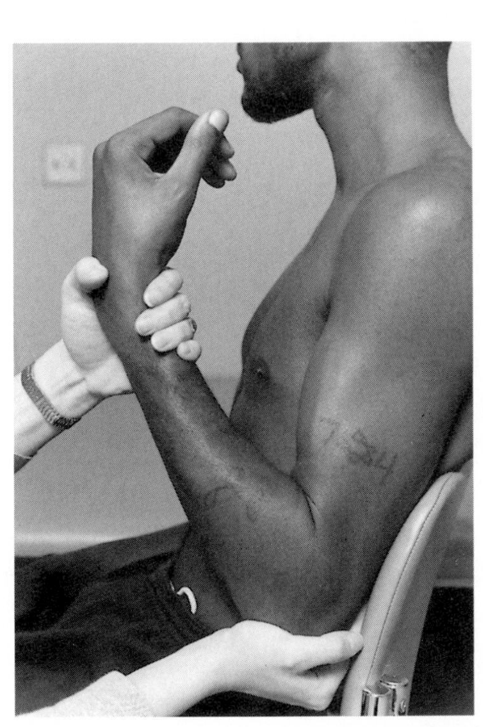

FIGURE 25–17. Muscle testing for elbow flexion (biceps) in the against-gravity position. (Courtesy of the Rehabilitation Institute of Chicago.)

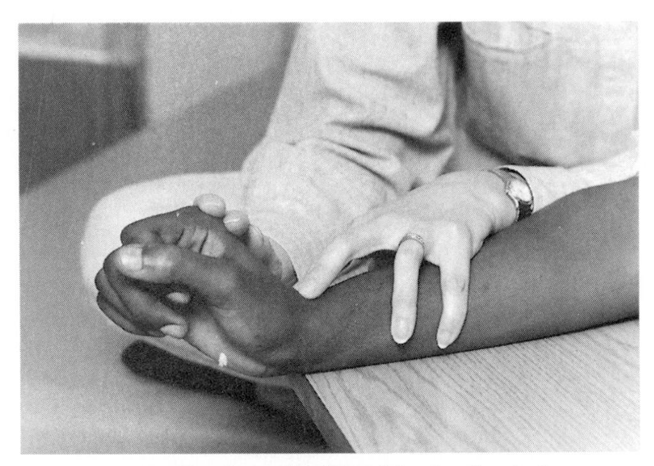

FIGURE 25–19. Muscle testing for wrist extension (extensor carpi radialis longus) in the against-gravity position. (Courtesy of the Rehabilitation Institute of Chicago.)

TABLE 25-7. **KENDALL MUSCLE GRADES**

Letter (% Grade)	Definition
N (100%)	Can hold against gravity and maximal resistance (defined as sufficient resistance to displace body weight proximal to tested part).
G, G+ (80–90%)	Can hold against gravity and moderate resistance.
F+, G−(60–70%)	Can hold against gravity and slight resistance.
F (50%)	Ability to hold test position.
F−(40%)	Gradual release from test position; ability to complete ROM with gravity eliminated.
P+ (30%)	Ability to move through moderate arch of ROM with gravity eliminated; can move into test position with moderate assistance.
P (20%)	Ability to move through minimal arch of ROM with gravity eliminated; can move into test position with maximum assistance.
P−/T (10–5%)	Muscle can be seen or palpated; no visible movement.

TABLE 25-8. **DANIELS AND WORTHINGHAM MUSCLE GRADES**

Letter Grade	Definition
N	Able to move part through full ROM against gravity and hold against maximal resistance at end of range (break test).
G	Able to move part through full ROM against gravity and take good resistance at end of range.
F+	Able to move through full ROM against gravity and take minimal resistance at end of range.
F	Able to move part through full ROM against gravity; not able to take any resistance at end of range.
F−	Able to move part through more than one half ROM against gravity.
P+	Able to move part through less than one half ROM against gravity.
P	Able to move part through full ROM in gravity-eliminated position.
P−	Able to move part through more than one half ROM in gravity-eliminated position.
T+	Able to move part through less than one half the ROM in gravity-eliminated position.
T	Contraction can be palpated—no movement of part.

TABLE 25-9. **SERRATUS ANTERIOR TESTING: COMPARISON OF TWO METHODS**

Testing Element	Kendall	Daniels and Worthingham
Client position (above fair)	Sitting	Supine (stabilize arm)
Palpation	Does not address	Does not address
Motion (above fair)	Abduction and lateral rotation of inferior angle of scapula through maintaining humerus at 120–130° flexion	Abduction and lateral rotation of interior angle of scapula (humerus flexed to 90°)
Resistance	Against lateral border of scapula, rotating, inferior angle medially and against shoulder in direction of extension	Grasp around forearm and elbow; pressure is downward and inward toward table
Substitution	Does not address	Does not address

TABLE 25-10. **RHOMBOID TESTING: COMPARISON OF TWO METHODS**

Testing Element	Kendall	Daniels and Worthingham
Client position		
• Above fair	Prone	Prone: head rotated to opposite side
• Below fair	Prone	Sitting: arm internally rotated, adducted across back (shoulder relaxed)
Palpation	Does not address	Angle formed by vertebral border of scapula and internal fibers of lower trapezius
Motion	Elbow flexed, humerus adducted in slight extension and lateral rotation	Adduction and medial rotation of inferior angle of scapula
Resistance	Examiner attempts to rotate laterally with one hand at shoulder, pushing in direction of shoulder depression and scapula lateral rotation	On vertebral border of scapula outward and slightly downward
Substitution	Does not address	Does not address

Oral Motor Control

Some occupational therapists evaluate and treat individuals with oral motor control problems. This can be done alone or in conjunction with a speech and language pathologist. In some work settings, occupational therapists do not address this area at all.

Dysphagia is defined as difficult in swallowing. Swallowing is a multistage sequence that, when normally elicited, momentarily blocks the opening to the respiratory tract as

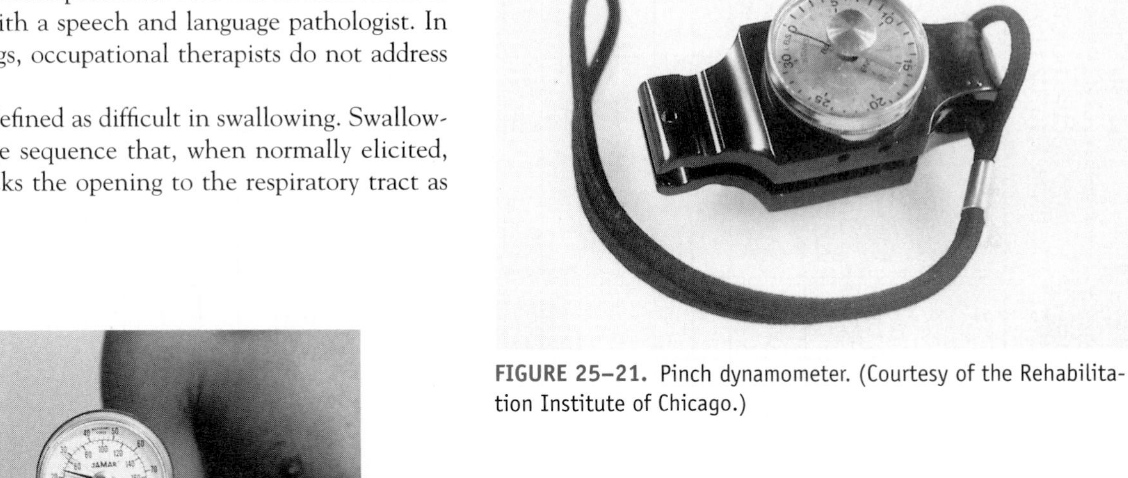

FIGURE 25-21. Pinch dynamometer. (Courtesy of the Rehabilitation Institute of Chicago.)

FIGURE 25-20. Dynamometer. (Courtesy of the Rehabilitation Institute of Chicago.)

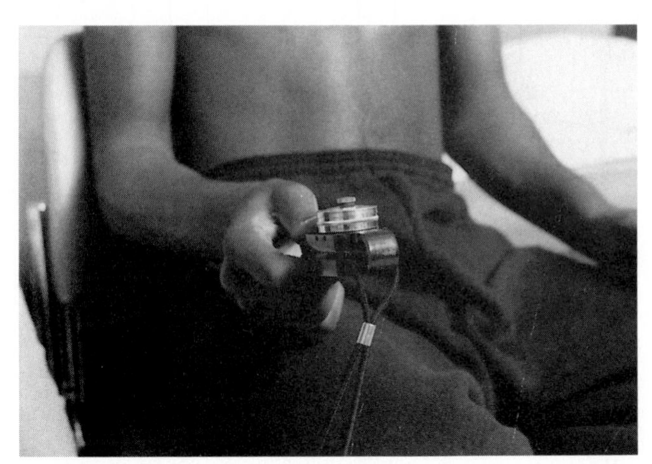

FIGURE 25-22. Measurement of lateral pinch. (Courtesy of the Rehabilitation Institute of Chicago.)

TABLE 25-11. **RESULTS OF UPPER EXTREMELY MUSCLE STRENGTH TESTING**[a]

REHABILITATION INSTITUTE OF CHICAGO OCCUPATIONAL THERAPY DEPARTMENT
FUNCTIONAL SKILLS/MOTOR FUNCTION

MANUAL MUSCLE EXAMINATION OF THE UPPER EXTREMITIES
GROSS / SPECIFIC (circle one)

Date	Date	Movement	Muscle	Level	Date	Date
		Abd/up rotation	Serratus anterior	C5-7		
		Elevation	Upper trapezius	C2-4		
		Add/Depression	Lower trapezius	C2-4		
		Adduction	Middle trapezius	C2-5		
		Add/down rotat.	Rhomboids	C5		
		SHOULDER				
		Flexion	Anterior deltoid	C5-6		
		Extension	Latissimus dorsi	C7-8		
		Abduction	Middle deltoid	C5-6		
		Horiz. abd.		C5-6		
		Horiz. add. Pect major (clavicular)		C5-7		
		Horiz. add. Pect major (sternal)		C7-T1		
		External rotator group		C5-6		
				C5-T1		
		ELBOW/FOREARM				
		Flexion	Biceps brachii	C5-6		
			Brachioradialis	C5-6		
		Extension		C(6)7-8		
		Supination		C5-6(7)		
		Pronation		C6-T1		
		WRIST				
		Flexion	Flexor carpi ulnaris	C7-8		
			Flexor carpi radialis	C6-8		
			Palmaris longus	C6-7		
		Ext.	Extensor carpi radialis longus	C6-7		
			Extensor carpi radialis brevis	C6-7		
			Extensor carpi ulnaris	C7-8		

Name:

RIC #:

Physician:

JOINT RANGE MEASUREMENTS

AROM	AROM	PROM	PROM				PROM	PROM	AROM	AROM
Date	Date	Date	Date				Date	Date	Date	Date
				< - Left	Right - >					
				Flexion	0-180	Shoulder				
				Extension	0-60	Shoulder				
				Abduction	0-180	Shoulder				
				External Rotation	0-90	Shoulder				
				Internal Rotation	0-70	Shoulder				
				Horiz. Abduction	0-90	Shoulder				
				Horiz. Adduction	0-45	Shoulder				
				Flexion	0-150	Elbow				
				Supination	0-80	Elbow				
				Pronation	0-80	Elbow				
				Flexion	0-80	Wrist				
				Extension	0-70	Wrist				
				Ulnar Dev.	0-30	Wrist				
				Radial Dev.	0-20	Wrist				
				M.P. Flexion	0-50	Thumb				
				I. P. Flexion	0-80	Thumb				
				Abduction	0-70	Thumb				

		FINGERS					
		1	MP Extension-Ext. digitorum communis				
		2	"		C7-8		
		3	"				
		4	"				
		1	DIP Flexion-Flex. digitorum profundus				
		2	"		C7-T1		
		3	"				
		4	"				
		1	PIP Flexion-Flex digit. superficialis				
		2	"		C6-8		
		3	"				
		4	"				
		1	MP Flexion	Lumbricales	C8-T1		
		2		Lumbricales			
		3		Lumbricales			
		4		Lumbricales			
		1	Adduction - Palmar Interoscous				
		2	"		C8-T1		
		3	"				
		1	Abduction - Dorsal Interoscous				
		2	"		C8-T1		
		3	"				
		4	"				

		THUMB				
		MP Flexion	Flex. Poll. brevis	C8-T1		
		IP Flexion	Flex. poll. longus	C8-T1		
		MP Extension	Ext. poll. brevis	C7-8		
		IP Extension	Ext. poll. longus	C7-8		
		Abduction	Abd. poll. brevis	C8-T1		
			Abd. poll. longus	C7-8		
		Adduction	Adductor pollicis	C8-T1		
		Opposition	Opponens policis	C8-T1		

Grade: N=Normal; G=Good; F=Fair; P=Poor; T=Trace; 0=Zero

				Motion	Range	Finger				
				M. P. Flexion	0-90	Index F.				
				M. P. Extension	0-45					
				P. I. P. Flexion	0-100					
				D. I. P. Flexion	0-80					
				M. P. Flexion	0-90	Long F.				
				M. P. Extension	0-45					
				P. I. P. Flexion	0-100					
				D. I. P. Flexion	0-90					
				M. P. Flexion	0-90	Ring F.				
				M. P. Extension	0-45					
				P. I. P. Flexion	0-100					
				D. I. P. Flexion	0-90					
				M. P. Flexion	0-90	Little F.				
				M. P. Extension	0-45					
				P. I. P. Flexion	0-100					
				D. I. P. Flexion	0-90					

PREHENSILE STRENGTH

	Date	Left	Right	Norm
Cylindrical Grasp				
3-Point Pinch				
Lateral Pinch				
9 Hole Peg Test				

Therapist   Date

[a]Reprinted with permission from the Rehabilitation Institute of Chicago.

food or beverage is passed through the pharynx and into the esophagus. Swallowing can occur either by willful cortical initiation or by a reflex, elicited independently from higher brain centers (Miller, Groher, Yorkston, & Rees, 1988). Swallowing has three phases:

- *Oral:* Preparation of the bolus or mass of chewed food.
- *Pharyngeal:* The bolus is propelled through the pharynx away from the airway.
- *Esophageal:* A primary peristaltic wave propels the bolus through the lower esophageal sphincter and into the stomach.

Nasal regurgitation is a symptom associated with weakness of the palatopharyngeal mechanism. Aspiration of food or liquid into the trachea ("windpipe") is a common complaint of clients with neurological impairment of the swallowing muscles. When there is difficulty swallowing solid food, a feeling of blockage is common.

When dysphagia is recognized or a swallowing complaint is registered, the examination should include the following: a complete medical history, a description of the complaint and associated symptoms, a physical examination of the peripheral deglutitive motor and sensory system, and motion radiographic studies (Avery-Smith, 2002; Avery-Smith, Rosen, & Dellarosa, 1997). Occupational therapy evaluation includes assessment of:

- Mental status.
- Strength of muscles of the face, mouth, neck, and trunk.
- Oral sensation.
- Primitive reflexes.
- Intraoral mucosa.
- Adequacy of swallowing.

Recording Results

Typically, a chart or grid is used to record muscle strength. Table 25-11 is a sample form for recording the results of upper extremity muscle strength testing. The timing of reevaluation may depend on the expected recovery rate, length of stay in therapy, and protocols of the setting. Therapists should keep in mind that the focus of therapy should be an increase in function, not necessarily an increase in the component area of strength.

Interpreting Results

Muscle testing is only one component of an evaluation. How the therapist interprets and uses the information is more important. The therapist should ask the following types of questions (Pedretti, 2001a). Is the problem one of strength, endurance, or a combination thereof? Endurance is the number of repetitions of muscle contraction before fatigue. If endurance is the issue, the therapist needs to emphasize repetitive movements (at less than maximal contraction) to increase it.

Are the results of the assessments influenced by impaired tactile sensation or proprioception? What is the diagnosis or expected course of the disease? Is there an expected recovery period? What is the progression of decline? Are there periods of exacerbation or remission?

The therapist should assess the degree of weakness, its distribution, and its pattern (e.g., generalized or specific). The muscle imbalance between agonists and antagonists suggest the type of intervention (e.g., resistive exercises, active assistive activities, orthotic intervention). The practitioner must coordinate the therapy program with other professionals so that the timing and type of appointments and goals are in line with other interventions.

REFLEX TESTING

"A reflex is an involuntary, stereotyped response to a particular stimulus" (Mathiowetz & Bass Haugen, 1995; p. 170). **Reflex** responses develop in utero and are clearly apparent in infancy. In normal development, primitive spinal and brainstem reflexes gradually become less obvious, and higher-level righting and equilibrium reactions become more obvious (Agostinucci, 1997; Mathiowitz & Bass Haugen, 2002; Preston, 2001). A reaction is a stereotyped, nonobligatory response to a particular stimulus.

After central nervous system injury or disease, the nervous system may exhibit more exaggerated reflexes. A reflex assessment is necessary to determine the status of the primitive reflex integration and of the righting and equilibrium reactions. The following principles should be noted when testing primitive reflexes (Agostinucci, 1997; Mathiowitz & Bass Haugen, 2002):

- Reflexes and responses should be tested in several developmental postures.
- Any stress can release elements of primitive postural reflexes in both the neurologically intact and the neurologically impaired population.
- Clients with chronic neuromotor disorders rarely demonstrate a primitive postural reflex in its pure form; usually, reflexes are combined so that clients demonstrate elements of several reflexes in one behavioral response.
- Reflexes are usually tested in developmental sequence.

The following is an overview of the various levels of reflex testing:

- *Innate primary reactions:* Primitive reflexes found in newborns, involving total patterns of flexion and extension (Table 25-12).
- *Automatic movement reflexes:* Produced by changes of the head's position in space (Table 25-13).
- *Spinal-level reflexes:* Phasic and basic to mobility motor patterns (Table 25-14).

TABLE 25–12. **INNATE PRIMARY REACTIONS**[a]

Reflex/Reaction	Age Range	Test Position	Stimulus	Response
Reflex stepping	Birth–3 months	Supported in upright position with some weight bearing on feet	Lean client forward; pressure of feet on supporting surface	Rhythmic, alternating stepping
Grasp reflex	Birth–3 to 4 months	Any—usually supine	Pressure in palm of hand or ulnar side	Flexing of fingers; grasping of stimulus object
Placing reaction	Birth–2 months	Sitting or supine	Brush dorsum of one of client's hands against under edge of a table or edge of a stiff cardboard	Flexion of arm with placement of the hand on tabletop
Sucking reflex	Birth–2 months	Any	Stimulation to lips. gums, or front of tongue	Sucking, swallowing motions
Rooting reflex	Birth–4 months	Any	Touch or stroke outward on corner of lips or on cheek	Lower lip, tongue, and head move toward stimulus

[a]Data from Mathiowetz and Bass Haugen (1995); Barnes, Crutchfield, Heriza (1982).

TABLE 25–13. **AUTOMATIC MOVEMENT REFLEXES**[a]

Reflex	Age Range	Test Position	Stimulus	Response
Moro reflex	Birth–5 months	Semireclining or supine	Dropping head backward from semisitting position or loud noise near the head	Extension or flexion and abduction of arms and spreading of fingers
Landau reflex	4–12 to 24 months	Prone, suspended in space with support under chest	Passive or active neck extension	Back and legs extend
Protective extensor thrust	6 months–death	Sitting or prone	Displace body forward, sideways and backward (separately)	Protective extension of limb to protect head

[a]Data from Mathiowetz and Bass Haugen (1995); Barnes, Crutchfield, Heriza (1982).

TABLE 25–14. **SPINAL-LEVEL REFLEXES**

Reflex	Age Range	Test Position	Stimulus	Response
Flexor withdrawal	Birth–2 months	Supine or sitting with head in midposition, legs extended	Stimulation to sole of foot	Uncontrolled flexion of stimulated leg
Extensor thrust	Birth–2 months	Supine or sitting with head in midposition; one leg is in extension and other is fully flexed	Pressure to ball of foot of flexed leg	Uncontrolled extension of stimulated leg
Crossed extension	Birth–2 months	Supine with head in midposition; one leg is in extension and other is fully flexed	Passively flex extended leg	Extension of opposite leg, with hip internal rotation and adduction

[a]Data from Mathiowetz and Bass Haugen (1995); Barnes, Crutchfield, Heriza (1982).

TABLE 25–15. **BRAINSTEM-LEVEL REFLEXES**[a]

Reflex	Age Range	Test Position	Stimulus	Response
Asymmetrical tonic neck reflex (ATNR)	Birth–4 to 6 months	Supine or sitting, with arms and legs extended; clients with minimal reflexes responses can be tested in quadruped	Passively or actively turn the head 90° to one side	Increase of extensor tone of limbs on face side and flexor tone of limbs on skull side
Symmetrical tonic neck reflex (STNR)	Birth–4 to 6 months	Sitting or quadruped	(1) Flex client's head and bring chin toward chest; (2) extend client's head	(1) Flexion of upper extremities and extension of lower extremity; (2) extension of upper extremities and flexion of lower extremities
Tonic labyrinthine reflex (TLR)	Birth–4 to 6 months	Prone with head in midposition	Test position is stimulus	Flexion of extremities or increase in flexor tone
TLR supine	Birth–4 to 6 months	Supine with head in midposition	Test position is stimulus	Extension of extremities or increase in extensor tone
Positive supporting reaction	Birth–4 to 6 months	Standing, supine, or sitting	Firmly contact ball of foot to floor; or footboard of bed and dorsiflex foot	Rigid extension of lower extremity owing to co-contraction of flexors and extensors of knee and hip joints
Associated reactions	Associated movements are normal throughout life when attempting strenuous activities; associated reactions are stereotyped tonic reactions by which one extremity influences posture of another extremity	Any position	Resist any motion or have client squeeze an object with unaffected hand	Motion used as a stimulus will be mimicked by other hand

[a]Data from Mathiowetz and Bass Haugen (1995); Barnes, Crutchfield, Heriza (1982).

TABLE 25–16. **MIDBRAIN-LEVEL REACTIONS**[a]

Reaction	Age Range	Test Position	Stimulus	Response
Neck righting	Birth–6 months	Supine with arms and legs extended	Passively turn head to one side and hold it there	Body rotates as a whole in direction to which head was turned
Labyrinthine righting acting on head	2 months–death	Prone, supine, or vertical positions in space; client's vision is occluded	Prone or supine positions are test stimuli, or in vertical position body is tilted laterally	Head seeks vertical position in space
Body righting acting on head	6 months–5 years	Client is blindfolded prone and supine	Asymmetric stimulation of pressure sense organs on anterior of body surface	Head is brought into a face-vertical position that orients it to surface with which client is in contact
Body righting on body	6–18 months	Supine with arms and legs extended	Passively or actively turn head to one side	Segmental rotation around body axis toward direction of head

[a]Data from Mathiowetz and Bass Haugen (1995); Barnes, Crutchfield, Heriza (1982).

TABLE 25-17. **CORTICAL REACTIONS**[a]

Reaction	Age Range	Test Position	Stimulus	Response
Optic righting	2 months–death	Prone or supine on a raised mat sitting with head laterally flexed; eyes open	Position of head in relation to landmarks in space	Head is raised upright in space
Equilibrium reaction	Depends on test position; throughout life	Supine (7–8 months); prone (5 months); quadruped (9–12 months); sitting (6 months); kneel-standing (15 months); standing (15 months)	Rocking client or supporting surface sufficiently to disturb balance	Automatic movements to maintain balance, right head and body; protective reactions

[a]Data from Mathiowetz and Bass Haugen (1995); Barnes, Crutchfield, Heriza (1982).

- *Brainstem-level reflexes:* Static, postural reflexes that cause a change in muscle tone throughout the body in response to a change of the head's position in space or in relation to the body, which activates the vestibular system; the changed tone is maintained as long as the stimulus is present (Table 25-15).
- *Midbrain-level reactions:* Permit the development of maturationally acquired motor milestones; righting reactions are integrated at this level and interact with one another to effect the normal head-to-body relation in space and to each other (Table 25-16).
- *Cortical reactions:* The result of the efficient interaction of the cerebral cortex, basal ganglia, and cerebellum (equilibrium reactions occur when muscle tone is normalized; enable the adaptation to changes in the body's center of gravity; and involve the integration of vestibular, visual, and tactile inputs) (Table 25-17).

Recording Results

Test position(s) should be noted. Results are usual recorded as to whether the client's response is positive or negative. Intensity (i.e., the speed of response and degree of change) as well as quality (i.e., which components of the response are present under which conditions) of responses should be documented.

Interpreting Results

Obligatory reflexive responses, such as domination of a postural reflex, indicates severe central nervous system abnormality. Disturbance of higher-integrating centers manifests by evidence of a reflex, but not complete domination (Agostonucci, 1997; Mathiowetz & Bass Haugen, 2002). For example, a weak reflex response would be tonal changes in the extremities as opposed to actual movement. This should not be confused with tonal changes in a stimulus-neutral condition. Problems with reflex integration result in decreased trunk segmentation, ability to perform isolated movement, adaptation of muscles to postural change, and function of antigravity muscles and increased synergistic movement. Formal evaluation should always be accompanied by observation of how reflexes affect motor and functional performance. For example, a positive asymmetric tonic neck reflex (ATNR) can interfere with rolling from supine to prone, due to scapular retraction on the skull-side extremity (which prevents bringing that arm across) and an extended arm on the face side.

ENDURANCE

Endurance can be defined as the ability to sustain a given activity over time. It is related to cardiopulmonary, biomechanical, and neuromuscular function (Asmussen, 1979; Farber, 1991a, 1991b; Lunsford, 1978; Trombly & Podolski, 2002). Endurance is a measure of stamina and fitness and can be compromised by inactivity, immobilization, cardiorespiratory deconditioning, muscular deconditioning, and diminished flexibility. Endurance is related to intensity, duration, and frequency of activity. It can be reported as a percentage of maximal heart rate, as a number of repetitions over time, or as the amount of time a contraction can be held (Trombly & Podolski, 2002).

Cardiorespiratory Endurance

Cardiorespiratory endurance is defined by the American College of Sports Medicine (1991) as "the ability to perform large-muscle, dynamic, moderate-to-high intensity exercises for prolonged periods" (p. 39). Cardiorespiratory endurance depends on the functional states of the respiratory, cardiovascular, and musculoskeletal systems. Maximal oxygen uptake ($\dot{V}O_2max$) is a standard measure of cardiorespiratory endurance. It is a measure of the maximal amount of oxygen that a person can take in and dispense during exercise and is related to a person's maximal metabolic equivalent (MET) capacity. "One MET is equivalent to an oxygen uptake of 3.5 [milliliters per kilogram body weight per minute]. It is conventional in exercise testing to

TABLE 25-18. **MET VALUES FOR SOME OCCUPATIONAL PERFORMANCE AREAS**[a]

METs	Oxygen Consumed (mL/kg/min)	Level of Activity	Self-Care Activities	IADL and Work Activities	Play and Leisure Activities
1.5–2.0	4–7	Very light, minimal	Eating, shaving, grooming, getting in and out of bed, dressing, undressing, standing, walking 1 km or 1.6 mph	Working at desk; typing; writing	Playing cards, sewing, knitting
2–3	7–11	Light	Showering in warm water; level walking 2 km or 3.25 mph	Ironing; light woodworking; using riding lawn mower	Level bicycling 8 km or 5 mph, playing billiards, bowling, golfing with power cart
3–4	11–14	Moderate	Walking 5 km or 3.5 mph	Cleaning windows; making beds; mopping floors; vacuuming; bricklaying; doing machine assembly	Bicycling 10 km or 6 mph, fly fishing standing in waders, horseshoe pitching
4–5	14–18	Heavy	Showering in hot water; walking 5.5 km or 3.5 mph	Scrubbing floors; hoeing; raking leaves; doing light carpentry	Bicycling 13 km or 8 mph, table tennis, doubles tennis
5–6	18–21	Heavy	Walking 6.5 km or 4 mph	Digging in garden; shoveling light earth	Bicycling 16 km or 10 mph, canoeing 6.5 km or 4 mph, ice or roller skating 15 km or 9 mph
6–7	21–25	Very heavy	Walking 8 km or 5 mph	Shoveling snow; splitting wood	Bicycling 17.5 km or 11 mph, light downhill skiing, ski touring 4 km or 2.5 mph

[a]Data from Ainsworth et al., 1998; Wilmore and Costill, 1999.

mL/kg/min, milliliters per kilogram body weight per minute; mph, miles per hour.

express $\dot{V}O_2$max in METs (e.g., $\dot{V}O_2$max of 35 [milliliters per kilogram body weight per minute] is equivalent to 10 METs)" (p. 16). The $\dot{V}O_2$max measurements require sophisticated equipment. Occupational therapists are not qualified to make these measurements without advanced training, but can use other indicators of cardiorespiratory endurance related to $\dot{V}O_2$max and MET levels of activity and heart rate responses to activity.

To measure MET levels of activities, the occupational therapist can consult a MET table, which indicates the average number of METs expended for given activities (Table 25-18). These tables report MET levels that have been established by exercise physiology research; the MET level values reported represent the average number of the METs expended by a 150-lb person. Heavier people will expend more METs, and lighter people will expend fewer METs than the indicated values for any given activity. In addition, MET levels vary with stress and environmental conditions (American College of Sports Medicine [ACSM], 1991). Therefore, a MET table figure represents only an approximate range of MET expenditure for any given activity and should be reported as such. For example, an occupational therapist could report that a client who was able to dress without experiencing shortness of breath or an increase in heart rate of more than 20 beats per minute (bpm) could tolerate activities of 2.5 to 3.5 METs (Trombly & Podolski, 2002).

Clients' specific heart rate responses to activity need to be recorded in addition to MET levels. Heart rate quantifies the physiological demand of an activity; in healthy individuals, higher heart rates correspond to higher oxygen consumption. This is not true for individuals with cardiopulmonary diseases, because these diseases disrupt normal physiological responses to activity (see Chapter 41). Heart rate responses to intervention activities can be related to a person's maximal heart rate as a percentage of maximum. For individuals who do not have cardiopulmonary disease, maximum heart rate can be determined by subtracting their age from 220 (220 − age). Clients who have cardiopulmonary disease should have their maximum heart rate determined by an exercise stress test administered by a cardiologist (ACSM, 1991).

Biomechanical and Neuromuscular Endurance

Biomechanical neuromuscular endurance refers to the capacity of a muscle or muscle group to sustain a contraction over time. In normal muscle, only a few of available motor units are needed at any one time, as active and resting units take turns. "However, if a person sustains a contraction that exceeds 15% to 20% maximum voluntary contraction (MVC) for the muscle group involved, blood flow to the working muscles will decrease, causing a shift to anaerobic metabolism which limits duration" (Dehn, 1980, cited in Trombly & Podolski, 2002, p. 132). Anaerobic metabolism can lead to an accumulation of lactic acid and slowed conduction velocity to muscle fibers, resulting in muscle fatigue, reduced tension development, and eventual inability to hold a contraction (Basmajian & DeLuca, 1985). Clients with poor neuromuscular endurance experience muscle fatigue sooner than those with good neuromuscular endurance.

Static endurance refers to the measure of sustained contractions. Isometric testing times how long an individual can maintain the tension of a maximum voluntary contraction, by using strain gauges, dynamometers, and some isokinetic equipment. Normally, a person can hold 25% MVC for 5 to 6 min, 50% MVC for 1 to 2 min, and 100% MVC only momentarily (Dehn & Mullins, 1977; Minor, 1991). People being tested should talk while doing an isometric contraction to preclude breath holding and a significant increase in blood pressure or additional stress to the cardiopulmonary system.

Clinical Functional Endurance

Perhaps the most pertinent clinical information on muscular endurance comes from monitoring client progress through an intervention program, as opposed to comparing scores to population norms. Therapists can evaluate and quantify endurance performance by applying the principles of the timed test of repetitions at a submaximal workload. Another method is to time how long clients can participate in activities such as dressing or light homemaking tasks before requiring a rest. To evaluate changes in activity tolerance, therapists can monitor clients' perception of how hard they are working or how tired they are after a given amount of time at a specified workload. One accepted scale is the Borg Scale of Rating of Perceived Exertion (RPE), which ranges from no work at all (0 on the scale) to very very heavy work (10) (Brannon, Foley, Starr, & Black, 1993; Minor, 1991). Studies have shown that standing endurance increases when performing personally meaningful as opposed to nonmeaningful tasks (Dolecheck & Schkade, 1999).

GROSS COORDINATION

Coordination is the combined activity of many muscles into smooth patterns and sequences of motion. Coordinated movement is characterized by rhythm, appropriate muscle tension, postural tone, refinement to the minimal number of muscle groups necessary to produce the desired movement, and equilibrium. Coordination is an automatic response that is monitored primarily through proprioceptive sensory feedback. Visual and tactile sensory feedback, body scheme, and ability to judge and move the body through space also affect overall coordination (Mathiowetz & Bass Haugen, 2002; Preston, 2001).

Incoordination is a broad term for extraneous, uneven, or inaccurate movements. Many types of lesions can produce disturbances of coordination. Cerebellar lesions, muscle or peripheral nerve disease or injury, lesions of the posterior column of the spinal cord, and lesions of the frontal or postcentral cortex can all cause incoordination.

The occupational therapist evaluates aspects of coordination that appear to interfere with function by using standardized tests and clinical observation. The neurologist or physiatrist usually performs the neurological examination. The physical therapist evaluates coordination as it relates to mobility. Occupational and physical therapy may compliment each other in so far as evaluating how gross coordination affects functional mobility, such as standing at the sink to perform oral–facial hygiene, gathering items and preparing a meal in the kitchen, bathing, and numerous other ADL (Mathiowetz & Bass Haugen, 2002; Preston, 2001). Several standardized tests for evaluating coordination are available (Table 25-19).

Cerebellar Dysfunction

Types of cerebellar dysfunction and methods of evaluating them are discussed in this subsection. *Intention tremor* occurs during voluntary movement, is less apparent or absent during rest, and intensifies at the termination of the movement. To test for this disorder, the therapist asks clients to touch alternately their own nose and then the therapist's finger, which is held in front of the client in various positions. Tremor can also be observed during performance of daily activities or during the finger-to-finger test. Similar to the finger-to-nose test, clients are asked to touch one of the examiner's fingers and then another held a distance away. Distance and target points are changed as the therapist notes tremor level, speed of response, and success rate.

TABLE 25–19. **STANDARDIZED TESTS OF GROSS MOTOR COORDINATION**[a]

Test	Age Level	Description
Bruininks-Oseretsky Test of Motor Proficiency	4.6–14.5 years	Assesses gross and fine coordination, dexterity, upper limb speed, visual motor control, muscle strength running, balance
Lincoln-Oseretsky Motor Development Scale	6–14 years	Assesses 36 motor tasks (e.g., one-foot standing, tapping rhythms, walking backward), speed of movement, and eye–hand coordination
Miller Assessment for Preschoolers	Preschool	Assesses 27 items (e.g., walking a line, stepping, hand-to-nose test) and gross motor assessment
Quick Neurological Screening Test	5 years–adult	Screens neurological integration (attention, balance, spatial organization, rate and rhythm of movement, motor planning, coordination)
Test of Motor Impairment	5–14 years	Assesses motor deficits (static and dynamic balance, manual dexterity, speed of movement, eye–hand coordination, problem-solving ability)

[a]Data from Farber (1991a).

Dysdiadochokinesia is a decreased ability to perform rapid alternating movements smoothly. Tests include having the client supinate and pronate the forearm, flex and extend the elbow, and grasp and release the hand. Other tests are alternate rotation of fully extended arms and tapping the table with extended fingers. These tests are performed bilaterally, and the therapist notes the number of alternations within a given time period and any differences between extremities.

Dysmetria is the inability to control muscle length, which results in overshooting or pointing past an object. The finger-to-nose and finger-to-finger tests are used to evaluate this. Functionally, clients may hit themselves in the face with a comb when attempting to comb their hair or overshoot and miss picking up the comb from the night stand.

Dyssynergia is a decomposition of movement. The lack of synergistic action between agonists and antagonists produces jerky movements. Dyssynergia can be observed in the alternating movement, finger-to-nose, and finger-to-finger tests.

Ataxic gait is often unsteady and wide based; clients with this disorder show a tendency to veer or fall toward the side of the lesion. The therapist can observe the client walking or ask the client to walk and turn quickly or walk heel to toe along a straight line.

Rebound phenomenon of Holmes is a lack of a check reflex to stop a motion to avoid striking something in the path of that motion. To test, the examiner resists the elbow flexion at the forearm and unexpectedly releases the resistance; the client's hand may hit his or her own chest, shoulder, or face if he or she is unable to check the motion.

Hypotonia is decreased muscle tone and decreased resistance to passive movement due to the loss of the cerebellum's facilitory influence on the stretch reflex. The therapist can observe hypotonia clinically and perform a quick stretch.

Posterior Column Dysfunction

The types of posterior column dysfunction and methods of evaluating them are discussed in this subsection. In this type of *ataxia* the wide-based gait results from loss of proprioception. Clients' ability to self-correct if they visually compensate as they watch the floor and the placement of their feet differentiates posterior column from cerebellar dysfunction. The *Romberg sign* is the inability to maintain standing balance with feet together and eyes closed. In posterior column deficit, dysmetria in the finger-to-nose test is exacerbated with the eyes closed.

Basal Ganglia Dysfunction

Types of basal ganglia dysfunction and methods of evaluating them are discussed next. *Athetosis* is a movement disorder characterized by slow, writhing, twisting, continuous, and involuntary movements, particularly of the neck, face, and extremities. These movements are not present during sleep. Muscles may have either increased or decreased tone. The therapist should note proximal or distal involvement, involved extremities, pattern of motions, and what stimuli increase or decrease the abnormal movements.

Dystonia is a form of athetosis that causes twisting movements of the trunk and proximal muscles of the extremities, distorted postures, and torsion spasms. *Choreiform movements* are irregular, purposeless, coarse, quick, jerky, and dysrhythmic. Muscles are hypotonic. Chorea may occur in sleep. *Hemiballism* is a rare, unilateral chorea that involves violent, forceful, sudden flinging movements of the extremities on one side of the body.

Resting tremors stop at the initiation of voluntary movement, but resume during the holding phase of a motor task, particularly when the client is tired or attention is diverted. An example is the pill-rolling tremor seen in Parkinsonism. *Bradykinesia* means poverty of movement.

Automatic movements, such as arm swinging during gait and facial expressions, are diminished (Copperman et al., 2002).

POSTURAL CONTROL

Before evaluation of postural control, the therapist needs to do an examination of posture. Posture is a composite of the positions of all the joints of the body at any given time. It is the static position assumed by any body part or by the body in general that requires muscular effort (Brooks, 1986; Farber, 1991a, 1991b; Kendall et al., 1993). In terms of kinesiology, the therapist must evaluate spinal alignment and curves, pelvis, trunk, head, neck, and upper extremity posture alone and in relation to each other in positions of standing, sitting, and lying down, if appropriate. Good body alignment occurs when the center of gravity of each body segment is located over the supporting base of the body. Structural problems and muscle strength deficits or imbalances can have a mechanical effect on postural control.

Postural adaptation refers to the ability of the body to maintain balance automatically and remain upright during alterations in position and challenges to stability (Woodson, 2002). There are several prerequisites for "normal" internal postural control. Clients need to be able to (Gilfoyle, Grady, & Moore, 1981):

- Produce movement through adequate ROM in the trunk and extremities.
- Differentiate body parts from one another (e.g., rotate the head independently of the shoulders).
- Stop and hold movement at the midrange of motion to stabilize against gravity, which is critical for transitional movement.
- Distribute normal postural tone in the body segments to support movement.
- Function symmetrically.

One difficulty in identifying the specific determinants of balance deficits is that balance behavior can be influenced by the somatosensory (proprioceptive, cutaneous, and joint), visual, and vestibular systems. Clients may show deficits in balance control during expected and unexpected perturbations, voluntary postural adjustments, or postural adjustments preceding voluntary limb movements. Valid conclusions about balance dysfunction require tests that differentiate among conditions that modify sensory inputs (DiFablo & Badke, 1990).

The therapist should note clinical observations of the client's ability to acquire and maintain the following developmental positions: prone, supine, sitting, crawling, standing, and walking, noting automatic responses in sagittal, frontal, and transverse body planes. Balance during various functional activities, such as reaching in the kitchen, tying shoes, and bathing, should be noted as well. There are several clinical assessment tools that evaluate postural control (Table 25-20).

TABLE 25–20. **POSTURAL CONTROL ASSESSMENTS**

Assessment	Description
Sensory Organization Test (SOT)	Defines six different sensory conditions or environments to measure postural sway; assesses influence of vision and somatic and vestibular sensory information.
Clinical Testing for Sensory Integration and Balance	A foam surface is used to disrupt somatic sensation; a visual conflict done with dots or lines is used to disrupt vision; measures client's ability to maintain balance under six conditions.
Functional Reach	Measures the distance between the anatomical reach and the maximal reach without slipping.
Tinetti's Balance and Gait Evaluation	Client is asked to do a variety of tasks (e.g., move from sitting to standing and ambulate); has high predictive validity for frail elderly at risk for falls.
Berg Balance Scale	Client is asked to complete 14 different tasks; each task is scored using a four-point scale.
Limits of Stability Test	Client stands and a computerized forceplated center of gravity is calculated; client volitionally shifts weight toward a series of targets; monitors movement for smoothness and accuracy of postural movements.
Fugl–Meyer Sensori-motor Assessment	Balance subtest measures the amount of assistance and time tolerated during static standing balance and tilting reactions.

See Appendix A for author, source, and description of assessments.

FINE COORDINATION AND DEXTERITY

Coordination can be defined as the smooth and harmonious action of groups of muscles working together to produce a desired motion. Dexterity is a type of fine coordination usually demonstrated in the upper extremity. There are several standardized tests that evaluate aspects of dexterity such as speed of object manipulation, accuracy of movement, grasp and release, prehension patterns, writing skills, and hand posture (Cooper, 2002; Preston, 2001). These tests are usually administered with the individual sitting with the arm supported. However, it is important to observe fine motor functioning in a variety of positions, with the arm supported and unsupported, as they occur in ADL. Functional tasks, such as buttoning, using scissors, handling coins, and writing, should be observed for the ease, accuracy, and timing of performance. The tests listed in Table 25-21 can be used to

TABLE 25-21. **FINE MOTOR COORDINATION TESTS**[a]

Dexterity Assessment	Description and Features
Crawford Small Parts Dexterity Test	• Measures eye–hand coordination and manipulation of small hand tools. • Designed for teenagers and adults. • Uses pins, collars, screws, tweezers, screwdriver. • Client is timed on tasks such as inserting pen in hole in metal plate with tweezers, covering with collar, threading screws.
Erhardt Developmental Prehension Assessment	• Measures components and skills of hand function development. • Designed for birth–6 years. • Uses variety of objects (e.g., small suitcase, plastic pail, toy hammer, key, beads, tin can, rubber ball, stacking rings) to measure grasp, reflex, and manipulation skills.
Fine Dexterity Test	• Assesses fine finger movements of adults.
Grooved Peg Board Test	• Measures eye–hand coordination and finger dexterity. • Client places grooved pegs in 25-hole peg board in various random positions.
Description and Test name	• Measures speed of eye–hand coordination and color matching for all age groups.
Purdue Peg Board Test	• Measures movements of arms, hands, fingers, and fingertip dexterity. • Normed for adults and children 5–15 years, 11 months. • Client places pins in peg board; assembles pins, washers, and collars.
Box and Block Test	• Tests manual dexterity. • Normed for children 7–9 years, adults, and adults with neuromuscular involvement. • Client picks up one block at a time and places it in attached compartment.
Nine Hole Peg Test of Fine Motor Coordination	• Measures fine dexterity. • Normed for adults >20 years. • Timed score to place nine 1¼-inch pegs in a 5 × 5-inch board and remove them.
Jebsen–Taylor Hand Function Test	• Evaluates functional capabilities. • Subtests include writing, card turning, picking up small objects, simulated feeding, stacking checkers, and picking up light and heavy objects.
Minnesota Rate of Manipulation Test	• Measures dexterity. • Assesses placing, turning, displacing, one-hand turning and placing, and two-hand turning and placing round blocks.

See appendix A for author, source, and descriptions of assessments.

identify specific dexterity difficulties as well as to monitor progress in a more standardized fashion.

Recording and Interpreting Results

Observation of functional abilities can be recorded directly on the initial evaluation. Results of standardized tests should be recorded according to the directions of each test.

Irregularity in rate of movement, excessive force, incorrect sequencing, and sudden corrective movements may indicate problems with coordination. Scores on standardized dexterity tests below norms also signal fine motor coordination problems. Determining the root(s) of the problem leads to an intervention plan. Several considerations should include sensory, specifically proprioceptive deficits, problems with body scheme, coordination of agonist and antagonist muscles, and ability to judge space accurately; cerebellar, spinal cord, posterior column, frontal, and postcentral cerebral cortex lesions also affect coordination. Again, the focus of intervention should be the functional implications of the performance deficit (Preston, 2001).

CONCLUSION

Evaluation is an ongoing process to gather data, formulate hypotheses, and guide clinical decisions. Although it is important to understand mechanics, such as administration protocols and diagnostic implications, evaluation is more than a compilation of technical information. Today's health-care environment necessitates that evaluation provide an overview and be prioritized based on how impairments affect occupational performance. The occupational therapist must integrate the information and focus on performance problems that are of most concern to the client and have the greatest bearing on desired occupations.

SECTION II

Perception and Cognition

KATHLEEN M. GOLISZ
JOAN PASCALE TOGLIA

WHY EVALUATE COGNITIVE–PERCEPTUAL FUNCTIONS?

"Thinking, remembering, reasoning, and making sense of the world around us are fundamental to carrying out everyday living activities" (Unsworth, 1999, p. 3). Cognition consists of interrelated processes, including the abilities to perceive, organize, assimilate, and manipulate information to enable the person to process information, learn, and generalize (Abreu & Toglia, 1987). Cognitive impairments may be seen as a result of developmental or learning problems, brain injury or disease, psychiatric dysfunction, or sociocultural conditions (American Occupational Therapy Association [AOTA], 1999). Cognitive impairments can result in significant activity limitations in all aspects of the client's life: ADL, instrumental activities of daily living (IADL), education, work, play and leisure, and social participation.

DEFINING THE EVALUATION OBJECTIVE

The evaluation process begins with an occupational profile that considers clients' typical routines and occupations (AOTA, in press). Clients are usually asked to identify everyday activities that they are most concerned about or would like to be able to do with greater ease. However, individuals with cognitive impairments often have limited awareness of their impairments and little understanding of the implications of these impairments. In some instances, cognitive impairments may not be readily apparent to significant others either.

Cognitive–perceptual symptoms can be easily misinterpreted and sometimes missed. This is particularly true when the client is in an inpatient setting and has not had the opportunity to experience or resume more complex activities. Observations of occupational performance within structured intervention environments may mask subtle cognitive deficits that are apparent only when the client has to plan and initiate complex activities in their natural contexts. For people with cognitive impairments, the occupational therapist needs to compare clients' perceptions of occupational performance to that of a significant other and to the practitioner's direct observations of performance. Discrepancies can reflect diminished self-awareness as well as decreased acceptance, defensive coping strategies, or lack of understanding of the nature of cognitive symptoms. Direct observation of occupational performance is guided by detailed information of clients' former occupations and expected roles and routines. If potential cognitive and perceptual symptoms are observed during performance, the therapist may need to administer specific cognitive–perceptual assessments to understand better the underlying nature of the impairment.

How does a therapist choose from the array of possible assessments and use the evaluation time most effectively? Occupational therapists must first decide what questions they have that need to be answered and then select an assessment that will address these questions. Based on the observation of the person engaged in an occupation, does the therapist need to clarify the presence of cognitive impairments? Does the therapist need to understand the effect of cognitive–perceptual impairments on occupational performance—for example, the activity limitation and participation restrictions from the International Classification of Functioning, Disability, and Health (ICF) (World Health Organization [WHO], 2001)? Does the therapist need information to guide treatment planning and intervention (e.g., conditions that increase or decrease cognitive symptoms)? Does the therapist need to establish a baseline as a measurement of change or outcome of intervention?

Determining the Presence of Impairments and Establishing Baselines for Change

Standardized assessments have specific administration guidelines and compare the client's performance to norms. They are static in nature, evaluating here-and-now performance. Standardized assessments can help the occupational therapist determine whether a cognitive impairment exists and quantify the severity of that impairment. These types of assessments are also useful as a baseline from which to measure changes over time. The occupational therapist should be wary in interpreting the functional implications of a particular standardized static assessment score.

Standardized cognitive and perceptual assessments typically have subtests that are divided into specific cognitive subskills, such as attention, visual processing, memory, and executive functions. Impaired performance on a specific task or subtest is typically assumed to define the impairment. For example, difficulty performing a figure-ground task (i.e., differentiating foreground objects or figures from background objects, such as picking up a white sock off a white sheet) would lead to the client being identified as having a figure-ground impairment (Zoltan, 1996). Examples of standardized assessments that can be used to identify impairments or measure change include mental status examinations and cognitive screenings.

The mental status examinations and screenings outlined in Table 25-22 focus primarily on the skills of **orientation, attention,** and **memory.** Cognitive-screening assessments are global and are designed to identify problems that need special or further attention. Many of the cognitive-screening assessments were designed for specific populations, such as clients with strokes (Hajek, Rutman, & Scher, 1989), multiple sclerosis (Rao, Leo, Bernardin, & Unverzagt, 1991), dementia (Mattis, Jurica & Leilten, 2001), or traumatic brain injury (Ansell & Keenan, 1989) or for elderly clients (Golding, 1989).

Occupational therapy practitioners should note that mental status examinations rely heavily on verbal skills, may not pick up subtle impairments, and have substantial false-negative rates. The deficits of clients with focal lesions, particularly right hemisphere lesions or mild diffuse cognitive disorders, are often missed (Nelson, Fogel, & Faust, 1986). Cognitive-screening assessments may also miss the deficits of clients with more subtle impairments displayed by clients with higher level cognitive skills as the breadth and depth of the item content are limited (Doninger, Bode, Heinemann, & Ambrose, 2000; Raskin & Mateer, 2000).

Occupational therapists also use cognitive–perceptual batteries like the Lowenstein Occupational Therapy Cognitive Assessment (LOTCA) to detect impairments (Katz, Itzkovich, Averbach, & Elazar, 1989). The LOTCA is a standardized, reliable, and valid battery that has a series of subtests for orientation, perception, visuomotor organization, and thinking skills. Attention and concentration are observed for all subtests. The LOTCA—G is a modification of the original assessment for use with geriatric clients with brain injury (Elazer, Itzkovich, & Katz, 1996). Performance on the LOTCA can predict ADL and IADL performance in clients who sustain right hemisphere strokes (Katz, Hartman-Maeir, Ring, & Soroker, 2000). The authors of the LOTCA are presently conducting research on a dynamic assessment

TABLE 25–22. **MENTAL STATUS EXAMINATIONS AND COGNITIVE-SCREENING ASSESSMENTS**[a]

Assessment	Subtest
Mental Status Examinations	
Mini Mental State Examination (Folstein, Folstein, & McHugh, 1975); Modified Mini-Mental Examination (Teng & Chui, 1987)	• Orientation (time and place), memory for three objects, attention, and calculation (serial 7s or spelling *world* backward), and language skills (naming objects, phrase repetition, following a three-step oral command and one-step written command, writing a sentence, and copying a design) • Has been used with a variety of populations • Modified examination includes an expanded number of items within each section and four new test items (semantic fluency, delayed memory, remote personal information, and abstraction)
Test of Orientation for Rehabilitation Patients (Deitz, et al, 1993)	• Questions are either open ended or recognition/multiple choice • Orientation to person and personal situation ("How old are you?"), place ("What is the name of the state we are in right now?"), time ("What year is it?"), schedule ("What is the first therapy you usually have in the morning?"), and temporal continuity ("What season comes after spring?") • Designed for adults and adolescents with brain injury in a rehabilitation setting
Galveston Orientation and Amnesia Test (Levin, et al, 1979)	• Orientation to person, place, time, and recall of events before (retrograde amnesia) and after (anterograde amnesia) injury ("What is the first event you can remember after the injury?") • Designed for use with patients after a coma
Cognitive-Screening Assessments	
Middlesex Elderly Assessment of Mental State (Golding, 1989)	• Consists of 12 subtests (orientation questions, recall of a name, recognition of pictures, comprehension, verbal fluency, arithmetic ability, spatial construction/line drawing, naming of objects, perception of fragmented letters and photos of objects from usual and unusual views, and motor perseveration) • Designed for ages 65+
Neurobehavioral Cognitive Status Screening Examination (Kiernan, Mueller, Longston, & VonDyke, 1987)	• Assesses intellectual functioning in the areas of: language (spontaneous speech, comprehension, repetition, and naming), constructions (concentration, visual memory, and constructional ability), memory, calculations, and reasoning (similarities and judgment) • Attention, level of consciousness, and orientation are independently scored • Norms available on ages 20–92
Cognitive Assessment of Minnesota (Rustad, DeGroot, Jungkunz, Freeberg, Borowick, & Wanttie, 1993)	• Consists of 17 subtests covering a wide range of skills (attention span, memory, orientation, mathematics, visual neglect, following directions, object identification, judgment, reasoning, and safety) • Tasks arranged to test the fund of knowledge, manipulation of knowledge, social awareness, judgment, and abstract thinking • Normed on ages 17–70.
Scales of Cognitive Ability for Traumatic Brain Injury (Adamovich & Henderson, 1992)	• Assesses the areas of perception and discrimination, orientation, organization, recall, and reasoning • Scores rate severity of impairments and can be charted to show progress during recovery • Progresses in difficulty to permit assessment of clients who functioned at very high levels before injury to be measured with the same instrument as they regain the use of higher-level abilities (e.g., complex organization and abstract reasoning)

[a]Adapted from Toglia (1996b).

version of the LOTCA for children (DOTCA-Ch) (Katz & Parush, 2001).

An alternative method used to identify cognitive–perceptual impairments is direct observation of function. A variety of standardized functional assessments, such as the Functional Independence Measure (FIM), rate performance, and the amount of physical assistance required on a numerical or descriptive scale (Granger, Cotter, Brown, & Fiedler, 1993). Other functional assessments, such as the Cognitive Performance Test (CPT; Allen, Earhart, & Blue, 1992), and the Rabideu Kitchen Evaluation (RKE-R; Neistadt, 1992), have been developed to identify cognitive–perceptual impairments that interfere with successful performance of tasks. Arnadottir's (1990) OT-ADL Neurobehavioral Evaluation (A-ONE) is an assessment that uses activity analysis to relate the results of an occupational therapy ADL evaluation to specific neurobehavioral impairments and to generate a hypothesis about the localization of cerebral dysfunction. For example, the activity of putting on a shirt is analyzed for the possible behavioral impairments of spatial-relation difficulties, unilateral spatial or body neglect, comprehension problems, ideational or ideomotor apraxia, tactile agnosia, organization and sequencing, attention impairments, and motivational impairments.

The Assessment of Motor and Process Skills (AMPS) is an attempt to analyze more systematically the process skills involved in the performance of functional activities (Fisher, 1993a, 1993b). Process skills—such as the client's ability to initiate, inquire, notice and respond, pace, sequence, organize, and terminate—are evaluated through the client's performance of functional activities.

Functional tasks require integration of a variety of performance skills, so it may be difficult to isolate specific problems interfering with function. These assessments tend to identify broad areas of cognitive and perceptual strengths and weaknesses by discovering the underlying processes that contribute to difficulty performing functional tasks. Subtle cognitive impairments may not be readily apparent in familiar activities. Functional assessments that simulate performance are structured by their very nature and may not predict performance in natural contexts, in which the person has to set goals, plan, initiate, perform, problem solve, and self-monitor performance. Novel and unpredictable situations that arise in real-world environments require higher-level cognitive–perceptual skills, which are difficult to capture in treatment environments. In hospital-based treatment settings the occupational therapist may not be able to create a close approximation of a real-world environment. Thus a bottom-up approach may identify potential cognitive–perceptual impairments that need to be further evaluated within real-world environments.

Evaluating to Guide Intervention

If cognition and perception are conceptualized in terms of hierarchically arranged distinct subskills, then the identification of specific deficits provides a foundation for intervention. Intervention addresses specific cognitive impairments and does not emphasize the quality of the client's performance or patterns of failure among several tests. For example, a client may perform poorly on assessments of both figure-ground and constructional skills because of a tendency to overattend to the details. In this evaluation approach, the client is classified as have impairments in both figure-ground and constructional praxis, although the cause of failure appears to be the same. In the clinical setting, practitioners rarely see isolated cognitive impairments. Cognitive problems overlap and are interrelated to one another, leading to questions of the benefit of applying a reductionistic approach to the evaluation process (Toglia & Golisz, 1990).

In functional approaches, information on the degree of assistance required to perform a task is sufficient. Most standardized functional assessments used in physical disabilities settings typically focus on the amount of physical assistance needed to perform the activity. Some functional assessments may contribute concrete information on potential safety problems and need for cues, assistance, or both.

Toglia (1998, 2001) offered a different perspective by describing cognitive dysfunction as inefficient use of processing strategies. Processing strategies are small units of behavior that enhance information processing and contribute to the effectiveness and efficiency of occupational performance (Toglia, 2001). This framework leads to cognition being conceptualized in terms of a dynamic interaction between the person, the activity and the context (Toglia, 1998, 2001). Figure 25-23 displays the components of Toglia's (1991b, 1998) Dynamic Interactional Model, which suggests that to understand cognitive function and dysfunction, the therapist must analyze the interaction among activity parameters, the context, and the person (i.e., internal processing strategies, self-awareness abilities, and personal characteristics). Self-awareness involves both knowledge of one's cognitive abilities and an ability to monitor performance of cognitive activities through recognizing and correcting errors and regulating activity performance.

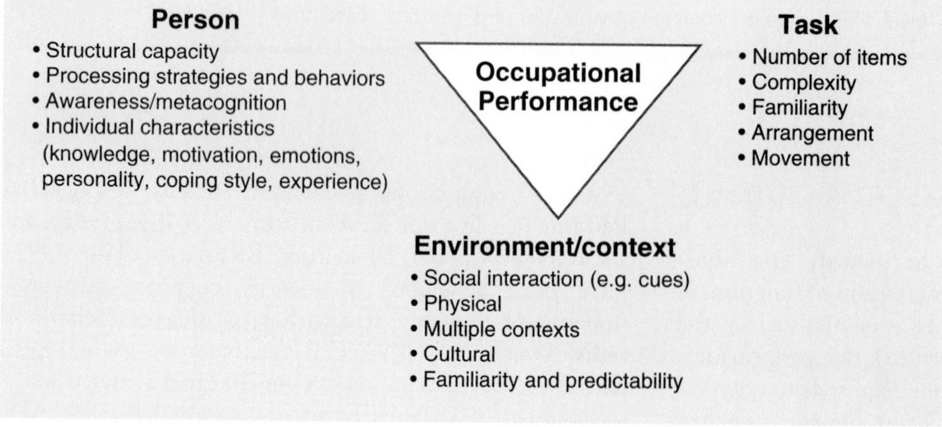

Person
- Structural capacity
- Processing strategies and behaviors
- Awareness/metacognition
- Individual characteristics (knowledge, motivation, emotions, personality, coping style, experience)

Occupational Performance

Task
- Number of items
- Complexity
- Familiarity
- Arrangement
- Movement

Environment/context
- Social interaction (e.g. cues)
- Physical
- Multiple contexts
- Cultural
- Familiarity and predictability

FIGURE 25–23. The Dynamic Interaction Model (From Toglia, J.P., 1998). A dynamic interactional approach to cognitive rehabilitation. In N. Katz (Ed.). Cognition and occupation in rehabilitation (pp. 5–50). Beshesda, MD: American Occupational Therapy Association. Reprinted with permission.

Cognition is not viewed as a static construct but as a dynamic interaction between the internal and external worlds. This conceptual framework leads occupational therapists to use a dynamic interactional evaluation approach and a dynamic intervention approach such as Toglia's (1998) Multicontext Approach (see Chapter 30, Section 5).

Dynamic evaluation includes an analysis of the strategies used in activity performance as well as the conditions that influence performance. Deficient cognitive functions represent areas of weakness and vulnerability. The extent to which symptoms are observed (and the cognitive strategies necessary to manage them) depend on the characteristics of the activity and the context in which they are performed.

Dynamic evaluation goes beyond observation of performance. It investigates a person's ability to learn certain tasks and identifies the conditions that facilitate such learning. During static standardized assessments, the client's response to test items are scored by the therapist without any attempt to intervene; however, during a dynamic evaluation, the therapist intervenes to change, guide, or improve the client's performance by providing graduated cues or modifications to the activity (Tzuriel, 2000). The aim is not normative comparison or diagnosis of dysfunction. The objective is to discover what the person is capable of doing with assistance or under favorable conditions. This may be useful in predicting a client's response to treatment and in discriminating differences in abilities not typically identified using conventional methods (Toglia, 1998).

The client's learning potential is evaluated through investigating the client's response to cues: Does the client detect errors? If errors are pointed out, does the client's performance improve? What happens if the therapist focuses the client's attention on a particular component of the assessment? If provided with a strategy to approach the activity, can the client improve performance? To use strategies effectively, the client must have an awareness of his or her current skills, be able to evaluate the level of activity difficulty, and recognize the need to use a strategy. The client must then choose the appropriate strategy and monitor its effectiveness.

Clients' use of strategies is investigated through clinical interview techniques that reflect or repeat clients' answers back to them for clarification or that present a hypothesis for verification. This type of interview reveals clients' cognitive style and strategies (Toglia, 1989a).

Toglia (1998) described a systematic cuing process used in a dynamic interactional assessment that moves from general to specific cuing. In this cuing sequence, clients may first be cued to check their answer. Next, the therapist might provide clients with more specific feedback that an error exists and follow-up with a cue that provides an approach to the activity. If cues appear to be ineffective at improving activity performance, the occupational therapist may investigate the impact of a modification of the activity (e.g., the number of items or the arrangement of the stimuli). Both qualitative and quantitative information gathered from clients' performance with the alteration of the activity can help the therapist gain insight into their impairments.

Toglia (1998) evaluates self-awareness by asking clients to predict performance before the initiation of the activity. Does clients' estimation match their performance on the activity? The occupational therapist is not aiming for clients to predict perfect performance but, rather, for them to have a clear understanding of their limitations and need to monitor strategy use and activity performance. After clients complete the activity, the therapist investigates self-awareness skills by asking them to rate their performance. Do the individuals have an accurate perception of how they did?

Dynamic assessments do not replace standardized tests. The information gathered and the questions answered are different. Dynamic assessments emphasize the processes involved in learning and change, whereas static assessments are product oriented (Grigorenko & Sternberg, 1998). Dynamic assessments have primarily been used with children. They are currently limited in number, and traditional psychometric-testing models do not easily accommodate dynamic testing procedures (e.g., cuing, greater client–practitioner interaction, or measurement of change within the testing session). Despite these limitations, dynamic assessment has "great potential for helping to understand people's potentials. . . . [Dynamic assessment's] potential has yet to be realized fully" (p. 75).

Measuring Change and Rehabilitation Outcomes

The increasing demands of third-party payers and a need to be accountable for the effectiveness of our services has encouraged occupational therapy practitioners to include measuring change and rehabilitation outcome as a goal of cognitive–perceptual evaluation. How a therapist defines *success* determines the outcomes he or she chooses to measure. Outcome is multidimensional and needs to include quantitative and qualitative measures of all three levels of the (ICF). Any single measure of outcome may show little change, but the combination of several outcome measures may hold key information on the effectiveness of treatment. Goal-attainment scales offer a concrete, individualized method of comparing changes in clients' goals related to performance of activities that require cognitive–perceptual skills (Malec, Smigielski, DePompoplo, 1991; Rockwood, Joyce, & Stolee, 1997).

The Community Integration Questionnaire (CIQ) quantifies social role limitations and community interactions of people with acquired brain injury (Willer, Rosenthal, Kreutzer, Gordon, & Rempel, 1993). The 30-item Mayo-Portland Adaptability Inventory (MPAI-3) was developed to measure long-term (postacute) outcome of acquired brain injury at both the impairment and societal participation levels of the ICF (Malec, Moessner, Kragness, & Lezak, 2000). Additional scales focusing on the activity limitation and participation restriction dimensions of the ICF can be located on the scales page of the Center for Outcome Measurement in Brain Injury's Web site (2002).

Considering Performance Contexts

It is important to remember the client's personal history and his or her natural social context and physical environment when performing a cognitive–perceptual evaluation (Diller, 1993). Cognitive–perceptual process skills cannot be evaluated or interpreted in isolation from the temporal, cultural, and environmental performance contexts. The client's age, developmental stage, and employment and educational history may influence his or her response to the evaluation process and performance on certain assessments. Practitioners should ensure that the assessments being administered are appropriate for each client's age and educational level; otherwise the results may be invalid. The acuteness or chronicity of the client's cognitive impairments should also be considered during the evaluation process. Will there be a need to frequently monitor the client for recovery of cognitive–perceptual functions (during the acute phase of recovery) or are the activity limitations considered stable?

Environmental contexts may also influence the client's performance on cognitive–perceptual assessments. Physical aspects of the environment, such as the room selected for testing (lighting, noise level, and such), may have an influence, but the social expectations and the cultural background of the client also need to be considered during interpretation of the assessment results. What was the client's previous quality or standard of work? Is the client from a different culture than the normative group of the assessment? Is the client of a different cultural background than the occupational therapy practitioner and thus is there is a potential for misinterpretation of responses and performance? What is normal within this client's culture?

OCCUPATIONAL THERAPY ROLE WITHIN A MULTIDISCIPLINARY TEAM

Currently, there is no single discipline responsible for the evaluation and treatment of cognitive–perceptual impairments. Neurologists, neuropsychologists, speech and language pathologists, occupational therapy practitioners, special educators, and cognitive therapists (specialists with 2- to 4-year degrees) all have the potential to make valuable contributions to understanding clients with a cognitive– perceptual impairment. Because of this overlapping responsibility for the cognitive–perceptual process skills there can be confusion and duplication of evaluation and intervention procedures. Intervention team members should discuss the philosophy of their respective disciplines and how their individual approaches to cognition and perception might complement each other. Although some cognitive assessments, like mental status examinations, can be administered by a variety of rehabilitation team members, other tests require specialized training or advanced degrees (typically relegated to team members with doctorates). Formal training in the test administration, advanced or continuing education, and supervision are necessities to provide quality cognitive–perceptual evaluation and intervention. Administration of cognitive assessments or any assessment by an untrained health professional is unethical and can invalidate the results (Stringer, 1996).

Occupational therapy practitioners provide a unique contribution to the evaluation and rehabilitation of cognitive perceptual process skills owing to their educational background, training in activity analysis, and ability to analyze how cognitive–perceptual symptoms change with different activity conditions. The role of the occupational therapist in evaluating cognition and perception is to provide clear, comprehensive information on the effect of cognitive–perceptual impairments on ADL, IADL, education, work, play and leisure, and social participation.

The work environment in which each practitioner practices may determine the depth of his or her involvement, depending on the nature of the practice setting and the client's length of stay. In acute care settings, the occupational therapist may focus on screening for potential impairments that should be followed up in rehabilitation settings or outpatient treatment. In rehabilitation settings, the occupational therapist may perform in-depth assessments and treatment. An occupational therapy assistant can contribute to the evaluation process by administering selected portions of cognitive assessments as directed by the occupational therapist, providing clinical observations, and completing behavioral checklists. These tasks are carried out under the supervision of the occupational therapist once the occupational therapy assistant has demonstrated service competency (AOTA, 1999).

EVALUATION OF SPECIFIC COGNITIVE AND PERCEPTUAL PROCESS SKILLS

Orientation

Orientation is the ability to understand the self and the relationship between the self and the past and present environment. Orientation depends on the integration of several mental activities, which are represented in different areas of the brain. Disorientation indicates that there are significant impairments in attention and memory (Lezak, 1995). Disoriented clients may think they are home in their own house rather than in a hospital. They may confuse the hospital staff with relatives, and they may believe each time they wake up from a short nap that it is a new day.

Evaluation of orientation traditionally includes the client's orientation to person, place, and time. Orientation to person involves both the self and others. Is the client able to report personal facts and events and describe his or her previous lifestyle? Does the client recognize people and associate them with their role and name? Orientation to place is demonstrated by the client's ability to understand the type of place he or she is in (e.g., a hospital), to report the name and location of the place, and to appreciate distance and direction. Orientation to time requires an ability to report the current point in time (month, year, date, day), to understand the continuity and sequence of time (estimation), and to associate events with time.

Topographical orientation is often considered a component of orientation to place. It is the ability to follow a familiar route or a new route once given an opportunity to become familiar with it. This skill involves the ability to describe the relationship of one place to another, as well as visuospatial skills (Benton, 1985). Topographical orientation also incorporates components of memory. Difficulties with the visual spatial and memory aspects of topographical orientation need to be distinguished during evaluation (Okkema, 1993). Can the client provide a verbal description of the location of the target site, but become confused and lost when attempting to follow a route to the site?

Orientation assessments are traditionally covered in mental status examinations. The Galveston Orientation Amnesia Test (GOAT; Levin, O'Donnell, & Grossman, 1979) and the Test of Orientation for Rehabilitation Clients (TORP; Deitz, Beeman, & Thorn, 1993) are two standardized screening tools for orientation. Both of these assessments are described in Table 25-22.

Occupational therapists frequently use nonstandardized measures of orientation, such as interviews with open-ended questions asked in a conversational or informal manner. Most practitioners use cues to determine the severity of the disorientation. If the client is unable to answer the questions independently, the practitioner may offer the client a multiple-choice array or offer verbal cues. Cues usually move from general or abstract cues initially to more concrete cues such as the severity of disorientation requires (e.g., "Today is the beginning of the work week" versus "Today is the day after Sunday"). The number and type of cues offer a method of scoring and monitoring progress. Fluctuations in orientation during the day should be noted, as clients may experience **sundowning** during which they become confused in the evening as a result of fatigue.

Insight and Awareness

Insight refers to the degree of awareness one has regarding his or her own physical or cognitive–perceptual impairments. Impaired awareness can significantly influence the outcome of rehabilitation (Katz & Hartman-Maeir, 1998; LaBuda & Lichtenberg, 1999). Clients with a decreased ability to recognize their strengths and weaknesses may develop a lack of motivation to adopt compensatory strategies during rehabilitation and may engage in poor judgment or have a tendency to attempt activities that are beyond their capabilities. For example, clients with poor awareness may attempt to transfer themselves independently to the toilet, despite dense hemiplegia and the need for physical assistance from a health-care worker. Lack of awareness differs from denial, which is a psychological defense mechanism characterized by overrationalization. Clients who are in denial are aware of but are unwilling to confront problems. They may become increasingly agitated when confronted with denied reality.

Crosson et al. (1989) described a hierarchical pyramid model of awareness, including intellectual, emergent, and anticipatory awareness. In the neurological literature, implicit knowledge of impairments has also been identified as a type of awareness. Clients' awareness of their impairments has implications for rehabilitation and their ability to function independently.

Intellectual awareness, according to Crosson et al. (1989), is present when the client has knowledge that a particular function is impaired but does not use this knowledge to monitor performance. The client may report he or she has difficulty remembering things, but when asked to bring certain items to the next treatment session does not attempt to initiate any strategy that could assist recall (e.g., writing the items down in a notebook or pocket calendar). Clients with only intellectual awareness of their impairments show significant safety risks, as they do not perform within their limitations.

Implicit knowledge of impairments is observed when clients deny the existence of an impairment but behave as though they have some knowledge of it. A client may deny memory problems but consistently write notes in a notebook. When questioned about the behavior, the client may report, "I just need to do this." Safety issues can arise for clients with this type of awareness, because they may be inconsistent in initiating compensatory strategies that demonstrate awareness. Clients may not admit to memory problems but be fairly consistent in checking that they turned off the stove. However, one slip in this behavior can threaten life and property.

A client who has the ability to recognize a problem only when it is actually happening has emergent awareness. For example, a client may estimate that an activity requiring significant organizational and problem-solving skills (both observed areas of difficulty for this person) will be easy. When faced with difficulty during the performance of the activity, the client with emergent awareness might state, "Everything is all messed up. I guess this is harder than I thought. Maybe I do have problems." For clients to be able to initiate the use of a strategy, they must have a minimum level of emergent awareness to be able to recognize problems and the need for compensatory strategies (Bruce, 1993). Clients with emergent awareness may not demonstrate a significant safety risk if they work within their limitations and recognize and correct errors. However, if they attempt tasks significantly outside their limits, they may end up in a situation where they are incapable of recognizing errors and making necessary corrections to ensure safety.

Anticipatory awareness is the ability to anticipate that a problem will likely occur as the result of an impairment, before performing the activity (Crosson et al., 1989). Clients with this type of awareness are excellent candidates for rehabilitation, for they comprehend the extent and implications of their impairments. Safety is typically not a major concern for these clients, because they have the ability to determine which tasks may be risky and to self-monitor their performance during the activity.

Toglia and Kirk (2000) proposed a dynamic model of awareness that includes self-knowledge and beliefs of one's abilities and limitations as well as self-monitoring and self-evaluation skills. This multidimensional view of awareness proposes that levels of awareness (intellectual, anticipatory, emergent, anticipatory) vary across different tasks and contexts within the same domain. A recent study by Abreu, Seale, Scheibel, Huddleston, Zhang, and Ottenbacher (2001) supported this nonhierarchical view of awareness. This dynamic model of awareness also distinguishes between awareness outside the context of an activity and that which is activated within the context of the activity (Toglia & Kirk, 2000).

Interview and rating scales for insight and awareness, such as the Self-Awareness of Deficits Interview (SADI; Fleming, Strong & Ashton, 1996), generally evaluate clients':

- Awareness of their limitations and strengths.
- Ability to generalize the impact of those limitations on functional tasks.
- Concern regarding their disability.
- Judgment skills.

A nonstandardized awareness interview typically asks clients questions about reason for hospitalization, physical and cognitive difficulties, and functional implications in a conversational or informal manner. Because awareness is not an all-or-nothing phenomenon, occupational therapists offer cues if a client is unable to answer independently. The questions should move from awareness of the limitations that impairments impose on general abilities (anticipatory awareness) to more specific questioning if the client does not appear to understand the functional implications of his or her impairments (e.g., "Why are you in the hospital?" to "Do you have difficulty writing?"). Generally worded or open-ended questions are less useful than specifically worded items for clients with cognitive impairments (Toglia & Kirk, 2000). Reality testing, by which clients are asked to perform the activity, is used to evaluate whether awareness emerges when clients experience difficulty with a particular activity that requires performance skills for which they are deficient.

The occupational therapist may use a formal rating scale that examines that discrepancy between client self-ratings and that of a clinician or significant other. For example, Prigatano's (1986) Competency Rating Scale requires the client and caregiver to independently rate (on a five-point scale) how easy or difficult it is to carry out each of 30 specific activities. The Contextual Memory Test (Toglia, 1993b) and the Toglia Category Assessment (Toglia, 1994) are two dynamic tests that evaluate the cognitive skills of memory and organization, respectively, but also include a format of test prediction within the context of an activity to evaluate clients' awareness. Clients are asked general and specific questions that require them to estimate performance before and after performing specific tasks. Differences between estimated performance before and after the task are compared with actual performance

Attention

Attention incorporates far more than the quantitative measure of the length of time a client can concentrate. It is a multidimensional capacity that involves several components: alertness (detection and reaction), selective attention, sustained attention, shifting of attention, and mental tracking. A client may be able to perform the lower-level tasks within each component of attention. However, this same client may have difficulty if requested to perform an activity that incorporates several different attentional components. Table 25-23 provides examples of basic and complex tasks for each component of attention.

Standardized tests such as the Digit Span (Lezak, 1995) and the Knox Cube Test (Stone & Wright, 1980) evaluate attention span and immediate recall of auditory and visual information, respectively. The Paced Auditory Serial Addition Test (PASAT; Gronwall, 1977) for adults and the children's version (CHIPASAT; Dyche & Johnson, 1991) detect subtle impairments in attention and speed of processing. Scores on the PASAT predict outcome after a traumatic brain injury (Gronwall, 1977). Functional observation of everyday activities, such as a multiple-component cooking activity or completion of a work task while carrying on a conversation, can be used to evaluate mental tracking abilities.

The Test of Everyday Attention (TEA) was designed to tap the different aspects of attention in higher-level clients (Robertson, Ward, Ridgeway, & Nimmo-Smith, 1994). It consists of eight subtests that use familiar, everyday materials, such as map and telephone book searching (i.e., selective visual attention and divided attention), counting elevator beeps on a tape (i.e., sustained attention and auditory selective attention), visual elevator floor counting (i.e., flexibility/switching attention), and lottery ticket reviews (i.e., sustained attention). There are three parallel versions of the TEA for test–retest that allows for easy retesting for change and norms for ages 18–80. A children's version of the TEA, the Test of Everyday Attention for Children (TEA–Ch) is normed for ages 6–16 (Manly, Robertson, Anderson, & Nimmo-Smith, 1999). The TEA is a valid and reliable assessment for use with people with more subtle attentional impairments (Chan, 2000; Crawford, Sommerville, & Robertson, 1997).

TABLE 25-23. **ASSESSMENT OF THE COMPONENTS OF ATTENTION**

Component	Basic Tasks	Complex Tasks
Detect/react	Detect and react to a gross change in the environment (e.g., telephone ringing or name being called)	Detect with increasing amounts of stimuli and with emphasis on speed (e.g., find the spelling errors on a page as quickly as possible)
Selection	Maintain visual fixation on a brightly colored pencil eraser while ignoring another pencil moved in visual field	Attend to target and inhibit competing distraction (e.g., attending to work activity and ignoring music playing, or people talking)
Sustain	Persist with a repetitive activity, such as bouncing a ball, over time	Persist and keep track of information (e.g., empty dishwasher top and bottom shelves, stuff envelopes, and keep track of the number completed)
Shifting attention	Follow one change in an activity (e.g., add numbers and then subtract numbers)	Shift back and forth between two task sequences (e.g., stop to answer telephone while filing and typing)
Mental tracking	Immediate recall (e.g., remembering a phone number just given on the telephone)	Keep track of two or more stimuli simultaneously (e.g., cooking while listening to the radio)

[a]Adapted from Toglia (1996b).

Visual Processing

Visual Discrimination

Clinical vision evaluation for oculomotor dysfunction should be performed before a visual-processing evaluation to screen out visual problems that will interfere with the accuracy of perceptual testing. Several clinical observations during functional tasks can alert occupational therapists to the need for a formal visual assessment: compensatory head movements and tilting, squinting, shutting of one eye, or a tendency to lose one's place while reading.

Whenever possible, the input of a neuro-ophthalmologist should be sought in the clinical evaluation of vision; however, a basic screening can be performed by the occupational therapist. Visual acuity should be measured for both near and distant vision with any corrective lens the client uses. Pupillary functions of size at rest, response to light, and visual accommodation need to be evaluated. The occupational therapist should assess the ROM of the eyes and ocular alignment. Visual field impairments are common after brain injuries or strokes and are best evaluated by an ophthalmologist or optometrist through perimeter testing. When this test is not available, the visual fields can be grossly evaluated using a confrontation method (described later). Last, visual pursuits (e.g., smooth tracking of moving objects), saccades (e.g., quick eye movements to place an object of interest in view), and visual-scanning functions should be evaluated. Any disruptions of these foundational performance skills, which are vulnerable to a wide range of neural injuries, affect all interpretations of higher-level visual-processing assessments (Warren, 1993).

The deficit-specific approach to visual processing categorizes visual perception into specific areas, such as figure-ground, position in space, form constancy, spatial relations, and visual recognition. An information-processing perspective conceptualizes visual perception as a process involving the reception, organization, and assimilation of visual information. Visual perception in the information-processing model is viewed on a continuum from simple to complex processing in each specific area.

When individuals process a simplistic visual scene (such as a familiar object or shape), they process the information globally at a fast speed with minimal effort. However, when processing a more complex visual array, with unfamiliar stimuli or the need for more subtle discriminations, their processing is slower and requires maximal effort. In this conceptualization, a visual-processing dysfunction is defined as a decrease in the amount that the visual system is able to assimilate at any one time (Toglia, 1989b). To understand the client's **visual perceptual** skills and the effects of impairments on functioning, the therapist must look at the activity conditions (complexity, amount, familiarity, and predictability) rather than the type of activity (visual spatial, visual discrimination, visual motor, or visual Gestalt). Simple visual-processing dysfunction may include the following:

- Difficulty in visual discrimination between objects, pictures of objects, colors, and basic shapes.
- Difficulty in detecting gross differences in size, position, direction, angles, and rotations.
- Decreased ability to locate visually single visual targets in space or to judge gross distances between two objects.
- Decreased ability to detect simple part–whole relationships in objects or basic shapes.
- Decreased ability to draw simple shapes or objects (e.g., geometric shapes or flowers).

An example of a therapist assessing client Mr. J's ability to recognize objects is given in What's a Practitioner to Do? 25-1.

Prerequisites to visual object assessment should include a visual screening, a discussion with the speech and language

WHAT'S A PRACTITIONER TO DO? 25-1
Identifying Objects

Mr. J is having difficulties locating objects in his bathroom closet and his bedside stand drawer. He will name what he wants to pick up but then reach for a different object.

Mr. J's ability to recognize objects was tested in the treatment room while he sat at a table covered with a white cloth. He was initially presented with single objects that were self-related and placed in a vertical arrangement. Mr. J. demonstrated no difficulty when asked, "Tell me what this object is." His ability remained constant, regardless of the number of objects (up to eight) presented in a horizontal line. When objects were presented in a scattered overlapping format, Mr. J. had a tendency to miss objects and misperceive components of objects as separate items. This tendency was even stronger when he was given unconventional objects and in increasing amounts. For example, he thought the handle of a small magnifying glass was an Allen wrench. He identified it as a magnifying glass only when the overlapping object was removed.

With all object identification tasks, Mr. J. demonstrated slow visual-processing time. Upon further testing, Mr. J's ability to imagine what an object looked like was deemed intact. He was able verbally to describe the critical features that could help him identify various objects.

The occupational therapist forms the hypothesis that Mr. J overfixates on individual features or parts of objects and misidentifies objects based on salient characteristics without integrating the elements (e.g., Mr. J's focus on the handle of the magnifying glass and subsequent misidentification of the object). The therapist initiates the cuing process by providing a prompt of repetition ("Look again, Mr. J."), which provides Mr. J. with the general feedback that his response was incorrect. Because this cue did not appear to assist Mr. J. in identifying previous misperceived objects, the occupational therapist decides to try another type of cue. The therapist believes cuing Mr. J. to perform a deeper analysis of the object, by focusing and describing properties of the object (weight, size, material, and such), will not improve his performance because he already overfocuses on features of the objects.

The occupational therapist next provides Mr. J. with specific perceptual cues to focus his attention on a critical detail of the object that should aid in identification, such as pointing to the lens of the magnifying glass and saying to Mr. J, "Look here." Additional items that overlap the target item may be removed to enable Mr. J. to see the target item as a continuous whole. Specific semantic cues that provide a multiple-choice array of possible categories that the object may belong to (e.g., "Mr. J, does this item belong to the category of tool, jewelry, or grooming item?") narrow the range of possible objects and, when combined with visual cues, aid in identification.

pathologist to rule out language impairments, and visual imagery questioning. A deficit-specific approach to object identification presents clients with actual objects or pictures of objects and asks them to identify each object. People who are unable to identify accurately the objects presented demonstrate visual agnosia.

The dynamic interactional approach to assessing visual object perception conceptualizes object recognition on a continuum and evaluates both conventional and unconventional objects under a variety of different activity conditions. Table 25-24 illustrates how an occupational therapist using this approach would analyze and systematically manipulate activity parameters and cue responses to investigate the use of strategies and to analyze fully why a client is having difficulty recognizing objects. Cues are used to facilitate object recognition when the client encounters difficulty. The Modified Dynamic Visual Processing Assessment (MDVPA) is an assessment that uses the dynamic interactional approach to evaluate visual processing (Toglia & Finkelstein, 1991).

Complex visual perceptual skills require a high degree of integration and analysis and typically involve visually confusing environments; abstract, unfamiliar, or detailed visual information; or conditions under which the distinctive visual features are partially obscured (e.g., constructing a three-dimensional object that cannot be rotated). Dysfunction of complex visual perceptual skills may include decreased ability to detect subtle differences in abstract shapes and objects or angles, size, distance, and position. A client may have difficulty making sense out of ambiguous, incomplete, fragmented, or distorted visual stimuli. As with Mr. J, the complexity of object recognition increases when distinctive features of objects are partially obscured (e.g., unconventional views, figures concealed in a complex pattern). One might expect Mr. J also to have difficulty performing functional tasks such as finding items on a crowded refrigerator shelf, closet, or supermarket shelf or locating key information on a bill or map. Safety risks may be present if Mr. J misperceives items in the kitchen or bathroom.

Visual Motor

Visual motor skills may include drawing tasks (e.g., drawing a map to a specific location) or construction of three-dimensional figures (e.g., assembling a coffee pot).

TABLE 25–24. **DYNAMIC ASSESSMENT OF OBJECT IDENTIFICATION**[a]

	Task Parameters					
Task Grading	**Environment**	**Familiarity of Objects**	**Directions**	**Number of Objects Present**	**Spatial Arrangement**	**Response Rate per Object (sec)**
Least difficult	Normal context	Self-related (e.g., toothbrush)	"What is this?"	1–5	Linear, nonrotated	< 0.8
Moderately difficult	Associated context	Non-self-related (e.g., pen)	"Find the [object]"	10	Scattered, rotated	1.1
Most difficult	Out of context	Unconventional (e.g., pen shaped like a candy cane)	"Tell me what you see."	20	Scattered, rotated, overlapping	1.3

[a]Reprinted with permission from Toglia (1989b).

These skills involve visual discrimination, motor-planning abilities, and other cognitive–perceptual skills. Clients may demonstrate difficulty on these types of tasks for many reasons. For example, a client may have difficulty constructing a block design because of:

- Poor scanning of the complete design.
- Decreased planning and organization.
- Unilateral neglect.
- Impaired discrimination of size, angles, and rotations.
- Constructional apraxia.

Clients are labeled as having constructional apraxia when they have difficulty performing drawing tasks or activities in which parts are put together to form a single entity or object and when this difficulty cannot be attributed to perceptual impairments, ideomotor apraxia, organizational impairments, or primary motor or sensory impairments (Benton, 1985). Constructional impairments may be seen in clients after damage to either parietal lobe, but the clinical presentation differs in spatial aspects, based on the hemisphere involved (Kramer, Kaplan, & Blusewicz, 1991; Robertson & Lamb, 1991). Several authors have found a close correlation between constructional abilities and ADL performance (Neistadt, 1992; Warren, 1981).

Both two-dimensional graphomotor tasks and three-dimensional object assembly have been used to evaluate visual motor skills. The sample activity may or may not be presented as a model, and the tasks themselves may vary in complexity. Two-dimensional free-drawing and copying tasks (e.g., draw a person or house) are frequently used. There is little standardization of scoring in these drawing tasks. The Benton Constructional Praxis Test is a classic standardized assessment of three-dimensional visual motor and constructional skills (Benton, Hamsher, Varney, & Spreen, 1983). This test correlated with performance in self-care activities in clients who sustained strokes (Titus, Gall, Yerxa, Roberson, & Mack, 1991). Nonstandardized construction tasks are also frequently used by occupational therapists, for example reproducing matchstick or toothpick designs, block designs, puzzles, and parquetry blocks. (Neistadt, 1989).

Unilateral Neglect

Unilateral neglect is a failure to orient to, respond to, or report stimuli presented on the side contralateral to the cerebral lesion in clients who do not have primary sensory or motor impairments (Heilman, Watson, & Valenstein, 1985). What's a Practitioner to Do? 25-2 describes Mr. Y, who shows many of the common problems associated with this condition.

The term *neglect* connotes a volitional component to the disorder, but this is a misnomer. Clients with unilateral neglect are unaware of the incompleteness of their perception and responses to the environment. Unilateral neglect can be a major disability in the acute phases of recovery from stroke and can impede later attempts to rehabilitate clients, and it has been identified as a major factor impeding functional recovery in clients who have sustained strokes (Chen Sea, Henderson, & Cermack, 1993; Cherney, Halper, Kwasnica, Harvey, & Zhang, 2001).

Occupational therapists evaluating clients with unilateral neglect must first distinguish between hemianopsia and unilateral neglect. Visual field cuts (hemianopsia) are hemiretinal, while neglect is hemispatial. Clients with visual field cuts typically have awareness of their visual field loss and make compensatory head movements and turns. Unilateral neglect may exist with or without hemianopsia, and one syndrome does not cause the other.

Unilateral neglect has been found to vary with stimulus characteristics. Clients may display asymmetry in functional activities, drawing tasks, reading, and writing, depending on the activity characteristics (Rizzolatti & Berti, 1993). Many clients with unilateral neglect exhibit anxiety or flattened affect and appear to deny the presence of their impairments. This lack of awareness can result in a display of anger when challenged about the presence of difficulties.

WHAT'S A PRACTITIONER TO DO? 25-2
Unilateral Neglect

Mr. Y recently sustained a right hemisphere stroke and presents with many of the typical clinical symptoms of unilateral neglect. He requires cues in the dining room to locate items on the left side of his food tray. If not cued, Mr. Y eats the food from only the right side of his plate. During morning self-care, Mr. Y shaves only the right side of his face and combs only the right side of his hair. He gropes for his left arm when dressing and needs cues to straighten his shirt on his left shoulder. When pushing his wheelchair he constantly veers toward the left and bumps into walls.

In the acute phase, unilateral neglect is often characterized by a marked deviation of the head, eyes, and trunk away from the left hemispace. Mr. Y appears to be magnetically drawn toward stimuli and activities located on his right side. It is not uncommon to see Mr. Y looking under his wheelchair on the right for a voice that is coming from the person sitting on his left. Mr. Y, unlike some clients with severe cases of unilateral neglect, does recognize his left-sided extremities as his own and has not attempted to fling the "unknown person" out of his bed.

Traditional evaluation of unilateral neglect has involved tasks of extinction and confrontation, line bisection, cancellation, and drawing tests. Tests of extinction and confrontation evaluate the sensory component of unilateral neglect (e.g., when two things are presented at the same time, the client attends only to the right-sided stimuli). For example, the occupational therapist may evaluate visual extinction by holding both arms at shoulder height in the client's intact visual fields and move a finger on one or both hands. Clients with visual extinction will report the single stimulus in each visual field, but only the right-sided stimulus when simultaneous stimuli occur. Before beginning tests for extinction the examiner must ensure that basic sensation for each modality is intact bilaterally.

Line bisection tasks require the client to estimate and mark the midpoint of lines. A deviation toward the ipsilesional side is considered a demonstration of unilateral neglect. Testing should be done with lines in horizontal and vertical orientations, as differences can be seen. There are numerous variations of line bisection tasks that manipulate the activity demands or stimulus parameters: length of the line (usually the longer the line, the greater the inattention), anchors at the end of the line (e.g., a red line drawn down the left-side margin), direction of visual scanning, different orientations of the lines, and different positions in space.

Researchers have also explored the performance of clients with unilateral neglect on line extension and line erasure tasks (Ishiai, 1994). In line extension tasks, the client is asked to extend a horizontal line leftward to double its original length. This activity directs attention toward the left not the right, and thus clients display less neglect than on traditional line bisection tasks. Line erasure tasks require the client to erase the line to midpoint. The gradual decrease in the amount of right stimuli leads to less demonstration of unilateral neglect.

Cancellation tests have been traditionally used to detect the presence of neglect. These tasks require the ability to locate and cancel, or mark, target stimuli from among a series of stimuli. The stimuli may be arranged in random or structured, linear formation, such as the Verbal and Nonverbal Cancellation Tasks (Mesulam, 1985), and include lines, letters, numbers, stars or other shapes such as bells (Gauthier, Dehaut, & Joanette, 1989). Cancellation tasks may vary in how easily the targets can be discriminated from the background stimuli. For example, it is simpler for a client to select red socks from a table scattered with white socks than to select dinner forks of a particular silverware pattern from a tabletop scattered with forks of four or more patterns. The second activity requires focal attention and subtle discriminations. Search time would be expected to increase with increases in amount or display size, owing to the slow, analytical search that must be conducted.

Drawing tests have been traditionally used to assess unilateral neglect. Clients with unilateral neglect typically have difficulty producing symmetrical drawings of objects such as daisies or clocks. The type and distribution of errors have been scored and analyzed, but there is no reported normative data, reliability, or validity. The Parietal Lobe Test of the Boston Diagnostic Aphasia Examination is an example of a standardized assessment with specific criteria for scoring drawings (Goodglass, & Kaplan, 1972). Copying asymmetric nonsense figures may be more sensitive than copying well-known symmetric objects.

Functional performance measures have also been used to evaluate unilateral neglect. Reading tests such as the Caplan (1987) Indented Paragraph Test, checklists, and semistructured ADL scales have been used to examine the relationship between scores on traditional tests of neglect and ADL performance. Reliability and validity of these nonstandardized ADL measures have not been examined.

The Behavioral Inattention Test (BIT) was designed to include both conventional tests of neglect and tests of everyday performance skills to provide more comprehensive information for developing rehabilitation programs (Wilson, Cockburn, & Halligan, 1987). It includes the conventional subtests of line crossing, letter cancellation, star cancellation, figure and shape copying, line bisection, and representational drawing. Behavioral subtests include picture scanning, telephone dialing, menu reading, telling and setting time, coin sorting, address copying, and map following. The BIT has two parallel versions that allows for retesting for improvements in the neglect symptoms.

A study by Hartman-Maeir and Katz (1995) explored the validity of the behavioral subtests of the BIT. Seven of the nine behavioral subtests differentiated significantly between subjects with visual neglect and those without neglect. The article reading and time-telling subtests appear to lack sufficient sensitivity to detect neglect, and educational background influenced performance on the article reading. Six of the nine behavioral subtests correlated significantly with parallel functional tasks or ADL checklist items, supporting the predictive validity of the BIT behavioral subtests as functional measures of neglect. Picture scanning and map navigation did not correlate significantly with parallel functional measures, suggesting that they are not valid measures of eating and mobility. The authors provided a framework for analyzing qualitative aspects of performance and suggested that the client's response to cuing has potential implications for treatment planning. Further studies are needed on the cuing aspect of this version of the BIT; however, Hartman-Maeir and Katz's study supports Toglia's (1991b) argument that it is not enough to know that unilateral neglect is present or absent on different tasks; we need to understand which activity characteristics change the magnitude of neglect.

During a dynamic assessment of neglect, cues are used to explore and facilitate performance after a baseline performance is established. Cues question clients' awareness or detection of errors by providing them with feedback on their performance (e.g., "How do you think you did?" "Was the activity difficult?" "Do you think you got all the information on the left side of the paper?"). Cues may also direct clients' attention to the essential features of the activity (e.g., "I want you to look over to where your left hand is on the edge of the paper." "See if you find any other information that you may have missed.") or probe strategy use to gain insight into clients' cognitive style and activity approach (e.g., "What did you do to make sure you were looking over to your left?").

Cues may present a hypothesis for verification (e.g., "It seems you had a hard time bringing your eyes and attention over toward the left.") or provide clients with strategies for performing the activity (e.g., "Let's try this again; but this time, I want you to make sure you touch your left hand as you look toward that left side of the paper to make sure you are all the way over on the left.").

Using a dynamic approach to evaluating unilateral neglect, the occupational therapist makes a hypothesis about the person's performance and tests the hypothesis by repeating the activity with modifications. Some activity components will be held constant while one activity parameter is varied. For example, if it is hypothesized that the client is neglecting greater information because of the arrangement of the information (scattered vs. linear), then the arrangement of the information is changed while the amount and complexity of the material stay the same (Toglia, 1998).

Motor Planning

Motor planning, or praxis, is the ability of individuals to figure out how to get their body to do what they want it to do (Lane, 1991). Apraxia is a narrower component of motor planning impairments and is defined as a disorder of skilled movement that cannot be adequately accounted for by incoordination, sensory loss, visual spatial problems, language comprehension difficulties, or cognitive problems alone (Heilman & Rothi, 1985). What's a Practitioner to Do? 25-3 shows how apraxia can affect even familiar task performance.

Motor planning has been viewed as a broad skill that involves the integration of a number of different processes: vision and perception, cognition, tactile-kinesthetic sensation, language, and selection and organization of movements. Motor planning involves the cognitive formulation of intending to move, selecting a goal, planning the movement, and anticipating the end result. Knowledge of the functional properties of objects, actions, and action sequences is necessary, as are attentional processes that enable the person to analyze the activity demands and attend to relevant environmental activity cues. Skilled movement also requires the integration of tactile-kinesthetic information, such as where the body is in space, how the parts of the body relate to each other during movement, and how the body and limbs are positioned. Vestibular functions provide a sense of body position and movement in space that help make postural adjustments during the execution of movement. Visual spatial information about size, spatial position, orientation, shape, and texture of objects helps guide the selection of motor patterns. Linguistic skills aid the person in translating verbal commands into action or using action and movement to convey meaning. The sequencing of the movement requires selection and pretuning of the order and configuration of muscles to be activated as well as the speed and amplitude of both the initial movement and the transition from one movement to another (Lane, 1991).

Damage to the association areas of the brain (affecting the cognitive aspects of motor control) is thought to cause apraxia (Kertesz, 1982). Apraxia may be seen after strokes to either brain hemisphere, although it is more commonly seen in clients who have sustained a left hemisphere lesion (Heilman & Rothi, 1985). These clients often display related impairments of aphasia, gesture recognition, and sequencing impairments (Harrington & Haaland, 1992). The related impairments, however, do not appear to be the primary cause of the client's inability to produce skilled movement. The presentation of apraxia differs among clients with left versus right strokes (York & Cermak, 1995). Individuals

WHAT'S A PRACTITIONER TO DO? 25-3
Apraxia

Mrs. H is a typical client with apraxia. She sustained a burst cerebral aneurysm in the left parietal region and, although she sustained no gross language, physical, or cognitive impairments, she appears to be having problems in the performance of functional tasks.

During a meal-preparation activity of making a grilled cheese sandwich, Mrs. H. is able to describe verbally the sequence of completing the activity; but when she attempts the activity, she is observed placing the cheese on the toaster-oven tray without the bread, which is still on the countertop. Mrs. H states, "I know that's wrong." During the activity of making muffins, she has significant difficulty placing the rotary blades into the mixer. She appears frustrated and says, "This shouldn't be so difficult." When asked to stop and to pantomime the sequence of making the muffins, Mrs. H tends to report her intended actions verbally rather than physically demonstrate them. When encouraged to act out the procedure, Mrs. H is observed using her hand as the motion of the mixer and many of her motor acts appear to be clumsy and perseverative (repetitive). If she weren't verbally reporting what she was pantomiming, the observer would not be able to identify the act of baking.

The occupational therapist decides to bypass verbal cuing because Mrs. H's narration of the sequence does not appear to be improving her performance. The therapist cues Mrs. H by asking her to imagine the sequence visually or to watch a demonstration of the correct action sequence. Tactile cues, such as performing hand over hand through the activity, might also be attempted to evaluate their effect on Mrs. H's motor performance.

with apraxia can improve performance of skilled movement over time (Basso, Burgio, Paulin, & Prandoni, 2000); however, they frequently continue to have significant functional limitations in both the learning of new motor tasks, such as one-handed shoe tying (Poole, 1998), and the performance of motor acts to verbal command or demonstration (Poole, 2000).

Roy (1978) identified two major subsystems in apraxia: the conceptual and the production. The symptoms of apraxia may reflect disorders in one of these subsystems or in both. The production aspect of motor planning concerns generating the action plan, sequencing and organizing the appropriate elements, and carrying out the plan (e.g., reaching for a glass of water to take a drink). This is thought of as the executive aspect of movement. The traditional term used to describe production errors is *ideomotor apraxia*. Production errors may be spatial (e.g., reaches with the right hand to the left side of the glass) or temporal (e.g., perseverative or repetitive). The greatest difficulty is observed when the client is asked to perform transitive pantomimes that are the pretended use of a tool or object (e.g., "Show me how you use a toothbrush.") or to perform an intransitive limb gestures (e.g., "Show me how you wave good-bye."). Perseveration, or repetition, of component movements may be seen, or the client may use a body part as the object (e.g., use a finger as a toothbrush). Some improvement may be seen when the client is asked to imitate the motion or to perform the motion with the actual object, but the movement is still imprecise. The client makes spatiotemporal errors when required to perform a series of actions (e.g., pour coffee into a cup, add sugar and milk, stir, and drink it).

The conceptual aspect of motor planning includes knowledge about the functional properties of an object, the object action, and the sequence of action (Roy, 1978). Conceptual errors, traditionally called ideational apraxia, involve object function (e.g., using a knife as a spoon), action knowledge (e.g., match demonstrated gesture to picture or object), and knowledge of sequence (e.g., brushing one's teeth). Some authors have questioned whether ideomotor and ideational apraxia are distinct disorders representing unique underlying neuropsychological impairments or a single underlying disorder along a continuum of severity (Belanger, Duffy, & Coelho, 1994).

The clinical assessment of apraxia has varied greatly and is primarily subjective. Evaluation typically involves observation of the client's performance of different types of movements, the method of evocation (e.g., command, imitation, or object use; Belanger, et al., 1994), and the type of errors made (e.g., position, orientation, target, body part as object, perseveration, delay, or clumsiness; Haaland, 1993). The evaluation of apraxia may also include the recognition and discrimination of gestures by having clients observe videotapes of gestures and select a picture of the pantomimed object or asking them to discriminate between well-performed and poorly performed pantomime acts (Heilman, Rothi, & Valenstein, 1982; Rothi, Heilman, & Watson, 1985). The evaluation of apraxia is difficult to score reliably, as item difficulty and familiarity, as well as sequential requirements, vary with each assessment.

When evaluating the client for motor-planning abilities, it is important to conduct a thorough neurological assessment, since apraxia is defined by exclusionary criteria. Clients may display motor-planning problems owing to significant sensory loss or incoordination, but clients with apraxia display motor-planning problems when free of significant sensory or motor impairments and incoordination.

TABLE 25-25. **CATEGORIES OF MOTOR PLANNING TASKS**[a]

Category of Movement[b]	Verbal Command
Proximal transitive	Show me how you would bounce a basketball
Proximal intransitive	Show me how you stop traffic
Distal transitive	Show me how you dial a phone
Distal intransitive	Show me how you snap your fingers
Oral nonrespiratory	Show me how you lick a lollipop
Oral respiratory	Show me how you sniff a flower

[a]Adapted from Helm-Estabrooks (1992).

[b]*Transitive,* movements involving use of an object; *intransitive,* movements involving limb gestures without objects.

Because many clients with apraxia are also aphasic (both disorders are typically seen after left hemisphere dysfunction), information on the client's language skills should be obtained from the speech and language pathologist or screened for by testing for yes or no comprehension and ability to follow one-step commands. Many clients with right hemiparesis and apparent apraxia will attribute their "clumsiness" to the use of their nondominant hand. Standardized assessments of gesture tend to be narrow and restrictive in scope and should be supplemented with evaluation of whole-body movements and functional movements, both on request and within an automatic context. Assessments for apraxia typically ask the client to perform or imitate a gesture, use an actual object, or imitate the examiner using an object. The movements are either performed using a limb or the face (buccofacial).

The Test of Oral and Limb Apraxia (TOLA) was designed to evaluate ideomotor, limb, and oral apraxia (Helm-Estabrooks, 1992). Limb apraxia tasks distinguish between distal and proximal gestures and intransitive and transitive (pretend object use) gestures. Table 25-25 describes some of the movements requested in the TOLA. All tasks are assessed both to command and to imitation. In addition, a gestured pictures subtest probes the ability to produce a gesture appropriate for a pictured object. Borod, Fitzpatrick, Helm-Estabrooks, and Goodglass (1989) found that there was a significant relationship between praxis performance and gestural communication in naturalistic settings.

A broader approach to kinematic analysis has been developed using videotapes of clients' movements (Poizner, Mack, Verfoellie, Rothi, & Heilman, 1990). Some researchers have used videotapes of ADL performance to code a client's movements quantitatively and qualitatively (Schwartz, Mayer, Fitzpatrick, DeSalme, & Montgomery, 1993). Occupational therapy practitioners may ask the client or family if there are any videos of the client's movement before the injury that can help the therapist to select familiar movement subroutines at rates and rhythms that approximate the client's typical movement patterns. It may be helpful to visit work sites and home when possible to be sure to evaluate movements in the contexts that the client typically performs them.

Fisher (1993a, 1993b) supported the use of the AMPS to observe the actions a person uses to move the body or activity objects during the performance of all daily living tasks. The AMPS simultaneously assesses motor and process skills involved in motor-planning functional tasks. Abreu (1994) had a broader view of motor planning and recommended including evaluation of gestures, timing of movement, object manipulation, and block construction in her assessment of apraxia.

An occupational therapist employing a dynamic assessment method would attempt to identify the activity conditions under which the limb apraxia symptoms emerge, the client's response to cuing, and the client's awareness of his or her activity performance. The client is asked to predict performance and then to perform a variety of movement tasks. A series of cues (visual, verbal, or tactile) may be used if the client experiences difficulty performing a requested movement. The cues are not arranged in any particular order. The degree to which the cue is effective depends on the nature of the error and the underlying difficulty (Toglia, 1998).

Memory

Memory gives individuals the ability to draw on past experiences and learn new information (Toglia, 1993a). This provides people with a sense of continuity in the environment and frees them from dependency in here-and-now situations. Memory is conceptualized in several models. The stage model describes memory as a multistep process involving encoding, storage, and retrieval (Squire & Butters, 1984). Memory has also been described in terms of sensory memory, working or immediate memory, and long-term memory. Table 25-26 defines types of memory, typical assessment tasks, and functional implications. Working memory temporarily holds information in the mind, internalizes information, and uses that information to guide behavior without the aid of external cues (Goldman-Rakic, 1993). Long-term memory holds an unlimited amount of information in a permanent state for hours or years. Long-term memory is usually divided into categories of semantic or episodic. Long-term memory may also be classified into categories of declarative memory (i.e., information that can be verbally stated, and the instance in which it was learned can be recalled) or procedural memory (i.e., performance of an activity displays learning occurred, but there is no recall of how the information was acquired or how the activity was learned) (Squire, 1992).

Typical clinical manifestations of clients with memory dysfunction include rapid forgetting, normal short-term capacity, and preserved skill acquisition. There is frequently

TABLE 25–26. **TYPES OF MEMORY TASKS**[a]

Types of Memory	Definitions	Typical Assessments	Functional Implications
Immediate memory	• Recall of information immediately after presentation or exposure (within 60 sec after stimulus presentation)	• Client is asked to recall a list of words just read • Client is asked to recall 10 objects just shown to him or her	• Looses track of instructions or rules of the activity
Delayed memory (declarative long-term memory)—semantic vs. episodic	• Recall of previously presented material any time minutes to hours after presentation • *Semantic:* Recall of knowledge such as major world events, famous people, and general facts • *Episodic:* Recall of personally experienced events	• Client is asked to perform above tasks after a delay of 20 min • *Semantic:* Client is asked to recall historical facts (e.g., London is in England). • *Episodic:* Client is asked autobiographical information (e.g., How did you spend last New Years?).	• Forgets conversation that took place 30 min ago. • Forgets dates of wedding anniversary, birthdays of family members, and such • Knows date of wedding anniversary but is unable to relate personal experience of event
Skill or procedural learning	• Ability to remember how to perform an activity or procedure • Memory for an action sequence, rather than a set of facts	• Client is shown a magic trick and asked to demonstrate it immediately and after a delay	• Knows how to ride a bicycle or perform correct sequence of ambulation with a walker
Prospective memory	• Ability to respond to cues, such as an alarm, that remind client to perform a particular activity at a future time	• Client is asked to remember to bring a specific object to next session, to mail a letter when passing a mailbox, or to return a phone call in 20 min	• Forgets appointments, dates to pay bills, phone calls to make, and such

[a]Adapted from Togila, J.P. (1996a). *Application of the multicontext treatment approach to disorders in attention, memory and executive function* [Supplement manual to workshop held at Rehabilitation Institute of Chicago]. New York: Author.

greater ability in recognition tasks than in tasks requiring free recall and improved performance when provided with retrieval cues. Table 25-27 describes the different types of retrieval tasks a client may be asked to perform.

A comprehensive evaluation of memory—whether static or dynamic—must address the different types of memory and methods of retrieval. It is important to evaluate both verbal and visual representations of events, as they are believed to be independently coded. Evaluation of memory impairments should explore performance on the different aspects of memory as well as modality-specific impairments and the presence of retrograde and anterograde amnesia (see GOAT in Table 25-22). Memory assessments must take into consideration the qualitative aspects of performance, such as the effects of associated cognitive impairments, activity demands, rate of forgetting, and amount and type of information that can be retained. The demands of the assessment activity itself may influence memory and should be considered during evaluation. Factors include the following:

- The modality in which the information is presented (auditory or visual).
- The type of instructions (general or specific).
- The amount of stimuli presented.
- The familiarity and meaningfulness of the information.
- The presence of contextual cues during the storage and recall phases.
- The type of information to be remembered (factual or skill related).
- The length of retention.

Memory questionnaires and ratings of memory problems in everyday life, such as Sunderland and Harris's (1984) Everyday Memory Questionnaire, explore a client's general awareness of memory capabilities and knowledge about the functioning of memory and memory strategies. These questionnaires also examine the frequency and type of forgetting. The Rivermead Behavioral Memory Test (RBMT) tests both visual (mainly recognition) and verbal memory (mainly recall) (Wilson, Cockburn, & Baddeley, 1985). The RBMT was designed to predict everyday memory tasks that are difficult for clients with memory impairments. Tasks include remembering a name, a hidden belonging, an appointment, a paragraph, or a route and delivering a message; recognizing pictures and faces; and answering orientation questions. There are four equivalent versions for retesting and norms on ages 16–96. A pediatric version of the RBMT-C exists for children between the ages of 5 and

TABLE 25–27. **TYPES OF MEMORY RETRIEVAL**[a]

Type of Recall	Definition	Sample Assessment Tasks
Free	Ability to recall information when no specific retrieval cues are provided	Client is asked to remember a list of words read or an array of objects shown (may be increasing amounts of information)
Cued	Ability to recall information when provided with cues (first letter, category, context, etc.) during either the encoding or the retrieval phase	Client is shown photo of musical instruments and cued to think about category items fit into
Recognition	Ability to recognize previously presented information	Multiple-choice format in which client is shown 10 photos of faces, then asked to pick those faces from an array of 20 faces; client is read a sentence, then asked to pick that sentence from a choice of three sentences

[a]Reprinted with permission from Toglia (1996b).

10 years (Aldrich & Wilson, 1991; Wilson, Ivani-Chalian, Besag, & Bryant, 1993), and the RBMT-E, an extended version was developed to enhance the sensitivity of the assessment and to broaden the cultural sensitivity of the test (Wilson, Clare, Cockburn, Baddeley, Tate, & Watson, 1999).

Prospective memory involves remembering to complete an activity at a future time. Examples of prospective memory tasks include remembering to mail a letter or to take medications. Prospective memory may be evaluated informally by asking the client to perform an activity at a future time, such as remembering to ask when the next appointment is at the end of the session. The Prospective Memory Screening (PROMS) is a standardized prospective memory assessment that requires clients to perform a variety of tasks at specified time intervals, ranging from 1 min to 24 hr (Sohlberg, White, Evans, & Mateer, 1992). The extent to which everyday memory problems are related to failure to recall a past conversation or event versus a failure to carry out a future activity is important to distinguish and provides implications for treatment strategies.

Dynamic assessment of memory, such as Toglia's (1993b) Contextual Memory Test (CMT), incorporates evaluation of awareness of memory capabilities, knowledge of and spontaneous use of strategies. The CMT begins by having clients answer general questions about their memory functioning and estimate their score before and immediately after activity performance. Recall of a page of 20 line-drawn objects related to a common theme are tested immediately after a 90-sec exposure and after a 15- to 20-min delay under various conditions (free recall, cued recall, and recognition). The clients' use of strategies for encoding and retrieval are probed. If clients have difficulty, an alternate version is given and they are provided a cue during the encoding phase to facilitate recall (e.g., "When you look at the pictures, think about what happens when you go to a restaurant."). The CMT is not intended to be a comprehensive memory assessment but a test to screen for memory impairments and to provide information for treatment planning. Josman, Berney, and Jarus (2000a) found the CMT to be a valid measure of memory abilities in children with traumatic brain injury. In addition they found that children with brain injuries demonstrated impaired self-awareness and a tendency to overestimate their performance, similar findings to those seen in adults with brain injuries (Toglia, 1993b). In both studies, the non-brain-injured control groups tended to slightly underestimate performance.

Executive Functions, Organization, and Problem Solving

Executive functions are a broad band of performance skills that allow a person to engage in independent, purposeful, self-directed behavior. Organization and problem-solving skills are specific higher-level cognitive functions that fall under the umbrella of executive functions. Impairments in executive functioning are often seen after frontal lobe injuries and involve a cluster of deficiencies, of which one or two may be especially prominent (Lezak, 1995). Lezak identified four primary components of executive functions: volition, planning, purposeful action, and self-awareness and self-monitoring. Volition is the capacity to formulate an intention or goal and to initiate action. The planning component of executive functioning involves the ability to organize efficiently the steps or elements of the behavior or activity. Planning also requires the ability to look ahead, anticipate consequences, weigh and make choices, conceive of alternatives, sustain attention, and sequence the activity. Purposeful action is the translation of an intention or plan into the activity—the carrying out of plans. This requires the ability to initiate switch and stop sequences (flexibility) as well as self-regulation. The individual's understanding of impairments and how they affect functioning (self-awareness) and the ability to monitor, self-evaluate, and correct performance (self-monitoring) are also considered executive functions.

WHAT'S A PRACTITIONER TO DO? 25-4
Executive Dysfunction

Chris is 26 years old and sustained a traumatic brain injury from a car accident approximately 6 months ago. Before the accident, Chris was employed as a certified public accountant. He is presently receiving outpatient therapy and has not returned to work. Physical impairments are subtle balance problems, and the neuropsychologist reports that Chris scores within normal ranges on all cognitive–perceptual tests except in the area of executive functions.

Chris's parents, with whom he lives, report that his personality has changed dramatically. Before the accident, Chris was an active, friendly person with a good sense of humor. He was a self-starter, who was well organized and able to handle many different tasks. Now Chris spends most of his day watching television. He does not shower or participate in family activities unless pushed to do so. He appears passive, rarely initiates conversation, appears to have lost his sense of humor, is disorganized, and is unable to get things done once cued to start tasks. Chris's parents are afraid to let him drive or leave the house on his own.

Chris shows many of the typical difficulties seen in clients with executive function disorders. He demonstrates decreased initiation, decreased ability to carry out established plans, poor planning and organizational skills, and poor self-awareness. Owing to problems in initiation, Chris appears passive, disinterested, apathetic, and unmotivated. Chris demonstrates poor initiation and requires prompts to engage in activities, because he does not appear to recognize the need for action. The occupational therapist needs to distinguish behaviors that result from the executive dysfunction from those that may have psychological causes (e.g., depression), as the behaviors may look similar clinically.

Executive dysfunction syndromes may significantly influence performance of ADL no matter how well preserved the person's other cognitive process skills may be (Lezak, 1995). Measures of executive functioning can better predict functional outcomes than many other cognitive tests, as they more accurately reflect real-world behaviors required for community reintegration (Hanks, Rapport, Millis, & Deshpande, 1999). What's a Practitioner to Do? 25-4 describes a young client with executive function impairments.

Clients with poor planning and organizational skills have a tendency to develop unrealistic goals and to underestimate the time required for activity completion. Impairments in other cognitive process skills, such as attention and memory, may affect the ability to perform organizational tasks. For example, a client may sort items incorrectly because of an inability to attend to critical details or an inability to recall the sorting principle. Concrete thinking may also be seen when the client overfocuses on one aspect of the object or situation and has difficulty gathering, consolidating, or sorting information. For example, when asked to sort a grocery list to make shopping easier, a client with concrete thinking might place the lemons separately from other produce items because they are sour.

Clients displaying executive dysfunction may demonstrate their greatest difficulty in problem-solving tasks. Decreased ability to carry out established plans may be clinically seen as decreased flexibility or impulsivity in carrying out activities. Often the client's approach is perseverative, concrete, or rigid. Poor self-awareness may need to be addressed early in the treatment process as the client with poor self-awareness shows an inability to profit from feedback and may have significant safety risks owing to poor detection of errors.

Problem-solving tasks may be graded on a continuum that considers the demands of the activity and the environment to determine the amount of effort and the extent to which different cognitive and perceptual process skills are needed. In basic tasks, the problem is clear and readily identified. All the relevant information is present and limited in amount. The therapist also limits irrelevant information, the number of factors that can influence the outcome, as well as possible choices and solutions. The solutions typically involve only one to three steps and incorrect solutions are readily apparent, for they may prevent success in resolution of the problem.

Complex problem-solving tasks require sorting out information to determine where the real problem exists (e.g., the checking account statement does not match the client's personal records). Analysis of the problem requires searching large amounts of information for additional information needed to solve the problem. This searching involves sorting out the irrelevant information and keeping track of a large number of factors that can influence outcome. Solving the complex problem requires the ability to plan, test, and reject different hypotheses and the skill to formulate alternatives to the problem. Execution of the plan entails carrying out several steps, and incorrect solutions are not readily apparent. Verification that the problem has been solved involves actively comparing the solution with the original problem. Clients with executive dysfunction syndromes appear to have difficulty with complex problem-solving tasks owing to the more abstract and ambiguous nature of these tasks.

Bransford and Stein (1984) identified the components of the IDEAL problem solver. The IDEAL problem solver *i*dentifies the problem, *d*efines the problem precisely, *e*xplores possible strategies, *a*cts on the chosen strategy, and *l*ooks at the effects to determine if the problem has been solved. Adults with brain injury tend to show typical patterns of breakdown at different stages of the problem-solving process, often caused by impairments in executive functions. Identification of the problem involves attention and awareness of the environment and an exploration of the environment and activity. Some clients do not recognize that a problem or obstacle exists; thus they do not engage in a problem-solving process. Clients who have difficulty understanding cause and effect may be unable to predict the consequences of an obstacle or action.

Defining the problem precisely requires analyzing the conditions of the problem and constructing a meaningful internal representation of it. How the client defines the problem is important in determining how the problem-solving process proceeds. Often clients perform an incomplete analysis of the problem and omit critical details. They may overattend to one aspect of the problem or engage in concrete thinking, in which they interpret the issues literally and fail to see the whole picture.

Exploring possible strategies involves the ability to formulate a plan, try alternate strategies, and test hypotheses. Clients with executive dysfunction syndromes caused by brain injury tend to approach problems in a haphazard, trial-and-error manner. Often they have difficulty deciding how to approach the problem and choose inefficient strategies. When their chosen strategy is obviously ineffective, they may still have difficulty letting go of a hypothesis and generating an alternative one.

When required to carry out the strategy or plan, some clients have difficulty initiating, persisting, or remembering and following the plan owing to executive skill dysfunction. Looking at the results of completion of the strategy or plan requires that the client compare the final solution with the original conditions of the problem. Some clients with brain injury forget this vital step of self-monitoring because of problems in executive functions.

Disorders in executive functions are most apparent in situations that are novel and require a deviation from the routine or when the tasks are unstructured and the client has to initiate, plan, and prioritize. Most standardized cognitive assessments are structured and do not adequately examine the area of executive functions; therefore, impairments in executive functions can easily be missed. Several assessments for executive functions have been recently developed. Although these assessments appear more ecologically valid (i.e., able to predict behavior in everyday situations), further research data on the reliability and validity of these assessment tools is needed (Sbordone, 1996).

The Executive Function Route Finding Task (EFRT) requires clients to find their way from a starting point to a predetermined location within the building (Boyd & Sautter, 1993). Clients must provide their own plan and structure and modify them according to feedback from the environment. While accompanying clients, the examiner rates them in the following areas:

- Understanding the task.
- Seeking information.
- Remembering instructions.
- Detecting errors.
- Correcting errors.
- Ability to stick with the task (or task behavior).

General or specific cues are provided if needed. The Profile of Executive Control System (PRO-EX) is a rating scale that rates behaviors in seven areas: goal selection, planning, sequencing, initiation, time sense, awareness of impairments, and self-monitoring while the client is performing an unstructured activity, such as organizing the contents of a desk drawer or finding out how to register to vote (Branswell et al., 1992). The Multiple Errands Test has high ecological validity, is completed in a community shopping area, and requires nonroutine problem solving, planning, organization, and initiation (Shallice & Burgess, 1991). The time needed for the preparation and administration of the Multiple Errands Test, however, may not make it practical for most clinicians to administer.

The Behavioral Assessment of the Dysexecutive Syndrome (BADS) was developed to predict everyday problems related to dysexecutive syndrome (Wilson, Alderman, Burgess, Emslie, & Evans, 1996). It taps different aspects of executive functioning and is particularly relevant to treatment planning. Parallel versions of the assessment can be used for measuring outcome. The BADS contains six subtests and a 20-item questionnaire that samples the range of problems commonly associated with executive dysfunction (emotional or personality changes, motivational changes, behavioral changes, and cognitive changes). The BADS is a valid and reliable assessment of subtle difficulties in executive skills in people who appear to be cognitively well preserved and who function well in structured situations (Norris & Tate, 2000; Wilson, Evans, Emslie, Alderman, & Burgess, 1998).

The Toglia Category Assessment (TCA) is a dynamic assessment of category flexibility that uses 16 plastic utensils of different sizes and colors (Toglia, 1994). Once the utensils are grouped according to one attribute the client is asked to sort the items again in a different way. This is repeated a third time, with the examiner asking the client after each trial to explain how the groups differ. A deductive-reasoning component consists of a questioning activity that investigates the client's ability to formulate and test different hypotheses. The client must determine which of the utensils the examiner is thinking of with the fewest number of yes-or-no questions and the least amount of guessing possible. The examiner uses a set of standard sequential cues with each subtest if the client encounters difficulty identifying the target item in the minimum number of questions that should be needed. The TCA is a reliable and valid assessment of categorization skills in both adults (Josman, 1998) and children (Josman, Berney, & Jarus, 2000b).

Nonstandardized evaluation of executive function, organizational, and problem-solving skills may include unstructured functional tasks. For example, clients can be asked to organize and sequence a day filled with multiple errands, stating the time they would leave home and the sequence in which the errands would be completed (Toglia, 1991a). Clients can be given tasks within the hospital environment that require seeking information (e.g., find out the location of the library or recreation area). Information-seeking tasks can also involve use of the telephone (e.g., call three local banks to find out their hours and fees for checking and use of an ATM card). Therapists should also introduce functional problem-solving tasks that require identifying the lack of necessary information (e.g., "You just bought a new hat for $12.60. When you received your change you realized that you did not receive the correct amount. How much change should you have received?") or organizing and planning (e.g., "You are organizing a breakfast meeting for 14 people. Coffee is 90¢ each, tea is 85¢ each, bagels are 65¢ each, doughnuts are 75¢ each, and Danishes are $1 each. You have $22. What could you buy?").

An occupational therapist using a dynamic interactional approach to the evaluation of executive functions, organizational, and problem-solving skills would pose questions to investigate the client's executive skill performance on all cognitive–perceptual assessments not just those deemed as problem-solving or executive function assessments. The questions should explore the client's

- Awareness.
- Ability to perform new versus rote, routine tasks.
- Need for prompts to start or complete simple activities (e.g., brushing teeth, getting a snack).
- Ability to deal with the unexpected in simple, everyday tasks (e.g., does the client take action if the toothpaste tube is empty?).
- Ability to stay on the activity and not get sidetracked by irrelevant information.

FACTORS THAT MAY AFFECT EVALUATION

Psychosocial Factors

Occupational therapy practitioners need to consider not only their clients' cognitive status but also their coping capacities and the changing context of their lives as a result of the injury or disease (Fine, 1993). The reaction to a brain injury may be immediate, with changes in personality and behavior as well as cognitive–perceptual abilities. These changes affect clients' perceptions of themselves and relationships with others. The psychosocial response to brain damage and cognitive impairments is a major life transition that involves stages of adjustment (Diller, 1993).

One of the most common secondary emotional responses to brain injury is depression. Occupational therapy practitioners need to understand the cognitive changes that may result from depression because many depressed clients display behavior patterns that appear similar to dementia. Depression may be exhibited in perseverative thoughts, poor initiation, slowed reaction times, and poor ability to predict the quality of activity performance. There are differences in clinical presentation; depressed clients are more likely to be aware of their impaired cognitive process skills and have a tendency to significantly underestimate performance both before and after the activity. Clients with brain injury will overestimate activity performance and show limited awareness (Squire & Zouzounis, 1988).

Clients' poor performance on cognitive-based testing may be greatly influenced by psychological factors. The secondary depression may make the cognitive impairments appear greater and prevent clients from initiating the use of coping strategies. Cognitive deficits can also exacerbate depression. Recognizing and appraising the situation requires attention, memory, and self-awareness. Coping with the situation involves initiative, decision making, flexibility, persistence, self-control, and self-regulation. These are the very skills that may be limited by the cognitive or executive skill dysfunction and thus may make the depression more evident and difficult to treat (Fine, 1993).

Language Impairments

Occupational therapy practitioners working with clients with language impairments will need to use keen observational skills and deductive reasoning to understand clients' cognitive–perceptual strengths and weaknesses. Information is often needed on the cognitive and perceptual abilities of clients with aphasia to determine the extent to which any impairment may interfere with the ability to successfully use an alternative communication system. To use a basic communication board requires clients to have awareness that an alternate communication system is needed, as well as the skills in visual attention, visual scanning, object identification, matching of line drawing or words to real objects, and association or categorization.

Whenever possible, the occupational therapy practitioner should consult with the speech and language pathologist to gain a better understanding of the client's level of comprehension and the most reliable method of expression. If information on the client's receptive and expressive language skills are not available, occupational therapy practitioners should first gain an understanding of yes-and-no reliability by evaluating the client's ability to follow simple commands. Such reliability is demonstrated when the client responds accurately to a series of single-statement questions (e.g., "Are you a woman?" "Is it snowing?"). The client may be able to handle multiple-choice questions with four or five choices, if the therapist can establish yes-and-no reliability.

The ability to comprehend simple written commands can be screened by having the client read and follow one- to two-step directions. It is important for the occupational therapist not to provide any gestural cues during this assessment to determine accurately if the client can follow the written direction. If the client cannot read, the command may be presented orally. Motor-planning impairments frequently co-exist with language impairments and need to be ruled out as interfering factors. The ability to imitate or follow gestural directions must be evaluated if the client cannot follow verbal one-step commands. Tactile cues may be necessary during this assessment.

If the client does not demonstrate yes-or-no reliability and is unable to follow one-step commands, cognitive–perceptual process skills cannot be accurately evaluated through formal methods. Most occupational therapy practitioners faced with this situation will take a functional approach to both evaluation and treatment. When basic communication skills of yes-and-no reliability and following simple commands are intact, cognitive–perceptual testing should still be adapted to minimize speech and language requirements. Assessments that can be answered by a yes- or-no response or multiple choice questions are recommended. In all assessments, the directions should be brief, accompanied by gestures, and have at least three trials with corrections and assistance before the actual testing to ensure that the client understands the directions.

Sensory Impairments

Evaluating a client with primary sensory loss (vision or hearing) is a challenge to occupational therapists. Therapists will need to focus their evaluation on the sensory modality that is intact by modifying existing assessments or selecting assessments that do not tap the impaired sensory modality. For example, the client who has a hearing impairment may be provided with written directions to follow, and the client with visual impairments may be presented with enlarged stimuli. Qualitative analysis along with clinical observations are needed to interpret the client's performance. Documentation of the results should clearly describe the modifications and means of evaluation.

INTERPRETATION AND DOCUMENTATION OF RESULTS

Differences in Evaluation Purpose Are Reflected in Documentation

The approach an occupational therapist takes to the process of evaluating cognitive–perceptual dysfunction guides the documentation process. When the evaluation method incorporates primarily static cognitive screening tools or a deficit-specific approach, the documentation typically includes a statement regarding the purpose of the evaluation, the name, a brief overview of the assessment or battery administered, the results, and the recommendations (Box 25-1).

When a dynamic interactional assessment has been conducted, the documentation reflects the focus on reporting the activity conditions that influenced cognitive–perceptual symptoms and the client's awareness of the impairments and use of processing strategies. The documentation describes each activity and the conditions that either increased or decreased the symptoms; the client's response to cuing; the client's awareness or ability to detect, predict, monitor, explain, or correct errors; and a summary to establish relationships to ADL, IADL, education, work, play and leisure, and social participation (Box 25-2).

Relating Results to Function

Occupational therapy practitioners have expertise in analyzing a person's performance in everyday activities and identifying the cognitive–perceptual facilitators or barriers

BOX 25-1 DOCUMENTATION EXAMPLE: MEAMS

Mr. B was given the Middlesex Elderly Assessment of Mental State (MEAMS), which was designed to screen for gross impairment of specific cognitive skills in elderly clients (age 65 and older). Subtests include orientation, name learning, naming, comprehension, remembering pictures, arithmetic, spatial construction, fragmented letter perception, unusual views, usual views, verbal fluency, and motor perseveration.

Mr. B scored 6 out of a possible score of 12 on the pass-or-fail screening format. This indicates the need for more detailed investigation and evaluation of cognitive–perceptual functioning. Subtests that were performed with 100% accuracy included orientation, arithmetic, comprehension, and motor persistence. Subtests that Mr. B had the most difficulty with were unusual views of objects, fragmented letter perception, and spatial construction.

The occupational therapist made the following recommendations: Further testing in the areas of difficulty. Follow-up and education to caregivers regarding possible difficulties.

BOX 25-2 DOCUMENTATION EXAMPLE: VISUAL DISCRIMINATION

Terry demonstrates no difficulty in attentional or visual discrimination tasks that involve 8 to 10 items. When presented with tasks that involve greater amounts of information, she demonstrates increasing disorganization and difficulty keeping track of the information. Terry has no difficulty sorting items into self-established categories when the activity involves 8 to 10 items. However, when presented with more items (25 picture cards), she requires assistance to structure categories and complete the activity. She appears to lose track of her categories and changes her sorting principle.

On the CMT (20 line drawings of items related to a restaurant), Terry initially recalled only 7 items and did not appear to use any strategy for grouping the information. She did not identify that the items were related to a restaurant. When provided with the theme of the items in part II of the test (a morning scene), Terry's performance improved to 14 out of 20 items.

The occupational therapist summarized the findings as follows: Throughout all tasks, Terry did not consistently check her work for errors; although when questioned, she did report that since her accident she has experienced problems in memory and concentration. Despite this vague understanding of her problems, Terry frequently overestimated her activity performance before beginning tasks. Terry had the most difficulty with tasks that required attention to detail and tracking and organizing larger quantities (> 10) of information. Performance generally improved when she was provided with one to two cues to structure the information or when the information was limited (< 10 items). Terry appears to have the ability to successfully use strategies when they are provided. Terry will be vulnerable to performance breakdown in tasks such as organizing monthly bills or performing a multiple-step cooking activity that requires the use of two or more cooking appliances and three or more foods.

to a person's engagement in meaningful occupations (AOTA, in press). Therapists are able to link the potential effect of the identified cognitive–perceptual impairments with the demands of activity performance. Occupational therapy practitioners should broadly define the concept of function and consider the effect of the observed cognitive–perceptual impairments on the multiple activities required for the client's successful engagement in both present and future occupational roles and the subsequent impact of these impairments on health, well-being, and life satisfaction (AOTA, in press). Activity performance needs to be evaluated in a variety of contexts that more closely resemble the demands of real-world behavior. Practitioners should consider that the structured, yet unfamiliar, hospital environment may either facilitate or impede performance. Documentation of the functional implications of the cognitive–perceptual impairments is vital for occupational therapy practitioners to demonstrate their valuable contribution to the health-care team in the evaluation and rehabilitation of cognitive and perceptual dysfunction and to ensure that third-party payers recognize this contribution.

Goal Setting

Goals addressing cognitive–perceptual impairments and their influence in activity performance require the same components as any goal. The goal should describe the behavior that is targeted for treatment, the conditions under which the behavior should be displayed, and the expected level of performance. Cognitive goals that address improved safety awareness and safe, independent performance of functional activities should be documented. Long-term cognitive–perceptual goals should address general cognitive–perceptual areas and the functional level of performance—for example, "Client will demonstrate increased awareness of impairments so that the client can successfully use compensatory strategies for independence in self-care by discharge." Short-term goals typically target more specific cognitive–perceptual process skills that are necessary steps to achieving improved functional performance—for example, "As a prerequisite to independence in basic self-care skills, the client will demonstrate the ability to use an organized scanning approach to locate target items in a crowded array (refrigerator shelf, drawer, telephone book, etc.) five times during a 30-min session, within 2 weeks." Or "As a prerequisite to independence in the community, the client will demonstrate increased simultaneous attention, as evidence by ability to perform multiple-step cooking tasks with only one to two verbal cues, within 2 weeks." Cognitive goals, like all goals, should be behavioral and clearly written, so if given to another practitioner he or she will know when the established goal has been achieved.

CONCLUSION

The AOTA (1999) stated, "occupational therapy practitioners have an important role in promoting maximal levels of performance in persons with cognitive impairments" (p. 601). Occupational therapy practitioners unique educational background in biological and behavioral sciences, activity analysis, and human occupations allows them to understand how performance of ADL is affected by cognitive and perceptual impairments. With a particular client in mind, the occupational therapist can select an approach and assessments to evaluate the impact of cognitive–perceptual impairments on functional performance and then use this information to plan and carry out an intervention plan.

SECTION III

Communication/ Interaction Skills and Socioemotional Factors

KATHLEEN DOYLE LYONS

Holistic occupational therapy evaluation includes assessment of the psychosocial aspect of clients' lives. This section reviews the importance of evaluating **communication/interaction skills** and **socioemotional factors** and presents models and tools that can be used by therapists.

WHAT ARE COMMUNICATION/ INTERACTION SKILLS AND SOCIOEMOTIONAL FACTORS?

Distinction between Skills and Factors

Skills are observable behaviors that have functional purposes and are manifested during occupational engagement (Kielhofner, 2002). Factors are underlying body functions and structures that reside within a person and have the potential to influence occupational performance (AOTA, in press). Factors are functions that are part of a person, whereas skills are purposeful and observable actions that a person uses to engage in occupation.

Definitions

Communication and interaction skills are observable acts or processes that convey intentions and needs and coordinate social behavior during interactions with others (Kielhofner, 2002). In this section, the term *socioemotional factors* is used to describe client factors that relate to socioemotional health. Socioemotional factors include temperament and personality, energy and drive, and emotional functions.

RELEVANCE OF COMMUNICATION/ INTERACTION SKILLS AND SOCIOEMOTIONAL FACTORS TO OCCUPATIONAL THERAPY

The first step in evaluation is to develop an understanding of the client as an individual and an occupational being (Hocking, 2001). Practitioners using a client-centered approach focus evaluation and intervention on client priorities and values (Dunn, 1998). Such an approach necessitates an understanding of the client's identity.

Identity is a theory of an individual that describes and interrelates his or her features, characteristics, and experiences (Schlenker, 1984). Identity can be thought of as the evolving life story an individual tells to make sense of and define the self (McAdams, 1996). Occupational therapy practitioners frequently elicit life stories in evaluation and intervention, and these stories can guide clinical reasoning (Burke & Kern, 1996; Mattingly & Fleming, 1994). Researchers have asserted that a person's identity, or sense of self, may be threatened by aging (Christiansen, 1999), physical illness (Charmaz, 1991), or mental illness (Estroff, 1989). As reconstructing a satisfactory identity is often part of becoming well (Davidson & Strauss, 1992; Strong, 1998), all occupational therapy practitioners need to be attuned to the potentially vulnerable identities of their clients (Christiansen, 1999).

Occupational therapy practitioners need to attend to communication/interaction skills because it is through these skills that a person conveys identity as well as needs, thoughts, and emotions, to others. Furthermore, communication/interaction skills are necessary to perform the many occupations that are not solitary in nature but rather occur in the presence of or with the cooperation of others. Socioemotional factors are important to occupational therapy practitioners because they help shape a person's identity. Socioemotional factors, such as personality and energy, and drive, also affect an individual's choice and subjective experience of occupations, and persistence in sustaining occupational behavior. For these reasons, communication/interaction skills and socioemotional factors should be considered in every occupational therapy evaluation. They should not be seen as issues that are relevant only to practitioners working with people who have psychiatric diagnoses.

When evaluating a client, the occupational therapist decides which assessments and methods to use based on the client's articulated needs and the therapist's professional judgment. The therapist might choose to assess communication/interaction skills and socioemotional factors formally or may decide to assess them informally and simply note these skills and factors as facilitators or barriers to occupational performance. The therapist may also use information collected from other disciplines, such as rehabilitation counseling or neuropsychology, to guide occupational therapy intervention planning. Thus communication/interaction skills and socioemotional factors should be considered, but may not be formally assessed, in each occupational therapy evaluation.

EVALUATING COMMUNICATION/ INTERACTION SKILLS

In evaluating communication/interaction skills, the therapist assesses whether the client's skills enable successful and personally fulfilling social interactions within occupations. During evaluation, the therapist contemplates the following questions:

- Is the client satisfied with his or her social occupational performance and interpersonal relationships?
- Are other people satisfied with the client's interactions and relationships with them?
- Do the communication/interaction skills facilitate the successful completion of occupations?
- Do the communication/interaction skills encourage effective and satisfactory interpersonal relationships?

The first two questions address whether the client and other people are satisfied with interpersonal relationships and the actual performance of occupations. The answers to these questions determine whether there is a need to evaluate communication/interaction skills formally. The last two questions center on how the skills themselves contribute to successful or unsuccessful relationships and occupational performance. The answers to the latter two questions help the occupational therapist determine the skills that may require therapeutic intervention.

Models of Communication/Interaction Skills in Occupational Therapy

Occupational therapy practitioners have only recently begun to develop a language to describe communication and interaction skills as they relate to occupational performance (Doble & Magill-Evans, 1992; Fisher et al., 1995). Doble and Magill-Evans (1992) proposed a model of social interaction to help practitioners organize their knowledge regarding socially oriented occupational behavior. Doble and Magill-Evan's Model of Social Interaction describes the process of receiving, interpreting, planning, and executing social behavior. In the model, sensory organs, cognitive abilities, emotional state, volitional traits, and interactional style all influence social enactment skills. Social enactment skills refer to the observable output of the social interaction process and include acknowledging skills, sending skills, timing skills, and coordinating skills.

Taxonomy of Communication and Interaction Skills

Forsyth, Salamy, Simon, and Kielhofner (1998) proposed a taxonomy of communication and interaction skills. Forsyth et al.'s taxonomy considers skills as they relate to three domains that must be managed during interactions: physicality, information exchange, and relations.

Physicality

Physicality refers to using the body to communicate with others. This dimension of communication/interaction skills involves contacts (touching or physically contacting others), gazes (using eye movement and gaze to communicate), gestures (using body movements to indicate, demonstrate, or add emphasis), maneuvers (moving the body in relation to others), orients (positioning the body in relation to a task or others), and postures (assuming physical positions).

Information Exchange

Information exchange refers to the giving and receiving of information within an occupation. Information exchange skills include articulates (produces clear, intelligible speech), asserts (expresses desires, refusals, and requests), asks (requests information), engages (initiates interactions), expresses (displays appropriate affect/attitude), modulates (displays volume and vocal inflection in speech), shares (provides factual or personal information), speaks (makes oneself understood through language), and sustains (maintains speech for appropriate durations).

Relations

Relations refer to the maintenance of appropriate relationships within an occupation. In this category are skills such as collaborates (coordinates actions with others in pursuit of a goal), conforms (follows social norms), focuses (directs behavior and conversation to ongoing social action), relates (attempts to establish rapport with others), and respects (accommodates to others' responses and requests).

Assessment Tools for Communication/ Interaction Skills

Many assessments of overall functioning include some items related to communication/interaction skills, for example, the FIM (Center for Functional Assessment Research, 1990) and the Behavioural Assessment Scale (BAS; Ritchie & Ledesert, 1991). The following subsections briefly highlight tools that have communication/interaction skills as their primary focus. Absent from the discussion are the many tools that have been developed for specific populations, such as the Matson Evaluation of Social Skills in Individuals with Severe Retardation (MESSIER; Matson & LeBlanc, 1999). Readers are encouraged to explore the research on social skills assessments for further information.

Adult Assessments

Adult assessments include the following. The Assessment of Communication and Interaction Skills (ACIS; Forsyth et al., 1998) is a criterion-referenced observational tool that is based on the taxonomy presented above. The ACIS is designed to assess the communication/interaction skills of adults who have physical or mental illness. When using the ACIS, the therapist observes the client engaging in an occupation that requires interacting with others. The therapist rates the client on each of the 20 skills listed in the taxonomy using a four-point scale.

The Social Interaction Scale (SIT) is an assessment of social competence (Trower, Bryant, & Argyle, 1978). It is used to rate social behavior that is exhibited during a semi-structured interview. The SIT contains 29 items that are grouped into subscales of voice quality, nonverbal, and conversation. An observer of the interview rates each behavior item on a five-point Likert scale, from good to very poor.

The Social Interaction Scale of the Bay Area Functional Performance Evaluation (BaFPE) is a standardized assessment of social behavior and competency (Williams & Bloomer, 1987). Practitioners rate interaction skills based on observation of occupational performance in five social situations.

Child Assessments

Child assessments include the following. The Child and Adolescent Social Perception Measure (CASP) is designed to assess a child's ability to use nonverbal cues to identify another person's emotions (Magill-Evans, Koning, Cameron-Sadava, & Manyk, 1995). The CASP derives its theoretical orientation from Doble and Magill-Evans's (1992) model of social interaction. The CASP consists of 10 videotaped scenes in which the verbal content is filtered so as to be unintelligible. Children are asked to identify the emotion that is being displayed in the scene and the nonverbal cues that suggest that emotion.

For further information, see Ghuman, Peebles, and Ghuman's (1998) comprehensive review of social interaction assessments used with infants and preschool children. Education literature is also replete with tools that use parent, teacher, and/or child report to identify social skills and behaviors of children, for example, the Child Behavior Checklist (Achenbach, 1991), and the Preschool and Kindergarten Behavior Scales (PKBS; Merrell, 1996). Demaray and Ruffalo (1995) reviewed six tools for assessing social skills of preschool and school-aged children.

EVALUATING SOCIOEMOTIONAL FACTORS

Definitions

Temperament and Personality

Temperament refers to the constitutional disposition of a person that encourages him or her to react to situations in a particular way. **Personality** describes the set of characteristics that make a person unique (World Health Organization [WHO], 2001). Personality researchers generally use the Five Factor Model as a coherent system for organization and description of personality traits in adults (McCrae & Costa, 1986). The five factors are continua of traits along which a person is rated. McCrae and Costa describe the five factors as:

- *Neuroticism:* Related to worrying, insecurity, self-consciousness, and chronic emotional distress; the other end of the continuum is emotional stability.
- *Extraversion:* Extraverts are described as sociable, fun-loving, friendly, and talkative; its opposite pole is labeled introversion.
- *Openness to experience:* The hardest factor to describe and interpret; characterized by originality, imagination, daring, and having broad interests; it is correlated with, but separate from, intelligence.
- *Agreeableness:* Related to traits such as trust, warmth, and sympathy; the opposite end of the continuum is antagonism.
- *Conscientiousness:* Typically hardworking, ambitious, energetic, and persevering; the other end of the continuum is undirectedness.

Other Functions

Energy and drive functions refer to psychological or physiological mechanisms that cause a person to attempt to satisfy certain needs and goals in a persistent manner (WHO, 2001). Included are functions such as motivation, appetite, energy level, and craving for substances.

Emotional functions are mental functions that relate to feelings and affective components of the mind (WHO, 2001). Aspects to consider are the range, appropriateness, and regulation of emotions such as sadness, happiness, love, fear, anger, hate, tension, anxiety, joy, and sorrow.

Assessment and Relevance to Occupational Therapy

Typically, other members of the interdisciplinary team are responsible for evaluating socioemotional factors.

BOX 25-3 VOLITION

Occupational therapy practitioners are interested in volition, which is a construct loosely related to the concept of motivation. As articulated in the Model of Human Occupation (Kielhofner, 1995), volition refers to cognitive and emotional orientations, combined with self-knowledge, that enable a person to seek out, experience, and interpret various occupations. Researchers have developed tools to measure and describe volition, including the Assessment of Occupational Functioning (Watts, Hinson, Madigan, McGuigan, & Newman, 1999), the Occupational Circumstances Assessment—Interview and Rating Scale (Haglund, Henriksson, Crisp, Friedhiem, & Kielhofner, 2001), and the Occupational Performance History Interview II (Kielhofner et al., 1998).

Haglund, L., Henriksson, C., Crisp, M., Friedhiem, L., & Kielhofner, G. (2001). *The Occupational Circumstances Assessment-Interview and Rating Scale (OCAIRS) (Version 2.0)*. Chicago: Model of Human Occupation Clearinghouse, Department of Occupational Therapy, University of Illinois.

Kielhofner, G., Mallinson, T., Crawford, C., Nowak, M., Rigby, M., Henry, A., & Walens, D. (1998). *A user's manual for the Occupational Performance History Interview (2nd version)*. Chicago: Model of Human Occupation Clearinghouse, Department of Occupational Therapy, University of Illinois.

Watts, J. H., Hinson, R., Madigan, M. J., McGuigan, P. M., & Newman, S. M. (1999). The Assessment of Occupational Functioning—Collaborative Version. In B. J. Hempill-Pearson (Ed.). *Assessments in occupational therapy in mental health* (pp. 193–203). Thorofare, NJ: Slack.

Occupational therapists most often collaborate with other professionals who are trained to evaluate socioemotional factors; consequently, therapists need to understand how to use the information about socioemotional factors to plan intervention. For example, a therapist may want to consider a client's level of extraversion when determining the balance of group versus individual intervention sessions. An introvert is less likely to thrive and be stimulated when around other people and may desire more time in solitary or one-on-one occupations than would an extraverted client.

It is important to realize that occupational therapy intervention is not aimed at changing or manipulating socioemotional factors—that is, it is not appropriate to set an outcome goal related to helping someone be more extraverted. However, occupational therapy practitioners might use information about socioemotional factors to plan intervention or to educate a client. For example, a practitioner might help a client understand how personality factors, such as extraversion and openness, contribute to the selection of occupations in daily life. The client then ideally can use that information to choose a balance of occupations that best contributes to his or her well-being.

KEY POINTS TO CONSIDER IN EVALUATION OF COMMUNICATION/ INTERACTION SKILLS AND SOCIOEMOTIONAL FACTORS

Communication/Interaction Skills Are Culture Specific

Each culture has its own set of display rules; these are the taken-for-granted norms that govern how people express emotions and interact with each other (Ekman & Friesen, 1969). Therapists should interpret a client's communication/interaction skills from the standpoint of the client's, not the therapist's, culture.

Evaluation Is an Interactive Process

Evaluation is a complex, dynamic process that is shaped by both the client and the therapist (Hinojosa & Kramer, 1998b). Therapists need to become aware of their presuppositions and to understand how their assumptions influence the interpretation of client actions (Kramer & Hinojosa, 1998). Therapists also need to be aware of what social psychologists call the *expectancy effect:* an evaluator's expectations for success or failure can be subtly communicated to another person, thereby influencing that person's behavior (see DePaulo & Friedman, 1998, for brief review). Thus if a practitioner expects a client to struggle with a particular task, the practitioner may be nonverbally communicating that expectation to the client and negatively influencing the client's performance.

First Impressions Should Be Treated as Hypotheses

In everyday social interactions, human beings form impressions of others quickly and often nonconsciously (Ambady, Bernieri, & Richeson, 2000). These first impressions become anchors from which subsequent judgments are made. Practitioners need to make a conscious effort to use their first impressions as hypotheses and not to treat them as if they were infallible and accurate judgments.

Some diseases create behaviors that are easily misinterpreted by others. For example, to the naive observer the Parkinson's disease symptom of bradykinesia (slowness of movement) can appear to be a sign of tentativeness, reluctance, or laziness (Pentland, 1991). Adults tend to use nonverbal cues more than verbal cues to determine a behavior's social meaning, especially when the nonverbal and verbal messages conflict (Burgoon, 1994). A verbal/nonverbal message conflict occurs, for example, if the client states in a slow and weary tone "I don't mind going to therapy now" and is slow to initiate rising out of the chair. In this situation, it is a natural but harmful mistake for the practitioner to attribute the client's slowness to lack of motivation, rather than to acknowledge it as a sign of a neurological disease.

Practitioners need to test the hypotheses formed by their first impressions and actively seek evidence that has the potential to disconfirm each hypothesis. It is also important to remember that evaluation continues informally throughout intervention, so practitioners always need to be alert to new information that could contradict their initial impressions of the client.

Context Shapes Behavior

Social behavior is shaped by the situation in which it occurs. Yet social psychologists have found that people tend to underestimate the influence of the situation when interpreting the behaviors of others, assuming instead that a person's behavior is a direct function of that person's traits and personality. This is known as the "fundamental attribution error" (Ross, 1977). Therapists need to be cognizant of this aspect of human nature when evaluating communication/interaction skills.

Evaluation methods should allow the therapist to observe the client engaging in occupations in multiple settings and with different people so that the therapist can determine how context influences the use of skills. Similarly, the use of multiple assessment tools and methods provide the deepest understanding of the client's skills, strengths, and problems (Hinojosa & Kramer, 1998a; Royeen & Richards, 1998). Assessment findings should not be considered in isolation but rather should be used to confirm and disconfirm each test's results (Duncan, 1998).

Strengths and Limitations of Self-Report

Occupational therapy practitioners advocate the use of client-centered or person-centered approaches to evaluation and intervention (AOTA, in press; Dunn, Brown, & McGuigan, 1994). This involves talking to clients, their families, and supportive others to obtain each person's perspective on the client's occupational needs. In the area of communication/interaction skills and socioemotional factors, it is important for therapists to be aware of the limitations of self-report. A person's perceived success in communication may not correspond to actual success as rated by peers (Riggio, Widaman, & Friedman, 1985). Because people do not always get clear, direct feedback regarding the effectiveness of their communication skills (Goffman, 1959), clients may not recognize communication as problematic for them.

This is not to say that a therapist should refrain from asking a client about his or her perception of communication/interaction skills and socioemotional factors; the client's perception of these issues is always important. However, the therapist needs to use language that the client can understand—that is, not ask about temperament but instead ask about the behavioral manifestations of temperament. And the therapist needs to supplement self-report methods with opportunities to engage clients in occupations so that the therapist can actually see the skills being used.

CONCLUSION

Occupational therapy practitioners are interested in how communication/interaction skills and socioemotional factors support and hinder a client's successful occupational performance. These skills and factors are important aspects of a holistic occupational therapy evaluation. They can be evaluated formally or informally, depending on the needs and priorities of the client. Other professionals, such as rehabilitation counselors and speech and language pathologists, can contribute to the occupational therapy practitioner's understanding of a client's communication skills and socioemotional factors. When evaluating communication/interaction skills and socioemotional factors, therapists need to be sensitive to cultural norms and contextual features that influence social interaction. Therapists must also be aware that while occupational therapy intervention programs may focus on improving communication/interaction skills, they should not be directed toward changing or manipulating socioemotional factors.

References

Abreu, B. C. (1994). Perceptual motor skills: Assessment and intervention strategies. In C. B. Royeen (Ed.). *AOTA self-study series: Cognitive rehabilitation* (pp. 1–48). Rockville, MD: American Occupational Therapy Association.

Abreu, B. C., Seale, G., Scheibel, R. S., Huddleston, N., Zhang, L., & Ottenbacher, K. J. (2001). Levels of self-awareness after acute brain injury: How patients' and rehabilitation specialists' perceptions compare. *Archives of Physical Medicine and Rehabilitation, 82*, 49–56.

Abreu, B., & Toglia, J. P. (1987). Cognitive rehabilitation: A model for occupational therapy. *American Journal of Occupational Therapy, 41*, 439–448.

Achenbach, T. M. (1991). *Manual for the Child Behavior Checklist/4-18 and 1991 profile*. Burlington: Psychiatry Department, University of Vermont.

Adamovich, B. B., & Henderson, J. (1992). *Scales of Cognitive Ability for Traumatic Brain Injury (SCATBI)*. Austin, TX: Pro-Ed.

Agostinucci, J. (1997). Upper motor neuron syndrome. In J. Van Deusen & D. Brunt (Eds.). *Assessment in occupational and physical therapy* (pp. 271–293). Philadelphia: Saunders.

Ainsworth, B., Haskell, W., Leon, A., Jacobs Jr., D., Montoye, H., Sallis, J., & Paffenbarger, R. Jr., (1998). Compendium of physical activities: Classification of energy costs of human physical activities. In J. Roitman (Ed.), *ACSM's resource manual for exercise testing and prescription* (pp. 657–665). Baltimore: Williams & Wilkins.

Aldrich, F. K., & Wilson, B. A. (1991). Rivermead Behavioural Memory Test for Children (RBMT-C): A preliminary evaluation. *British Journal of Clinical Psychology, 30*, 161–168.

Allen, C. K., Earhart, C. A., & Blue, T. (1992). *Occupational therapy treatment goals for the physically and cognitively disabled*. Rockville, MD: American Occupational Therapy Association.

Ambady, N., Bernieri, F. J., & Richeson, J. A. (2000). Toward a histology of social behavior: Judgmental accuracy from thin slices of the behavioral stream. *Advances in Experimental Social Psychology, 32*, 201–271.

American College of Sports Medicine (1991). *Guidelines for exercise testing and prescription* (4th ed.). Philadelphia: Lea & Febiger.

American Occupational Therapy Association (1999). Management of occupational therapy services for persons with cognitive impairments [Statement]. *American Journal of Occupational Therapy, 53*, 601–607.

American Occupational Therapy Association—Commission on Practice (1995). Clarification of the use of the terms assessment and evaluation. *American Journal of Occupational Therapy, 49*, 1072–1073.

American Occupational Therapy Association (In press). Occupational therapy practice framework: Domain and process. *American Journal of Occupational Therapy*.

American Society for Hand Therapists (1981). *Clinical assessment recommendations*. Indianapolis: Author.

American Spinal Injury Association [ASIA]. (2000). International Standards for Neurological Classification of Spinal Injury Patients. Chicago: Author.

Ansell, B. J., & Keenan, J. E. (1989). The Western Neuro Sensory Stimulation Profile: A tool for assessing slow-to-recover head injured patients. *Archives of Physical Medicine and Rehabilitation, 70*, 104–108.

Arnadottir, G. (1990). *The brain and behavior: assessing cortical dysfunction through activities of daily living*. St. Louis: Mosby.

Ashworth, B. (1964). Preliminary trial of carisoprodol in multiple sclerosis. *Practitioner, 192*, 540–542.

Asmussen, E. (1979). Muscle fatigue. *Medical Science and Sports, 11*, 313–321.

Atchison, B. (1995). Cardiopulmonary diseases. In C. A. Trombly (Ed.). *Occupational therapy for physical dysfunction* (4th ed., pp. 875–892). Philadelphia: Williams & Wilkins.

Avery-Smith, W. (2002). Dysphagia. In C. A. Trombly & M. V. Radomski (Eds.). *Occupational therapy for physical dysfunction* (5th ed., pp. 1091–1109). Philadelphia: Lippincott, Williams & Wilkins.

Avery-Smith, W., Rosen, A. B., & Dellarosa, D. M. (1997). *Dysphagia evaluation protocol*. San Antonio, TX: Therapy Skill Builders.

Ayres, J. (1989). *Sensory Integration and Praxis Tests manual*. Los Angeles: Western Psychological Services.

Barnes, M. R., Crutchfield, C. A., & Heriza, C. B. (1982). The neurophysiological basis of patient treatment. Vol. II: Reflexes in motor development. Atlanta, GA : Stokesville Publishing Co.

Barrows, H. (1980). *Guide to neurological assessment*. Philadelphia: Lippincott.

Basmajian, J. V., & DeLuca, C. J. (1985). *Muscles alive: Their functions revealed by electromyography* (5th ed.). Baltimore: Williams & Wilkins.

Basso, A., Burgio, F., Paulin, M., & Prandoni, P. (2000). Long-term follow-up of ideomotor apraxia. *Neuropsychological Rehabilitation, 10*, 1–13.

Belanger, S. A., Duffy, R. J., & Coelho, C. A. (1994). An investigation of limb apraxia regarding the validity of current assessment procedures. *Clinical Aphasiology, 22*, 191–201.

Bellace, J. V., Healy, D, Besser, M. P., Byron, T., & Hohman, L. (2000). Validity of the Dexter Evaluation System's Jamar dynamometer attachment for assessment of hand grip strength in a normal population. *Journal of Hand Therapy, 13*(1), 46–51.

Benton, A. (1985). Visoperceptual, visuospatial, and visuoconstructive disorders. In K. M. Heilman & E. Valenstein (Eds.). *Clinical neuropsychology* (pp. 151–185). New York: Oxford University Press.

Benton, A. L., Hamsher, K. de S., Varney, N. R., & Spreen, O. (1983). *Contributions to neuropsychological assessment: Clinical manual*. New York: Oxford University Press.

Bentzel, K. (2002) Assessing abilities and capacities: Sensation. In C. A. Trombly & M. V. Radomski (Eds.). *Occupational therapy for physical dysfunction* (5th ed., pp. 159–175). Philadelphia: Lippincott, Williams & Wilkins.

Bobath, B. (1978). *Adult hemiplegia: Evaluation and treatment* (2nd ed.). London: Heinemann.

Bohannon, R., & Smith M. (1987). Interrater reliability of a modified Ashworth scale of muscle spasticity. *Physical Therapy, 87*, 206–207.

Borod, J. C., Fitzpatrick, P. M., Helm-Estabrooks, N., & Goodglass, H. (1989). The relationship between limb apraxia and the spontaneous use of communicative gesture in aphasia. *Brain and Cognition, 10*, 121–131.

Boyd, T. M., & Sautter, S. W. (1993). Route-finding: A measure of everyday executive functioning in the head-injured adult. *Applied Cognitive Psychology, 7*, 171–181.

Brannon, F. J., Foley, M. W., Starr, J. A., & Black, M. G. (1993). *Cardiopulmonary rehabilitation: Basic theory and application* (2nd ed.). Philadelphia: Davis.

Bransford, J. D., & Stein, B. S. (1984). *The ideal problem solver*. New York: Freeman.

Branswell, D., Hartry, A., Hoornbeek, S., Johansen, A., Johnson, L., Schultz, J., & Sohlberg, M. M. (1992). *The Profile of Executive Control System*. Puyallup, WA: Association for Neuropsychological Research and Development.

Brennan, J. (1959). Clinical method of assessing tonus and voluntary movement in hemiplegia. *British Medical Journal, 1*, 767–768.

Brooks, V. B. (1986). *The neural bases of motor control*. New York: Oxford University Press.

Bruce, M. G. (1993). Cognitive rehabilitation: Intelligence, insight, and knowledge. In C. B. Royeen (Ed.). *AOTA self-study series: Cognitive rehabilitation* (pp. 1–48). Rockville, MD: American Occupational Therapy Association.

Burgoon, J. K. (1994). Nonverbal signals. In M. L. Knapp & G. R. Miller (Eds.). *Handbook of interpersonal communication* (2nd ed., pp. 229–285). Thousand Oaks, CA: Sage.

Burke, J. P., & Kern, S. B. (1996). Is the use of life history and narrative in clinical practice reimbursable? Is it occupational therapy? *American Journal of Occupational Therapy, 50*, 389–392.

Caplan, B. (1987). Assessment of unilateral neglect: A new reading test. *Journal of Clinical and Experimental Neuropsychology, 9*, 359–364.

Center for Functional Assessment Research. (1990). *Guide for use of the Uniform Dataset for Medical Rehabilitation including the Functional Independence Measure (FIM)*. Buffalo: State University of New York.

Center for Outcome Measurement in Brain Injury. (2002). Scales. Available at: www.tbims.org/combi/list.html. Accessed August 2, 2002.

Chan, R. C. (2000). Attentional deficits in patients with closed head injury: A further study to the discriminative validity of the test of everyday attention. *Brain Injury, 14*, 227–236

Charmaz, K. (1991). *Good days, bad days: The self in chronic illness and time*. New Brunswick, NJ: Rutgers University Press.

Chen Sea, M. J., Henderson, A., & Cermack, S. A. (1993). Patterns of visual spatial inattention and their functional significance in stroke patients. *Archives of Physical Medicine and Rehabilitation, 74*, 355–360.

Cherney, L. R., Halper, A. S., Swasnica, C. M., Harvey, R. L., & Zhang, M. (2001). Recovery of functional status after right hemisphere stroke: Relationship with unilateral neglect. *Archives of Physical Medicine and Rehabilitation, 82*, 322–328.

Christiansen, C. H. (1999). Defining lives: Occupation as identity: An essay on competence, coherence, and the creation of meaning. [Eleanor Clarke Slagle Lecture]. *American Journal of Occupational Therapy, 53*, 547–558.

Chusid, J. G., & DeGroot, J. (1988). *Correlative neuroanatomy* (20th ed.). East Norwalk, CT: Appleton & Lange.

Compton, C. (1984). *A guide to 75 tests for special education*. Belmont, CA: Fearon Education.

Cooper, C. (2002). Hand impairments. In C. A. Trombly & M. V. Radomski (Eds.). *Occupational therapy for physical dysfunction* (5th ed., pp. 927–963). Philadelphia: Lippincott, Williams & Wilkins.

Copperman, L., Forwell, S., & Hugos, L. (2002). Neurodegenerative diseases. In C. A. Trombly & M. V. Radomski (Eds.). *Occupational therapy for physical dysfunction* (5th ed., pp. 885–908). Philadelphia: Lippincott, Williams & Wilkins.

Crawford, J. R., Sommerville, J., & Robertson, I. H. (1997). Assessing the reliability and abnormality of subtest differences on the Test of Everyday Attention. *British Journal of Clinical Psychology, 36*, 609–617.

Crosson, C., Barco, P. P., Velozo, C., Bolesta, M. M., Cooper, P. V., Werts, D., & Brobeck, T. C. (1989). Awareness and compensation in postacute head injury rehabilitation. *Journal of Clinical and Experimental Neuropsychology, 2*, 355–363.

Daniels, L. & Worthingham, C. (1986). *Muscle testing—Techniques of manual examination* (5th ed.). Philadelphia: Saunders.

Davidson, L., & Strauss, J. S. (1992). Sense of self in recovery from severe mental illness. *British Journal of Medical Psychology, 65*, 131–145.

Dehn, M. M. (1980). Rehabilitation of the cardiac patient: The effects of exercise. *American Journal of Nursing, 80*, 435–440.

Dehn, M. M., & Mullins, C. B. (1977). Physiologic effects and importance of exercise in patients with coronary artery disease. *Cardiovascular Medicine, 2*, 365–371, 377–387.

Deitz, T., Beeman, C., & Thorn, D. (1993). *Test of orientation for rehabilitation patients*. Tucson, AZ: Therapy Skill Builders.

Demaray, M. K., & Ruffalo, S. L. (1995). Social skills assessment: A comparative evaluation of six published rating scales. *School Psychology Review, 24*, 648–672.

DePaulo, B. M., & Friedman, H. S. (1998). Nonverbal communication. In D. T. Gilbert, S. T. Fiske, & G. Lindzey (Eds.). *The handbook of social psychology* (4th ed., vol. 2, pp. 3–40). New York: McGraw-Hill.

DiFablo, R. P., & Badke, M. B. (1990). Relationship of sensory organization to balance function in patients with hemiplegia. *Physical Therapy, 70*, 342–548.

Diller, L. (1993). Introduction to cognitive rehabilitation. In C. B. Royeen (Ed.). *AOTA self-study series: Cognitive rehabilitation* (pp. 1–36). Rockville, MD: American Occupational Therapy Association.

Doble, S. E., & Magill-Evans, J. (1992). A model of social interaction to guide occupational therapy practice. *Canadian Journal of Occupational Therapy, 59*, 141–150.

Dolecheck, J. B., & Schkade, J. (1999). The extent dynamic standing endurance is effected when CVA subjects perform personally meaningful activities rather than nonmeaningful tasks. *Occupational Therapy Journal of Research, 19*(1), 40–54.

Doninger, N. A., Bode, R. K., Heinemann, A. W., & Ambrose, C. (2000). Rating scale analysis of the Neurobehavioral Cognitive Status Examination. *Journal of Head Trauma Rehabilitation, 15*, 683–695.

Duncan, M. (1998). Interpretation and application. In J. Hinojosa & P. Kramer (Eds.). *Evaluation: Obtaining and interpreting data* (pp. 145–164). Bethesda, MD: American Occupational Therapy Association.

Dunn, W. (1991). Assessing sensory performance enablers. In C. Christiansen & C. Baum (Eds.). *Occupational therapy. Overcoming human performance deficits* (pp. 471–505). Thorofare, NJ: Slack

Dunn, W. (1998). Person-centered and contextually relevant evaluation. In J. Hinojosa & P. Kramer (Eds.). *Evaluation: Obtaining and interpreting data* (pp. 47–76). Bethesda, MD: American Occupational Therapy Association.

Dunn, W., Brown, C., & McGuigan, A. (1994). The ecology of human performance: A framework for considering the effect of context. *American Journal of Occupational Therapy, 48*, 595–607.

Dyche, G., & Johnson, D. (1991). Development and evaluation of CHIPASAT, an attentional test for children. II: Test-retest reliability and practice effect for a normal sample. *Perceptual Motor Skills, 72*, 563–572.

Ekman, P., & Friesen, W. V. (1969). The repertoire of nonverbal behavior: Categories, origins, usage, and coding. *Semiotica, 1*, 49–98.

Elazer, B., Itzkovich, M., & Katz, N. (1996). *Loewenstein Occupational Therapy Cognitive Assessment for geriatric population*. Pequannock, NJ: Maddak.

Estroff, S. E. (1989). Self, identity, and subjective experiences of schizophrenia: In search of the subject. *Schizophrenia Bulletin, 15*, 189–196.

Farber S. D. (1991b). Neuromotor dimensions of performance. In C. Christiansen & C. Baum (Eds.). *Occupational therapy. Overcoming human performance deficits* (pp. 259–282). Thorofare, NJ: Slack.

Farber, S. D. (1991a). Assessing neuromotor performance enablers. In C. Christiansen & C. Baum (Eds.). *Occupational therapy. Overcoming human performance deficits* (pp. 507–521). Thorofare, NJ: Slack.

Fess, E. E. (1995). Guidelines for evaluating assessment instruments. *Journal of Hand Therapy, 8*, 144–148.

Fine, S. (1993). Interaction between psychological variables and cognitive function. In C. B. Royeen (Ed.). *AOTA self-study series: Cognitive rehabilitation* (pp. 1–40). Rockville, MD: American Occupational Therapy Association.

Fisher, A. G. (1993a). Functional measures: Part 1: What is function, what should we measure and how should we measure it? *American Journal of Occupational Therapy, 46*, 183–185.

Fisher, A. G. (1993b). Functional measures: Part 2: Selecting the right test, minimizing the limitations. *American Journal of Occupational Therapy, 46*, 278–281.

Fisher, A., Kielhofner, G., Bernspang, B., Bryze, K., Doble, S., Englund, B., Salamy, M., & Simon, S. (1995). Skill in occupational performance. In G. Kielhofner (Ed.). *A model of human occupation* (2nd ed., pp. 113–137). Baltimore: Williams & Wilkins.

Fleming, J. M., Strong, J., & Ashton, R. (1996). Self-awareness of deficits in adults with traumatic brain injury: How best to measure? *Brain Injury, 10*, 1–15.

Flowers, K. R., Stephens-Chisar, J., LaStayo, P., & Grakante, B (2001). Intrarater reliability of a new method and for measuring passive supination and pronation. A preliminary study. *Journal of Hand Therapy, 14*(1), 30–35.

Folstein, M. F., Folstein, S. E., & McHugh, P. R. (1975). Mini-mental state: A practical method for grading the cognitive state of patients for the clinician. *Journal of Psychiatric Research, 12*, 189–198.

Forsyth, K., Salamy, M., Simon, S., & Kielhofner, G. (1998). *Assessment of Communication and Interaction Skills (Version 4.0 ed.)*. Chicago: Model of Human Occupation Clearinghouse, Department of Occupational Therapy, University of Illinois.

Fugl-Meyer, A., Jaasko, L., Leyman, I., Olson, S., & Steglind, S. (1975). The post-stroke hemiplegic patient: A method for evaluation of physical performance. *Scandinavian Journal of Rehabilitation Medicine, 7*, 13–31.

Gauthier, L., Dehaut, F., & Joanette, Y. (1989). The Bells Test: A quantitative and qualitative test for visual neglect. *International Journal of Clinical Neuropsychology, 11*, 49–54.

Ghuman, J. K., Peebles, C. D., & Ghuman, H. S. (1998). Review of social interaction measures in infants and preschool children. *Infants and Young Children, 11*(2), 21–44.

Gilfoyle, E. M., Grady, A. P., & Moore, J. C. (1981). *Children adapt*. Thorofare, NJ: Slack.

Gillam, J., & Barstow, I. (1997). Joint range of motion. In J. Van Deusen & D. Brunt (Eds.). *Assessment in occupational and physical therapy* (pp. 49–77). Philadelphia: Saunders.

Goffman, E. (1959). *The presentation of self in everyday life*. Garden City, NY: Anchor.

Golding, E. (1989). *The Middlesex Elderly Assessment of Mental State*. Bury St. Edmands, UK: Thames Valley Test.

Goldman-Rakic, P. S. (1993). Specification of higher cortical functions. *Journal of Head Trauma Rehabilitation, 8*, 13–23.

Goodglass, H., & Kaplan, E. (1972). *Assessment of aphasia and related disorders*. Philadelphia: Lea & Febiger.

Granger, C., Cotter, A. C., Brown, B. B., & Fiedler, R. C. (1993). Functional assessment scales: A study of persons after stroke. *Archives of Physical Medicine and Rehabilitation, 74*, 133–138.

Gregson, J., Leathley, M., Moore, P., Sharma, A., Smith, T., & Watkins, C. (1999). Reliability of the tone assessment scale and the Modified Ashworth Scale as clinical tools for assessing poststroke spasticity. *Archives of Physical Medicine and Rehabilitation*. 80, 1013–1016.

Grigorenko, E. L., & Sternberg, R. J. (1998). Dynamic testing. *Psychological Bulletin, 124*, 75–111.

Gronwall, D. M. A. (1977). Paced Auditory Serial Addition Task: A measure of recovery from concussion. *Perceptual and Motor Skills, 44*, 367–373.

Haaland, K. Y. (1993, March). *Assessment of limb apraxia*. Paper present at the AOTA Neuroscience Institute Treating Adults with Apraxia, Baltimore.

Hajek, V. E., Rutman, D. L., & Scher, H. (1989). Brief assessment of cognitive impairment in patients with stroke. *Archives of Physical Medicine and Rehabilitation, 70*, 114–117.

Hamilton, A., Balnare, R. & Adams, R. (1994). Grid strength testing reliability. *Journal of Hand Therapy, 7*(3), 163–70.

Hanks, R. A., Rapport, L. J., Millis, S. R., & Deshpande, S. A. (1999). Measures of executive functioning as predictors of functional ability and social integration in a rehabilitation sample. *Archives of Physical Medicine and Rehabilitation, 80*, 1030–1037.

Harrington, D. L., & Haaland, K. Y. (1992). Are some cognitive deficits specific to limb apraxia? *Brain, 115*, 857–874.

Hartman-Maeir, A., & Katz, N. (1995). Validity of the Behavioral Inattention Test (BIT): Relationships with functional tasks. *American Journal of Occupational Therapy, 49*, 507–516.

Heilman, K. M., & Rothi, L. J. (1985). Apraxia. In K. M. Heilman & E. Valenstein (Eds.). *Clinical neuropsychology* (pp. 131–150). New York: Oxford University Press.

Heilman, K. M., Rothi, L. G., & Valenstein, E. (1982). Two forms of ideomotor apraxia. *Neurology, 32*, 342–346.

Heilman, K. M., Watson, R. T., & Valenstein, E. (1985). Neglect and related disorders. In K. M. Heilman & E. Valenstein (Eds.). *Clinical neuropsychology* (pp. 400–426). New York: Oxford University Press.

Helm-Estabrooks, N. (1992). *Test of Oral and Limb Apraxia (TOLA)*. Chicago: Riverside.

Hinojosa, J., & Kramer, P. (1998). Evaluation—Where do we begin? In J. Hinojosa & P. Kramer (Eds.). *Evaluation: Obtaining and interpreting data*. Bethesda, MD: American Occupational Therapy Association.

Hinojosa, J., & Kramer, P. (1998b). *Evaluation: Obtaining and interpreting data*. Bethesda, MD: American Occupational Therapy Association.

Hislop, H., Montgomery, J., Connelly, B., & Daniels (1995). *Daniels and Worthingham's muscle testing: Techniques of manual examination*. Philadelphia: Saunders.

Hocking, C. (2001). Implementing occupation-based assessment. *American Journal of Occupational Therapy, 55*, 463–469.

Ishiai, S. (1994). Unilateral spatial neglect. *Neuropsychological Rehabilitation, 4*, 143–146.

Iyer, M. B., & Pedretti, L. W. (2001). Evaluation of sensation and treatment of sensory dysfunction. In L. W. Pedretti & M. B. Early (Eds.). *Occupational therapy: Practice skills for physical dysfunction* (5th ed., pp. 422–443). St. Louis: Mosby.

Jebsen, R. H., Taylor, N., Trieschmann, R. B., Trotter, M. J., & Howard, L. A. (1969). An objective and standardized test of hand function. *Archives of Physical Medicine and Rehabilitation, 50*, 311–319.

Jacobs, K. (1999). *Quick reference dictionary for occupational therapy* (2nd ed). Thorofare, NJ: Slack.

Josman, N. (1998). Reliability and validity of the Toglia Category Assessment Test. *Canadian Journal of Occupational Therapy, 66*, 33–42.

Josman, N., Berney, T., & Jarus, T. (2000a). Performance of children with and without traumatic brain injury on the Contextual Memory test (CMT). *Physical and Occupational Therapy in Pediatrics, 19*, 39–51.

Josman, N., Berney, T., & Jarus, T. (2000b). Evaluating categorization skills in children following severe brain injury. *Occupational Therapy Journal of Research, 20*, 241–255.

Katz, N., & Hartman-Maeir, A. (1998). Metacognition: The relationships of awareness and executive functions to occupational performance. In N. Katz (Ed.). *Cognition and occupation in rehabilitation* (pp. 323–342). Bethesda, MD: American Occupational Therapy Association.

Katz, N., & Parush, S. (2001, April). *Dynamic occupational therapy cognitive assessment for children*. Paper presented at the meeting of the American Occupational Therapy Association, Philadelphia.

Katz, N., Hartman-Maeir, A., Ring, H., & Soroker, N. (2000). Relationships of cognitive performance and daily function of clients following right hemisphere stroke: Predictive and ecological validity of the LOTCA battery. *Occupational Therapy Journal of Research, 20*, 3–17.

Katz, N., Itzkopvich, M., Averbuch, S., & Elazar, B. (1989). Lowenstein Occupational Therapy Cognitive Assessment (LOTCA) battery for brain-injured patients: Reliability and validity. *American Journal of Occupational Therapy, 43*, 184–192.

Katz, R. T., Rovai, G. P., Brait, C., & Rymer, W. Z. (1992). Objective quantification of spastic hypertonia: Correlation of clinical findings. *Archives of Physical Medicine and Rehabilitation, 73*, 339–347.

Katz, R., & Rymer, W. (1989). Spastic hypertonia: Mechanisms and measurement. *Archives of Physical Medicine and Rehabilitation, 70*, 144–155.

Kendall, F. P., McCreary, E. K., & Provance, P. G. (1993). *Muscles testing and function* (4th ed). Baltimore: Williams & Wilkins.

Kertesz, A. (1982). *Western Aphasia Battery*. San Antonio, TX: The Psychological Corporation.

Keyser, D. J., & Sweetland, R. C. (Eds.). (1984). *Test critiques*. Kansas City: Test Corporation of America.

Kielhofner, G. (1995). *A model of human occupation: Theory and application* (2nd ed.). Baltimore: Williams & Wilkins.

Kielhofner, G. (2002). Dimensions of doing. In G. Kielhofner (Ed.). *A model of human occupation* (3rd ed.). Philadelphia: Williams & Wilkins.

Kiernan, R. J., Mueller, J., Langston, J. W., & Von Dyke, C. (1987). The Neurobehavioral Cognitive Status Examination: A brief but differentiated approach to cognitive assessment. *Annals of Internal Medicine, 107*, 481–485.

Killingsworth, A. P., & Pedretti, L. W. (2001). Functional mobility assessment. In L. W. Pedretti & M. B. Early (Eds.). *Occupational therapy: Practice skills for physical dysfunction* (5th ed., pp. 279–284). St. Louis: Mosby.

King, T. (1987). A scale for more definitive measurement of hypertonicity. *Occupational Therapy Forum, 2*, 9–12.

King-Thomas, L., & Hacker, B. J. (Eds.). (1987). *A therapist's guide to pediatric assessment*. Boston: Little, Brown

Kramer, J. H., Kaplan, E., & Blusewicz, M. J. (1991). Visual hierarchical analysis of block design configural errors. *Journal of Clinical and Experimental Neuropsychology, 13*, 455–465.

Kramer, P., & Hinojosa, J. (1998). Theoretical basis of evaluation. In J. Hinojosa & P. Kramer (Eds.). *Evaluation: Obtaining and interpreting data* (pp. 17–28). Bethesda, MD: American Occupational Therapy Association.

LaBuda, J., & Lichtenberg, P. (1999). The role of cognition, depression, and awareness of deficit in predicting geriatric rehabilitation patients' IADL performance. *Clinical Neuropsychologist, 13*, 258–267.

Lamb, R. (1985). Manual muscle testing. In J. Rothstein (Ed.). *Measurement in physical therapy* (pp. 47–55). New York: Churchill Livingstone.

Lane, S. (1991). Motor planning. In C. B. Royeen (Ed.). *AOTA self-study series: Neuroscience Foundations of human performance* (pp. 1–36). Rockville, MD: American Occupational Therapy Association

LaStays, P., & Wheeler, D. (1994). Reliability of passive wrist flexion and extension goniometric measurements: A multicenter study. *Physical Therapy, 74*, 162–174.

Levin, H. S., O'Donnell, V. M., & Grossman, R. G. (1979). The Galveston Orientation and Amnesia Test: A practical scale to assess cognition after head injury. *Journal of Nervous and Mental Diseases, 167*, 675–684.

Lezak, M. D. (1995). *Neuropsychological assessment* (3rd ed.) New York: Oxford University Press.

Lunsford, B. R. (1978). Clinical indicators of endurance. *Physical Therapy, 58*, 704–709.

Magill-Evans, J., Koning, C., Cameron-Sadava, A., & Manyk, K. (1995). The child and adolescent social perception measure. *Journal of Nonverbal Behavior, 19*, 151–169.

Malec, J. F., Moessner, A. M., Kragness, M., & Lezak, M. D. (2000). Refining a measure of brain injury sequelae to predict postacute rehabilitation outcome: Rating scale analysis of the Mayo-Portland Adaptability Inventory. *Journal of Head Trauma Rehabilitation, 15*(1), 670–682.

Malec, J. F., Smigielski, J. S., & DePompolo, R. W. (1991). Goal attainment scaling and outcome measurement in postacute brain injury rehabilitation. *Archives of Physical Medicine and Rehabilitation, 72*, 138–143.

Manly, T., Robertson, I., Anderson, V., & Nimmo-Smith, I. (1999). *The Test of Everyday Attention for Children*. Bury St. Edmunds, UK: Thames Valley Test.

Mathiowetz, V., & Bass-Haugen, J. B. (2002). Assessing abilities and capacities: Motor behavior. In C. A. Trombly & C. Podolski (Eds.). *Occupational therapy for physical dysfunction* (5th ed., pp. 137–158). Philadelphia: Williams & Wilkins.

Mathiowetz, V., & Bass Haugen, J. B. (1995). Evaluation of motor behavior: Traditional and contemporary views. In C. A. Trombly (Ed.), *Occupational therapy for physical dysfunction* (4th ed.) (pp. 157–185). Philadelphia: Lippincott Williams & Wilkins.

Matson, J. L., & LeBlanc, L. A. (1999). Reliability of the Matson Evaluation of Social Skills in Individuals with Severe Retardation (MESSIER). *Behavior Modification, 23*, 647–662.

Mattingly, C., & Fleming, M. H. (1994). *Clinical reasoning: Forms of inquiry in a therapeutic practice*. Philadelphia: Davis.

Mattis, S., Jurica, P. J., & Leilten, C. L. (2001). Dementia Rating Scale-2 (DRS-2). San Antonio, TX: The Psychological Corporation.

McAdams, D. P. (1996). Personality, modernity, and the storied self: A contemporary framework for studying persons. *Psychological Inquiry, 7*, 295–321.

McCrae, R. R., & Costa, P. T., Jr. (1986). Clinical assessment can benefit from recent advances in personality psychology. *American Psychologist, 41*, 1001–1002.

Merrell, K. W. (1996). Social-emotional assessment in early childhood: The Preschool and Kindergarten Behavior Scales. *Journal of Early Intervention, 20*, 132–45.

Mesulam, M. (1985). Attention, confusional states and neglect. In: M. Mesulam (Ed.). *Principles of behavioral neurology* (pp. 125–168). Philadelphia: Davis.

Mielke, K., Novak, C. B., Mackinnon, S. E., & Feely, C. A. (1996). Hand sensibility measures used by therapists. *Annals of Plastic Surgeyr*, 36(3), 292–296.

Miller, R., Groher, M., Yorkston, K., & Rees, T (1988). Speech, language, swallowing and auditory rehabilitation. In J. DeLisa (Ed.). *Rehabilitation medicine principles and practice* (pp. 116–139). Philadelphia: Lippincott.

Minor, M. (1991). Assessing the physiological enablers of performance. In C. Christiansen & C. Baum (Eds.). *Occupational therapy. Overcoming human performance deficits* (pp. 455–468). Thorofare, NJ: Slack.

Mitchell, J. V (Ed.). (1985). *The ninth mental measurement yearbook*. Lincoln, NE: Buros Institute of Mental Measurements

Neistadt, M. E. (1989). Normal adult performance on constructional praxis training tasks. *American Journal of Occupational Therapy, 43*, 448–455.

Neistadt, M. E. (1992). The Rabideau Kitchen Evaluation—Revised: An assessment of meal preparation skill. *Occupational Therapy Journal of Research, 12*, 242–255.

Neistadt, M. E. (2000). *Occupational therapy evaluation for adults*. Baltimore: Lippincott, Williams & Wilkins.

Nelson, A., Fogel, B. S., & Faust, D. (1986). Bedside cognitive screening instruments: A critical assessment. *Journal of Nervous and Mental Disease, 174*, 73–83.

Norris, G., & Tate, R. L. (2000). The Behavioural Assessment of the Dysexecutive Syndrome (BADS): Ecological, concurrent and construct validity. *Neuropsychological Rehabilitation, 10*, 33–45.

Okkema, K. (1993). *Cognition and perception in the stroke patient*. Gaithersburg, Maryland: Aspen.

Oxford, K. L. (2000). Elbow positioning for maximum grip performance. *Journal of Hand Therapy, 13*(1), 33–36.

Pedretti, L. W. (2001a). Joint range of motion. In L. W. Pedretti & M. B. Early (Eds.). *Occupational therapy: Practice skills for physical dysfunction* (5th ed., pp. 285–315). St. Louis: Mosby.

Pedretti, L. W. (2001b). Muscle strength. In L. W. Pedretti & M. B. Early (Eds.). *Occupational therapy: Practice skills for physical dysfunction* (5th ed., pp. 316–359). St. Louis: Mosby.

Pentland, B. (1991). Body language in Parkinson's disease. *Behavioural Neurology, 4*, 181–187.

Poizner, H., Mack, L., Verfaellie, M., Rothi, L. J., & Heilman, K. M. (1990). Three dimensional computer graphic analysis of apraxia: Neuronal representation of learned movement. *Brain, 113*, 85–101.

Poole, J. L. (1998). Effect of apraxia on the ability to learn on-handed shoe tying. *Occupational Therapy Journal of Research, 18*, 99–104.

Poole, J. L. (2000). A comparison of limb praxis abilities of persons with developmental dyspraxia and adult onset apraxia. *Occupational Therapy Journal of Research, 20*, 106–120.

Preston, L. A. (2001). Motor control. In L. W. Pedretti & M. B. Early (Eds.). *Occupational therapy: Practice skills for physical dysfunction* (5th ed., pp. 360–385). St. Louis: Mosby.

Prigatano, G. P. (1986). *Neuropsychological rehabilitation after brain injury*. Baltimore: Johns Hopkins University Press.

Rao, S. M., Leo, G. J., Bernardin, L., & Unverzagt, F. (1991). Cognitive dysfunction in multiple sclerosis. *Neurology, 41*, 684–691.

Raskin, S. A., & Mateer, C. A. (2000). *Neuropsychological management of mild traumatic brain injury*. New York: Oxford University Press.

Richards, L. G., Olson, B., & Palmiter-Thomas, P. (1996). How forearm position affects grip strength. *American Journal of Occupational Therapy*, 50(2), 133–138.

Riddle, D. (1992). Measurement of accessory motion: Critical issues and related concepts. *Physical Therapy, 72*, 865–874.

Riggio, R. E., Widaman, K. F., & Friedman, H. S. (1985). Actual and perceived emotional sending and personality correlates. *Journal of Nonverbal Behavior, 9*, 69–83.

Ritchie, K., & Ledesert, B. (1991). The measurement of incapacity in the severely demented elderly: The validation of a behavioural assessment scale. *International Journal of Geriatric Psychiatry, 6*, 217–226.

Rizzolatti, G., & Berti, A. (1993). Neural mechanisms of spatial neglect. In I. H. Robertson & J. C. Marshall (Eds.). *Unilateral neglect: Clinical and experimental studies* (pp. 87–105). Hillsdale, NJ: Erlbaum.

Robertson, I. H., Ward, T., Ridgeway, V., & Nimmo-Smith, I. (1994). *The Test of Everyday Attention (TEA)*. Bury St. Edmunds, UK: Thames Valley Test.

Robertson, L., & Lamb, M. R. (1991). Neuropsychological contributions to theories of part/whole organization. *Cognitive Psychology, 23*, 299–230.

Rockwood, K., Joyce, B., & Stolee, P. (1997). Use of goal attainment scaling in measuring clinically important change in cognitive rehabilitation patients. *Journal of Clinical Epidemiology, 50*, 581–588.

Ross, L. (1977). The intuitive psychologist and his shortcomings: Distortions in the attribution process. In L. Berkowitz (Ed.). *Advances in experimental social psychology* (vol. 10, pp. 173–220). San Diego, CA: Academic Press.

Rothi, L. G., Heilman, K. M., & Watson, R. T. (1985). Pantomime, comprehension and ideomotor apraxia. *Journal of Neurology, Neurosurgery, and Psychiatry, 48*, 207–210.

Roy, E. A. (1978). Apraxia: A new look at an old syndrome. *Journal of Human Movement Studies, 4*, 191–210.

Royeen, C. B., & Richards, J. (1998). Non-standardized assessments. In J. Hinojosa & P. Kramer (Eds.). *Evaluation: Obtaining and interpreting data* (pp. 107–125). Bethesda, MD: American Occupational Therapy Association.

Rustad, R. A., DeGroot, T. L., Jungkunz, M. L., Freeberg, K. S., Borowick, L. G., & Wanttie, A. M. (1993). *The Cognitive Assessment of Minnesota*. Tucson, AZ: Therapy Skill Builders.

Sabari, J. (1997). Motor control. In J. Van Deusen & D. Brunt (Eds.). *Assessment in occupational and physical therapy* (pp. 249–272). Philadelphia: Saunders.

Sattler, J. M. (1982). *Assessment of children's intelligence and special abilities* (2nd ed.). Boston: Allyn & Bacon

Sbordone, R. J. (1996). Ecological validity: Some critical issues for the neuropsychologist. In R. J. Sbordone and C. J. Long (Eds.). *Ecological validity of neuropsychological testing* (pp. 15–41). Delray Beach, FL: St. Lucie.

Schlenker, B. E. (1984). Identities, identifications, and relationships. In V. J. Derlega (Ed.). *Communication, intimacy, and close relationships* (pp. 71–104). Orlando, FL: Academic.

Schwartz, M. F., Mayer, N. H., Fitzpatrick-DeSalme, E. J., & Montogomery, M. W. (1993). Cognitive theory and the study of everyday action disorders after brain damage. *Journal of Head Trauma Rehabilitation, 8*, 59–72.

Sehgal, N. & McGuire, J. (1998). Beyond Ashworth. Electrophysiologic quantification of spasticity. *Physical Medicine and Rehabilitation Clinics of North America*, 9(4), 949–979.

Shallice, T., Burgess, P. (1991). Deficits in strategy application following frontal lobe damage in man. *Brain, 114*, 727–741.

Simmonds, M. (1997). Muscle strength. In J. Van Deusen & D. Brunt (Eds.). *Assessment in occupational and physical therapy* (pp. 27–48). Philadelphia: Saunders.

Smidt, G., & Roger M. (1982). Factors contributing to the regulation and clinical assessment of muscle strength. *Physical Therapy, 62*, 1283–1290.

Sohlberg, M. M., White, O., Evans, E., & Mateer, C. (1992). An investigation of the effects of prospective memory training. *Brain Injury, 6*, 139–154

Squire, L. R. (1992). Declarative and nondeclarative memory: Multiple brain systems supporting learning and memory. *Journal of Cognitive Neuroscience, 4*, 232–243.

Squire, L. R., & Butters, N. (Eds.). (1984). *Neuropsychology of memory*. Hillsdale, NJ: Erlbaum.

Squire, L. R., & Zouzounis, J. A. (1988). Self-ratings of memory dysfunction: Different findings in depression and amnesia. *Journal of Clinical and Experimental Neuropsychology, 10*, 727–738.

Stone, M. H., & Wright, B. D. (1980). *Knox Cube Test*. Chicago: Stoelting.

Stringer, A. Y. (1996). *A guide to adult neuropsychological diagnosis*. Philadelphia: Davis.

Strong, S. (1998). Meaningful work in supportive environments: Experiences with the recovery process. *American Journal of Occupational Therapy, 52*, 31–38.

Sunderland, A., & Harris, J. (1984). Failures in everyday life following sever head injury. *Journal of Clinical Neuropsychology, 6*, 127–142.

Sweetland, R. C., & Keyser, D J. (1986). *Tests*. Kansas City: Test Corporation of America.

Teng, E., & Chui, H. (1987). The Modified Mini-Mental State (3MS) Examination. *Journal of Clinical Psychiatry, 48*, 314–318.

Titus, M. N. D., Gall, N. G., Yerxa, E. J., Roberson, T. A., & Mack, W. (1991). Correlation of perceptual performance and activities of daily living in stroke patients. *American Journal of Occupational Therapy, 45*, 410–418.

Toglia, J. P. & Finkelstein, N. (1991). *Manual for the Dynamic Visual Processing Assessment*. Unpublished manuscript.

Toglia, J. P. (1989a). Approaches to cognitive assessment of the brain injured adult: Traditional methods and dynamic investigation. *Occupational Therapy Practice, 1*, 36–57.

Toglia, J. P. (1989b). Visual perception of objects: An approach to assessment and intervention. *American Journal of Occupational Therapy, 43*(9), 587–595.

Toglia, J. P. (1991a). Generalization of treatment: A multicontext approach to cognitive perceptual impairment in adults with brain injury. *American Journal of Occupational Therapy, 45*, 505–516.

Toglia, J. P. (1991b). Unilateral visual inattention: Multidimensional components. *Occupational Therapy Practice, 3*(1), 18–34.

Toglia, J. P. (1993a). Attention and memory. In C. B. Royeen (Ed.). *AOTA self-study series: Cognitive rehabilitation* (pp. 1–72). Rockville, MD: American Occupational Therapy Association.

Toglia, J. P. (1993b). *The Contextual Memory Test*. Tucson, AZ: Therapy Skill Builders.

Toglia, J. P. (1994). *Toglia Category Assessment (TCA)*. Paquannock, NJ: Maddak.

Toglia, J. P. (1996a). *Application of the multicontext treatment approach to disorders in attention, memory and executive function* [Supplement manual to workshop held at Rehabilitation Institute of Chicago]. New York: Author.

Toglia, J. P. (1996b). A multicontext approach to cognitive rehabilitation [Supplement manual to workshop held at New York Hospital-Cornell Medical Center]. New York: Author.

Toglia, J. P. (1998). A dynamic interactional approach to cognitive rehabilitation. In N. Katz (Ed.). *Cognition and occupation in rehabilitation* (pp. 5–50). Bethesda, MD: American Occupational Therapy Association.

Toglia, J. P., & Golisz, K. (1990). *Cognitive rehabilitation: Group games and activities*. Tucson, AZ: Therapy Skill Builders.

Toglia, J. P., & Kirk, U. (2000). Understanding awareness deficits following brain injury. *NeuroRehabilitation, 15*, 57–70.

Toglia, J. P. (2001, April). The multicontext approach to cognitive rehabilitation. Paper presented at the Educational Special Interest Section Workshop at the meeting of the American Occupational Therapy Association, Philadelphia.

Trombly, C. A. & Podolski, C. R. (2002). Assessing abilities and capacities: Range of motion, strength and endurance. In C. A. Trombly & M. V. Radomski (Eds.), *Occupational therapy for physical dysfunction* (5th ed., pp. 47–136). Philadelphia: Lippincott, Williams, & Wilkins.

Trower, P., Bryant, B., & Argyle, M. (1978). *Social skills and mental health*. London: Methuen.

Tzuriel, D. (2000). Dynamic assessment of young children: Educational and intervention perspectives. *Educational Psychology Review, 12*, 385–435.

Unsworth, C. (1999). Introduction to cognitive and perceptual dysfunction: Theoretical approaches to therapy. In C. Unsworth (Ed.). *Cognitive and perceptual dysfunction* (pp. 1–41). Philadelphia: Davis.

VanDeusen, J., & Foss, J. (1997). Sensory processing. In J. Van Deusen & D. Brunt (Eds.). *Assessment in occupational and physical therapy* (pp. 295–301). Philadelphia: Saunders.

Warren, M. (1981). Relationship of constructional apraxia and body scheme disorders to dressing performance in CVA. *American Journal of Occupational Therapy, 35*, 431–442.

Warren, M. (1991). Strategies for sensory and neuromotor remediation. In C. Christiansen & C. Baum (Eds.). *Occupational therapy. Overcoming human performance deficits* (pp. 633–662). Thorofare, NJ: Slack.

Warren, M. (1993). A hierarchical model for evaluation and treatment of visual perceptual dysfunction in adult acquired brain injury, Part 1. *American Journal of Occupational Therapy, 47*, 42–54.

Wei, S., McQuade, K., & Smidt, G. (1993). Three dimensional joint range of motion measurements from skeletal coordinate data. *Journal of Physical Therapy, 18*, 687–691.

Wheatley, C. J. (2001). Evaluation and treatment of perceptual and perceptual motor deficits. In L. W. Pedretti & M. B. Early (Eds.). *Occupational therapy: Practice skills for physical dysfunction* (5th ed., pp. 444–455). St. Louis: Mosby.

Willer, B., Rosenthal, M., Kreutzer, J., Gordon, W., & Rempel, R. (1993). Assessment of community reintegration following rehabilitation for traumatic brain injury. *Journal of Head Trauma Rehabilitation, 8*, 75–87.

Williams, S., & Bloomer, J. (1987). *Bay Area Functional Performance Evaluation (BaFPE)*. Pequannock, NJ: Maddak.

Wilmore, J. H., & Costill, D. L. (1999). *Physiology of Sport and Exercise* (2nd ed.). Champaign, IL: Human Kinetics.

Wilson, B., Alderman, N., Burgess, P., Emslie, H., & Evans, J. (1996). *Behavioural Assessment of the Dysexecutive Syndrome*. Bury St. Edmunds, UK: Thames Valley Test.

Wilson, B., Clare, L., Cockburn, J., Baddeley, A., Tate, R., & Watson, P. (1999). *The Rivermead Behavioral Memory Test—Extended Version*. Bury St. Edmunds, UK: Thames Valley Test.

Wilson, B., Cockburn, J., & Baddeley, A. (1985). *The Rivermead Behavioral Memory Test*. Bury St. Edmunds, UK: Thames Valley Test.

Wilson, B., Cockburn, J., & Halligan, P. (1987). *Behavioral Inattention Test (BIT)*. Bury St. Edmunds, UK: Thames Valley Test.

Wilson, B., Evans, J., Emslie, H., Alderman, N., & Burgess, P. (1998). The development of an ecologically valid test for assessing patients with a dysexecutive syndrome. *Neuropsycholigical Rehabilitation, 8*, 213–228.

Wilson, B., Ivani-Chalian, R., Besag, F. M., & Bryant, T. (1993). Adapting the Rivermead Behavioural Memory Test for use with children aged 5 to 10 years. *Journal of Clinical and Experimental Neuropsychology, 15*, 474–486.

Woodson, A. M. (2002). Stroke. In C. A. Trombly & M. V. Radomski (Eds.), Occupational therapy for physical dysfunction (5th ed.) pp. 817–853.

World Health Organization. (2001). International classification of functioning, disability, and health. Geneva, Switzerland: Author.

Worley, J., Bennett, W., Miller, G., Miller, M., Walker, B., & Harmon, C. (1991). Reliability of three clinical measures of muscle tone in the shoulders and wrists of post-stroke patients. *American Journal of Occupational Therapy, 45*, 50–58.

York, C. D., & Cermak, S. A. (1995). Visual perception and praxis in adults after stroke. *American Journal of Occupational Therapy, 49*, 543–550.

Zoltan, B. (1996). *Vision, perception, and cognition: A manual for the evaluation and treatment of the neurologically impaired adult* (3rd ed.). Thorofare, NJ: Slack.

CHAPTER 26

EVALUATION OF PERFORMANCE CONTEXTS

JEAN COLE SPENCER

MEANINGS AND SIGNIFICANCE OF CONTEXT

The occupational therapy practice framework identifies contexts as sources of facilitators or barriers to performance in areas of occupation (American Occupational Therapy Association [AOTA], in press). The framework addresses physical, social, cultural, virtual, and spiritual contexts, each of which is examined in this chapter. The term *context* is derived from the Latin word *contexere*, meaning "to weave together," suggesting a holistic view of "the whole situation, background, or environment relevant to a particular event, personality, or creation" (Neufeldt et al., 1994, p. 301.)

Emphasis on the context of occupational engagement represents a shift in perspective away from the historical view that problems of individuals with disabilities are solely the result of some defect or malfunction within the person. In the last several decades of the twentieth century, a number of social movements contested this individual-centered view of disability, asserting that the environment is at least as powerful a determinant of the lives and functioning of people with disabilities as their individual impairments. This change in perspective began with the normalization movement (Wolfensberger, 1972), the independent living movement (DeJong, 1979), and the movement for inclusion of children with disabilities in regular schools (Gliedman & Roth, 1980). A conceptualization of human functioning based on the interaction between people and their environmental contexts has been incorporated in the new International Classification of Functioning, Disability, and Health of the World Health Organization (WHO; 2001). A person–environment perspective is also reflected in many practice models in occupational therapy, as exemplified by the Model of Human Occupation (Kielhofner, 2002), the ecology of human performance (Dunn, Brown, & McGuigan, 1994), the Canadian person–environment–occupation model (Law, Cooper, Strong, Stewart, Rigby, & Letts, 1996), and occupational adaptation (Schkade & Schultz, 1992).

FOUR TRADITIONS OF EVALUATION: ASSESSMENT TOOLS IN THE CONTEXT OF THEORY AND RESEARCH

The purpose of this chapter is to present a variety of approaches and tools that can be used to evaluate aspects of context. Rather than providing an exhaustive list of all available tools, I examine connections between selected tools and the contexts from which they came. This involves examining theoretical perspectives that identify factors to which therapists should pay attention as well as describing methods by which various domains of context can be studied. The focus is on conceptualization of evaluation goals and strategies rather than on critiques of the measurement properties of specific tools, which are available elsewhere (Asher, 1996; Forer, 1996; Letts, Law, Rigby, Cooper, Stewart, & Strong, 1994; Plake & Impara, 2001). The assessments cited have been selected to illustrate four major traditions of evaluation, which have contrasting purposes and methods (Table 26-1).

CONTEXTUAL DOMAINS

The occupational therapy practice framework (AOTA, in press) defines five domains of context:

- *Physical contexts:* The nonhuman aspects of contexts, including accessibility to and performance within environments that have natural terrain, plants, animals, buildings, furniture, objects, tools, and/or devices.
- *Social contexts:* The availability and expectations of significant individuals, such as a spouse or partner, friends, and caregivers, including larger social groups that are influential in establishing norms, role expectations, and social routines.
- *Cultural contexts:* The customs, beliefs, activity patterns, behavior standards, and expectations accepted by the society of which the individual is a member, including political aspects, such as laws, that affect access to resources or affirm personal rights.
- *Virtual contexts:* The environments in which individuals or objects are not actually present in the immediate physical space but that are experienced through the senses by electronic means. Virtual reality, a related term, is defined as a realistic simulation of an environment, including three-dimensional graphics created by a computer system and interactive software and hardware.
- *Spiritual contexts:* The fundamental orientation of a person's life, that which inspires and motivates the individual, including beliefs about the ultimate issues of life and death, the meaning and purpose of individual and collective existence, and a moral code of responsibility to self and others that guides day-to-day behavior. It also includes processes and practices that foster presence, transcendence, self-mastery, and a deep connection with self, others, and the earth as well as with the past, present, and future and with a higher cosmic reality. Secular spiritual contexts involve philosophical literature, principles, and shared purposes; religious spiritual contexts involve doctrines, myths, ethics, rituals, experiences, and institutions.

TABLE 26–1 **THE FOUR MAJOR TRADITIONS OF EVALUATION**

Type	Description
Experimental tradition	Based on performance of standardized tasks; high degree of examiner control over testing situation
Behavior observation	Documentation of natural behavior in real-world settings, usually on a time-sampling basis
Survey tradition	Use of written or oral questionnaires to document self-reported practices or opinions of respondents
Qualitative tradition	Participant observation and interviews with open-ended questions designed to capture an insider's view of activity and its meaning to participants

CONTEXTUAL SCALES

Each of these environmental domains is examined at different levels, or scales, moving from those closest to the individual to those that are more remote. These scales are defined in ways that make sense as recognized entities by individuals who inhabit environments at each level. The concept of environmental scale is important not only because it draws attention to different kinds of influences on occupational engagement but also because it has important implications for who controls the environment and, therefore, the processes by which environmental change might occur.

- *Immediate scale contexts:* Include surroundings that are in close and direct contact with the individual (e.g., a computer workstation) or that involve direct personal interactions (e.g., between caregiver and care recipient). Typically evaluation at this level involves close examination of a single occupation. Clients or their advocates are usually able to exert relatively direct influence to make changes in these contexts.
- *Proximal scale contexts:* Include surroundings at the level of a single behavior setting (e.g., kitchen, office, playground, or occupational therapy clinic), which can typically be traversed by walking or simple mobility devices. Such settings usually contain interactive occupations of several individuals. Clients may have substantial influence in making decisions about these contexts, but these settings are often shared with other individuals who also influence decisions.
- *Community scale contexts:* Include geographic neighborhoods or communities as defined and known personally by inhabitants, that are often traversed by more complex modes of transportation than required in single behavior settings, and that typically contain the overall constellation of occupations that are part of an individual's usual daily routine. Clients may have difficulty altering these contexts, but they can choose to move to a more compatible environment or participate in social processes to advocate for community change.
- *Societal scale contexts:* Include public policies, widely held beliefs and attitudes, and major social institutions (e.g., transportation, health care, and educational systems). Clients have little direct control over these contexts, but they can participate actively in social or public policy processes to advocate for change at this level.

PHYSICAL CONTEXTS

Theories that have shaped views of physical aspects of contexts in occupational therapy have come both from social science disciplines, such as ecological psychology and geography, and from applied fields, such as architecture and urban planning. Some of these fields are concerned with how physical settings shape naturally occurring activity and social interaction and with the symbolic meaning attached to places. Others are concerned with how buildings and public spaces should be designed to facilitate movement of people and performance of activities or how objects and tools should be designed to make them easier to use (Fig. 26-1).

Immediate

Studies of immediate scale physical contexts include research in ergonomics and industrial design, which typically use experimental methods to examine the usability of particular tools and equipment. Such methods are frequently employed for work capacity evaluation (Burke, 1998; International Labour Office, 1996; Jacobs, 1999). The Baltimore Therapeutic Equipment (BTE) Work Simulator exemplifies tools used in such evaluations (Neimeyer, Matheson, & Carlton, 1989). The BTE Work Simulator evaluates upper extremity function by using alternative devices, such as a knob, screwdriver, lever, or steering wheel, attached to an electrically controlled brake that permits adjustment of resistance to measure the amount of force produced during simulated tasks. This equipment allows practitioners to determine whether clients have the capabilities to return to work tasks they have done previously or to perform simulated tasks that may have lesser demands. If increased strength is required for task performance, the simulator allows therapists to pinpoint specific upper extremity areas in which improved performance is needed.

Experimental methods also underlie rehabilitation engineering evaluations of how individuals with disabilities perform when using assistive technology, such as seating and positioning equipment, various kinds of switches, or alternative computer interface technologies. Cook and Hussey (1995) developed a comprehensive framework for organizing an assistive technology evaluation process. This tool is based on a human activity assistive technology model that includes the human, an activity, assistive technology, and the context in which the client seeks to function. A background-information questionnaire documents demographic and referral information, medical and health information, sensory and perceptual abilities, activities of daily living (ADL), social interaction, learning and behavior, functional abilities, motor skills, mobility and positioning, and communication skills. Evaluation forms provide standardized tasks for evaluating (1) motor abilities (grasp, hand range, body part movement and control, foot range, and head control), and (2) symbol location, type, and size. The framework also provides the Communication Prosthesis Payment Review Summary and Seating/Wheeled Mobility Payment Review Summary. With this holistic evaluation process, practitioners can consider assistive technology as an extrinsic enabler that allows an individual to maximize efficient performance of activities and can also provide rationale for the selection of particular devices to justify reimbursement.

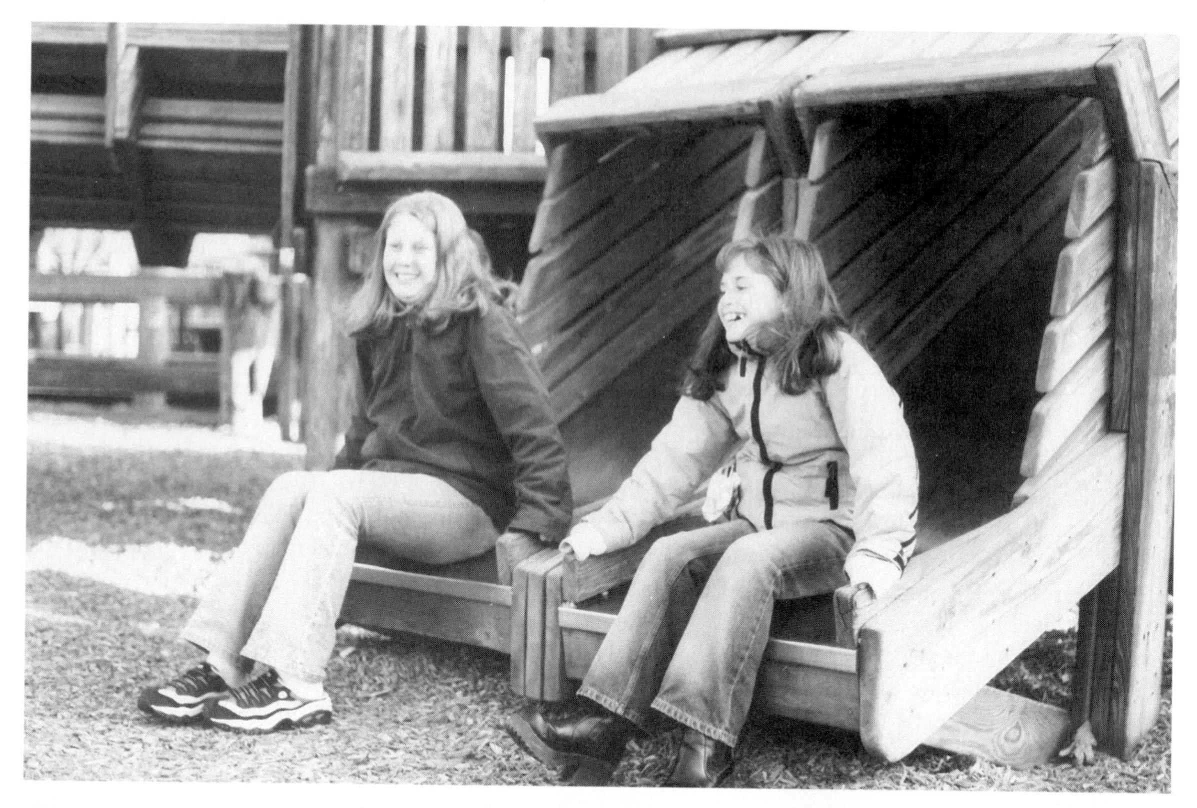

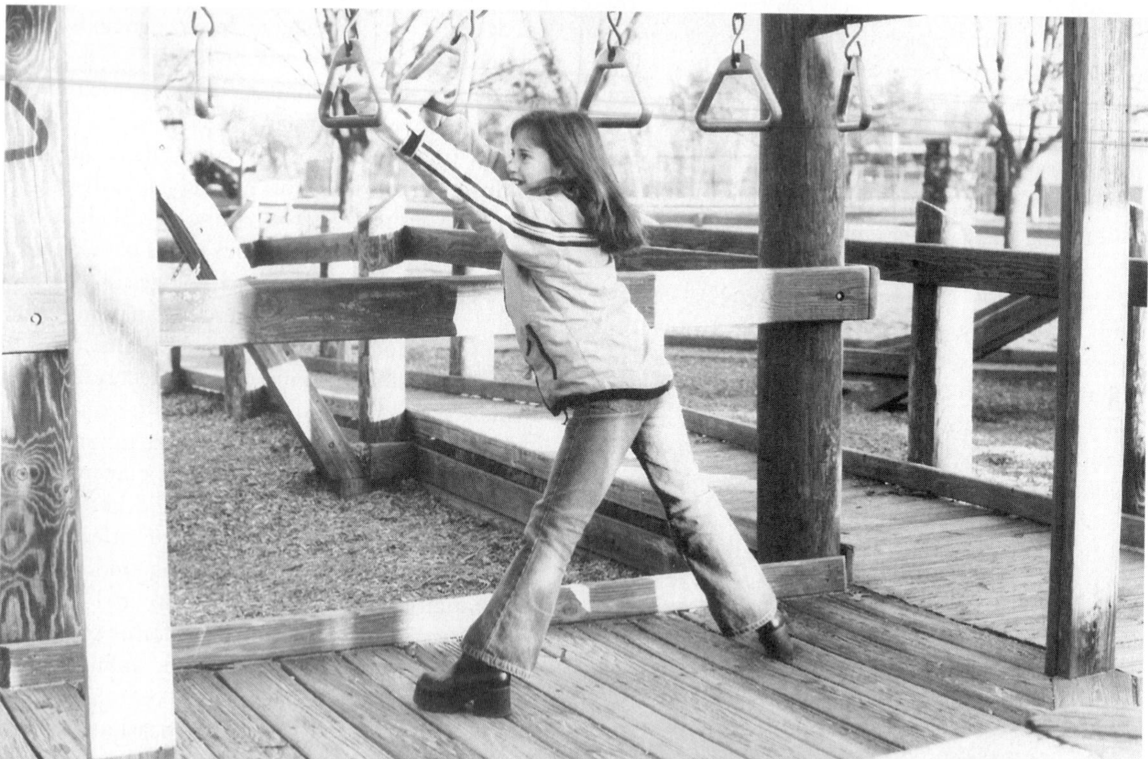

FIGURE 26–1. Children playing at an adapted community playground. The ramps and boardwalk provide access for all children. **(A)** Two girls sitting on the end of a slide. **(B)** Child reaching for rings. (Courtesy of E. Cohn.)

In contrast to an experimental approach, naturalistic behavior observation methods have been used to document how clients use naturally occurring objects and spaces. This approach is exemplified by a history of studies of free play of infants and children with objects in home and playground settings. Studies in the behavior observation tradition have used structured behavior checklists and time-sampling procedures to document manipulation of a variety of toys and objects, allowing therapists to make inferences about the development of hand skills and other more abstract capabilities, such as understanding cause-and-effect relations (Yarrow, Rubenstein, & Pederson, 1975).

The behavior observation approach has been used in occupational therapy to develop a format for studying fine motor tasks in classroom settings. The Fine Motor Task Assessment groups tasks into four categories (McHale & Cermak, 1992): fine motor tasks (require major use of hands), integrated fine motor tasks (fine motor and other academic tasks occur simultaneously), other academic tasks (frequent use of hands not required), and nonacademic activities (functional or transitional rather than instructional). The duration of time spent on specific tasks is recorded during an established observation period. Fine motor tasks are described in detail (academic subject, precise task, materials used), which facilitates task analysis in terms of kinds of tools required, degree of student control, and other dimensions. This assessment provides an in-depth picture of the kinds of interactions expected of children and the tools and objects in their immediate physical environment, which can be used by practitioners to cultivate required skills in children or to consult with teachers on how to make environmental demands more manageable for children with fine motor problems.

In addition to studies focusing on the effect of physical environments on task performance, symbolic aspects of immediate scale physical contexts have also received some attention in occupational therapy. Bates, Spencer, Young, and Rintala (1993) used in-depth ethnographic interviews and chart review to examine the process by which an iron worker with a spinal cord injury adapted during his rehabilitation to use of a wheelchair, which would become a lasting part of his immediate physical environment. Initially, this young man hated the wheelchair, thinking of it as a symbol of disability and helplessness, which was in dramatic contrast to the views of the health-care staff, who considered it a useful tool for mobility. This study, which identified both pragmatic and emotional adaptation processes, indicated that assistive technology may have meanings to users that differ from those of occupational therapy practitioners.

A similar difference in meanings of assistive devices was reported by Covington (1998), who discussed his initial aversion and later acceptance of a white cane, needed because of his visual impairment. Research indicates that individuals with disabilities frequently discard assistive devices for a variety of reasons, ranging from lack of acceptability to failure of the device to improve their functional abilities (Brooks, 1991; Garber & Gregorio, 1990). Attention to the meaning of devices and equipment to clients can have important implications for their acceptance and use over time.

Proximal

In studying physical environments of proximal scale behavior settings, therapists have frequently turned their attention toward wheelchair accessibility of home and work settings. Much of the current research in this area is guided by the concept of universal design, which is based on the premise that ordinary physical spaces and objects can be designed to be usable by people with a wide range of capabilities (Mace, Hardie, & Place, 1991). Several accessibility checklists have been developed for use in home settings, such as the Home Modification Workbook (Adaptive Environments Center, 1988) and the Source Book (Kelly & Snell, 1989). Others have been developed to address workplace or public settings, such as the Workplace Workbook (Mueller, 1990) and the Americans with Disabilities Act Accessibility Guidelines Checklist for Buildings and Facilities (U.S. Architectural and Transportation Barriers Compliance Board, 1992).

In occupational therapy, accessibility and safety issues in home environments have commonly been addressed through ADL assessments to help rehabilitation clients anticipate how they will be able to perform specific self-care or housekeeping activities in their home bathrooms or kitchens (Christiansen, 1994). Frequently, such assessments are performed in clinic settings designed to simulate the kitchen or bathroom spaces of clients' homes. However, the assumption that performance in a simulated setting is a good indicator of performance in the real-world proximal environment of the home has been questioned (Park, Fisher, & Velozo, 1994). With the trend toward home health care and community-based practice, occupational therapists have often been conducting such assessments directly in clients' homes. Some tools for home use address safety as well as accessibility, as exemplified by the Safety Assessment of Function and the Environment for Rehabilitation (SAFER).

The SAFER was developed by Community Occupational Therapists and Associates in Toronto, Canada to evaluate home safety for elders (Oliver, Blathwayt, Brackley, & Tamaki, 1993). Safety is broadly conceptualized to include personal safety, peace of mind, freedom from risk, and access to emergency services and health care. This tool evaluates risks in various room of the house; general risks, such as fire hazards; and safety issues in how the client performs self-care and household tasks. It also examines the client's potential for wandering and the use of memory aids and identifies how help could be summoned. The assessment of these domains in home-based consultation fosters the development of goals for improving environmental safety and supportiveness.

Historically, many ADL assessments have been developed by specific facilities or agencies rather than a few well-developed standardized assessment tools that are widely used. An exception is The Enabler, which has been systematically evaluated by occupational therapists in homes of clients in Sweden, demonstrating good usability and reliability (Iwarsson & Isacsson, 1996). This tool first documents functional limitations and use of assistive devices by a particular individual and then documents a list of potential environmental barriers inside and outside the home, such as irregular walking surfaces. These two checklists are then combined in a cross-cutting matrix to identify potential problems, known problems, severe problems, and impossibility of use for a particular client. Use of this tool in home-based consultation permits matching client capabilities and environmental features to allow successful occupational engagement.

Proximal physical contexts of work settings have been extensively studied in the field of ergonomics, a growing area of practice in occupational therapy (Jacobs, 1999). Assessments in this area are exemplified by the Risk Factor Checklist developed by the National Safety Council (1998). This tool identifies specific workplace risks, including repetitive movements, lifting requirements, pushing and pulling requirements, carrying requirements, awkward postures, use of power tools, pressure points, maintenance of same position, environmental features (cold/hot, light/glare, and vibration), continuous keyboard use, and incentive work and level of worker control over the job pace. These risks are weighted according to how much time during the day they are experienced by workers. The format also prompts identification of changes to reduce specific risks that could be recommended by practitioners in workplace consultation.

Although much of the research on proximal scale physical contexts has used concrete observations of activity performance, some authors have recognized the symbolic importance of behavior settings for users. For example, Bates (1994) cited the circumstances of a woman who chose not to make her recently redecorated bathroom wheelchair accessible, despite the fact that it would have made self-care tasks much easier. This choice reflected her personal value of appearance over function. Geographer Rowles (1991) eloquently urged practitioners to recognize the meaning of place as a component of occupational therapy, a view that is consistent with the growing emphasis on the importance of the meaning of occupations as well as their performance requirements (Trombly, 1995).

Architect Lifchez (1987) addressed these issues when examining how designers of the built environment can come to understand what he called the "quality of experience" of individuals with disabilities. Lifchez's Interview-in-Place is based on qualitative methodology. Clients are asked to select a place (a room at home, cafe, workplace) in which they feel comfortable speaking about that place as a physical and social setting. The setting itself generates a variety of topics for discussion: "What physical and social factors make the setting noteworthy for you?" "How do you feel being in this setting and going to and from it?" Additional questions allow generalization to other spaces: "What places outside home do you regularly visit?" "How do you get there?" "What sorts of activities do you need help with in those settings?" "What places would you most like to visit?" "What prevents you from going there?" This methodology is based on the premise that being in clients' commonly used settings prompts them to articulate personal environmental meanings and priorities in ways that are not evoked in the foreign setting of an architect's office or occupational therapy clinic. This premise has been supported by Lifchez's research on interactions between architecture students and people with physical disabilities. This assessment approach could be particularly useful for practitioners in community-based practice, for which being in the client's territory is a natural occurrence to develop understanding of how environmental features and symbolic meanings shape occupational performance.

Community

It is surprising that, although community scale physical contexts are frequently studied in fields such as architecture and urban planning, they have received relatively little attention in occupational therapy. This is surprising because many clients have mobility impairments that may constrain their ability to move easily around the neighborhood and community, thus limiting their access to resources. Some therapists have become involved in surveying the accessibility of neighborhood and community scale environments for features such as curb cuts and the slope of ramps, which potentially influence use of spaces by individuals with disabilities. Various accessibility checklists for evaluating community scale environments are available, such as the Readily Achievable Checklist (Cronberg, Barnett, & Goldman, 1991) and the Accessibility Checklist (Goltsman, Gilbert, & Wohlford, 1992).

Beyond surveys of specific environmental features that limit the ability of individuals with disabilities to use neighborhood spaces, there has been some research that examines actual use of neighborhood and community spaces by elderly persons. In a classic study, Cantor (1979) conducted a large-scale survey of white, African-American, and Hispanic elderly persons in inner city neighborhoods in New York City and mapped their mobility spheres and use of resources, such as grocery stores. Cantor found that, rather than being isolated and homebound, many older individuals in this inner city environment frequently traveled within a 10-block radius by walking to visit valued destinations.

Her study methodology forms the groundwork for the Neighborhood Mobility Survey. Although designed for research rather than clinical use, this survey tool provides a framework for evaluating how far and by what methods people travel on a regular basis to reach important resources in the environment. A list of resources is provided, which includes grocery stores and other shops, banks, restaurants, health services, churches and synagogues, and recreational facilities such as parks. Respondents are asked how often they visit these resources, how far they travel in blocks (which could be converted to miles), and what methods of mobility or transportation they use. The findings are portrayed by the use of concentric circles that represent commonly used distances, such as 1–2 blocks, 2–6 blocks, and 6–10 blocks, depending on the use patterns of particular individuals. At each level of the person's mobility sphere, frequently used resources are listed. Other research supports the importance of mobility to many elders. Rush and Ouellet (1998) found six critical qualities of mobility: ease and freedom of movement, independence, automaticity, purposefulness or goal directedness, awareness of self in relation to the environment, and continuity in activity patterns. Evaluating mobility issues has important implications for practitioners in working with clients who are planning where to live, shop, and work after the onset of disabilities. Having resources within walking or wheelchair-rolling distance can minimize the need for formal transportation systems that generally remain inadequate for persons with disabilities in most communities, despite progress in recent decades to improve availability of this service.

Societal

Societal scale physical contexts are generally not evaluated by occupational therapists as part of routine clinical practice. However, it is important for practitioners to be knowledgeable about broad public policies and their influence on the lives of clients. These policies can have major implications for the usability of physical environments by clients with disabilities. Examples include public policies concerning accessibility of transportation systems and policies concerning availability of housing and assistive technology (National Council on Disability, 2000).

The Disability Rights Guide is a tool designed to identify problems affecting people with disabilities in accessing community and broader-scale resources (Goldman, 1991). The guide is a self-report questionnaire that is contained in a textbook with content based on the Americans with Disabilities Act. The questionnaire is useful for community planning and advocacy for public policies that support the rights of persons with disabilities, activities that are identified in the Occupational Therapy Code of Ethics (see Appendix C) as appropriate concerns for practitioners who are committed to improving opportunities for clients in ways beyond intervention at an individual or family level.

SOCIAL CONTEXTS

In occupational therapy, theories have been borrowed from the social sciences, including social psychology, anthropology, and sociology, about how human interaction is organized and patterned. Role theory has been particularly influential as a way in which therapists have conceptualized how occupations are selected and their performance organized. The Occupational Performance Model (Christiansen and Baum, 1997) and the Model of Human Occupation (Kielhofner, 2002) are two practice models in occupational therapy that view roles as central organizing ideas.

Immediate

In social contexts of immediate scale, in-depth attention is focused on social interaction between dyads of two individuals. Application of these approaches in occupational therapy often involves evaluation of the interaction between clients and their caregivers. Several different methods have been used to study close human interactions, including behavior observation, as illustrated by studies of interaction between mothers and children with disabilities (Barrera & Vella, 1987), qualitative interviews used to study ethical dilemmas and decision making between elders and their caregivers (Hasselkus, 1989), and textual analysis of interactions between therapists and clients in studies of clinical reasoning (Crepeau, 1991; Mattingly & Fleming, 1994). These studies show that caregivers or service providers can have a powerful effect on occupational performance that is encouraged or allowed for individuals with disabilities and, likewise, that the behavior of care recipients influences the interaction in significant ways. McCuaig and Frank's (1991) research on ways a woman with cerebral palsy managed independent living indicated that a central focus of her efforts was convincing people with whom she interacted that she was an intelligent and competent person, despite major mobility and speech impairments. These issues are of great importance to practitioners who are often in a position to influence the ways in which families or other providers interact with persons with disabilities.

The Mother-Child Interaction Checklist (Barrera & Vella, 1987) provides a structured format for detailed observations of interactions between mothers and children that has been used in comparisons of children with disabilities and those without disabilities. The observation format specifies the following:

- Maternal behaviors, including vocalization, verbalization, question, command, praise, regard, and interactive play.
- Infant behaviors, including vocalization, negative response, regard, visual orientation toward the face of the mother, independent play, interactive play, and looking away.
- Reciprocal behaviors, including particular sequences of maternal and child behaviors.

Research has indicated that mothers of disabled infants engaged in less eye contact and vocalizations than mothers of nondisabled peers. Using findings from the assessment of interaction patterns between mothers and infants with disabilities, practitioners could encourage parents to behave in ways that promote optimal participation by infants in their proximal social environments.

The Cost of Care Index was developed as a case-management tool to help health-care professionals identify issues in families in which care is provided to elders (Kosberg & Cairl, 1986). There are 20 items that address five domains: personal and social restrictions, physical and emotional health, value placed on care giving, characteristics of the care recipient that may evoke negative responses, and economic costs of care giving. In using this tool from the survey tradition, clients respond to statements using a Likert format, ranging from strongly agree to strongly disagree. Scores for each domain highlight potential problem areas that can be addressed in intervention with caregivers or care recipients.

Proximal

Social contexts of proximal scale have been studied using the concept of social roles attached to particular behavior settings, such as classrooms, workplaces, and clinical settings. The concept of *role* refers to defined social positions that have attached expectations for behavior. Roles organize the ways individuals with different social positions interact in a particular setting, as illustrated by the roles of students and teachers organizing the ways they interact in classroom settings or by the roles of clients and practitioners organizing who does what in clinical settings.

The Family Assessment Device is based on the McMaster model of family functioning (Epstein, Baldwin, & Bishop, 1983). It is a self-administered questionnaire with 53 items grouped into seven subscales: general family functioning, problem solving, communication, roles, affective responsiveness, affective involvement, and behavior control. This tool has been used to evaluate adaptation to having a child with head injury (Rivara, Jaffe, Polissar, Fay, Liao, & Martin, 1996). Research on families that include children with disabilities indicates that strong support systems, involvement in outside activities, good communication and problem-solving skills, low levels of family conflict and stress, and positive belief systems are predictors of positive adjustment over time (Beavers, Hampson, Hulgas, & Beavers, 1986; Hauser, Jacobsen, Wertlieb, Weiss, Follansbee, & Wolfselorf, 1986; Rivara et al., 1996). These are resources and skills that practitioners can seek to cultivate in families that include a child with a disability.

Brown, Hamera, and Long (1996) developed an assessment that examines engagement of individuals with mental illness in proximal scale social settings and social systems. In addition to self-care tasks commonly included in ADL evaluations, the Daily Activities Checklist also has subscales for community living skills, socialization, and quality of daily life. Sample items ask respondents "Did you go anywhere today?" (with possible responses being a community-support program, coin laundry, store, bank, job for the center, job outside the center, restaurant, and visiting friends and family). Items also address various forms of social interaction, including talking in person, talking on the telephone, helping someone, and doing something with a group of people.

Research using this tool found that it can be completed accurately by persons with mental illness living in the community, and that it identifies differences in environmental engagement between people who are working and those who are not. This tool provides practitioners with an assessment approach that uses consumer-oriented methods and recognizes the importance of context in daily life for individuals with mental illness who might be expected to have difficulties with social interaction.

In examining proximal scale social contexts, Moos (1974) and his associates originally coined the term *social climate* to convey the expectations associated with roles in various clinical settings. His initial work using this concept involved development of two survey instruments called the Ward Atmosphere Scale and Community Oriented Programs Evaluation Scale. Using these scales, Moos had staff and clients of psychiatric facilities rate 10 dimensions: involvement, support, spontaneity, autonomy, practical orientation, personal problem orientation, anger, aggression, order, and organization. In occupational therapy, Kannegeiter (1987) used the work of Moos to develop the Environmental Assessment Scale for psychiatric clinical facilities. This method for evaluating social climate of proximal social environments has been applied to many other kinds of settings, including college dormitories, military units, and workplaces.

The Work Environments Scale, based on the social climate tradition, provides a list of statements about the interpersonal environment of a workplace that address 10 dimensions in three broad areas of relationships, personal growth, and system maintenance and change (Moos, 1981). Employers and workers indicate their agreement or disagreement with a set of statements that can be used to compare perceptions of different participants in the setting. Similar to Moos's (1974) previous scales, which were initially designed for evaluating treatment environments, this scale can also be rated according to perceptions of the actual environment in contrast to perceptions of what employers and workers feel would be an ideal environment. Differences between perceptions of actual and ideal environments can be used as a stimulus for planning change in work settings.

An additional method that has been used to study roles and social climate in clinical settings is ethnographic participant observation, developed in the discipline of anthropology. Rather than using rating scales or structured survey instruments, this qualitative method uses the researcher as a participant observer, who interacts with the setting and documents both how people interact and how various participants understand the social processes. A classic study using this method—called the Psychiatric Hospital as a Small Society—was completed by Caudill (1953). He found many social mechanisms that distanced the roles of clients from those of various kinds of staff. A recent study in occupational therapy examined the social relationships among clients and between clients and staff in a rehabilitation hospital (Spencer, Young, Rintala, & Bates, 1995). Important differences were found in how these groups thought about the purposes and methods of rehabilitation.

The social systems of proximal scale environments have major implications for how individuals with disabilities are incorporated into, or distanced from, the usual rounds of activity. They thus become a potential focus for occupational therapy practitioners who see their role as fostering engagement of clients in daily life opportunities.

Community

Community scale social contexts involve human interaction over wider distances than particular behavior settings. The concept of social support has frequently been used in studies of community-level social environments (McCubbin, Cauble, & Paterson, 1982; Moos, 1986). There are many measures of social support that use structured questionnaires to gather information on the types of assistance exchanged and kinds of people who provide and receive assistance. The social support assessment cited below by Rowles (1983) also incorporates analysis of geographic factors that shape how social support exchanges operate at a community level. In an extensive study of the ways elders function within the social system of a small community in Appalachia, Rowles (1983) found that different types and intensities of support were derived from different spatial zones, which led to the concept of sociospatial support systems.

The Sociospatial Support Inventory identifies a spatial hierarchy of the following seven zones: home, surveillance, vicinity, community, subregion, region, and nation (Rowles, 1983). Rowles used time–space diaries, in which respondents recorded trips outside of home, all visits, and telephone calls made and received, to identify the kinds of support received by elders within these zones. The home was a major source of assistance with daily activities for individuals who lived with a companion, although many elderly people and those with disabilities often lived alone.

The surveillance zone, which can be seen from the respondent's home, was an important source of "watchful reciprocity" with neighbors, who monitored daily routines and departures from routine as a signal of potential trouble. Within the vicinity (up to a ½-mile radius), neighbors and family members provided frequent functional support, such as buying groceries or providing a ride to church. At the level of community, elders interacted frequently with fellow members of the "society of the old," used many formal resources such as stores or banks, and exchanged frequent telephone calls. Less frequent support was provided through formal resources and through family in the subregion, region, and national zones.

The concept of sociospatial support systems allows evaluation not only of the kinds of assistance received but also of the logistical issues, such as transportation, involved in provision of support. Practitioners could use this assessment tool to help elders or persons with disabilities examine alternative ways in which they might manage community living support arrangements under the circumstances of a particular geographic context in which they currently live or to which they might move.

In contrast to an emphasis on informal social support, another view of community scale social environments conceptualizes the community as a network of formal (organizationally based) resources and services. This view is illustrated by a history of research using the Older Americans Resources and Services model, originally developed to study community support service packages, which could be coordinated to prevent unnecessary institutionalization of elders (Duke University Center for the Study of Aging and Human Development, 1978). The Multidimensional Functional Assessment Questionnaire, developed through this project, has been widely used for clinical program intake, population surveys, and longitudinal studies. This tool is a structured questionnaire consisting of Part A, which examines the functional level of the individual, and Part B, which examines community service use and perceived need for services. Dimensions in Part A include mental health, physical health, economic resources, social resources, and ADL and are rated on a six-point scale. Part B documents actual use of, and perceived need for, a list of 24 community services (transportation; social and recreational services; various kinds of employment, education, and training services; mental health services; personal care; nursing, medical, and physical therapy services; supportive devices and prostheses; supervision; homemaker–household and meal preparation services; checking services, legal protection services; financial assistance; assistance with food and groceries; housing or relocation services; and information and referral). Although designed for use with elders, this structured questionnaire could be used by practitioners to evaluate services use and needs of a variety of clients with physical or mental disabilities in many service-delivery settings to plan optimal community living arrangements. The ways that elders and individuals with disabilities make decisions about when to use formal support services and how these decisions are related to their informal support systems are important issues (Groger, 1993; Soldo, Agree, & Wolf, 1989).

Societal

At a societal scale, various methods have been used to study ways in which individuals with disabilities are included or excluded from social systems. There is a long history of studies of attitudes toward persons with disabilities that use survey questionnaire methods (Antonak, 1981; Yuker, 1988). One approach within this tradition uses the concept of social distance to examine levels of social interaction that people would find acceptable or unacceptable with specific types of other individuals, rather than examining attitudes toward people with disabilities in general.

The Disability Social Distance Scale was originally developed to determine whether attitudes toward individuals with disabilities are affected by type of disability (Tringo, 1970). A list is provided of 21 disabilities, or "anomalous social conditions." The list includes hidden disabilities, such as diabetes and ulcers, and potentially visible disabilities, such as cerebral palsy and stroke. Also on the list are mental retardation, mental illness, alcoholism, and a criminal record. For each of these social groups, respondents are asked to specify one of nine levels of social interaction they would find acceptable: would marry, would accept as a close kin by marriage, would have as a next-door neighbor, would accept as a casual friend, would accept as a fellow employee, would keep away from, would keep in an institution, would send out of the country, and would put to death.

Recent studies using this tool have found that occupational therapy students do not differ substantially from other students in their preferences for social interaction with individuals who have hidden disabilities, followed by visible physical disabilities; the least preferred group includes those who have "disorders of the mind" such as mental retardation, psychiatric disorders, alcoholism, and a criminal record (Lyons & Hayes, 1993). Such findings about how students view individuals with disabilities have important implications for socialization of students to values of the profession (Eberhardt & Mayberry, 1995).

Social processes involving people with disabilities have also been studied using ethnographic participant observation to examine their interactions with other members of society. Anthropologist Murphy (1990), who himself became disabled by a spinal tumor, used the concept of liminality (meaning an in-between state) to describe the lack of clear social status and consequent uncertain social processes surrounding persons with physical disabilities in our society (Murphy, Scheer, Murphy, & Mack, 1988). Although usually not evaluated in structured ways, social processes are often observed by practitioners who go with clients into community settings where they interact with the general public on trips to restaurants or recreational activities. Informal evaluation of such experiences with clients can become useful avenues for discussion of strategies clients can use to interact successfully in society.

CULTURAL CONTEXTS

Although there are many definitions of culture, in general this term refers to the shared way of life of a group of people. The group may be as small as a family or as large as an ethnic group. Increasing attention is being given in occupational therapy to the importance of culture in shaping human occupational life (Krefting & Krefting, 1992). Current definitions of culture emphasize its importance in providing established patterns for how things are done as well as systems of beliefs and values for interpreting the meanings of what is done by various participants in the action (Geertz, 1983). This attention to meaning makes the concept of culture particularly useful in occupational therapy because of growing emphasis on understanding occupation as meaningful units of activity and the belief that engagement in human occupation is therapeutic in part because of its meaning (Clark, 1993; Trombly, 1995).

The concept of culture provides a way to examine meanings that are shared within a group, in contrast to personal meanings based on individual experience. Medical anthropologist Kleinman (1992) coined the term *local worlds* to describe the shared culture attached to local settings in which people live their daily lives, such as the culture of a large household, the culture of a workplace, and the culture of a school or of a neighborhood. In each of these settings there are established patterns of activity and agreed-on ways of understanding motivations that prompt people to do what they do and how behavior is interpreted. For example, in a small-town restaurant, greeting the children of strangers might be interpreted by fellow diners as a friendly gesture; whereas in the local world of a city restaurant, this same action might be interpreted as unwanted familiarity and a hazard to the safety of the children.

Cultures have typically been studied using the classic ethnographic methods developed in anthropology of participant observation, in-depth interviews, and sometimes document review. These methods, which rely heavily on the perceptiveness and skill of the researcher as the main instrument of study, were originally developed for use by full-time researchers who visited remote cultures and spent months or years conducting research. Adapting these methods for applied use in the health-care professions has required some modification. However, the essence of the approach, designed to capture the insiders' perspective of participants in the culture rather than the mindset of outside researchers, has continued in ethnographic studies of the influence of culture on occupational life at many levels (Krefting & Krefting, 1992).

An ethnographic assessment process for use in occupational therapy has been developed in a way that can be applied to a variety of local worlds to study cultural environments of differing scales. The Ethnographic Assessment Process (Spencer, Krefting, & Mattingly, 1993) involves a sequence of four steps:

- Define the unit of study, which could be a single behavior setting, such as a workplace or day-care center, or the neighborhood or community in which a person's daily round of occupations occurs.
- Describe the culture of this unit, including the material domain (how occupations are regularly performed), the social domain (the roles and relationships that organize performance of these occupations), and the

ideological domain (the meaning and value of occupations to various participants).

- Analyze the functioning of the individual according to expectations within the context.
- Develop intervention goals for the person or the environmental context.

Participant observation and conversations with people involved in the context are major methods of data collection. This assessment allows practitioners to evaluate occupational performance according to standards and expectations within the local world of the client and thereby avoid imposing personal goals valued by practitioners on clients who may value other ways of organizing their occupational lives. For example, in a local world that values interdependence and cooperative performance of tasks, emphasis on independence by the practitioner may be incongruent.

Immediate

In occupational therapy, the general methods of ethnography have been applied to a number of particular evaluation problems. Studies of immediate scale cultural environments have demonstrated the usefulness of this approach for understanding how culture shapes interaction between a practitioner and client (Crepeau, 1991) and how cultural beliefs about independence and competence shape the ways in which a woman with cerebral palsy manages her attendant assistance to live independently (McCuaig & Frank, 1991).

A method for understanding how the culture of a household shapes care giving was developed for use in the local world of elders' homes. The Home-Based Intervention for Caregivers of Elders with Dementia involves a series of five home visits and an evolving process of evaluation and intervention centered on caregiver use of the environment to manage behavioral problems common among persons with dementia (Corcoran & Gitlin, 1992). Visit one involves building rapport, identifying problem areas, and establishing goals. The second visit involves specifying environmental influences on the problems identified previously, introducing information on dementia management, and developing a plan to address specific problem behaviors of the elderly persons with dementia. Visit three involves review of the plan and initial implementation by the caregiver and refinement or modification of planned management strategies. The fourth visit focuses on the transfer of greater decision making and problem solving to the caregiver and generalization of the problem-solving process to other problems. The last visit involves a final review of the problem-solving process, final modification of specific strategies, and discussion of applying environmental management strategies to future problems. Use of this method can be thought of as a strategy for modifying the culture of the household to support optimal occupational performance of both elderly persons and caregivers.

The Test of Environmental Supportiveness is another tool designed to evaluate the influence of immediate scale cultural contexts on occupational performance (Bundy, 1999). It was designed for use in conjunction with the Test of Playfulness (by the same author) and assesses the extent to which elements of a particular environment support an individual's play. This tool identifies 17 environmental elements: the caregiver's actions and the rules and boundaries they establish, peer playmates' use of cues and domination of interaction, older playmates' use of cues and domination of interaction, younger playmates' use of cues and domination of interaction, natural and fabricated objects, amount and configuration of space, sensory environment, safety of space, and accessibility of space. A four-level scale is provided for rating the extent to which a particular element supports or hinders playfulness of the individual being evaluated. This tool can be used by practitioners when consulting with managers of immediate scale environments, such as parents and day-care personnel, to explore ways the culture in which a child interacts might be modified to encourage greater playfulness.

Proximal

The concept of culture is well suited to studying the local worlds of proximal behavior settings of living environments, classroom and work settings, and clinical environments. For example, Suto and Frank (1994) examined the culture of board and care homes for persons with schizophrenia and how their occupational routines and belief systems shaped the time use and future time perspectives of residents. Dyck (1992) studied the effects of the culture within a fish-packing work setting on the ways in which a Chinese woman managed her arthritis. Griswold (1994) studied the cultures of classroom settings that shaped occupational performance of students and led to development of a tool for use in school-based practice.

The Classroom Observation Guide examines three domains of classroom settings—activities, people, and communication (Griswold, 1994). Dimensions of activities are purpose, objects used, time required, space required, and type of learning. The dimensions of the people domain are roles and interaction. And those of the communication domain are who is giving information; to whom information is given; the purpose, context, and words used; nonverbal communication; and the consequences of communication. Observation is used as a data collection method. Griswold's research provides examples of contrasting classroom cultures that have important implications for how children with disabilities are able to function. Use of this tool can allow practitioners to think about classroom cultures and to suggest activities and strategies to enhance the development and functioning of children with special needs.

The Community Adaptive Planning Assessment (CAPA) was developed to examine the major occupations of an individual at times of expected change and how present and future engagement in the occupation is shaped by environmental influences (Spencer & Davidson, 1998). This tool identifies the following:

- Activities involved in the occupation.
- The people involved and roles of each.
- The physical setting and how the individual gets to that location.
- The value of the occupation to self and others.

Semistructured interview questions organize documentation of information on how the occupation was performed before expected changes, which is recorded on a card for each major occupation. Optional quantitative ratings, using a scale from 1 to 10, may be used to document satisfaction with time spent on the occupation, satisfaction with the individual's level of participation, negotiability of the environment, and value of the occupation.

The heart of the CAPA planning process is collaborative problem solving between practitioner and client to identify expected losses (things that can no longer be performed as in the past) and expected gains (new ways highly valued occupations might be performed with changes in the social or physical environment). The format also has a column for later documentation of the extent to which expected gains (goals) were reached, which has been used in follow-up studies of the CAPA as a discharge planning tool from various kinds of programs and for individuals who have a variety of disabilities (Spencer & Davidson, 1998).

Community

The cultures of community scale contexts have also been studied in occupational therapy in terms of their effects on the life experience of individuals with disabilities. Kielhofner (1981) examined the community experience of deinstitutionalized adults with mental retardation and found that, although these individuals were living in community settings, they were excluded from many of the routine activities and taken-for-granted meanings of events that went on there. Similarly, Krefting (1989) studied the experience of people with head injury living in the community and found that they worked very hard to conceal their disabilities and to revise the generally accepted meanings of key cultural concepts such as *work* and *independence*. Such research clearly suggests that the cultures of community scale environments may not readily incorporate persons with disabilities, a finding that has major implications for the lives of many occupational therapy clients.

A striking exception to the commonly found isolation or liminality of people with disabilities (Murphy et al., 1988) was studied by Groce (1985) in a remarkable community on Martha's Vineyard in which congenital deafness is historically very prevalent. Because individuals with hearing impairments are a taken-for-granted part of the community, use of sign language by everyone is part of the shared culture on this island, which allows individuals with disabilities to participate fully in the family, school, work, recreational, and social life of the community. Groce's work provides striking evidence for the cultural influence of a local world on the lives of individuals with disabilities.

Assessments have been developed to evaluate the involvement of persons with disabilities in community scale environments. The Craig Handicap Assessment and Report Technique (CHART) is based on the original model of disablement developed by the WHO to evaluate the concept of handicap. In contrast to impairments and disabilities that occur at a personal level, handicap involves disadvantages that limit or prevent the fulfillment of a role that would be considered normal for an individual in his or her culture (Whiteneck, Charlifue, Gerhart, Overholser, & Richardson, 1992). (In the revised WHO model these terms have been changed to positive terms such as the body, activities, and social participation.) Six dimensions identified by the WHO model that were used to develop the CHART are orientation, physical independence, mobility, occupation, social integration, and economic self-sufficiency.

The CHART is an interview tool with items that identify behaviors, rather than perceptions or attitudes. Examples include hours per day someone provides physical assistance (physical independence); time out of the house and use of transportation (mobility); time spent in employment, school, homemaking, recreation, and self-improvement activities (occupation); family, friends, and associates (social integration); and household income (economic self-sufficiency). The instrument is intended to document "absence of handicap" in a number of ways on each subscale, which can be interpreted to mean active engagement in the culture of the community and in roles expected within that culture.

The Community Integration Questionnaire (CIQ) was specifically designed as a simple and efficient tool for use with individuals who have brain injury living in the community (Willer, Rosenthal, Kreutzer, Gordon, & Rempel, 1993). It contains 15 items that evaluate participation in household activities, shopping, errands, leisure activities, visiting friends, social events, and productive activities. These are grouped into three dimensions: home integration, social integration, and productive activities. This tool has been used as a measure of community integration in the Model Traumatic Brain Injury Systems as well as in other research. Practitioners could use the CHART or CIQ to help clients examine the extent of their community participation and to identify goals and problem-solving strategies to increase involvement in local worlds of the community.

Societal

Finally, cultural contexts have been studied at a societal level in terms of their effect on people with disabilities. Shapiro (1993) traced historic changes in how these individuals have been viewed in our society, articulating a general trend from a cultural view of such people as objects of charity and pity to a view that emphasizes their civil rights as citizens who make important contributions to society. Research has used media images as ways of examining how persons with disabilities are viewed culturally (Biklen, 1986; Clogston, 1990; Haller, 1995; Zola, 1985).

Although not designed as a clinical assessment, Haller's (1995) models of media representation can provide a framework for evaluating aspects of cultural context at a societal level. Models of Media Representation of Disability identifies four traditional and four progressive models. The traditional models are as follows:

- *Medical model:* People with disabilities are perceived as having an illness or malfunction.
- *Social pathology model:* People with disabilities are presented as disadvantaged and needing support, which is regarded as a gift rather than a right.
- *Supercrip model:* People with disability are portrayed as deviant because they perform superhuman feats in spite of their disability.
- *Business model:* People with disabilities are thought of as costly to society.

The progressive models are as follows:

- *Minority–civil rights model:* People with disabilities are seen as members of a disability community that has legitimate political grievances based on denial of civil rights.
- *Legal model:* People with disabilities may not, by law, be treated in certain ways.
- *Cultural pluralism model:* People with disabilities are seen as multifaceted individuals and their disabilities do not receive undue attention.
- *Consumer model:* People with disabilities are seen as an untapped consumer group.

Practitioners could use these models to identify subtle ways in which general societal beliefs and values shape their own views. The models could also be used to help clients anticipate and deal with how they may be viewed when they reenter society after onset of a new identity as a person with a disability.

VIRTUAL CONTEXTS

Virtual contexts are a new component of the occupational therapy practice framework (AOTA, in press). Use of computer technology by occupational therapists is growing rapidly for a variety of purposes, including clinical and reimbursement documentation, evaluation, treatment, and student and patient education (Hammel & Smith, 1993). Use of the Internet by the general public grew dramatically in the 1990s, from an estimated 8.4 million adults using this technology in 1995 compared to 40 million adults in 1999 (Stokols, 1999).

Concern has been raised about the growing disparity in opportunities for persons with and without access to computers, particularly children living in affluent circumstances versus those living in poverty. This technology offers a wealth of opportunities for access to a great diversity of information, distance learning opportunities, and the capacity to communicate with known and unknown persons. However, according to some research, this technology also offers the potential for stimulation overload and distraction from important tasks and actual experiences (Hartig, Mang, & Evans, 1991). Concerns have also been raised about the questionable authenticity of information posted on the World Wide Web (Stoll, 1995).

It is noteworthy that computer use by individuals with disabilities is significantly lower than use by other members of society. Recent research on people 15 years of age and older from the 1998 Current Population Survey indicates that less than one quarter of individuals with disabilities (23.9%) have access to a computer at home, compared to just over one half (51.7%) of their nondisabled counterparts (Kaye, 2000). And one tenth (9.9%) of those with disabilities used the Internet, compared to four tenths (38.1%) of those without disabilities. Despite these findings, access to virtual environments provides an important resource that is potentially available to persons who may have difficulty getting to or participating in other environmental contexts.

Immediate

Research on assessment of immediate scale virtual contexts has involved studies of attitudes toward computers and how these affect use of computer-based technology (Gardner, Discenza, & Dukes, 1993). One scale used for this purpose is the Computer Attitude Scale (Loyd & Gressard, 1984). Subscales include confidence, liking, and anxiety. This tool has 40 items to which persons respond using a four-point Likert scale ranging from strongly agree to strongly disagree. Items address general attitudes toward computers, use of computers in particular situations such as work, and approach toward solving computer problems. Practitioners might use this tool as they introduce use of computerized virtual environments to clients or students.

Research in this area has also used questionnaires to examine satisfaction with software interface systems (Chin, Diehl, & Norman, 1988). An evaluation system that examines both overall systems and more specific scenarios is the Computer System Usability Questionnaire (Lewis, 1995). This tool has 19 items on aspects of software design of which respondents rate using a seven-point Likert scale ranging from strongly agree to strongly disagree. This questionnaire also includes two open-ended questions about features that were most negative and most positive. Research indicates that components of this scale measure three factors—usefulness, information quality, and interface quality. Practitioners could use this tool to evaluate specific software programs for use with clients or students.

Usability of software programs has been evaluated by various methods other than user questionnaires (Chapanis, 1991). In a study of heuristic, think-aloud, and performance testing methods, heuristic methods based on evaluation by software design experts were found to detect usability problems most efficiently (Virzi, Source, & Herbert, 1993). However, experiential evaluation by potential users of the software was also an effective method of identifying and correcting usability problems. In the think-aloud protocol method, respondents are asked to use a software program and talk on an ongoing basis as they work through its procedures (Wright & Monk, 1991). During this process, users are observed or videotaped to identify features of using the system that are problematic or desirable. This open-ended qualitative method captures the perspective of users, which may differ from that of designers or experts in system evaluation. These methods offer practitioners alternative ways to assess software programs they are developing.

Proximal

Research on proximal scale virtual contexts has examined ways in which individuals respond to different methods of knowledge representation in such environments. Dual coding theory identifies verbal and nonverbal (imaginal) encoding systems (Paivio & Harshman, 1983; Clark & Paivio, 1991). Use of both forms of knowledge representation in combination has been shown to increase recall of information (Rieber & Kini, 1991; Mayer & Sims, 1994). Differences among persons in the use of these two modes of knowledge representation have been assessed using the Individual Differences Questionnaire originally developed by Paivio (1971). This tool is an 86-item questionnaire that asks respondents to rate items on a five-point Likert scale. Subscales address imagery and verbal thinking habits and skills. Use of this tool can help practitioners identify or create virtual contexts that are usable by individuals with different thinking and learning styles.

Proximal scale virtual contexts have been used to provide health care in client homes and other settings via virtual visits in the fields of medicine (Friedman, Stollerman, Mahoney, & Rozenblyum, 1997) and nursing (Lindberg, 1997; Rooney, Studenski, & Roman, 1997). Use of virtual visits has sometimes been based on relatively simple telephone technology. For example, Friedman et al. evaluated a system for telephone-linked care (TLC) to monitor patients with chronic illnesses, check on targeted health behaviors, and provide caregiver support in 29 communities in the Boston area. This study evaluated the virtual visit approach based on weekly telephone visits using clinical outcomes to compare medication adherence and blood pressure levels in clients with hypertension who used TLC to those who received only regular care. Both medication adherence and blood pressure levels were significantly better for the TLC participants. The TLC approach was also found to improve health behaviors, as documented by decreased cholesterol levels and increased time spent walking among individuals who received weekly virtual visits by telephone. A user satisfaction questionnaire indicated that most clients found the TLC system easy to use (94%), made them more aware of their health problems (95%), and relieved their worries (79%).

Video technology has also been used to provide virtual visits through an interactive home-based health-care program in rural Kansas (Lindberg, 1997). Clients in home settings who have 13-in. color televisions with video cameras mounted on top can communicate interactively with nurses in four base locations about management of a variety of health problems such as diabetes, chronic obstructive pulmonary disease, and Parkinson's disease. Evaluation of the system has included client status logs, which document the functional, mental, and nutritional status of clients; their medication use; and their use of services. Evaluation of the system also includes use of questionnaires documenting client and provider satisfaction. Practitioners could use virtual visits using simple telephone technology or more sophisticated computer systems to maintain and evaluate contact with clients in the community on an ongoing basis.

Community

Community scale virtual contexts include systems for interacting with communities of persons who have common interests, such as mailing lists, chat rooms, and bulletin boards identified with a particular topic or organization. Such computer networks have been used effectively to provide support systems for caregivers (Brennan, Moore, & Smyth, 1995; Gallienne, Moore, & Brennan, 1993). A formal evaluation of a computer network for caregivers of people with Alzheimer's disease was based on an experimental design that compared decision-confidence, decision skill, and social isolation among users of the computer network with those of other caregivers who were not a part of the system (Brennan et al., 1995). A significant difference between users of the network and nonusers was found in decision confidence. Established scales were used to evaluate outcomes, including the Decision-Confidence Scale, which has 14 items that are rated using a five-point Likert format. Items include statements such as "Access to ComputerLink helped me better understand my choices." The Network Monitoring System documented ways in which the network was used by members, including mutual support (37%), discussion of the care recipient's situation (24%), the emotional impact of care giving (19%), use of outside support (13%), interpersonal relationships (4%), self-care (3%), and home care (2%). Practitioners could use such networks to provide ongoing support to clients and their families.

A network system has also been used to connect a community of cancer facilities (London, Morton, Marinucci, Catalano, & Comis, 1997). This system is designed to provide Web site information on clinical trials of cancer treatment that are currently being conducted. It also provides one-to-one video consultations that can be used by network health-care providers to evaluate whether particular clients would be appropriate for enrollment in specific clinical trials. Informal evaluation indicates that the system processes an average of 11.1 requests per day. Outcomes have not been formally evaluated.

Societal

Societal scale virtual contexts include systems for interacting with the world at large, such as Web systems. The Allen Semantic Differential Scale (ASDS) was used to evaluate responses to health-care intervention based on Web site use (Allen 1986). The ASDS has 14 bipolar adjective pairs grouped into subscales for comfort, creativity, and function. The items are pleasant–unpleasant, comfortable–uncomfortable, threatening–nonthreatening, and overpowering–easy to control (comfort subscale); rigid–flexible, stimulating–boring, creative–unimaginative, and impersonal–personal (creativity subscale); and useful–useless, meaningless–meaningful, valuable–worthless, efficient–inefficient, inappropriate–appropriate, and time saving–time consuming (function subscale). Practitioners could use this tool to evaluate user responses to Web page interventions.

A Web system has been developed as a collaborative effort at the University of Cincinnati to provide health information to users from 29 counties in three states (Morris et al., 1997). Access to the system is by Internet, regional free Nets, and 43 public-access sites in libraries and clinics. This system is targeted particularly for individuals termed information have-nots who, for socioeconomic or geographical reasons, may not have regular access to computer technology. Content includes consumer-oriented information about drugs and diseases, physician referral, wellness information, alternative therapies, insurance information, and professional health literature. Quantitative analysis of this system includes transaction log analysis as well as an online survey to document user responses. Future evaluation plans include monitoring community health data and qualitative interviews to determine what users have done with the information from the Web system.

The influence of information from Web sites has been studied using qualitative interviews in a comparative study of how hope evolves over time in occupational therapy clients in contrasting clinical settings (Davidson, White, & Spencer, 2000). In this study, a woman who had a brain tumor used Web pages to find information about alternative clinical facilities where she might be seen, information that shaped where she sought treatment. She also used Web site information to become more knowledgeable about the prognosis of others with her condition, which she then discussed with care providers at the specialized facility where she became a patient. A new role for practitioners may be helping clients make sense of information they have obtained from Web site use.

SPIRITUAL CONTEXTS

Spiritual contexts are a new addition to the occupational therapy practice framework (AOTA, in press). As in other health-care professions (Dyson, Cobb, & Foreman, 1997; Pulchalski, 1998), spirituality is gaining increasing attention in occupational therapy as an essential aspect of humanity and as a source of meaning that influences occupational lives (Christiansen, 1997; Collins, 1998; Egan & DeLaat, 1997; Peloquin, 1997). In spite of these developments and the inclusion of spiritual contexts in the new occupational therapy practice framework, one survey found that some occupational therapists are unsure of the place of spirituality in the profession and how it might be integrated into practice (Engquist, Short-DeGraff, Gliner, & Oltjenbruns, 1997). A review indicated that much of the literature on spirituality in occupational therapy is philosophical, with relatively few empirical studies (Schulz, 1999). Spirituality is thus an area in which exploration is likely to continue both in practice and in research.

Immediate

At an individual level, there are several assessments from the survey tradition designed to evaluate aspects of spirituality. These include the Materialism-Spiritualism Scale (Mathew, Mathew, Wilson, & Georgi, 1995), the Spiritual Involvement and Beliefs Scale (Hatch, Burg, Naberhaus, & Hellmich, 1998), and the Spiritual Well-Being Scale (Bufford, Paloutzian, & Ellison, 1991).

The Spiritual Well-Being Scale is a 20-item instrument intended for use in the general population. It is based on a conceptualization of two basic dimensions of spirituality—a direct personal relationship with God (religious well-being) and a perception that life has meaning and purpose without reference to any particular religion (existential well-being). Respondents indicate the extent of their agreement with a series of statements using a four-point Likert scale ranging from not at all to very much. Examples of statements included on the scale are "I believe that God loves me and cares about me." (religious) and "I feel a sense of well-being about the direction my life is headed in." (existential). Research among individuals with a variety of chronic conditions, including amputation, polio, spinal cord injury, breast cancer, and prostate cancer found that individuals clustered into a religious group, an existential group, and a nonspiritual group (Riley, Perna, Tate, Forchheimer, Anderson, & Luera, 1998). In this study, members of the religious and existential groups reported significantly higher levels of quality of life and life satisfaction than persons in the nonspiritual group.

Qualitative interviews are also a useful way to examine spirituality in clients after the onset of disability or other major life changes. In a study of adaptation to disabling hand injury based on a combination of qualitative and quantitative methods, participants often spoke of the meaning of their injury experience in spiritual terms (Chan & Spencer, 2001). For example, a factory worker with a crush injury caused by a falling piece of sheet metal said "I have always been religious and everything I believe happens for a reason, so you just sort of take it even if it sets you back a little bit." An engineer whose thumb was injured in a construction accident expressed a similar view: "I think still that God has great power. It's just according to His will whether things happen the way they do. I think that prayer has great power to change God's mind, but I can accept whatever He puts forth still." Practitioners frequently see clients at times of major life disruptions that may have long-term implications, and they could use information from structured questionnaires or qualitative interviews to explore spiritual beliefs about life changes and their personal significance.

Proximal

At a proximal scale, spiritual contexts include the ways spirituality is reflected or enacted in settings of daily life. The connection between spirituality and people's daily occupations is explored in a variety of ways in a special issue of *The American Journal of Occupational Therapy* that is devoted to occupation, spirituality, and life meaning (Peloquin & Christiansen, 1997).

A questionnaire designed to capture an occupational therapy view of spirituality is the OT-Quest (Schulz, 2000). It is based on a definition of spirituality as "feeling a meaningful connection to our core self, other humans, the world and/or a greater power as expressed through our reflections, narratives, and actions" (p. 5). The emphasis on expression indicates that in this view spirituality has a *doing* component. The first section of this tool contains 11 questions, each on a visual analog scale, to indicate the extent to which the item characterizes the respondent. The second section contains 12 sentence-completion questions to yield qualitative as well as quantitative information. Examples of sentence-completion questions that document how spirituality is expressed in contexts of daily life are "I am most engaged in an activity when . . ." and "I am most able to express myself when the environment . . ." A study to evaluate the initial research version of this questionnaire identified several issues to be incorporated in a revised version, such as use of time and the value of struggle or challenge. Tools such as the OT-Quest can assist practitioners in exploring how clients incorporate spirituality in daily life settings and occupations.

Qualitative interviews have also been used to examine spiritual occupations performed in daily life settings. Frank, et al., (1997) interviewed couples about how they expressed their Orthodox Jewish beliefs in daily practices, which included observing the Sabbath, studying and praying, and keeping a Kosher home.. Similarly, elders who had to relocate to new living arrangements after a hospitalization also spoke frequently in qualitative interviews about the daily occupation of prayer and how it fostered a sense on continuity in their new homes (Spencer et al., 2001). One participant spoke of the importance of this occupation as "I couldn't live without prayer every day." Another described what she did during prayer: "All you have to do is ball it up and put it in His hands and leave it there. When you give Him something, you have to leave it alone. And that's what I do." Qualitative interviews provide a valuable means for practitioners to address the spiritual significance of occupations and how they are enacted on a daily basis.

Community

Community scale spiritual contexts involve engagement in spiritual life as part of a community. This may include religious observances of organizations such as churches, synagogues, or mosques. It may also include activities of such communities that are not directly religious, as illustrated by the concept of interfaith care teams that are organized to assist people with various illnesses such as dementia or AIDS (Jacobs, 1997; Shelp, DuBose, & Sunderland, 1990).

Spiritual aspects of communities have been studied using the concept of rituals that occur in secular and religious organizations. Norris (2000) used ethnographic participant observation and semistructured interviews with residents and staff to study the use and significance of rituals in a transitional residential program for people with brain injury. The study examined rituals of the everyday and larger ceremonial practices using these methods. Norris saw rituals as part of a continuum, with habits or routines at one end, rituals of the everyday in the middle, and ceremonial rituals at the other end. All of these forms involve structured action with increasing symbolism, a longer time frame, and a more conscious element of performance as one moves on the continuum toward ceremonial rituals. A major ceremonial ritual at the transitional learning community studied by Norris was the graduation ceremony for which residents prepare throughout their stay in the program, culminating in writing and delivering a speech about how their lives are changing and about their plans for the future. Outcomes for residents of the graduation process include developing a new narrative or life story, learning to deal with a socially stigmatizing condition, and establishing connections with others who share their condition—all of which can be interpreted as aspects of their spiritual lives as part of a community. Norris advocated for more conscious awareness of ritual in occupational therapy practice in a variety of settings as a potentially powerful way to evoke and represent meaning for clients.

Societal

Spiritual contexts of societal scale refer to broadly shared belief systems. In some societies, such beliefs are more homogeneous than is the case in a multicultural society such the United States. There is a history of research on diverse societal scale belief systems and their significance for health and healing (Kleinman, 1980).

Child psychiatrist Coles (1990) studied spiritual belief systems among children from many populations, including Jewish, Islamic, Native American, Christian, and nonreligious groups. He used conversations with individual children and with groups of children about the universal questions and also had children create drawings and paintings of the spiritual aspects of their lives. Coles found that art is a valuable way of helping people express spiritual images and ideas that are difficult to express verbally. In his research, Coles found that location often made a substantial difference in what children told him or drew for him. For example, a Hopi child said very little when interviewed in her school run by white personnel but expressed much about her spiritual beliefs when she was walking outdoors with Coles, where natural environments prompted her reflections about nature and its significance in the Hopi way of life. Practitioners can draw on the history of therapeutic use of art in occupational therapy to explore spiritual issues with children or other clients.

SUMMARY OF CONTEXTUAL ASSESSMENT STRATEGIES

The array of tools described in this chapter illustrate alternative ways of evaluating contexts at immediate, proximal, community, and societal scales (Table 26-2). These tools

TABLE 26-2. **TOOLS FOR ASSESSING CONTEXTS**

Immediate Scale	Proximal Scale	Community Scale	Societal Scale
Physical Context			
BTE Work Simulator	Accessibility checklists	Accessibility checklists	Disability Rights Guide
Assistive technological evaluation	SAFER	Neighborhood Mobility Survey	
Fine motor task evaluation	Risk Factor Checklist		
Ethnographic interviews	The Enabler		
	Interview-in-Place		
Social Context			
Mother-Child Interaction Checklist	Family Assessment Device	Sociospatial Support Inventory	Disability Social Distance Scale
Cost of Care Index	Daily Activities Checklist	Multidimensional Functional Assessment Questionnaire	Ethnographic participant observation
	Work Environments Scale Ethnographic participant observation		
Cultural Context			
Ethnographic Assessment Process	Classroom Observation Guide	CHART	Models of Media Representation of Disability
Home-Based Intervention for Caregivers of Elders with Dementia	CAPA	CIQ	
Test of Environmental Supportiveness			
Virtual Context			
Computer Attitude Scale	Individual Differences Questionnaire	Decision-Confidence Scale	ASDS
Computer System Usability Questionnaire	Virtual visits—clinical outcomes	Network Monitoring System	Transaction log analysis
Think-aloud protocol	Client status logs		Qualitative interviews
Spiritual			
Spiritual Well-Being Scale; qualitative interviews	OT-Quest; qualitative interviews	Ethnographic participant observation	Drawings and paintings

employ a variety of methods, including formal measurements of quantitative variables (e.g., distance), behavior observation (using coding checklists and time-sampling procedures to document how environments are naturally used in daily life), self-report questionnaires or scales (to document how aspects of environments are perceived by users), and qualitative methods (e.g., ethnography, participant observation, and conversations with individuals about occupational patterns and their meanings). Each of these methods offers strengths and weaknesses, and collectively they can be viewed as complementary approaches for understanding relevant features of environmental contexts that reflect the richness of possible perspectives on context. As many others have pointed out, having a clear sense of what questions to ask should precede decisions about the best tools to use for a particular purpose (Davidson, 1992; Letts et al., 1994; Ottenbacher, 1992).

CONCLUSION

The studies reported in this chapter indicate that contexts indeed have a powerful influence on occupational engagement. Therefore, wise use of tools for evaluating context can become an important aspect of a practice grounded in the daily life experience of clients. Yerxa (1994) asserted that occupational therapy practitioners are particularly well equipped to help clients bridge the gap between their experience in health care or other service-delivery settings and the local worlds of their daily lives. In an era in which there are many pressures to standardize treatment, practitioners are challenged to maintain the relevance of therapy to the lives of clients and to maintain their beliefs in the personal, social, cultural, and spiritual meaning of human occupation as a major aspect of its therapeutic potential.

ACKNOWLEDGMENTS

My ideas about the significance of environmental contexts in occupational therapy have been shaped by professional interactions and collaborative research with many colleagues and students. Most significant among these has been my evolving work with faculty colleagues Josephine Chan, Harriett Davidson, Gayle Hersch, and Virginia White. In preparation of this chapter, I drew on ideas and work by doctoral students Teresa Norris and Emily Schulz as well as that of a number of master's degree students.

References

Adaptive Environments Center (1988). *Home modification workbook*. Boston: Author.

Allen, L. (1986). Measuring attitudes toward computer assisted instruction: The development of a semantic differential tool. *Computers in Nursing, 4*(4), 144–151.

American Occupational Therapy Association (in press). Occupational therapy practice framework: Domain and process. *American Journal of Occupational Therapy*.

Antonak, R. (1981). Prediction of attitudes toward disabled persons: A multivariate analysis. *Journal of General Psychology, 104*, 119–123.

Asher, I. (1996). *Occupational therapy assessment tools: An annotated index* (2nd ed.). Bethesda, MD: American Occupational Therapy Association.

Barrera, M., & Vella, D. (1987). Disabled and nondisabled infants' interactions with their mothers. *American Journal of Occupational Therapy, 41*, 168–172.

Bates, P. (1994). The self-care environment: Issues of space and furnishings. In C. Christiansen (Ed.). *Ways of living: Self-care strategies for special needs* (pp. 423–451). Rockville, MD: American Occupational Therapy Association.

Bates, P., Spencer, J., Young, M., & Rintala, D. (1993). Assistive technology and the newly disabled adult: Adaptation to wheelchair use. *American Journal of Occupational Therapy, 47*, 1014–1021.

Beavers, J., Hampson, R., Hulgas, Y., & Beavers, W. (1986). Coping in families with a retarded child. *Family Process, 25*, 365–378.

Biklen, D. (1986). Framed: Journalism's treatment of disability. *Social Policy, 16*, 45–51.

Brennan, P., Moore, S., & Smyth, K. (1995). The effects of a special computer network on caregivers of persons with Alzheimer's disease. *Nursing Research, 44*(3), 166–172.

Brooks, N. (1991). Users' responses to assistive devices for physical disability. *Social Science and Medicine, 32*, 1417–1424.

Brown, C., Hamera, E., & Long, C. (1996). The Daily Activities Checklist: A functional assessment for consumers with mental illness living in the community. *Occupational Therapy in Health Care, 10*(3), 33–44.

Bufford, R., Paloutzian, R., & Ellison, C. (1991). Norms for the Spiritual Well-Being Scale. *Journal of Psychology and Theology, 19*, 56–70.

Bundy, A. (1999). *Test of environmental supportiveness*. Fort Collins: Department of Occupational Therapy, Colorado State University.

Burke, M. (1998). *Ergonomics tool kit: Practical applications*. Gaithersburg MD: Aspen.

Cantor, M. (1979). Life space and social support. In T. Byerts, S. Howell, & L. Pastalan (Eds.). *Environmental context of aging: Lifestyles, environmental quality, and living arrangements* (pp. 33–61). New York: Garland.

Caudill, W. (1953). *The psychiatric hospital as a small society*. Cambridge, MA: Harvard University Press.

Chan, J., & Spencer, J. (2001). *Holistic examination of adaptation to hand injury*. Unpublished manuscript.

Chapanis, A. (1991). *Human factors for informatics usability*. New York: Cambridge University Press.

Chin, J., Diehl, V., & Norman, K. (1988). *Development of an instrument measuring user satisfaction of the human-computer interface*. Paper presented at ACM CHI '88.

Christiansen, C. (Ed.). (1994) *Ways of living: Self-care strategies for special needs*. Rockville MD: American Occupational Therapy Association.

Christiansen, C. (1997). Acknowledging a spiritual dimension in occupational therapy practice. *American Journal of Occupational Therapy, 51*, 169–172.

Christiansen, C., & Baum, C. (Eds.). (1997). *Occupational therapy: Enabling Occupational Performance*. New York: McGraw Hill.

Clark, F. (1993). Occupation embedded in real life: Interweaving occupation science and occupational therapy. [Eleanor Clarke Slagle Lecture]. *American Journal of Occupational Therapy, 47*, 1067–1078.

Clark, J., & Paivio, A. (1991). Dual coding theory and education. *Educational Psychology Review, 3*, 149–210.

Clogston, J. (1990). *Disability coverage in 16 newspapers*. Louisville: Advocado Press.

Coles, R. (1990). *The spiritual life of children*. Boston: Houghton Mifflin.

Collins, M. (1998). Occupational therapy and spirituality: Reflecting on quality experience in therapeutic interventions. *British Journal of Occupational Therapy, 61*, 280–284.

Cook, A., & Hussey, S. (1995). *Assistive technologies: Principles and practice*. St. Louis: Mosby.

Corcoran, M., & Gitlin, L. (1992). Dementia management: An occupational therapy home-based intervention for caregivers. *American Journal of Occupational Therapy, 46*, 801–808.

Covington, G. (1998). Cultural and environmental barriers to assistive technology: Why assistive devices don't always assist. In D. Gray, L. Quatrano, & M. Lieberman (Eds.). *Designing and using assistive technology: The human perspective*. Baltimore: Brookes.

Crepeau, E. (1991). Achieving intersubjective understanding: Examples from an occupational therapy treatment session. *American Journal of Occupational Therapy, 45*, 1016–1026.

Cronburg, J., Barnett, J., & Goldman, N. (1991). *Readily achievable checklist: A survey for accessibility*. Washington, DC: National Center for Access Unlimited.

Davidson, H. (1992). Assessing environmental factors. In C. Christiansen & C. Baum (Eds.). *Occupational therapy: Overcoming human performance deficits* (pp. 427–452). New York: McGraw Hill.

Davidson, H., White, V., & Spencer, J. (2000). *How hope develops over time following onset of disability*. Unpublished manuscript.

DeJong, G. (1979). Independent living: From social movement to analytic paradigm. *Archives of Physical Medicine and Rehabilitation, 60*, 435–446.

Duke University Center for the Study of Aging and Human Development. (1978). *Multidimensional functional assessment: The OARS methodology*. Durham, NC: Author.

Dunn, W., Brown, C., & McGuigan, A. (1994). The ecology of human performance: A framework for considering the effect of context. *American Journal of Occupational Therapy, 48*, 595–607.

Dyck, I. (1992). Managing chronic illness: An immigrant woman's acquisition and use of health care knowledge. *American Journal of Occupational Therapy, 46*, 696–705.

Dyson, J., Cobb, M. & Forman, D. (1997). The meaning of spirituality: A literature review. *Journal of Advanced Nursing, 26*, 1183–1188.

Eberhardt, K., & Mayberry, W. (1995). Factors influencing entry-level occupational therapists' attitudes toward persons with disabilities. *American Journal of Occupational Therapy, 49*, 629–636.

Egan, M., & DeLaat, M. (1997). The implicit spirituality of occupational therapy practice. *Canadian Journal of Occupational Therapy, 64*, 115–121.

Engquist, D., Short-Degraff, M., Gliner, J., & Oltenbruns, K. (1997). Occupational therapists' beliefs and practices with regard to spirituality and therapy. *American Journal of Occupational Therapy, 5*, 173–180.

Epstein, N., Baldwin, L., & Bishop, D. (1983). The McMaster family assessment device. *Journal of Marital and Family Therapy, 9*, 171–180.

Forer, S. (1996). *Outcome management and program evaluation made easy: A toolkit for occupational therapy practitioners*. Bethesda MD: American Occupational Therapy Association.

Frank, G., Bernardo, C., Tropper, S., Noguchi, F., Lipman, C., Maulhardt, B., & Weitz, L. (1997). Jewish spirituality through actions in time: Occupations of young orthodox Jewish couples in Los Angeles. *American Journal of Occupational Therapy, 51*(3), 199–206.

Friedman, R., Stollerman, J., Mahoney, D., & Rosenblyum, L. (1997). The virtual visit: Using telecommunications technology to take care of patients. *Journal of the American Medical Informatics Association, 4*(6), 413–425.

Gallienne, R., Moore, S., & Brennan, P. (1993). Alzheimer's caregivers: Psychosocial support via computer networks. *Journal of Gerontological Nursing, 19*(12), 15–22.

Garber, S., & Gregorio, T. (1990). Upper extremity assistive devices: Assessment of use by spinal cord injured patients with quadriplegia. *American Journal of Occupational Therapy, 44*, 126–131.

Gardner, D., Discenze, R., & Dukes, R. (1993). The measurement of computer attitudes: An empirical investigation of available scales. *Journal of Educational Computing Research, 9*(4), 487–507.

Geertz, C. (1983). *Local knowledge: Further essays in interpretive anthropology*. New York: Basic Books.

Gliedman, J., & Roth, W. (1980). *The unexpected minority: Handicapped children in America*. New York: Harcourt Brace Jovanovich.

Goldman, C. (1991). *Disability rights guide: Practical solutions to problems affecting people with disabilities*. Lincoln NE: Media.

Goltsman, S., Gilbert, T., & Wohlford, S. (1992). *The accessibility checklist: An evaluation system for buildings and outdoor settings*. Berkeley, CA: M.I.G. Communications.

Griswold, L. (1994). Ethnographic analysis: A study of classroom environments. *American Journal of Occupational Therapy, 48*, 397–402.

Groce, N. (1985). *Everyone here spoke sign language: Hereditary deafness on Martha's Vineyard*. Cambridge, MA: Harvard University Press.

Groger, L. (1993). *African-American elders' choices for long-term care: An exploratory study*. Oxford, OH: Scripps Gerontology Center, Miami University.

Haller, B. (1995). Rethinking models of media representation of disability. *Disability Studies Quarterly, 15*(2), 26–30.

Hammel, J., & Smith. R. (1993). The development of technology competencies and training guidelines for occupational therapists. *American Journal of Occupational Therapy, 47*(11), 970–979.

Hartig, T., Mang, M., & Evans, G. (1991). Restorative effects of natural environment experiences. *Environment and Behavior, 23*, 3–26.

Hasselkus, B. (1989). The meaning of daily activity in family caregiving for the elderly. *American Journal of Occupational Therapy, 43*, 649–656.

Hatch, R., Burg, M., Naberhaus, D., & Hellmich, L. (1998). The Spiritual Involvement and Beliefs Scale: Development of a new testing instrument. *Journal of Family Practice, 46*(6), 476–486.

Hauser, S., Jacobsen, D., Wertlieb, B., Weiss, P., Follansbee, D., & Wolfselorf, J. (1986). Children with recently diagnosed diabetes: Interaction with their families. *Health Psychology, 5*, 273–276.

International Labour Office (1996). *Ergonomic checkpoints: Practical and easy-to-implement solutions for improving safety, health, and working conditions*. Geneva: Author.

Iwarsson, S., & Isacsson, A. (1996). Development of a novel instrument for occupational therapy assessment of the physical environment in the home: A methodologic study on "The Enabler." *Occupational Therapy Journal of Research, 16*(4), 227–244.

Jacobs, K. (1999). *Ergonomics for therapists* (2nd ed.). Boston: Butterworth Heinemann.

Jacobs, S. (1997). *A descriptive study of volunteers' use of activities to provide support for Alzheimer's patients and their families*. Unpublished thesis. Denton, Texas: Texas Woman's University.

Kannegeiter, R. (1987). The development of the environmental assessment scale. *Occupational Therapy in Mental Health, 6*, 67–83.

Kaye, H. (2000, July). *Disability and the digital divide*. *Disability Statistics Abstract*. Washington, DC: U.S. Department of Education.

Kelly, C., & Snell, K. (1989). *The source book: Architectural guidelines for barrier free design*. Toronto, ON, Canada: Barrier-Free Design Centre.

Kielhofner, G. (1981). An ethnographic study of deinstitutionalized adults: Their community settings and daily experiences. *Occupational Therapy Journal of Research, 1*, 125–142.

Kielhofner, G. (2002). *A model of human occupation* (3rd ed.). Baltimore: Lippincott Williams & Wilkins.

Kleinman, A. (1980). *Patients and healers in the context of culture*. Berkeley: University of California Press.

Kleinman, A. (1992). Local worlds of suffering: An interpersonal focus for ethnographies of illness experience. *Qualitative Health Research, 2*, 127–134.

Kosberg, J., & Cairl, R. (1986). The cost of care index: A case management tool for screening informal care providers. *Gerontological Society of America, 26*, 273–278.

Krefting, L. (1989). Reintegration into the community after head injury: The results of an ethnographic study. *Occupational Therapy Journal of Research, 9*, 67–83.

Krefting, L., & Krefting, D. (1992). Cultural influences on performance. In C. Christiansen & C. Baum (Eds.). *Occupational therapy: Overcoming human performance deficits* (pp. 101–122). New York: McGraw Hill.

Law, M., Cooper, B., Strong, S., Stewart, D., Rigby, P., & Letts, L. (1996). The person-environment-occupation model: A transactive approach to occupational performance. *Canadian Journal of Occupational Therapy, 3*(1), 9–23.

Letts, L., Law, M., Rigby, P., Cooper, B., Stewart, D., & Strong, S. (1994). Person-environment assessments in occupational therapy. *American Journal of Occupational Therapy, 48*, 608–618.

Lewis, J. (1995). IBM computer usability satisfaction questionnaire: Psychometric evaluation and instructions for use. *International Journal of Human-Computer Interaction, 7*(1), 57–78.

Lifchez, R. (1987). *Rethinking architecture: Design students and physically disabled people*. Berkeley: University of California Press.

Lindberg, C. (1997). Implementation of in-home telemedicine in rural Kansas: Answering an elderly patient's needs. *Journal of the American Medical Informatics Association, 4*(1), 12–17.

London, J., Morton, D., Narinucci, D., Catalano, R., & Comis, R. (1997). Telemedicine within a community cancer network. *Journal of the American Medical Informatics Association, 4*(1), 18–24.

Loyd, B., & Gressard, C. (1984). Reliability and factorial validity of computer attitude scales. *Association for Educational Data Systems Journal, 17*, 67–77.

Lyons, M., & Hayes, R. (1993). Student perceptions of persons with psychiatric and other disorders. *American Journal of Occupational Therapy, 47*, 541–548.

Mace, R., Hardie, G., & Place, J. (1991). Accessible environments: Toward universal design. In W. Preisler, J. Vischer, & E. White (Eds.). *Design intervention: Toward a more human architecture*. New York: Van Nostrand Reinhold.

Mathew, R., Mathew, V., Wilson, W., & Georgi, J. (1995). Measurement of materialism and spiritualism in substance abuse research. *Journal of the Study of Alcoholism, 56*(4), 470–475.

Mattingly, C., & Fleming, M. (1994). *Clinical reasoning: Forms of inquiry in a therapeutic practice*. Philadelphia: Davis.

Mayer, R., & Sims, V. (1994). For whom is a picture worth a thousand words? Extensions of a dual-coding theory of multimedia learning. *Journal of Educational Psychology, 86*(3), 389–401.

McCuaig, M., & Frank, G. (1991). The able self: Adaptive patterns and choices in independent living for a person with cerebral palsy. *American Journal of Occupational Therapy, 45*, 224–234.

McCubbin, H., Cauble, A., & Patterson, J. (1982). *Family stress, coping, and social support*. Springfield, IL: Thomas.

McHale, K., & Cermak, S. (1992). Fine motor activities in elementary school: Preliminary findings and provisional implications for children with fine motor problems. *American Journal of Occupational, 46*, 898–903.

Moos, R. (1974). *Evaluation of treatment environments: A sociological approach*. New York: Wiley.

Moos, R. (1981). *Work environment scale manual*. Palo Alto, CA: Consulting Psychologists Press.

Moos, R. (Ed.) (1986). *Coping with life crises: An integrated approach*. New York: Plenum.

Morris, T., Guard, J., Marine, S., Schick, L., Haag, D., Tsipsis, G., Kaya, B., & Shoemaker, S. (1997). Approaching equity in consumer health information delivery: NetWellness. *Journal of the American Medical Informatics Association, 4*(1), 25–30.

Mueller, J. (1990). *The workplace workbook: An illustrated guide to job accommodation and assistive technology*. Washington, DC: Dole Foundation.

Murphy, R. (1990). *The body silent*. New York: Norton.

Murphy, R., Scheer, J., Murphy, Y., & Mack, R. (1988). Physical disability and social liminality: A study in the rituals of adversity. *Social Science and Medicine, 26*, 235–242.

National Council on Disability. (2000). *National disability policy: A progress report*. Washington, DC: Author.

National Safety Council. (1998). *Risk factor checklist*. Washington, DC: Author.

Neimeyer, L., Matheson, L., & Carlton, R. (1989). Testing consistency of effort: BTE work simulator. *Industrial Rehabilitation Quarterly, 2*, 5–32.

Neufeldt et al. (1994). *Webster's New World Dictionary* (3rd ed.). New York, Prentice-Hall.

Norris, T. (2000). *Placing ritual within occupational therapy: A phenomenological study of ceremonial rituals and rituals of the everyday*. Unpublished doctoral dissertation, Denton, Texas: Texas Woman's University.

Oliver, R., Blathwayt, J., Brackley, C., & Tamaki, T. (1993). Development of the Safety Assessment of Function and the Environment for Rehabilitation (SAFER) Tool. *Canadian Journal of Occupational Therapy, 60*(2), 78–82.

Ottenbacher, K. (1992). Confusion in occupational therapy research: Does the end justify the method. *American Journal of Occupational Therapy, 46*, 871–874

Paivia, A., & Harshman, R. (1983). Factor analysis of a questionnaire on imagery and verbal habits and skills. *Canadian Journal of Psychology, 37*, 461–483.

Paivio, A. (1971). Coding distinctions and repetition effects in memory. *Psychology of Learning and Motivation, 9*, 179–214.

Park, S., Fisher, A., & Velozo, C. (1994). Using the assessment of motor and process skills to compare occupational performance between clinic and home settings. *American Journal of Occupational Therapy, 48*, 697–709.

Peloquin, S. (1997). The spiritual depth of occupation: Making worlds and making lives. *American Journal of Occupational Therapy, 51*, 167–168.

Peloquin, S., & Christiansen, C. (Eds.). (1997). Special issue on occupation, spirituality, and life meaning. *American Journal of Occupational Therapy, 51*(3), 165–234.

Plake, B., & Impara, J. (Eds.). (2001). *Mental measurements yearbook* (14th ed.). Lincoln: University of Nebraska Press.

Pulchaski, C. (1998). Spirituality and medicine. *World & I, 13*, 180–185.

Rieber, L. & Kini, A. (1991). Theoretical foundations of instructional applications of computer-generated animated visuals. *Journal of Computer-Based Instruction, 18*(3), 83–88.

Riley, B., Perna, R., Tate, D., Forchheimer, M., Anderson, C., & Luera, G. (1998). Types of spiritual well-being among persons with chronic illness: Their relation to various forms of quality of life. *Archives of Physical Medicine and Rehabilitation, 79*, 258–264.

Rivara, J., Jaffe, K., Polissar, N., Fay, G., Liao, S., & Martin, K. (1996). Predictors of family functioning and change three years after traumatic brain injury in children. *Archives of Physical Medicine and Rehabilitation, 77*, 754–764.

Rooney, E., Studenski, S., & Roman, L. (1997). A model for nurse case-managed home care using televideo. *Journal of the American Geriatric Society, 45*, 1523–1528.

Rowles, G. (1983). Geographical dimensions of social support in rural Appalachia. In G. Rowles & R. Ohta (Eds.). *Aging and milieu: Environmental perspectives on growing old* (pp. 111–130). New York: Academic Press.

Rowles, G. (1991). Beyond performance: Being in place as a component of occupational therapy. *American Journal of Occupational Therapy, 45*, 265–272.

Rush, K. & Ouellet, L. (1998). An analysis of elderly clients' views on mobility. *Western Journal of Nursing Research, 20*(3), 295–311.

Schkade, J., & Schultz, S. (1992). Occupational adaptation: Toward a holistic approach for contemporary practice, Part 1. *American Journal of Occupational Therapy, 46*, 829–837.

Schulz, E. (1999). *Spirituality and disability: A literature review*. Unpublished manuscript, Texas Woman's University, Denton, Texas.

Schulz, E. (2000). *The OT Quest: A spirituality and quality of experience assessment tool*. Unpublished manuscript, Texas Woman's University, Denton, Texas.

Shapiro, J. (1993). *No pity: People with disabilities forging a new civil rights movement*. New York: Times Books/Random House.

Shelp, E., DuBose, E., & Sunderland, R. (1990). The infrastructure of religious communities: A neglected resource for care of people with AIDS. *American Journal of Public Health, 80*, 970–972.

Soldo, B. J., Agree, W. M., & Wolf, D. A. (1989). The balance between formal and informal care. In J. Ory & K. Bond (Eds.). *Aging and health care: Social science and policy perspectives* (pp. 193–216). New York: Routledge.

Spencer, J., & Davidson, H. (1998). The Community Adaptive Planning Assessment: A clinical tool for documenting future planning with clients. *American Journal of Occupational Therapy, 52*(1), 19–30.

Spencer, J., Hersch, G., Schulz, E., Wiley, A., Schwartz, M., Kearney, K., McDonald, F., McGaugh, S., & Tegethoff, S. (2001). *Adaptation to relocation by elders following hospitalization: Evaluation of a model*. Unpublished manuscript.

Spencer, J., Krefting, L., & Mattingly, C. (1993). Incorporation of ethnographic methods in occupational therapy assessment. *American Journal of Occupational Therapy, 47*, 303–309.

Spencer, J., Young, M., Rintala, D., & Bates, S. (1995). Socialization to the culture of a rehabilitation hospital: An ethnographic study. *American Journal of Occupational Therapy, 49*, 53–62.

Stokols, D. (1999). Human development in the age of the Internet: Conceptual and methodological horizons. In S. Friedman & T. Wachs (Eds.). *Measuring environment across the lifespan* (pp. 327–356). Washington, DC: American Psychological Association.

Stoll, C. (1995). *Silicon snake oil: Second thoughts on the information highway*. Garden City NY: Doubleday.

Suto, M., & Frank, G. (1994). Future time perspective and daily occupations of persons with chronic schizophrenia in a board and care home. *American Journal of Occupational Therapy, 48*, 586–589.

Tringo, J. (1970). The hierarchy of preference toward disability groups. *Journal of Special Education, 4*, 295–306.

Trombly, C. (1995). Occupation: Purposefulness and meaningfulness as therapeutic mechanisms. [Eleanor Clarke Slagle Lecture]. *American Journal of Occupational Therapy, 49*, 960–972.

U.S. Architectural and Transportation Barriers Compliance Board. (1992). *Americans with Disabilities Act accessibility guidelines checklist for buildings and facilities*. Washington, DC: Author.

Virzi, R., Sorce, J., & Herbert, L. (1993). A comparison of three usability evaluation methods: Heuristic, thing-aloud, and performance testing. In *Proceedings of the Human Factors and Ergonomics Society* 37th Annual Meeting (pp. 309–313). Monterey, CA: Human Factors and Ergonomics Society.

Whiteneck, G., Charlifue, S., Gerhart, K, Overholser, J., & Richardson, G. (1992). Quantifying handicap: A new measure of long-term rehabilitation outcomes. *Archives of Physical Medicine and Rehabilitation, 73*, 519–526.

Willer, B., Rosenthal, M., Kreutzer, J., Gordon, W., & Rempel, R. (1993). Assessment of community integration following traumatic brain injury. *Journal of Head Trauma Rehabilitation*, 8(2), 75–87.

Wolfensberger, W. (1972). *Normalization: The principle of normalization in human services*. Toronto, ON, Canada: National Institute on Mental Retardation.

World Health Organization [WHO]. (2001). *International classification of functioning, disability and health (ICF)*. Geneva: Author.

Wright, P., & Monk, A. (1991). The use of think-aloud evaluation methods in design. *SIGCHI Bulletin, 23*, 55–57.

Yarrow, L. Rubenstein, J., & Pederson, F. (1975). *Infant and environment: Early cognitive and motivational development*. New York: Wiley.

Yerxa, E. (1994). Dreams, dilemmas, and decisions for occupational therapy practice in a new millennium: An American perspective. *American Journal of Occupational Therapy, 48*, 586–589.

Yuker, H. (1988). *Attitudes toward persons with disabilities*. New York: Springer.

Zola, I. (1985). Depictions of disability—Metaphor, message, and medium in the media: A research and political agenda. *Social Science Journal, 22*(4), 5–17.

CASE ANALYSIS: UNIT VII

MAUREEN E. NEISTADT

In Chapter 4, you met Mary Weber and her occupational therapist, Anna Deane Scott. Anna Deane's evaluation process was exactly what Mary needed. Let's look at why Anna Deane's evaluation was successful in relation to what you have read in this unit: "Occupational Therapy Evaluation."

Anna Deane did not choose to use any formal, standardized assessments of occupational performance. There were two reasons for this. First, for the first 6 months that Anna Deane worked with her, Mary was crying and having too many seizures to participate in formal assessments. Mary was grieving the loss of her life as she had known it before her injury. Her activity tolerance was severely restricted by the seizure disorder and mental fatigability that resulted from her traumatic head injury. When Mary became mentally fatigued, she could not process information to engage in conversation or activity. Under these conditions, formal assessments of occupational performance would have to have been done in incremental pieces over several sessions. The end result of that testing would have been to tell Anna Deane what she already knew from Mary's friend Sally—that Mary was having tremendous difficulty in her day-to-day occupations. Mary was already at home and was often unsafe owing to her occupational performance problems. Time spent on formal assessments would be lost time from helping Mary problem solve strategies for safer day-to-day functioning. So Anna Deane chose to use observation and activity analysis as her primary evaluation tools.

Second, when Anna Deane began working with Mary in the late 1970s there were no standardized occupational therapy assessments available for Mary's primary body function deficits—perception and cognition. Anna Deane felt she needed more in-depth information about Mary's perceptual and cognitive abilities than nonstandardized assessments could provide. So when Mary was able to participate in testing, Anna Deane arranged for her to have neuropsychological testing at home. This neuropsychological testing confirmed the hypotheses Anna Deane had formed about Mary's abilities, based on her observation of Mary's participation in desired occupations. The testing provided additional information as well. For example, the neuropsychology testing indicated that Mary was experiencing right frontal and left parietal lobe dysfunction. This information helped Anna Deane think of additional strategies Mary might use to perform her daily occupations safely.

During the first session, Anna Deane interviewed Mary (see Chapter 4). That interview started with Mary "sitting in the dark on a couch, crying." Anna Deane took her cues from this situation; she understood that Mary might need the darkness to keep her sensory stimulation to a minimum and to prevent a seizure. She respected Mary's sadness and the darkness and sought to talk with Mary about something clearly of value to her—her dogs. When you visit Mary, you cannot miss her dogs and cats. They are numerous and friendly. As a dog owner, Anna Deane understood how important one's pets can be. So she talked of dogs to form a bond that might help ease Mary's sadness. And in the process, she would have been able to evaluate Mary's ability to engage in conversation, to concentrate on a topic, to recall dog stories, and to talk abstractly about people's attachment for their pets. When Mary called Anna Deane after their first meeting, Anna Deane was genuine and empathetic, telling Mary she "felt sad" during their first meeting. This genuineness and empathy led Mary to feel she could trust Anna Deane; therapeutic collaboration is built on trust.

After the first meeting, Anna Deane would listen to Mary identify day-to-day problems and observe Mary try the occupations she identified. By listening to Mary describe her problems and by watching how Mary attempted important occupations, Anna Deane was able to hypothesize about potential barriers to successful performance and suggest solutions to overcome those problems, solutions that built on Mary's assets. Sometimes the solutions needed to be modified. Here again, Anna Deane used the process of listening, observation, and activity analysis to figure out how unsuccessful solutions could be modified to be more effective.

In Mary's case observation and activity analysis were the primary occupational therapy evaluation tools. Evaluation was an ongoing aspect of the intervention and progress was measured in Mary's increased ability to complete her valued daily occupations. Although the occupational therapy evaluation in this story was informal, nonetheless, it was rigorous and successful. The therapist in this story also sought consultation from other professionals (neuropsychologists), as needed, to supplement her evaluation information. This sharing of evaluation information among the professionals involved in a client's care yields a rich composite picture of an individual's strengths and areas for change and avoids costly duplication of assessments.

Some of your future clients will, like Mary, need informal evaluation procedures. Others may need more formal evaluations, especially at the beginning, midpoint, and end of intervention. All practitioners should be using Anna Deane's methods of listening, observation, and activity analysis throughout the intervention process to fine tune intervention in response to clients' changes.

UNIT *eight*

Occupational Therapy Intervention

Learning Objectives

After completing this unit, readers will be able to:

- Describe how to plan occupational therapy intervention based on an understanding of client interests and concerns, occupational performance assets and limitations, and the evidence relevant to intervention options.
- Differentiate among intervention types and approaches.
- Recommend intervention approaches based on analysis of the transaction between the person (client) and the environment as evidenced by the client's occupational performance.
- Describe the relative advantages and disadvantages of top-down versus bottom-up intervention strategies.
- Choose interventions based on client values and activity performance relative to independence, safety, and adequacy for occupational performance areas of the following:
    - Activities of daily living
    - Instrumental activities of daily living
    - Education
    - Work
    - Play
    - Leisure
    - Social participation
- Select and justify interventions focused on the client's personal skills and abilities.
- Select and justify interventions focused on contextual factors and adaptations influencing occupational performance.

This unit describes the variety of intervention strategies occupational therapy practitioners use to address client problems identified from the occupational therapy evaluation. The ultimate goal of occupational therapy intervention is to help clients become as proficient as they desire in their valued life activities. The methods that practitioners use fall into three general categories: (1) training designed to improve skill and performance in selected occupational performance areas, (2) activities and exercises to improve targeted client factors and prevent problems that interfere with desired occupational performance, and (3) environmental adaptations that make performance of occupational activities easier.

Occupational therapy services are provided to individuals and to groups. Often, a blend of intervention strategies is needed to meet the needs of clients. The mix of intervention approaches depends on a variety of factors, including the client's particular problem and intervention preferences, the nature of the impairment or environmental limitation, the potential for improvement, the anticipated length of intervention, the practitioner's knowledge, and the resources available in the practice setting.

Occupational therapy intervention is highly customized, because no single intervention strategy or combination of strategies is appropriate for all clients. Effective intervention requires an understanding the each client's occupational abilities and concerns, knowledge of the relevant theories and related research, and proficiency in a range of therapeutic skills designed to help clients gain mastery over their occupational lives. The theoretical bases for intervention were discussed in earlier units. This unit provides a variety of strategies and guidelines, which are further exemplified in later units that focusing on common conditions affecting the occupational performance of children, adults, and older adults. (Note: Words in **bold** type are defined in the Glossary.)

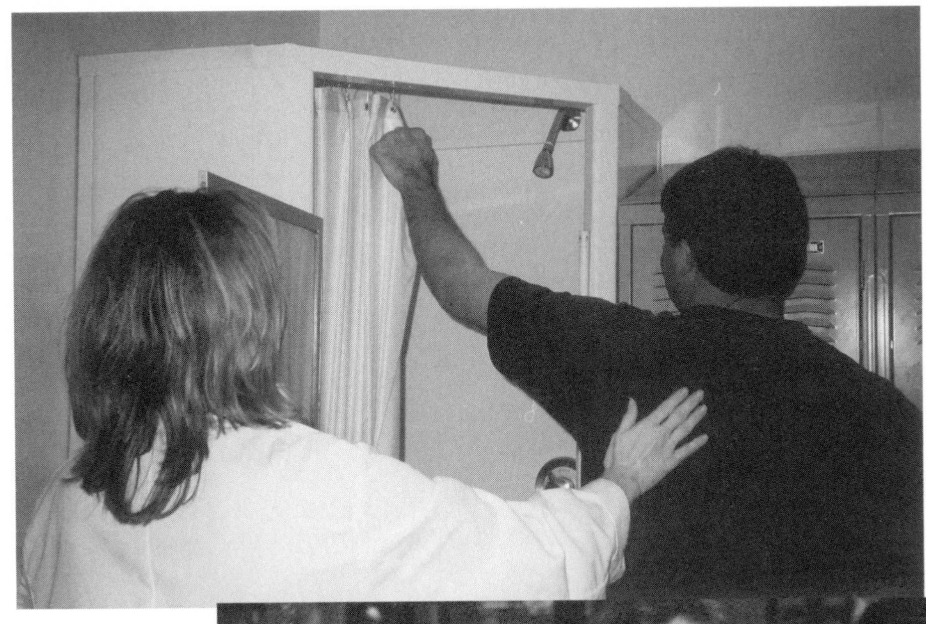

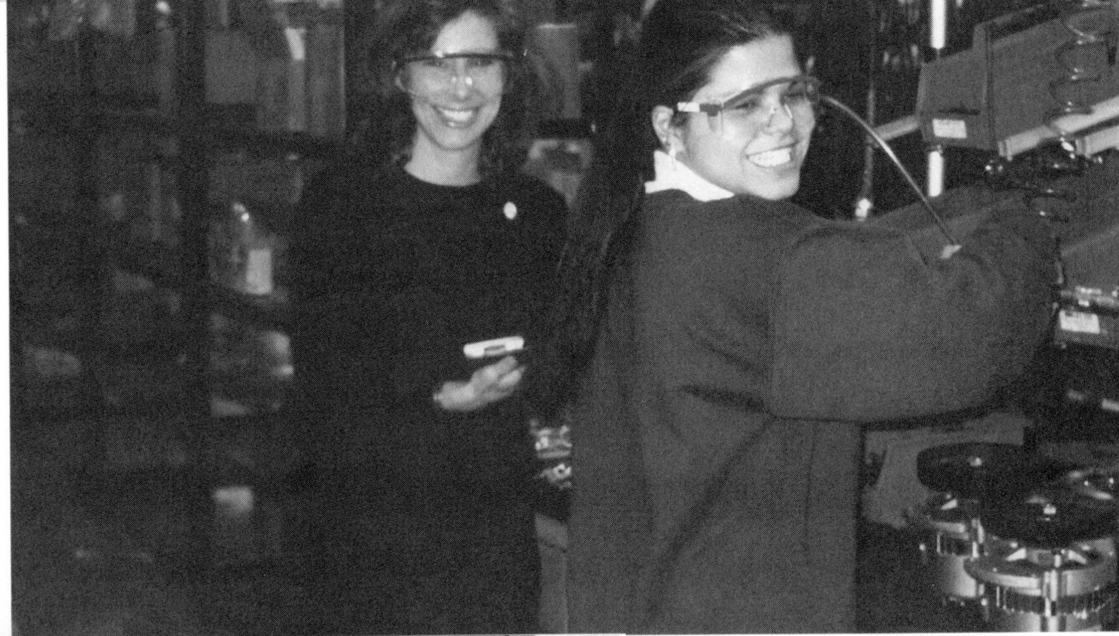

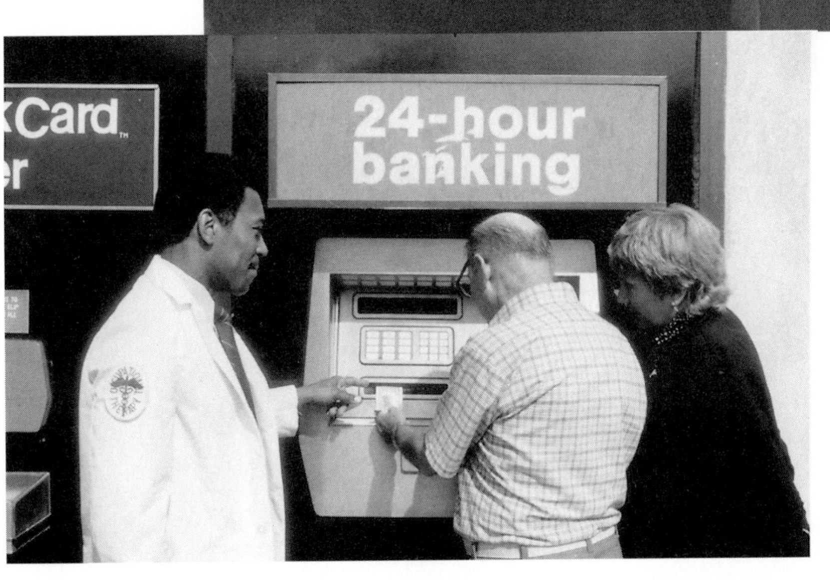

Occupational therapy practitioners help people gain skills in the contexts of daily life and community environments. (*top*) A man working on having the motor control needed to close a shower curtain. (Courtesy of Massachusetts General Hospital.) (*middle*) An occupational therapist observes a worker as she demonstrates how she can now safely use the tools required in her job. (Courtesy of S. Fenton.) (*bottom*) Learning to use an ATM is part of a community-skills training program for a client with persistent mental illness. (Courtesy of the archives of the American Occupational Therapy Association, Bethesda, MD.)

CHAPTER 27

OVERVIEW OF INTERVENTION

SECTION I: Occupational Therapy Intervention
SECTION II: Person–Task–Environment Interventions: A Decision-Making Guide

SECTION I

Occupational Therapy Intervention

BARBARA A. BOYT SCHELL
ELIZABETH BLESEDELL CREPEAU
ELLEN S. COHN

Occupational therapy **intervention** is the term used for the processes and methods that occupational therapy practitioners use to help their clients achieve desired occupational performance in their valued activities. These include personal and instrumental **activities of daily living** (ADL), education, work, play and leisure, and social participation (American Occupational Therapy Association—Commission on Practice [AOTA], in press). Section I provides an overview of intervention and the factors affecting intervention choices (Fig. 27-1). In Section 2 of this chapter, Holm, Rogers, and Stone provide a guide to intervention that is based in the person–task–environment transaction. Subsequent units apply these intervention methods to meet the needs of children and adults. Although practitioners design intervention for groups and whole populations, this section focuses primarily on intervention planning for individuals. Similar planning and approaches can also be used for groups.

Occupational therapy interventions occur in medical, educational, and a variety of community settings (Table 27-1). Each of these settings has particular characteristics that influence intervention. These are physical resources (such as tools, activities, and spaces available) as well as social factors (such as the policies guiding intervention, payment resources, and availability of personnel). In addition, intervention is influenced by the relative **acuity** versus **chronicity** of the person's health condition and the presence of supportive versus high-risk contextual factors.

The intervention process is integrally related to evaluation. Figure 27-1 provides an overview of the occupational therapy process, showing the interactive relationship among client concerns, evaluation, and intervention. Although both occupational therapists and occupational therapy assistants may implement interventions, the occupational therapist is responsible for ensuring that interventions are grounded in

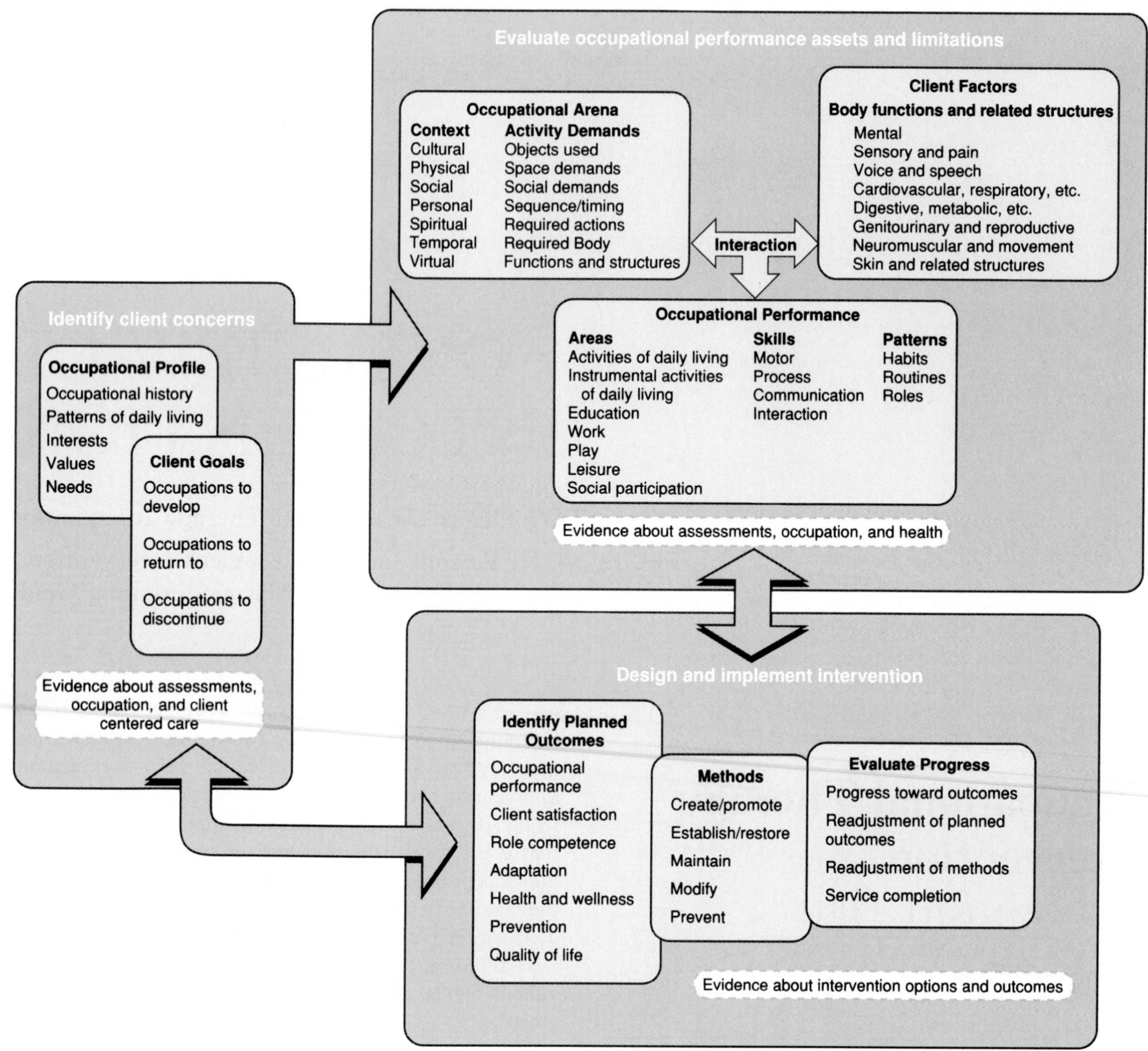

FIGURE 27–1. The occupational therapy process involves understanding the client's occupational concerns, evaluating occupational performance, and using occupational therapy interventions that address the identified concerns.

sound clinical reasoning and provided according to professional standards (Hinojosa, & Blount, 1998; Moyers, 1999).

IDENTIFY CLIENT CONCERNS

Occupational therapy practitioners base their intervention on an understanding of the client as a person with a unique history of life activities, patterns of daily living, values, and interests. Client goals are elicited by systematically interviewing the client and relevant others about how the client's occupations have been disrupted, threatened, or inadequately enacted. This information provides the basis for knowing where to focus attention and is the foundation for generating ideas about intervention.

EVALUATE OCCUPATIONAL PERFORMANCE ASSETS AND LIMITATIONS

Therapists evaluate occupational performance, focusing on the previously identified areas of concern. Beyond the

TABLE 27-1. **INTERVENTION TYPES**[a]

Type	Definition
Therapeutic use of self	Practitioners' planned use of their personality, insights, perceptions, and judgments as part of the therapeutic process
Therapeutic use of occupations & activities	Occupations/activities selected to meet specific therapeutic goals; categories include the following: • Occupational activities • Purposeful activities • Preparatory methods
Consultation process	Practitioners' use of knowledge and expertise to collaborate with clients in identifying problems and effective solutions, which are then implemented primarily by clients
Education process	Imparting knowledge and information about occupation and activity to the client

[a]Adapted from AOTA (in press).

client's actual performance, therapists may assess the context in which the client lives and works, the activity demands of this context, and specific aspects of the individual (such as strength, coordination, and mental functions that might influence performance).

Therapists are also concerned with the adequacy of the transactions between individuals and their contexts and how these transactions influence clients' ability to carry out their day-to-day lives. Using the World Health Organization's (WHO, 2001) classification of function, this means occupational therapists look at the impact of individual capacities (body functions and structures) on desired activity and participation. Simultaneously, occupational therapists also consider the impact of the context (environmental and personal factors) on activity and participation. A careful appraisal of the interaction among these factors allows therapists to identify both person-based and context-based limitations that contribute to clients' occupational performance concerns. Equally important, these analyses identify assets that can serve to promote occupational health.

Although it is critical to base intervention on careful evaluation, therapists often interweave the evaluation and intervention processes (Rogers, Holm, & Stone, 1997). There are several reasons for this.

- *Intervention is needed to explore a person's performance potential more fully*. For example a therapist might receive a referral for a client with cerebral palsy who needs to use assistive technology at his work site. While conducting the initial evaluation, the therapist notes that the client is not well positioned in his wheelchair. The therapist switches to an intervention of providing a firmer seat and trunk supports to help stabilize the client before proceeding with the rest of the evaluation related to assistive technology.
- *Critical concerns must be addressed to prevent further decline in function*. An example of this is the fabrication of a protective splint for a client recovering from a wrist fracture before beginning work on self-care and home management concerns.
- *New observations of occupational performance prompt further investigation*. For example, a practitioner working in a public school may observe that a child is able to initiate interactions with peers in the classroom after a participating in a social skills group led by an occupational therapist. However, after observing the child struggle to keep up with peers in a kick-ball game on the playground, the therapist decides that an evaluation of motor skills is also indicated. In this case, even though intervention was well under way, new data prompted further evaluation.

In whatever sequence, the occupational therapist is responsible for using the information from the evaluation process in combination with the best evidence available to recommend intervention options for the client (Holm, 2000). These intervention options should be related to the anticipated outcomes that will occur as a result of the intervention.

DEVELOP INTERVENTION PLAN

A well-stated intervention plan includes two components: the anticipated outcomes and the methods the therapist and client will use to achieve those outcomes (AOTA, in press; Moyers, 1999). Stated outcomes are necessary to help therapist and client clarify the focus of intervention. Outcomes should do the following:

- Relate to the client's goals and desired occupational performance.
- Be measurable, so that it is evident when the outcome has been achieved.

- Be accompanied by an estimated time frame for intervention

Practitioners routinely document expected intervention outcomes, although the documentation form varies greatly, depending on the setting.

The intervention plan states the methods the practitioner will use to meet the outcomes. Occupational therapists must be explicit about the underlying assumptions guiding their decision making. There must be a logically justifiable chain of reasoning and evidence that undergirds the therapist's evaluation findings and selection of intervention methods.

IMPLEMENT INTERVENTION

Once the therapist and the client agree on an intervention plan, it is implemented. Intervention approaches can address the person's skills and patterns during occupational performance or they can focus more on the activity demands and performance context. Often several are addressed simultaneously. (Section 2 provides many examples of the different variations associated with intervention focus.)

Interventions also can be characterized by the how closely they connect to the person's occupations (Fisher, 1998). Fisher described several ways to think about this issue:

- *Ecological relevance:* Is the intervention a contrived exercise or a more naturalistic occupation?
- *Purpose and meaning:* Do the purpose and related meanings come primarily from the therapist (e.g., "Do this because it is good for you.") or do they come from the client (e.g., "This is something I want or need to do.").
- *Focus of intervention:* Is the activity designed to remediate or improve some aspect of the client's abilities (such as a body function) or is it focused on improving occupational performance directly?

Occupational, Purposeful, and Preparatory Activities

New practitioners often struggle with how to select interventions, perhaps because they are overwhelmed with all the factors that must be considered. A good place to start is to attend carefully to the person's valued **occupations.** Often the best thing to do is to work directly on the occupational performance concern, using those valued occupations as the methods (Gray, 1999; Trombly, 1995). Table 27-2 shows the range of choices that practitioners have to focus on when selecting an occupational approach. For example, when trying to help a child with developmental disabilities learn to feed herself in a socially acceptable manner, the therapist would be focusing on an ADL. The therapist could focus on skills, such teaching the child the correct methods of using eating utensils to bring the food to her mouth. Alternatively, the therapist could work with the child's mother and the child to develop good eating habits, such as alternating drinking liquids with eating solid foods, to help the child swallow and avoid food spillage from her mouth. The therapist could change the activity demands by having the child's mother present only one food item at a time. Or the therapist could increase the social demand by having the child eat in a restaurant. Finally, selected client factors could be addressed. For example, if the child is overly excitable, part of the intervention plan might be to introduce chewy foods first as a form of proprioceptive input that would have a calming effect on her nervous system.

Using relevant occupational activities as the intervention works because clients attach meaning to these occupational activities, which in turn help them develop or regain their identities (Christiansen, 1999). The practitioner must carefully analyze and grade the relevant activity. Practitioners also need to collaborate with the client to create circumstances that permit the activity to occur in its natural context. Alternatively, the client may need to bring in relevant tools or materials from home, work, or school to the intervention setting. Using these approaches, clients

TABLE 27-2. **INTERVENTION CHOICES**

	Skills	Habits and Routines	Context	Activity Demand	Client Factors
ADL					
IADL					
Education					
Work					
Play					
Leisure					
Social Participation					

Occupational performance concerns, related assets, and limitations form the basis for selecting the focus of intervention.

gradually develop or regain the desired skills as a function of gradually engaging in occupation activities.

In other situations, clients learn new or adaptive skills. Occasionally, clients resist attempting occupational activities, either because the feel they cannot perform as well as they did in the past or because they fear failure in the future. In these situations, practitioners need to identify alternative activities that share some similar characteristics as the occupational activities but that do not pose a threat, because the person has no internalized image of competence relative to this new activity. These are sometimes referred to as **purposeful activities.** This term can be confusing, as it is used in different ways (American Occupational Therapy Association [AOTA], 1993, 1995). All interventions have a purpose, in that they are selected for their likelihood of helping the client attain valued occupational outcomes. Occupational activities are selected because they have inherent meaning to the person and can be customized to meet specific aims, such as increasing concentration, coordination, or social skills. Purposeful activities are selected because they are congruent with the person's general interests and because they promote specific outcomes.

In addition to occupational and purposeful activities, practitioners also use **preparatory** and **adjunctive methods** (AOTA, in press; Moyers, 1999). Practitioners use preparatory methods to facilitate performance by helping some part of the client's body or mind perform more effectively in preparation for engaging in an activity. For instance, a client might be encouraged to practice visualization techniques to promote better performance in high stress activities, such as taking a test or going to a job interview. Another client might be encouraged to use a hot pack or to take a hot shower in the mornings to reduce morning stiffness from arthritis, thus improving mobility for household chores or gardening.

As discussed in the next section, there are differing views in the field about the appropriate sequencing of occupational and purposeful activities and the use of preparatory and adjunctive methods. We suggest that preparatory or adjunctive interventions be nested within therapy that always includes either occupational or purposeful activity. This is for two reasons. First, current research about motor and cognitive learning supports the need for individuals to use knowledge in the context of daily activities for the most effective gains to occur (see Chapters 21 and 30). Second, by consistently using occupation or purposeful activities as therapy, it is easier for clients and other interested parties to understand the unique contribution of occupational therapy to health.

Intervention Monitoring and Service Completion

Practitioners monitor the client's responses to intervention as therapy proceeds. Therapists systematically evaluate progress toward outcomes and adjust interventions as needed. For instance, some goals may be met and new ones emerge. Alternatively, some clients may not respond to the intervention as planned, and the methods may need to be changed. Eventually, clients reach a point at which outcomes have been met or continued therapy services are unlikely to substantially benefit them. At this point, services are discontinued. There are also circumstances in which the client chooses to discontinue services or in which there are not sufficient resources to support continued intervention. In the latter situation, therapists should seek alternatives to meet the needs of clients who wish to receive intervention.

CONCLUSION

Occupational therapy intervention is highly customized, taking into account the client's occupational profile and concerns, the evaluation findings, and the range of intervention options most likely to be successful in meeting desired outcomes. The use of occupational and purposeful activities during intervention serves the dual purpose of harnessing the client's values and interests and illustrating occupational therapy's unique contribution to health care.

HISTORICAL NOTE 27–1

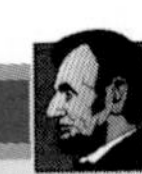

Susan Tracy's Vision: The Need to Focus on Meaning

SUZANNE M. PELOQUIN

Susan E. Tracy started a program of manual arts at the Adams Nevine Asylum in Boston, the first course designed to train nurses as crafts instructors. She left a legacy of her views in a book published years before the founding of the Society for the Promotion of Occupational Therapy.

Tracy (1913) thought that the crafts teacher had to be "thoughtful of the deeper needs of her patient" (p. 10). She believed that an instructor who met those needs realized larger gains:

> *If a nurse can prove to the patient who chafes against his limitations that there is really a broad highway of usefulness opening before him of which he knew not, the mental friction is diminished and satisfaction steals in, while the whole physical organism prepares to respond by improved conditions. (p. 171)*

Tracy's vision of broad pathways to usefulness is an inspiring one. It reminds therapists today to explore those treatments that press past impaired sensation or limited motion to reach their clients' more basic needs for satisfaction and meaning.

Tracy, S. E. (1913). *Studies in invalid occupation: A manual for nurses and attendants*. Boston: Whitcomb & Barrows.

SECTION II

Person–Task–Environment Interventions: A Decision-Making Guide

MARGO B. HOLM
JOAN C. ROGERS
RONALD G. STONE

Historically, occupational therapy practitioners have been recognized for expertise in the direct observation of clients' performance of the everyday tasks that define and bring meaning to their clients' lives (Booth, Davidson, Winstanley, & Waters, 2001; Fisher & Short-DeGraff, 1993; Guralnik, Branch, Cummings, & Curb, 1989; Hilton, Fricke, & Unsworth, 2001). The unique contribution of occupational therapy, as a profession, is at the level of societal participation and activity capacity and performance, namely the person–task–environment (PTE) transaction. In considering function at this level, practitioners bring cognizance of the factors within the client (body functions and structures; personal capacities) during the client's transaction with specific tasks and task environments.

This section is divided into six major subsections. The first subsection begins with a brief review of occupational therapy frames of references that highlight PTE transactions. The review documents the increasing attention that is being given to explaining the way in which humans influence their environments and the way in which environments influence humans. The PTE transaction is then described in terms of its component parts and their synergistic interactions. This discussion provides needed background for understanding the PTE transaction in health and disease/disorder—that is, in function and dysfunction. In the second subsection, the PTE transaction is placed in the context of rehabilitation and occupational therapy theoretical perspectives. This discussion provides core concepts for understanding occupational therapy approaches to managing performance discrepancies. In the third subsection, the two major approaches to managing performance discrepancies—bottom-up and top-down—are defined and described. The top-down approach is selected as the approach of choice for meeting the challenges of the emerging practice areas and managed health care. The subsection concludes with a discussion of the nature of performance discrepancy. Thus the third subsection sets the stage for the delineation of decision points for occupational therapy interventions.

The fourth subsection discusses the nature of performance discrepancy and presents a clinical decision–making guide. The fifth subsection uses the clinical decision-making guide for determining whether performance discrepancies originate from deficits in skills or habits. This determination aids occupational therapy practitioners in understanding the nature of a performance discrepancy and thereby in planning appropriate interventions. The last major subsection concentrates on the establishment of target functional outcomes and their management through environmental interventions. In this subsection, five intervention strategies are defined and illustrated through clinical cases.

PTE TRANSACTION MODELS

Safe, adequate, and independent performance of ADL, instrumental ADL (IADL), work/school, and play and leisure tasks depends on a successful PTE transaction. Ecological models, those concerned with interactions between people and their environments, address the PTE transaction. Occupational therapists have historically acknowledged the contribution of the environment to task performance, with early leaders Slagle (1922), Meyer (1922), and Haas (1944) suggesting the adaptation of environmental characteristics as one means of improving the function of clients. However, serious attempts to translate this philosophy into practice models are of more recent origin. Since the 1980s, several ecological models have been presented in the occupational therapy literature to assist practitioners' understanding of the PTE transaction.

In 1982, Rogers borrowed concepts from the behavioral sciences to modernize and enrich the fundamental premises about the link between function and the environment articulated in occupational therapy's early philosophy. Independent behavior was viewed as a function of the competence and autonomy of the person and the behavior-evoking aspects of the physical, social, and temporal environment. Normally, habits of daily living enable humans to respond automatically and appropriately to a variety of environmental demands. The balance between person capacities and environmental demands may be disrupted by impairment-associated or age-related physical, cognitive, and affective deficits. A fundamental therapeutic strategy for raising capacity, reduced by impairment, is to lower environmental demands and then raise them gradually as competence improves. Kiernat (1982) further articulated the concept of the environment as a therapeutic modality.

Barris (1982) developed the concept of environment in conjunction with the Model of Human Occupation proposed by Kielhofner and Burke (1980). Accordingly, individuals choose environments to become involved with based on such environmental properties as novelty, complexity, and compatibility with interests and values. Environmental demands for performance, which are associated with the people and objects available in the environment, strongly influence the development of roles, habits, and skills. The development of competence involves the ability to interact successfully with an increasingly broader range of environments. Thus the model clarifies environmental properties and their influence on people.

Howe and Briggs (1982), like Barris, used general systems theory to describe the person–environment relationship. In their Ecological Systems Model, humans and their environments shape each other. People are at the center of the ecosystem and are surrounded by three interacting environment layers—the immediate setting, social networks and institutions, and ideology. These layers make up the life space for the performance of life tasks and roles. Behavior is functional if person–environment interactions enable individuals to achieve goals that are consonant with their views of quality of life.

When defining occupation, Nelson (1988) made a distinction between occupational form and occupational performance. He argued that occupational performance, or action, can be understood only in the context of occupational form—that is, "an objective set of circumstances, independent of and external to a person" (p. 633). One dimension of occupational form involves the physical stimuli present in the environment, including the materials used, the surrounding environment, the human context, and temporal relationships. A second dimension of occupational form is the sociocultural milieu. The first dimension focuses on the doing aspect of performance, while the second dimension emphasizes the symbolic aspect (e.g., values and norms). According to Nelson, occupational performance, then, is the action elicited, guided, or structured by an occupational form.

Holm and Rogers (1989) described the PTE transaction as a relationship between the capacities required of a task performer and the inherent properties, procedures, equipment, and materials involved in functional activities. Emphasis was placed on the natural setting, as opposed to the clinical setting, as a means of eliminating contrived environmental influences. Subsequently, Rogers and Holm (1991a) adapted Lawton's (1982) ecological model of aging to explicate further the PTE transaction. Lawton described behavior (B) as a function (f) of person capacities (P) and environmental demand (E)—or $B = f(P, E)$—and noted that as a person's capacities become impaired, the influence of the environment (i.e., environmental press) on behavior increases. By implication, then, activity performance depends on the match between the capacities of the person and the demands that the environment places on these capacities.

Rogers and Holm (1991a) revised Lawton's formula to highlight the role of nonhuman environmental elements in task performance by including assistive technology devices (ATDs) for the person, objects in the environment (OE), and/or the structural environment (SE) into the equation, as a method of equalizing the person capacity–environmental demand relationship. The formulas are as follows:

$$B = f[(P + \text{ATD}) \times \text{OE} \times \text{SE}] \quad \text{(ATD for the person, such as a listening device)} \tag{27-1}$$

$$B = f[P \times (\text{OE} + \text{ATD}) \times \text{SE}] \quad \text{(ATD for a task object, such as a built-up spoon)} \tag{27-2}$$

$$B = f[P \times \text{OE} \times (\text{SE} + \text{ATD})] \quad \text{(ATD for a structural environment, such as a ramp)} \tag{27-3}$$

By incorporating assistive technology devices into the equation, task performance becomes a function of person capacities, which may be enhanced by ATDs interacting with environmental demands, which may be reduced by the ATDs. Another ecological model was introduced by Christiansen (1991) and Baum, namely, the Person–Environment–Performance model. In their model, person factors (e.g., motivation, experience, beliefs, abilities, and skills) are viewed as intrinsic enablers of performance. Performance includes activities, tasks, and roles of occupations, and the environment includes physical, social, and cultural factors. A unique contribution of this model is the emphasis of person capacities as enablers of activity and task performance.

In the University of Southern California (USC) Model of Human Subsystems That Influence Occupation, occupational behavior is portrayed as emerging from six internal subsystems—physical, biological, information processing, sociocultural, symbolic-evaluative, and transcendental (Clark et al., 1991). These human subsystems interact with the external environment, which is comprised of the sociocultural context and the person's history.

The Occupational Adaptation frame of reference includes the person, the occupational environment, and the interaction of these factors during occupation (Schkade & Schultz, 1992; Schultz & Schkade, 1992). This frame of reference focuses on the client's experience of self in relevant occupational contexts and the use of meaningful occupations to affect the client's internal adaptation process rather than outward measures of performance (Dolecheck & Schkade, 1999; Gibson & Schkade, 1997). Desired outcomes of the occupational adaptation model are effective, efficient, and satisfying responses to the demands posed by the environment.

The Ecology of Human Performance (EHP) framework, proposed by the occupational therapy faculty of the University of Kansas differentiates between a task and the person's performance of the task, thus adding one more dimension to a person capacity–environmental demand model (Dunn, Brown, & McGuigan, 1994). The EHP defines person, task, performance, and context, using the "Uniform Terminology for Occupational Therapy—Third Edition" (Uniform Terminology; AOTA, 1994), and describes possible relationships among the four components. In addition, five collaborative approaches to intervention (establish/restore, alter, adapt, prevent, and create) that incorporate all four components of the EHP framework are described.

In a further theoretical development of the Model of Human Occupation, Kielhofner (1995) identified the environment as influencing occupational behavior through affording and pressing. In the former, the environment affords opportunities for performance; whereas in the latter, it presses for certain types of behavior. The physical environment was conceptualized as being composed of natural and built environments and objects. The social environment consists of social groups and occupational forms—that is, rule-bound action sequences. The physical and social environments intertwine to create occupational behavior settings, or meaningful contexts for occupational performance.

Similar to the EHP framework, the Person–Environment–Occupation model also separates the concept of occupation from the performance of the occupation and emphasizes the consequences to occupational performance when there is any change in the person, the environment, or the occupation (Law et al., 1996; Strong et al., 1999). The model is designed to help occupational therapy practitioners take into consideration the temporal aspects of occupational routines, not only on a daily, weekly or monthly basis but also from a lifespan development perspective.

Finally, task analysis, which is essential to occupational therapy practice, merits recognition as an ecological conceptual framework. In essence, task analysis defines the relationship between the person and the environment as an action (e.g., reaches) oriented toward an object (e.g., into the cupboard). As a theoretical approach, task analysis has been highly developed in human factors engineering (Militello, 1998; Militello & Hutton, 1998; Pelland & McKinley, 2001; Schaafstal, Schraagen, & van Berlo, 2000; Yu, Hwang, & Huang, 1999). A human factors approach to capacity-demand models uses task analysis to divide tasks into discrete sequential steps and then defines the physiological (e.g., actions, postures, grasps), sensory (e.g., feels, sees), and cognitive (e.g., searches, scans) requirements for successful task completion (Faletti, 1984). The occupational therapy practitioner then compares the demands of each step of the task, including environmental demands, with the capacities of the person. When the task-environmental demands are greater than the person's capacities, the specific area for intervention is targeted (Clark, Czaja, & Weber, 1990; Czaja, Weber, & Nair, 1993).

This brief review of ecological models indicates that the PTE transaction has been described from numerous perspectives and with different emphases on the various components. A common theme emerging from them is that clients use their capacities to accomplish a task at a given time, using the objects available, in a specific place. The **outcomes** of a person's performance in terms of parameters such as independence, safety, and adequacy depend on the transactions between and among the capacities of the person; the demands of the task; and the demands of the physical, social, cultural, and temporal context in which the task takes place. Just as therapists' attempts to understand the occupational functioning of clients have led to a delineation of the factors within clients, so too, their attempts to understand the interface between individuals with activity limitations and their life demands will lead to a delineation of the factors outside clients that are critical for social participation.

As used in this section, a performance transaction implies a negotiation or arrangement among three factors: person capacities, environmental demands at the task level, and environmental demands at the physical and social levels. After defining and describing each of these factors separately, we view them in concert in the discussions of the transaction and of performance discrepancy.

Person (Client) Capacities

Person capacities include inherent generic abilities and task-specific skills. Mental, sensory, and neuromuscular capacities and other bodily functions and structures underlie, support, and enable the performance of multiple tasks (AOTA, in press). Examples of these capacities are attention, proprioception, and joint mobility. Generic capacities coalesce into unique combinations to form task-specific performance skills and habits. Task-specific skills and habits emerge to affect the performance and participation in real-life occupations, such as dressing, meal preparation, Web-site designing, and playing wheelchair basketball. Task-specific skills are developed through training and practice—that is, through the learning and repetition of the PTE transaction in standardized and real-life situations (Giles, Ridley, Dill, & Frye, 1997; Ma & Trombly, 1999; Mathiowetz & Wade, 1995; WHO, 2001)

Environmental Demands

Environmental demands are extrinsic to person capacities. These demands occur at two levels: the level of the task and the level of the surrounding physical, social, cultural, spiritual, and virtual environment (AOTA, in press).

Task Demands

Client capacities are challenged by the requirements of tasks, which are usually referred to as task demands (Johnson, 2000; Seki, Ishiai, Koyama, & Sato, 1999; Steptoe, Cropley, & Joekes, 2000). Task demands are identified through **task analysis,** which is the analytic process of breaking tasks down into discrete, sequential steps (Creighton, 1992; Cynkin, 1979). Task analysis identifies the actions that clients are to perform in relation to objects. For example, to make a cup of tea, clients must do the following:

Action	Object
Locate	Tea bag and drinking container
Place	Tea bag in drinking container
Obtain	Container for water
Obtain and heat	Water
Pour	Water over tea bag
Remove	Tea bag

The actions making up task performance are highly influenced by the objects used to perform them, which include the task materials, tools, and equipment. Task objects have inherent properties that influence the strength or force of the task demand. For instance, pancake batter presents less resistance when stirred than a stiff cookie dough, a plastic garbage bag placed on a car seat provides less resistance than cloth seat covers when transferring into and out of a car, and an overhead knit shirt has stretch capabilities whereas an overhead cotton weave shirt does not stretch when it is donned.

When calculating the demand properties of a task, the nature of the inherent properties of task objects must be analyzed. For example, one method practitioners can use to analyze the properties of task objects is based on the effect the properties have on the senses. When touched, lifted, carried, pushed, or pulled, task objects can be slick, sticky, wet, dry, greasy, crumbly, hard, soft, warm, cold, sharp, scratchy, smooth, heavy, and light. When visualized, they can be large, small, colorful, bright, dull, far, and near and have distinct shapes and patterns. When listened to they can produce loud, soft, irritating, soothing, and inaudible sounds. Task objects can taste sweet, sour, salty, and bitter and emanate odors that are pleasant, noxious, or unnoticeable. In some environments, the inherent properties of objects may also be hazardous to health, such as certain chemicals, solvents, heavy metals, and radiation materials (Brigham, Engelberg, & Richling, 1996). Task materials (e.g., bread, shirt, shampoo bottle), tools (e.g., fork, drill, ice-cream scoop), and equipment (e.g., computer, stove, work bench) vary based on their function, design, size, and shape (Cynkin, 1979; Demore-Taber, 1995; Hagedorn, 1995a; Levine & Brayley, 1991; Rogers & Holm, 1991a).

The properties of task objects can be used to increase and decrease task demands. For example, if practitioners consider the actions required and the properties of task objects described above, the task demands for making a cup of tea can vary greatly. Heating water for a cup of tea can be accomplished by heating the water in a teapot or pan on the stovetop, heating a cup of water in a microwave, using an electric kettle, or placing an electric heating element into the cup. The tea leaves can be loose in a can, contained in a tea bag, or ground into powder for instant tea. The tea can be served in a ceramic mug, a plastic mug, a china cup, or the lid of a thermos. Thus the task steps, and inherent properties and design of specific task objects used to perform a task have a strong influence on the task demands and performance outcomes.

Surrounding Physical and Social Environment Demands

In addition to the demands inherent in tasks performed with available objects, task performance is also influenced by the surrounding physical and social environments (Christiansen, 1991; Dunn et al., 1994; Iwarsson, Isacsson, & Lanke, 1998; Law et al., 1996; Letts, law, Rigby, Cooper, Stewart, & Strong, 1994; Rogers, 1982). The properties of the physical environment usually include space, arrangement, equipment controls, surface heights, lighting, temperature, noise, humidity, vibration, and ventilation (Demore-Tabor, 1995; Hagedorn, 1995a; Jacobs, 1999; Raschko, 1991). Each of these properties has been further delineated in architectural (Raschko, 1991; Stamps, 2000), anthropometric (Baker, 1999; Diffrient, Tilley, & Bardagjy, 1974; Pheasant, 1998), ergonomic (Jacobs, 1999; Kroemer & Grandjean, 1997; Rice, 1998), and occupational health and safety literature (Brigham et al., 1996; Carson, 1994; Kroemer & Grandjean, 1997; Moore & Garg, 1995). Not only are there static aspects of the physical environment to be considered but there are also the dynamic aspects: machines that have moving parts, temperatures that fluctuate, noise levels that rise and fall, humidity that rises and falls, and ventilation that fluctuates. Moreover, some environments, including new office buildings and homes, are referred to as sick environments because of how they affect the performance of those who work or live in them (Arcury, Quandt, Cravey, Elmore, & Russell, 2001; Kopias, 2001; Rosenberg, Barbeau, Moure-Eraso, & Levenstein, 2001). These environments are deemed sick because of inadequate ventilation systems, asbestos insulation, radon, improperly functioning cooling systems, or old plumbing systems that deliver water tainted with lead (Brigham et al., 1996).

The demands of the physical environment may compound those of the task. If a toilet is on the second floor of a two-story house and a client cannot climb stairs, the client will not be able to get to the toilet to use it. A portable toilet may need to be purchased or rented and installed in a first-floor bedroom or closet to reduce the demands of physical structures. Furthermore, if space in the bedroom is restricted, or if there is no lighting in the closet, the safety of toilet transfers may be compromised, and adaptations may need to occur to reduce the negative effect of environmental demand.

Often environmental demand is viewed solely in terms of the physical environment. However, the social environment also influences role and task performance (Woodward, Hales, Litidamu, Phillips, & Martin, 2000). The social environment includes more than the mere number of persons in the home, school, or workplace. The knowledge, skills, habits, expectations, values, attitudes, and motivations of these people create a social climate that fosters or hinders task performance (MacDonald, Karasek, Punnett, & Scharf, 2001; Seki et al., 1999; Walker, Goodwin, & Warren, 1995). Cultural beliefs, norms, customs, and practices also influence the social environment (Hagedorn, 1995a). The temporal environment, or the ebb and flow of task performance, is also an environmental demand. Moreover, people arrange their physical, social, and temporal environments. They select and place task objects, organize and govern social groups, and establish daily schedules and the pacing of tasks (MacDonald et al., 2001). In so doing, they set the overall level of stimulation (e.g., too much, just right, too little) surrounding them during task performance (Christiansen, 1991; Gerdner, Hall, & Buckwalter, 1996; Keuter, Bryne, Voell, & Larson, 2000). At any given time, a person can have numerous roles (e.g., worker, parent, husband, grandparent, co-worker, volunteer, client, and social activist), each of which has unique task demands that occur in separate or overlapping physical and social environments.

The Transaction

Clients are not passive recipients of the effects of their environments. Rather, they act on, as well as are acted on, by task and physical and social environmental forces. This creates a transactional relationship that is characterized as an interdependence between person capacities and the demands of the task and the task environment (Dunn et al., 1994; Law et al., 1996; Lawton, 1982; Rogers, 1982). For example, a client who is unable to get up the stairs to the bathtub may install a shower on the first floor of the home, provide a stair lift to the second level, or bathe at the kitchen sink. Each of these decisions changes the task objects and the task environment, and, in turn, these environmental changes alter the PTE transaction.

When Demands Exceed Capacities: Performance Discrepancy

When the capacities of a client are sufficient to manage the demands of the task and the surrounding environment, the client's performance and the level of performance that is expected, required, or desired are congruent. However, when demands exceed capacities, task performance is compromised, and there is a **performance discrepancy** between actual performance and the performance skills or habits that are expected, required, or desired (Lawton, 1982; Mager & Pipe, 1984; Mangino, 2000). The performance discrepancy can be reduced, eliminated, or prevented by establishing or restoring capacities, by reducing task or environmental demands, or by using a combination of these two methods (Holm, Santangelo, Fromuth, Brown, & Walter, 2000; Law et al., 1996; Mathiowetz & Matuska, 1998; Rogers et al., 1999; Rogers et al., 2000; van Heugten et al., 1998). With the diminishment of their capacities through impairment, trauma, developmental delay, age-related decrements, psychological maladaptation, or environmental deprivation, clients become more susceptible to environmental influences. They have fewer internal resources and less energy to resist environmental forces or to devise adaptive strategies to counteract them (Lawton, 1982). By designing a therapeutic environment to accommodate diminished capacity, practitioners may be able to improve task performance (Close et al., 1999; Cummings et al., 1999; Mee & Sumsion, 2001; Rogers et al., 1999, 2000).

THE PTE TRANSACTION AND MODELS OF FUNCTION AND DYSFUNCTION

The **PTE transaction** is a composite of person capacities influencing and being influenced by the demands of objects and the ambient physical and social environment. Now that we have reviewed the PTE transaction, but before we examine further the nature of performance discrepancies, we will consider the PTE transaction from the overall perspective of rehabilitation and occupational therapy science. This perspective assists in understanding occupational therapy approaches to fostering competent PTE transactions.

Clients are referred for occupational therapy services primarily because there is a discrepancy in current activity or social participation performance compared to the performance that is expected of, required of, or desired by them. These performance discrepancies are usually the

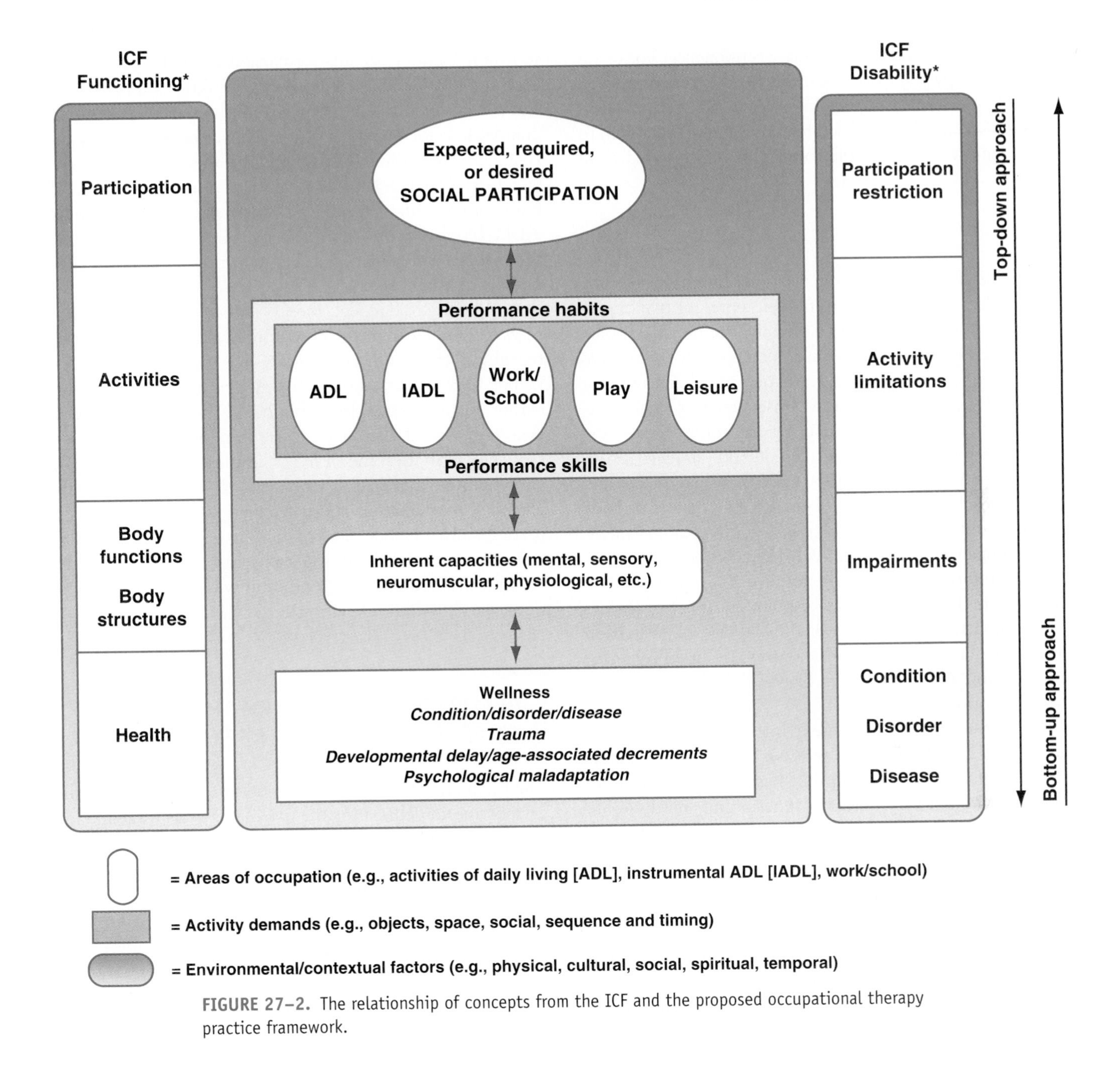

FIGURE 27–2. The relationship of concepts from the ICF and the proposed occupational therapy practice framework.

result of a specific disease or disorder and its consequences for daily living. The International Classification of Functioning, Disability and Health (ICF; WHO, 2001) defines health as having two parts—part 1 concerns functioning and disability, and part 2, contextual factors. Part 1 focuses on positive and negative aspects of body functions and structures and on activities and participation. Part 2 focuses on the positive and negative impact of environmental factors (i.e., the external environmental) and less so on personal factors (i.e., personal characteristics not part of a current health condition, such as upbringing and education). Positive aspects of health are referred to as *functioning*, and the negative aspects as *disability*. There are similarities and differences between the hierarchy of the ICF and that implicit in the occupational therapy practice framework (AOTA, in press), which are depicted in Figure 27-2.

As seen in Figure 27-2, the ICF hierarchy of functioning is built on a foundation of health, indicative of "functional and structural integrity" of body functions and body structures (WHO, 2001). In the health condition, generic activities (i.e., tasks and actions executed by a person) are not limited. When activities are carried out in a standardized environment, meaning that the influence of the environment on the task has been neutralized, it is referred to as *activity capacity*. When activities are carried out in the real-life environment, it is known as *activity performance*. For occupational therapy practitioners, this is the difference between an activity performed in the clinic versus one performed in the client's home. When discrete activities are combined to enact social roles in real-life situations, it is referred to as *participation* in the ICF model.

ICF

Figure 27-2 also shows the ICF disability hierarchy. Disease and disorder, according to this model, represent two opposing explanations of disability—namely, the medical model and the social model. The medical model views disability as a consequence of factors within the person, whereas the social model views disability as a consequence of factors extrinsic to the person. ICF, in using the terms *disease* and *disorder*, captures the perspectives of both models into a biopsychosocial approach (WHO, 2001). When disease and disorder negatively affect a person, change or loss of body functions and structures can occur, leading to impairment. In turn, impairment can negatively influence activity capacity and performance, yielding activity limitations. When one or more discrete activities are limited, this can lead to reduced involvement in everyday life situations, or participation restriction. Neither functioning nor disability occur in a vacuum. As illustrated in Figure 27-2, both are influenced by contextual factors.

ICF further delineates context into environmental factors (e.g., physical, social, attitudinal), and personal factors (e.g., attributes of the person that have an effect on functioning or disability). Therefore, functioning and disability are always embedded in a context that interacts with components of each hierarchy.

Occupational Therapy Practice Framework Model

The occupational therapy practice framework (OTPF) is also embedded in a context (AOTA, in press) (Fig. 27-1). Thus contextual factors, such as the physical environment, social, and cultural environments, influence clients at all levels of being. The OTPF is silent on disease and disorder, so we have also incorporated the ICF biopsychosocial approach as the lowest level on the OTPF hierarchical scheme. In the OTPF model, wellness, disease, or disorder can positively or negatively have an effect on a client's capacities (e.g., mental, sensory, neuromuscular). In wellness, a person's capacities support the development of performance skills necessary for everyday occupations, and as routines are developed in the performance of those skills, performance habits emerge.

As people fulfill the social roles that are expected, required, or desired by them, they combine the performance skills and habits of occupations such as ADL, IADL, work and school tasks, play, and leisure into a broader engagement in everyday life situations, known as social participation. As part of an occupational profile, practitioners routinely evaluate clients for capacities unaffected by disease and disorder as well as unaffected skills and habits because they constitute a client's strengths and can be used to compensate for or replace those capacities that are negatively affected. When disease and disorder have a negative effect on a client's capacities, then performance skills and habits used when carrying out everyday occupations (e.g., ADL, IADL, leisure) can also be negatively affected. In turn, social participation roles may not be fulfilled adequately or at all.

Unlike the ICF model, the OTPF model not only recognizes the influence of the contextual environment but also recognizes that each occupation has unique activity demands (e.g., objects, space, sequence of steps), as discussed earlier in this chapter. In both models, the PTE transaction becomes particularly salient at the third level of the hierarchy (i.e., activities and activity limitations, occupations), and maintains significance at the fourth level of the hierarchy (i.e., participation and participation restriction, social participation). Hence, factors that are essential to the PTE transaction, although external to clients, must be taken into account when intervening for disability (i.e., activity limitations, participation restriction).

OCCUPATIONAL THERAPY APPROACHES TO PERFORMANCE DISCREPANCY

The hierarchy of occupational functioning provides a useful perspective for delineating the two major evaluation and intervention approaches for performance discrepancies used in occupational therapy. Trombly (1993, 1995) labeled these the bottom-up and top-down approaches.

Bottom-Up Approach to Performance Discrepancy

Occupational therapy practitioners, when using a *bottom-up approach*, focus evaluation and intervention on the client's generic abilities (i.e., body functions and structures and related impairments according to the ICF model; or client factors and performance skills using the OTPF). For Mrs. Fisher, a 63-year-old client who sustained a right cerebrovascular accident (CVA), the practitioner might focus the evaluation on muscle tone, reflexes, postural control, visual motor integration, and short-term memory. Interventions are remedial in nature with the intent of restoring body functions and structures lost secondary to stroke.

The rationale underlying the bottom-up approach is that body structures and functions support task performance in all occupational areas and that by restoring these abilities to their normal state, task performance, which was previously dysfunctional, automatically becomes functional, because the skills and habits needed to perform these tasks are once again intact. Once generic abilities are restored, some remedial interventions may be devised for activity performance to reintegrate newly restored generic abilities into everyday performance of the client's ADL, IADL, work, and play or leisure activities. This intervention would not need to be extensive, however, because the "cure" of impairments reestablishes the client's capacities, and task reactivation occurs rapidly, particularly for well-learned and well-practiced everyday skills. Hence, the bottom-up approach to performance discrepancy is efficient because the restoration of task abilities returns clients to their premorbid (pre-disease, predisorder) condition, and activities and participation are resumed at their prior level.

The bottom-up approach permits the occupational therapy practitioner to focus the evaluation and intervention on discrete client capacities without initially having to consider activity demands or the surrounding physical and social environment. Mrs. Fisher's muscle tone, reflexes, and postural control can be evaluated on a mat table and her visual-motor integration and short-term memory can be evaluated through tests as she sits in her wheelchair. Neurodevelopmental interventions to normalize tone, inhibit abnormal reflex patterns, and improve postural control can also be implemented with Mrs. Fisher on the mat table. Interventions to resolve problems in form constancy, visual closure, figure-ground perception, and short-term memory can be implemented through paper-and-pencil exercises done on a lapboard. For the most part, environmental interactions are limited to test and intervention objects and instructions.

The demands of real-life situations are introduced into the intervention plan once generic capacities have been restored or their improvement has plateaued. For example, because Mrs. Fisher has not achieved full voluntary control of her affected left extremities and cannot perform transfers in a typical manner, her occupational therapy practitioner practices bed and toilet transfers with her to help her integrate postural control techniques and inhibition of abnormal tone and reflexes into these procedures.

Top-Down Approach to Performance Discrepancy

The second major approach to occupational therapy evaluation and intervention—the *top-down approach*—begins by establishing performance discrepancies at the highest level—that is, the ICF level of social participation/restriction. It then moves to the tasks necessary to sustain valued social roles—that is, to the ICF level of activities/activity limitations or to the OTPF level of occupations and related performance skills and patterns. Finally, the focus is transferred to generic capacities that support activities and social role performance, or to the ICF level of body functions and structures/impairments or the OTPF level of inherent client factors. The fundamental rationale underlying the top-down approach is that even though impairments cannot always be cured, activities and social participation can be improved through adapted performance of tasks and actions associated with these activities and social roles. The following logic undergirds this rationale (Mathiowetz, 1993; Trombly, 1993, 1995):

- Evaluation and intervention begin with tasks that are of value to clients (i.e., necessary for carrying out valued activities and social roles).
- Factors external to clients that contribute to performance discrepancies can be identified during task performance.
- Inferences about probable external causes of performance discrepancies can be verified by changing the activity or environmental demands during task performance, thereby reducing or resolving the performance discrepancy.
- The contribution of capacities and impairments can be observed as they interact synergistically in the performance of real-life activities and social roles.
- A more focused evaluation of impairments can occur in the context of task performance to formulate appropriate intervention strategies to restore, establish, or prevent loss of generic capacities.

For Mrs. Fisher, who sustained a right CVA, the occupational therapy practitioner begins by evaluating Mrs. Fisher's participation in the social roles that would most likely be restricted after a stroke. Mrs. Fisher values most her roles as a wife and homemaker. She enjoys cooking for her husband and baking for her grandchildren, who visit her every Tuesday. She is also concerned about her role as a self-carer. In addition to walking, feeding, bathing, toileting, dressing, and hygiene, Mrs. Fisher expresses concern about medication management and emergency communication when her husband is not home.

Once the most salient activities comprising each social role have been identified, performance-based evaluation is initiated to identify activity performance that is unaffected as well as activity limitations. In-depth evaluations are needed to identify the specific point in an activity sequence where breakdown occurs, as well as the activity demands, and to develop clinical hypotheses about the impairments responsible for this breakdown. Intervention strategies to reduce activity and environmental demands involving compensatory methods of activity performance, the use of adaptive equipment, and modification of the ambient physical and social environmental may be implemented. These compensatory strategies may resolve performance discrepancies relatively quickly, and they may be temporary or permanent solutions to performance discrepancies. If temporary solutions, they are usually implemented to enable adapted activity performance while impairment-oriented interventions are instituted later to restore person capacities.

The top-down approach to performance discrepancies permits the occupational therapy practitioner initially to focus evaluation and intervention on the social roles and responsibilities that define a client's participation in the home and community. Knowledge of activity demands and the physical and social environment are integral to the occupational therapy process from the beginning.

Mrs. Fisher, for example, indicated that her present concerns center on her roles as self-carer, wife, grandparent, and homemaker. She is anxious about her ability to carry out these roles since her stroke. Ideally, evaluation of the critical tasks that constitute her homemaker role (e.g., meal preparation, household maintenance, clothing care) and her self-carer role (e.g., bathing, toileting, dressing) would be carried out in her home so that information obtained about the PTE transaction is accurate and valid. Under less-than-ideal conditions, these tasks are evaluated in an occupational therapy clinic. Accuracy and validity of information are increased under clinical conditions by simulating as much as possible the activity and environmental demands that Mrs. Fisher will face in her home at discharge.

For example, because the bathroom in the Fisher home is too narrow to allow Mrs. Fisher to turn her wheelchair around in the bathroom while she is sitting in it, the occupational therapy practitioner trained Mrs. Fisher to back her wheelchair into the clinic bathroom, thus simulating how she would have to perform this maneuver at home. This procedure enabled Mrs. Fisher to practice transfers to the tub bench as well as the toilet, toward the stronger, unaffected right side of her body. She then learned to collapse the wheelchair and reposition it in the opposite direction before transferring out of the bathtub. Turning the chair allowed her to again transfer toward her stronger, unaffected side. The space needed to turn the chair is less when she is not in the chair because her thigh length does not need to be taken into account. In addition to the compensatory approaches, neurodevelopmental interventions (i.e., restorative) to improve postural control by normalizing muscle tone and inhibiting abnormal reflex patterns would be incorporated into transfer practice exercises.

Advantages and Disadvantages of the Two Approaches to PTE Transaction Discrepancies

The Bottom-Up Approach

An advantage of the bottom-up approach to PTE discrepancies is that intervention aimed at establishing or restoring generic capacities may benefit many tasks. For example, increasing muscle strength or range of motion (ROM) in the upper extremities will facilitate all tasks for which these abilities were deficient. Similarly, reducing apathy will foster reengagement in previously neglected occupational areas. Likewise, correcting visual-sequencing deficits will enhance the performance of all tasks negatively affected by this impairment. Thus, potentially, by remediating neuromuscular, mental, or psychological impairments, multiple task disabilities can be treated simultaneously.

Because the bottom-up approach emphasizes performance factors that are internal to clients, consideration of external, environmental factors is extremely limited. Therefore, the approach is economical to administer because occupational therapy practitioners do not need to assess or manage the demands of activities and the surrounding physical and social environment, or how they impinge on the client's capacities.

Nonetheless, an inherent disadvantage of the bottom-up approach is that improvements in generic capacities may not generalize to generic activities (ADL, IADL) or their specific tasks (e.g., dressing, medication management) or actions (e.g., buttoning, sorting medications). Generalization may not occur for several reasons. First, capacities-oriented interventions concentrate on the body functions and structures that are common to many activities and tasks. However, task performance requires the application of these common abilities to the specific demands of individual tasks. Improvements in visual figure-ground perception demonstrated on paper-and-pencil tests, using black-and-white stimulus materials, may not enable clients to identify hazards, such as water spills, on a multicolored and patterned vinyl floor surface. Second, when capacities are exercised in isolation from tasks, they are not integrated with the other capacities that are also needed to perform these tasks (Ma & Trombly, 1999; Trombly & Wu, 1999). In other words, discrete capacities-oriented interventions do not acknowledge either the interaction between task-related abilities or their coalescence in the PTE transaction in which the discrete capacities will be used. Perceiving a water spill on the floor must be accompanied by the decisional capacity to motor plan to avoid the spill and the neuromuscular strength and endurance to execute walking around it. Finally, generalization may not occur because although capacities may be improved, they may not be improved sufficiently to meet task demands. An increase in ROM of 10° at the shoulder joint is still inadequate for grooming if 25° more motion is needed to comb the hair on the back of the head.

The bottom-up approach may also result in the identification and treatment of impairments that may not actually be causing performance dysfunctions. A deficit score on a test of visual figure-ground perception may not translate into performance deficits on well-learned daily living skills. Without assessing the PTE transaction during tasks, the meaning of impairments for performance is vague.

The bottom-up approach is generally initiated with the intent to switch to the top-down approach if full recovery does not occur or once maximum benefit is obtained from restorative interventions. The danger in this tactic is that too much intervention time may be spent on remediating impairments. At the outset of intervention, it is difficult to predict if full recovery will be achieved, and occupational therapy practitioners are prone to persist in restorative interventions as long as gains are being made. Unfortunately, if full recovery is not achieved, there may be little intervention time left for addressing activity limitations or participation restrictions. Clients may then be deprived of independent, safe, and adequate activity performance that could have been achieved—or achieved more readily—through compensatory interventions. The risk of clients being discharged from therapy before maximum improvement in task performance has been achieved has been intensified by managed care and reduced time allocations for rehabilitation (Angelelli, Wilber, & Myrtle, 2000; Banja & DeJong, 2000).

Another disadvantage of the bottom-up approach, is that clients may not see the connection between interventions aimed at discrete impairments (e.g., motor control exercises, visual-scanning programs on a computer, stacking cones) and improvement of their ADL and social participation. Hence, they may be less motivated to participate in occupational therapy. However, by educating clients and their families about the connection between impairment reduction and activity improvement, this disadvantage may be overcome.

The Top-Down Approach

A primary advantage of the top-down approach is that evaluation and intervention center on social role participation and activity performance that is meaningful to clients, yet discrepant with the level of performance that is expected, required, or desired (Trombly, 1993). Consistent with this advantage are two additional benefits. First, because the occupational therapy process focuses on social role participation and activity performance that is meaningful to clients, the relevance of therapy for improving daily life is readily apparent to clients (Trombly, 1993). Thus motivation to participate in therapy is heightened. Second, social role and activity performance are influenced directly by the intervention. Real-life performance is both the medium and the outcome of therapy (Dirette & Hinojosa, 1999; Dolecheck & Schkade, 1999; van Heugten et al., 1998).

The top-down approach also has the advantage of reinforcing and expediting an approach that people often implement naturally when problems are experienced in task performance (Fried, Herdman, Kuhn, Rubin, & Turano, 1991; Yakobina, Yakobina, & Tallant, 1997). When difficulties are encountered in doing tasks, people tend to seek the assistance of others, use a tool to help themselves, or try a different way of performing the task. These compensatory procedures foster task completion. Because the top-down approach enhances procedures that humans turn to naturally when problems are encountered, it is familiar to clients, and hence it is likely to be well accepted by them.

The top-down approach provides a further advantage at the point when intervention switches from a social role participation or activity focus to an impairment orientation. The top-down approach facilitates the identification of impairments in the context of social roles and the activities; consequently, the relevance of impairments for social roles and their activities is known. In contrast, in the bottom-up approach, by which impairments are evaluated in isolation, their relevance for social roles and activities can only be inferred. The visual-perceptual impairments identified through a paper-and-pencil test may or may not impair social roles and activities. The identification of role and activity-related impairments, in turn, enables a more targeted evaluation of impairments as well as more precisely directed restorative interventions.

The disadvantage of the top-down approach is that evaluation and intervention are social role and activity specific, with no or minimal transfer from one task to another. Moreover, for intervention to be maximally effective, it must occur in the occupational context in which the client lives, works, or plays. Thus the approach requires the occupational therapy practitioner to take into account the complexity of environmental factors that impinge on performance.

INTERVENTION APPROACH FOR THE TWENTY-FIRST CENTURY

The predominant approach to the occupational therapy process over the past several decades has been the bottom-up approach and restorative interventions. Nonetheless, even with its disadvantages, the top-down approach, and its concomitant compensatory interventions, is the best fit for the emerging system of health-care delivery. Leaders within occupational therapy, the Centers for Medicare and Medicaid Services, and consumers have promoted this reversal of emphasis.

Within occupational therapy, Dunn (1993), in an article titled "Measurement of Function: Actions for the Future," proposed the following:

> *We need to consider the fact that a contextual approach to assessment provides an opportunity to identify what the person needs or wants to do. It is essential for occupational therapy to begin assessment at this level and to create goals for services from this list of expressed needs. This strategy has the advantage of engaging the person's motivational system, providing another mechanism to facilitate a successful outcome. (p. 357)*

Rogers and Holm stressed the pivotal position of task performance and compensatory interventions for maximizing performance gains (Holm & Rogers, 1989, 1991; Rogers & Holm, 1989; Rogers et al., 1997). Mathiowetz (1993), in a discussion of neuromuscular capacity evaluation and intervention for function, noted that it is possible for some clients to have grip or pinch strength within normal limits but not be able to accomplish necessary functional tasks and for others to have grip or pinch strength below normal limits and yet be able to accomplish all their functional tasks. He further pointed out that the kinesiology literature suggests that motor learning is task specific, with little carryover to other tasks, and thus the best way to improve motor function is to practice the task for which it is required. According to Trombly (1993), "we have no definitive study in occupational therapy that indicates that a person's occupational functioning is better as a result of restorative therapy rather than adaptive therapy" (p. 255), and Wood (1996) summarized concerns about a singular use of the bottom-up approach to PTE transaction discrepancies (Humphrey, Jewell, & Rosenberger, 1995; Neistadt, 1994a, 1994b; Trombly, 1995) by noting that there "has been increasing evidence that improvements in performance components do not necessarily translate into competent functioning in everyday life" (p. 631).

More compelling arguments for the top-down approach have come from health insurance companies because they can define acceptable outcomes of therapy through their reimbursement practices. For example, Blue Cross of California defined a meaningful outcome of therapy as "one in which the activity level achieved by the patient . . . is that level necessary for the patient to function most effectively at home or at work" (Stewart & Abeln, 1993, p. 213). Another parameter of acceptability, a utilitarian outcome of therapy, is defined as a functional outcome that is economically and efficiently achieved (Eastwood, 1999; Stewart & Abeln, 1993).

Finally, the disability rights movement has also promoted compensatory approaches that focus on environmental adaptation, because the compensatory approach does not assume that there is something wrong with the person with a disability that needs to be fixed or changed. Instead, the compensatory approach concentrates on the environment and its demands, probing to identify how it affects performance and then seeking to work around it or capitalize on it (Dunn, 1993; Verbrugge, 1990). As Verbrugge (1990) noted, the request of advocacy groups for persons with disabilities is: "Change the milieu, not me" (p. 68).

Performance Discrepancy: Person Capacity Versus Environmental Demand

This subsection focuses on disease or disorder experienced at the level of activity limitation—that is, ADL, IADL, work/school, play, or leisure. This is a pivotal level that stands at the interface between social role participation and a person's inherent capacities. The fulfillment of societal roles depends on a client's ability to perform a unique combination of ADL, IADL, work/school, and play and leisure tasks. The ability to carry out everyday tasks safely, adequately, and independently depends, in turn, on the neuromuscular, mental, sensory, and physiological capacities of the client.

The role of the environment in activity performance becomes more salient as one moves up the hierarchy from inherent person capacities to societal participation. At the level of activities and social participation, the environment, in terms of objects, structures, and people, is inextricably linked to client performance. Numerous methods of adapting a client's performance environment to achieve, restore, or improve function and to prevent dysfunction are available. Rather than devising an approach to environmental modifications for each disease/disorder, impairment, and activity limitation or participation restriction experienced by clients, we chose to develop a clinical decision-making guide to help occupational therapy practitioners systematically determine the nature of the performance discrepancy. This evaluation provides the basis for determining the most appropriate type of environmental modification. The guide, consisting of a series of questions, is used to determine the nature of a client's performance discrepancy, specifically, if it is a skill or habit deficit, and to formulate intervention strategies that will meet target outcomes within the constraints of the health-care service delivery system (Fig. 27-3).

In this subsection, we emphasize the decision-making process leading to environmental adaptations for enhancing the PTE transaction rather than present a compendium of adaptive environmental solutions, which are prone to change rapidly as technologies improve. We use case examples to illustrate the guide. (See Appendix F for more practical information on specific technologies and services.) Concepts included in the decision-making guide are based on the ICF (WHO, 2001), the proposed OTPF (AOTA, in press), human factors methodologies (Czaja et al., 1993; Faletti, 1984), the EHP framework (Dunn et al., 1994), the Model for Skill and Habit Acquisition (Rogers & Holm, 1991b), and the Model of Occupational Functioning (Trombly, 1995).

Two approaches to managing performance discrepancies were described: bottom-up and top-down (Trombly, 1993). Employing the top-down approach to clinical problem solving suggested by Trombly (1993), the clinical decision-making guide presented in Figure 27-3 begins with the identification of the discrepancy between a client's current societal role participation and activities performance and that which is expected, required, or desired (Mager & Pipe, 1984; Rogers & Holm, 1991b).

For example, parents may indicate that their son does not interact with toys, children, or adults in the same manner that their other children did at age 3½ and that the preschool that they wish their son to attend requires age-appropriate dexterity and social skills. A worker who sustained a rotator cuff injury wishes to return to work but finds that he cannot sustain the motions required for operating the surge machine for 2 hr consecutively, the minimum standard required by the Occupational Health and Safety Office. A middle-aged adult with developmental delay who was moved into a group home 1 week after the death of his surviving parent refuses to come out of his room and is aggressive with staff. The group home's admission criteria stipulate that residents must participate in daily activities and chores and must not exhibit aggressive or self-destructive behaviors. An older adult wishes to return to her senior apartment after a stroke, but she is unable to meet two of the residency criteria: managing her medications and preparing two light meals per day.

In each of these situations, there is a discrepancy between the client's current performance and the demands of

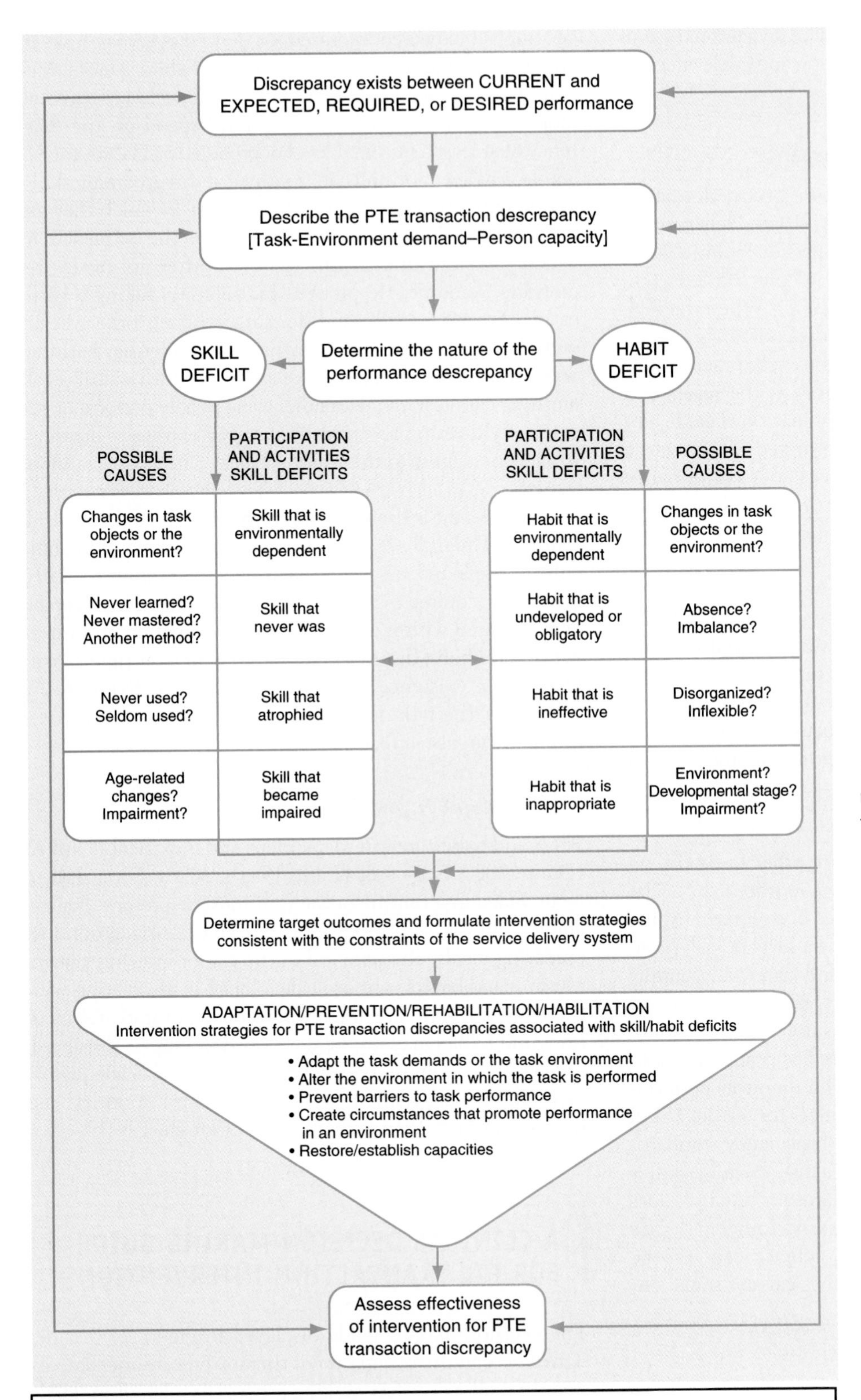

Key:
PTE=Person-Task-Environment
Participation=Societal role participation
Activities=Tasks and actions associated with activities of daily living (ADL), instrumental ADL, work/school, play and leisure activities
Impairment=Significant deviation, loss or problem in body functions or structures
Environment=Physical, cultural, social, spiritual, temporal, or virtual contexts

FIGURE 27–3. A clinical decision-making guide for PTE transaction interventions.

the physical or social environment. The specific nature of the discrepancy helps focus the evaluation and guide effective intervention.

Nature of the Performance Discrepancy

Two broad categorizations of the nature of a performance discrepancy are skill deficit (Fleishman, 1966; Fleishman & Quaintance, 1984; Gentile, 1987; Rogers & Holm, 1991b, 2000) and habit deficit (Dunn, 2000; Poole, 2000; Reich, 2000; Rogers, 2000; Rogers & Holm, 2000). When the PTE transaction is unsafe, inadequate, or dependent on others, the decision-making guide is designed to help practitioners ascertain if the performance discrepancy is the result of a skill or a habit deficit. Once this determination is made, environmental adaptations can be incorporated to reduce the environmental demand to match the client's performance level. If the probable cause of the performance discrepancy is a skill deficit, environmental adaptations can be incorporated that reduce environmental demand, thereby potentiating the client's level of skill. Likewise, if the probable cause is a habit deficit, short-term environmental adaptations can be incorporated, which substitute for habit acquisition and reduce the performance discrepancy until enough time has passed to develop or restore routines and habits. (For intervention approaches that focus on development and restoration of person capacities, see Chapter 30.)

Skill and Skill Deficit

Skill is a task-specific ability to perform proficiently the requirements of a task (Fleishman, 1966; Gentile, 1987). The standards for proficiency are determined both internally and externally. Internally, people determine a level of skill proficiency that is acceptable to them, and externally, family members, teachers, friends, employers, and co-workers establish skill proficiency levels for tasks that are adequate to meet societal standards. Skill is acquired by practicing tasks under the supervision of an expert, who monitors performance and provides corrective guidance for errors. Skill deficit is a lack of ability to meet the proficiency standards set by oneself or others for performing a task. Because skill is task specific, failure to meet the standards for one task does not necessarily mean that the standards for other tasks are not being met. In addition, skill proficiency can also be influenced by task demands and the physical and social environments.

Habit and Habit Deficit

Several skills linked together into a sequence constitute a routine; routines linked together constitute a **habit** (Clark, 2000). Habits are usually developed over time as a means of making performance more efficient (Dunn, 2000; Kielhofner & Burke, 1985; Rogers 1986; Rogers & Holm, 1991b). Habits are patterns of daily living that are unique to each person and are labor-saving mechanisms that enable humans to accomplish expected, required, or desired everyday tasks in an efficient manner. The acquisition of habits is more difficult than the acquisition of skills, because habits involve more complex units of behavior and depend on the existence of at least a minimal level of proficiency. Habits, for example, involve morning care routines versus grooming skills. While skills are individualized by the style in which they are performed, habits are individualized by the sequence in which tasks are linked into routines. After arising in the morning, some people proceed by toileting, taking a bath, eating, brushing teeth, and dressing, whereas others begin with brushing teeth and then move to toileting, bathing, dressing, and eating. Habits are also embedded within each morning care task. For example, some people perform upper extremity dressing first and then lower extremity dressing, while others dress in the reverse order or in a more random fashion.

Habit deficit is the cessation or disruption of daily living routines. The individuality of habits makes them more difficult to assess and treat than skill deficits. Similar to skills, habits are acquired over time, but unlike skills, which can be demonstrated within a single session, evaluation and intervention for habit discrepancies must occur over time to validate their existence, consistency, and effectiveness. As with skills, the task demands and physical and social environment can also affect habits.

Relationship between Skills and Habits

Skills and habits are interdependent and inextricably linked (Dunn, 2000; Rogers & Holm, 1991b, 2000). For a skill to be included in a routine or habit, it must be present. For example, unless a person possesses skill in dressing, grooming, preparing meals, changing oil in the car, or mowing a lawn, routines and habits cannot be developed in association with these tasks. If skills are absent, inadequate, or impaired, routines and habits may not be developed or may be disrupted. Likewise, skills must be used frequently to be adequately maintained and refined or developed into routines and habits (Mager & Pipe, 1984; Rogers & Holm, 1991b).

A CLINICAL DECISION-MAKING GUIDE FOR PTE TRANSACTION INTERVENTIONS

The decision-making guide displayed in Figure 27-3 is designed to lead the occupational therapy practitioner step by step through a decision-making process to rule out probable causes of performance discrepancy during a PTE transaction. The top-down approach was chosen because it enables the occupational therapy practitioner to begin with social roles and activities that are meaningful to the client and because observation of the PTE transaction at the participation or activities level incorporates both person capacities and environmental demands.

The decision-making guide prompts examination of discrepancies in performance from the perspective of skill deficits or habit deficits. Skill and habit were chosen because clients with neuromuscular impairments most often exhibit problems with skills, whereas clients with mental and psychological impairments may also exhibit problems with habits. Skill deficits are examined first, because skills are requisite for habit development and maintenance. Skills that may be environmentally dependent are discussed first, because unfamiliar task objects or surrounding environments can negatively affect a client's performance, even if no impairments are present. Subsequently, the guide helps practitioners explore whether the skill was ever learned, never used, or seldom used. Finally, the guide prompts practitioners to examine age-related changes in the client or impairments as probable causes of skill deficits.

If skill deficits are ruled out or resolved and a performance discrepancy remains, the guide begins with consideration of whether the habit is environmentally dependent. If task objects or physical and social environments change, habits and routines can be disrupted and thus be a source of performance discrepancies. The guide goes on to encourage examination of whether habits were ever developed, are obligatory in nature, are ineffective, or are socially inappropriate. Once the nature of the performance discrepancy is established, the guide prompts for the establishment of target outcomes and consideration of appropriate intervention strategies to reduce environmental demand.

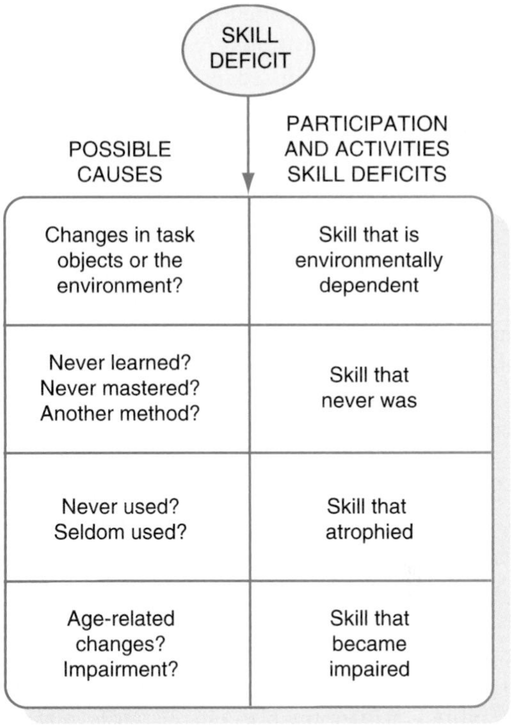

SKILL DEFICIT

POSSIBLE CAUSES	PARTICIPATION AND ACTIVITIES SKILL DEFICITS
Changes in task objects or the environment?	Skill that is environmentally dependent
Never learned? Never mastered? Another method?	Skill that never was
Never used? Seldom used?	Skill that atrophied
Age-related changes? Impairment?	Skill that became impaired

FIGURE 27–4. Skill deficits influencing the PTE transaction and their possible causes.

Is It a Skill Deficit?

There are several types of skill deficits (Fig. 27-4). As indicated in the decision guide, these deficits can be grouped into four general categories: skills that may be environmentally dependent, skills that were never learned or mastered, skills that are never or seldom used, and skills that are impaired.

Changes in Task Objects or Environment?

Is performance discrepant because of changes in task objects or the surrounding environment? When occupational therapy practitioners evaluate task performance, they establish the conditions under which this takes place. They select the task objects to be used during the evaluation, establish the interpersonal climate, and determine the level and kind of help that will be offered during the evaluation. Except when the evaluation takes place in the naturalistic setting—that is, in the client's home, school, or workplace—they also select the physical environment (e.g., the occupational therapy clinic or the client's room in a hospital or rehabilitation center). The evaluation conditions may facilitate or hinder task performance or may be neutral to it, depending on a client's capacities. Hence, these conditions are one possible cause of a performance deficit.

During an occupational therapy evaluation, for example, Ms. Chu, a single 67-year-old female with macular degeneration who is recovering from a below-the-knee amputation of her right leg secondary to diabetic neuropathy, is unable to interpret a utility bill or write out a check. The amputation is healing well, and she was alert and oriented immediately after surgery and thereafter. Ms. Chu reports that she always took care of her own finances and balanced her checkbook before coming into the hospital. At home, however, Ms. Chu uses enlarged checks and a template to locate the lines on the check. After completing the check, she uses a high-intensity halogen lamp and a magnifying glass to check her work. Without her usual task objects and intensified lighting, as much as she tries to please the occupational therapy practitioner, she is unable to complete the checking tasks. Ms. Chu is rated as having a skill deficit by the occupational therapy practitioner, who did not explore the implications of the evaluation materials on the client's task performance, and the practitioner documented the possible emergence of mental impairment.

Skill deficits similar to those induced by occupational therapy evaluation objects may occur when clients change their living, learning, working, or playing environments. Mrs. Wallen, for example, calls the Geriatric In-Home Assessment Program because she noted that her mother, who had recently moved to a senior apartment, was burning food quite frequently and seemed to be storing "garbage" in the refrigerator. The evaluation reveals that the client is having difficulty learning to use the electric stove because she has cooked on a gas stove for the past 64 years. Furthermore, she is storing leftover food temporarily in the refrigerator because the garbage container is located in the basement, 10 floors down, and this is too far to go every day.

Skill deficits may be induced by social as well as physical environments and objects. The mere presence of the occupational therapy practitioner overseeing task performance during an occupational therapy evaluation may be sufficient to disrupt performance, because the feeling of being observed and evaluated may make clients nervous or anxious. People in the environment may also be remiss in their responsibility for arranging task objects. For example, clients with moderate dementia can often perform tasks when they are reminded to do so by being given task objects by their caregivers (e.g., cereal, bowl, and milk left on the kitchen counter). Without this reminder from caregivers, however, task performance may not occur.

A change of environment, either temporarily or permanently, challenges clients' adaptive capacities. Skill deficits may occur in a new environment because task performance was environmentally dependent on specific task objects or physical or human environments in the usual performance setting. Occupational therapy practitioners need to be sensitive to skill deficits that may be environmentally induced so that ratings of performance are not artificially lowered because clients are not using their usual task objects or performing in their usual environments. Ascertaining the degree of difference between usual and clinic task objects and arrangements helps discern if the skill deficit is the result of environmental dependence. If performance does not seem to be affected by environmental factors, perhaps the skill was never learned or mastered, is not used frequently, or has not been required recently.

Never Learned or Mastered?

Is performance discrepant because a skill was never learned or mastered? Before a determination can be made that the performance discrepancy is caused by the pathologies or impairments, it is necessary to ascertain if the skill was ever learned or mastered (Mager & Pipe, 1984; Rogers & Holm, 1991b). For instance, if Mrs. Siburg, a 68-year-old widow who sustained a right CVA, has difficulty writing out a check and balancing a checkbook ledger, it is important to ascertain if she knew how to do these tasks before she had her stroke. Mrs. Siburg reports that she always used cash and money orders before she was married. Mr. Siburg handled all the family finances until his death 2 years ago, and Mrs. Siburg's daughter has taken over her finances since then. Thus her inability to do these tasks is most likely owing to a skill deficit caused by lack of learning.

A skill that was never learned or never mastered requires habilitation, not *re*habilitation. More important, however, is the need to determine if the skill is even needed and, if it is needed, the proficiency level that will be required. After a traumatic injury or the onset of a deteriorating neurological condition, for example, a move to a new apartment, assisted living center, or group home may require skills that are deficient owing to lack of learning or mastery. Such lifestyle changes may also require the use of previously learned, but never or seldom used, skills.

Is performance discrepant because another method was learned or mastered? Another factor to consider at this point is whether the client uses a method different from the one required in the evaluation to accomplish the same task. As part of an evaluation protocol, an occupational therapy practitioner may ask a client to review a utility bill, write a check for the amount on the bill, and balance the checkbook ledger. The client, however, may always use money orders to pay bills and thus have adequate money management skills, even though check-writing skills are deficient. If it is determined that the relevant skill (ability to pay bills) was learned and mastered, and that another method of task performance is familiar to the client, then changes in task objects or the task environment are logical factors to consider as precipitating a skill deficit.

Never or Seldom Used?

Is performance discrepant because the skill is never or seldom used? Skills may not be demonstrated or may be inadequate or unsafe because they have been dormant for months or years. Meal preparation and laundry skills are often atrophied in married males of the World War II generation, because their wives have been doing these tasks for them since they were discharged from the armed forces some 60 years ago. Widows of the same generation frequently report that they have not managed finances since their marriage because their husbands did this. Thus data about a client's task performance history are required to determine the frequency and recency of skill use. Again, if a skill has not been adequately practiced, perhaps habilitation is needed, not rehabilitation. If the practitioner can rule out, however, that the performance discrepancy is not due to the result of a lack of opportunity to use it frequently or recently, then age-related sensory, mental, psychosocial, or neuromuscular or physiological changes or recent impairments may impede skill performance.

Age-Related Changes or Impairments?

Is performance discrepant because of age-related changes? In older adults, normal age-related changes in inherent capacities may interfere with task performance. The effects of these age-related changes may be compounded by new and preexisting disease or disorder-associated impairments. Identifying the contribution of aging and pathology to skill deficits requires good observation skills against a background of knowledge of normal aging and the classical manifestations of diseases/disorders.

Mr. Rowland, a 67-year-old farmer who required a left above-elbow amputation in 1953 owing to a Korean War injury, is seen in the outpatient clinic after surgery for a herniated lumbar disk. He reports that many of the problems he currently experiences with bending, lifting, pulling, and pushing were not apparent even 10 years ago when he was younger and stronger. At 67 years, however, Mr. Rowland notes that he does not have the strength he had previously, and he can no longer use brute force and one-handed lifting as he used to do. With decrements in functioning associated with the normal aging process, people usually make gradual accommodations in how they carry out tasks. If these accommodations no longer enable safe or adequate performance, however, it may be necessary to reduce the environmental demands to match current client capacities.

Is performance discrepant because of impairments? Impairments reflect the expression of disease and disorder on body functions and structures (WHO, 2001). Mr. Baker, a 46-year-old self-employed electronics sales representative who sustained a left CVA, has difficulty writing out checks and balancing a checkbook ledger. Before his stroke, however, Mr. Baker managed the family's finances, as well as the financial aspects of his business. Hence, the most likely causes of his skill deficits are the residual impairments from his stroke. Although he is left-hand dominant and can manipulate a pen adequately, his aphasia and impulsivity impair the quality of his financial skills. Even though the classic impairments and activity limitations associated with disorders such as CVAs and multiple sclerosis are enumerated in medical textbooks, the classic pattern is rarely exhibited in individual clients, and the occupational therapy practitioner must be sensitive to unique manifestations. Moreover, skill deficits may arise from a combination of new and preexisting impairments.

Is It a Habit Deficit?

After it has been ascertained that a performance discrepancy may not be attributable to a skill deficit, evaluation of habit deficits is begun. As indicated on the decision guide, habit deficits generally fall into four categories: those that are environmentally dependent, those that are undeveloped or obligatory, those that are ineffective, and those that are inappropriate (Fig. 27-5).

Changes in Task Objects or the Environment?

Is performance discrepant because of changes in task objects or the surrounding environment? Habits that are environmentally dependent can be triggered by task objects (e.g., toothbrush, zipper, blouse with buttons down the front), physical environments (e.g., bathroom, lunchroom, assembly workstation), and social environments (e.g., baseball practice, religious services). When PTE transactions do not reveal any obvious routines or habits, before concluding that these have not been developed, it is appropriate to determine if the environment precludes a client from maintaining usual routines and habits. Hospitals and long-term care facilities (LTCFs) are often unsupportive of habit acquisition and maintenance because they are organized around the routines

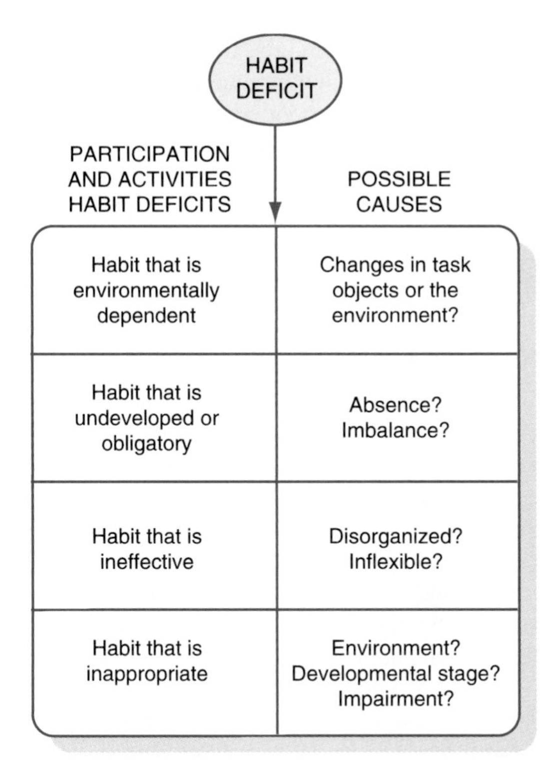

FIGURE 27–5. Habit deficits influencing the PTE transaction and their possible causes.

established by staff. The schedules of hospital clients and LTCF residents revolve around nursing shifts and dietary schedules. Hospitalized clients are not allowed to self-medicate, thus eliminating the opportunity to demonstrate the habits that support their medication management skills. Residents of LTCFs who toileted independently at home but are considered mobility impaired by facility criteria may become incontinent while waiting for assistance to ambulate to the bathroom. Mental health settings provide disincentives to habit maintenance and encourage dependency on staff with policies that require the removal of razors, fingernail polish, and manicure scissors for safety reasons and the locking up of watches, money, and denture tablets for security purposes.

Because habits can be environmentally dependent (e.g., the drawer a person automatically reaches for to obtain toothpaste), a move to a new room within a hospital or LTCF—and certainly a move to a new home—can cause a temporary disruption or cessation of intact habits and routines.

For example, during an evaluation of meal preparation, Mrs. Odden seems confused. Even though she had been oriented to the kitchen in the occupational therapy department, she opens and closes doors and drawers trying to locate items and repeatedly turns appliances on and off. However, an alternate explanation to confusion is that her cooking habits are somewhat attached to the kitchen in which she has cooked for 52 years, including the location of utensils and food supplies and the equipment controls. Clarification of the usual task environment, as well as the usual patterns and routines the client engages in, can help the occupational therapy practitioner arrange the task environment and provide the relevant task objects necessary for efficient and adequate task performance. If such accommodations are made, and performance is still discrepant, perhaps the habits are undeveloped.

Absence or Imbalance?

Is performance discrepant because of an absence of habits? The absence of habits and routines reflects a lifestyle that lacks sufficient structure and is relatively unpredictable. In young children, there may be an absence of self-initiated habits, but even toddlers quickly accommodate to routines and habits established by family members and day-care staff. When habits and routines are absent in their environments, children may not develop age-appropriate skills and may experience difficulty adjusting to preschool or school environments (Kramer & Hinojosa, 1993). Furthermore, if regular attendance at school is not in a child's repertoire, skill development is likely to be negatively influenced. For adolescents and adults in the work environment, the absence of habit patterns that support on-time arrival at the workplace, follow-through with assigned tasks, and adherence to safety procedures can negatively influence the ability to obtain or retain a job, even when the worker is highly skilled (Barris, et al., 1985). If habits have been in place, but are suddenly disrupted because of a major illness in the family, relocation, or the apathy associated with depression, a performance discrepancy may also become evident (Kramer & Hinojosa, 1993).

With the reduced time for rehabilitation in managed care, it is difficult to help clients develop routines that may become habits over time. Furthermore, in the inpatient setting, the usual physical and social environments that trigger and support a habit are not found. This affords the opportunity to use educational techniques creatively to help clients develop routines and habits for organizing their lives and making tasks more efficient. If habits and routines are present, but performance is still discrepant, then habit imbalance is possible.

Is performance discrepant because of an imbalance of habits? Habit imbalance can take the form of routines lacking in number, diversity, type, and pacing of activities (Cubie & Kaplan, 1982; Florey & Michelman, 1982; Kielhofner & Burke, 1985; Rogers, 1986; Rogers & Holm, 1991b) as well as an obligatory adherence to habits and routines (Barris et al., 1985). Neuromuscular, sensory, and psychological impairments can cause clients to restrict severely the type of activities they pursue and the frequency with which they pursue them.

For example, before an automobile accident that resulted in central cord syndrome and paresis in all four extremities, Mr. Jotel, a 48-year-old divorced male, jogged every morning and lifted weights five nights a week. Although he recently returned to his position as a tax auditor for the Internal Revenue Service, he is dissatisfied with his present lifestyle. During a on-site job analysis, he reports that he spends all his waking hours performing either self-care or work tasks and, further, that "if this is all that my life is going to be from now on, it isn't worth it."

Imbalance can also take the form of habits or routines that clients treat as obligatory (du Toit, van Kradenburg, Niehaus, & Stein, 2001; Rapport, 2001). Impairments associated with dementia and obsessive-compulsive disorders can result in this type of imbalance.

Mr. Goldman, who is 84 and has moderate cognitive impairment from dementia of the Alzheimer type, spends many hours each day watching Lawrence Welk videotapes. Some days, he will watch the same tape 8 to 10 times. Whereas he used to be quite social, Mrs. Goldman is unable to coax him to go out to visit with relatives or accompany her to the store. Mrs. Goldman has difficulty scheduling meals so that they coincide with the ending of the videotapes, and her husband gets upset if she turns them off to have him come into the kitchen to eat.

In obsessive-compulsive disorders, habit imbalance usually takes the form of rituals, such as hair pulling or hand washing (du Toit et al., 2001). Because these rituals are repeated often, such as hand washing every 15 min, they tend to disrupt the normal rhythm of social participation and everyday activities. Changes in either the physical or social environment may serve to trigger new routines, serve as distracters from obligatory habits, or prevent the carrying out of routines due to lack of trigger stimuli or presence of new stimuli. If discrepant performance cannot be attributed to an imbalance in habits and routines, perhaps disorganization or inflexibility of response is affecting performance.

Disorganization or Inflexibility?

Is performance discrepant because of habit disorganization? When a smooth rhythm of daily routines is not evident in the client's PTE transactions, habit disorganization may be the reason. Pathologies such as traumatic brain injury, stroke, depression, attention deficit disorder, and bipolar affective disorder can result in impaired attention span, decreased ability to concentrate, impulsiveness, indecisiveness, and apathy, all of which can contribute to habit disorganization. Clients with habit disorganization tend to focus on the here and now and fail to plan for upcoming events, making them absent, unprepared, or late for appointments.

For example, during the evaluation of personal care tasks, the occupational therapy practitioner observes that although Mr. Takada prepares for bathing and shaving by collecting his soap, towel, and razor, he leaves them on his dresser when he goes into the bathroom. When he returns to his side of the room, presumably to get the bathing and shaving materials, he notices his clothes, which had been stacked on the bed by the nursing aide. He then proceeds to dress. And when finished dressing, he puts his razor, soap, and towel in his dresser.

For habits to become automatic as well as purposeful, practice in planning, organizing, and implementing efficient routines is needed (Bransford & Stein, 1984). Habits that are only partially in place or disorganized yield ineffective performance, as do inflexible habit patterns.

Is performance discrepant because of inflexible habit patterns? Inflexibility of response can also disrupt habits and routines (Kielhofner & Burke, 1985). Characteristics of inflexibility are the inability to change routines to accommodate unanticipated or changing circumstances as well as an inability to adjust emotionally when routines are changed. For clients who cannot vary routines or habits when necessary or who become upset, agitated, angry or confused when habits are disrupted, role and task performance may be discrepant because of inflexible habit patterns (Rogers & Holm, 1991b). A wife who still cooks her husband's favorite high-calorie, high-fat food, even though he is now on a low-cholesterol, diabetic diet demonstrates inflexible habit patterns. A client who has recently undergone a coronary artery bypass graft after years of high fat and cholesterol intake and complies with his severe dietary restrictions while complaining through every meal, is an example of someone who becomes upset when habits are changed.

Social support for changes in habits can aid adjustment when changes need to occur that are difficult for clients to accept. However, inflexible habit patterns can also serve as an adaptive response for skill deficits, by conserving the response repertoire. Some inflexible habits are adaptive, rather than maladaptive, and it is critical for the occupational therapy practitioner to gather sufficient information about clients to be able to make this distinction. A client who checks every electrical outlet and touches the rim of each burner on an electric range before leaving the house may have developed this routine because of short-term memory deficits. It may be an effective adaptive strategy designed to prevent fires that was developed after having left a burner or an iron on when out of the house. If the client's habits or routines seem ineffective, but not due to disorganization or inflexibility, then perhaps they are just inappropriate for the time or situation in which they occur.

Inappropriate Environment?

Is performance discrepant because the habit is enacted in the wrong environment? Many everyday tasks are linked to specific environments such as bathrooms, kitchens, and bedrooms. Clients with mental or psychological impairments may carry out acceptable habits in an inappropriate environment, thus making them unacceptable.

Julian, an ambulatory 18-year-old male with severe developmental delay, recently began to masturbate during mealtimes when in the dining room of the group home. Although this habit is appropriate in the privacy of his bedroom or in the bathroom, Julian enacts this habit in the wrong environment; therefore, his performance is discrepant with social norms.

Cues from significant members of the client's social environment may be needed to clarify behaviors that are acceptable and unacceptable in a specific environment. If a discrepancy is not due to performance in the wrong environment, it may be developmentally inappropriate.

Developmental Stage?

Is performance discrepant because the habit pattern is inconsistent with the client's developmental stage? Although exceptions are made based on pathology and impairment, society has certain expectations of appropriate behavior based on a person's age and stage of development (Eisenberg, Sutkin, & Jansen, 1984). A 12-year-old girl who sucks her thumb when stressed or tired runs the risk of ridicule by peers, because this performance is age inappropriate. Similarly, adults who have the habit of pouting or sulking in the workplace also display a performance discrepancy. Whereas such behavior is frequently observed in children and teenagers, it is inappropriate for adults and is usually not tolerated by co-workers in the work environment. Again, cues from peers or supervisors in the social environment are helpful for eliminating developmentally inappropriate habits and supporting those that are consistent with a person's age and stage. If routines and habits are still discrepant, but not because they are inconsistent with a client's age or developmental stage, then impairment must be considered as a probable cause.

Impairment?

Is performance discrepant because of impairment? Many diseases/disorders can result in impaired judgment, leading to occasional or chronic socially inappropriate behavior (Eisenberg et al., 1984; Reed, 2000).

Since she sustained a left CVA, 71-year-old Sister Mary Joseph has had expressive aphasia. When she does speak, she repeats a phrase, consisting of several four-letter words, that would have brought her ruler down on the knuckles of any child she taught who uttered even one of them. In the room next to Sister Mary Joseph is Mr. Graves, a 57-year-old longshoreman. Mr. Graves has also sustained a left CVA, and every time he has visitors he cries. Mrs. Graves had never seen her husband cry before, and she is particularly concerned about his crying because some of their friends have mentioned that they stopped visiting because they were embarrassed by his outbursts and did not know how to respond to them. The nursing staff had to explain to Mrs. Graves about emotional lability (i.e., rapidly changing emotions) and its relationship to stroke.

Another client, 43-year-old Mr. Jackson, sustained a traumatic brain injury in a car accident 2 months ago and repetitively touches his crotch every 2–3 min. His family is embarrassed by his actions, and friends and co-workers have stopped visiting him.

In each of these instances, impairments have resulted in routine responses that are inconsistent with the clients' premorbid personalities and are viewed by friends and family in the social environment as inappropriate.

APPROACHES TO ACHIEVING TARGET OUTCOMES

We have focused on one systematic clinical decision-making guide for identifying the nature of performance discrepancies and their probable causes. Once the client or the client's advocates have identified the level of task performance that is required, desired, or expected for each discrepant PTE transaction, target functional outcomes can be established (Fig. 27-6). The client and the occupational therapy practitioner then need to establish collaboratively the rank order in which target outcomes will be addressed and the performance discrepancies to be resolved (Cipriani et al., 2000; McAndrew, McDermott, Vitzakovich, Warunek, & Holm, 2000), taking into account the severity of the client's impairments and the constraints of the service delivery system (Evans, Small, & Ling, 1995; Hagedorn, 1995b). As some performance discrepancies are resolved, others may be identified, and further evaluation may be needed to assess sensory, mental, neuromuscular, psychosocial, or physiological impairments and develop long-term outcomes aimed at establishing or restoring generic capacities (Rogers et al., 1997; Trombly, 1993, 1995).

The EHP model identifies five intervention strategies that incorporate the environment (Dunn et al., 1994). By using the utilitarian parameters of economy and efficiency to guide intervention, we organized the intervention strategies into the top-down approach shown in Figure 27-6. Therefore, we begin discussion at the top with the adapt strategy, because of its potential for an immediate resolution of the performance discrepancy, and end with the establish/restore strategy, which may delay resolving the performance discrepancy until generic capacities are developed or redeveloped. Each intervention strategy is first defined and then illustrated with case scenarios involving skill and habit deficits.

Adapt

Adapt contextual features and task demands so they support performance in context. Therapeutic interventions can adapt contextual features and task demands so they are more supportive to the person's performance. In this intervention, the therapist changes aspects of context and/or tasks so performance is more possible. This can include enhancing some features to provide cues, or reducing other features to reduce distractibility (Dunn et al., 1994, p. 606).

Case Examples: Adapt Environment for Skill Deficit

Mrs. Hill is a 63-year-old female with a 20-year history of multiple sclerosis that has resulted in bilateral numbness and weakness below the hips, decreased sensation in the hands, and low back pain with prolonged sitting. Because of several recent falls from her wheelchair when transferring,

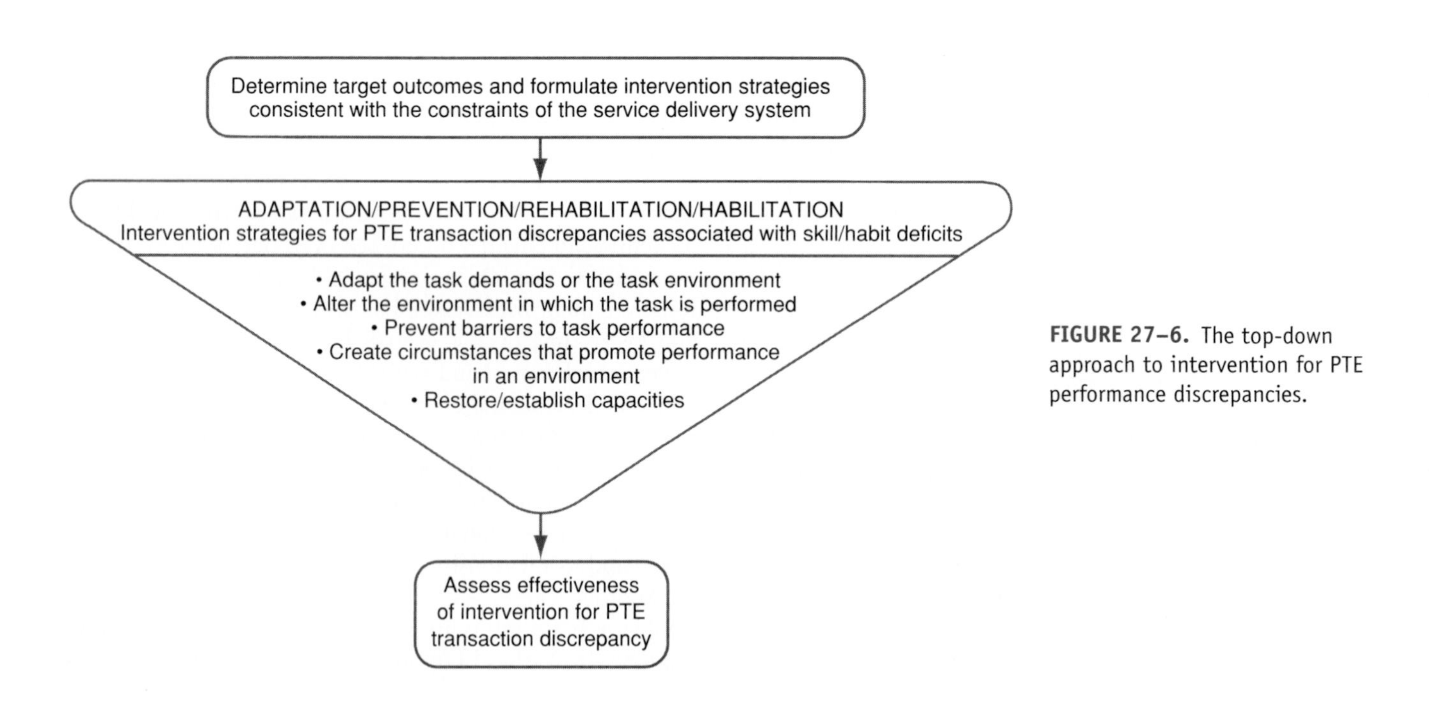

FIGURE 27–6. The top-down approach to intervention for PTE performance discrepancies.

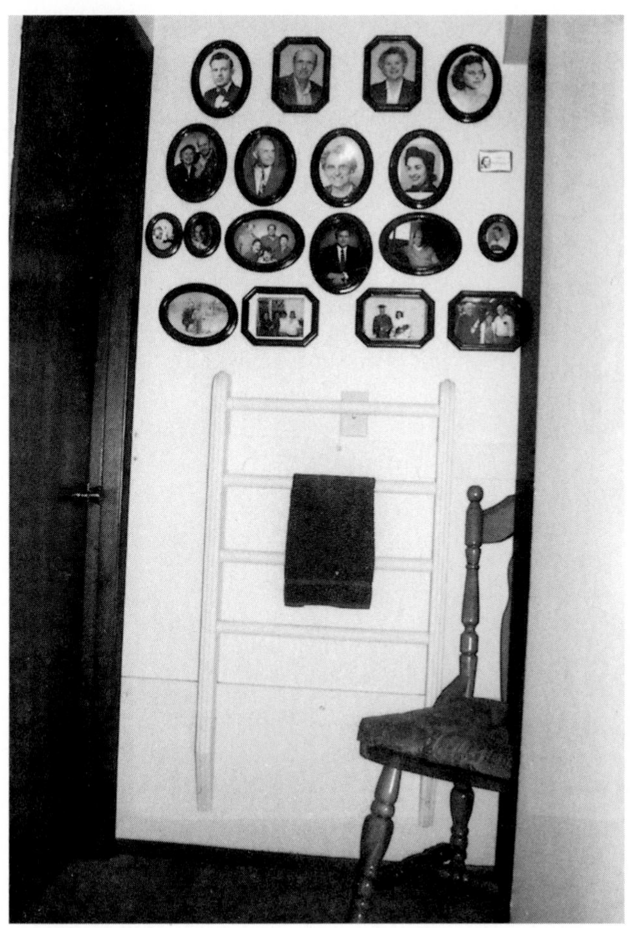

FIGURE 27–7. A wall ladder designed to blend in with the decor of the home environment.

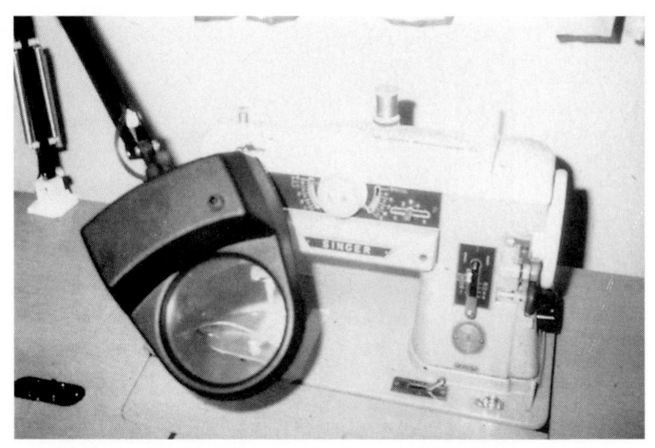

FIGURE 27–8. A lighted magnifier used to adapt a sewing task.

her family members want her to have an attendant while her husband is at work. She adamantly rejects their suggestion. Because Mrs. Hill had used a ladder successfully in the physical therapy clinic to get back into her chair, the occupational therapy practitioner recommends that a similar ladder be installed in the home. A suitable site was located, and when Mrs. Hill slips to the floor during a transfer from bed to wheelchair, she is able to crawl to the ladder, pushing her wheelchair ahead of her, and to use the ladder successfully to get back in her chair (Fig. 27-7).

Mrs. Rogers is an 83-year-old female with a 5-year history of macular degeneration, resulting in loss of central vision and fluctuating acuity in her peripheral vision. She has always enjoyed sewing items for craft fairs, but she can no longer see to thread the needle on her sewing machine, even when she uses a wire needle threader. She also cannot see the tension and stitch settings on the machine. The occupational therapy practitioner suggests a lighted magnifier, which has enabled Mrs. Rogers to continue a meaningful pastime (Fig. 27-8).

Matt is a 7-year-old male with multiple pterygium syndrome as well as arthrogryposis. The result is severe limitations in all joints, contractures, and deformities. He uses a custom ramp (mounted on a rolling library stool), designed by his occupational therapy practitioner, to access any area that he cannot get up to, such as the couch, bed, tub, dining room chair, or toilet (Fig. 27-9).

Keenan is a 3-year-old boy with a closed head injury. His occupational therapy practitioner adapted Bigfoot (a motorized ride-on vehicle) with hand controls so the boy could have functional mobility in his yard and neighborhood (Fig. 27-10).

Other modified ride-on toy vehicles are shown in Figures 27-11 and 27-12. One has been adapted by adding a positioning chair and a lever switch to move the vehicle forward. The other has been adapted with the addition of a car seat for postural stability and has been fitted with a joy stick for vehicle control. The ride-on toy vehicles are battery operated, can be purchased in any major toy store, and enable children with mobility impairments to explore their environments and enjoy functional mobility with their peers. The vehicles were adapted by an occupational therapy practitioner and are fitted with a safety control so that the practitioner or parent can override the system and stop the car.

Case Examples: Adapt Environment for Habit Deficit.

Ms. Desai is a 26-year-old female who is confined to bed and has an organic brain disorder secondary to a brain tumor. Unable to communicate her wants and needs, she learned to scream to get assistance from the LTCF staff. Eventually, she began to scream all the time when left alone. Because of her screaming, other residents avoided her and the staff placed her in her room with the door shut to reduce the disturbance to others. The occupational therapy practitioner suggests using an audiocassette tape player and headset with tapes of music that Ms. Desai liked in the past (Casby & Holm, 1994). The family brought in the tapes, and within 1 week, Ms. Desai's screaming was reduced to only one or two cycles a day.

Gary is a 17-year-old male with cerebral palsy (hemiplegia) and moderate mental retardation. As part of his individualized

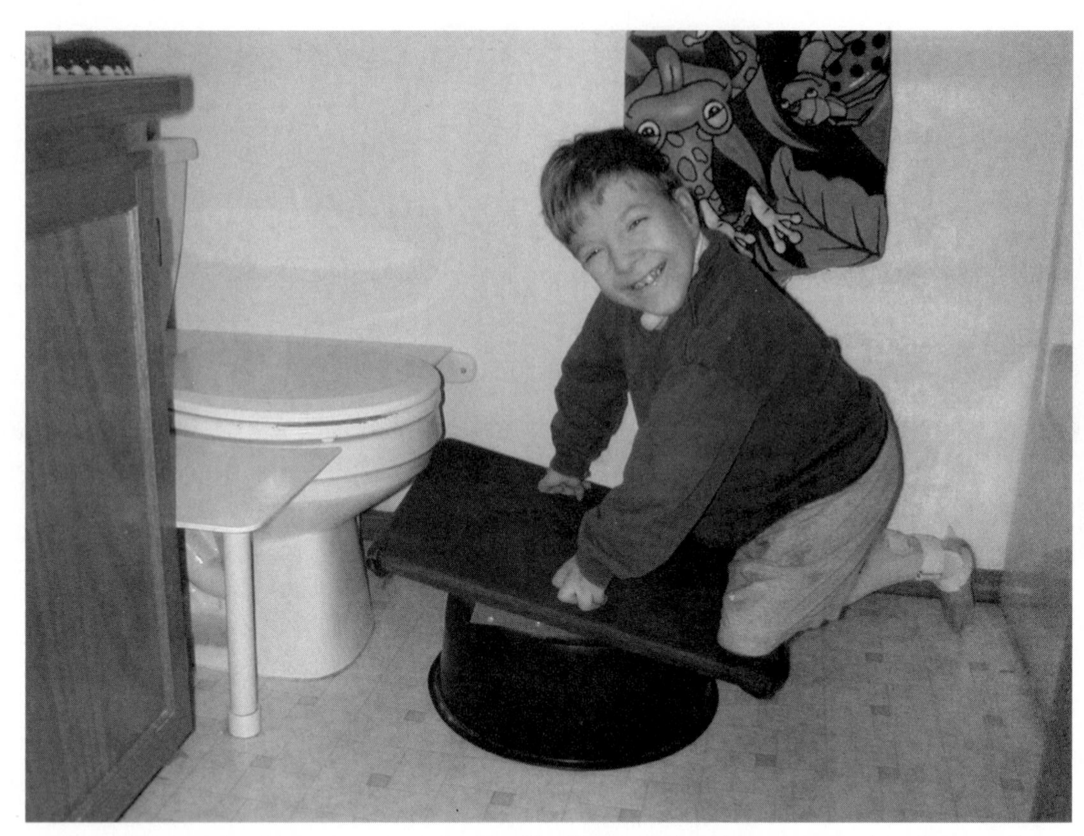

FIGURE 27–9. A custom ramp mounted on a rolling library stool enables access to the toilet as well as to the couch, bed, tub, and chairs. (Built by S. Shores, Good Samaritan Hospital, Puyallup, WA.)

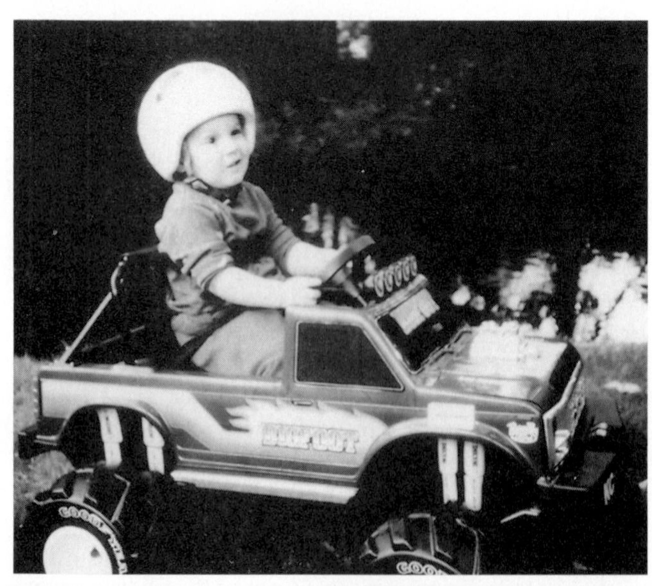

FIGURE 27–10. Adapted motorized vehicles, such as this Bigfoot, enable functional mobility and exploration capabilities for children with motor impairments. (Vehicle adapted by S. Shores, Good Samaritan Hospital, Puyallup, WA.)

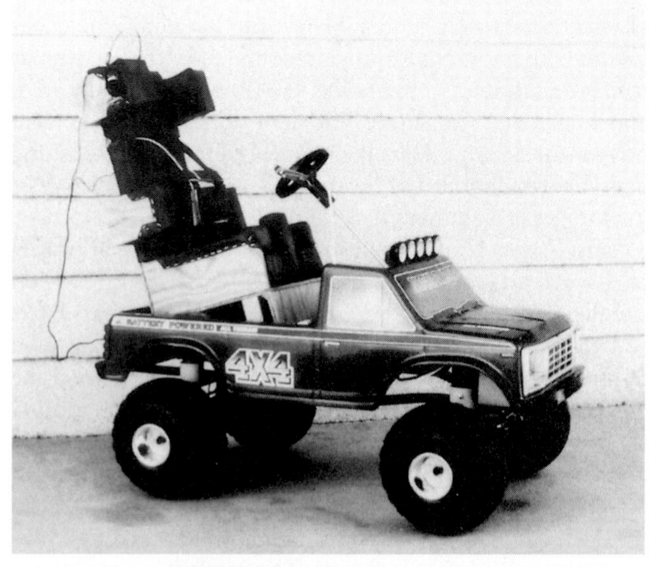

FIGURE 27–11. Adapted motorized toy vehicle with an added-on positioning chair. (Vehicle adapted by S. Shores, Good Samaritan Hospital, Puyallup, WA.)

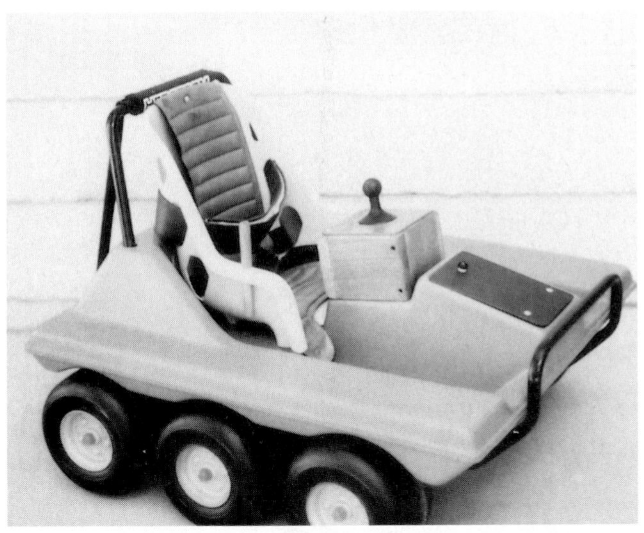

FIGURE 27–12. Motorized toy vehicle with an added-on car seat and joy stick. (Vehicle adapted by S. Shores, Good Samaritan Hospital, Puyallup, WA.)

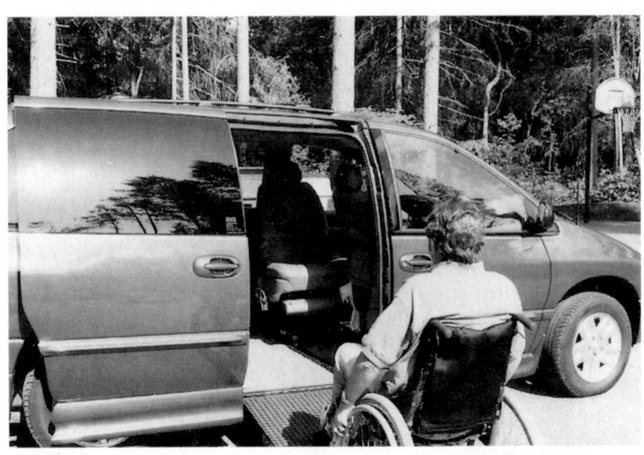

FIGURE 27–14. This adapted van allows the driver to open the door with a remote control and then enter the van via a ramp. The ramp folds into the door when it closes, and the driver transfers into the bucket seat and engages the hand controls.

vocational plan, he spends 3 hr each day in a work program. He is assigned to the lawn decorations assembly crew so he can develop work habits. The special education teacher notifies the occupational therapy practitioner that Gary does not maintain a good posture while working and that he has difficulty assembling the pinwheel pieces in the correct order.

The occupational therapy practitioner adapts the task routines by breaking them into several extra steps that Gary can manage. She put nails in a board so that Gary can sort the pinwheel pieces in the basket by color in the correct sequence for assembly, then pick up the pieces from the nail board in correct sequence and assemble them onto a jig for the next student to continue the assembly.

In regard to posture, the occupational therapy practitioner observes that once Gary becomes engaged in his tasks, he forgets about his posture. To solve this problem, a tape player with one of Gary's favorite tapes is attached to a switch plate (Fig. 27-13). To trigger the switch plate, Gary has to have most of his hand on the switch; to accomplish this, he must develop the habit of sitting upright instead of listing to the left with his shoulder protracted, elbow flexed, and wrist flexed.

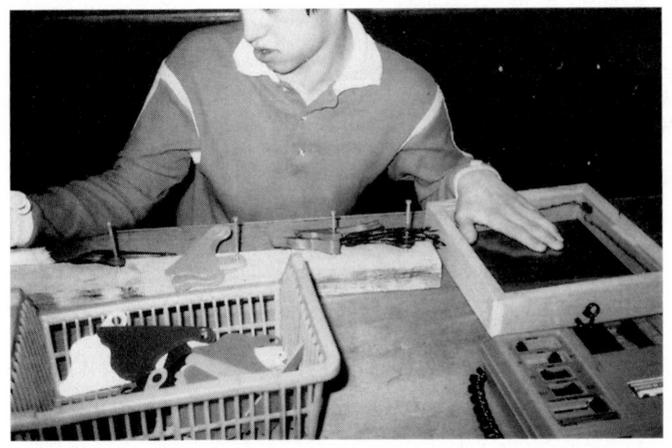

FIGURE 27–13. A switch plate adapted to trigger a tape player when the student's hand is placed firmly on the switch.

Mr. Jakke is a 48-year-old male with a 10-year history of multiple sclerosis, resulting in bilateral lower extremity weakness and numbness, decreased balance, and decreased sensation in his hands. After the last exacerbation of symptoms, Mr. Jakke has been unable to transfer independently into his car, and the family decided to invest in a car that will suit his needs. The occupational therapy practitioner refers them to a company that specializes in adapting vehicles to meet the needs of the user. Mr. Jakke's van has a remote control for opening the door, closing the door, and positioning the driver's seat, thus enabling him to transfer easily in and out of the van (Fig. 27-14). The van also features hand controls. While these adaptations do not seem economical, they enable Mr. Jakke to take his children to school and transport them to and pick them up from social activities. He can also take himself to therapy and support groups while his wife is at work. If Mr. Jakke could not drive, the costs to him (in isolation, loss of therapy, and loss of support) and to his family (in loss of normative activities and routines for his children and time lost from work for his wife) could easily be more in the long term than the adaptations to the van.

Mark is an 18-year-old male whose diagnosis is undifferentiated schizophrenia. An occupational therapy practitioner has seen him as an outpatient as part of a supported employment program. Mark is being placed in a fast-food restaurant and is assigned to work in the supply room and on the grill. To develop appropriate work habits, Mark is supplied with a Neuropage System (Hersh & Treadgold, 1994) that is programmed to get him up in the morning, cue him

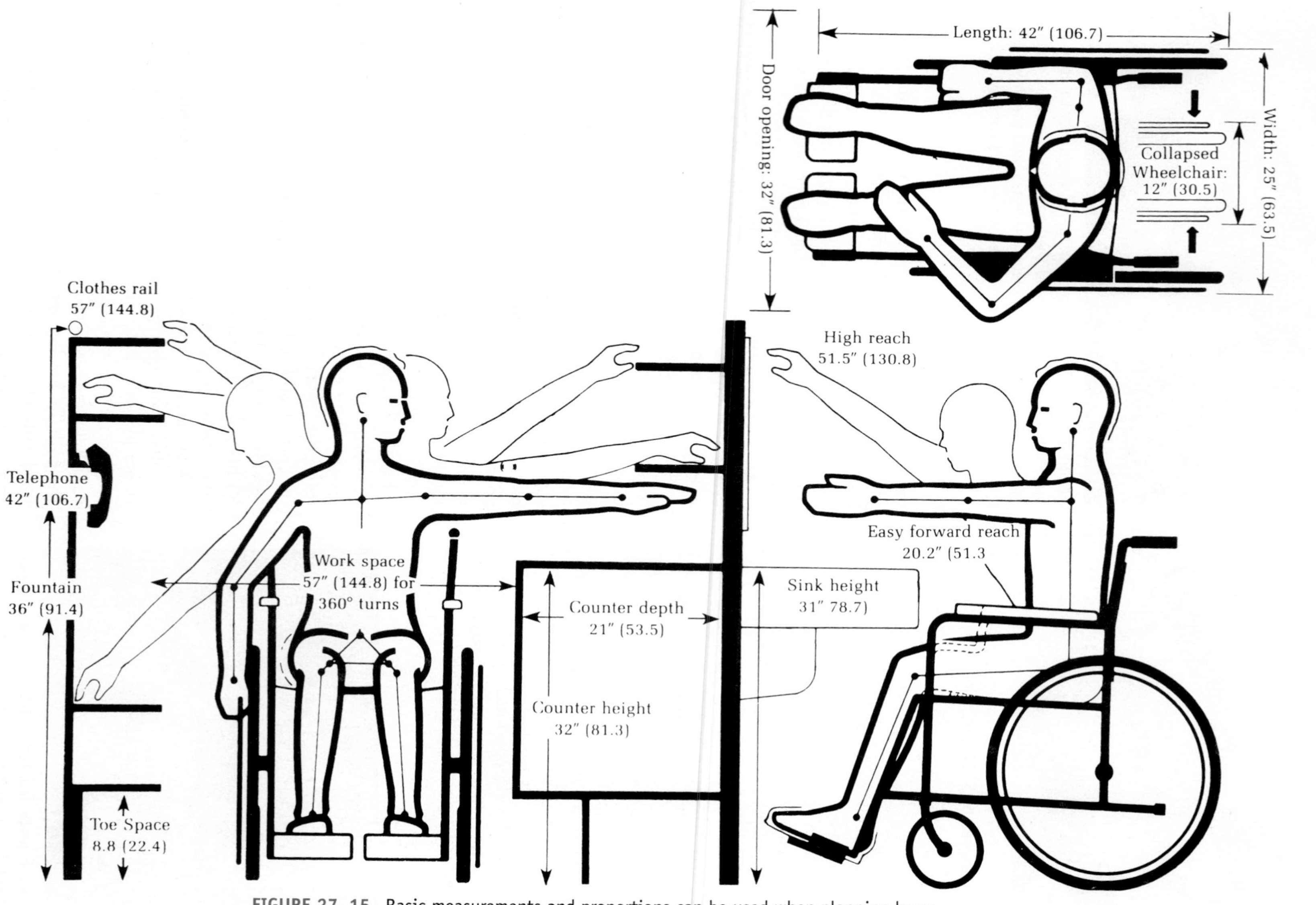

FIGURE 27–15. Basic measurements and proportions can be used when planning home modifications. Measurements are given in inches and centimeters. (Adapted from Diffrient, Tilley, & Bardagjy, 1974.)

about items to bring to work, and cue him about which medications are to be taken when the pager activates. The target outcome is to decrease Mark's reliance on the paging system to make him be on time for work and keep his medication blood levels within the therapeutic window.

Alter

> *Alter actual context in which people perform. Therapeutic interventions can alter the context within which the person performs. This intervention emphasizes selecting a context that enables the person to perform with current skills and abilities. This can include placing the person in a different setting that more closely matches current skills and abilities, rather than changing the present setting to accommodate needs (Dunn et al., 1994, p. 606).*

Case Example: Alter Environment for Skill Deficit

Before Mr. Jakke and his family moved into their new home, several alterations were made to enable successful PTE transactions using a wheelchair. Mr. Jakke (a contractor) reviewed the relevant dimensions (Fig. 27-15). and made several alterations to the physical environment The plumbing was recessed under the bathroom sink to allow Mr. Jakke to roll under the sink without worrying about burning his insensate lower extremities on the pipes, and two drawers were made into one deep drawer so that items could be obtained and stored easily from a seated position (Fig. 27-16). The standard 15-in.-high toilet was replaced with an 18-in.-high toilet for easier transfers. The oak grab bars for standing pivot transfers, which are next to the toilet, double as towel racks (Fig. 27-17). In the kitchen, static shelves were replaced with pull-out drawers for easier access to items (Fig. 27-18). The microwave oven was placed by the cutting board to facilitate the transfer of hot dishes to the table (Fig. 27-19). This setup allows Mr. Jakke, who has weakness and some loss of sensation in his hands, to transfer a hot dish from the microwave to the counter, reposition it, move it from the counter to the cutting board, reposition it, and then move it from the cutting board to the table. Finally, a counter was built in

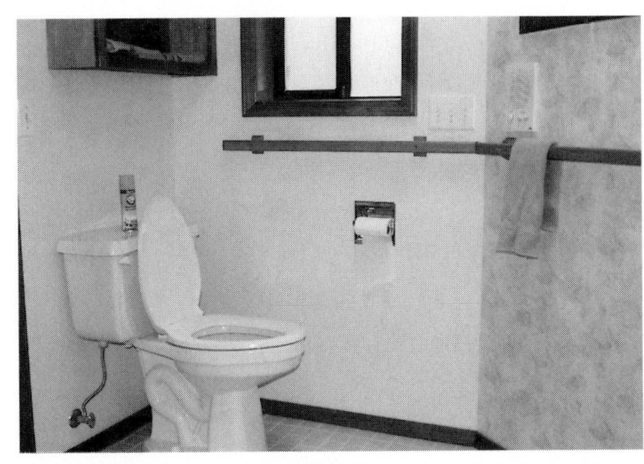

FIGURE 27–17. The oak grab bars also serve as a towel rack, and the extra-high toilet enables an easy side-to-side transfer from a wheelchair.

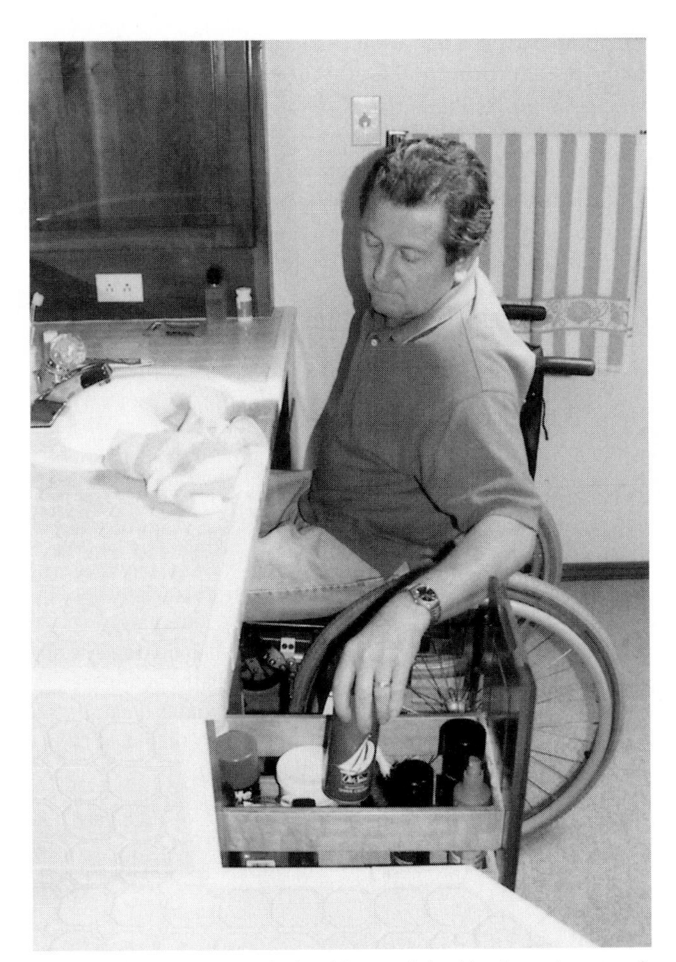

FIGURE 27–16. Recessed plumbing and double-deep drawers allow easy access to the sink area from a seated position.

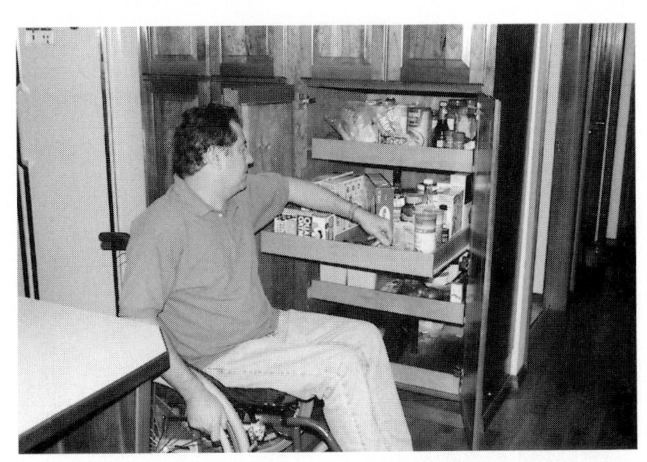

FIGURE 27–18. Shallow drawers on gliders make all goods accessible from a seated position.

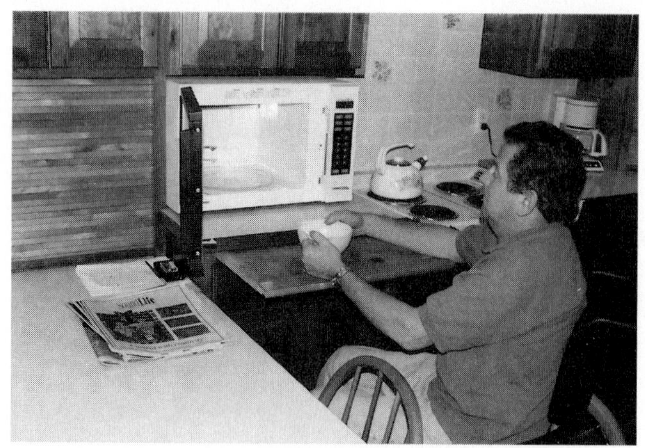

FIGURE 27–19. The placement of the microwave enables hot items to be stepped down to the cutting board and then transferred to the table with ease.

the laundry room to enable Mr. Jakke to fold laundry while seated in his wheelchair (Fig. 27-20).

Case Example: Alter Environment for Habit Deficit

Mr. Bitner is a 68-year-old male with dementia of the Alzheimer type (DAT). He is a retired pharmaceutical company executive, and he and his wife, Anne, enjoy entertaining family and friends in their home. Mr. Bitner's current stage of DAT includes increased memory loss resulting in continuous repetitive questioning of Mrs. Bitner, difficulty concentrating, loss of interest in previous activities secondary to memory loss and depression, withdrawal from social activities, and constant pacing. Mrs. Bitner has tried to rearrange their home to accommodate her husband's new habit of pacing, but 2 weeks ago Mr. Bitner sustained bilateral Colles' fractures when he tripped over a coffee table in the family room. After assisting Mrs. Bitner with suggestions for her husband's personal care, the occupational therapy practitioner also provided her with information about an adult day-care program for persons with dementia that would provide her husband with a low-stimulus environment designed for his current level of functioning. Moreover, it would also provide Mrs. Bitner, his caregiver, some respite from his other new habit of asking questions and repeating phrases.

Prevent

> *Prevent the occurrence or evolution of malpractice [sic] performance in context. Therapeutic interventions can prevent the occurrence or evolution of barriers to performance in context. Sometimes, therapists can predict that certain negative outcomes are likely without intervention to change the course of events. Therapists can create intervention to change the course of events. Therapists can create interventions that address person, context, and task variables to change the course, thus enabling functional performance to emerge (Dunn et al., 1994, p. 606).*

Case Examples: Prevent Skill Deficit by Changing Environmental Demand

Mr. Ibrahim is a 72-year-old male with a 30-year history of rheumatoid arthritis and a 10-year history of type 2 diabetes who has incurred a mild right CVA. His wife is now concerned about how she will manage him during bathtub transfers. Mr. Ibrahim likes to soak twice a day in the bathtub to relieve his arthritis pain. The home-health occupational therapy practitioner recommends a spring-loaded mechanical bathtub seat that allows Mr. Ibrahim to transfer safely into the bathtub, move down to and up from the bottom of the bathtub, and transfer out of the bathtub, thus preventing falls (Fig. 27-21).

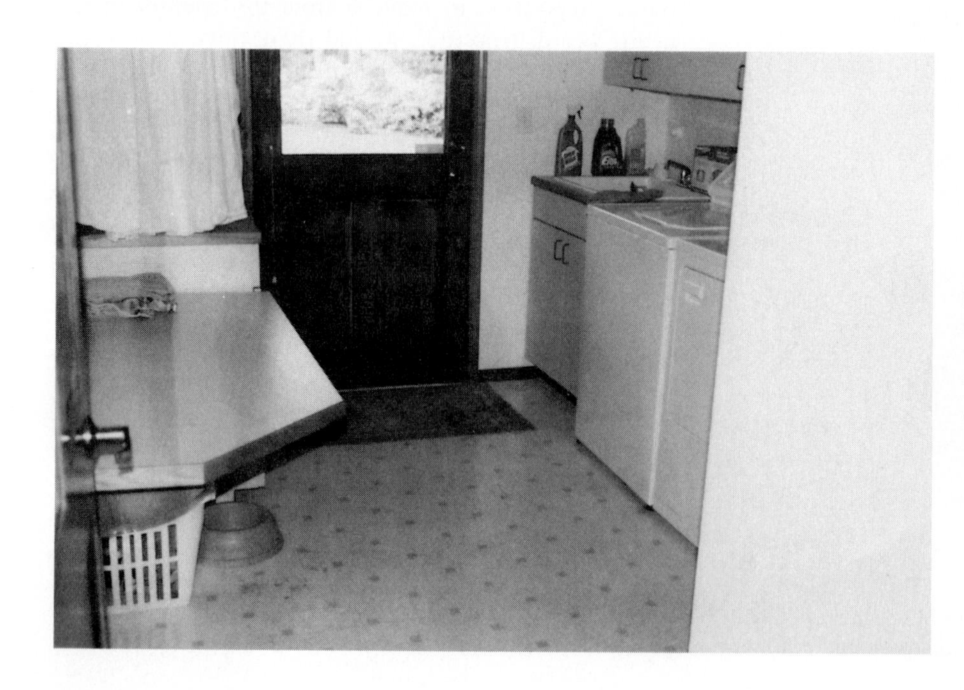

FIGURE 27–20. The laundry table is angled to allow a clear pathway for the wheelchair, and the counter height is 32 in. for ease of use when seated, with clear access underneath.

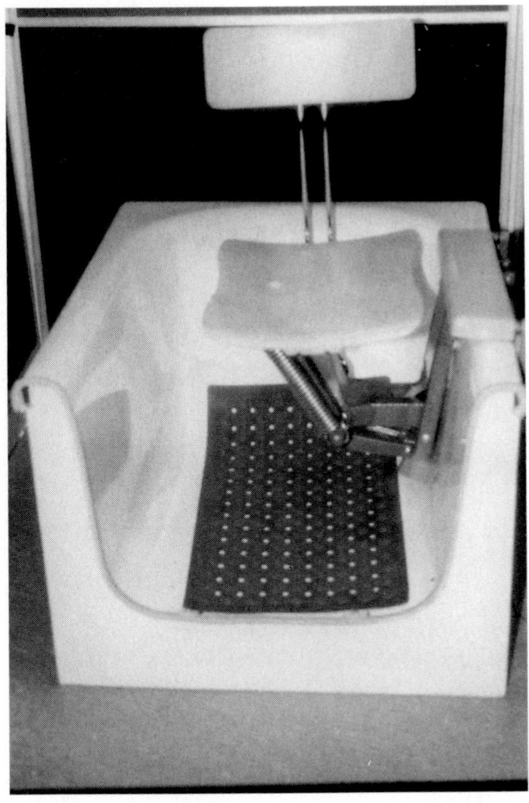

FIGURE 27–21. The mechanical tub seat is spring loaded and raises from the tub bottom with a weight shift and a simultaneous pushing up on the tub edges.

Mrs. Prescott is a 51-year-old with a fast-progressing dementing illness of unknown origin. She was hospitalized in a psychiatric unit after she lost 30 lb in 2 months, exhibited apraxia during everyday tasks, and became extremely labile. At discharge, she is unable to dress herself, cannot remember how to use silverware, and is incontinent. Her family wishes to care for her at home and has hired a live-in attendant. The occupational therapy practitioner meets with the family and the attendant to demonstrate a hierarchy of assists that are available to them to maintain the skills Mrs. Prescott still retains and to provide the necessary support as her capacities decrease. The occupational therapy practitioner shows them a videotape he made while assisting Mrs. Prescott during a meal. As they watch the tape, the therapist identifies lower-level verbal cues, middle-level gestural cues, and higher-level physical assists (physical guidance and total assistance) as each is given. He then discusses using lower-level assists before higher level assists, the need to vary the type of assists from day to day as Mrs. Prescott's performance fluctuates, and the increased use of higher-level assists as her dementia progresses. The practitioner gives each caregiver a list of the types of assists that Mrs. Prescott has required for personal care tasks, explaining each one and then responding to questions. Although Mrs. Prescott's progressive deterioration of skill deficits cannot be prevented, the appropriate level of cues from the social environment can prevent a faster rate of skill deterioration (Rogers et al., 2000).

Case Example: Prevent Habit Deficit by Changing Environmental Demand

The Reverend Tengesdal is an 83-year-old with profound deafness, which is corrected slightly with his hearing aid. He is the visiting pastor of a large church and is having difficulty hearing some of the frail home-bound parishioners he visits as well as his wife's soft voice. Recently, he got in the habit of removing himself from conversations with more than one person because he can no longer hear. His daughter, an occupational therapy practitioner, prescribes a Pocket Talker with a magnetic loop to enhance his hearing aids and an attached microphone (Fig. 27-22). The Pocket

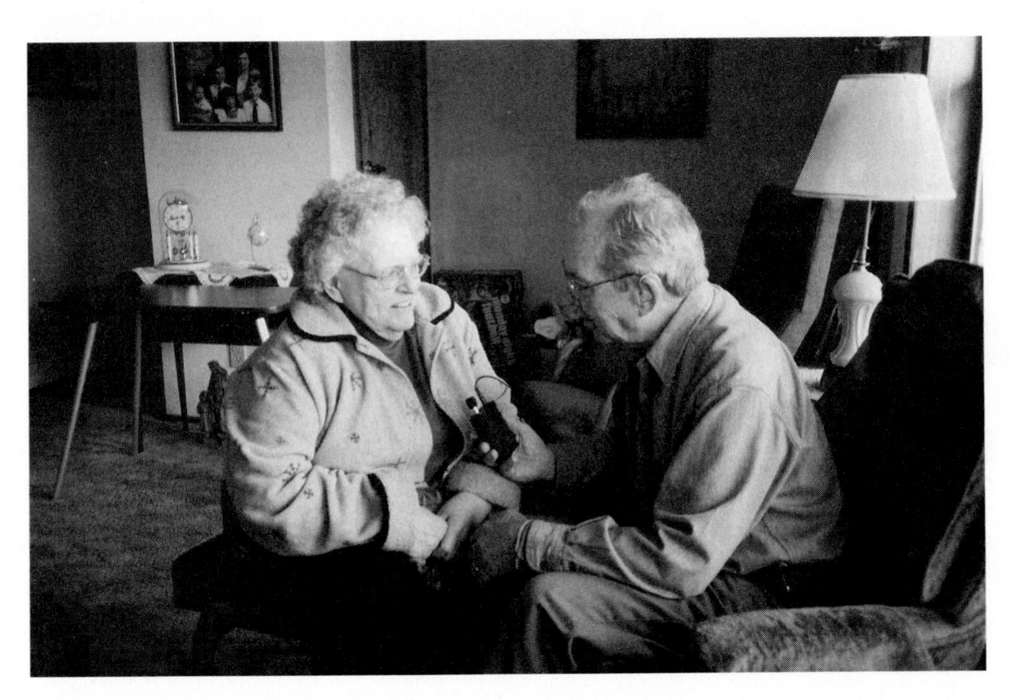

FIGURE 27–22. The Pocket Talker has a magnetic loop that the user wears around the neck to enhance the magnification of sound in the hearing aid, which allows easier communication with those in the social environment.

Talker allows him to hear clearly the voice of his bride of 50 years, as well as those of his parishioners—individually or in groups.

Create

> *Create circumstances that promote more adaptable/complex performance in context. Therapeutic interventions can create circumstances which promote more adaptable performance in context. This therapeutic intervention does not assume a disability is present or has the potential to interfere with performance. This therapeutic choice focuses on providing enriched contextual and task experiences that will enhance performance (Dunn et al., 1994, p. 606).*

Case Examples: Create Environments That Enhance Skill

Ms Yi-Sun is the occupational therapy practitioner at Vintage LTCF. She is asked by the administration to create an environment that will be safe for residents with dementia to wander and pace when they become anxious (Hall & Buckwalter, 1987). With the assistance of students from the nearby educational program for occupational therapy assistants, she designs stations in a hallway where residents can stop and wind pocket watches, fold towels, sort and stack heavy plastic dishes, watch fish in an eye-level aquarium, and pick up finger foods. Outside, in the fenced-in patio area, they build raised plant boxes that can be tended without bending and place fencing around areas where the ground is uneven or there are tripping hazards that could place residents at risk for falls (Fig. 27-23). All the staff and residents enjoy the patio on nice days, creating a positive environment for everyone.

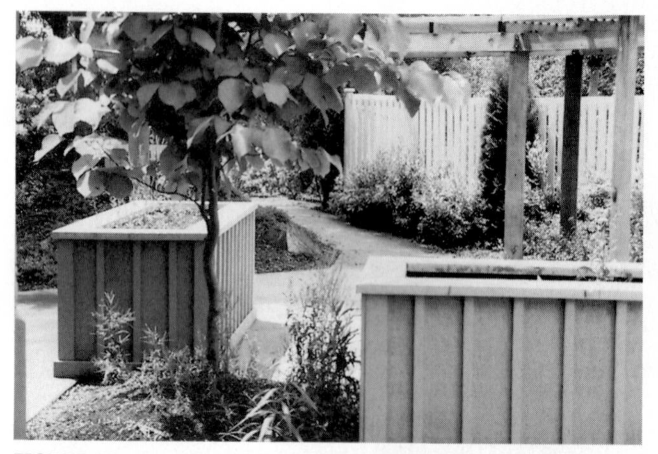

FIGURE 27–23. The wandering paths and built-up planter enable nursing home residents to pace and wander in a safe and attractive environment.

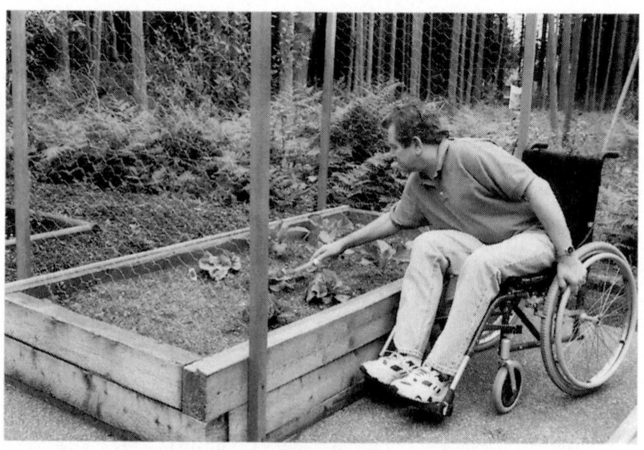

FIGURE 27–24. The raised gardens enable clients to tend plants from a seated position.

Case Example: Create Environments That Enhance Habit

Mr. Jakke has always liked being outdoors. Several years ago he took up gardening and was accustomed to spending about 2 hr each morning tending his vegetables, flowers, and bonsai trees. He previously used a portable kneeler/bench that provided support for kneeling or sitting. However, he is no longer able to use this device because of increased lower extremity spasticity. Hence, his morning gardening routine has come to a halt. The occupational therapy practitioner suggests raised gardens for his vegetables and flowers (Fig. 27-24) and a fence with shelves to tend and display his bonsai trees.

As illustrated through the cases of Ms. Yi-Sun and Mr. Jakke, a distinguishing feature of creating environments, as opposed to altering environments, is building new structures or developing new social settings.

Establish/Restore

> *Establish/restore a person's abilities to perform in context. Therapeutic intervention can establish or restore person's [sic] abilities to perform in context. This emphasis is on identifying a person's skills and barriers to performance, and designing interventions that improve the person's skills and experiences (Dunn et al., 1994, p. 606).*

Case Example: Establish/Restore Skill for Performance in a Specific Environment

Mrs. Kochinski is an 86-year-old female with multi-infarct dementia, who currently resides in an assisted living center. Because she is having difficulty locating her room after meals and other activities, the occupational therapy practitioner helps her put some favorite pictures of herself and her husband (circa 1940) on her door and then cues her to find the door with her pictures after each meal and activity

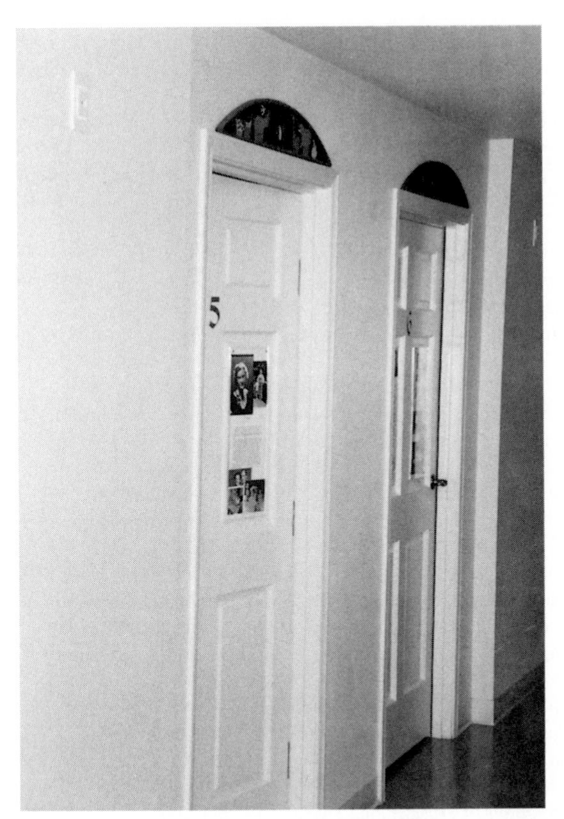

FIGURE 27–25. Familiar cues in a new environment help nursing home residents find their way home.

session (Fig. 27-25). In 3 days, her way-finding skills are established for her new environment.

Case Example: Establish/Restore Habit for Performance in a Specific Environment

Andrew is a 13-year-old male who has a diagnosis of attention deficit disorder. He has his own room with a desk for studying, but he becomes easily distracted and rarely completes his homework. Andrew's psychologist works with an occupational therapy practitioner consultant, whom he asked to evaluate Andrew and make recommendations. The therapist recommends the following:

> *After removing all items from Andrew's desk except the desk lamp, and all posters from the walls surrounding his desk, have Andrew study in a dark room with only the desk lamp on and the items necessary for a particular assignment on his desk. In addition, have Andrew wear a Walkman that plays a tape of "white noise." This will help to reduce environmental stimulation. Have Andrew study at the same time every evening, and go through the same routines to set up his study area until habit patterns are established and maintained.*

The intervention is successful.

CONCLUSION

Occupational therapy practitioners have expertise in the analysis of performance discrepancies in the PTE transaction that occurs when clients engage in meaningful tasks in relevant environments. Practitioners' knowledge base, derived from the biological, physical, behavioral, and occupational sciences, also prepares them to identify and implement efficient and economical interventions that will enable clients to perform meaningful tasks in a safe, independent, and adequate manner.

The clinical decision-making guide presented in this section was designed to prompt practitioners to consider a top-down approach to the evaluation of skill and habit performance discrepancies. Moreover, given the need to achieve functional outcomes in limited time frames (Angelelli et al., 2000; Banja & DeJong, 2000; Christiansen, 1993, 1996; Cope & Sundance, 1995; Eastwood, 1999), we recommend several of the compensatory environmental intervention strategies delineated by Dunn et al. (1994) as the initial approach to performance discrepancy, followed by restorative strategies.

In the appendices are several resource compendiums. They are not meant to be exhaustive listings but rather to provide examples of resources that are available to occupational therapy practitioners and their clients. The appendices are meant to stimulate further research for resources by providing sample categories and examples of what is available in the private and public sectors. Consistent with the decision-making guide, appendices contain resource for person support; task-environment adaptation; and resources for family members, advocates, caregivers, employers, co-workers, and/or friends in the client's environment.

In summary, the guide presented in this section is meant to provide a pathway through the decision-making processes required to enhance person capacities and reduce or change environmental demands to enable clients to achieve successful PTE transactions. The following chapters address a variety of specific intervention strategies to promote participation and to improve skills and abilities, either directly or through the use of assistive technology.

References

American Occupational Therapy Association [AOTA]. (1993). Purposeful activity. *American Journal of Occupational Therapy*, 47, 1081–1082.

American Occupational Therapy Association [AOTA]. (1994). Uniform terminology for occupational therapy—Third edition. *American Journal of Occupational Therapy*, 48, 1047–1059.

American Occupational Therapy Association [AOTA]. (1995). Occupation. *American Journal of Occupational Therapy*, 49, 1015–1018.

American Occupational Therapy Association (in press). Occupational therapy practice framework: Domain and process. *American Journal of Occupational Therapy*.

Angelelli, J., Wilber, K., & Myrtle, R. (2000). A comparison of skilled nursing facility rehabilitation treatment and outcomes under Medicare managed care and Medicare fee-for-service reimbursement. *Gerontologist, 40*, 646–653.

Arcury, T., Quandt, S., Cravey, J., Elmore, R., & Russell, G. (2001). Farmworker reports of pesticide safety and sanitation in the work environment. *American Journal of Industrial Medicine, 39*, 486–498.

Baker, N. A. (1999). Anthropometry. In K. Jacobs (Ed.). *Ergonomics for therapists* (2nd ed., pp. 49–84). Boston: Butterworth-Heinemann.

Banja, J., & DeJong, G. (2000). The rehabilitation marketplace: Economics, values, and proposals for reform. *Archives of Physical Medicine and Rehabilitation, 81*, 233–240.

Barris, R., (1982). Environmental interactions: An extension of the model of human occupation. *American Journal of Occupational Therapy, 36*, 637–644.

Barris, R., Kielhofner, G., Neville, A. M., Oakley, F. M., Salz, C., & Watts, J. H. (1985). Psychosocial dysfunction. In G. Kielhofner (Ed.). *A model of human occupation* (pp. 248–305). Baltimore: Williams & Wilkins.

Booth, J., Davidson, I., Winstanley, J., &Waters, K. (2001). Observing washing and dressing of stroke patients: Nursing intervention compared with occupational therapists. What is the difference? *Journal of Advanced Nursing, 33*(1), 98–105.

Bransford, J. D., & Stein, B. S. (1984). *The ideal problem solver*. New York: Freeman.

Brigham, C., Engelberg, A. L., & Richling, D. E. (1996, February 16). The changing role of rehab: Focus on function. *Patient Care*, 144–184.

Carson, R. (1994). Reducing cumulative trauma disorders: Use of proper workplace design. *AAOHN Journal, 42*, 270–276.

Casby, J., & Holm, M. B. (1994). The effect of music on repetitive disruptive vocalizations of persons with dementia. *American Journal of Occupational Therapy, 48*, 883–889.

Christiansen, C. (1991). Occupational therapy intervention for life performance. In C. Christiansen & C. Baum (Eds.). *Occupational therapy: Overcoming human performance deficits* (pp. 3–43). Thorofare, NJ: Slack.

Christiansen, C. (1993). Continuing challenges of functional assessment in rehabilitation: Recommended changes. *American Journal of Occupational Therapy, 47*, 258–259.

Christiansen, C. (1996). Managed care: Opportunities and challenges for occupational therapy in the emerging systems of the 21st century. *American Journal of Occupational Therapy, 50*, 409–412.

Christiansen, C. H. (1999). Defining lives: Occupation as identity: An essay on competence, coherence and the creation of meaning. [Eleanor Clark Slagle Lecture]. *American Journal of Occupational Therapy, 53*, 547–558.

Cipriani, J., Hess, S., Higgins, H., Resavy, D., Sheon, S., Szychowski, M., & Holm, M. B. (2000). Collaboration in the therapeutic process: Older adults' perspectives. *Physical and Occupational Therapy in Geriatrics, 17*(1), 43–54.

Clark, F. A. (2000). The concepts of habit and routine: A preliminary theoretical synthesis. *Occupational Therapy Journal of Research, 20*(Suppl. 1), 123S–137S.

Clark, F. A., Parham, D., Carlson, M. E., Frank, G., Jackson, J., Pierce, D., Wolfe, R. J., & Zemke, R. (1991). Occupational science: Academic innovation in the service of occupational therapy's future. *American Journal of Occupational Therapy, 45*, 300–310.

Clark, M. C., Czaja, S. J., & Weber, R. A. (1990). Older adults and daily living task profiles. *Human Factors, 32*, 537–549.

Close, J., Ellis, M. Hooper, R., Glucksman, E., Jackson., S., & Swift, C. (1999). Prevention of falls in the elderly trial (PROFET): A randomised controlled trial. *Lancet, 353*, 93–97.

Cope, D. N., & Sundance, P. (1995). Conceptualizing clinical outcomes. In P. K. Landrum, N. D. Schmidt, & A. McLean (Eds.). *Outcome-oriented rehabilitation* (pp. 43–56). Gaithersburg, MD: Aspen.

Creighton, C. (1992). The origin and evolution of activity analysis. *American Journal of Occupational Therapy, 46*, 45–48.

Cubie, S., & Kaplan, K. (1982). A case analysis method for the model of human occupation. *American Journal of Occupational Therapy, 36*, 645–656.

Cummings, R. G., Thomas, M., Szonyi, G., Salkeld, G., O'Neill, E., Westbury, C., & Frampton, G. (1999). Home visits by an occupational therapist for assessment and modification of environmental hazards: A randomized trial of falls prevention. *Journal of the American Geriatrics Society, 47*, 1397–1402.

Cynkin, S. (1979). *Occupational therapy: Toward health through activities*. Boston: Little, Brown.

Czaja, S., Weber, R. A., & Nair, S. N. (1993). A human factors analysis of ADL activities: A capability-demand approach. *Journals of Gerontology, 48*, 44–48.

Demore-Taber, M. (1995). Americans with Disabilities Act work site assessment. In K. Jacobs & C. Bettencourt (Eds.). *Ergonomics for therapists* (pp. 229–244). Boston: Butterworth-Heinemann.

Diffrient, N., Tilley, A., & Bardagjy, F. (1974). *Humanscale 1/2/3*. Cambridge, MA: MIT Press.

Dirette, D., & Hinojosa, J. (1999). The effects of a compensatory intervention on processing deficits of adults with acquired brain injuries. *Occupational Therapy Journal of Research, 19*, 223–240.

Dolecheck & Schkade, J. (1999). The extent dynamic standing endurance is effected when CVA subjects perform personally meaningful activities rather than nonmeaningful tasks. *Occupational Therapy Journal of Research, 19*, 40–54.

du Toit, P., van Kradenburg, J., Niehaus, D. J., & Stein, D. J. (2001). Characteristics and phenomenology of hair-pulling; An exploration of subtypes. *Comprehensive Psychiatry, 42*, 247–256.

Dunn, W. (1993). Measurement of function: Actions for the future. *American Journal of Occupational Therapy, 47*, 357–359.

Dunn, W. (2000). Habit: What's the brain got to do with it? *Occupational Therapy Journal of Research, 20*(Suppl. 1), 6S–20S.

Dunn, W., Brown, C., & McGuigan, M. (1994). The ecology of human performance: A framework for considering the effect of context. *American Journal of Occupational Therapy, 48*, 595–607.

Eastwood, E. A. (1999). Functional status and its uses in rehabilitation medicine. *Mt. Sinai Journal of Medicine, 66*, 179–187.

Eisenberg, M. G., Sutkin, L. C., & Jansen, M. A. (1984). *Chronic illness and disability through the life span: Effects on self and family*. New York: Springer.

Evans, R. W., Small, L., & Ling, J. S. (1995). Independence in the home and community. In P. K. Landrum, N. D. Schmidt, & A. McLean (Eds.). *Outcome-oriented rehabilitation* (pp. 95–124). Gaithersburg, MD: Aspen.

Faletti, M. V. (1984). Human factors research and functional environments for the aged. In I. Altman, M. P. Lawton, & J. F. Wohlwill (Eds.). *Elderly people and the environment* (pp. 191–237). New York: Plenum.

Fisher, A. G. (1998). Uniting practice and theory in an occupational framework. [Eleanor Clarke Slagle Lecture]. *American Journal of Occupational Therapy, 52*, 509–521.

Fisher, A. G., & Short-DeGraff, M. (1993). Improving functional assessment in occupational therapy: Recommendations and philosophy for change. *American Journal of Occupational Therapy, 47*, 199–201.

Fleishman, E. A. (1966). Human abilities and the acquisition of skill. In E. A. Bilodeau (Ed.). *Acquisition of skill* (pp. 147–167). New York: Academic Press.

Fleishman, E. A., & Quaintance, M. K. (1984). Taxonomies of human performance. Orlando, FL: Academic Press.

Florey, L. L., & Michelman, S. M. (1982). Occupational role history: A screening tool for occupational therapy. *American Journal of Occupational Therapy, 36*, 301–308.

Fried, L. P., Herdman, S. J., Kuhn, K. E., Rubin, G., & Turano, K. (1991). Preclinical disability. *Journal of Aging and Health, 3*, 285–300.

Gentile, A. M. (1987). Skill acquisition: Action, movement, and neuromotor processes. In J. H. Carr & R. B. Shepherd (Eds.). *Movement science foundations for physical therapy in rehabilitation* (pp. 93–154). Rockville, MD: Aspen.

Gerdner, L. A., Hall, G. R., & Buckwalter, K. C. (1996). Caregiver training for people with Alzheimer's based on a stress threshold model. *Image: Journal of Nursing Scholarship, 28*, 241–246.

Gibson, J., & Schkade, J. (1997). Occupational adaptation intervention with patients with cerebrovascular accident: A clinical study. *American Journal of Occupational Therapy, 51*, 523–529.

Giles, G., Ridley, J., Dill, A., & Frye, S. (1997). A consecutive series of adults with brain injury treated with a washing and dressing retraining program. *American Journal of Occupational Therapy, 51*, 256–266.

Guralnik, J. M., Branch, L. G., Cummings, S. R., & Curb, J. D. (1989). Physical performance measures in aging research. *Journal of Gerontology, 44*, 141–146.

Haas, L. (1944). *Practical occupational therapy*. Milwaukee: Bruce.

Hagedorn, R. (1995a). Environmental analysis and adaptation. In R. Hagedorn (Ed.). *Occupational therapy: Perspectives and processes* (pp. 239–257). Melbourne, Australia: Churchill Livingstone.

Hagedorn, R. (1995b). Intervention. In R. Hagedorn (Ed.). *Occupational therapy: Perspectives and processes* (pp. 175–195). Melbourne, Australia: Churchill Livingstone.

Hall, G. R., & Buckwalter, K. C. (1987). Progressively lowered stress threshold: A conceptual model for care of adults with Alzheimer's disease. *Archives of Psychiatric Nursing, 1*, 399–406.

Hersh, N., & Treadgold, L. (1994). Neuropage: The rehabilitation of memory dysfunction by prosthetic memory and cuing. *NeuroRehabilitation, 4*, 187–197.

Hilton, K., Fricke, J., & Unsworth, C. (2001). A comparison of self-report versus observation of performance using the Assessment of Living Skills and Resources (ALSAR) with an older population. *British Journal of Occupational Therapy, 64*(3), 135–143.

Hinojosa, J. & Blount, M. F. (1998). Professional competence. *American Journal of Occupational Therapy, 52*, 698–701.

Holm, M. B. (2000). Our mandate for the new millennium: Evidence-based practice. [Eleanor Clark Slagle Lecture]. *American Journal of Occupational Therapy, 54*, 575–585.

Holm, M. B., & Rogers, J. C. (1989). The therapist's thinking behind functional assessment, II. In C. Royeen (Ed.). *Assessment of function: An action guide* (pp. 1–34). Rockville, MD: American Occupational Therapy Association.

Holm, M. B., & Rogers, J. C. (1991). High, low, or no assistive technology devices for older adults undergoing rehabilitation. International Journal of Technology and Aging, 4, 153–162.

Holm, M. B., Santangelo, M., Fromuth, D., Brown, S., & Walter, H. (2000). Effectiveness of everyday occupations for changing client behaviors in a community living arrangement. *American Journal of Occupational Therapy, 54*, 361–371.

Howe, M. C., & Briggs, A. K. (1982). Ecological systems model for occupational therapy. *American Journal of Occupational Therapy, 36*, 322–327.

Humphrey, R., Jewell, K., & Rosenberger, R. C. (1995). Development of in-hand manipulation and relationship with activities. *American Journal of Occupational Therapy, 49*, 763–771.

Iwarsson, S., Isacsson, A., & Lanke, J. (1998). ADL dependence in the elderly population living in the community: The influence of functional limitations and physical environmental demand. *Occupational Therapy International, 5*, 173–193.

Jacobs, K. (Ed.). (1999). *Ergonomics for therapists* (2nd ed.). Boston: Butterworth-Heinemann.

Johnson, D. N. (2000). Task demands and representation in long-term repetition priming. *Memory and Cognition, 28*, 1303–1309.

Keuter, K., Byrne, E., Voell, J., & Larson, E. (2000). Nurses' job satisfaction and organizational climate in a dynamic work environment. *Applied Nursing Research, 13*(1), 46–49.

Kielhofner, G. (1995). Environmental influences on occupational behavior. In G. Kielhofner (Ed.). *A model of human occupation: Theory and application* (2nd ed.. pp. 91–111). Baltimore: Williams & Wilkins.

Kielhofner, G., & Burke, J. P. (1980). A model of human occupation, Part I. Conceptual framework and content. *American Journal of Occupational Therapy, 34*, 572–581.

Kielhofner, G., & Burke, J. P. (1985). Components and determinants of human occupation. In G. Kielhofner (Ed.). *A model of human occupation* (pp. 12–36). Baltimore: Williams & Wilkins.

Kiernat, J. M. (1982). Environment: The hidden modality. *Physical and Occupational Therapy in Geriatrics, 2*(1), 3–12.

Kopias, J. A. (2001). Multidisciplinary model of occupational health services: Medical and non-medical aspects of occupational health. *International Journal of Occupational Medicine & Environmental Health, 14*(1), 23–28.

Kramer, P., & Hinojosa, J. (1993). *Frames of reference for pediatric occupational therapy*. Baltimore: Williams & Wilkins.

Kroemer, K. H., & Grandjean, E. (1997). *Fitting the task to the human: A textbook of occupational ergonomics* (5th ed.). London: Taylor & Francis.

Law, M., Cooper, B., Strong, S., Stewart, D., Rigby, P., & Letts, L. (1996). The person-environment-occupational model: A transactive approach to occupational performance. *Canadian Journal of Occupational Therapy, 63*, 9–23.

Lawton, M. P. (1982). Competence, environmental press, and the adaptation of older people. In M. P. Lawton, P. G. Windley, & T. O. Byerts (Eds.). *Aging and the environment: Theoretical approaches* (pp. 33–59). New York: Springer.

Letts, L, Law, M., Rigby, P., Cooper, B., Stewart, D., & Strong, S. (1994). Person-environment assessments in occupational therapy. *American Journal of Occupational Therapy, 48*, 608–618.

Levine, R. E., & Brayley, C. R. (1991). Occupation as a therapeutic medium. In C. Christiansen & C. Baum (Eds.). *Occupational therapy: Overcoming human performance deficits* (pp. 591–631). Thorofare, NJ: Slack.

Ma, H., & Trombly, C. (1999). The effect of context on skill acquisition and transfer. *American Journal of Occupational Therapy, 53*, 138–144.

MacDonald, L., Karasek, R., Punnett, L., & Scharf, T. (2001). Covariation between workplace physical and psychosocial stressors: Evidence and implications for occupational health research and prevention. *Ergonomics, 10*, 696–718.

Mager, R. F., & Pipe, P. (1984). *Analyzing performance problems* (2nd ed.). Belmont, CA: Lake.

Mangino, M. (2000). The aging employee: The Impact on occupational health. *AAOHN Journal, 48*, 349–357.

Mathiowetz, V. (1993). Role of physical performance component evaluations in occupational therapy functional assessment. *American Journal of Occupational Therapy, 47*, 225–230.

Mathiowetz, V., & Matuska, K. (1998). Effectiveness of inpatient rehabilitation on self-care abilities of individuals with multiple sclerosis. *Neuro Rehabilitation, 11*, 141–151.

Mathiowetz, V., & Wade, M. (1995). Task constraints and functional motor performance of individuals with and without multiple sclerosis. *Ecological Psychology, 7*(2), 99–123.

McAndrew, E., McDermott, S., Vitzakovich, S., Warunek, M., & Holm, M. B. (2000). Therapist and patient perceptions of the occupational therapy goal setting process: A pilot study. *Physical and Occupational Therapy in Geriatrics, 17*(1), 55–63.

Mee, J., & Sumsion, T. (2001). Mental health clients confirm the motivating power of occupation. *British Journal of Occupational Therapy, 64*(3), 121–128.

Meyer, A. (1922). The philosophy of occupational therapy. *Archives of Occupational Therapy*, 1, 1–10.

Militello, L. G., & Hutton, R. J. (1998). Applied cognitive task analysis (ACTA): A practitioner's toolkit for understanding cognitive task demands. *Ergonomics, 41*, 1618–1641.

Militello, L. G., & Hutton, R. J. (1998). Learning to think like a user: Using cognitive task analysis to meet today's health care design challenges. *Biomedical Instrumentation and Technology, 32*(5), 535–540.

Moore, J. S., & Garg, A. (1995). The strain index: A proposed method to analyze jobs for risk of distal upper extremity disorder. *American Industrial Hygiene Journal, 56*, 443–456.

Moyers, P. A. (1999). The guide to occupational therapy practice. *American Journal of Occupational Therapy, 53*(3), 247–322

Neistadt, M. E. (1994a). Perceptual retraining for adults with diffuse brain injury. *American Journal of Occupational Therapy, 48*, 225–233.

Neistadt, M. E. (1994b). The effects of different treatment activities on functional fine motor coordination in adults with brain injury. *American Journal of Occupational Therapy, 48*, 877–882.

Nelson, D. L. (1988). Occupation: Form and performance. *American Journal of Occupational Therapy, 42*, 633–641.

Pelland, L, & McKinley, P. (2001). The Montreal rehabilitation performance profile: A task-analysis approach to quantify stair descent performance in children with intellectual disability. *Archives of Physical Medicine and Rehabilitation, 82*, 1106–1114.

Pheasant, S. (1998). *Bodyspace: Anthropometry, ergonomics, and the design of work* (2nd ed.). London: Taylor & Francis.

Poole, J. (2000). Habits in women with chronic disease: A pilot study. *Occupational Therapy Journal of Research, 20*(Suppl. 1), 112S–118S.

Rapport, M. (2001). Bridging theory and practice: Conceptual understanding of treatments for children with attention deficit hyperactivity disorder (ADHD), obsessive-compulsive disorder (OCD), autism, and depression. *Journal of Clinical Child Psychology, 30*(1), 3–7.

Raschko, B. B. (1991). *Housing interiors for the disabled and elderly*. New York: Von Nostrand Reinhold.

Reed, K. L. (2000). *Quick reference to occupational therapy* (2nd ed.). Gaithersburg, MD: Aspen.

Reich, J. W. (2000). Routinization as a factor in the coping and the mental health of women with fibromyalgia. *Occupational Therapy Journal of Research, 20*(Suppl. 1), 41S–51S.

Rice, V. (Ed.). (1998). *Ergonomics in health care and rehabilitation*. Boston: Butterworth-Heinemann.

Rogers, J. C. (1982). The spirit of independence: The evolution of a philosophy. *American Journal of Occupational Therapy, 36*, 709–715.

Rogers, J. C. (1986). Occupational therapy assessment for older adults with depression: Asking the right questions. *Physical and Occupational Therapy in Geriatrics, 5*, 13–33.

Rogers, J. C. (2000). Habits: Do we practice what we preach? *Occupational Therapy Journal of Research, 20*(Suppl. 1), 119S–122S.

Rogers, J. C., & Holm, M. B. (1989). The therapist's thinking behind functional assessment, I. In C. Royeen (Ed.). *Assessment of function: An action guide* (pp. 1–29). Rockville, MD: American Occupational Therapy Association.

Rogers, J. C., & Holm, M. B. (1991a). Task performance of older adults and low assistive technology devices. *International Journal of Technology and Aging, 4*, 93–106.

Rogers, J. C., & Holm, M. B. (1991b). Teaching older adults with depression. *Topics in Geriatric Rehabilitation, 6*(3), 27–44.

Rogers, J. C., & Holm, M. B. (2000). Daily-living skills and habits of older women with depression. *Occupational Therapy Journal of Research, 20*(Suppl. 1), 68S–85S.

Rogers, J. C., Holm, M. B., & Stone, R. G. (1997). Evaluation of daily living tasks: The home care advantage. *American Journal of Occupational Therapy, 51*, 410–422.

Rogers, J. C., Holm, M. B., Burgio, L. D., Granieri, E., Hsu, C., Hardin, J. M., & McDowell, B. J. (1999). Improving morning care routines of nursing home residents with dementia. *Journal of the American Geriatrics Society, 47*, 1049–1057.

Rogers, J. C., Holm, M. B., Burgio, L. D., Hsu, C., Hardin, J. M., & McDowell, B. (2000). Excess disability during morning care in nursing home residents with dementia. *International Psychogeriatrics, 12*, 267–282.

Rosenberg, B., Barbeau, E., Moure-Eraso, R., & Levenstein, C. (2001). The work environment impact assessment: A methodologic framework for evaluating health-based interventions. *American Journal of Industrial Medicine, 39*, 218–226.

Schaafstal, A., Schraagen, J., & van Berlo. (2000). Cognitive task analysis and innovation of training: The case of structured troubleshooting. *Human Factors, 42*(1), 75–86.

Schkade, J. K., & Schultz, S. (1992). Occupational adaptation: Toward a holistic approach for contemporary practice, part 1. *American Journal of Occupational Therapy, 46*, 829–837.

Schultz, S. & Schkade, J. K. (1992). Occupational adaptation: Toward a holistic approach for contemporary practice, part 2. *American Journal of Occupational Therapy, 46*, 917–925.

Seki, K., Ishiai, S., Koyama, Y., & Sato, S. (1999). Unassociated responses to two related task demands: A negative factor for improvement of unilateral spatial neglect. *Neuropsychologia, 37*(1), 75–82.

Slagle, E. C. (1922). Training aides for mental patients. *Archives of Occupational Therapy, 1*, 11–17.

Stamps, A. E. (2000). Evaluating architectural design review. *Perceptual & Motor Skills, 90*, 265–271.

Steptoe, A., Cropley, M., & Joekes, K. (2000). Task demands and the pressures of everyday life: Associations between cardiovascular reactivity and work blood pressure and heart rate. *Health Psychology, 19*(1), 46–54.

Stewart, D. L., & Abeln, S. H. (1993). *Documenting functional outcomes in physical therapy*. St. Louis: Mosby.

Strong, S., Rigby, P., Stewart, D., Law, M., Letts, L., & Cooper, B. (1999). Application of the person-environment-occupation model. *Canadian Journal of Occupational Therapy, 66*(3), 122–133.

Trombly, C. (1993). Anticipating the future: Assessment of occupational function. *American Journal of Occupational Therapy, 47*, 253–257.

Trombly, C. (1995). Occupation: Purposefulness and meaningfulness as therapeutic mechanisms. [Eleanor Clarke Slagle Lecture]. *American Journal of Occupational Therapy, 49*, 960–972.

Trombly, C., & Wu, C. (1999). Effect of rehabilitation tasks on organization of movement after stroke. *American Journal of Occupational Therapy, 53*, 333–344.

van Heugten, D., Dekker, J., Deelman, B., van Dijk, A., Stehmann-Saris, J., & Kinebanian, A. (1998). Outcome of strategy training in stroke patients with apraxia: A phase II study. *Clinical Rehabilitation, 12*, 294–303.

Verbrugge, L. M. (1990). The iceberg of disability. In S. M. Stahl (Ed.). *The legacy of longevity: Health and health care in later life* (pp. 55–75). Newbury Park, CA: Sage.

Walker, B. Jr., Goodwin, N., & Warren, R. C. (1995). Environmental health and African Americans: Challenges and opportunities. *Journal of the National Medical Association, 87*(2), 123–129.

Wood, W. (1996). Legitimizing occupational therapy's knowledge. *American Journal of Occupational Therapy, 50*, 626–634.

Woodward, A., Hales, S., Litidamu, N., Phillips, D., & Martin, J. (2000). Protecting human health in a changing world: The role of social and economic development. *Bulletin of the World Health Organization, 78*, 1148–1155.

World Health Organization [WHO]. (2001). *International classification of functioning, disability and health (ICF)*. Geneva: Author.

Yakobina, Y., Yakobina, S., & Tallant, B. K. (1997). I came, I thought, I conquered: Cognitive behavior approach applied in occupational therapy for the treatment of depressed (dysthymic) females. *Occupational Therapy in Mental Health, 13*(4), 59–73.

Yu, F., Hwang, S., & Huang, Y. (1999). Task analysis for industrial work process from aspects of human reliability and system safety. *Risk Analysis, 19*, 401–415.

CHAPTER 28

INTERVENTIONS FOR DAILY LIVING

SECTION I: Interventions for Activities of Daily Living
SECTION II: Home Management
SECTION III: Sexuality and Disability
SECTION IV: Childrearing and Care Giving

SECTION I

Interventions for Activities of Daily Living

MARGO B. HOLM
JOAN C. ROGERS
ANNE BIRGE JAMES

The occupational therapy practitioner and the client must carefully craft an intervention that meets the individual needs and goals of the client (Corring & Cook, 1999; Sumsion & Smyth, 2000; Wilkins, Pollock, Rochon, & Law, 2001). The specific intervention strategies available to the occupational therapy practitioner are endless, and many of these are described in detail in subsequent chapters.

Before selecting intervention strategies, however, the practitioner must determine the appropriate intervention approach for each client. Several approaches are available to select from, and they may be used singly or in combination. Because of the complexity of human behavior, the employment of standardized (i.e., nonindividualized) intervention strategies will likely fail to meet the needs of most clients. Similar to the ubiquitous "one size fits all" garment, which may be donned by all but fits no one well, standardized intervention strategies may make intervention planning easier and faster for the occupational therapy practitioner, but this may be at the expense of the client, whose potential may not be realized. In a health-care era in which occupational therapy practitioners must meet high demands for productivity, it is easy to fall into intervention planning ruts. These ruts may be caused by adopting standardized protocols or by using the same intervention strategies with all clients, because they have worked well in the past and the practitioner is efficient and comfortable in using them.

This section is designed to assist practitioners in planning client-centered interventions for deficits in activities of daily living (ADL) and hence to prevent them from falling into planning ruts.

The section is divided into two major subsections. In the first, the parameters used to describe and measure activity performance (introduced in Chapter 24, Section 1) are revisited and discussed in relation to establishing target intervention outcomes. Target intervention outcomes are a necessary prerequisite to planning an intervention because, as the old adage says, "If you don't know where you are going, you will not know how to get there or when you have arrived." In the second subsection, three approaches to treating ADL limitations—namely, restoration, compensation, and education—are presented. Under each of these approaches, strategies for promoting independent, safe, and adequate task performance are outlined.

PARAMETERS USED FOR ESTABLISHING TARGET INTERVENTION OUTCOMES

The critical first step in planning an intervention is establishing reasonable, attainable, functional outcomes, or goals that are to be achieved through occupational therapy. This requires analysis of the evaluation profile in conjunction with additional factors influencing outcome, namely, the client's ability to learn, the client's prognosis, the time allocated for intervention, the client's discharge disposition, and the client's ability to follow through with new routines or techniques. Synthesizing this vast amount of information into a meaningful, individualized intervention plan is a complex cognitive task and can be overwhelming for the student or new occupational therapy practitioner. A closer look at the implications of interventions, focused on the multiple factors influencing outcomes, may help guide novice practitioners in clinical reasoning and structure the problem-solving process for more experienced practitioners, especially when they are managing particularly complex or challenging clients.

The Influence of Task Parameters on Intervention Planning

In Chapter 24, Section 1, the evaluation of ADL and instrumental activities of daily living (IADL) was described relative to four parameters: **value** of the activity to the client, level of **independence** in performing the task, **safety** of activity performance, and **adequacy** of activity performance. Adequacy of task performance involved **difficulty, pain, fatigue** and dyspnea, **duration** (efficiency), **societal standards, satisfaction, experience, resources,** and **aberrant task behaviors.** A comprehensive evaluation addresses all these parameters, and each parameter is viewed from the perspective of the known or anticipated performance environment before decisions regarding outcomes and intervention strategies are finalized.

Value

Identification of a client's social role restrictions and the activities that comprise those roles is an essential component of the occupational therapy evaluation and should be the first consideration in establishing outcomes. Evaluation using a top-down approach (Fisher, 1998; Trombly, 1995a) begins with the identification of the client's social role participation, including the relative value each role has in the client's life, the roles that are most restricted, and the client's priorities for resuming those roles after discharge (Clark, 1993; Neistadt, 1995; Pollock, et al., 1990; Trombly, 1995a). Because the specific activities and tasks that make up a role vary considerably from person to person, these must also be identified by clients (Canadian Association of Occupational Therapists, 1991). For example, two young men with similar spinal cord injuries may both identify being the father of a young son as a significant life role. However, activities that define the role of father may be different for each of them. For one father, coaching Little League, hiking, and camping are essential activities, whereas for the other father, teaching computer skills and going to the science museum assume priority. The intervention strategies for these two fathers need to be quite different if each is to successfully return to his role of father.

The value clients place on a given activity influences the motivation for participation in any intervention aimed at improving performance for that activity. Because many occupational therapy interventions require the acquisition of new skills through practice, motivation can greatly influence the ultimate functional outcome. Clients who put little value on the activity being addressed during an intervention are unlikely to follow through with the home program necessary for improving skill in that activity.

Whenever possible, occupational therapy practitioners should work within the values defined by their clients. This requires a collaborative approach between the client and the occupational therapy practitioner as the details of the intervention plan are established (Cipriani et al., 2000; McAndrew, McDermott, Vitzakovich, Warunek, & Holm, 2000). Priorities for activities to be included in an intervention must be established by the client under the guidance of the practitioner, who needs to elicit sufficient data about a client's values and preferences to devise an individualized plan. One life role commonly omitted by clients is the self-care role. The role of self-carer—typically developed by the age of 6—becomes so habituated by adulthood that adults often neglect to mention it as a valued role. Self-care is highly valued by most adults, because of the dependency on others that accompanies role dysfunction (Robinson-Smith, Johnston, & Allen, 2000). However, people with severe activity limitations may need to or want to accept assistance from others in ADL, so that they can conserve energy to perform other activities.

This is the situation with Mr. Fritz, a 32-year-old with a recently sustained spinal cord injury, resulting in C6 quadriplegia. He is married with three small children and is self-employed as a tax accountant. His wife works part-time as a nurse and takes care of their children before and after school. The family depends on Mr. Fritz's income, and he has no disability insurance coverage. Although outcomes in ADL are initially established for Mr. Fritz, it soon becomes apparent that attempts at self-care retraining are being met with resistance and frustration. Further discussion of the targeted intervention outcomes reveal that Mr. Fritz is anxious to return to work and that he can do this if he can use the computer in his home office. Although he expresses an interest in becoming independent in self-care, he feels that the best option for him is to return to work as quickly as possible to minimize the financial burden on his family from his current inability to work. His wife is able and willing to help him with self-care tasks when he returns home. The couple feels that self-care retraining can be delayed until the family business is again operational. With intervention outcomes refocused on activities most valued by Mr. Fritz—namely computer access and home mobility—he becomes highly motivated to participate in therapy.

Some clients may identify reasonable intervention outcomes, but establish priorities that make the intervention process inefficient and potentially ineffective (Cipriani et al., 2000). Particularly when dealing with severe disorders of sudden onset (e.g., stroke, traumatic injury), self-care training often helps clients develop capacities and problem-solving skills that can later be applied to activities that are more complex than self-care. For example, suppose Mr. Fritz needs to drive to get to work, an ultimately realistic goal for his injury. Different intervention priorities are established. Initiating intervention with driver training is impractical, because he lacks the prerequisite functional mobility skills. Functional mobility skills must be developed to an adequate level before driver training can begin. ADL training—involving bathing, dressing, transferring, and wheelchair mobility—facilitates the development of functional mobility skills. Such training, therefore, logically precedes driver training. In this situation, having someone assist Mr. Fritz with financial planning and educating him about the commonalities among the skills needed for both self-care and driving, may best meet his needs. This plan recognizes his valued roles and progresses him to the desired outcome in the most efficient way possible.

When the most valued activities and roles are beyond the potential skill level of clients, the occupational therapy practitioner helps clients refocus their priorities so that the intervention plan is realistic and outcomes are achievable. If Mr. Fritz were the owner–cook of a small restaurant, for example, it is unlikely that he would meet the essential job requirements of a short-order cook, even if the kitchen were adapted for wheelchair accessibility and use, because activities must be done quickly. It is possible, however, that he could perform the activities of restaurant owner. For example, he could manage personnel, handle the finances, operate the cash register, and seat customers. In this and similar situations, occupational therapy practitioners assist clients in establishing realistic outcomes for intervention by using their expertise in activity analysis and functional adaptation (Liddle & McKenna, 2000).

Independence

The parameter most commonly focused on in occupational therapy interventions is independence in activity performance. The targeted outcome is generally to increase the level of independence (Croser, Garrett, Seeger, & Davies, 2001; Evans, Small, & Ling, 1995; Ford, Haug, Stange, Gaines, Noekler, & Jones, 2000; Healy & Rigby, 1999; Nyland, Quigley, Huang, Lloyd, Harrow, & Nelson, 2000; Rogers & Holm, 2000). This may be accomplished in various ways, including changing activity materials (e.g., using pullover instead of button-down garments), teaching adapted techniques (e.g., dressing an impaired extremity before a nonimpaired one), and prescribing assistive technology (e.g., providing a shoehorn with an extended handle). The occupational therapy practitioner may also structure activity performance so that progressively less human assistance is given as recovery of function occurs. For example, as muscle strength increases, the amount of physical assistance provided by the practitioner is decreased. Alternately, rather than changing the amount of assistance, the type of human assistance may change, with less powerful assists replacing more powerful ones. For example, as muscle strength increases verbal cuing may replace physical assistance.

Activity performance may be divided into three phases: initiation of a task, continuation of a task, and completion of a task. Initiation is an aspect of activity performance that is frequently overlooked when intervention outcomes are established, in part, because it is difficult to evaluate and treat. The very presence of the occupational therapy practitioner may be a cue to initiate a task and certainly a greeting, such as, "Good morning Mrs. Smith, today we will work on dressing," serves as a prompt for action. Adults are typically expected to initiate self-care and home management activities independently. Expectations for children also exist, depending on the children's ages and skills and the division of task responsibilities among family members. Impairments in activity initiation may occur as a result of many diseases and disorders, such as dementia, depression, schizophrenia, brain injury from trauma or stroke, multiple sclerosis, and Parkinson disease.

Family members generally find it frustrating to have to cue (constantly nag) a client with an initiation impairment for each aspect of a daily routine. In addition, lack of initiation severely limits a client's ability to find and retain employment, engage in leisure, and participate in meaningful social roles and relationships. Training in the use of memory aids, such as memory notebooks, checklists, cue cards, and electronic cuing devices may be viable for these clients (Knoke, Taylor, & Saint-Cyr, 1998; Parenté & Herrman, 1996; Schwartz, 1995; Thompson, 1998).

Perceived self-efficacy—that is, clients' beliefs about their ability to perform activities—influences both the initiation and performance of self-care activities (Gage, Noh, Polatajko, & Kaspar, 1994; Holm, Rogers, & Kwoh, 1998; Robinson-Smith et al., 2000). Clients may overestimate or underestimate their skill level. The primary concern with clients who overestimate their skill level is safety (addressed later). Those who underestimate their skill level may impose activity limitations on themselves even though they have the capacity to be safe, independent, and adequate in performing an activity.

For example, Mrs. Jasper slipped on the ice last winter and fractured her left hip. Surgery was required to stabilize the fracture, but she recovered quickly and returned to her home, where she lives alone. Before her fall, she was independent in shopping, which she did in a small grocery store one block from her home. The physical therapy discharge summary from home health care indicated that Mrs. Jasper could ambulate independently without a walking aid on a variety of indoor and outdoor walking surfaces. She was advised to use a cane if it made her feel more secure. However, since her accident, Mrs. Jasper has had a persistent fear of falling and believes that she cannot walk safely outdoors. Hence, she continues to be dependent in shopping, relying on her daughter to shop for her. In this case, an activity limitation in shopping is caused by a perceived incapacity to walk safely outdoors, not by actual walking skills. This client is unlikely to meet the otherwise realistic intervention outcome of independence in shopping unless the intervention includes strategies to alleviate her fear of falling and her perceived incompetence.

Caregiver training may be implemented to maximize a client's functional outcome while minimizing the efforts of the caregiver (Bogardus, et al., 2001; Hepburn, Tornatore, Center, & Ostwald, 2001; Miller & Butin, 2000). For example, Mr. Ford sustained a left cerebrovascular accident (CVA) and required minimal physical assistance with verbal cuing from the occupational therapy practitioner for wheelchair transfers. Mrs. Ford was physically able to help her husband but had no prior experience in transferring a person with hemiparesis. One day, she decided to help her husband move from his hospital bed to the chair. Because she did not block his right knee or tell him to wait for her cue before standing, they both fell onto the bed while attempting to execute the transfer. Fortunately, no one was hurt. As a consequence of this experience, Mrs. Ford was convinced she could not care for her husband at home. At the same time, she was distressed by the thought of having to admit him to a long-term care facility. She was receptive to receiving transfer training from the occupational therapy practitioner and was delighted to find that by using the proper physical and verbal techniques, she could easily and safely assist her husband. In this case example, caregiver training increased the client's level of independence and the probability that he could go home at discharge.

Safety

During the occupational therapy evaluation, it is recommended that two parameters of activity performance—safety and independence—be rated separately to ensure that deficits in safety are clearly identified. Because safety is a quality of the person–task–environment transaction, however, it cannot be observed or treated in isolation from independence (Anemaet & Moffa-Trotter, 1999; Letts, Scott, Burtney, Marshall, & McKean, 1998; Unsworth, 1999). Although the intervention outcomes of safety and independence are inextricably linked, it is often advisable to list them as separate outcomes because clients can be independent but not safe. A comparison of two clients with T4 paraplegia, secondary to spinal cord injury, who are learning independent transfers illustrates this point.

Ted and Ryan were both recently injured and are learning sitting balance and mobility skills. Ted demonstrates good judgment and a realistic perception of his skills. He has learned to transfer safely by following certain guidelines (e.g., position wheelchair at a 45° angle to the bed; secure brakes on wheelchair; ascertain that bed height is level with the wheelchair); he follows these guidelines consistently and hence is allowed to do bed–chair transfers independently. Ryan's spinal cord injury is similar to Ted's, but he also incurred a mild brain injury. Although Ryan's motor skills are comparable to Ted's, Ryan has difficulty recalling the guidelines for transfers. Hence he is not considered independent in transfers, because his performance is inconsistent; and when he fails to implement the guidelines, he places himself at risk for falling out of his wheelchair. Both Ted and Ryan have the motor capacity to perform transfers independently; however, Ted consistently performs them safely, whereas Ryan does not meet this criterion. Ryan continues to require supervision and occasional verbal cuing for safety. Ryan's intervention outcomes may need to be adjusted to reflect realistically his capacity for safe as well as independent transfers.

Although occupational therapy practitioners agree that safety is an intervention priority, there is less consensus about specific activity behaviors that are safe or unsafe. A wide range of behaviors fall into a questionable zone, in which activities may be rated as safe by some and unsafe by others. For example, few people would disagree that it is unsafe to drive on an urban interstate at 110 miles per hour (mph), even when traffic is light and road conditions are excellent. With a posted speed limit of 65 mph, however, most would agree that driving 70 mph is still within the safety margin. So, what speed would mark the transition from safe to unsafe? Ask 10 people and you would probably get 10 different answers. Occupational therapy practitioners must frequently address questions of safe and unsafe behaviors. The attitudes of clients, caregivers, and families may be helpful in determining the level of risk that is viewed as acceptable.

When determining acceptable risk, it is useful to consider clients' comfort level with risk, their ability to analyze the risks associated with a particular activity and devise a plan for managing them, and, most important, their ability to implement the plan expeditiously despite impairments. For example, rock climbing has obvious inherent risks, but the skilled mountaineer knows how to analyze situations to minimize the potential for accidents and has a repertoire of rescue and emergency skills that facilitate a safe outcome, even when things go wrong. Novices who opt to climb without this bag of tricks may find themselves in difficulty. Occupational therapy clients have varying abilities to adapt to situations that have inherent risks or present unexpected hazards. At times, the level of independence in activity performance may need to be sacrificed for safety. A person who is independent in ambulation but has delayed and impaired balance reactions may need to restrict walking to smooth, level walking surfaces. This restriction may significantly limit independence in community mobility. The inability to adapt to unexpected events (e.g., regain balance after being bumped) makes it necessary to limit independence to maximize safety.

Analysis of a client's risk orientation can provide valuable insight into the tendency to engage in risky behaviors before disability. Many clients find themselves in need of occupational therapy services because of risky behaviors: for example, a client with traumatic brain injury from a motor vehicle accident that occurred while driving under the influence of drugs or alcohol, a client with AIDS who reports having multiple sexual partners without protection; and a teenager with multiple fractures and skin abrasions who rode a skateboard through rush-hour traffic in downtown Manhattan. Intervention goals aimed at identifying the potential risks inherent to specific behaviors and the consequences of risky behavior may be appropriate to establish for these clients.

Clients who tend to overestimate their abilities may present occupational therapy practitioners with challenging safety issues. Activities that were previously performed by clients may continue to be perceived as doable, despite newly acquired limitations that make such activities unsafe. The nature of the activity itself and the consequences of limited capacity in performing the activity are important considerations. Activities that require mobility, including walking and transferring, are common examples of activities that may be unsafe when attempted by those with insufficient skill. A likely consequence of the skill deficit in this instance is a fall. For other activities, skill deficit may lead to unsuccessful performance but present no hazard to clients or others. For example, activity limitations in eating may result in soiled clothing, but clients are unlikely to injure themselves attempting this activity, unless the food is quite hot or swallowing is impaired.

The activity performance environment must also be taken into account when considering safety. Clients with reasonable judgment may be forced to engage in risky behavior if the performance environment does not accommodate alterations in activity performance to ensure safety (Cummings et al., 1999). For example, Mrs. Ethridge has rheumatoid arthritis and requires a walker for safe ambulation since her recent hospitalization for a medication reaction. She is discharged to her home where she lives alone. When she returns home, she discovers that her walker does not fit into her bathroom. Thus she has to walk the length of the bathtub to get to the toilet, holding onto the shower curtain to help maintain her balance. Although she recognizes that this is unsafe, she sees no other options.

Intervention for limitations in safe activity performance is often aimed at adapting the activity or the environment so that performance can be improved as soon as possible. (Close et al., 1999; Cummings et al., 1999). In contrast, improvement in independence can occur over time, as long as adequate assistance is available. Education for clients and their caregivers should be a component of intervention for safety, because clients relearn familiar activities with reduced levels of capacity and often within new and unfamiliar performance environments.

Adequacy

Several aspects of activity performance contribute to the adequacy or quality of the action or outcome. Most standardized assessment tools do not include measures of adequacy, although these parameters may be instrumental in motivating clients to follow through with activities. This may be particularly important for clients who are independent and safe with their performance but who feel dissatisfied with the process or the outcome. Without measurement of these qualitative deficits and the establishment of outcomes that include adequacy parameters, the justification for funding additional intervention is lacking. Nine adequacy parameters are discussed: difficulty, pain, fatigue and dyspnea, duration, societal standards, satisfaction, experience, resources, and aberrant task behaviors. Some of these parameters may be interdependent within a single client. For instance, pain may lead to changes in duration of activity performance (e.g., takes longer) as well as the ability to meet normative standards and personal satisfaction.

Difficulty

The perceived ease with which a client completes an activity and the projected difficulty that will remain after intervention are important to incorporate into intervention outcomes (Fried, Herdman, Kuhn, Rubin, & Turano, 1991; Thornsson & Grimby, 2001; Verbrugge, 1990). The occupational therapy practitioner, who is skilled in activity analysis and has knowledge of pathology and impairment, must determine the prognosis for functional difficulty. This prognosis must then be communicated to clients so that decisions about acceptable levels of difficulty can be made collaboratively. Clients set intervention priorities, in part, by weighing the projected level of difficulty within the context of value—that is, how much difficulty they are willing to tolerate to be independent in an activity?

For example, Mrs. Hernandez lives alone in an apartment in a retirement community. Her sister and brother-in-law also reside in the community, and she has many close friends there. She has had multiple sclerosis for many years, with some weakness and spasticity, but she remained independent in her ADL until a recent exacerbation, which required hospitalization. An increase in lower extremity spasticity and decrease in strength resulted in the need for physical assistance with ADL and the need for a wheelchair for mobility. Strength, endurance, and balance may improve somewhat over time; however, it is anticipated that she will need a wheelchair indefinitely. The retirement community requires Mrs. Hernandez to be independent in ADL and able to prepare breakfast and a light evening snack. A hot meal is provided at midday. The occupational therapy practitioner explained to Mrs. Hernandez that, although independence in ADL is a reasonable goal, completing her ADL will likely be time-consuming and may leave her little energy for other activities. Mrs. Hernandez is enthusiastic about beginning therapy, indicating that she is willing to face the difficulty associated with these activities because independence will enable her to remain in the retirement community with family and friends.

A different scenario plays out with Mrs. McKay, who also has multiple sclerosis. Similar to Mrs. Hernandez, she has had a recent exacerbation that caused a functional decline and a poor prognosis for independent functioning. Mrs. McKay works full-time as a programmer for a local radio station and is the mother of two young children. Mrs. McKay perceives her role as a self-carer to be important, along with those of worker and mother. However, when it became apparent that independence in ADL would significantly interfere with her ability to perform her work and parenting roles, she opted to hire a personal care attendant.

The frequency with which an activity is performed should also be considered when establishing intervention outcomes that reflect the level of difficulty. In general, for activities that need to be done routinely, a higher level of proficiency or ease of performance is needed, whereas for activities that are done only occasionally, a lower level of proficiency or ease of performance may be acceptable. However, the risk associated with a lower performance standard also needs to be taken into account.

For example, Mr. James has a spinal cord injury resulting in C8 quadriplegia. He has a neurogenic bladder and requires intermittent catheterization. He identified self-catheterization as a critical task for fulfilling his roles as self-carer and worker, because he is away from home for 9 hr daily. The occupational therapy practitioner is working with Mr. James and the nursing staff to adapt this task so he can complete it accurately and efficiently. Repetition is a critical intervention strategy, as is completing the activity in the performance environment—a bed and a wheelchair. Another client, Mr. Frank, also has a C8 quadriplegia from spinal cord injury. He can typically get adequate emptying of his bladder without self-catheterization and wears a condom catheter. On rare occasions, however, Mr. Frank has episodes of urinary retention, requiring catheterization within about 1 hr of experiencing symptoms. Mr. Frank lives alone and works at home. He works with the occupational therapy practitioner and nursing staff to learn self-catheterization. The activity is tedious for him and must be done in bed. The process he uses is safe and clean, and the outcome—bladder emptying—is met. Although the activity remains extremely difficult for him, his skill level is adequate for meeting his needs, because he does not have to catherize himself often.

Pain

Pain, either during or following an activity, can also negatively influence performance, even if the activity is completed independently (Birkholtz & Blair, 2001a, 2001b; Mullersdorf, 2000a, 2000b). The source of pain and the prognosis for it must be carefully considered when establishing outcomes and selecting an intervention approach. Activity modification to minimize or eliminate pain is an obvious first choice for intervention, although the cause of the pain or the nature of the activity may not make this feasible. Clients may use a variety of modalities for pain management, including medication, massage, transcutaneous electrical nerve stimulation (TENS), visual imagery, relaxation techniques, yoga, and chiropractic care (Birkholtz & Blair, 2001a, 2001b; Strong, 1998). The role of the occupational therapy practitioner is to integrate successful pain management modalities with the performance of ADL to minimize pain during activity performance, thereby enhancing the adequacy of performance. Collaboration with each professional(s) who prescribed the pain intervention modalities is essential so that safe and effective follow-through with each modality is maintained. Intervention outcomes must include an index of pain so that intervention remains focused on achieving the projected level of independence while simultaneously reducing the influence of pain.

For clients with certain disorders, pain is a signal to stop or restrict a movement or activity. For example, in people with rheumatoid arthritis who have erosion of the joint capsule, pain may indicate that action is causing further destruction of the bony surfaces and hastening joint deformity. Activity modification is an important intervention strategy with these clients, because intervention aimed only at pain reduction may enable clients to participate in potentially harmful activities. In addition, outcomes must be established that reflect the client's capability to follow through with tasks while respecting pain by altering performance to minimize further impairment (Lorig & Fries, 1990).

Fatigue and Dyspnea

Fatigue, the sensation of tiredness experienced during or following an activity, and dyspnea, difficult or labored breathing, may interfere with activity performance (Breslin, 1992; Fuchs-Climent et al., 2001; Liao & Ferrell, 2000; Robichaud-Ekstrand, 1991). Both fatigue and dyspnea are likely to be exacerbated by activity performance. Activity analysis takes into account the effort required to perform a task and its typical duration. In addition, the client's entire daily routine must be examined so that the energy demands of one activity can be weighed in relation to the client's other activities (Mathiowetz, Matuska, & Murphy, 2001). Assisting clients to examine the physical demands of their preferred activities can help them prioritize activities so that appropriate outcomes can be established. Similar to budgeting money, clients must be encouraged to look at their energy dollars and decide how they wish to spend them. The occupational therapy practitioner contributes to this decision-making process by bringing valuable information about options for activity adaptation that may reduce the energy demands of activities, thereby saving clients' energy for other tasks.

Diagnosis is important to consider when intervention outcomes are formulated relative to fatigue and dyspnea. Overexertion may exacerbate symptoms or even the disease process itself for conditions such as cardiac disease and multiple sclerosis. Prognosis is another important diagnostic consideration, especially when deciding on specific activity adaptations or the advisability of interventions focused on impairments. Clients with chronic obstructive pulmonary disease are likely to become worse; therefore, activity adaptations that accommodate a decline in function are appropriate. With paraplegia secondary to spinal cord injury, however, fatigue from poor endurance is likely a result of having to use and develop the smaller muscles of the upper extremity for wheelchair mobility to compensate for the larger lower extremity muscles previously used for walking. For clients with paraplegia, endurance is likely to improve and interventions should be graded to require increasing endurance to facilitate progress (Gift & Pugh, 1993; McDowell & Newell, 1996; Tack, 1991).

Duration

The length of time required to complete activities is typically thought of as a reflection of efficiency. Although measuring performance time may be a relatively simple activity, interpreting time data in a meaningful way is often difficult. The duration of daily living activities depends highly on the nature of the activity and the task objects people choose to use in performing the activity. It takes longer to prepare dinner than it does to fix a light snack. Most of us spend more time dressing when we are going out to dine in an elegant restaurant than we do we when are going to a fast-food establishment. Thus it is difficult to establish meaningful norms for ADL, and IADL.

Establishing acceptable time frames for specific ADL must be done with clients and their significant others and should be reflected in the functional outcomes. For example, Dan, a 12-year-old with cerebral palsy, is independent in dressing; but dressing takes almost 90 min to complete. He needs to be on the school bus at 7:15 A.M. It is not practical for Dan or his parents to arise at 5:00 A.M. to enable Dan to dress independently. Instead, Dan's parents assist him with dressing on school days. To increase efficiency for some dressing components, Dan is expected to manage his clothing during toileting and for donning and doffing his jacket, because these skills are needed in school. To increase efficiency for the entire activity, however, he is encouraged to dress independently on days he is not going to school. This schedule enables Dan to increase his dressing efficiency in a way that best meets his and his family's needs. By taking into account a client's disease or disorder, functioning, disabilities, and intervention options, the occupational therapy practitioner can offer expertise in functional rehabilitation by predicting a likely outcome for the duration of a specific activity.

When analyzing activity performance that seems too short, safety, independence, and adequacy all come into play. Clients may be at increased risk when they rush through activities. Professional caregivers may limit the independence of activity performance by giving overcare to meet their own productivity requirements (Rogers et al., 1999; Rogers et al., 2000). Clients may also neglect performance standards just to get activities done quickly. Activity performance that seems too long also needs to be evaluated in reference to safety, independence, and adequacy. Clients with swallowing deficits, for example, may need to eat slower than those without such deficits to avoid choking. People with poor fine motor coordination or sensory deficits may need to slow down when using a sharp knife to improve control of the knife and prevent injury. However, slower activity performance is not necessarily safer. Crossing a street, for example, must occur within the time allowed by the traffic light, or safety is compromised.

Societal and cultural standards also need to be taken into consideration when establishing outcomes for activity duration. In the United States, timeliness is highly valued, and efficient performance in community skills is expected. Shoppers generally become irritated when they are standing in a checkout line behind a customer who takes several minutes to identify and count currency. In other countries, this delay may go unnoticed. An American with cognitive or visual impairments that interfere with the ability to count currency may need to decrease the time required for this activity to reduce embarrassment when shopping. The intervention outcome, then, needs to include an efficiency measure to reflect this activity parameter. A client from a culture that measures time in hours, rather than minutes, may believe that intervention focused on increasing speed is unnecessary.

Societal Standards

Performance standards, determined by the society and culture in which the client lives, are likely to exist for outcomes in terms of both the end result and the process through which this is achieved. As discussed in Chapter 24, the line between acceptable and unacceptable performance is likely to be thick rather than narrow, and may vary considerably, depending on characteristics such as age, gender, and cohort (generation) membership.

Societal standards exist, for example, for neatness. A client may dress safely and independently, but if the color of clothing clashes and appearance is disheveled (the end product), the client's dressing may not meet societal standards. If the client is a teenager, this appearance is likely to be considered acceptable. However, if the client is a public relations manager going to work, it is likely to be labeled unacceptable and could well put the client's job in jeopardy. An example of varied societal standards for process is evident in expectations for eating behavior. Stuffing down a hot dog in record time while waiting for a subway is unlikely to draw attention from fellow passengers, as long as the person does not choke, does not spill food on clothing or on others, and disposes of litter properly. Displaying this same process as a bridal attendant seated at the head table at a wedding reception is considered ill-mannered.

Evaluation of societal standards must take into account who established the standards and the environment in which specific performance behaviors are to occur. It is critical to identify the most relevant societal standards for inclusion in intervention outcomes and when planning an intervention, to keep the focus manageable. Whereas consideration of societal standards may seem subjective and difficult, the use of indicators of societal standards is critical for establishing outcomes, justifying interventions, establishing intervention strategies, and documenting changes in performance. From the foregoing example, the intervention outcome may be that, when eating during a social event, Ms. Lee will demonstrate appropriate pacing as evidenced by completing a meal in no less than 15 min, swallowing each bite before putting additional food in her mouth, and conversing between bites of food.

Satisfaction

In addition to societal standards, clients have their own standards of acceptable performance, and these standards also need to be incorporated into functional outcomes (Natterlund & Ahlstrom, 1999). Mr. Bruce, for example, is always losing things. He never seems to know where his wallet and keys are, and he is always searching for something. Nonetheless, items seem to turn up, and he sees no reason to go to the trouble of organizing his apartment better to help him keep track of his belongings. Mr. Johns, however, has always been meticulously neat and could put his hands on items the minute he wanted them. Recently, he sought medical attention for memory problems. He complained that he needed to search for items because he failed to put them in their usual places. He was particularly concerned about his memory problem because of a family history of Alzheimer disease. He was referred to occupational therapy to learn strategies to help him remember where items are placed. Objectively, Mr. Johns is not performing any worse than Mr. Bruce; however, he interprets his performance as impaired, and, furthermore, he is dissatisfied with his performance.

People with acquired impairments may set high standards for satisfaction in the performance of activities that they performed well before incurring impairment. In a study that surveyed the significance of sea kayaking in people with spinal cord injuries, one female participant identified its significance in terms of it being a new skill (Taylor & McGruder, 1996). Because sea kayaking was new to her, she did not have preconceived ideas about how well she should perform. Before her injury, she had been a basketball player. Although she had tried wheelchair basketball, she found it extremely dissatisfying because she could not meet her preinjury standards. Hence, she chose to abandon basketball and exchange it for a new sport, sea kayaking, because of the satisfaction it gave her.

When establishing client satisfaction, it is necessary to elicit this objectively from the client. During the evaluation as well as the intervention, the practitioner should keep questions open ended and focused on clients' feelings about activity performance. When trying to understand the satisfaction or dissatisfaction that clients experience from activities, occupational therapy practitioners should refrain from giving their observations about clients' performance and their projections about the extent to which performance might be improved through training.

Experience

Information gathered in the evaluation regarding a client's past and recent experience with an activity is important to consider so that relevant and attainable outcomes are established and effective intervention strategies for attaining them are identified. Recent experience may facilitate progress in reestablishing independence in an activity because the client is learning a new way to do the activity rather than developing a new skill. For example, Mrs. McCarthy needs to relearn cooking skills following a CVA. She uses a wheelchair for mobility and has minimal use of her right, dominant, hand. Her cognitive skills are intact, and she can easily follow a recipe. Furthermore, she demonstrates good problem-solving skills in adapting cooking activities to improve her performance. Like Mrs. McCarthy, Miranda, a 12-year-old with spastic hemiplegia secondary to cerebral palsy, has limited use of one hand and uses a wheelchair for mobility. She wants to cook simple meals and bake cookies. Her intervention is likely to require more time and guidance than Mrs. McCarthy's intervention, because she has to learn basic cooking skills along with the activity adaptations required to compensate for her impairments.

At times, adults are also confronted with needing to learn new activities. Some of these activities relate to skills needed to manage impairments, such as performing self-catheterization, donning pressure garments, or learning to operate an environmental control unit. New learning may also be needed when new roles are assumed; for example, when a spouse becomes disabled or dies and the partner has to take on new responsibilities. Whenever a skill is unfamiliar to clients, additional intervention time and education from the occupational therapy practitioner may be needed for basic skill acquisition.

Resources

Established functional outcomes must be achievable within the client's available resources, including social and financial (Seigley, 1998). The social environment is particularly salient to consider when human assistance is needed for the performance of essential ADL. Some families may be able to provide the level and type of assistance needed, whereas other families may be unable or unwilling to do this. When activity adaptations or assistive devices are beneficial, the client's ability to pay for them must be appraised. Some activity adaptations and assistive devices are expensive and may not be covered by the client's insurance carrier. If the client does not have the financial resources to pay for needed items, interventions and outcomes may need to be appropriately adjusted.

Aberrant Task Behaviors

Functional outcomes and interventions must address any aberrant task behaviors that interfere with activity performance (Rogers et al., 2000). Criterion-referenced measures are often the easiest to use when aberrant task behaviors are a problem, because they can include criteria that require the reduction or elimination of the anomalous behaviors if outcomes are to be reached. Intervention strategies to eliminate such behaviors vary greatly, depending on the nature of the target behavior. Behavior modification techniques may be useful for aberrant behaviors under volitional control, like stuffing food into the mouth. Unwanted movements, such as athetoid movements, are typically involuntary and modification of the environment through proper seating and positioning may be required for their reduction or elimination. Exploration of the underlying cause of the aberrant task behavior facilitates the establishment of realistic outcomes and the selection of effective intervention strategies.

Client's Capacity for Learning

The client's capacity for learning must be evaluated, because intervention often requires learning new methods of completing activities (Fuhrer & Keith, 1998). Fewer intervention options exist for clients with limited learning capacity, and the duration of the intervention may need to be longer. Clients with a good capacity for learning and an openness to alternative methods may be able to address more task deficits because of increased intervention options and the reduced time required for learning. It is important to view capacity for learning on a continuum because clients may fall between the extremes, and capacity may be better for some tasks than for others. A client may be capable of learning the relatively simple task adaptation of using a joy stick to drive a wheelchair but be unable to master a more complex environmental control system, even one that relies on the same movements used to control the joy stick.

Prognosis for Impairments

The client's potential for improvement of body function and structure impairments must be examined within the context of any existing disease or disorder and resulting impairments (Hansen & Atchison, 1993; Ostchega, Harris, Hirsch, Parsons, & Kington, 2000). First, the practitioner must consider any precautions or contraindications pursuant to the diagnosis that may preclude the use of certain intervention strategies. Compare, for example, two clients whose endurance significantly limits their performance. Mr. Bell has multiple sclerosis, a disorder that may worsen if he becomes overfatigued. An aggressive program to increase endurance is contraindicated for him, so alternative intervention strategies should be explored. Mr. Jones, who sustained multiple injuries in a motor vehicle accident, has had several surgeries and has been primarily confined to bed for 7 weeks. Although his medical problems have been resolved, he is deconditioned. A program to extend the limits of his endurance may be an efficient way to increase endurance, thereby enhancing performance of functional activities.

Second, the prognosis for improvement of impairments, given the client's diagnosis (i.e., disease, disorder, or condition), must be considered. Increasing impairment is expected in progressive disorders, such as Alzheimer disease, amyotrophic lateral sclerosis, and rheumatoid arthritis. Hence, intervention outcomes must be established with these potential declines in mind, so that they are realistic. Occupational therapy practitioners must evaluate each impairment separately, however, because progressive diseases may not affect all bodily structures and functions directly. This point is illustrated by Jonathan, a teenager who has muscular dystrophy. He has significant muscle weakness in the trunk and all four extremities and has developed some limitations in pelvic and ankle range of motion (ROM) that preclude maintaining an optimal position for functioning from his wheelchair. His muscle strength is expected to decline, even with intervention. His ROM restrictions, however, are secondary to the muscle weakness, not a direct result of the muscular dystrophy. Intervention gains can be expected in ROM, despite the overall prognosis. In turn, increased ROM can enhance function by increasing the options available for functional positioning in his wheelchair.

Stable or diminishing impairments may be anticipated in many disorders and after injury. Pharmacological intervention, for example, may improve the impairments associated with depression, so that occupational therapy intervention can be focused on transferring gains made in mental and psychological capacities into performance. Typically, clients who have had CVAs can expect some spontaneous return of motor function in the early stages of recovery. Projected intervention outcomes take into account the typical improvements for this diagnosis.

Time for Intervention

The projected timeline for occupational therapy may be influenced by multiple factors, including the functional prognosis, the client's motivation for improvement, and the client's finances. In managed health care, it is becoming common for health insurance carriers to set the number of visits or length of stay (DeJong & Sutton, 1995; Kramer et al., 2000). To a considerable extent, the occupational therapy intervention program must be tailored to meet the client's needs as much as possible within the time allotted. Nonetheless, it must also be recognized that best practice takes into account all the client's needs. Often, with clear and complete documentation of adequate progress toward established outcomes, additional occupational therapy visits can be approved by third-party payers. Occupational therapy practitioners need to be aware of their professional responsibility to clients to request intervention extensions and to support these requests through detailed documentation.

Expected Performance Environment: Discharge Setting

Clients' expected discharge environments must be considered when establishing outcomes and selecting interventions that are to be relevant to the environment in which clients will ultimately perform tasks (Cox, 1996; Dunn, 1993; Dunn, Brown, & McGuigan, 1994; Law et al., 1996). The human environment is critical for clients who require assistance from others after discharge. Clients' needs vary broadly in terms of the type and duration of assistance required. Some clients need only supportive services, such as help with shopping or housecleaning. Those with significant activity limitations and intact cognition may require considerable physical assistance, but can be left alone once ADL are completed, they have eaten, and they are mobile in their wheelchairs. Clients with cognitive impairments do not always need physical assistance but may need verbal cuing to maintain activity performance, and this assistance may need to be constant. Inadequate support in the client's expected environment may necessitate a change in the discharge plan.

The physical environment must also be considered in intervention planning (Gill, Williams, Robison, & Tinetti, 1999; Gitlin, Corcoran, Winter, Boyce, & Hauck, 2001; Gitlin, Miller, & Boyce, 1999; Hagedorn, 1995). For example, Mr. Flora has been progressing with his bathing skills during his hospital-based rehabilitation and is now independent with a bath bench, a hand-held shower hose, and a grab bar. The occupational therapy practitioner wants to order this equipment for him. However, Mr. Flora reports that he must shower in a 3 × 3-ft. shower stall because the only bathtub is on the second floor and he cannot manage stairs. This shower will not accommodate the transfer tub bench he requires for safe transfers and balance during showering. An alternative approach to bathing should have been explored at the beginning of intervention so that Mr. Flora's program focused on developing skills he could use at home, such as managing a rolling chair for the shower stall, or sponge bathing at the sink.

The actual adaptability of the discharge environment must also be explored. A house that is high above the street with 21 steps to the front door makes the installation of a properly graded ramp extremely difficult. Wall grab bars cannot be installed on fiberglass tub surrounds, making a safety rail placed on the side of the bathtub the only feasible option, regardless of where the client really needs the most support. Clients living in rental units may be unable to make structural alterations as desired because they do not own the unit.

Last, the client's expected discharge environments must be explored if activities are likely to be performed in more than one place. Clients in a hospital-based setting may be primarily focused on returning home, but most people do not confine themselves to a single environment. Hence, at some point, intervention must address performance of tasks across environments. Adaptations for toilets, such as raised toilet seats and toilet armrests, are commonly used for people with limited mobility. Home adaptations are easily made, but clients may often be in environments that have not been adapted, such as public buildings, friends' homes, airplanes, hotels, and portable toilets at the local fair. If clients are likely to be in these environments, their intervention plan must incorporate these varied environmental features if independence is to be enhanced.

Projected Follow-Through with Home Program

Efforts to contain health-care costs have led to increasingly shorter lengths of stay in hospitals and rehabilitation centers and a reduction in outpatient and home-health visits. Clients are expected to take a more active role in their therapy programs and to supplement formal interventions with self-directed intervention (e.g., home programs). Intervention outcomes, therefore, need to be established with some estimate of the client's capacity to follow through with a self-directed program, as this will greatly influence the success of any intervention (Cope & Sundance, 1995).

Several of the activity parameters previously delineated can give the occupational therapy practitioner guidance in this area. Clients have more motivation for programs aimed at activities that they highly value than those they do not value, making a client-centered approach critical for success. In addition, activity parameters such as difficulty, fatigue, pain, and satisfaction must be graded so that self-directed programs are manageable within the context of the client's daily routines. *Manageable* must be established by clients in consultation with the occupational therapy practitioner and should take into consideration clients' daily activities and responsibilities, tolerance for frustration, and perseverance.

Many clients require some assistance to practice activities, and the occupational therapy practitioner must be sure that these resources are available. This assistance may include setting up an activity, providing assistance for specific activity steps, and allowing ample time (as prescribed) for effective practice. It is important to remember that many impairments affect the ability to initiate or persevere with everyday activities. For these clients, assistance is needed for initiation and follow-through in the home program. This responsibility often falls on family members and occupational therapy practitioners need to interact with and educate family members about their critical role (DaCunha & Tackenberg, 1989).

INTERVENTION IMPLEMENTATION

The selection of specific intervention strategies is guided in large part by the frame(s) of reference selected by the occupational therapy practitioner for each client. Specific frames of reference are beyond the scope of this chapter, but can be found in Unit VI. The following subsection focuses on broader intervention approaches and their related strategies. It includes a discussion of grading activities to progress clients to the established outcomes and concludes with outlines of intervention strategies for several prototypical activity limitations.

Selection of an Intervention Approach

Intervention approaches for limitations in activity performance fall into three broad categories: compensation, restoration, and education. Frames of reference tend to focus on either compensation or restoration. The rehabilitation frame of reference relies on compensatory techniques to accommodate or compensate for impairments that hinder task performance and is a compensatory approach. The biomechanical and sensory integrative frames of reference are restoration approaches because they focus on restoring capacities that are impaired, with the assumption that gains made in a person's generic capacities will be transferred into everyday tasks. However, both the compensatory and restorative approaches need to be combined with an educational approach to ensure carryover of the program to functional activities (Trombly, 1995b).

Compensation

Activity performance can be enhanced through **compensation** for activity limitations, rather than restoration of previous capacities. This is often necessary when restoration is not an option; at this time in history, a client with a complete C5 quadriplegia will not regain previous hand function, regardless of the restorative approach used. Compensation for impairments is needed. Even in clients for whom restoration is possible, a compensatory approach may be more appropriate if time limitations or client motivation would lead to less than optimal outcomes. Compensatory strategies may also be warranted when some but not full restoration of function is achieved. Generally, compensatory strategies require less intervention time for achieving functional outcomes compared with restorative strategies.

Three intervention strategies may be employed under the compensatory approach. The activity or task method may be altered, the task objects may be adapted, or the environment may be modified (Tables 28-1 to 28-9). Combinations of these methods may be used to maximize client performance.

Alter the Task Method

When the task method is altered, the same task objects are used in the same environment, but the method of performing the task is altered to make the task feasible given the client's impairments. Many one-handed techniques for tasks that are normally done with two hands use this strategy, including one-handed dressing, one-handed shoe tying (Fig. 28-1), and one-handed typing techniques. To master an altered task method successfully, clients require the capacity to learn. The level of learning capacity necessary depends on the complexity of the method that is to be learned. Practice is a necessary component of learning, so good follow-through with a training program is needed to meet adequacy parameters, such as difficulty, satisfaction, and duration. Lengthy practice is required if the desired outcome is habituation of the skill for routine performance.

Adapt the Task Objects or Prescribe Assistive Devices

The objects used for the task may be altered to facilitate performance; for example, handles can be built up on utensils for clients with decreased finger ROM. For many tasks, adaptation of the task objects does not significantly alter the task method, so the need for learning is less than when the method is altered. When this is the case, the need for practice is reduced. Examples of simple adaptations include utensils with enlarged or extended handles, a cutting board with nails to stabilize food while cutting, and elastic shoelaces.

The prescription of assistive devices must simultaneously take into account the client's capabilities and the features of the device. With the proliferation of assistive

(text continues on page 507)

TABLE 28-1. **INTERVENTION STRATEGIES FOR ACTIVITY LIMITATIONS ASSOCIATED WITH VISUAL IMPAIRMENT**[a]

Baseline Status	*Potential Approaches and Strategies for Intervention*					*Outcome Status*
	Compensation Approach					
Activity Limitations Identified during Evaluation	**Alter Task Method**	**Adapt Task Objects; Use Assistive Devices**	**Modify Environment**	**Restoration Approach (Restore/Establish)**	**Education Approach**	**Target Outcomes at Discharge**
Grooming, Oral Hygiene, Bathing, Showering						
Client may walk into open drawers, and doors left ajar Client may have difficulty with sharp objects (razors, fingernail scissors) Client may have difficulty locating or discerning among bathing, grooming, and oral hygiene task objects Client may have difficulty applying makeup accurately, and shaving evenly Client may neglect aspects of task performance not in visual field (one side, peripheral visual field) Client may experience fatigue and decreased endurance during task performance Task outcomes may not meet acceptable societal standards Client may express dissatisfaction with task outcomes Client may initially demonstrate aberrant task behaviors (spray deodorant on hair)	Always close drawers and leave doors fully closed or open Rely on tactile cues in addition, or in lieu of visual cues Store task objects in same place Adhere to routines and patterns that make these tasks more efficient Use only level of assistance that is needed; do not remove client's right to participate in task if it is not harmful Do not rush task Simplify hair style Use electric razor Grow beard Simplify makeup Use clippers	Replace overhead incandescent lights with fluorescent lights Label like containers with large black letters or with tactile labels (raised print letters, braille, or special glue dots) Use pump-action containers of different shapes for soap, toothpaste, and shampoo Use plastic tape in a color that contrasts with countertop to mark small items (clippers) Float bright object in tub to see water height Use soap-on-a-rope	Increase amount of light available (overhead fluorescent lights; incandescent or halogen task lights close to task) Decrease glare with amber tint on overhead light fixtures or by installing a dimmer switch in bathroom Keep task materials in same place on counter and keep materials for like tasks together (in caddy) Install tap water overflow alarm Mount magnifying mirror on wall with an extension arm Reset water temperature to <120°F Install wall-to-wall or indoor/outdoor carpeting in bathroom to prevent slipping on spills that cannot be seen	Sensory training to enhance tactile sensibility Establish routines Develop memory aids (two rubber bands means container holds shampoo) Train client to scan through total range (one-sided neglect) Train client to use peripheral vision Recommend evaluation by low-vision specialist	Instruct family members about necessity of closing drawers, fully opening or closing doors, and returning task objects to a designated place Demonstrate restorative and adaptive strategies (sample marking systems for memory aids) and have client do a return demonstration Provide a handout or other resources with drawings or pictures of strategies (suggested lighting), directions, and a number to call for assistance Provide video of suggested strategies with client as subject if possible and practitioner as caregiver if appropriate	Increased level of independence Improved safety Improved adequacy of performance: Decreased difficulty Decreased fatigue Increased endurance Increased approximation to societal standards Increased satisfaction Decreased aberrant behavior

			Install grab bars around tub or shower Place contrasting bath mat over tub edge to increase its visibility Use nonskid mat of contrasting color so foot placement is accurate			
Toileting						
Client may walk into open drawers and doors left ajar Client may have difficulty positioning self onto toilet seat Client may have difficulty determining if cleansing is adequate after bowel movement Task outcomes may not meet acceptable societal standards (fecal matter on cuff of sleeve after cleansing) Client may initially demonstrate aberrant behavior (inadequate cleansing of hands after toileting)	Replenish supplies on routine basis Use toilet paper, moistened wipes, and then toilet paper to ensure adequate cleansing	Use color contrasting tissue	Provide storage space for toilet paper and moistened wipes within arm's reach while seated on toilet Use color contrasting toilet seat Use toilet seat frame with arms if client also has difficulty raising or lowering self or has balance problems	Sensory training	Instruct family members about necessity of closing drawers, fully opening or closing doors, and returning task objects to designated place Provide handout with enlarged drawings or pictures of technique or adaptations, sequential directions, and number to call for assistance Provide audiotape with suggestions, including phone numbers and item numbers for vendors (toilet frame with arms)	Increased level of independence Improved safety Improved adequacy of performance: Decreased difficulty Increased approximation to societal standards Decreased aberrant behavior

Continues

TABLE 28–1. **INTERVENTION STRATEGIES FOR ACTIVITY LIMITATIONS ASSOCIATED WITH VISUAL IMPAIRMENT[a]** *(Continued)*

Baseline Status	***Potential Approaches and Strategies for Intervention***					***Outcome Status***
	Compensation Approach					
Activity Limitations Identified during Evaluation	**Alter Task Method**	**Adapt Task Objects; Use Assistive Devices**	**Modify Environment**	**Restoration Approach (Restore/Establish)**	**Education Approach**	**Target Outcomes at Discharge**
Dressing						
Client may have difficulty selecting clothing that matches Client may walk into open drawers and doors left ajar Client may experience fatigue and decreased endurance during task performance Task outcomes may not meet acceptable societal standards (client may not see stains on front of clothing) Client may express dissatisfaction with task outcomes (client may have difficulty differentiating like outfits of different colors) Client may initially demonstrate aberrant task behaviors (not notice necktie is label side out)	Hang matching outfits on the same hanger or on adjacent hangers with clothespins to connect them Ask another person to spot-check clothing for stains on a routine basis	Keep upper body clothing buttoned except at neck (easier one-step over-head donning and keeps items on hangers) Use washable textile puff paints to put color system, dots, or letters on clothing items	Have client arrange drawers, closets, and cupboards based on logical system for client Install automatic, or pull-chain wall lights inside closets and cupboards in position that casts few shadows and little glare	Sensory training Establish routines Develop behavioral memory aids Recommend evaluation by low-vision specialist	Instruct family members about necessity of closing drawers, fully opening or closing doors, and returning task objects to designated place Help client decide on memory aid system that will work to distinguish among like clothing items Provide audiotape with suggestions, organization strategies, and memory aids, including number to call for assistance	Increased level of independence Improved safety Improved adequacy of performance: Decreased difficulty Decreased fatigue Increased endurance Increased approximation to societal standards Increased satisfaction Decreased aberrant behavior
Feeding and Eating						
Client may not know what is on plate if someone else served food Task outcomes may not meet acceptable societal standards (client	Place food groups in same place on plate consistently Use systematic approach to arrangement and	Use "clock" method to identify where food is located Use contrasting dinnerware if food is	Set table consistently, with glasses, cups, and other spillable items always located in same place	Sensory training Develop behavioral memory aids	Demonstrate restorative/adaptive strategies (clock method); have client or caregiver	Increased level of independence Improved safety Improved adequacy of performance:

may bump and spill items when reaching) Client may initially demonstrate aberrant task behaviors (spoon sugar onto table instead of in coffee cup)	placement of food and tableware	primarily light or dark in color Use small separate dishes for food items			do return demonstration Provide handout with enlarged drawings or pictures of technique (suggested position of tableware to avoid bumping, spilling), adaptations, sequential directions, and number to call for assistance Provide audiotape of suggested adaptations	Decreased difficulty Increased approximation to societal standards Decreased aberrant behavior
Medication Management						
Client may not be able to see directions on medication container Client may have difficulty determining time for taking medication Client may have difficulty telling pills apart if they are spilled or out of container Client may demonstrate unsafe aberrant task behaviors (distribute wrong medication into organizer)	Organize medications so that they are always in same place (alphabetical order) Organize medicine cabinet so other health supplies and over-the-counter medications are always in same place Use medication syringe for liquids instead of spoon for both client and caregiver administration	Have pharmacist put only non-childproof lids on pill bottles Use medication organizer for daily medications; fill organizer on first or last day of month Use Daytime™ appointment alarm to signal medication schedule (can set up to 31 alarms per day) Label pill bottle with a black marker and a single large letter for easy identification (*P* for Prozac™)	Place medications out in logical place where they are easy to retrieve at time they are to be taken (kitchen counter, bedside table) if client is responsible for medication management	Sensory training Develop behavioral memory aids	Demonstrate medication management routines and have client or caregiver do return demonstration Provide audiotape with adaptive strategies	Increased level of independence Improved safety Improved adequacy to performance: Decreased difficulty Decreased aberrant behavior

Continues

TABLE 28–1. **INTERVENTION STRATEGIES FOR ACTIVITY LIMITATIONS ASSOCIATED WITH VISUAL IMPAIRMENT**[a] *(Continued)*

Baseline Status	***Potential Approaches and Strategies for Intervention***					***Outcome Status***
	Compensation Approach					
Activity Limitations Identified during Evaluation	**Alter Task Method**	**Adapt Task Objects; Use Assistive Devices**	**Modify Environment**	**Restoration Approach (Restore/Establish)**	**Education Approach**	**Target Outcomes at Discharge**
Functional Mobility						
Client may walk into open drawers, and doors left ajar Client may be unsafe when ambulating (unable to avoid clutter left in traffic areas or on stairs) Client may be unsafe at top and bottom of stairs Client may experience fatigue and decreased endurance Client may be unable to find way around home or community Client may express dissatisfaction with task performance Client may demonstrate aberrant and unsafe behaviors (bump into things, hesitant gait, walk into wrong room, walk in wrong direction, become disoriented)	Have client wear sturdy, low, and broad-heeled shoes if gait is unsteady Have client walk next to and slightly behind caregiver, holding onto caregiver's elbow (especially in community or on uneven ground) Have caregiver accompany client until way finding is mastered	Use cane holder to keep cane near and easy to locate Use tape of contrasting color to make cane easy to locate	Stabilize furniture near natural traffic routes that can be used as tactile guide Remove low coffee tables Repair walking surfaces so they are even and remove tripping hazards Provide lighted pathway from bedroom to bathroom (night light) so client does not need to turn on/off bright light and wait for eyes to accommodate Make stairways safe: Sturdy handrails on both sides Uniform stair height and tread widths Clearly discernable tread edges Top and bottom landings marked with different color or surface Add lighting to area at top and bottom of stairways	Sensory training Develop behavioral memory aids Recommend evaluation by mobility specialist	Instruct family members about necessity of closing drawers, fully opening or closing doors, returning furniture to designated place, and keeping traffic areas free of clutter Provide catalog with relevant assistive devices marked Provide handout with enlarged drawings or pictures of technique or adaptations (stair safety guidelines) and a number to call for assistance Provide audiotape of suggested adaptations	Increased level of independence Improved safety Improved adequacy to performance: Decreased difficulty Decreased fatigue Increased endurance Increased approximation to societal standards Increased satisfaction Decreased aberrant behavior

[a]*Impairment:* low vision, absence of vision, or visual-perceptual deficit. *Common diseases/disorders:* macular degeneration, glaucoma, cataracts, diabetic retinopathy, corneal disease, retinitis pigmentosa, stroke, trauma, or congenital blindness.

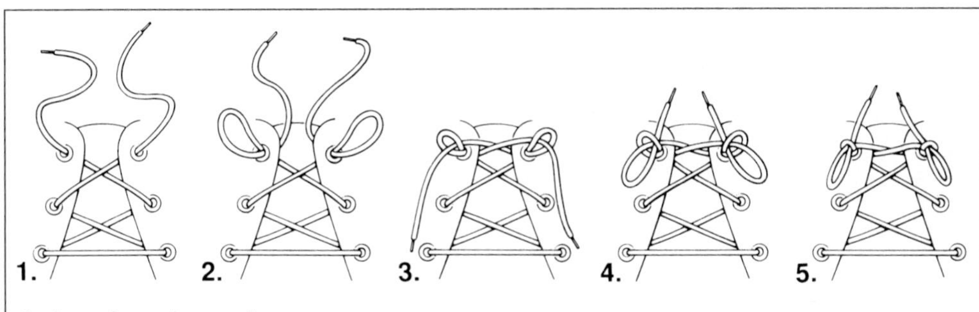

1. Lace laces in usual way.
2. Put both lace ends back through the holes they exited until the loops formed are small.
3. Put the lace ends through the opposite loops and pull to tighten loops, allowing just enough room to put the lace end back through the loop.
4. Put lace ends back through the loops, forming another loop.
5. Pull on these loops alternately to tighten.

FIGURE 28–1. One-handed shoe-tying method. (Reprinted with permission from Davis, 1977.)

devices, however, there has not always been accompanying information about the features of the device, including weight of the model and exact dimensions (Rogers & Holm, 1991). The prescription of an assistive device is frequently oversimplified. Figure 28-2 emphasizes the complexity of the decision-making process by highlighting potential decisions involved in prescribing an adapted spoon. Although many assistive devices prescribed by occupational therapy practitioners are quite simple mechanically, some are sophisticated and include complex electronics, circuits, and microprocessors, such as environmental control units that interact with smart houses.

Just as the prescription of assistive devices seems deceptively simple, so do task adaptations. Some task adaptations, however, significantly alter task performance and require considerable learning on the part of clients. For example, a system of Morse code may be used with a sip-and-puff switch for typing on a computer. However, such an adaptation requires that the client have good cognitive skills and considerable patience to practice and master this adaptation efficiently.

One disadvantage of adapting task objects is if the adaptive equipment must be available to clients whenever and wherever they engage in the task. This may or may not pose a problem, depending on the task and the adaptation. Clients who use a memory book at work to compensate for cognitive impairments may incorporate the structure and cues needed into a daily planner or a handheld personal data assistant—a strategy that was used before the impairment. If a client requires built-up utensils for eating, however, and wishes to eat at a restaurant, the utensils must be taken along. This is cumbersome, and some clients find it embarrassing.

Finally, some clients find that the use of adaptive equipment reduces satisfaction with task performance. To enhance personal satisfaction with task performance, they may be willing to cope with the increased difficulty of doing a task without adapted tools. For example, a female client with multiple sclerosis found that her mobility was safer and easier in a wheelchair, but she preferred to walk when out in the community. Her dissatisfaction with the wheelchair overrode other considerations.

Modify the Task Environment

Modification of the environment itself may be used to facilitate task performance (Dunn et al., 1994). Typically, when the environment is modified, the demand for learning and practice is less than that required for learning an alternative method or using adapted task objects. Environmental modifications are often fixed in place so clients do not need to remember to bring along the necessary adaptations and the adaptations cannot be easily displaced (e.g., they cannot be dropped out of reach). Usually, the task method is unchanged, or only minimally changed, so that clients can rely on previous experience. Examples include installing a wheelchair ramp, installing grab bars and a floor-to-ceiling pole in the bathroom (Fig. 28-3), recessing plumbing under the sink to accommodate a wheelchair user, increasing available light, removing cupboard doors for easy access, and installing a toilet seat frame.

The biggest drawback of environmental modifications is that clients may become limited in terms of performance context. They must do the task in the modified environment or in one that has been similarly modified, because the modifications are not easily transportable and may be custom designed for a specific setting.

Restoration

A **restoration** approach typically focuses intervention at the impairment level with the aim of restoring or establishing

(text continues on page 515)

TABLE 28-2. **INTERVENTION STRATEGIES FOR ACTIVITY LIMITATIONS ASSOCIATED WITH UNILATERAL IMPAIRMENTS**[a]

Baseline Status	*Potential Approaches and Strategies for Intervention*					*Outcome Status*
	Compensation Approach					
Activity Limitations Identified during Evaluation	**Alter Task Method**	**Adapt Task Objects; Use Assistive Devices**	**Modify Environment**	**Restoration Approach (Restore/Establish)**	**Education Approach**	**Target Outcomes at Discharge**
Grooming, Oral Hygiene, Bathing, Showering						
Client may be unable to reach, hold, manipulate, adjust, open or close task objects that require use of both hands or bilateral coordination, thus preventing task initiation, continuation or completion Client may be unable to sustain grooming or oral hygiene actions long enough to complete tasks adequately (decreased endurance) Task performance may be unsafe (tub transfers, use of straight-edge razor with nondominant hand) Client may experience pain, fatigue, or lack of satisfaction with task performance Task outcomes may not meet acceptable societal standards	Use unaffected extremity to assist or compensate for affected or missing extremity Use affected extremity to stabilize objects, unaffected extremity to manipulate objects Use mouth to stabilize or open containers Stabilize task objects on nonskid surfaces or on towels Stabilize task objects between knees Rest elbow of affected extremity on counter edge so unaffected hand is free to apply deodorant, shave armpit Use electric razor Simplify hairstyle Use beauty salon Grow beard	Use pump-action containers for soap, toothpaste, and shampoo Use suction devices to hold soap in place Use suction brushes for nails and dentures Use soap-on-a-rope or place soap into an old nylon and secure it to shower head or faucet Stabilize fingernail clipper to board and extend lever arm of clipper for easier use with one hand Use fliptop lipsticks Use mirror that can be hung around neck	Clear shelf or counter so that all items for each task can be stored on counter or shelf in basket (handle over forearm) or plastic container that can be transported to task site with one hand Remove cupboard door for easier access Make space for stool or chair near counter so that surfaces (counter, lap) can be used Mount hairdryer on wall so that it does not have to be held Install mirror with extension arm on wall Install grab bars around tub/shower area for safety and stability when entering and exiting or turning Install bath bench that extends over tub edge for safer transfers	PROM Active assistive, active, or resistive exercises for strengthening Continuous passive motion Inhibitory or tacilitatory treatment Motor learning Transfer of dominance training Splinting Casting Desensitization program Sensory reeducation Prosthetic training	Demonstrate restorative strategies (self-ranging, PROM by caregiver before grooming, bathing); have client or caregiver do return demonstration Demonstrate adapted methods; have client or caregiver do return demonstration Demonstrate proper use of adapted task objects; have client or caregiver do return demonstration Provide handout with drawings or pictures of strategies or adaptations, sequential directions, and number to call for assistance Provide video of suggested strategies with client as subject if possible and practitioner as caregiver if appropriate	Increased level of independence Improved safety Improved adequacy of performance: Decreased difficulty Decreased pain Decreased fatigue Increased endurance Increased approximation to societal standards Increased satisfaction Decreased aberrant behavior

			Install shower caddy for holding items Install hand-held flexible shower hose with on/off switch that can be controlled at shower head			
Toileting						
Client may be unable to lower self, raise self, or transfer onto toilet safely Client may have difficulty doffing and donning clothing associated with toileting Client may be unstable (unsafe) when reaching for toilet paper or reaching to cleanse Client may have difficulty manipulating toilet paper roll or separating paper from roll Client may experience pain or fatigue during task performance	Use unaffected upper extremity to assist or compensate for affected or missing extremity Use extra-wide base of support to prevent slacks, underpants from dropping to floor Position head against wall to maintain balance while pulling up clothing with one hand Wrap end of toilet paper stream around dispenser edge or nearby towel rack to make it easier to rip off paper Maintain extra broad base of support while seated on toilet to prevent imbalance or falls while reaching for toilet paper or cleansing self	Substitute free-standing toilet roll holder that positions roll vertically or put tissue in basket next to toilet Use reacher to get clothes up from floor Attach suspender to slacks on affected side to bring lower body clothing up while coming to stand and while securing fasteners Use slacks with elastic in waistband or with hook closures for easier manipulation with one hand	Install grab bars for raising and lowering from toilet if stability is problem Install floor-to-ceiling pole for transfer; lean into it while adjusting clothing with one hand Install waist-high bar to lean into while doffing and donning clothing Install commode at bedside for night use Place urinal next to bed for night use	Postural stability Weight-shifting exercises Balance exercises Transfer of dominance training Motor learning PROM Active assistive, active, or resistive exercises for strengthening Inhibitory or facilitatory treatment Motor learning Prosthetic training	Demonstrate restorative strategies (weight shifting, balance); have client or caregiver do return demonstration Demonstrate adapted methods (positioning and repositioning wheelchair by toilet); have client or caregiver do return demonstration Demonstrate proper use of adapted task objects and assistive devices; have client or caregiver do return demonstration Provide handout with drawings or pictures of technique or adaptations, sequential directions, and number to call for assistance Provide catalog with relevant assistive devices Provide video of suggested strategies with client as subject if possible and practitioner as caregiver if appropriate	Increased level of independence Improved safety Improved adequacy of performance: Decreased difficulty Decreased pain Decreased fatigue Increased endurance Increased approximation to societal standards Increased satisfaction Decreased aberrant behavior

Continues

TABLE 28–2. **INTERVENTION STRATEGIES FOR ACTIVITY LIMITATIONS ASSOCIATED WITH UNILATERAL IMPAIRMENTS**[a] *(Continued)*

Baseline Status	*Potential Approaches and Strategies for Intervention*					*Outcome Status*
	Compensation Approach					
Activity Limitations Identified during Evaluation	**Alter Task Method**	**Adapt Task Objects; Use Assistive Devices**	**Modify Environment**	**Restoration Approach (Restore/Establish)**	**Education Approach**	**Target Outcomes at Discharge**
Dressing						
Client may be unsafe during task performance (unable to simultaneously maintain balance and reach or manipulate task items) Client may have difficulty donning and doffing clothing items on unaffected side Client may be unstable when reaching to don or doff lower body clothing items Client may have difficulty manipulating and securing fasteners Client may be unable to tie laces on shoes Client may experience pain or fatigue during task performance Client may express lack of satisfaction with results of task performance or time necessary to complete task performance Task outcomes may not meet acceptable societal standards (fasteners not secured)	Use unaffected upper extremity to assist or compensate for affected or missing extremity Don and doff clothing using methods suggested in Tables 28-3 to 28-5 Sit on bed with pillows on either side for added stability when dressing Lie on bed to don lower body garments and bridge using unaffected lower extremity to pull up garments Lie on bed to don lower body garments and roll from side to side while pulling up Use extra-wide base of support to prevent slacks, underpants from dropping to floor while donning in a standing position	Keep upper body clothing buttoned except at the neck, for easier over-head donning Use elastic on buttoned cuffs to allow hands to move through easily Use button hook with suction at end for buttons on sleeve on unaffected side Trap button hook in drawer or between knees for stability while using it to button sleeve on unaffected side Use reacher to get clothes up from the floor or to pull on pant loops Attach suspender to slacks on affected side to bring lower body clothing up while coming to stand and while securing fasteners Use slacks with elastic in waistband or with hook closures for easier manipulation	Place stable chair with arms near bed to use for dressing Install floor-to-ceiling pole by bed for transfer, and to lean into while adjusting clothing with one hand	PROM Active assistive, active, or resistive exercises for strengthening Continuous passive motion Inhibitory or facilitatory treatment Motor learning Transfer of dominance training Splinting Casting Desensitization program Sensory reeducation Prosthetic training	Demonstrate restorative techniques (weight shifting exercises); have client or caregiver do return demonstration Demonstrate adapted dressing methods; have client or caregiver do return demonstration Demonstrate proper use of adapted task objects and assistive devices; have client or caregiver do return demonstration Provide handout with drawings or pictures of technique (one-handed shoe tying method) or adaptations, sequential directions, and number to call for assistance Provide catalog with relevant assistive devices	Increased level of independence Improved safety Improved adequacy of performance: Decreased difficulty Decreased pain Decreased fatigue Increased endurance Increased approximation to societal standards Increased satisfaction Decreased aberrant behavior

Client may demonstrate aberrant task behaviors (tries to dress only unaffected side)	Position head against wall, if unsteady when standing, to achieve stability while pulling up clothing with one hand Use one-handed shoe tying method	Use clothing items that stretch (knits) and elastic shoelaces or shoes with hook and loop closure			Provide video of suggested strategies with client as subject if possible and practitioner as caregiver if appropriate	
Feeding and Eating						
Client may have difficulty swallowing liquids and solids Client may aspirate liquids and solids Client may have difficulty cutting food Client may have difficulty scooping up food Client may experience pain, fatigue, and inadequate endurance to complete task performance Task performance may not meet societal standards (client may drool) Client may express lack of satisfaction with task performance (food does not taste good, takes too much effort to eat) Client may initially demonstrate aberrant task behaviors (food may accumulate in cheek of affected side)	Position client with chin slightly tucked, trunk aligned and upright, hips flexed, and feet supported Use unaffected upper extremity to assist or compensate for affected or missing extremity Support affected extremity Have caregiver cut food Prepare food of optimal consistency (thickened; cold versus room temperature; ground beef versus steak)	Add Thickit™ or similar thickening agent to liquids Change food consistency so that bolus is easily formed Provide straw for liquids to enable easy handling in upright position Use Knifork with unaffected side Use rocker knife Use plate guard, soup bowl, or plate with raised edge to enable easier scooping Place nonslip placemat under plate to prevent plate from moving or consider dishes with nonslip surfaces underneath Provide lap board for wheelchair Consider suspension sling for affected extremity to remove effect of gravity	Provide stable chair that accommodates positioning devices Adjust table height to accommodate wheelchair	Oral motor stimulation Recommend swallowing evaluation Fine motor dexterity exercises for nondominant hand Transfer of dominance training Motor learning Sensory reeducation Prosthetic training	Demonstrate restorative techniques (stimulation of tongue); have client or caregiver do return demonstration Demonstrate feeding methods; have client or caregiver do return demonstration (to ensure that caregiver is not using "bird" feeding technique) Demonstrate proper use of adapted task objects and assistive devices; have client or caregiver do return demonstration Provide handout with drawings or pictures of technique (suggested position of tableware to avoid bumping, spilling), adaptations, sequential directions, and number to call for assistance Provide catalog with relevant assistive devices marked	Increased level of independence Improved safety Improved adequacy of performance: Decreased difficulty Decreased pain Decreased fatigue Increased endurance Increased approximation to societal standards Increased satisfaction Decreased aberrant behavior

Continues

TABLE 28–2. **INTERVENTION STRATEGIES FOR ACTIVITY LIMITATIONS ASSOCIATED WITH UNILATERAL IMPAIRMENTS**[a] *(Continued)*

Baseline Status	***Potential Approaches and Strategies for Intervention***					***Outcome Status***
	Compensation Approach					
Activity Limitations Identified during Evaluation	**Alter Task Method**	**Adapt Task Objects; Use Assistive Devices**	**Modify Environment**	**Restoration Approach (Restore/Establish)**	**Education Approach**	**Target Outcomes at Discharge**
Feeding and Eating (Contd.)						
					Provide video of suggested strategies with client as subject if possible and practitioner as caregiver if appropriate (positioning client who needs to be fed)	
Medication Management						
Client may have difficulty opening pill bottles, removing lids from liquid medication containers, and removing pills from medication organizer compartments Client may have difficulty opening medication patch packaging and separating patch from protective liner Client may have difficulty pouring liquid medication into spoon without spilling Client may express dissatisfaction with task performance (time needed to complete task; number of errors made)	Use unaffected extremity to assist or compensate for affected or missing extremity Stabilize bottles on nonskid surfaces or between knees to open lids Use medication syringe for liquids instead of spoon Sort medications into nut cups that can be easily picked up and emptied	Have pharmacist put only non-childproof lids on pill bottles Put liquid medicine into squeeze bottle and label Use rubber circle to increase resistance on liquid medicine bottles Stabilize liquid medicine bottle between knees and use jar opener Use Daytimer™ appointment alarm to signal medication schedule (can set up to 31 alarms per day)	Place medications out in logical place where they will be constantly noticed and easy to access (kitchen counter) if client is responsible for medication management Install jar opener on wall or under cupboard	Fine motor dexterity exercises for nondominant hand Transfer of dominance training Active assistive, active, or resistive exercises for strengthening Inhibitory or facilitatory treatment Motor learning Prosthetic training	Demonstrate one-handed methods for manipulating containers and bottles; have client or caregiver do return demonstration Demonstrate proper use of adapted task objects and assistive devices; have client or caregiver do return demonstration Provide catalog with relevant assistive devices marked	Increased level of independence Improved safety Improved adequacy of performance: Decreased difficulty; Increased approximation to societal standards; Increased satisfaction

Functional Mobility						
Client may be unable to move safely, efficiently or without difficulty or pain during bed mobility/wheelchair transfers (to/from bed, toilet, bathtub bench, easy chair, car) Client may be unable to transfer objects while ambulating Client may be unable to manipulate objects while standing Client may experience pain, fatigue, and inadequate endurance for task performance (transferring in and out of bathtub) Client may experience dissatisfaction with performance (feels unsteady or unsafe) Client may demonstrate aberrant task behaviors (forget to lock knee before beginning to ambulate)	Standing pivot transfer Standing pivot transfer with assistance Bobath transfers	Insert rail on one side of bed so client can use it to pull against when positioning self in bed, lowering into and raising up from bed Attach overhead trapeze bar on bed Use denser foam cushion in wheelchair to raise seat for easier transfers Use portable dense foam cushion to place in easy chairs to make them same height as wheelchair Use plastic garbage sacks on car seats to ease shifting and turning Use wheeled cart to transfer task objects if ambulatory Use walker bag or tray to transfer task objects Use wheelchair bag or lapboard to transfer task objects	Ensure distance from floor to all surfaces for transfers (toilet seat, tub bench, easy chair) is no greater than distance between floor and 2 in. below midpoint of client's patella when client is seated Install grab bars by toilet and in tub area as needed Install floor-to-ceiling pole by bed on client's unaffected side	Postural control exercises Weight-shifting exercises Balance exercises Active assistive, active, or resistive exercises for strengthening Inhibitory or facilitatory treatment Motor learning Transfer of dominance training Prosthetic training	Demonstrate restorative techniques; have client or caregiver do return demonstration Demonstrate proper use of adapted task objects and assistive devices (bed rail); have client or caregiver do return demonstration Provide catalog with relevant assistive devices marked Provide handout with drawings or pictures of technique or adaptation, sequential directions, and number to call for assistance Provide video of suggested strategies with client as subject if possible and practitioner as caregiver if appropriate (use of floor-to-ceiling pole, car transfers)	Increased level of independence Improved safety Improved adequacy of performance: Decreased difficulty Decreased pain Decreased fatigue Increased endurance Increased satisfaction Decreased aberrant behavior

[a]*Impairment:* one upper extremity or one upper extremity and lower extremity (one body side); PROM, AROM, or strength impairment, with or without sensory loss. *Common diseases/disorders:* cerebrovascular accident, traumatic brain injury, unilateral amputation, cerebral palsy (hemiplegia), peripheral nerve injury, tendon laceration.

PROM, passive range of motion.

TABLE 28–3. UPPER BODY DRESSING FOR CLIENTS WITH IMPAIRED UPPER EXTREMITY PROM AND AROM

Method 1
Donning Garment Over Head

1. Place shirt (over head or cardigan) face down on lap, with sleeves and collar near knees.
2. Slide arms through shirt into sleeves and push sleeves over elbows.
3. Gather shirt back and lift over head (may rest elbows on knees or table and bend head down to push through shirt collar).
4. Protract, retract, elevate, and depress shoulders to get shirt over shoulders, or push shirt over one shoulder and then other with opposite upper extremity.
5. Retract shoulder while leaning forward slightly to get shirt down in back.
6. Pull shirt front panels near bottom to straighten and bring down fully (cardigan).
7. Place hands inside shirt front and pull slightly away from body, down and toward sides, to bring shirt down fully (over-head clothing).

Doffing Garment

- Place hand inside over-head shirt toward opposite sleeve, and pull sleeve opening over elbow. Repeat for other sleeve and remove over head.
- Push collar area of cardigan back over shoulders, extend upper extremity, and retract shoulders to help sleeve drop below elbow, pull arm from sleeve. Or push one sleeve off shoulder, reach opposite upper extremity to sleeve hole and hold while elevating shoulder, extending arm and flexing elbow to remove arm from sleeve. Then pull shirt around back to other side with arm still in sleeve and slide arm out.
- Unbutton using hand to stabilize shirt against body and thumb or knuckle to push button through hole while opposite thumb pushes fabric up over bottom.

Method 2 (cardigan)

For patients with good trunk and lower extremity mobility but limited upper extremity strength and or ROM (e.g., upper extremity amputees, burn patients); garment must fit loosely.

1. Place cardigan garment faceup on bed.
2. Place one upper extremity in sleeve, and lie down using friction of shirt against bed to hold garment while sliding arm in.
3. Once one arm is all the way in and collar is up over shoulder, start other arm in sleeve and sit up to work arm into sleeve.

Method 3 (pullover)

For use with over-head clothing.

1. Put head through neck hole first.
2. Place hand in sleeve and push arm all the way into sleeve.

PROM, passive range of motion; *AROM,* active range of motion.

TABLE 28–4. UPPER BODY DRESSING FOR CLIENTS WITH IMPAIRMENT OF A SINGLE UPPER EXTREMITY OR BODY SIDE

Donning Garment
Method 1 (cardigan)

1. Place garment on lap with front up, collar toward knees, and opening for sleeve for affected side exposed between legs.
2. Place affected upper extremity into sleeve, leaning forward to drop into sleeve as far as possible.
3. Pull sleeve up affected arm, at least above elbow.
4. With unaffected hand, grasp collar and sleeve that are to be put on that side.
5. Lift unaffected arm over head, pulling shirt around back.
6. While pulling shirt around back, slip unaffected arm in sleeve, letting shirt fall onto arm, and pushing arm into sleeve as shirt is pulled around.

Method 2 (cardigan)

1. Place garment on lap with front up, collar near thighs, and opening for sleeve for affected side exposed between legs.
2. Place affected upper extremity in sleeve opening, leaning forward to drop it in as far as possible.
3. Pull sleeve up affected arm, at least above elbow, preferably up to axilla.
4. Place unaffected upper extremity in its sleeve.
5. Grasp collar, gather up back material, and lift over head.

Method 3 (pullover)

1. Place shirt collar down on lap, and open bottom of shirt to expose sleeve openings.
2. Place affected upper extremity in its sleeve opening, and pull garment on to above elbow.
3. Place unaffected upper extremity in its sleeve opening.
4. Grasp back collar, gather back fabric with unaffected upper extremity, and lift over head.

Doffing Garment
Cardigan

1. Pull fabric toward unaffected side to make it as loose as possible.
2. Grasp unaffected side of unbuttoned garment, reach back and to the side to get it off shoulder. Then pull it down, and wriggle elbow out of shirt. Or grasp sleeve of unaffected side with that hand, and gradually pull it down until elbow can be worked out of sleeve.
3. Pull fabric to affected side, and remove affected upper extremity.

Pullover

1. Pull fabric toward unaffected side to loosen.
2. Pull bottom of shirt on unaffected side down, squeeze elbow through sleeve hole, and remove unaffected upper extremity from sleeve.
3. Gather fabric, and grasp collar to lift garment over head. Or grasp collar near nape of neck, gather back fabric with hand, and pull back over head.
4. Remove unaffected upper extremity from sleeve.
5. Remove sleeve from affected upper extremity.

TABLE 28–5. LOWER BODY DRESSING FOR CLIENTS WITH IMPAIRMENT OF A SINGLE UPPER EXTREMITY OR BODY SIDE

Donning Pants

1. Sit on bed at side or in chair or wheelchair that allows feet to be firmly positioned on floor. Sitting on bed is preferable if client is unable to stand to pull up pants, because client can lie back down on bed to roll and pull pants over hips.
2. Cross affected leg over unaffected leg.
3. Place garment over foot, and pull up to or over knee, making sure foot is through bottom of leg opening.
4. Replace foot on floor.
5. Hold garment near waist with unaffected upper extremity, and reach down to allow lifting of unaffected lower extremity into opening.
6. Pull garment up over thighs as far as possible while sitting.
7. Use affected upper extremity if possible to hold pants up while coming to stand, or hold pant waist with unaffected hand while using affected upper extremity as support while coming to stand.
8. Stand to pull pants over hips, leaning against wall, bed, or other stable object if necessary.
9. Attach fasteners while standing, because clothing is looser if this can be done safely; if not, wear looser clothing and fasten while sitting.

Doffing Pants

1. Unfasten in seated position.
2. Allow garment to drop from hips while coming to stand.
3. Remove unaffected leg first and then affected leg by letting garment drop to floor and lifting affected leg out while holding garment on floor with unaffected leg or by crossing affected leg over unaffected leg.

Donning Socks and Shoes

1. Put on loose socks by putting unaffected hand in sock opening and spreading fingers to start sock over toes.
2. Place affected foot on a footstool or lift to opposite knee to stabilize it.
3. Once socks are over toes, pull up using unaffected upper extremity.
4. Put shoes on unaffected side without adaptation.
5. Put shoes on affected side by lifting foot to opposite knee or by crossing affected leg over unaffected leg; then, using unaffected upper extremity, place shoe on foot. (For some styles, place shoe on floor and lift affected foot into it; push on affected knee to place heel into shoe.)

Donning Ankle–Foot Orthoses[a]

1. Open the laces wide, and fold tongue back over laces.
2. Lay brace on the floor between feet with shoe directly under knees.
3. Lift affected foot into shoe.
4. Pick up brace by calf band or metal upright, and slide shoe onto foot while moving it into position flat on the floor. Use unaffected foot to prevent heel of affected foot from slipping backward out of shoe.
5. Push on knee of affected leg to slide heel into shoe.

Doffing Ankle–Foot Orthoses[a]

1. Loosen straps and laces.
2. Hold heel of shoe down with unaffected foot while lifting affected heel out; then push on calf band to push shoe off. Or cross affected leg over unaffected leg, and lever shoe off foot by pushing on calf band.

[a]For more methods, see Trombly and Radomski (2002).

the capacities that are needed for functional tasks (Bendix, Bendix, Labriola, Haestrup, & Ebbeh, 2000; Dunn et al., 1994; Trombly, 1995a). Intervention may be used to restore capacities such as strength, endurance, ROM, short-term memory, visual figure-ground, and interests. More information regarding specific techniques may be found in the chapters that follow. Regardless of the specific frame of reference or techniques used, however, one must always establish the link between the impairment and the resulting activity limitations. Careful documentation of the evaluation assists other health professionals and third-party payers to understand the connection between the intervention and the established functional outcomes. Clients must also be educated regarding the relationship between their inherent capacities and the everyday tasks they pursue so that they

(text continues on page 523)

TABLE 28-6. **INTERVENTION STRATEGIES FOR ACTIVITY LIMITATIONS ASSOCIATED WITH UPPER AND LOWER BODY IMPAIRMENTS**[a]

Baseline Status	*Potential Approaches and Strategies for Intervention*					*Outcome Status*
	Compensation Approach					
Activity Limitations Identified during Evaluation	**Alter Task Method**	**Adapt Task Objects; Use Assistive Devices**	**Modify Environment**	**Restoration Approach (Restore/Establish)**	**Education Approach**	**Target Outcomes at Discharge**
Grooming, Oral Hygiene, Bathing, Showering						
Client may be unable to safely initiate, continue, or complete all aspects of task performance (transfers) Client may be unable to reach, hold, manipulate, adjust, lift, open or close task objects, thus preventing task initiation, continuation, or completion Client may be unable to sustain grooming or oral hygiene actions long enough to complete tasks adequately Client may be unable to get into or out of tub/shower Client may be unable to reach all body parts for grooming or bathing Client may experience pain, fatigue, or inadequate endurance necessary for task performance	Use one extremity to assist another Use tenodesis action to pick up small items Use both hands to hold objects Use mouth to stabilize or open containers Stabilize task objects on damp towels Stabilize task objects between knees Rest elbows on counter edge to apply deodorant, shave armpits Use electric razor Simplify hairstyle Use a beauty salon Grow beard Use terry cloth robe as towel	Use splints for wrist stability and functional hand position Use pump-action containers for soap, toothpaste, and shampoo Use adapter for spray deodorant Use nonskid materials to stabilize items (nail file, dentures) Use soap-on-a-rope Stabilize fingernail clipper on board, and extend lever arm Use fliptop lipsticks Use adapted or loop handles, special holders, universal cuffs, or extended handles on brushes, razors, etc. Use electric toothbrush or Waterpik™ Use wash mitt Use sponge with dorsal hand band	Store task items on counter or shelf in a basket (handle over forearm) or plastic container that can be transported to task site easily Remove cupboard door for easier access Make sink area wheelchair accessible (remove cupboard bottom, recess or insulate plumbing) Mount hairdryer on wall Install mirror with extension arm on wall Install single-lever faucets Install grab bars around tub/shower area Install bath bench that extends over tub edge for safer transfers	PROM Continuous passive motion Splinting Casting Prosthetic training Active assistive, active, or resistive exercises for strengthening Inhibitory or facilitatory treatment Motor learning Sensory reeducation	Demonstrate restorative strategies (self-ranging, PROM by caregiver before grooming, bathing); have client or caregiver do return demonstration Demonstrate adapted methods (bathing strategies); have client or caregiver do return demonstration Demonstrate proper use of adapted task objects (deodorant adapter); have client or caregiver do return demonstration Provide handout with drawings or pictures of strategies or adaptations, sequential directions and number to call for assistance Provide video of suggested strategies with client as subject if possible	Increased level of independence Improved safety Improved adequacy of performance: Decreased difficulty Decreased pain Decreased fatigue Increased endurance Increased satisfaction

Client may express dissatisfaction with effort and time necessary to complete task performance		Use long-handled lightweight sponge with loop handle for back, feet Suction long-handled sponge to wall or wedge in grab bars to wash underarms Use long-handled mirror for skin inspection	Install shower caddy for holding items Install hand-held flexible shower hose with on/off switch that can be controlled at shower head Install nonskid surface/mat on tub or shower bottom Use portable shampoo basin		and practitioner as caregiver if appropriate (bathtub transfers)	
Toileting						
Client may not always be able to reach bathroom in time Client may be unable to lower self, raise self, or transfer onto toilet safely Client may have difficulty managing catheter valve Client may have difficulty doffing and donning clothing associated with toileting Client may be unstable or have difficulty when reaching for or manipulating toilet paper roll or separating paper from roll Client may be unstable when reaching to cleanse body parts Client may need assistance with catheterization or bowel program	Maintain extra-broad base of support while seated on toilet to prevent imbalance or falls while reaching for toilet paper, cleansing self, or being cleansed Wrap end of toilet paper stream around dispenser edge or nearby towel rack to make it easier to rip off paper Wrap toilet paper around hand Eliminate underwear Plan ahead for adequate hydration Plan ahead for incontinence emergencies	Substitute free-standing toilet roll holder that positions roll vertically rather than horizontally Put tissue in hanging basket next to toilet Use reacher to get clothes up from floor Use slacks with elastic waistband for easier donning and doffing Use slacks with hook-and-loop tape at leg seams for easy access to catheter and quick removal Wear rings on fingers to create friction on catheter tubes, etc. Use incontinence garment Use long-handled toilet aid or tongs	Install grab bars for raising and lowering from toilet if stability is problem Install elevated toilet seat (client or caregiver should be able to reach under for bowel program) Install toilet frame that can provide security for client with poor trunk control Install bidet Install commode near bed for night use Install urinal near bed for night use	PROM Postural stability Weight-shifting exercises Balance exercises Active assistive, active, or resistive exercises for strengthening Training in self-catheterization, bowel stimulation	Demonstrate restorative strategies (weight shifts) and adaptive strategies (applying condom catheter); have client or caregiver do return demonstration Demonstrate proper use of adapted task objects and assistive devices; have client or care- giver do return demonstration Provide handout with drawings or pictures of the strategies (changing catheter from bed bag to leg bag), adaptations, sequential directions, and number to call for assistance Provide catalog with relevant assistive devices marked	Increased level of independence Improved safety Improved adequacy of performance: Decreased difficulty Decreased pain Decreased fatigue Increased endurance Increased satisfaction

Continues

TABLE 28–6. **INTERVENTION STRATEGIES FOR ACTIVITY LIMITATIONS ASSOCIATED WITH UPPER AND LOWER BODY IMPAIRMENTS**[a] *(Continued)*

Baseline Status	***Potential Approaches and Strategies for Intervention***					***Outcome Status***
	Compensation Approach					
Activity Limitations Identified during Evaluation	**Alter Task Method**	**Adapt Task Objects; Use Assistive Devices**	**Modify Environment**	**Restoration Approach (Restore/Establish)**	**Education Approach**	**Target Outcomes at Discharge**
Toileting (Contd.)						
Client may experience pain, fatigue, or inadequate endurance for task performance Client may express dissatisfaction with effort required and time necessary to complete task performance Client may initially demonstrate aberrant task behaviors (inadequately seal condom catheter)		Use assistive devices for bowel/bladder care Catheter-insertion device Device to prepare and apply external catheter Adapted urinary drainage bag valve Labia spreader Suppository inserter Digital stimulator			Provide video of suggested strategies with client as subject if possible and practitioner as caregiver if appropriate	
Dressing						
Client may be unable or have difficulty lifting clothing items or body parts Client may be unable or have difficulty donning and doffing clothing items Client may be unable to reach all body parts (feet, back) Client may be unstable when reaching to don or doff lower body clothing items	Dress in bed Dress in wheelchair Don and doff clothing using methods suggested in Tables 28-7 and 28-8 Position bed against two walls and wedge self into corner for stability when dressing Place clothing for next day near bed Alter dressing sequence to accommodate donning	Keep upper body clothing buttoned except at neck, for easier over head donning Use elastic on buttoned cuffs to allow hands to move through easily Use clothing items that stretch (knits) Order special clothing designed to meet needs of clients in wheelchairs or with ROM restrictions	Place stable chair with arms near bed, to use for dressing Install trapeze bar or rope ladder to shift body weight and position self Install bed rails Order bed with elevating head Install floor-to-ceiling pole	Postural stability Weight-shifting exercises Balance exercises Fine motor dexterity exercises Train client in use of tenodesis action Prosthetic training	Demonstrate restorative strategies (weight-shifting exercises); have client or caregiver do return demonstration Demonstrate adapted dressing methods (dressing in wheelchair); have client or caregiver do return demonstration Demonstrate proper use of adapted task objects (loops on	Increased level of independence Improved safety Improved adequacy of performance: Decreased difficulty Decreased pain Decreased fatigue Increased endurance Increased satisfaction

Client may have difficulty manipulating and securing fasteners Client may be unable to tie shoelaces Client may not be able to stand or sit unsupported while dressing Client may experience pain, fatigue, or inadequate endurance for task performance Client may express dissatisfaction with effort required and time necessary to complete task performance	and doffing of upper and lower body prosthetics, ankle–foot orthoses, and splints Lick palm for friction when donning socks Wear slip-on shoes (nonambulatory)	Use baggy over foot to decrease friction when donning pants Sew loops on clothing for better grasp Wear rings on fingers for friction when changing catheter tubes, etc. Use assistive devices for dressing Reacher Dressing stick Long shoehorn Clothing ladder Sock aid Zipper pull Hook-and-loop tape closures Button hook Elastic shoelaces Rubber palm for friction Leg lifters Use splints for wrist stability or functional hand position			clothing) and assistive devices (rope ladder); have client or caregiver do return demonstration Provide handout with drawings or pictures of the strategies (plastic bags on socks), sequential directions, and number to call for assistance Provide a catalog with relevant assistive devices marked Provide video of suggested strategies with client as subject if possible and practitioner as caregiver if appropriate (dressing in wheelchair)	
Feeding and Eating						
Client may be unable or have difficulty grasping utensils Client may have difficulty cutting food Client may have difficulty scooping up food and reaching to get food to mouth Client may aspirate liquids or solids Client may be unable or have difficulty grasping finger foods	Position client with chin slightly tucked, trunk aligned and near upright, and feet supported Support extremities Use one extremity to assist others Weave utensil handles through fingers Use tenodesis action to pick up light objects and larger finger foods	Add Thickit™ or similar thickening agent to liquids Place nonslip placemat under plate to prevent plate from moving; consider dishes with nonslip surfaces underneath Use mobile arm supports Use suspension sling or other antigravity device to support	Provide stable chair that accommodates positioning devices Add lapboard to wheelchair Add water bottle setup and straw to wheelchair to encourage hydration	Oral motor stimulation Recommend a swallowing evaluation Training in use of tenodesis action Prosthetic training Active assistive, active, or resistive exercises for strengthening PROM	Demonstrate restorative strategies (tenodesis action); have client or caregiver do return demonstration Demonstrate feeding methods; have client or caregiver do return demonstration (to ensure caregiver is not using "bird" feeding techniques)	Increased level of independence Improved safety Improved adequacy of performance: Decreased difficulty Decreased pain Increased satisfaction

Continues

TABLE 28-6. **INTERVENTION STRATEGIES FOR ACTIVITY LIMITATIONS ASSOCIATED WITH UPPER AND LOWER BODY IMPAIRMENTS**[a] *(Continued)*

Baseline Status	*Potential Approaches and Strategies for Intervention*					*Outcome Status*
	Compensation Approach					
Activity Limitations Identified during Evaluation	**Alter Task Method**	**Adapt Task Objects; Use Assistive Devices**	**Modify Environment**	**Restoration Approach (Restore/Establish)**	**Education Approach**	**Target Outcomes at Discharge**
Feeding and Eating (Contd.)						
Client may be unable to lift drink Client may experience pain, fatigue, or inadequate endurance necessary for task performance Client may express dissatisfaction with effort and time necessary to complete task performance	Use both hands to hold objects Cut finger foods so they can be eaten with utensils	weight of upper arm and enable hand-to-mouth motion Use splints for wrist stability or functional hand position Use universal cuff for utensils if grasp is absent or inadequate Use built-up handles if grasp is incomplete or weak Use swivel utensils or extended utensils if excursion is inadequate Use plate guard, soup bowl, or plate with raised edge to enable easier scooping Use Swedish knife™ Use extra-long straw and straw holder			Demonstrate proper use of assistive devices (utensils); have client or caregiver do return demonstration Provide handout with drawings or pictures of strategies (position mobile arm support), sequential directions, and number to call for assistance Provide catalog with relevant assistive devices marked Provide video of suggested strategies with client as subject if possible and practitioner as caregiver if appropriate (use of mobile arm support for eating)	
Medication Management						
Client may be unable to open pill bottles, remove lids from liquid medication containers and	Use medication syringe for liquids instead of spoon Sort medications into nut cups that can	Use splints for wrist stability or functional hand position Have pharmacist put only non-childproof lids on pill bottles	Place medications out in logical place where they will be used (kitchen table if medications are	Use of tenodesis action Prosthetic training Fine motor dexterity training	Demonstrate system for organizing medications; have client or caregiver do return demonstration	Increased level of independence Improved safety

remove pills from medication organizer compartments Client may be unable to open medication patch packaging or separate patch from protective liner Client may have difficulty pouring liquid medication into spoon without spilling Client may be unable or have difficulty getting spoon with medication to mouth Client may experience pain trying to open medication containers Client may express dissatisfaction with effort required and time needed for task performance	be easily picked up and emptied into mouth	Use rubber circle to increase resistance on liquid medicine bottles Stabilize liquid medicine bottle between knees and use jar opener Use Daytimer™ appointment alarm to signal medication schedule (can set up to 31 alarms per day)	taken at mealtime, bathroom or bedside if medications are taken at bedtime) if client is responsible for medication management	Active assistive, active, or resistive exercises for strengthening PROM	Demonstrate proper use of adapted task objects and assistive devices; have client or caregiver do return demonstration Provide catalog with relevant assistive devices marked	Improved adequacy of performance: Decreased difficulty Decreased pain Increased satisfaction
Functional Mobility						
Client may be unable to move safely, efficiently, or without difficulty or pain during bed mobility Client may be unable to move safely, efficiently or without difficulty or pain during wheelchair transfers to and from Bed Toilet Bathtub bench Easy chair Car	Dependent transfer Standing pivot transfer Standby assist Independent transfer	Sliding board transfer Standing pivot Insert rail on one side of bed so client can use it to pull against when positioning self in bed, lowering into bed, and raising up from bed Use gel or foam cushion in wheelchair to raise seat for easier transfers Use portable cushion to place in easy chair to make it	Ensure that distance from floor to all surfaces for transfers (toilet seat, tub bench, easy chair) is no greater than distance between floor and 2 in. below midpoint of client's patella when client is seated Attach overhead trapeze bar on bed Attach rope ladder to bed to help with positioning	Postural control exercises Weight-shifting exercises Balance exercises Prosthetic training Active assistive, active, or resistive exercises for extremity strengthening	Demonstrate restorative strategies and proper use of adapted task objects and assistive devices (rope ladder); have client or caregiver do return demonstration Provide catalog with relevant assistive devices marked Provide handout with drawings or pictures of strategies or adaptations	Increased level of independence Improved safety Improved adequacy of performance: Decreased difficulty Decreased pain Decreased fatigue Increased endurance Increased satisfaction

Continues

TABLE 28-6. **INTERVENTION STRATEGIES FOR ACTIVITY LIMITATIONS ASSOCIATED WITH UPPER AND LOWER BODY IMPAIRMENTS**[a] *(Continued)*

Baseline Status	*Potential Approaches and Strategies for Intervention*					*Outcome Status*
	Compensation Approach					
Activity Limitations Identified during Evaluation	**Alter Task Method**	**Adapt Task Objects; Use Assistive Devices**	**Modify Environment**	**Restoration Approach (Restore/Establish)**	**Education Approach**	**Target Outcomes at Discharge**
Functional Mobility (Contd.)						
Client may experience fatigue or inadequate endurance during task performance Client may express dissatisfaction with effort required and time needed to complete task performance		same height as wheelchair Use plastic garbage sacks on car seats to ease shifting and turning Order wheelchair with removable armrests	Install grab bars by toilet and in tub area as needed Arrange spaces so that wheelchair can be placed in optimal position for transfers		(transfers), sequential directions, and number to call for assistance Provide video of suggested strategies with client as subject if possible and practitioner as caregiver if appropriate (car transfers)	

[a]*Impairment:* upper and lower extremity passive range of motion (PROM) and active range of motion (AROM) or strength impairment, with or without sensory loss. *Common diseases/disorders:* quadriplegia, arthritis, multiple sclerosis, burns, cerebral palsy, multiple amputation, traumatic brain injury, orthopedic trauma.

TABLE 28–7. **LOWER BODY DRESSING FOR CLIENTS WITH IMPAIRED UPPER AND LOWER EXTREMITY PROM AND AROM**

Method 1

1. Sit with legs extended in bed, with or without back support, with clothing nearby on bed or chair.
2. Use weak grasp or drape garment over hand to hold it in preparation for putting it over foot.
3. Pull leg with forearm, lift under knee to bend leg, and bring foot up to opposite knee.
4. Drape garment over foot through leg opening and pull it up to knee.
5. Lift leg and push on knee to extend.
6. Pull trousers over foot and up to knee during same step as underwear or use same method for trousers as for underwear after underwear is pulled to waist.
7. Once garment is pulled to knees, pull it partly over thighs by pulling on crotch of pants with forearm and pulling with hand in pocket of pants, or use both hands together to grasp and pull.
8. Lie down and roll side to side, pulling pants up over hip that is on top with each roll. Pull pants up using hand in pocket, thumb in belt loop, or hand inside pants under waistband.
9. Elastic waistbands can eliminate need to use equipment to fasten garment.
10. Reverse process to remove clothing.

Method 2

1. Leave legs extended in bed, separated slightly.
2. Reach forward to feet, and place one wrist under ipsilateral heel.
3. Drape garment leg opening over toes, and pull garment over heel while lifting upper extremity under heel slightly.
4. Continue as in Method 1

Method 3

1. Place pants face up with waist just above knees and under legs.
2. Lift legs up with forearm one at a time, and place feet in leg openings.
3. Exert pressure on knee to cause leg to extend into trouser.
4. Continue as in Method 1

PROM, passive range of motion; *AROM,* active range of motion.

understand how the intervention will ultimately lead to improved task performance.

All intervention programs designed to restore or establish inherent capacities must provide clients with a structured opportunity to transfer the gains made in these capacities to relevant functional tasks. This ensures that the intervention outcome is functional, and helps maintain gains made through increasing capacity and reducing impairment, by providing an opportunity for practice within the daily routine. For example, intervention resulting in increased right shoulder flexion capacity should be accompanied by functional tasks that require movement into the newly acquired range, such as using the right upper extremity to reach into kitchen cabinets or resuming swimming or yoga practice.

Intervention aimed at restoration is often most efficient for clients for whom a few impairments affect many tasks and for whom diminished capacities can be expected to improve. For example, Mr. Stapinski has had postcircumferential second-degree burns to both upper extremities. The resulting bilateral restrictions in elbow flexion prevent him from completing most ADL due to an inability to reach his

TABLE 28–8. **LOWER BODY DRESSING FROM WHEELCHAIR FOR CLIENTS WITH IMPAIRED MOBILITY**

1. Sit on low bed, wheelchair, or standard chair with feet firmly on floor.
2. Cross one leg over other to start garment and put on socks and shoes.
3. To pull garment over hips in wheelchair or bed (if unable to stand), lean far to one side to pull garment over opposite thigh and buttock; repeat for opposite side. In wheelchair, support weight on elbows and lean on back of chair, bridging to lift buttocks from chair and pull pants up.
4. To stand to pull up garment, stabilize with one upper extremity on ambulation aide, or grab bar while pulling up garment with other upper extremity, alternating sides. Or stabilize against wall, bed, or grab bar while pulling garment up.

(text continues on page 530)

TABLE 28–9. **INTERVENTION STRATEGIES FOR ACTIVITY LIMITATIONS ASSOCIATED WITH COGNITIVE IMPAIRMENT**[a]

Baseline Status	***Potential Approaches and Strategies for Intervention***					***Outcome Status***
	Compensation Approach					
Activity Limitations Identified during Evaluation	**Alter Task Method**	**Adapt Task Objects; Use Assistive Devices**	**Modify Environment**	**Restoration Approach (Restore/Establish)**	**Education Approach**	**Target Outcomes at Discharge**
Grooming, Oral Hygiene, Bathing, Showering						
Client may use poor judgment with sharp objects (razors, fingernail scissors) Client may fear or resist bathing, grooming, and oral hygiene tasks or insist tasks were just completed Client may use poor judgment around water (turn on faucet and leave it running, run water that is too hot) Client may have difficulty getting into and out of tub Client's dentures may become loose and cause mouth sores after weight loss Client may lose dentures or retainers Client may be at risk for falls due to poor judgment Task outcomes may not meet acceptable societal standards (body odor from inadequate bathing)	Adhere to routines and patterns that reinforce timing and occurrence of grooming, hygiene, and bathing tasks Use only level of assistance that is needed; do not remove client's right to participate in task if it is not harmful Explain each step to client before proceeding so that there are no surprises Do not rush task Change to client's preferred time if possible Monitor bathing and showering at all times Partially fill tub before entering bath area with client so there is no waiting State "Bath is ready" if client thinks bath has already been completed	Use hand-held shower if caregiver is assisting Mark dentures and retainers with client's name Place rubber mesh in sink bottom when client brushes dentures in case dentures are dropped Use foaming gel spray on washcloth if client gets agitated with water running Place checklist in bathroom to be marked when each task is completed	Keep task materials in same place and keep materials for like tasks together Install nonskid bath mat in tub or shower Install grab bars around tub or shower Reset water temperature <120°F Install tap water overflow alarm Keep sharp and toxic (nail polish) items in a locked cabinet, if necessary Label drawers and cupboards with contents Remove clutter from task performance area	Cognitive retraining Establish routines Observe for client preferences so that these can be built on Develop behavioral memory aids for use until routines and habits are established	Demonstrate restorative and adaptive strategies (hierarchies of assistance); have caregiver do return demonstration Demonstrate proper use of distraction to avoid confrontation; have caregiver do return demonstration Provide handout with drawings or pictures of strategies or adaptations, sequential directions, and number to call for assistance Provide video of suggested strategies with client as subject if possible and practitioner as caregiver if appropriate	Increased level of independence Improved safety Improved adequacy of performance: Decreased difficulty Decreased pain Decreased fatigue Increased endurance Increased approximation to societal standards Increased satisfaction Decreased aberrant behavior

Client may demonstrate aberrant task behaviors (may swallow toothpaste rather than spit it out)	Bathe at sink Let client hold washcloth and scrub one area while caregiver washes another Provide toothpaste that can be swallowed Use electric razor Use clippers Turn nail care into a time to be pampered					
Toileting						
Client may be incontinent of bladder and bowel Client may not make it to bathroom in time Client may not remember what to do when brought to bathroom Client may not want to stay seated on toilet Client may forget to cleanse self after toileting Client may have difficulty doffing and donning clothing associated with toileting Client may be at risk for falls due to poor judgment Task outcomes may not meet societal standards (client may soil self in toileting process) Client may demonstrate aberrant task behaviors (stuff toilet	Adhere to routines and patterns that reinforce timing and occurrence of toileting Take client to bathroom; do not ask Within a task, explain next step to client before proceeding so there are no surprises Do not rush task Remove items that client tends to urinate in Help initiate toileting by: Pulling down client's clothing Have client sit on toilet Run water in sink Give water to drink Rub lower back Pour warm water over perineum into the toilet	Use clothing and underwear that is easy to remove Use incontinence garments Use protective sheet on bedding Use foaming gel spray to cleanse fecal matter and urine from client if bathing is not possible Place checklist in front of toilet with reminders about washing hands and flushing	Keep task materials stocked and within arm's reach so one hand can be on client while other is reaching for wipes, etc. Use raised toilet seat if client has difficulty lowering or raising self Use padded toilet seat if client needs to sit for extended periods Label drawers and cupboards with contents	Cognitive retraining Establish routines Develop behavioral memory aids for use until routines and habits are established	Demonstrate restorative and adaptive strategies (hierarchies of assistance; behavioral signs that client needs to use toilet); have caregiver do return demonstration Demonstrate proper use of distraction to avoid confrontation; have caregiver do return demonstration Provide handout with drawings or pictures of strategies or adaptations, sequential directions, and number to call for assistance Provide video of suggested strategies with client as subject if possible and practitioner as caregiver if appropriate	Increased level of independence Improved safety Improved adequacy of performance: Decreased difficulty Increased approximation to societal standards Decreased aberrant behavior

Continues

TABLE 28-9. **INTERVENTION STRATEGIES FOR ACTIVITY LIMITATIONS ASSOCIATED WITH COGNITIVE IMPAIRMENT**[a] *(Continued)*

Baseline Status	***Potential Approaches and Strategies for Intervention***					***Outcome Status***
	Compensation Approach					
Activity Limitations Identified during Evaluation	**Alter Task Method**	**Adapt Task Objects; Use Assistive Devices**	**Modify Environment**	**Restoration Approach (Restore/Establish)**	**Education Approach**	**Target Outcomes at Discharge**
Toileting (Contd.)						
paper into toilet, leave water running in sink)	Give client magazine to hold Allow up and down, if necessary					
Dressing						
Client may be unable to select appropriate clothing Client may wear same outfit day after day Client may have difficulty sequencing donning and doffing of clothing Client may have difficulty manipulating and securing fasteners Client may have difficulty attending to task Client may be unable to tie shoelaces Client may be unstable when donning or doffing clothing Task outcomes may not meet societal standards (client may layer clothing inappropriately) Client may demonstrate aberrant task behaviors (may remove clothing at inappropriate times)	Force clothing options by limiting clothing available in closet or drawers Buy several outfits that are alike if client has distinct preference Remove extra clothing from closets and drawers if client layers Ascertain if client is warm enough if layering persists Keep only seasonally appropriate clothing in closet and drawers Have client sit while dressing Arrange clothing in stack, in the order that it is to be donned Use clothes that are difficult to remove	Keep upper body clothing buttoned except at neck, for easier one-step over-head donning Use elastic on buttoned cuffs to allow hands move through easily Adapt clothing for easier donning and doffing (hook-and-loop tape fasteners, zipper pulls, large buttons) Develop checklists for donning and doffing clothing (hang up or put in laundry basket)	Place stable chair with arms near bed to use for dressing Label drawers, cupboards, closets with contents	Cognitive retraining Establish routines Develop behavioral memory aids for use until routines and habits are established	Demonstrate restorative and adaptive strategies (routines, use of memory aids); have client or caregiver do return demonstration Provide handout with drawings or pictures of strategies or adaptations (setting up clothing for donning), sequential directions, and number to call for assistance Provide video of suggested strategies with client as subject if possible and practitioner as caregiver if appropriate	Increased level of independence Improved safety Improved adequacy of performance: Decreased difficulty Increased endurance Increased approximation to societal standards Decreased aberrant behavior

	if client doffs clothing in inappropriate places Use clothing items that stretch and are washable (knits) Use clothing that is easy to don or doff Use shoes with hook-and-loop tape closures					
Feeding and Eating						
Client may forget to eat or drink Client may not initiate self-feeding or may not continue Client may have difficulty managing utensils Client may have difficulty cutting food Client may have difficulty scooping up food Client may forget to chew Client may eat nonfood items Client may choke on liquids Client may be distracted or inattentive during mealtime Task outcomes may not meet acceptable societal standards (client may drool) Client may demonstrate aberrant task behaviors (may refuse to open mouth or may stuff food in cheeks)	Set alarm to remind client it is time to fix food or to eat or drink Position client upright with feet supported Monitor fluid intake Place only small amounts of food in front of client at one time Provide food that smells appetizing Point out each type of food and put a small amount on client's lips to stimulate opening of mouth Ask client to say "ah" (and demonstrate), instead of saying, "open your mouth" Cut food into small bites Use finger foods and tolerate finger feeding Tolerate declining table manners	Place nonslip placemat under plate to prevent plate from moving; consider dishes with nonslip surfaces underneath Use small plastic glasses or cups and then refill Use Thickit™ or other thickening agent in liquids Develop checklists for using the microwave, putting away food, etc.	Provide suitable stable chair Label drawers, cupboards, and closets with contents Lock cupboards that contain sharp or inedible items (detergent), if necessary	Cognitive retraining Oral stimulation Develop behavioral memory aids for use until routines and habits are established Recommend a swallowing evaluation	Demonstrate restorative strategies (oral stimulation); have client or caregiver do return demonstration Demonstrate feeding methods; have client or caregiver do return demonstration (to ensure that caregiver is not using "bird" feeding techniques) Demonstrate proper use of adapted task objects and assistive devices; have client or caregiver do return demonstration Provide handout with drawings or pictures of strategies or adaptations (suggested position of tableware to avoid bumping, spilling), sequential directions, and number to call for assistance	Increased level of independence Improved safety Improved adequacy of performance: Decreased difficulty Increased endurance Increased approximation to societal standards Decreased aberrant behavior

Continues

TABLE 28–9. **INTERVENTION STRATEGIES FOR ACTIVITY LIMITATIONS ASSOCIATED WITH COGNITIVE IMPAIRMENT**[a] *(Continued)*

Baseline Status	***Potential Approaches and Strategies for Intervention***					***Outcome Status***
	Compensation Approach					
Activity Limitations Identified during Evaluation	**Alter Task Method**	**Adapt Task Objects; Use Assistive Devices**	**Modify Environment**	**Restoration Approach (Restore/Establish)**	**Education Approach**	**Target Outcomes at Discharge**
Feeding and Eating (Contd.)						
	Remind client to chew and swallow after each bite and stroke client's throat gently Demonstrate chewing Serve soft foods Avoid sticky food and food that is hard Put hand on client's arm to block movement if client is stuffing food in mouth; remove extra food If client lives alone, check refrigerator for spoiled food				Provide video of suggested strategies with client as subject if possible and practitioner as caregiver if appropriate (managing client during mealtime)	
Medication Management						
Client may not remember to take medications Client may not interpret medication directions correctly Client may not remember that medications were taken and take extra doses Client may have difficulty opening medication containers Client may refuse medication	Use medication syringe for liquids instead of spoon for ease of administration for both client and caregiver Check with nurse or pharmacist about which medications can be crushed and mixed into applesauce or other soft foods Sort medications into nut cups, envelopes,	Have pharmacist put only non-child proof lids on medication bottles if client is managing medications Use medication organizer that is acceptable to client Use Daytimer™ appointment alarm to signal medication schedule (can set up to 31 alarms per day)	Lock medications in cupboard if client is likely to take medications inappropriately Place medications out in logical place where they will be constantly noticed (kitchen counter) if client is responsible for medication management	Cognitive retraining Develop behavioral memory aids for use until routines and habits are established Recommend swallowing evaluation	Demonstrate medication management routines; have client or caregiver do return demonstration Provide catalog with relevant assistive devices marked	Increased level of independence Improved safety Improved adequacy of performance: Decreased difficulty Decreased aberrant behavior

Client may demonstrate aberrant task behaviors (may spit out pills)	or saucers that are labeled with day and time so that client knows when to take medications and if medications were not taken					
Functional Mobility						
Client may be unable to find way around home or community Client may move in unsafe and awkward manner (bump into things, unsteady gait, trip over items) Client may have difficulty getting up from bed or chair Client may pace and wander Client may not remember limitations, precautions, or how to use assistive device for ambulation and thus be at risk for falls (especially if client has concomitant physical impairment) Client may demonstrate aberrant task behaviors (pick up walker and carry it around)	Have client wear sturdy, low- and broad-heeled shoes if gait is unsteady Have client walk beside caregiver, holding onto arm Have caregiver accompany client until way finding is mastered Write out directions for community way finding and provide easy-to-follow map	Insert rail on one side of bed so client can use it to hold onto when positioning self in bed, lowering into and raising up from bed Use portable dense foam cushion to place in easy chairs to make it easier to raise self Use chair with arms Evaluate ability to use walking aids if gait is unsteady Install gates by stairs if necessary	Add lighting to areas where client is likely to trip Provide lighted pathway from bedroom to bathroom Repair walking surfaces so they are even Remove tripping hazards Stabilize furniture near natural pathways Make stairways safe: Sturdy handrails on both sides Make stair height and tread widths uniform Mark tread widths and top and bottom landings marked with a different color or surface Provide safe environment for wandering (natural, clear pathways)	Postural control exercises Balance exercises Cognitive retraining Develop behavioral memory aids for use until routines and habits are established Practice way finding with client	Demonstrate restorative strategies and proper use of adapted task objects and assistive devices (walking aid); have client or caregiver do return demonstration Provide catalog with relevant assistive devices marked Provide handout with drawings or pictures of strategies or adaptations (stair safety guidelines), sequential directions, and number to call for assistance Provide video of suggested strategies with client as subject if possible and practitioner as caregiver, if appropriate (indoor safety for wandering pathways)	Increased level of independence Improved safety Improved adequacy of performance: Decreased difficulty Decreased aberrant behavior

[a]*Impairment:* cognitive (attention span, memory, sequencing, problem solving, generalization, initiation and termination of task). *Common diseases/disorders:* cerebrovascular accident, traumatic brain injury, dementia, mental retardation.

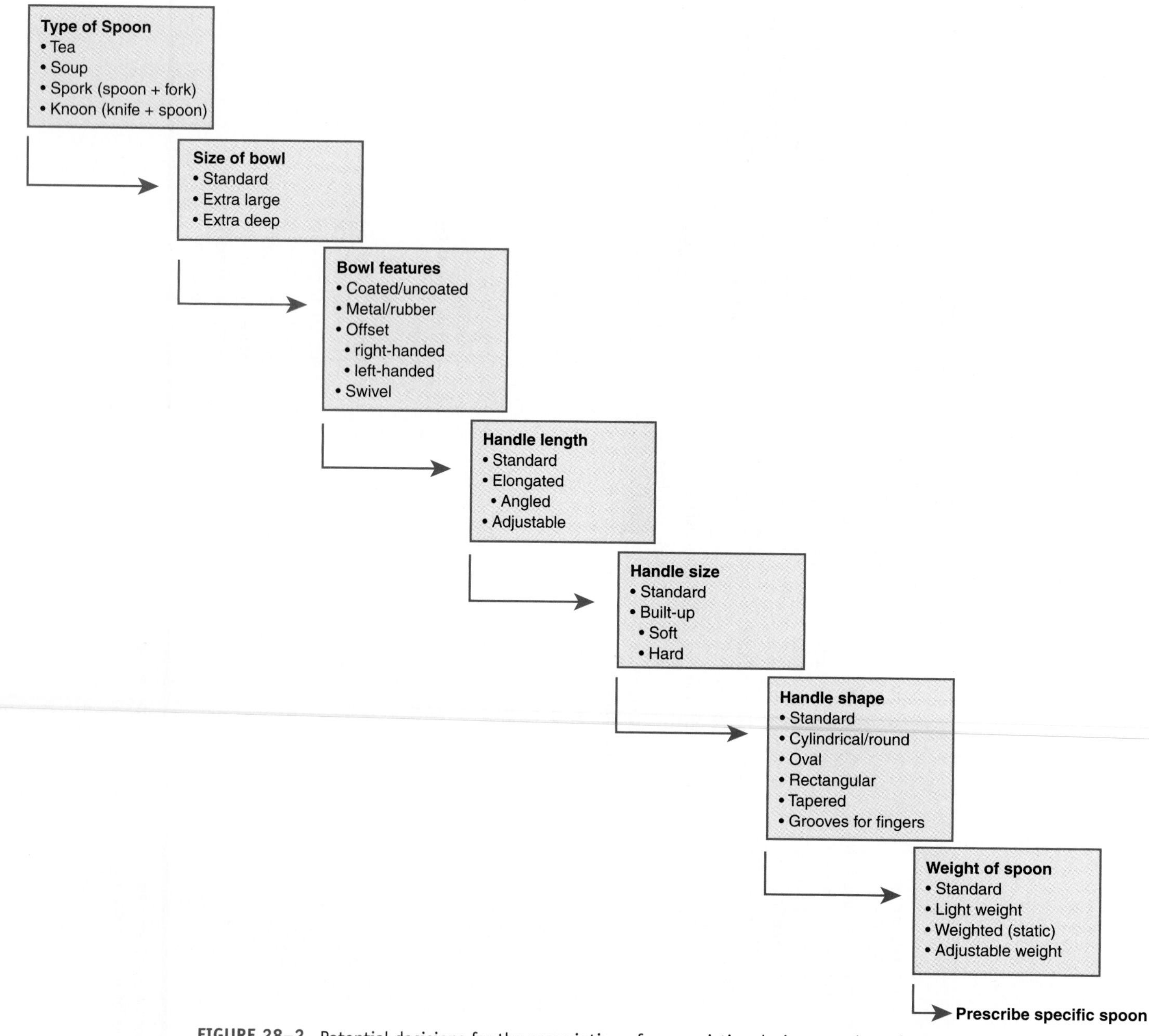

FIGURE 28–2. Potential decisions for the prescription of one assistive device: an adapted spoon.

face, head, or trunk. Tasks can be easily adapted by using long-handled devices, but extended tools would likely be needed for all ADL tasks (e.g., eating utensils, toothbrush, comb, brush, bath sponge). Because clients with b urns can be expected to increase elbow flexion with passive stretching, scar management, and exercise, intervention will be most efficient if it is aimed at increasing ROM. Whereas adapting task objects improves his ADL performance in the short term, the long-term goal of restoring Mr. Stapinski's capacity to flex his elbows will enhance function across many different tasks.

A restorative approach may be appropriate for some clients with progressive disorders even though their capacities are expected to deteriorate, given the typical course of the condition. The focus, however, becomes slowing the decline of specific capacities and skills. For example, clients with Parkinson disease may slow the progression of the effects of bradykinesia and difficulty in initiating and ceasing movement with the use of a movement exercise program.

For many impairments, carefully structured everyday activities can restore or establish capacities while permitting

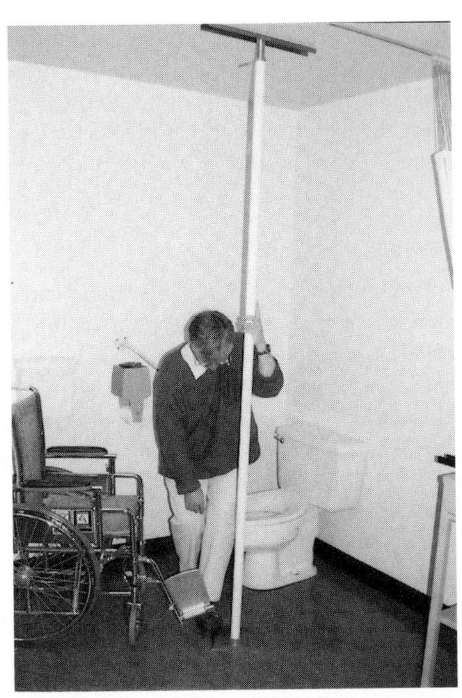

FIGURE 28–3. A floor-to-ceiling pole that can be used to facilitate stability during transfers.

the practice of the activities. Clients who are severely deconditioned may find their activity level limited by poor endurance. For example, intervention could be aerobic exercise to increase cardiopulmonary endurance, with the goal of participating in functional activities when an adequate increase in cardiopulmonary capacity is achieved. Instead, an intervention that graded the intensity and duration of daily activities could be as effective in increasing cardiovascular fitness, while enabling the client to participate in desired tasks. In addition, gains made in endurance are immediately transferred into functional activities.

The nature of the specific capacity that needs restoration warrants attention because the restoration of some capacities does not result in generalization of the newly gained skills to functional activities. Visual-perceptual skills, such as visual scanning, figure-ground perception, right–left discrimination, and topographical orientation are often treated with exercises outside of the context of daily activities. Few studies have been done to support the efficacy of this approach for improving functional performance (Quintana, 1995). In one study, Ross (1992), examined the outcome of a computer-based intervention to enhance visual scanning skills on the ability to locate items on a grocery shelf. She found that clients demonstrated improvement in scanning skills during the computer task, but that these skills did not improve the grocery store scanning task. Higher-level cognitive skills also require practice within the natural environment of an activity, because clients must learn to interpret and use relevant environmental cues for problem solving and these cues are activity dependent.

Recent studies in motor learning support the treatment of sensorimotor skills within the context of functional activities because of the importance of environmental cues and the task specificity of motor control (Horak, 1991, Mathiowetz & Bass Haugen, 1995; Shumway-Cook & Woollacott, 1995). It is important for tasks to be structured to challenge the client's motor skills, so careful grading of functional activities is critical. Grading of tasks is also used with constraint-induced movement therapy (CIMT) for clients who have incurred a stroke. CIMT requires constraint of the nonaffected upper extremity while the client undergoes intensive training and massed practice, using the affected extremity (Taub, Uswatte, & Pidikiti, 1999). Compensation with the uninvolved nondominant hand (transfer of dominance) may also facilitate activity performance, but would not be consistent with the restorative approach for improving motor control.

Depending on the nature of the performance discrepancy and the degree of impairment, the intervention time needed when using restorative approaches may be longer than that required for compensatory approaches. This increased time must be taken into consideration, particularly in managed care settings. In addition, clients must recognize that the rehabilitation period may be longer, and that follow-through with a home program is vital if gains are to be made.

Integrating Intervention for Impairments and Activity Limitations

At first glance, it may seem that restoration and compensation are mutually exclusive intervention approaches—that is, the outcome is either to restore the impaired capacity or to compensate for it. Using both approaches simultaneously may seem a bit like using a belt and suspenders. A carefully crafted program, however, enables clients to be more functional through the use of compensatory strategies while at the same time working to restore functional capacities. It is critical that the occupational therapy practitioner reduce the use of compensatory strategies as clients make gains in skill performance.

For example, Mr. Stapinski, whose burns resulted in bilateral limitations in elbow flexion, may benefit from utensils with extended handles. With the extended handles on the utensils, he can feed himself independently during the 2–3 weeks that it takes to increase his elbow flexion sufficiently for him to feed himself without these utensils. The extended handles should be fabricated to require him to flex fully within his available range and should be shortened as gains in ROM are made, so that the new range is incorporated into the feeding task.

Whenever task or environmental adaptations are anticipated to be temporary, it is necessary to consider cost in relationship to the anticipated time the equipment will be needed, and the potential benefit to clients. Thermoplastic or wood extensions can be added temporarily to the handles of regular utensils rather than prescribing the more costly commercially available utensils with elongated handles. For some tasks, safety concerns supersede cost considerations. Using a collapsible lawn chair in the shower would be an inexpensive alternative to a shower chair, but it would not provide adequate stability.

Education of the Client or Caregiver

Instructional Methods

A variety of instructional methods are available for client and caregiver **education** (Fuhrer & Keith, 1998), and methods should be selected that best meet the needs of the person (Tables 28-1 to 28-9). When a facility has a homogeneous client population, group instruction can be an efficient and effective method for providing basic education. Many arthritis centers provide group instruction in joint-preservation techniques. Teaching a group is cost-effective and, when well structured, can facilitate learning through peer interaction. For caregiver groups, the contact with others who are experiencing similar problems in their caregiving roles can provide valuable emotional support and an opportunity for constructive group problem solving.

Some type of individualized instruction is typically needed to complement group instruction so that information can be tailored to meet the specific and unique needs of each person. If group instruction has preceded the individualized instruction, the client-specific sessions can be relatively short and focused on application of the information learned in the group to the client's particular circumstances. For example, clients would be taught how to apply proper lifting techniques to the objects and dimensions of their own homes.

Individualized instruction is more appropriate for many clients and caregivers because the personal nature of the tasks that need to be learned does not lend itself to group instruction (e.g., bathing). Furthermore, in intervention settings serving a diverse case mix, the opportunity for group instruction rarely occurs. One-to-one client or caregiver education and training enables the occupational therapy practitioner to obtain immediate feedback from the person as the session progresses and to alter the amount and focus of learning accordingly.

A vast array of media are available to occupational therapy practitioners to facilitate the learning process. Written materials may be developed specifically for a client or caregiver, or published materials may be used, if appropriate ones are available. Videocassette recorders are widely available, even in clients' homes, and custom or commercially made videotapes can be effective teaching tools. Audiotapes can also be effective, particularly when visual input would be distracting. For example, an audiotape may be used to facilitate visual imagery for relaxation or stress reduction. The Internet is becoming increasingly accessible to the general population and many occupational therapy clinics have Internet access. A wealth of information about a variety of disorders is available that is specifically geared toward clients and caregivers through the World Wide Web . Clients may also find peer support groups through chat rooms or list servers.

Caregiver Training

In addition to evaluating clients' learning capacity, the learning capacity of their caregivers needs to be appraised. Similar to clients, caregivers also have varied learning styles and capacities. In many situations, the caregiver is a family member who is still coping with the emotional impact of having a family member with a disability, whether it is a new mother with a child with cerebral palsy or the spouse of a woman who had a CVA. Particularly in situations in which the person is new to the caregiver role, time must be taken to assess the caregiver's capacity to understand and apply the information necessary for safe and effective management of the client's needs. People under emotional stress may need more time and repetition to process information accurately (Blake & Lincoln, 2000). When caregivers are expected to assist clients physically, their physical capacity for providing this assistance also warrants evaluation.

Caregivers have varied learning styles, and instruction that caters to their preferred style is likely to be the most efficient and effective (Banford et al., 2001). Some people, for example, are kinesthetic learners. They learn most quickly through doing. Visual learners may prefer to watch a demonstration of the activity several times before attempting it themselves. Others may prefer written instructions. All learners benefit from the opportunity to ask questions to clarify instructions. Media that support teaching by a practitioner can be a great asset. Videotapes, for example, provide caregivers with an excellent visual image of how an exercise or activity is to be done. Often, home- or clinic-made videotapes can be made of a client's activity performance. These productions add little time to the intervention session, because they are recorded as activities are practiced during regular therapy. They have the advantage of providing richer and more detailed information than is feasible in oral or written instructions.

When caregivers are helping to carry out an intervention program, the outcome and general intervention strategies should be made clear to them. For restoration programs, clients may need assistance with implementing specific exercises or grading of activities in a way that will help to restore skills. Caregivers need to learn specific cuing strategies so that home programs, whether these are carried out in clients' homes, group homes, or long-term care settings, are carried out accurately. Caregivers are often pivotal in motivating clients. Motivating clients who have disorders that impair motivation, such as depression, can be particularly challenging. Helping caregivers understand that disinterest and lack of motivation are a part of the disorder and providing concrete strategies for managing the "getting going" phase of the home program will foster its success (Resnick, 1998). For clients with behavior problems, such as the catastrophic reactions that often accompany Alzheimer disease, teaching caregivers behavior management strategies that defuse potentially volatile situations can be invaluable to their success as caregivers.

Caregiver training for assisting clients with functional activities should focus first on safety for clients and caregivers. The occupational therapy practitioner should emphasize components of the activity that promote safety, such as locking the wheelchair brakes or blocking the client's knee to prevent buckling when transferring to and from the wheelchair. As intervention progresses, the occupational therapy practitioner should inform caregivers of the activities that are safe and unsafe to perform outside of the therapy situation. For example, although a client may be working on bathtub transfers during therapy, skilled facilitation to get in and out safely may be required, making it premature for the client to practice these transfers at home.

When caregivers need to provide physical assistance, they should be trained in using proper body mechanics. Training should include body mechanics for transfers or bed mobility and also for wheelchair positioning. Assisting a client in a wheelchair with ADL, such as brushing teeth or feeding, while standing, can fatigue lower back muscles. Taking care of the caregiver is frequently overlooked in occupational therapy interventions and is an essential component of the person–task–environment transaction, particularly when it is anticipated that the client will require assistance over a long period of time.

Grading the Intervention Program

Intervention programs should never be static. It is important to progress the client continually toward the established intervention outcomes. The specific means of grading intervention when a restoration approach is being implemented depends on the impairments and the intervention strategies being used. (The chapters on restoration of impairments provide more specific guidance.) If the intervention plan uses both restoration and compensation, the program can be graded by reducing the amount of task and environmental adaptations as clients' capacities are restored. Intervention for activity limitations can be graded by modifying many of the activity parameters described earlier in the chapter, including increasing the level of independence, taking more responsibility for safety, enhancing personal satisfaction, reducing the level of difficulty or required exertion, and decreasing the duration or the occurrence of aberrant task behaviors.

Grade Task Progression from Easier to Harder

One means of grading an intervention program is to begin with easier tasks and progress to more difficult ones. This progression will be relative to the client's activity limitations. Money management may be relatively easy for a client with quadriplegia to perform once the use of a writing tool is mastered, whereas lower extremity dressing is much more difficult. Conversely, a client with a head injury that resulted in significant cognitive impairment with relatively preserved motor skills is likely to find lower extremity dressing to be relatively easy but money management extremely difficult.

Increase Complexity within the Task

Rather than progressing only from easier to harder activities, intervention may also be graded by increasing the complexity within an activity, or by progressing from simple to more complex ways of doing it. Cooking skills may extend from simple preparations such as cold sandwiches to more complex, multicourse dinners. Even seemingly simple tasks can often be graded. A sock donning intervention, for example, might be scaled from using looser, ankle socks to tighter, knee socks, and finally to Ted™ hose.

Same Task in Varied Performance Environments

A critical part of a graded intervention program involves progression from the intervention environment to the real-life environment in which the activity will actually be performed. This may involve transfer from a clinic to a home setting or the more subtle dynamics associated with the transfer of help from the occupational therapy practitioner to the natural caregiver. The client may be independent in donning a jacket sitting on a mat table in the clinic, but may be unable to do so when sitting on a chair with a back, or standing (the way a jacket is typically donned by ambulatory persons). Providing practice in increasingly demanding performance environments can facilitate the generalization of skills, thereby enhancing the client's functional flexibility.

CONCLUSION

In this section, three broad approaches to occupational therapy intervention for activities of daily living were discussed: compensation, restoration, and education. We discussed the necessity of establishing target outcomes for activity performance that address value of the activity to the client, level of independence in performing the activity, safety of activity performance, and adequacy of activity performance. Adequacy of activity performance included the parameters of difficulty, pain, fatigue and dyspnea, duration (efficiency), societal standards, satisfaction, experience, resources, and aberrant task behaviors. Other factors influencing target outcomes and choice of intervention approaches were also presented, including the client's ability to learn, the client's prognosis, the time allocated for intervention, the client's discharge disposition, and the client's ability to follow through with new routines or techniques.

SECTION II

Home Management

KATHLEEN HILKO CULLER

Home maintainer is one of the major roles a person may have during a lifetime. A home maintainer is a person who has responsibility, at least once a week, for home management tasks (Oakley, 1986). The occupational practice framework (AOTA, in press) includes different categories relating to the area of home making. The categories are home establishment and management, meal preparation and cleanup, and safety procedures and emergency responses. Successful performance of home management tasks is required for independent community living and requires higher-level organizational and planning skills than performance of self-care tasks (Lawton & Brody, 1969). A major focus of occupational therapy is to assist a client to assume or return to the occupational role of home maintainer or to activities pertinent to the client's lifestyle. These activities can include cooking, laundry, cleaning, home and yard maintenance, money management, and the ability to recognize and act on safety hazards in the home.

LIFESTYLE VARIATIONS

Adults have varied responsibilities in the areas of home management. Therefore, occupational therapy practitioners help clients perform tasks and levels of task performance pertinent to their lifestyles. The Rehabilitation Institute of Chicago (RIC) Functional Assessment Scale (1998) recognizes varying levels of performance for each IADL. For instance, meal preparation and cleanup has five levels of complexity, from easiest to hardest: preparation of self-serve, such as a salad from a grocery store salad bar; cold meals, such as sandwiches; hot beverages, soups, or prepared foods, such as frozen dinners; hot one-dish meals, such as baked macaroni; and hot multi-item meals such as baked chicken with potatoes and vegetables. Each successive level requires progressively more sophisticated cognitive, perceptual, and motor skills and abilities. The level of complexity for any given client depends on his or her lifestyle before intervention and the levels of cognitive, perceptual, and motor skills he or she is likely to achieve by the end of therapy. Intervention goals and activities for home management should be consistent with the client's lifestyle, priorities, and anticipated abilities.

INTERVENTION STRATEGIES FOR HOME MANAGEMENT

There are four types of intervention strategies used for clients who demonstrate deficits in home management:

- Establishing or restoring areas of occupation, performance skills, and client factors.
- Teaching new methods for modifying task performance to compensate for deficient areas of occupation, performance, and client factors.
- Suggesting environmental modifications to make occupational activities easier.
- Educating clients and families to support occupational engagement or to prevent future problems.

Restoration

The focus of the restorative approach is to develop client skills and abilities or restore the client's performance to preintervention levels. A restorative approach is appropriate when a client's condition or diagnosis (e.g., generalized weakness or deconditioning, acute arthritis) or deficits in skills or abilities are likely to improve enough to achieve preintervention task proficiency. For example, a practitioner may teach clients with arthritis exercises to improve their shoulder ROM so that they could perform meal preparation tasks, such as reaching into a cabinet for cooking supplies or dishes. Table 28-10 provides an overview of the parameters to be considered when analyzing homemaking and grading the task for client success.

Grading Activities

Various parameters need to be considered when grading activities and measuring the effectiveness of intervention using a restorative approach. These parameters include the following.

- *Physical assistance*. There should be an inverse correlation between the amount of ability demonstrated by the client and the amount of physical help or assistance provided by the practitioner or caregiver. That is, as a client displays

TABLE 28–10. **PARAMETERS TO CONSIDER WHEN ANALYZING HOME MANAGEMENT ACTIVITIES**

Activity			*Therapist or Caregiver Role*			*Environment*	
				Supervision or Verbal Assist			
Sequencing	**Type**	**Demands**	**Physical Assist**	**Number of Cues**	**Type of Cue**	**Familiarity**	**Stimulation**
Multiple tasks Entire task Increasing portion Small portion	Unfamiliar, unstructured Familiar or structured	High cognitive, high motor Low cognitive, high motor *or* high cognitive, low motor Low cognitive, low motor	Independent Independent: • with modified environment • with equipment • but slow Minimal assist Moderate assist Maximal assist Dependent	None Occasional Frequent Consistent	Written Tactile Verbal: Indirect Direct	New or unfamiliar Familiar	High stimulation Low stimulation

increased skill in completing a task, the practitioner or caregiver should intervene less frequently.

- *Supervision and cuing*. Supervision and cuing can include the number of cues given, in addition to the types of cues used. Written materials (booklets, handouts, written home programs with illustrations or pictures) can reinforce teaching that has occurred during therapy. Tactile cues can be used to modify or guide client performance (e.g., stroking a client's involved arm to cue a reach for a glass in a cabinet). Verbal cues can affect client performance. For example, while in the grocery store, a direct cue provides the client with a specific instruction, such as, "The spaghetti is here," as the practitioner points to the aisle where spaghetti is located. An indirect verbal cue provides assistance to the client in a less directive manner, such as, "Can you find the foods listed on your grocery list?"
- *Activity demands*. The amount of cognitive and physical skill required to perform the activity affects the quality of client performance. In selecting the type of activity, the therapist should consider the complexity of performance skills demanded by the activity. As a general rule, for clients with neurological deficits, it is better to select an activity with low-motor and high-cognitive demands or with high-motor and low-cognitive demands (Chapparo, 1979) and then to progress to increasing levels of cognitive and motor demands simultaneously. For example, participating in a community outing may be a high-cognitive demand activity for a client who has had a stroke. In addition, the client's mobility may be compromised. Thus the client may initially ambulate for a short amount of time, but as the quality of the client's gait decreases, the client may need to complete the community outing in a wheelchair (high-cognitive, low-motor demand).
- *Sequencing of activity*. Increasing the number of steps or tasks that a client needs to complete can indicate increased proficiency. During a community outing, a client may be able to progress from completing one errand in 1 hr to completing three errands in 1 hr.
- *Type of activity*. Cognitive activities can be graded from routine and familiar to unfamiliar or new. For example, it is less demanding for a client to cook a familiar recipe from memory than to follow a new recipe from a cookbook. An activity organized by the client without assistance from the practitioner demands a high level of performance.
- *Environment*. A familiar environment, such as the client's home kitchen, is less demanding than a new environment, such as the clinic's kitchen (Robbins & Goldstein, 1998). In addition, the type of stimulation can vary from a quiet, nondistracting environment, such as a room with no noise or other people, to a distracting, busy environment, such as the community. For clients who use wheelchairs, lack of wheelchair accessibility can prohibit the client's ability to access services (banks, restaurant, stores) in the community. By altering the various parameters in therapy, an activity can be upgraded or downgraded to provide a difficult, but not overwhelming, challenge that results in a successful experience for the client.

Modification, Compensation, Adaptation

The modification, compensation, adaptation approach focuses on using the client's remaining abilities to achieve the highest level of functioning possible in the areas of homemaking. If the client cannot perform these activities in the usual manner, then adapted techniques or equipment are used to maximize performance. This strategy

TABLE 28-11. **HOME MANAGEMENT FOR ONE-HANDED PERFORMANCE**

ADL Area	Adaptive Equipment	Adaptive Techniques
Meal preparation and cleanup	Use adapted cutting board with stainless-steel or aluminum nails for cutting or peeling; raised corners on the board can stabilize bread to spread ingredients or make sandwich Use sponge, Dycem, or suction devices to stabilize bowls or dishes during food preparation. Use pot stabilizer Use adapted jar openers Electric appliances (food processor, hand mixer) to save time and energy; *Note:* Client safety and judgment must be considered when electrical appliances are considered Use a rocker knife Use a whisk to mix food Compensate for impaired standing tolerance and/or mobility by use of utility cart to transport objects If cooking is done at wheelchair level or seated, use angled mirror over rangetop to watch food on burner Use hand-held spray for rinsing dishes Place rubber mat at bottom of sink to reduce breakage Use suction-type brush to clean glassware	Use knees to stabilize objects Slide pots and pans across counters, rather than lift Open jar by placing it in drawer; then lean against it to stabilize it before opening Use scissors to open plastic bags Use fork prongs to open milk carton Crack egg by holding it in palm of hand, hitting it against edge of bowl, and separating eggshell with index and middle fingers Compensate for impaired standing tolerance and/or mobility by doing tasks while seated Soak dishes before washing Allow dishes to air dry
Clothing management (laundry, clothing repair)	Laundry can be transported to and from washer and dryer in wheeled cart	
Housecleaning	Use tank-type vacuum so client can sit and reach areas to be cleaned Use long-reach duster Use long-handled dustpan and brush Use self-wringing mop	Save energy by making bed completely at each corner before progressing to next corner Install no-wax flooring Some floor care can be managed from seated position

can be used when a client's condition is temporary, such as for hip replacement; when precautions need to be taken; when the condition is not amenable to restoration; and when task speed and proficiency are greatly improved by use of adaptive equipment or adaptive techniques. Use of adaptive techniques is preferable to use of equipment, because techniques allow the client more flexibility. Use of adaptive equipment is less preferable because of the cost incurred for equipment purchase and maintenance and the inconvenience of having to transport the equipment for task performance (Barnes, 1991; Klinger, 1978; Pedretti, 1996; Trombly, 1995c).

Clients with the following impairments and related diagnoses are likely to benefit from adaptive techniques and equipment which are listed in Tables 28-11 through 28-14.

- *One-handed performance*. Clients with hemiplegia resulting from a CVA, unilateral trauma or amputation, or temporary conditions such as burns or peripheral neuropathy may need to learn how to complete activities with one hand. The recommended strategies given in Table 28-11 focus on stabilizing objects for task completion and compensating for loss of balance or mobility.
- *Reduced upper extremity ROM and strength*. Clients with quadriplegia, burns, arthritis, upper extremity amputation, multiple sclerosis, amyotrophic lateral sclerosis, and orthopedic and other traumatic injuries may need to learn how to compensate for lack of reach or hand grip, lack of strength, or decreased tolerance for prolonged activity. The recommended strategies given in Table 28-12 focus on using gravity to assist with activity completion.
- *Incoordination of upper extremities*. Clients with head injury, cerebral palsy, CVA, multiple sclerosis, tumors, or other neurological condition may need learn how to compensate for poorly controlled movement. The recommended

TABLE 28–12. **HOME MANAGEMENT FOR CLIENTS WITH REDUCED UPPER EXTREMITY ROM AND STRENGTH**

ADL Area	Adaptive Equipment	Adaptive Techniques
Meal preparation and cleanup	Use adapted jar opener Use foam or built-up handles on utensils Use universal cuff to hold utensils to compensate for reduced grip Use long-handled reacher to obtain lightweight objects from high or low places Use wheeled cart to transport objects Use adapted cutting board Add loop handles to utensils to substitute for reduced grasp Use walker basket to transport objects	Use joint protective measures for rheumatoid arthritis Position electrical appliances within easy reach, to help conserve energy Work at a seated position to conserve energy Use teeth to open containers Purchase convenience foods to eliminate food preparation Use tenodesis action (wrist extension and finger flexion; wrist flexion and finger extension) to pick up lightweight objects Use fork prongs to open milk carton Use lightweight pots, pans, and utensils
Laundry	If client is ambulatory, use top-loading washer to avoid need to bend Push-button controls on washer and dryer are easier to use than knobs; adapt knobs if necessary If client chooses to iron, set iron at a low temperature; place asbestos pad at the end of ironing board to eliminate need to stand iron up	Use premeasured packages of soap or bleach to avoid handling large containers (or buy large containers and have someone else measure soap or bleach into single packets) Place hangers near dryer to hang permanent-press items as they come out of dryer Remain seated when ironing Replace sheets on bed immediately after coming out of dryer to avoid folding Place dirty clothing into different bins so it is ready for laundering and can be transported in small quantities
Housecleaning	Use long-handled reacher to pick up objects from floor Use long-handled sponge to clean bathtub Use self-wringing mop Use lightweight tools (sponge mops and brooms) for floor care	Use aerosol cleaners to dissolve dirt before cleaning surfaces When making bed, do not tuck in sheets

strategies listed in Table 28-13 focus on stabilizing proximal portions of limbs and reducing movements distally by using weights to stabilize objects to avoid breakage or accidents with sharp utensils or hot foods or equipment.

- *Lower extremity mobility impairment*. Clients with paraplegia, osteoarthritis, lower extremity amputation, burns, and leg and knee fractures and replacements may need to learn how to compensate for lack of accessibility and endurance. The recommended strategies given in Table 28-14 focus on mobility from a wheelchair; work heights; maneuverability; and access to storage, equipment, and supplies.

Energy Conservation and Work Simplification Techniques

Energy conservation and work simplification techniques can help clients perform home management tasks in spite of the mobility and endurance problems imposed by many disabilities (American Heart Association, n.d.; Pedretti, 1996; RIC, 1988; Trombly, 1995c). These techniques require that the practitioner and client address the following points:

- Determine what tasks need to be improved (i.e., according to the client, what tasks take too long, cause fatigue, or take too much energy).
- List all the steps of the task, including setup, performance, and cleanup.
- Analyze the activity (see Chapter 16.)
- Develop a new method of performing the task; consider eliminating unnecessary steps, combining motions and activities, rearranging the sequence of the steps, and simplifying the details of the task by taking the following steps:
  - Use the correct work height to reduce fatigue and promote good posture (correct work height while

TABLE 28–13. **HOME MANAGEMENT FOR CLIENTS WITH INCOORDINATION OF THE UPPER EXTREMITIES**

ADL Area	Adaptive Equipment	Adaptive Techniques
Meal preparation and cleanup	Use heavy cookware and ironstone dishes to aid with distal stabilization Use pots and casseroles with double handles to provide greater stability Weighted wrist cuffs may reduce tremors Use nonslip materials, such as Dycem, to provide stability Use adapted cutting board to stabilize food while cutting Serrated knives are less likely to slip than straight-edged knives Use frying basket to cook foods such as vegetables, for safe removal and reduced chance of burns Freestanding appliances, electric skillet, and countertop mixer, are safer than transferring objects out of oven or using hand-held mixer Use milk carton holder with handles to pour milk Use stove with front controls so client does not need to reach over hot pots to the back of stove Transport food with weighted wheeled cart Place rubber mat or sponge cloth at the bottom of the sink to cushion dishes when washing up	Stabilize arms proximally to reduce tremors during food preparation, such as cutting and peeling Start rangetop after food has been placed on burner Slide food and dishes over counter rather than lifting them Avoid breakage by soaking dishes, rinsing with hand sprayer, and air drying
Laundry		Use premeasured soap and bleach to eliminate spills Use permanent-press or no-iron materials to eliminate ironing Use stabilizing measure, such as holding upper arms close to body and sitting while working
Housecleaning	Use heavier work tools Use dust mitt instead of duster Use fitted sheets	Eliminate or store excess household decorations to reduce dusting

standing is 2 in. below the bent elbow; while sitting, clients should avoid positions that require lifting the shoulders or winging out the elbows).

- Position supplies and equipment in work areas; clear the area of unnecessary items (e.g., to pay bills, obtain needed supplies, such as calculator, bills, and stamps, before beginning task).
- Organize the work center; having the necessary supplies and equipment increases productivity with less effort (e.g., place the can opener near the canned goods; place the most frequently used items within easy reach on counters or shelves immediately above or below counter height).
- Use labor-saving devices (e.g., use wheels for transport; in the kitchen, use an electric mixer and food processor; for outdoors, use an electric garage door opener and motorized lawn mower).
- Schedule regular rest breaks; fatigue can result in poor body mechanics and reduced safety awareness; clients should alternate light and heavy tasks throughout the day and week; heavy work tasks (e.g., oven cleaning, stripping, and waxing floors,

TABLE 28–14. **HOME MANAGEMENT FOR CLIENTS WITH IMPAIRMENT OF LOWER EXTREMITY MOBILITY**

ADL Area	Adaptive Equipment	Adaptive Techniques
Meal preparation and cleanup	Transport items using a wheelchair laptray Use laptray as work surface to protect lap from hot pans Use stove with controls at front Use angled mirror above range to see contents of pots	Remove cabinet doors to eliminate need to maneuver around them Place frequently used items on easy-to-reach shelves, above and below countertop level Increase height of wheelchair to allow use of standard-height countertops
Laundry	Use front-loading washer and dryer	
Housekeeping	Use self-propelled lightweight vacuum	

doing yard work) should be delegated to another family member or a paid professional.

- Use proper body mechanics (e.g., use a wide base of support, use both sides of the body, keep objects close to the body, face objects when reaching or lifting to avoid twisting or pushing rather than pulling, and alternate positions and motions to avoid fatigue).

Environmental Modifications

Environmental modifications are considered a modification, compensation, adaptation strategy. Compared to restoration and compensation, in which the practitioner directly influences client functioning, environmental modification is a means of indirectly maximizing client function. Modifications can range from extensive home modifications to make a home wheelchair accessible to low-cost strategies, such as removing obstacles to make a household safer for an older person who has impaired vision and mobility.

Education of Client and Family

Client and family education is a key feature of occupational therapy because the approaches of restoration, compensation, and prevention involve learning new strategies and, more important, incorporating these strategies into client and family habits and lifestyles. In some circumstances, the practitioner may provide education to the family in addition to client education or in place of client education.

Guidelines for Client and Family Education

The following guidelines are central to effective client and family education (Bowling, 1981; Kautzman, 1991):

- *Develop a clear plan and purpose for the teaching session.* Clear goals for teaching can assist both the practitioner and client regarding expectations and anticipated outcome. Based on client and family motivation, cognitive status, the skill level needed to be achieved, and the time available for the teaching and learning processes, the expected outcomes or goals may vary. The three levels of goals are knowledge, application, and problem solving. At the level of knowledge, a client is asked to recall basic facts presented by the practitioner. For example, the practitioner may ask a client to name the five techniques used for good body mechanics. At the application level, the client and family are shown ways of incorporating this information into home management. The practitioner may demonstrate how to use body mechanics when retrieving food from the oven during meal preparation and then ask the client to incorporate the same strategy while performing the task. At the level of problem solving, the client is asked to use information in new situations that have not been demonstrated by the practitioner. For example, the practitioner may ask the client to demonstrate how to use good body mechanics when shoveling snow.
- *Present information that is appropriate to the clients' educational and emotional levels.* The choice of terminology used with a client who has had few years of formal education should vary from that used with a client who has a college education. Client readiness to receive information will vary. The client may be overwhelmed with life changes caused by the disability and unable to concentrate on issues that the practitioner feels should be addressed. Therefore, for a task that a client may not be concerned with, but that will be needed at home, the inpatient practitioner may try to increase client awareness by introducing appropriate adaptive equipment. Once the client has returned home, the motivation to perform in this area may increase. Then the outpatient practitioner can promote client application and problem solving in the outpatient occupational therapy program.
- *Clear instructions increase the possibility of client carryover.* For example, instead of telling a client to use proper body mechanics for all activities, it is preferable and more realistic to begin with having the client identify one or two activities that require these techniques. Another strategy for increasing carryover is to explain the rationale for the therapy recommendations.
- *Ask open-ended questions to ensure client understanding.* For example, ask, "Why is it important for you to incorporate proper body mechanics into your day-to-day activities?"
- *Use the client's response to determine the amount of information presented during a session.* If the client's attention is waning or if the client's learning ability is decreased, termination of the teaching session is recommended. If the amount of information is extensive, it may be preferable to present it over several sessions. Taking the added time to ensure client competence in performance is time well spent.
- *Promote the highest level of learning possible, preferably at the problem-solving level.* Involve the clients by asking questions about how information presented might affect their lifestyles. For example, a practitioner may ask of a client with arthritis, "Which joint protection techniques do you think you would use at home? How could you use those techniques while cooking?" It is preferable to follow this up with client demonstration to ensure that the client has integrated the information into pertinent tasks.
- *Illustrate or demonstrate the points being taught.* Use of aids such as demonstration, pictures, videotapes, and handouts reinforce teaching and help the client and family remember the information presented. A study of client–doctor visits found that clients remembered only half of the information covered (Ley, 1972). Some of the ways of reinforcing teaching include repeating information throughout the session and allowing adequate time for practice by the client or family members to ensure that they are comfortable with and capable of using the information outside the therapy situation. If the client or family

member cannot gain adequate competency or perform the task in a safe manner, then other options, such as a paid caregiver or identifying community support (e.g., home health aide) need to be considered.

SAFETY PROCEDURES AND EMERGENCY RESPONSES

The occupational practice framework (AOTA, in press) defines safety procedures and emergency responses as "knowing and performing preventive procedures to maintain a safe environment and recognizing sudden, unexpected hazardous situations and initiating emergency action to reduce the threat to health and safety" (pg. 35). Interventions for safety procedures and emergency responsiveness include restoration of deficient client skills and abilities, environmental or task adaptation, and provision of safety education to both client and caregiver. To differentiate between safe and unsafe behavior, Holm, Rogers. and James (see Section 1) suggest that the occupational therapy practitioner explore the attitudes of the client, caregiver, and family to determine the level of risk acceptable to each person. Additional considerations include the client's comfort level with risk, the client's ability to analyze risk associated with a specific task and ability to devise a plan for managing that risk, and the client's ability to quickly implement an appropriate response to a safety issue. Finally, the practitioner needs to consider his or her perspective regarding the presence of an unsafe behavior and if or when an intervention needs to be provided. For example, two practitioners might observe the same client perform a homemaking task such as preparing an omelet. If there is smoke coming from the pan, one practitioner may feel comfortable waiting for a longer period of time to see if the client, although slowly, comes to recognize a safety situation and acts to resolve it. Another practitioner might intervene more quickly, negating the clients' opportunity to demonstrate appropriate safety behaviors.

Pedretti (1985) and Okkema (1993) noted that impulsiveness, decreased insight into disability, impaired judgment, impaired memory, poor attention to the environment, limited ability to process all information relevant to a situation, difficulty anticipating the consequences of a particular action or breakdown in any part of the problem-solving process might compromise an individual's safety awareness. For example, a client with traumatic brain injury with moderate cognitive limitations may lack insight into his or her disability that results in unsafe behavior.

To enhance client's insight, the practitioner might ask the client to predict how well he or she might perform a task such as preparing an omelet. The practitioner could videotape the client's performance and review the tape with the client to determine which aspects of his or her behavior reinforced safe behavior and which ones needed to be changed to enhance safe performance. Since there are a number of client factors that could result in unsafe behavior, the selection of appropriate restorative interventions is based on which client factor is compromised. Chapter 30, Section 5 offers additional intervention strategies.

For the older client, normal physical and sensory changes of aging can affect safe and efficient performance, and environmental changes in an individual's home may be indicated. For instance, an 85-year-old requires three times the amount of light for functional vision as does a younger individual (Schreter, 1991). Sources for making home modifications include the American Association of Retired Persons (n.d.) and the American Occupational Therapy Association (n.d.). Environmental adaptations are related to appropriate identification of client skills and abilities and can vary from low- or no-cost considerations (removing area rugs to prevent falls) to expensive alternatives (making a home wheelchair accessible). Chapter 31, Section 2 discusses assistive technology to promote safe environments. One example is an emergency call system available on a rental basis. The service provides a pendant with a telephone dialing mechanism. If there is no verbal response from the client, an ambulance or other identified contact is called.

Dutton (1995) noted that safety education might allow an individual to be discharged to a less restrictive environment. However, clients do not always see the need for safety education. Safety education requires vigilant application of abstract concepts and may be problematic when a client exhibits cognitive impairments. For example, it may be difficult for a client with memory problems to attend to hip precautions when performing homemaking tasks. The practitioner often suggests changes in habit and must be sensitive to the challenges of behavior change and must identify strategies that will increase compliance and promote safety in the home. The practitioner might ask the client to identify potential safety concerns in the home and use that conversation as the starting point to increase client compliance in adhering to safety precautions. Allen and Blue (1998) designed a checklist of safety precautions that a caregiver can use to promote safe functioning of daily living and household tasks.

Training Apartment

A training apartment, available in many health-care settings, can be used to simulate the experience of returning home to explore potential issues that may need further consideration. The time spent in a training apartment may range from a 1-hr individual session to a 1- to 2-night stay. Given the anticipated living circumstances, the client and family members (if appropriate) can attempt personal care and home management tasks that will be required after discharge. This simulation provides an opportunity to identify areas in which the client and family members feel comfortable and issues that need further consideration.

The practitioner then can design intervention strategies to prepare for discharge to home.

HOME VISITS

After hospitalization, a question often arises about whether the client will be safe at home. Home visits are conducted to evaluate the client's level of functional independence and safety at home and to provide the client and family with recommendations concerning accessibility, safety, and home modifications. During the home visit, the client completes activities that typically are performed at home, such as making a bed, transferring in and out of the tub, moving on and off the toilet, and preparing food in the kitchen. The tasks should be relevant to anticipated home responsibilities as well as to client and family experiences. Anderson and Ross (1992) provided a sample home-evaluation questionnaire.

The results of the home visit and recommendations should be discussed with the client and family. Recommendations are then written to reinforce the discussion. When a home visit is not feasible, obtaining information from the client or family member about to the discharge environment is a useful option.

CONCLUSION

The occupational therapy practitioner plays a major role in facilitating a client's return to the role of home manager. Intervention strategies include restoration, compensation, environmental modification, and education. The practitioner selects the intervention strategies on the basis of factors such as client and family goals, client condition, anticipated length of intervention, interdisciplinary goals, and the practitioner's professional judgment about skills needed to perform pertinent home management.

SECTION III

Sexuality and Disability

KRYSS McKENNA

Attitudes and Values
Communication Skills
Service Delivery Model
Permission
Limited Information
Specific Suggestions
Intensive Therapy
Illness, Disability, and Sexual Problems
Problem-Solving Solutions to Sexual Dysfunction
Work Simplification and Energy Conservation
Adaptive Techniques for Specific Deficits
Use of Adjunct Modalities and Technologies
Other Advice and Suggestions
Sexual Education and Counseling Programs
Contraception and Sexually Transmitted Diseases
Menstruation, Pregnancy, and Childbirth
Conclusion
Acknowledgments

Sexuality develops throughout life in response to a person's physical, psychological, and social development (Sipski & Alexander, 1997a). It is part of everyday thoughts, feelings, behaviors and relationships, shaping gender identity and contributing to self-esteem and social roles (Katchadourian, 1989). Sexuality is fundamental to human life and "all people are sexual by virtue of being human" (Linton & Rousso, 1988, p. 115). Illness, disability, and some treatments can affect sexual function and the way that people express their sexuality (Couldrick, 1998a).

Linton and Rousso (1988) asserted that people with disabilities have sexual needs and concerns that are more similar to than different from those of people without disabilities. The most significant problem people with disabilities confront has been stereotypical and discriminatory attitudes (Couldrick, 1998a). Because society has traditionally placed such emphasis on physical perfection, people with disabilities were once viewed as unattractive, lacking in wholeness, and not in need of closeness and sexual expression (Linton & Rousso, 1988). However, with the liberalization of societal attitudes, sexuality is now accepted as being integral to human existence and is a recognized component of quality of life (Bowling, 1991). Thus sexuality has a fundamental place in the rehabilitation process (Sipski & Alexander, 1997a) and is an important concern of occupational therapy practitioners. With knowledge of anatomy, physiology, and disability and an ability to assess and treat areas of function that affect occupational roles, occupational therapy practitioners are in an ideal position to provide clients with intervention related to sexuality (Couldrick, 1998b).

ATTITUDES AND VALUES

Sexuality is an intimate issue and occupational therapy practitioners can feel uncomfortable addressing this topic with clients. Reasons for this include a lack of training in sexuality education and counseling during professional education and the fact that sexuality is a value-laden area, heavily influenced by a person's attitudes, life experiences, culture, and religion (Couldrick, 1998b). While the majority of occupational therapy practitioners acknowledge sexuality as a legitimate area of concern for them as professionals, fewer address sexuality with clients (Agnew, Poulsen, & Maas, 1985; Conine, Christie, Hammond, & Smith, 1979; Evans, 1985; Novak & Mitchell, 1988). By failing to address sexuality with clients, practitioners can reinforce the societal myth that people with an illness or disability are asexual (Gender, 1992).

Practitioners must examine both societal attitudes toward people with disabilities and their own beliefs, values, and attitudes about sexuality. Cultural and religious biases must be put aside, and there must be an acknowledgment that there is no universal agreement about acceptable or unacceptable, right or wrong sexual behavior (Couldrick, 1999). Practitioners need to be sensitive to others' perspectives and nonjudgmentally discuss sexual preferences and activities that differ from their own.

Clients can be emotionally vulnerable and begin to assign sexual feelings to a therapeutic relationship, particularly in settings where there is a lengthy stay and extensive physical contact during therapy sessions (Dunn, 1997). Blurring of personal and professional relationships can be damaging for both clients and practitioners; therefore, maintenance of appropriate personal boundaries and consideration of sexual ethics are vital (Alexander, 1997).

COMMUNICATION SKILLS

Knowing how to initiate the topic of sexuality with clients and being able to recognize cues that a client is ready to discuss these issues help practitioners invite clients to explore potential issues in a nonintrusive and respectful manner (Couldrick, 1999; Herson, Hart, Gordon, & Rintala, 1999). To engage in a discussion of sexual issues, there is also a need to be confident and fluent in the terminology and language appropriate to the interaction. Practitioners must be sensitive to clients' needs for privacy and must demonstrate respect for confidentiality (Couldrick, 1999).

SERVICE DELIVERY MODEL

A model that is extensively used in sexuality counseling is the Permission, Limited Information, Specific Suggestions, and Intensive Therapy (PLISSIT) model (Annon, 1976). The first three levels are appropriate for intervention by occupational therapy practitioners; the fourth level requires referral to a specialist in sexual counseling (Neistadt, 1986).

Permission

The permission level acknowledges the client's sexuality, gives legitimacy to his or her concerns, and validates communication about sexuality (Gender, 1992). An atmosphere of acceptance can be achieved in a number of ways. Open responses can be given to clients' direct questions or to their subtle cues related to sexuality. The occupational therapy practitioner can introduce the topic in a nonthreatening way. For example, during an interview with the client, a gradual approach to the introduction of the topic of sexuality can be used, moving from general to more specific and from less to more personal topics (Dunn, 1997). Alternatively, a general statement can be made as a lead-in, such as, "Many people who have had a heart attack have concerns about being able to be close to someone again. Is this a concern of yours?" (Waldman & Eliasof, 1997). Another approach is to introduce the topic of sexuality when explaining the role of occupational therapy or the content of a rehabilitation program to a client. By assisting the client to dress and groom in a way that expresses his or her sexuality, the occupational therapy practitioner can endorse sexuality as a legitimate concern of the client (Dunn, 1997).

Limited Information

The limited information level focuses on providing clients with general, factual information. This can include details about the anatomy and physiology of the sexual organs and contraception, the effect of medications on sexuality, problem-solving strategies found to be useful by clients with a similar illness or disability, and the dispelling of myths and misconceptions (Dunn, 1997).

Specific Suggestions

The third level of the PLISSIT model is more client centered, focusing on clients' specific sexuality concerns or problems (Summerville & McKenna, 1998). The occupational therapy practitioner and client work together to set goals and explore individualized ways to solve problems (Dunn, 1997). This level requires more specific knowledge and skills, which the occupational therapy practitioner can acquire from postgraduate courses, continuing self-education.

Intensive Therapy

To provide intensive therapy, the expertise of a specialist sexuality counselor is required. This can include, for example, relationship counseling or the management of infertility or severe mental health problems (Summerville & McKenna, 1998).

ILLNESS, DISABILITY, AND SEXUAL PROBLEMS

Illness and disability can affect sexuality in a number of ways. Disruption to the vascular, neurological, or **endocrine** systems can have a physiological impact on the sex organs and sexual response cycle. Sexuality can be impeded by disorders that affect mobility, sensation, energy levels, communication, and bodily comfort (Linton & Rousso, 1988). Secondary complications such as **rigidity, spasticity,** pressure sores, and **contractures** can interfere with sexual expression (Sipski & Alexander, 1997b).

Treatment modalities can also affect sexual function. For example, pelvic irradiation can lead to vaginal dryness and antidepressant medication can lower interest in sex (Sipski & Alexander, 1997b). Aside from physical problems, psychological issues such as depression, anxiety, low self-image, and role disruption can interfere with sexual expression (Sipski & Alexander, 1997b). Thus the reasons for sexual dysfunction in clients with disabilities can be multifactorial, representing an interplay between physiological, physical, and psychological factors. All of these aspects—as well as the client's and his or her partner's needs, values, and priorities—must be considered when dealing with sexuality.

Illnesses or disabilities that directly affect the sexual organs or sexual response cycle are spinal cord injuries, traumatic brain injury, and cancer. Depending on the type and level of spinal cord injury, sensory and motor loss in the limbs, trunk, and genitalia can alter a client's physiological and physical capacity for sexual activity (Drench, 1982).

In males, spinal cord injury can affect the ability to achieve an erection and ejaculation and can affect fertility. Males with a complete spinal cord lesion can retain the ability to achieve a reflex but not a psychogenic erection. Reflex erections are produced by direct tactile stimulation of the penis and occur independently of erotic stimuli or thoughts. They are mediated by the parasympathetic nervous system and require intact sacral reflexes (S2 to S4). Therefore, reflex erections are usually preserved in spinal cord lesions above the L2 level (Smith & Bodner, 1993). However, reflex erections may not occur when required, may be insufficient for penetration, and may be transitory in nature (Yarkony & Chen, 1995). Psychogenic erections originate from impulses in the hypothalamus and limbic system, precipitated by thoughts and erotic stimuli, often in the absence of direct tactile stimulation (Smith & Bodner, 1993). Ejaculation is a complex physiological process, mediated by the sympathetic nervous system and thoracolumbar spinal segments. Ejaculation is more common with more **caudal** lesions, although the ejaculate can have decreased volume, sperm counts, and sperm motility (Yarkony & Chen, 1995).

In females with spinal cord injury, sensory loss and decreased lubrication can reduce the possibility of achieving orgasm, although fertility is often preserved after a period of amenorrhea. According to Yarkony and Chen (1995), "[V]aginal lubrication may occur reflexly with lesions at T9, not at all with lesions between T10 and T12, and psychogenic lubrication may occur in lesions below T12" (p. 335).

The sexual organs and their neurovascular supply can be directly affected by cancer. For example, prostate and ovarian cancers are common forms of cancer (Waldman & Eliasof, 1997). Treatments such as chemotherapy, radiotherapy, and surgery can produce sexual impairment. In particular, chemotherapy and radiotherapy can cause either temporary or permanent loss of fertility in both men and women (Waldman & Eliasof, 1997).

The effect of traumatic brain injury on sexuality has not been extensively researched. The percentage of clients who report sexual dysfunction after brain injury is varied, most likely owing to the heterogeneity of the samples included in different studies (Sandel, 1997). Losses of libido, erectile dysfunction, and the decline in orgasm have been reported after brain injury (Sandel, 1997). Frontal lobe lesions have been linked to hypersexuality and disinhibited behavior. Endocrine disturbances can occur after brain injury. Posttraumatic **hypopituitarism** with permanent hypogonadotropic **hypogonadism** can result in loss of libido and impotence (Sandel, 1997). Temporal lobe seizure disorders can directly affect the sex organs, causing impotence in males and reproductive dysfunction in females. This occurs because the temporal lobes exert a modulatory influence on the hypothalamic regulation of the pituitary gland (Sandel, 1997).

After a CVA, a marked decline in sexual activity has been reported. In addition, diminished libido, arousal problems, erectile dysfunction, reduced vaginal lubrication, and difficulties with ejaculation and orgasm have been noted (Korpelainen, Nieminen, & Myllyla, 1999). The cause of these changes may have less to do with the stroke itself and more to do with the loss of independence that occurs after stroke, as well motor, sensory, cognitive, psychological, and communication deficits (Buzzelli, di-Francesco, Giaquinto, & Nolfe, 1997). Sensory loss, muscle weakness, changes in muscle tone, and bladder and bowel incontinence can affect the client's ability to participate in sexual activity. In other illnesses and disabilities, motor symptoms and complications can also affect sexual function. For example, in spinal cord injury, lower extremity spasms and flexor tone, contractures, and pressure sores can cause difficulties with positioning and mobility. Loss of ROM, stiffness, and pain can cause similar difficulties in clients with arthritis, as can loss of motion and balance in clients who have undergone amputation.

For clients who have coronary artery disease or chronic obstructive pulmonary disease, symptoms such as chest pain, lack of cardiac reserve, breathlessness, and coughing can affect sexual function. Therefore, there are physiological reasons for a sexual impairment. although there is no direct effect on the sexual organs. While varying rates of sexual dysfunction, such as erectile failure, have been reported, it is more likely that this is to the result of anxiety, misconceptions, depression, and avoidance (Krukofsky, 1988).

Sex is a less physiologically demanding activity than has previously been believed (Stitik & Benevento, 1997). According to Masters and Johnson (1966), peak heart rates between 110 and 180 beats per minute (bpm) have been recorded in males and females during orgasm. In men, systolic blood pressure can rise 40–100 millimeters of mercury (mm Hg) and diastolic blood pressure can rise 20–50 mm Hg; in females, the elevations are almost as high (Hellerstein & Friedman, 1970). In terms of metabolic equivalents (METs), orgasm requires 4–6 METs for a brief period (Cohen, 1986), while the overall energy expenditure for sexual activity is around 3.7 METs (Cole, Levin, Whitley, & Young, 1979). Climbing two flights of stairs and completing 20 steps in 10 sec is a task that requires similar levels of energy expenditure. Indeed, it has been argued that a rough estimate of a client's readiness for safe return to sexual activity can be made by having the client complete a two-flight of stairs test (Stitik & Benevento, 1997). A more reliable indicator is the client's performance on an exercise stress test.

Psychological symptoms can have a profound effect on sexuality. The onset of a disability or chronic illness can be a catastrophic event, derailing not only the client's life but also that of his or her partner and family. Major depression, anger, anxiety, and withdrawal from life can affect the way that clients define themselves, causing them to feel diminished self-worth and to have a negative view of their sexual selves (Krukofsky, 1988). Role disruption can also accompany the onset of disability and chronic illness, with the client's partner being required to take on a caring role. Clients can feel a loss of control over their lives, which can negatively affect their sense of competence, including their sexual competence (Waldman & Eliasof, 1997).

Clients who must depend on their partner to manage their basic needs have reported more sexual problems than clients who are independent (Monga & Kerrigan, 1997). Disfigurement and altered body image, fear of rejection or of a recurrence of the event, and partner reluctance and protectiveness can all have a negative impact on sexual expression (Thurer, 1992).

PROBLEM-SOLVING SOLUTIONS TO SEXUAL DYSFUNCTION

Applying the PLISSIT model to the conditions just discussed, clients and partners should first be provided with permission to discuss sexuality as part of the education or, if in place, total rehabilitation program. It should never be assumed that a client is too sick or too old to have sexual concerns (Krukofsky, 1988). Failure to invite openness to discuss sexual issues can cause clients to repress or deny their sexual expression or to make decisions based on their own understandings or misconceptions (Krukofsky, 1988).

The content of the second phase, limited information, is specific to the disease or condition in question. For example, for clients with cardiac or pulmonary disorders, general information can be provided regarding the timing of resumption of sexual activity. To minimize cardiac workload, clients should be advised that sexual activity is best undertaken after resting, when relaxed, in cooler environments and at least 2 to 3 hr after a heavy meal or alcohol consumption (Krukofsky, 1988). In addition to these precautions, clients with chronic obstructive pulmonary disease are advised to avoid sex immediately on waking because of the likelihood of a build up of secretions that can precipitate coughing. Furthermore, participation in a prescribed exercise program can increase overall tolerance for activity and improve sexual function (Stitik & Benevento, 1997).

In the specific suggestions phase, advice and assistance are individually tailored to clients' particular goals and problems. However, a number of problem-solving principles apply.

Work Simplification and Energy Conservation

It is important that clients conserve energy during sexual activity and do not become overstressed or fatigued. For example, sitting and side lying require less energy and upper limb strength than traditional positions, and the use of a waterbed or rocking chair can assist with achieving a momentum during sex (Stitik & Benevento, 1997). Medications can be used prophylactically to reduce symptoms such as chest or joint pain.

Adaptive Techniques for Specific Deficits

For clients with chronic obstructive pulmonary disease, positions that put pressure on the chest need to be avoided (Stitik & Benevento, 1997). The same is true for clients with arthritis, for whom positions that place prolonged pressure on painful, inflamed joints are not recommended (Buckwalter, Wernimont, & Buckwalter, 1982). The partners of clients who have had a stroke can be advised of the areas of the client's body without sensory loss that can be touched or kissed (Monga & Kerrigan, 1997). Clients with stroke who do not have shoulder pain can be advised to assume a side lying position on the affected side to leave the unaffected arm free for use during sex (Monga & Kerrigan, 1997). If hip adductor spasticity is an issue, rear vaginal entry requires only minimal hip abduction (Monga & Kerrigan, 1997). For clients with above-knee amputations, use of pillows can help maintain stability; and for those with above-elbow amputations, side lying is the most viable option (Buckwalter et al., 1982).

Use of Adjunct Modalities and Technologies

Clients with arthritis may benefit from applying a hot pack or taking a warm bath before sex to achieve more pain-free motion (Buckwalter et al., 1982). After sex, the application of ice can reduce inflammation in affected joints. In male clients with spinal cord lesions, advice regarding the treatment of erectile dysfunction can include the surgical implantation of a penile prosthesis or the use of vacuum erection devices or intracorporeal injection therapy (Smith & Bodner, 1993). Electrovibration and electroejaculation are methods that can be used to obtain semen (Yarkony & Chen, 1995), although specialist referral may be required when clients want to learn more about these options.

Other Advice and Suggestions

Occupational therapy practitioners can discuss alternative means of expressing sexuality with clients. Sexuality is more than physical contact and exploration of alternatives may provide couples with other ways to engage in sexual expression. It may also be appropriate to encourage partners to take a more active role in the expression of the couple's intimacy (Linton & Rousso, 1988).

SEXUAL EDUCATION AND COUNSELING PROGRAMS

Although sexual education and counseling in the rehabilitation of clients with illness or disability are important, how best to deliver these services is an open question. One option is to provide clients and their partners with written or audiovisual information that they can consider in the privacy of their own environment. Afterward, they can meet with the practitioner to address any further concerns. Alternatively, clients and their partners can participate in group sessions or support groups, in which group members are able to benefit from sharing in others' experiences. According to Tepper (1992), clients with spinal cord injury indicated that the most valuable source of sexual information and advice was other clients with the same disability who had more sexual experience. A final option is to offer a formal sexuality program. Programs for clients with head injuries and developmental disabilities (Dunn, 1997), spinal cord injuries (Tepper, 1992), and chronic obstructive pulmonary disease (Spica, 1992) are described in the literature.

The timing of the provision of sexual education and counseling has been debated in the literature. Tepper (1992) suggested that a discussion of sexuality should be initiated early, even if only to provide the client with permission to raise issues in this area. Waldman and Eliasof (1997) suggested that a client's sexual health be determined during an initial interview, ascertaining relationship status, sexual history, prior dysfunctions, and the importance of sexuality in his or her life. Others have argued that these discussions are best left until a strong rapport has been established between client and therapist, although with shortened hospital stays, this may mean that the topic goes unaddressed (Dunn, 1997). Alternatively, discussion of this topic may coincide with the client going home on a weekend pass, after other more immediate concerns have been resolved (Monga & Kerrigan, 1997). The consensus seems to be that while each client's needs should be managed individually, discussions about sexuality should not be delayed but offered early in the recovery process (Monga & Kerrigan, 1997).

CONTRACEPTION AND SEXUALLY TRANSMITTED DISEASES

Sexuality education should include information about contraception and prevention of sexually transmitted diseases. Not all contraceptive methods are suitable for clients with illnesses or disabilities for a number of reasons. Some require the ability to plan and make judgments, others necessitate manual dexterity, and the oral contraceptive pill may be contraindicated for certain conditions (Kewman, Warschausky, Engel, & Warzak, 1997).

MENSTRUATION, PREGNANCY, AND CHILDBIRTH

For some clients, such as those with traumatic brain injury and developmental delays, occupational therapy practitioners may be involved in providing menstrual hygiene training. For clients with loss of upper limb function, practitioners may provide advice to assist with the placement or application of sanitary products.

A woman with a chronic illness or disability needs to consider the effect that pregnancy will have on her condition and the possible effect her condition will have on the pregnancy. For example, women with a spinal cord injury are more likely to experience urinary tract infections, pulmonary distress, and anemia during pregnancy than other women (Sipski, 1997). Occupational therapy practitioners have a role in addressing the functional concerns of clients during pregnancy and childbirth, including the following (Freda, Cioschi, & Nilson, 1989; Neistadt & Freda, 1987):

- Mobility and balance problems owing to increased weight and shift in center of gravity.
- Joint instability caused by hormonal changes and the softening of ligaments and tendons.
- Increased pain as a result of weight gain and other bodily changes.
- Decreased transfer independence caused by weight gain and unequal distribution of weight.
- Decreased independence in manual wheelchair mobility.
- Decreased endurance secondary to diminished respiratory capacity caused by increased uterus size.

- Decreased independence in ADL (especially lower extremity hygiene and dressing).
- Decreased independence in homemaking owing to decreased mobility.
- Positioning difficulties for labor and delivery because of spasticity, contracture, or other deformities.

CONCLUSION

Occupational therapy practitioners can play an important role in sexuality education and counseling for clients with chronic illnesses or disabilities. They can help clients explore their sexuality, problem solve ways that they can express themselves sexually, and assist them to achieve fulfilling lives.

ACKNOWLEDGMENTS

This section was adapted from the section by Maureen Freda that appeared in the 9th edition of this book. Freda's work provided the structure for this section as well as some of its content. This is gratefully acknowledged.

SECTION IV

Childrearing and Care Giving

ELLEN S. COHN
ALEXIS D. HENRY
KIMBERLY MARKS

Childrearing and **care giving,** essential relationships to the continuity of life, are common yet highly complex occupations. Both public and private, these occupations are intensely personal, openly shared, and socially constructed. In this chapter, the terms *childrearing* and *care giving* are used interchangeably to describe the occupation of nurturing the well-being of others. Understanding the meaning, ideals, and values of childrearing and care giving from societal and individual perspectives is essential to occupational therapy practice.

Historically, intervention focused primarily on parents whose child had a disability. Interventions were typically designed to help parents support the development of children with disabilities, and limited attention was given to helping parents create sustainable routines to enhance **family** priorities and lifestyles. In fact, Llewellyn (1994) stated that the occupations of childrearing and care giving were "neglected human occupations". Also overlooked by occupational therapy are caregivers who have a disability themselves. Accordingly, this chapter focuses on childrearing and care giving occupations, caring for individuals with disabilities across the life course, being a caregiver with a disability, and interventions for caregivers.

CHILDREARING AND CARE-GIVING OCCUPATIONS

Childrearing and care giving take place in multiple environments and can be conceptualized using ecological (Bronfenbrenner, 1979), developmental (Olson et al. 1984), and occupation-centered (Jackson, 1998) perspectives. Ecological perspectives recognize the numerous factors influencing caregiver's ideals, decisions, and actions. The family—defined as "a group of people living together or in close contact to take care of each other and provide guidance for their dependent members" (Wood, 1995, p. 437)—is the center of the ecological system, supporting the growth of family members. Personal factors such as family member characteristics (age, education, and socioeconomic status) and characteristics of the care recipient (age, type of disability) influence how a family conceptualizes parenting, disability, and the role of services (Luster & Okagaki, 1993).

Cultural and societal factors also influence care-giving actions. In Asian cultures, the elderly are cared for within the family; thus, alternative living situations may not be accepted options (Spector, 1996). In the Hmong culture, epilepsy is seen as a gift possessed only by the respected shaman. This cultural belief is contradictory to the medical model in Western societies, which holds that epilepsy is a disease to be treated with medication. Such clashing worldviews have major implications for practitioners striving to support people in their childrearing and care-giving occupations (Fadiman, 1997). Only when the influence of cultural beliefs is examined is it possible to understand caregivers' actions and goals for intervention. A societal influence on childrearing and care giving is the shifting role of fathers. In earlier generations, fathers had limited participation in the daily lives of children, but fathers today are often active participants in childrearing and care giving (Lamb, 2000). Thus childrearing and care giving are viewed as gender-neutral occupations.

Extended family, neighborhoods, co-workers, and other parents may be integral components of a caregiver's personal social network, therefore influencing the attitudes and beliefs of caregivers (Dyck, 1990). This social network can provide childrearing assistance and support for care givers. Although social networks are typically a source of support for care givers, for some, extended family members may undermine the confidence of a struggling parent.

Another factor influencing caregivers and families is the developmental concept of the family life cycle. Olson, et al. (1984) proposed a model to conceptualize and describe the family life cycle that includes specific phases or life events and challenges to be confronted at each point in the cycle. For example, families make a transition when a child is old enough to be launched from the immediate family system and live on his or her own or in a new setting. Developmental trajectories intersect with other family dynamics, and as families' progress over time, changes occur in both structure and function. Practitioners need to understand and consider the impact of the major events that families may be experiencing at any given time.

Along with ecological and developmental perspectives, scholars in occupational science advocate for an occupation-centered perspective. Rather than focusing on specific tasks or activities in isolation, separate from an understanding of the meaning of tasks, an occupation-centered analysis focuses on the overarching occupation itself. Ruddick's (1989) analysis of mothering helps explain the meaning associated with childrearing across cultures and countries. Although Ruddick focused on mothering, her analysis is applicable to fathers as well. According to Ruddick, the work of parenting includes protection, nurturance, and training. Protection requires scrutiny of the child and the environment, coupled with an acceptance that a child will inevitably be subjected to minor and major mishaps that parents cannot control. Parents must accept their own limits as protector and still continue with the intent of keeping their child safe. Protection falls on a continuum from a lack of protection to overbearing. Nurturance, or fostering growth, refers to developing a child's body and spirit. Fostering growth requires the ability to change as the child grows. A caregiver provides the conditions for growth, and these conditions vary among cultures, socioeconomic levels, and other environmental factors. Training involves teaching the child behaviors and values necessary to achieve acceptance by family and society. Along with protection, nurturance, and training, parents of a child with disabilities identify advocacy and obtaining appropriate resources as critical aspects of parenting (Landsman, 1998).

Jackson (1998) addressed the "enfolded nature of occupations" (p. 57), which also honors the multiple factors that influence occupations. DeVault's (1991) research suggested that parents are often not delineating their childrearing and care-giving tasks; rather they are enfolding them within one another. DeVault's example of feeding the family illustrated that parents provide sustenance to the child while simultaneously fostering social communication skills for acceptance into society. Dyck's (1990) analysis of working parents offers another example of enfolded occupations. Dyck proposed that women develop strategies for remaining a good mother while participating in the labor force. Strategies might involve hiring an after-school baby-sitter to drive a child to activities so the parent can work while the child engages in developmentally stimulating programs. An occupation-centered analysis directs practitioners to consider the social, symbolic, and interpersonal meaning associated with childrearing and care giving. (Jackson, 1998).

CARING FOR INDIVIDUALS WITH DISABILITIES ACROSS THE LIFE COURSE

Parenting a Child with a Disability

When parents learn their child has a disability, they may feel anger and may need to mourn the loss of the idea of a "perfect" child. Initially, parents may have feelings of shock and denial, followed by anger and depression. Parents may repeat the process of mourning as they encounter unexpected discrepancies between reality and their hopes and expectations. Among and within families, there may be great variability in reactions to and perceptions of the family member with a disability. Mothers of children with disabilities report more stress than fathers, whereas fathers report more trouble forming bonds with their children (Beckman et al. 1991). Services need to be tailored to meet the different needs of each family member.

Parenting a child with a disability does not always result in long-term negative effects on family members. Rather, the lives of many parents, across socioeconomic classes and in families with children with various disabilities, are positively changed as a result of the birth of a child with a disability (Scorgie & Sobsey, 2000). Some parents may reexamine their expectations, with a transformation of values, resulting in a new sense of what really matters. In one study (Scorgie & Sobsey, 2000), parents report acquiring new life-enriching roles, such as being a parent group leader, writer, or speaker at conferences. Some parents learned better communication skills and used these skills to foster open, supportive family relationships. Scorgie and Sobsey recommended that practitioners avoid catastrophizing the effects disability can have on a family. Rather, parents should be made aware that initial feelings of grief are common but that many families adapt to disability in the family. Connecting parents in the initial stages of coping with parents who have adapted positively to life with a child with a disability can aid families in forming a positive outlook for the future.

Caring for an Adult with a Disability

Parents of a child with disabilities often continue parenting throughout the child's life into adulthood (Hodapp, Dykens, Evans, & Merighi, 1992). Adolescence is often a time when caregivers realize the permanence of the child's disabilities and begin to worry about the future. The features of the disability may change as the child ages and grows (Seltzer, Krauss, Orsmond, & Vestal, 1997). As the caregiver ages, his or her health needs may change. Aging can have an effect on community involvement, leading to increased social isolation and stress for both the person with a disability and the caregiver. Practitioners may address the caregiver's physical and psychological well-being by providing additional supports in the home and community, making referrals for respite services, and, if appropriate, providing strategies to minimize behavioral difficulties (Biegel, Sales, & Schulz, 1991).

Middle-aged adults—often described as the sandwich generation—may face the simultaneous demands of parenting adolescents or young adults and caring for their elderly parents (Sorensen & Zarit, 1996). Family caregivers are the primary source of support for frail older people, and 80% of all family caregivers for the elderly provide unpaid help 7 days a week (Hasselkus, 1989). Hasselkus's research with family caregivers for frail older people living in the community suggested that caregivers are focused on getting things done to sustain the family system, achieving a sense of well-being for the care receiver, and achieving a sense of well-being for themselves. Hasselkus recommended collaborative intervention in which the practitioner strives to understand the meaning caregivers attach to their role and supports the caregiver to balance daily occupations.

BEING A CAREGIVER WITH A DISABILITY

Adults with disabilities experience the same desires to form intimate relationships and to have and raise children as do adults without disabilities. Estimates on the prevalence of disability suggest that there are millions of families in the United States in which one or both parents have a disability (LaPlante, Carlson, Kaye, & Bradsher, 1996; Nicholson, Biebel, Hinden, Henry, & Stier, 2001). Moreover, families in which an adult has a disability have an increased likelihood of having at least one child with a disability (LaPlante et al., 1996). Caregivers with disabilities and/or persistent illness have not historically received services from occupational therapy practitioners or other rehabilitation providers. Despite a functional approach, few rehabilitation providers have been responsive to an individual's needs as a parent. For example, one cancer survivor reported that none of her health care providers asked her if she had any children (Tannen, 2000).

Caregivers with disabilities face the same daily responsibilities and stresses associated with childrearing as those without disabilities. Having a disability adds additional challenges, and limitations associated with a disability may affect a caregiver's ability to perform daily occupations. Caregivers may have physical, cognitive, or psychiatric disabilities. Other factors that may put an individual at risk for difficulty in care giving include being a teen parent, having a history of substance abuse, having been abused in childhood, domestic violence, and divorce (Huxley & Warner, 1993; Kowal, Kottmeier, Ayoub, Komives, Robinson, & Allen, 1989; Panzarine, 1988). Moreover, to the extent that disability and other risk factors are associated with poverty, a lack of knowledge of and access to supports and resources, a lack of education and skills, and a limited life experience, parents with disabilities may face even more daunting challenges (Whitman & Accardo, 1993).

Current research on the effects of disability and persistent illness on parenting is limited. Disability or illness is often viewed as the predominant characteristic of the individual. Emerging from this perception of disability are numerous stereotypes concerning parents with disabilities and illness. These stereotypes include the idea that parents with disabilities are too immersed in their own self-care to adequately care for their children, children are used to satisfy the personal needs of parents with disabilities, parental tasks cannot be performed effectively by parents with disabilities, and parents with disabilities pass on a negative self-image to their children. These stereotypes cannot be challenged without interventions to support parents (Tannen, 2000).

Parents with Physical Disabilities

Parents with physical disabilities may have compromised mobility, movement, and/or stamina, which present challenges to the physical demands of parenting. A report of the National Task Force on Parents with Disabilities and Their Families (Through the Looking Glass [TLG], 2001) indicates that parents with physical disabilities encounter multiple barriers to parenting and have service needs across several areas. Many parents reported needing adapted baby- and child-care equipment; barriers to obtaining equipment included lack of availability and cost. A majority of parents reported using personal assistance services for help with care giving, yet many felt that these services interfered with their role as parents. Parents also reported difficulty in obtaining affordable accessible housing, needing assistance in recreation with their children, and encountering problems with transportation that interfere with or prevent routine childcare activities (TLG, 2001).

Thus parents with physical disabilities may be helped by environmental modifications that allow them to participate fully in their role as parents (Farber, 2000). Parents with conditions characterized by periods of symptom exacerbation and diminution, such as multiple sclerosis or rheumatoid arthritis, may need assistance in planning for these periods and in accessing community support services that will be useful during exacerbations (Crist, 1993). Women with physical disabilities who are planning pregnancy may need to consider the possible medical complications that can occur with disability. These prospective mothers need practitioners with positive attitudes and expertise in managing pregnancy in women with physical disabilities (TLG, 2001).

Parents with Cognitive Disabilities

Parents with cognitive disabilities may lack knowledge and skill in specific areas of parenting, such as providing for a child's safety, nutrition, or daily routine care. These parents may have difficulty with problem solving, social skills, and advocacy for family needs. For example, a woman with a traumatic brain injury, which can cause cognitive and social skill deficits, may have a difficult time assisting her 12-year-old daughter in solving social problems between friends at school (Uysal, Hibbard, Robillard, Pappadopulos, & Jaffe, 1998).

Parents with cognitive disabilities may have difficulty following directions or learning new skills. They may tend to overgeneralize skills and problem-solving strategies to contexts that require different or more complex skills. Individuals with cognitive disabilities have greater success in learning when strategies are broken down into steps; are demonstrated, modeled, and practiced; and are paired with rewards. Because of difficulties with generalization, skills-training services to parents with cognitive disabilities should be provided in naturally occurring environments, such as the home and community (Bakken, Miltenberger, & Schauss, 1993).

Parents with Psychiatric Disabilities

The stigma associated with mental illness is probably the most pervasive factor affecting access to and participation in services among parents with psychiatric disabilities. Because of the presumption that individuals with psychiatric disabilities are compromised in their ability to parent, many parents do not seek support services because they fear the loss of custody of their children. Parents with psychiatric disabilities (and those with developmental disabilities) are at an increased risk of custody loss; yet many parents with psychiatric disabilities are raising or helping to raise their children (Nicholson, Biebel, Hinden, Henry & Stier, 2001; Wong, 1995).

The needs of a family in which a parent has a psychiatric disability are often not addressed until the child is in need of services. When services are provided they are often child-centered and provided by clinicians who are not trained to work with adults. Moreover, services tend to be problem focused and deficit based rather than preventative or strengths based (Nicholson, Geller, Fisher, & Dion, 1993). Across the United States, only a few programs have been developed that specifically target the needs of parents with psychiatric disabilities and their children (Nicholson, et al., 2001).

Parents with psychiatric disabilities may benefit from parenting skills training and from training in strategies to cope with exacerbations in symptoms. For example, parents may need help in planning for care for their children during times they need to be hospitalized. Parents can also benefit from training in ways to advocate for services for themselves and their children. Peer support groups can provide opportunities to build social networks and decrease isolation. A strong social support network can act as a mediator of stress, increasing the parent's functioning during stressful times. Because parents with psychiatric disabilities may have had disrupted relationships with their families of origin, extended family members may be of limited support. Many parents worry about their children's understanding of mental illness; practitioners can help parents develop ways of talking with children about mental illness that are age appropriate (Nicholson, Henry, Clayfield, & Phillips, 2001).

INTERVENTIONS FOR CAREGIVERS

The first step in developing interventions for parents and family caregivers is to gain an understanding of the daily experiences and responsibilities of individuals in these roles. Assessment should be family centered and collaborative, with a goal of identifying family strengths, priorities, and values as well as daily challenges associated with care giving. Occupational therapy can involve the provision of direct or indirect services. In partnership with parents and caregivers, practitioners can provide direct services in skills training, environmental adaptations, and/or support services.

Areas of skills training may include the following:

- Teaching parenting skills (e.g., home maintenance, time and money management, child behavior management, and advocacy for services).
- Teaching parents to support their child's development and to nurture their relationship with their child.
- Helping parents communicate with children about disability.

Environmental adaptations may include the following:

- Creating play spaces in the home that are accessible for family members with disabilities.
- Helping parents access human and nonhuman resources.
- Designing adapted baby-care equipment.
- Designing environments to minimize fatigue.

Support services may include the following:

- Providing support groups for family caregivers or parents with disabilities.
- Accessing naturally occurring resources (e.g., friends, neighbors, and community services).

In addition to direct services, practitioners can provide indirect services, such as advocacy for the needs of families in which a member has a disability or referral to a range of community-based services that may be available for parents and caregivers. Examples are formal services, such as mental health and substance abuse services; early intervention and Head Start programs; school-based services; and respite services. In addition, there are a variety of informal services that may benefit parents and caregivers: national self-help and support groups such as Children and Adults with Attention Deficient/Hyperactivity Disorder (CHADD), the National Depressive and Manic Depressive Association, and the Alzheimer's Association. Many of these national groups have local chapters. Finally, there are many community support systems, such as faith-based institutions, community centers, and libraries that provide assistance to parents and caregivers.

CONCLUSION

Childrearing and care giving are complex lifelong occupations. Across the life course, individuals are likely to engage in parenting and or caring for other family members. People engaged in these occupations might benefit from direct or indirect interventions that support their nurturing role.

References

Agnew, P. J., Poulsen, A., & Maas, F. (1985). Attitudes and knowledge of occupational therapy clinicians and students regarding the sexuality of disabled people. *Australian Occupational Therapy Journal, 32,* 54–61.

Alexander, C. J. (1997). Ethical concerns. In M. L. Sipski & C. J. Alexander (Eds.). *Sexual function in people with disability and chronic illness: A health professional's guide* (pp. 403–412). Gaithersburg, MD: Aspen.

Allen, C., & Blue, T. (1998). Cognitive disabilities model: How to make clinical judgments. In N. Katz (Ed.). *Cognition and occupation in rehabilitation* (pp. 225–279) Bethesda, MD: American Occupational Therapy Association.

American Association of Retired Persons. (n.d.). *The doable renewable home stock* [#D12470]. Washington, DC: AARP.

American Heart Association. (n.d.). *Five step plan for work simplification* [Handout]. AHA.

American Occupational Therapy Association. (n.d.). *Home assessment checklist for fall hazards and information needs in designing accessible environments.* Bethesda, MD: Author.

American Occupational Therapy Association. (In press). Occupational therapy practice framework: Domain and process. *American Journal of Occupational Therapy.*

Anderson, B., & Ross, J. (1992). Smoothing the transition. *Home Clinical Management, 12*(5), 46–52.

Anemaet, W., & Moffa-Trotter, M. (1999). Promoting safety and function through home assessments. *Topics in Geriatric Rehabilitation, 15*(1), 2655.

Annon, J. S. (1976). The P-LI-SS-IT model: A proposed conceptual scheme for the behavioural treatment of sexual problems. *Journal of Sexuality Education Therapy, 2,* 1–15.

Bakken, J., Miltenberger, R. G., & Schauss, S. (1993). Teaching parents with mental retardation: Knowledge versus skills. *American Journal of Mental Retardation, 97,* 405–417.

Banford, M., Kratz, M., Brown, R., Emick, K., Ranck, J., Wilkins, R., & Holm, M. B. (2001). Stroke survivor caregiver education: Methods and effectiveness. *Physical and Occupational Therapy in Geriatrics, 19*(1), 37–51.

Barnes, K. (1991). Modification of the physical environment. In C. Christiansen & C. Baum (Eds.). *Occupational therapy overcoming human performance deficits* (pp. 701–746). Thorofare, NJ: Slack.

Beckman, P. J., Barnwell, D., Horn, E., Hanson, M. J., Gutierrez, S., & Leiber, J. (1998). Communities, families, and inclusion. *Early Childhood Research Quarterly, 13,* 125–150.

Bendix, T., Bendix, A., Labriola, M., Haestrup, C., & Ebbeh, N. (2000). Functional restoration versus outpatient physical training in chronic low back pain: A randomized controlled comparative study. *Spine, 25,* 2494–2500.

Biegel, D. E., Sales, E., & Schulz, R. (1991). Common factors affecting family caregivers. In D. E. Biegel, & R. Schulz (Eds.). *Family caregiver application series.* Vol. 1: *Family caregiving in chronic illness* (pp. 199–214.). London: Sage.

Birkholtz, M., & Blair, S. (2001a). Chronic pain—The need for an eclectic approach: Part 1. *British Journal of Therapy and Rehabilitation, 8*(2), 68–73.

Birkholtz, M., & Blair, S. (2001b). Chronic pain—The need for an eclectic approach: Part 2. *British Journal of Therapy and Rehabilitation, 8*(3), 96–99.

Blake, H., & Lincoln, N. B. (2000). Factors associated with strain in co-resident spouses of patients following stroke. *Clinical Rehabilitation, 14,* 307–314.

Bogardus, S., Bradley, E., Williams, C., Jaciejewski, P, van Doorn, C., & Inouye, S. (2001). Goals for the care of frail older adults: Do caregivers and clinicians agree? *American Journal of Medicine, 110,* 97–102.

Bowling, A. (1991). *Measuring health: A review of quality of life measurement scales.* Milton Keynes, [England], Philadelphia: Open University Press.

Bowling, B. (1981). *Effective patient education techniques for use with aging patient.* Lexington: University of Kentucky.

Breslin, E. (1992). Dyspnea-limited response in chronic obstructive pulmonary disease: Reduced unsupported arm activities. *Rehabilitation Nursing, 17*(1), 12–21.

Bronfenbrenner, U. (1979). *The ecology of human development: Experiments by nature and design.* Cambridge, MA: Harvard University Press.

Buckwalter, K. C., Wernimont, T., & Buckwalter, J. A. (1982). Musculoskeletal conditions and sexuality (Part II). *Sexuality and Disability, 5,* 195–207.

Buzzelli, S., di-Francesco, L., Giaquinto, S., & Nolfe, G. (1997). Psychological and medical aspects of sexuality following stroke. *Sexuality and Disability, 15,* 261–270.

Canadian Association of Occupational Therapists. (1991). *Guidelines for the client-centered practice of occupational therapy.* Toronto, ON, Canada: Author.

Chapparo, C. (1979). *Sensory integration for adults.* Workshop sponsored by Illinois Occupational Therapy Association, Glen Ellyn, Illinois.

Cipriani, J., Hess, S., Higgins, H., Resavy, D., Sheon, S., Szychowski, M., & Holm, M. B. (2000). Collaboration in the therapeutic process: Older

adults' perspectives. *Physical and Occupational Therapy in Geriatrics, 17*(1), 43–54.
Clark, F. (1993). Occupation embedded in a real life: Interweaving occupational science and occupational therapy. *American Journal of Occupational Therapy, 47*, 1067–1078.
Close, J., Ellis, M., Hooper, R., Glucksman, E., Jackson, S., & Swift, C. (1999). Prevention of falls in the elderly trial (PROFET): A randomised controlled trial. *Lancet, 353*, 93–97.
Cohen, J. A. (1986). Sexual counseling of the patient following myocardial infarction. *Critical Care Nurse, 6*, 18–29.
Cole, C. M., Levin, E. M., Whitley, J. O., & Young, S. H. (1979). Brief sexual counseling during cardiac rehabilitation. *Psychological Aspects of Critical Care, 8*, 124–129.
Conine, T. A., Christie, G. M., Hammond, G. K., & Smith, M. F. (1979). An assessment of occupational therapists' roles and attitudes toward sexual rehabilitation of the disabled. *American Journal of Occupational Therapy, 33*, 515–519.
Cope, D. N., & Sundance, P. (1995). Conceptualizing clinical outcomes. In P. K. Landrum, N. D. Schmidt, & A. McLean (Eds.). *Outcome-oriented rehabilitation* (pp. 43–56). Gaithersburg, MD: Aspen.
Corring, D. J., & Cook, J. V. (1999). Client-centred care means that I am a valued human being. *Canadian Journal of Occupational Therapy, 66*, 71–82.
Couldrick, L. (1998a). Sexual issues: An area of concern for occupational therapists? *British Journal of Occupational Therapy, 61*, 493–496.
Couldrick, L. (1998b). Sexual issues within occupational therapy. Part 1: Attitudes and Practice. *British Journal of Occupational Therapy, 61*, 538–544.
Couldrick, L. (1999). Sexual issues within occupational therapy, Part 2: Implications for education and practice. *British Journal of Occupational Therapy, 62*, 26–30.
Cox, C. (1996). Discharge planning for dementia patients: Factors influencing caregiver decisions and satisfaction. *Health and Social Work, 21*(2), 97–104.
Crist, P. (1993). Contingent interaction during work and play tasks for mothers with multiple sclerosis and their daughters. *American Journal of Occupational Therapy, 47*, 121–131.
Croser, R., Garrett, R., Seeger, B., & Davies, P. (2001). Effectiveness of electronic aids to daily living: Increased independence and decreased frustration. *Australian Occupational Therapy Journal, 48*, 35–44.
Cummings, R., Thomas, M., Szonyi, G., Salkeld, G., O'Neill, E., Westbury, C., & Frampton, G. (1999). Home visits by an occupational therapist for assessment and modification of environmental hazards: A randomized trial of falls prevention. *Journal of the American Geriatrics Society, 47*, 1397–1402.
DaCunha, J. P., & Tackenberg, J. (Eds.). (1989). *How to teach patients*. Springhouse, PA: Springhouse.
Davis, J. (1997). *NDT Certification Course*, Harmarville, PA.
DeJong, G., & Sutton, J. P. (1995). Rehab 2000: The evolution of medical rehabilitation in American health care. In P. K. Landrum, N. D. Schmidt, & A. McLean (Eds.). *Outcome-oriented rehabilitation* (pp. 3–42). Gaithersburg, MD: Aspen.
DeVault, M. (1991). *Feeding the family*. Chicago: University of Chicago Press.
Drench, M. E. (1992). Impact of altered sexuality and sexual function in spinal cord injury: A review. *Sexuality and Disability, 10*, 3–13.
Dunn, K. L. (1997). Sexuality education and the team approach. In M. L. Sipski & C. J. Alexander (Eds.). *Sexual function in people with disability and chronic illness: A health professional's guide* (pp. 381–402). Gaithersburg, MD: Aspen.
Dunn, W. (1993). Measurement of function: Actions for the future. *American Journal of Occupational Therapy, 47*, 357–359.
Dunn, W., Brown, C., & McGuigan, A. (1994). The ecology of human performance: A framework for considering the effect of context. *American Journal of Occupational Therapy, 48*, 595–607.
Dutton, R. (1995). *Clinical reasoning in physical disabilities*. Baltimore: Williams & Wilkins.
Dyck, L. (1990). Space, time, and renegotiating motherhood: An exploration of the domestic workplace. *Environment and Planning D: Society and Space, 8*, 459–483.
Evans, J. (1985). Performance and attitudes of occupational therapists regarding sexual habilitation of paediatric patients. *American Journal of Occupational Therapy, 39*, 664–670.
Evans, R. W., Small, L., & Ling, J. S. (1995). Independence in the home and community. In P. K. Landrum, N. D. Schmidt, & A. McLean (Eds.). *Outcome-oriented rehabilitation* (pp. 95–124). Gaithersburg, MD: Aspen.
Fadiman, A. (1997). *The spirit catches you and you fall down*. New York: Noonday.
Farber, R. S. (2000). Mothers with disabilities: In their own voice. *American Journal of Occupational Therapy, 54*, 260–268.
Fisher, A. G. (1998). Uniting practice and theory in an occupational framework. [Eleanor Clark Slagle Lecture]. *American Journal of Occupational Therapy, 52*, 509–521.
Ford, A. B., Haug, M. R., Stange, K. C., Gaines, A. D., Noekler, L. S., & Jones, P. K. (2000). Sustained personal autonomy: A measure of successful aging. *Journal of Aging and Health, 12*, 470–489.
Freda, M., Cioschi, H., & Nilson, C. (1989). Childbearing issues for women with physical disabilities. *Physical Disabilities Special Interest Section Newsletter, 12*, 1–4.
Fried, L. P., Herdman, S. J., Kuhn, K. E., Rubin, G., & Turano, K. (1991). Preclinical disability: Hypotheses about the bottom of the iceberg. *Journal of Aging and Health, 3*, 285–300.
Fuchs-Climent, D., Le Gallais, D., Varray, A., Desplan, J., Cadopi, M., & Prefaut, C. G. (2001). Factor analysis of quality of life, dyspnea, and physiological variables in patients with chronic obstructive pulmonary disease before and after rehabilitation. *American Journal of Physical Medicine and Rehabilitation, 80*, 113–120.
Fuhrer, M., & Keith, R. (1998). Facilitating patient learning during medical rehabilitation: A research agenda. *American Journal of Physical Medicine and Rehabilitation, 77*, 557–561.
Gage, M., Noh, S., Polatajko, H. J., & Kaspar, V. (1994). Measuring perceived self-efficacy in occupational therapy. *American Journal of Occupational Therapy, 48*, 783–790.
Gender, A. R. (1992). An overview of the nurse's role in dealing with sexuality. *Sexuality and Disability, 10*, 71–79.
Gift, A. G., & Pugh, L. C. (1993). Dyspnea and fatigue. *Nursing Clinics of North American, 28*, 373–384.
Gill, T. M., Williams, C. S., Robison, J. T., & Tinetti, M. E. (1999). A population-based study of environmental hazards in the homes of older persons. *American Journal of Public Health, 89*, 553–556.
Gitlin, L. N., Corcoran, M., Winter, L., Boyce, A., & Hauck, W. W. (2001). A randomized controlled trial of a home environmental intervention: Effect on efficacy and upset in caregivers and on daily function of persons with dementia. *Gerontologist, 41*, 4–14.
Gitlin, L. N., Miller, K. S., & Boyce, A. (1999). Bathroom modifications for frail elderly renters: Outcomes of a community-based program. *Technology and Disability, 10*, 141–149.
Hagedorn, R. (1995). Environmental analysis and adaptation. In R. Hagedorn (Ed.). *Occupational therapy: Perspectives and processes* (pp. 239–257). Melbourne, Australia: Churchill Livingstone.
Hansen, R. A., & Atchison, B. (1993). *Conditions in occupational therapy: Effect on occupational performance*. Baltimore: Williams & Wilkins.
Hasselkus, B. R. (1989). The meaning of daily activity in family caregiving for the elderly. *American Journal of Occupational Therapy, 43*, 649–656.
Healy, H., & Rigby, P. (1999). Promoting independence for teens and young adults with physical disabilities. *Canadian Journal of Occupational Therapy, 66*, 240–249.
Hellerstein, H. K., & Friedman, E. H. (1970). Sexual activity and the post-coronary patient. *Archives of Internal Medicine, 125*, 987–999.
Hepburn, K., Tornatore, J., Center, B., & Ostwald, W. (2001). Demential family caregiver training: Affecting beliefs about caregiving and caregiver outcomes. *Journal of the American Geriatrics Society, 49*, 450–457.

Herson, L., Hart, K. A., Gordon, M. J., & Rintala, D. H. (1999). Identifying and overcoming barriers to providing sexuality information in the clinical setting. *Rehabilitation Nursing, 24*, 148–151.

Hodapp, R. M., Dykens, E. M., Evans, D. W., & Merighi, J. R. (1992). Maternal emotional reactions to young children with different types of handicaps. *Developmental and Behavioral Pediatrics, 13*, 118–123.

Holm, M. B., Rogers, J. C., & Kwoh, C. K. (1998). Predictors of functional disability in patients with rheumatoid arthritis. *Arthritis Care and Research, 11*, 346–355.

Horak, F. (1991). Assumptions underlying motor control for neurologic rehabilitation. In Foundation for Physical Therapy (Ed.). *Contemporary management of motor problems: Proceedings of the II Step Conference* (pp. 11–27). Alexandria, VA: Editor.

Huxley, P., & Warner, R. (1993). Primary prevention of parenting dysfunction in high-risk cases. *American Journal of Orthopsychiatry, 63*, 582–587.

Jackson, J. (1998). Is there a place for role theory in Occupational Science? *Journal of Occupational Science, 5*, 56–65.

Katchadourian, H. (1989). *Fundamentals of human sexuality*. Orlando: FL: Holt, Rinehart & Winston.

Kautzman, L. (1991) Facilitating adult learning in occupational therapy patient education programs. *Occupational Therapy Practice, 2*, 1–11.

Kewman, D., Warschausky, S., Engel, L., & Warzak, W. (1997). Sexual development of children and adolescents. In M. L. Sipski & C. J. Alexander (Eds.). *Sexual function in people with disability and chronic illness: A health professional's guide* (pp. 355–378). Gaithersburg: MD: Aspen.

Klinger, J. (1978). *Mealtime manual for people with disabilities and the aging* (2nd ed.). Camden, NJ: Campbell Soup Co.

Knoke, D., Taylor, A. E., & Saint-Cyr, J. A. (1998). The differential effects of cueing on recall in Parkinson's disease and normal subjects. *Brain and Cognition, 38*, 261–274.

Korpelainen, J. T., Nieminen, P., & Myllyla, V. V. (1999). Sexual functioning among stroke patients and their spouses. *Stroke, 30*, 715–719.

Kowal, L. W., Kottmeier, C. P., Ayoub, C. C., Komives, J. A., Robinson, D. S., & Allen, J. P. (1989). Characteristics of families at risk of problems in parenting: Findings from a home-based secondary prevention program. *Child Welfare, 68*, 549–538.

Kramer, A. M., Kowalsky, J. C., Lin, M., Grigsby, J., Hughes, R., & Steiner, J. F. (2000). Outcome and utilization differences for older persons with stroke in HMO and fee-for-service systems. *Journal of the American Geriatrics Society, 48*, 726–734.

Krukofsky, B. (1988). Sexuality counseling of people with chronic illness. In E. Weinstein & E. Rosen (Eds.). *Sexuality counseling: Issues and implications* (pp. 259–273). Pacific Grove, CA: Brooks/Cole.

Lamb, M. (2000). The history of research on father involvement: An overview. In *Fatherhood: Research, Interventions, and Policies*, 23–41.

Landsman, G. H. (1998). Reconstructing motherhood in the age of "Perfect" babies: Mothers of infants and toddlers with disabilities. *Signs: Journal of Women in Culture and Society, 24*, 69–99.

LaPlante, M. P., Carlson, D., Kaye, H. S., & Bradsher, J. E. (1996). *Families with disabilities in the United States* [Report 8]. San Francisco: Disability Statistics Center, University of California.

Law, M., Cooper, B., Strong, S., Stewart, D., Rigby, P., & Letts, L. (1996). The person–environment–occupation model: A transactive approach to occupational performance. *Canadian Journal of Occupational Therapy, 63*, 9–23.

Lawton, M. P., & Brody, E. (1969). Assessment of older people: Self-maintaining and instrumental activities of daily living. *Gerontologist, 9*, 179–186.

Letts, L, Scott, S., Burtney, J., Marshall, L., & McKean, M. (1998). The reliability and validity of the safety assessment of function and the environment for rehabilitation (SAFER Tool). *British Journal of Occupational Therapy, 61*, 127–132.

Ley, P. (1972). Comprehension, memory and the success of communications with the patient. *Journal of Instructional Health Education, 10*, 23–29.

Liao, S., & Ferrell, B. (2000). Fatigue in an older population. *Journal of the American Geriatrics Society, 48*, 426–430.

Liddle, J., & McKenna, K. (2000). Quality of life: An overview of issues for use in occupational therapy outcome measurement. *Australian Occupational Therapy Journal, 47*, 77–85.

Linton, S., & Rousso, H. (1988). Sexuality counseling for people with disabilities. In: E. Weinstein & E. Rosen (Eds.). *Sexuality counseling: Issues and implications* (pp. 114–134). Pacific Grove, CA: Brooks/Cole.

Llewellyn, G. (1994). Parenting: A neglected human occupation. Parents' voices not yet heard. *Australian Occupational Therapy Journal, 41*, 173–176.

Lorig, K., & Fries, J. F. (1990). *The arthritis helpbook* (3rd ed.). New York: Addison-Wesley.

Luster, T., & Okagaki, L. (1993). *Parenting: An ecological perspective*. Hillsdale, NJ: Erlbaum.

Mathiowetz, V., & Bass Haugen, J. (1995). Remediation of motor behavior: Contemporary task oriented approach. In C. A. Trombly (Ed.). *Occupational therapy for physical dysfunction* (4th ed., pp. 510–527). Baltimore: Williams & Wilkins.

Mathiowetz, V., Matuska, K. M., & Murphy, M. E. (2001). Efficacy of an energy conservation course for persons with multiple sclerosis. *Archives of Physical Medicine and Rehabilitation, 82*, 449–456.

McAndrew, E., McDermott, S., Vitzakovich, S., Warunek, M., & Holm, M. B. (2000). Therapist and patient perceptions of the occupational therapy goal setting process: A pilot study. *Physical and Occupational Therapy in Geriatrics, 17*(1), 55–63.

McDowell, I., & Newell, C. (1996). *Measuring health: A guide to rating scales and questionnaires* (2nd ed.). New York: Oxford University Press.

Miller, P. A., & Butin, D. (2000). The role of occupational therapy in dementia: COPE (Caregiver options for practical experiences). *International Journal of Geriatric Psychiatry, 15*, 86–89.

Monga, T. N., & Kerrigan, A. J. (1997). Cerebrovascular accidents. In M. L. Sipski & C. J. Alexander (Eds.). *Sexual function in people with disability and chronic illness: A health professional's guide* (pp. 189–219). Gaithersburg, MD: Aspen.

Mullersdorf, M. (2000a). Factors indicating need of rehabilitation: Occupational therapy needs among persons with long-term and/or recurrent pain. *International Journal of Rehabilitation Research, 23*, 281–294.

Mullersdorf, M. (2000b). The actual state of the effects, treatment, and incidence of disabling pain in a gender perspective: A Swedish study. *Disability and Rehabilitation, 15*, 840–854.

Natterlund, B., & Ahlstrom, G. (1999). Problem-focused coping and satisfaction with activities of daily living in individuals with muscular dystrophy and postpolio syndrome. *Scandanavian Journal of Caring Sciences, 13*(1), 26–32.

Neistadt, M. E. (1995). Methods of assessing clients' priorities: A survey of adult physical dysfunction settings. *American Journal of Occupational Therapy, 49*, 428–436.

Neistadt, M. E. (1986). Sexuality counseling for adults with disabilities: A module for an occupational therapy curriculum. *American Journal of Occupational Therapy, 40*, 542–545.

Neistadt, M. E., & Freda, M. (1987). *Choices: A guide to sex counseling with physically disabled adults*. Malabar, FL: Krieger.

Nicholson, J., Biebel, K., Hinden, B., Henry, A., & Stier, L. (2001). *Critical issues for parents with mental illness and their families*. Washington, DC: U.S. Department of Health and Human Services Administration, Center for Mental Health Service.

Nicholson, J., Geller, J. L., Fisher, W. H., & Dion, G. L. (1993). State policies and programs that address the needs of mentally ill mothers in the public sector. *Hospital and Community Psychiatry, 44*, 484–489.

Nicholson, J., Henry, A. D., Clayfield, J., & Phillips, S. (2001). Parenting well when you're depressed. A complete resources for maintaining a healthy family. Oakland: New Harbinger.

Novak, P. P., & Mitchell, M. M. (1988). Professional involvement in sexuality counseling for patients with spinal cord injuries. *American Journal of Occupational Therapy, 42*, 105–112.

Nyland, J., Quigley, P., Huang, C., Lloyd, J., Harrow, J., & Nelson, A. (2000). Preserving transfer independence among individuals with spinal cord injury. *Spinal Cord, 38*, 649–657.

Oakley, F., Kielhofner, G., Barris, R., Reichler, R. K. (1996). The role checklist: Development and empirical assessment of reliability. *Occupational Therapy Journal of Research, 6(3)*, 157–170.

Okkema, K. (1993). *Rehabilitation Institute of Chicago: Cognition and perception in the stroke patient: A guide to functional outcomes*. Gaithersburg, MD: Aspen.

Olson, D. H., McCubbin, H. I., Barnes, H., Larson, A., Muxen, M., & Wilson, M. (1984). *One thousand families: A national survey*. Beverly Hills, CA: Sage.

Ostchega, Y., Harris, T. B., Hirsch, R., Parsons, V. L., & Kington, R. (2000). The prevalence of functional limitations and disability in older persons in the United States: Data from the National Health and Nutrition Examination Survey III. *Journal of the American Geriatrics Society, 48*, 1132–1135.

Panzarine, S. (1988). Teen mothering. *Journal of Adolescent Health Care, 9*, 443–448.

Parenté, R., & Herrman, D. (1996). *Retraining cognition: Techniques and applications*. Frederick, MD: Aspen.

Pedretti, L. (1996). *OT practice skills for physical dysfunction*. St. Louis: Mosby.

Pollock, N., Baptiste, S., Law, M., McColl, M. A., Opzoomer, A., & Polatajko, H. (1990). Occupational performance measures: A review based on the guidelines for the client-centered practice of occupational therapy. *Canadian Journal of Occupational Therapy, 57*, 77–81.

Quintana, L. A. (1995). Remediating perceptual impairments. In C. A. Trombly (Ed.). *Occupational therapy for physical dysfunction* (4th ed., pp. 529–537). Baltimore: Williams & Wilkins.

Rehabilitation Institute of Chicago [RIC]. (1988). *Occupational therapy work simplification/energy conservation principles* [Handout]. Chicago: Author.

Rehabilitation Institute of Chicago [RIC]. (1998). *Rehabilitation Institute of Chicago Functional assessment scale* (version V). Chicago: Author.

Resnick, B. (1998). Motivating older adults to perform functional activities. *Journal of Gerontological Nursing, 24*(11), 23–30.

Robichaud-Ekstrand, S. (1991). Shower versus sink bath: Evaluation of heart rate, blood pressure, and subjective response of the patient with myocardial infarction. *Heart and Lung: Journal of Critical Care, 20*, 375–382.

Robins, N., & Goldstein, K. (1998) Home advantage. *OT Practice, 3*, 8, 41–42.

Robinson-Smith, G., Johnston, M. V., & Allen, J. (2000). Self-care self-efficacy, quality of life, and depression after stroke. *Archives of Physical Medicine and Rehabilitation, 81*, 460–464.

Rogers, J. C., & Holm, M. B. (1991). Task performance of older adults and low assistive technology devices. *International Journal of Technology and Aging, 4*, 93–106.

Rogers, J. C., & Holm, M. B. (2000). Daily-living skills and habits of older women with depression. Habits I Conference (January 1999). *Occupational Therapy Journal of Research, 20*(Suppl. 1), 68S–85S.

Rogers, J. C., Holm, M. B., Burgio, L. D., Granieri, E., Hsu, C., Hardin, J. M., & McDowell, B. J. (1999). Improving morning care routines of nursing home residents with dementia. *Journal of the American Geriatrics Society, 47*, 1049–1057.

Rogers, J. C., Holm, M. B., Burgio, L. D., Hsu, C., Hardin, J. M., & McDowell, B. (2000). Excess disability during morning care in nursing home residents with dementia. *International Psychogeriatrics, 12*, 267–282.

Ross, F. (1992). The use of computers in occupational therapy for visual scanning training. *American Journal of Occupational Therapy, 46*, 314–322.

Ruddick, S. (1989). *Maternal thinking: Toward a politics of peace*. Boston: Beacon.

Sandel, M. E. (1997).Traumatic brain injury. In M. L. Sipski & C. J. Alexander (Eds.). *Sexual function in people with disability and chronic illness: A health professional's guide* (pp. 221–245). Gaithersburg, MD: Aspen.

Schreter, C. (1991, April). The perfect fit remodeling for changing needs. *Retired Officer Magazine*, 28–31.

Schwartz, S. M. (1995). Adults with traumatic brain injury: Three case studies of cognitive rehabilitation in the home setting. *American Journal of Occupational Therapy, 49*, 655–657.

Scorgie, K., & Sobsey, D. (2000). Transformational outcomes associated with parenting children who have disabilities. *Mental Retardation, 38*, 195–206.

Seigley, L. (1998). The effects of personal and environmental factors on health behaviors of older adults. *Nursingconnections, 11*(4), 47–58.

Seltzer, M. M., Krauss, M. W., Orsmond, G. I., & Vestal, C. (1997). Families of adolescents and adults with autism: Uncharted territory. *International Review of Research in Mental Retardation, 20*, 267–294.

Shumway-Cook, A., & Woollacott, M. H. (1995). *Motor control: Theory and practical applications*. Baltimore: Williams & Wilkins.

Sipski, M. L. (1997). Spinal cord injury and sexual function: An educational model. In M. L. Sipski & C. J. Alexander (Eds.). *Sexual function in people with disability and chronic illness: A health professional's guide* (pp. 149–188). Gaithersburg, MD: Aspen.

Sipski, M. L., & Alexander, C. J. (1997a). Introduction. In M. L. Sipski & C. J. Alexander (Eds.). *Sexual function in people with disability and chronic illness: A health professional's guide* (pp. xxi–xxiv). Gaithersburg, MD: Aspen.

Sipski, M. L., & Alexander, C. J. (1997b). Impact of disability or chronic illness on sexual function. In M. L. Sipski & C. J. Alexander (Eds.). *Sexual function in people with disability and chronic illness: A health professional's guide* (pp. 3–12). Gaithersburg, MD: Aspen.

Smith, E. M., & Bodner, D. R. (1993). Sexual dysfunction after spinal cord injury. *Urology Clinics of North America, 20*, 535–542.

Sorenson, S., & Zarit, S. H. (1996). Preparation for care giving: A study of multigeneration families. *International Journal of Aging and Human Development, 42*, 43–64.

Spector, R. E. (1996). *Cultural diversity in health and illness* (4th ed.). Stamford, CT: Appleton & Lange.

Spica, M. M. (1992). Educating the client on the effects of COPD on sexuality: The role of the nurse. *Sexuality and Disability, 10*, 91–101.

Stitik, T. P., & Benevento, B. T. (1997). Cardiac and pulmonary diseases. In M. L. Sipski & C. J. Alexander (Eds.). *Sexual function in people with disability and chronic illness: A health professional's guide* (pp. 303–335). Gaithersburg, MD: Aspen.

Strong, J. (1998). Incorporating cognitive-behavioral therapy with occupational therapy: A comparative study with patients with low back pain. *Journal of Occupational Rehabilitation, 8*(1) 61–71.

Summerville, P., & McKenna, K. (1998). Sexuality education and counselling for individuals with a spinal cord injury: Implications for occupational therapy. *British Journal of Occupational Therapy, 61*, 275–279.

Sumsion, T., & Smyth, G. (2000). Barriers to client-centredness and their resolution. *Canadian Journal of Occupational Therapy, 67*, 15–21.

Tack, B. B. (1991). *Dimensions and correlates of fatigue in older adults with rheumatoid arthritis*. Unpublished doctoral dissertation, University of California at San Francisco.

Tannen, N. (2000). *The impact of parental illness on the child and family: Implications for system change*. Washington, D.C.: The National Technical Assistance Center for Children's Mental Health, Georgetown University Child Development Center.

Taub, E., Uswatte, G., & Pidikiti, R. (1999). Constraint-induced movement therapy: A new family of techniques with broad application to physical rehabilitation—A clinical review. *Journal of Rehabilitation Research and Development, 36*, 237–251.

Taylor, L. P., & McGruder, J. E. (1996). The meaning of sea kayaking for persons with spinal cord injuries. *American Journal of Occupational Therapy, 50*, 39–46.

Tepper, M. S. (1992). Sexual education in spinal cord injury rehabilitation: Current trends and recommendation. *Sexuality and Disability, 10*, 15–31.

Thompson, K. M. (1998). Early intervention services in daily family life: mothers' perceptions of "ideal" versus "actual" service provision. *Occupational Therapy International, 5*, 206–221.

Thornsson, A., & Grimby, G. (2001). Ability and perceived difficulty in daily activities in people with poliomyelitis sequelae. *Journal of Rehabilitation Medicine, 33*, 4–11.

Through the Looking Glass [TLG]. (2001). Keeping our families together. A report of the national task force on parents with disabilities and their families. Available at: www.lookingglass.org/taskforce.html. Accessed on June 18, 2001.

Thurer, S. L. (1992). The long-term sexual response to coronary bypass surgery: Some preliminary findings. *Sexuality and Disability, 5*, 208–211.

Trombly, C. (1995a). Occupation: Purposefulness and meaningfulness as therapeutic mechanisms. [Eleanor Clarke Slagle Lecture]. *American Journal of Occupational Therapy, 49*, 960–972.

Trombly, C. (1995b). Planning, guiding, and documenting therapy. In C. A. Trombly (Ed.). *Occupational therapy for physical dysfunction* (pp. 3–40). Baltimore: Williams & Wilkins.

Trombly, C. (Ed.). (1995c). *Occupational therapy for physical dysfunction.* (4th ed.). Baltimore: Williams & Wilkins.

Trombly, C. & Radomski, M. (Eds.). (2002). *Occupational therapy for physical dysfunction* (5th ed.). Baltimore: Lippincott Williams & Wilkins.

Unsworth, G. (1999). Living with epilepsy: Safety during home, leisure and work activities. *Australian Occupational Therapy Journal, 46*(3), 89–98.

Uysal, S., Hibbard, M. R., Robillard, D., Pappadopulos, E., & Jaffe, M. (1998). The effect of parental traumatic brain injury on parenting and child behavior. *Journal of Head Trauma Rehabilitation, 13*(6), 57–1.

Verbrugge, L. M. (1990). The iceberg of disability. In S. M. Stahl (Ed.). *The legacy of longevity: Health and health care in later life* (pp. 55–75). Newbury Park, CA: Sage.

Waldman, T. L., & Eliasof, B. (1997). Cancer. In M. L. Sipski & C. J. Alexander (Eds.). *Sexual function in people with disability and chronic illness: A health professional's guide* (pp. 337–354). Gaithersburg, MD: Aspen.

Whitman, B. Y., & Accardo, P. J. (1993). The parent with mental retardation: Rights, responsibilities, and issues. *Journal of Social Work and Human Sexuality, 8*, 123–136.

Wilkins, S., Pollock, N., Rochon, S., & Law, M. (2001). Implementing client-centered practice: Why is it so difficult to do? *Canadian Journal of Occupational Therapy, 68*(2), 70–79.

Wong, K. (1995, March–April). Dependency proceedings show biases against mentally disabled parents. *Youth Law News*, 13–16.

Wood, B. L. (1995). A developmental biopsychosocial approach to treatment of chronic illness in children and adolescents. In R. H. Midesell & P. Lusterman (Eds.). *Integrating family therapy: Handbook of family psychology and systems theory* (pp. 437–455). Washington, DC: American Psychological Association.

Yarkony, G. M., & Chen, D. (1995). Sexuality in patients with spinal cord injury. *Physical Medicine and Rehabilitation: State of the Art Reviews, 9*, 325–344.

CHAPTER 29

INTERVENTIONS TO PROMOTE PARTICIPATION

SECTION I: Work
SECTION II: Education
SECTION III: Play and Leisure
SECTION IV: Community Integration

SECTION I

Work

SHERLYN FENTON
PATRICIA GAGNON
DONALD G. PITTS

HISTORICAL OVERVIEW

In the late 1700s, one of two men credited with conceiving the moral treatment movement, Phillippe Pinel, used "work treatment" for the "insane." He used the occupations of physical exercise, work, farming, music, and literature in his treatment approaches (Sabonis-Chafee & Hussey, 1998). Since that time, occupational therapy practitioners have been involved in helping individuals with a wide variety of impairments caused by developmental disabilities, injuries, and illnesses engage or reengage in work. This section focuses on industrially related work programs as one of the more common examples of the occupational therapy roles associated with assisting people to engage in work.

Clinical programming as related to industrial rehabilitation has been greatly influenced in the United States by the legislative and political environments. Laws, such as the federal Industrial Rehabilitation Act of 1923, required all general hospitals in the United States that treated individuals who had industrial accidents or illnesses to offer occupational therapy. Global politics also played an integral role in the development of occupational therapy in work programs. The late 1940s post–World War II era emphasized retraining and reeducation of injured soldiers. After World War II, the industrial economy was growing. Because of the limited number of able-bodied workers, industries modified work environments to accommodate employees with disabilities. The adoption of the Vocational Rehabilitation Amendments in 1954 further bolstered professional interest in work-related programs.

Throughout the following two decades, the economy in the United States shifted from manufacturing industries to service industries. The passing of the Occupational Safety and Health Act in 1970, workers' compensation legislation, and the rising cost of vocational rehabilitation programs created opportunities for occupational therapy practitioners to address the safety and rehabilitation issues of injured workers.

The 1980s brought unparalleled growth and expansion in the rehabilitation of injured workers. Programs called **work hardening,** functional restoration, industrial rehabilitation, and return-to-work therapies are all synonymous with the term *work programs*. This area of specialization employed occupational therapy practitioners, and work programs were an increasingly popular approach to bridging the gap between acute rehabilitation and meaningful levels of function.

In 1988, both the Commission on Accreditation of Rehabilitation Facilities (CARF) and the National Advisory Committee on Work Hardening established guidelines for work hardening programs. The committee presented the following definition:

> *Work hardening is a highly structured, goal oriented, individualized treatment program designed to maximize the individual's ability to return to work. Work-hardening programs, which are interdisciplinary in nature, use real or simulated work activities in conjunction with conditioning tasks that are graded to progressively improve the biomechanical, neuromuscular, cardiovascular/metabolic and psychosocial functions of the individual. Work hardening provides a transition between acute care and return to work while addressing the issues of productivity, safety, physical tolerances, and worker behaviors. (Ogden-Niemeyer, & Jacobs, 1989, p. 1)*

As an occupational performance area, work encompasses activities related to employment, volunteerism, and retirement planning (American Occupational Therapy Association in press). Individuals engaging in work as an occupational activity may be both a medium and a goal of occupational therapy.

Occupational therapy practitioners continue to play an integral role in work hardening programs. Lost work time, lost dollars, and restricted worker abilities have encouraged employers to become more involved and knowledgeable about the care and management of their injured workers. Injury-prevention programs and worker education training are receiving greater emphasis today than in the past. Occupational therapy practitioners of the 1990s were essential in addressing the occupational health needs of clients, industries, and insurance companies alike. Moreover, the Occupational Safety and Health Administration (OSHA) turned to occupational therapists as the first experts when seeking feedback on the proposed ergonomics standard (Gourley, 2000).

INDUSTRIAL REHABILITATION REFERRAL PROCESS

An accident is an unanticipated, sudden event that results in injury or illness. Injury is physical damage to body tissues caused by an accident or by exposure to environmental stressors. Many work injuries result from accidents; however, some work-related injuries are caused by normal work activities that are repetitive in nature. Not all injuries are clearly identified as work related. So who is appropriate to receive occupational therapy services in a specialized work program setting? Occupational therapy is recommended when an individual experiences limitation in the performance area of work.

If improved occupational performance is the desired outcome, there are no limits to the scope of diagnoses appropriate for referrals to a work program. If the existing condition limits an individual's ability to perform one or more of life's major functions, a functional restoration program is an appropriate referral whether the injury or illness is acute or chronic. Laborer, homemaker, electrician, computer analyst, and student are all descriptions of occupations, each with unique characteristics. Individuals engaged in these occupations may require graduated approaches to wellness.

"I used to have my own law practice. Now I deliver newspapers. The truth is, this job is saving my life" (Norlen, 1999, p. 12). In a 1999 *Newsweek* article titled "Healing Myself with the Power of Work," Norlen candidly described his experience with depression. He informed readers that through the vehicle of work, he provided himself with therapy. Moreover, he reminded practitioners that many types of illness and injuries are best approached and treated through the medium of purposeful and productive activity.

The sources of referrals for work programs vary as much as the clients do. Physicians, occupational medicine nurses, insurance case managers, therapy practitioners, vocational counselors, attorneys, rehabilitation personnel, employers, and the clients themselves are some of the many referral sources. A work program may be the last stage of a therapeutic process to integrate an individual back into the workforce or may serve as an isolated therapeutic approach to determine a worker's functional and physical capacity. Program objectives identify occupational performance capabilities rather than emphasize the extent of pain and disability. Program outcomes highlight workers' behavioral performance and their ability to accomplish occupational tasks.

Many programs in the United States require a physician's order and a payment agreement before clients can begin. Each facility determines admission policies according to state legislation and professional licensure standards. Once the referral process has been completed, the occupational therapist is responsible for the initial client screening. Ongoing litigation and behavioral, psychological, or social factors may delay or prevent commencement of program participation.

The advent of managed care has altered the sequence of the admissions process and programming in the United States. Programs must operate from a prospective, not a retrospective, reimbursement system. Instead of having a client in a therapy program and then measuring the outcome, the managed care approach defines the medical necessity of the program goals, predetermines the services to be rendered and the duration of treatment, and ultimately the reimbursement schedule. This utilization review process has led many clinics in highly industrial areas that specialize in work programs to diversify their clientele or to close their doors altogether. This is an example of how reimbursement methods have a direct effect on intervention regimes as well as access to rehabilitative services.

The criteria for admission vary, depending on the program and client goals. Criteria may include the client's use of pain medications, the required healing period to ensure skin integrity before prosthetic retraining, and any surgical intervention to augment rehabilitative services and allow increased function (e.g., a tendon release to increase active range of motion after a burn injury). Programs must consider individual circumstances and client goals rather than following a narrow selection process designed merely to support successful program outcomes.

The sooner the injured worker participates in rehabilitation, the more successful the outcome. Frymoyer found that only 40% of clients with low back pain returned to work after having been disabled for 6 months; for those who were disabled 1 year, this figure dropped to 20%, and after 2 years, the chances of return to work were nil (cited in Niemeyer, Jacobs, Reynolds-Lynch, Bettencourt, & Lang, 1994). These findings suggest that clients who enter a work hardening program at ≤6 weeks after injury have an 80–90% expectation of return to work, whereas those who enter a program after 6 months have an expectation of only 20–40% (Niemeyer et al., 1994). Managed care approaches that have determined preferred providers can quickly initiate evaluation and programming to maximize the client's perceived role of worker and to facilitate return to work.

THE INDUSTRIAL REHABILITATION TEAM

A comprehensive, interdisciplinary team is required when the injured client's many roles are affected (worker, parent, spouse, teammate, homemaker). While collaborating with professionals from other disciplines, occupational therapists provide clients with the following:

- Quantifiable evaluations of occupational performance status.
- Analysis of both client and environmental factors that affect occupational performance.
- Intervention planning, implementation, and progression.
- Documentation according to governmental, reimbursement, and licensure standards.
- Discharge planning.

The certified occupational therapy assistant often plays a significant role in work programming. The occupational therapist focuses on problem identification, problem analysis, and the planning required for problem solution. The occupational therapy assistant focuses on delivery of direct services and documenting client response and progress (Larson, 2001).

Exercise physiologists have an excellent understanding of how the body responds physiologically to the effects of activity and exertion. They can play an integral role in the work conditioning phase of a functional restoration program (Hardway, 1993).

The Commission on Accreditation of Rehabilitation Facilities (CARF) has mandated that psychological services be offered in a return-to-work program. Upon admission, clients complete a battery of psychological screenings that assess attitudes, experiences, motivation, and pain tolerances. When the psychologist does intervene directly with a client in work hardening, therapy must be focused directly on the barrier identified. Interventions should be time limited and goal oriented, such as relaxing training, education on strategies to manage pain, and counseling to help the client adjust to the disability (Young 1993).

Work program clients may have their own attending physicians, but it is helpful to have a program medical director who is a physiatrist to address the immediate rehabilitation concerns of clients. Physiatrists also provide a medical sounding board for team members. The physiatrist often approves the clinical evaluation and signs off on an individual's impairment rating. Finally, the incorporation of physiatry in the clinical setting increases the timeliness of client care efficiency in report distribution to the appropriate parties.

Physical therapists, prosthetists, occupational health nurses, rehabilitation counselors, insurance case managers, social workers, vocational counselors, and medical specialists all are professionals who may play a role in the functional restoration rehabilitation team.

WORK PROGRAM EVALUATION

Work evaluations administered by an occupational therapist are called functional capacity evaluations (FCEs), and vary in length. The most reliable format occurs over two consecutive days, and the most critical items are presented on the second day. The evaluation time may be longer on the initial day than on the second, or it may be divided equally between the two days. The two-day format allows for retesting for accuracy and for evaluating the effect of the first day's work on the client. In some cases, the evaluation on the second day will reveal that the client has increased physical symptoms (muscle spasm, joint swelling) from work done on the first day. In other cases, the client may show increased abilities on the second day (because he or she has worked through the fears and caution) or may be consistent with the first day's performance. Therefore, the second test day is highly important for evaluating the effects of work so that recommendations for day-to-day work activity can be made (Iserhagen, 1988). Fiscal constraints may disallow a two-day evaluation. Therefore, therapists must gather more baseline information as the client begins participating in the actual program.

A referral for a FCE may be made solely to determine the individual's current physical demand level according to the *Dictionary of Occupational Titles* (U.S. Department of Labor, 1991). The results of this test may define the worker's capability to perform a specific job, may investigate effort and present abnormalities, or may be a prescreening to determine a prework physical. The FCE usually defines a baseline for the beginning of a functional restoration work program.

Functional capacity evaluations are often administered in a clinical setting, with specific equipment and control of external variables that might influence the test results. Because standardization is an important aspect of the FCE, the equipment and its placement are important. Selection of the items to be tested and the arrangement of all testing equipment should be done in advance of an assessment. One of the growing services, however, is on-site evaluation and rehabilitation. Hyland and Ruggles (2001) reported that their practice saw a tripling in amount of interest in on-site work injury management services since the mid-1990s.

The use of job-specific equipment or tools has become essential with the implementation of the Americans with Disabilities Act (ADA). This policy dissuades the evaluator from using high-technology, generic equipment to determine job-specific capabilities (see Chapter 24, Section 3). Evaluation of client factors that affect performance uses job-specific equipment. "The type of testing that I am suggesting is not computerized lifting evaluation but rather one that uses real and simulated work to determine objectively whether a person has the physical abilities to perform the job" (Fontana 1999, p. 2).

JOB SITE ANALYSIS

Job site analysis (JSA) plays a critical role in the success of the functional restoration program and is completed for several different reasons. A JSA may help the therapist understand the exposures of a specific job, which may increase the understanding of the client's disorder. A JSA also allows the therapist to design an accurate environment to simulate the job-specific tasks. Finally, the JSA establishes the job performance criteria and clinical reasoning on which program goals are based (Fig. 29-1). The client's

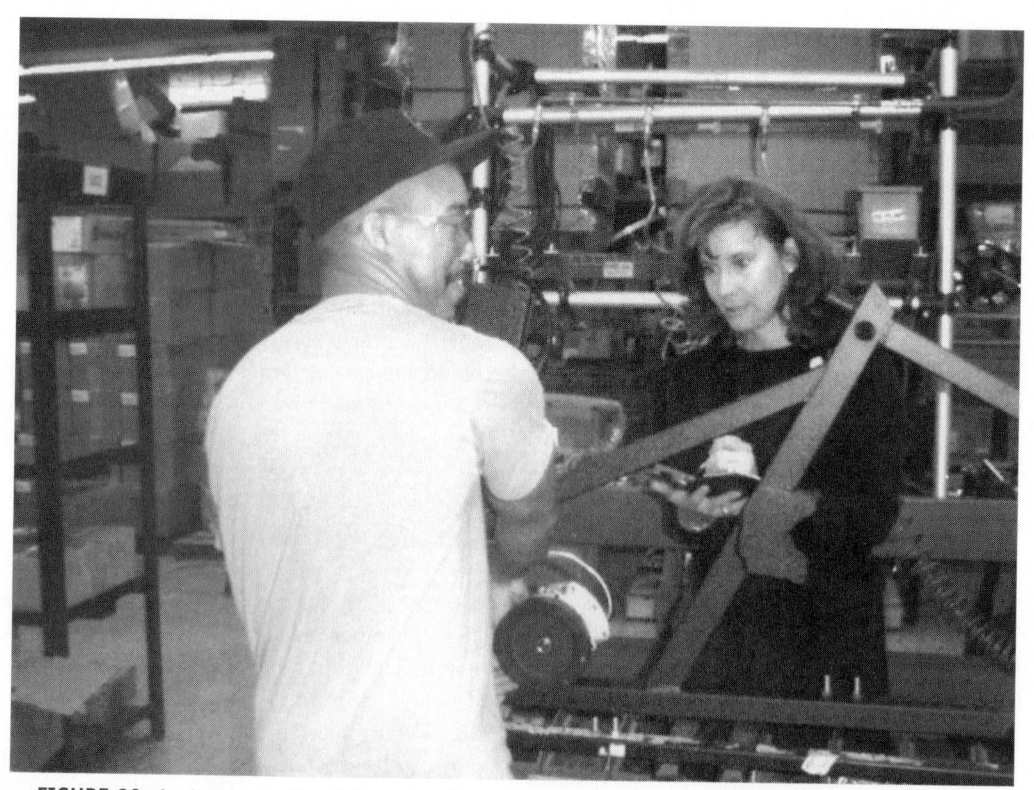

FIGURE 29–1. An occupational therapist observes an injured worker as he returns to his job. Through job site analysis, she can monitor how well her client can handle work demands. (Photo courtesy Sherlyn Fenton, Holliston, MA)

performance relative to these goals is analyzed so that the therapist can make discharge recommendations, which may consist of the following options:

- Return to work (full duty, modified duty, reasonable accommodations).
- Further vocational exploration and retraining.
- Additional medical investigation for unresolved symptoms.

The JSA is one of the most effective ways to engage the employer in the work program philosophy and process. It often offers opportunity to request the loan and use of actual tools and materials that are appropriate to be transferred to and used in the clinical setting. Whether it is approached from a work methods analysis or an ergonomic perspective, JSA is a valuable tool in providing a comprehensive work program.

WORK PROGRAM INTERVENTION

Frequency and Duration

Intervention frequency may vary according to the client's program goals. A client may attend therapy daily and progress from a 2-hr to a 6-hr and then to an 8-hr day. However, if clients are currently at their jobs with restrictions, they may attend in conjunction with work hours. Clients participating in full-time light-duty work may augment their normal work schedule with a program to increase specific performance areas to transition into full-time unrestricted work.

The classification of *material handler* is often used when discussing client job requirements. The term is commonly used to describe an individual who must rely on physical capacity to accomplish job demands. Often caregivers and laypeople mistakenly perceive strength as the primary factor required to accomplish job tasks; however, the rate and duration demands are equally significant components (Botehlo, Fenton, Jones, Meedzan, & Meyers, 1993).

Intervention duration depends on the individual's goals; ability to progress to meet the work demands of load, pace, and duration; opportunity to return to the desired occupational role; and ability to obtain program reimbursement. Moreover, the severity of injury and the time between injury and program admission may be the most influential factors when considering the treatment duration required to effect a successful discharge outcome (Joe, 1995). Occupational therapists use their knowledge of anatomy, physiology, and the effects of pathology, along with careful analysis and grading of occupational performance tasks, to maximize function and encourage safe work practice.

Work Conditioning and Work Hardening

A functional restoration program is often made up of two components: work conditioning and work hardening. The work conditioning portion of the program consists of a fitness program and nonspecific, job-simulated work tasks. Strengthening and flexibility through spinal stabilization, lumbar retraining, and cardiovascular exercise all make up a good fitness regimen. Nonspecific job tasks include lifting at various levels, carrying, pushing, and pulling. These adjunct activities are part of a progressive schedule to increase strength and endurance, preparing the client for an occupational role to be determined after completion of the functional restoration program.

When the client has occupational goals with well-defined physical and psychological demands, work hardening is appropriate. Job-specific enabling activities incorporate work tasks that progress the client to the physical demand levels of the actual job as described within the employer's functional job description instead of with the demands listed in the *Dictionary of Occupational Titles* (U.S. Dept. of Labor, 1991). These activities require great collaboration among the practitioner, client, and employer to obtain the accurate equipment, tools, materials, and criteria to establish a simulated work environment.

Job simulation allows clients a good opportunity to test their abilities to sustain work-related practices while in a noncompetitive setting. The simulated environment should mimic factors such as noise, lighting, timing, and safety issues of the actual workplace as closely as possible. Simulation provides the practitioner and client with an opportunity to consider and trial necessary adaptations or modified work practices.

Since the implementation of the ADA, more workers are able to return to their desired jobs with some type of reasonable accommodation. Just a few years ago such accommodation would not have been considered worth the effort or expense; now employers are realizing that their most valuable asset is their workforce.

Specialized Protocols

Traditionally, acute industrial injuries far surpassed other diagnoses treated in functional restoration programs. Yet over the past decade with advancements in technology, new risk factors have led to an increase in soft tissue, musculoskeletal disorders. Carpal tunnel syndrome and chronic cervical tension are just two of the work-related complaints caused by prolonged use of computer workstations, which require employees to engage in awkward and often repetitive movements. "As noted, musculoskeletal discomfort is ubiquitous, and ergonomists concede it has many causes other than work. It occurs (and dissipates) naturally and is correlated with aging, obesity, and genetic predisposition, among other things" (Kolber, 2001, p. 26). These clients may share similar conditions and objectives, so that they can be appropriately treated in a group approach.

In contrast, clients with limitations secondary to burns, electrocution, amputation, and systemic disease present with special circumstances that require therapists to consider individual programs with less focus on physical demand levels of a specific job and more emphasis on the restoration of the performance areas. Program goals may initially include both personal and instrumental activities of daily living, while deferring vocational goals until the client is deemed medically stable and at a physical end point for joint range of motion (ROM), prosthetic fitting, and pain management techniques.

For injured workers who require the use of their upper extremities and specifically their hand function, the incorporation of a certified hand therapist (CHT) is an appropriate referral. These specialists (most of whom are occupational therapists) are often recommended after a surgical procedure to facilitate therapeutic techniques such as dynamic splinting and closely monitored hierarchical progressions while reestablishing function. For all industrial rehabilitation programs, a keen knowledge of neuromuscular control is essential for establishing clinical reasoning to better facilitate client recovery while documenting program duration validity.

Body Mechanics

While posture can reflect attitudes, it also can be the cause of discomfort and pain (Turner, 2000). Many programs include short courses in proper body mechanics. This information covers anatomy, anthropometrics, and the physiology of healthy movement practices. Clients increase their understanding of the mechanical structures and the risk factors they are exposed to while in and out of the workplace. Body mechanics training can minimize and, at times, eliminate the risk of injury. Although there are other factors that reduce clients' risk of reinjury, knowledge of proper body mechanics in conjunction with good fitness are the first steps to reaching program objectives.

Documentation

Well-established documentation systems are an integral function of any successful work program. Practitioners must document their work clearly and concisely throughout the work program process. The purpose of an effective documentation system is for the reader to be able to discern easily and quickly the client's occupational tolerances. From initial evaluation responses to daily documented program reactions, written records provide the practitioners, clients, and other involved parties with insight and direction for programming and discharge planning.

As important as objective measurements are in this type of setting to quantify decision making, skilled, subjective observations and interpretations often qualify future planning. In this area, however, it is imperative for practitioners to maintain documented perceptions in measurable terminology. A good example of this practice is the issue of determining the feasibility of a client's returning to work. Client attendance, timeliness, ability for transition between program tasks, and the willingness to complete the scheduled day can all be described in the feasibility evaluation checklist (FEC; Ogden-Niemeyer & Jacobs, 1989).

The client is also expected to self-report such items as work task progression, pain levels, and reactions to the therapeutic program on a daily basis. At discharge, the report should contain input from both client and therapist and include the results from standardized and nonstandardized tests, a summary of what goals have been achieved, a comparative analysis of the client's performance from admission to discharge, and any recommendations for accommodations and job modifications (Hertfelder & Gwin, 1989).

The client generally engages in specific job simulation tasks for 1 to 2 weeks before program discharge. When recommending discharge and documenting release to return to a specific job, the rehabilitation team must be able to document the client's ability in relation to the job requirements. For those clients with no specific job to return to, the team must demonstrate either achievement of work-related rehabilitation goals or a plateau in progress (Frantzlett, McCabe, Tramposh, & Tate-Henderson, 1988). The more the practitioner communicates with the involved parties before discharge, the smoother the client's return to work.

Vocational Counseling

If a client cannot return to the (1) same employer, same job; (2) same job, different employer; or (3) same employer, different job, the client should be referred for vocational counseling, as previously described. Clients can improve job-seeking skills, scholastic aptitudes, and interviewing techniques through combined efforts with the rehabilitation staff and the vocational counselor. They can also explore transitional skills and retraining opportunities that will enhance their current vocational potential.

Prework Screening

Employers often ask therapists to perform physical screenings to determine if a prospective employee is appropriate to complete a specific job. The employer concerns include soaring workers' compensation costs, lost workdays and productivity, and worker protection. Yet issues of discrimination, disclosure, liability in the failure to identify a potential problem, and the questionable predictive validity of these tests are equally important and should be of significant concern to the therapist. Detailed functional job descriptions and adequate training periods provided to returning or new workers are alternatives to these screenings.

Prevention Education

Injury is epidemic in America and most other industrialized nations and is one of America's greatest health problems. This scenario not only creates incentive for employers to incorporate safety prevention and rehabilitation programs but also mandates it. In 1999, back injuries accounted for 46% of lost workday injuries among nurse assistants and orderlies, according to the U.S. Bureau of Labor Statistics (Childs, 2001).

In a study reported by Cooper, Tate and Yassi (1997), work assessment and work hardening were components of a comprehensive interdisciplinary program to prevent and manage back injury in nurses in a large tertiary-care hospital. The results support the concept of maintaining individuals with back injury in the workplace by providing early on-site intervention that includes work hardening and modified work.

Prevention programs should incorporate a variety of media to address the various learning styles of the workforce. A 2-hr session may include the following: a simple anatomy review, descriptions of common workplace injuries, a short video on proper body mechanics, an explanation of ergonomic controls (worker, engineering, and administrative), and a clinical practice session. If the therapist avoids playing the role of expert and allows audience members to have input from their own experiences, program participation is facilitated and participants more readily buy into new knowledge and methods of safe work practices. This approach ultimately fosters safe work practice compliance on the job.

CONCLUSION

To ensure successful outcomes in work programming, the occupational therapy practitioner needs to be cognizant of an ever-changing environment. Moreover, the therapist must be able to consider all aspects of the case management team and adapt effective client treatment approaches according to criteria that are often set by someone other than an attending physician. "Returning to work following an injury has changed considerably over the past decade. From 'must be at 100%' to 'light duty,' the wide range of options for workers can pose challenges to the health care provider who needs to offer appropriate recommendations. Solutions must be as unique as each injury case and job" (Griffin, 2000, p. 30). Meeting the goals of the worker, employer, and third-party payer can be challenging; yet with good communication and well-defined program objectives, this area of specialty is a rewarding career path for an occupational therapy practitioner.

SECTION II

Education

YVONNE L. SWINTH

OVERVIEW

Generally, within public school settings, the interventions provided by occupational therapy practitioners are guided by the most current reauthorization of the Individuals with Disabilities Education Act (IDEA). (The background and guiding philosophical assumptions of this federal legislation were discussed in Chapter 24, Section 4.) The purpose of the legislation is to provide a free and appropriate public education (FAPE) in the least restrictive environment (LRE) to those students who need special education services. The IDEA also mandates **related services,** such as occupational therapy, when needed as part of the individualized education program (IEP) for student success.

Occupational therapy practitioners also may provide services in the public schools and other educational settings (e.g., private schools, universities, adult education centers) under § 504 of the Rehabilitation Act (1973) as well as under the ADA. The ADA is a civil rights act and provides protection to individuals with disabilities similar to protections provided to individuals on the basis of race, color, sex, national origin, age, and religion. The ADA supports the notion that individuals with disabilities should have equal opportunities to live, work, and play within society.

In addition, the primary work setting for an occupational therapy practitioner may be a hospital or private clinic, and a therapist may contract services to an educational setting. In rare instances, occupational therapy practitioners may be hired by a public school district to provide services to any student who may need their support (special education or general education). Table 29-1 provides an overview of the legislation and funding that support occupational therapy services in educational settings.

The occupational therapy practitioner in the educational setting is primarily concerned with students' occupations

TABLE 29-1. **OCCUPATIONAL THERAPY SERVICES IN EDUCATIONAL SETTINGS**[a]

Legislation or Sources of Funding	Population Served	Role of Occupational Therapy
IDEA[b]	• Students who are eligible for special education and require the related service of occupational therapy to receive FAPE in the LRE	• To collaborate with the IEP Eteam to determine the students' needs and to provide services as outlined in the IEP to support student performance relevant to the educational environment
§ 504 of the Rehabilitation Act	• Students who have a disability, a history of a disability, or a perceived disability that affects their performance in school. (In the public schools, generally students who are not eligible for special education) • Students who meet the definition *of individual with a disability* (i.e., have a physical or mental impairment that substantially limits one or more major life activities)	• To collaborate with the § 504 team to provide the accommodations and adaptations needed by students to access the school environment and services
ADA	• Ensures equal opportunity for individuals with disabilities in employment, state and local government services, public accommodations, commercial facilities, and transportation. • A civil rights legislation that supports participation in the educational setting by students who have a disability	• To provide support through consultation and monitoring to ensure that students have access to and can participate in the educational setting. • Often involves working with environmental adaptations, accommodations, and assistive devices
Other funding sources[c]	• Any student who may need the support of an occupational therapy practitioner	• To support student performance in occupations relevant to the educational environment

[a]Adapted from Swinth, Chandler, Hanft, Jackson, and Shepherd (in press).

[b]IDEA is applicable only for students (ages 0–21) who receive special education services through their public school setting.

[c]For example, general education funds (for public schools), private insurance, private agencies (e.g., United Cerebral Palsy), and state agencies (e.g., Division of Vocational Rehabilitation).

relevant to the educational environment, regardless of which legislation is guiding practice. Occupational therapy service may address a student's performance in education, work, play/leisure, and social skills, with outcomes that are directed toward improved student participation in the curriculum, access to the school environment, and participation in extracurricular activities. Thus, within educational settings, occupational therapy practitioners need to be familiar with and understand the educational environment in which they work as well as what legislation and/or funding source(s) support their involvement in that setting.

FACTORS INFLUENCING OCCUPATIONAL THERAPY INTERVENTIONS IN EDUCATIONAL ENVIRONMENTS

There are a variety of factors that affect the planning and implementation of intervention by occupational therapy practitioners within educational environments. Some of the factors include the makeup of the educational team, how decisions are made, and the unique characteristics of the system. Since a majority of practitioners work in schools under the IDEA requirements, this section focuses on the intervention considerations and requirements related to this legislation. However, the principles and strategies discussed are applicable to all students who occupational therapy practitioners may serve in any educational setting.

Educational Teams

The concept of teaming, or collaborating as a team, to make decisions about the program and services to be provided has been a guiding principle of special education law since its inception. With the reauthorization in 1997, the IDEA became more explicit regarding the emphasis on teaming and collaboration among professionals and families to make effective decisions about student need(s). The IDEA (1997) clearly specifies that whenever decisions are made about a student, the parents or caregivers must be involved.

There are two types of teams specified in the IDEA: the evaluation team and the IEP team. Both teams must include qualified professionals who are knowledgeable about the student and his or her need(s). If a decision is being made about occupational therapy involvement in a student's program, then an occupational therapist must be involved in the teaming process. In the public schools, the specific makeup of each team is driven by the student's needs and may include general and special education teachers, therapists (physical, occupational, and speech), psychologists, counselors, parents, the student, and different community members. The focus of the team decision-making process must be on student outcomes and performance with an emphasis on the general education environment whenever possible.

Team Decision Making

Effective and efficient delivery of services, in the school environment, requires a systematic process for team decision making and problem solving. There is a tendency for professionals to identify a need and immediately start proposing and implementing solutions without first identifying the necessary outcomes required for the student to participate in the educational environment. Educational teams employ a variety of tools that support a systematic process of decision making. Many of the process-oriented assessments described earlier in the book (Chapter 24, Section 4)—such as the McGill Action Planning System (MAPS) and Choosing Outcomes and Accommodations for Children (COACH)—can be used in this manner, since they help support the team decision-making and problem-solving processes. For example, the MAPS consists of seven specific questions that support the planning process and identification of team-generated outcomes for students with disabilities (O'Brien & Forest, 1989). The questions are as follows:

- What is the student's history?
- What are your dreams for the student?
- What are your fears for the student?
- Who is the student? (One word statements that describe the student.)
- What are the student's strengths, gifts, and abilities?
- What are the student's needs?
- What would the student's ideal day at school look like and what must be done to make it happen?

A typical MAPS planning session can take up to 2 hr. The entire team (parents, students, therapists, and teachers) as well as other invited members (siblings, other family members, or community members) provide input to each question. The questions are not quick or easy to answer, but the result of a good planning session is a strong foundation from which to develop the student's IEP. The process focuses on the value of the integration of the student in neighborhood schools and in general education classes to develop friendships and to ensure a quality education for the child (Vandercook & York, 1988). By the time the team is addressing question six (What are the student's needs?), it has the background to be able to establish both short-term and long-term outcomes. These outcome goals are then used to guide a discussion regarding the student's ideal day and how to get there.

Range of Services

There is a range of services occupational therapy practitioners provide in educational environments. Intervention may include one-on-one services or collaborating with other team members to identify and implement environmental adaptations and modifications to the physical layout of the school campus or the classroom. Regardless of how services are provided, practitioners must be aware of curricular issues such as education reform, standards-based assessment, and the requirements of general education. The IDEA requires that students with disabilities be considered for and have access to the general education curriculum whenever possible and to be included in education reform and statewide assessments. Thus occupational therapy service may address the requirements of general education as well. For example, in some states, occupational therapists are being asked to address alternative assessments for students with severe disabilities and are involved in making decisions about reasonable testing accommodations for students with learning disabilities. To fully participate in these discussions and to support the implementation of the recommendations, the occupational therapist must have a basic understanding of the identified educational outcomes and testing requirements within his or her system.

REFERRAL PROCESS

When a classroom teacher is concerned about a student, initial interventions should be developed and implemented through a collaborative team process. Increasingly, occupational therapy practitioners are involved with the planning and implementation of prereferral interventions. In some cases, effective prereferral interventions, such as the use of a move-and-sit cushion for a fidgety student or the development and implementation of a handwriting curriculum, may successfully support the student within the educational environment and further intervention may not be needed.

If the prereferral interventions are not effective, the student is then referred to an evaluation team. The evaluation team determines if the special education process, as outlined in the IDEA, should be initiated or if the student should be referred for some other type of support, such as what is provided under § 504 of the Rehabilitation Act. For example, if a student requires only additional accommodations or adaptations and does not require specially designed instruction to meet educational outcomes, then the evaluation team may not recommend a full special education evaluation. They would instead refer the student to the school's 504 team. If the evaluation team feels that the student may need specially designed instruction (special education) to receive FAPE in the LRE, then the special education evaluation process would be initiated.

Ideally, the therapist should be involved throughout the teaming and decision-making process, if the evaluation team feels that the student may require services by an occupational therapy practitioner or that the student has needs that may require the input from an occupational therapist. Once the student is referred to special education and it is determined that the referral is appropriate, a team of qualified professionals design and initiate the evaluation. The team should be knowledgeable about the student and the suspected areas of disability. The purpose of the evaluation is to determine if the student has a disability, whether the disability adversely affects his or her educational performance in the general education curriculum, and to make a determination of the nature and extent of the student's need for specially designed instruction and any necessary related services (see Chapter 24, Section 4).

DEVELOPMENT OF THE INDIVIDUALIZED EDUCATION PROGRAM

Once the evaluation is completed, the IEP team collaborates to design the student's program (Giangreco, 2001). First, the IEP team, which includes the parents and student (if old enough), reviews the evaluation results and writes a summary of the student's educational performance, called **present levels of education performance (PLEPs).** The PLEPs describe the student's strengths and areas of concern in relation to the expectations of the general education curriculum. The IEP team then develops the student's goals and objectives based on the data summarized in the PLEPs and the agreed-on outcomes identified by the team.

Different settings have different requirements for how goals and objectives are written. Under the IDEA, the objective is that goals and objectives are developed as a team. Thus there may not be an occupational therapy goal page in the IEP. This is particularly common in some early intervention settings and is becoming increasingly common across all ages. Generally, it is expected that goals and objectives identify a functional outcome, state what the student will do and under what conditions the skill or behavior will be performed, and include a timeline for completion (Borcherding, 2000).

Collaborating with the team is an important aspect of occupational therapy service delivery in the schools. This collaboration sets the stage for focusing intervention strategies on specific student outcomes. Since parents (and older students) are involved in the team planning and decision-making process their perspectives are well represented in the occupational profile developed by the occupational therapist. Throughout the collaborative process, the occupational therapist identifies where he or she may be able to support the student's occupational performance in the educational environment. Box 29-1 provides an example of the goal setting documentation for Susie, a sixth-grade student with spina bifida.

After the goals and objectives have been developed, the team discusses which professional(s) should address which particular goals (e.g., teacher and occupational therapist or, maybe, occupational therapist and speech pathologist), when they will be addressed (e.g., during physical education, during art, or when walking in the hall) and where (e.g., in the general education classroom, in the cafeteria, or on the playground). Each of these decisions are made based on student need, not the personal preferences of professionals. Thus, if needed, the occupational therapist designs the occupational therapy intervention plan based on the outcomes identified by the entire educational team.

OCCUPATIONAL THERAPY INTERVENTION PLAN

Once the IEP team has developed the program and determines that a student would benefit from receiving occupational therapy as a related service, the occupational therapy practitioner develops a specific occupational therapy intervention plan to reach anticipated outcomes. The intervention plan addresses the occupational performance areas as well as the performance skill or student factor that is affecting the student's ability to participate fully in the educational environment. Occupational areas that an occupational therapist may address in the school setting are given in Table 24-2.

As in other settings, the occupational therapy practitioner considers student factors such as motor skills, process skills, and communication/interaction skills when determining student needs. In addition, the practitioner considers performance patterns, such as habits and routines, the activity demands in the school setting, and the entire school context. Keeping occupational performance as the core, a variety of conceptual frameworks for practice and frame of references guide the interventions in educational settings. The primary perspectives may include occupational behavior, developmental, neurodevelopmental, learning, biomechanical, sensory integration, and coping (Kramer & Hinojosa, 1999).

SERVICE DELIVERY

Planning Intervention

When planning the intervention implementation, occupational therapists must consider the LRE requirement of IDEA: "to the maximum extent appropriate, children with disabilities are to be educated with children who are not disabled. . . . [R]emoval of these children from the general educational environment occurs only when the nature or severity of the disability is such that education in regular classes with the use of supplementary aids and services cannot be achieved satisfactorily (Least Restrictive Environment)" (§ 300.550). Thus occupational therapy is provided

BOX 29–1 GOAL SETTING DOCUMENTATION FOR SUSIE

Susie is in the sixth grade at the Norwood Middle School. Susie has spina bifida and some cognitive delays. The school psychologist, Susie's teacher, the occupational therapist, the physical therapist, and the speech therapist each completed an individualized evaluation. The occupational therapy evaluation included an occupational profile and an analysis of Susie's occupational performance in her educational setting. Based on the individual assessments, an evaluation report was written. The following are some of the strengths and concerns that were identified.

STRENGTHS

- Able to move independently about the school in her wheelchair.
- Social skills with peers.
- Verbal expressive language.
- Creativity.

CONCERNS

- Easily distracted in the classroom.
- Cannot transfer in and out of her wheelchair independently.
- Receptive language.
- Written language.
- Fine and gross motor skills.

EXCERPTS FROM SUSIE'S PRESENT LEVELS OF EDUCATIONAL PERFORMANCE

Susie currently participates in her general education classroom throughout her day. Her assignments are modified so that she can complete them within the same amount of time as her peers. Noise and visual stimuli can easily distract Susie within her classroom environment. She goes to the resource room for assistance with math and written language when she cannot complete the assignment independently in her general education classroom.

Susie can move about her school environment, without assistance, using her manual wheelchair. In the classroom, she requires physical assistance to transfer from her wheelchair to the desk chair and back. She has difficulty with fine and gross motor skills. Her difficulty with fine motor skills affects her ability to complete written assignments and art projects with her peers. Her delays in gross motor skills affects her ability to participate in physical education and recess activities.

Susie demonstrates good adaptive skills during social interactions with her peers. However, she is becoming increasingly aware of her disability and limitations. This awareness has caused some episodes of depression and has resulted in extended absences from school. Susie demonstrates emerging self-determination skills in other areas as well. She can describe potential accommodations/adaptations that she would like to her parents and other familiar adults, but she does not advocate for herself during school.

GOALS

Psychosocial Skills

Susie will demonstrate improved self-determination and self-advocacy by collaborating with her therapists and teachers to identify and implement any needed modifications and adaptations into her educational program from <50% of the time to 90% of the time, as measured by therapist and teacher data, by June.

Written Language

Susie will use identified accommodations/adaptations and/or assistive technology (e.g., word processor, spell checker, adapted writing utensil) to complete her classroom assignments within the general education setting and within the same amount of time as her peers from 75% of the time to 100% of the time, as measured by therapist and teacher data by June.

OUTLINE OF OCCUPATIONAL THERAPY INTERVENTION PLAN

Using the team-identified goals and objectives as a guide, Susie's occupational therapist developed an intervention plan. This plan included some direct therapy to identify any needed accommodations/adaptations and to teach Susie how to implement them and how to use any assistive technology. The occupational therapist also worked with Susie to teach other school district personnel about her accommodations/adaptations and assistive technology. Ongoing consultation and monitoring were also included to ensure that Susie was able to participate within her educational environment. Finally, since Susie also received therapy from a community-based occupational therapist, the school therapist contacted the community therapist at least every 6 months to discuss Susie's program.

in the student's typical environment to the extent possible. Such environments may include the classroom, lunchroom, bathroom, or playground.

Service Delivery Models

Many different service delivery models are used within the educational setting. The IDEA defines four different categories for service delivery:

- Specially designed instruction.
- Related services.
- Supplemental aids and services.
- Services on behalf of the child.

In most educational settings, occupational therapists provide related services, supplemental aid and service, and services on behalf of the child. Depending on the rules and regulations within a particular state, an occupational therapist may provide the specially designed instruction. Generally, it is rare for an occupational therapist to be the only professional providing special education services to a student with a disability. However, a student with normal cognition but significant motor delays (e.g., muscular dystrophy, spina

TABLE 29–2. **OCCUPATIONAL THERAPY INTERVENTIONS IN SCHOOL SETTINGS**[a]

Performance Skill	Examples	Student Interventions	Educational Staff Interventions	Systems Intervention
Process skills	Energy, knowledge, temporal, orientation, organizing space and objects, adaptation	• Learning about self-regulation, levels of arousal and attention • Use of sensory media during intervention • Sensory integrative techniques • Initiates activities and sustains attention to complete them • Organization of desk and other work areas • Accommodates/adapts to changes in the routine • Work on visual perceptual skills • Orientation to time and place • Problem solving • Self-determination • Behavior management	• Teach staff how to use sensory processing techniques in the classroom • Provide in-services on programs such as the Alert Program[b] to help students recognize how alert they are feeling and to identify sensorimotor experiences that can be used to change the level of alertness • Training and collaborative program development	• Participate on curriculum committees • Educate the system in specific environmental factors that support self-regulation and arousal in the school • Environmental modifications
Motor skills	Posture, mobility, coordination, strength and effort, energy	• Participation in physical education and recess activities • Participation in classroom activities such as written work • Posture/body alignment during school activities • Mobility within the school environment • Accessing assistive technology • Teach energy-conservation techniques	• Training on use of adaptive equipment and accommodations and modifications • Training on positioning, lifting, and transferring	• Work with the system to adopt a handwriting curriculum • Application of universal design to physical environment and the curriculum • Ordering appropriate adaptive equipment (e.g., lifts) for staff safety • Proper use of backpacks campaign • Adapted equipment (e.g., weight-training machines)
Communication and interaction skills	Physicality, information exchange, relations	• Social skill development • Psychosocial skill development • Peer interactions • Development of self-determination skills	• Training and collaborative program development	• Staff development activities • Participation on curriculum committees

[a]This is not an inclusive list; rather, it suggests some possibilities for intervention. Specific needs of the student, staff, and system help define the particular interventions to be used.

[b]Williams and Shellenberger (1994).

bifida, cerebral palsy) may require more support than just accommodations or adaptations to participate within the educational setting.

The occupational therapist may choose to use a variety of service models specified in IDEA. However, student need is the driving factor when deciding how services should be provided. The three most commonly described models in the occupational therapy literature are direct services, monitoring, and consultation (Dunn, 1988; Hanft & Place, 1996; Case-Smith, Rogers, & Johnson, 2001). Direct service, one of the most common models, is when the practitioner meets directly with the student or group of students on a regular basis. Monitoring is when the practitioner identifies the student's needs and designs appropriate interventions but another person implements the plan. The practitioner meets with the student regularly to monitor progress. Consultation uses the specialized expertise of the practitioner to improve the educational environment and train the teacher and the parents to implement interventions for the student. The practitioner does not work directly with the student. The consultative therapy model is increasing in popularity, as practitioners, parents and teachers are becoming more educated and are recognizing the importance of communication among all team members in achieving desired outcomes (Sandler, 1997).

Often the different service delivery models are presented as a continuum and in a linear fashion. As a result, the assumption is made that consultation is less restrictive than direct services, and thus the goal is to move toward a consultative or monitoring type of service delivery. However, for some students, the opposite may be true. Therefore, it may be more appropriate to view all the service delivery models as pieces of a pie. Each service delivery model is important and valuable. Usually, therapy practitioners working in the schools use a variety of service delivery models (e.g., some one on one, some small groups, and some consultative services) to meet a student's identified need(s).

Inherent to service delivery in any setting is the documentation of services. Documentation serves as a communication tool to the students and families regarding the individualized program. In addition to the development of the IEP, documentation includes regular reporting of progress and describing the services delivered.

In addition to providing services on behalf of a specific student, some occupational therapy practitioners also may provide services to the educational staff, parents, and/or the educational system. If the services are provided on behalf of a specific student, then they are documented on the IEP as consultation. However, if occupational therapy practitioners are providing general services, then the recipient of services (or client) may actually be the educational staff, parents, or the system. Table 29-2 provides example of the range of interventions provided by an occupational therapy practitioner in the school setting.

Interagency Collaboration

Another an important aspect of occupational therapy service delivery in educational settings includes collaboration between school personnel and staff from any clinic a child might be attending, as well as collaboration with other agencies. Interagency collaboration is particularly necessary if the occupational therapy practitioner is providing services for students using assistive technology or during transition planning for older students.

Periodic Review

All decision making about occupational therapy intervention in the schools should be based on data. IDEA requires that the IEP be reviewed at least annually, with regular updates to the family regarding the student's progress. (IDEA requires that updates regarding student progress on IEPs must be at least at the same intervals as general education report cards.) However, the occupational therapist should consistently (more often than quarterly) reevaluate the intervention plan to ensure that the student is moving toward achieving targeted outcomes. If needed, the occupational therapy intervention plan, or even the IEP, may need to be modified before the annual review.

CONCLUSION

Occupational therapy intervention in the schools is guided by the IDEA. Practitioners working in the schools collaborate with the IEP team to determine student needs and targeted outcomes. Once these needs and outcomes have been defined on the IEP and the team determines that occupational therapy services are needed, then the occupational therapist designs the specific intervention plan. Occupational therapy intervention in the schools focuses on the occupational performance of the student within the educational environment. Practitioners may also provide services directed to the needs of the educational staff, parents, or system.

SECTION III

Play and Leisure

LOREE A. PRIMEAU

PLAY AND LEISURE IN OCCUPATIONAL THERAPY

Occupational therapy has a long tradition of incorporating **play and leisure** into intervention (Parham & Primeau, 1997). In the founding years of the profession, the play spirit was seen as essential for living a worthwhile life (Saunders, 1922; Slagle, 1922; Ziegler, 1924). Over time, as occupational therapy practitioners became increasingly concerned with scientific and technical aspects of intervention, play and leisure were thought to be unscientific and inappropriate for use in practice. Late in the twentieth century, scholars in occupational therapy and occupational science reclaimed play and leisure (Bundy, 1993; Canadian Association of Occupational Therapists [CAOT], 1996; Parham, 1996; Parham & Fazio, 1997; Primeau, 1996; Reilly, 1974; Suto, 1998). To explain play and leisure in intervention, I present a conceptual framework based on the work of Blanche (1997) and Pierce (1997). Play and leisure in intervention may be lures or rewards, means to achieve intervention goals, and ends or intervention outcomes.

PLAY AND LEISURE AS LURES OR REWARDS

Practitioners use play and leisure as *lures* or *rewards* to motivate clients to participate in therapeutic activities or to reward them for their participation in intervention (Blanche, 1997; Pierce, 1997). A survey of 222 occupational therapists working with preschool-aged children indicated that all respondents regarded play as important in motivating children to participate in intervention; 91% reported that it was very important (Couch, Deitz, & Kanny, 1998). Pierce (1997) described the use of play with a toy as a therapy lure when it is presented out of reach of a child. The child is then encouraged to move toward the toy and, when successful, is allowed to play with it. Another example of play and leisure as lures is practitioners' frequent use of a playful attitude in their interactions with clients to draw them into intervention activities. Practitioners have historically attended to this affective aspect of therapy by creating intervention settings that are infused with feelings of cheerfulness, an esprit de corps, and hope (Kielhofner & Burke, 1983).

Play and leisure as *rewards* are also frequently employed in intervention. Of 203 occupational therapists working with preschool-aged children, 99% reported their use of play as a reinforcer; 40% indicated this use in >50% of their caseload (Couch et al., 1998). Play as reinforcer is typically used when practitioners provide an opportunity for children to engage in free-play activities during or at the conclusion of an intervention session. Blanche (1997) urged those who use play to reinforce children's specific actions to allow time for play consistently throughout a session, rather than banishing it to the end of a session. The common practice of timing opportunities for free-play at the end of a session leaves it open to interruption or postponement, suggesting that it is less important than other intervention activities, and disregards children's view of play as one of primary importance (Blanche, 1997). Leisure is also used as a reinforcer, particularly when participation in specific leisure activities is the culmination of intervention sessions in which clients planned and organized these activities.

PLAY AND LEISURE AS MEANS

Play and leisure as *means* refers to their use in intervention as therapeutic media or modalities to achieve specific intervention goals. Clients' engagement in play and leisure is the method or process through which change occurs (Gray, 1998; Trombly, 1995). Practitioners employ play and leisure as means to target change in client factors and performance skills (underlying all areas of occupation) and two specific areas of occupation (play and leisure).

Means to Address Client Factors and Performance Skills

Play and leisure as means are frequently used to address impairments in clients' body functions and structures and limitations in their performance skills. Practitioners engage their clients in play and leisure activities that are designed to facilitate their achievement of intervention goals related to those impairments and limitations. Survey results indicated that 100% of 212 occupational therapists working with preschool-aged children used play as a therapeutic modality to enhance motor, sensory, or psychosocial outcomes; 92% indicated this use in >50% of their caseload (Couch et al., 1998). These results resonate other occupational therapy literature in which play is typically described as a means to facilitate children's development of their physical, cognitive, and psychosocial abilities and their acquisition of motor, process, and communication and interaction skills (Blanche, 1997; CAOT, 1996; Morrison & Metzger, 2001; Parham & Primeau, 1997; Pierce, 1997).

Although descriptions of leisure as means in the occupational therapy literature are limited (Bundy, 1993; Suto, 1998), other literature indicates that it is used to achieve physical, cognitive, psychological, social, and spiritual benefits (Driver, Brown, & Peterson, 1991). Occupational therapy practitioners often employ leisure activities, such as games or crafts, as means to improve their clients' manual dexterity, increase their attention to task, develop their social skills, or enhance their feelings of self-efficacy and self-esteem.

Means to Enhance Areas of Occupation: Play and Leisure Performance

Play and leisure as means can target change in two specific areas of occupation: play and leisure. They are used to address limitations in clients' play and leisure performance (what they actually do and their experience while doing it). Practitioners engage their clients in play and leisure activities to achieve intervention goals related to their competence in and experience of these activities. Intervention provides opportunities for clients to practice specific play and leisure activities, explore new ones, or enhance their experience while engaged in them (Bundy, 2001; Gray, 1998; Morrison & Metzger, 2001).

When clients demonstrate problems with competence in their chosen play and leisure activities, practitioners can provide opportunities for them to practice play and leisure activities in a positive and safe environment or to explore alternate play and leisure activities in which they can experience higher levels of competence. For example, intervention for a boy with developmental dyspraxia who has difficulty playing soccer with his peers can include sessions in which he actually plays soccer so that he can practice the skills and tasks required for success in a safe and positive environment with no serious consequences for failure (Morrison & Metzger, 2001). In addition, based on evaluation of this boy's activity interests and activity choices, the practitioner can address the mismatch among his interest in and choice of soccer and his limited competence in it by engaging him in other sport activities that may provide a better match.

When clients report problems with their experience of play and leisure, practitioners can design and adapt play and leisure activities and the environments in which they occur (Bundy, 2001; Morrison & Metzger, 2001) to facilitate their clients' experience of playfulness, positive affect, personal meaning, and overall satisfaction with their play and leisure experience. For example, an elderly woman reported that the leisure experience she had previously obtained through cooking was no longer satisfying and personally meaningful secondary to her physical impairments related to a cerebrovascular accident (Bundy, 2001). The practitioner adapted the leisure activity of cooking and designed the kitchen environment to facilitate her performance in such a way that her leisure experience during cooking was enhanced. Rather than focusing intervention on her body functions and structures and performance skills in the context of remediation of motor control, the practitioner used the client's leisure activity of cooking as means to enable her to regain the experience of leisure.

PLAY AND LEISURE AS ENDS: PLAY AND LEISURE PARTICIPATION

Play and leisure as *ends* refers to clients' participation in play and leisure as the goal or outcome of intervention (Gray, 1998; Trombly, 1995). Intervention focuses on their ability to engage in play and leisure occupations that are typically expected of and available to people of the same age and culture in home, school, work, and community settings (Coster, 1998; Primeau & Ferguson, 1999). Practitioners who address clients' play and leisure as ends promote clients' play and leisure participation for its own sake, not as a means to some other end (Blanche, 1997; Bundy, 1993; Parham & Primeau, 1997).

Although occupational therapy claims to value play and leisure as ends, the literature does not support this claim. Practitioners who address play as ends are rare (Pierce, 1997), as indicated by a survey finding that only 2% of 205 occupational therapists focused on preschool-aged children's participation in play as an outcome of intervention (Couch et al., 1998). In addition, a search through issues of two major occupational therapy journals from the 1980s and 1990s identified less than eight articles related to leisure (Suto, 1998).

Literature outside occupational therapy, dating back to the 1970s, demonstrates a high correlational relationship between leisure satisfaction and overall life satisfaction (Parker, Gladman, & Drummond, 1997). Even though issues of causality in these studies are inconclusive (Headey, Veenhoven, & Wearing, 1991), they indicate that leisure participation can have significant repercussions on overall life satisfaction and quality of life (Brown & Frankel, 1993; Lloyd, 1996; Marans & Mohai, 1991), leading some authors to suggest that play and leisure participation has a direct role in prevention, health promotion, and population health initiatives (Caldwell & Smith, 1988; Coleman & Iso-Ahola, 1993).

Practitioners promote clients' play and leisure as ends through their use of the therapeutic methods of areas of occupation as means, teaching and education, problem solving, and environmental design and modification.

Areas of Occupation as Means

Play and leisure as means can be used to facilitate clients' play and leisure as ends. As described previously, they are means to address clients' impairments and limitations in body functions and structures, performance skills, and play and leisure performance. Other areas of occupation are also means to enhance play and leisure as ends. For example, practitioners may engage in their clients in activities of daily living (ADL), such as dressing or toileting, or in instrumental activities of daily living (IADL), such as driving or money management, to improve their ability to participate in play and leisure in home, school, work, and community settings.

Teaching and Education

Teaching and education are therapeutic methods that are used with clients, family members, friends, teachers, co-workers, or other people of significance to clients. Practitioners use a variety of strategies to promote skill acquisition and structure the teaching-learning situation (Poole, 1995). They teach their clients skills that are required for play and leisure participation, such as how to throw and catch a ball or how to access leisure opportunities in the community. They teach other people (parents, other family members, teachers, peers) how to facilitate clients' play and leisure participation by modeling playful interactions (CAOT, 1996). Practitioners also teach clients and others how to use adaptive equipment in play and leisure, such as computer games, toys with switches, and adaptive sports equipment (Deitz & Swinth, 1997). Leisure education programs educate clients about leisure, its potential benefits, and personal and community resources for and barriers to leisure and how to access or overcome them (Bundy, 2001).

Problem Solving

Problem solving is a therapeutic method in which practitioners collaborate with clients and others in their home, school, work, and community settings to identify issues that affect their successful participation in play and leisure and then to plan solutions that address those issues (Barris, Kielhofner, & Watts, 1988). The focus is on clients' participation in play and leisure outside of therapy in the context of their daily lives (Kielhofner, 1997). Leisure counseling, a specific type of problem solving, helps clients identify and clarify leisure values, interests, and attitudes; determine their abilities and skills for leisure participation; improve or refine their skills as needed; and locate and access community resources for leisure (Barris et al., 1988; Caldwell & Smith, 1988).

Environmental Design and Modification

Environmental design and modification is a therapeutic method through which practitioners address contextual factors (physical, social, cultural, attitudinal, organizational) that facilitate or hinder clients' successful participation in play and leisure in home, school, work, and community settings (Cooper, Rigby, & Letts, 1995). As consultants and advocates for change (Law, Stewart, & Strong, 1995), practitioners advise, coordinate, educate, and collaborate with clients and others to remove barriers and shape supportive environments that facilitate clients' access to and inclusion in play and leisure opportunities (CAOT, 1996). For example, practitioners advocate for accessible community playgrounds; collaborate with parents, teachers, and other adults to facilitate children's inclusion in play with peers and to ensure protected play time (Blanche, 1997); and advise employers on the requirement of the ADA to include clients with disabilities in all employment-related activities, including holiday parties, sports events, and business trips (Crist & Stoffel, 1992).

CONCLUSION

Play and leisure in intervention may be lures or rewards, means, or ends. As lures, they motivate clients to engage in therapeutic activities; as rewards, they reinforce their participation in intervention. They are therapeutic means to achieve intervention goals related to clients' impairments and limitations in body functions and structures, performance skills, and play and leisure performance. Play and leisure as ends are the goals or outcomes of intervention when practitioners promote clients' play and leisure participation for its own sake, not as a means to some other end. Areas of occupation as means, teaching and education, problem solving, and environmental design and modification are therapeutic methods to facilitate clients' play and leisure as ends. Practitioners choose among these purposes of play and leisure as lures or rewards, as means, or as ends to design interventions that lead to outcomes directly related to clients' participation and occupational engagement in home, school, work, and community settings.

ACKNOWLEDGMENT

I acknowledge Janice M. Ferguson, MS, OT(C), for her contributions to our previous conceptualization of occupation as ends, which is the basis for this discussion of play and leisure as ends.

SECTION IV

Community Integration

BRIAN J. DUDGEON

To design goals and interventions that promote participation in communities, it is important to consider concerns for specific individuals as well as the needs of the entire community. This distinction acknowledges differences between **client-centered approaches** and **community-centered approaches.** In promoting participation, both client and community approaches are used, as they share common issues and goals; but each has distinct intervention strategies. In this section, I review the continuum of client-centered and community-centered interventions to facilitate participation for people with disability.

On an individual basis, intervention may focus on community integration of a child with disability or reintegration of an adult with onset of disability. This client-centered approach emphasizes developing, restoring, or adapting the individual's skills, as well as organizing and using assistance available in natural supports from family and friends (Law & Mills, 1998). It also includes the creation of accessible environments that promote the individual's membership, belonging, and sense of having a constructive role.

On a population or community basis, intervention emphasizes accessibility and acceptance within physical, social, and cultural environments. Community-centered approaches generally involve advocating, creating universal or accessible design throughout the community, and promoting understanding and inclusion of those with differing characteristics or abilities.

PARTICIPATION IN COMMUNITY: DEFINITIONS

Difficulty in carrying out activities is regarded as disability, and various impairments of body systems can contribute to an individual's inability to carry out activities in an expected or accepted manner. While many activities are private, disability is also associated with problems in participation, or an individual's involvement in life situations in communities. Activity limitations as well as environmental barriers may contribute to restrictions in participation. Environmental factors include the physical, social, and attitudinal settings in which people live and conduct their lives (World Health Organization, 2001).

Definitions of community include a group of people's sharing of an area (e.g., locality, district, government), as well as interests and interactions, and perhaps a sense of shared identity (*Oxford English Dictionary*, 2001). Community is also defined by the designation of rural, suburban, and urban, which are based on metropolitan statistical area or measurements of population density. These designations are sometimes used to contrast communities in terms of resource availability, lifestyle, and diversity (Fazio, 2001).

Traditional views of community are helpful in conceptualizing both the needs of individuals as well as groups within the community. Toennies (1957) used the German term **Gemeinschaft** to characterize the relationships among individuals that are private and based on shared interests with kin or family, neighborhoods, and groups of friends. Such community elements were contrasted with **Gesellschaft,** the term used to characterize social actions that are a public expression or response to a duty or to an organization within society. While both Gemeinschaft and Gesellschaft are present in contemporary societies, urban settings are often viewed as having less Gemeinschaft or fewer psychosocial supports in place (Christenson, 1979). The rural versus urban and personal versus systemic contrasts may be overly simplistic, particularly in modern times, because intentional or virtual communities form on the basis of shared interests and identity, with connections that are electronic and not dependent on shared geography (Rheingold, 1998; Fellowship for Intentional Community, 1996).

Nevertheless, these definitions of community remind practitioners to draw on natural helpers and supports in the environment (Gemeinschaft elements), while also informing clients about their rights, responsibilities, and entitlements to draw on community programs and systems (Gesellschaft elements). The use of natural helpers and supports is a hallmark of community integration and can play a key role in assessment and intervention planning (Israel, 1985; Hagner, Rogan, & Murphy, 1992).

Another traditional characterization of community is found in Bronfenbrenner's (1977) model that recognizes the interdependencies that exist among people and their social settings. According to Bronfenbrenner, the individual lives in a microsystem; the immediate settings that involve factors of place, time, physical features, activity, participants, and roles. Interrelations among microsystems such as home, school, and workplaces are designated as a *mesosystem*, which includes personal groupings such as family and friends, schoolmates, and co-workers. Formal and informal social systems at the local level are termed *exosystems* and include influences of neighborhood, mass media, agencies of government, business, communication and transportation systems, and other social networks. At the societal level is the *macrosystem*, the overarching patterns of the culture or subculture that often guide or organize the economy and educational, social, legal, and political systems.

The complex interdependence among individuals and their environmental surroundings is important for understanding and developing interventions to include all levels of community. Client-centered approaches focus on microsystems (e.g., the home), and community-based approaches include mesosystems as well (e.g., local stores, school, work settings). Community-centered approaches are focused on exosystems (e.g., public health programs) and macrosystems (e.g., public policy, rules, and regulations) that may optimize accessibility and acceptance within communities. An individual's success with a transition toward community participation will likely involve change at both the individual and the community levels and points to a necessary blending of client-centered and community-centered approaches.

The term *community (re)integration* suggests that a poor fit exists between the individual and the community in which he or she seeks a connection. The individual may feel different, excluded, and perhaps not welcomed. Therapeutic and social efforts seek to afford individuals a right to become members within a community and guidance in understanding responsibilities and duties to the community. When successful, integration allows unrestricted and equal association, access, and acceptance into a community. Inclusion may be used to describe a person's presence in a group or an opportunity to participate fully. With a strong understanding of person–environment interactions, occupational therapy practitioners are well prepared to promote community integration (Collins, 1996).

For occupational therapists and other practitioners, tension exists between the scope of practice and the context of practice. There has been a move from institutional to center-based care to community-based care. Institutional-care, now generally frowned on, began as a thoughtful strategy to congregate and protect individuals who were perceived as being vulnerable. However, protection resulted in segregation, alienation, and stigmatization (Preistly, 1999). The moves toward deinstitutionalization lead to center-based care, in which buildings were created for the purposes of congregating services, with an effort made to have centers be considered a part of the regional or local community. Dissatisfaction still exists with these centers because of the perceived disconnection with natural contexts. So now a community-based orientation is promoted, with a focus on actual environments of function and participation (e.g., homes, schools, businesses, parks, and transportation) (Law & Mills, 1998; McColl, 1998).

Client-centered and family-centered approaches can be community based (Scaffa, 2001), but are distinct from community-centered approaches, by which community systems, places, or attitudes are addressed. These approaches have specific focuses of concern and different evaluation and intervention practices.

Client-Centered Approaches

Concern for the individual's community participation typically involves analysis of personal environments, such as home accessibility, safety, supervision needs, and personal as well as social engagements. Reorganization of such environments, additions of durable medical equipment, and architectural modifications are sometimes necessary, as are family training and counseling. Client or family-centered approaches may include accessing, advising, and/or training to support performance in local community settings such as the grocery store, movie theater, or park and/or use of community transportation systems. Sometimes attention is focused specifically on performance and participation in educational programs, volunteer or paid work settings, or involvement with organized city or county recreational facilities and programs. Citizenship activities such as access to voting also may be addressed.

The individual's and family's means of making changes in the home, communication systems, means of transportation, and returning or new participation in community activity is planned with and around the client and his or her resources. Values that are supported in that effort are client specific and culturally sensitive. For some people, independence and a reduced care and/or economic burden on his or her personal network (e.g., family) are priorities. Sometimes the choices and ultimate decisions made by clients and families might differ from practitioner recommendations, but in client-centered care the authority and preferences of clients are supported by the practitioner's teaching and guidance rather than his or her directing or commanding (Scaffa, 2001).

The practitioner uses a nondirective style and a phenomenological approach in having individuals describe their experiences and their reality (Law & Mills, 1998). Respect for the client and families and making sure that enough time is devoted to active listening are essential components of a client-centered approach. Self-efficacy is also at the core of client-centered practice (Baum, 1998), but clients and families will differ in how much they want to participate in the partnership. Regardless, being treated with respect and receiving information that will help decision making are likely to increase client and family satisfaction.

Community-Centered Approaches

Concerns for integration of all community members with disability calls for different orientations and intervention strategies. I review community-focused strategies below, but first, I discuss the community participation challenges experienced by people with disabilities, because it is helpful for the purposes of understanding needs and setting priorities.

A survey reported that 53 million people (20% of the U.S. population) age 15 years or older have a disability or limitation in one or more ADL or IADL (McNeil, 1997). More than 12% of the U.S. population has what is regarded as a severe disability, and almost 4% need personal assistance during their daily lives. IADL problems outnumber ADL difficulties for people with disability, who are most often challenged by problems of mobility; cognition; manipulation; and activities involving vision, hearing, and communication. Another common characteristic of people in the community with disability is unemployment. For many groups with disability, the communitywide rate of unemployment is well over 60% and the poverty rate for people age 25–64 with severe disability is nearly 28%, compared to 8% for those without disability. Although older age and residing in a rural setting indicate greater rates and severity of disability, the prevalence of disability appears to be on the increase in all age groups (Kroll, McNeil, Palsbo, & DeJong, 2001).

A move from a client-centered focus to a community-centered orientation to health and well-being brings attention to the reality that, while health is a personal issue, the individual's health status and functional well-being dynamically interact with personal factors as well as community factors. The later can be explored by addressing the **independent living movement (ILM)** practices of public health and other efforts to create healthy communities.

Independent Living Movement

During the later half of the twentieth century as more individuals with disability sought opportunities within communities, the ILM was created and gave rise to a number of public changes in views about disability (DeJong, 1979). For example, the ADA 1990 brought forth a sense of civil rights to all communities, an extension of the rights previously associated only with government programs (e.g., the Rehabilitation Act of 1973 and the Education for All legislation of 1975). The ILM is a social movement conceived and aimed toward a better quality of life for people with disability. The

ILM is heavily indebted to other contemporary social movements, such as civil rights, consumerism, self-help, demedicalization of self-care, and deinstitutionalization.

The self-empowerment of people with disability is credited with a shifting of traditional policy values to integrated living values. Examples include shifts from concepts of care to participation, segregation to integration, normalization to self-determination, charity to civil rights, and caseload to citizenship (Priestly, 1999). The ILM recognizes that

> *Each person has the right to independence through maximum control over his or her life, based on an ability and opportunity to make choices in performing everyday activities. These activities include: managing one's personal life; participating in community life; fulfilling social roles, such as marriage, parenthood, employment, and citizenship; sustaining self-determination; and minimizing physical or psychological dependence on others. Community integration incorporates ideas of both place and participation, so that a person is physically located in a community setting, and participates in community activities. Issues of consumer direction and control also are integral to concepts of community integration. (National Center for the Dissemination of Rehabilitation Research, n.d.)*

The ILM continues to be a social force that acknowledges changing community systems. For example, during the rise in health-care costs nationwide, those with disability are particularly put at risk. Medical expenditure per capita for people reporting two or more disabling chronic conditions can be five times the amount incurred by those with no limiting conditions and almost twice the amount incurred by those with one limiting condition (Rice & LaPlante, 1992). Individuals with disabilities caused by chronic conditions have higher-than-average health-care costs and are considered a high-risk population, which calls for rehabilitation specialists to partner with consumers to advocate effectively (Batavia, 1999). Moves toward managed care has put a squeeze on individuals and groups of people with disability and results in Medicaid (i.e., publicly funded health insurance) being the single largest provider of health-care financing for these people (Kroll et al., 2001).

Public Health Perspective

Financial dilemmas associated with health-care costs and particular challenges associated with disability raise another important community orientation. A **public health** perspective recognizes the value of medical care as only one level of intervention, bringing attention to prevention of communitywide health challenges. In public health, the **target condition** is the health or disease outcome that the preventive care intervention avoids (primary prevention) or identifies early (secondary prevention) or treats effectively (tertiary prevention). **Risk factors** are the attributes associated with the target condition and may include demographic variables, behavioral risk factors, and environmental factors.

The most promising role for prevention in current practice may lie in changing the personal health behaviors of individuals before disease or injury onset. For example, about half of all disability and deaths may be attributed to factors such as tobacco, alcohol, and illicit drug use; diet and activity patterns; motor vehicles; and sexual behavior. Prevention practice can involve all health and education professionals (U.S. Preventive Services Task Force, 1996).

Although public health practices are found in various agencies outside of hospitals or other health-care settings, important roles for all practitioners are acknowledged. Physicians, for example, are encouraged to provide brief advice during routine visits and to refer clients to allied health professionals with special counseling skills in their areas of expertise (e.g., occupational therapy for automobile driver safety). For all practitioners, principles of prevention include the following:

- Assisting individuals to assume greater responsibility for their own health and personal health practices.
- Seeing individuals as the principal agents in primary prevention and empowering and counseling individuals to change health-related behaviors.
- Understanding that when people have the confidence to affect their health, they are more likely to do so than when they do not have this confidence (Schwarzer, 1992).
- Shared decision making and respect for values about possible outcomes.
- Education and consideration of choices, preferences, and uncertainty as part of decision making are preferred over a uniform policy for all people.

Every opportunity should be taken to deliver preventive services, especially to individuals with limited access to care. Delivering preventive services at every visit is recommended. For some health problems, community-level interventions may be more effective than clinical preventive services. An important role for clinicians is their participation in community systems that address various types of health problems.

Public health practices are often described by an analogy of a continuously flowing river (Orleans, Gruman, Ulmer, Emont, & Hollendonner, 1999). Downstream tactics or programs seek to make a change in individual behaviors of those in targeted groups at risk and sometimes in all groups within communities. Midstream strategies are designed to influence those who may have an influence on individuals. Physicians and other health practitioners as well as educators may be recruited to deliver prevention practice information. Upstream concerns confront public policy and regulatory mechanisms that have a population focus. Examples include pollution and other environmental issues as well as roadway safety and manufacturing of devices common to public use.

Healthy People 2010

Within the United States, public health strategies are a part of the development of national health priorities. Sponsored by the U.S. surgeon general and building from previous national health priorities, Healthy People 2010 identifies 10 public health priorities for the country (Office of Disease Prevention and Health Promotion, 2000). Healthy People 2010 seeks to augment the health of each individual, the health of communities, and the health of the nation. The report serves as a basis for developing community plans to address two paramount goals for individuals of all ages: increase quality and years of healthy life and eliminate health disparities that exist within the population.

Stark differences in health exist based on gender, race or ethnicity, education or income, disability, geographic locations, and sexual orientation. Healthy People 2010 designated 10 health indicators to serve as targets for individual and community action. Focus areas call for specific attention to key activities to reduce or eliminate illness, disability, and premature death among individuals within communities.

Public Health Challenge Targets

- Promote regular physical activity.
- Promote healthier weight and good nutrition.
- Prevent and reduce tobacco use.
- Prevent and reduce substance abuse.
- Promote responsible sexual behavior.
- Promote mental health and well-being.
- Promote safety and reduce violence.
- Promote healthy environments.
- Prevent infectious disease through immunization.
- Increase access to quality health care.

Health promotion and disease prevention activities have long been advocated within occupational therapy, and Healthy People 2010 calls for community-centered application of those ideals (Hildenbrand & Froehlich, 2002).

National organizations, such as the American Occupational Therapy Association (AOTA), are called on to develop programs that empower individuals to make informed health-care decisions and promote communitywide safety, education, and access to health care, such as backpack safety for school-aged children (AOTA, 2001). Primary prevention is a priority for community action. To address Healthy People 2010 objectives, places for programmatic interventions include school settings; work-site settings; health-care settings; the community-at-large through public facilities, local government agencies, social services; and faith-based and civic organizations to reach people where they live, work, and play.

EVALUATION AND INTERVENTION TO ENABLE COMMUNITY PARTICIPATION

Evaluation and intervention services can be provided on a continuum using both client-centered and community-centered perspectives. Intervention initially may focus on the individual and a shifting from institution or clinical context of care to the client's own community. This shift moves intervention to natural environments in which clients conduct their lives and encounter and adapt to realities of physical, social, and political contexts. At the other end of the continuum, intervention may focus primarily on the community, where individuals take action to change community systems to enable full participation by all people, including those with disability.

Client-Centered Evaluation and Intervention

Evaluation of the individual includes a traditional approach of addressing the client's skills and needs, but also includes people who are in the client's personal network (e.g., family, friends, neighbors). An individual's place of residence (e.g., home assessment) as well as the local settings in the community and transportation systems are also assessed. Examples of interviews or survey instruments available to appraise an individual's views about connecting to community are the Community Integration Questionnaire (Sander, Fuchs, High, Hall, Kreutzer, & Rosenthal, 1999), the Community Integration Measure (McColl, Davies, Carlson, Johnston, & Minnes, 2001), and the Craig Handicap Assessment and Reporting Tool (Whiteneck, Charlifue, Gerhart, Overholser, & Richardson, 1992).

Shifting from a center-based to a community-based approach requires shifting practice environments as well as shifting philosophy. Practitioners must be expert in consultation and program development and focus on broader issues than in typical direct service (Dudgeon & Greenberg, 1998). Working through teachers in schools, supervisors in jobs, and other natural supports in the community may be necessary and effective. In transitioning to community-based practice, Fazio (2001) suggested that natural settings may be the most effective arena for service delivery. Community-based approaches, such as evaluating people's needs in their homes, are encouraged (Freeman, 1997; Sabari, Meisler, & Silver, 2000) and are sometimes found to be effective for stroke rehabilitation and for individuals with brain injury (Anderson, Rubenach, Mhurchu, Clark, Spenser, & Winsor, 2000; Willer, Button, & Rempel, 1999).

Community-Centered Evaluation and Involvement

Community assessment may involve exploration of incidence and prevalence of occupational dysfunction needs with populations. However, assessing dysfunction could backfire and not support a community, because it focuses on deficiency rather than potential. Kretzmann and McNight (1993) suggested that therapists need to move away from focusing on community deficiencies (e.g., unemployment, crime, illiteracy, gangs, and dropouts). Instead, therapists should move toward recognizing and using the relationships among community assets, including those that exist within individuals (e.g., elderly, youth, artists), citizen organizations (e.g., cultural groups, churches), and local institutions (e.g., schools, businesses, parks, hospitals). A needs survey may be seen as a deficiency inventory, but a capacity inventory can be seen as means to empower communities. McKnight (1994) argued that health-care organizations can behave as community members (e.g., through advocacy, financing, volunteerism, and space availability) and address community needs by focusing not on an epidemiological or diagnostic ideology but on an individual, family, or community capacities and assets.

Kretzmann (2000) contended that health is a product of four determinants: the behavior of the individual, the strength of individual social relationships, the healthfulness of the physical environment, and the economic status of the individual. He proposed "asset-based community assessment and development" (p. 42). Skills of local residents; power of voluntary citizen's associations; and resources of public, private, and nonprofit institutions should be harnessed to promote health within a community. For example, to address the influence of local associations, practitioners might explore partnerships with schools, youth organizations, and local business and associations that promote participation by those with disability. Such partnerships may include collaborations with Coalitions of Citizens with Disability, the National Alliance for the Mentally Ill, ARCR (the national organization of and for people with mental retardation and related developmental disabilities and their families), the Arthritis Foundation, or other support and advocacy organizations.

Occupational therapy practitioners have much to contribute to community accessibility and acceptance of people with disabilities. Contributions may involve developing community partnerships with a "new cadre of colleagues including people with disabilities, engineers, architects, personal assistants, independent living counselors, recreation and exercise personnel, city planners, law enforcement, and transportation specialists" (Baum & Law, 1997, p. 280).

Advocacy about Accessibility

Advocacy, a key element of community-centered care, brings attention to issues and educates potential members of a community, ultimately drawing them into problem-solving actions that may resolve or lessen barriers to participation. At the community level, advocacy may focus on accessibility and acceptance. Community accessibility involves the application of accessible design rules, established over the years at federal, state, and local levels through building codes. In both new construction and remodeling, accessibility guidelines help create access for those challenged with mobility, cognition, manipulation, hearing, vision, and/or communication. Access applies to the building environment as well as products and other community systems, such as transportation, communication, and information systems. For example, for those with any combination of sensory, motor, or cognitive difficulties, access to the Internet is challenged by Web design problems that restrict accessibility options and may restrict such individuals from access to information and participation in virtual communities (World Wide Web Consortium, 2001).

While accessibility guidelines have been in place for several decades, some dissatisfaction continues to exist with design because building codes dictate a minimal approach to access rather than a universal application of design that may apply to a more-inclusive community. **Universal design** concepts and principles suggest that environments and products be designed to be usable by all people, to the greatest extent possible, without the need for special arrangements, adaptations, or greater cost (Center for Universal Design, 1997).

Accessible and universal design needs to have advocates in the community. While many people with disability do advocate on behalf of themselves and others, greater community awareness and improved timing of attention to accessibility must occur. Both design and manufacturing of buildings and other systems are expensive ventures, and a lack of attention to access or universal design becomes cost prohibitive if applied too late. As advocates, therapists need to practice what they preach. Such an attitude may include doing business with those who provide access and boycotting those who fail to address accessibility. Therapists can also apply accessibility and universal design to their own environments.

In recent years, the concept of visitability has been suggested and is sometimes mandated (disAbility Resource Center, 2001). Visitability applies simple design elements to residential settings. The concept and practice creates at least one level entrance to a dwelling and access (e.g., 32 in. wide) to one bathroom on that level. Other suggestions for universal design in homes are the creation of both floor space for toilet and tub transfers as well as structural supports in the walls for mounting grab bars, which may become necessary for safety and independence. A shortage of accessible living settings in neighborhoods is a recognized problem, and creation of visitability may help overcome such shortages.

Advocacy about Acceptance

Addressing community acceptance of people with disability may be a harder advocacy role to assume. The differentness that disability entails often creates mystery and uneasiness. Comfort within a community is sometimes based on similarity rather than on differentness (Whyte & Ignstad, 1995). A more accessible environment may provide people with disability a greater feeling of acceptance, but disability also can evoke feelings of blame, shame, pity, and avoidance. Physical, cognitive, sensory, and behavioral differences may need to be addressed by educating for understanding and the practice of inclusion in residential, educational, employment, and recreational settings.

One of the hallmarks of community-based rehabilitation, is the recognition that barriers to full participation exist in the community and that individuals can increase community awareness of the needs of members with disability and provide changes that create occupational opportunities (Baker & Brownson, 1999). Access to opportunities for citizenship, housing, employment, transportation, education, and other social structures enable people with disabilities opportunities to be successful.

Occupational therapy practitioners can support the initiatives of people with disabilities or advocacy groups that promote social development and help create an institutional, political, and social framework that supports full participation. For example, practitioners can hold forums to educate employers in the local community about workplace accommodations most useful to people with psychiatric disabilities. Unlike a physical accommodation, such as a wheelchair ramp, accommodations for people with psychiatric disabilities are often social in nature and need ongoing attention and retraining.

CONCLUSION

Community well-being is both behavioral and social in nature and includes individual lifestyle behaviors; the environment; socioeconomic factors; and local, state, and federal regulations and policies. One way to conceive of community care is to apply a public health model, with practitioners providing midstream and upstream interventions.

Primary prevention measures are those that prevent the onset of a targeted condition (e.g., antismoking, promotion of activity and fitness). Such practices may be advocated and taught in community centers, senior programs, schools, and workplaces. Secondary prevention measures identify and treat asymptomatic people who have developed risk factors or preclinical disease before the condition is clinically evident. Examples include backpack safety for schoolchildren, ergonomics for at-risk workers, and fall prevention among the elderly. Tertiary prevention measures focus on intervention with people with clinical illnesses or health conditions.

Traditionally, occupational therapy practitioners focused on development, recovery, or adaptation; prevention of secondary complications; and maintenance of skills in community living. More recently, practitioners are shifting their focus to include community-centered intervention approaches to promote participation for all people, regardless of their ability status.

References

"community, *n*." *Oxford English Dictionary*. Ed. John Simpson. 3rd. ed. *OED Online*. Draft Mar. 2000. Oxford University Press. 16 Apr. 2000. <http://dictionary.oed.com/cgi/entry/00045243>

American Occupational Therapy Association (2002). Backpack Strategies for Schools: Help Students Ease the Backpack Burden. Available at: http://www.aota.org/backpack/links/schlfact.asp. Accessed September 12, 2002.

American Occupational Therapy Association (in press). Occupational therapy practice framework: Domain and process. *American Journal of Occupational Therapy*.

American with Disabilities Act of 1990 [ADA], 42 U.S.C. § 12134. (1990).

Anderson, C., Rubenbach, S., Mhurchu, C.N., Clark, M., Spencer, C., & Winsor, A. (2000). Home or hospital for stroke rehabilitation? Results of a randomized controlled trial 1: Health outcomes at 6 months [approx. 29 paragraphs]. *Stroke* [on-line version], *31*. Available: stroke.ahajournals.org

Baker, E. A., & Brownson, R. C. (1999). Defining characteristics of community-based health promotion programs. In R. C., Brownson, E. A. Baker, & L. F. Novick (Eds.). *Community-based prevention: Programs that work* (pp. 7–19). Gaitherburg, MD: Aspen.

Barris, R., Kielhofner, G., & Watts, J. H. (1988). *Occupational therapy in psychosocial practice*. Thorofare, NJ: Slack.

Batavia, A. I. (1999). Independent living centers, medical rehabilitation centers, and managed care for people with disabilities. *Archives of Physical Medicine and Rehabilitation*, 80, 1357–1360.

Baum, C. (1998). Client-centered practice in a changing health care system. In M. Law (Ed.). *Client-centered occupational therapy* (pp. 29–45). Thorofare, NJ: Slack.

Baum, C., & Law, M. (1997). Occupational therapy practice: Focusing on occupational performance. *American Journal of Occupational Therapy, 51*, 277–288.

Blanche, E. I. (1997). Doing with—Not doing to: Play and the child with cerebral palsy. In L. D. Parham & L. S. Fazio (Eds.). *Play in occupational therapy for children* (pp. 202–218). St. Louis: Mosby-Year Book.

Borcherding, S. (2000). *Documentation manual for writing SOAP notes in occupational therapy*. Thorofare: NJ: Slack.

Botehlo, K., Fenton, S., Jones, V., Meedzan, N., & Meyers, P. (1993). Rehabilitation of the heavy manual laborer. In S. Hochschuler, H. Cotler, & R. Guyer (Eds.). *Rehabilitation of the spine science and practice* (pp. 659–665). Boston: Mosby.

Bronfenbrenner, U. (1977). Toward an experimental ecology of human development. *American Psychologist, 32*, 513–531.

Brown, B. A., & Frankel, B. G. (1993). Activity through the years: Leisure, leisure satisfaction, and life satisfaction. *Sociology of Sport Journal, 10*, 1–17.

Bundy, A. C. (1993). Assessment of play and leisure: Delineation of the problem. *American Journal of Occupational Therapy, 47*, 217–22.

Bundy, A. C. (2001). Leisure. In B. R. Bonder & M. B. Wagner (Eds.). *Functional performance in older adults* (2nd ed., pp. 196–217). Philadelphia: Davis.

Caldwell, L. L., & Smith, E. A. (1988). Leisure: An overlooked component of health promotion. *Canadian Journal of Public Health, 79*, S44–S48.

Canadian Association of Occupational Therapists [CAOT]. (1996). Practice paper: Occupational therapy and children's play [Insert]. *Canadian Journal of Occupational Therapy, 63*, 1–20.

Case-Smith, J., Rogers, J., & Johnson, J. H. (2001). School-based occupational therapy. In J. Case-Smith (Ed.). *Occupational therapy for children* (4th ed., pp. 757–779). Philadelphia: Mosby.

Center for Universal Design (1997, April 1). What is universal design? North Carolina State University, Center for Universal Design. Available at: www.design.ncsu.edu:8120/cud/univ_design/ud.htm. Accessed May 7, 2001.

Childs, N. (2001, February). The hidden insurance crisis. *Provider*, 22–34.

Christenson, J. A. (1979). Gemeinschaft and Gesellschaft: Testing the spatial and communal hypothesis. *Social Forces*, *63*, 160–168.

Coleman, D., & Iso-Ahola, S. E. (1993). Leisure and health: The role of social support and self-determination. *Journal of Leisure Research*, *25*, 111–128.

Collins, L. F. (1996). Easing client transition from facility to community. *OT Practice*, *1*, 36–39.

Cooper, B., Rigby, P., & Letts, L. (1995). Evaluation of access to home, community, and workplace. In C. A. Trombly (Ed.). *Occupational therapy for physical dysfunction* (4th ed., pp. 55–72). Baltimore: Williams & Wilkins.

Cooper, J., Tate, R., & Yassi, A. (1997). Work hardening in an early return to work program for nurses with back injury. *Work: A Journal of Prevention, Assessment and Rehabilitation*, 8(2), 149–156.

Coster, W. (1998). Occupation-centred assessment of children. *American Journal of Occupational Therapy*, *52*, 337–344.

Couch, K. J., Deitz, J. C., & Kanny, E. M. (1998). The role of play in pediatric occupational therapy. *American Journal of Occupational Therapy*, *52*, 111–117.

Crist, P. A. H., & Stoffel, V. C. (1992). The Americans with Disabilities Act of 1990 and employees with mental impairments: Personal efficacy and the environment. *American Journal of Occupational Therapy*, *46*, 434–443.

DeJong, G. (1979). Independent living: From social movement to analytic paradigm. *Archives of Physical Medicine and Rehabilitation*, *60*, 435–446.

Dietz, J. C., & Swinth, Y. (1997). Accessing play through assistive technology. In L. D. Parham & L. S. Fazio (Eds.). *Play in occupational therapy for children* (pp. 219–232). St. Louis: Mosby Year Book.

disAbility Resource Center. (2000). Housing is major unmet need. Available at: www.wa-ilsc.org/housing_visitability.html Accessed August 15, 2001.

Driver, B. L., Brown, P. J., & Peterson, G. L. (Eds.). (1991). *Benefits of leisure*. State College, PA: Venture.

Dudgeon, B. J., & Greenberg, S. L. (1998). Preparing students for consultation roles and systems. *American Journal of Occupational Therapy*, *52*, 801–809.

Dunn, W. (1988) Models of occupational therapy service provision in the school system. *American Journal of Occupational Therapy*, *42*(11), 718–723.

Fazio, L. S. (2001). *Developing occupation-centered programs for the community: A workbook for students and professionals*. Upper Saddle River, NJ: Prentice-Hall.

Fellowship for Intentional Communities (1996, October). What's true about intentional communities: Dispelling the myths. Available at: www.ic.org/pnp/myths.html. Accessed August 15, 2001.

Fontana, P. (1999). Preventing industrial injuries and return-to-work programs: A road map for success. *Work Programs Special Interest Section Quarterly*, *13*(3), 1–4.

Frantzlett, C., McCabe, N., Tramposh, A., & Tate-Henderson, S. (1988). Components of functional capacity evaluations. In S. J. Iserhagen (Ed.). *Work injury management and prevention* (pp. 216–223). Baltimore: Aspen.

Freeman, E. A. (1997). Community-based rehabilitation of the person with a severe brain injury. *Brain Injury*, 11, 143–153.

Giangreco, M. F. (2001). Guidelines for making decisions about I.E.P. services [60 pages]. Available at: www.uvm.edu/~cdci/iepservices/pdfs/decision.pdf. Accessed August 10, 2002.

Gourley, M. (2000, September 11). Refining OT's edge in ergonomics. *OT Practice*, 14–17.

Gray, J. M. (1998). Putting occupation into practice: Occupation as ends, occupation as means. *American Journal of Occupational Therapy*, *52*, 354–364.

Griffin, J. (2000). Return to work review. *Rehabilitation Management*, 30–34.

Hagner, D., Rogan, P., & Murphy, S. (1992). Facilitating natural supports in the workplace: Strategies for support consultants. *Journal of Rehabilitation*, *58*, 29–34.

Hanft, B. E., & Place, P. A. (1996). *The consulting therapist: A guide for OTs and PTs in schools*. San Antonio, TX: Therapy Skill Builders.

Hardway, J. (1993). The exercise physiologist on the work hardening team. *Rehabilitation Management*, 73.

Headey, B., Veenhoven, R., & Wearing, A. (1991). Top-down versus bottom-up theories of subjective well-being. *Social Indicators Research*, *24*, 81–100.

Hertfelder, S., & Gwin, C. (1989). *Work hardening guidelines*. *Occupational therapy in work programs*. Rockville, MD: American Occupational Therapy Association.

Hildenbrand, W. C., & Forehlich, K. (2002). Promoting health: Historical roots, renewed vision. *OT Practice*, *7*(5), 10–15.

Hyland, M., & Ruggles, J. (2001). Industrial expansion. *Rehabilitation Management*, *14*(6), 32–60.

Iserhagen, S. (1988). *Functional capacity evaluation parameters*. *Work injury management and prevention*. Baltimore: Aspen.

Israel, B. A. (1985). Social networks and social support: Implications for natural helpers and community level interventions. *Health Education Quarterly*, *12*(1), 65–80.

Joe, B. (1995). Effective work programs. *OT Week*, 9(48), 12–13.

Kielhofner, G. (1997). *Conceptual foundations of occupational therapy* (2nd ed.). Philadelphia: Davis.

Kielhofner, G., & Burke, J. P. (1983). The evolution of knowledge and practice in occupational therapy: Past, present, and future. In G. Kielhofner (Ed.). *Health through occupation: Theory and practice in occupational therapy* (pp. 3–54). Philadelphia: Davis.

Kolber, E. (2001). The battle to protect American workers. *Rehabilitation Management*, *14*(1), 24–65.

Kramer, P., & Hinojosa, J. (1999). *Frames of reference for pediatric occupational therapy* (2nd ed.). Philadelphia: Lippincott, Williams & Wilkins.

Kretzmann, J. P. (2000). Co-producing health: Professionals and communities build on assets. *Health Forum Journal*, *43*, 42.

Kretzmann, J. P., & McKnight, J. L. (1993). *Building communities from the inside out: A path toward finding and mobilizing a community's assets*. Evanston, IL: Northwestern University.

Kroll, T., McNeil, M. J., Palsbo, S. E., & DeJong, G. (2001, July). New challenges for health care and society in the management and rehabilitation of disability [Health and Disability Issue Brief; Emerging Disabilities Series]. Available at: www.nrhchdr.org/NewChalg-IssueBrief.pdf. Accessed August 2, 2001.

Larson, B. (2001). Work injury activities. In S. Ryan & K. Sladyk (Eds.). *Ryan's occupational therapy assistant* (3rd ed.). Thorofare, NJ: Slack.

Law, M., & Mills, J. (1998). Client-centered occupational therapy. In M. Law (Ed.). *Client-centered occupational therapy* (pp. 1–18). Thorofare, NJ: Slack.

Law, M., Stewart, D., & Strong, S. (1995). Achieving access to home, community, and workplace. In C. A. Trombly (Ed.). *Occupational therapy for physical dysfunction* (4th ed., pp. 361–375). Baltimore: Williams & Wilkins.

Lloyd, K. (1996). Planning for leisure: Issues of quality of life. *Social Alternatives*, *15*, 19–22.

Marans, R. W., & Mohai, P. (1991). Leisure resources, recreation activity, and the quality of life. In B. L. Driver, P. J. Brown, & G. L. Peterson (Eds.). *Benefits of leisure* (pp. 351–363). State College, PA: Venture.

McColl, M. A. (1998). What do we need to know to practice in the community? *American Journal of Occupational Therapy*, *52*, 11–18.

McColl, M. A., Davies, D., Carlson, P., Johnston, J., & Minnes, P. (2001). The community integration measure: development and preliminary validation *Archives of Physical Medicine and Rehabilitation*, *82*, 429–434.

McKnight, J. L. (1994). Hospitals and the health of their communities. *Hospitals and Health Networks*, *68*, 40–41.

McNeil, J. (2001). Americans with Disabilities: 1997 [Current Population Reports P70-73]. Available at: www.census.gov/hhes/www/disable/sipp/disab97/asc97.html. Accessed August 2, 2001.

Morrison, C. D., & Metzger, P. (2001). Play. In J. Case-Smith (Ed.). *Occupational therapy for children* (4th ed., pp. 528–544). St. Louis: Mosby.

National Center for the Dissemination of Rehabilitation Research. (n.d.). NIDRR's long range plan—Independent living and community integration research (Section 2, Chapter 6). Available at: www.ncddr.org/rpp/ilcir/lrp_ov.html. Accessed July 19, 2001.

Niemeyer, L., Jacobs, K., Reynolds-Lynch, K., Bettencourt, C., & Lang, S. (1994). Work hardening: Past, present and future—The work programs special interest section national work hardening outcome study. *American Journal of Occupational Therapy* , *48*, 327–329.

Norlen, M. (1999, October 25). Healing myself with the power of work. *Newsweek*, 12.

O'Brien, J., & Forest, M. (with Snow, J., & Hasbury, D.). (1989). *Action for inclusion*. Toronto, ON, Canada: Frontier College Press.

Office of Disease Prevention and Health Promotion. (2000, November). Healthy people 2010: Understanding and improving health (2nd ed.). Available at: www.health.gov/healthypeople. Accessed July 15, 2001.

Ogden-Niemeyer, L., & Jacobs, K. (1989). *Definition and history of work hardening. Work hardening: State of the art (p.1)*. Thorofare, NJ: Slack.

Orleans, C. T., Gruman, J., Ulmer, C., Emont, S. L., & Hollendonner, J. K. (1999). Rating our progress in population health promotion: Report card on six behaviors. *American Journal of Health Promotion, 14*, 75–82.

Parham, L. D. (1996). Perspectives on play. In R. Zemke, & F. Clark (Eds.). *Occupational science: The evolving discipline* (pp. 71–80). Philadelphia: Davis.

Parham, L. D., &. Fazio, L. S. (Eds.). (1997). *Play in occupational therapy for children*. St. Louis: Mosby-Year Book.

Parham, L. D., & Primeau, L. A. (1997). Play and occupational therapy. In L. D. Parham & L. S. Fazio (Eds.). *Play in occupational therapy for children* (pp. 2–21). St. Louis: Mosby-Year Book.

Parker, C. J., Gladman, J. R. F., & Drummond, A. E. R. (1997). The role of leisure in stroke rehabilitation. *Disability and Rehabilitation, 19*, 1–5.

Pierce, D. (1997). The power of object play for infants and toddlers at risk for developmental delays. In L. D. Parham & L. S. Fazio (Eds.). *Play in occupational therapy for children* (pp. 86–111). St. Louis: Mosby-Year Book.

Poole, J. L. (1995). Learning. In C. A. Trombly (Ed.). *Occupational therapy for physical dysfunction* (4th ed., pp. 265–276). Baltimore: Williams & Wilkins.

Priestly, M. (1999). *Disability politics and community care*. Philadelphia: Kingsley.

Primeau, L. A. (1996). Work and leisure: Transcending the dichotomy. *American Journal of Occupational Therapy, 50*, 569–577.

Primeau, L. A., & Ferguson, J. M. (1999). Occupational frame of reference. In P. Kramer & J. Hinojosa (Eds.). *Frames of reference for pediatric occupational therapy* (2nd ed., pp. 469–516). Philadelphia: Lippincott, Williams & Wilkins.

Reauthorization of the Individuals with Disabilities Education Act of 1990. Pub. L. 105-17, 20 U.S.C. (1997).

Rehabilitation Act of 1973, 29 U.S.C. § 504 (1973).

Reilly, M. (1974). An explanation of play. In M. Reilly (Ed.). *Play as exploratory learning: Studies of curiosity behavior* (pp. 117–149). Beverly Hills, CA: Sage.

Rheingold, H. (1998). The virtual community, Homesteading on the electronic frontier. Available at: www.rheingold.com/vc/book. Accessed May 15, 2001.

Rice, D. P., & LaPlante, M. P. (1992). Medical expenditures for disability and disabling comorbidity. *American Journal Public Health, 82*, 739–741.

Sabari, J. S., Meisler, J., & Silver, E. (2000). Reflections upon rehabilitation by members of a community based stroke club. *Disability Rehabilitation, 22*, 330–336.

Sabonis-Chafee, B., & Hussey, S. (1998). *Introduction to occupational therapy*. St. Louis: Mosby-Year Book.

Sander, M., Fuchs, K., High, W., Hall, K., Kreutzer, J., & Rosenthal, M. (1999). The Community Integration Questionnaire revisited: An assessment of factor structure and validity. *Archives of Physical Medicine and Rehabilitation*, 80, 1303–1308.

Sandler, A. G. (1997) Physical and occupational therapy services: Use of a consultive therapy model in the schools. *Preventing School Failure, 41*(4) 164–167.

Saunders, E. B. (1922). Psychiatry and occupational therapy. *Archives of Occupational Therapy, 1*, 99–114.

Scaffa, M. (2001). *Occupational therapy in community-based practice settings*. Philadelphia: Davis.

Schwarzer, R. (1992). Self-efficacy in the adoption and maintenance of health behaviors: Theoretical approaches and a new model. In R. Schwarzer (Ed.). *Self-efficacy: Thought control of action* (pp. 217–243). Washington, DC: Hemisphere.

Slagle, E. C. (1922). Training aides for mental patients. *Archives of Occupational Therapy, 1*, 11–17.

Swinth, Y. L, Chandler, B., Hanft, B., Jackson, L., & Shepherd, J., (In press). Personnel issues in school-based occupational therapy: supply and demand, preparation, and certification and licensure. Center on Personnel Studies in Special Education, University of Florida.

Suto, M. (1998). Leisure in occupational therapy. *Canadian Journal of Occupational Therapy, 65*, 271–278.

Toennies, F. (1957). *Community and society* (C. P. Loomis, Trans.). New Brunswick, NJ: Transaction.

Trombly, C. A. (1995). Occupation: Purposefulness and meaningfulness as therapeutic mechanisms. *American Journal of Occupational Therapy, 49*, 960–972.

Turner, C. (2000). Posture perfect. *Advance for Directors in Rehabilitation*, 9(5), 53–54.

U.S. Department of Labor. (1991). *Dictionary of occupational titles* (4th ed.). Washington, DC: Author

U.S. Preventive Services Task Force. (1996). *Guide to clinical preventive services* (2nd ed., Stock No. 017001005258). Washington, DC: U.S. Department of Health and Human Services. Information at: odphp.osophs.dhhs.gov/pubs/guidecps. Accessed July 19, 2001.

Vandercook, T., & York, J. (1988). Integrated education: MAPS to get you there. *IMPACT Newsletter, 1*(2), 17–??.

Whiteneck, G. G., Charlifue, S. W., Gerhart, K. A., Overholser, J. D., & Richardson, G. N. (1992). Quantifying handicap: A new measure of long-term rehabilitation outcomes. *Archives of Physical Medicine and Rehabilitation, 73*, 519–526.

Whyte, S. R., & Ingstad, B. (1995). Disability and culture: An overview. In B. Ingstad & S. R. Whyte (Eds.). *Disability and culture* (pp. 3–32). Berkeley: University of California Press.

Willer, B., Button, J., & Rempel, R. (1999). Residential and home-based postacute rehabilitation of individuals with traumatic brain injury: A case control study. *Archives of Physical Medicine and Rehabilitation, 80*, 399–406.

Williams, M. S., & Shellenberger, S. (1994). The alert program for self-regulation. *Sensory Integration Special Interest Section Newsletter, 17*(3).

World Health Organization [WHO]. (2001). *International classification of functioning, disability and health (ICIDH-2)* (final draft, full version). Geneva: Author.

World Wide Web Consortium [W3C]. (2001, September 14). Web accessibility initiative (WAI). Available at: www.w3.org/WAI/. Accessed October 1, 2001.

Young, D. (1993). Psychological services in work-hardening programs. *Work Programs Special Interest Section Quarterly, 47*(3), 2–??.

Ziegler, L. H. (1924). Some observations on recreations. *Archives of Occupational Therapy, 3*, 255–265.

CHAPTER 30

INTERVENTIONS TO IMPROVE PERSONAL SKILLS AND ABILITIES

SECTION I

Sensory Reeducation

JANET WAYLETT-RENDALL

Sensory reeducation is a combination of techniques used to teach those with peripheral nerve injuries how to interpret and make functional use of the abnormal impulses that injured nerves relay to the brain (Dellon, 1981). Sensory reeducation also assists these people in learning to interpret the altered profile of impulses reaching the conscious level (Dellon, 1981). Repetition, practice, and structured use of the involved hand are integral aspects of sensory reeducation (Byl & Merzenich, 1997).

SENSORY REEDUCATION AND PERIPHERAL NERVE INJURY

Reinnervation at the periphery can occur but never achieves prior injury function, especially in adults with nerve laceration (Dagum, 1998; Lundborg, 2000). Peripheral nerves do regenerate, but the physical structures laid down during regeneration are affected in the following ways:

- Axon regeneration may be blocked by scar tissue or compressed by neuroma formation.
- Sensory end organs, found in the fingertips, may survive years of denervation; however, endoneurial tubes (which contain the nerve fascicles) shrink, making it difficult for regenerating fascicles to enter the appropriate tube.
- Motor nerve injuries have an added problem of resulting muscle atrophy and fibrosis, especially if denervation is >6 months.

The central nervous system (CNS), specifically at the somatosensory cortex, is affected by loss of peripheral innervation or imperfect reinnervation (Lundborg, 2000; Merzenich & Jenkins, 1993). Nonhuman primate studies show that sensory input that is altered by peripheral nerve injury causes the corresponding somatosensory cortex representation to become inactive (Byl & Merzenich, 1997; Merzenich & Jenkins, 1993). Reinnervation at the peripheral level causes a reorganization of the somatosensory cortex; however in adult nonhuman primates, the injured nerve never regains its normal representation in the cortex. Parallel human perceptual changes mirror findings from the nonhuman primate population. Specifically, children <9 years of age can experience complete recovery from large nerve lesions of the hand; however, only a small percentage of adults are can expect such an excellent outcome. The plasticity of the CNS in children is believed to cause these differing outcomes.

GOALS OF SENSORY REEDUCATION

The ultimate goal of sensory reeducation is to improve or enhance useful sensation. Corollary goals include the prevention of burns and other injuries and the improvement of functional hand use.

The first level of sensory reeducation is to teach the client how to compensate for a lack of protective sensation. This involves both temperature recognition (often the only sensory impairment the person is aware of) and pressure recognition. Decreased touch pressure thresholds combined with diminished proprioceptive input affects hand use. These individuals use excessive force during prehension and manipulation of tools and objects to gain sensory feedback. Over time, this excessive force causes overuse injuries to muscles, tendons, and joints. In neuropathies such as Hansen disease (leprosy), overuse injuries are common. People with peripheral nerve injuries are also more susceptible to skin injuries. Damage to the autonomic nerve fibers of the peripheral nerves results in loss of sweating, causing the skin to become dry and thus more susceptible to injury. Dry and cracked skin is more easily broken than normal skin, which is kept moist by sweat.

In addition to using injury prevention strategies, people with sensory loss are more functional if they can learn how to use their bodies without relying on visual input. For example, removal of screws from casings without vision may be a necessary job task if the person's hands are working inside or behind equipment. Another example is that most adults need to be able to feel keys or coins to identify and remove them from a pocket or purse.

EVALUATION RELATED TO SENSORY REEDUCATION

Before providing sensory reeducation intervention, occupational therapists need to perform a thorough evaluation of the skin and muscles denervated by nerve damage (see Chapter 25, Section 1). Two issues specific to sensory reeducation evaluation are hypersensitivity and stereognosis.

Hypersensitivity

People who are recovering from peripheral nerve injuries experience varying degrees of hypersensitivity during reinnervation. One explanation for this may be related to enlarged cortical representation of adjacent skin regions representing uninjured nerves (Merzenich & Jenkins, 1993). If the hypersensitivity is severe, it can be a serious detriment to sensory reeducation. Therefore, occupational therapists need to evaluate the degree of hypersensitivity to see if a given client is appropriate for sensory reeducation training.

Clients with severe hypersensitivity need to receive desensitization training before beginning a sensory reeducation program. Desensitization involves graded and repetitious application of physical stimuli to the affected body part (Waylett-Rendall, 1995). For example, clients may first be asked to touch soft objects, such as cotton balls or a terry cloth towel. When touching these objects becomes tolerable, the person is asked to rub the soft objects over the affected skin in a slow, rhythmic fashion. To progress further, the client follows this same sequence with smooth, hard objects such as books, tool handles, or utensils. Finally, the person should be able to touch rough, hard objects, such as sandpaper or a scouring pad, without discomfort.

Stereognosis

Stereognosis is the ability to recognize familiar objects by tactile exploration. It is the highest level of discriminative sensory function (Dannebaum & Jones, 1993). As such it is an important indicator of the success of a sensory reeducation program. Stereognosis requires the integration of temperature sensation, proprioception, texture, weight, and shape recognition.

Since sensory reeducation and desensitization both affect the reorganization of the somatosensory cortex, the results of these two treatments may have almost identical outcomes at that level of CNS functioning (Carter-Wilson, 1991).

SENSORY REEDUCATION INTERVENTIONS

The best candidates for sensory reeducation are individuals with good cognitive function and high levels of motivation. The first level of sensory reeducation is to teach the person how to compensate for a lack of protective sensation (e.g., pain and temperature sensation) by using vision and recruiting any residual sensory function. To wean away from these compensatory techniques, clients then need to engage in a program that combines graded sensory stimulation and the use of the affected hand in functional activities.

Treatment sessions focusing on sensory stimulation should last 10–15 minutes for optimum concentration by the client. A suggested sequence of activities is as follows (Callahan, 1995):

1. Initiate localization of moving touch, since it returns before constant touch. The therapist touches the client's finger or an area on the hand with a fingertip or the eraser end of a pencil. This is done first with the client's eyes open and then, in the same place, with the client's eyes closed. In the eyes-closed condition, the client concentrates on remembering the sensory and visual images of the application and tries to point to the area of the skin just touched.
2. Progress to localization of constant touch.
3. Work on discriminatory touch to help clients determine the tactile similarities and differences among objects. Commercially available training programs are available for teaching shape, texture, and object identification. Grades of cloth (highly textured to finely woven), sandpaper, metal (rough to smooth), or wood can also be used for discrimination training.
4. Stereognosis is treated last through structured and repetitive practice in recognizing graded, meaningful objects with vision occluded.

It is important to document baseline deficits or abilities and to reevaluate at least once every 4 weeks to track progress and make adjustments to the treatment program.

Clinicians have noted the most dramatic functional improvement in sensibility occurs in individuals who actively use the involved extremity during their daily occupational activities and routines, such as activities of daily living (ADL) and work. Use of the affected extremity in leisure activities also helps normalize sensory input. Meaningful leisure activities can harness a high level of motivation so they might be substituted for ADL or work simulation early in treatment. If clients are discouraged or self-critical of their occupational performance, purposeful activities such as crafts or games they are unfamiliar with can encourage hand use, since there should be no preconceived expectation for performance. If return to work is the goal, therapy should begin with the critical job demands that allow vision to substitute for imperfect sensation. Therapists can then gradually introduce critical job demands that require visual occlusion for hand use.

CONCLUSION

Sensory reeducation after peripheral nerve injuries can prevent disability by helping individuals adjust to and use their postinjury sensation during their day-to-day activities. For further details on sensory retraining, see specialty texts on this topic, such as the ones listed in the references.

SECTION II

Strengthening

DEBORAH PINET O'MAHONY

Deficits in **strength** can affect a person's ability to complete ADL, instrumental activities of daily living (IADL), work, social, and leisure pursuits. Without adequate strength, a client may have difficulty engaging in meaningful areas of occupation. Factors such as pain, edema, **adhesions** and **contractures,** abnormal tone, and sensory deficits, limit muscle function and result in strength problems. Decreased strength can also lead to joint deformity, owing to imbalances between agonist and antagonist muscles. If the strength impairment is not addressed, dysfunction in occupations can occur because the client does not have the sufficient strength to complete activities such as bathing, carpentry, or tennis.

Strength impairments can also affect the client's role performance. An individual's successful participation in roles such as parent, worker, student, partner, or athlete may depend, in part, on sufficient muscle strength. A client with muscle weakness may have difficulty accomplishing the tasks required of identified roles or may need to accomplish them in an altered manner. Strength deficits can also affect how an individual functions within specific environments or contexts whether in the home, at a job site, or on a tennis court.

DESCRIPTION OF STRENGTH

"Strength is the ability of a muscle or muscle group to produce tension and a resulting force in one maximal effort, either dynamically or statically, in relation to the demands placed upon it" (Kisner & Colby, 1996, p. 14). Skeletal muscles are made up of many individual muscle fibers, which act as contracting units. Muscle fiber contraction requires stimulation by a motor neuron. One motor nerve and all the attached muscle fibers form a **motor unit.** Stimulation of the motor unit occurs via the motor end plate, which is an enlargement at the end of the nerve fiber. At this neuromuscular junction, a neurotransmitter is released, which causes the muscle fibers to contract as a motor unit. When the muscle fibers contract, they generate an amount of tension or force that is applied to the muscle, its tendon, and the bone to which the tendons are connected. This force can either promote movement of the attached bones or provide stability and maintenance of a position. The amount of force produced is related to the number of motor units being stimulated. The greater the number of motor units firing, the stronger the tension, as more muscle fibers are contracting (Kisner & Colby, 1996).

TYPES OF MUSCLE CONTRACTIONS

There are two basic categories of muscle contractions, **isometric** and **isotonic** (Breines, 2001). During an isometric muscle contraction, the motor units stimulate the muscle fibers to increase the tension in the muscle, but the muscle does not shorten for joint movement. Stability at the joint occurs, as the force generated in the muscle is equal to gravity or any other applied resistance. An example of an isometric contraction is maintaining a grasp on a blow dryer (finger flexors and thumb opposition).

Isotonic contraction of a muscle involves changes in the muscle fiber's length resulting in joint movement. This contraction can occur with or without resistance. Two types of isotonic contractions are possible, **concentric** or **eccentric.** During concentric contraction, the muscle shortens to allow motion. The force generated in the muscle is increased to overcome resistance to movement. A concentric contraction of the biceps (elbow flexors) occurs when a person raises a blow dryer to dry the wet hair. The tension in the biceps increases to move the forearm up against the resistance of gravity. During eccentric contraction, the muscle fibers of an already shortened muscle lengthen to resist a force and produce a controlled joint motion. An eccentric contraction occurs at the biceps, when a person slowly lowers the blow dryer after drying the hair (Breines, 2001; Jackson, Gray, & Zemke, 2002). Both isometric and isotonic muscle contractions are needed to engage in occupations.

FACTORS AFFECTING MUSCLE STRENGTH

Edema, adhesions and **contractures,** abnormal muscle tone, and sensory deficits all influence the muscle's ability to contract. Edema and adhesions are associated with the inflammatory response that occurs whenever there is trauma to the body. During inflammation, the blood vessels dilate sending additional white blood cells to the damaged area. This results in swelling, or edema, of the tissues surrounding the muscles. Fibrin, a sticky substance, is deposited to clot the blood and reduce the edema in the area. Fibrin also causes the development of adhesions, or the holding together of two superficial surfaces. The stronger the adhesions, the greater the chances of muscle atrophy, because they prevent the muscle from lengthening or shortening to generate an adequate contraction. The edema, if left untreated, can place pressure on nerves, blood vessels, and various joint structures, delaying healing and causing pain and stiffness. Expedient prevention and treatment of edema are critical for maintaining joint integrity and optimal muscle functioning. Active range of motion (ROM) for fluid absorption and soft tissue mobility, elevation of the edematous extremity, compression of the tissues through retrograde massage, wrapping or pressure garments, and the use of ice for vasoconstriction are all interventions that address edema (Kasch & Nickerson, 2001).

Abnormalities in muscle tone, or tightness, can lead to contractures. A contracture occurs when there is permanent shortening of a muscle owing to spasm or paralysis (Thomas, 1997). The shortened muscle fibers limit joint ROM and can negatively affect participation in areas of occupation. Contractures can cause pain and sensory changes as well, because of the immobility. Contractures can be prevented through stretching and protection of unstable joints by maintaining soft tissue length. Splints and positioning can be used to facilitate normal muscle tone and tissue mobility. Muscle strengthening is not focused on until normal muscle tone is achieved (Preston, 2001). (Sections 3 and 4 discuss specific motor control and sensorimotor techniques.)

Accurate sensory processing contributes to coordinated movement. The inclination to move is based on sensory feedback. Without adequate sensation, movement can be ineffective, despite recovery of motor functioning. A thorough sensory evaluation must be done in conjunction with an assessment of active range of motion (AROM) and manual muscle testing. Observation and analysis of the client's participation in activities requiring strength and sensation are also necessary to identify problems and targeted outcomes. Treatment of sensory deficits can be remedial or compensatory in nature, depending on the cause of the impairments. (See Sections 1 and 4 for details regarding this topic.) When sensory deficits are present, a strengthening program should include modifications to prevent injury from lack of sensory feedback to the muscle.

PRINCIPLES AND CHARACTERISTICS OF STRENGTHENING ACTIVITIES

Resistance

Once a strength deficit is detected, the occupational therapist, in conjunction with the client, designs an intervention plan to increase the strength needed for the identified areas of occupation. According to the **overload principle,** to increase strength, the load or force applied to the muscle must exceed the capacity of that muscle, causing recruitment of more motor units. Resistance is often used to stimulate muscle contraction. The greater the intensity or the amount of resistance applied, the more motor units are recruited (Kisner & Colby, 1996). The intensity of the load, rather than the number of completed repetitions, has the most influence on the development of muscle strength. More motor units firing cause a larger force in muscle tension, which means more muscle strength. Carrying a grocery bag with 6 lb of food recruits more muscle fibers than carrying a bag with 3 lb of groceries and making two trips from the car (Hamill & Knutzen, 1995; Lillegard & Terrio, 1994; Umphred, 1995b).

Gravity is one force that places a load on muscles during contraction. The amount of this force depends on the plane of movement, either against or with gravity. Muscles have to work harder to move a body part against gravity than to move it in a horizontal or gravity-eliminated plane. The muscle grade awarded through manual muscle testing determines the plane of movement for muscle strengthening. Muscles should be able the move joints through the full available ROM in a gravity-eliminated and then against-gravity plane before external loads or forces are applied to them.

Types of Muscle Contraction

The type of muscle contraction stimulated influences the development of strength. "A muscle produces the most force output when contracting eccentrically (lengthening) against resistance. The muscle produces slightly less force when contracting isometrically (holding) and the least force when contracting concentrically (shortening) against a load" (Kisner & Colby, 1996, p. 15).

Most occupational activities require a combination of muscle contractions. Muscle groups respond in different patterns, depending on the demands of specific tasks. These response patterns can be classified as open or closed chains of movement or kinetic links. The chain is considered closed when the distal end of an extremity is bearing weight. When the extremity is free distally, the chain is considered open to a variety of movement possibilities (Goldstein, 1995). A closed-chain movement uses eccentric and concentric muscle contractions and the force of the person's body weight to add a load to the muscle. An example is using a transfer board to move from a bed to a wheelchair. The upper extremities are extended down against the board while the person's body weight is shifted along the board until the transfer is completed. An example of an open-chain movement is bringing a hot cup of coffee to the mouth to take a drink and then carefully lowering it back down to the table. Eccentric and concentric contractions are also used in this example. Closed-chain movements are more representative of the muscle functioning needed in ADL (Hamill & Knutzen, 1995).

Speed of Contraction

The speed of muscle contraction affects strengthening. Greater forces or torques are produced at slower speeds of movement, as there is more time to recruit additional motor units. This results in greater strength (Kisner & Colby, 1996). Factors such as the frequency of the program, the number of repetitions performed, the duration of activities, and the rest periods also influence successful muscle strengthening. (Specific strengthening programs are discussed below.)

Endurance of Muscle Contraction

Muscle endurance is needed for maximal participation in everyday tasks. Muscle endurance is related to strength, because it is "the ability to contract repeatedly or generate tension and sustain that tension over a prolonged period of time" (Kisner & Colby, 1996, p. 16). Muscle endurance is developed through high repetitions and low-stress load to the muscle (<50% of maximal intensity). As endurance increases, a muscle is able to perform a greater number of contractions or hold against a load over an extended period of time. This enables longer participation in chosen activities.

Standing at the kitchen sink to wash dishes facilitates prolonged muscle tension in the lower extremities and trunk, increasing muscle endurance (Buchner & Coleman, 1994).

DESCRIPTION OF SPECIFIC EXERCISE PROGRAMS

Exercise in occupational therapy is used to facilitate sensory and motor functioning for performing selected occupations. **Therapeutic exercise** is defined as "any body movement or muscle contraction to prevent or correct a physical impairment, improve musculoskeletal function and maintain a state of well-being" (Breines, 2001, p. 513). Exercise programs are designed based on a number of factors. The occupational therapist considers the muscle grade and muscle endurance levels, precautions for movement, prognosis, and activity demands of the individual's preferred areas of occupation. Exercise programs used in occupational therapy can be described as passive, isotonic active assistive, isotonic active, isometric without resistance, isotonic resistive, isometric resistive, and isokinetic (Breines, 2001; Jackson et al., 2002).

Passive Exercise

Passive exercise involves passive range of motion (PROM) and passive stretching of tight soft tissue. No active muscle contraction occurs. Therefore, these activities are not used for strengthening. The purpose is to achieve joint flexibility by maximally stretching the muscle fibers to prevent any loss of AROM.

The stretching is done by the practitioner, who applies a force to the limited soft tissue while moving the joint through the full ROM. The stretching is done in the opposite direction of the tightness and is completed slowly to allow the tight structures to lengthen without rupturing. The practitioner holds the joint at the end range of motion for 15-30 sec to stretch the tissue effectively (Kisner & Colby, 1996). Stretching can also be done by machines, which, when attached to joints, continually move the joint through a preset ROM. When only one upper extremity is affected, PROM and stretching can be accomplished by using overhead pulleys; the unaffected upper extremity actively pulls the affected extremity through the available ROM.

Passive range of motion and stretching should be done cautiously when there is inflammation, limited sensory feedback for pain detection, and prolonged immobilization, which can lead to osteoporosis or tendon and ligament tears. Positioning of the joints to avoid deformity development should also be done in conjunction with a passive exercise program (Buckner, 2001).

Isotonic Active Assistive Exercise

Isotonic active assistive exercise requires isotonic muscle contractions. It is used for clients who have muscle grades of trace, poor minus, and fair minus. The client actively moves the joint as far as possible, and then some kind of outside force assists with moving the joint through the remainder of the ROM. Either the client or the practitioner can provide the affected extremity with manually additional assistance. Another option is the use of equipment, such as a pulley system, mobile arm supports, overhead suspension slings, or a tabletop upper extremity skateboard to assist in obtaining maximal ROM.

Active assistive exercise in a gravity-eliminated plane is used when the muscle grades are trace to poor minus, whereas active assistive exercise in an against-gravity plane is appropriate for fair minus muscle grades. As the client gains more strength, there is less reliance on the outside assistance. The person participates in an active assistive exercise program until full AROM is achieved.

Isotonic Active Exercise

Isotonic active exercise also requires isotonic muscle contractions; however, the client moves fully through the available ROM without any assistance or additional force applied to the joint (Lillegard & Terrio, 1994). A client who has muscles grades of poor to fair can participate in this type of program. Active exercise in a gravity-eliminated plane is used when muscle grades are poor to fair minus, and active exercise in an against-gravity plane is appropriate for fair muscle grades. The goal is to increase strength by increasing the frequency, repetitions, or duration of the exercises or by changing the plane in which the exercises are performed.

Isometric without Resistance Exercise

Isometric without resistance exercises are useful when AROM is not possible or is prohibited after surgery or a flair-up of rheumatoid arthritis. The goal is to maintain muscle strength through isometric muscle contractions. The client contracts the muscle, increasing the tension, and holds the joint in a stable position for approximately 5 sec. Then the muscle is relaxed and the procedure is repeated. Isometric muscle contraction causes an increase in both systolic and diastolic blood pressures; therefore, it is not recommended for clients who have cardiac conditions (Breines, 2001; Lillegard & Terrio, 1994).

Isotonic Resistive Exercise

Once a client is able to move the joint through the full range of motion against gravity, the next step for improving muscle strength and endurance is to add an extra load to the muscle. During isotonic resistive strengthening exercises, the load is applied to the muscle contraction by using a number of different items, including weights and dumbbells, springs, pulleys, rubber bands, resistive putty, strengthening machines, and everyday objects (Figs. 30-1 and 30-2). The client should have muscle grades of fair plus to participate in this type of program. Isotonic muscle contractions are used

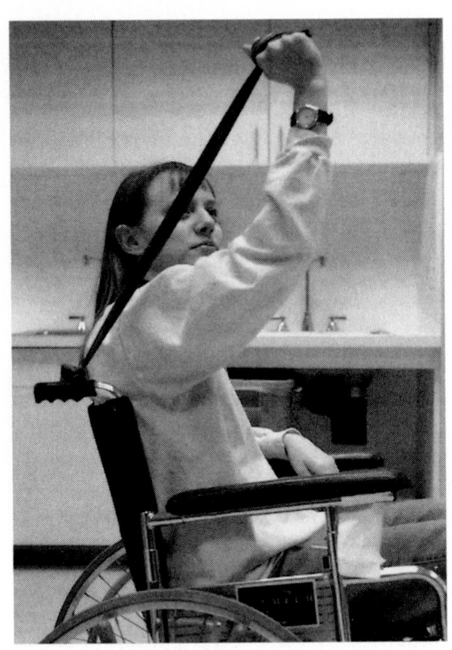

FIGURE 30–1. Use of an elastic band provides isotonic resistive against-gravity exercise for the triceps.

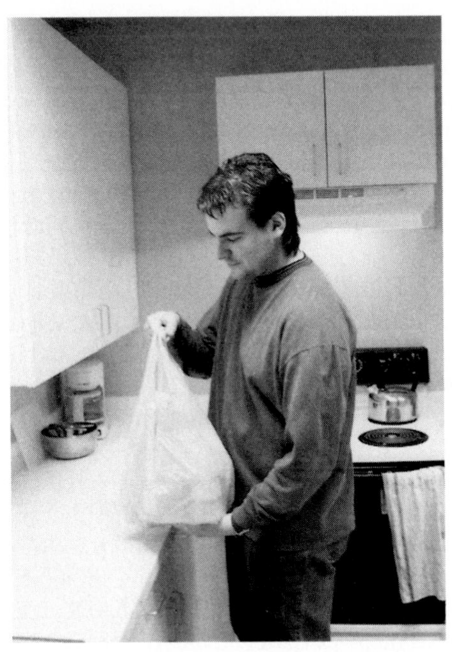

FIGURE 30–2. An applied load to biceps contraction occurs when lifting groceries against gravity.

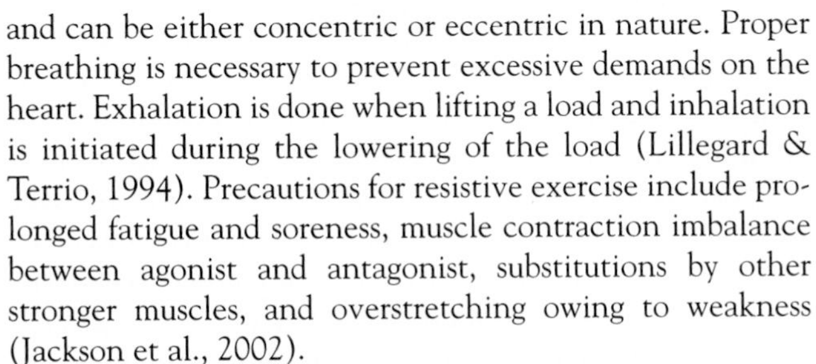

and can be either concentric or eccentric in nature. Proper breathing is necessary to prevent excessive demands on the heart. Exhalation is done when lifting a load and inhalation is initiated during the lowering of the load (Lillegard & Terrio, 1994). Precautions for resistive exercise include prolonged fatigue and soreness, muscle contraction imbalance between agonist and antagonist, substitutions by other stronger muscles, and overstretching owing to weakness (Jackson et al., 2002).

There are two specialized resistive exercise programs: the DeLorme method of progressive resistive exercise (PRE), and the Oxford technique of regressive resistive exercise (RRE). These exercises should be completed once a day, four or five times per week (Breines, 2001). In the DeLorme method, the muscle is allowed a warmup period leading to full muscle contraction. The first step involves determining the maximal load or weight the client can lift through the entire ROM for 10 repetitions. Then a program is designed in which the person completes 10 repetitions with a weight that is 50% of the maximal load, progresses to 10 repetitions using a weight that is 75% of the maximal load, and finishes with 10 repetitions using the maximal weight. The client rests for 2–4 min between progressions with the different weights.

The Oxford technique is basically the reverse approach of the DeLorme method. The client begins at maximal weight and lifts a lesser load with each set of 10 repetitions. The reasoning behind this approach is that the muscle fatigues with more contractions; therefore, the muscle cannot effectively contract to respond to the increased loads. This approach may be more useful in the beginning of therapy, until the muscle can make more gains in recruiting motor units (Breines, 2001).

Isometric Resistive Exercise

Isometric resistive exercise, no joint motion occurs, because the muscle is contracting isometrically against some additional force. The outside force can be applied by the occupational therapist pushing against the held contraction or the client can hold a weight distally while maintaining a stable proximal joint position. These exercises have the same uses and precautions as isometric without resistance exercises.

Isokinetic Exercise

Isokinetic exercise combines the characteristics of both isometric and isotonic resistive exercise. Equipment such as an isokinetic dynamometer is used to control the speed of movement, the amount of load on the muscle, and the stimulation of motor units through the full ROM (Lillegard & Terrio, 1994; McArdle, Katch, & Katch, 1996). The use of isokinetic exercise equipment is generally part of a physical therapy treatment program and not an exercise modality typically used by occupational therapists.

OCCUPATIONAL THERAPY INTERVENTION OPTIONS

The occupational therapist identifies strength deficits through analysis of occupational performance and assessment of client factors. A client-centered plan of intervention is designed to address deficits in areas of occupations. The practitioner and the client develop a plan of activities and methods that fall within a continuum. The continuum represents four approaches characterized by the types of activities used during recovery. They are adjunctive methods, enabling activities, purposeful activity, and occupational performance and occupational roles. Practitioners may use any of these intervention types to address strength impairments, depending on the severity of the deficit and the impact on the performance areas (Pedretti & Early, 2001). Neistadt and Seymour's (1995) survey of occupational therapists working in adult physical rehabilitation facilities found that the four most frequently selected treatment activities were self-care tasks, upper extremity exercise, functional mobility and neuromuscular training. Recent research on motor control supports the use of purposeful and task-oriented approaches (see Section 3).

In the early stages of strength recovery, the practitioner may use adjunctive methods or procedures that prepare the client for participation in meaningful activities. Muscle weakness, pain, edema, or limitations in joint range of motion prevent maximal performance of ADL, IADL, work, and leisure. The practitioner focuses on treating these client factors using exercise, joint positioning and splinting, edema control, neurosensory stimulation, and physical agent modalities (Pedretti & Early, 2001). It is important for the practitioner to help the client enfold adjunctive approaches into his or her occupational routines for optimum healing and pain control and to promote a sense of self-efficacy.

The challenge for the therapist in the early stages of recovery is to identify activities that promote interest and quantitative improvements in movement. The use of meaningful objects in treatment has been shown to facilitate increased repetitions and duration of movement compared to rote exercise alone. (Thomas, 1996; Zimmerer-Branum & Nelson, 1995). Having two people play a game of balloon volleyball encourages upper extremity ROM, strengthening, and endurance as well as socialization and concentration.

Enabling activities such as this can be thought of as prerequisites or stepping-stones to other more difficult or complex tasks (Pedretti & Early, 2001). Likewise, purposeful activities may be selected that relate to the client's interests and that are carefully matched to the client's therapy needs. For example, a client might not have adequate strength for performing previous carpentry activities. But by completing a simple woodworking project using sanding blocks of differing weights, the client is able to increase strength, enabling future resumption of meaningful work roles.

In occupation-based approaches, the occupational therapy practitioner helps the client directly engage in activities, habits, and routines identified from the client's occupational profile (American Occupational Therapy Association—Commission on Practice [AOTA], in press). These tasks are chosen to improve areas of occupation and roles specific to that person (Fig. 30-3). Giving choices is thought to improve the quality of performance and encourage a sense of self–efficacy and dignity (LaMore & Nelson, 1993). The activities at this stage may be graded to increase in difficulty and/or adaptive equipment can be provided to facilitate successful completion of tasks. The carpenter can use lightweight tools to construct a bookcase. The weight of the tools, the plane of movement, and the length of time spent working on the project can be increased to achieve the strength required for the worker's role.

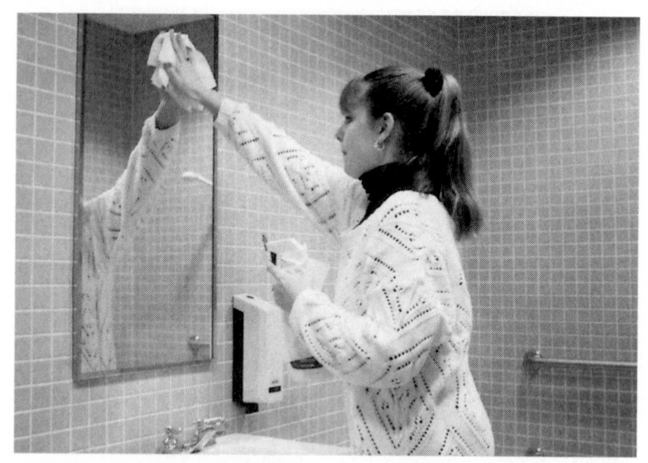

FIGURE 30–3. Home management activity for upper extremity strengthening and resumption of previous roles.

Clients do not always achieve the outcomes of the designed interventions. Strong collaboration with the client right from the start helps the client assume an active role in the intervention process, which is critical for effectiveness and positive outcomes. The therapist needs to provide clear information about the purpose and benefit of the interventions while structuring the environment for success and carryover of techniques (Chen, Neufield, Feely, & Skinner, 1999). The emphasis is on maximum functioning and resumption of roles in the selected environment. For example, the client with strength impairments may participate in a work hardening program to improve endurance for return to the carpentry job. If the person has reached a plateau in the strengthening program, the practitioner focuses on educating the client in job modifications. Using these different intervention options, the occupational therapy practitioner can simultaneously address the client's impairment in strength and the resultant impact on areas occupational performance.

CONCLUSION

Adequate muscle strength is important for satisfactory participation in many occupational activities. Through various occupational therapy approaches, clients can regain or maximize strength to perform activities that give meaning to their lives. The focus of any strengthening intervention program in occupational therapy should incorporate a client-centered approach to facilitate successful outcomes for occupational engagement and participation.

SECTION III

Motor Control Theories and Models Guiding Occupational Performance Interventions Principles and Assumptions

CLARE G. GIUFFRIDA

The field of motor control and learning tries to explain both the regulation and control of normal movements as well as the factors and processes involved in normal motor learning. More specifically, motor control involves the study of the nature, cause, and mechanisms of posture and movement control (Rose, 1997). Through scientific inquiries, the multiple determinants of movement—such as the physiological, biomechanical, neurological, psychological, and environmental factors—can be investigated (Shumway-Cook & Woollacott, 2001). However, the practitioner in therapy focuses on the client's posture and movement while the client is engaged in different tasks. This enables the practitioner to understand better how different tasks influence and regulate the client's posture and movement control in different contents.

In the movement sciences, a thorough understanding of motor control implies knowing about what is controlled and how the various processes influencing control are organized (Horak, 1991, Rose, 1997). Likewise, motor control involves a person's ability to regulate or direct the mechanisms essential to posture and movement. However, an individual's goal-directed movements emerge in many contexts through the efforts of many brain structures and processes, including the individual's perception, cognitive, and action systems. Accordingly, movement is described and studied within the context of accomplishing a particular activity. Therefore, motor control needs to reflect an understanding of movement control in relation to the person's specific goals, movement activities, or contextual demands.

For movement science, Rosenbaum (1991) has proposed that the central issues in motor control revolve around the multiple factors determining movement selection, movement sequencing, and the coordination of perception and action in goal-directed activities. For instance, a fundamental question for motor control theorists is how stability is maintained and controlled while the individual acts in and on the environment. In the context of occupational performance, this question becomes, "How is postural stability and movement regulated and controlled for an individual engaged in an everyday activity, such as dressing while sitting on a stable or unstable surface, such as a chair or soft mattress?"

Motor learning, in contrast to motor control, is directed more to understanding how movements are acquired and modified with practice. Schmidt and Lee (1999) defined motor learning as a set of processes associated with practice or experience leading to permanent changes in the capability for skilled acts. Shumway-Cook and Woollacott (2001) proposed that motor learning develops from a complex set of perceptual, cognitive, and action processes developed in response to individual– task–environment interactions.

The field of motor control and learning provides occupational therapy with new ideas for understanding the nature, cause, acquisition, and modification of movement supporting optimal occupational performance. The motor control approaches used in occupational therapy reflect an integration of ideas that explain the nature and regulation of movement. There is not one singular motor control theory of occupational therapy, but several applied motor control approaches and models with different principles and assumptions. These approaches are supported with motor control research drawn from the movement and therapeutic sciences and can provide evidence supporting different occupational therapy interventions.

The following subsection provides a synopsis of the prevailing motor control theories and their implications for occupational therapy treatment. Theories are organized according to whether the control is centralized within the CNS or dispersed throughout the CNS and or other systems. See Burtner & Woollacott (1996) and Bate (1997) for other organizational frameworks for motor control theories. Chapter 21, Section 6 contains more detail about motor learning principles, which are integrated into many models of motor control underlying current therapeutic practice.

MOTOR CONTROL MODELS

Central or Peripheral Nervous System Control

Reflex Model

Description

The classic experiments of Sherrington (1947) provided the basis for the **reflex model of motor control.** In these experiments, nervous system processes were inferred by motor outputs in response to sensory inputs given to unconscious anesthetized animals. By stimulating specific sensory receptors, Sherrington induced a variety of distinct stereotyped movements in animal preparations.

Reflexes are the basis for all movements in this model of motor control (Easton, 1972). This model and therapeutic approaches derived from it assume that sensory input controls motor output. This view of motor control is *peripheralist,* as it posits that motor control depends on peripheral sensory input controlling the motor response. The nervous system, therefore, is a passive recipient of sensory stimuli, which trigger, coordinate, and activate muscles that can excite more sensory systems to activate more muscles (Horak, 1991). This sensory motor input–output relationship became incorporated into therapeutic techniques to cause or induce movement with clients who demonstrate limited movement patterns.

Therapeutic Implications

Horak (1991) proposed several clinical implications from this model. The first involves the role of the therapist in identifying reflexes in their clients and predicting from the client's quality of motor function. This is seen in therapeutic approaches in which therapists identify reflexes in young children and adults with CNS disorders. Second, this model implies that stereotypic reflex responses can be elicited if appropriate stimulation is provided. In therapy, this occurs when therapists elicit righting reactions by moving a child or adult on a therapy ball or rocker platform.

Limitations

In the reflex model of motor control, the reflex is the basic building block for coordinated behavior. Considerable evidence now exists to show that coordinated movement is not controlled by a series of integrated reflexes (Bradley & Beckoff 1989; Towen, 1984). Deafferentation studies by Polit and Bizzi (1979) support the hypothesis that sensory feedback is not necessary, as originally thought, for accurate movement production. For example, a concert pianist can move so rapidly from one key to another key that there is no time for sensory information from one stroke to activate the next. Sensory feedback, however, is necessary for adjusting to environmental demands and in movement learning (Horak, 1991, Shumway-Cook & Woollacott, 2001). This model also cannot account for novel movements or variations in movements owing to changes in task demands (Shumway-Cook & Woollacott, 2001).

Hierarchical Model of Motor Control

Description

Jackson in 1932 articulated the **hierarchical model of motor control** (Foerster, 1977). In this model, control of movement is organized hierarchically from the lowest levels in the spinal cord to intermediate levels in the brainstem to the highest levels in the cortex. This model provides a central view of motor control in that normal movements are governed by CNS motor programs that were originally conceived of as specifying muscle activation patterns. Keele (1968) defined motor programs as a set of muscle commands that are structured before a movement sequence begins and allow the sequence to be carried out uninfluenced by peripheral feedback.

Although there continues to be considerable controversies about what constitutes motor programming, the hierarchical model clearly separates high-level movement control and low-level reflexive control. This model, along with the reflex model, became further articulated as the reflex hierarchical model and/or programming model of motor control, which also serves as the basis for neurotherapeutic approaches (Mathiowetz & Haugen, 2002).

Clinical Implications

Two key occupational therapy approaches—the neurodevelopmental and sensory integration approaches—are based on this model of hierarchical organization in the CNS (Montgomery, 1991). Also, many forms of central nervous system dysfunction are considered disruptive to higher-level control of movement. Released reflexes are thought to interfere with or block coordinated movement patterns. Therefore, a reasonable goal for therapy is to identify and prevent primitive reflexes from dominating or interfering with higher-level goals. Strategies designed to enhance control are seen in the neurorehabilitation approaches. These strategies can include sensory-integration procedures and neurodevelopment facilitation as well as inhibition and handling techniques. Both are hypothesized means of developing more control in the system. However, research evidence in support of hierarchical control is limited.

Limitations

In light of contemporary evidence for motor behavior, there are several limitations to this model. For example, low levels of control, such as seen in spinal cord control, dominates motor control when necessary. Also, lower levels of control are evident in cats walking on a treadmill, despite total transactions preventing control from higher centers. Coordinated reflexive locomotor movement patterns such as walking, trotting, and galloping appear not to require top-down control and presents evidence against motor control being top-down.

Also challenged in light of recent research is the assumption that motor development and recovery of functions follows a stepwise or hierarchical progression from reflex-driven movements to internally commanded movements. Studies demonstrate that motor development does not always follow a set sequence. In addition, learning to reach and to kick seem to begin with predictive self-generated movements that become increasingly responsive to ongoing sensory feedback (Thelen, Kelso, & Fogel, 1987; von Hofsten, 1980) and are not reflexively controlled.

There are other limitations evident in this model, such as its inability to account for both reflexive and voluntary control seen in a variety of situations. Furthermore, it cannot account for instances in which reflexive control dominates. For example, stepping on a pin results in immediate withdrawal of the leg and is evidence for lower-level control dominating and being adaptive for the person in a particular context. Also, this model cannot account for the adjustment of reflexive control being monitored by voluntary control or modified by conscious commands or instructions. For example, instructions to release or resist a movement are shown to modify unexpected perturbations to the limb (Shumway-Cook & Woollacott, 2001).

Motor Programming Theories

Description

In **motor programming models of movement control,** movements depend on a motor program, such as a central pattern generator or an abstract code in the system, that allows a movement to be carried out by any effector system (Shumway-Cook & Woollacott, 2001). These theories were proposed to explain how movements could be generated without reflexive action, and they have considerable experimental support.

For example, studies in the early 1960s showed that the timing of the locust's wing beat depended on a rhythmic pattern generator. In these studies, wing beat prevailed in spite of the sensory nerves being cut. Sensory input was not necessary to drive the output but was shown to contribute to modulating the action. Central processes drive the central motor pattern. Further work, done by Grillner (1981) with cats, also demonstrated that locomotion could occur without sensory input or descending patterns from the brain. Changes in stimuli intensity to the spinal cord of the cat were shown to produce walking, trotting, or galloping. These studies are now being used to support treadmill training in patients with stroke and spinal cord injury by which different patterns of gait are induced by different speeds on the treadmill.

Besides motor programs induced by central pattern generators, the term *motor programming* is also used to describe the higher-level motor programs that represent actions in abstract terms or codes within the CNS. Research in the fields of psychology and motor learning support this idea. The motor programming concept allows for the storing of rules for generating movements so that tasks can be performed by any effector system. For example, the motor programming concept is used to explain people's ability to write their name with any extremity. In this case, elements of the signature— regardless of the extremity used— remain constant.

Limitations

The concept of central pattern generators allows therapists to expand their understanding of movement control. It was not intended, however, to deny that sensory control could also be important. Neither the concept of central pattern generators nor motor program takes into account other factors that may also influence the production of the movement.

Implications

Motor program theories allow therapists to move beyond the reflexive explanations of movement control. In therapy, atypical control can be a function of central pattern disturbance as well as problems with the rules for movement. If patients have higher levels of motor programming affected, the therapist can then help them relearn the rules for action.

Distributed and Systems Models of Motor Control

Distributed Models of Motor Control

Description

In **distributed models** of motor control, control of movement is not peripheral or central. As scientists looked at different motor behaviors and other characteristics of the movement system, a concept of distributed control of movement emerged, which considered the internal and external forces acting on this system (Keshner, 1991). Distributed models of motor control are not unidirectional. Rather, they allow for communication within the nervous system to take place in ascending, descending, and lateral arrangements. The control hierarchy is not perceived as a descending chain of command but as an overlapping circular network in which each level influences those above and below it. Various sites within and throughout the system are part of the process underlying and controlling movement. Some models of distributed control, however, minimize the relevance of the nervous system. Others, such as neural network models, continue to rely heavily on processing units consisting of neurons and their extensive system of linked dendrites (Bate, 1997). Control of movement in these models is seen as distributed throughout many working systems, which can include mechanical and environmental factors as well as nervous system factors. There are several different theories about distributed control of movement.

Systems Theory Bernstein, a Russian scientist, was among the first to look at internal and external forces acting on the body to understand the characteristics of the system being moved. The body was regarded as a mechanical system with mass and that was subject to external forces, like gravity, as well as inertial- and movement-dependent forces. Bernstein asked questions related to the function of the system in a continually changing environment, the properties of the initial conditions affecting movement, and the body as a mechanical system influencing the control process (Shumway-Cook & Woollacott, 2001).

Bernstein was also responsible for identifying what is known as the degrees-of-freedom problem. In describing the mechanics of the system, Bernstein noted that many degrees of freedom need to be controlled for coordinated movement to occur. For example, there are many joints that can flex, extend, and/or rotate, and these options complicate the control of movement. Motor control, therefore, involves converting the body into a controllable system (Schmidt & Lee, 1999).

Bernstein's solution to this problem was to propose that hierarchical control exists to simplify the body's multiple degrees of freedom. He believed that groups of muscle were constrained to act together as a unit and that these units were activated at lower levels in the system.

Dynamic Action Theory (Synergetics) The **dynamic action theory** comes from the study of dynamics or synergetics, the study of how parts of systems work together. Dynamic action theory asks two fundamental questions: How do patterns and organization emerge from orderless parts? How do systems change over time? A fundamental principle of this theory is self-organization. This principle states that when a system of individual parts comes together, its collective elements behave in an ordered fashion. With respect to motor control, there is no need to have a higher center issuing commands to achieve coordinated output (Rosenbaum, 1991).

Descriptions of these self-organizing systems are expressed mathematically, and the critical features of the system are nonlinear properties. Nonlinear behavior is described as a situation in which one parameter is altered to reach a critical value, causing the system to go into a different behavioral pattern. For example, as an animal walks faster and faster, there is a point at which it breaks into a trot and later a gallop. The parameter being altered is walking speed and the accompanying behavioral changes are the animal's gait: walking, trotting, and galloping.

Dynamic Pattern Theory Dynamic pattern theory is an operational approach to the study of coordinated movement (Keshner, 1991) used in the movement sciences. The impact of this theory is seen in a variety of research areas, including development (Thelen & Smith, 1994), aging (Green & Williams, 1996), rehabilitation (Scholz, 1990), and coordination research (Lee, 1998; Sternad, 1998; Walter, 1998). Dynamic pattern theory incorporates aspects of Bernstein's systems theory and dynamic action theory. It is an attempt to define terms and provide behavioral and mathematical predictions for coordinated movement patterns. The following five basic concepts are fundamental to many dynamic systems approaches and motor control research.

First, the human system exhibits self-organizing behavior. Second, the human system is a many-element system that can be described by a few elements, which are referred to as collective variables. Collective variables are the fewest number of variables that completely describe a behavior (Heriza, 1991). For example, Heriza proposed that, for humans, walking is a highly complex behavior characterized by a specific movement pattern. The new walker compresses the many degrees of freedom available from the muscles, bones, joints, tendons, neurons, and motor units to the relatively few degrees of freedom observed in walking. In this example, a complex behavior, walking, becomes characterized by a description of the behavior, the specific movement pattern.

Third, collective variables characterize movement patterns and capture the systems, cooperating to produce the movement, since movement is more than just muscles and motor neurons. For example kicking, stepping, and throwing a ball are examples of coordinated movement patterns. Again, an example by Heriza (1991) helps clarify this. In intralimb coordination, such as seen within one limb in kicking or stepping, the identified collective variables are the timing of the individual movement phases (flexion and extension), phase lags, (the time between the onset of movement of one joint with respect to another joint), and the relationship of individual joints to each other.

Fourth, the identification of phase transitions is basic to understanding behavior. **Control parameters** are variables that shift the movement from one movement form to another form. Control parameters reorganize the system. In the example of intralimb coordination and in interlimb coordination, behavioral states can drive the system. For instance, when an infant is asleep or drowsy, little kicking is noted. If the infant is aroused, the spatial and temporal pattern of kicking is observed. If the infant is in a crying state, a new pattern emerges, which is described as a rigid coactivation of all the muscles into stiff mobility. Therefore, control parameters can be defined as essential components but nonspecific to the movement behavior. In this example, the control parameters can reside in the individual (e.g., behavioral state), in the environment (e.g., gravity), in the social environment (e.g., caretaker), or in the goal or in the task. New coordinated patterns emerge because old patterns become unstable and the system is driven to a new state. Changes in the control parameters push the system to a new state. During these shifts in phase, or phase transitions, the prevailing movement pattern becomes less stable and more easily perturbed by the control parameter (Heriza, 1991).

The final concept is that the study of the stability or instability of behavior during transition periods is essential for understanding pattern change in complex systems. In this approach, movement behavior and control can be aptly described by a set of collective variables and control variables associated with phase transition (Haugen, Mathiowetz, & Flinn, 2002).

Implications

Dynamic systems are systems in which behaviors evolve over time and are marked by their capacity to change states.

Systems theories take into account factors other than the nervous system in regulating movement, for example, physical characteristics, such as the mass of the system being moved. These theories have enlarged the understanding of the multiple factors responsible for controlled movement. The individual is seen as active within the environment, and movement is an emergent product of many systems. These theories may be helpful in taking into account the passive components of a patient's biomechanics and factoring these components into explanations for movement stability and instability (Bate, 1997).

Limitations

The role of the nervous system is minimized in these theories. Transitions in movement patterns are explained in terms of physical causality, mathematical functions, and variables. These theories primarily seek physical factors that contribute to movement characteristics and thus seem more aligned with biomechanical interpretations of movement. However, several reviews of motor control theories suggest that dynamic motor control views and alternate information processing views are not necessarily mutually exclusive (Walter, 1998). Furthermore, Walter contended that the relative role, as well as the strengths and weaknesses, of each theoretical account of motor control needs to be determined.

Parallel Distributed Processing Theory

Description

Computer analysis and simulations also provide models and theories for motor control. These are relatively recent efforts undertaken to try to develop models of higher-level processes that are based in an understanding of neural processing and patterns of neural activity provided by imaging studies. These attempts start by asking how the brain might achieve a higher level of processing rather than asking how the brain actually achieves such processing. Modeling starts from a basic understanding of how neurons work and asks how higher-level function could be achieved by connecting basic elements, like neurons, together (Anderson, 1995).

The **parallel distributed processing (PDP)** theory of motor control describes how the nervous system as a network processes information for action. It reflects current knowledge in neuroscience about the serial and parallel processing of the nervous system. Serial processing is processing of information through a single pathway, whereas parallel processing is processing information through many pathways (Kandel, Schwartz, & Jessell 1991). Parallel distributed processing is unique in its emphasis on explaining neural mechanisms associated with motor control. Neural modeling, or computer simulation of nervous system functioning, has correctly predicted aspects of processing in both the perception and the action systems. As neural modeling develops, it may provide further knowledge as to how the nervous system solves particular problems.

Implications

Modeling of function and dysfunction can be integrated into clinical practice. Shumway-Cook and Woollacott (1995) proposed that a PDP model could be used to predict how changes within the nervous system affects function. As an example, the theory predicts that parallel redundant pathways exist so that a loss of a few elements will not necessarily affect function. The loss of additional elements or once a certain threshold is attained, however, may affect the capacity of the system to function. This idea of a threshold of dysfunction is demonstrated in many pathological states, such as in Parkinson disease.

Limitations

PDP is a tool to help researchers think about the way in which the nervous system works. Some of the proposed functions are not replicated in nervous system processing, and modeling cannot fully account for what is known about nervous system processing.

Ecological Theory

Ecological theory, developed by Gibson (1966), explores the interaction between the motor (action) system and goal-directed behavior. Gibson's research focused on how humans detect environmental information and how they use that information to control their movements. Environmental information is seen as relevant to action in the environment. Perception rather than sensation is important to the individual acting on the environment. From this perspective, determining how the individual detects information in the environment, the form of this environmental information, and how this information is used to modify and control movement are important.

In ecological theory, the organization of movement depends on the active exploration of tasks, the environment, and the individual's multiple ways to accomplish a task. Perception guides action, and action guides perception. Therefore, movement disorders not only are the consequences of structural changes but also can be understood as an atypical spatial temporal organization in the perception–action coupling and in movement coordination (Wagenaar & van Emmerik, 1996).

This approach has broadened therapists' understanding of nervous system function from depending on sensory motor control to that of a more global perception action system that actively explores the environment to satisfy its goals. Likewise, disordered motor control is a disruption in the perception action system and not at the level of the CNS.

Implications

A major contribution of this perspective is seeing the individual as active in the environment and the environment as crucial in determining movements. Active exploration of the environment allows the individual to develop multiple ways to accomplish a task.

Limitations

This approach has enlarged the understanding of the interaction between the organism and environment. Research is at the level of the organism–environment interface. Ecological theory has contributed less to the knowledge of the organization and function of the nervous system, which is a primary concern of therapists intervening in motor control problems, based on traditional neurotherapeutic approaches.

Task-Oriented Theories

In task-oriented theories, motor control is understood by identifying what problems the CNS system has to solve to accomplish a motor task. By *task,* Greene (1972) meant the fundamental problems, such as the degrees-of-freedom problem described by Bernstein, that the central nervous system is required to solve to accomplish a motor task. Greene proposed that this approach could provide the basis for a coherent picture of the motor system.

Implications

The task-oriented perspective suggests practicing functional tasks for retraining in therapy. It acknowledges the role of perceptual, cognitive, and action systems to accomplish tasks (Greene, 1972). It requires an understanding of motor strategies used to accomplish a task as well as an understanding of the perceptual basis for action and the cognitive contributions to actions.

Limitations

There is a lack of agreement on the fundamental tasks of the CNS. There is also lack of agreement on the essential elements being controlled within a task. For example, in studying postural control, some scientists believe the essential goal of the postural system is to control head position. Other scientists think that controlling the center of mass position to attain body stability is the essential goal of postural control (Shumway-Cook & Woollacott, 1995).

MOTOR CONTROL APPROACHES PROPOSED FOR THERAPEUTIC INTERACTION

New approaches to intervening with motor performance deficits that affect occupational performances have evolved as models of motor control have evolved. These therapeutic approaches are based more solidly on the more contemporaneous models of how movement is controlled rather than on the models guiding earlier neurotherapeutic approaches still used by practitioners.

Task-Oriented Models

Description

Task-oriented models target both peripheral and central control systems (Gordon, 1987; Horak, 1991; Shumway-Cook & Woollacott, 2001). In line with system models of motor control, the task-oriented model assumes that control of movement is organized around goal-directed functional tasks. Clients are taught to accomplish goals for functional tasks. By practicing a wide variety of movements, the client solves different types of motor problems.

The assumptions listed in Table 30-1 guide treatment. Along with these assumptions and guidelines, Horak (1991)

TABLE 30–1. **ASSUMPTION'S GUIDING TASK-ORIENTED APPROACH**[a]

Assumptions	Treatment Principles
• Movement is controlled by the individual's goals • A wide variety of movement patterns can be accomplished by a task • Facilitation of normal movements is not necessary • The nervous system adapts continually to its environment and musculoskeletal constraints • The nervous system is not a passive recipient of sensory stimuli but actively seeks to control its own perception and actions • Voluntary and automatic control systems are interrelated • Multiple system involvement results in movement • The nervous system is exposed to its own specific environment • The nervous system seeks to accomplish goals with remaining systems after injury	• The goal of therapy is to teach clients to accomplish goals for functional tasks • Therapists do not treat or limit therapy to one normal movement pattern • Therapists try to teach the client's nervous system how to respond to and solve different motor problems by practicing in a wide variety of situations • Therapist seek to manipulate these environmental and musculoskeletal systems to allow for efficient purposeful behavior • Clients must practice motor behaviors and be motivated by the goal of task accomplishment • Clients are encouraged to assist voluntarily in accomplishing a motor behavior with therapist's encouragement • The therapist and the environment provide feedback • Therapists must design interventions in which practice of controlled movements is outside structured sessions • Therapists help clients identify and use compensatory strategies

[a]Data from Horak (1991) and Gordon (1987).

suggested that the therapist use organizing questions around several areas in treating clients with motor performance deficits. These areas are the client's behavioral goals, movement strategies, musculoskeletal constraints, compensatory strategies, and need for adaptations. Examples of questions for these areas follows:

- *Behavioral goals:* Are the therapist's and client's goals the same?
- *Movement strategy:* What are the organizing principles of a normal movement strategy?
- *Musculoskeletal constraints:* How much of the motor deficit in a person with neurologic impairments is caused by a deficit in the musculoskeletal system rather the neural components?
- *Compensatory strategies:* Has the client found the most effective strategy?
- *Adaptation:* How must a movement strategy be adapted to accomplish a task in a new environmental context?

Carr and Shepherd's Approach

Description

The Carr and Shepherd framework for reestablishing motor control depends on a synthesis of the prevalent dynamic systems theory of motor control, an understanding of the plasticity of the CNS, and recognition of maladaptive changes that occur after CNS injury (Carr & Shepherd, 2000, Sabari, 2002). To maximize the client's recovery of function, principles of motor learning guide the therapist's interventions. This approach is more specific to the rehabilitation of clients after stroke than are other motor control approaches.

Carr and Shepherd's approach uses a framework for assessing and improving four categories of motor performance: standing up and sitting down, walking, reaching, and manipulation (Sabari, 2002). In reviewing this approach, Sabari proposed the following guidelines as central for the therapist when designing interventions within this framework:

- Anticipate, prevent, and reduce mechanical constraints that are likely to interfere with performance.
- Understand the kinematics and the kinetics that research has shown to accompany typical performance by individuals with intact musculoskeletal function.
- Understand how research has shown the kinematics and kinetics of performance differ in individuals with CNS dysfunction.
- Understand how postural adjustments are integrated into efficient task performance.
- Structure activities to provide graded challenge to anticipatory and ongoing postural adjustments.
- Structure activities to help patients develop a kinesthetic understanding of fundamental movement strategies.
- Structure activities that help patients develop motor task analysis and problem-solving skills.

In this program, intervention is directed to relearning of control rather than to activities that incorporate exercise or neurotherapeutic techniques (Sabari, 2002). It is directed to enhancing motor performance, and emphasis is on practice of specific tasks, the training of controllable muscle action, and control over the movement components of these tasks. The major assumptions about motor control and recovery underlying this approach are listed in Table 30-2.

Occupational Therapy Task-Oriented Approach

Description

Haugen et al. (2002) proposed a client-centered and task-oriented approach based on a systems model of motor control that is influenced by contemporary developmental and motor learning (skill acquisition) theories. This model takes into account the interaction between the personal characteristics or systems of the client, such as the sensory-motor system or the cognitive system, and the client's performance context. To enable optimal occupational functioning, the interventions used in this approach need to address both the personal and the environmental systems affecting the person's activities and participation in different physical and social environments.

In this approach, recovery from brain damage is defined as the client's discovery of what skills remain to perform tasks

TABLE 30-2. **ASSUMPTIONS ABOUT MOTOR CONTROL GUIDING: CARR AND SHEPHERD'S APPROACH**[a]

- Recovery does not necessarily precede in a proximal-to-distal sequence; therapists and patients need to monitor emerging and changing strength in all segments of the limb
- Shoulder stability and control do not have to occur before therapeutic challenges to hand function are incorporated in the intervention session; incorporating hand function into therapeutic activities may also help organize shoulder function
- Spasticity does not have to be inhibited before making therapeutic challenges to active limb use
- There are no universal linkages of muscle groups that occur with recovery of function after brain injury; rather, research supports the idea that abnormal patterns of motor performance are related to each patient's distribution of muscle weakness, combined with the demands of different tasks

[a]Modified from Sabari, J. S. (2002). Optimizing motor control using the Carr and Shepherd approach. In C. A. Trombly & M. V. Radomski (Eds.). *Occupational therapy for physical dysfunction* (5th ed., pp. 501–519) Philadelphia: Lippincott Williams & Wilkins.

TABLE 30–3. ASSUMPTIONS GUIDING OCCUPATIONAL THERAPY TASK-ORIENTED APPROACH[a]

- Functional tasks help organize motor behavior
- Occupational performance emerges from the interaction of multiple systems that constitute the unique characteristics of the person and the environment
- After CNS damage or other changes in personal or environmental systems, clients' behavioral changes reflect attempts to achieve functional goals
- Practice and active experimentation with varied strategies and in varied contexts are needed to find the optimal solution for a motor problem and to develop skill in performance

[a]Adapted with permission from Bass-Haugen, J., Mathiowetz, V., & Flinn, N. (2002). Optimizing motor behavior using the occupational therapy task-oriented approach. In C. A. Trombly and M. V. Radomski (Eds.). *Occupational therapy for physical dysfunction* (5th ed., pp. 481–499). Philadelphia: Lippincott Williams & Wilkins.

TABLE 30–4. TREATMENT PRINCIPLES OF A TASK-ORIENTED APPROACH

Client-Centered Focus

- Adopt a client-centered focus in treatment
- Elicit active participation of the client in treatment

Occupation-Based Focus

- Use functional tasks as the focus in treatment
- Select tasks that are meaningful and important in the client's role
- Analyze the characteristics of the tasks selected for treatment
- Describe the movements used for task performance
- Determine whether the movement patterns are stable or in transition
- Analyze the movement patterns and functional outcomes of task performance

Person and Environment

- Identify the personal and environmental factors that serve as major influences on occupational performances
- Anticipate that the personal and environmental variables influencing occupational performance will change
- Address critical personal and environmental systems to cause change in occupational performance
- Treat neural and nonneural factors of the sensorimotor system that interfere with occupational performance
- Adapt the task or broader environment to promote occupational performance
- Use natural objects and natural environments

Practice and Feedback

- Structure practice of the task to promote motor learning
- Design the practice session to fit the type of task and learning strategies
- Provide feedback that facilitates motor learning and encourages experimentation with solutions to occupational performance problems
- Optimize occupational performance given the constraints on the person and environment

General Treatment Goals

- Discover the optimal movement patterns for task performance
- Achieve flexibility, efficiency, and effectiveness in task performance
- Develop problem-solving skills in clients so they can identify their own solutions to occupational performance problems in home and community environments

[a]Adapted with permission from Bass-Haugen, J., Mathiowetz, V., & Flinn, N. (2002). Optimizing motor behavior using the occupational therapy task-oriented approach. In C. A. Trombly and M. V. Radomski (Eds.). *Occupational therapy for physical dysfunction* (5th ed., pp. 481–499). Philadelphia: Lippincott Williams & Wilkins.

(Haugen et al., 2002). The role of the therapist in this approach is to take into account all systems as potential variables to explain the behavior of each client at a specific time. For example, the flexor pattern of spasticity seen with clients after a cerebrovascular accident (CVA) can be the result of more than neural components; therefore, more than the sensory motor system needs to be evaluated by the therapist. Each client is seen as unique, with his or her own course of recovery that reflects the specific problems and environmental demands concerning his or her functions in a unique environment. The assumptions and treatment principles given in Tables 30-3 and 30-4 are proposed to guide treatment.

CONCLUSION

Models of motor control and learning can guide occupational therapy interventions for clients with motor performance deficits. More detail on the models presented here can be found in the sources in the reference list. Practitioners need to be aware that as scientific knowledge about movement evolves, new models of practice may emerge. Practitioners have a responsibility to keep up to date on motor control and learning research, so that they can provide clients with the most effective treatment possible for motor deficits.

SECTION IV

Sensorimotor Techniques

CATHY DOLHI
MARY LOU LEIBOLD
JODI SCHREIBER

Rehabilitation pioneers such as Bobath (1990), Kabat (1950), and Rood (1956), who did their original work in the 1940s and 1950s, developed intervention approaches to use for people with sensorimotor impairments. Practitioners continue to find these approaches helpful (Umphred, 1995a), although (as discussed in the previous section) our understanding of why and how well they work is far from complete. When used appropriately with the client who has a neurological impairment, these strategies and techniques seem to aid in supporting the person's motor system for more effective performance, thus improving occupational performance capabilities.

The ways these approaches are used can be characterized along the continuum from adjunctive to occupation based (Pedretti & Early, 2001). **Adjunctive strategies** are actions taken by the therapist to prepare the client for activity. **Enabling activities** are exercises or drills that require client involvement but are not activity based. Purposeful activities are tasks with apparent goals but that may not have particular meaning to the person beyond the therapy setting or that are done out of context of usual performance. **Occupational** activities are a naturally occurring part of a person's life and have inherent meaning to the individual. These categories are used to organize the case studies accompanying this section.

ROOD APPROACH

In the 1940s, Rood (1954) used controlled multisensory input combined with normal developmental positioning and purposeful activity to yield desired motor output. The use of sensory input to stimulate a motor response was a key component of the Rood approach (Gentile & Iyer, 2001). As such, Rood identified a number of **inhibition** and **facilitation** techniques, which are summarized in Table 30-5 (Royeen, Duncan, & McCormack, 2001;

TABLE 30–5. **ROOD'S INHIBITION AND FACILITATION TECHNIQUES**

Inhibition Techniques		*Facilitation Techniques*	
Technique	**Description**	**Technique**	**Description**
General	• Physical handling techniques should include touch that is slow, deep, and continual to promote a calming, relaxing effect • Treatment should occur in quiet setting with minimal distractions • Therapist's use of quiet, soothing voice and calm, slow movements aids in inhibition	General	• Physical handling techniques should include touch that is light and quick • Treatment environment should heighten client's awareness of self and surroundings but not be distracting • Intonation and volume of therapist's voice should be stimulating to client

Continues

TABLE 30–5. **ROOD'S INHIBITION AND FACILITATION TECHNIQUES** *(Continued)*

Inhibition Techniques		*Facilitation Techniques*	
Technique	**Description**	**Technique**	**Description**
Neutral warmth	• Noninvasive, nonthreatening approach of wrapping targeted body part or entire body in blanket, towel, or sheet for 5–10 min • Client feels light pressure and warmth of wrap and often feels relaxed, resulting in decreased tone	Light moving touch	• Stimulation applied by fingertips, cotton ball, or camel-hair brush • Limited to three to five strokes with 30-sec intervals between applications
Gentle rocking or shaking	• Rhythmical, controlled rocking or shaking movement that incorporates joint approximation and distraction • Commonly used at head, shoulder, forearm, pelvis, and lower extremities • Precise hand placement and manipulation skills are necessary	Fast brushing	• Use of battery-operated brush over dermatomal area supplying muscle to be stimulated • Application limited to 3–5 sec with 30-sec intervals between applications
Slow stroking	• Application of firm, direct pressure to both sides of spinous processes (primary posterior rami) from occiput to coccyx for up to 3 min, with client in prone • May be accomplished with index and long digits in V position, stroking down the spine • As one hand reaches coccyx area, alternate hand begins to repeat stroking from occipital area to ensure continuous pressure	Icing	• Three different application techniques to stimulate client's level of alertness, postural responses, and/or parasympathetic responses • Powerful, potentially unpredictable results may occur
Slow rolling	• Slow, passive rolling of client by therapist from side lying toward prone • May include slow manual rotation of pelvis and trunk • Technique should be completed on each side	Heavy joint compression	• Pressure greater than body weight applied through longitudinal axis of bone • Most commonly used through long bones (humerus, femur) • May be accomplished in combination with developmental positions (prone-on-elbows, quadruped, standing)
Deep tendon pressure	• Deep, direct pressure at tendon insertion site of targeted muscle	Quick stretch	• Accomplished by providing a quick stretch movement to limb in opposite direction of desired movement just distal to joint while stabilizing proximally
Joint compression	• Application of pressure less than or equal to body weight to move bones on either side of a joint closer together • Commonly performed at shoulder followed by moving humerus in small circles, resulting in decreased pain and stiffness • May also be accomplished by client in weight-bearing positions in which pressure is less than body weight	Pressure	• Rubbing belly of muscle being facilitated with fingertips of index, long, and ring fingers
Maintained stretch	• Maintenance of affected muscle in elongated position	Stretch pressure	• Manual stretching of belly of muscle being facilitated with fingertips while applying pressure
		Tapping	• Tapping three to five times over belly of muscle being facilitated with fingertips before or during muscle contraction
		Vibration	• Use of small hand-held vibrator parallel to muscle fibers on belly of muscle being facilitated • Contraindicated in young children

CASE STUDY 30-1

Jacob: A Man with a Recent Stroke

Occupational profile: Jacob is a 57-year-old married policeman with three grandchildren; he is concerned about his ability to return to work.

Diagnosis: Subarachnoid hemorrhage, hypotonic distal right upper extremity.

Selected skill deficit: Low tone and limited AROM of involved right upper extremity.

Treatment focus: Increase tone and AROM of involved right upper extremity for use in daily occupations.

Approach used: Rood, neurodevelopmental treatment.

Techniques chosen: Tapping, vibration, manual guiding, proper positioning in seated position.

Treatment environment: Inpatient rehabilitation unit, bright lighting, comfortable but slightly louder and quicker tone of voice, busy but nondistracting environment.

ACTIVITY CONTINUUM

Adjunctive: Tapping and/or vibration of wrist extensors and finger flexors completed one at a time. Jacob sits in midline in a chair with a back, bilateral arm supports, firm seat, and back support. His pelvis is in slight anterior tilt with hips, knees, and ankles at 90°.

Enabling: Jacob reaches and picks up soup cans from the tabletop to promote improved gross grasp. The therapist stands at Jacob's involved side and provides tapping and/or vibration one at a time as Jacob completes the task.

Purposeful: Jacob reaches and picks up soup cans and places them in a grocery bag to promote improved gross grasp and release. The therapist stands at his involved side and provides tapping and/or vibration one at a time as he completes the task.

Occupation-based: Jacob holds onto the phone receiver with his dominant (right) hand and dials the phone with his left hand. He calls his wife at home. The therapist stands at Jacob's involved side and provides tapping and/or vibration one at a time as he completes the task.

Trombly, 2002). Case Study 30-1 shows how a therapist can blend these techniques into an occupational therapy program for someone with a fairly acute problem. Case Study 30-2 demonstrates how a client with long-standing problems might be helped.

PROPRIOCEPTIVE NEUROMUSCULAR FACILITATION

Proprioceptive neuromuscular facilitation (PNF) principles evolved from the study of normal movement patterns, normal motor development, and normalization of muscle tone (Kabat, 1950). The basic techniques build on the use of two diagonal movement patterns referred to as diagonal 1 (D1) and diagonal 2 (D2). The diagonals are seen in both arm and leg motions. Figure 30-4 summarizes the components of each diagonal of the upper extremities and provides examples of the diagonals typical in daily occupational activity.

Each diagonal involves a flexion (✓) and an extension (/) component as well as a rotational element. In the examples provided here, the execution of the patterns is not pure during the performance of routine activities and occupations. Rather, many actions use movement patterns that contain major components of the diagonals (Pope-Davis, 2001).

PNF Elements and Techniques

The PNF approach uses several modes of sensory input, referred to as elements, in conjunction with handling techniques to further enhance motor performance. The elements are used simultaneously with the techniques to increase strength, increase or decrease abnormal muscle tone, increase available ROM, increase postural stability, and increase or maintain balance (Adler et al., 1993; Voss et al., 1985). All of these strategies are applied within the general diagonal patterns. Table 30-6 summarizes the elements used in the PNF approach, and Table 30-7 illustrates their use with the techniques.

Integration into Occupational Therapy Intervention

Therapists must use ingenuity to incorporate PNF patterns effectively into intervention by structuring the environment and objects required for the therapeutic task. For example, a therapist may engage a homemaker experiencing right shoulder weakness in a task such as putting groceries away in an

CASE STUDY 30-2

Faye: A Woman Who Had a Stroke Many Years Ago

Occupational profile: Faye is a 35-year-old single dental receptionist, who lives in an apartment; she has a cat and is actively involved in her church.

Diagnosis: 15 years post CVA.

Selected skill deficit: High tone in left affected side, use of left upper extremity restricted to stabilizing assist.

Treatment focus: To perform tone management techniques independently in the work setting.

Approach used: Rood and neurodevelopmental treatment.

Techniques chosen: Warmth, weight bearing, self-range of motion (SROM), positioning and repositioning, body symmetry in stance and while seated, creating and using environmental workplace adaptations to promote normal movement patterns.

Treatment environment: Reception area in dentist's office.

ACTIVITY CONTINUUM

Adjunctive: Faye takes a warm shower before work.

Enabling: Faye completes SROM after her shower and before going to work. At work, Faye periodically bears weight on her involved upper extremity throughout the day (on forearm placed on desk when seated and on extended upper extremity on desk surface when standing).

Purposeful: Not needed, as goal is to incorporate strategies into receptionist's occupational duties.

Occupation-based: Workplace modifications for Faye include positioning while seated and standing and placement of needed supplies and equipment to promote normal movement patterns.

Habit pattern: Faye creates a habit pattern to incorporate tone management methods while using environmental modifications in her daily work flow. This habit pattern includes (1) answering the phone and writing appointments with her right hand (dominant), (2) weight bearing on her involved left forearm while using it as a stabilizing assist, (3) breaking from activity and completing SROM exercises with her left arm with emphasis on scapular protraction, and (4) alternating between sitting and standing to promote proper and symmetrical posture.

TABLE 30-6. **ELEMENTS USED IN PNF**[a]

Element	Practitioner's Action
Manual contact	The physical placement of the therapist's hands on the muscles requiring facilitation for guiding and facilitation
Maximal resistance	The amount of pressure placed on the client's extremity throughout the pattern; refers to the maximal amount of resistance that can be applied to an active contraction while allowing full ROM to occur or applied to an isometric contraction without breaking the client's hold; typically used for attempting to increase strength, endurance, and stability
Verbal cues	Speed, intonation, and volume of the therapist's voice can directly influence the desired motor outcome and should be monitored by the therapist; should be short and precise to allow the client to develop internal motor planning (e.g., "Up and out" when moving from D2 [/] into D2 [✓])
Visual tracking	Involves the client watching (tracking with head and eyes) each component of the pattern as it is being completed; can encourage trunk rotation and direct attention toward areas of neglect (body and/or environment)
Verbal meditation	Refers to the client repeating the steps of the pattern and tasks aloud to facilitate motor learning
Quick stretch	Applying a quick stretch to the muscle needing facilitation to cause proprioceptors to respond for movement
Timing	Relearning of a movement pattern should be focused on completing the occupation at the standard speed and timing

[a]Data from Adler, Beckers, and Buck (1993); Loomis and Boersma (1982); Pope-Davis (2001); and Voss et al. (1985).

Diagonal	Position of upper extremity	Diagonal illustration	Examples of daily occupations
D1 (✔)	thumb adduction; finger flexion and adduction; wrist flexion and radial deviation; forearm supination; elbow in slight flexion; shoulder flexion, external rotation, and adduction; scapular elevation and abduction	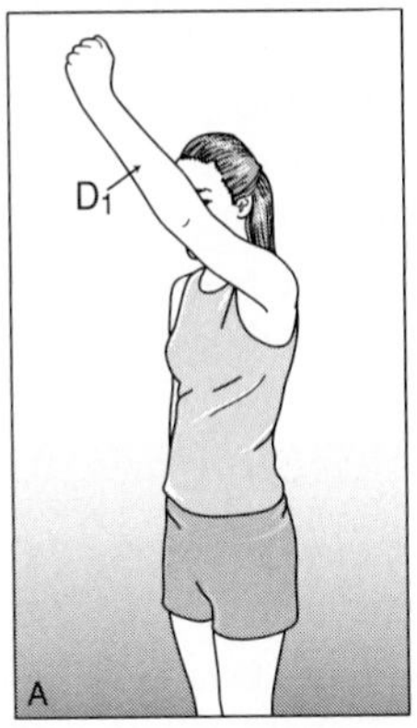 A (D_1)	Combing the left side of the hair, shaving, or applying make-up to the left side of face with the right hand; Removing a pullover shirt; Pushing a desk chair into the desk while standing behind it
D1 (/)	thumb abduction; finger extension and abduction; wrist extension and ulnar deviation; forearm pronation; elbow extension; shoulder internal rotation, abduction, and extension; scapular depression and adduction	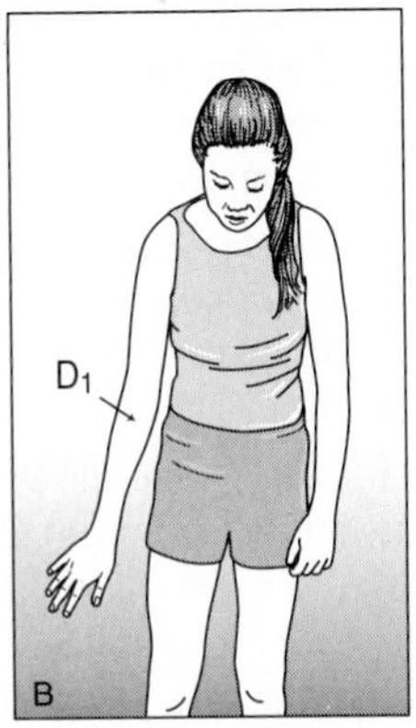 B (D_1)	Reaching down to pick a briefcase up from the floor; Pushing a car door closed while walking away; Pulling a shirt down toward the waist
D2 (✔)	thumb extension; finger extension and abduction; wrist extension and radial deviation; forearm supination; elbow in slight flexion; shoulder external rotation, abduction, and flexion; scapular adduction and elevation	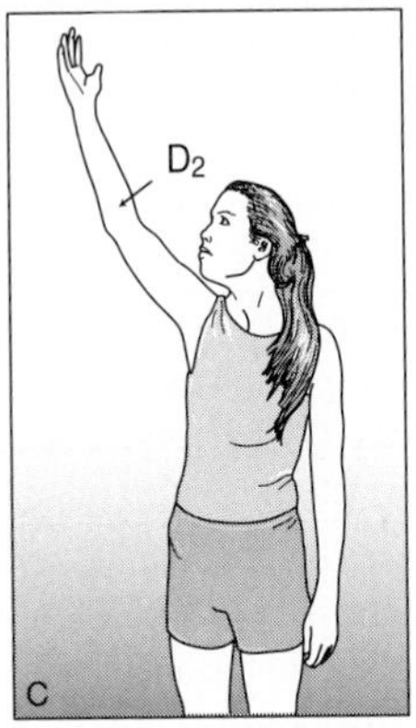 C (D_2)	Brushing the right side of the hair with the right hand; Carrying a serving tray on the right shoulder
D2 (/)	thumb opposition; finger flexion and adduction; wrist flexion and ulnar deviation; forearm pronation; elbow flexion; shoulder extension, adduction, and internal rotation; scapular depression an abduction	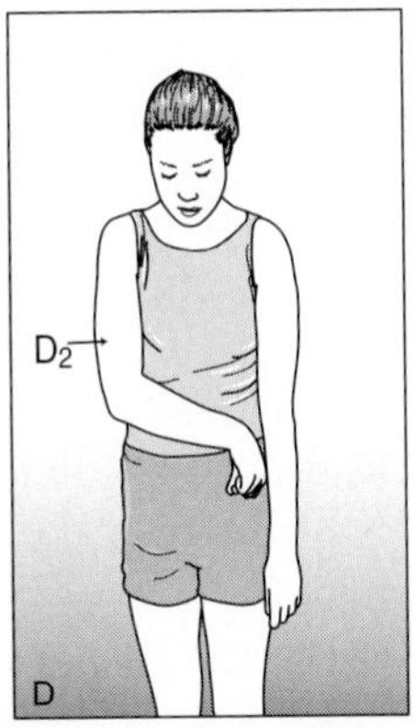 D (D_2)	Beginning to thread a belt into the left side belt loops with the right hand; Sweeping with a broom from left to right; Fastening pant closures

FIGURE 30–4. PNF Diagonals and examples. (Data from Pope-Davis, 2001, and Voss et al., 1985.)

TABLE 30–7. **EXAMPLES OF PNF TECHNIQUES**[a]

Technique	Description	Purpose
Slow reversal	• Isotonic contraction of the antagonist followed by the agonist using MC throughout the entire D1 or D2 pattern • Uses isotonic muscle contractions	To teach pattern and gain mobility
Slow reversal hold	• Contraction of the antagonist followed by the agonist using MC and MR throughout the entire D1 or D2 pattern with an added isometric hold at the end range of flexion followed by a QS; then MR throughout the extension diagonal followed by a QS before returning to the flexion component • Facilitates isotonic → isometric → QS → isotonic → isometric → QS → isotonic muscle contractions	To increase mobility, stability, endurance, and strength
Timing for emphasis	• Contraction of the antagonist followed by the agonist using MC and MR throughout the entire D1 or D2 pattern with an added isometric hold at the point when one muscle or muscle group weakens followed by a QS of the weak muscle only; then continue to complete the pattern with MR • Facilitates isotonic → isometric of part of the pattern → QS to part of the pattern → isotonic to complete the pattern	To increase mobility, stability, and strength when one part of pattern is weak
Rhythmic rotation	• Client is moved passively through the pattern with MC on the neutral borders of the hand and elbow; when resistance is evident, the limb is rotated slowly and rhythmically; once relaxed, PROM is continued through new, available range	To decrease high tone or spasticity; not used for increasing strength or AROM
Rhythmic initiation	• Technique begins with passive movement through either the D1 or D2 diagonal; can move through increments of the pattern • Can proceed from PROM → AAROM → AROM → slight resistance • VC set rhythm of movement	To teach pattern and inhibit increased muscle tone; avoid use of QS
Repeated contractions	• Contraction of the agonist followed by the antagonist using MC and MR throughout the entire D1 or D2 pattern with an added isometric hold at the point that the entire pattern becomes weak; isometric hold is followed by QS of the entire pattern proceeded by completing the movement pattern • Facilitates isotonic → isometric of entire pattern → QS to entire pattern → isotonic to complete pattern	To increase mobility, stability, and strength when the entire motor pattern is weakened
Chop[b]	• Client actively performs the D1 (/) with the right UE; at the same time, the client's left hand grasps right wrist and follows the right UE; as the right UE performs the D1 (/) pattern, the left UE is simultaneously performing the D2 (/) pattern	To strengthen abdominal muscles
Lift[b]	• Similar to the chop, the client actively moves the right UE into D2 (✓) while grasping the right wrist with the left UE; this leads to the left UE performing a D1 (✓) movement simultaneously with the right UE D2 (✓).	To increase truck extension and rotation

[a]Data from Pope-Davis (2001) and Voss et al. (1985).

[b]Chop and lift techniques may begin with right or left UE; right and left are noted for illustration only. Both the chop and the lift may be used or only one technique may be indicated, depending on the needs of the client.

MC, manual contacts; *MR,* maximal resistance; *QS,* quick stretch; *UE,* upper extremity; *VC,* verbal cues.

overhead kitchen cabinet while standing. The chosen PNF diagonal for this activity could be either D1 or D2, depending on the height of the cabinet and the person's available AROM. In this example, the D2 (✓) pattern is used. To facilitate shoulder ROM and strength, the occupational therapist may have the client perform the slow reversal hold technique using maximal resistance before asking the client to participate in the purposeful activity. To enhance the therapeutic effectiveness of this task, the groceries are placed on the counter to the client's left and the client moves them to the cabinet on the right. In addition, the D1 (/) pattern could be used by the therapist to facilitate eccentric muscle control of the shoulder by having the client transfer items from the overhead cabinets on the left side to the right side of the counter. Case Study 30-3 and What's a Practitioner to Do? 30-1 illustrate other clinical applications.

CASE STUDY 30-3

Patricia: A Homemaker with Parkinson's Disease

- *Occupational profile:* Patricia is a 64-year-old widow, primary homemaker, who needs to be independent to return home alone.
- *Diagnosis:* Parkinson's Disease.
- *Selected skill deficit:* Decreased trunk rotation, rigidity.
- *Treatment focus:* Increase trunk rotation and decrease rigidity for improved mobility during daily routine.
- *Approach used:* PNF D2 diagonal.
- *Techniques chosen:* Rhythmic initiation, rhythmic rotation, and slow reversal with visual tracking.
- *Treatment environment:* Son's home, soft music, quiet and distraction free, soft lighting.

ACTIVITY CONTINUUM

- *Adjunctive:* The therapist stands on Patricia's right side and teaches slow reversal D2.
- *Enabling:* Patricia uses a D2 diagonal to exercise.
- *Purposeful:* Patricia reaches toward targets throughout the range.
- *Occupation-based:* Patricia hangs laundry using the D2 movement pattern.

WHAT'S A PRACTITIONER TO DO? 30-1

Mike: A Man with Left Hemiplegia

Mike is 65 years old and has no significant past medical history but has sustained a right CVA with resultant left hemiparesis. At 5 days after his stroke, he is referred to occupational therapy for "evaluation and treatment as indicated."

SESSION 1

The occupational therapy initial evaluation is completed at the client's bedside in the acute care hospital with his wife present. Findings include the following:

Occupational Profile

Mike lives at home with his wife who is in good health. Before his CVA, he was independent with all his daily activities and was an avid golfer, reader, woodworker, and cook. He also maintained his own lawn as well as the lawns of some of his neighbors. Mike's wife is supportive and anxious to help. He plans to return home.

Occupational Performance Observations

Mike is alert but oriented to name only. He has moderate left-sided neglect. Tone throughout the left side of the body is low. Mike is beginning to display a flexor synergy pattern in his left arm; however, the extremity is nonfunctional during daily occupations. Mike requires moderate assistance from the therapist to maintain static sitting balance on the edge of the bed, because he leans to the left and in a forward direction. He displays an uncoordinated swallow of pureed foods with honey-thick liquids and requires 50% assistance with eating and feeding. Mike requires maximum assistance for the remainder of his basic ADL.

Intervention

At this time, the focus of treatment is on performance skills and their influence on Mike's ability to engage in ADL. In this acute care setting, occupational therapy is allocated for six treatment sessions at 45–60 min per session. Treatment during this session includes the following:

- Orientation.
- Proper positioning in bed and wheelchair.
- Training in SROM.
- Tone facilitation.
- Activities to increase sitting balance on the edge of bed.
- A simple ADL such as combing his hair or shaving with an electric razor while seated on the edge of the bed.

Adjunctive interventions are used at the beginning of the treatment session with Mike seated on the edge of the bed and the therapist on his left side. His legs are positioned with hips, knees, and ankles at 90°. The therapist instructs Mike and has him perform both a chop and lift PNF technique to increase trunk stability and strength for improving sitting balance during the

Continued

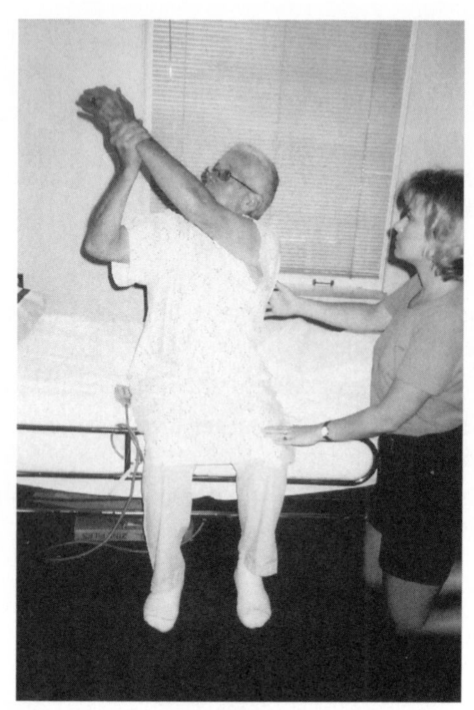

FIGURE 30–A. Mike does the PNF lift.

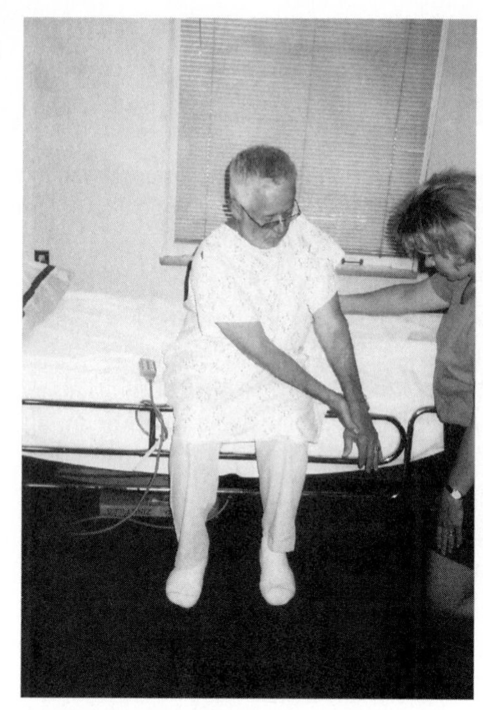

FIGURE 30–B. Mike does the PNF chop.

treatment session. Mike is also instructed to include the visual tracking element to the lift and chop techniques to promote awareness of his involved side (Figs. 30-A and 30-B).

Next, the therapist incorporates the enabling strategy of guiding the affected upper extremity during the occupation of shaving. Mike holds the electric razor with his left, dominant hand, which was affected by the stroke. The therapist's hand is placed over top of Mike's hand to aid with grasp (Fig. 30-C). The occupational therapist manually facilitates proper trunk alignment and upright posture while guiding Mike's left arm through the normal movement patterns used in shaving. In addition, the therapist may tap intermittently on the biceps to promote elbow flexion during shaving (Fig. 30-D).

SESSIONS 2 AND 3

Intervention is again completed at the bedside. The nursing staff has completed most of Mike's morning self-care for him, and he is resting in bed when the therapist arrives for the midmorning session. The therapist starts each session by engaging Mike in casual conversation to build rapport and check his level of orientation. For example, the therapist talks with Mike about things such as the weather, today's date, television, visitors, and events of the previous evening. To support his orientation, the therapist hangs a calendar in Mike's room, within his field of vision and instructs team members and visitors to use it with Mike.

The therapist next works with Mike on his ability to move around in and get out of bed. This involves rolling side to side and moving supine to sit. These purposeful activities promote his awareness of his left side, body symmetry, and proper positioning and end with Mike sitting on the edge of the bed. At this stage, sitting unsupported can be a challenge. Mike works on improving his sitting balance on the edge of the bed by properly positioning his body with hips and knees all positioned at 90°. The therapist encourages Mike to sit erect with his

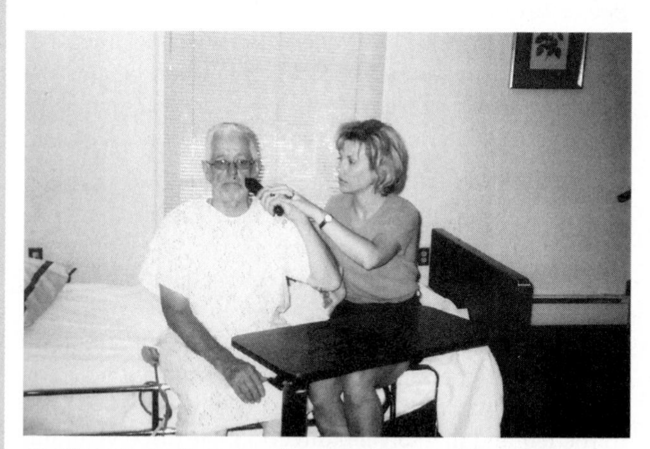

FIGURE 30–C. Hand-over-hand assistance with shaving.

Continues

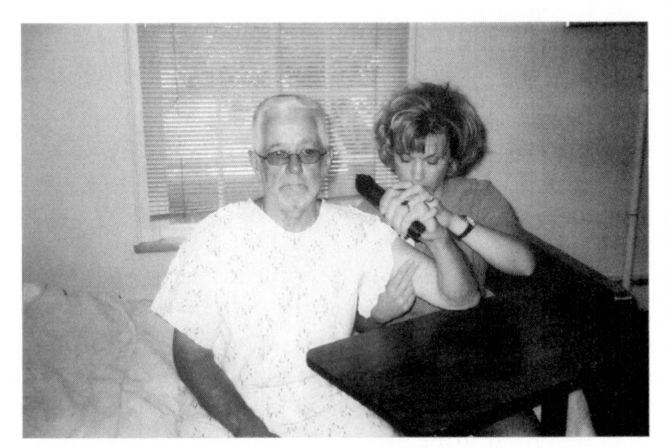

FIGURE 30–D. The therapist taps on Mike's biceps to facilitate muscle contraction.

trunk at midline and helps Mike rest his arms on an over-the-bed table to promote symmetry.

If Mike had trouble maintaining this posture, it might be necessary to incorporate enabling strategies to facilitate erect posture. These strategies include manually supporting Mike into an anterior pelvic tilt and/or using the PNF chop and lift to improve trunk extension. In a consistent client-centered approach, all of these efforts are designed to help Mike succeed in an activity that he either wants or needs to do.

It is important that the intervention culminate in Mike actually doing the desired activity. In this case, Mike looks through the TV program guide (Fig. 30-E). Other activities of interest are reviewing and completing menus for upcoming meals, opening mail, and using the telephone. All of these are activities that Mike has an interest in doing and that can facilitate orientation, provide some minimal challenge to his sitting balance, and improve sitting tolerance.

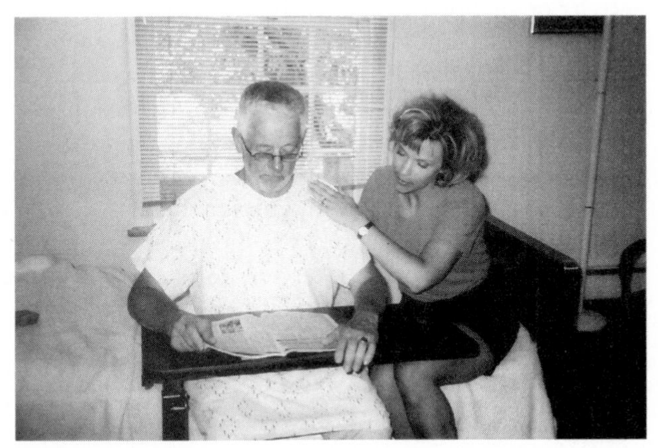

FIGURE 30–E. The therapist cues Mike to maintain good symmetry while sitting.

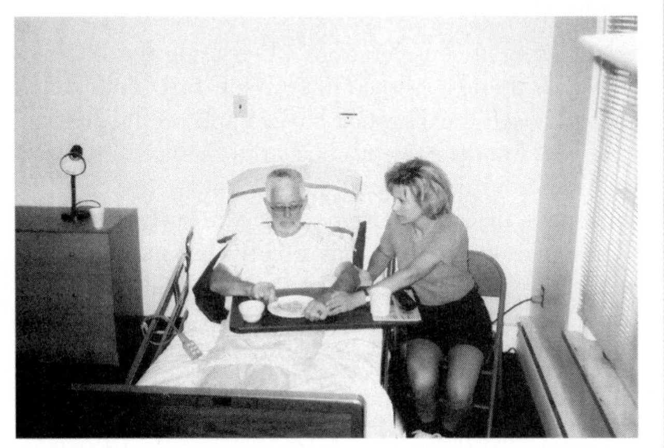

FIGURE 30–F. Mike bears weight on his left (involved) arm, using it to stabilize the plate while eating lunch.

SESSION 4

The occupational therapy session is scheduled to begin 30 min before the arrival of Mike's lunch tray in his room. The therapist initiates the treatment session by orienting him through conversation and by using the calendar. Mike is in bed, and the practitioner coaches and assists him to move his body up to the head of the bed, which is then raised in anticipation of the meal. Mike can long sit in bed with the back of bed elevated so as not to challenge balance and excessively fatigue him during eating (Fig. 30-F). The therapist asks Mike to demonstrate his SROM program; when it is completed, the therapist encourages him to position his left arm on the over-the-bed table for weight bearing while he is eating. Mike eats lunch with the tray on the over-the-bed table while long sitting in bed.

SESSIONS 5 AND 6

OT is again scheduled 30 min before the arrival of Mike's lunch tray in his room. The interventions include a series of activities beginning with bed mobility, balance activities while seated at the edge of the bed, and transferring from the bed to a chair with arms. After he is properly positioned, Mike performs his upper extremity SROM routine. The sessions end with Mike eating his lunch from a seated position while the practitioner incorporates appropriate sensorimotor techniques to facilitate proper posture and enhance upper extremity function.

QUESTIONS AND EXERCISES

1. What are some ways the practitioner can communicate with nursing and other team members about recommended positioning for Mike?
2. What are some factors in the environment that might affect Mike's attention and muscle tone?
3. What might you change to help Mike's performance?

Considerations for Application

There are special considerations when using the PNF approach. The therapist should not inhibit the client's ability to move through the diagonal. For example, as the diagonal moves away from the client's body, the therapist must also move away from the body to allow room for the client to complete the diagonal pattern. This can easily be accomplished if the therapist stands slightly behind the upper extremity involved in the diagonal (Voss et al., 1985). In addition, correct hand placement by the therapist is crucial for enhancing the client's ability to perform the desired movement. Improper sliding or positioning of the therapist's hands may cause co-contraction of both agonist and antagonist muscles, leading to isometric versus isotonic muscle contraction (Adler et al., 1993).

The inflection, speed, and volume of the therapist's voice may also affect the client's performance (Adler et al., 1993). As noted in the Rood approach, the environment and the therapist's therapeutic use of self can either facilitate or inhibit the body's reaction. For example, shouting may increase muscle tone, whereas speaking softly and slowly may promote muscle relaxation. Also, the therapist must try to promote client learning through the therapeutic procedures. To enhance the learning effect, it may be beneficial to keep verbalizations to a minimum, as lengthy instructions and commands may interfere with the client's ability to develop a movement scheme.

Finally, and perhaps most important, the client needs to do the work, because the PNF approach emphasizes the use of active muscle contractions to affect the client's body (Adler et al., 1993). It is a common mistake for therapists using PNF to move the client passively through the diagonal. Muscles cannot increase in strength and control if they are not actively contracting. Thus the client must actively move through the diagonal pattern. The therapist may, in addition, employ the strategies discussed earlier to improve AROM and/or strength.

NEURODEVELOPMENTAL TREATMENT

Neurodevelopmental treatment (NDT) is based on the therapist's working knowledge of **postural symmetry,** normal movement, and **tone management.** The therapist evaluates the neuromuscular factors contributing to abnormal posture and movements that are considered likely to impede occupational performance. Intervention is then directed toward the management or remediation of the identified impairments. The theoretical constructs of NDT are reviewed in Chapter 20; additional resources are Bobath (1990), Davis (2001), and Levit (2002).

NDT emphasizes the facilitation of normal movement by focusing on the quality of movement at all times. The quality of movement throughout the process of completing a task is considered crucial to developing normal movement patterns. The therapist provides a variety of opportunities for the client to move through normal movement patterns. This might include hands-on, guided practice in which the therapist literally moves the person's body or extremity through the normal movement pattern. In all cases, the therapist engages the client in individually designed activities that promote normal movement.

To illustrate, consider an occupational therapist and a woman standing in front of the side-by-side washer and dryer in the woman's laundry room. The occupational therapist assists in the maintenance of symmetrical stance and facilitates bilateral lower extremity weight bearing and weight shifting while the woman reaches into the washer to retrieve the wet laundry. In addition, the woman is instructed to place her affected arm on top of the washer so that weight bearing to the upper extremity may occur during the activity. As each item is retrieved from the washer, the client places it on top of the dryer. This task requires trunk rotation and weight shifting, which the therapist facilitates while the woman accomplishes the task. As this example illustrates, there is a careful choreographing of movements as the therapist provides needed cues and support.

Similar to Rood and PNF techniques, NDT principles can be used as adjunctive methods or in conjunction with enabling or purposeful activities. The research on motor learning suggests that NDT principles are most effective when integrated into client-centered, meaningful occupations. The NDT approach can be used with clients in various stages of recovery. The incorporation of a variety of NDT techniques within the activity continuum and across the continuum of care is illustrated in Case Studies 30-1 and 30-2.

Clients who are more capable can take a more active role in managing their tone and movement patterns. Those who are more severely impaired may rely more heavily on the therapist's providing treatment or setting up a therapeutic activity or guiding them through an activity to accomplish its therapeutic purpose. It is proposed that continual normal posture and frequent repetition of normal movement patterns, as initially facilitated and guided by the therapist, will enhance the client's potential to develop optimal movement patterns and neuromuscular performance (Davis, 2001). Using this approach requires the therapist to be continually cognizant of how and why the client is moving in a particular manner and to intervene to break up abnormal movement patterns and facilitate normal movement as needed.

Tone Management

Because normal movement cannot be superimposed on abnormal muscle tone, 24-hr tone management becomes a priority. This includes management of tone at rest and during activity. Weight bearing is one of the most effective

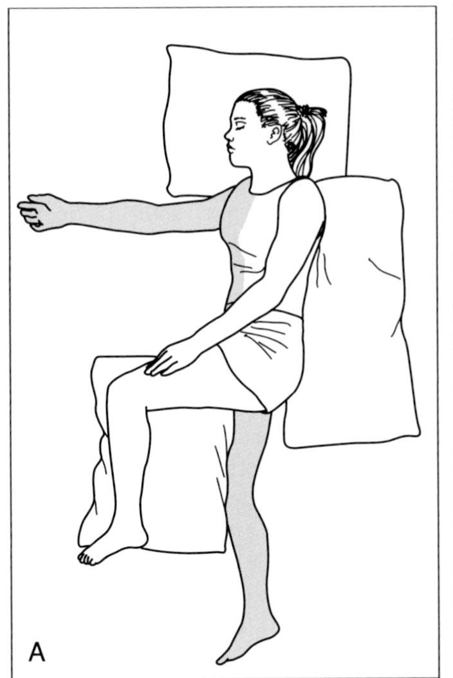

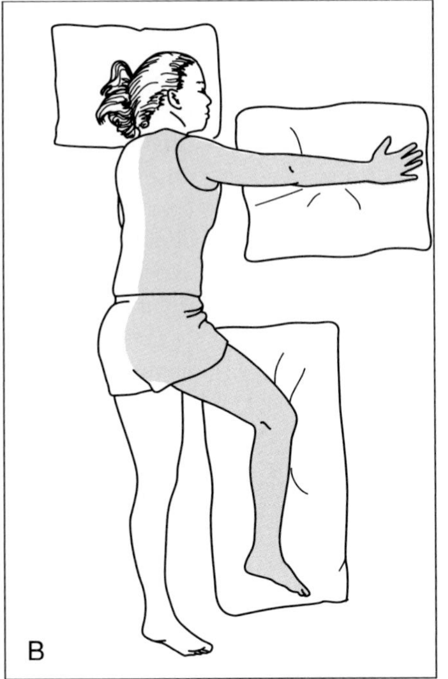

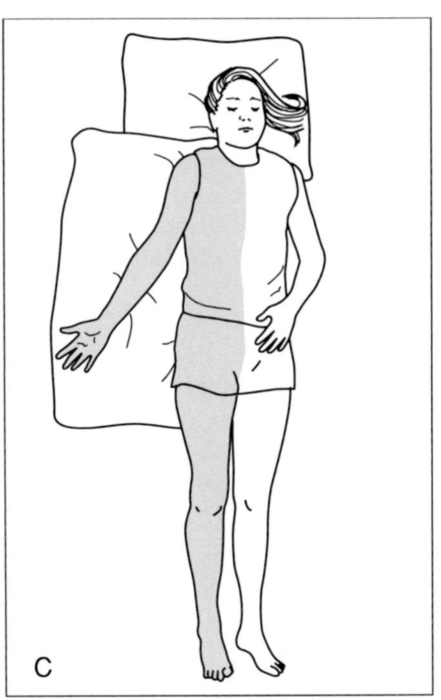

FIGURE 30–5. NDT approaches to positioning in bed. **A,** Lying on the involved side. **B,** Lying on the uninvolved side. **C,** Lying supine. (Adapted from Healthsouth Harmarville Rehabilitation Hospital, Pittsburgh, PA.)

strategies for managing tone (Davis, 2001). It can be used as a facilitation technique for the client with low tone as well as an inhibition technique for the client with high tone. Because many clients with neurological impairments may spend a considerable amount of time either in bed or in a seated position, these areas are addressed in detail.

Bed Positioning

When a client is lying in bed, there are three primary options for positioning (Fig. 30-5). These include lying on the involved side, lying on the uninvolved side, and lying supine. In all positions, the head is supported in midline with pillows. Proximal musculature is positioned first, since these efforts influence the tone in the distal musculature.

When a client is lying on the involved side, the scapula should be protracted, the shoulder flexed to approximately 90° and externally rotated, and the elbow fully extended when possible. The involved lower extremity is positioned with the hip in neutral and the knee slightly flexed. The uninvolved lower extremity is positioned in flexion at the hip and knee and supported with a pillow between the legs. This position facilitates weight bearing over the key points of control in the upper and lower extremities on the involved side. To maintain this position, a pillow is placed behind the back. The uninvolved upper extremity is positioned alongside the trunk and anteriorly at the hip (Fig. 30-5A).

When a client is lying on the uninvolved side, the body is positioned toward prone to achieve optimal positioning. The entire involved arm is supported on a pillow with the scapula protracted; shoulder flexed to approximately 90°; and elbow, wrist, and fingers extended. The entire involved leg is supported on a pillow with the hip and knee flexed to approximately 45°. The uninvolved arm is positioned underneath the pillow supporting the involved arm. The uninvolved leg is positioned with hip and knee in slight flexion (Fig. 30-5B).

When lying in supine, a pillow is positioned under the client's involved scapula and hip to prevent retraction in these areas. The shoulder of the involved arm is slightly abducted and externally rotated with the elbow, wrist, and fingers extended on a pillow. The involved leg is positioned with the both the hip and knee extended in midline. An additional pillow might be positioned alongside the client's leg to keep the hip from externally rotating. Placing a pillow directly behind the knee is avoided, as this may contribute to a knee flexion contracture or a deep vein thrombosis (Fig. 30-5C).

Typically, a client's position is changed every 2 hr initially to promote skin integrity. Restless clients may also need frequent repositioning. Variations in positioning can be used to enhance the client's comfort or to accommodate special needs of the individual. The most desirable bed position for many clients is on the involved side as it promotes proper positioning away from spastic patterns as well as promotes tone management through weight bearing on the involved side. In addition, it can minimize a stretch weakness of the musculature that may result from prolonged abnormal positioning. Finally, this position can enhance sensory awareness of the involved hemibody by adding continual proprioceptive input through weight bearing.

Sitting

The goal in sitting is to achieve a symmetrical upright midline posture. This promotes readiness for the client to move in a normal manner as well as increases the client's level of alertness. It also facilitates appropriate position in space and the manner in which the client views and interacts with the environment. The type of chair and amount of support provided are critical. A firm seating surface with back support and bilateral arm supports promotes optimal trunk positioning and provides a safe position for clients with decreased balance. Firm seat boards or cushions are recommended to prevent the hips from internally rotating in wheelchair seats that tend to sling. Clients typically sit directly on some type of cushion to prevent skin breakdown if seated in a wheelchair for long periods of time. A lumbar support may be used to promote anterior tilt of the pelvis to enhance proper alignment of the spine and promote an individual's readiness to move.

The legs should be positioned with hips, knees, and ankles at 90° of flexion, while the client is sitting on the wheelchair cushion. Footstools; adjustable leg rests; and adaptive devices such as wedge cushions, straps, and pommel cushions may be used to achieve and maintain this position. For the person with low arm tone, equipment options include a wider wheelchair armrest, lapboard, bedside table, or other padded surface that promotes symmetrical posture and support at the shoulder. The client with increased tone in the arm may not use an arm support and can rest the arm in the lap to allow gravity to assist with elongation of the musculature. However, the arm may be positioned on a solid surface, such as a table, to facilitate weight bearing through the arm as a tone reduction method. Consistent proper positioning by all members of the care team is promoted for 24-hr follow-up. The occupational therapist often plays a significant role in the education of other staff, clients, and family about positioning.

Proper positioning is considered critical for effectively addressing the client's identified goal areas. Once this is done, principles of NDT can be incorporated throughout the occupational therapy intervention in several ways. The therapist may set up the desired activity in a way that minimizes tone, promotes symmetry, and/or promotes normal movement. The therapist also may physically guide the client through movement patterns so that the client may experience normal movement, which he or she is unable to do unaided. The therapist continually observes the quality of the client's movement and intervenes as abnormal movement patterns occur by redirecting and guiding the client. Finally, the therapist may engage the client in tone management techniques such as weight bearing before, during, and after an activity so that optimal performance and reinforcement of techniques are realized.

What's a Practitioner to Do? 30-1 describes the clinical reasoning of one therapist as she uses NDT principles along with Rood and PNF during occupational therapy interventions with a man in an acute care setting. As you read that case study, see if you can identify what sensorimotor techniques or principles the therapist is using.

CONCLUSION

Rood, PNF, and NDT are all approaches used by occupational therapy practitioners to improve an individual's motor skills during occupational performance. The primary focus of these approaches is at the body functions level, with goals directed toward improving strength, ROM, quality of movement, and tone management. The literature does not reveal strong evidence in the efficacy of these approaches (Dobkin, 1996; Levit, 2002), yet personal experience and anecdotal reports by occupational therapy practitioners indicate that they can be useful.

In practice, occupational therapists must first understand the basic tenets of each theorist. They can then apply theories singularly or in combination to determine the usefulness with individual clients. Further research is needed for stronger population-based evidence of the effectiveness of each approach. To develop mastery in using these approaches, practitioners require continuing education along with supervised practice. Although these approaches are primarily used within the field by occupational therapists, experienced occupational therapy assistants can follow through with methods deemed most effective for a particular client.

SECTION V

Cognitive–Perceptual Retraining and Rehabilitation

JOAN PASCALE TOGLIA

OVERVIEW OF INTERVENTION APPROACHES

Cognitive–perceptual difficulties can significantly affect a person's abilities to perform everyday tasks, fulfill former roles, and maintain personal and social relationships. The aim of occupational therapy intervention for people with cognitive–perceptual dysfunction is to decrease activity limitations and enhance participation in everyday activities.

Although the ultimate goal of intervention with this population is clear, there are different perspectives concerning the means by which this can best be accomplished. For example, occupational therapy intervention can emphasize the underlying impairments as a prerequisite for occupational performance or can focus directly on occupation-based activity. The former approach seeks to restore or remediate the impaired cognitive–perceptual skills, whereas the latter approach focuses directly on areas of occupation. Within each of these approaches, there are significant differences in the areas targeted for intervention as well as in underlying assumptions concerning individuals' abilities to learn and generalize information. The characteristics of different intervention approaches as well as the underlying assumptions are explored in this section. Factors that are critical in influencing selection of intervention approaches are discussed and methods for systematically integrating intervention approaches are illustrated. Finally, the application of different intervention methods to specific areas of cognitive perceptual dysfunction is described.

CAPITALIZING ON THE ASSETS: THE FUNCTIONAL APPROACH

The functional approach capitalizes on the person's assets to improve occupational performance. The emphasis is on reducing activity limitations and participation restrictions rather than on restoring impaired skills. The functional approach can be subdivided into three different intervention techniques: adaptation of the activity or context, functional task training, and compensation.

Adaptation of the Task or Environment

Adaptation involves changing, altering, or structuring the activity demands or context to prevent disruptive behaviors or accidents; minimize cognitive or perceptual demands of a task, minimize caregiver burden, and maintain the clients level of functioning (Radomski, Dougherty, Fine, & Baum, 1993). Adaptations may be fixed, such as installing an alarm on a door to prevent wandering, or they may require ongoing implementation and monitoring, such as preselecting clothes from the closet on a daily basis. In the latter case, implementation depends on the ability, consistency, and reliability of another person.

A significant other may be trained to alter or structure the activity demands or context to maintain the person's performance capabilities. For instance, the person may not be able to attend to the task of preparing a meal, but may be able to perform individual components such as mixing the salad and folding napkins in half for the table setting. Engagement in meaningful activity components can maintain the client's performance capabilities and prevent disruptive behaviors (Radomski et al., 1993). Allen (1993) discussed a cognitive disability approach that provides guidelines for matching and adapting the individual's cognitive level with activity demands.

Adaptations seek to change the activity or context, rather than the person (Toglia, 1993). Therefore, the focus is on providing support, education, and training to the caregiver, family, or employer instead of direct treatment to the client. Adaptations should directly address the problems and needs identified by the client or significant others and should be designed in collaboration with them (Campbell, Duffy, & Salloway, 1994).

Adaptations can produce rapid changes in function. However, the effects of adaptation are limited to the activity or environment adapted, and success often depends on the extent to which others are able consistently to follow through with the adaptations.

Functional Task Training

Giles (1998) described a neurofunctional approach that emphasizes the use of task specific training within natural contexts. Task-specific training involves rote repetition of a specific task with gradually fading cues. Emphasis is on the mastery of a specific task rather than on the underlying skills needed to perform the task. Behavioral techniques, including positive reinforcement, contingent reinforcement, and backward chaining, are often incorporated into structured and repetitive training of an action sequence. Intervention involves breaking down a functional task into small subcomponents and systematically recording the number of prompts or assistance required for each subcomponent (Giles, 1998; Glisky, Schacter, & Butters, 1994). Gradually, the number of cues provided by the practitioner is reduced. Rote repetition of the activity capitalizes on procedural learning or memory for the actual performance of tasks, not the memory of a specific set of facts (Glisky, 1995).

A slightly different approach to teaching task-specific skills involves errorless learning. In addition to receiving a sequence of fading cues, the person is prevented from making mistakes during the learning process (Wilson & Evans, 1996). There is evidence that suggests that the task and context determine whether errorless learning is more effective than trial-and-error learning (Evans et al., 2000).

Functional task training requires learning from the individual; however, the learning expected is primitive or associative. In **association learning,** individuals' behaviors are a direct response to environmental stimuli; thus learners are unable to deal with more then minor changes in the task stimuli or environment. Learning is characterized by hyperspecificity (Neistadt, 1994a). Glisky et al. (1994) found evidence that considerable overlearning of a specific task may increase the ability of severely amnesic individuals to transfer and perform the task with greater variations.

Functional task training has been demonstrated through case studies to produce significant changes in ADL and work tasks in clients with severe impairments (Giles, 1998; Giles & Clark-Wilson, 1988; Giles, Rideley, Dill, & Frye, 1997; Giles & Shore, 1989; Glisky et al., 1994, Wehman, 1991). However, intervention addresses only one task or routine at a time. Extensive training, time, and effort may be required to achieve success within one task sequence and environment. Proponents of this method have argued that treatment of people with cognitive impairment should take place in the natural context in which they will function, because these people are unable to **generalize** learning (Giles, 1998; Glisky et al., 1994; Mayer, Keating, & Rapp, 1986). However, if the person is unable to cope with minor unforeseen events or slight changes in routine, even performance within the same context will be compromised. The ability to cope with minor changes, minor disruptions in routines, and unforeseen circumstances is a part of daily life, even within the same context.

Compensation

Compensation teaches the person to bypass or minimize the effects of the impairment by modifying the method used to perform an activity. The client is expected to initiate and implement use of an external aid or strategy to enhance occupational performance in a variety of different situations (American Occupational Therapy Association [AOTA], 1999). This requires some awareness and acceptance as well as the ability to generalize use of a learned strategy (Toglia, 1993a). An example is use of a memory notebook to compensate for memory loss. Independent use requires that the client recognize that he or she is having difficulty with his or her memory and perceives the need to write things down as a help in remembering. In addition, it requires initiation of use of the book in a variety of different situations.

Summary of the Functional Approaches

The different techniques within the functional approach inherently contain different requirements and assumptions concerning learning. For example, adaptation seeks to change the activity demands or context rather than the person. Functional task training requires a primitive level of learning, which is hyperspecific to the task and environment, whereas compensation often requires the person to apply a learned strategy to a variety of situations. The three techniques can be viewed on a continuum from those that do not expect the client to change or learn to those that do require learning and generalization. The assumptions and requirements of different treatment techniques need to be matched with the abilities of the client (AOTA, 1999).

ADDRESSING THE IMPAIRMENT

In contrast to the functional approach, which minimizes use of the impaired skill, remedial approaches place an emphasis on restoring the underlying cognitive and perceptual skills. Demands are placed directly on the impaired skill (Raskin & Mateer, 2000). Learning and generalization are expected to occur. Remedial approaches seek to change the person's skills rather than manipulate the activity demands or context (Neistadt, 1990; Zoltan, 1996). The conceptualization of cognition and perception determines what is addressed in treatment.

Three different remedial approaches have been described: the Affolter approach, cognitive remediation, and the multicontext approach. Each of these approaches reflects different conceptualizations of the underlying cognitive perceptual impairment.

Sensory Motor Deficits: The Affolter Approach

Sensory motor approaches view cognitive–perceptual symptoms as reflections of inadequate assimilation and integration of vestibular, tactile, proprioceptive, and kinesthetic information. They are based on the assumption that the development of sensory motor skills provides a foundation for the development of complex cognitive and perceptual skills.

The Affolter method views cognitive–perceptual problems as a reflection of inadequate tactile–kinesthetic input and environmental interaction. The tactile–kinesthetic perceptual system is considered to be essential for "adaptation and the development of more complex performances" (Davies, 1985, p. 2). It is assumed that clients who fail in complex behaviors receive inadequate tactile–kinesthetic input. Therefore, intervention consists of guiding or tactile–kinesthetic stimulation to facilitate interaction between the environment and the person. Therapy focuses on the input of tactile–kinesthetic information rather than on production or performance.

Specific cognitive perceptual skills are not addressed. Instead, there is an emphasis on improving information processing by guiding the person through problem-solving interactions with tasks and the environment. During guiding, the practitioner places his or her hand over the dorsal aspect of the client's hands and guides movement as the client performs a purposeful activity (Davis, 1992; Rubio, 1998). Effective guiding emphasizes constant contact with surfaces to maximize tactile and kinesthetic input and interaction with the environment, rather than moving in free space. Examples of activities that may be used are peeling a banana, cutting an apple, dialing a telephone, and setting a table.

Guiding enables the client to experience successful performance. The practitioner does not let the client fail. There is an assumption that learning takes place through repeated successful experiences. During guiding there is no verbal instruction or feedback. Signs of effectiveness of guiding include increased attention span, increased eye contact, changes in facial expressions, and improved initiation and problem solving (Davies, 1985; Davis, 1992).

The Affolter approach differs from traditional remedial approaches in that it uses purposeful or occupation-based activities. It is considered remedial because treatment aims to improve underlying sensory motor abilities to enhance the ability of the person to take in and process information.

The Affolter approach provides an alternative to treatment, particularly for clients with aphasia or apraxia. Although the Affolter approach emphasizes errorless learning and successful experiences, it should be kept in mind that in some situations, learning is enhanced when the person is given the opportunity to initiate the activity, make errors, and learn from mistakes (Evans et al., 2000; Poole, 1991; Sabari, 1991). At this time, there are no research studies that have systematically investigated effectiveness of the Affolter approach.

Cognitive–Perceptual Remediation: Specific Skill Training

In traditional cognitive–perceptual remedial approaches, cognitive skills are conceptualized in terms of higher cortical skills, which are hierarchal and divided into discrete subskills, such as attention, discrimination, memory, sequencing, categorization, concept formation, and problem solving. Lower-level skills provide the foundation for more complex skills and behaviors (Toglia, 1998). For example, attention skills are addressed before higher-level cognitive skills such as problem solving. Intervention emphasizes practice of the specific cognitive or perceptual skills that have been identified as being deficient. For example, if the person demonstrates impaired selective attention, intervention involves repetitive practice with tabletop or computerized exercises that are graded to place increasing demands on selective attention (Raskin & Mateer, 2000).

In cognitive–perceptual remediation, there is an assumption that improvement in underlying cognitive or perceptual skills will have a greater influence on behavior than direct functional task training, because learning will spontaneously generalize to a wider range of activities. For example, if block design construction improves during remedial treatment it is assumed that there will also be improvement on a wide range of other tasks involving constructional skills, such as dressing or making a sandwich. Remedial treatment aims to influence a wide range of everyday activities by improving underlying cognitive–perceptual subskills. This has also been referred to as the transfer training approach (Toglia, 1998).

Cognitive–perceptual remediation is based on the assumption that direct practice of the impaired skill promotes recovery or reorganization of that skill. Information on functional reorganization and adult brain plasticity supports this view. For example, it has been postulated that some parts of the brain may take over new functions or may work together in different ways as a result of environmental experiences (Luria, 1973). Functional neuroimaging tools provide preliminary support for this premise (Grady & Kapur, 1999; Laatsch, Pavel, Jobe, Lin, & Quintana, 1999). However, as Neistadt (1994b) observed, "because both remedial and adaptive treatment approaches both stimulate clients to learn new behaviors, neither approach can claim to take advantage of adult brain plasticity more than the other" (p. 426).

Most outcome studies on cognitive remediation have been conducted with the adult brain-injured population. Recently, there has been interest in applying cognitive remediation programs to the schizophrenic population (Bennet, Davalos, Green, & Rial, 1999; Hayes & McGrath, 2001; Suslow, Schonauer, & Arolt, 2001; Wykes, 2000). Several studies demonstrated changes in cognitive–perceptual skills as a result of focused cognitive training (Ben-Yishay, Piasetsky, & Rattok, 1987; Palmese & Raskin, 2000; Ruff et al., 1989; Sohlberg, McLauglin, Pavese, Heidrich, & Posner, 2000); however, few studies have directly explored the extent to which these improvements generalize to everyday function (Cicerone et al., 2000).

In addition, there are few studies that have actually compared the results of different treatment approaches. One study that compared remedial intervention with a functional approach for adult men with head injuries found that task-specific learning occurred in both groups (Neistadt, 1992). Another study, compared remedial and compensatory interventions in people with acquired brain injury and found that both groups improved and that there were no significant differences between the two treatment approaches. However, the study also found that clients in the remedial intervention group initiated use of compensatory strategies; thus the authors concluded that compensatory and remedial treatment approaches are not mutually exclusive (Dirette & Hinojosa, 1999).

Although it is unclear whether remedial intervention improves function, awareness and insight may improve as a result of remedial intervention. Because remediation emphasizes repetitive practice of the impaired skill, clients' awareness and insight into their deficits may increase as a secondary effect. This awareness is necessary for sustained participation and motivation in treatment and may eventually allow some individuals to initiate use of compensatory strategies. Several authors have observed a positive relationship between awareness and functional outcome (Katz & Hartman-Maeir, 1998; Prigatano & Wong, 1999; Sherer, Bergloff, Levin, High, Ogen & Nick, 1998).

Inefficient Use of Processing Strategy: Strategy Training

Strategy training focuses on teaching clients to change their approach, style, or technique for a wide variety of tasks. In dynamic approaches to intervention, cognitive–perceptual problems are conceptualized in terms of deficiencies of processing strategy. Processing strategies are defined as small units of behavior that enhance information processing and contribute to the effectiveness and efficiency of occupational performance (Toglia, 2001). Deficiencies in processing strategies account for difficulties on several different activities. For example, a tendency to overfocus on details may interfere with a meal preparation activity, shopping, or preparing bills (Toglia, 1998).

An example of an approach that uses processing strategies is the multicontext approach described in Chapter 21. Treatment targets a processing strategy that interferes with a variety of different tasks and is most responsive to cuing. This strategy is identified with the dynamic assessment procedures described in Chapter 25, Section 2. If a person requires cues more than 25% of the time, then the activity chosen may be too difficult for the client.

Separate cognitive perceptual skills are not addressed in the multicontext approach. For example, the client may demonstrate a tendency to miss important details in tasks that are unfamiliar and include 15–20 pieces of information. He or she may be taught to highlight important information with a color highlighter (external strategy) and to remember to choose important information before making a decision or attempting to solve the problem (internal strategy). The person then practices the application of the targeted strategies within a variety of purposeful and occupation-based activities. Activity demands are increased after application of the targeted strategy has been observed in a variety of different situations.

The multicontext approach focuses on both impaired skills and areas of strength and thus contains both compensatory and remedial components (Toglia, 1991a). This approach assumes that transfer of learning will occur in some clients only if it is directly addressed during treatment. There are several case reports that support the use of strategy training in brain-injured individuals (Cicerone & Wood, 1987; Neimeier, 1998; Nelson & Lenhart, 1996; Trexler, Webb, & Zappala, 1994).

AN INTEGRATED MODEL OF TREATMENT: MIXING AND MATCHING TREATMENT TECHNIQUES

Although the different treatment approaches have different requirements and underlying assumptions, they are not mutually exclusive. In clinical practice, both functional and remedial approaches are often used together (Blundon & Smits, 2000). Abreu (1998) discussed an integrated and holistic approach to treatment referred to as the quadraphonic approach. The quadraphonic approach uses both a microperspective and a macroperspective for treatment. The microperspective emphasizes treatment of cognitive impairments, whereas the macroperspective emphasizes functional performance and real-life occupations (Abreu, 1998, 1999).

The different approaches may be used sequentially or concurrently. Remediation may be used in preparation for occupation-based activities. Averbuch and Katz (1998) described a cognitive retraining program with two phases. The first phase focuses on strengthening cognitive impairments

TABLE 30-8. **INTEGRATION OF TREATMENT APPROACHES: THE MATCH BETWEEN INDIVIDUAL, TASK, AND ENVIRONMENT FOR PUTTING ON A BUTTON-DOWN SHIRT**[a]

Activity Components That Are Difficult for Client	Improve Underlying Skills (remedial)	Use a Different Task Method (compensation)	Adaptation of Task (others change task)	Adaptation of Environment (others change environment)
Difficulty selecting clothes from closet (requires excessive time; often mis-matched)			Garments preselected	Garments removed from busy closet and placed on hanger outside the closet
Puts on shirt quickly without proper positioning (puts hand in wrong end of sleeve)	Practice monitoring pacing speed of performance; scan entire garment	Use strategy of finding label to check proper orientation before putting garment on.	Solid garments without distracting patterns	
Tends to visually focus on parts of objects and fails to appreciate the whole	Practice getting an impression of the whole prior to locating the pieces			
Loses track of sequence of steps (especially when interrupted or distracted)	Practice attending to all aspects and monitoring distractions	Remember to read each step on checklist before execution; check off each step after completion	Checklist provided by caregiver	Quiet environment; telephone, radio turned off

[a]Adapted from Toglia (1996).

with remedial exercises, and the second phase focuses on adaptation to the environment. Neistadt (1994b) suggested that different treatment approaches may be appropriate at different stages of recovery or severity. For clients with severe impairments, adaptation or functional task training may be most effective; for those with milder deficits, remediation may be effective. In addition, different intervention approaches may be used to address different areas of dysfunction in the same individual. For example, a practitioner may choose to use a compensatory approach or adaptive approach to address the individual's memory deficits and a remedial approach to address visual scanning and unilateral neglect problems.

The Dynamic Interactional Model of Cognition provides a framework for simultaneously using and integrating remedial and functional approaches (Toglia, 1998). Table 30-8 illustrates how different intervention methods can be used simultaneously within a functional activity by emphasizing the interaction of the person, the activity, and the context Therapists need to begin activities at the performance capabilities of the client. This may require breaking down the steps of an activity and adapting some features of the context and activity while simultaneously emphasizing practice of a targeted strategy or cognitive subskill.

The question of whether occupational therapy intervention should focus on restoring the impaired cognitive–perceptual skills or on capitalizing on the person's assets should be rephrased to the following set of questions: How much change is expected from the person? How much learning and generalization are expected? How much do the activity demands or context need to be changed or altered to meet the person's capabilities? Is the person aware of his or her difficulties?

Factors Important in Selecting and Choosing Treatment

As you read the scenario in What's a Practitioner to Do? 30-2, think about the intervention approach that you would emphasize.

Performance Context

The context of the person's life, including the person's daily routines, roles and occupations, personality, interests, premorbid level of functioning, length of time since the onset of cognitive impairments, available external supports and resources, the culture, and family values are all performance context factors that need to be considered in treatment (AOTA, 1999). A person who lives alone requires a different set of skills than one who is married and has three small children. A person who previously worked as a lawyer requires a different set of cognitive skills to return to work than one who previously worked as a janitor. The cognitive and perceptual skills needed to return to former roles and occupations are individual in nature and vary tremendously.

WHAT'S A PRACTITIONER TO DO? 30-2
Cognition and Performance Contexts

SCENARIO 1

Mr. X is a 24 year old with a 10-year history of attention and memory problems related to a head trauma sustained at age 14. He has difficulty recalling conversations and events that occurred just hours before. During performance of a task he easily loses track of the steps and repeats some steps twice, while omitting other steps altogether. Mr. X. denies any difficulty with his concentration or memory and would like to return to school. He currently lives at home with his parents who care for him.

SCENARIO 2

Mr. Z is a 64 year old with attention and memory problems related to a head trauma sustained 3 weeks earlier. He has difficulty recalling conversations and events that occurred just hours before. During performance of a task he easily looses track of the steps and repeats some steps twice, while omitting other steps altogether. Mr. Z is well aware of his difficulties and is depressed by them. For example, he states, "I can't even remember what I ate for breakfast. What good am I? If I have to give up my business, my life is over." Mr. Z was recently widowed and lived alone before his accident.

QUESTIONS AND EXERCISES

The two scenarios describe the same clinical symptoms, but the performance contexts are different.

1. How do the differences in context influence the emphasis in treatment that you would use?
2. What influenced your selection?

DISCUSSION

There are no absolute right or wrong answers to these questions. In scenario 1, Mr. X is 10 years postinjury, so the potential for change in the underlying cognitive skills is assumed to be minimal. A remedial approach that focuses on improving memory and attention skills would not be warranted unless there were some evidence of potential for further improvement. Compensatory strategies, such as use of a memory notebook or a checklist could be considered; however, Mr. X denies any difficulty in memory or attention. This lack of self-awareness will present a major obstacle to independent initiation and use of compensatory strategies.

Caregiver training, task, and environmental adaptation, and the possibility of functional skill training to increase performance on a specified task appear to be the most appropriate areas for intervention. Techniques to increase awareness may be attempted as a prerequisite for using compensatory aids. External memory aids, such as memory notebook training, may be introduced using task-specific training methods in combination with maximum prompts and external cues for their use; however, success likely depends on Mr. X's ability to gain some awareness and acceptance of his disability.

In scenario 2, Mr. Z is only 3 weeks postinjury, so that the potential for change in the underlying skills is presumably present. In addition, Mr. Z is well aware of his problems. This would appear to make him a prime candidate for remedial techniques; however, he is also depressed by his deficits. He may not be able to cope emotionally with an approach that focuses on the impairment.

An approach that will provide greater opportunities for success and control over his environment may be the initial intervention emphasis. For example, adaptive techniques in which the caregiver or practitioner presents one-step directions at a time may make it easier for Mr. X. to follow task instructions. Training in use of compensatory strategies, such as use of a memory notebook to keep track of daily events and conversations and in use of a checklist to assist in keeping track of task steps that have already been completed, may enhance task performance. As Mr. X. gains self-confidence and control, remedial tasks that focus on improving attention may be gradually introduced if he is able to tolerate them.

The practitioner must analyze the skills and activity demands of expected roles and occupations. This analysis provides the context for goal setting and treatment

Emotional and Personality Characteristics: Obstacles to Treatment

There are several personality and emotional characteristics that can present obstacles to some of the treatment approaches described in the foregoing. Some of these characteristics may be part of a reaction to the illness and are thus temporary, whereas others may be part of the person's premorbid personality. In either case, these personality blocks need to be identified and the practitioner, along with the team, needs to determine if treatment should assist the client in working through the obstacle or in bypassing it. These characteristics and the effect that they may have on treatment selection are described in the following subsections.

Premorbid Personality Characteristics

Some people may have a lifelong pattern of personality characteristics that may present obstacles to intervention. For example, consider the person who has always been resistant to change, has always been set in his or her ways of doing things, and has been unable to modify or change his or her style even when that style has been unsuccessful. It may be particularly difficult for this type of person to adopt compensatory strategies (Gross & Schutz, 1986). Compensation requires modification of a routine or task. It involves a willingness to change the way one has done something for the past 20 years and adopt a new method.

Similarly, consider the person who has always been fearful of failure. He or she may have a lifelong pattern of avoidance or withdrawal from difficult situations. Mistakes may have always been accompanied by a defensive position or rationalization. This person may not be emotionally capable of dealing with interventions that emphasizes the areas of weakness or impairments. Intervention may need to emphasize opportunities for success and control.

Secondary Psychological Reactions

Secondary psychological reactions after brain injury can cause significant stress, anxiety, and depression, all of which further diminish cognitive functioning. The person with brain injury may experience repeated failures, a loss of hope, a sense of vulnerability and helplessness, a loss of productivity, uncertainty about the future, constant comparison to premorbid functioning by others, a loss of mastery over the environment, a loss of self-esteem, a loss of autonomy, low frustration tolerance, loneliness, and a sense of social isolation. All of these factors can lead to significant despair and depression (Fine, 1993; Sbordone, 1991). A person who is having difficulty in psychologically coping with his or her deficits and is overwhelmed by them may not be able to deal emotionally with tasks that focus on the deficits (e.g., remedial approach). Although the person may have the physical and cognitive potential to progress, he or she may not be emotionally ready to participate in an approach that brings out the areas of weakness. Rather than choosing a remedial approach, therapists may initially emphasize a functional approach aimed at providing opportunity for success and control and increasing self-esteem and a sense of self-worth.

Helpless Adjustment Style

Some individuals appear to seek dependency, rather than independence. They may not be motivated to learn strategies that would allow them to be independent in self-care skills. For example, a client may state, "I am old and I have done everything for everyone else for years. It is time for my family to take care of me." The appearance of helplessness may effectively attract positive attention from family members and friends. A sense of self-esteem may be based on the ability to attract help from others (Gross & Schutz, 1986). This lack of desire for independence may be either a maladaptive coping style or a value that is shared by the individual's culture or family system. Intervention may need to deemphasize independence in self-care skills and emphasize function in other areas, such as leisure activities. It is essential that the caregiver or family is involved in the goal-setting and treatment-planning process.

Learned Helplessness

Some people may desire independence but state, "Whatever I do, things won't change. No matter how hard I try, my situation will remain the same." The person who perceives a loss of control over their situation may not persist or actively participate in treatment (Gage & Polatajko, 1994). Treatment for **learned helplessness** may need to emphasize techniques that help the client gain some insight and sense of control over difficulties.

Awareness

Lack of awareness is a major obstacle to several of the treatment approaches discussed earlier. It results in poor motivation and compliance, lack of sustained effort and persistence, unrealistic expectations, incongruence between goals of the client and the family, impaired judgment and safety, and inability to use compensatory strategies efficiently (Barco, Crosson, Bolesta, Werts, & Stout 1991; Sherer, Oden, Bergloff, Levin, & High, 1998; Toglia & Kirk, 2000). "Clients who lack awareness of their deficits may, if compliant, go through the motions of rehearsing a strategy, but are clearly not engaged in the process. Consequently, the likelihood of the client putting the strategy to functional use is minimal" (Ylvisaker, Szekeres, Sullivan, & Wheeler, 1987, p. 140). A number of studies support the association between awareness and functional outcome (LaBuda & Lichtenberg, 1999; Malec & Moessner, 2000; Prigatano & Wong, 1999; Sherer, Bergloff, et al., 1998; Tham, Ginsberg, Fisher, & Tegner, 2001).

A lack of understanding of personal strengths and limitations prevents an individual from choosing goals that are realistic and attainable. If self-awareness is limited, a close relative or friend should participate in identifying concerns and priorities for intervention. Intervention should be directed toward narrowing any discrepancy between the client's perceptions of his or her abilities and those of the significant other. The practitioner should assist the client in focusing on skills needed for the here and now.

Structured methods of breaking down the client's broad or unrealistic goals into more realistic subgoals can be used to help him or her focus on current strengths and limitations. As awareness increases, the client gradually assumes a greater role in the goal-setting and treatment-planning process. "The power of a close therapeutic alliance cannot be underestimated in helping persons with brain injury to recognize and accept their difficulties" (Toglia & Kirk, 2000, p. 67).

The practitioner needs enthusiastically to create a supportive and nonthreatening atmosphere that allows the client to gain self-awareness without accompanying frustration, anxiety, and depression. The way in which treatment sessions are presented sets a tone and atmosphere that can be effective in enhancing active participation in treatment. The following statement is an example of introducing the purpose of cognitive rehabilitation to a client.

> *After a brain injury, it is common to have changes in the ability to quickly think and organize information. At times, things may seem like a jumbled jigsaw puzzle. It takes time to sort things out and to recognize the changes that have occurred. The first step in getting better is recognizing and understanding some of the changes that have occurred and getting to know your limits. If you know what type of difficulties that you may run into, it will be easier to stay a step ahead. As we do different activities, I can help you see some the areas that may give you difficulty so that you can stay a step ahead. This will not be easy, but if you are willing to give this a try, I believe it will make it easier for you to function.*

Awareness training involves helping a person with brain injury adjust and learn about the changes that have occurred. It involves helping clients get to know themselves again. Intervention should be directed toward helping people with cognitive–perceptual deficits self-discover their own errors. This is most likely to occur in tasks that are familiar so that individuals have a basis for comparison of performance. In addition, activities should be at a just right challenge level so that the person is able to integrate and assimilate the experience.

Directly pointing out errors or telling clients that they have problems is least effective in increasing awareness. Direct confrontation tends to elicit defensive reactions (Toglia & Kirk, 2000). There may be times when a person demonstrates strong denial and rationalizations of his or her mistakes. For example, a client may say, "Yes, I know my memory is not like it used to be, but a lot of people have bad memory. It won't interfere with my ability to work. My memory was never that good. . . . If I forget what I was supposed to do, I'll just ask someone else. What is the big deal?" The type of person who overrationalizes errors is difficult to engage in treatment. Strong denial may be more related to premorbid personality characteristics and use of defensive coping methods rather than decreased awareness resulting from brain injury (Prigatano, 1999). Deficits should be introduced slowly and indirectly within structured experiences while simultaneously emphasizing strategies to control and monitor the emergence of cognitive symptoms.

Over the past several years, the interest in the area of awareness and awareness training has significantly increased. However, this is still a relatively new area of investigation.

Few attempts have been made to address the issues of awareness in treatment systematically, although initial studies indicate that direct intervention may be effective in some groups of clients (Cicerone & Giacino, 1992; Schlund, 1999; Tham & Tegner, 1997; Tham et al., 2001). The following is a description of some of the techniques that can be used within a wide range of activities to enhance awareness.

Self-Prediction

Self-prediction involves asking the person to anticipate difficulties or predict his or her performance on a task. The client may be asked to indicate on a rating scale whether the activity will be easy or hard or to predict specific parameters of performance. For example, the accuracy of performance, the time required to complete the task, the amount of verbal cues required, or the type of difficulties that one may encounter may be estimated and discussed before actually performing the activity.

Immediately after performance, the actual results are compared with predicted results and any discrepancies are discussed (Toglia, 1991a, 1998). Case studies using self-prediction have been reported on clients with executive dysfunction, memory disorders, and unilateral neglect (Cicerone & Giacino 1992; Rebmann & Hannon, 1995; Schlund, 1999; Tham et al., 2001).

Specific Goal Ratings

Daily or weekly self-ratings of clearly defined behaviors or targeted strategies can be used to help a person focus on what he or she can do in the present. Goal attainment scales offer a concrete, individualized focus that can increase self-awareness and realistic goal orientation (Malec, Smigielski, & DePompoplo, 1991; Rockwood, Joyce, & Stolee, 1997). Client self-ratings of goal attainment can be compared to the ratings of the practitioner or of a significant other, and any discrepancies can be discussed. For example, a client with moderate memory deficits continually relies on others to remember events and does not use a memory notebook. If the targeted behavior is to rely less on others for information, the client may be asked to rate himself or herself weekly, on a scale of 1 (relies on others all the time or does not use book), to 5 (does not rely on others for information or consistently uses book). The client's rating can be compared to the rating of a significant other and any discrepancies can be discussed. Self-ratings can be charted or graphed over time and tracked to improve awareness (Sohlberg, 2000).

Videotape Feedback

A videotape of a client that illustrates problems in performing a task may be used to enhance awareness. Videotape feedback is concrete, and it allows clients to reexperience their performance and evaluate their difficulties as they are occurring rather than discussing them after the fact. Videotape feedback has been used successfully in clients with stroke (Paul, 1997; Soderback, Bengtsson, Ginsburg, & Ekholm 1992; Tham & Tegner, 1997) and head injury (Boake, 1991). Videotape feedback has been demonstrated to be more effective in enhancing awareness than verbal feedback in individuals with unilateral neglect (Tham & Tegner, 1997).

Self-Evaluation

The practitioner provides a structured system—such as a set of questions, a checklist, or a rating system—that the client uses as a guide to evaluate his or her performance. (Toglia, 1991a, 1998). Sample self-evaluation questions are, "Have I attended to all the necessary information?" "Did I check over my work?"

Self-Questioning

Questions that are designed to cue the client to monitor his or her behavior may be written on an index card or memorized. At specific time intervals during the task, the client is expected to stop and answer the same two or three questions, such as: "Am I sure that I am looking all the way to the left?" "Am I paying attention to the details?" "Am I going too quickly?" (Fertherlin & Kurland, 1989).

Journaling

The client keeps a journal in which activity experiences and performance results are recorded. The client is encouraged to reflect on and interpret activity experiences, think about what he or she has learned about himself or herself, and summarize strengths and weaknesses (Tham et al., 2001; Ylvisaker & Feeney, 1998).

WORKING WITH A MULTIDISCIPLINARY TEAM

A strong interdisciplinary approach is needed to address the complexity of issues that arise from cognitive–perceptual problems. In addition to the occupational therapy practitioner, the intervention team may include a neuropsychologist or psychologist, social worker, speech and language pathologist, recreational therapist, and physical therapist. Other disciplines may be nursing, psychiatry, special education, and optometry. Each discipline brings its own perspective and philosophy to the treatment team. It is important that the team members discuss their different viewpoints and agree on an overall team philosophy to provide a well-integrated program. Team goals and specific discipline goals should be identified. The family and client are also members of the team and should be involved in team discussions and provide input into the overall intervention plan.

The multicontext treatment framework can be used to guide an interdisciplinary intervention program. The team should emphasize the same major goals during treatment rather than working on separate skills. For example, the speech and language pathologist may address attention problems within the context of language material, such as listening to tapes or conversations; the neuropsychologist may use remedial attentional exercises; the physical therapist may reinforce attention through motor tasks; and the occupational therapy practitioner may address attentional strategies within the contexts of self-care, leisure, community, or work activities. Although the activities vary, the skills and strategies emphasized may remain similar across the different disciplines as described in the multicontext approach.

Some teams choose to give the responsibility of training specific cognitive and perceptual skills to specific disciplines. For example, the occupational therapy practitioner addresses visual perceptual problems, whereas the speech and language pathologist addresses language problems, and the psychologist addresses higher-level cognitive problems. Although this clearly delineates roles and prevents duplication of services, it is clearly fragmented and may be more comfortable for the different professionals than for the client. The client with brain injury is struggling to make sense out of the chaos and confusion in his or her mind. A strong integrated approach that assists the person in seeing patterns of behaviors across different activities is strongly advocated, rather than one that only reinforces the fragmentation that the client already perceives.

The **occupational therapy assistant** works in cooperation with the occupational therapist to implement aspects of the occupational therapy intervention plan. Once the targeted behaviors for treatment have been clearly identified, the occupational therapy assistant and occupational therapist collaborate to choose a variety of different activities that can be used to reinforce the desired behaviors. For example, if the use of a checklist to perform multistep activities has been determined to be an emphasis in the treatment program by the occupational therapist, the occupational therapy assistant may reinforce the use of this strategy during a variety of different activities, such as a trip to the supermarket, planning a meal, or organizing a calendar. The results are discussed with the occupational therapist. Together, the occupational therapist and the occupational therapy assistant may decide to modify the strategy (decrease the size of the checklist, reduce the number of steps listed on a key outline, or eliminate the need to check off each step as it is completed) or upgrade the complexity of the treatment activities (AOTA, 1999).

ADDRESSING THE COGNITIVE–PERCEPTUAL FUNCTIONS AND SKILLS

This subsection reviews techniques for improving specific cognitive–perceptual skills. These techniques need to be embedded within the context of an intervention program that is tailored to the client's interests, daily occupations, and lifestyle. Each area describes techniques that target change in the person (specific skill training and strategy training) and change in the task and environment (adaptation). Specific skill training generally uses remedial exercises in preparation for purposeful and occupation-based activities. Strategy training involves training use of a strategy across a wide range of purposeful activities and occupation-based activities, whereas adaptation focuses on modifying a specific natural context or occupation based activity (AOTA, in press).

Although these techniques are separated for the purpose of discussion, intervention should simultaneously incorporate both areas to meet the information processing abilities of the client, as discussed earlier in this section. Awareness and self-monitoring techniques should be integrated within intervention approaches that seek to change the client, because the effective use of strategies requires awareness and self-monitoring skills. The Affolter approach and the functional task training approach are not addressed in this section, because they are used in the same way with a wide range of cognitive perceptual impairments; however, they should be kept in mind as options for intervention.

Disorientation

Disorientation and confusion are symptoms of severe attention and memory problems and can overshadow performance on all tasks. Intervention can be approached from different perspectives.

Specific Skill Training

Reality orientation programs involve reviewing specific information concerning person, place, and time. The key intervention principles are structure and consistency. The same orientation questions or facts should be reviewed several times a day according to an established routine or time schedule.

Orientation to person is addressed before orientation to place or time. In cases of severe disorientation, the same three or four key personal facts may be reviewed in the form of multiple-choice questions several times a day. If the client has difficulty, additional cues or multiple-choice answers may be provided. For example, if the client does not accurately recall his or her grandchildren's names, pictures of the grandchildren can be shown or the first letter of the names can be provided. Gradually, the amount and type of information the person is asked to recall may be expanded. The emphasis is on increasing the client's ability to retrieve correct orientation facts through repeated questioning. Retrieval of the same information over and over is hypothesized to strengthen the retrieval pathways and increase the likelihood of accurate recall (Harrell, Parente, Bellingrath, & Lisicia, 1992).

A reality orientation program aims to help the person feel connected to who he or she is. Family members should be asked to bring in a tape of the client's favorite music, a picture album with labels showing family events and holidays, favorite magazines or books, or videotapes of family members or family events. An audiotape or videotape can also be created by a family member to review orientation information and explain what has happened and why the person is in the hospital. These items can be used to assist in cuing the person to retrieve accurate facts.

Structured orientation review sessions may also be conducted within a group setting. A group setting may enhance attention, motivation, and participation in some clients. Group projects, such as a collage that involves a holiday theme or season, may be used to improve orientation.

Orientation questions can also be incorporated into a bean bag toss game, a board game, or a *Family Feud*–style game (Toglia & Golisz 1990). Each game format places different demands on attention, memory and orientation. For example, the *Family Feud*–style format requires a quick speed of response, whereas the board format requires the ability to keep track of whose turn it is, the playing pieces, and positions on the board. The cognitive demands of each playing format need to be matched with the abilities of the group.

Strategy Training

Strategy training for disorientation consists of teaching the person to use external cues to reduce confusion. The client is trained to look for cues when he or she is feeling confused or is having difficulty recalling orientation information. For example, an information poster that contains orientation facts can be placed on a wall, closet, or eventually inside a notebook. When the client is asked orientation information, he or she is expected to locate the information poster to verify responses or to find the correct answers. A memory book that includes pictures and names of familiar people, important life events, and such can also be placed in a key location within the room. An alarm preprogrammed to ring several times a day can be used to cue the person to read his or her orientation fact book.

A calendar posted on the wall or closet may be helpful in orienting the person to time. If the client has poor selective attention, a single piece of paper with the day and date written daily, rather than a monthly calendar, may be needed.

To assist the client in finding his or her room, directional arrows may be placed in the hallway, and tape indicating the route to his or her room can be placed on the floor. Key landmarks can be pointed out and made more salient with arrows or colored tape.

The practitioner needs immediately to reinforce initiation or use of any of these external cues by praising the client. The practitioner should keep track of each time the client initiates use of an external cue by recording it on a chart or visual graph. In addition, points can be used to reinforce the desired responses. The frequency of use of external cues should be tracked and gradually faded until the orientation information is internalized. In addition, the person should be trained to look for orientation cues (clocks, calendars, etc.) in different environments.

Adaptations of Task or Environment

An alarm clock or talking watch that automatically announces the date and time on an hourly basis may be used to assist a person in maintaining orientation to time. In addition, large brightly colored clocks can be placed in the person's room or a large brightly colored sign with the day and date can be placed on the closet door. A large colored sign with the client's name can be placed on door to reduce the likelihood of him or her entering the wrong room. The saliency of these key items is likely automatically to capture the client's attention without effort. The color and location of the cue signs may need to be changed periodically to prevent habituation (Giles & Wilson, 1993). In addition to the use of external cues, the caregiver may be trained to structure each day with a set routine. Daily repetition of the same schedule may assist in decreasing confusion.

Attention

Specific Skill Training

In remedial training, specific components of attention are addressed in a hierarchical manner, so that intervention tasks gradually place greater demands on attention. Table 30-9 presents a sample attention remedial program. In general, remedial studies of attention have shown improvements in neuropsychological test results in both brain-injured and schizophrenic populations (Ben-Yishay et al., 1987; Brown, Harwood, Hays, Heckman, & Short, 1993; Palmese & Raskin, 2000; Sohlberg et al., 2000; Suslow et al., 2001). Although several authors have observed generalization to functional activities, it has not been directly measured in the majority of studies. Recently, Sohlberg et al. (2000) provided support for generalization of an attention training program and found that the program influenced self-reports of daily living concerns.

A review of the literature concerning remediation of attention deficits after stroke concluded that there is some indication that training in attention improves alertness and sustained attention, but there is no evidence to support or refute remediation of attentional deficits to improve functional independence (Lincoln, Majid, & Weyman, 2000). A review of the literature in remediation of attention deficits in persons with traumatic brain injury and stroke by Cicerone et al. (2000) found level 2 evidence to support the effectiveness of attention training and recommended attention training as a practice guideline during the postacute phase of recovery. However, they indicated that this intervention appears to be more effective when it includes use of self-monitoring techniques, strategy training, and functional activities.

In addition to remedial tabletop and computer tasks, gross motor activities such as ball throwing and hitting a balloon have also been used to increase alertness and reaction time. Shimelman and Hinojosa (1995) found no significant differences on test scores measuring attention after gross motor activity; however, they did note positive changes in attention behaviors, such as scanning and self-checking.

Strategy Training

In strategy training, the emphasis is not on training specific attentional skills but on training use of a strategy to control the emergence of attentional symptoms, such as distractibility, impulsivity, or a tendency to lose track or

TABLE 30–9. **ATTENTIONAL PROCESS TRAINING PROGRAM**[a]

Attentional Components	Sample Treatment Tasks
Sustained attention (concentration)	• Shape and number cancellation worksheets: Find the target number(s) or shape(s) • Listen for a target number or letter on a tape
Selective attention (focusing attention on selected stimuli)	• A distractor overlay is placed over number and shape cancellation worksheets to make it more difficult to identify the relevant targets • Listen for target letters or numbers on a tape with the addition of background noise
Alternating attention (switching attention from one stimuli to another)	• Cancellation worksheet; the client is asked to alternate between canceling odd and then even numbers in response to the examiner saying "Change" • Worksheet requiring adding or subtracting pairs of numbers in response to the examiner saying "Change"
Divided attention (paying attention to more than one stimuli at a time)	• Client performs a cancellation worksheet while listening and responding to target numbers or letters on a tape
	• Sort cards by suit while turning over any card that contains a target letter in the spelling of its name

[a]Adapted from Toglia, J. (1993, Dec). Treating individuals with constructional apraxia, AOTA Advanced Apraxia Institute: Assessing and Treating Adults, Denver, CO.

overfocus on details. Intervention strategies that may be emphasized include the following:

- Taking time-outs from a task when concentration begins to fade.
- Remembering to get a sense of the whole situation before attending to the parts.
- Monitoring a tendency to become distracted by either internal thoughts or external stimuli.
- Remembering to look all over and actively search for additional information before responding.
- Self-instruction.
- Time pressure management strategies.

Self-instruction involves saying each step of a task aloud to focus attention on the task and inhibit distractions and stereotypical behaviors. It may also involve saying self-cues or task instructions out loud. Gradually, the client is trained to say these cues silently rather than out loud (Webster & Scott, 1983). Time pressure management involves teaching the client strategies to prevent and manage time pressures that result from decreased rate of processing (Fasotti, Kovacs, Eling, & Brouwer, 2000).

Strategy training can be integrated within a wide range of everyday activities. During activity performance, the practitioner assists the client in monitoring use of the targeted strategy or behavior by recording the frequency with which the strategy is initiated and used across different activities.

Adaptations of Task or Environment

Adaptations designed to minimize attention demands involve reducing or limiting the amount of information presented to the client at any one time. Examples include the following (Toglia, 1993):

- Simplifying task instructions so that only one step is presented at a time.
- Reducing the number of items or choices presented to the client at any one time.
- Preselecting relevant objects needed for tasks.
- Task segmentation or presenting only one component of a task at a time.

Moulton, Taira, and Grover (1995) found that segmenting the task of eating and presenting one food item at a time to dementia clients, rather than presenting a cluttered food tray, decreased the amount of assistance required, improved food and fluid intake, and qualitatively improved behavior.

The enhancement or reduction of salient visual cues in the environment can be used to promote desired behaviors. For example, limiting clutter and distraction in the environment, closing the window, or turning off the radio can prevent a person from getting sidetracked off a task. In the task of brushing teeth, for example, unnecessary items should be removed from the sink, and the items required for use should be made salient with contrasting colors. The contrasting colors of the toothpaste, toothbrush, and cup provide a cue to assist the client in attending to the different items.

Visual Foundation Skills

Treatment of visual foundation skills such as visual acuity, contrast sensitivity, oculomotor skills, and visual fields generally involves adaptations and compensation; however, remedial exercises may be recommended for individuals with oculomotor deficits or visual field deficits.

Specific Skill Training

Oculomotor Skills

Range of motion eye exercises to the involved muscle have been advocated for individuals with eye muscle paresis. For example, if the lateral rectus muscle of the right eye is weakened, the client may be asked to move the eyes as far as possible to the right and hold that position for a few seconds. Optometrists who specialize in vision therapy may recommend specific eye exercises for oculomotor deficits that can be reinforced during occupational therapy sessions and real-life tasks (Chaikin, 2001).

Visual Fields

There is some evidence that deficits in visual fields can be decreased with intensive stimulation and training in saccadic eye movements (Warren 1993; Zihl, 1981). Kerkhoff, MunBinger, and Meier (1994) found that systematic training of saccadic eye movements in clients with visual field deficits increased visual search field sizes, restored oculomotor functions, and improved performance in functional visual activities. Williams (1995) described a person with a scotoma in the central field who demonstrated functional gains with a visual scanning program. Occlusion of the intact visual field with eye patching has also been used to force use of the impaired visual field (Warren, 1993).

Adaptations of Task or Environment

Visual Acuity

Deficits in visual acuity are frequently addressed with corrective lenses; however, adaptation to the environment may also be helpful, particularly if eyeglasses are not able to correct acuity. Adaptations that may be beneficial include the following:

- Large print reading materials.
- Talking watch or clock.
- Talking calculator.
- Telephone with preprogrammed numbers.
- Telephone with voice recognition.
- Dialing feedback or large numbered buttons.
- Talking books.

- Adaptations to the computer (working with large fonts, using talking word-processing programs).
- Colored knobs on cabinets or door handles.
- Magnifiers.

In addition, use of halogen and florescent light provide high-intensity light with minimal glare. The contrast between objects within a task or the environment should be increased whenever possible (Warren, 1993; Zoltan, 1996). For example, finding a white toothbrush on a white shelf is much more difficult than locating a red toothbrush on a white shelf. Pouring coffee into a white cup may be much safer than pouring coffee into a black cup.

Oculomotor

An optometrist or ophthalmologist may recommend different types of eye patching for double vision. One type of eye-patching regimen is to alternate a patch on each eye on a daily or hourly basis. When the eye patch is on, double vision is eliminated. Time without the patch may be recommended so that the eyes will attempt to gain fusion. Some eye specialists do not advocate eye patching at all because it may contribute to eye weakness and discourage any attempt by the brain to overcome the double vision. Fresnel prisms, applied to the client's eyeglasses, may be recommended as an alternative to eye patching to reduce or eliminate double vision (Chaikin, 2001).

Visual Field Deficits

Prisms place a peripheral image to a more central area of the retina. Rossi, Kheyfets, and Reding (1990) found that prisms improved visual perceptual test performance in stroke clients with visual field cuts or unilateral neglect. However, scores on a functional assessment did not improve. The effectiveness of prisms and its carryover to function needs further study. Prisms distort the visual world, and they may be difficult to adjust to in patients who have accompanying visual perceptual problems.

Unilateral Neglect

Specific Skill Training

Visual scanning training is also used to remediate unilateral neglect. However, for this problem, the emphasis is not on the preciseness and speed of eye movements but on increasing awareness and attention to the affected side. In unilateral neglect, it has been observed that clients demonstrate a decrease in eye movements to the affected side. This decrease in eye movements reflects a decrease in attention to one side of the environment (Antonucci, Guariglia, Magnotti, Paolucci, Pizzamiglio, & Zoccolotti, 1995; Pizzamiglio, Antonucci, Judica, Montenero, Razzano, & Zoccolotti, 1992; Toglia, 1991b).

A scientific literature review by Cicerone et al. (2000) concluded that there is level 1 evidence to support use of visuospatial interventions, which include practice in visual scanning, because it improves compensation for unilateral neglect and generalizes to everyday activities. Therefore, they recommended visuospatial rehabilitation with visual scanning as a practice standard for clients with visual neglect after right hemisphere stroke. Intervention appears to be most effective when a wide combination of intervention activities, including everyday tasks is used (Antonucci et al., 1995; Pizzamiglio et al., 1992). Programs with greater levels of intensity have generally produced more positive outcomes. However, even with intensive training, it has been demonstrated that individuals with unilateral neglect have poorer functional outcome than others with stroke (Paolucci, Antonucci, Grasso, & Pizzamiglio, 2001).

Scanning activities usually involve locating specific items from an array of stimuli within small- and large-size spaces. Remedial exercises include cancellation tasks, such as putting a line through all the letter A's on a page or circling all the *the*'s in a paragraph. Large-size scanning boards can be constructed or purchased that require scanning and reaching in larger space. Computerized scanning programs are available that involve quickly locating or matching a shape, letter, or number that appears on the screen in random locations. These programs generally provide information on the time it takes for the individual to locate targets in different quadrants of the visual field. Isolated use of microcomputer visual scanning training exercises has not been found to be effective (Cicerone et al., 2000).

Electronic scanning devices, such as the Dynavision 2000, have also been used to practice quickly locating and following targets in the visual fields. The Dynavision 2000 is a large electronic scanning board in which the user has to hit lighted target buttons before they are extinguished. The apparatus can generate a variety of different type of scanning and reaction time tasks (Klavora & Warren, 1998). Klavora et al. (1995) found that visual reaction time and scanning training with the Dynavision 2000 improved driving performance in stroke clients with marked visual and attentional difficulties.

Because unilateral neglect is hypothesized to be related to decreased level of arousal on the affected side, gross motor activities that increase general arousal and alertness have been used in combination with scanning activities to increase attention to the affected side. Vestibular input increases gaze and attention to the affected field (Cappa, Sterzi, Vallar, & Bisiach, 1987). Tactile input such as encouraging physical manipulation of scanning material may also aid in visual scanning (Warren, 1993).

Weinberg et al. (1977) designed systematic training techniques that incorporated a combination of remedial and strategy training methods during reading and scanning tasks. For example, they used graded anchoring, pacing the speed of scanning, feedback, and decreasing the density of the stimulus. Anchoring involves placing a vertical line in the left-hand margin of the page to serve as a cue to attend to the left. The person is instructed to find the anchor before reading each line. Initially, a red line may be used to capture attention to the left side. Gradually, the saliency of the cue may be faded, and a thin pencil line can be used as an anchor. Each line may also be numbered sequentially on both sides to assist the client in orienting himself or herself spatially to a page and in moving from one line to another without skipping lines (Weinberg et al., 1977).

Robertson, Tegner, Tham, Lo, and Smith (1995) taught clients with chronic unilateral neglect to tell themselves to pay attention. Although the focus was on the general ability to sustain attention, rather than on directly addressing visual scanning, significant improvements in unilateral neglect as well as sustained attention were found. This suggests that unilateral neglect may be remediated by techniques aimed at general attentional skills rather than focused visual scanning training.

Other alternatives to visual scanning training for clients with unilateral neglect include the use of limb activation methods and visual occlusion techniques. The effectiveness of a limb activation program using a "neglect alert device" was described by Robertson, Hogg, and McMillan (1998). Treatment involved repeated use of the left upper extremity within left-sided space to turn off a buzzer at 8-sec intervals during a variety of different tasks (ADL, reading, card sorting). Active limb movements on the side contralateral to the lesion or within contralateral space have been found to increase visual attention to the left side of space. (Lin, 1996; Robertson, North, & Geggie. 1992).

Partial visual occlusion methods attempt to force the client to use the neglected visual field by patching the eye ipsilateral to the lesion (Butter & Kirsch, 1992), patching the nonneglected half field of eyeglasses (Beis, Andre, Baumgarten, & Challier, 1999), or darkening the nonneglected half field of eyeglasses (hemispatial sunglasses) (Arai, Ohi, Sasaki, Nobuto, & Tanaka, 1997). Beis et al. (1999) found that right CVA subjects with a patch on the right half field of eyeglasses demonstrated greater functional outcome compared to those who received monocular right eye patching. One of the benefits of partial visual occlusion techniques is that they can easily be incorporated into ADL and home programs (Freeman, 2001).

Recently, a computerized assisted training program consisting of a series of complex visuospatial tasks, including several tasks in which clients with unilateral neglect simulated operation of a wheelchair through an obstacle course, was studied. Trained subjects performed better on a real-life wheelchair obstacle course and had fewer accidents than control subjects. The use of virtual reality–based technology appears to show potential for clients with unilateral neglect (Webster, McFarland, Rapport, Morrill, Roades, & Abadee, 2001).

Strategy Training

Scanning strategies vary with the demands of activities. Table 30-10 describes activity parameters that can be used as a guide in grading the difficulty of visual scanning treatment activities. During intervention, some activity parameters are held constant while others are changed. For example, the number of items and the horizontal arrangement may be held constant while the activity is graded in difficulty by narrowing the spacing between items. This requires strategies aimed at pacing speed of visual scanning and paying attention to details. On the other hand, changing the arrangement of items from a horizontal predictable pattern to an unpredictable scattered pattern requires a more systematic and organized approach to the task. Intervention should include practice in identifying situations that require different scanning strategies or that place greater demands on scanning.

The visual search strategies described in the foregoing can be integrated within a wide variety of tasks. For example, the client can practice scanning or locating specific information in train schedules, spreadsheets, the telephone book, menus, calendars, movie clocks, or maps. He or she may practice finding specific items in a draw, on a shelf, or in a magazine; scanning for a particular type of a greeting card; and locating items within a certain price range in a food circular. The movement pattern, context, and content of the activities should vary while the same strategy is practiced repeatedly in tasks that match the abilities of the client. (Toglia, 1991b).

Individuals with unilateral neglect do not always know when they are attending to the left side. They frequently think that they are looking to the left when, in fact, they are not. Intervention needs to assist clients in finding external cues that will provide feedback about when they are indeed attending to the left. An emphasis in treatment should be teaching the client to find the edges of a page or the periphery of stimuli *before* beginning a task and to mark it with an anchor, such as colored tape, a colored highlighter, a bright object, or the placement of his or her arm. For example, clients with unilateral neglect may be told, "Look for your left hand as you are doing the task. When you see your left hand, then you know you are on the left side."

Worthington (1996) found that a strategy that involved training the individual to locate the left edge of the page was superior to teaching the person a nonvisual limb activation strategy of opening and closing the left fist in the task of reading. The use of auditory cuing has also been used successfully to decrease unilateral neglect. In a case report described by Seron, Deloche, and Coyette (1989), a beeper or alarm device was placed in the client's left pocket. The client was required to scan space and attend to the left to turn off the sound.

Other intervention strategies for unilateral neglect include tactile search and use of mental imagery. Tactile search involves teaching the client to feel the left side of the space with eyes closed or to feel the left edges of objects before visual search. Visual imagery teaches imagining and describing familiar scenes or routes and using mental images

TABLE 30–10. **GRADING VISUAL SCANNING ACTIVITIES**

Activity Parameter	Easy (less attention and effort)	Difficult (more attention and effort)	Demands with Increased Complexity
Discriminability	Target items are easy to discriminate and grossly different from surrounding items	Target items are more detailed and similar to the surrounding items	Greater demands on visual acuity, contrast sensitivity, selective visual attention, ability to recognize distinctive cues, pattern recognition
Arrangement	Organize into predictable format such as horizontal rows	Randomly scattered and/or overlapping so that some features of objects are partially obscured	Greater demands on saccadic eye movements, strategies to keep track of visual stimuli, ability to change search pattern
Spacing between stimuli	Even spaces between each item and each line	Items are close together and/or unevenly spaced	Greater demands on saccadic eye movements and focal attention
Amount	Only one or two items are presented at any one time	Increased amount of items are presented simultaneously	Greater demands on selective attention, strategies to keep track of visual stimuli
Predictability	The client knows the exact number of targets that need to be found	The number of targets is unknown	Greater initiation of exploration and search in peripheral fields
Timing	Untimed	Timed limit for search	Greater demands on reaction time, sustained attention, and speed of oculomotor skills
Meaningfulness	Meaningful and familiar stimuli provide a context that cues visual search	Unfamiliar or meaningless stimuli (random string of numbers, pictures, words)	Greater demands on initiation and visual search; fewer cues to direct eye movements and visual search
Number of targets and rules	Find one target item	Find two or more different items (cross out the letters *A* and *H* when they are preceded by the letter *O*)	Greater demands on visual memory, ability to keep track of visual information
Size of space	Space for scanning is large (not always easier)	Space for scanning is small (this is not necessarily harder)	Greater dependence on peripheral fields and visual search; requires initiation of active visual exploration
Sample activity	Four objects on the bathroom counter (cup, toothbrush, comb and razor); find the toothbrush (objects are grossly different)	Look at a large menu; identify the number of meat items between $8 and $11	Nearly all task parameters are changed to illustrate simple and complex visual scanning tasks; in treatment, only one or two task parameters should be changed at any one time

during movement of limbs or visual scanning (Niemeier, 1998; Smania, Bazoli, Piva, Guidetti, 1997). For example, reduction in neglect symptoms and increased performance on functional tasks was reported after a mental imagery program that involved teaching clients with neglect to imagine their eyes as sweeping beams of a lighthouse from left to right across the visual field. Clients were cued to use this mental image during functional and therapy training tasks (Niemeier, 1998; Niemeier, Cifu, & Kishore, 2001).

Unilateral neglect is frequently accompanied by disturbances in awareness (Tham et al., 2001). Awareness training techniques, such as those described earlier, need to be deeply embedded within treatment (Toglia, 1991b).

Adaptations of Task or Environment

To minimize the need to attend to the left, it has been suggested that the environment be rearranged so that key items such as the telephone, nurse call button, bedside table, and radio or TV are on the unaffected side. However, a study by Kelly and Ostreicher (1985) found no significant difference in functional outcome in clients whose hospital rooms were rearranged in this way.

Lennon (1994) described the successful use of large colored paper markings on the edges of tables, corners, and elsewhere to prevent collision in clients with unilateral neglect. The client was trained to look for these markers. Markers were gradually faded. Performance improved and was maintained with removal of markers; however, effects did not generalize to other environments.

Calvanio, Levine, and Petrone, (1993) described the use of an adapted plate to increase feeding skills in a client with a severe case of left inattention and a dense left hemianopia. The authors devised a sectioned plate, with raised edges, that was mounted on a lazy Susan so that it could be rotated. As the client pushed at her food with the fork, the plate rotated so that all the food eventually came into view. This eliminated the need for scanning or head turning to the left. Other environmental adaptations include placing red tape on the client's wheelchair brakes or placing brightly colored objects such as a napkin or cup on the left side (Golisz, 1998).

Visual Discrimination, Visual Spatial, and Visual Constructional Skills: Specific Deficits

Specific Skill Training

The remedial approach to visual perception addresses deficits in specific visual perceptual skills through graded tabletop or computerized exercises and practice drills (Zoltan, 1996). Examples include practice in identifying and matching objects or designs that have subtle differences in size, position, or shape; finding objects or shapes embedded within an array of other items; identifying objects or shapes that are partially hidden; and copying the position and arrangement of objects or designs. Computerized tasks have the advantage of providing a controlled rate of stimulus presentation, an objective record of the client's accuracy and speed of discrimination, and objective feedback (Ross, 1992). There is currently no evidence to demonstrate that training on visual perceptual worksheets, block designs, parquetry blocks, or computerized visuospatial exercises generalizes to function.

Strategy Training

Some strategies that may be used to maximize the client's ability to process visual information are getting a sense of the whole before looking at the parts, teaching the person to partition space before localizing details, using a finger to trace visual stimuli and to focus attention on details, covering or blocking out visual stimuli when too much information is presented at once, verbalizing salient visual features or subtle differences, and mentally visualizing a particular item before looking for it (Toglia, 1989, 1998).

Different activity parameters can be manipulated to emphasize different aspects of visual processing. Tables 30-11 and 30-12 illustrate this and provide guidelines for grading visual discrimination activities. Intervention involves careful manipulation of activity parameters, holding some parameters constant while systematically changing others to emphasize specific aspects of visual processing in a wide variety of everyday activities.

Adaptation of Task or Environment

The key guideline in minimizing the effects of visual perceptual difficulties is to make the distinctive features of objects more salient with color cues. An example is placing color tape on buttons to operate appliances or using salient

TABLE 30–11. **VISUAL DISCRIMINATION: ACTIVITY GRADING**[a]

Activity Parameters	Simple (less attention and effort)	Complex (greater attention and effort)	Demands with Increased Complexity
Familiarity of stimuli	Familiar stimuli (simple shapes, everyday objects, letters, words)	Less familiar (unusual objects, abstract unfamiliar shapes)	More difficult to pick up distinctive features
Directions	Structured (matching or point to specific items)	Unstructured ("Tell me what you see")	Requires initiation and organized visual search strategies
Distinctive features	Readily apparent (regular pen; pen point is the distinctive feature)	Obscure or partially hidden features (novelty pen that looks like a candy cane)	Greater visual attention; more difficult to recognize objects; increased likelihood of misperception
Degree of detail	Little to no detail	Fine detail	Greater demands on visual attention
Contrast	High contrast (red sock with white socks)	Low contrast (light beige and white socks)	Harder to determine where one item ends and another begins; greater demands on selective attention
Background	Soft backgrounds, solids, nonpatterned	Confusing and distracting backgrounds, patterns	Greater visual selective attention
Context	Within environmental context (grooming item in bathroom)	Outside of context (grooming item in therapy area)	Greater visual attention to critical features; fewer cues for recognition

[a]Task parameters such as the amount and arrangement (see Table 30-10) are also applicable to visual discrimination.

TABLE 30–12. **CONSTRUCTIONAL ACTIVITY GRADING**[a]

Activity Parameters	Simple	Complex	Demands with Increased Complexity
Model	Three-dimensional model to copy	No model; figure out how the pieces fit together	Greater demands on planning and problem-solving strategies
Familiarity	Prior experience	Unfamiliar	Greater visual analysis and discrimination
Number of pieces, lines or details	1–2	>12	Greater selective attention and discrimination
Spatial alignment	Nonprecise	Precise placement and orientation of angles, pieces	Greater attention to detail
Regularity of pieces	All same size and shape	Pieces are different sizes and shapes	Greater discrimination
Color	Different colored pieces	Pieces are all the same color	Less contrast, greater spatial analysis
Choose stimuli	Preselected pieces; design provides outline for placement of each piece	Decide and find pieces from a large array	Greater demands on visual search, discrimination, planning, and decision making
Error feedback	Immediate feedback with errors (pieces do not fit together or construction collapses)	Requires close inspection to detect errors	Greater self-monitoring; harder to recognize and detect errors

[a]Adapted from Toglia (1993b).

color cues on objects to make them easier to locate and discriminate (e.g., bright pink tape on a medication bottle to make it easier to identify in the medicine cabinet). Cues such as colored marks or tape at spatial landmarks (tape recorder, wheelchair foot rests), reduces spatial demands and makes it easier to orient and align pieces together.

Written material can be perceived with greater ease if there are spaces between lines and a felt tip pen is used to provide greater contrast instead of a pencil. Paper with raised lines makes it easier for clients with spatial difficulties to maintain alignment of lines during writing.

Visual stimuli—such as items on a shelf or sentences on a page—that are large in size and arranged in an organized manner with large spaces between items are easy to perceive. Consistent locations for objects in the refrigerator, closet, or drawer increase predictability and provide contextual cues for recognition.

Significant others should be instructed to decrease visual distractions in the room or within a task by limiting designs and patterns and by using solid colors with high contrast. Patterns, designs, and decorations make it harder to select and recognize critical features of an object. For example, Mr. D saw a paper clip with a bright pink decorative heart decal on it. He looked at the object and thought it was something rather peculiar. He did not recognize it as a paper clip. When the practitioner covered the decoration, he immediately recognized the object. The brightly colored decoration had captured his visual attention and made it difficult for him to recognize the distinctive features. Although intervention focused on recognizing critical features of objects, the use of patterns and designs was avoided on clothes to enhance his ability to dress.

Significant others should also be trained to introduce only a small amount of visual information at one time. For example, during grooming, a caregiver may be instructed to have no more than two objects on the sink or counter at one time. When the client is finished with the first two objects needed for the task, the caregiver introduces the next two objects.

Motor Planning

Specific Skill Training

Interventions to overcome motor planning deficits may emphasize either the production aspect or the conceptual aspect of motor planning (Roy, 1985). Techniques that address the orientation of an object or limb in space or the timing, sequence, and organization of the motor elements aim to enhance the production aspect of motor planning. For example, if a movement pattern is performed in an awkward or clumsy manner with unnecessary fixation or movements, the practitioner may provide physical contact to limit the inappropriate or extraneous movements while simultaneously using guiding methods to facilitate a smooth motor pattern. Hand-over-hand assistance or a light touch may be used to guide a movement pattern along a specific trajectory pattern or to guide the manipulation of objects (Okkema, 1993). Through repeated practice in different tasks, such as reaching for an object on a shelf or washing the face, the client begins to learn the movement patterns that feel right, and the practitioner gradually withdraws assistance. For some clients, light touch on the distal components of the extremity may be more effective in guiding

TABLE 30-13. **ACTIVITY GRADING FOR MOTOR PLANNING**[a]

Simple	Complex
Automatic, overlearned tasks	Unfamiliar tasks
Everyday objects	Less familiar objects
Single gestures	Gestures involving multiple movement elements
Meaningful gestures	Meaningless gestures
Transitive gestures (brushing teeth)[b]	Intransitive gestures (salute)[b]
One to two steps	Multiple steps
Imitation	Movement to command
Small object or target	Large object or target
Total body movements	Discrete smaller movements
Movement toward body	Movement away from body
Bilateral	Unilateral
Proximal movements required	Distal movements
Symmetrical	Asymmetrical
Repetitive actions, movements	Nonrepetitive
In context	Out of context
Stable, predictable, stationary environment	Changing, unpredictable, moving environment
Closed loop	Open loop
Fixed posture (stationary)	Dynamic posture (in motion)

[a]Adapted from Toglia (1993b).

[b]Transitive gestures involve pretended object use; intransitive gestures do not involve pretended object use.

motor patterns, whereas for others heavier contact and deep pressure may be more effective. It should be kept in mind that deep proprioceptive input and contact have an inhibitory effect on normal people, whereas light touch tends to have a more facilitatory effect (Farber, 1993).

Familiar tasks that are performed in context are easier for people with motor planning disorders, because the context provide cues that facilitate the desired action. Interventions can be graded by gradually introducing activities and environments that have less stability and predictability, such as negotiating around obstacles in a crowded store. Table 30-13 provides guidelines for grading and manipulating task parameters in treatment. In grading motor planning tasks, it is suggested that only one or two task parameters are changed at a time while the other parameters are held constant. However, the context in which the task is performed should vary widely. Clients who use a lot of extra fixation, co-contraction, or proximal movements may benefit from biofeedback or sensory feedback to limit extraneous movements and inhibit unnecessary fixation patterns.

Intervention addressing the conceptual aspect of motor planning focuses on facilitating the client's understanding of how an object is used or a gesture is performed. Remedial techniques involve practicing the ability to use gestures, objects, or pantomime according to a hierarchical treatment sequence and have been described in the literature (Cubelli, Trentini, & Montagna, 1991; Helm-Estabrooks, 1982; Pilgrim & Humphreys, 1994; Smania, Girardi, Domenicali, Lora, & Aglioti, 2000).

Strategy Training

Clients may be taught to use verbal, visual, or tactile cues to enhance movement. For example, the client may be taught a mental practice strategy. Before performing an activity, the client imagines himself or herself performing the activity in a smooth, accurate, and coordinated manner. Asking the client to arrange a picture or action sequence of the activity may enhance visual imagery or mental practice. In addition, the person may be asked to imagine how an object should look in his or her hand before picking it up. For example, imagine the orientation of the object, the way the fingers should be positioned, and so forth. Incorrect patterns of movement, such as holding an object the wrong way, can also be visualized with an emphasis on having the client mentally practice correcting the movement.

In addition to visual mental practice, the person can be taught to verbally rehearse an action sequence by going over the steps out loud and then gradually whispering the steps and then saying them silently. Self-monitoring strategies can be used to teach a client to monitor unnecessary cocontraction, incomplete actions, or difficulty in switching direction of movements.

Another strategy is to teach the client to associate the movement pattern with a rhyme, rhythm, musical tune, visual image, or word. Initially, the musical tune or rhythm may be provided externally; then, gradually, the client should imagine the rhythm or tune silently to himself or herself while performing the activity.

Adaptation of Task or Environment

Attention to the critical features of an activity can facilitate action and motor planning. Techniques that increase the saliency of critical features include the following:

- Colored tape on the handle of a drawer, utensil, or faucet to assist the client in proper grasp placement.
- Use of a florescent colored ball to make it easier to catch or hit.
- Use of a colored nail to make it easier to hit with a hammer.

Attention to the wrong cue or less important cues can result in an inappropriate motor response and can interfere with actions. Thus patterns and designs on utensils, clothing, or other items should be avoided. In addition, tool use should be minimized or eliminated (Poole, 2000).

Other adaptations include training the caregiver to modify instructions so that the activity is broken into one command at a time (Lamm-Warburg, 1988). Simple whole commands (e.g., "Get up") may put the activity on an automatic level and effectively enhance motor planning (Zoltan, 1996).

Adaptive equipment should be selected with caution for the apraxic client. For example, some adaptations—such as a button hook, one-handed can opener, reacher, one-handed shoe tying, and one-arm drive wheelchair—may be confusing for clients with apraxia and may place greater demands on motor planning abilities. Other adaptations—such as elastic-waist trousers, elastic buttons, hook-and-loop tape fasteners, wash mitts, slip on shoes, and elastic shoelaces—may simplify the task or motor pattern required to manipulate or hold objects, reduce the number of steps, and facilitate function in the client with apraxia.

Memory

Specific Skill Training

Tabletop or computerized **memory** exercises and drills have been used to attempt to remediate memory. Although memory has been shown to improve on specific training tasks, there is no evidence that repetitive practice of word lists or objects, generalizes to other material (Cicerone et al., 2000).

Memory deficits can be closely related to other cognitive deficits, particularly attention. Some investigators have suggested that an indirect approach that addresses other cognitive skills, such as attention or organization, rather than memory itself, may be most effective. Although intervention does not directly address memory, it is expected to increase as a result of improvement in other cognitive skills (Toglia, 1993). For example, Sohlberg and Mateer (1989a) reported improvement in memory function after a remedial attentional program. In addition to remedial approaches, functional skill training and errorless learning, as described in the beginning of this section, have been used successfully to teach clients with severe memory disorders to complete rote but complex tasks.

Strategy Training

Another method commonly used to address memory problems is the training of internal strategies. Memory strategies may be directed primarily at encoding operations (getting information in) or the retrieval phase of memory (getting information out). Encoding strategies include the following:

- Chunking or grouping similar items together.
- The story method or linking a series of facts or events into a story.
- Rehearsal or repeating information over and over silently.
- Rhymes or recalling a fact by changing the fact into a rhyme.
- Visual imagery.

Retrieval strategies include the following:

- Alphabetical searching or going through the alphabet letter by letter attempting to find the first letter of a forgotten item.
- Retracing one's steps to find a missing object or to recall an event.
- Thinking of associated information to cue the recall of a new fact or event.

Training in internal strategies is most appropriate for people with mild memory deficits or those who have other areas of cognition intact (Tate, 1997). The client needs to practice using one or two targeted memory strategies in a variety of different tasks, such as remembering a telephone number, news headlines or events, items that need to be bought in a store, stories, or instructions to an activity (Harrell et al., 1992). During practice on different memory tasks, a variety of self-monitoring techniques may also be used (Toglia, 1993).

Memory External Strategies and Aids

External aids such as notebooks, tape recorders, and computers store information that the person may have difficulty remembering. Other aids, such as pagers or alarm signals, serve to remind a person to perform an action. External memory aids include the following:

- Timers.
- Tape recorders.
- Devices with preprogrammed alarms or alarm messages.
- Electronic devices such as pagers, cell phones, and pocket computers.
- Computers.
- Pill box organizers.
- Lists.
- Daily planners.
- Notebooks.

Case studies have documented the effectiveness of external aids (Kim, Burke, Dowds, & George, 1999; Wade & Troy, 2001; Wilson, Emslie, Quirk, & Evans, 2001). A review of the literature concluded that there is level 1 evidence that demonstrates that compensatory memory training in individuals with mild memory impairments reduces everyday memory failures. Intervention is most effective when the client is motivated, involved in identifying the memory problem, and is fairly independent in daily function (Cicerone et al., 2000).

Recently, the success of a paging system in significantly reducing everyday memory failures in clients was demonstrated in a randomized control trial (Wilson et al., 2001). In addition, evidence obtained from case studies supports the use of memory notebooks and other external aids for those with moderate to severe memory impairments (Cicerone et al., 2000, Kerns & Thomson, 1998; Kim et al., 1999; Wade & Troy, 2001). However, the successful use of

TABLE 30–14. **OBSTACLES TO THE USE OF A MEMORY BOOK AND TECHNIQUES FOR OVERCOMING THEM**[a]

Obstacle	Techniques
Decreased insight into memory problems	• Use book that looks normal or inconspicuous • Write explanation for book and place inside cover of book • Videotape or audiotape discussion involving importance of book • Highlight forgotten information during rereading • Use of prediction and estimation techniques
Initiate carrying memory book	• Book is kept in a consistent location • Signs in room, on door, etc. say "Take book" • Book is a distinctive color (yellow, orange) • Positive reinforcement, praise, or points for carrying book
Difficulty initiating writing and rereading memory book	• Preprogrammed message alarms • Posted signs ("Read book") • Positive reinforcement; scoring system • Use during therapy—not after • Consistent daily time schedule for writing or rereading book • Log in immediately after an event or session—gradually lengthen time of entries
Difficulty finding the correct place to write in the book	• A system for discarding old or useless information • Daily review of notebook sections • Start with only one or two color-coded sections • Bookmark sticky note to mark the page and date to write on
Difficulty including the relevant information	• Structured note taking; each page contains an outline; gradually reduce the structure • Practice asking others to clarify or summarize conversations to assist journal entry • Increase effectiveness and efficiency of note taking; practice summarizing; identifying the main point of articles and conversations • Place check mark or star next to "good" entries • Practice in reducing notes to key retrieval cues; single words or short phrases

[a]Adapted from Toglia (1996).

an external memory aid may require extensive training. The client needs to practice initiating and using the aid in a variety of different situations.

The use of external aids may need to be graded during intervention. In the initial stages, the client may be expected to use the aid only when its use is initiated by another person. Gradually, the client may be trained to initiate the use of the aid independently. The number of times the person initiates or carries the external aid can be charted, graphed, or awarded points to provide concrete positive feedback and enhance motivation. The most commonly used external memory strategy is the memory notebook. The memory notebook needs to be designed with the person's needs and lifestyle in mind. Sample sections in a memory notebook are as follows:

- Personal facts.
- Names of people to remember.
- Calendar and schedule.
- Things to do (daily, within next week).
- Daily log of important events.
- Conversations.
- Important upcoming events.
- Summary of readings (articles, newspaper).
- Medication schedule.
- Directions to frequently traveled places.

Initially, the notebook should begin with one or two sections and gradually increase if the client is able to handle it. Table 30-14 lists some of the common obstacles that need to be addressed during memory notebook training.

Memory notebook training needs to take place within the context of a variety of everyday activities. Therapy sessions should include role playing and practice in use of the notebook. For example, the client may be asked to:

- Summarize simulated or actual conversations.
- Take telephone messages.
- Listen and summarize the news or an interview on the radio or television.
- Summarize an article.
- Summarize the key steps in a new recipe, game, or activity.

In addition, the client may be asked questions that involve reviewing and rereading the memory notebook.

Specific memory notebook training protocols have been described in the literature (Donaghy & Williams 1998; Sohlberg & Mateer 1989b).

Adaptations of Task or Environment

Tasks and environments can be rearranged so that they place fewer requirements on memory:

- Cue cards or signs in key places (e.g.. sign on door to be read before leaving: "Take keys and . . .")
- Labeling the outside of drawers or closets to minimize the need to recall the location of items.
- Providing step-by-step directions to reduce memory demands.
- Providing checklists to assist in keeping track of task steps.

Significant others can be trained to use methods that increase the likelihood that the client will remember material, such as asking the client to repeat any instructions or important information in his or her own words; encouraging the client to ask questions; and presenting material in small groups, clusters, or categories (Wilson, 1995).

Executive Functions: Higher-Level Cognitive Functions

Specific Skill Training

Executive functions are best addressed with unstructured tasks that require the person to initiate and plan goals, monitor time, make choices, and establish priorities. Commercial games such as MasterMind, Sequence, and Othello can be modified and graded to address planning skills, cognitive flexibility, and problem solving. Typical remedial tasks include logic worksheets, logic grids, and puzzles such as the Tower of London and Tower of Hanoi.

Strategy Training

Verbal mediation has been reported to be an effective strategy in improving executive function and self-regulation deficits (Van Cramon, Matthes-Von Cramon, & Mai, 1991). For example, Cicerone and Wood (1987) reported the successful use of a self-instructional procedure in a client with impaired planning ability and poor self-control secondary to brain injury. Intervention involved requiring the client to verbalize a plan of action before and during execution of a task. Gradually, the client was instructed to whisper, rather than talk aloud, and eventually to talk silently to himself. Generalization to real-life situations was observed after an extended period of time that included training in self-monitoring.

Training in problem-solving strategies involves teaching the client to break down complex activities into smaller and more manageable steps. Strategies may also aim to help the person maintain the focus of goals and intentions (Levine et al., 2000). A literature review by Cicerone et al. (2000) concluded that there is level 2 evidence to support the use of formal problem-solving training with application to everyday activities. The authors recommended such training as a practice guideline for individuals with stroke or traumatic brain injury during postacute rehabilitation (Cicerone et al., 2000). The intervention goal is to replace an impulsive and disorganized approach with a systematic and controlled approach to planning activities, maintaining goal intentions, and solving problems. The steps of the problem–solving process are reinforced with use of self-questioning techniques. For example, self-questioning cue cards with the following types of questions can be used during problem-solving tasks:

- What do I need to do?
- Do I need more information?
- What do I have to do next?
- Am I getting stuck in one approach?
- Have I identified all the critical information?
- Do I understand the problem?
- Am I getting side tracked by irrelevant details?
- What are all the possible solutions? Did I choose the best one?

These problem-solving strategies can be practiced in simulated or actual everyday problem-solving situations. Table 30-15 provides a description of the features of simple and complex problem-solving tasks.

Broad checklists or task guidance systems are commonly used to assist the client in initiating, planning, and carrying out an activity systematically. Checklists may be specific to a particular activity (e.g., checklist for making a salad) or they may be designed broadly so that they can be used in a variety of similar activities (e.g., checklist for food preparation or cooking activities).

Intervention should incorporate practice in identifying the situations or activities in which use of a checklist may be helpful. The client may be given the opportunity to practice the same activity with and without the use of a checklist to enhance awareness. Initially, the goal may be to have a client follow a checklist established by the practitioner or significant other. Eventually, the client may be given checklists with missing steps, and asked to review the lists to identify the missing components. Finally, the client may be required to create a checklist independently. Burke, Zencius, Wesolowskis, and Doubleday (1991) described four cases of individuals with executive dysfunction for whom checklists were successfully used to improve the ability to carry out routine vocational tasks.

Decreased initiation, one of the hallmark features of executive dysfunction, can significantly interfere with the ability to use and apply a learned strategy. For example, a person with deficits in executive functions may use a strategy effectively when cued but may not use the strategy spontaneously because of a failure to initiate its use. External cues such as alarm

TABLE 30–15. **ACTIVITY GRADING FOR PROBLEM SOLVING**[a]

Activity Parameter	Simple	Complex	Demands with Increased Complexity	Complex Treatment Tasks
Identify problem	Immediate problem is clear and readily apparent (shampoo bottle is empty; toaster is unplugged)	Requires sorting out information to determine where the real problem exists	Places greater demand on initiation, exploration, attention to the environment and the ability to predict ahead and establish goals	Emphasis on problem recognition or selection of goals; recognize that a bill entry is missing in a checkbook activity
Define problem precisely	All the necessary information is presented; small amount of information relevant to the problem is presented	Requires searching for additional information needed to solve the problem; large amount of information—both relevant and irrelevant—is included	Greater demands on selective attention strategies, choosing priorities, simultaneously attending to details, and keeping the whole situation in mind; requires processing of multiple information and strategies for keeping track of a large number of factors	Emphasis on discriminating between relevant and irrelevant information (identifying relevant information in a travel advertisement or "Find the two least-expensive restaurants that deliver lunch in the area.")
Explore possible strategies	Limited choices and solutions; problem may be approached in only one or two ways; can be solved with trial and error	Many different possibilities	Requires ability to generate, plan, test, and reject different hypotheses and formulate alternative solutions; greater demands on flexibility and abstract thinking	Generation of ideas and alternatives ("How many different combination of coins can make 65¢?" "You are going to visit a friend in another state for 2 weeks. List everything you will need to do before you leave." "Now you are going away for 3 months. How would you revise your list?")
Act	One to three steps; external time monitor	Multiple steps; internally monitoring time	Greater demands on self-regulation and self-monitoring of behaviors and time	Set a time goal and ask client to monitor time during an activity
Look at the effects	Incorrect solution is readily apparent and prevents success	Incorrect solution is not readily apparent; requires actively comparing solution with original problem	Requires greater self-monitoring strategies.	Have client fill out a structured self-evaluation rating form or checklist; gradually reduce the structure of the rating form

[a]Adapted from Toglia (1996).

signals may be used to prompt the client to initiate a task or use a particular strategy within an activity (Evans, Emslie, & Wilson, 1998). An alarm signal programmed to go off every 10 or 15 min can cue the individual to use a checklist or to self-evaluate his or her work before continuing. Preprogrammed alarm messages (on a watch or electronic scheduler) can cue the client to initiate an errand, make an important telephone call, take mediations, or go to an appointment.

Adaptations of Task or Environment

Adaptations that minimize demands on executive functions and problem-solving skills include training a significant other to preorganize an activity or activity materials. For example, all the items needed for grooming can be prearranged on the sink in the sequence in which they are used. As an alternative, one task step can be introduced at a time. These adaptations limit the need for planning and organization (Mateer, 1999).

People who have difficulty with initiation, organization, and decision making require structure. Open-ended questions such as "What do you want to eat?" should be avoided. Clients who have difficulty in initiation have a great deal of difficulty in answering open-ended questions. Questions should provide a limited number of choices whenever feasible.

A predictable and structured daily routine enhances the client's ability to initiate tasks and should be established and monitored by a significant other. Audiotape instructions that cue the client to initiate an activity and perform each step at a time in its proper sequence have been reported to be successful. Schwartz (1995) described the use of a tape recorder with a personalized message and automatic timer to prompt a client with executive dysfunction to begin his morning routine. The tape included questions that elicited verbal responses such as, " When you see the three S's [shower, shave and shampoo] what do you do?" To reinforce the tape message, written cues were placed on the bedroom door directing the client to the bathroom. After 3 months, the client completed two to three of the five morning activities daily. Eventually, the tape-recorded message was discontinued, and the client was effectively able to progress to a checklist.

CONCLUSION

The different intervention approaches discussed in this section all ultimately aim to enhance engagement and participation in occupation(s). Some of the approaches seek to do this by emphasizing change in the activity demands and context, and others seek to change the client's behavior or skills. The extent to which learning and awareness are required for success differs among the approaches and needs to be considered in designing intervention. In clinical practice, a combination of techniques that aim to change the person, activity, and context is recommended. However, at times it may be appropriate to emphasize one aspect more than another. The decisions about what to treat and how to treat it constitute complex clinical reasoning processes that depend on the practitioner's conceptualization of cognitive function and dysfunction as well as the client's level of awareness, potential for learning, and emotional-psychological characteristics and the performance context.

Intervention for people with cognitive–perceptual impairments has moved away from the use of isolated tabletop and computerized remedial exercises. Newer approaches such as the quadraphonic approach (Abreu, 1998, 1999) and the multicontext approach (Toglia, 1991a, 1998) have emerged that encourage the practitioner to integrate information regarding the person's personality, interests, daily occupations, and lifestyle into an individually tailored treatment program. The focus on identifying and treating separate cognitive perceptual skills has diminished in favor of an information-processing perspective.

There is documentation that supports the effectiveness of strategy training (Cicerone, et al., 2000; Fasotti, et al., 2000; Landa-Gonzalez, 2001; Niemeier et al., 2001; Trexler et al., 1994). The role of awareness and meta-cognitive training has been increasingly emphasized within cognitive rehabilitation since the 1990s (Barco et al., 1991; Katz & Hatrman-Maier, 1998; Prigatano, 1999; Tham et al., 2001). In addition, studies in cognitive rehabilitation reflect a trend toward incorporating a wider variety of intervention tasks, including practice within functional contexts (Antonucciet et al., 1995; Levine et al., 2000; Niemeier et al., 2001). Finally, there is an acknowledgment that the different intervention approaches are not mutually exclusive but can be integrated and used simultaneously to promote engagement in occupations.

SECTION VI

Process Skills

ROBIN T. UNDERWOOD

DEFINITION OF SKILLS

To perform daily occupations successfully, an individual must perform certain actions. The observable elements of these actions, which have implicit functional purposes, are referred to as skills. Fisher and co-workers described both

BOX 30–1 KEY CONCEPTS PROCESS SKILLS DOMAINS AND SKILLS[a]

Energy pertains to sustained and appropriately allocated mental energy.
Paces: Maintains a rate or tempo of performance across an entire task.
Attends: Maintains attention focused on the task.

Knowledge is the ability to seek and use knowledge.
Chooses: Selects appropriate tools and materials.
Uses: Employs tools and materials according to their intended purposes.
Handles: Supports, stabilizes, and holds tools and materials in an appropriate manner.
Heeds: Uses goal-directed task performance that is focused toward the completion of the intended task.
Inquires: Seeks appropriate spoken or written information by asking questions or reading directions.

Temporal organization pertains to the beginning, logical ordering, continuation, and completion of the steps and action sequences of a task.
Initiates: Starts or begins doing an action or step without hesitation.
Continues: Performs an action sequence of a step without unnecessary interruption and as an unbroken, smooth progression.
Sequences: Performs steps in an effective or logical order for efficient use of time and energy.
Terminates: Finishes or brings to completion single actions or steps without perseveration, inappropriate persistence, or premature cessation.

Organizing space and objects pertains to skills for organizing space and objects.
Searches/locates: Looks for and locates tools and materials through the process of logical searching.
Gathers: Collects together needed or misplaced tools and materials.
Organizes: Logically positions or spatially arranges tools and materials in an orderly fashion and in between appropriate workspaces.
Restores: Returns and puts away tools and materials and restores immediate workspaces to original condition.
Navigates: Modifies the movement of the arm, body, or wheelchair to avoid or to maneuver around existing obstacles that are encountered in the course of moving the arm, body, or wheelchair through space.

Adaptation relates to the ability to anticipate, correct for, and benefit by learning from the consequences or errors that arise in the course of action.
Notices/responds: Responds appropriately to nonverbal environmental and perceptual cues that provide feedback regarding task progression.
Accommodates: Modifies action or location of objects within the work space in course of anticipation or in response to circumstances or problems that might arise in the course of action or to avoid undesirable outcomes.
Adjusts: Changes environmental conditions in anticipation of or in response to circumstances and problems that arise in the course of action or to avoid undesirable outcomes.
Benefits: Anticipates and prevents undesirable circumstances or problems from recurring or persisting.

[a]Reprinted with permission from Fisher and Kielhofner (1995).

motor and process skills, which they identified through a review of information processing, sensory integration, and motor control literature (Fisher & Kielhofner, 1995). Fisher's (1999) work eventually led to the development of the Assessment of Motor and Process Skills (AMPS). Motor skills and their underlying constituents are discussed in several other sections of this text. Process skills are the focus of this section. The following definitions and descriptions of process skills are based on the work of Fisher, Kielhofner, and their co-workers (Fisher & Kielhofner, 1995; Fisher, Liu, Velozo, & Pan, 1992; Nygard, Bernspang, Fisher, & Windblad, 1994; Pan & Fisher, 1994; Park, Fisher, & Velozo, 1994).

DEFINITION OF PROCESS SKILLS

Process skills are the skills that humans use in managing and modifying actions during the completion of daily occupations. Process skills are observable actions related to underlying attentional, conceptual, organizational, and adaptive capacities of the person. (Fisher & Kielhofner, 1995). They are related to cognitive skills, but they are not the same. Process skills are observable actions carried out in a definitive manner, which leads to accomplishment of an occupational form. Cognitive skills are underlying and unobservable processes such as memory, attention, and problem solving that vary across process skills and the tasks performed. When an occupational therapy practitioner is working with a client on process skill improvement, the attention is focused on the actual doing or the performance versus the amount of underlying capacity. There are five domains of process skills, and each domain has several skills within it (Box 30-1).

PROCESS SKILL DOMAINS

Energy

The energy domain is included in both the motor and process skill performance areas, but within the process skill area, it is defined as the sustained and appropriately allocated mental energy skills. Paces and attends are the skills within this domain. The skill of paces is observed when the client maintains a rate or tempo of performance across an entire task. The skill of attends is demonstrated when the client maintains attention focused on the task. For example, when doing a budget, the client is not distracted from the task by other stimulation and does not focus too much on certain parts of the budget while ignoring others.

Knowledge

Skills within the knowledge domain relate to the ability to seek and use knowledge that will yield goal-directed task performance. A person has to understand or be able to conceptualize the task and determine the necessary objects and actions that will result in successful task performance. The different skills under this domain are chooses, uses, handles, heeds, and inquires. The skill of chooses is defined as the selection of appropriate tools and materials. The skill of uses is observed when a person employs the tools and materials according to its intended purposes. Handles refers to the skill when the tools and materials are supported, stabilized, and held in an appropriate manner. Heeds is the skill demonstrated when a person uses goal-directed task performance that focuses on the completion of the intended task. The skill of inquires is when the appropriate oral or written information is sought by asking questions or by reading directions.

Temporal Organization

The skills in the domain of temporal organization relate to the beginning, logical ordering, continuity, and completion of the steps and action sequences of a task. The process skill of initiates relates to the start or beginning of the performance of an action or step without hesitation or delays. The skill of continues is observed when an action sequence of a step is performed without unnecessary interruption and as an unbroken, smooth progression. Sequences is the skill by which the steps of a task are performed in an effective or logical order for efficient use of time and energy. The skill of terminates is demonstrated when the actions or steps are completed without perseveration, inappropriate persistence, or premature cessation.

Organizing Space and Objects

The organizing space and objects domain includes skills for performance of occupations within a physical world. This includes finding and arranging necessary materials and tools, negotiating the body among the physical objects, and terminating an occupation by putting away tools and materials. The skill of searches/locates relates to the ability to look for and locate tools and materials through a process of logical searching. Gathers is the skill of collecting together needed or misplaced tools for task performance. The skill of organizing relates to the logical positioning or the spatial arrangement of tools and materials in an orderly fashion and in between appropriate workspaces. Restores is the skill of returning/putting away tools and materials and restoring the workspace to the condition before the task performance. The skill of navigation is the modification of movement patterns of the body or wheelchair to avoid or to maneuver around existing obstacles that are encountered as moving through space during task performance.

Adaptation

The process skill domain of adaptation relates to the ability to anticipate, correct for, and benefit by learning from the consequences or errors that arise in the course of action. The process skill of notices/responds is defined as the appropriate response to nonverbal environmental/perceptual cues that provide feedback regarding the progression of the task. Accommodates is the skill of modifying actions or the location of objects within a workspace in anticipation of, or in response to, circumstances or problems that might arise during action and/or to avoid undesirable outcomes. The skill of adjusts is observed when the environmental conditions are changed in anticipation of, or in response to circumstances or problems that may arise during action and/or to avoid undesirable outcomes. Finally, the skill of benefits relates to the anticipation and prevention of undesirable circumstances or problems from recurring or continuing.

INTERVENTIONS FOR IMPROVING PROCESS SKILLS

Intervention is based on the client's concerns along with the therapist's evaluation findings and involves planning, implementation, and review. The following subsections describe the stages along with strategies to use during each one. Refer to Case Study 30-4 which provides background information about Mrs. Thomas. Determine the process skills that Mrs. Thomas exhibits and the ones that she has difficulties performing. Then think about what methods are appropriate for each stage of her intervention.

Stage 1: Intervention Plan

Activity Analysis

An activity analysis before the client performs the occupation is essential when working with a client on process skill improvement. For the occupational therapy practitioner to determine if the client is performing these skills effectively, the therapist must understand all aspects of the occupation (see Chapter 16). In the case of Mrs. Thomas, the occupational therapist goes to the assisted living center to analyze the task of getting food from the buffet table. She notes noise and activity during the meal and gets clarification

CASE STUDY 30-4

Mrs. Thomas: In an Assisted Living Center

Mrs. Thomas is 80 years old and has been living alone in her own home for the 20 years, since her husband died. Her son and daughter note that she has had increasing difficulty performing her homemaking tasks over the past 6 months. They are also concerned about Mrs. Thomas's social isolation and some periodic incidences of confusion. When they have taken her out to events where there are a large number of people, they have observed Mrs. Thomas having difficulties navigating through the crowds and paying attention. They suggest that their mother consider entering an assisted living center, and Mrs. Thomas has agreed to this plan.

The staff members at the assisted living center evaluate Mrs. Thomas for admission, but they are concerned about her being able to perform the required tasks independently. For example, Mrs. Thomas has to serve herself meals from a buffet table and she has to be independent in social participation in the dining room and during community outings. Before the decision regarding admission to the center is made, an occupational therapy assessment is requested to determine whether Mrs. Thomas can perform these tasks.

The occupational therapist observes Mrs. Thomas on two different occasions while she is serving herself from a buffet table at the assisted living center. Mrs. Thomas was instructed to go through the buffet line and to serve herself food. The following are the therapist's observations of Mrs. Thomas's performance of this task:

SESSION 1: IN THE DINING AREA

Mrs. Thomas appeared hesitant to begin gathering up a plate and utensils, requiring encouragement from the therapist to begin the task. She independently chose her plate and used the spoons correctly for serving herself from the serving containers. She demonstrated difficulty with reaching under the buffet hood to scoop up food when the container was far away from her. She gave up attempting to place certain foods on her plate after having difficulties a couple of times. She became distracted frequently, especially when other people moved around her. She appeared to take a few minutes to recall what she had been doing, and then she attended to the food again. She was given several reminders to continue going through the buffet line. She did read the labels on the salad dressings before deciding which dressing to place on her salad. She overfilled her plate and periodically dropped food items on the buffet table or floor. She did not seem to notice this. After her plate was completely full of salad items, she then stated that she wanted to have a meat item also and that she did not know what to do about this. She needed verbal cues to put the salad plate down at her table and to then get another plate for the meat.

SESSION 2: IN THE DINING AREA

Mrs. Thomas performed the task much the same as she did the first time. She made the same error of filling up her plate with salad and then wanting a meat dish also. Again, she looked toward the therapist to direct her regarding what to do about this.

QUESTIONS AND EXERCISES

1. Which processing skills appear to be intact for Mrs. Thomas?
2. Which processing skills are problematic for Mrs. Thomas?

about the performance expectations that the assisted living center staff have for their residents.

Context

When attempting to facilitate improvement of process skills, considerations of cultural, physical, social, temporal, and spiritual contexts are extremely important. Lave's (1988) research on learning in everyday life indicates that actions represent a complex interaction of the person acting and the setting in which he or she is performing. Physical context considerations are highlighted in this section because they relate to decisions about the location of the performance of the occupation. Clients' process skills performance may be different in different physical contexts or settings.

In a study designed specifically to look at process skills, researchers found a significant difference between process skills exhibited by older adults performing IADL within their own homes and those within clinic environments (Park et al., 1994). These findings support the hypothesis that process skills abilities are affected by the environment more than motor skill abilities. The implication is, when possible, the occupational therapy practitioner should have the client perform in his or her natural environment. In Mrs. Thomas's case, this is at the assisted living center dining room during mealtime.

The location of the intervention also influences the degree to which the individual can demonstrate existing skills and can learn new skills. Furthermore, the ability to generalize these skills and develop solutions that can be applied in a variety of situations often requires that interventions be practiced in a variety of contexts. When newly learned skills or strategies are applied to multiple situations or environments, research suggests that there is greater facilitation of learning transfer (Detterman & Sternberg, 1994; see also Chapter 21). Therefore, if transfer and generalization of process skills are the objectives of the intervention, facilitation of the performance of targeted process skills within multiple tasks and in multiple settings needs to be part of the intervention. In Mrs. Thomas's situation, facilitation of process skills may also be done in her apartment, in a restaurant, or in another community setting.

Determination of Intervention Strategies

When planning the intervention strategy for facilitation of process skill performance, the therapist must decide whether to use restoration, adaptation, or a combination of both approaches. The focus of restoration is on restoring or remediating impairments as opposed to adaptation, in which the focus is on changing the task or the environment (Moyers, 1999; see also Chapter 27).

Decisions regarding the intervention approaches are driven by multiple factors, including frames of reference, diagnostic issues (diagnosis and prognosis), venue of care, (hospital versus home or community setting), and pragmatic constraints (payment options, limited time of intervention, and the intervention environment) (Moyers, 1999). Another important consideration when planning the intervention is whether to use the occupation as both a means and an end. Occupation is used as a means when it is acting as a therapeutic change agent to remediate the process skill deficits. It is an end when the practitioner organizes the meaningful task for successful completion (Trombly, 1995). An example of this is working with Mrs. Thomas on increasing her independence in the dining room. While she practices the occupation, she also improves her ability to attend, pace, etc. If transfer and generalization of learning are desired, then it makes sense to use the occupation as both a means and an end.

Stage 2: Intervention Implementation

Restoration

If remediation of skills or restoration is the focus, the occupational therapist plans methods for facilitating the development of process skills and related performance of the occupation. Within this intervention strategy, the occupational therapy practitioner may attempt to first change the biological, psychological, or neurological processes to facilitate improved performance (Moyers, 1999). For example, the sensory stimulation from the center exercise group provides Mrs. Thomas with visual, auditory, proprioceptive, vestibular, and kinesthetic stimulation. This, it is hoped, will yield improved alertness so that she can demonstrate increased pacing and attending during the task.

Restoration strategies also include teaching the skills to the client. This strategy is appropriate when working on process skill improvement, because the focus is on changed behaviors and, therefore, recognizable actions. Occupational therapy practitioners use behavioral, cognitive behavioral, and information-processing theories of learning.

Occupational therapy practitioners have an important role in providing the opportunities for clients to learn process skills. Some clients may have difficulty performing process skills related to certain occupations because they have had little or no opportunity to perform them. This would seem to be the true in Mrs. Thomas's case, due to her increased social isolation. According to the International Classification of Function (World Health Organization, 2001), this is an example of a participation restriction.

When doing skill training as an intervention, occupational therapy practitioners may need to need to sit on their hands while their clients struggle with the performance of a certain skill or while clients take time to figure out how to perform the skill. In these cases, it is imperative that practitioners do not step in to assist clients prematurely. During these sessions, practitioners often take on the role of a coach during client performance of process skills. To facilitate learning, practitioners watch the performance and determine when to give cues or prompts or demonstrations for enhanced skill performance. Throughout the performance, practitioners give clients positive reinforcement and feedback about their skills.

Compensation

An adaptation approach involves adapting the task objects, changing the task methods, modifying the environment, and/or training the family or caregiver (Moyers, 1999). The occupational therapy practitioner may wait to introduce compensation techniques until remediation/restoration has been exhausted. However, compensatory techniques may be used immediately if the practitioner thinks that there is little chance for remediation/restoration or if there is a limited time for the client to do something independently. In Mrs. Thomas's case, a combination of intervention strategies is used because of the potential for skill improvement and the limited time before she enters the assisted living center.

Stage 3: Intervention Review

Throughout the coaching of skill performance, occupational therapy practitioners are continually assessing the client's ability to perform process skills. Practitioners make note of client successes and how much cuing, prompting, teaching, and encouragement have to be done during skill performance. Also, practitioners reflect on the amount of task and/or environmental adaptations used during skill building. Practitioners perform these analyses to decide whether the client is making progress and to analyze what intervention strategies facilitated the skill improvement. Based on these factors, practitioners decide what strategies to use during subsequent intervention sessions. If continued skill improvement is indicated, the practitioner may decide to grade the task during the next session, to make it more of a skills challenge for the client. The practitioner may also decide that a compensation strategy is indicated and may intersperse this with the remediation strategies. Any changes in intervention strategies are discussed with the client during future sessions.

CONCLUSION

Many factors need to be considered when planning and implementing interventions to facilitate client improvement in process skills. The occupational therapy practitioner must plan interventions that are meaningful to the client and that will facilitate generalization of learning. Both restoration and adaptation strategies may be used to promote improved process skill performance and independence in desired occupations.

SECTION VII

Pain Management

JOYCE M. ENGEL

The problem of chronic **pain** has reached outrageous proportions and exhausts great economic resources. Recent statistics indicate 50 million Americans experience chronic pain and most are significantly disabled by it, sometimes permanently (American Academy of Pain Medicine [AAPM], 2001; Brownlee & Schrof, 1997). Approximately 45% of all Americans pursue care for persistent pain at some point in their lives (AAPM, 2001). The economic impact of **chronic pain** is alarming. Back pain, migraine headaches, and arthritis alone account for medical costs of $40 billion annually, and pain is the cause of 25% of all sick days taken yearly. The annual total cost (direct medical expenses, lost income, lost productivity, compensation payments and legal fees) of all chronic pain syndromes is at least $100 billion. Moreover, the costs of suffering cannot be estimated.

Despite the magnitude of suffering, chronic pain is often undertreated. The reasons for this include the low priority of pain relief in the health-care system, lack of knowledge of pain interventions among clients and health professionals, and fear of opioid addiction (American Academy of Pain Medicine and American Pain Society [AAPM], 1997; Brownlee & Schrof, 1997). Unrelieved pain has many negative consequences, including a decline in a person's occupational performance, and may compromise role competence.

DEFINING PAIN

Pain has typically been conceptualized as a neurophysiological event that involves a complex pattern of emotional and psychological arousal. By definition, "Pain is an unpleasant sensory and emotional experience associated with actual or potential tissue damage or described in terms of such damage" (International Association for the Study of Pain—Ad hoc Subcommittee for Occupational Therapy/Physical Therapy Curriculum [IASP], 1979). This definition emphasizes the multidimensional nature as well as the inherent subjectivity of pain. Individual variables, such as mood, prior pain experiences, and culture, are known to affect an individual's perception of pain (Turk & Melzack, 1992). It should be noted that an inability to communicate in no way negates the possibility that an individual is experiencing pain and is in need of appropriate pain-relieving intervention.

Although definitions of pain vary, most authors agree that acute and chronic pain should be differentiated. Differentiating acute from chronic pain is essential for using the appropriate evaluation and intervention strategies. Pain associated with tissue damage, irritation, inflammation, or a disease process that is relatively brief (hours, days, weeks), regardless of intensity, is referred to as **acute pain** (e.g., post-surgical pain). Acute pain serves a biological or adaptive purpose by directing attention to injury, irritation, or disease and by signaling the necessity for immobilization and protection of an injured area, such as a fracture. Fortunately, acute pain usually responds to medication and treatment of the underlying cause of pain (Hawthorn & Redmond, 1998).

In contrast, pain that persists for extended periods of time (months or years), that accompanies a disease (e.g., arthritis pain), or is associated with an injury that has not resolved within the expected time frame (e.g., low back pain) is referred to as chronic pain (Turk & Melzack, 1992). This pain serves no biologic purpose. Chronic pain typically produces significant changes in personality, lifestyle, and occupational performance (Hawthorn & Redmond, 1998).

OCCUPATIONAL THERAPY EVALUATION OF PAIN

Pain is a primary reason for seeking health care. A referral for occupational therapy evaluation is made when pain interferes with the client's mood and performance of occupations. Occupational therapy practitioners focus evaluation on psychosocial and environmental factors that contribute to the client's pain perception and the effects of pain on occupational performance. Proper evaluation requires the use of valid and reliable instruments for determining pain interference before and after intervention. Several methods for pain evaluation have been used to assess chronic pain.

Behavioral

Behavioral evaluation is used to identify behaviors in need of change and to identify environmental variables that trigger specific pain behaviors (Fordyce, 1976).

Overt

Overt behaviors, or observable pain behaviors, are commonly targeted in evaluation. Such pain behaviors include guarded movement, bracing, posturing, limping, rubbing, and facial grimacing, all of which suggest discomfort (Keefe & Block, 1982). The Pain Behavior Checklist is an example of a standardized rating scale that is valid, reliable, and easy to use for documenting overt pain behaviors (Turk, Wack, & Kerns, 1985). Analysis of the client's overt behaviors before, during, and after intervention can provide valuable information about the role of environmental and learned factors in that individual's pain perception and responses to intervention. Merskey (1992), however, cautions clinicians not to provide treatment for reducing overt pain behaviors in lieu of attempts at alleviating pain. Evaluation that focuses solely on observable pain behaviors may lead to the inaccurate conclusion that pain behavior suggests malingering, lack of motivation, or hypochondriasis.

Covert

Covert behaviors or self-reports of pain are also assessed, since pain is believed to be a private experience. The clinical interview focuses on the client's identification of pain onset, location, intensity, frequency, duration, exacerbating and relieving pain factors, past and current pain interventions, mood, occupational performance, and goals. Self-report is considered the gold standard for the assessment of pain. The Descriptive Pain Intensity Scale, 0–10 Numeric Pain Intensity Scale, or Visual Analog Scale can be used in assessing self-reports of pain. All of these scales are easy to use and can be adapted to the client's vocabulary (Jensen & Karoly, 1992).

Occupational performance is the primary focus of the occupational therapy practitioner. The client may complete daily activity diaries as an assessment technique and outcome measure (Follick, Ahern, & Laser-Wolston, 1984). After extensive training, the client makes hourly entries of time spent sitting, standing, reclining, and other productive activities, which may be corroborated by trained personnel. The Brief Pain Inventory is a valid and reliable instrument that may also be used to measure how much pain interferes with occupational performance and mood (Cleeland, 1991). Clients rate on an ordinal scale of 0 (does not interfere) to 10 (completely interferes) how much pain interferes with general activity, mood, walking, work, social activity, relations with others, and sleep. This information may be helpful in collaborating with the client on occupational performance goals.

Cultural, Familial, and Spiritual

Cultural, familial, and spiritual influences are other important factors to be considered in evaluation and intervention, especially when the cause of the pain is unclear (Chapman & Turner, 1990; MacRae & Riley, 1990). Each culture, family, and religion has its own system of values and attitudes about pain (Niemeyer, 1990). Depending on the culture, the individual may be rewarded, ignored, or punished for emitting pain behaviors.

OCCUPATIONAL THERAPY PRACTITIONER'S ROLE IN PAIN MANAGEMENT

Intervention goals related to health and occupations necessitate and are enriched by collaborative interdisciplinary relationships. As interdisciplinary team members, physicians, psychologists, physical therapy practitioners, and occupational therapy practitioners work together with the client to reduce discomfort and associated disability, promote optimal occupational performance, and enable meaningful interpersonal relationships (IASP, 1994).

Communication of Pain

Discrimination training is directed at enhancing stimulus control so that the client discusses pain with appropriate people (such as health-care providers) at appropriate times and places. People interacting with the person experiencing chronic nonmalignant pain are instructed to avoid giving attention and sympathy for either verbal or nonverbal expressions of pain and to praise the client's achievements and efforts to cope with pain. Social skills training (expressing feelings) may also be used by the occupational therapy practitioner, during which the client is taught and reinforced for using behaviors not revolving around the pain experience in social contexts. Involvement of the partner or significant other in stress or anger management, resolution of sexual dysfunction, and goal setting may make up part of the total treatment package (Fordyce, 1990; Turk, Meichenbaum, & Genest, 1983).

Physical Activity

Increasing the client's activity level is the cornerstone of most chronic pain management treatment programs and is a major area of occupational therapy intervention. Intervention involves positively reinforcing the client's attempts at participation. When the client exhibits pain behaviors, treatment staff withdraw attention. Activity increases are done on a gradual basis, and the client works to tolerance (gradual increase in task demands) as opposed to pain before a scheduled rest break. Resting at the time of the pain onset or elevation is avoided because it may reinforce the pain behaviors (Fordyce, 1976). Group or individual progressive mobility, strengthening, and endurance activities are routinely scheduled daily to assist the client in achieving maximal functional status. Modalities (heat or cold) may be applied to prepare the client for exercise.

Proper use of posture, body mechanics, energy conservation, and joint protection techniques are also emphasized as a means of pain reduction (Caruso & Chan, 1986; Giles & Allen, 1986). Adaptive equipment and splinting may be prescribed to enhance independent performance of ADL (Tyson & Strong, 1990).

Relaxation Training

There is strong evidence for the efficacy of relaxation training for reducing chronic pain (National Institutes of Health, 1995). Relaxation training may involve teaching the client to contract and relax the major skeletal muscle groups systematically **(progressive muscle relaxation),** to repeat silently phrases about the ideal psychophysiological state **(autogenic training),** or to use purposeful images to achieve a desired goal **(guided imagery).** The potential benefits of these approaches are the reduction of anxiety, distraction from pain, alleviation of skeletal muscle tension, reduction of fatigue, improved sleep, enhancement of other pain relief measures, and a sense of control over pain (Turner & Chapman, 1982). Research suggests that relaxation rehearsal may be helpful in the reduction of the person's perceived pain frequency, intensity, or duration and in the achievement of occupational goals (Engel & Rapoff, 1990; Strong, Cramond, & Mass, 1989).

Biofeedback

Biofeedback is a treatment procedure by which the occupational therapy practitioner monitors, with the help of a machine, bodily functions that the client is usually unaware of. The practitioner then feeds back this information to the client, usually through an auditory modality such as a tone that goes higher or lower, depending on the activity of the bodily function being monitored. The combination of this feedback with verbal prompting to alter the feedback in the desired direction (e.g., lower the tone) usually results in the client learning to alter the target body function (e.g., to decrease muscle activity in the area monitored by the electromyographic (EMG) machine. Biofeedback-assisted relaxation training is a common treatment for individuals with chronic pain conditions and has been consistently shown in controlled trials to reduce headache and back pain (Blanchard, Kim, Hermann, & Steffek, 1993; Newton-John, Spence, & Schotte, 1995).

Cognitive Restructuring

Numerous studies have shown that individuals' pain-related cognitions (the meaning of pain, expectations regarding control over pain) beliefs, and coping strategies are associated with their pain intensity, physical functioning, psychological status, and disability. Cognitive interventions aim to identify and modify clients' maladaptive cognitions and beliefs regarding pain and disability. Cognitions can be modified directly by cognitive restructuring techniques (e.g., attention diversion) or indirectly by the modification of maladaptive thoughts, feelings, and beliefs. In a variety of populations for which chronic pain is the primary disability, cognitive behavioral interventions have been effective in improving physical and psychosocial functioning (Jensen, Romano, Turner, Good, & Wald, 1999).

Distraction

Increased pain awareness may result from a lack of distracting occupations. Therefore, it is advantageous for clients experiencing pain to learn how to distract themselves more effectively when exposed to noxious stimuli (painful medical or rehabilitation procedures) and during periods of minimal activity. Clients cannot attend to pain when concentrating on something other than pain (engaging in an occupation) or focusing inward (reminiscing), but not directly on the pain. Involvement in purposeful activity has been demonstrated to improve pain tolerance (Heck, 1988; McCormack, 1988). A balance of occupations is of value in distracting attention away from pain (Heck, 1988).

Social Support

The importance of social support in facilitating behavior change cannot be underestimated. Support groups may assist people suffering from pain by helping them realize that others have endured similar circumstances, may provide a neutral place to express feelings, and may provide opportunities for learning coping strategies. Support groups can ease the transition from terminating treatment to self-management and the maintenance of behavioral change. Patrick and D'Eon (1996) reported that clients whose spouses were emotionally supportive had higher physical performance levels.

CONCLUSION

Occupational therapy practitioners have a core role in providing therapeutic activities that enable the client with pain to develop the skills and tolerances necessary for occupational performance. Because of the complex nature of pain, a cure is not readily available. Consequently, intervention cannot simply emphasize the reduction of the pain experience. Ideally, interventions focus on improving functional levels and coping strategies, while being sensitive to the client's belief and value systems.

SECTION VIII

Stress Management

GORDON MUIR GILES

Stress is the collection of physical and psychological changes that occur in response to perceived challenge or threat; it is the outcome of an interaction between the person and the environment. People's resources (e.g., personality factors, social support), their appraisal of situations, and their capacity to handle those situations influence their stress reactions and the effects that stress can have on their health. This section describes the physiological and psychological effects of stress, common stressors, factors that mediate the effects of stress on the individual, and stress management techniques.

PHYSIOLOGICAL RESPONSE TO STRESS

The General Adaptation Response

Selye (1978) described the body's stress reaction as the **general adaptation response.** This response occurs in three stages: the alarm reaction, the adaptive or resistive stage, and the exhaustion stage. Not everyone experiences all three stages. The exhaustion stage is reached only when the person either gets stuck in the alarm stage or goes through the alarm and adaptive stages too often.

Alarm Reaction

The alarm reaction is the fight-or-flight response that prepares a person to meet a challenge or threat (Cannon, 1939). During this stage, the cerebral cortex activates the reticular-activating system to increase general alertness. The cortex also activates the autonomic nervous system (ANS) and endocrine systems by way of the hypothalamus. The sympathetic branch of the ANS increases heart rate, blood pressure, perspiration, muscle tone, and cell metabolism. Blood vessels just under the skin constrict, and digestion is slowed. The endocrine system releases hormones from the adrenal and thyroid glands that increase the supply of glucose and accelerate cell metabolism. In addition, the hypothalamus triggers the release of β-endorphins from the pituitary gland, which are endogenous opiate proteins that elevate mood and decrease pain perception. They have also been linked to immune system suppression (Shavit, Terman,

Martin, Lewis, Liebeskind, & Gale, 1985). It is the combination of nervous system and endocrine system response that leads to the neuroendocrine stress reaction.

Adaptive or Resistive Stage

In the adaptive or resistive stage, the body returns to its pre-excited state and recovers from the physiologic strains of the alarm stage. Stress-prone or overstressed individuals, who interpret even normal events as negative stressors, are often unable to reach this stage. Such individuals develop an extended alarm reaction until their bodies enter the exhaustion phase. People who are able to move successfully to the adaptive stage may also reach the exhaustion phase if they experience too many stressors.

Exhaustion Stage

The exhaustion stage is a reaction to the constant high metabolic demands of the alarm stage. During the exhaustion stage, the neurophysiological ability to respond effectively to stressors is abolished.

Chronic Stress

The physiologic demands of chronic stress have been linked to many disorders. Chronic stress has been linked to hypertension, cardiac arrest, alcoholism, pain, and numerous other medical conditions (Mandle, Jacobs, Arcari, & Domar, 1996). Chronic stress can depress immune functioning, increase vulnerability to disease, and compromise recovery.

The Immune System and Stress

Immune responses are part of the acute phase response to infection or injury that involve the body diverting resources from routine activities to overcome illness. Behaviors associated with the acute phase response include a decrease in overall activity (e.g., exploration, social interaction, and intake of food and water) and increased sleep. The behaviors associated with stress (fight-or-flight) are the opposite of those associated with the acute phase immune response. During fight-or-flight, it is adaptive to mobilize energy for combat or escape and to reduce immune responses. Chronic overarousal from stress is associated with reduced activity in the immune system, potentially rendering the individual at increased risk for infection (Kiecolt-Glasser, Fisher, Ogrocki, Stout, Speicher, & Glasser, 1987) and other illness (Fawzy et al., 1990).

PSYCHOLOGICAL RESPONSES TO STRESS

The Interaction of Person and Stressors

Stress arises from an imbalance between the requirements of the environment and the person's appraisal of his or her ability to cope with those demands. Individual differences in motivation and cognition lead to markedly different reactions to potential stressors. For example, developing relationships with co-workers at a new job might be exciting for one person and distressing for another. The recognition that a stressor can mean different things to different people has led to recognition that there may be positive outcomes from stress (Park, Cohen, & Murch, 1996). Exposure to chronic stressors may lead to psychological growth and positive reappraisal of life goals and events (Folkman & Moskowitz, 2000).

Types of Stressors

Any agent or circumstance capable of triggering a stress reaction is called a stressor (Selye, 1978). Knowing the sources of stress can help predict and control the amount of stress a person feels. Clients can be taught to monitor physical and psychological markers of stress and to use these as cues to implement stress reduction techniques. Here, I discuss categories of stressors—such as physical or environmental stressors, major life events, chronic strains, and hassles—and mediating factors—that is, factors that modify the effect of the stressor on the person (personality factors, behaviors, occupation, social support, and sociocultural factors).

Environmental Stressors

Physical or environmental stressors include noise, crowding, poor lighting, inadequate ventilation, and environmental pollutants. Excessive or continuous noise (≥90 dB) can increase blood pressure and cause hearing loss (Raloff, 1982a, 1982b). Crowding increases irritability and aggression (e.g., road rage). Poor lighting and ventilation can cause eye irritation, headaches, nausea, and drowsiness in workers (Raloff, 1981a, 1981b). Daily exposure to environmental stressors makes a baseline coping demand on a person's nervous system, reducing the reserve capacity available for coping with other forms of stress.

Major Life Events

Major life events can be divided into extreme or nonnormative events such as natural or human-made disasters (e.g., fires, floods, tornadoes, earthquakes, war) and normative major life changes (e.g., marriage, illness, bereavement). Reactions to major life events can be acute, chronic, or both. If a person is exposed to an event that involves serious threat (e.g., actual or threatened death or serious injury to themselves or a loved one) they may experience posttraumatic stress disorder (PTSD). The symptoms associated with extreme trauma include persistent reexperiencing of the event, avoidance of stimuli associated with the event, a numbing of responsiveness, or persistent overarousal (American Psychiatric Association, 2000). The management of individuals with PTSD is a specialized area of practice and is beyond the scope of this section. However, many of the techniques used in stress management are appropriate for use in an integrated PTSD program.

Major life changes that alter social roles and relationships (e.g., marriage, divorce, job change, serious illness, death of a loved one) can increase susceptibility to stress, especially when several of these changes occur within a brief period of time. Multiple major life changes within 1 year correlate with a higher risk of injury or illness (Holmes & Rahe, 1967; Rahe, 1979). Although both positive and negative life events do seem to have an effect, there is increasing evidence that it is not change per se but the quality of the change that is potentially damaging to people; specifically, it is events that are undesired, unscheduled, nonnormative, and in which the individual has no control that are detrimental (Folkman & Moskowitz, 2000; Somerfield & McCrae, 2000).

Chronic Strain

An aspect of **chronic strain** that has received considerable attention is the effect of employment on health. High-stress occupations have been defined as those with high psychological demands and limited decision-making freedom (Karasek, 1979). Psychological strain, increased cardiovascular risk, and decreased general health have been linked to high-stress occupations (Karasek, Theorell, Schwartz, Schall, Pieper, & Michela, 1988; Siegrist, Peter, Junge, Cremer, & Seidel, 1990).

Many health-care workers seem to be at risk because of the long hours and frequent changes in shifts that lead to disruptions in the sleep–wake cycles (Czeisler, Moore-Ede, & Coleman, 1982). Such schedule irregularities have been correlated to a high number of stress related errors on the job (Hilts, 1980). Caregiver burden has also associated with stress (Mitchell, 2000; Steffen, 2000).

Hassles

Minor changes or day-to-day aggravations can act as stressors. These hassles can have cumulative effects that are magnified during periods of major life change. Major life changes, in addition to their immediate impact, can create a ripple effect of continuing minor hassles. For example, providing care to an impaired loved one may be stressful in itself, but it may also interfere with employment and produce economic problems as secondary stressors.

Mediating Factors

Mediating factors seem either to aggravate or to diminish the effect of stressful events or life circumstances and provide avenues for intervention to minimize the effect of stress on health.

Personality Factors

Personality type has been associated with different responses to stress. Cardiovascular reactivity to stress is higher among people with type A behavior pattern (TABP; Friedman, 1969). TABP is a risk factor for the development of coronary artery disease (CAD; Mathews, 1988; Rosenman, Brand, Jenkins, Friedman & Wurm, 1975). Among individuals with CAD, TABP is a risk for sudden cardiac death (Case, Heller, Case & Moss, 1985; Shekelle, Gale, & Norusis, 1985; Shekelle et al., 1985). Counseling specifically directed at TABP components has been shown to decrease hostility, time urgency, anger, impatience, and depression and to increase **social support** (Mendes de Leon, Powell, & Kaplan, 1991; Nunes, Frank, & Kornfeld, 1987).

Other personality factors influence an individual's response to stress. Stress-prone people see change as a threat, feel helpless in controlling their environment, and have a sense of alienation about their lives. Personality factors associated with poor responses to stress include anger, cynicism, external locus of control, neuroticism, depression, and irrational beliefs (McNaughton et al., 1995).

Personality traits that appear to be associated with resilience (resistance to stress) include constructive thinking (Epstein & Meier, 1989), hardiness (Hills & Norvell, 1991), dispositional optimism (Scheier & Carver, 1987), hope (Snyder et al., 1991), positive affect (Folkman & Moskowitz, 2000), self-efficacy, mastery/internal locus of control, and possibly conscientiousness (Friedman et al., 1995). Many of these traits tend to be stable response characteristics (Somerfield & McCrae, 2000).

Behaviors

Behaviors with potential health consequences—such as alcohol use, smoking, and drug abuse—can be regarded as part of an individual's attempt to manage stress (Bradstock et al., 1988; Gottleib & Green, 1984) but may also exacerbate stress-related problems and may inhibit the adoption of more effective stress-management strategies. Psychological factors such as self-efficacy (Grembowski et al., 1993) and positive affect (Griffin, Friend, Eitel, & Lobel, 1993) are associated with increased levels of positive **health behaviors.** Social support and the existence of a social network are associated with lower negative health behaviors (Gottleib & Green, 1984).

Social Support

The degree to which a person is connected to others may influence health in a more fundamental way than by reducing negative health practices. There is a relationship between social support and health and mortality (Hibbard & Pope, 1992; Vogt, Mullooly, Ernst, Pope, & Hollis, 1992). Berkman and Syme (1979) found that people who lacked social support were more likely to die than those with social support, and the association between social ties and decreased mortality was found to be independent of socioeconomic status, health practices, obesity, physical activity, or the use of preventative health services. Social support has many dimensions, including emotional, material assistance, and information and referral.

Occupations

The potential role of meaningful occupations in mediating stress has received little attention in the stress and coping literature. Familiar and routine occupations (e.g., gardening, fishing) that are removed from stressful events may facilitate mature defense mechanisms and assist individuals in self-soothing. Occupational therapy assists in maintaining the health and well-being of community dwelling elders and engagement in meaningful occupation is associated with increased longevity (Clark et al., 1998; Glass, Mendes de Leon, Marottoli, & Berkman, 1999).

Sociocultural Factors

Larger sociocultural factors (e.g., overcrowding) may complicate other types of stressors. Low income may force people to live in an unsafe neighborhood, placing them under chronic stress. Unemployment is a risk factor for mortality even when socioeconomic factors are accounted for (Moser, Fox, & Jones, 1984). It is interesting that the risk extends to the wives of unemployed men, who also show a raised risk of mortality. Mortality has been found to be particularly high from malignant neoplasms, accidents, poisonings, and violence (Moser et al., 1984).

Types of Coping

Coping appears to be highly contextual, depending on the type of stressor, the environmental conditions, and the state of the person under stress. Lazarus (1993) suggested that the type of coping employed depends on the appraisal of whether or not anything can be done to change the situation. Lazarus described two basic types of coping responses: problem-focused coping and emotion-focused coping. If the person believes that something can be done, problem-focused coping predominates. The person is likely to interact actively with the environment and attempt to gain mastery and to change the situation so that it becomes less stressful. If people believe that nothing can be done to change the situation, they are likely to use emotion-focused coping, which involves changes in the way the stress is attended to or changes in the way the event is understood and integrated into their lives.

Unconscious defense mechanisms play important roles in helping individuals manage stress. The role of psychological defense is to avoid unwanted emotional experiences and to maintain adequate levels of personality functioning (Cramer, 2000). Denial may be effective as an emergency coping technique but may be detrimental in the long term if it interferes with adaptive behaviors.

STRESS AND OCCUPATIONAL THERAPY

Individuals who receive occupational therapy are particularly prone to stress. Illness and disability are major life changes, can cause social role changes, and generate a host of changes in daily activities. Learning the culture of the hospital can be extremely stressful to some clients (Spencer, Young, Rintala, & Bates, 1995). Changes in appearance or behavior can render a client constantly fearful of rejection.

On the other side of the therapeutic relationship, practitioners have to manage job-related stressors that can lead to burnout, chronic fatigue, and irritability. Time pressures are intense in many settings, and demands for direct intervention, documentation, interdepartmental and intradepartmental communication, and staff training may be made constantly and simultaneously.

Stress-Management Techniques

Stress-management techniques have been developed to help relieve chronic stress and its consequences. These techniques are learned behaviors that interrupt the nervous system's stress reactions. Central to many of the techniques is the relaxation response, described as the physiological opposite of the fight-or-flight response (Benson, 1975). The relaxation response is marked by a decrease in pulse, respiratory rate, blood pressure, and metabolism. Practitioners use a variety of techniques intended to prevent excessive stress via behavioral and lifestyle changes and to promote relaxation. A brief description of some techniques and recommendations about teaching them follow. Resources that describe these techniques in more detail are available (Benson, 1975; Jacobsen, 1938; Kabat-Zinn, 1990; McCormack, 1993; Pelletier, 1977).

Coping Skills Training

Coping skills training is a multimodal approach to helping individuals who have stress related problems. It involves both cognitive and behavioral techniques and usually occurs in a group format. A typical coping skills training program might include the management of physiological arousal (relaxation training), time management training (to help the individual develop a daily schedule with both work and leisure time activities), cognitive restructuring (in which individuals identify cognitive distortions associated with stressful events; see Section 5), and social skills or assertiveness training. In coping skills training clients are encouraged to work on specific stressful events and to recognize how they can effect change in their lives (Meichenbaum & Cameron, 1983).

Aerobic Exercise

Aerobic exercise involves, repetitive, rhythmic contractions of the large muscles of the legs and arms. Examples are walking, running, bicycling, and swimming (Cooper, 1977). Aerobic exercise has been demonstrated to be effective in the relief of pain and stress-related disorders (Wigers, Stiles, & Vogel, 1996). Anyone planning to start an aerobic exercise program should first be seen by a physician for a complete physical examination; all exercise programs should begin gradually and work slowly toward increased difficulty. Specific guidelines for developing individualized aerobic exercise programs are available (American College of Sports Medicine, 1991). Some other forms of exercise such as yoga and tai-chi share aspects of meditation and may facilitate the relaxation response (Mandel et al., 1996).

Communication Skills

Both psychiatric and medical disorders can be exacerbated by stressful communication with others (Ehlers, Osen, Wenninger, & Gieler, 1994). Practicing effective communication skills such as clarifying expectations, defining needs honestly, and providing tactful and constructive feedback can decrease the number of stressful misunderstandings. Social skills training and assertiveness training programs are important parts of stress management for certain client populations (e.g., persons with chronic pain).

Laughter

The healing power of humor has been recognized by healthcare professionals (Vergeer & MacRae, 1993). Some writers have suggested that laughter may stimulate the release of endorphins, thereby helping to alleviate pain and stress (Cousins, 1979). Practitioners should remember that therapy does not have to be solemn to be effective.

Time Management

Time management techniques include realistically scheduling and organizing time, setting priorities about task accomplishments, making lists, setting limits, and accepting that everything cannot be done at once. An appropriate schedule should include both work and leisure time activities.

Verbalization

Talking to friends and acquaintances about stressors can help reduce stress. Friends can offer different perspectives, new suggestions, and support, all of which are helpful in extricating a person from feeling stuck with a problem situation (Rippere, 1977).

Engagement in Meaningful Occupation

Developing a balanced routine of occupations that involves both work and diverse social and recreational activities that have meaning for the individual is important for the management of stress. Engagement in meaningful occupation rather than activity per se seems to be important in maintaining health and life quality (Clark et al., 1998). Many individuals have difficulty including pleasant diversional activities in their daily routine and fail to notice that all of their activities are *musts* rather than *wants*. Participation in meaningful occupations is associated with improved health status (Glass et al., 1999).

Deep Breathing

Deep (diaphragmatic) breathing involves slowly inhaling and exhaling to reduce tension in the shoulders, trunk, and abdomen. The process begins with focusing on normal breathing in a quiet and comfortable place. This is followed by a period of deep inhalation and slow exhalation. During inhalation, the abdominal muscles should be relaxed. During exhalation, the abdominal muscles should be contracted. It is often helpful to rest a hand lightly on the abdomen during this process.

Deep breathing is relatively easy to learn, requires no equipment, and can be done anywhere. Deep abdominal breathing has been demonstrated to reduce physiological responsiveness (Forbes & Pekala, 1993).

Autogenic Training

Autogenic training uses autosuggestion or self-hypnosis and mental imagery to achieve relaxation. Autosuggestion typically involves imagining sensations of physical heaviness and warmth to achieve muscle relaxation and vasodilatation. Imagining oneself in settings in which one would feel warm, comfortable, and heavy can facilitate these autosuggestion. Learning this process requires considerable practice and is not recommended for people who are agitated or actively psychotic (Courtney & Escobedo, 1990). Controlled trials suggest that autogenic training is an effective adjunctive treatment for stress related conditions (Ehlers, Stangier, & Giles, 1995).

Progressive Relaxation Exercises

Progressive relaxation exercises involve tensing and relaxing muscle groups, one group at a time, from head to foot. This technique teaches the difference between muscle tension and muscle relaxation by exaggerating the contrast between the two tone states. The learning sequence for this technique is (1) systematic tensing and relaxing of muscle groups to verbal cues, (2) systematic relaxing of muscle groups to verbal cues, and (3) relaxation of muscle groups by autosuggestion. Progressive relaxation exercises require discipline and practice and can take months to learn completely (Jacobsen, 1938).

Progressive relaxation is not recommended for clients with upper motor neuron lesions and spasticity. Because these exercises involve isometric muscle contractions, they are not recommended for clients with hypertension or cardiac disease (Courtney & Escobedo, 1990; Smith & Lukens, 1983). Progressive relaxation appears to be effective in regulating mood (Thayer, Newman, & McClain,

1994) and has been shown to increase skin temperature and decrease pulse rate, suggesting that it can reduce physiological reactivity (Forbes & Pekala, 1993).

Meditation

Meditation involves focusing attention on a rhythmic, repetitive word, phrase, or sensation (e.g., breathing, heart rate) to achieve relaxation. Benson (1975) suggested that this mental process blocks the stress response of the sympathetic nervous system by activating the anterior hypothalamus, which controls the parasympathetic nervous system. These techniques require considerable practice and can take many months to learn.

General Guidelines for Choice of Technique

Self-Assessment

Guided self-assessment of individual stressors and stress reactions is the first step in designing an appropriate stress management program. The guiding can be done by the practitioner or by structured self-administered questionnaire. The Holmes-Rahe Life Change Index (Holmes & Rahe, 1967) or the Stress Management Questionnaire (Stein & Nikolic, 1989) can help identify stressors. Other questionnaires are available to help people assess their physical, emotional, and behavioral stress responses (Vitaliano, Russo, Carr, Maiuro, & Becker, 1985).

General factors

Some stresses can be avoided; others cannot. The foregoing discussion has highlighted the importance of individualized assessment and training (Van Fleet, 2000). A first step may be to evaluate whether the person is currently using counterproductive techniques (e.g., overeating, abusing alcohol, or caffeine) and encouraging the person to discontinue these maladaptive responses. Some general factors to consider in suggesting stress management techniques for people or when deciding on such techniques for oneself are how long does it take to master the stress reduction technique versus how much time is available, the nature of the individual's lifestyle and daily routine, the level of financial and interpersonal support available to the person, and the person's commitment to change.

For example, meditation takes many months to learn and cannot be taught during a short hospital stay. Deep breathing techniques, on the other hand, are relatively easy to learn, require no outside equipment, and can generally be taught quickly.

Exercise is probably the easiest and single most effective stress reduction strategy, but in the long term, there may be low levels of compliance. To be effective in the long term, overall lifestyle changes and reprioritizations may be indicated. Practitioners intent on helping clients change behavior patterns may use techniques such as motivational interviewing (Miller & Rollnick, 1991) and the development of implementation intentions (Gollwitzer, 1999).

CONCLUSION

Although not everyone needs formal stress management training, it is important to remember that most clients seen in occupational therapy are in stressful situations by virtue of illness or disability. Effective stress management programs can be part of individual or group therapy sessions and are particularly helpful for those with stress related illnesses or with high stress levels that seriously impede their functional progress. More research examining the daily process of adaptation to stress is needed (Somerfield & McCrae, 2000).

References

Abreu, B. C. (1998). The quadraphonic approach: Holistic rehabilitation for brain injury. In N. Katz (Ed.). *Cognition and occupation in rehabilitation: Cognitive models for intervention in occupational therapy* (pp. 51–97). Bethesda, MD: American Occupational Therapy Association.

Abreu, B. C. (1999). Evaluation and intervention with memory and learning impairments. In C. Unsworth (Ed.). *Cognitive and perceptual dysfunction* (pp. 163–207). Philadelphia: Davis.

Adler, S. S., Beckers, D., & Buck, M. (1993). *PNF in practice: An illustrated guide*. New York: Springer-Verlag.

Allen, K. C. (1993). Lesson 11: Creating a need—Satisfying, safe environment management and maintenance approaches. In C. B. Royeen (Ed.). *Cognitive rehabilitation* [AOTA Self–Study Series] (pp. 1–36). Rockville, MD: American Occupational Therapy Association.

American Academy of Pain Medicine and American Pain Society [AAPM]. (1997). The use of opioids for the treatment of chronic pain. *Clinical Journal of Pain, 13*, 6–8.

American Academy of Pain Medicine [AAPM]. (2001). FAQs about pain. Available at: www.painmed.org/faqs/pain_faqs.html. Accessed 5/13/01

American College of Sports Medicine. (1991). *Guidelines for exercise testing and prescription* (4th ed.). Philadelphia: Lea & Febiger.

American Occupational Therapy Association [AOTA]. (1999). Management of occupational therapy services for persons with cognitive impairments (statement). *American Journal of Occupational Therapy, 53*, 601–607.

American Occupational Therapy Association [AOTA] (in press). Occupational therapy practice framework: Domain and process. *American Journal of Occupational Therapy*.

American Psychiatric Association. (2000). *Diagnostic and statistical manual of mental disorders* (4th ed.). Washington, DC: Author.

Anderson, J. R. (1995). *Cognitive psychology and its implications*. New York: Freeman.

Antonucci, G., Guariglia, A., Magnotti, l., Paolucci, S., Pizzamiglio, L., & Zoccolotti, P. (1995). Effectiveness of neglect rehabilitation in a randomized group study. *Journal of Clinical and Experimental Neuropsychology, 17*, 383–389.

Arai, T., Ohi, H., Sasaki, H., Nobuto, H., & Tanaka, K. (1997). Hemispatial sunglasses: Effect on unilateral spatial neglect. *Archives of Physical Medicine and Rehabilitation, 78*, 230–232.

Averbuch, S., & Katz, N. (1998). Cognitive rehabilitation: A retraining model for clients following brain injuries. In N. Katz (Ed.). Cognition and occupation in rehabilitation: Cognitive models for intervention in occupational therapy (pp. 99–123). Bethesda, MD: American Occupational Therapy Association.

Barco, P. P., Crosson, B., Bolesta, M. M., Werts, D., & Stout, R. (1991). Training awareness and compensation in postacute head injury rehabilitation. In J. S. Kreutzer & P. H. Wehman (Eds.). *Cognitive rehabilitation for persons with traumatic brain injury* (pp. 129–146). Baltimore: Brookes.

Bate, P. (1997). Motor control theories—Insights for therapists. *Physiotherapy, 83*, 397–305.

Beis, J., Andre, J., Baumgarten, A., & Challier, B. (1999). Eye patching in unilateral spatial neglect: Efficacy of two methods. *Archives of Physical Medicine and Rehabilitation, 80*, 71–76.

Bennet, T. L., Davalos, D. B., Green, M., & Rial, D. (1999). Addressing executive functioning and cognitive rehabilitation in the treatment of schizophrenia. *Rehabilitation Psychology, 44*, 403–410.

Benson, H. (1975). *The relaxation response*. New York: Avon.

Ben-Yishay, Y., Piasetsky, E. B., & Rattok, J. (1987). A systematic method for ameliorating disorders in basic attention. In M. Meir, A. Benton & L. Diller (Eds.). *Neuropsychological rehabilitation* (pp. 165–181). New York: Guilford.

Berkman, L., & Syme, S. L. (1979). Social networks, host resistance, and mortality: a nine-year follow-up study of Alameda County residents. *American Journal of Epidemiology, 109*, 186–204.

Blanchard, E. B., Kim, M., Hermann, C. U., & Steffek, B. D. (1993). Preliminary results of the effects on headache relief of perception of success among tension headache patients receiving relaxation. *Headache Quarterly, 4*, 249–253.

Blundon, G., & Smits, E. (2000). Cognitive rehabilitation: A pilot survey of therapeutic modalities used by Canadian occupational therapists with survivors of traumatic brain injury. *Canadian Journal of Occupational Therapy, 67*, 184–196.

Boake, C. (1991). Social skills training following head injury. In J. S. Kreutzer & P. H. Wehman (Eds.). *Cognitive rehabilitation for persons with traumatic brain injury* (pp. 181–190). Baltimore: Brookes.

Bobath, B. (1990). *Adult hemiplegia: Evaluation and treatment* (3rd ed.). Oxford, UK: Butterworth-Heinemann.

Bradley, N. S., & Beckoff, A. (1989). Development of locomotion: animal models. In. Woollacott M., Shumway-Cook (Eds.). *The Development of posture and gait across the life span* (pp 48–73). Columbia: University of South Carolina Press.

Bradstock, K., Forman, M. R., Binkin, N. J., Gentry, E. M., Hogelin, G. C., Williamson, D. F., & Trowbridge, F. L. (1988). Alcohol use and health behavior lifestyles among U.S. women: The behavioral risk factor survey. *Addictive Behaviors, 13*, 61–71.

Breines, E. B. (2001). Therapeutic occupations and modalities. In L. W. Pedretti & M .B. Early (Eds.). *Occupational therapy: Practice skills for physical dysfunction* (5th ed., pp. 503–528). St. Louis: Mosby.

Brown, C., Harwood, K., Hays, C., Heckman, J., & Short, J. E. (1993). Effectiveness of cognitive rehabilitation for improving attention in patients with schizophrenia. *Occupational Therapy Journal of Research, 13*, 71–86.

Brownlee, S., & Schrof, J. M. (1997, March 17). The quality of mercy. *U.S. News and World Report*, 55–57, 60–62, 65, 67.

Buchner, D. M., & Coleman, E. A. (1994). Exercise considerations in older adults: Intensity, fall prevention and safety. *Physical Medicine and Rehabilitation Clinics of North America, 5*, 357–375.

Buckner, W. S. (2001). Infection control and safety issue in the clinic. In L. W. Pedretti & M. B. Early (Eds.). *Occupational therapy: Practice skills for physical dysfunction* (5th ed., pp. 101–115). St. Louis: Mosby.

Burke, W. H., Zencius, A. H., Wesolowskis, M. D., & Doubleday, F. (1991). Improving executive function disorders in brain injured clients. *Brain Injury, 5*, 241–252.

Burtner, P. & Woollacott, M. (1996). Theories of motor control, In C. M. Fredericks and L. K. Saladin (Eds.). *Pathophysiology of the motor system* (pp. 217–234). Philadelphia: Davis.

Butter, C. M., & Kirsch, N. (1992). Combined and separate effects of eye patching and visual stimulation on unilateral neglect following stroke. *Archives of Physical Medicine and Rehabilitation, 73*, 1133–1139.

Byl, N., & Merzenich, M. (1997) Neural consequences of repetition: clinical implications of a learning hypothesis. *Journal of Hand Therapy, 10*(2), 160–174.

Callahan, A. (1995) Methods of compensation and reeducation for sensory dysfunction. In J. M. Hunter, E. J. Mackin, & A. D. Callahan (Eds.). *Rehabilitation of the hand* (4th ed., pp. 701–715). St. Louis: Mosby.

Calvanio, R., Levine, D., & Petrone, P. (1993). Elements of cognitive rehabilitation after right hemisphere stroke. *Neurologic Clinics, 11*, 25–57.

Campbell, J. J., Duffy, J. D., & Salloway, S. P. (1994). Treatment strategies for patients with dysexecutive syndromes. *Journal of Neuropsychiatry and Clinical Neurosciences, 6*, 411–418.

Cannon, W. B. (1939). *The wisdom of the body*. New York: Norton.

Cappa, S., Sterzi, R., Vallar, G., & Bisiach, E. (1987). Remission of hemineglect and anosognosia during vestibular stimulation. *Neuropsychologia, 25*, 775–782.

Carr, J. H., & Shepherd, R. B. (2000). A motor learning model for rehabilitation. In J. Carr & J. Shepherd (Eds.). *Movement science, foundations for physical therapy in rehabilitation* (pp. 33–110). Gaithersburg, MD: Aspen System.

Carter-Wilson, M. (1991). Sensory reeducation. In R. H. Gelberman (Ed.). *Operative nerve repair and reconstruction* (pp. 827–844). Philadelphia: Lippincott.

Caruso, L. A., & Chan, D. E. (1986). Evaluation and management of the patient with acute back pain. *American Journal of Occupational Therapy, 46*, 347–351.

Case, R. B., Heller, S. S., Case, N. B., Moss, A. J., and the Multi-center Post-infarction Research Group. (1985). Type A behavior and survival after acute myocardial infarction. *New England Journal of Medicine, 312*, 737–741.

Chaikin, L. E. (2001). Disorders of vision and visual-perceptual dysfunction. In D. A. Umphred (Ed.). *Neurological rehabilitation* (4th ed.; pp. 821–852). St. Louis: Mosby.

Chapman, C. R., & Turner, J. A. (1990). Psychologic and psychosocial aspects of acute pain. In J. J. Bonica (Ed.). *The management of pain* (2nd ed., pp. 122–132). Philadelphia: Lea & Febiger.

Chen, C. Y., Neufield, P. S., Feely, C. A., & Skinner, C. S. (1999). Factors influencing compliance with home exercise programs among patients with upper extremity impairment. *American Journal of Occupational Therapy, 53*, 171–180.

Cicerone, K. D., Dahlberg, C., Kalmar, K., Langenbahn, D. M., Malec, J. F., Bergquist, T. F., Felicetti, T., Giacino, J. T., Harley, J. P., Harrington, D. E., Herzog, J., Kneipp, S., Laatsch, L., & Morse, P. A. (2000). Evidence-based cognitive rehabilitation: Recommendations for clinical practice. *Archives of Physical Medicine and Rehabilitation, 81*, 1596–1615.

Cicerone, K. D., & Giacino, T. J. (1992). Remediation of executive function deficits after traumatic brain injury. *NeuroRehabilitation, 2*(3), 12–22.

Cicerone, K. D., & Wood, J. C. (1987). Planning disorder after closed head injury: A case study. *Archives of Physical Medicine and Rehabilitation, 68*, 111–115.

Clark, F., Azen, S. P., Zemke, R., Jackson, J,. Carlson, M., Mandel, D., Hay, J., Josephson, K., Cherry, B., Hessel, C., Palmer, J., & Lipson, L. (1998). Occupational therapy for independent-living older adults. A randomized controlled trial. *Journal of the American Medical Association, 279*, 1321–1326.

Cleeland, C. S. (1991). Research in cancer pain: What we know and what we need to know. *Cancer, 67*, 823–827.

Cooper, K. (1977). *The aerobics way*. New York: Bantam.

Courtney, C., & Escobedo, B. (1990). A stress management program: Inpatient to outpatient continuity. *American Journal of Occupational Therapy, 44*, 306–311.

Cousins, N. (1979). *Anatomy of an illness as perceived by the patient*. New York: Bantam.

Cramer, P. (2000). Defense mechanisms in psychology today: Further processes for adaptation. *American Psychologist, 55*, 637–646.

Cubelli, R., Trentini, P., & Montagna, C. G. (1991). Re-education of gestural communication in a case of chronic global aphasia and limb apraxia. *Cognitive Neuropsychology, 8*, 369–380.

Czeisler, C. A., Moore-Ede, M. C., & Coleman, R. H. (1982). Rotating shift work schedules that disrupt sleep are improved by applying circadian principles. *Science, 217*, 460–463.

Dagum, A. B. (1998) Peripheral nerve regeneration, repair, and grafting. *Journal of Hand Therapy, 11*(2), 111–117.

Dannebaum, R. M., & Jones L. A. (1993). The assessment and treatment of patients who have sensory loss following cortical lesions. *Journal of Hand Therapy*, 6(2), 130–139.

Davies, P. M. (1985). *Steps to follow*. New York: Springer-Verlag.

Davis, J. Z. (1992). The Affolter method: A model for treating perceptual disturbances in the hemiplegic and brain-injured patient. *Occupational Therapy Practice: Is That OT?* 3(4), 1–88.

Davis, J. Z. (2001). Neurodevelopmental treatment: The Bobath approach. In L. W. Pedretti & M. B. Early (Eds.). *Occupational therapy practice skills for physical dysfunction* (5th ed., pp. 624–640). Philadelphia: Mosby.

Dellon, A. L. (1981) *Evaluation of sensibility and reeducation of sensation in the hand*. Baltimore: Williams & Wilkins.

Detterman, D. K., & Sternberg, R. J. (1994). Transfer on trial. In D. K. Detterman & R. J. Sternberg (Eds.). *Transfer on trial: Intelligence, cognition and instruction* (p. 1–24). Norwood, NJ: Ablex

Dirette, D. K., & Hinojosa, J. (1999). The effects of a compensatory intervention on processing deficits of adults with acquired brain injuries. *Occupational Therapy Journal of Research, 19*, 223–240.

Dobkin, B. H. (1996). *Neurologic rehabilitation*. Philadelphia: Davis.

Donaghy, S., & Williams, W. (1998). New methodology: A new protocol for training severely impaired patients in the usage of memory journals. *Brain Injury, 12*, 1061–1076.

Easton, T. (1972). On the normal use of reflexes. *American Scientist, 60*, 591–599.

Ehlers, A., Osen, A., Wenninger, K., & Gieler, U. (1994). Atopic dermatitis and stress: The possible role of negative communication with significant others. *International Journal of Behavioral Medicine, 1*, 107–121.

Ehlers, A., Stangier, U., & Gieler, U. (1995). Treatment of atopic dermatitis: A comparison of psychological and dermatological approaches to relapse prevention. *Journal of Consulting and Clinical Psychology, 63*, 624–635.

Engel, J. M., & Rapoff, M. A. (1990). A component analysis of relaxation training for children with vascular, muscle contraction, and mixed-headache disorders. In D. C. Tyler & E. J. Krane (Eds.). *Advances in pain research therapy* (Vol. 15, pp. 273–290). New York: Raven.

Epstein, S., & Meier, P. (1989). Constructive thinking: A broad coping variable with specific components. *Journal of Personality and Social Psychology, 57*, 332–350.

Evans, J. J., Emslie, H., & Wilson, B. A. (1998). Case study: External cueing systems in the rehabilitation of executive impairments of action. *Journal of the International Neuropsychological Society, 4*, 399–408.

Evans, J. J., Wilson, B. A., Schuri, U., Andrade, J., Baddeley, A., Bruna, O., Canavan, T., Sala, S. D., Green, R., Laaksonen, R., Lorenzi, L., & Taussik, I. (2000). A comparison of "errorless" and "trial-and-error" learning methods for teaching individuals with acquired memory deficits. *Neuropsychological Rehabilitation, 10*(1), 67–101.

Farber, S. (1993, March). *OT intervention for individuals with limb apraxia*. Paper presented at the American Occupational Therapy Association Neuroscience Institute: Treating Adults with Apraxia, Baltimore.

Fasotti, L., Kovacs, F., Eling, P., & Brouwer, W. H. (2000). Time pressure management as a compensatory strategy training after closed head injury. *Neuropsychological Rehabilitation, 10*, 47–65.

Fawzy, I. F., Kemeny, M. E., Fawzy, N. W., Elashoff, R., Morton, D., Cousins, N., & Fahey, J. L. (1990). A structured psychiatric intervention for cancer patients: II Changes over time in immunological measures. *Archives of General Psychiatry, 47*, 313–319.

Fertherlin, J. M., & Kurland, L. (1989). Self-instruction: A compensatory strategy to increase functional independence with brain injured adults. *Occupational Therapy Practice, 1*(1), 75–78.

Fine, S. (1993). Lesson 3: Interaction between psychosocial variables and cognitive function. In C. B. Royeen (Ed.). *Cognitive rehabilitation* [AOTA Self–Study Series] (pp. 1–40). Rockville, MD: American Occupational Therapy Association.

Fisher, A., &, Kielhofner, G (1995). Skill in occupational performance. In G. Kielhofner (Ed.). *A model of human occupation theory and application* (2nd ed., pp. 113–137). Baltimore: Williams & Wilkins.

Fisher, A. G. (1999). *Assessment of motor and process skills* (3rd ed.). Ft. Collins, CO: Three Star.

Fisher, A., Liu, Y., Velozo, C., & Pan, A. W. (1992). Cross-cultural assessment of process skills. *American Journal of Occupational Therapy, 46*, 876–884.

Foerster, O. (1977). The motor cortex in man in light of Hughlings Jackson's doctrines. In: O. D. Payton, S. Hirt, & R. Newman (Eds.). *Scientific basis for neurophysiologic approaches to therapeutic exercise* (pp. 13–18). Philadelphia: Davis.

Folkman, S., & Moskowitz, J. T. (2000). Positive affect and the other side of coping. *American Psychologist, 55*, 647–654.

Follick, M. J., Ahern, D. K., & Laser-Wolston, N. (1984). Evaluation of a daily activity diary for chronic pain patients. *Pain, 19*, 373–382.

Forbes, E. J., & Pekala, R. J. (1993). Psychophysiological effects of several stress management techniques. *Psychological Reports, 72*, 19–27.

Fordyce, W. E. (1976). *Behavioral methods for chronic pain and illness*. St. Louis: Mosby.

Fordyce, W. E. (1990). Contingency management. In J. J. Bonica (Ed.). *The management of pain* (2nd ed., pp. 1702–1710). Philadelphia: Lea & Febiger.

Freeman, E. (2001). Unilateral spatial neglect: New treatment approaches with potential application to occupational therapy. *American Journal of Occupational Therapy*, 55(4), 401–408.

Friedman, H. S., Tucker, J. S., Schwartz, J. E., Martin, L. R., Tomlinson-Keasey, C., Wingard, D. L., & Criqui, M. H. (1995). Childhood conscientiousness and longevity: Health behaviors and cause of death. *Journal of Personality and Social Psychology*, 68, 696–703.

Friedman, M. (1969). *Pathogenesis of coronary artery disease*. New York. McGraw-Hill.

Gage, M., & Polatajko, H. J. (1994). Enhancing occupational performance through an understanding of perceived self efficacy. *American Journal of Occupational Therapy, 48*, 783–790.

Gentile, P. A., & Iyer, M. B. (2001). Traditional sensorimotor approaches to treatment: An overview. In L. W. Pedretti & M. B. Early (Eds.). *Occupational therapy practice skills for physical dysfunction* (5th ed., pp. 567–575). Philadelphia: Mosby.

Gibson, J. J. (1966). *The senses considered as perceptual systems*. Boston: Houghton Mifflin.

Giles, G. M. (1998). A neurofunctional approach to rehabilitation following severe brain injury. In N. Katz (Ed.). *Cognition and occupation in rehabilitation: Cognitive models for intervention in occupational therapy* (pp. 125–147). Bethesda, MD: American Occupational Therapy Association.

Giles, G. M., & Allen, M. E. (1986). Occupational therapy in the treatment of the patient with chronic pain. *British Journal of Occupational Therapy, 49*, 4–9.

Giles, G. M., & Clark-Wilson, J. (1988). The use of behavioral techniques in functional skills training after severe brain injury. *American Journal of Occupational Therapy, 42*(10), 658–669.

Giles, M. G. & Wilson, C. J. (1993). Brain injury rehabilitation: A neurofunctional approach. East Sussex, UK: Chapman and Hall.

Giles, G. M., Ridley, J. E., Dill, A., & Frye, S. (1997). A consecutive series of adults with brain injury treated with a washing and dressing retraining program. *American Journal of Occupational Therapy, 51*(4), 256–266.

Giles, G. M., & Shore, M. (1989). A rapid method for teaching severely brain injured adults how to wash and dress. *Archives of Physical Medicine and Rehabilitation, 70*, 156–158.

Glass, T. A., Mendes de Leon, C., Marottoli, R. A., & Berkman, L. F. (1999). Population based study of social and productive activities as predictors of survival among elderly Americans. *British Medical Journal, 319*, 478–483.

Glisky, E. L. (1995). Computers in memory rehabilitation. In A. D. Baddeley, B. A. Wilson, & F. N. Watts (Eds.). *Handbook of memory disorders* (pp. 557–575). New York: Wiley.

Glisky, E. L., Schacter, L. D., & Butters, A. M. (1994). Domain-specific learning and remediation of memory disorders. In M. J. Riddoch & G. W. Humphreys (Eds.). *Cognitive neuropsychology and cognitive rehabilitation* (pp. 527–548). East Sussex, UK: Erabaum.

Goldstein, T. S. (1995). *Functional rehabilitation in orthopaedics*. Gaithersburg, MD: Aspen.

Golisz, K. M. (1998). Dynamic assessment and multicontext treatment of unilateral neglect. *Topics in Stroke Rehabilitation, 5*, 11–28.

Gollwitzer, P. M. (1999). How can good intentions become effective behavior change strategies. *American Psychologist, 54*, 493–503.

Gordon, J. (1987). Assumptions underlying physical therapy intervention: Theoretical and historical perspectives. In. J. H. Carr, R. B. Shepherd, J. Gordon, A. M. Gentile, & J. M. Held (Eds.). *Movement science: Foundation for physical therapy in rehabilitation* (pp. 1–30). Rockville, MD: Aspen Systems.

Gottlieb, N. H., & Green, L. W. (1984). Life events, social network, lifestyle, and health: An analysis of the 1979 national survey of personal health practices and consequences. *Health Education Quarterly, 11*, 91–105.

Grady, C. L., & Kapur, S. (1999). The use of neuroimaging in neurorehabilitative research. In D. T. Stuss, G. Winocur, & I. H. Robertson (Eds.). *Cognitive neurorehabilitation* (pp. 47–58). Cambridge, UK: Cambridge University Press.

Green, L. S. & Williams, H. G. (1996). Aging and coordination from the dynamical pattern perspective. In A. M. Ferrandez & N. Teasdale (Eds.). *Changes in sensory motor behavior in aging* (pp. 89–131). Amsterdam: Elsevier.

Greene, P. H. (1972). Problems of organization of motor systems. In R. Rosen & F. M. Snell (Eds.). *Progress in theoretical biology* (pp. 304–338) San Diego: Academic.

Grembowski, D., Patrick, D., Diehr, P., Durham, M., Beresford, S., Kay, E., & Hecht, J. (1993). Self-efficacy and health behavior among older adults. *Journal of Health and Social Behavior, 34*, 89–104.

Griffin, K. W., Friend, R., Eitel, P., & Lobel, M. (1993). Effects of environmental demands, stress, and mood on health practices. *Journal of Behavioral Medicine, 16*, 643–661.

Grillner, S. (1981). Control of locomotion in bipeds, tetrapods, and fish. In V. B. Brooks (Ed.). *Handbook of physiology: The nervous system. Volume 2: Motor control* (pp. 1179–1236). Baltimore: Wilkins & Wilkins.

Gross, Y., & Schutz, L. E. (1986). Intervention models in neuropsychology. In B. Uzzell & Y. Gross (Eds.). *Clinical neuropsychology of intervention* (pp. 179–204). Boston: Nijhoff.

Hamill, J., & Knutzen, K. M. (1995). *Biomechanical basis of human movement*. Baltimore: Williams & Wilkins.

Harrell, M., Parente, F., Bellingrath, E., & Lisicia, K. (1992). *Cognitive rehabilitation of memory: A practical guide*. Gaithersburg, MD: Aspen.

Haugen, J., Mathiowetz, V., & Flinn, N. (2002). Optimizing motor behavior using the occupational therapy task oriented approach. In. C. Trombly & M. V. Radomski (Eds.). *Occupational therapy for physical dysfunction* (pp. 481–500). Philadelphia: Lippincott, Williams & Wilkins.

Hawthorn, J., & Redmond, K. (1998). *Pain causes and management*. Malden, MA: Blackwell Science.

Hayes, R. L., & McGrath, J. J. (2001). *Cognitive rehabilitation for people with schizophrenia and related conditions* [Cochrane Library, Issue 3]. Oxford, UK: Update Software.

Heck, S. A. (1988). The effect of purposeful activity on pain tolerance. *American Journal of Occupational Therapy, 42*, 577–581.

Helm-Estabrooks, N. (1982). Visual action therapy for global aphasics. *Journal of Speech and Hearing Disorders, 47*, 385–389.

Heriza, C. (1991). Motor development: Traditional and contemporary theories. In M. Lister (Ed.). *Contemporary management of motor control problems* (pp. 99–126) Alexandria, VA: American Physical Therapy Association.

Hills, H., & Norvell, N. (1991). An examination of hardiness and neuroticism as potential moderators of stress outcomes. *Behavioral Medicine, 17*, 31–38.

Hilts, P. (1980). The clock within. *Science, 80*, 61–67.

Holmes, T. H., & Rahe, R. H. (1967). The social readjustment rating scale. *Journal of Psychosomatic Research, 11*, 213–218.

Horak, F. (1991). Assumptions underlying motor control for neurological rehabilitation. In M. Lister (Ed.). *Contemporary management of motor control problems* (pp. 11–28). Alexandria, VA: American Physical Therapy Association.

International Association for the Study of Pain [IASP]. (1979). Pain terms: A list with definitions and notes on usage. *Pain, 6*, 249–252.

International Association for the Study of Pain—Ad hoc Subcommittee for Occupational Therapy and Physical Therapy Curriculum [IASP]. (1994 Nov/Dec). Pain curriculum for students in occupational therapy or physical therapy. *International Association for the Study of Pain Newsletter*, 3–8.

Jackson, J., Gray, J. M., & Zemke, R. (2002). Optimizing abilities and capacities: Range of motion, strength, and endurance. In C. A. Trombly & M. V. Radomski (Eds.), *Occupational therapy for physical dysfunction* (5th ed., pp. 463–480). Philadelphia: Lippincott, Williams & Wilkins.

Jacobsen, E. (1938). *Progressive relaxation*. Chicago: University of Chicago Press.

Jensen, M. P., & Karoly, P. (1992). Self-report scales and procedures for assessing pain in adults. In D. C. Turk & R. Melzack (Eds.). *Handbook of pain assessment* (pp. 135–151). New York: Guilford.

Jensen, M. P., Romano, J. M., Turner, J. A., Good, A. B., & Wald, L. H. (1999). Patient beliefs predict patient functioning: Further support for a cognitive-behavioural model of chronic pain. *Pain, 81*(1–2), 95–104.

Kabat, H. (1950). Studies in neuromuscular dysfunction, XIII: New concepts and techniques of neuromuscular reeducation for paralysis. *Perm Foundation Medical Bulletin*, 8(3), 121–143.

Kabat-Zinn, J. (1990). *Full catastrophe living*. New York: Delta.

Kandel, E., Schwartz, J. H., & Jessel, T. M. (Eds.). (1991). *Principles of neuroscience* (3rd ed.). New York: Elsevier.

Karasek, R. A. (1979). Job demand, job decision latitude and mental strain: implications for job redesign. *Administrative Science Quarterly, 24*, 285–308.

Karasek, R. A., Theorell, T. T., Schwartz, J., Schall, P., Pieper, C., & Michela, J. L. (1988). Job characteristics in relation to the prevalence of myocardial infarction in the US HES and HANES. *American Journal of Public Health, 78*, 910–918.

Kasch, M. C. & Nickerson E. (2001). Hand and upper extremity injuries. In L. W. Pedretti & M. B. Early (Eds.). *Occupational therapy: Practice skills for physical dysfunction* (5th ed., pp. 833–866). St. Louis: Mosby.

Katz, N., & Hartman-Maeir, A. (1998). Metacognition: The relationship of awareness and executive functions to occupational performance. In N. Katz (Ed.). *Cognition and occupation in rehabilitation: Cognitive models for intervention in occupational therapy* (pp. 323–342). Bethesda, MD: American Occupational Therapy Association.

Keefe, F. J., & Block, A. R. (1982). Development of an observation method for assessing pain behavior in chronic low back pain patients. *Behavior Therapy, 13*, 363–375.

Keele, S. (1968). Movement control in skilled motor performance. *Psychological Bulletin, 70*, 387–403.

Kelly, M., & Ostreicher, H. (1985). Environmental factors and outcomes in hemineglect syndromes. *Rehabilitation Psychology, 30*, 35–37.

Kerkhoff, G., MunBinger, U., & Meier, E. K. (1994). Neurovisual rehabilitation in cerebral blindness. *Archives of Neurology, 51*, 474–481.

Kerns, K. A., & Thomson, J. (1998). Case study: Implementation of a compensatory memory system in a school age child with severe memory impairment. *Pediatric Rehabilitation*, 2(2), 77–87.

Keshner, E. (1991). How theoretical framework biases evaluation and treatment. In M. Lister (Ed.). *Contemporary management of motor control problems* (pp. 37–49). Alexandria, VA: American Physical Therapy Association.

Kiecolt-Glaser, J. K., Fisher, L. D., Ogrocki, P., Stout, J. C., Speicher, C. E., & Glaser, R. (1987). Marital quality, marital disruption, and immune function. *Psychosomatic Medicine, 49*, 13–25.

Kim, H. J., Burke, D. T., Dowds, M. M., & George, J. (1999). Utility of a microcomputer as an external memory aid for a memory-impaired head injury patient during in-patient rehabilitation. *Brain Injury, 13*(2), 147–150.

Kisner, C., & Colby, L. A. (1996). *Therapeutic exercise: Foundations and techniques*. Philadelphia: Davis.

Klavora, P., Gaskovski, P., Martin, K., Forsyth, D. R., Heslegrave, J. R., Young, M., & Quinn, P. R. (1995). The effects of Dynavision rehabilitation on behind-the-wheel driving ability psychomotor abilities of persons after stroke. *American Journal of Occupational Therapy, 49*(6), 534–542.

Klavora, P., & Warren, M. (1998). Rehabilitation of visuomotor skills in poststroke patients using the Dynavision apparatus. *Perceptual and Motor Skills, 86*, 23–30.

Laatsch, L., Pavel, D., Jobe, T., Lin, Q., & Quintana, J. C. (1999). Incorporation of SPECT imaging in a longitudinal cognitive rehabilitation therapy programme. *Brain Injury, 13*, 555–570.

LaBuda, J., & Lichtenberg, P. (1999). The role of cognition, depression, and awareness of deficit in predicting geriatric rehabilitation patients' IADL performance. *Clinical Neuropsychologist, 13*(3), 258–267.

Lamm-Warburg, C. (1988). Assessment and treatment strategies for perceptual deficits. In S. O'Sullivan & T. J. Schmitz (Eds.). Physical rehabilitation: Assessment and treatment (2nd ed., pp. 93–120). Philadelphia: Davis.

LaMore, K. L., & Nelson, D. L. (1993). The effects of options on performance of and art project in adults with mental disabilities. *American Journal of Occupational Therapy, 47*, 635–637.

Landa-Gonzalez, B. (2001). Multicontextual occupational therapy intervention: A case study of traumatic brain injury. *Occupational Therapy International, 8*(1), 49–62.

Lave, J. (1988). *Cognition in practice: Mind, mathematics and culture in everyday life*. Cambridge, UK: Cambridge University Press.

Lazarus, R. S. (1993). From psychological stress to the emotions: A history of a changing outlook. *Annual Review of Psychology, 44*, 1–21.

Lee, T. D. (1998). On the dynamics of motor learning research. *Research Quarterly for Exercise and Sport, 69*, 334–343.

Lennon, S. (1994). Task specific effects in the rehabilitation of unilateral neglect. In M. J. Riddoch & G. W. Humphreys (Eds.). *Cognitive neuropsychology and cognitive rehabilitation* (pp. 187–203). East Sussex, UK: Erlbaum.

Levine, B., Robertson, I. H., Clare, L., Carter, G., Hong, J., Wilson, B. A., Duncan, J., & Stuss, D. (2000). Rehabilitation of executive functioning: An experimental-clinical validation of goal management training. *Journal of International Neuropsychological Society, 6*, 299–312.

Levit, K. (2002). Optimizing motor behavior using the Bobath approach. In C. A. Trombly & M. V. Radomski (Eds.). *Occupational therapy for physical dysfunction* (5th ed., pp. 521–541). Philadelphia: Lippincott, Williams & Wilkins.

Lillegard, W. A., & Terrio, J. D. (1994). Appropriate strength training. *Medical Clinics of North America, 78*, 457–477.

Lin, K. C. (1996). Right-hemispheric activation approaches to neglect rehabilitation poststroke. *American Journal of Occupational Therapy, 50*, 504–515.

Lincoln, N. B., Majid, M. J., & Weyman, N. (2000). *Cognitive rehabilitation for attention deficits following stroke* [Cochrane Library, Issue 4]. Oxford, UK: Update Software.

Loomis, J. E., & Boersma, F. J. (1982). Training in right brain damaged patients in wheelchair task: Case studies using verbal mediation. *Physiotherapy* [Canada], *34*(4), 204–208.

Lundborg, G. (2000). A 25 year perspective of peripheral nerve surgery: Evolving neuroscientific concepts and clinical significance. *Journal of Hand Surgery* [America], *25*(3), 391–407.

Luria, A. R. (1973). *The working brain* (B. Haigh, Trans.). New York: Basic.

MacRae, A., & Riley, E. (1990). Home health occupational therapy for the management of chronic pain: An environmental model. *Occupational Therapy Practice, 1*(3), 69–76.

Malec, J. F., & Moessner, A. M. (2000). Self–awareness, distress, and postacute rehabilitation outcome. *Rehabilitation Psychology, 45*(3), 227–241.

Malec, J. F., Smigielski, J. S., & DePompolo, R. W. (1991). Goal attainment scaling and outcome measurement in postacute brain injury rehabilitation. *Archives of Physical Medicine and Rehabilitation, 72*, 138–143.

Mandle, C. L., Jacobs, S. C., Arcari, P. M., & Domar, A. D. (1996). The efficacy of relaxation response interventions with adult patients: A review of the literature. *Journal of Cardiovascular Nursing, 10*(3), 4–26.

Mateer, C. A. (1999). Executive function disorders: Rehabilitation challenges and strategies. *Seminars in Clinical Neuropsychiatry, 4*(1), 50–59.

Mathews, K. A. (1988). Coronary heart disease and Type A behaviors: Update on and alternative to the Booth-Kewley and Friedman (1987) quantitative review. *Psychological Bulletin, 104*, 373–380.

Mathiowetz, V., & Haugen, J. (2002). Assessing abilities and capacities: motor behavior. In C. Trombly & M. V. Radomski (Eds.). *Occupational therapy for physical dysfunction* (pp. 157–187). Philadelphia: Lippincott, Williams & Wilkins.

Mayer, N. H., Keating, D. J., & Rapp, D. (1986). Skills, routines, and activity patterns of daily living: A functional nested approach. In B. P. G. Uzzell, Y. (Ed.). *Clinical neuropsychology of intervention* (pp. 205–222). Boston: Nijhoff.

McArdle, W. D., Katch, F. I., & Katch, V. L. (1996). Exercise physiology: Energy, nutrition and human performance (4th ed.). Malvern, PA: Lea & Febiger.

McCormack, G. L. (1988). Pain management by occupational practitioners. *American Journal of Occupational Therapy, 42*, 582–590.

McCormack, G. L. (1993). *Pain management: Mindbody techniques for treating chronic pain syndromes*. Tucson, AZ: Therapy Skill Builders.

Meichenbaum, D (1985). *Stress innoculation training*. New York: Pereamon.

McNaughton, M. E., Patterson, T. L., Smith, T. L., & Grant, I. (1995). The relationship among stress, depression, locus of control, irrational beliefs, social support and health in Alzheimer's disease caregivers. *Journal of Nervous and Mental Disease, 183*, 78–85.

Mendes de Leon, C. F., Powell, L. H., & Kaplan, B. H. (1991). Change in coronary-prone behaviors in the Recurrent Coronary Prevention Project. *Psychosomatic Medicine, 53*, 407–419.

Merskey, H. (1992). Limitations of pain behavior. *American Pain Society Bulletin, 1*, 101–104.

Merzenich, M., & Jenkins, W. (1993). Reorganization of cortical representations of the hand following alterations of skin inputs induced by nerve injury, skin island transfers and experience. *Journal of Hand Therapy, 6*(2), 89–105.

Miller, W. R., & Rollnick, S. (1991). *Motivational interviewing*. New York: Guildford Press.

Mitchell, E. (2000). Managing carer stress: An evaluation of a stress management programme for carers of people with dementia. *British Journal of Occupational Therapy, 63*, 179–184.

Montgomery P. (1991). Neurodevelopmental treatment and sensory integrative theory. In M. Lister (Ed.). *Contemporary management of motor control problems* (pp. 135–137). Alexandria, VA: American Physical Therapy Association.

Moser, K. A., Fox, A. J., & Jones, D. R. (1984). Unemployment and mortality in the OPCS longitudinal study. *Lancet, 2*, 1324–1329.

Moulton, H. J., Taira, E. D., & Grover, R. (1995, November). *Utilizing occupational therapy and families at mealtimes with nursing home residents with dementia*. Paper presented at the Annual Conference of the Gerontological Society on Aging, Los Angeles.

Moyers, P. (1999). The guide to occupational therapy practice. *American Journal of Occupational Therapy, 53*, 247–322.

National Institutes of Health. (1995, October). *Integration of behavioral and relaxation approaches into the treatment of chronic pain and insomnia*. Statement from the NIH Technology Assessment Conference, Bethesda, MD.

Neistadt, M. E. (1990). A critical analysis of occupational therapy approaches for perceptual deficits in adults with brain injury. *American Journal of Occupational Therapy, 44*, 299–304.

Neistadt, M. (1992). Occupational therapy treatments for constructional deficits. *American Journal of Occupational Therapy, 46*(2), 141–148.

Neistadt, M. (1994a). The neurobiology of learning: Implications for treatment of adults with brain injury. *American Journal of Occupational Therapy, 48*, 421–430.

Neistadt, M. (1994b). Perceptual retaining for adults with diffuse brain injury. *American Journal of Occupational Therapy, 48*, 225–233.

Neistadt, M. E., & Seymour, S. (1995). Treatment activity preferences of occupational therapists in adult physical dysfunction settings. *American Journal of Occupational Therapy, 49*, 437–443.

Nelson, D. L., & Lenhart, D. A. (1996). Resumption of outpatient occupational therapy for a young woman five years after traumatic brain injury. *American Journal of Occupational Therapy, 50*, 223–228.

Newton-John, T. O., Spence, S. H., & Schotte, D. (1995). Cognitive-behavioral therapy versus EMG biofeedback in the treatment of low back pain. *Behaviour Research and Therapy, 33*, 691–697.

Niemeier, J. P. (1998). The lighthouse strategy: use of a visual imagery technique to treat visual inattention in stroke patients. *Brain Injury, 12*(5), 399–406.

Niemeier, J. P., Cifu, D. X., & Kishore, R. (2001). The lighthouse strategy: Improving the functional status of patients with unilateral neglect after stroke and brain injury using a visual imagery intervention. *Topics in Stroke Rehabilitation*, 8(2), 10–18.

Niemeyer, L. O. (1990). Psychologic and sociocultural aspects of responses to pain. *Occupational Therapy Practice, 1*(3), 11–20.

Nunes, E. V., Frank, K. A., & Kornfeld, D. S. (1987). Psychologic treatment for the type A behavior pattern and for coronary heart disease: A meta analysis of the literature. *Psychosomatic Medicine, 48*, 159–173.

Nygard, L., Bernspang, B., Fisher, A., & Winblad, B (1994). Comparing motor and process ability of person with suspected dementia in home and clinic settings. *American Journal of Occupational Therapy*, 48, 689–696.

Okkema, K. (1993). *Cognition and perception in the stroke patient*. Gaithersburg, MD: Aspen.

Palmese, C. A., & Raskin, S. A. (2000). The rehabilitation of attention in individuals with mild traumatic brain injury, using the APT-II programme. *Brain Injury, 14*(6), 535–548.

Pan, A. W., & Fisher, A. (1994). The assessment of motor and process skills of persons with psychiatric disorders. *American Journal of Occupational Therapy, 48*, 775–782.

Paolucci, S., Antonucci, G., Grasso, M. G., & Pizzamiglio, L. (2001). The role of unilateral spatial neglect in rehabilitation of right brain-damaged ischemic stroke patients: A matched comparison. *Archives of Physical Medicine and Rehabilitation, 82*, 743–749.

Park, C. L., Cohen, L. H., & Murch, R. L. (1996). Assessment and prediction of stress related growth. *Journal of Personality Assessment, 64*, 71–105.

Park, S., Fisher, A., & Velozo, C. (1994). Using the assessment of motor and process skills to compare occupational performance between clinic and home settings. *American Journal of Occupational Therapy*, 48, 697–709.

Patrick, L., & D'Eon, J. (1996). Social support and functional status in chronic pain patients. *Canadian Journal of Rehabilitation, 9*, 195–201.

Paul, S. (1997). The effects of video assisted feedback on a scanning kitchen task in individuals with left visual neglect. *Canadian Journal of Occupational Therapy*, 64(2), 63–69.

Pedretti, L. W., & Early, M. B. (2001). Occupational performance and models of practice for physical dysfunction. In L. W. Pedretti & M. B. Early (Eds.). *Occupational therapy: Practice skills for physical dysfunction* (5th ed., pp. 3–11). St. Louis: Mosby.

Pelletier, K. (1977). *Mind as healer, mind as slayer*. New York: Delta.

Pilgrim, E., & Humphrey's, G. W. (1994). Rehabilitation of a case of ideomotor apraxia. In M. J. Riddoch & G. W. Humphreys (Eds.). *Cognitive neuropsychology and cognitive rehabilitation* (pp. 271–315). East Sussex, UK: Erlbaum.

Pizzamiglio, L., Antonucci, G., Judica, A., Montenero, P., Razzano, C., & Zoccolotti, P. (1992). Cognitive rehabilitation of the hemineglect disorder in chronic patients with unilateral right brain damage. *Journal of Clinical Experimental Neuropsychology*, 14(6), 901–923.

Polit, A., & Bizzi, E. (1979). Characteristics of motor programs underlying arm movements in monkeys. *Journal of Neurophysiology, 42*, 183–194.

Poole, J. L. (1991). Application of motor learning principles in occupational therapy. *American Journal of Occupational Therapy, 45*, 531–537.

Poole, J. L. (2000). A comparison of limb praxis abilities of persons with developmental dyspraxia and adult onset apraxia. *Occupational Therapy Journal of Research*, 20(2), 106–120.

Pope-Davis, S. A. (2001). Proprioceptive neuromuscular facilitation approach. In L. W. Pedretti & M. B. Early (Eds.). *Occupational therapy practice skills for physical dysfunction* (5th ed., pp. 606–623). St. Louis: Mosby.

Preston, L. A. (2001). Motor control. In L. W. Pedretti & M. B. Early (Eds.). *Occupational therapy practice skills for physical dysfunction* (5th ed., pp. 360–386). St. Louis: Mosby.

Prigatano, G. P. (1999). *Principles of neuropsychological rehabilitation*. New York: Oxford University Press.

Prigatano, G. P., & Wong, J. L. (1999). Cognitive and affective improvement in brain dysfunctional patients who achieve inpatient rehabilitation goals. *Archives of Physical Medicine and Rehabilitation*, 80, 77–84.

Radomski, V. M., Dougherty, M. P., Fine, B. S., & Baum, C. (1993). Lesson 10: Case studies in cognitive rehabilitation. In C. B. Royeen (Ed.). *Cognitive rehabilitation* [AOTA Self–Study Series] (pp. 4–68). Rockville, MD: American Occupational Therapy Association.

Rahe, R. H. (1979). Life change events and mental illness: An overview. *Journal of Human Stress, 5*, 2–9.

Raloff, L. (1981a). Basement parking and high rise CO_2. *Science News, 120*, 316.

Raloff, L. (1981b). Building illness. *Science News, 120*, 316.

Raloff, L. (1982a). Occupational noise—The subtle pollutant. *Science News, 121*, 347–350.

Raloff, L. (1982b). Noise can be hazardous to your health. *Science News, 121*, 377–380.

Raskin, S. A. & Mateer, C. (2000). *Neuropsychological management of mild traumatic brain injury*. New York: Oxford University Press.

Rebmann, M. J., & Hannon, R. (1995). Treatment of unawareness of memory deficits in adults with brain injury: Three case studies. *Rehabilitation Psychology*, 40(4), 279–287.

Rippere, V. (1977). "What is the thing to do when you are feeling depressed?" A pilot study. *Behavior Research and Therapy, 15*, 185–191.

Robertson, I. H., North, N. T., & Geggie., C. (1992). Spatiomotor cueing in unilateral left neglect: Three single case studies of its therapeutic effects. *Journal of Neurology, Neurosurgery & Psychiatry, 55*, 799–805.

Robertson, I. H., Hogg, K., & McMillan, T. M. (1998). Rehabilitation of unilateral neglect: Improving function by contralesional limb activation. *Neuropsychological Rehabilitation*, 8(1), 19–29.

Robertson, I. H., Tegner, R., Tham, K., Lo, A., & Smith, N. I. (1995). Sustained attention training for unilateral neglect: Theoretical and rehabilitation implications. *Journal of Clinical Neuropsychology, 17*(3), 416–430.

Rockwood, K., Joyce, B., Stolee, P. (1997). Use of goal attainment scaling in measuring clinically important change in cognitive rehabilitation patients. *Journal of Clinical Epidemiology; 50*, 581–588.

Rood, M. S. (1954). Neurophysiological reactions as a basis for physical therapy. *Physical Therapy Review, 34*, 444–449.

Rood, M. S. (1956). Neurophysiological mechanisms utilized in the treatment of neuromuscular dysfunction. *American Journal of Occupational Therapy, 10*, 220–225.

Rose, D. (1997). *A multilevel approach to the study of motor control and learning*. Needham Heights, MA: Allyn & Bacon.

Rosenbaum, A. (1991). *Human motor control*. San Diego: Academic Press.

Rosenman, R. H., Brand, R. J., Jenkins, C. D., Friedman, M., & Wurm, M. (1975). Coronary heart disease in the Western Collaborative Group Study: Final follow-up experience of eight and one half years. *Journal of the American Medical Association, 233*, 872–877.

Ross, F. (1992). The use of computers in occupational therapy for visual scanning. *American Journal of Occupational Therapy, 46*, 314–322.

Rossi, W. P., Kheyfets, S., & Reding, J. M. (1990). Fresnel prisms improve visual perception in stroke patients with homonymous hemianopia or unilateral visual neglect. *Neurology, 40*, 1597–1599.

Roy, E. A. (1985). *Neuropsychological studies of apraxia and related disorders*. Amsterdam: Elsevier Science.

Royeen, C. B., Duncan, M., & McCormack, G. (2001). The Rood approach: A reconstruction. In L. W. Pedretti & M. B. Early (Eds.). *Occupational therapy practice skills for physical dysfunction* (5th ed., pp. 576–587). Philadelphia: Mosby.

Rubio, K. B. (1998). Treatment of neurobehavioral deficits: A function-based approach. In G. Gillen & A. Burkhardt (Eds.). *Stroke rehabilitation: A function-based approach* (pp. 334–352). St. Louis: Mosby.

Ruff, R. M., Baser, C. A., Johnston, J. W., Marshall, L. F., Klauber, S. K., Klauber, M. R., & Minteer, M. (1989). Neuropsychological rehabilitation: An experimental study with head injured patients. *Journal of Head Trauma Rehabilitation, 4*, 20–36.

Sabari, J. S. (1991). Motor learning concepts applied to activity-based intervention with adults with hemiplegia. *American Journal of Occupational Therapy, 45*, 523–536.

Sabari, J. (2002). Optimizing motor control using the Carr and Shepherd approach. In. C. Trombly & M. V. Radomski (Eds.). *Occupational therapy for physical dysfunction* (pp. 501–520). Philadelphia: Lippincott, Williams & Wilkins.

Sbordone, R. J. (1991). Overcoming obstacles in cognitive rehabilitation of persons with severe traumatic brain injury. In J. S. Kreutzer & P. H. Wehman (Eds.). *Cognitive rehabilitation for persons with traumatic brain injury* (pp. 105–116). Baltimore: Brookes.

Scheier, M. F., & Carver, C. S. (1987). Dispositional optimism and physical wellbeing: The influence of generalized outcome expectancies on health. *Journal of Personality, 55*, 169–210.

Schlund, M. W. (1999). Self awareness: effects of feedback and review on verbal self reports and remembering following brain injury. *Brain Injury, 13*(5), 375–380.

Schmidt, R. A. & Lee, T. D. (1999) . *Motor control and learning; A behavioral emphasis*. Champaign, IL: Human Kinetics.

Scholz, J. (1990). Dynamic pattern theory—Some implications for therapeutics. *Physical Therapy, 70*, 827–843.

Schwartz, M. S. (1995). Adults with traumatic brain injury: Three case studies of cognitive rehabilitation in the home setting. *American Journal of Occupational Therapy, 49*, 655–668.

Selye, H. (1978). *The stress of life*. New York: McGraw–Hill.

Seron, X., Deloche, G., & Coyette, F. (1989). A retrospective analysis of a single case of neglect therapy: A point of theory. In X. Seron & G. Deloche (Eds.). *Cognitive approaches in neuropsychological rehabilitation*. Hillsdale, NJ: Erlbaum.

Shavit, Y., Terman, G. W., Martin, F. C., Lewis, J. W., Liebeskind, J. C., & Gale, R. P. (1985). Stress, opioid peptides, the immune system and cancer. *Journal of Immunology, 135*, 834s–837s.

Shekelle, R. B., Gale, M., & Norusis, M. (1985). Type A score (Jenkins Activity Survey) and risk of recurrent coronary heart disease in the Aspirin Myocardial Infarction Study. *American Journal of Cardiology, 56*, 221–225.

Shekelle, R. B., Hulley, S. B. Neaton, J. D., Billing, J. H., Borhani, N. O., Gerace, T. A., Jacobs, D. R., Lasser, N. L., Mittlemark, M. B., & Stamler, J. (1985). The MRFIT behavioral pattern study, I: Type A behavior pattern and risk of coronary death in MRFIT. *American Journal of Epidemiology, 122*, 559–570.

Sherer, M., Bergloff, P., Levin, E., High, W. M., Oden, K. E., & Nick, T. G. (1998). Impaired awareness and employment outcome after traumatic brain injury. *Journal of Head Trauma Rehabilitation, 13*, 52–61.

Sherer, M., Oden, K., Bergloff, P., Levin, E., & High, W. M. (1998). Assessment and treatment of impaired awareness after brain injury: implications for community reintegration. *NeuroRehabiliation, 10*, 25–37.

Sherrington, C. S. (1947). *The integrative action of the nervous system*. New Haven, CT: Yale University Press.

Shimelman, A., & Hinojosa, J. (1995). Gross motor activity and attention in three adults with brain injury. *American Journal of Occupational Therapy, 49*, 973–978.

Shumway-Cook, A., & Woollacott, M. (1995). *Motor control: Theory and practical application*. Baltimore: Williams & Wilkins.

Shumway-Cook, M. & Woollacott, M. (2001). *Motor control: Theory and practical applications*. Baltimore: Williams & Wilkins.

Siegrist, J., Peter, R., Junge, A., Cremer, P., & Seidel, D. (1990). Low status control, high effort at work and ischemic heart disease: Prospective evidence from blue-collar men. *Social Science and Medicine, 31*, 1127–1134.

Smania, N., Bazoli, F., Piva, D., & Guidetti, G. (1997). Visuomotor imagery and rehabilitation of neglect. *Archives of Physical Medicine and Rehabilitation, 78*, 430–436.

Smania, N., Girardi, F., Domenicali, C., Lora, E., & Aglioti, S. (2000). The rehabilitation of limb apraxia: A study in left-brain-damaged patients. *Archives of Physical Medicine and Rehabilitation, 81*, 379–388.

Smith, D. A., & Lukens, S. A. (1983). Stress effects of isometric contraction in occupational therapy. *Occupational Therapy Journal of Research, 3*, 222–242.

Snyder, C. R., Harris, C., Anderson, J. R., Holleran, S. A., Irving, L. M., Sigmon, S. T., Yoshinobu, L., Gibb, L., Langelle, C., & Harney, P. (1991). The will and the ways: Development and validation of an individual-differences measure of hope. *Journal of Personality and Social Psychology, 60*, 570–585.

Soderback, I., Bengtsson, I., Ginsburg, E., & Ekholm, J. (1992). Video feedback in occupational therapy: Its effect in patients with neglect syndrome. *Archives of Physical Medicine and Rehabilitation, 73*, 1140–1146.

Sohlberg, M. M. (2000). Assessing and managing unawareness of self. *Seminars in Speech and Language, 21*,135–150.

Sohlberg, M. M., & Mateer, A. C. (1989b). Training use of compensatory memory books: A three stage behavioral approach. *Journal of Clinical Neuropsychology, 11*, 871–891.

Sohlberg, M. M., & Mateer, C. A. (1989a). *Attention process training*. San Antonio, TX: Psychological Corporation.

Sohlberg, M. M., McLaughlin, K. A., Pavese, A., Heidrich, A., & Posner, M. I. (2000). Evaluation of attention process training and brain injury education in persons with acquired brain injury. *Journal of Clinical and Experimental Neuropsychology, 22*, 656–676.

Somerfield, M. R., & McCrae, R .R. (2000). Stress and coping research: Methodological challenges, theoretical advances and clinical applications. *American Psychologist, 55*, 620–625.

Spencer, J., Young, M. E., Rintala, D., & Bates, S. (1995). Socialization to the culture of a rehabilitation hospital: An ethnographic study. *American Journal of Occupational Therapy, 49*, 53–62.

Steffen, A. M. (2000). Anger management for dementia caregivers: A preliminary study using video and telephone interventions. *Behavior Therapy, 31*, 281–299.

Stein, F., & Nikolic, S. (1989). Teaching stress management techniques to a schizophrenic person. *American Journal of Occupational Therapy, 43*, 162–169.

Sternad, D. (1998). A dynamical systems perspective to perception and action. *Research Quarterly for Exercise and Sport, 69*, 319–325.

Strong, J., Cramond, T., & Maas, F. (1989). The effectiveness of relaxation techniques with patients who have chronic low back pain. *Occupational Therapy Journal of Research, 9*, 184–192.

Suslow, T., Schonauer, K., & Arolt, V. (2001). Attention training in the cognitive rehabilitation of schizophrenic patients: A review of efficacy studies. *Acta Psychiatrica Scandinavica, 103*, 15–23.

Tate, R. L. (1997). Subject review: Beyond one-bun, two-shoe: Recent advances in the psychological rehabilitation of memory disorders after acquired brain injury. *Brain Injury, 11*(12), 907–918.

Tham, K., Ginsburg, E., Fisher, A., & Tegner, R. (2001). Training to improve awareness of disabilities in clients with unilateral neglect. *American Journal of Occupational Therapy, 55*(1), 46–54.

Tham, K., & Tegner, R. (1997). Video feedback in the rehabilitation of patients with unilateral neglect. *Archives of Physical Medicine and Rehabilitation, 78*, 410–413.

Thayer, R. E., Newman, R., & McClain, T. M. (1994). Self-regulation of mood: Strategies for changing a bad mood, raising energy and reducing tension. *Journal of Personality and Social Psychology, 67*, 910–925.

Thelen, E., Kelso, J., & Fogel, A. (1987). Self-organizing systems and infant motor development. *Developmental Review, 7*, 39–65.

Thelen, E., & Smith, L. B. (1994). *A dynamic system approach to the development of cognition and action*. Cambridge, MA: Bradford.

Thomas, C. L. (Ed.). (1997). *Taber's cyclopedic medical dictionary* (18th ed.). Philadelphia: Davis.

Thomas, J. J. (1996). Materials-based, imagery-based, and rote exercise occupational forms: effect on repetitions, heart rate, duration of performance, and self–perceived rest periods in well elderly women. *American Journal of Occupational Therapy, 50*, 783–789.

Toglia, J. P. (1989). Visual perception of objects: An approach to assessment and intervention. *American Journal of Occupational Therapy, 43*(9), 587–595.

Toglia, J. P. (1991a). Generalization of treatment: A multicontextual approach to cognitive perceptual impairment in the brain injured adult. *American Journal of Occupational Therapy, 45*(6), 505–516.

Toglia, J. P. (1991b). Unilateral visual inattention: Multidimensional components. *Occupational Therapy Practice, 3*(1), 18–34.

Toglia, J. P. (1993). Lesson 4: Attention and memory. In C. B. Royeen (Ed.). *Cognitive rehabilitation* [AOTA Self–Study Series] (pp. 4–72). Rockville, MD: American Occupational Therapy Association.

Toglia, J. (1993, December). Treating individuals with constructional apraxia, Handouts from presentation at American Occupational Therapy Association (AOTA) Advanced Apraxia Institute: Assessing and Treating Adults. Denver, CO.

Toglia, J. (1996). A multicontext approach to cognitive rehabilitation. [Supplement manual to workshop held at New York Hospital-Cornell Medical Center, New York], New York: Author.

Toglia, J. P. (1998). A dynamic interactional model to cognitive rehabilitation. In N. Katz (Ed.). Cognition and occupation in rehabilitation: Cognitive models for intervention in occupational therapy (pp. 5–50). Bethesda, MD: American Occupational Therapy Association.

Toglia, J. P. (2001, April). *The multicontext approach to cognitive rehabilitation*. Paper presented at the Educational Special Interest Section Workshop at the meeting of the American Occupational Therapy Association, Philadelphia.

Toglia, J. P., & Golisz, K. M. (1990). *Cognitive rehabilitation: Group games and activities*. Tucson, AZ: Therapy Skill Builders.

Toglia, J., & Kirk, U. (2000). Understanding awareness deficits following brain injury. *NeuroRehabilitation, 15*, 57–70.

Towen, C. L. (1984). Primitive reflexes—Conceptual or semantic problems? *Clinics in Development Medicine, 94*, 115–125

Trexler, L. E., Webb, P. M., & Zappala, G. (1994). Strategic aspects of neuropsychological rehabilitation. In A. L. Christensen & B. P. Uzzell (Eds.). *Brain injury and neuropsychological rehabilitation: International perspectives* (pp. 99–123). Hillsdale, NJ: Erbaum.

Trombly, C. (1995). Occupation: Purposefulness and meaningfulness as therapeutic mechanisms. *American Journal of Occupational Therapy, 49*, 960–972.

Trombly, C. A. (2002). Managing deficit of first-level motor control capacities. In C. A. Trombly & M. V. Radomski (Eds.). *Occupational therapy for physical dysfunction* (5th ed., pp. 571–584). Philadelphia: Lippincott, Williams & Wilkins.

Turk, D. C., Meichenbaum, D., & Genest, M. (1983). *Pain and behavioral medicine*. New York: Guilford.

Turk, D. C., & Melzack, R. (1992). The measurement of pain and the assessment of people experiencing pain. In D. C. Turk & R. Melzack (Eds.). *Handbook of pain assessment* (pp. 3–12). New York: Guilford.

Turk, D. C., Wack, J. T., & Kerns, R. D. (1985). An empirical examination of the "pain behavior" construct. *Journal of Behavioral Medicine, 8*, 119–130.

Turner, J. A., & Chapman, C. R. (1982). Psychological interventions for chronic pain: A critical review. I. Relaxation training and biofeedback. *Pain, 12*, 1–21.

Tyson, R., & Strong, J. (1990). Adaptive equipment: Its effectiveness for people with chronic lower back pain. *Occupational Therapy Journal of Research, 10*, 111–121.

Umphred, D. A. (1995a). Introduction and overview: Multiple conceptual models: frameworks for clinical problem solving. In D. A. Umphred (Ed.). *Neurological rehabilitation* (3rd ed., pp. 3–32). St. Louis: Mosby.

Umphred, D. A. (1995b). *Neurological rehabilitation* (3rd ed.). St. Louis: Mosby.

Van Cramon, D. Y., Matthes-Von Cramon, G., & Mai, N. (1991). Problem solving deficits in brain injured patients: A therapeutic approach. *Neuropsychological Rehabilitation, 1*, 45–64.

Van Fleet, S. (2000). Relaxation and imagery for symptom management: Improving patient assessment and individualizing treatment. *Oncology Nursing Forum, 27*(3), 501–510.

Vergeer, G., & MacRae, A. (1993). Therapeutic use of humor in occupational therapy. *American Journal of Occupational Therapy, 47*, 678–683.

Vitaliano, R., Russo, J., Carr, J., Maiuro, R., & Becker, J. (1985). The ways of coping checklist: Revisions and psychometric properties. *Multivariate Behavioral Research, 20*, 3–26.

Vogt, T., Mullooly, J., Ernst, D., Pope, C., & Hollis, J. (1992). Social networks as predictors of ischemic heart disease, cancer, stroke and hypertension: incidence, survival and mortality. *Journal of Clinical Epidemiology, 45*, 659–666.

Von Hofsten, C. (1980). Predictive reaching for moving objects by human infants. *Journal of Experimental Psychology, 30*, 383–388.

Voss, D. E., Ionta, M. K., & Myers, B. J. (1985). *Proprioceptive neuromuscular facilitation: Patterns and techniques* (3rd ed.). Philadelphia: Harper & Row.

Wade, T. K., & Troy, J. C. (2001). Mobile phones as a new memory aid: A preliminary investigation using case studies. *Brain Injury, 15*(4), 305–320.

Wagenaar, R., & van Emmerik, R. E. (1996). Dynamics of movement disorders. *Human Movement Science, 15*, 161–175.

Walter, C. (1998). An alternative view of dynamical systems concepts in motor control and learning. *Research Quarterly for Exercise and Sport, 69*, 326–333.

Warren, M. (1993). Lesson 7: Visuospatial skills: Assessment and intervention strategies. In C. B. Royeen (Ed.). *Cognitive rehabilitation* [AOTA Self–Study Series] (pp. 1–76). Rockville, MD: American Occupational Therapy Association.

Waylett-Rendall, J. (1995) Desensitization of the traumatized hand. In J. M. Hunter, E. J. Mackin, & A. D. Callahan (Eds.). *Rehabilitation of the hand* (4th ed., pp. 693–700). St. Louis: Mosby.

Webster, J .S., McFarland, P. T., Rapport, L. J., Morrill, B., Roades, L. A., & Abadee, P. S. (2001). Computer-assisted training for improving wheelchair mobility in unilateral neglect patients. *Archives of Physical Medicine and Rehabilitation, 82*, 769–775.

Webster, J. S., & Scott, R. R. (1983). The effects of self-instructional training on attentional deficits following head injury. *Clinical Neuropsychology, 5*, 69–74.

Wehman, P. H. (1991). Cognitive rehabilitation in the workplace. In J. Kreutzer & P. H. Wehman (Eds.). *Cognitive rehabilitation for persons with traumatic brain injury* (pp. 269–288). Baltimore: Brookes.

Weinberg, J., Diller, L., Gordon, W. A., Gerstman, L. J., Lieberman, A., Lakin, P., Hodges, G., & Ezrachi, O. (1977). Visual scanning training effect on reading related tasks in acquired right brain damage. *Archives of Physical Medicine and Rehabilitation, 58*, 479–486.

Wigers, S. H., Stiles, T. C., & Vogel, P. A. (1996). Effects of aerobic exercise versus stress management treatment in fibromyalgia. *Scandinavian Journal of Rheumatology, 25*, 77–86.

Williams, T. A. (1995). Low vision rehabilitation for a patient with a traumatic brain injury. *American Journal of Occupational Therapy, 49*, 923–926.

Wilson, B. A. (1995). Management and remediation of memory problems in brain—Injured adults. In A. D. Baddeley, B. A. Wilson, & F. N. Watts (Eds.). *Handbook of memory disorders* (pp. 451–479). Chichester, UK: Wiley.

Wilson, B. A., Emslie, H. C., Quirk, K., & Evans, J. J. (2001). Reducing everyday memory and planning problems by means of a paging system: a randomised control crossover study. *Journal of Neurology, Neurosurgery & Psychiatry, 70*(4), 477–482.

Wilson, B. A., & Evans, J. J. (1996). Error free learning in the rehabilitation of individuals with memory impairments. *Journal of Head Trauma Rehabilitation, 11*, 54–64.

World Health Organization. (2001). *International classification of functioning, disability and health (ICF)*. Geneva: Author.

Worthington, A. D. (1996). Cueing strategies in neglect dyslexia. *Neuropsychological Rehabilitation, 6*, 1–17.

Wykes, T. (2000). The rehabilitation of cognitive deficits. *Psychiatric Rehabilitation Skills*, 4(2), 234–248.

Ylvisaker, M., & Feeney, T. J. (1998). *Collaborative brain injury intervention*. San Diego, CA: Singular.

Ylvisaker, M., Szekeres, S. F., Sullivan, D. M., & Wheeler, P. (1987). Topics in cognitive rehabilitation therapy. In M. Ylvisaker & E. M. R. Gobble (Eds.). *Community re-entry for head injured adults* (pp. 137–215). Boston: College-Hill Press.

Zihl, J. (1981). Recovery of visual functions in patients with cerebral blindness: Effects of specific practice with saccadic localisation. *Experimental Brain Research, 44*, 159–169.

Zimmerer-Branum, S., & Nelson, D. L. (1995). Occupationally embedded exercise versus rote exercise: A choice between occupational forms by elderly nursing home residents. *American Journal of Occupational Therapy, 49*, 397–402.

Zoltan, B. (1996). Vision, perception and cognition: *A manual for the evaluation and treatment of the neurologically impaired adult* (3rd ed.). Thorofare, NJ: Slack.

CHAPTER 31

CONTEXTUAL MODIFICATION AND ASSISTIVE TECHNOLOGY

SECTION I: Manual Wheelchair Seating and Mobility
SECTION II: Assistive Technology in Occupational Therapy
SECTION III: Splinting and Orthotics

SECTION I

Manual Wheelchair Seating and Mobility

MARY ELLEN BUNING
MARK R. SCHMELER

INTRODUCING WHEELED MOBILITY AND POSITIONING

The wheelchair has long been viewed as a symbol of illness and loss. For this reason, many people avoid using a wheelchair even when upright ambulation is no longer safe and efficient. While ambulation is undeniably useful there are many examples today of people who use wheelchairs to achieve occupational competence and contribute to their communities. They have learned to substitute wheelchair use for ambulation.

Occupational therapy practitioners are naturally interested in assistive devices, especially ones that support occupational performance across life domains. Practitioners also bring empathy and understanding of the adaptation process and the reacquisition of a positive self-image in the face of disability. This understanding, combined with acquired knowledge about wheelchairs and positioning and mobility options, makes occupational therapy practitioners well suited to help clients move beyond negative stereotypes. When clients received well-fitted, comfortable wheelchairs appropriate for their environments they are able to escape the constraint of impaired ambulation and return to valued life activities. As a foundation for developing this knowledge and skill, this section covers manual wheelchairs and seating to manage posture, pressure, and comfort.

A Manual or a Power Wheelchair?

Let's quickly look at the choice between manual or powered mobility. The past practice was to insist on **manual propulsion** if a client had the ability to do it. Wheelchair propulsion was viewed as exercise or, for children, a training regimen. This practice is now under fire as long-term users develop repetitive strain injuries (RSIs) and rotator cuff tears that not only end their days of manual wheelchair propulsion but also constrain them for transfers, lifting, and reaching (Boninger, Baldwin, Cooper, Koontz, & Chan, 2000). Children left behind in the effort of manual propulsion are slow to initiate interactions or satisfy their curiosity (Butler, 1986b). More can be learned about clients who are best suited for powered mobility in Section 3.

Starting with the Client

A number of diagnoses are associated with wheelchair use: amputation, amyotrophic lateral sclerosis (ALS), cerebral palsy, muscular dystrophy, multiple sclerosis (MS), postpolio, rheumatoid arthritis, spina bifida, spinal cord injury (SCI), stroke, and traumatic brain injury (TBI). Though clients with diagnoses such as SCI require wheelchair use, those with other diagnoses may need a wheelchair only at later stages or in certain contexts. For example, a wheelchair may be useful for long distances or when efficiency and the desire to focus on occupation rather than ambulation are important.

Evaluating for a manual wheelchair begins with interviewing the client or a family member about the client's interests and occupations, mobility needs, and contexts. A mat examination may follow (described later). The information gained guides the development of intervention goals and the selection of the wheelchair type and/or external postural supports or **pressure reducing cushions.** These goals also guide interaction with the certified rehabilitation technology supplier (CRTS). This professional is an expert on current products and is able to suggest components and features. The CRTS may be able to set up a chair for trial use to ensure satisfaction, comfort, and accurate fit. The CRTS and the occupational therapy practitioner work together with the client to suggest options and to provide a wheelchair that enables return to occupational performance.

SEATING BIOMECHANICS BASICS

The human body is not well suited for maintaining a seated position for prolonged periods of time across a variety of tasks. Yet, for people who use wheelchairs, sitting is their only option. To better understand this dilemma, look at the seated body from a biomechanical perspective. In a seated position the body is an unstable structure. The base of support is the pelvis, which is essentially an inverted pyramid. On this is stacked a tower of blocks (vertebrae) topped with a large sphere (head). At the bottom of the pelvis are support points, including the ischial tuberosities, coccyx, and the hip joints. Prolonged and continuous pressure on these points can lead to sores or cause the femoral head to migrate out of the acetabulum, causing the pelvis to tilt. The role of the occupational therapist is to recognize this dilemma and to develop and implement seating and positioning strategies that accommodate the functional and physiological needs of the seated person.

Finding Balance and Stability

The human body maintains balance and structure through connective tissue, the nervous system, and coordinated muscle contractions. On a micro level the seated body continuously co-contracts groups of muscles to maintain balance and function. On a macro level, an individual automatically shifts body position periodically to relieve pressure, rebalance and stabilize, obtain comfort, and gain better function.

Human bodies uses some basic behaviors to find stability, comfort, or function:

- Shifting the pelvis into a posterior tilt and leaning the trunk back into a back support.
- Shifting the pelvis into an anterior position, leaning the trunk forward, and resting the arms on a surface such as a table or lap tray.
- Tilting the pelvis to one side and leaning the trunk laterally into a surface.

Other behaviors include crossing the arms to gain additional trunk stability and crossing the legs to lock and stabilize the pelvis.

The ability to adjust position and maintain balance and stability becomes limited for people with diagnoses such as those named earlier. For example, external stability can be gained by tilting the pelvis and relaxing the trunk muscles (i.e., slouching), which requires less work. However, over time this posture leads to collapse of the spine and the development of spinal deformities such as kyphosis, scoliosis, and its combinations. These deformities can be painful and debilitating and can compromise vital organ capacity. External stabilizers, such as seat and back supports, offer those with poor trunk muscle control a means to compensate for their inability to actively maintain a functional seated position. These stabilizers are referred to as **adaptive seating systems.**

Different Postures for Different Activities

Different tasks require different postures and, therefore, different postural supports. Consider these two examples:

- *A person sits at a workstation and types on a computer:* The body is relatively upright with the trunk stabilized to allow for distal function of the hands. Trunk stability first comes from pelvic stabilization and then either co-contraction of the trunk muscles or a well-designed back support. The arms may also be rested on a wrist support to provide further anterior trunk support. The body works hard to maintain this posture and attend to the task at hand. During this active posture, the body rests by changing position.
- *A person sits to watch a movie in a theater:* For this leisure activity, the pelvis tilts back and the trunk sinks into the backrest. The arms are on the armrests and the legs might cross. This posture requires less work and, therefore, can be maintained for long periods of time, until pressure and discomfort prompt the body to reposition.

The practitioner's challenge is to identify seating interventions that accommodate a variety of postural needs. Some of these interventions will be identified later.

A Common Fallacy of Seating

Many practitioners falsely believe that a client with good wheelchair sitting posture sits with a vertical trunk, 90° of flexion at the hips and knees, and neutral position of the ankles. This is a posture that is not tolerated by many, or not for very long. Put yourself in this position as you read this text without leaning forward or resting your arms on the table and hold it for as long as you can. Then consider the client who is forced by the design of a prescribed seating system to sit this way continuously. This awareness helps a practitioner recognize the postural behaviors clients use to get comfortable, reduce pressure, or find a new functional position. It is important to understand that there is no one ideal posture and several dynamic variables should be considered when recommending seating systems.

Seating Assessment

Before designing a seating system, a practitioner needs to conduct a thorough physical motor assessment on a therapy mat table. This involves the assessment of transfers, sitting balance, lateral symmetry, and range of motion (ROM). It is also important to assess factors that will affect sitting: tone, spasticity, primitive reflexes, and cognitive–perceptual awareness. ROM in the hips and knees is especially important when considering what seat-to-back angle and footrest positions will be tolerated. A seating system needs to accommodate these variables and limitations. Consider these examples:

- A client measured with 75° of bilateral hip flexion will not be comfortable or sit well in a wheelchair seat with a 90° seat-to-back angle.
- A person with tight hamstrings and limited knee extension will not be comfortable or sit well in a wheelchair with footrests that require at least 70° of knee extension.
- A person with insufficient trunk balance will not be comfortable or sit well in a fully upright back support.

Clients placed in these seats will assume a posterior pelvic tilt, slide forward in their seat, and will be less able to propel themselves or use their hands for functional activities.

Goals of Seating and Positioning

Seating goals exist on two levels: one related to medical and physiological considerations and the other, to functional and lifestyle considerations. It is important to prioritize the goals of the client, because these goals can conflict with one another. Table 31-1 lists common considerations when setting goals.

TABLE 31–1. **CONSIDERATIONS FOR SEATING GOALS**

Medical	Functional	Personal and Lifestyle
• Reduce the potential for deformities • Maintain vital organ capacity • Reduce strain on soft tissue • Reduce pain and maximize comfort	• Increase tolerance to activities • Maximize functional independence • Increase distal motor control • Increase attention • Increase communication	• Facilitate participation in the community and society • Facilitate fulfillment of life goals and roles • Facilitate the ability to get around • Facilitate personal productivity • Compatible with other requirements in the environment

SEATING SYSTEMS

Intervention goals like those listed in Table 31-1 guide the occupational therapist in selecting the components of seating systems. Customized seating meets the specific medical, functional, and occupational needs of the client.

Soft Tissue Management

Many people who use manual wheelchairs sit in them for extended periods of time and need to be aware of the threat of soft tissue injury. Since the cost of treatment or repair of a pressure ulcer is substantial and does not include time lost to healing it is important to prevent rather than treat them (Allman, Goode, Burst, Bartolucci, & Thomas, 1999). Everyone, but especially those with impaired sensation and/or weakness that prevents postural shifts, needs to be aware of the causes of pressure ulcers. Some are extrinsic such as excessive, prolonged pressure from bony areas in the direction of gravity, which impedes cellular function and damages soft tissue. In addition, friction or shear generated by external sources, as well as the build up of heat and moisture, contribute to the damage. Intrinsic factors include the inability to move, poor nutrition, and the loss of soft tissue elasticity with aging. The loss of sensation is a key factor, since discomfort is the usual trigger for shifting and moving. Since the causes of pressure ulcer vary, the choice of cushion is based on each client's risk factors and the characteristics of the cushion.

It is also worth noting that the fit of the wheelchair contributes to soft tissue management too. Properly adjusting footrests and armrests and modifying the seat angle can reduce pressures on the ischial tuberosities.

Cushions and Pelvic Supports

For some clients, protecting the soft tissue may be an important seating goal, but for others, the issue is postural control, alignment, or stability. Cushions accomplish this by providing external support for weak musculature or by resisting the forces of spasticity or fluctuating tone. Molded systems can accommodate fixed skeletal deformities, whereas viscous fluids provide the pelvic stabilization needed to support trunk and upper extremity function. Cushions with a slight posterior tilt can be used to reduce sliding or to diminish extensor tone. Pelvic belts keep the pelvis positioned, when needed for stability and performance.

Matching Material Properties and Cushion Types to Client Needs

Cushions are chosen based on their characteristics, which are related to the properties of their materials. Such properties include the following:

- *Density:* The ratio of mass or quantity of material to the cubic area of the cushion (e.g., a honeycomb cushion has a low density).
- *Stiffness:* The strength of the resistance to compression (e.g., egg-crate foam has low stiffness and does not resist body weight).
- *Thermal characteristics:* The ability of the material to insulate or conduct (e.g., dense foam cushions hold in body heat).

RESEARCH NOTE 31–1

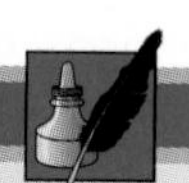

How Do We Know if New Interventions Are Better?

Methods of treatment change over time in all areas of health care. Practitioners assume that the evolution of treatment methods results in new interventions and assistive devices that are more effective, efficient, and safer than those used previously. But how do we know this? How do systems of treatment change? More important, how do we know that the new or revised methods (or devices) are more effective, efficient, and safer?

Ideally, new treatment activities are based, at least in part, on research findings from systematic comparisons. Change is progress only if it can be demonstrated that the change (new treatment or device) produces better results. Research is one of the tools practitioners use to make the distinction between change and true progress. Shechtman, Hanson, Garrett, and Dunn (2001) conducted such a study when they compared six wheelchair cushions for effectiveness of pressure relief and comfort in a sample of 40 adult wheelchair users. The six cushions represented a variety of construction materials and price. Some were new models, whereas others had been available to rehabilitation practitioners for many years. The investigators systematically measured the ability of each cushion to relieve pressure in the subjects and collected information on perceived comfort for each cushion. There were differences in effectiveness of pressure relief across the conditions, depending on the subject's body mass index. One type of cushion was consistently rated as the most comfortable.

Comparison studies such as the one by Shechtman et al. (2001) provide therapists and consumers with information essential for determining if changes in treatment represent genuine improvements in client performance.

Shechtman, O., Hanson, C. S., Garrett, D., & Dunn, P. (2001). Comparing wheelchair cushions for effectiveness of pressure relief. *Occupational Therapy Journal of Research, 21,* 29–38.

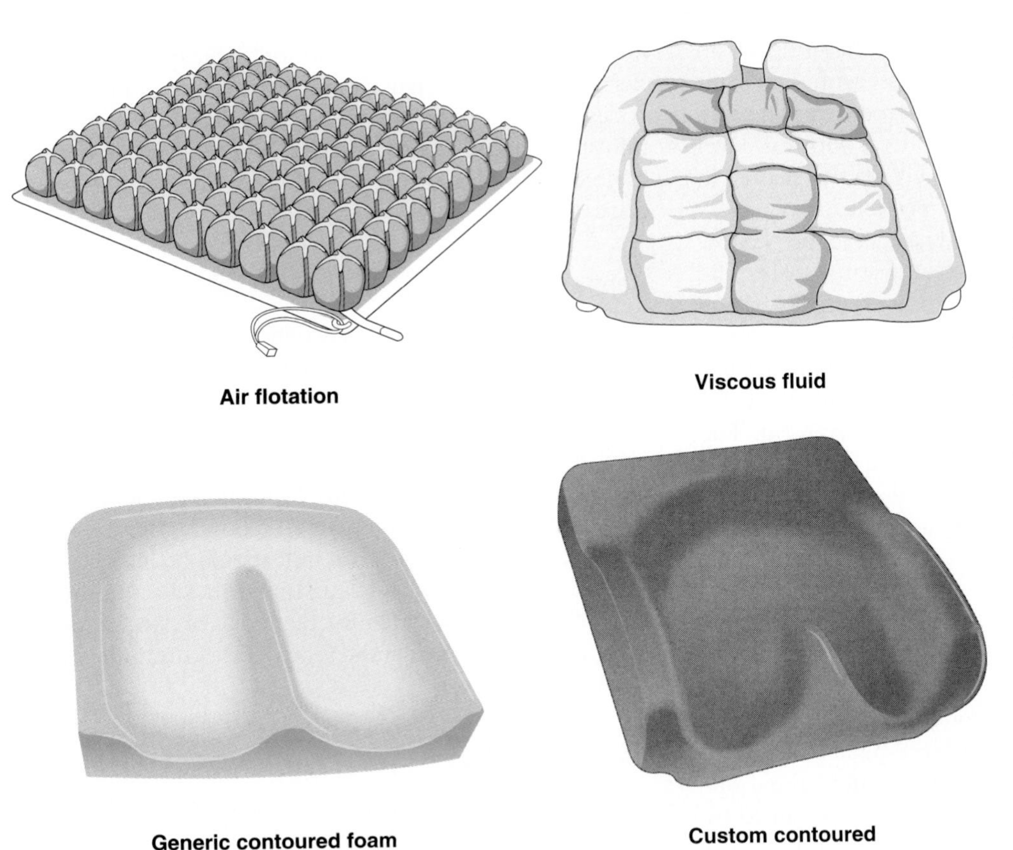

FIGURE 31-1. Cushion properties are matched to the client's seating goals and needs, because many factors contribute to pressure and posture problems. Cushions should be covered with a washable low-shear material. **A,** Air floatation. **B,** Viscous fluid. **C,** Generic contoured foam. **D,** Custom contoured.

- *Friction:* The ability to maintain position and to reposition if needed (e.g., cushions with slick covers make sliding in lateral transfers easy).

Manufacturers make cushions that possess these qualities by using flat and contoured foams, air-filled bladders, combinations of air and foam, viscous fluids, contoured plastic honeycombs, custom-contoured foam, and alternating pressure systems (Fig. 31-1). These cushions vary in efficacy of pressure distribution, provision of postural stability, ability to insulate or conduct heat, and the reliability of their performance over time. The seating specialist (often the occupational therapist) seeks out knowledge of current products and their properties. For example, finding a cushion with good airflow and pressure distribution is important for an immobile client who perspires heavily. Alternately, for a client prone to pressure ulcers, the practitioner would identify cushions with optimal distribution of peak forces. If all the needed features cannot be found in one cushion, trade-offs are necessary. Research evidence supports that properly fitted pressure reducing cushions (compared to low-cost foam cushions) reduce the incidence of pressure sores. (Brienza, Karg, Geyer, Kelsey, & Trefler, 2001; Conine, Herschler, Deachsel, Peel, & Pearson, 1994).

Pressure Mapping

Pressure mapping technology estimates interface pressure. A mat with pressure sensors is placed between the client and the seating surface. The mat connects to a computer and presents data in graphical and numerical forms. As part of a skilled clinical assessment it can predict potential risk for pressure sores (Brienza et al., 2001; Conine et al., 1994). This technology can help practitioners decide which cushion provides the best pressure distribution for a particular client. It is also important to remember that pressure mapping devices do not measure shear forces, heat, moisture, postural stability, or maintenance of the cushion. These factors must also be considered.

Back Support

A back support should support the spinal curves and allow movement. The spine stabilizes the trunk, supports the head and is the basis for upper extremity function. The typical back support in a folding-frame wheelchair is sling upholstery, not because it provides a good back support but because it collapses. Like cushions, wheelchair backs are chosen based on the client's seating goals. For example, an active user with a lumbar SCI may prefer a low back on a manual wheelchair to allow full arm mobility and rotation and leaning with the upper spine. It comes with the trade-off of reduced stability; being able to lean and reach changes the center of gravity and can cause tipping.

For clients with muscle weakness in the trunk, the stability from a high and contoured backrest with good lateral support is needed to maintain head and neck movement.

Some clients may need only the soft contouring of an adjustable-tension sling backrest, but those with significant **kyphoscoliosis** may need a custom-contoured backrest to enable sitting in an upright posture. Clients with this level of weakness or deformity will most likely use this seating in a power mobility base as described in Section 2.

Again, the CRTS becomes a good partner for an occupational therapy practitioner with clear seating goals. The range of products is large and constantly expanding. Some back systems are modular and adjustable, and custom-contoured systems require high-level skills to form and finish. New products combine features like a high back for stability with scapular cutouts to allow arm movement. The advent of modular and dynamic seating components allows for improved customization with off-the-shelf products. This can be useful for a client with fluctuating tone and/or changing postural needs.

Head Supports and Other Options

Clients with significant weakness and motor control problems may need external support for their heads, arms and legs. This need may arise with high-level spinal cord injury, ALS, or advanced MS. Other clients may need these options because they have high or fluctuating tone caused by cerebral palsy or TBI. Keeping body parts safe and in good alignment contribute to safety and pressure management.

Recline and Tilt in Space

Recline and tilt in space technologies relieve pressure, manage posture and comfort, and help with personal-care activities. *Recline* changes the seat-to-back angle. In manual wheelchairs, this is typically an attendant-controlled system, but power wheelchairs allow the user to control this feature. Because reclining the seat back creates shear, practitioners must take care that antishear mechanisms are installed or that caregivers are aware of skin care. Recline helps stretch hip flexors and allows clients to attend to catheters and toileting. *Tilt in space* keeps the hip and knee angles constant while inclining the client to the rear. While tilted (up to 80°), gravity pulls on the hips, trunk, and shoulders and assists in repositioning. As with recline, tilt in space greatly reduces pressure on the ischial tuberosities by temporarily shifting the pressure to the torso. Both systems require head support to protect the head. Research supports the use of these interventions (Sprigle & Sposato, 1997).

TYPES OF MANUAL WHEELCHAIRS

In general, all wheelchairs have seats, backs, footrests, and casters. The presence of other features, like push handles, wheel locks, and large rear wheels with pushrims, depends on the purpose of the chair. Manual wheelchairs are classified in several ways. The Centers for Medicare and Medicaid Services (CMS) assign manual wheelchairs one of nine codes, based on their features (Health Care Finance Administration and United HealthCare, 1998). We use this CMS code to categorize wheelchair systems in the following discussion.

Dependent Systems

Dependent manual wheelchairs are not designed for occupant control. A dependent system is appropriate only for situations in which the user does not have the cognitive, perceptual, or physical capabilities to operate any type of manual or powered mobility system. They might also be appropriate as backup systems or in environments where using the primary self-propelled or powered chair is not feasible. Otherwise, every attempt should be made to provide clients with a wheelchair that will give the highest level of independent mobility. Examples of dependent systems, along with their indications and contraindications, follow.

Adaptive Strollers

Adaptive strollers are appropriate for young children who cannot propel any other type of manual wheelchair and cannot operate a power wheelchair. They are lightweight and reasonably easy to fold or disassemble for transportation in a vehicle. Adaptive seating systems are also available, and some models allow for transfer of the seating system off the stroller base for use as a car seat or highchair.

Transport Wheelchairs

Transport wheelchairs are simple folding wheelchairs generally equipped with a sling seat and back upholstery, fixed-position arm and foot supports, small rear wheels, and small front casters. Transport wheelchairs weigh less than other chairs and fold easily for stowing in a vehicle. The sling seating provides no support, and passengers should sit in them only for short periods of time. Poor posture, slouching, and other complications (discussed earlier) will follow if the wheelchairs are used for longer periods. Furthermore, they are not designed for self-propelling. Similar to strollers, these systems are ideal as backup devices, however for an adult population.

Standard Weight Wheelchairs

Standard weight wheelchairs (coded K0001 and K0002) are similar to transport wheelchairs, except they have large rear wheels, giving the perception they are suitable for self-propulsion. Their folding frame design was introduced in the 1930s, and the design has not changed significantly since. The design uses the concept of the folding cross-frame deck chair with sling-style upholstery. Unfortunately, upholstery stretches over time, and the design promotes a slouched posture. Furthermore, they are heavy, have no adjustability, and are difficult to self-propel, leaving folding for storage and stowing in a car trunk as their only advantages.

When these chairs are ordered with a lower seat-to-floor height, they are referred to as *hemi wheelchairs*. Theoretically, this allows a person with hemiplegia to propel with one arm and leg; however, the chair weight and lack of adjustability make it a poor choice for self-propulsion.

Standard wheelchairs, sometimes called *depot chairs*, come in a limited number of sizes, which implies a one-size-fits-all concept. They might be appropriate for short-term use with a fractured foot and for long-distance attendant-pushed transportation in an airport or mall. They should not be used as a ongoing solution, especially in long-term care facilities where they are often provided for residents.

Self-Propelled Systems

An important goal when prescribing manual wheelchairs is to reduce the amount of stress applied to the upper extremities. Evidence supporting the importance of this goal is growing (presented later). Types of self-propelled systems and their indications and contraindications are discussed next.

Standard Lightweight Wheelchairs

Standard lightweight wheelchairs (coded K0003) are identical to standard manual wheelchairs, except they are slightly lighter with frame weight of less than 36 lb. There is no adjustability, and utility is limited.

High-Strength Lightweight Wheelchairs

The frames of the high-strength lightweight chairs (coded K0004) weigh less than 34 lb, and they have limited adjustability. These chairs come in more sizes than the standard chairs and are well designed to accept specialized seating components. The seat-to-floor height can be lowered to allow foot propulsion if indicated.

Ultra-Lightweight Manual Wheelchairs

The ultra-lightweight manual wheelchairs (coded K0005) are preferable to the previously mentioned wheelchairs, because they have more usability features. They are easier to propel, as they are constructed of stronger, lighter materials (e.g., titanium) with frames weighing less than 30 lb. The most important feature they offer is the ability to adjust the fore/aft position of the rear axle.

Rigid Frame Wheelchairs

Rigid frame wheelchairs are similar to and often classified the same as ultra-lightweight systems. A rigid frame wheelchair does not fold, though it can be made more compact by releasing the large wheels and folding the seat back forward. A rigid frame further increases propulsion efficiency, as the energy dissipated in the flex of a cross frame is transferred to forward propulsion. These are significantly lighter (some weigh less than 25 lb) and stronger than standard chairs, especially when constructed of materials such as titanium.

Recreational Wheelchairs

There are a multitude of specially designed recreational type wheelchairs that allow people who use wheelchairs to engage in leisure activities. Wheelchairs have been specially designed for tennis, basketball, rugby, racing, and ice hockey. Hand-cycles are also available for recreational riding and may be beneficial to people who are prone to RSI (Fig. 31-2).

Prevention of Repetitive Stress Injuries

Wheelchair adjustability offers two things, both of which are important in preventing RSI. The rear axle can be aligned directly below the shoulder, allowing a balance of muscles to engage in propulsion and improving access to the pushrims throughout the stroke. Second, it increases the rate and efficiency of strokes on the pushrims. The result is fewer strokes per distance traveled, and fewer repetitions means a decreased likelihood of RSI. A disadvantage of forward axle position is decreased stability, making it easier to tip backward. Installing rear antitippers and training the user in wheelchair propulsion skills is advised. Ideally, this type of wheelchair should be considered for long-term users. These chairs are lighter, easier to propel, and adjustable to accommodate varying needs.

It is well documented in the literature that there is a 49–73% incidence of carpal tunnel syndrome (CTS) in manual wheelchair users (Boninger et al., 2000; Boninger, Cooper, Baldwin, Shimada, & Koontz, 1999). CTS is a serious concern for manual wheelchair users, as they depend on their upper extremities not only for propulsion but also for transfers and other activities of daily living (ADL). Chronic CTS can further lead to the need for costly medical and surgical interventions and loss of productivity. It may also result in the need to convert to the use of powered mobility and, therefore, the need for significant lifestyle changes (Buning, Angelo, & Schmeler, 2001).

The body of scientific evidence favoring ultra-lightweight manual wheelchairs is growing. A research study by Boninger et al. (2000) found that wheelchair rear axle position relative to shoulder position was correlated with median nerve injuries. Furthermore, the study concluded that providing clients with adjustable rear axle position wheelchairs, as well as properly fitting clients to the wheelchair, improved propulsion biomechanics and helped reduce injury. At this time, ultra-lightweight wheelchairs are the only type of manual wheelchairs equipped with an adjustable rear axle, although new options may soon emerge.

Ultra-lightweight wheelchairs are also associated with improved ride comfort. In a comparison of ultra-lightweight versus standard wheelchairs used on a driving course, riders

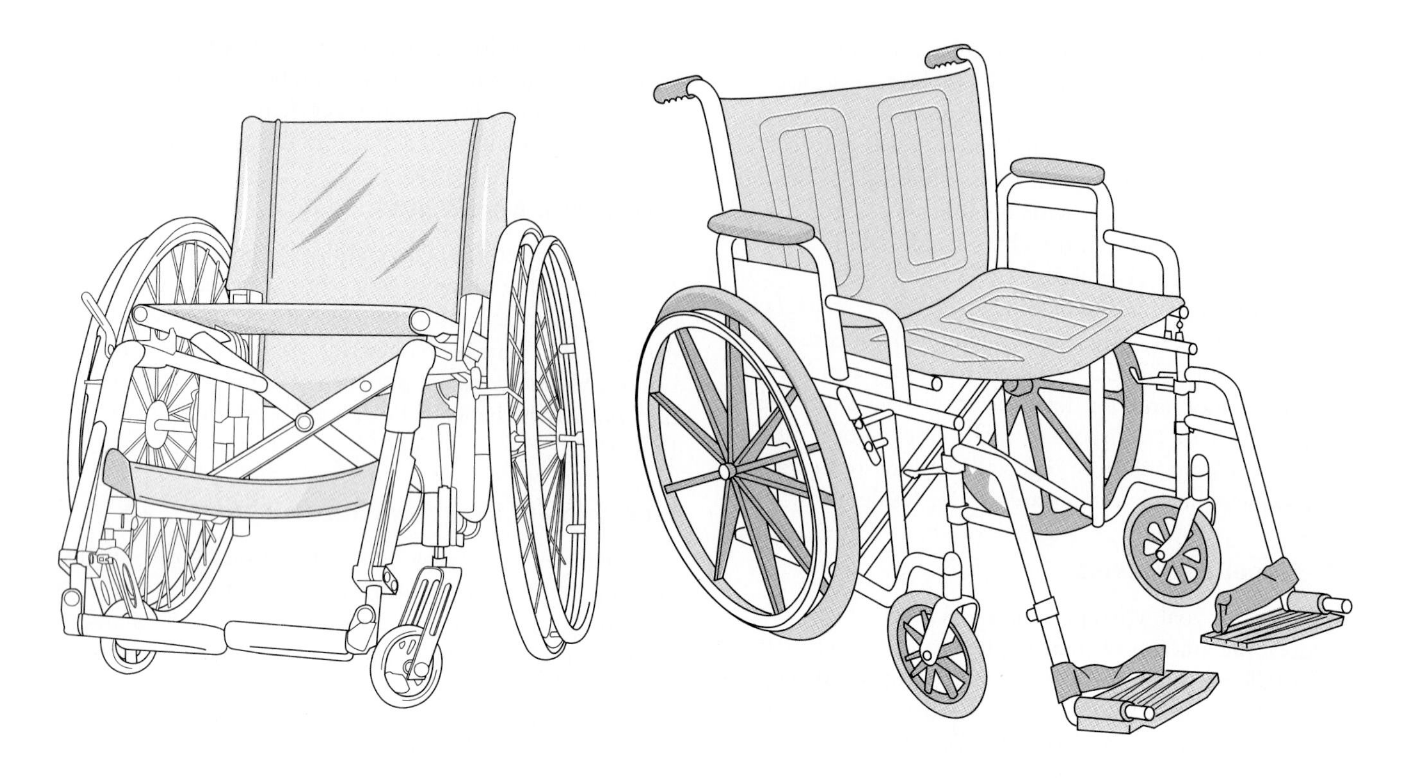

FIGURE 31–2. Many benefits are associated with the use of a rigid ultra-lightweight (**A**) compared to a standard wheelchair (**B**).

reported a significant positive difference in perceived comfort (DiGiovine, Cooper, Boniger, Lawrence, VanSickle, & Rentschler, 2000). In addition, when both standard and ultra-lightweight wheelchairs were tested in a manner to simulate normal use, the ultra-lightweight chairs proved more durable (Cooper, Boninger, & Rentschler, 1999; Cooper, Gonzalez, Lawrence, Rentschler, Boninger, & VanSickle 1997). Using cost and durability data, Cooper found ultra-lightweight wheelchairs averaged 673 cycles/dollar, compared to standard wheelchairs, which averaged only 78 cycles/dollar.

DELIVERING THE SERVICES RELATED TO WHEELCHAIRS

As in other aspects of occupational therapy, there are unique considerations associated with the service-delivery process.

Interdisciplinary and Client Focused

Effective occupational therapy practice in seating and manual wheelchair mobility requires an interdisciplinary team effort. Since the solutions sought are driven by consumer needs and goals, the client holds the key position. The team works in a consultant role to suggest solutions and options. A CRTS or rehabilitation engineer contributes information about rapidly changing products and technologies. This technical information is used to evaluate options and allow for informed decisions.

Environmental Issues

The Americans with Disabilities Act (ADA) of 1990 did much to increase wheelchair access to public buildings, transportation, and community facilities. Regardless, a client's home may be far from accessible. An occupational therapy practitioner should always ask a new wheelchair user about interior and exterior accessibility for home or daily environments. Consultation or a referral for accessibility modifications may be needed.

Transportation is essential in American life. Public transit or paratransit provides transportation for many people. Others use private vehicles, as either drivers or passengers. Because private vehicles travel at high speeds, clients need information about how to restrain both themselves and their wheelchair safely. Four-point tie-downs provide inexpensive, crash-tested safety in both private and public transportation vehicles.

Documentation

The process of recording client needs and goals and data from a mat assessment provides the documentation needed for funders to see the relationship between the client's physical status and the request. Practitioners need to assume that the funder knows nothing about their service and has every incentive to deny it. Describe and justify each part, referring back to the clinical assessment for rationale. Funders are more likely to finance the wheelchair or seating requested when practitioners concisely document a methodical decision-making process. In the United States, documentation is so related to reimbursement that practitioners unwilling to do it well should not even do assessments. They will be wasting their time!

Follow-Up

When the chair is delivered the client should return to the occupational therapy practitioner to ensure optimal adjustment and to resolve any issues caused by a change in status. This is a time when a good relationship with a CRTS shows its value—during problem resolution. If training is needed, it should be provided at this time. Following up with clients lets the practitioner know how he or she is doing. It is especially important when serving clients with progressive conditions. The practitioner should let these consumers know that they plan to recall them in 6 months to see how they are doing.

CONCLUSION

This section discusses interviewing, establishing goals, assessment, mat evaluation, working with a CRTS, creating opportunities for trial use, home and transportation assessment, and documentation to support reimbursement. Practitioners working in seating and manual wheeled mobility services provide an important service. This tool for adaptive mobility has immediate and tangible results, allowing clients to access the community and regain independence in occupational environments.

This section provides only a brief introduction to seating and manual wheelchair mobility. Novice practitioners need to work closely with an expert or seek out continuing education and self-directed learning opportunities. They must learn more about evaluation and matching product features to consumer needs, increasing funding approvals, and providing consumer training and follow-up. Additional resources are listed in Appendices I and L.

SECTION II

Assistive Technology in Occupational Therapy

BEVERLY K. BAIN

For most people technology makes things easier. For people with disabilities, however, technology makes things possible. (Radabough, 1990)

As society has moved into the technological age, so too has the profession of occupational therapy. Historically, occupational therapy has used adaptive equipment to help clients enhance their functional abilities in self-care, school, work, and leisure. With advances in technology have come new assistive devices that can increase functional abilities and offer independence for clients of all ages at various functional levels. Technological devices, such as **powered wheelchairs** and remote **electronic aids for daily living (EADLs)**—formerly known as **environmental control systems (ECUs)**—are used by physically and sensory impaired clients to perform activities of daily living not possible a decade ago; specially adapted computers and **augmentative and alternative communication system (SAAC)** now make it possible for severely disabled, nonverbal children to participate in classrooms; for adults with impaired hand functions to become gainfully employed; and for individuals with physical, sensory, or psychosocial disabilities to enjoy leisure-time activities in the community.

The Technology Related Assistance for Individuals with Disabilities Act (TRAIDA; 1988, amended in 1994) defines an **assistive technology device (ATD)** as "any item, piece of equipment, or product system, whether acquired commercially off-the-shelf, modified, or customized, that is used to increase, maintain, or improve the functional capabilities of individuals with disabilities." This broad definition includes low-technology devices that can be purchased from electronic or specialty stores, such as a simple attachment to a standard lamp that allows a person to turn on a lamp with the touch of a hand, rather than fumbling with a hard-to-find small switch. The definition also includes complex high-technology devices, such as a powered computerized wheelchair that enables a person to control the chair, turn on and off lights and appliances, use the telephone, and operate an AAC and a computer through one integrated system. The ATDs addressed here are switches, powered wheelchairs, powered scooters, adapted vehicles, verbal communication aids, AACs, and EADLs.

The knowledgeable occupational therapy practitioner can use these advanced devices to increase, maintain, and improve the functional capabilities of many clients. Assistive technology services are also mandated by the TRAIDA and include "any service that directly assists an individual with a disability in the selection, acquisition, or use of assistive technology services." The competent therapist must be able to do the following:

- Assess the client; the client's tasks, needs, and goals; the technological device; and the environments in which the device will be used.
- In collaboration with other interdisciplinary team members, assist the client to select the most effective and cost-efficient devices to meet the his or her needs and abilities.
- Train the client and caregiver in the use and maintenance of the device.
- Document the client's abilities and needs, the selected devices, and all the environments in which the devices will be used.
- Periodically reevaluate the client, the tasks, all devices, and environments.
- Contribute to the development, research, and field testing of new devices.
- Serve as consultants to other professionals and caregivers.

For more details see Hammel (1995).

Assistive technology can be viewed as a system of four integrated and interdependent components: the client, the tasks and goals that the client needs to accomplish, the device(s), and the environments (Fig. 31-3).

Each component must be evaluated in the context of the others, selected on the basis of how it interfaces with the others, and applied as it interacts with the others. Devices are being developed rapidly, and some are extremely expensive; many are purchased only once, and too frequently they are underused or abandoned (Batavia & Hammer 1990; Phillips, 1992; Phillips & Zhao, 1993). Occupational therapists should carefully evaluate the appropriateness of each new device in light of each client's unique needs.

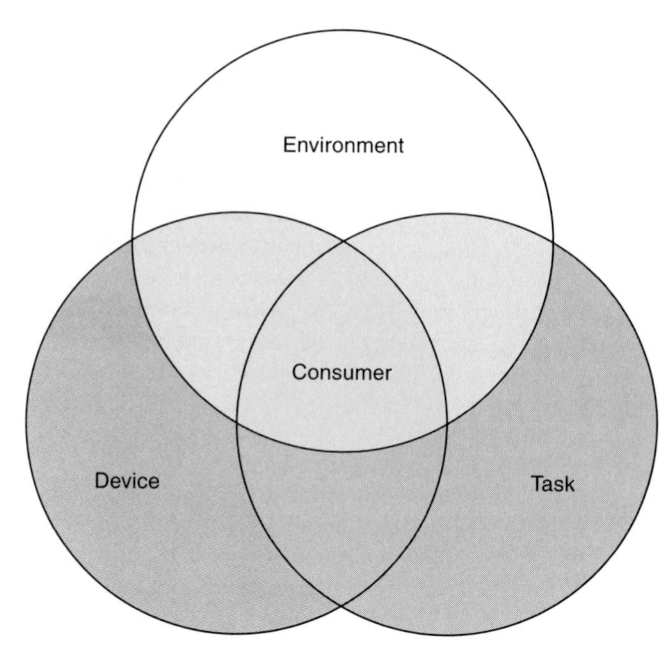

FIGURE 31–3. Consumer, task, environment, and device model.

Since the provision of an ATD begins with the client, each client must be asked about the tasks he or she desires to do and the goals to be achieved. This, in turn, requires that the client be evaluated and trained from a holistic perspective, with input from an interdisciplinary team. Both the immediate and the future environments must be considered, if the client is to accomplish the desired tasks and achieve his or her goals. Given the rapid pace of development, occupational therapy practitioners need to know the therapeutic concepts and principles related to technology that are built on the profession's body of knowledge, because these remain constant.

THERAPEUTIC FOUNDATION

In the area of occupational therapy assistive technology practice, the therapeutic foundation is based mainly on the following frames of reference: biomechanical, specifically the work simplification and energy conservation principle; acquisitional, the learning and maturation theories; and rehabilitation, for adaptations of devices and environmental modifications (see Unit VI).

Biomechanical work simplification and energy conservation principles are the basis for prescribing battery-powered wheelchairs for individuals with spinal cord injuries to reduce the physical energy needed for wheelchair movement and to increase the energy available for

ADL, work, play, and leisure activities. EADL and computers are used to control lights and appliances, simplify work, and conserve energy for clients with low physical tolerance, including those with MS, muscular dystrophy, ALS, arthritis, cardiac disease, or burns. In the future, robots, as they become less expensive, can be used to conserve the energy of both the user and the caregiver in the home and workplace.

The acquisitional frame of reference relates to learning the "specific skills needed for successful interaction in the environment" (Mosey, 1986, p. 433). For example, clients with lower extremity impairments can learn to interact successfully in their environments by learning to use powered wheelchairs and adapted vans to solve their mobility problems. Children with severe, multiple disabilities can learn to participate in activities and games by using a switch to control appliances or toys.

The major learning theories relevant to the occupational therapy process are described in Chapter 21. When teaching a client to use an ATD, the therapist may use one learning theory or a combination. For example, an augmentative communication aid is prescribed for a person who is severely cognitively impaired and nonverbal. This client might randomly press keys on the aid. If he or she happens to strike a certain key and hears the communication aid speak the word *food* and then strikes the key again and the response is repeated, the person has learned through conditioning that pressing a designated key gives a definite response. Alternatively, another client with intact cognitive skills may learn to use ATDs best through opportunities to explore the uses of devices at home, school, or work.

The rehabilitation frame of reference includes the use of adaptive equipment and modification of the environment to help clients compensate for physical and sensory impairments or deficits. Assistive technology devices are a new dimension of adaptive equipment. Through the use of devices such as power scooters and EADL, many environments require fewer adaptations. The technologic and ergonomic advances in tool and work environment designs and the emerging developments in universal design have also enhanced environmental modifications.

Technology is congruent with the philosophic assumption that "rehabilitation must be dynamic and keep in step with both scientific advances and changes in society" (Hopkins & Smith, 1983, p. 135). Based on rehabilitation assumptions, an occupational therapy intervention program for a client with a C4 quadriplegia, for example, would be to teach the person to use an EADL to compensate for the lack of hand manipulative skills; a powered wheelchair to foster independent mobility; and a computer to increase possible educational, leisure, and vocational activities, enabling the client to be involved in the community. In addition, the intervention process may include technological adaptations of the home, school, and workplace environments to help the client live a more purposeful and satisfying life.

The occupational performances of ADL, instrumental activities of daily living (IADL), work/school, play, leisure, and social participation can be enhanced through the use of assistive technology. Powered wheelchairs, computers, EADL, and AAC can increase a client's function in each area. However, the client's motor, sensory, cognitive, psychological, and social abilities must be carefully evaluated before the selection or application of any technological device. For example, each ATD must be activated, which requires some form of motor function (this can be in the form of pressing a switch, blinking an eye, or saying a command); each device has some form of feedback, which is usually visual or auditory, requiring sensory integration; and each device requires a certain amount of cognitive ability, such as learning sequencing to control an EADL or computer. In addition, the client must be motivated to use the equipment for any device to be effective.

The occupational therapist's fundamental concern is ensuring the client's capability throughout the life span to perform with satisfaction those tasks and roles essential to productive living and to the mastery of self and environment. Technology can be used throughout the life span; for example, infants at risk or severely disabled children can operate toys that allow them to interact and learn from the environment, and the elderly can use powered scooters and EADL to increase their independence in performing tasks safely.

Technology, however, should not be considered the only solution. Rather, technology provides an extension of the abilities of clients treated by a reflective therapist who has thoroughly assessed each component, the various ATDs, and the environments in which the individuals will use them.

EVALUATION OF CLIENTS, TASKS, DEVICES, AND ENVIRONMENTS

A primary responsibility of the occupational therapist is to complete a holistic evaluation of the client; the needs, tasks, and goals of the clients; various ATDs; and possible environments in which the devices will be used. Basic evaluation tenets should be practiced in the ongoing process with special attention to the characteristics of the device(s). A structured evaluation is necessary in view of:

- The proliferation of available devices.
- The increasing number of clients being referred to occupational therapy for aids.
- The price range of different devices.
- The greater level of participation in community life by people with disabilities, as more architectural and social barriers are removed.

Practitioners must systemically evaluate each client's functional need for each device and all possible environments in which the client will use the device.

A valid assistive technology evaluation should be a collaborative team effort that includes input from the client, physician, occupational therapist, physical therapist, speech pathologist, social worker, teacher, rehabilitation technology supplier, and caregiver. The occupational therapist contributes valuable and unique professional skills to the evaluation team, such as assessment of factors affecting client performance, analysis of skills required to use an ATD successfully, and the ability to assist clients with positioning to maximize performance.

Most devices are activated by switches; therefore, the optimal control sites (the anatomic parts of the body that are used to activate the switches) can best be determined by a therapist who evaluates a client's motor abilities. For example, a client who has motor control impairments of the upper and lower extremities may use the head, neck, or breath to activate the switches that propel the powered wheelchair. In addition, the therapist must evaluate the client's spatial and depth perception abilities as well as cognitive ability. Furthermore, an experienced practitioner is cognizant of the psychological implications of adaptive equipment for a client and can determine the best time to introduce ATDs into the intervention program.

For severely involved clients who require complex technology systems, an occupational therapist with specialty skills related to assistive technology is consulted by the primary occupational therapist. The primary therapist gathers data about the client's background and needs, evaluates the client's abilities, and relates this information to an occupational therapy technology specialist. The specialist should have knowledge of and experience with various devices, evaluate the client with several devices before recommending the appropriate ATD, continue to evaluate both the client and assistive technology system during the training process, teach the client all applications and maintenance of the ATD, and coordinate the integration of all technologic and standard equipment that the client requires. In settings in which off-the-shelf ATDs are used, an occupational therapy assistant, consulting with a specialist, is able to follow through with the application of the ATD and report when reevaluation of the client or ATD is needed, or maintenance of the ATD is required.

A structured assessment instrument has been developed and field tested with various populations, including adults and children with severe physical disabilities, sensory impairments, and developmental disabilities (Bain, 1997). The primary areas to consider in the problem-solving approach to the evaluation of clients for ATDs by the entry-level therapist are presented in this subsection, along with specific guidelines for switches, powered wheelchairs, AACs, EADL, and adapted computers.

Each part of the technology system must be evaluated to ensure that the most appropriate device is selected and used effectively by the client. The four major areas of assessment of clients for ATDs are data collection of the client's background and needs; evaluation of client's abilities, including positioning; planning with the client, caregivers, and rehabilitation team members; and selection of appropriate ATDs that will enhance the client's functional abilities throughout the day and in a variety of environments. As with all assessments for any assistive or adaptive equipment, a problem-solving approach is essential. The following guidelines have proved to be effective (Table 31-2):

- What are the client's needs and goals?
- What are the client's abilities?
- What ATDs would be appropriate based on the client's needs, goals, and abilities, considering
  - The input, processing, output, and display characteristics.
  - The commercial availability of an ATD or the adaptability of a commercial ATD.
  - Safety and reliability.
  - Practicality.
  - Affordability.
- Where will the ATD be used? (Consider all present and possible future environments).
- Where can the ATD be ordered and will it need to be adapted?
- Who will train the client to use the ATD and how many training sessions will be required?
- Who will document the assessment and where?
- When should the client, the ATD, and the environment be reevaluated and by whom?

Therapists should remember that, based on the evaluation of the client, the ATD, and the environments in which the ATD will be used, the client should try a variety of ATDs. Most rehabilitation technology suppliers and manufacturers of ATDs will lend therapists equipment for their clients to use on a trial basis. These guidelines may be modified to meet the intervention setting and the qualifications of the rehabilitation technology team members. Many sites will not have all members of the desired team, and frequently the occupational therapist will be responsible for the coordination of the team evaluation.

As noted earlier, technological devices are usually ordered only once, some are expensive, and often they are discarded or underused. Therefore, a precise, structured evaluation of each part of the system is worthy of professional time and effort, often requiring two or more sessions. Also, the clinical judgment of the therapist and members of the rehabilitation team should take precedence over the salesmanship of suppliers or manufacturers, who may try to influence the selection of devices.

The best ATD is the one that best facilitates the client's functional abilities. It may be an expensive, high-technology, integrated system or it may be an affordable, low-technology, single piece of equipment. In either case, the decision must be based on clinical knowledge of the entire team, which includes the client and caregiver. For details, see Hammel

TABLE 31–2. **STEPS IN A PROBLEM-SOLVING APPROACH TO THE EVALUATION OF CONSUMERS FOR ASSISTIVE TECHNOLOGY DEVICES (ATDs)**

Steps	Part of System	Problem	Action
1.	Task	Identify the tasks the consumer needs to accomplish with the ATD Communication Mobility Environmental controls Computer adaptation Switch interface	Review records Interview consumers, caretakers, and family
2.	Consumer or user	Identify the consumer's abilities in lying, sitting, and standing positions	Observation Formal testing: Motor MMT, reflexes, ROM Coordination Endurance Sensory Psychosocial Cognitive Social Interview Observation
3.	ATD	Based on 1 and 2, identify possible devices	Characteristics: Input, processing, output, display Commercial availability Safety and reliability Practicality Affordability
4.	Environment	Present and future: Bed or chair Home School or work Community	Interview Observation On-site visits
5.	All	Trial period	Try various devices in a variety of environments
6.	ATD	Selection	Order, adapt, or fabricate
7.	Consumer or user	Application	Train in use and maintenance
8.	All	Documentation	Record in all intra- and interdepartmental files
9.	All	Reevaluation	Periodically consumer, ATD, environment, and task(s)

(1995), and for assessments of acute and rehabilitation centers see the AOTA *Technology Special Interest Section Newsletters* for March and June 1995.

Currently there is not one comprehensive interdisciplinary evaluation especially designed for assistive technology. There are separate evaluations for powered wheelchairs, ACAs (Fishman, 1987), EADL (Bain, DiSalvi, Gold, Kollodge, & Schein, 1993), and computers (Anson, 1997; Fraser, McGregor, Arango, & Kangas, 1995; Lee & Thomas, 1990). *OT Fact*, a software assessment tool developed by Smith (1990, personal communication, 1994), has two sections that are relevant to assistive technology: the use of environment-free scoring behavior and the use of environmental-adjusted behavior. Other assistive technology assessments that should be reviewed are by Cook and Hussey (1995), Galvin and Scherer (1996), Lee and Thomas (1990) and Williams, Stemach, Wolfe, and Stanger (1993).

SWITCHES, CONTROL INTERFACES, AND INPUT DEVICES

Each assistive technology system has four parts: the input, known as the *switch* or *control interface* that activates the device; the throughput, or processing unit of the device; the *output*, which is the result of a successful operation; and a *display*, which is the visual, auditory, or tactile feedback that informs the operator that the system was activated. When a person turns on a light by pushing or twisting a switch (input), the electrical current in the building is the throughput and the light turning on is the output and also the visual display.

Switches enable people with disabilities to interact with their environments, to increase functional activities, and to extend their capabilities. The purpose of switches is to control devices; therefore, in the technology literature they are usually referred to as control interfaces. It has often been said that the most magnificent technological device or the simplest toy is underused or useless if the person cannot efficiently operate it; it can also be the most frustrating experience for the client, caregiver, and therapist. Thus the therapist must be certain that the client can readily and efficiently activate the switch or control interface.

Because switch selection and mounting for ATDs are usually the responsibility of the occupational therapist, the therapist first evaluates several control sites to determine the most accurate, reliable, and efficient movement that the client can make (Wright & Nomura, 1990). Next, the therapist determines the proper mounting system for the switch, which depends both on where the switch will be used and on which devices it will interface with. For example, an EADL or AAC needs to be controlled when the user is in bed as well as when the user is in a wheelchair. The trend toward integrated technology warrants the use of one switch to control many ATDs in different modes.

The technology specialist should be able to select two or three possible control sites at which the client demonstrates purposeful movement by reviewing the physical abilities assessment, by interviewing the client, and by observing the client's voluntary motion in various environments. Almost any part of the body can be used as an optimal control site; for individuals with severe impairments that might be the head, eyes, tongue, chin, breath, or voice as well as the leg or foot.

A wide variety of switches and control interfaces are commercially available. Some can readily be fabricated by the therapist, other clients, family members, or caregivers. The most commonly used switches include the following (Webster, Cook, Tompkin, & Vanderheiden, 1985):

- *Mechanical switches:* joysticks, cushions, treadles, rockers, and pneumatic switches (e.g., sip and puff switches).
- *Electromagnetic switches:* light beam infrared switches, light emitting diode (LED) detectors, and optical head pointers.
- *Electromyographic switches:* those used to control myoelectric prosthesis.
- *Sonic switches:* ultrasound and voice switches that convert sound levels to switch closure.

People with different disabilities require different types of switches. A client with a spinal cord injury who has limited motion and muscle power requires a sensitive switch (sip and puff), whereas a client with poor gross motor control may require a strong pressure switch with individual slots, to restrict inadvertent selection.

Single, dual, and multiple switches are used to operate technical aids: For a simple on-or-off toy, a single cushion switch may be used; for an EADL that requires scanning and then selection, a dual pneumatic switch may be needed; for a powered wheelchair that moves in many directions, a multiple joystick may be required. Switches operate in momentary or latching modes. A momentary switch activates the device only as long as pressure or contact is being applied—for example, a car horn, an electric bed, or a powered wheelchair switch. A latching switch requires one motion to turn on the device, which remains on until the switch is reactivated, disengaging the latch to the off position—for example, a wall light switch or the power switch of a computer. A momentary switch mode can be changed to a latching mode with an inexpensive interface available from most switch suppliers. Most powered wheelchairs and scooters use switches that allow a smooth gradual acceleration, known as proportional switches.

Switches act as the interface between the person and the device; they activate or deactivate the device and control the device by direct selection, scanning, or certain encoding techniques. Direct selection is the most frequently used and efficient selection technique. It can require more motor control than scanning, which requires higher cognitive and visual tracking skills. Two types of scanning are linear scanning and row-column scanning. In linear scanning, each element is sequentially pointed to; in row-column scanning, first the row or column is selected, followed by the linear scanning of each element in the selected row or column. The later technique reduces time and effort. Encoding can be used with both direct selection and scanning techniques, and it usually requires multiple selections such as Morse Code. Encoding is an abbreviation or acceleration selection technique. When recommending a switch or control interface, the therapist should take into consideration which selection technique will be used for each device to integrate the total assistive technology system. For example, many EADL and AACs require scanning techniques, but some powered wheelchairs do not; therefore, whenever possible, all devices should be integrated to use the same switches or control interface with a compatible selection technique.

In communication, for instance, a client using a picture communication board who wishes to convey the desire for a glass of water can indicate that desire by pointing directly to the appropriate picture on the board. If the client is using a more complex communication device that has letters of the alphabet in rows of eight letters per row, however, the client may point first to the third row, where the letter *W* appears, then to each letter in that row until *W* is selected. Speed is an important factor and should be taken into account when choosing the appropriate technical aid. When the message sender can reduce the effort and time it takes to make a selection, the communication becomes more effective. An example of the increased communication speed of high technology might be a computerized communication aid that has been programmed so that when a nonverbal client points at two or three icons, the computerized voice says, "I want a drink of water, please." This communication aid has switch encoded selection ability, whereby one or more symbols, letters, or words can be coded to convey a complete phrase or sentence.

Most switches require some form of mounting to keep the switch within reach and to allow for effective operation. Some switches can be kept in place on tabletops, wheelchair trays, or bed rails using hook-and-loop tape with adhesive backing or clamps, a single or multiple joint mounting arm, and a mounting clamp. There are rigid stainless-steel tubular mounting arms and flexible gooseneck or caterpillar arms. Switches can also be mounted directly on the client, including the head, chin, over any muscle on the client's chest, or on the roof of the mouth. A rehabilitation engineer may assist the therapist if a customized mounting system is necessary.

The variety of available interface systems and the range in prices warrant that a therapist check various suppliers' catalogs, carefully evaluate the client's abilities and all the environments in which the switch will be used, and integrate the switch and mounting system with the other ADL and hospital equipment the client may use. A primary consideration when selecting a control interface should always be the client's position in lying or sitting, so that reflexes or poor postures are not elicited. If a complex system is used, the occupational therapist should draw a diagram or take pictures so all caregivers mount the switch correctly.

In summary, it should be noted that

- The selection of the switch or control interface is crucial to the operation of all ATDs.
- The occupational therapist is primarily responsible for selecting the switch and mounting system, but collaboration with other team members is essential.
- One switch or control interface system requires less physical motion but higher cognitive abilities to integrate all the client's ATDs.

The following case study illustrates the importance of proper evaluation. Susan is 4 years old and is visually impaired. She can learn her ABCs and listen to stories by pressing a large switch connected to a tape recorder. The occupational assistive technology specialist has evaluated Susan's needs, tried various switches, and taught her certified occupational therapist assistant and caregivers how to insert the switch into the tape recorder. A tape recorder is only the first switch Susan will learn to use; as she matures, she can learn to use switches to control her voice-activated computer or EADL.

BOX 31-1 GUIDELINES FOR SWITCH OR CONTROL INTERFACE SELECTION

- Discuss with the client or significant others their thoughts, opinions, and desires.
- Establish the optimal position for the client, noting all other functions, especially ADL.
- Determine what ATDs the client needs the switch to interface with (toy, wheelchair, EADL, ACA, computer, or other).
- Evaluate the client's physical abilities, considering the sensorimotor, cognitive, and psychosocial components (voluntary control, action, ROM, endurance, speed of response, vision, reflexes).
- Note all precautions (seizures, respiration, endurance/fatigue, visual fields).
- Test the client for two or three possible control sites by observing, formal testing, interviewing, and reviewing the initial assessment (if the client cannot communicate, be sure to observe all voluntary motions that are accurate, reliable, and efficient).
- Interview the caregiver.
- Evaluate the operational features of the switch (activation, force requirements, distance the switch must travel, size of the control surface, durability, feedback, connector type, momentary or latching mode).
- Analyze the selection technique required by the ATD (direct selection, scanning, or encoding).
- Determine where the switch will be used (in bed, on wheelchair, at a workstation, or other).
- Mount the switch temporarily. Do not hold the switch.
- Try the switch with a temporary mounting. If this is not successful, try another switch or change the mounting; if successful, mount the switch permanently and note the position in writing (draw a picture) so all caregivers will be informed.
- Reevaluate periodically.

AUGMENTATIVE AND ALTERNATIVE COMMUNICATION

The basic areas of communication are verbal, conversational, written, and gesturing. Historically, the occupational therapist and the classroom teacher have screened, evaluated, and trained children in the area of written communication. Today, there is an increasing use of computers as writing and drawing aids for the all students, as well as those with disabilities. This subsection focuses on verbal communication and the vital role of the occupational therapist in collaborating with the speech pathologist, who is usually the technology coordinator of AACs.

Communication aids are defined by the American Speech-Language-Hearing Association (ASHA; 1991) as "physical objects or devices used to transmit or receive messages (e.g. a communication book, board, chart, mechanical, or electrical device or computer)" (p. 10). Augmentative and alternative communication (AAC) systems "attempt to compensate (either temporarily or permanently) for the impairment and disability pattern of individuals with severe expressive communication disorders" (ASHA, 1989, p. 107).

The term *augmentative communication* is defined as some way of communicating that does not require speech. If someone has a severe physical disability, this communication may be through gesturing, facial expressions, body or sign language, or through the use of picture, letter, and word boards, commonly known as communication boards. When clients with physical impairments lack the motor ability to convey a message, an AAC system is required. When a communication aid is used, the speed at which the user can locate and select a key, the number of required selections before the aid offers an output, and the quality of the output must be considered. The most frequently used nonelectronic communication system requires the user or communication partner to point to choices to convey messages. Pointing by the user may be done with the hand, with a head pointer, a light beam pointer, or with the eyes.

An electronic AAC system uses a form of electronic technology as throughput. The input can be a single pressure switch, a dual rocker-level switch, a joystick, an optical pointer, a keyboard, an eye blinking switch, or any other control interface that is properly mounted and readily accessible to the user. The output can be by spelling; abbreviation; pictures; coding of words, phrases, and sentences by synthesized speech; visual display; printed copy; or a combination of these.

A communication evaluation should begin by identifying all the tasks, needs, and goals of the client and communication partners. The client's cognitive, motor, and hearing abilities that should be assessed for the elements of communication are sender–receiver–feedback. In addition, the client's language and educational skills need to be considered. The environment where the AAC system is used should be assessed for proper mounting, whether in bed or in a wheelchair.

The key characteristics of any communication system are as follows (Church & Glennen, 1992; Fishman, 1987; Flippo, Inge, & Barcus, 1995; Mann & Lane, 1995):

- Rate or speed that a message can be conveyed.
- Portability of the aid.
- Accessibility to the user in various positions.
- Dependability of both manual and electronic power sources.
- Quality of the output.
- Durability.
- Independence of the user.
- Vocabulary flexibility (programmable or fixed).
- Time required for repairs and maintenance of the aid.

Team cooperation is required to deliver the appropriate augmentative communication services to a client. In the service delivery of electronic communication, the four substantial contributions of the occupational therapist are the following (Angelo & Smith, 1989; Church & Glennen, 1992; Fishman, 1987):

- Holistically evaluating the client, including physical factors (e.g., seating and positioning, ROM, coordination, reflexes) as well as cognitive and perceptual factors.
- Evaluating and recommending the most effective control interface and selection technique.
- Training the client to access the aid.
- Collaborating with other team members.

The speech therapist usually evaluates the client's communication needs, assesses the client's language ability, collaborates in the selection of an aid, and trains the client and his or her major communication partners. Other professional members of the team may include a physician, who is required to sign orders for equipment; a social worker, who may counsel the client and family; a rehabilitation engineer, who may modify the control interface and mounting system; the rehabilitation technology supplier, who designs and produces the electronic aid; and the special education teacher, who will be responsible for language development and implementation of the aid in the school setting.

To be effective, this professional team must work closely with the nonverbal client and the client's communication partners. As with all ATDs, the optimum approach to AAC systems includes the following:

- The aid meets the client's needs.
- The client, various aids, and all environments in which the aids will be used are carefully evaluated.
- The selection is the result of collaboration between the client and the rehabilitation technology team members.
- A backup, standard, nonelectric aid is also available to the client.
- The AAC system can be integrated with all other ATDs.
- The aid does not interfere with ADL.

The occupational therapy technology specialist needs to be aware of various AACs, from simple, small battery-operated aids that can be used bedside for nonspeaking persons (e.g., people with diagnoses such as muscular dystrophy (MS) amyotrophic lateral sclerosis (ALS), cerebrovascular accident (CVA), and laryngectomy), to complex, programmable, wheelchair-mounted systems that integrate with computers and EADL. For additional information, speech pathologists, rehabilitation technology suppliers, and manufacturers are available for in-services, workshops, and training institutes. Three valuable comprehensive resources are the ASHA (1995); the International Society for Augmentative and Alternative Communication's (ISAAC) journal, which includes proceedings of its biennial conference; and Borden, Lubich, and Vanderheidwen (1996). Also check the Internet and World Wide Web for current information from suppliers or professional organizations.

The occupational therapist needs to know what equipment is available and the most appropriate control interface. The speech pathologist is responsible for evaluating the client's language communication abilities, and an interdisciplinary team approach should enable the client to effectively use the AAC device(s). A case study illustrates these points.

James is a nonverbal, 11-year-old, with severe athetoid motion of all four extremities, who also needs a powered wheelchair. Before any assistive technology equipment is ordered, the occupational therapy assistive technology specialist and James's primary therapist evaluate him for the most appropriate switch control site. The speech pathologist collaborates with the occupational therapist, the seating specialist, the physical therapist, and a rehabilitation engineer to design an assistive system that will enable James to control his AAC device through his powered wheelchair using his head as the control site. The rehabilitation engineer designs a secure mounting for the AAC device that can be readily removed when James needs ADL care.

POWERED MOBILITY

Powered mobility is the ATD that liberates individuals with physical impairments and enables them to move about the home environment and into the community. Various powered mobility aids are available; those most frequently used are three-wheeled battery-powered scooters, adapted vehicles, powered wheelchairs, and adapted farm vehicles. Powered mobility is a system that begins with proper positioning of the client in an appropriate powered wheelchair or scooter that is maneuverable in accessible environments and is transportable in a car, van, train, plane, and bus. Each part of the mobility system depends on the other for functional mobility. The salient characteristics that are desirable for a powered mobility device include safety, comfort, dependability, portability for long-range transportation, ease of maintenance, ease in operation for user and caregivers, and compatibility with other ATDs (AACs, ventilators, EADL) (Axelson & Chesney, 1995; Ramsey, 1999; Warren, 1990).

The occupational therapist is a valuable member of the technology rehabilitation team that selects and then trains clients who need powered mobility. The clients most frequently referred for powered mobility are those with cervical-level spinal cord injuries (C4 and above); those with advanced muscle weakness caused by such diseases as ALS, MS, and muscular dystrophy; and those with poor coordination in all extremities such as those with cerebral palsy. Clients of all ages who have to travel long distances and have low levels of endurance usually need powered wheelchairs or scooters. In addition, as discussed earlier, there is increasing evidence that other clients may benefit from powered mobility to avoid repetitive motion injuries. However, they will also need a standard wheelchair as backup when their powered chair is being recharged or repaired and for those times when a powered chair cannot be transported.

Since 1980, an increasing number of young children have been referred for powered mobility, but always with two main concerns: safety for the user and others and the potential adverse effects on the child's physical development. The limited research in powered mobility for young children with disabilities indicates there is improvement in the child's social, cognitive, and communication development when provided with early powered mobility (Butler, 1986a Verburg, 1987). Trefler (Trefler, Kozole & Snell, 1986) and Taylor (1995) reported positive psychosocial effects for early powered mobility, such as improved self-image, attitudes toward approaching new tasks and participation in educational programs. Specialists agree that a comprehensive evaluation of each child's proper positioning, cognitive and perceptual development, and all possible environments in which the chair will be used is crucial (Barnes, 1991; Furamaso, 1997; Jaffe, 1987; Kangas, 1993; Trefler, et al., 1986; Warren, 1990).

Members of the technology rehabilitation team most responsible for the optimum powered wheelchair system are occupational therapists, physical therapists, rehabilitation engineers, rehabilitation technology suppliers, family members or caregivers, and social service professionals. The occupational therapist has a vital role in evaluating the client holistically, collaborating on the selection of a powered wheelchair system, verifying the chair prescription with the user, training the user and caregivers, and following-up periodically—especially as children grow and adults' physical conditions change. The client's primary therapist and the occupational therapy technology specialist can collaborate on the holistic evaluation of the client's positioning, physical ability to access the control interface, cognitive ability to follow instructions and use judgment, perceptual skills (especially spatial relations and figure-ground perception), and motivation. Powered wheelchairs are discussed here; Section 1 provides information on manual wheelchairs.

The designing of a total mobility system requires the occupational therapist either to have advanced knowledge about seating or to consult with an occupational or physical therapist who is a seating specialist. These professionals work with the client and caregivers to determine the best seating position before selecting any mobility device. In addition to evaluating the user and the environment, the occupational therapy technology specialist should carefully assess the numerous powered wheelchairs that are now available. Some have power that allows the user to tilt in space, some allow the user to recline completely, a few allow the user to stand, and some standard wheelchairs can be converted to motorized wheelchairs by adding a power pack to the back of the chair.

The power base is the first portion of the chair that is selected, with special consideration given to types of batteries (usually gel), safety brakes, and any additional powered equipment (e.g., as powered recliners, ventilators, phrenic nerve stimulator platforms). The output from the controller is connected to the user's external device (e.g., AAC system EADL). With a switch, the user transfers the output of the controller from the motors to the AAC system or EADL, which allows for direct scanning (Cook & Hussey, 1995).

The technology specialist must also assess the user's optimum control site because power mobility in particular requires accurate, reliable, and efficient user control. In addition, the technology specialist is usually responsible for evaluating and recommending the switch control method and mounting system. The most frequently used power wheelchair controlled method is the hand-controlled proportional joystick. A proportional joystick allows for graduation in speed and for smooth acceleration. For individuals with limited motion, a proportional joystick can be adjusted with a short throw feature that requires approximately 50% less movement than the standard proportional device setting. For clients who have short, jerky, uncoordinated movements, the proportional joystick can be adjusted with a tremor-dampening feature. Other control methods include the following (Ramsey, 1999):

- *Pneumatic switches* (sip-and-puff breath controls for individuals with limited upper extremity functional movements).
- *Multiple single* switches (mounted on laptrays or headrests for on–off, forward–backward, and right–left movements).
- *Microswitches* that can be programmed to integrate with EADL and AAC systems and to control speed.

Another responsibility of the technology specialist is to collaborate on a detailed wheelchair prescription with other team members. Most wheelchair vendors have worksheets or prescription forms; however, it is recommended that each wheelchair clinic develop its own forms, which should be completed by the clinic coordinator and the vendor, who ideally is a CRTS. It is imperative that the rehabilitation technology team work with a reliable, reputable, dependable vendor who will service the powered chair after it is purchased. Once the chair has been delivered, the therapist should carefully check each part against the prescription and test drive the chair before training the user.

Powered wheelchairs are delivered 4–6 months after they are ordered. Clients must receive training in powered wheelchair use before the chair arrives. Begin training in a large space by having the client go forward and stop, reverse and stop, turn right and left, and make circles. Then the client should practice going around an obstacle course. Training sessions may vary, depending on the age, cognitive ability, and physical function of the user.

Clients who receive powered wheelchairs that are equipped with AAC systems, EADL, computer interfaces, and ventilators need to be trained in the entire integrated control system by all team members. As stated before, an integrated control system uses a single input device (switch) to operate other ATDs. For example, a joystick on a wheelchair can be programmed through the controller to operate an AAC device, a computer, a power recliner, and an EADL. In addition to training the user with controls, the therapist should train the user in various environments, including rough and smooth surfaces, indoors and outdoors, inclines and declines, large and small spaces (most powered wheelchairs have a turning radius of 30 in.) and in different climatic conditions.

With the passage of the ADA (1990), there was an increase in public accommodations, public transportation, and employment opportunities for individuals with disabilities. The primary occupational therapist or occupational therapist assistant is qualified to assess the architectural barriers in the user's home, school, work, and community. For example, consider a farmer with no function in his or her lower extremities. This client uses a standard wheelchair around a barrier-free home with smooth surfaces. But when the farmer goes outside to work, the surface may have sand, gravel, mud, or loose soil and the climatic conditions vary. The farmer will have to transfer from a standard wheelchair to a hand-controlled truck or tractor or an all-terrain vehicle (Freeman, Brushingham , & Field, 1992).

Consider a child who has limited functioning of all extremities and must travel to school in a wheelchair on a bus that cannot accommodate a powered wheelchair. This child may need a standard chair with tie-downs on the bus, but to keep pace with other children in the school building and on the playground, he or she will need a powered chair. Rehabilitation Engineering and Assistive Technology Society of North America (RESNA) developed guidelines for transporting people with disabilities, and Snell (1999) provided guidelines for safely transporting people in wheelchairs.

Another means of power mobility is the scooter. A powered scooter requires the user to have good sitting balance, good eye–hand coordination, adequate spatial and figure-ground perception, and good judgment (Bain, 1997; Warren, 1990). Scooters can be used by people who have limited stamina in conjunction with walkers, canes, or standard wheelchairs in the home, in the workplace, or when traveling in the community. Some scooters can be transported on car racks, and some can be dismantled for ease in transporting.

Adapted cars and vans are another source of powered mobility for those with limited function of both lower and upper extremities, with only one arm or one leg, with restricted joint motion, or with no lower extremities. The occupational therapist and the driving specialist must do scrupulous evaluation before the client is trained and issued a license (see Chapter 24, Section 2). The entry-level therapist should be aware of various vehicle adaptations, including proportional steering and hand controls, braking systems and safety back-up systems, auxiliary control boxes, and hydraulic lifts. Vans with lifts are the preferred means of transportation for powered wheelchairs with batteries that weigh between 25 and 50 lb and can carry people who weigh up to 250 lb. Lifts can conserve energy and the time required for the client to transfer into a car and push or disassemble the powered wheelchair before placing it into a car.

Wheelchair and power wheelchair standards have been developed by the Americans National Standards Institute (ASNI) and RESNA committee. These standards provide the user and professional with information on how products measure in durability and performance. Powered wheelchair evaluation criteria have also been developed by the National Rehabilitation Hospital. For additional information on powered mobility see Trefler et al. (1986) as well as Digman (1996), Jaffe (1987), Kreutz (1998), Nead (1997), and Warren (1990).

ELECTRONIC AIDS FOR DAILY LIVING

Occupational therapists play a primary role in helping clients identify, evaluate, and use EADLs. An EADL is defined as:

> *a means to purposefully manipulate and interact with the environment by alternately accessing one or more electrical devices via switches, voice activation, remote control, computer interface and other technologic adaptations. The purpose of an EADL is to maximize functional ability and independence in the home, school, work, and leisure environment."* (Bain, DiSalvi, Gold, Kollodge, & Schein, 1991, p. 55)

Since the late 1980s, there has been a technology explosion in commercially available, convenient remote controls

BOX 31–2 CLASSIFICATION OF ENVIRONMENTAL CONTROL UNITS

CLASSIFICATION OF ECUs

Level I

- Devices are available off-the-shelf
- Devices do not require an adaptive switch
- Devices use direct selection and may be used with adaptations, such as mouthstick, typing pegs, hand splints, and so forth
- Devices offer primarily latching control; but very limited momentary control
- Devices allow control of on or off functions of appliances and lights (which can also be brightened and dimmed); includes telephones, multiple stand-alone devices, or small units that will control more than one appliance
- Devices may use infrared and radio frequency remote controls

Level II

- Devices are available through specialty equipment manufacturers
- Devices are controlled by an adaptive switch
- Devices use direct selection or scanning
- Devices offer primarily latching control
- Devices allow control of on or off functions of appliances, lights (including brightening and dimming), television, VCR, and so forth, and adapted access to telephone functions
- Devices may use remote control through infrared, radio frequency and ultra sound transmissions

Level III

- Devices are available through specialty equipment manufacturers
- Devices are controlled by an adaptive switch
- Devices use scanning, with the exception of voice activation
- Devices offer both latching and momentary control
- One system allows control of all functions of multiple devices, including full telephone and bed control
- Devices may use remote control through infrared, radio frequency, and ultrasound transmissions

Level IV

- Devices are available through specialty equipment manufacturers
- Devices are controlled by adaptive switch
- Devices use scanning
- Devices offer both latching and momentary control
- One system allows control of all functions of multiple devices, including full telephone and bed control
- Devices incorporate integration with other electrical devices, such as augmentative and alternative communication aids, power wheelchair electronics, and computers using the same switch to access all functions

Level V

- Future developments integrating technology into the community for television, lights, telephones, emergency calls, door locks and openers, temperature regulators, and other appliances in the home and workplace. Some are simple systems that control two or three appliances; others are more complex and control more than 200 appliances; some can be integrated with AAC systems, power wheelchairs, computers, and telephones.

For a person with poor hand skills, EADL can be operated with switches; for a person with low physical stamina, tasks can be completed with greater speed and less energy; for a person with pulmonary and cardiac complications who needs constant monitoring, an EADL can be a safety device; and for the caregiver, an EADL saves time and energy by increasing the client's self-reliance, self-confidence, and independence. EADL can be used by clients of all ages and with a variety of levels of function. Some require limited cognitive ability, whereas others require problem-solving, sequencing, memory, and concept-formation abilities. Most EADL have auditory, visual, or tactile feedback and, therefore, can be used by clients with sensory or motor impairment.

Each EADL consists of the four standard assistive technology parts: input (buttons, switches, computer commands, or voice), throughput or transmission (batteries, household current, household current plus module, radio waves, ultrasound, or infrared); output (on–off control), and feedback (auditory, visual, or vibrating cues) (Fig. 31-4).

The evaluation of a client for an EADL begins with an assessment of the client's needs and functional abilities; next, all environments where the EADL will be used must be considered, especially to determine if a portable system is required. Evaluation of the EADL should include the user's access method, feedback requirements, integration with other equipment, expandability for future use, flexibility (e.g., adjustable rate and method of scanning), installation, and cost (Fig. 31-5; Bain, 1996; Bain et al., 1991; Cook & Hussey, 1995).

There are several levels of EADL (Box 31-2). The selection of an EADL begins with commercially available devices that can readily be purchased from a local electronics store. Some EADL remote controls have small input buttons that can be adapted with dime-size felt pads or grids made of plastic strips. Mouth sticks, universal cuffs, or splints can be used for access if a person has limited hand manipulation skills (level 1). If a person needs a switch,

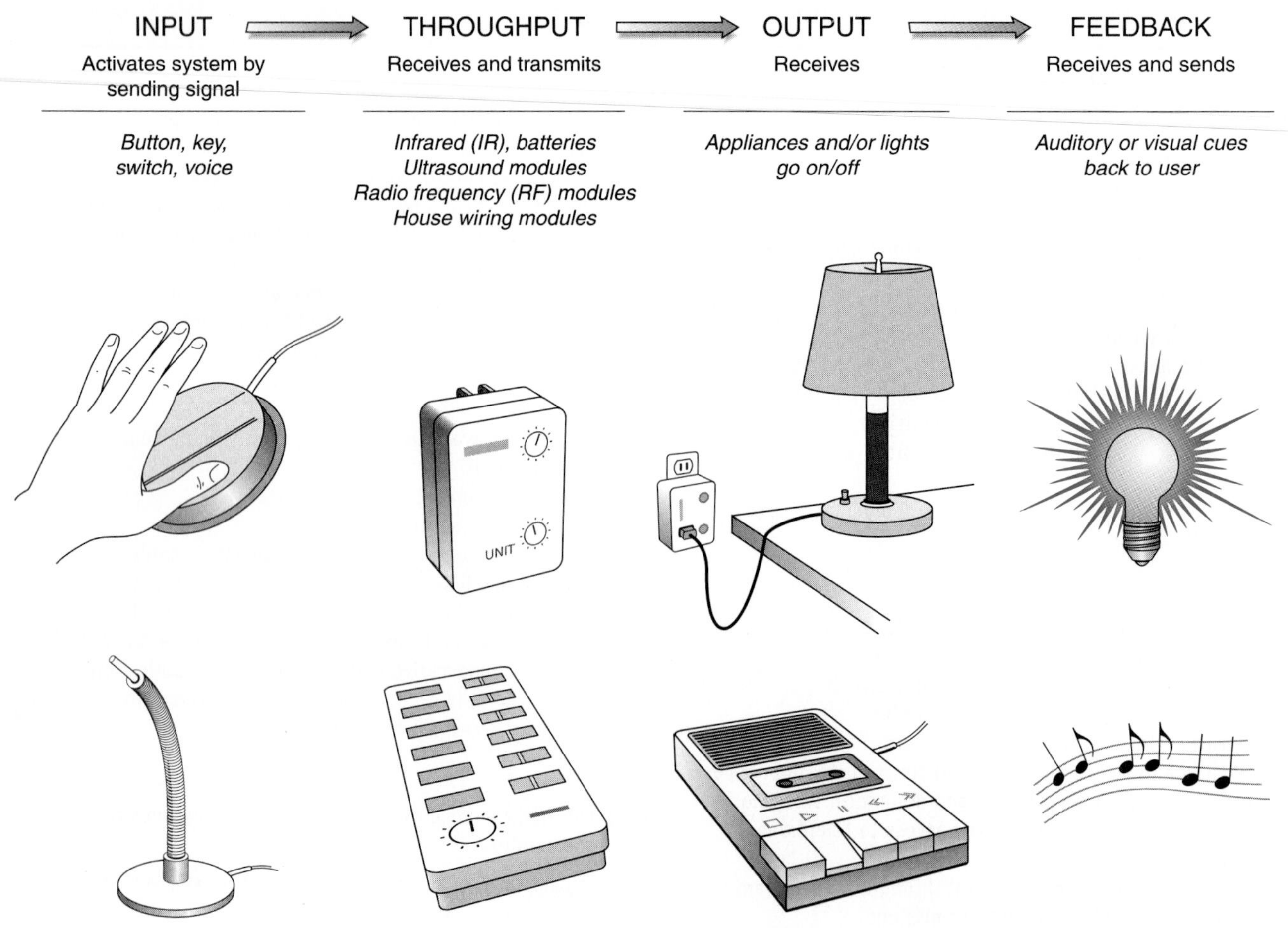

FIGURE 31–4. EADL control sequence.

Electronic aids for daily living: evaluation

Name ______________________ Date __________ Age ______ Sex ______
Date of onset ______________ Diagnosis ______________________
Reason for referral ______________________________________
Major functional problem areas: Communication ______________ Manipulation ______________
Motor ______________ Other ______________

Devices To be controlled	Location					Feedback			Transmission			
	Bed	Wheel-chair	School	Work place	Other	Auditory	Visual	Tactile	AC	IR	RF	Ultrasound or voice
Call bell												
Emergency call system												
Telephone												
Intercom												
Lights: Lamps												
Overhead												
Bed control												
Television												
VCR												
Stereo												
Radio												
Tape recorder												
Fan												
Temperature												
Computer												
Page turner												
Door opener												
Door lock												
OTHER:												

Access methods: Direct selection ☐ Indirect selection ☐ Scanning ☐ Encoding ☐ Voice ☐

Switch(s) ______________________ **Mounting** ______________________

Integration: Wheelchair ☐ Computer ☐ AAC ☐ Other ☐

Funding ______________________________________

Comments: ______________________________________

Evaluator ______________________ **Date** ______________

Revised Bain, 2001, from Bain, Disalvi, Gold , Kollodge, Schein, AOTA Institute 6/1/91

FIGURE 31–5. EADL assessment form. *AC,* alternating currency; *IR,* infrared; *RF,* radiofrequency.

then level 2, 3, and 4 EADL are recommended. Switch-activated EADL are available from special assistive technology rehabilitation suppliers. Transmission can be from AC (household current), infrared, ultrasound, voice, or radiofrequency. Most use infrared or ultrasound transmissions; some can operate telephones; and some can scan TV channels, operate a VCR, and activate appliances in and outside a building.

Note that ultrasound waves are not transmitted through walls, radiowaves have a greater transmission distance, and household AC current has the greatest transmission distance. Infrared signals transmit in direct-line of sight; however, one infrared device can teach other infrared devices. For example, there are infrared ATDs that can teach a television remote control infrared receiver to accept signals. In addition, some infrared ATDs can send signals to an infrared receiver that converts the signal to house current to operate other appliances. There are also devices that can extend the length of infrared signals from one room to another. For a comparison of different transmission systems, see Bain (1996, 1997) and Lange (1996).

Planning is a crucial step in the selection process for present and future EADLs. To illustrate, consider that a person with a C4 spinal cord injury will need a level 3 EADL when in bed for calling a nurse, scanning TV channels, and making telephone calls. Portability is important when the user is in a wheelchair at home, in school, at work, or in the barrier-free community. A compact system can be used to control lights and electrical appliances (e.g., tape recorder, rotating file system, computer, mail opener, letter folder).

EADL are not usually funded, and if they are, they will usually be purchased only once. Therefore, the therapist must consider all present and future environments in which the EADL will be needed and how much support will be provided by caregivers. Currently, there are some systems at level 2, 3, or 4 that can accomplish all of the aforementioned tasks. Therefore, sometimes it may be necessary to purchase a level 3 or 4 device for hospital and/or home, and a Level 2I EADL for school and/or workplace.

In the future, as robots become less expensive, they may be the EADL of choice. A robotic arm is currently available that is mounted on a powered wheelchair and can pick up a pill from the floor, put it in a person's mouth, reach up to get a glass out of the cupboard, fill it with water, and deliver the water to the person. There are also workstation (desktop) designs and mobile robots with computer controllers (Bain, 1996; Cook & Hussey, 1995).

After the EADL system has been evaluated and the selection has been completed, the next step is helping the client and all caregivers learn how to use the device. Usually, this is part of the occupational therapist's role. It is important that both the client and caregivers know how to assemble the system, understand all its capabilities, know about the routine maintenance, and know where repairs can be made. When a client is in the hospital, it is advisable for the therapist to place drawings or pictures of all connections near the person's bed and to give in-service training to the staff. Before leaving the hospital or rehabilitation center, the person and/or caregiver should demonstrate to the therapist how to assemble, operate, and maintain the system. Most assistive technology suppliers have catalogs on the EADL application and some will supply videos to the user.

Because insurance and vocational rehabilitation agencies rarely reimburse the cost of an EADL, another responsibility for the occupational therapist working in conjunction with the social worker and client/family is to find funding for the EADL system that best meets the client's needs. Sometimes this may mean beginning with an affordable ($50–100), off-the-shelf commercially available unit purchased by the family or friends and then progressing to a more comprehensive system as funding becomes available. Another plan is to purchase software that enables a user to control the EADL system through a computer or AAC aid, which frequently are funded by schools or vocational rehabilitation agents.

When requesting funding for EADL, rehabilitation technology team members need to include in their calculations the hours and cost of attendant care that will be saved when the client can be independent because of the EADL. At present, there are not sufficient research data to validate these savings (Mann & Lane 1995; Petra, 1996). The occupational therapist can wisely spend time by searching electrical specialty shops and trade magazines and by attending workshops to find affordable off-the-shelf EADL.

Other important factors to consider when prescribing an EADL are its safety features, its durability, and the reliability of the manufacturer. It is frustrating to the client, caregivers, and therapist when the system needs constant repairs or when the manufacturer is not reliable.

Telephones

Telephones mean safety as well as convenience and leisure for people with disabilities. Numerous technologic telephone advances have been made that benefit people with hearing, speaking, visual, and motor impairments. For the visually impaired, there are telephones with enlarged numbers, and enlarged stick-on numbers can be applied to any phone. In addition, telephone bills can be printed in braille. Another useful aid for people with visual impairments and for people with motor impairments is to dial the operator (0), who will then assist by dialing the desired number.

For people who need assistance dialing 0, there is an overlay that fits over the buttons and requires only a gross motion to push down the correct button. Other telephone aids for people with motor impairments include telephones that can be controlled by switches or interfaced with an EADL; portable, lightweight headset telephones; telephones with four-button emergency attachments; memory storage; battery backup; conference calls; and redial capabilities. For people with weak voice quality, there are telephones that amplify the voice, and for those with poor voice volume, there are electronic artificial larynxes.

Great advances have been made in technology to increase the telephone capabilities of people with hearing impairments and those who are deaf, including fax and e-mail. People with hearing impairments can attach small amplifiers to any handset or purchase a handset with adjustable amplification built-in. Deaf or speech-impaired people can call person-to-person to another deaf person or to anyone, any time of the day, any day of the year, through the use of a telecommunications device for the deaf (TDD) and the telephone company dual relay system (check the local telephone directory for details). Section IV of the ADA ensures that interstate and intrastate telecommunications relay services are available to hearing- and speech-impaired people.

Monitoring Systems

Personal-response systems are technologic devices that are worn or carried by people who wish to live alone or who are left alone, such as the frail elderly, people with physical disabilities, or children who are old enough to care for themselves after school, but who need help if there is an emergency. These devices can be activated by various switches; for people with severe impairments, sip and puff, light pressure, or eyebrow switches are usually used. The switch sends a signal to a monitoring center, which then puts the user in touch with a relative, friend, neighbor, or an emergency service. Most users with cardiac problems are linked directly to hospital monitoring centers. Such devices can be cost-effective in reducing nursing home or hospital stays while granting safe independence to the user and comfort to relatives who are unable to offer constant care (Joe, 1990). Another means of monitoring people in the same house is an inexpensive (<$50) baby monitor, which is sensitive enough to hear breathing anywhere in the house.

The therapist must be cognizant of the client's tolerance to equipment and the psychological implications of being dependent on aids. Every effort should be made to recommend only the EADL that will enhance the client's functional abilities and improve or maintain the client's independence. Often, the most efficient solution is for the therapist to suggest architectural changes in the environment.

For additional EADL information refer to the numerous specialty resources: American Occupational Therapy Association (AOTA; 1996); Kreutz (1998); Church and Glennen (1992) for excellent drawings and clear descriptions of EADL; Mann and Lane (1995) for several pictures and a list; Lange (1996) for a comprehensive selection chart; and Cook and Hussey (1995) for charts, drawings, and use of robots.

COMPUTERS

Computers have become an integral part of everyone's lives. For many people with disabilities, computers have enhanced their functional abilities, increased their independence, and improved their quality of life. To illustrate, children with cerebral palsy can learn to count or play games using a computer with auditory feedback; a high school student with a learning disability can use a computer to prepare written assignments correctly and to practice math problems; a young adult with a high level spinal cord injury can become gainfully employed using a computer to draw architectural designs; a young mother with MS can conserve her energy by grocery shopping online; and a grandmother with severe arthritis can send e-mail letters to her grandson in college. These are some ways that computers have become an important part of client's lives in all performance areas. For occupational therapy practitioners, computers have become valuable tools.

Evaluation

Therapists should be aware of a few assessment instruments that are valuable for evaluating a client's abilities to use computers effectively. Anson's (1997) nonstandardized access guide to computer selection uses a decision tree method to guide the therapist through the process of evaluating clients who have physical or sensory limitations. The Physical Characteristics Assessment (PCA) is a standardized checklist for computer access for individuals with cerebral palsy. The PCA has been statistically studied for validity and interrater reliability and is reported to be a valid instrument when used by professionals and educators (Fraser, McGregor, et al., 1995; Fraser, Bryen, & Morano, 1995). Lee and Thomas (1990) provide another comprehensive assessment manual, which contains a systematic overview for the selection of access systems to control computer-based technology, including computers, powered mobility, and AAC systems. It can be used as a guide for professionals and nonprofessionals and is a valuable learning tool. Struck and Corfman (1994) described a model for evaluating school-based students using a problem-solving approach. The student's needs and goals are the core of the evaluation, which also includes curriculum requirements, characteristics of the ATD, and environmental concerns (Struck, 1995; Struck & Corfman, 1994).

The first step in the evaluation process is to determine what tasks, needs, and goals the client wants to accomplish with a computer. Before assessing computer needs, the primary therapist should complete, a holistic evaluation of the client's physical, cognitive, psychological, and sensorimotor abilities. Evaluation of the client's physical abilities should begin with positioning. Special attention is given to seating the client with the pelvis secure and stable in the seat, shoulders in front of the trunk, arms and hands visible, head free to rotate, and the feet flat on the floor or supported.

Reflexes should be observed during computer use and avoided when possible. The client's ROM, muscle tone, strength, endurance, and gross and fine coordination should be part of the physical evaluation. If the client needs to use a switch, the primary therapist and technology specialist should collaborate on selecting several possible control sites that can be used. The client's cognitive abilities are important factors to evaluate, including cause and effect, attention span, ability to follow directions, sequencing, problem solving, and memory. The psychological abilities required for computer use are motivation, behavior readiness, a high level of coping skills, and a lack of computer phobia. A crucial area to evaluate carefully is the client's sensorimotor abilities, including visual acuity, figure-ground, right or left neglect, depth perception, and spatial relations. Tactile and auditory abilities and deficits also need to be evaluated for computer use.

Once the client's abilities have been assessed, the next step is to consider all environments in which the computer will be used (in a wheelchair, at a desk, at home, school, workplace, or in the community). Note that several different environments may be used. For example, a student uses a computer in school at a desk, but at home, the family's computer work area prevents proper positioning of the student. The therapist suggests several modifications, such as using a thick telephone book to support the child's feet. Other environmental factors to note include the light and noise levels.

A comprehensive computer characteristics evaluation should be completed by the technology occupational therapy specialist, in collaboration with a computer specialist when necessary. The input (means of activating the computer) can be via the keyboard, mouse, on-screen keyboard, switch(es), or voice. The throughput is the central processing unit (CPU), which is the controlling motor of the computer, operated with power supplied by house current or computer battery. The output can be the monitor, hardcopy, Braille hardcopy, or synthesized voice. Visual, auditory, tactile, or a combination are the possible feedback methods. Peripherals are both input devices (e.g., keyboards) and output devices (e.g., monitors and printers) (Anson, 1997; Fraser, McGregor et al., 1995; Kollodge, 1997; Lee &

TABLE 31–3. **SUGGESTIONS FOR COMPUTER MODIFICATIONS**[a]

Problem Area	Possible Solution(s)[b]
Visual	
Acuity	Large, contrasting colored stickers on keys
Figure/ground	Enlarge font size and style
Light sensitivity	Large, magnified, anti-glare monitor
Lateral neglect	Right or left Dvorak keyboard; Braille keyboard
Legally blind	Voice-controlled software; screen reading software (text to speech)
Cognitive (use "Help" key)	
Attention span	Word prediction
Short-term memory	Written sheet of step-by-step directions
Following directions	Graded from one step to multiple steps
Sequencing	Abbreviation expansion; macros; specially designed software; synthesized speech
Motor	
Limited reach	Mouth stick; head or chin pointer; universal cuff; splint; infrared light pointer; ultrasound system; mini keyboard; on-screen keyboard; touch window; track ball
Limited hand coordination	Key guard; mitten with one finger exposed; expanded keyboard; alternative keyboard; switches (head, elbow, shoulder, knee, foot, sip and puff with computer access interface) track ball; numeric pad for mouse directions; voice-controlled software
Excessive hand motions (good head control)	Switch control with head (infrared, laser, or ultrasound); voice software (consistent speech patterns required); place hands under laptray/table; repeat or delay keyboard
One handed	Key latch for simultaneous key strokes; right or left Dvorak keyboard; mouse keys with *Windows,* sticky keys

[a]Data from Anson (1997), Bain (1997), Lange (2001), Kollodge (1997), Bain (2001).

[b]Resources: ABLEDATA (www.abledata.com), Microsoft Accessibility and Disabilities Group (www.microsoft.com/enable/; "Accessibility" in the "Help" menu in *Windows* 95, 98, and 2000), Apple/Disability (www.apple.com/disability/easyaccess.html), catalogs, conferences and workshops, other computer users.

Thomas, 1990). Another hardware component of a computer is the modem (modulator/demodulator), a device that allows one computer to exchange information with another over telephone lines. Modems allow computer users to access the Internet and send faxes.

Intervention

A carefully planned therapeutic computer program with definite outcomes should be based on sound occupational therapy practice principles. Some examples are activities that can be graded, beginning with a simple task such as a greeting card project using a drawing software program for an adult with limited computer skills. Computer activities should be age appropriate: A computer program designed for a 2-year-old is colorful and has musical feedback to encourage the child's active involvement. Word processing can enhance the functional abilities of people with limited motor control who cannot write by hand legibly or for individuals who have learning disabilities.

A person with a visual impairment can learn to use a voice-activated software program as part of his or her prevocational program. Note that consistent speech patterns are required to successfully use voice-activation software, and the person must have the cognitive ability to learn the system. In addition, the training environment must be conducive to hearing the synthesized voice and quiet enough not to interfere with the voice commands.

A computer program for use in a school needs to address the objectives as stated in the individualized education program (IEP; e.g., writing or math). For a young adult, a computer program might relate to work exploration; for an older person, the program might have home management or leisure objectives. These are only a few examples of how useful computers are in a therapeutic program.

Modification

Each part of the assistive technology system can be modified (Table 31-3). As with all ATDs, begin with standard, commercially available, simple devices using direct selection access. Next, adapt the device or change the environment, such as covering the keys with large letters or tilting the keyboard (low technology). If the client needs switch selection, some computers require a switch interface, and some will accept a switch plugged into the computer's serial port (high technology). If a person is unable to reach all the keys on a standard keyboard, a simple mouthstick (low tech) might be used, or a mini keyboard (high tech) can be adapted to bring the most frequently used keys within easy reach. A combination of low and high technology might include the use of a universal cuff to access a touch screen keyboard.

To summarize, the computer, as well as all other ATDs, is a therapeutic tool that can increase the functional independence of a variety of clients when used in a planned program with definite client goals and objectives. The occupational therapist can collaborate with other team members in the evaluation of the client, analyzing the tasks and selecting the most appropriate devices. Practitioners may be responsible for the training of the client and others, including the teacher, employer, or family members.

CONCLUSION

Since the late 1980s, occupational therapists have learned to use assistive technology to extend the abilities of clients of all ages and with varying degrees of function. It is the intent of this section to encourage practitioners to seek additional information, knowledge, skills, and competency by attending workshops, enrolling in technology courses, and networking with other professional groups.

The AOTA has a number of resources to support practitioners, including the Technology Special Interest Section, as well as regular continuing education events. Another informative interdisciplinary professional group is the RESNA, which also has publications, conferences, and continuing education opportunities. See Appendix F for these and other resources.

As with any specialty area, assistive technology builds on the body of professional occupational therapy knowledge. It is advisable to first learn about switches and control interfaces and then to progress to an area relevant to your practice, such as toys, wheelchairs, EADL, or computers. At first, it may seem impossible to keep up to date with the rapid advances in technology, but networking with occupational therapists, other professionals, and users is beneficial.

Assistive technology is one of many tools of the occupational therapy profession. Attempts should be made to avoid inappropriate application of high technology when it is not needed and to use it only when its application is beneficial to the client. Assistive technology can make many tasks possible for many clients when it is based on sound therapeutic foundations, an ongoing comprehensive evaluation of all parts of the system, an interdisciplinary team (including the client and caregiver) to make decisions on the selection of ATDs with a focus on the individual client's needs and goals.

ACKNOWLEDGMENTS

I gratefully acknowledge the professional contributions of Margy DiSalvi-Wolf, Judy Gold, Barbara Kollodge, and Ronnie Schein; the editing and reviewing of Dawn Leger; the graphics of Rani Bandaru; and those faculty and students who assisted me at New York University and at the Matheny School and Hospital in New Jersey.

SECTION III

Splinting and Orthotics

SUSAN EMERSON
ALICE SHAFER

Occupational therapists in many settings are expected to evaluate, fabricate, and modify splints. The term **splint,** or **orthotic device,** is generally used to describe an external device applied to the body that is designed to immobilize or restrain injured tissues, align or correct deformity, or improve function (Anderson, Anderson, & Glanze, 1998; O'Toole, 1997). The terms *splint* and *orthotic device* may be used interchangeably in practice; but technically, a splint is a temporary device that is part of an intervention program to facilitate recovery from an injury or enhance function. An orthotic device is usually a more permanent device intended to substitute for or replace loss of muscle function. Generally, orthotic devices are made or provided by an orthotist and fabricated of high-temperature materials or metal. Splints associated with the practice of occupational therapy are generally made of low-temperature thermoplastic materials, high-density foams, and various types of fabrics. A splint may be needed for a wide variety of reasons but the most frequent may include the following:

- Support healing tissue and bone during the healing process.
- Control pain.
- Augment or restrict muscle actions.
- Substitute for loss of active motion.
- Increase ROM.

The occupational therapist is responsible for determining effective splint options and assessing splint fit and use. Either the therapist or the occupational therapy assistant may fabricate splints.

When the need for a splint has been identified, practitioners may fabricate a splint or custom-fit a pre-formed splint. Splints may be needed by clients with:

- Central nervous system (CNS) problems, such as stroke, spinal cord injuries, and coma.
- Traumatic peripheral injuries, such as fractures, tendon lacerations, and crush injuries.
- Following surgical procedures, such as joint replacement.
- Repetitive stress injuries, such as carpal tunnel syndrome and lateral epicondylitis.

Although occupational therapists may fabricate splints for any part of the body, this chapter focuses on hand splints, as they are a common part of interventions for those practitioners working with physically disabled individuals.

CRITICAL CONSIDERATIONS

The nature of the injury or level of client cooperation may limit or prohibit observation of function as a method of determining the appropriate type of splint. In some situations, the therapist providing a hand splint may have to depend on referral and diagnostic information rather than on observation of functional task performance to guide splinting interventions. For example, a diagnosis of an acute tendon injury may require construction of a complex custom-fabricated splint designed to accommodate the site of surgical repair, the postsurgical intervention protocol, and the level of tendon repair. Box 31-3 provides guiding questions that can

BOX 31–3 QUESTIONS THAT ASSIST WITH SPLINT CHOICE AND DESIGN

- What hand anatomy and biomechanics are relevant to this diagnosis?
- What functional loss is implied by the specific diagnosis? How does this affect the type of splint needed?
- What intervention theories support the use of a splint for this diagnosis?
- What is the purpose of the splint?
- What is the expected duration of use?
- Can the client properly apply and use the device?
- Is a custom-fabricated or a custom-fitted prefabricated splint more appropriate? Which is more cost-effective?
- What is the skill level needed to construct the splint? Is there adequate supervision if it is needed?

BOX 31-4 BASIC ANATOMICAL AND BIOMECHANICAL CONSIDERATIONS

- Preserve palmar arches.
- Use hand creases as landmarks for splint design and molding.
- Maintain antideformity position.
- Properly position and tighten straps to allow blood flow or venous return.
- Properly contour splints.
- Avoid or minimize pressure over bony prominence.
- Allow motion out of the splint when possible.

help therapists ensure that the optimal splint is provided to the client to maximize functional outcome.

Anatomical and Biomechanical Considerations

Understanding basic hand anatomy is necessary for effective splint design and application. Proper application of basic biomechanical principles that apply to splint design protects the person's hand from injury caused by a poorly designed or fitted splint (Box 31-4).

Identify Creases and Preserve Arches of the Hand

The creases of the hand reflect normal joint mobility, muscle function, and grasp patterns and are important anatomical landmarks in splint design. Hand creases identify the relative position of the underlying bony joints and should always be considered as the therapist designs and fabricates or custom-fits a splint.

There are three palmar creases: two horizontal and one vertical (Fig. 31-6). The distal palmar crease, one of the two horizontal creases, identifies the location of the metacarpal phalangeal (MP) joints. Note that the distal palmar crease slants diagonally across the palm. Splints meant to allow MP joint motion must fit below this crease to ensure that motion at those joints is unencumbered. The second horizontal crease is the proximal palmar crease. This crease is often used to identify the optimal location for the distal radial edge of splints that stabilize the wrist.

The vertical palmar crease is the thenar crease, which may be traced proximally from the proximal palmar crease medially and around the thenar eminence to the mid-proximal palm. Therapists designing splints to allow thumb carpometacarpal joint motion should use this crease as a guide to allow clearance for thenar motion.

The distal and proximal wrist creases, located on palmar side of the hand, identify the articulation point of the radiocarpal joint and proximal border of the carpal bones. Any splint that allows wrist motion must fully clear the wrist creases.

The digital palmar creases are titled distal, middle, and proximal to reflect their anatomical location, and they represent the distal interphalangeal (DIP), proximal interphalangeal (PIP), and MP joints, respectively. Any splint that is designed to support one of these joints must include the bones proximal and distal to these creases. Conversely, a splint designed to allow motion at one of these joints must allow the crease and corresponding joint to be free (Coppard, 2001a; Fess & Phillips, 1987).

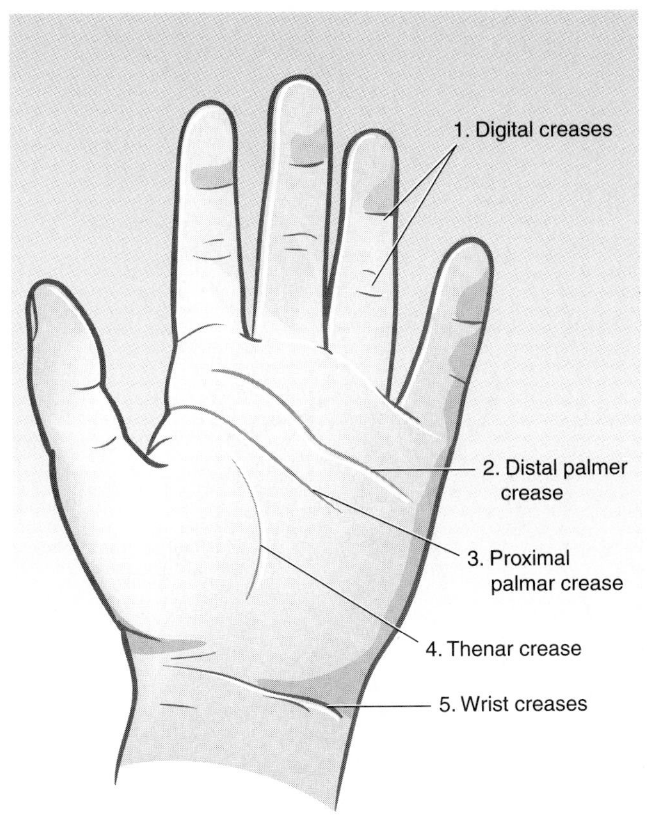

FIGURE 31-6. The creases of the palm. *1,* Digital creases: distal, middle, and proximal; *2,* distal palmar crease; *3,* proximal palmar crease; *4,* thenar crease; *5,* distal wrist creases. (Adapted from Trombley and Fadonski, 2001.)

The bones and articulations of the hand and wrist joints are arranged to form three arches that allow strong functional grasp; they must be preserved when splints are applied to the hand (Fig. 31-7) (Coppard, 2001a). If a person's hand is placed in a splint that is not contoured to match these arches, future function may be severely compromised.

The proximal transverse arch formed by the distal row of carpal bones acts as the stable pivot point among the wrist, the forearm, and the digits (Coppard, 2001a). The distal transverse arch, which identifies the position of the metacarpal heads, is mobile and critical to hand grasp and function. By flexing and extending the digits of the hand, it is possible to observe the distal transverse arch. Note that the fourth and fifth metacarpals have the most mobility. Achievement of a full fist depends on the mobility of the transverse palmar arch (Coppard, 2001a; Fess & Phillips, 1987).

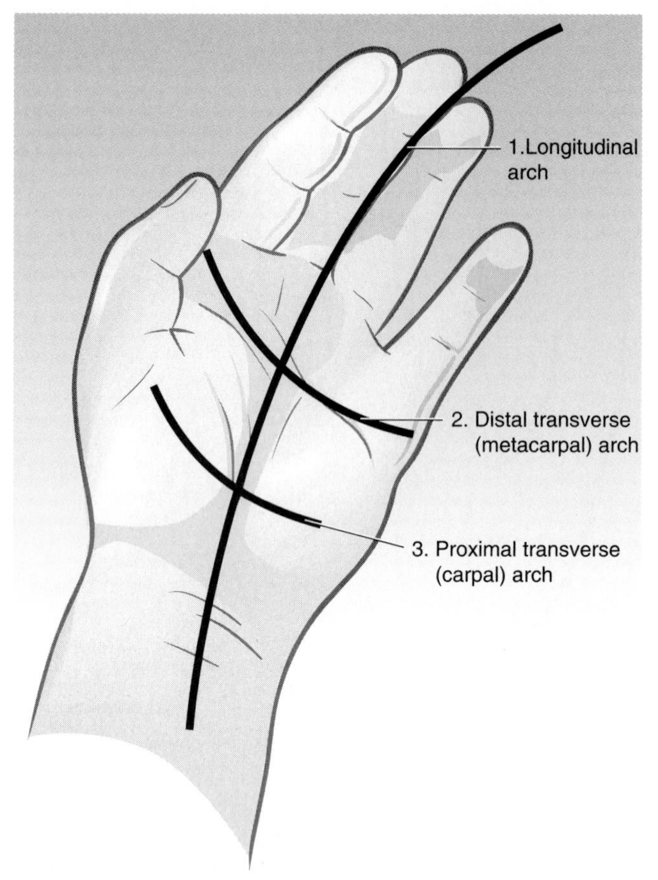

FIGURE 31–7. The arches of the hand. *1,* Longitudinal arch; *2,* distal transverse arch; *3,* proximal transverse arch. (Adapted from Trombley and Fadonski, 2001.)

The longitudinal arch, which connects the two transverse arches, may be thought of as having a stable center unit and two adjacent mobile units. The center unit of this arch is the relatively rigid second and third metacarpals. The thenar muscles move the thumb metacarpal and the fourth and fifth metacarpals around the rigid center unit. The rigid portion of this arch is the stable base against which an object is held while the mobile units and their corresponding digits move to manipulate or securely grasp the item. Any hand splint incorporating these arches must preserve the arches to protect future function (Coppard, 2001a).

Antideformity Positions

In the event of hand trauma and consequent edema, the unsupported hand typically adopts a position of wrist flexion, MP extension, interphalangeal (IP) flexion, and thumb adduction. If allowed to remain in this posture, connective tissue, particularly ligaments, may remodel and become shortened and fibrotic, limiting motion and function (Fess & Kiel, 1998; Schultz-Johnson, 1996; Brand, 1985). Careful consideration of joint position during periods of immobilization minimize these consequences.

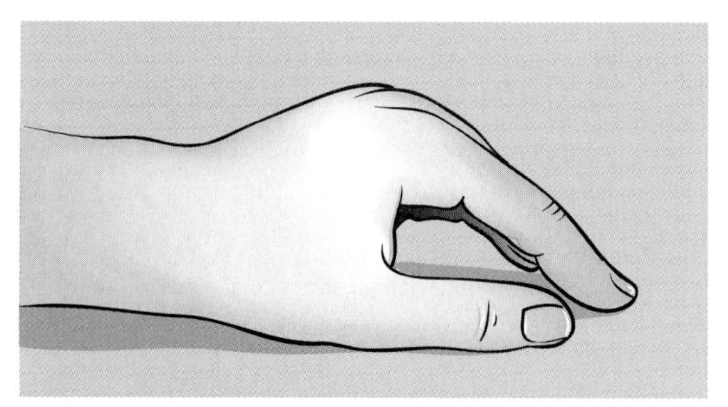

FIGURE 31–8. The antideformity or safe position, used to protect joints and preserve function while the hand is splinted (Adapted from Trombley and Fadonski, 2001.)

When possible, splints involving the whole hand should incorporate a position that puts the wrist in neutral to slight extension, the MP joints in 70–90° of flexion, the IP joints in extension, and the thumb in abduction; a position also known as the safe or *antideformity position* (Fig. 31-8) (Coppard, 2001b; Strickland, 1987). The differences in the recommended positions for the MP and IP joints reflect their unique anatomical configurations. Function is most easily obtained when motion is resumed from the antideformity position.

Position Straps to Allow Blood Flow and Venous Return

Straps should be carefully applied to prevent constriction of blood flow and venous return. Interstitial fluid is reabsorbed into the body's vascular system through the lymphatic vessels located on the dorsal hand. If splint straps are too tight or inappropriately placed or if the hand is left in a dependent posture below the level of the heart, circulation is compromised. If a client is not able to monitor the status of his or her arm and hand, caregivers should be instructed to examine the person's arm regularly for evidence of edema between straps or in the digits.

Contour Splints and Minimize Pressure over Bony Prominences

Splints should be carefully contoured around bony structures for proper support and to avoid uneven distribution of pressure over bony prominences. Material that is rounded and not flat has improved strength and disperses pressure more evenly (Fess & Phillips, 1987). Furthermore, splints that are too high or tight on the either side of the wrist may impinge on the radial or ulnar styloid processes. Splints that include or approximate the scaphoid at the base of the thumb, the head of the index metacarpal, or lateral aspects of the finger joints should also be carefully contoured to avoid pressure in these locations.

Allow Appropriate Motion

Movement of the hand prevents muscular atrophy, soft tissue adhesion and shortening, and limits deformity (Malick, 1974). Whenever possible, the client should be encouraged to remove a splint and perform active and or passive range of motion of the involved tissues. Splint dependency and consequent deconditioning may occur if the client unnecessarily limits use. This, of course, depends on specific diagnostic intervention protocols and requires client instruction.

Wound Healing

Understanding the implications of the biological process of wound healing is critical to determining the appropriate type of splint and its use in the continuum of therapeutic intervention. Any type of trauma to tissue initiates an organized and predictable cellular response that is essential to healing. However, scar can be deleterious to hand function if stiffness and decreased ROM result from excessive restrictive scar. For a detailed explanation of the phases of wound healing, see Hardy (1989) and Smith (1995).

Redness, heat, and edema mark the inflammatory phase of wound healing, which usually lasts 4–5 days from the time of injury. During this phase, the healing tissue is fragile and usually requires immobilization for protection. Proper positioning of the involved parts is tissue and protocol specific and critical to the ultimate functional outcome. The inflammatory phase is immediately followed by the fibroplastic or rebuilding phase, which usually lasts 5–21 days. Splinting during this phase generally consists of a balance between sessions of limited and guarded motion and judicious use of splints that protect the healing tissues and guard against the development of deformity. The remodeling phase, the last phase of wound healing, determines the final configuration of the scar. Prudent use of splints that apply gentle and prolonged force to maintain tissue at its available end range may assist with improved ROM and function.

SPLINT REFERRAL AND PRESCRIPTION

The professionals who refer clients for splinting vary greatly in their understanding of splinting options and related functional implications. Ideally, the referral includes the diagnosis, the specific body parts to include in the splint, and instructions about the purpose of the splint. Occasionally, the specific splint referral, in the therapist's opinion, does not reflect the optimal solution for the client's problem. In this situation, the therapist should initiate a discussion with the referring professional to clarify the request, describe options, and arrive at the best solution.

For example, a client with a diagnosis of wrist tendonitis was referred for a custom-fabricated thermoplastic wrist cock-up splint to wear at her job as a computer data entry operator. While a wrist splint is indicated for individuals with this diagnosis, a thermoplastic splint would be awkward to wear when using a computer keyboard. In this situation, the therapist called the referring physician and suggested a soft fabric splint with an internal stay to support the wrist.

Occasionally, the therapist is asked to fabricate a splint that is beyond his or her skills and experience. In most situations, it is best to advise the referral source that the requested device cannot be made and the client should be either referred to a more experienced therapist or rescheduled for a time when supervision can be provided to ensure that the prescription is completed appropriately.

TYPES OF SPLINTS

Hand splints are broadly classified into two groups: mobilizing and immobilizing splints. An immobilizing splint may be designed to support healing tissue, prevent motion, or prevent the development of deformity. Mobilizing splints are usually more complicated and are designed to assist weak or absent active motion or to exert a force on joints and tissue that have limited ROM and function. Either type of splint is appropriate for clients with hand impairments resulting from CNS injuries or diseases, with peripheral major traumatic injuries, and with repetitive **microtrauma,** depending on the stage of wound healing.

Immobilizing Splints

The most common type of immobilizing splint is the **static splint.** Static splints are generally simple splints that are usually removable and by definition do not have any moving parts. Static splints are appropriate for use during the inflammatory phase of a healing wound to support injured structures as the tissue begins to mend. For people with CNS impairments, a static splint maintains sufficient ROM to allow hygienic care and prevents deformity from developing by supporting the hand until recovery is maximized. The most common types of static splints are the wrist cock-up splint, the thumb spica splint, and the hand-resting splint. Figure 31-9 shows these splints and lists common diagnoses for which they might be appropriate.

Another type of immobilizing splint with a different purpose is the **serial static splint** used when adaptive shortening has occurred. **Adaptive shortening** occurs when tissue remodels to a shortened length because the joint is immobilized in a position in which the surrounding tissue is slack and deprived of the stress that occurs with normal motion (Schultz-Johnson, 1996). This could happen with prolonged positioning resulting from a CNS diagnosis such as head trauma or after immobilization from a major trauma such as a burn or crush injury. If adaptive shortening occurs, joint

Splint type	Associated diagnoses
Wrist cock up 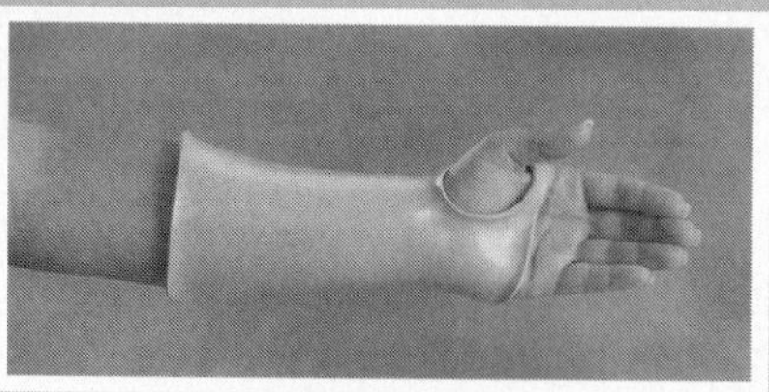	Carpal tunnel syndrome Radial nerve palsy Tenosynovitis/tendinitis Wrist fractures Rheumatoid arthritis Osteoarthritis Relfex sympathetic dystrophy Wrist sprains
Resting splint 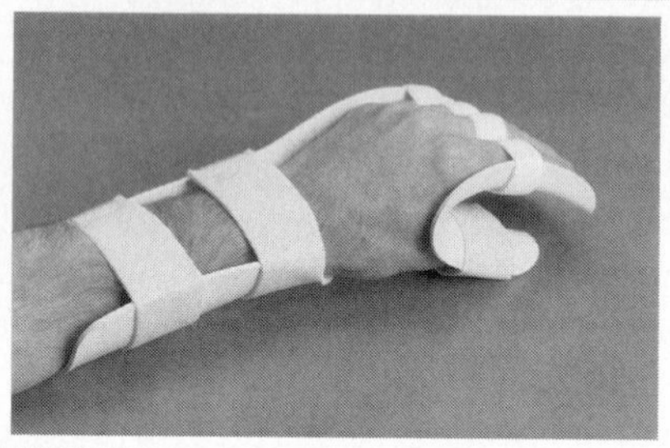	Rheumatoid arthritis Traumatic injuries: crush, contusion Burns Tendon injuries Stroke Spinal cord injury Central nervous system disease and injury Post op Dupuytren's Infections
Thumb spica 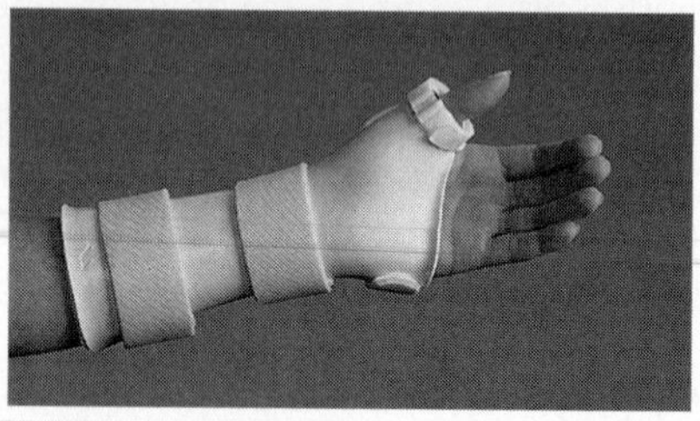	Dequervain's tendonitis Degenerative arthritis/basilar joint arthritis Rheumatoid arthritis Thumb sprains Median nerve injuries

FIGURE 31–9. Common static splints and associated diagnostic conditions. (Photos courtesy of the Rehabilitation Division of Smith+Nephew, Germantown, WI.)

mobility and ROM may be improved or restored through the use of serial splinting.

Serial splinting works on the principle that cells can be realigned, permitting more tissue flexibility, when tissue is held in maximum extension (Bell-Krotoski, 1995). A serial static splint may be made of thermoplastic materials or plaster of Paris (Fig. 31-10). The splint is either frequently and gradually remolded or applied to hold the tissue at the end of the available ROM until maximum range of motion occurs or there is a plateau in progress. The serial static splint is considered appropriate for musculotendinous tightness, for adhesions associated with fractures and tendon injuries, and for situations that have resulted in moderate-to-severe joint contractures (Tribuzi, 1995).

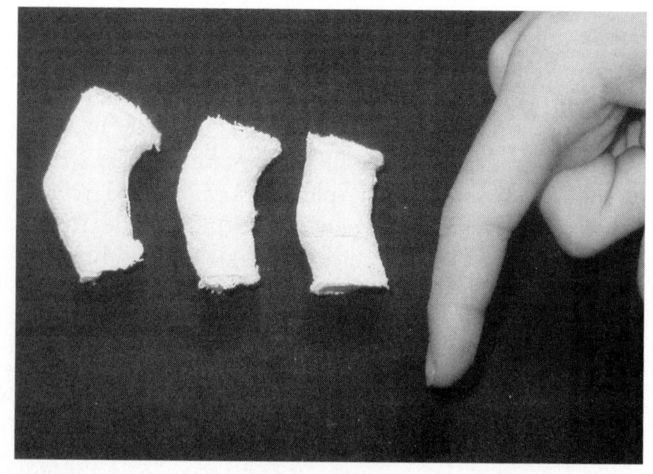

FIGURE 31–10. Progressive casting is used to increase joint and soft tissue ROM.

Mobilizing Splints

There are two types of mobilizing splints: **dynamic splints** and **static progressive splints.** Both types of splints affect

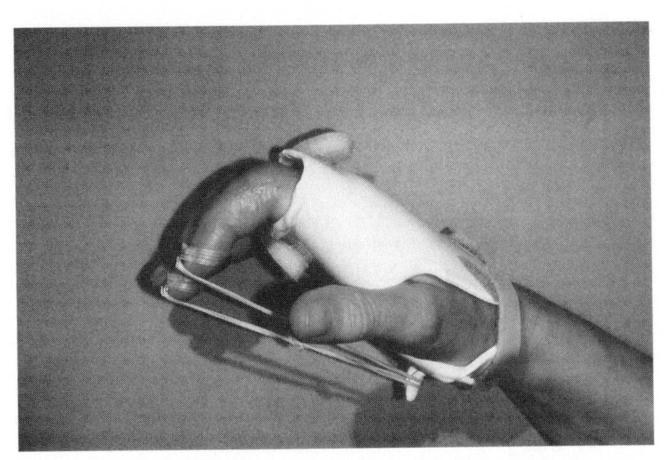

FIGURE 31–11. A dynamic splint that might be used to improve flexion of the PIP and DIP joints.

tissue by application of force through the use of an adjustable component part attached to a static splint base. Splint selection and design must be carefully matched to the state of tissue healing. A dynamic splint generally consists of a splint base with straps, an outrigger that properly aligns the force applied to the affected structures, finger loops or finger hooks to connect the force to the digit or joint, and a force coupler such as a rubber band (Fig. 31-11). Dynamic splints may be requested after surgical procedures such as tendon repairs or joint replacements. They are also used to improve grasp and function and to augment weak muscle function. For example, a wrist tenodesis splint may be appropriate for improving hand function for a quadriplegic client.

Static progressive splints are similar to dynamic splints, but the force application is constant, not dynamic (Fig. 31-12). The joint is positioned at its end range and held in that position for a prolonged period of time to encourage tissue growth and lengthening. The splint incorporates a component that allows slight increases in tension controlled by the client. Hook and loop tape or commercially available turn screw–type components attached to the splint base are adjusted to increase tension on the finger loops, resulting in a gradual increase in force application. These splints are most helpful when significant resistance is felt at the end range of the joint (Colditz, 1995).

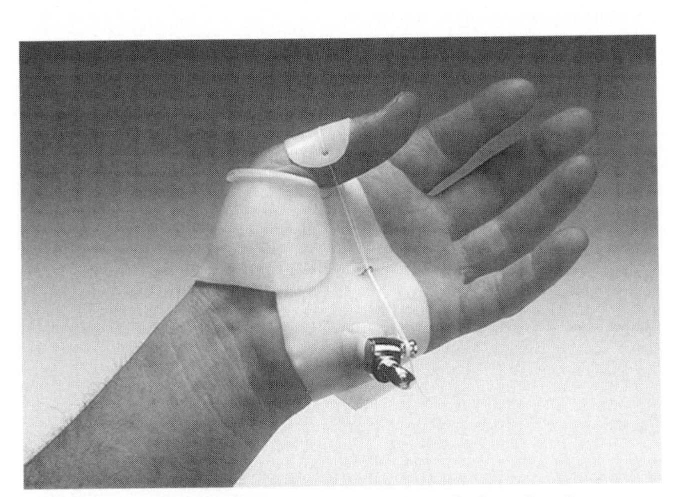

FIGURE 31–12. A static progressive splint designed to improve thumb MP range of motion. (Courtesy K. Schultz-Johnson, UE Tech, MERIT™, A trademark of UE Tech, Edwards, Colorado.)

For an occupational therapist to function in the specialty setting in which the use of dynamic and static progressive splinting is common, advanced training in design, fabrication, application, and modification of mobilizing splints is essential and beyond the scope of this chapter. Attending continuing education courses and working with the close supervision of an experienced therapist are the best methods of developing the skills necessary to determine and fabricate appropriate mobilization splints.

FABRICATING A THERMOPLASTIC STATIC SPLINT

Fabricating any splint is a multistep process that requires practice to become proficient. Making many splints for a colleague's hand or for your own nondominant hand (using a one-handed approach) is the most effective way to develop fabrication skills.

Choosing Splint Material

There are many high-quality low-temperature thermoplastic materials currently available, all of which share common characteristics. All thermoplastics become soft and pliable when heated in water as directed by the manufacturer. Splints made of low-temperature thermoplastic retain their shape when fully cooled; however, these splints lose their shape if left in hot cars or near heat sources, such as on radiators.

Understanding the properties of the various types of low-temperature splinting materials ensures a quality finished product (Breger-Lee & Buford, 1992). Low-temperature thermoplastic materials can be generally classified into two broad categories (Breger-Lee & Buford, 1992): those with a plastic base (e.g., Polyform) and those with a rubber base or rubber-like base (e.g., Orthoplast and Ezeform). Within these groups, there are important differences in how the materials should be handled to obtain a good result.

Plastic-based materials drape and shape easily when pliable. Because these materials stretch more easily than rubber-based materials, optimal application occurs when the material can be draped over the involved extremity. When using a plastic-based material, the client should be positioned so that the effect of gravity can assist with the fabrication process. Wraps should not be used to hold the material in place because unattractive demarcations result. When fabricating a splint that requires anatomical detail, such as matching the shape of a client's palmar arch, a plastic-based material is a good choice.

Rubber-based materials are particularly appropriate for large splints, because they are easier to control and less apt to overstretch. They are better than plastic based materials if the client is unable to position the extremity in a position that allows draping. It is possible to use an elastic wrap to hold rubber-based materials in place during the forming process without introducing unsightly marks on the splint. On the other hand, anatomical details will not be as evident because rubber materials are less malleable than plastic-based materials (Coppard & Lynn, 2001).

No thermoplastic materials should be overheated. Manufacturer's directions for proper heating are helpful, but if they are not available, most plastic-based materials will be ready to use after 30–45 sec of exposure to 120–170°F water (Breger-Lee & Buford, 1992). It is always better to underheat than to overheat splint materials, particularly plastic-based materials, because they will stretch and become difficult to control if heated too long. Overheating materials may also reduce durability and increase the possibility that the splint will break at stress points. Rubber-based materials tend to retain heat longer than plastic-based materials and can cause a superficial burn if applied when too hot. Use of a thermal barrier, such as a stockinette, and properly heating the material help protect the client. Note, too, that both rubber- and plastic-based materials are difficult to shape if inadequately heated. Practice is the best method for determining optimal management of thermoplastic materials.

Making a Splint

The process for making any static, static progressive, or dynamic splint begins with making a custom pattern and ends with applying straps to the finished product. Information on specific pattern designs and construction methods is available from the numerous books (Coppard & Lohman, 2001; McKee & Morgan, 1998) and continuing education courses.

BOX 31–5 DECIDING FACTORS FOR PRE-FORMED VERSUS CUSTOM-FABRICATED SPLINTS

- Does the practitioner have the skills necessary to custom fabricate a splint?
- Does client's anatomy allow use of a pre-formed splint or is a custom-fabricated splint mandated?
- Does the diagnosis allow use of a pre-formed splint or is a custom-fabricated splint mandated?
- Is there adequate time to custom fabricate a splint?
  - Is an appropriate fit achievable with custom fitting?
  - Can the splint be adapted in areas where adaptation is needed?
  - Are uninvolved joints free to move through full ROM?
  - Are involved joints adequately supported?
  - Are straps adequate to close the splint?
  - Do the splint edges meet appropriately? Is there a gap or do they overlap?
  - Is the splint the proper length?
- The wrist cock-up splint:
  - Does the distal edge angle match the transverse metacarpal arch angle?
  - Can the angle of the dorsal or volar wrist stay be correctly fitted to contact and stabilize the wrist?
  - Can the thumb move freely?
  - Is there pressure over the radial styloid?
- Which splint will the patient most readily accept?
- Will the client wear the splint full time, part time, at home, at work, at play?
- Which splint will be most appropriate to the expected duration of use?

PRE-FORMED SPLINTS

Since the mid-1980s, a wide variety of pre-formed and precut static and dynamic hand splints have become commercially available. It is now possible to substitute a well-designed off-the-shelf product for a custom-fabricated splint in many situations, if the pre-formed splint is chosen for appropriate reasons and the splint is correctly fitted to the client.

Selecting and custom-fitting pre-formed splints often becomes the responsibility of the occupational therapist. It is important to understand the features of particular products as well as the function of the splint within the total context of client rehabilitation and management. This knowledge, combined with an understanding of the client's occupational performance needs, allows the therapist to match effectively a particular problem to an appropriate product. Once selected, the splint is custom-fitted or formed. The therapist then provides instructions in relevant activities, exercises, and splint wearing schedules.

Fabricating Versus Using Pre-Formed Splints

The decision to use a pre-formed or a custom-fabricated splint is the result of a variety of factors, summarized in Box 31-5. The therapist must evaluate the client's needs specific to the impairment, accepted intervention protocols, and occupational performance concerns. Based on an understanding of these issues, the therapist determines the splint configuration indicated and then decides if there is a pre-formed splint to match those needs.

Custom-Fitting a Pre-Formed Splint

The adage "One size fits no one" might apply to pre-formed splints that are issued to a client without custom fitting. Common methods to custom-fit pre-formed splints are outlined in Figure 31-13.

Splint	Method	Example
Wrist cock up (Fabric with volar metal stay) 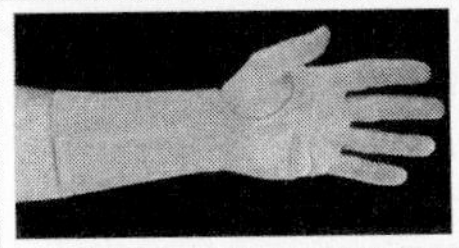	• Bend stay to fit wrist • Instruct client to attach distal straps, then slide hand into splint, then secure wrist strap to optimize fit	Diagnosis: Carpal tunnel syndrome Purpose: Night use Rationale: Adjust splint to contour to wrist; support in neutral wrist position
Wrist cock-up (Neoprene with dorsal thermoplastic stay) 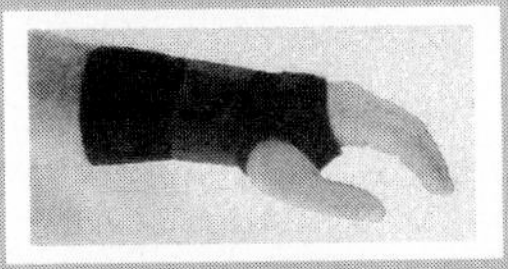	• Trim distal end and thumb-hole to maximize range of motion of uninvolved joints • Heat splint in convection oven and remold dorsal stay	Diagnosis: Wrist tenosynovitis Purpose: Wear at computer work station to train to maintain neutral wrist position Rationale: Adjust splint to allow free motion and stabilize wrist while working
Long thumb spica (Closed cell foam) 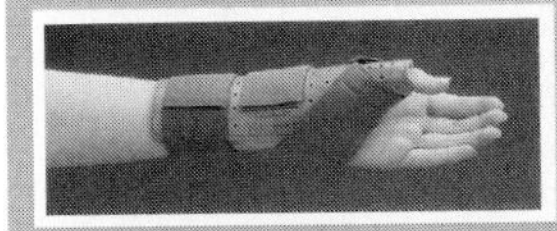	• Spot heat web area to avoid abrasion when using • Reheat and remold splint to improve contour and fit	Diagnosis: Dequervain's tendonitis Purpose: Prevent full thumb ROM Rationale: Adjust to eliminate pressure over radial styloid/first dorsal compartment
Resting (Thermoplastic) 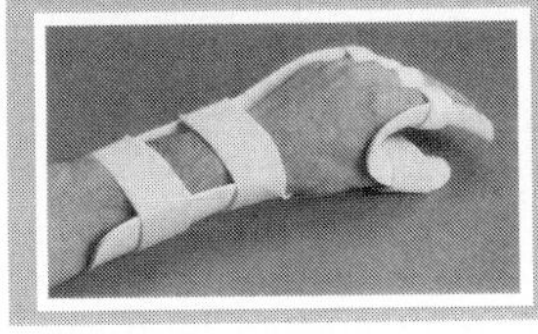	• Remold splint to reduce angle and properly seat wrist in splint • Adjust thumb angle to increase thumb extension	Diagnosis: CVA with returning tone Purpose: Protect position of function, decrease tone Rationale: To support wrist and thumb

FIGURE 31–13. Common methods for custom-fitting preformed splints. (Photos of wrist cock-up and resting splints courtesy of AliMed, Dedham, MA; photo of long thumb spica splint courtesy of the Rehabilitation Division of Smith+Nephew, Germantown, WI.)

INSTRUCTIONS FOR USE AND CARE OF A SPLINT

Clients must be instructed in the appropriate use and care of their splints. Instruction should include the purpose and benefits of the splint, safety precautions, and specific wearing schedules. The client or caregiver must be instructed to monitor the involved hand for edema or redness, because abrasion or unevenly distributed pressure could lead to tissue breakdown. If appropriate, frequency of splint removal and a home exercise program should be reviewed.

It is important to ask the client or caregiver to verbalize instructions and demonstrate correct application of the splint. Written instructions, including the name of the splint and specific directions, are a helpful reminder should the client or caregiver have questions later (Box 31-6).

Appropriate methods for cleaning and caring for the splint should be provided, as well-worn splints sometimes become unsightly and smelly. Most thermoplastic custom-fabricated splints can be washed with cool water and a soft toothbrush and common household cleaners, such as toothpaste. The client may be issued a cotton or polyester stockinette liner that is used to reduce sweating under the splint and improve comfort and compliance. Some types of stockinette can be washed; others are discarded after 1 or 2 day's use.

A splint used by a resident of an institutional setting, such as a nursing home or rehabilitation facility, should be marked with the client's name and room number and, possibly, right/left and top/bottom. This may be done with indelible ink or marked on a piece of tape that can be removed on discharge. If it appears that the client may have difficulty remembering the proper position of the splint or location of straps or if there are multiple caregivers responsible for applying the splint, a photograph of the splint helps ensure proper positioning and use. Asking the caregiver to demonstrate how to put on and remove the splint may be appropriate. In a situation in which the client is nonverbal, as with an infant or an aphasic client, caregivers should be advised to remove the splint and check the skin condition every half hour for at least the first day of use and regularly thereafter.

BOX 31–6 SAMPLE SPLINT INSTRUCTION SHEET

Client name: ____________ Date: ____________
At your health-care provider's request, you have been issued a ____________ splint

GENERAL INSTRUCTIONS

- Do not pull the straps too tightly or you may decrease circulation to your arm. If you see swelling between the straps or in your fingers, loosen the straps slightly and elevate your arm above heart level for ____________ minutes.
- Do not place your splint near anything hot or leave it in the sun or in your car. It may melt and lose its shape.
- Watch for any red spots on your skin and note any places that hurt that might be from the fit of the splint. If you have a problem with your splint, let us know, and we will adjust the splint.

WEARING SCHEDULE

____________ Full time; do not remove splint
____________ At night
____________ Day/Night: Remove splint to eat, bathe, when relaxing, when exercising (circle appropriate)
____________ Perform attached exercises ____________ times per day.

SPECIFIC PRECAUTIONS

CARE OF YOUR SPLINT

____________ Wash with cool water and common household cleansers. Rinse and dry thoroughly before reapplication.
____________ Stockinette may be washed by hand and air-dried
____________ Stockinette should be discarded after use
____________ Other
Therapist: ____________ Phone number: ____________

DOCUMENTATION

As with all services provided to clients, the therapist must carefully document the splinting process and outcome. Splint notes should include the following:

- Basic client information such as name, age, gender, and hand dominance.
- Confirmation of referral information that demonstrates knowledge of the diagnosis, splint purpose, and type of splint requested and provided.
- Relevant evaluation data that affected choice of splint design and materials.
- Modifications to the splint, and rationale for these (appropriate in follow-up notes).
- Wearing schedule.
- Instructions provided and to whom.

ETHICS NOTE 31–1

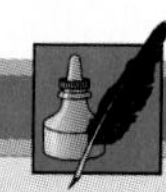

What Should a Practitioner Tell Clients about Colleagues?

Jackie is an occupational therapist with 12 years of practice experience. She is a certified hand therapist (CHT). She is aware that a new hand therapy clinic is opening in the area. They do not, at present, have any CHTs on staff. One of Jackie's clients tells her that his insurance will not longer cover Jackie's treatment. The insurance, however, will cover treatment at the new hand therapy clinic. Jackie's client asks for her opinion of the new clinic and the caliber of the staff.

QUESTIONS AND EXERCISES

1. **Is it legally and ethically appropriate to share your personal views about other professionals with a client? If so, under what circumstances?**
2. **What methods should a practitioner use to determine whether a professional colleague is competent?**
3. **Does advanced certification or credentialing ensure competence to practice? What are the limits to this interdependence?**

- Concerns about client understanding of the splint purpose, methods of use, care, and compliance.

Careful documentation of the splinting process enhances communication with other health-care providers, facilitates third-party reimbursement, helps track the efficacy of treatment, and protects the therapist in the unlikely situation of litigation.

CONCLUSION

The occupational therapist involved in splint fabrication and provision may choose from a wide variety of splint types, including custom-fabricated and commercially available static, static progressive, and dynamic splints. A splint may be used in many ways, with the ultimate goal of regaining function and improving occupational performance. The therapist must integrate the functional purpose of the splint with issues of wound healing, diagnosis-related protocols, patient compliance and acceptance, and the effect of the splint on functional performance.

References

Allman, R. M., Goode, P. S., Burst, N., Bartolucci, A. A., & Thomas, D. R. (1999). Pressure ulcers, hospital complications, and disease severity: impact on hospital costs and length of stay. *Advances in Wound Care, 12*(1), 22–30.

American Occupational Therapy Association [AOTA]. (1995). Assessment of assistive technology. *Technology Special Interest Section Newsletter*, 5, 1, 2.

American Occupational Therapy Association [AOTA]. (1996). *Assistive technology and occupational therapy: A link to function* [Self-Paced Clinical Course]. Rockville, MD: Author.

American Speech-Language-Hearing Association [ASHA]. (1989). Report: Competencies for speech-language pathologists providing services in augmentative communication. *American Speech-Language-Hearing Association, 31*, 107–110

American Speech-Language-Hearing Association. [ASHA]. (1991). Report: Augmentative and alternative communication. *American Speech-Language-Hearing Association, 33*(4, Suppl. 5), 9–12.

Americans with Disabilities Act. (1990). Public Law 101-336, 42, U.S.C. 12101.

Anderson, K., Anderson, L., & Glanze, W. (Eds.). (1998). *Mosby's medical, nursing and allied health dictionary* (5th ed.). St. Louis: Mosby.

Angelo, J., & Smith, R. O. (1989). The critical role of occupational therapy in augmentative communication services. In American Occupational Therapy Association (Ed.). *Technology Review '89: Perspectives on occupational therapy practice* (pp. 49–54) Rockville, MD: Editor.

Anson, D. (1997). *Alternative computer access: A guide to selection*. Philadelphia: Davis.

Axelson, P., & Chesney, D. (1995). Potential hazards of wheelchair lapbelts. In *Proceedings of the Rehabilitation Engineering and Assistive Technology Society of North America Conference* (pp. 314–316). Arlington, VA: Resna Press.

Bain, B. K. (1996). Lesson 7: Environmental controls and robots. In J. Hammel (Ed.). *Technology and occupational therapy: A link to function* (pp. 1–44). Bethesda, MD: American Occupational Therapy Association.

Bain, B. K. (1997). *Evaluation*. In B. K. Bain & D. Leger (Eds.). *Assistive technology: An interdisciplinary approach* (pp. 17–35). New York: Churchill Livingstone.

Bain, B., DiSalvi, M., Gold, J., Kollodge, B., & Schein, R. (1991, June). *Environmental control systems: Assessment, selection, and training*. Paper presented at the American Occupational Therapy Association annual conference, Cincinnati.

Bain, B., DiSalvi, M., Gold, J., Kollodge, B., & Schein, R. (1993). Technology. In H. Hopkins & H. Smith, (Eds.). *Willard and Spackman's occupational therapy* (9th ed., pp. 498–513). Philadelphia: Lippincott.

Barnes, K. H., (1991). Training young children for powered mobility. *Developmental Disabilities Special Interest Section Newsletter, 14*, 1–2.

Batavia, A., & Hammer, G. (1990). Toward the development of consumer-based criteria for the evaluation of consumer-based criteria for the evaluation of assistive devices. *Journal of Rehabilitation Research and Development, 27*, 425–435.

Bell-Krotoski, J. (1995). Plaster cylinder casting for contractures of the interphalangeal joints. In J. Hunter, E. Mackin, & A. Callahan (Eds.). *Rehabilitation of the hand: Surgery and therapy* (4th ed., pp.1609–1616). St. Louis: Mosby.

Boninger, M. L., Baldwin, M., Cooper, R. A., Koontz, A., & Chan, L. (2000). Manual wheelchair pushrim biomechanics and axle position. *Archives of Physical Medicine and Rehabilitation, 81*(5), 608–613.

Boninger, M. L., Cooper, R. A., Baldwin, M. A., Shimada, S. D., & Koontz, A. (1999). Wheelchair pushrim kinetics: Body weight and median nerve function. *Archives of Physical Medicine & Rehabilitation*, 80(8), 910–915.

Borden, P., Lubich, J., & Vanderheiden, G. (1996). *Trace resource book: 1996–97 edition*. Madison, WI: Trace Research and Development Center

Brand, P. (1985). *Clinical biomechanics of the hand*. St. Louis: Mosby.

Breger-Lee, D., & Buford, W. (1992). Properties of thermoplastic splinting materials. *Journal of Hand Therapy*, 5(4), 202–211.

Brienza, D. M., Karg, P. E., Geyer, M. J., Kelsey, S., & Trefler, E. (2001). Relationship between pressure ulcer incidents and buttock seat cushion interface pressure in at-risk elderly wheelchair users. *Archives of Physical Medicine and Rehabilitation, 82*(4), 529–533.

Buning, M. E., Angelo, J. A., & Schmeler, M. R. (2001). The transition to powered mobility and occupational performance: A pilot study. *American Journal of Occupational Therapy*, 55(4), 339–344.

Butler, C. (Ed.). (1986a). *Effects of powered mobility on self-initiated behaviors of two and three-year old children with neuromuscular skeletal disorders*. Washington, DC: Rehabilitation Engineering and Assistive Technology Society of North America.

Butler, C. (1986b) Effects of powered mobility on self-initiated behaviors of very young children with locomotor disability. *Developmental Medicine and Child Neurology 28*, 325–332.

Church, C., & Glennen, S. (1992). *The handbook of assistive technology*. San Diego: Singular.

Colditz, J. (1995). Therapist's management of the stiff hand. In J. Hunter, E. Mackin, & A. Callahan (Eds.). *Rehabilitation of the hand: Surgery and therapy* (4th ed., pp. 1141–1159). St. Louis: Mosby.

Conine, T. A., Herschler, C., Daechsel, D., Peel, C., & Pearson, A. (1994). Pressure ulcer prophylaxis in elderly patients using polyurethane foam or Jay wheelchair cushions. *International Journal of Rehabilitation Research, 17*(2), 123–137.

Cook, A., & Hussey, S. (1995). *Assistive technologies: Principles and practice*. New York: Mosby.

Cooper, R. A., Boninger, M. L., & Rentschler, A. (1999). Evaluation of selected ultralight manual wheelchairs using ANSI/RESNA standards. *Archives of Physical Medicine and Rehabilitation*, 80(4), 462–467.

Cooper, R. A., Gonzalez, J., Lawrence, B., Rentschler, A., Boninger, M. L., & VanSickle, D. P. (1997). Performance of selected lightweight wheelchairs on ANSI/RESNA tests. *Archives of Physical Medicine and Rehabilitation, 78*(10), 1138–1144.

Coppard, B. (2001a). Anatomical and biomechanical principles of splinting. In B. Coppard & H. Lohman (Eds.). *Introduction to splinting: A critical-thinking and problem-solving approach* (2nd ed., pp. 34–72). St. Louis: Mosby.

Coppard, B. (2001b). Hand immobilization splints. In B. Coppard & H. Lohman (Eds.). *Introduction to splinting: A critical-thinking and problem-solving approach* (2nd ed., pp. 185–218). St. Louis: Mosby.

Coppard, B., &, Lohman, H. (Eds.). (2001). *Introduction to splinting: A critical-thinking and problem-solving approach* (2nd ed.). St. Louis: Mosby.

DiGiovine, M. M., Cooper, R. A., Boninger, M. L., Lawrence, B. M., VanSickle, D. P., & Rentschler, A. J. (2000). User assessment of manual wheelchair ride comfort and ergonomics. *Archives of Physical Medicine and Rehabilitation, 81*(4), 490–494.

Digman, G. H. (1996) Lesson 4. In J. Hammel (Ed). *Technology and Occupational Therapy: a link to function*, (pp 1–47) Bethesda, MD: American Occupational Association.

Fess, E., & Kiel, J. (1998). Neuromuscular treatment: Upper extremity splinting. In M. Neistadt & E. Crepeau, E. (Eds.). *Willard and Spackman's occupational therapy* (9th ed., pp. 406–421).
Philadelphia: Lippincott.

Fess, E., &, Philips, C. (1987). *Hand splinting principles and methods*. St. Louis: Mosby.

Fishman, I. (1987). *Electronic communication aids*. Boston: College-Hill Press.

Flippo, K., Inge, K., & Barcus, J. (1995). *Assistive technology: A resource for school, work, and community*. Baltimore: Brookes.

Fraser, B. A., Bryen, D., & Morano, C. K. (1995). Development of a physical characteristics assessment (PCA): A checklist for determining appropriate computer access for individuals with cerebral palsy. *Assistive Technology, 7*, 26–33.

Fraser, B. A., McGregor, G., Arango, G. A., & Kangas, K. (1995). *Physical characteristics assessment: Computer access for individuals with cerebral palsy*. Poster Presentation at annual meeting of ISAAC, Philadelphia.

Freeman, S., Brushingham, D., & Field, W. (1992). Selecting mobility aids for farmers and ranchers with physical disabilities. *Technology and Disability, 4*, 63–67.

Furamaso, J. (Ed.). (1997). *Pediatric powered mobility: Developmental perspectives technical issues clinical approaches*. Arlington, VA: Rehabilitation Engineering and Assistive Technology Society of North America.

Galvin, J., & Scherer, M. (1996). *Evaluating, selecting and using appropriate assistive technology*. Gaithersburg, MD: Aspen.

Hammel, J. (Ed.). (1995) *Assistive technology competencies for occupational therapy practice*. Rockville, MD: American Occupational Therapy Association.

Hardy, M. (1989). The biology of scar formation. *Physical Therapy, 69*, 1014–1024.

Health Care Finance Administration and United HealthCare. (1998). Medicare supplier *Manual: Region A DMERC* (rev. no. 008). Wilkes Barre, PA: United HealthCare Insurance.

Hopkins, H. L., & Smith, H. D. (Eds.). (1983) *Willard and Spackman's occupational therapy* (6th ed.). Philadelphia: Lippincott.

Jaffe, K. (Ed.). (1987). *Childhood powered mobility: Developmental technical, and clinical perspectives*. Washington, DC: Rehabilitation Engineering and Assistive Technology Society of North America.

Joe, B. E. (1990). International symposium focuses on emergency response devices. *Occupational Therapy Week, 4*, 45.

Kangas , K., (1993). *Assessment and treatment strategies for pediatric power mobility*. Paper presented at the Ninth International Seating Symposium, Memphis, TN.

Kollodge, B. (1997). Specialized computer applications. In B.K. Bain & D. Leger (Eds.) *Assistive technology: An interdisciplinary approach* (pp. 149–165). New York: Churchill Livingstone.

Kreutz, D. (1998). Characteristics of seating and positioning technologies. *Fundamentals in assistive technology* (2nd ed., pp. 1–20). Arlington, VA: Rehabilitation Engineering and Assistive Technology Society of North America.

Lange, M. (1996). Selecting environmental controls. In J. Hammel (Ed.). *Assistive technology and occupational therapy: A link to function* (pp. 35–39). Bethesda, MD: American Occupational Therapy Association.

Lang, M. (2001, Jan) Windows accessibility features, OT Practice.

Lee, K., & Thomas, D. (1990). *Control of computer-based technology for people with physical disabilities*. Toronto, ON, Canada: Toronto Press.

Malick, M. (1974). *Manual on dynamic hand splinting with thermoplastic materials*. Pittsburgh: Harmarville Rehabilitation Center.

Mann, W. C., & Lane, J. P. (1995). *Assistive technology for persons with disabilities*. Bethesda, MD: American Occupational Therapy Association.

McKee, P., &, Morgan, L. (1998). *Orthotics in rehabilitation: splinting the hand and body*. Philadelphia: Davis.

Mosey, A. C. (1986). *Psychosocial components of occupational therapy*. New York: Raven.

Nead, R. W. (1997). Behind-the-wheel driver training. In B.K. Bain & D. Leger (Eds). *Assistive technology: An interdisciplinary approach* (pp. 209–223). New York: Churchill Livingstone.

O'Toole, M. (Ed.). (1997). *Miller and Keane encyclopedia and dictionary of medical nursing and allied health* (6th ed.). Philadelphia: Saunders.

Petra, E. (1996). *The "director": Its effectiveness in reducing need for attendant care and increasing independent control of home appliances in adults with developmental disabilities*. Unpublished masters thesis, New York University.

Phillips, B. (1992). Technology abandonment from the consumer point of view. *NARIC Quarterly, 3*, 2–3.

Phillips, B., & Zhao, H. (1993). Predictors of assistive technology abandonment. Assistive technology. *Rehabilitation Engineering and Assistive Technology Society of North America, 5*, 36–45.

Radabough, M. P. (1990, June). Keynote address presented at the Rehabilitation Engineering and Assistive Technology Society of North America Conference, Washington, DC.

Ramsey, C., (1999). Power mobility access methods. AOTA *Technology Special Interest Section Quarterly, 9*, 1–3.

Schultz-Johnson, K. (1996). Splinting the wrist. *Journal of Hand Therapy*, 9(2), 165–176.

Smith, K. (1995). Wound care for the hand patient. In J. Hunter, E. Mackin, & A. Callahan (Eds.). *Rehabilitation of the hand: Surgery and therapy* (4th ed., pp. 237–250). St. Louis: Mosby.

Smith, R. (1990). *Administration and scoring manual: OT Fact*. Rockville, MD: American Occupational Therapy Association.

Snell, M. A. (1999, June). Guidelines for safely transporting wheelchair users. *OT Practice*, 35–38.

Sprigle, S., & Sposato, B. (1997). Physiologic effects and design considerations of tilt and recline wheelchairs. *Orthopedic Physical Therapy Clinics of North America*, 6(1), 99–122.

Strickland, J. W. (1987) Biological basis for hand splinting. In E. E. Fess & C. A. Phillips (Eds.). *Hand splinting: Principles and methods* (2nd ed., pp. 43–70). St. Louis: Mosby.

Struck, M. (1995). Augmentative and alternative communication and computer access. In P. Allen & J. Case-Smith (Eds.). *Occupational therapy for children* (3rd ed., pp. 545–561). St. Louis: Mosby.

Struck, M., & Corfman, S. K. (1994). Strategies for integration of adapted computer use. *AOTA School System Special Interest Section Newsletter, 1*(3), 3–4.

Taylor, S. J. (1995). Powered mobility evaluations and technology: *Journal of Spinal Cord Injury Rehabilitation, 1*, 22–36.

Technology Related Assistance for Individuals with Disabilities Act [TRAIDA]. (1988,1994). 29 U.S.C. 2202 (2) and (3).

Trefler, E., Kozole, K., & Snell, E. (Eds.). (1986). *Selected readings on powered mobility for children and adults with severe physical disabilities*. Washington, DC: Rehabilitation Engineering and Assistive Technology Society of North America.

Tribuzi, S. (1995). Serial plaster splinting. In J. Hunter, E. Mackin, & A. Callahan (Eds.). *Rehabilitation of the hand: Surgery and therapy* (4th ed., pp. 1599–1608) St. Louis: Mosby.

Trombley, K. A., & Fadonski, M. V. (Eds.). (2001). *Occupational therapy for physical dysfunction* (5th ed.). Philadelphia: Lippincott, Williams & Wilkins.

Verburg, G. (1987). Predictors of successful powered mobility control. In Jaffee (Ed.). *Childhood powered mobility: Developmental, technical and clinical perspectives. Proceedings of the RESNA conference* (pp. 10–104). Washington, DC: Rehabilitation Engineering and Assistive Technology Society of North America.

Warren, C. G. (1990). Powered mobility and its implications. In S. P. Todd (Ed.). *Choosing a wheelchair system* (pp. 74–85). Washington DC: Veterans Health Services and Research Administration.

Webster, J. G., Cook, A. M., Tompkins, W. J., & Vanderheiden, G. C. (Eds.). (1985). *Electronic devices for rehabilitation*. New York: Wiley.

Williams, B. W., Stemach, G., Wolfe, S., & Stanger, C. (1993). *Lifespace access profile: Assistive technology planning for individuals with severe or multiple disabilities*. Sebastopol, CA: Authors.

Wright, C., & Nomura, M. (1990). *From toys to computers: Access for the physically disabled child* (2nd ed.). San Jose, CA: Authors.

CASE ANALYSIS: UNIT VIII

MAUREEN E. NEISTADT AND BARBARA A. BOYT SCHELL

In Chapter 4, you met Mary Feldhaus-Weber and her occupational therapist, Anna Deane Scott. Anna Deane's intervention was extremely effective in helping Mary become more independent in her valued day-to-day activities. Mary said, "In the year that I worked with her I could see small changes in my life and as I got greater control over the details of my life again, the person who I had been started to reemerge." Let's look at why this intervention program was so effective in light of what you have read in this unit.

First of all, Anna Deane directed intervention toward occupational goals that Mary thought were important. Mary said, "Anna Deane felt her role was not to tell me what to do, but to work with me, to empower me. She asked me constantly what was important to me. What did I think of something? What did I want to do? And she LISTENED to me." This is a good example of what being client-centered looks like in practice. It also shows how important Anna Deane's therapeutic use of self was in building an alliance with Mary.

Anna Deane chose to work directly on the occupational performance activities that Mary identified as priorities. Though Mary had significant cognitive problems, Anna Deane did not offer Mary remedial skills for her impairments. One reason for this was that Mary was experiencing such serious memory problems; it was unlikely she would be able to transfer learning from remedial drills to real-life activities. Second, remedial drills—such as practicing recalling lists of words to improve memory—would have reminded Mary of her sense of loss. Third, and most important, Mary was already at home, and often unsafe because of her occupational performance problems. Focusing directly on Mary's occupational performance activities was the quickest way to improve her safety. Anna Deane was concerned about Mary's safety with:

- Personal care, especially in the bathroom.
- Kitchen activities.
- Medication management.
- Telephone use.
- Setting of household temperature controls.
- Community activities, such as grocery shopping.

For Mary's most dangerous activities, Anna Deane adapted the task and the environments. For example, Mary reports, "I was afraid of falling in the shower when I was getting spacey from a seizure, so we got a shower chair and a metal bar on the wall and rubber rugs inside the tub and outside the tub. . . . I was also afraid of burning myself on the flames of my gas stove if I was feeling confused, so we got a large electric hot plate and I could heat something up without being afraid of lighting myself or my clothes on fire." In both of these examples, the environment was changed to compensate for Mary's impairments and increase her safety.

Other times, Anna Deane taught Mary a strategy for particular tasks, such as unlocking her front doors.

> *Anna Deane watched me try to get into the house and said she understood what the problem was. She said when I couldn't get in the outside door with one key, that I should try the other key. It had not occurred to me to try to the other key. I would stand endlessly with the wrong key doing it over and over again, but when I had this new strategy, it freed me to get into my own house, and each time I opened the door myself it was such a victory. And I began to feel hope for myself.*

In this case, Mary learned a new approach to the task of unlocking her front doors. Sometimes, for extremely difficult tasks, such as grocery shopping, the strategy was for Mary to have someone do the task for her. In working with Mary, Anna Deane observed and analyzed Mary's occupational activity demands. In the front door example, Mary says, "Anna Deane watched me try to get into the house." Anna Deane was able to hypothesize what Mary's difficulty with this task was by watching how she did the task. By Mary's account, she "would stand endlessly with the wrong key, doing it over and over again." This behavior of repeating the same thing over and over again is called perseveration. Anna Deane noted this behavior and suggested a strategy to get around it: "She said when I couldn't get in the outside door with one key, that I should try the other key." This strategy worked; therefore, it was unnecessary to try to modify the front door system of Mary's apartment.

By studying the neuropsychology test results and keeping careful track of which strategies worked and which did not, Anna Deane discerned the kind of cuing Mary needed to learn. Mary says, "Anna Deane and I discovered that while it was impossible for me to just follow or understand verbal directions, if I could also watch someone do a task, listen to the directions, even place my hands on the things at the same time, I could after a number of tries, do it again myself." Once Anna Deane knew that this combination of demonstration with verbal explanation and hand-over-hand practice worked for Mary, she was able to use it for all the activities Mary wanted to master. Throughout the intervention process, Mary and Anna Deane worked together to discover and build on Mary's strengths. The interweaving of intervention and evaluation is characteristic of occupational therapy.

The empowerment and careful trial-and-error experimentation of this intervention process are central components of all effective intervention. Scientific evidence can assist clients and therapists to choose options that are likely to be effective. However, practitioners need to understand that intervention is not a series of unending successes, but a series of successes and failures that collectively move clients toward their goals.

UNIT *nine*

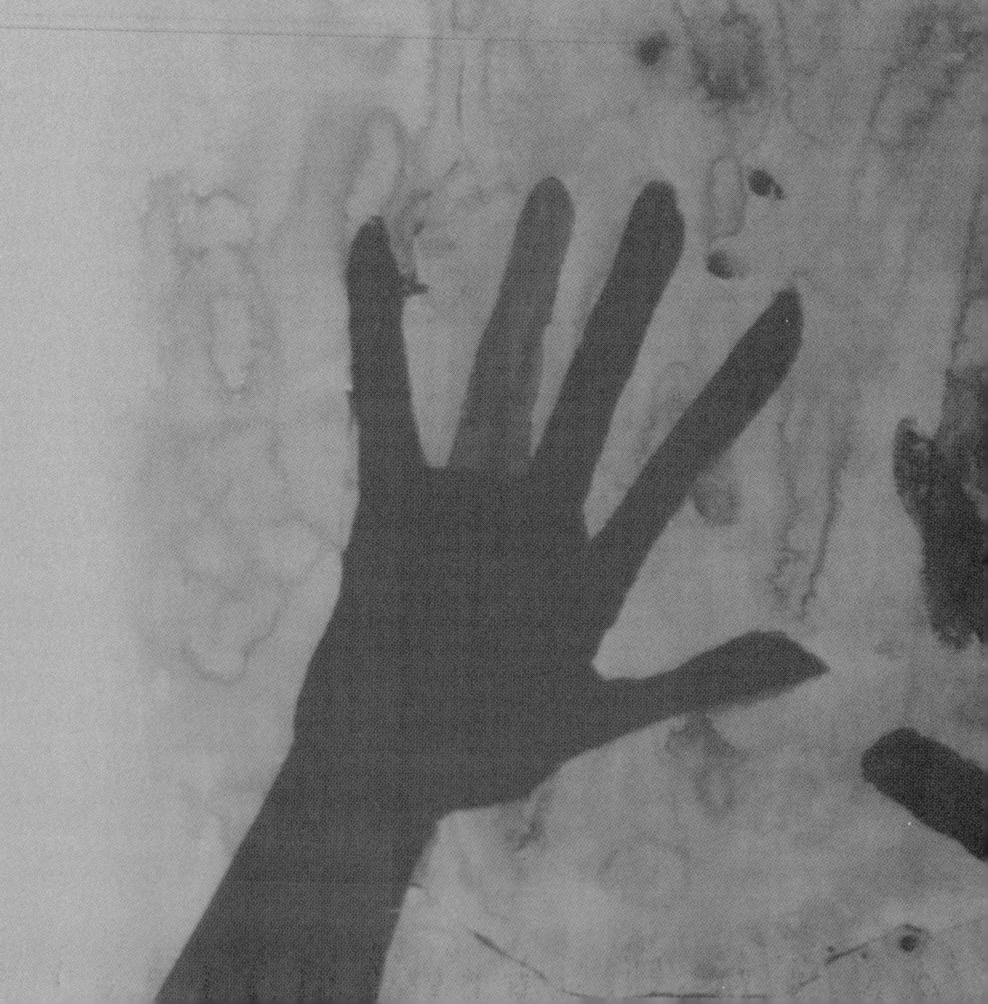

Diagnostic Considerations for Infants, Children, and Adolescents

Learning Objectives

After completing this unit, readers will be able to:

- Describe the population served by occupational therapy practitioners working with infants, children, and adolescents.
- Summarize key U.S. legislative acts guiding occupational therapy practice with infants, children, and adolescents.
- Define common diagnostic conditions of infants, children, and adolescents receiving occupational therapy and the effect of these conditions on occupational performance:
  - Neurological dysfunction (cerebral palsy, learning and attention disorders, developmental disabilities, and pervasive developmental disorders, spinal cord injury, and traumatic brain injury)
  - Cardiopulmonary dysfunction (asthma, cystic fibrosis, and bronchopulmonary dysplasia)
  - HIV and AIDS
  - Psychosocial dysfunction (attention deficit hyperactivity disorder)
  - Conduct disorders, mood disorders, pervasive developmental disorders
  - Child abuse and neglect
- Define and explain evaluation and intervention strategies for infants, children, and adolescents receiving occupational therapy intervention.

Occupational therapy services for infants, children, and adolescents spans the full spectrum of care from medically focused acute care for children with AIDS, cystic fibrosis, and other conditions to community-based services in schools, homes, and community recreation facilities. Legislation has stimulated the expansion of services for infants, children, and adolescents to include early intervention programs, equal opportunity, and inclusion for all children and adolescents in public school settings; modifying environments to facilitate performance; and working with systems, administrators, and legislators to promote change. The influence of families on development is acknowledged in the emphasis on family-centered care in providing services. Family-centered care involves meeting family concerns, building on family strengths, respecting family diversity and cultural backgrounds, sharing information, promoting partnerships and collaboration, and encouraging social support.

Unit IX builds on previous units in the book that provided information about the people who seek occupational therapy, occupational therapy practitioners, the conceptual bases for practice, and the principles of occupational therapy evaluation and intervention. This unit begins with description of a diverse group of infants, children, and adolescents, all of whom may benefit from occupational therapy intervention. The story of Patrice, a 9-year-old boy who sustained a closed head injury, is introduced. Chapters 33 through 37 focus on specific conditions and evaluation and intervention strategies commonly used by practitioners working with infants, children, and adolescents. The unit closes with an analysis of Patrice's condition and the intervention plan developed by the interdisciplinary educational team at his school. Appendix A summarizes assessments commonly used by occupational therapists working with infants, children, and adolescents. (Note: Words in **bold** type are defined in the Glossary.)

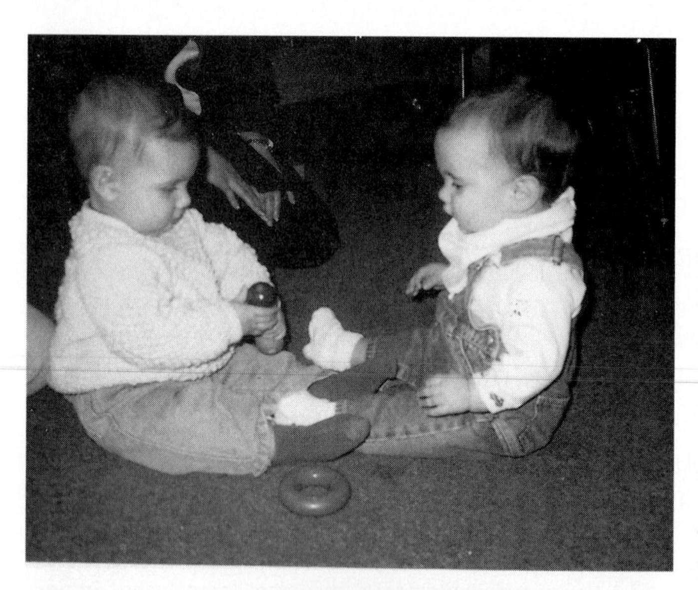

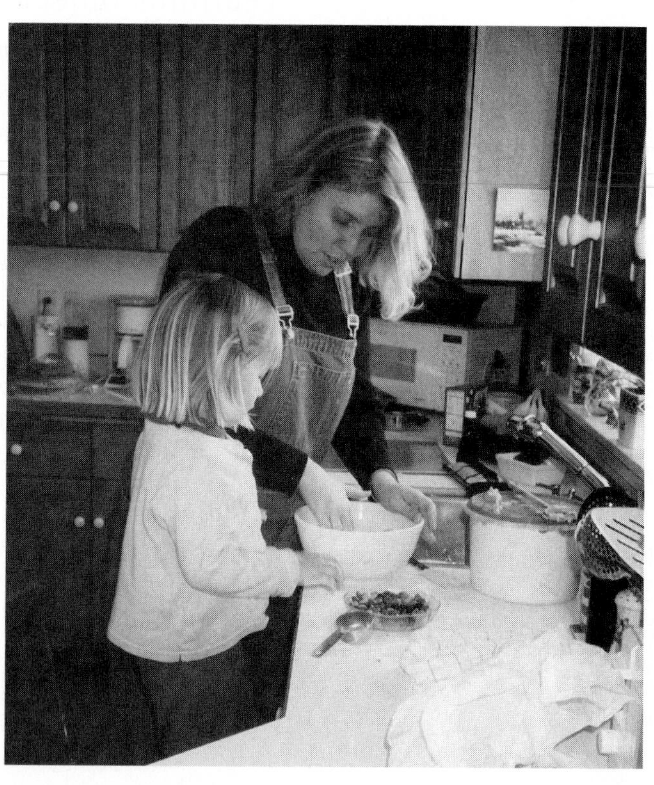

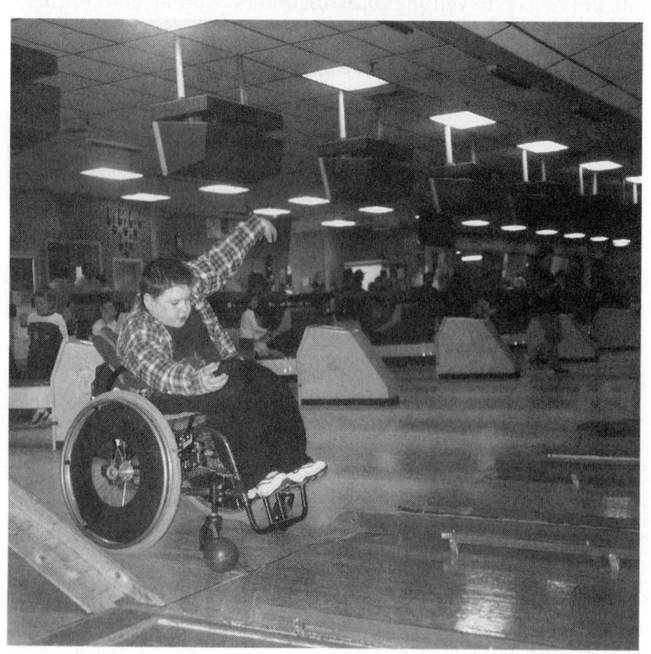

Occupational therapy practitioners promote the development of occupational performance in infants, children, and adolescents. (*top*) Two babies are playing with rings (Photo courtesy of Olga Baloueff, Arlington, MA). (*middle*) A woman and child are cooking together (Photo courtesy of Elizabeth Crepeau, Newmarket, NH). (*bottom*) A boy in a wheelchair is bowling (Photo courtesy of Stacey Lehrer, Durham, NH).

CHAPTER 32

INTRODUCTION TO THE INFANT, CHILD AND ADOLESCENT POPULATION

OLGA BALOUEFF and ELLEN S. COHN

- Sashsa was born 6 weeks early and spent the first 2 months of her life living in an intensive care nursery hooked up to monitors.
- Lucille is a 3-year-old who enjoys teasing her younger brother and carving pumpkins with her father. She uses a wheelchair for mobility because she has cerebral palsy characterized by spastic quadriplegia.
- Simon, only 4 years old and living in a rural community with his aunt and two older sisters, spends his time watching TV and playing video games. He does not engage in physical activity because he is extremely overweight. Other children make fun of him, and he is at risk for premature cardiovascular disease.
- Isaac, age 8, hopes to be a professional hockey player someday and is happiest when he can go to the ice rink to practice power drills. School is quite challenging for him because he has attention deficit hyperactivity disorder and finds it difficult to avoid blurting out all his creative ideas and answers to his teacher's questions.
- Joseph lives with his mother, maternal grandmother, aunt, uncle, and two cousins in a housing project in a busy city. He was diagnosed with AIDS 4 years ago and does not want the kids at school to know, for fear of rejection. He frequently visits the nurse to take midday naps.
- Nicole is a fifth grader at the Moon Hill Elementary School. A full-time aide spends the school day with Nicole because she has spinal bifida and is unable to take care of her toileting and hygiene needs independently. She is thinking about going to middle school next year and expressed a desire to go to school without an aide.
- Adrienne, Jenny, and Jessica are seventh graders at the Clarke Middle School. They sling their backpacks over one shoulder and usually carry 1-in. binders, science, math, history, and grammar textbooks—which together weigh about 25 lb.
- Chris, Don, and Bob attend the local middle school, have few friends, and often sit alone during lunchtime

at school. All three boys live with single parents whose histories include maltreatment as children and drug abuse; they are now living in poverty.

- Michael, a 19-year-old, received special education services throughout his public school career. His education focused on basic academics, some school- and home-based training in independent-living activities, and vocational preparation that included community-based instruction. Michael has moderate mental retardation and hopes to work in a local restaurant after graduating from high school.

These diverse groups of infants, children, and adolescents have something in common: They can all benefit from occupational therapy services. The overarching goal of occupational therapy is to facilitate overall well-being and quality of life by supporting people's ability to engage in important and meaningful occupations (American Occupational Therapy Association—[AOTA], in press). Services for individuals from birth to 21 years old are provided in a range of settings, from hospitals and clinics to school systems and community agencies (e.g., early childhood programs, after-school programs, homeless shelters, and home settings). Within these settings, services may include direct intervention focused on changing the biological, physiological, psychological, or neurological processes of the infant, child, or adolescent. Intervention may also include teaching clients news skills, habits, or behaviors to enable their participation in relevant contexts. Teaching or consulting with the child's caregivers or other adults who are with the child on a daily basis is an essential component of intervention with this age group. Sometimes intervention focuses on compensation, adaptation, or changing the context, and the practitioner may suggest adapting the task requirements, using adaptive equipment, or using assistive technology (Hanft & Pilkington, 2000).

Disability prevention, education, and health promotion designed to help people avoid the onset of unhealthy conditions, diseases, or injuries are essential for this developing age group (American Occupational Therapy Association [AOTA], 2001). For example, to prevent back injuries to the middle school girls with the heavy backpacks described above, occupational therapy practitioners may educate the girls about the proper ways to load and wear a backpack. Practitioners may help Simon, the 4-year-old who is obese, engage in physically demanding activities to strengthen his cardiovascular capacity and reduce his weight. Many of these services are provided through consultation to clients, families, care providers, teachers, other health professionals, organizations, communities, and government policy makers (Moyers, 1999).

Since the 1980s, occupational therapy services for infants, children, and adolescents have grown in size and complexity. More than one third of occupational therapy practitioners in the United States work with this age group and, of them, more than half practice in schools (AOTA, 2001; Rainville, Cermak, & Murray, 1996). This chapter focuses on four themes common to all areas of occupational therapy intervention with infants, children, and adolescents:

- Promoting participation in desired activities and occupations.
- Understanding U.S. legislation related to services for this age group.
- Providing **family-centered** intervention that honors the dynamic family system.
- Providing **evidence-based** intervention that "integrates individual clinical expertise with the best available external clinical evidence from systematic research" (Sackett, Richardson, Rosenberg, & Haynes, 1997, p. 2).

PROMOTING SOCIAL PARTICIPATION

As therapists' understanding of disability has shifted from a medical model focused on illness, physical incapacitation, and symptoms to a social model focused on access and participation in activity, there is increasing recognition that participation in daily activities is vital to children's development. Acknowledging that disability is a social process, the World Health Organization (2001) defined participation for people of all ages as "the nature and the extent of a person's involvement in life situations." Coster (1998) offered a view of social participation specific to children: "The extent to which a child is able to orchestrate engagement or participation in occupations in a given context that is positive (which for a developing child would often include growth enhancing), personally satisfying, and acceptable to the adults in society who are responsible for children" (p. 341). Law and Dunn (1993) provided a contextual view of social participation by proposing that the physical environment, attitudes of the society, and policies can either facilitate or act as barriers to social participation. Social participation enables children to grow and develop; to understand the expectations of society; and to gain the skills needed to be included in their homes, schools, and communities. Infants, children, and adolescents with disabilities are at risk for lower participation in daily activities; and as they grow, they may be at increased risk for decreased participation in adult occupations (Brown & Gordon, 1987).

In the social model of disability, the nature and the extent of participation is likely to vary as a function of the interactive process among the environment, the occupation, and personal factors, including—but not limited to—the nature and severity of the individual's disability. Thus occupational therapy interventions are based on determining whether limits in social participation relate to the client's person factors, the demands of the occupation, or the external factors in the environment.

UNDERSTANDING FEDERAL LEGISLATION RELATED TO INFANTS, CHILDREN, AND ADOLESCENTS

In the United States, federal legislation has greatly influenced the provision of health care, education, and social services for children and adolescents. The first of such laws, the Sheppard-Towner Act (a plan for the "public protection of maternity and infancy") was written in 1921 (Meisels & Shonkoff, 2000). Since then, numerous legislative policies have been enacted to support the provision and delivery of comprehensive services to children and their families.

In 1975, the Education of the Handicapped Act (EHA; PL 94-142) revolutionized the educational system by ruling that no child (aged 5–21) with a disability could be excluded from public education. The EHA required that education be individualized and achieved through an **individualized education program** (IEP) in the least restrictive environment (LRE) (Mellard, 2000). Multidisciplinary evaluation and intervention to support the children's level of educational performance opened opportunities for occupational therapy practitioners to work in the school system, supporting the inclusion of students with disabilities into the general curriculum (Mellard, 2000).

Part B of the Education of the Handicapped Amendments of 1986 (PL 99-457) extended educational services to include children from the ages of 3 to 5. Part H of the 1986 law provided financial incentives to the states to develop and provide family-focused early intervention services for children with, or at risk for, developmental deviations. To ensure the parents' central role in the planning and administration of their child's program of services, the law requires the development of a family-centered service plan called the **individualized family service plan** (IFSP) (Mellard, 2000). Since the passage of these two pioneering laws, new laws and their subsequent reauthorizations have been enacted. The most recent, the Individuals with Disabilities Education Act (IDEA) Amendments of 1997 (PL 105-17), provides a concept of service continuum for infants, children, and youths with disabilities: Part B provides guidelines for educational services for children aged 3–21, and Part C provides guidelines for early intervention for infants and toddlers (Maruyama, Chandler, Clark, West, Lawlor, & Jackson, 1999). The IDEA amendment further specifies that all special education students 14 years of age and older must have individualized transition plans that include specific goals to facilitate their success as adults. The focus of transition services on helping students with disabilities acquire essential skills needed for meaningful and productive adult lives is consistent with occupational therapy's focus on promoting social participation and overall well-being.

ETHICAL NOTE 32–1

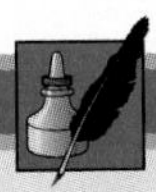

Is Intervention a Right or a Privilege?

The Lopes family lives in a rural area. Their 3-year-old daughter, Maria, has severe athetosis with quadriplegic involvement. The parents want her to receive occupational, physical, and speech therapy in their home. The local school administrator says that the school cannot afford to provide early intervention in the home. The best that the school district can offer is to provide therapy in a school that is 70 miles from the Lopes' home.

QUESTIONS AND EXERCISES

1. **Do the parents have the right to expect or demand these services?**
2. **Does the school have any legal or ethical obligation to provide these services?**
3. **Are there other possible service delivery options that might work?**
4. **Is treatment for Maria a right or a privilege?**

Occupational therapy practitioners who work with children must keep informed about laws regulating their services in schools and early intervention programs (Muhlenhaupt, Miller, Sanders, & Swinth, 1998). A summary of U.S. legislation since 1975 that affects the civil rights and education of children with disabilities and their key issues are presented in Table 32-1. Table 32-2 compares Parts B and C of IDEA and addresses several issues related to service provisions.

FAMILY-CENTERED SERVICES

Families are the primary social context in which children live and receive care and nurturing; consequently, they provide the central influence in the lives of children. Services to children with disabilities and the nature of parent–professional relationship have changed drastically since the late 1970s. Intervention for children with chronic health problems and developmental disabilities used to be child centered, with doctors and therapists setting goals for the child. In this model, parents were often bystanders and were ordered to follow-up with treatment recommendations (Rosenbaum, King, Law, King, & Evans, 1998). The implementation of the EHA and IDEA amendments supports the belief that parents are the primary decision makers concerning the care of their children, thus giving rise to family-centered services.

"At the core of a family-centered approach is the recognition of the centrality of the family—not just the mother—in the life of the child" (Turnbull, Turbiville, &

TABLE 32–1. **U.S. FEDERAL LEGISLATION SINCE 1975 THAT AFFECTS OCCUPATIONAL THERAPY SERVICES FOR CHILDREN**[a]

Year Enacted	Public Law Number	Title	Key Issues
1975	PL 94-142	EHA	Free appropriate education in the LRE for all children with "handicaps," ages 5–21 Occupational therapy as a related service to support special education Established IEP Child-centered and educational
1978	PL 95-602	Developmental Disability Amendments of 1978	Persons with developmental disabilities have the right to appropriate treatment, services, and habilitation in the LRE to maximize their full potential
1986	PL 99-457	Amendments to EHA	Part B: programs for preschoolers (3–5 years) with handicaps; occupational therapy as a related service to special education Part H: statewide systems of early intervention for infants and toddlers (0–3 years) at risk for or with disabilities Established IFSP Provision of services in natural environment Family focused Occupational therapy included in direct and primary services
1990	PL 101-392	Carl D. Perkins Vocational and Applied Technology Educational Act	Full vocational educational opportunity for youths with disabilities
1990	PL 101-476	IDEA	Reauthorization of EHA Amendments for Part H Part B: educational services for children 3–21 years with identified disabilities is permanently reauthorized Autism and traumatic brain injury added to definition of children with disabilities Wording change from *handicapped* to *individuals with disabilities* Transition and assistive technology services to be included in IEP
1990	PL 101-336	Americans with Disability Act (ADA)	Mandate making all facets of the public and private sector accessible to persons with disabilities
1991	PL 102-119	IDEA Amendments	Reauthorizes early intervention Mandates Interagency Coordinating Council (ICC) for each state, establishing comprehensive system (16 components) of early intervention services
1992	PL 102-569	Rehabilitation Act Amendments	Transition planning at high school graduation, includes coordination of assistive technology services and rehabilitation system
1994	PL 103-227	Goals 2000: Educate America Act	Hallmark of education reform and basis of all future education legislation Eight educational goals designed to help all students reach academic and occupational standards
1994	PL 103-252	Head Start Reauthorization Act of 1994	Amendments to Head Start Creates Early Head Start, providing services for infants and toddlers of low-income families, including young children with disabilities
1994	PL 103-239	School-to-Work Opportunities Act of 1994	Statewide school-to-work transition systems for preparing students to move into the workforce
1997	PL 105-17	IDEA Amendments of 1997	Restructuring IDEA into four parts Part B: in addition to the 10 categories of disability, states have option to service children 3–9 years with developmental delay Part C (formerly Part H): reaffirms natural environment for early intervention services and transition planning

[a]Data from Fischer (1994), Maruyama et al. (1999), and Mellard (2000).

TABLE 32-2. **COMPARISON OF PARTS B AND C OF IDEA 1997**[a]

Feature	Part C: Early Intervention Services	Part B: Education Services
Age	Birth–3 years	3–21 years
Eligibility	Children <3 years experiencing developmental delays in one or more of these areas: cognitive physical, communication, social or emotional adaptive or Have a diagnosed physical or medical condition with a high probability of resulting in developmental delay and At state's discretion, may include children who are at risk of experiencing substantial developmental delays if EI services are not provided	Children with a disability in any of 10 categories—mental retardation, hearing impairments, speech or language impairments, visual impairments, autism, serious emotional disturbance, traumatic brain injury, orthopedic impairments, other health impairments, and specific learning disabilities—and who because of these impairments need special education and related services At state's discretion, may include children ages 3–9 who are experiencing developmental delays, as defined by the state and LEA
Service document	IFSP Emphasizes family-centered approach	IEP Emphasizes educational approach
Timelines	Evaluation and IFSP to be completed in 45 calendar days	Evaluation and IEP must be developed in 40 school days
Services	EI services designed to enhance the family's ability to meet their child's needs and enhance the child's development Occupational therapy is one of the primary services	Special education and general education with related services, aids, and supports Occupational therapy is one of the related services
Transitions services	Beginning 6 months before 3rd birthday, transition process is addressed in IFSP	Beginning at age 14, and by 16, statement of transition services, including interagency responsibilities, is added to IEP
Environment	Natural environments typical of children of that age in which children without disabilities participate	LRE with children without disabilities Removal from the regular educational environment occurs only when the nature or severity of disability is such that participation in regular education with use of supplemental aids and service cannot be achieved satisfactorily
Parental involvement	Central to all facets of IFSP including assessment	Collaborative goal setting for IEP

[a]Data from IDEA (1997), Maruyama et al. (1999), Mellard (2000), Muhlenhaupt et al. (1998).

EI, early intervention; *LEA*, local education agency.

Turnbull, 2000, p. 638). A family-centered approach also acknowledges that the relationships between individual family members and the community have an effect on the family functioning and the development of the child (Rosenbaum et al., 1998; Schultz-Krohn, 1997; Turnbull et al., 2000). The goal of family-centered intervention is to improve the well-being of the family as a whole (Rosenbaum et al., 1998; Turnbull et al., 2000). Delivery of services in family-centered intervention is based on family choice, or the opportunity for the family to decide the level of involvement they wish in decision making for their child (Rosenbaum et al., 1998; Turnbull et al., 2000). The other guiding principle for service delivery is the adoption of a family strengths perspective, focusing on the family's abilities and resources (Case-Smith, 1998; Turnbull et al., 2000).

Viscardis (1998), the mother of a child with special needs, provided the following definition of a family-centered approach:

> *It begins with the child's and family's strengths, needs and hopes, and results in a service plan which responds to the needs of the whole family. It involves education, support, direct services and self-help approaches. The role of the service provider is to support, encourage and enhance the competence of parents in their role as caregivers. (p. 44)*

The challenge for all health professionals is to understand not only the principles of family-centered care but also how to develop a spirit of collaboration with families. Parent–professional relationships are greatly enhanced when professionals respect family diversity and cultural backgrounds, communicate clearly, listen to and support

CASE STUDY 32-1

Patrice's Story: A Client and Family Narrative

OLGA BALOUEFF

Today, 1 month after the start of school, Susan, a registered occupational therapist, and Mary, a certified occupational therapy assistant, meet with the director of special education, the classroom resources teacher, the physical therapist, the speech therapist, the school psychologist, and Mr. and Mrs. Douce, the parents of a third-grade student named Patrice. As a team, they will discuss Patrice's IEP.

Patrice is a 9-year-old boy, the middle child in a family of three children. He has an 11-year-old sister, Marie, and a 7-year-old brother, Justin. Patrice and his family immigrated to the United States from Haiti 3 years ago. They left Haiti as political refugees and came to the Boston area, where they knew a few people, including the father's brother and his family.

The children have integrated well into their community and school, but it has been much harder for the parents who had to learn English, find new resources and support, and secure employment. Both parents work, Mrs. Douce as a nurse's aide on the afternoon shift in a nursing home and Mr. Douce at the Haitian Resources Center. Patrice's parents describe him as handsome, vivacious, and energetic with an interest in sports, particularly basketball. He is a good student, is a quick learner who enjoys reading and art projects, and excels in spelling and arithmetic skills. But this was before an accident that changed the family's life.

On a sunny afternoon in early May after school, Patrice took his bike, but not his bicycle helmet, and went to his friend Bruce's house. Both boys biked to the local playground to play basketball with their friends. The boys had a good time; but, suddenly, in the middle of the game, the players began to argue about the rules of the game and about the fact that Patrice had been pushed by another boy and forced to drop the ball. In the middle of the argument, Patrice became angry, kicked the ball into the bushes, jumped on his bike, and pedaled furiously home. At a road intersection, he ignored the traffic signal and did not see a car coming in his direction. The driver of the car tried to avoid Patrice. Unfortunately, it was too late, and Patrice was hit by the car and thrown from his bike. He lay unconscious on the pavement as the driver of the car and passers-by anxiously waited for the ambulance and the police to arrive.

Emergency medical technicians arrived within minutes of the accident and attended to Patrice right at the scene and in the ambulance. He was transported to a local pediatric trauma center. On arrival at the hospital, the trauma team immediately attended to him. Patrice was diagnosed as suffering from closed head trauma, multiple fractures, and contusions. His family was notified of the accident. When the parents arrived at the emergency room, they were informed of their son's condition by the doctor and were assisted by a nurse and a social worker. They saw Patrice lying unconscious, pale, and hooked up to life support units as he was wheeled into the operating room.

Patrice survived the surgery to relieve the intracranial pressure, but his prognosis remained extremely guarded for the following 5 days. He lay in a coma, showing at first only a generalized response to sensory stimuli and pain and facial grimaces in response to light touch and loud sounds. The first 10 days were most stressful for Patrice's parents. Their feelings ranged from the initial shock to fear to hope, guilt, and confusion as they saw their son hooked up to a respirator and other life support units monitoring every facet of his body. Patrice's mother recalled, "All I could do in the beginning was cry."

The family received enormous support from friends, their church, the parent–teacher organization (PTO) at their children's school, and from the hospital pediatric staff. Through the PTO, meals were brought to the family. The other two children stayed at friends' homes after school until the parents came home after visiting Patrice at the hospital. Members of the church offered their prayers and rides to the hospital.

Patrice's primary nurse, the doctor, his occupational therapist, and physical therapist encouraged the parents to talk to him about his life, about who he was, what he liked to do; to touch him; and to hug and kiss him. His parents were told that a person in a coma absorbs familiar sounds and people's voices. The staff encouraged Mr. and Mrs. Douce to tape the voices of Patrice's sister, brother, and classmates and to play them back to him at different times during the day. The medical team actively involved the family in the care of their son and gave them emotional support.

After 12 days, Patrice came out of the coma and was taken off of the respirator; 3 weeks after the accident, he was finally medically stable. A family conference with his pediatric team was scheduled to discuss his progress and to plan his discharge to a pediatric rehabilitation center. At that time, the boy had language problems, such as being slow to respond, speaking unclearly, and having difficulty with finding the right words. He also had behavioral problems, exemplified by being emotionally labile, anxious, argumentative, and irritable. Patrice seemed unaware of his difficulties. He

Continues

wanted to go home and cried each time his parents left his room. He was still totally dependent on assistance for self-care activities, and his left leg and arm were in casts. He was able to sit in a chair for only 20 min at a time and was on phenytoin for seizures.

Patrice spent 21/2 months in a rehabilitation hospital. A multidisciplinary team of clinicians worked with him to help him regain function and go back home and to school. Finally, at the end of August, Patrice went home, to his overjoyed family and friends. He had made an excellent recovery, but his therapists warned his parents that Patrice still had some lingering problems that would affect his performance in daily living, educational, and play activities. However, over time, and with the support of his family and the school team, he would be expected to do well.

In early September, Patrice entered Ms. Fowler's third-grade class with several of his previous classmates. This teacher knew the Douce family well because Patrice's sister, Marie, had been in her class when the family first arrived at the school. She is a warm, well-organized teacher who keeps regular contact with her pupils' parents and who values the services of the special educational team. The classroom is on the first floor, with direct access to the playground.

Physically, Patrice walks independently, with a slight limp on the left side. His balance is fairly good, unless he is tired or runs. Because of poor stamina and difficulty in anticipating the position of the ball or the players on the field, participation in recreational activities with his peers is still limited. This is frustrating to him. He dresses himself independently and takes care of his toileting needs and grooming, but he is somewhat slow. Patrice's speech is somewhat laborious at times. He seems to stumble on words, forgets them, and stutters when he is tired. Once this made his classmates laugh, and he became upset.

In class, at midday he often becomes withdrawn, apathetic, and distracted, especially when the classroom atmosphere is noisy and the children are moving about. He has difficulty with arithmetic and spelling, frequently forgetting a letter or the place of a number. When his teacher corrects him, he often reacts with a temper outburst. Once he threw his papers on the floor and accused Mrs. Fowler of picking on him unfairly. Mr. and Mrs. Douce remark that their son has similar tantrums at home, especially if they give him verbal instructions regarding various tasks. This is upsetting to the whole family, because they expect the boy to be well behaved and to be polite with them and his teachers.

Finally, Patrice's written work, which had always been well organized and neatly done, is now sloppy. He often forgets to do his homework for the next day. At this point, Mr. and Mrs. Douce are becoming worried about their son's behavior at school and at home. Their other two children are resentful of the long disruption in the family's routine. They also do not understand why their brother has changed so much, although he looks well and is able to walk. After speaking with Mrs. Fowler, it is clear to Mr. and Mrs. Douce that their son needs help with his behavior at home and to keep up with school work.

To provide quality care in pediatrics, occupational therapy practitioners must recognize the issues affecting each family and must become familiar with federal regulation that shapes the delivery of health and educational services. Parent–professional interactions are central to the quality of interventions given to children. Patrice's story reflects the complexity of the issues surrounding children who need occupational therapy intervention and their families. Patrice's occupational therapy evaluation and intervention in his school setting are the focus of the Case Analysis at the end of Unit IX.

families, and believe and trust parents (Case-Smith, 1998; Rosenbaum et al., 1998). Families who identify a high degree of satisfaction with the services they receive indicate that "their families' choices and decisions are respected and that services are planned with families' scheduling needs in mind" (Viscardis, 1998, p. 49).

EVIDENCE-BASED PRACTICE

To provide a respectful, collaborative relationship with clients and with those acting on their behalf, practitioners need to inform the people involved about the following:

- The nature of the client's occupational status.
- The relationship of that status to potential quality of life.
- The nature and quality of the assessments recommended.
- The nature of the quality and probable outcomes of relevant interventions.

Once informed, clients can choose to participate or not in occupational therapy assessment and intervention. Practitioners are responsible for providing information to clients based on a thorough review of the body of evidence available (Cermak & Vergara, 2001; Tickle-Degnen, 2000). Evidence-based practice involves a systematic search and analysis of the scientific literature to incorporate the best evidence into the clinical reasoning and decisions making for clients. Practitioners often search databases to find research studies relevant to a particular condition or intervention. Appendix F provides a list of a few Web sites with specific reviews of evidence related to children with disabilities.

CONCLUSION

To provide quality care for infants, children, and adolescents, occupational therapy practitioners must recognize client's unique concerns for participating in a range of contexts in their daily lives. Therapists must carefully listen to understand and design intervention to address the needs of the entire family system. To provide services within organized settings, practitioners must become familiar with the health policies influencing the delivery of health and educational services. In addition, effective practitioners use both individual clinical expertise and the best available external evidence to provide clients and those acting on their behalf with information for making decisions about whether to pursue occupational therapy intervention. Case Study 32-1, which tells Patrice's story, reflects the complexity of concerns surrounding children and their families who seek occupational therapy intervention. The Case Analysis at the end of Unit IX further explores Patrice's intervention.

References

American Occupational Therapy Association—[AOTA]. (In press). Occupational therapy practice framework: Domain and process. *American Journal of Occupational Therapy*.

American Occupational Therapy Association [AOTA]. (2001). *Member compensation survey*. Bethesda, MD: Author.

Brown, M., & Gordon, W. A. (1987). Impact of impairment on activity patterns of children. *Archives of Physical Medicine and Rehabilitation, 68*, 828–832.

Case-Smith, J. (1998). Foundations and principles. In J. Case-Smith (Ed.). *Pediatric occupational therapy and early intervention* (2nd ed., pp. 3–25). Boston: Butterworth-Heineman.

Cermak, S., & Vergara, E. (2001). Infusing evidence-based practice into the pediatric curricula. *Maternal and Child Health Bureau–Boston University Center for Leadership in Pediatric Occupational Therapy Education Newsletter, 5*, 1–4.

Coster, W. (1998). Occupation-centered assessment of children. *American Journal of Occupational Therapy, 52*(5), 337–344.

Hanft, B. E., & Pilkington, K. O. (2000). Therapy in natural environments: The means or end goal for early intervention? *Infants and Young Children, 12*(4), 1–13.

Law, M., & Dunn, W. (1993). Perspectives on understanding and changing the environment for children with disabilities. *Physical and Occupational Therapy in Pediatrics, 13*, 1–17.

Maruyama, E., Chandler, B. E., Clark, G. F., Dick, R. W., Lawlor, M. C., & Jackson, L. L. (1999). *Occupational therapy services for children and youth under the Individuals with Disabilities Education Act* (2nd ed.). Bethesda, MD: American Occupational Therapy Association.

Meisels, S. J., & Shonkoff, J. P. (2000). Early childhood intervention: A continuing evolution. In J. P. Shonkoff & S. M. Meisels (Eds.) *Handbook of early childhood intervention* (2nd ed., pp. 3–31). New York: Cambridge University Press.

Mellard, E. (2000). Impact of federal policy on services for children and families in early intervention programs and public schools. In W. Dunn (Ed.). *Best practice occupational therapy: In community service with children and families* (pp. 147–156). Thorofare, NJ: Slack.

Moyers, P. (1999). Guide to occupational therapy practice. *American Journal of Occupational Therapy, 53*, 247–322.

Muhlenhaupt, M., Miller, H., Sanders, J., & Swinth, Y. (1998). Implications of the 1997 Reauthorization of IDEA for school-based occupational therapy. *AOTA School System Special Interest Section Quarterly, 5*(3), 1–4.

Rainville, E. B., Cermak, S. A., & Murray, E. A. (1996). Supervision and consultation services for pediatric occupational therapists. *American Journal of Occupational Therapy, 50*(9), 725–731.

Reauthorization of the Individuals with Disabilities Education Act Amendments of 1997. Pub. L. 105–17, Proposed regulations for assistance to states for education of children with disabilities, 62 Fed. Reg. 55068.

Rosenbaum, P., King, S., Law, M., King, G., & Evans, J. (1998). Family-centered service: A conceptual framework and research review. *Physical and Occupational Therapy in Pediatrics, 18*(1), 1–20.

Sackett, D. L., Richardson, W. S., Rosenberg, W., & Haynes, R. B. (1997). *Evidence-based medicine*. New York: Churchill Livingstone.

Schultz-Krohn, W. (1997). Early intervention: Meeting the unique needs of parent-child interaction. *Infants and Young Children, 10*(1), 47–60.

Tickle-Degnen, L. (2000). Communicating with clients, family members, and colleagues about research evidence. *American Journal of Occupational Therapy, 54*, 341–343.

Turnbull, A. P., Turbiville, V., & Turnbull, H. R. (2000). Evolution of family-professional partnerships: Collective empowerment as the model for the early twenty-first century. In J. P. Shonkoff & S. M. Meisels (Eds.). *Handbook of early childhood intervention* (2nd ed., pp. 630–650). New York: Cambridge University Press.

Viscardis, L. (1998). The family-centered approach to providing services: A parent perspective. *Physical and Occupational Therapy in Pediatrics, 18*(1), 45–53.

World Health Organization. (2001). *ICF: International classification of functioning, disability, and health*. Geneva: Author. Available at www.who.int/icidh. 9/24/02.

CHAPTER 33

NEUROLOGICAL DYSFUNCTION IN CHILDREN

SUSAN COOK MERRILL and SHELLEY E. MULLIGAN

The scope of neurological dysfunction in children includes all conditions that affect child neurodevelopment. These conditions may be acquired before birth, in utero (e.g., drug exposure, congenital anomalies, or cerebral vascular accident); at the time of birth (e.g., cerebral palsy resulting from birth trauma or prematurity); or after birth (e.g., traumatic brain or spinal cord injury). Neurological conditions may also result from genetic disorders. This chapter focuses on specific considerations for children with neurological conditions commonly seen by occupational therapy practitioners, including cerebral palsy, learning disabilities, developmental disabilities, and pervasive developmental disorders. Many of the theoretical and intervention principles related to occupational therapy for adults with spinal cord injury and traumatic brain injury apply to children as well (see Chapter 39). Other neurological conditions less often seen by occupational therapy practitioners are also briefly discussed.

Neurodevelopment affects children's ability to participate in almost all childhood occupations. Childhood occupations typically include self-care or self-maintenance occupations, play, learning, family and peer interactions, and, for older children, community living and vocational occupations. Children with neurodevelopmental disabilities are situated in an ecocultural context with numerous adults nurturing their growth. Therefore, evaluation and intervention are conducted in collaboration with parents, educators, and other health-care personnel. Occupational therapy practitioners provide services for children with neurological conditions in a variety of settings (e.g., hospital intensive care units, rehabilitation units, early intervention community settings, homes, schools, psychiatric facilities), and the characteristics of these settings need to be considered in the evaluation and intervention process.

CLIENT FACTORS INFLUENCING THE OCCUPATIONAL PERFORMANCE OF CHILDREN WITH NEUROLOGICAL DYSFUNCTION

The analysis of occupational performance of children with neurological conditions requires knowledge of central nervous system (CNS) function, sensory processing and adaptation, development of motor control and an appreciation for the complexity of development in children. Development is a process in which neurological maturation (including motivation, arousal, and autonomic integrity) interacts with external environmental conditions (Gilfoyle, Grady, & Moore, 1990). These interactions between neurological systems and the environment create feedback loops that modify both. Development, therefore, proceeds based on previous experiences, genetic programming, and environmental influences. Movement (often disrupted in children with neurological disorders) allows children to interact with the environment and provides feedback to the CNS, promoting more mature movement patterns and providing a foundation for cognitive and social development (Alexander, Boehme, & Cupps, 1993).

Children with neurological conditions may experience a variety of deficits in sensorimotor, neuromusculoskeletal, cognitive, perceptual, and psychosocial areas. Such deficits often affect children's ability to develop or acquire the skills necessary for successful engagement in meaningful childhood occupations.

Sensorimotor Functions

Children with neurological conditions may experience specific sensory system deficits, such as visual loss or hearing impairment. Approximately 50% of children with cerebral palsy and 25% of children with mental retardation are estimated to have visual impairments (Pellegrino, 1997; Shapiro & Batshaw, 1993). Other children with neurological conditions may experience generalized difficulty in the processing of sensory information, without a specific sensory loss. The general ability to process sensations in an organized way may be viewed as a perceptual skill, affecting children's ability to make adaptive responses to environmental sensory experiences.

Perception involves recognizing and interpreting sensory information from the environment (Parham & Mailloux, 2001). For example, a child may overact to auditory or tactile sensory input by responding aggressively or withdrawing from the sensory stimuli. This behavior, sometimes referred to as sensory defensiveness, is hypothesized to be an overreaction of the CNS to the sensory input. Other children may not be able to discriminate types of tactile, visual, or auditory sensory information well, which may result in a variety of functional and/or academic difficulties.

Visual Processes

Visual impairment results from problems with any visual system component, including the eyes, eye muscles, optic nerve, and areas of the cerebral cortex that process visual information (Gersh, 1991). Optic nerve damage, visual field losses, and cataracts are common in premature infants with retinopathy. These infants may be partially or totally blind, owing to injury to visual pathways or the cerebral cortex. Children with neurological dysfunction may have problems with visual acuity and focusing, **oculomotor control,** or **visual perception,** and these deficits have a tremendous influence on all areas of occupation.

New diagnostic techniques are available for the testing of vision of young infants and children as well as children who are nonverbal. It is important for occupational therapists to inquire about visual testing that has been done by optometrists or ophthalmologists, and to screen for visual deficits.

Coordination of eye movements, called oculomotor ability, is related to neuromuscular function of the entire body, particularly of the vestibular system. Therefore, children with neuromuscular dysfunction, muscle tone abnormalities, and poor coordination may experience problems with oculomotor control. Oculomotor skills are essential for school-related activities, such as reading, writing, and computer use.

Visual perception includes visual discrimination, visual memory, spatial relationships, form constancy, sequential visual memory, figure-ground discrimination, and visual closure. Children with learning disabilities, traumatic brain injury, cerebral palsy, and neural tube defects with hydrocephalus often have visual perceptual deficits, commonly addressed by occupational therapy practitioners (see Chapter 30, Section 5).

Auditory Processes

Mild-to-profound auditory problems may result in sensorineural or conductive hearing impairments. Sensorineural loss results from damage to the inner ear, the auditory nerve, or both. It may be hereditary, congenital, or acquired later in childhood from meningitis, high fever, or medications.

Conductive loss is a result of anatomical malformation or frequent middle ear infections. Persistent middle ear fluid can cause temporary hearing loss, which may be a critical problem during early speech and language development (Gersh, 1991).

Despite normal hearing, some children with neurodevelopmental conditions, such as learning disorders or autism, may have auditory processing problems that impair their ability to follow complex directions and learn from verbal instruction. These children may also be overly sensitive to sounds so that loud noises are perceived as frightening or painful, or they may be distracted by subtle environmental noises. Such auditory processing problems affect children's ability to perform everyday tasks and, in particular, may negatively affect their ability to participate in school and other group situations. Consulting with speech pathologists to understand the specific auditory processing problems of children helps occupational therapy practitioners develop effective compensation strategies or adaptations to enhance children's ability to interact with others and perform meaningful activities.

Tactile Processes

Children with neurological impairments may experience problems with **tactile processing,** including both the discriminative (e.g., deficits in stereognosis and localization of touch) and the protective systems (e.g., tactile defensiveness) (Brasic-Royeen & Lane, 1991). Tactile receptors found throughout the skin are activated through touch, including pain, pressure, and temperature. Tactile discrimination is thought to be associated with the development of body scheme and motor planning abilities and is believed to contribute to the development of fine motor skill (Case-Smith, 1995). Children with tactile defensiveness often avoid activities heavily loaded with tactile stimuli, such as grooming tasks, manipulating art materials, and wearing certain fabrics, and may avoid contact with others or feel stressed when with others. Other children may seek out tactile stimuli and appear to be underresponsive to this type of sensory input (Dunn, 1999).

Vestibular-Proprioceptive Processes

The **vestibular system** includes neural receptors that are located in the semicircular canal, the utricle, and the saccule of the inner ear. This system is stimulated by movement of the head and is influenced by gravity. Vestibular functioning plays an important role in awareness of body position and movement in space and postural control. The components of postural control are muscle tone, equilibrium and balance, and stabilizing the eyes in space during head movements (Fisher, 1991). These areas are commonly affected in children with neurological impairment such as traumatic brain injury and cerebral palsy. Evaluation of vestibular processing should, therefore, include the assessment of postural control factors, including righting, equilibrium and protective reactions, muscle tone, and balance skills.

Proprioceptive processing refers to the functioning of specialized receptors located in the muscles and joints, which are stimulated through active movement. Proprioception gives individuals information about the spatial orientation of their body, the rate and timing of their movements, the amount of muscle force being exerted, and how fast and how much a muscle is being stretched (Fisher, 1991; Matthews, 1988). Proprioception plays an important role in the development of body awareness, motor planning, and accuracy of motor movements. Because it is difficult to separate the vestibular system from the proprioceptive system during motor performance, occupational therapy evaluation of these systems often occurs simultaneously. The ability to modulate sensory input from vestibular and proprioceptive systems also plays an important role in children's ability to maintain optimal levels of arousal for learning and performance (Fisher, 1991). Therefore, evaluating the effects of such stimuli on behavior is important.

Motor Skills

Reflexes that dominate infant movement and behavior largely characterize sensorimotor development in early infancy. Reflex behavior serves an important survival function for the infant and is primarily controlled by primitive CNS areas, including the spinal cord and brainstem (Mathiowetz & Haugen, 1995). For example, the infant's rooting reflex allows him or her to locate food. As the infant develops, primitive reflexes gradually disappear, most by the first year of life; and many are incorporated into more complex, voluntary actions. For example, the grasp reflex (with pressure into the palm of the hand, the infant curls the fingers inward and grabs onto the finger or object) predominates until 3–4 months of age, when the infant then becomes capable of voluntarily reaching out and opening the hand to grab desired objects.

It is important to examine reflex behavior in infants and children with suspected neurological impairment, because reflex behaviors serve as a window into children's CNS. Data describing these reflexes and when they tend to emerge and disappear provide the therapist with soft signs of neurodevelopmental maturation (Gilfoyle et al., 1990). The examination of reflex behavior is also important, because these reflexes greatly influence children's ability to perform functional motor skills. For example, if the grasp reflex persists, such children will have difficulty developing hand skills. Asymmetries in the performance of reflexes may also indicate pathology. Continuation of these reflexes is common in children with neurological conditions and may interfere with their ability to develop postural control and functional fine and gross motor skills (Campbell & Wilhelm, 1985).

Automatic or postural reactions such as righting and protective and equilibrium reactions develop as children begin to gain postural control for movement, and they are often impaired in children with neurological dysfunction. The development of these reactions has been reported to occur first in prone; then in supine, sitting, and quadruped (crawling on hands and knees) positions; and finally in standing (Bartlett, 1997; Chandler, Andrews, & Swanson, 1980). They serve as mechanisms for maintaining balance during active and passive movement. As with the primitive reflexes, automatic reactions provide information about quality of movement, children's ability to acquire increasingly complex motor skills, and neurodevelopmental maturation.

The development of postural control for movement requires the ability to move against gravity and requires stability at the proximal joints (e.g., pelvic and shoulder girdles) and is affected considerably by **muscle tone. Hypertonia,** or high muscle tone, results in slow, rigid movements and sometimes limited range of motion (ROM) as a result of excessive tension in the muscles. **Hypotonia,** or low muscle tone, is characterized by floppiness, or lack of tension in muscles when a body part is moved, and hyperextensibility. Low tone interferes with the balance between stability and mobility for almost all movement, especially antigravity motor control. Many children with neurological dysfunction have a combination of muscle tone and postural control deficits, which may be distributed in different parts of the body. The ability to develop, execute, and integrate reflexes, automatic reactions, and postural control provide a foundation for the development of fine and gross motor skills (Campbell & Wilhelm, 1985).

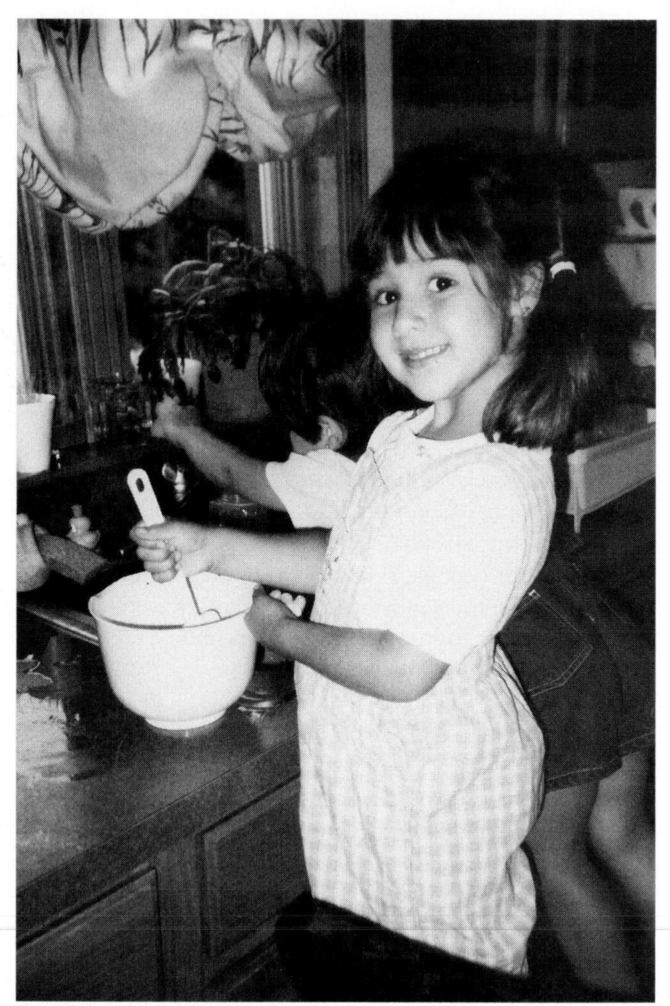

FIGURE 33–1. A cooking activity requires fine motor and sequencing skills. (Courtesy of P. Masciarelli-Patel, Wakefield, MA)

Gross, Fine, and Oral Motor Skills

The ability to learn to perform motor skills depends on a number of underlying client factors, including neuromusculoskeletal and movement functions, such as muscle strength, postural control and balance, muscle tone, ROM, agility, motor coordination, and **motor planning.** Sensory awareness and processing—particularly of the tactile, proprioceptive, and visual sensory systems—also contributes to motor skill performance. Cognitive functions such as attention and problem-solving abilities may be contributing factors as well as the psychological components, interests, and values. Environmental factors, such as a lack of experience with certain motor activities, may also affect children's level of competency in performing certain motor tasks. Gross motor skill acquisition is important for developing a functional means for mobility and for play, which is the primary occupation of children. Children's ability to move accurately throughout their environment and manipulate play materials provides them with many opportunities to engage in and learn from play. Therefore, it is important to provide adaptations for children with motor impairments so that they can play successfully (Morrison & Metzger, 2001).

The ability to learn and perform fine motor skills also depends on a number of client factors, including reach, grasp, release, dexterity, in-hand manipulation, bilateral hand use, and visual motor skills (Fig. 33-1). Skilled movement depends on the foundation of basic motor patterns acquired during early life. There are a number of typical motor sequential patterns that contribute to the ability to acquire increasingly complex fine motor skills over time. Generally, hand function progresses from gross to fine; proximal to distal, ulnar to radial, and more asymmetrical to more symmetrical patterns (Gilfoyle et al., 1990). However, the ability to perform a specific fine motor activity also depends on other factors such as the demands of the task, use of compensatory strategies, and motivation. Self-feeding, managing clothing fasteners, writing, and using typical classroom tools (glue, scissors) are examples of functional fine motor skills most school-aged children are expected to master (Coster, Deeney, Haltwanger, & Haley, 1998).

Visual motor integration is the ability of the eyes and hands to work together in smooth, efficient patterns. Controlled eye movements precede controlled hand movements. At the same time, coordinated hand movements influence the eyes, as both systems exchange information needed for

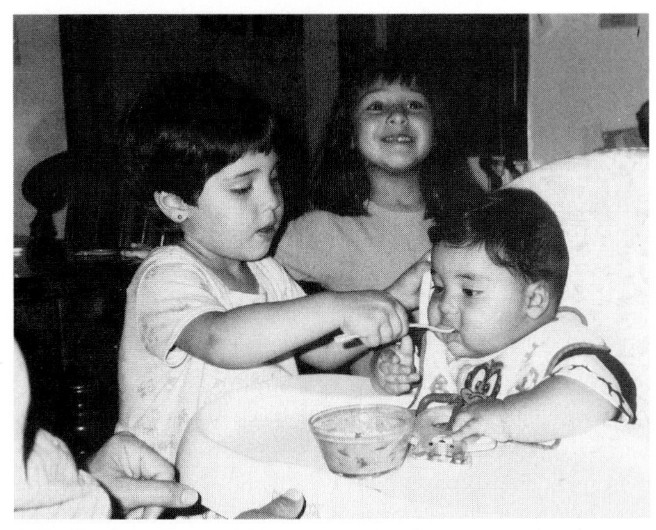

FIGURE 33–2. A proud big sister assists her younger brother with oral motor skills for mealtime occupations. (Courtesy of P. Masciarelli-Patel, Wakefield, MA)

adapting to environmental demands or tasks, such as scissor use or ball play (Erhardt, 1994). Coordination of hands and eyes depends also on head control, which enables the eyes to monitor the work of the hands.

The development of oral motor skills necessary for feeding and expressive language also may be considered a fine motor skill, as these movements are quite intricate (Fig. 33-2). Postural control factors such as the persistence of primitive reflex patterns, abnormal muscle tone, muscle weakness and incoordination, and oral hypersensitivities may all have a significant impact on a child's oral motor control (Logemann, 1983).

Cognitive Processes

A large percentage of children with neurological conditions have cognitive deficits related to the mental processes of thinking, understanding, and using the senses to gather information and make sense of the world (Rogers, Gordon, Schanzenbacher, & Case-Smith, 2001). It is often challenging to evaluate the cognitive skills of children with severe neuromotor dysfunction, particularly when they are nonverbal and/or not able to control their hand movements to respond. However, it is important to understand how cognitive abilities are influencing children's capability to perform functional skills and interact with others and objects in their environments. Some aspects of cognition addressed by occupational therapy practitioners include levels of arousal or consciousness (particularly for children with traumatic brain injury), orientation, memory, sequencing, problem solving, abstract thought, and judgment.

For example, a child's level of alertness and ability to attend must be taken into consideration when interpreting the results of evaluation procedures. Children's ability to generalize what is learned from one situation to the next is an important consideration for intervention planning. Visual cues, such as scheduling boards may be used as a compensatory strategy for children with memory deficits to help them anticipate their daily schedule of activities at school. Although other professionals such as psychologists conduct comprehensive evaluations of cognition, occupational therapy practitioners need to understand how cognition influences occupational performance.

Communication and Interaction Skills

The development of language is largely considered a cognitive skill; however, expressive language requires motor planning, sequencing, and coordination of intricate oral motor movements. Infants communicate primarily through crying and facial expressions; between 6 and 12 months, infants develop the use of gestures, such as pointing toward desired objects and waving good-bye. Then language development proceeds rapidly: The average 3-year-old uses 3000–4000 words (Miller, 1981), and language is typically well developed by 4 years (Sroufe, Cooper, & DeHart, 1992). It is essential for children with severe neurological conditions to find a means of communication, and occupational therapy practitioners often work with speech pathologists to prescribe augmentative communication devices for this purpose.

Children with neurological conditions often experience psychosocial and other emotional and behavioral difficulties as a part of their conditions (e.g., autism), or psychosocial-emotional difficulties may co-exist with physical or learning disorders. Infants and toddlers with neurological disorders may have difficulties with coping skills and self-regulatory behavior, affect and level of interest and engagement in social interaction, the development of healthy attachment with parents and caregivers, and self-expression and the beginning of development of self-concept. Disabilities in these areas can influence the children's ability to play, establish routines for eating and sleeping, learn new skills, and establish healthy relationships with caregivers and peers (Greenspan, & Weider, 1998).

For preschool and school-aged children with neurological dysfunction, naturalistic observations of behavior and interviews with children and families are important for understanding the affects of psychosocial-emotional functioning on these children's ability to succeed in valued occupations. Such information should address children's likes and dislikes; behavior in structured and nonstructured situations (attention span, ability to concentrate, aggressiveness, self-control, play preferences); responses to direct requests and challenges; interaction styles with peers, family members, and persons of authority; and coping skills. Mental status, thought processes, and affect should also be observed. Specific problem behaviors such as self-abusive or aggressive behaviors are common in children with severe impairments. When behavior problems exist, practitioners should consider the specific environmental and personal factors that may underlie the behavior as well as the consequences for the behavior when designing interventions

Adolescence is a time when those with and without neurological disabilities struggle to define their identities. Independence and peer acceptance become increasingly important. While adolescents without neurological conditions begin to develop greater independence, adolescents with mobility limitations may be at greater risk for social isolation (Brown & Gordon, 1987). Late adolescence is an important time for intervention as plans for life after high school and a new living situation may be considered. Feelings of self-worth and perceived level of competencies, ability to relate to others, and coping skills need to be considered as transition plans are developed. Other factors to consider include family support and peer relationships, community support networks, ability to find and use resources, and participation in valued occupations.

EVALUATION AND INTERVENTION OF CHILDREN WITH NEUROLOGICAL DYSFUNCTION

Evaluation

As with all clients, the evaluation process begins by developing an occupational profile: an understanding of children and their families, the daily activities that are important to them, and their values and interests. The goal of an evaluation is to understand children's strengths and challenges related to the contexts and occupations in which they participate. Family members, particularly parents, and other professionals, such as teachers, are integral to the evaluation process. Occupational profiles for children should also include children's likes and dislikes, temperament, important peer and family relationships, school program information and learning history, and extracurricular activities. Once an occupational profile has been identified, the next step is to conduct a thorough analysis of occupational performance, which considers the dynamic interaction among performance skills, patterns, contexts, activity demands, and client factors.

Evaluation information may be gathered from formal standardized assessments as well as from interviews, checklists, formal and informal observations of performance, and children's interactions with people and objects (Huber & King-Thomas, 1987). Information gathered from medical records and interviews with children and parents includes any major illnesses, diagnoses, and hospitalizations, relevant birth history information, sensory history, and when major developmental milestones (walking, saying first words) were achieved. To evaluate areas of occupation and client factors, such as level of participation in self-care activities and/or classroom behavior, checklists and interviews are commonly used. Some standardized assessments that measure performance skills of children with significant neurological impairment are the following:

- Pediatric Evaluation of Disability Inventory (PEDI; Haley, Coster, Ludlow, Haltiwanger, & Andrellos, 1992).
- Hawaii Early Learning Profile (Furuno, O'Reilly, Hosaka, Inatsuka, Allman, & Zeisloft, 1984).
- School Function Assessment (SFA; Coster et al., 1998).
- Vineland Adaptive Behavior Scales (Sparrow, Balla, & Cicchetti, 1984).

More specialized evaluation procedures may be used to evaluate specific skills, such as feeding and swallowing, seating and positioning, need for assistive technology, and handwriting. Consideration of the demands of valued occupations and the contexts in which they are performed are also important, as adaptations to the context or activity itself may be a useful intervention strategy for enhancing performance. Assessments such as the Home Observation and Measurement of the Environment (HOME) may be used to evaluate performance contexts (Caldwell & Bradley 1979; see also Chapter 26).

Following evaluation of children's performance skills and contexts, occupational therapists form hypotheses to explain why children are experiencing occupational performance problems. Client factors suspected of affecting performance are further assessed.

Sensory processing can be evaluated through observation of occupations, with attention given to the sensory opportunities provided by objects and activities and children's responses to the sensory input. Formal clinical observations, such as testing for eye tracking or checking if an infant responds to auditory stimulation by turning in the direction of a noise, may be conducted. Examples of standardized assessments available to measure sensory processing follow:

- Sensory Profile (Dunn, 1999).
- Sensory Integration and Praxis Tests (SIPT; Ayres, 1989).
- Erhardt Developmental Vision Assessment (Erhardt, 1990).

Tests of nonmotor visual perception often used by occupational therapists include the following:

- Test of Visual Perceptual Skills (Gardner, 1995b).
- Motor-Free Visual Perception Test—Revised (Colarusso & Hammill, 1995).

To evaluate neuromotor capacities in regard to reflexes, automatic reactions, and other postural control factors, many practitioners use a variety of structured and nonstandardized assessments of muscle tone, reflex patterns, and overall motor development (Cook, 1991; Nichols, 2000). Standardized neuromotor assessments used for this purpose include the following:

- Movement Assessment for Infants (MAI) (Chandler et al., 1980)

- Alberta Infant Motor Scales (AIMS) (Piper & Darrah, 1994)
- Toddler and Infant Motor Evaluation (TIME; Miller & Roid, 1994).
- Peabody Developmental Motor Scales—2 (Folio & Fewell, 2000).
- Bruininks-Oseretsky Test of Motor Proficiency (Bruininks, 1978).
- Bayley Scales of Infant Development (Bayley, 1993).
- Miller Assessment for Preschoolers (Miller, 1988).

Although psychologists commonly evaluate cognition, occupational therapy practitioners consider how cognitive capacities such as memory and attention affect children's ability to perform occupations. Occupational therapy practitioners monitor levels of consciousness in children with traumatic brain injury and others whose levels of arousal or ability to attend and concentrate may fluctuate. The Glasgow Coma Scale (Teasdale & Jennett, 1974), and its infant/toddler version (Gharai & Hariri, 1992) are often used for this purpose. These criterion-referenced tools use a behavioral rating scale to measure motor, verbal, and eye-opening responses.

The social interaction skills of children with neurological dysfunction can be evaluated using informal and formal observations during structured or nonstructured individual and group activities, as well as by standardized assessments. Examples of assessment tools that measure social and emotional functioning and behavior, include the following:

- Social Skills Rating System (Gresham & Elliot, 1990).
- Behavior Assessment System for Children (BASC; Reynolds & Kamphaus, 1992).
- Early Coping Inventory (Zeitlin, Williamson, & Szczepanski, 1998).

Although standardized assessments increase the reliability of the evaluator's judgment, few are designed for children with moderate-to-severe disabilities. Standardized testing may be difficult for children who are nonverbal or who have significant motor impairments and/or behavioral problems. Therefore, keen observations of children performing occupations in natural contexts provide valuable information. The final phase of the evaluation involves the synthesis or integration of all the information gathered with that from other team members and consideration of the children's and their family's goals and priorities.

Intervention

Effective intervention for children with neurological conditions is based on a synthesis of the information gathered in the evaluation and from other team members. Children must be considered within the social context of their families, their educational environments, and their communities. They must be viewed as unique, goal-oriented individuals who influence the world, are influenced by it, and who are intrinsically motivated to seek stimulation and interaction and to learn. In relation to occupational performance, practitioners consider the practice setting; roles and skills of other members of the team; access to space, materials, and therapy equipment; and the research evidence supporting the intervention considered.

Play, the primary occupation of children, is also the most common therapeutic activity used with children. Bundy (1991) stated, "If play is the vehicle by which individuals become masters of their environments, then play should be among the most powerful of therapeutic tools" (p. 61). For activities to be considered play, they must be intrinsically motivating, internally controlled by the child, and free from objective reality (Bundy, 1991). Play should be fun, somewhat spontaneous, interesting, and challenging but stress-free. According to Takata (1974), play is a set of behaviors characterized by a dynamic process that involves a particular attitude and action. Through play, infants and young children learn and practice new skills, refine others, experiment with social roles, experience emotions, and develop friendships. Children are intrinsically motivated to play. They are naturally inclined to explore environments, imitate, and create play situations, providing opportunities for experimentation and repetition of experience (see Chapter 24, Section 5 and Chapter 29, Section 3).

Other theoretical approaches to occupational therapy commonly used for children with neurological dysfunction are developmental (neurodevelopmental and sensory integration), rehabilitative (biomechanical and compensatory approaches), learning, and occupational behavior. Practitioners may use any combination of these approaches when intervening with an individual child.

Summary

Occupational therapy evaluation and intervention with children with neurological conditions is complex, as is the nature of the multifaceted conditions and challenges many of these children face. Practitioners must draw on their knowledge of neurodevelopment and multiple theoretical approaches to provide effective services for children and their families; they must also work collaboratively with others. It is important to consider children's strengths and challenges in the context of their environments and in relation to the roles and activities that are most important to them. The concerns and priorities of children and their families should be the driving force in determining evaluation and intervention techniques.

CEREBRAL PALSY

Cerebral palsy refers to a group of movement disorders caused by damage to the brain occurring before, during, or shortly after birth; these conditions are not caused by problems of nerves and muscles (National Institute of Neurological

Disorders and Stroke [NINDS], 2001). While postural and movement problems are the hallmarks of cerebral palsy, there are almost invariably secondary disorders. Visual and/or auditory deficits, seizures, cognitive impairment, learning disabilities, and oral motor and behavioral problems add further complications to the lives of children with cerebral palsy (Pelligrino, 1997).

Cerebral palsy may result from many conditions. Genetic abnormalities can lead to brain malfunction during embryonic development. Intrauterine infection, such as rubella, cytomegalovirus, and toxoplasmosis can damage the fetal nervous system. Rhesus blood antigen incompatibility, in which the mother's body produces antibodies that destroy the fetus's blood cells, can create too much bile pigment in the blood (jaundice). Untreated jaundice can cause brain damage. Anoxia, as a result of complications during labor and delivery, may deprive the fetal brain of vital blood and oxygen—a condition called hypoxic-ischemic encephalopathy. Coagulation disorders in the mother or infant can cause a stroke in the fetus or newborn. A healthy infant may develop symptoms of cerebral palsy after traumatic brain injury. The common factor in all these conditions is interruption of the developmental processes of the brain, resulting in brain damage (NINDS, 2001; Pelligrino, 1997).

Breech presentation, complicated labor and delivery, low birth weight, prematurity, low Apgar score, multiple births, late pregnancy complications (bleeding, proteinuria), and newborn seizures increase the possibility of cerebral palsy and long-term neurological problems (NINDS, 2001).

The symptoms of cerebral palsy vary widely (Table 33-1). Cerebral palsy may manifest in difficulty with fine motor skills, trouble with balance and walking, or uncontrollable body movements. Cerebral palsy is typically classified according to the type and severity of motor involvement children experience. The development and quality of movement patterns are affected by the location of brain damage or lesions (Miller & Clark, 1998).

TABLE 33-1. **CLASSIFICATION OF CEREBRAL PALSY**

Type	CNS Location	Muscle Tone and Movement
Spastic (hypertonic)	Motor cortex	Severity of tone and limb involvement varies among children; small, limited, midrange only
Athetoid (dyskinetic)	Basal ganglia	Tone fluctuates from low to high, child to child, and daily; rapid, random, and jerky movements or slow, writhing movements; difficulty with fixation; uses asymmetry to stabilize
Ataxia	Cerebellum	Tone low to normal; difficulty with voluntary movement for balance and control of trunk, head, and limbs

Children with cerebral palsy are at risk for the development of contractures and deformities over time. These deformities result from abnormalities in movement and muscle tone combined with the influences of body growth and gravity. Adults with cerebral palsy often find that the normal aging process leads to increased problems with performance and increased wear on joints, resulting in arthritic discomfort (Granet, Balaghi & Jaeger, 1997).

Language and other cognitive deficits often complicate development for 50–75% of children with cerebral palsy (NINDS, 2001). Approximately 35% of children with cerebral palsy have impaired speech and language. In addition to receptive problems, these children often have difficulty producing understandable speech, because of impaired tongue, lip, and respiratory movements (Pelligrino, 1997).

Eating problems are also associated with abnormal oral motor abilities. Children with cerebral palsy often have oral sensory disturbances, which result in hypersensitivity or hyposensitivity around and in the mouth. The infant with cerebral palsy may never develop the quality of sucking, swallowing, and chewing that promotes adequate nutritional intake. Often dietary supplements and specific eating techniques must be used. Children with cerebral palsy are commonly diagnosed with failure to thrive syndrome, owing to the combination of poor nutrition and damage to the brain centers that control growth and development (NINDS, 2001).

In addition to oral motor sensory disturbances, children with cerebral palsy may experience disturbances in other sensory systems. Nearly 25% of children with cerebral palsy have hearing loss for which hearing aides are required. Auditory perception can also be a problem. Visual deficits can include impaired acuity; limitations in tracking, movement, and coordination; and strabismus. Visual perceptual limitations are also common. Up to 50% of children with cerebral palsy have visual deficits (Pelligrino, 1997).

Children with cerebral palsy are at risk for psychosocial and behavioral problems and may experience isolation from peers because of their motor, cognitive, and sensory differences. Emotional support, socialization, and behavior management are often important for these children and their caretakers (NINDS, 2001).

Medical Intervention

Medical management of the tonal problems experienced by children with cerebral palsy includes medications for spasticity, rigidity, and choreoathetosis, although medications are not universally effective (Pranzatelli, 1996). Medications such as diazepam (relaxant), baclofen (CNS inhibitor), and dantrolene (calcium channel blocker) can reduce spasticity or rigidity for some children for short periods of time (Pelligrino, 1997). The side effects of some of these medications (e.g., drowsiness, nausea, headache, decreased blood pressure) may outweigh the benefits; therefore, medical management of tonal problems requires careful monitoring.

Nerve and motor point blocks are used to target spasticity in specific muscle groups (Koman, Mooney, & Smith, 1996). Nerve blocks carry the risk of damaging sensory nerve fibers that are bundled with motor fibers. Motor point blocks interrupt the nerve supply without damaging sensory fibers. Inhibition of spasticity using these techniques can last for several months, and the procedure can be repeated when the effect wears off. Often these blocking techniques are used to allow children to participate more fully in therapy and to postpone orthopedic surgery (NINDS, 2001).

Surgical intervention for children with cerebral palsy is of two types: neurosurgery and orthopedic surgery. The most accepted neurosurgical procedure is selective dorsal rhizotomy, which interrupts the overactive stretch reflex responsible for spasticity by cutting the afferent fibers that supply the muscles. Another neurosurgical procedure is implantation of a medical pump to deliver antispasticity medications directly into the spinal fluid to inhibit motor nerve conductivity. The long-term effects of this treatment are unknown. Since the pump is placed in the abdomen or lumbar spine, there are risks of mechanical failure and secondary medical problems (Miller & Clark, 1998; Pelligrino, 1997).

The purpose of orthopedic surgeries is to correct or prevent joint deformities. Deformities commonly occur from shortening or contracture of one or more groups of muscles around a joint. Surgery increases the joint ROM in one of three ways: by lengthening a tendon, by releasing (cutting through) a muscle or tendon, or by moving the point at which the tendon attaches to the bone. None of these procedures changes the primary problem of muscle tone, so repeated surgeries are often necessary. Children with cerebral palsy often have hip dislocations and scoliosis that may also require surgical intervention.

Specific Considerations for Occupational Therapy

Occupational therapy for children with cerebral palsy typically begins in the first few months after diagnosis is made, often in the first few months of life. Occupational therapy evaluations of children with cerebral palsy constitute an ongoing, fluid process that uses neurodevelopment and occupation frames of reference. Outcomes of initial evaluations include in-depth profiles of the occupations that are meaningful to children and their primary caretakers (Stewart, 2001).

Intervention

A primary intervention approach used by occupational therapists for children with cerebral palsy is **neurodevelopmental treatment** (NDT) (Figs. 33-3 and 33-4). This approach is designed to provide children with sensory motor experiences that enhance the development of normal movement patterns (Bobath, 1980; see also Chapter 20, Section 2). Using the motor learning and skills acquisition approaches, occupational therapy practitioners use activities from children's daily routines to provide learning opportunities that are meaningful to both children and caregivers.

Occupational therapy practitioners use a rehabilitation approach to prevent deformities and contractures. Splinting

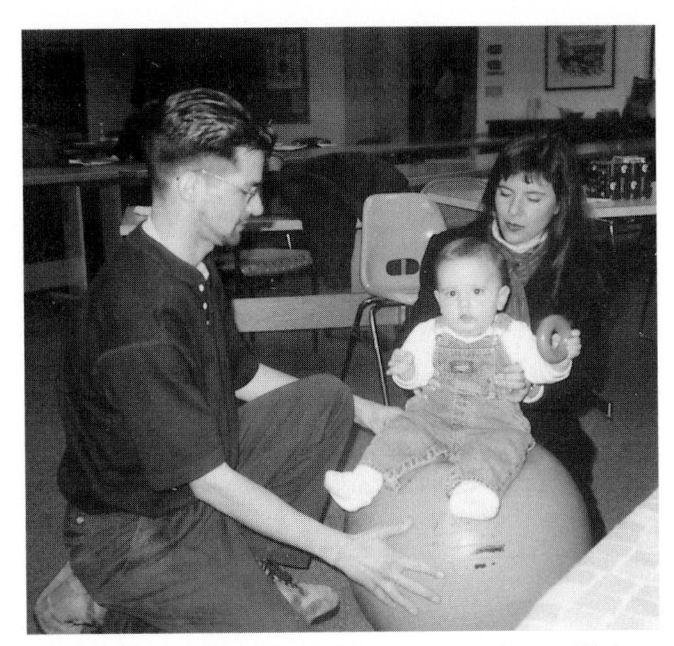

FIGURE 33–3. Sitting on a therapeutic ball requires equilibrium and balance.

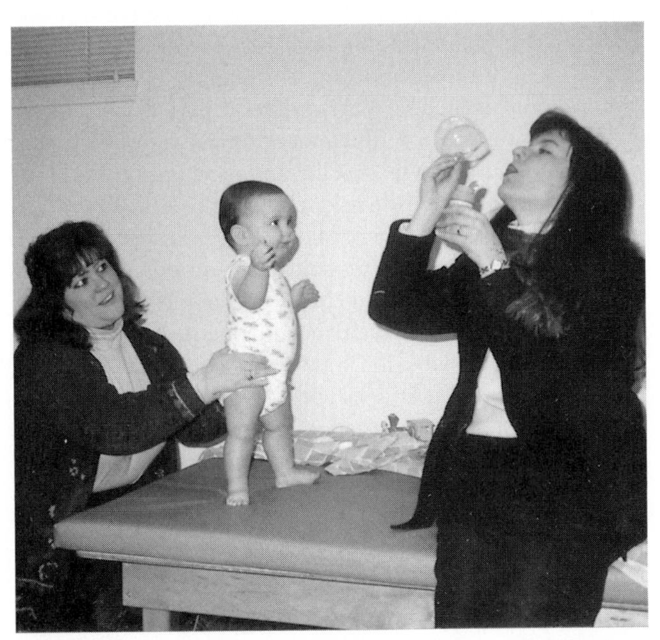

FIGURE 33–4. A practitioner provides support to a child while his mother engages him with bubbles.

and other orthopedic techniques in combination with positioning during activity are vital to the maintenance of ROM. Applying the principles of positioning to identify positions that promote participation in activities while supporting the child in ways that minimize the influences of pathological forces on the body is essential. Team members, including caregivers, develop positioning programs to ensure that recommended techniques are also compatible with established home and school routines and schedules (Dudgeon, 2001).

Occupational therapy practitioners also adapt the environment to enhance performance. Low technology can help children with cerebral palsy compensate for limitations in movement, balance, cognition, and communication. For example, a laptray on a wheelchair may help a child complete classroom activities.

Since the 1980s, high-technology has become increasingly important in most people's daily lives (Anson, 1997). From simple switches to complex robotics, high-technology provides unique opportunities for enhancing the lives of individuals with cerebral palsy. These technologies can enable children with limited motor control to have wonderful opportunities that otherwise might not be possible (Swinth & Case-Smith, 1993).

Self-Care

Therapy practitioners help parents understand atypical movement patterns and develop handling skills as part of their daily interactions with their children. Because managing self-care activities can be especially difficult for families, practitioners set up routines that are feasible for the family and that incorporate therapeutic goals.

Eating is an important social and emotional activity for families and in the larger society. The motor control and oral motor problems of children with cerebral palsy often make eating difficult and time-consuming. Common oral motor problems include increased or decreased muscle tone around mouth, poor coordination of tongue movement, and poor coordination of the swallowing mechanism. Early intervention can reduce the risk of long-term eating disorders, such as rejection of some or all foods or textures, failure to thrive, and strained parent–child interactions concerning food and eating (Humphrey, 1991; Logemann, 1983).

A broad range of adaptive equipment, typically low-technology, is available for those whose upper extremity and oral motor dysfunction does not allow them to put food in their mouths. A wide variety of dishes, bottles, cups, and spoons as well as more sophisticated food systems, when used properly, can promote active participation in eating and proper positioning for safety.

Hygiene includes bathing, toileting, and grooming. Examples of bathing aids that promote motor control are portable devices, bathtub and shower seats, and chairs and hydraulic lifts. For example, lightweight, portable bath chairs that provide head and trunk support and have suction cups on the legs for stability in the tub or shower can be useful for children with dyskinetic or ataxic cerebral palsy. Practical low-technology materials with suggestions for bathing children should be individualized and taught to caregivers by occupational therapy practitioners. For instance, children with poor hand control may be able to wash themselves using a bath mitt rather than a washcloth.

Many children with cerebral palsy are incontinent and remain so throughout their lives. Other children either can participate in a scheduled toileting program or be independently trained. Occupational therapy practitioners create toileting programs, such as devising schedules and recommending equipment. Adapted seats and chairs that provide motor control and comfort can make toileting easier and more effective.

Dressing activities provide a perfect opportunity for motor learning and skill acquisition. NDT handling principles—such as supporting the pelvis to promote the ability to reach upward to put an arm into a sleeve or downward to pull on socks—are particularly helpful for dressing. Occupational therapy practitioners also make recommendations for adapted clothing that make dressing easier, such as elastic shoelaces, pants with elastic waistbands, and pullover shirts.

Play

Children with cerebral palsy are often unable to participate in play experiences that promote development of motor control (Fig. 33-5). Barriers to adequate play include limitations imposed by caregivers who fear injury; physical limitations of children, which hinder exploratory play; environmental barriers at home, school and the community; and social barriers (Bundy, 1997; Morrison & Metzger, 2001; Pierce, 2000). Occupational therapy practitioners

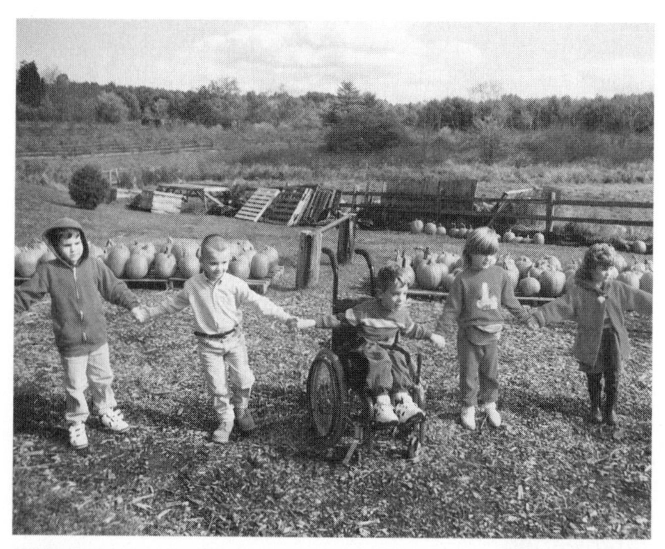

FIGURE 33–5. A child uses a wheelchair to participate with classmates during a preschool field trip. (Courtesy of L. McIntosh, Dover, NH)

can influence environmental and social barriers by evaluating school playgrounds and community buildings and making recommendations that allow access for children with cerebral palsy. Practitioners serve as advocates by teaching people in the community about the importance of inclusion of all children and by demonstrating the ways in which children with cerebral palsy can participate in social play.

By integrating NDT, motor control approaches, and assistive technology into play, therapy practitioners promote interaction with the environment and mastery of new skills. Children are given opportunities to develop risk-taking, problem-solving, and decision-making abilities (Reilly, 1974). Children absorbed in play are not focused on the specific motor demands of the activity and can be stimulated to use more appropriate movement to improve head, trunk, and extremity control. Practitioners' activity analysis skills are used continually to adapt the size, shape, or consistency of materials; the rules and procedures; the positions of children and materials; and the nature and degree of social interaction.

Orthotics

Orthotics may be considered part of the occupational therapy programs for children with neuromusculoskeletal deficits, such as ROM limitations (soft tissue integrity). The purpose of orthotics is to maintain (often postsurgically) joint position and integrity. The variety of thermoplastic materials used to fabricate customized orthotics provides many options for upper and lower extremities, as well as the trunk.

Soft splints, the least cumbersome and restrictive devices, can be constructed from neoprene, webbing, and hook-and-loop fastener material. These splints do not limit mobility and sensory input as much as thermoplastics. For children with moderate degrees of spasticity, stronger, molded thermoplastics materials are necessary to prevent contractures. Ankle–foot orthoses (AFO) and shoe inserts provide stability during standing and ambulating and are typically fabricated by physical therapists or orthotists. Spinal orthoses and seating orthoses can be used to support spinal curvatures such as scoliosis, kyphosis, and lordosis.

Practitioners have also found upper extremity casting—which provides prolonged, gentle stretching of spastic or contracted muscles—to be an effective adjunct to therapy. Casts position the extremity so that spastic muscles are lengthened. When children have contractures, casts are often applied serially to allow children to increase ROM gradually. Once maximal range and position have been gained, the cast is worn periodically to maintain the position. There is evidence that serial inhibitory casting improves hand use in children with cerebral palsy (Smelt, 1989; Yasukawa, 1990).

The central role of occupational therapy intervention for children with cerebral palsy is to facilitate their participation in meaningful occupations. Occupational therapy practitioners, using any or all of the methods described in this section, promote children's involvement in all the environments in which they live. When children participate in the world around them, they develop physically, socially, and cognitively and gain an understanding of their talents and abilities (Fig. 33-6).

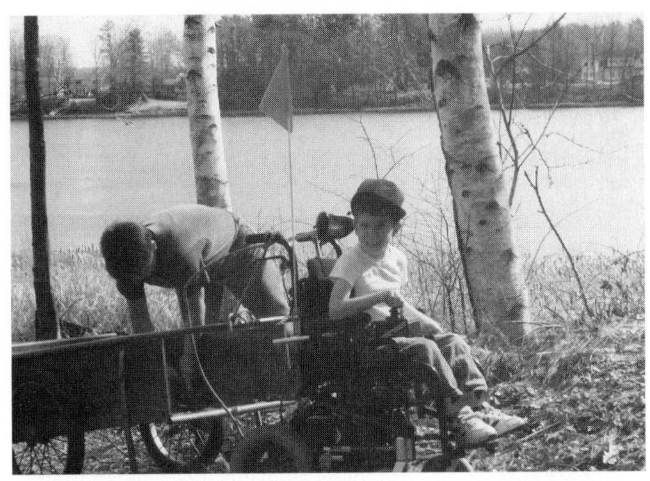

FIGURE 33–6. A child uses his powered wheelchair to pull a garden cart to help his mother with yard work. (Courtesy of L. McIntosh, Dover, NH)

LEARNING DISABILITIES AND ATTENTION DEFICIT-HYPERACTIVITY DISORDER

The term **learning disability** is used to describe a number of deficits related to interpreting visual or auditory information and/or the ability to link information from different parts of the brain. Such limitations may include problems with written and spoken language, motor coordination, and/or the ability to attend and concentrate. These impairments impede academic performance in areas such as reading, writing, and math (National Institute of Mental Health [NIMH], 1999). The *Diagnostic and Statistical Manual of Mental Disorders* (4th edition; American Psychiatric Association [APA], 1994) includes diagnostic criteria for a number of specific learning disorders, such as reading disorder and math disorder.

Most children with learning disabilities have average to above-average intelligence. They typically have a discrepancy between their cognitive abilities (as measured by IQ testing) and their academic performance (achievement in math, writing, or reading) that cannot be explained by environmental conditions, sensory impairments (visual or hearing loss), or other neurological diagnoses, such as traumatic brain injury. It is estimated that 4–5% of school-aged children have learning disabilities and that boys are more commonly affected than girls (4:1 ratio) (Church, Lewis, &

CASE STUDY 33-1

Sam: A Boy with Cerebral Palsy

Sam is a 10-year-old with cerebral palsy spastic diplegia. He was born 3½ months early and weighed 2 lb at birth. Sam received occupational and physical therapy periodically from 5 months of age. He had several surgeries and procedures to reduce muscle tone in his legs, including a selective posterior rhizotomy at age 4; *Botox* and phenol injections to his hip adductors; and orthopedic surgery to lengthen his adductors, heel cords, and hamstring tendons at age 6. At the time of this occupational therapy evaluation, he is receiving weekly physical therapy at home to address mobility and gross motor skills and consultative occupational therapy at school.

Sam lives at home with his parents and 14-year-old brother. His father is a computer consultant, and his mother is a nurse. His family members promote his independence at home and encourage and support his participation in family and community activities. Sam has average intelligence, but learning disabilities affect his math skills and memory. He is in a regular fourth grade class but receives help from the resource room teacher for math and from a classroom aide whenever necessary.

Sam was evaluated by the school occupational therapist in the spring as part of his 3-year evaluation, along with assessments by a regular educator, a special educator, a psychologist, and a physical therapist. This interdisciplinary evaluation was conducted to identify his levels of performance in school-related activities and to identify his educational programming needs. The next school year, he will attend the middle school.

The middle school environment is evaluated to determine accessibility issues (cafeteria, gym, classroom, lockers, outside areas) and to understand curriculum and fifth-grade program expectations. Interviews are conducted with Sam's current teacher and next year's teacher and with Sam and his parents to determine each person's priorities and concerns. Because Sam has special technology needs, an evaluation his of current technology and of his projected needs in the future is also conducted.

Sam's occupational therapy evaluation considers the educational system and setting and use of occupational, rehabilitation, and neurodevelopmental frames of references. The SFA is used to evaluate his performance in educationally relevant school activities (Coster, Deeney, Haltiwanger, & Haley, 1998). A co-evaluation with the physical therapist and parents is completed to examine wheelchair mobility, transfers, seating and positioning needs; toilet transfers, and ambulation with walker. Observations of other skills, such as eating and dressing, classroom behavior while sitting, computer use, and participation during group activities are made. Neuromuscular evaluation includes assessing Sam's upper extremity use, ROM, tone, coordination, strength, and postural control.

The evaluation reveals that Sam needs supervision when using his walker and with transfers, although he is able to move around the school and outside in his power wheelchair. Sam is able to dress his upper body independently, but needs help with managing his leg braces, shoes, and pulling up his pants. In the bathroom, Sam transfers out of his wheelchair or walker and grasps the bars on the toilet. He needs help pulling his pants down and up again, because he cannot let go of the bars without falling. He is able to wash his face and hands without assistance by leaning on the sink for balance. He is independent in the lunchroom, although he is slow to finish eating and occasionally requires help opening packages. His problems are largely the result of increased tone in his upper and lower extremities (there is significantly more involvement in the lower extremities and on the left side), poor balance and trunk control, and decreased upper extremity coordination.

In the classroom, Sam's aide often retrieves books and other items for him and helps him get things from his backpack. His aide takes dictation for most of his written assignments and does all writing for math. Sam often requires hands-on help with manipulatives during math and science activities.

Sam uses an IBM-compatible computer at home and at school and has good mouse control with his right hand. He types on a regular keyboard, although slowly (one key every 3 sec). He has deficits in visual tracking and convergence, but reads large-print materials adequately. Sam's speech is clear, although he speaks slowly. His mother and teacher feel it is important for Sam to become less reliant on his classroom aide. His teacher notes that he does much more for himself when his aide is absent.

Evaluation of the middle school indicates that Sam will have different teachers for each subject. Students keep their belongings in lockers with combination locks. The curriculum includes math, English, science, social studies, and health education. Fifth grade emphasizes working from outlines and writing research papers and includes more science experiences than in the lower grades.

Sam's parents would like Sam to be more independent in both academic and leisure activities and hope

Continues

that technology will address Sam's writing problems so that he can write independently. They would like Sam to become involved in more extracurricular activities and with peers, such as joining the drama club.

Sam likes computers and video games and being with friends and engaging in adapted skiing, swimming, and boating with his family. He is a social child who loves to tell jokes and be with his peers. He has a lot of friends at school but rarely gets invited to other children's homes. Occasionally, he has a friend over to play. Sam is in a club for children who use wheelchairs, and he enjoys the meetings, special trips, and sleep overs.

Based on this occupational therapy evaluation, it is recommended that Sam receive direct occupational therapy intervention to assist with his transition to middle school. Occupational therapy services assist in promoting independence and safety with mobility and self-care activities at school, particularly around accessing his belongings, managing his locker, moving safely around the school, and dressing and toileting. Because it has been determined that Sam's neuromuscular skills and abilities have plateaued, compensatory approaches are more appropriate than remedial ones.

Adapted devices and technology are suggested to increase his independence in school-related activities and to promote his participation in extracurricular and social activities. For example, a laptop computer with a voice synthesizer program is suggested to address his writing needs. By promoting his independence, Sam will require less time with a teacher's aide, which will also enhance his peer relationships and opportunities for socialization in privacy from adults.

Coster, W., Deeney, T., Haltiwanger, J., & Haley, S. (1998). *School function assessment (SFA)*. San Antonio, TX: Psychological Corporation.

Batshaw, 1997). Educational psychologists or neuropsychologists typically diagnose these disorders once children reach school age.

The causes of learning disability are largely unknown. However, evidence suggests a neurological origin that results in atypical integration of information from various brain areas. Learning disabilities are known to a have a genetic component, so that children are more likely to have learning disabilities if one of their parents, siblings, or close relatives is affected. Errors in fetal development, smoking and drug use by the mother during pregnancy, problems during pregnancy and delivery (e.g., prematurity), and toxins in the child's environment may increase his or her vulnerability to learning disorders (NIMH, 1999).

Learning disabilities often co-exist (about 20% of the time) with **attention deficit hyperactivity disorder** (NIMH, 1999), and both of these conditions are often associated with sensory integration dysfunction (Mulligan, 1996, 1998). Attention deficit hyperactivity disorder (ADHD) is the most frequently diagnosed neurobehavioral disorder in childhood, with prevalence estimates of 5–10% (Castellanos, 1997). Diagnostic criteria for ADHD provided in the *Diagnostic and Statistical Manual of Mental Disorders* (APA, 1994), suggest three hallmark features: inattention, impulsivity, and hyperactivity. Barkley (1997) described a somewhat different conceptual model of ADHD, emphasizing that it is primarily a deficit in behavioral inhibition, linked to problems with working memory, self-regulation, internalization of speech, and reconstitution of verbal and nonverbal behaviors.

Often children with learning disorders and ADHD experience academic and social problems that affect their relationships with their peers and family members, which may result in feelings of frustration and failure (Barkley, 1997). Although learning disorders and ADHD may be viewed as mild conditions, the long-term implications may be serious. Compared to their peers, these children are more likely to drop out of high school and have a higher risk of developing mental health problems in adulthood, including substance abuse, anxiety disorders, conduct disorders, depression, and suicide (Barkley, 1998). Interventions for children with ADHD commonly include the use of stimulant pharmacology (e.g., methylphenidate), behavioral interventions, and special education interventions.

Occupational therapy for children with ADHD and learning disability addresses co-existing physical or sensory integration concerns, such as motor planning, balance and coordination problems, and handwriting difficulties. Occupational therapy practitioners consider the effect that learning and attention problems have on children's ability to perform valued activities. Practitioners provide support to parents around behavior management and develop strategies to help parents help their children. Occupational therapy provides a unique service for these children, using occupation as the vehicle to promote health, and is one of the few disciplines that combine knowledge of psychological aspects of behavior and learning with sensory motor aspects. For example, intervention strategies that apply regular school activities for a young elementary school child who has a combination of motor coordination, attention, and learning problems may include the use of an air seat cushion to provide the child with subtle movement, a quiet work space or preferential seating away from distracting doors and windows to help the child focus, and permission for the child to stand for some seat work. Setting up fine and gross motor activity centers in the classroom provides ample opportunities for skill development in these areas. Handwriting accommodations, such as wide-lined paper with dark margins and a pencil grip, can be used to complete class assignments. School projects or assignments can incorporate the child's interests and be broken down into well-defined, small stages.

Like other areas of practice, the first step in the evaluation process of children with ADHD and/or learning disorders is to develop an occupational profile and to examine the children's ability to perform their everyday activities. Assessment tools such as the SFA (Coster et al., 1998) and naturalistic observations of functional activities and play are commonly helpful. Then the practitioner may take a closer look at child factors such as evaluations of sensory integration functions, visual perceptual skills, motor performance, behavior, and social skills. Some assessment tools commonly used by occupational therapists with this population include the following:

- Sensory Profile (Dunn, 1999).
- Sensory Integration and Praxis Tests (Ayres, 1989).
- Bruininks-Oseretsky Test of Motor Proficiency (Bruininks, 1978).
- Beery Test of Visual-Motor Integration (Beery, 1997).
- Test of Visual-Motor Skills—Revised (Gardner, 1995a).
- Test of Visual Perceptual Skills—Revised (Gardner, 1995b).
- Behavior Assessment System for Children (BASC; Reynolds & Kamphaus, 1992).
- Social Skills Rating System (Gresham & Elliot, 1990).

Skill-specific assessments, such as vocational and handwriting assessments, are also commonly used.

Depending on the child's identified strengths and challenges, intervention for this population typically includes techniques from **sensory integration,** motor learning and skill acquisition, rehabilitative, cognitive-behavioral approaches, and psychosocial approaches. Occupational therapy practitioners need to work closely with parents and teachers, because consistency of approaches and expectations are important to children's success across settings.

The role of occupational therapy for children who have learning and attention problems also depends somewhat on the child's age. With younger children, the focus may be on remediating sensory integration functions, motor, play, and self-help skills. With elementary school children, the focus may be on addressing visual perceptual skills, handwriting, and other important school-related tasks; process and communication/interaction skills; and compensating for and remediating sensory processing problems. For older children, occupational therapy practitioners may address vocational skills, study skills, community living, transition planning, and process and communication/interaction skills.

Consultative approaches are commonly used with children with learning disability and ADHD. Practitioners may assist teachers in developing environmental and curriculum modifications in the classroom to help minimize distractions and assist children in maintaining an optimal state for learning. A recent survey of elementary school teachers (Mulligan, 2001) found that simple environmental modifications, such as preferential seating, reducing the amount of visually distracting stimuli in the classroom, and using designated quiet work areas were helpful. Curriculum modifications were also identified as being helpful in enhancing student interest and attention, and the teachers emphasized classroom structure and routine as vital for promoting optimal behavior. Computer software such, as word-prediction programs, and keyboarding adaptations may be used to address writing needs.

Occupational therapy practitioners often help children with ADHD identify and use self-regulation strategies. For example, practitioners may develop a list of sensory-based activities (or a sensory diet) that helps children either increase or decrease their level of activity and help them stay focused. The Alert Program was designed by occupational therapists to help children become more aware of their states of arousal and to help them identify and use sensory-based strategies for maintaining optimal levels of alertness (Williams & Shellenberger, 1994).

Research evidence supporting the effectiveness of behavioral interventions for reducing the negative behaviors associated with ADHD is quite strong (Fiore, Becker, & Nero, 1993; MTA Cooperative Group, 1999). Behavioral strategies typically use contingencies, such as positive and negative reinforcement, to either increase or decrease the occurrence of targeted behaviors. Practitioners may assist others such as school psychologists to develop behavioral support plans for children with ADHD. Children with learning disability and/or ADHD may also benefit from assistance with developing social skills, peer relationships, and rewarding leisure activities.

PERVASIVE DEVELOPMENTAL DISORDERS, INCLUDING AUTISM

Pervasive developmental disorders (PDD) make up a group of conditions that share some general clinical features, in that they have their onset in early childhood and are associated with characteristic patterns of delay and qualitative differences that are pervasive across various domains of development. The most common of the pervasive developmental disorders are autism (see Chapter 36), Asperger syndrome, and pervasive developmental disorder not otherwise specified (PDD-NOS).

The sensory processing problems of children who have autism are well documented in occupational therapy literature (Ayres, & Tickle, 1980; Kientz & Dunn, 1997) and elsewhere (O'Neill & Jones, 1997). Children with autism often exhibit sensory registration and modulation difficulties. They may be capable of processing sensory information sometimes but not at other times and may be hyporesponsive or hyperresponsive to sensory stimuli (Ayres & Tickle, 1980; Kientz & Dunn, 1997).

The prognosis of children with autism is diverse, as is the range of severity. Some individuals live and work independently in the community, although they typically continue to experience difficulty with social skills and relationships. Others are fairly independent, needing only minimal support, and others may be totally dependent to manage even basic self-care needs. Prognosis as it relates to independent functioning appears to be closely related to intelligence and level of communication (Rogers et al., 2001).

The evaluation of children suspected of having autism is complex and requires an experienced team of professionals, including psychologists, pediatric neurologists, occupational therapy practitioners, and speech pathologists. The diagnosis is made based on observations of behavior rather than on specific medical tests. Although it is relatively uncommon for children to be diagnosed with autism before 3 years of age, current research indicates that a reliable diagnosis can be made before 18 months (Baron-Cohen et al., 1996). Children receiving early intervention services (by 3 years of age) have more positive functional and cognitive outcomes than children who receive services later; therefore, early intervention services are important for these children (Dawson & Osterling, 1997).

Occupational therapy evaluation of children with autism typically includes evaluation of structured and unstructured play and social skills, functional self-help skills, and evaluation of sensory-processing abilities and motor functions. Watling, Deitz, Kanny, and McLaughlin (1999) surveyed occupational therapy practitioners working with children with autism and reported the most common assessment tools and procedures as follows:

- Sensory profiles and sensory histories (Dunn, 1999).
- Self-care checklists (Rogers & D'Eugenio, 1981).
- Clinical observations (Ayres, 1981).
- Measures of motor performance.

Common frames of reference used with this population include sensory integration and other developmental and behavioral approaches. For example, an occupational therapy evaluation of a 3-year-old child suspected of having autism may entail motor testing with the Peabody Developmental Motor Scales (Folio & Fewell, 2000); clinical observations of play and interactions with peers and family members; and a structured parent interview set up specifically to gather detailed information about self-care skills, likes and dislikes, and sensory processing abilities. This evaluation would be considered along with evaluations from other team members, such as a pediatric neurologist, psychologist, and speech pathologist to make the diagnosis and to create collaboratively an appropriate intervention program.

A number of intervention approaches have been proposed for children with autism, although there is no agreement on the best method, and no method to date has been totally effective in treating autism. Generally, an interdisciplinary approach that combines behavioral intervention such as discrete trial training, special education, speech therapy, pharmacology, and family support interventions is commonly implemented (Mauk, Reber, & Batshaw, 1997). Occupational therapy practitioners may be involved in family support interventions and the development and delivery of special education programs. They may also provide direct services using sensory integration techniques for children with sensory modulation problems, and dyspraxia or other sensory motor deficits. It is important for occupational therapy practitioners to work closely with parents and other professionals to ensure consistency in the ways in which challenging behaviors are managed and in the use of strategies for promoting social communication and language and to be sure that all child and family goals are being addressed.

DEVELOPMENTAL DISABILITIES

Developmental disability (DD) is the term used to indicate atypical neurodevelopment that is not specific to one body system (Brown & Elksnin, 1994). Onset of DD can be prenatal, perinatal, or early childhood. Children with DD fail to achieve age-appropriate milestones. In the first months of life, inadequate sucking response, floppy or increased muscle tone, and/or lack of visual or auditory responsiveness often indicate DD. Later, motor delays in sitting and walking and absent or delayed language often suggest DD. Children with significant delays in all developmental spheres are usually diagnosed with mental retardation (Batshaw & Shapiro, 1997). Isolated mild delays in expressive language or motor abilities may resolve over time and are not considered developmental disabilities. They may, however, indicate that children are at risk for learning disabilities and that will become obvious when they are school aged. Although there are many causes of DD, the most common are **Down syndrome** and **fragile X.**

Down Syndrome

Down syndrome is the most common diagnosable form of DD. Down syndrome is one of several trisomy disorders, resulting from an excess of chromosomal material (Roizen, 1997). Down syndrome results from an additional chromosome 21 and is found in about 1 in 1000 births. More than half of all children with Down syndrome are male (March of Dimes, 2001).

The physical features of children with Down syndrome include a short, stocky stature with a small head and flattening of the back and of the face. The nose is recessed, and there is an upward slant to the eyes with epicanthal folds at the inner corners. The ears and mouth are small, as are the hands and feet. A simian crease in the palms is characteristic

(Roizen, 1997). While children with Down syndrome have been stereotyped as being amiable and happy, studies have shown their emotional profiles to be similar to typically developing children (Vaughn, Contreras, & Seifer, 1994).

Children with Down syndrome have an increased risk of abnormalities in almost every organ system. The most common complications are congenital heart disease, vision and hearing problems, congenital hypothyroidism, orthopedic problems (including atlantoaxial instability and hip dislocation) caused by ligamentous abnormalities, dental abnormalities, gastrointestinal malformations, seizures, and dermatological conditions (Roizen, 1997).

Children with Down syndrome have developmental disabilities in performance skills that support occupational performance, including deficits with communication and interaction and with motor and process skills. These children often have significant language delays, especially in expressive language. Coping skills and understanding the rules of social interaction are also delayed for children with Down syndrome. These children typically have generalized hypotonia that affects the achievement of motor milestones. Although gross motor development is affected, significant physical disabilities are uncommon.

Cognitive disabilities vary widely, but most often mental retardation is in the mild-to-moderate range. In the first 2 years of life, children with Down syndrome, because of social responsiveness may appear to have less cognitive impairment than actually exists. Visual motor skills may be a strength for children with Down syndrome. Adolescents with Down syndrome may demonstrate deterioration in cognitive or psychological functioning because of undiagnosed hyperthyroidism or depression. Medical intervention is effective in managing these problems.

Early intervention is important for children with Down syndrome. Occupational therapy practitioners in early intervention and school-based settings focus on sensory motor, cognitive, and communication/interaction skills and these children's ability to engage in meaningful occupations. With older children, the role of occupational therapy focuses on supporting community participation, including the development of vocational and life skills and building support networks.

Fragile X

Fragile X is the most common inherited cause of developmental disability (FraXa Research Foundation [FraXa], n.d.). Studies suggest that fragile X affects 1 in 2000 males and 1 in 4000 females of all races and ethnic groups (Bailey & Nelson, 1995). Fragile X is an X-linked disorder that is carried by 1 in 259 women. It affects the production of the protein FMRA, which is essential to early fetal brain development. The absence of FMRA appears to delay the development of neurons, rather than damage them (FraXa, n.d.).

Boys demonstrate a pattern of impairments; girls typically demonstrate less severe symptoms (Batshaw, 1997). A hallmark of fragile X is physical appearance. Boys have a characteristically elongated face with prominent jaw and forehead and protruding ears. Behavioral manifestations include mental retardation, vision problems (e.g., strabismus), communication disorders, hyperactivity, self-stimulatory behaviors, and impulsivity. For girls, the pattern of impairment includes learning disability, mild mental retardation, abnormal speech patterns, and emotional outbursts.

A reliable diagnostic test for fragile X became available in 1992 (FraXa, n.d.). This DNA-based blood test can detect both carriers and fully affected individuals and is being used more often for children with unexplained developmental delay or mental retardation. Experts have determined that 80–90% of people with fragile X are not yet correctly diagnosed.

There is no cure for fragile X syndrome and the long-term outcome is not known. Specialists agree that special education, behavioral management, social and life skills training, and pharmacotherapy can improve the quality of life for people with fragile X and their caregivers (Batshaw, 1997; FraXa, n.d.).

The occupational performance of children with fragile X shows persistent delays in self-care, school-related activities, and play because of the presence of stereotypic behaviors, poor eye contact, unusual sensory stimuli responses, and lack of social skills. Practitioners use remediation approaches (e.g., sensory integration) and compensation/adaptation approaches (e.g., cues and environmental modifications) in intervention programs with children who have this syndrome.

Occupational therapy practitioners have an important contribution to make to the transition of youths with developmental disabilities to adult roles, activities, and environments. Effective transitional services are characterized by collaborations that involve the student, family, and educational team and vocational, residential, and recreational adult service agencies.

ALCOHOL AND DRUG EXPOSURE

Fetal Alcohol Syndrome

Alcohol consumption during pregnancy is estimated to be the third leading cause of birth defects and a leading cause of developmental disability (Batshaw & Conlon, 1997). Alcohol is one of many teratogenic substances (such as aspirin, cortisone, caffeine, heroin, LSD, Dilantin, and tetracycline) that can cause a wide range of congenital defects. The effects of alcohol are generally categorized by severity: The term *fetal alcohol syndrome* (FAS) indicates severe developmental and physical problems that are often identifiable at birth, and the term *fetal alcohol effects* (FAE) indicates more subtle problems that may go undetected until children are school aged. At least 1200 children each year are born with FAS, and even more are born with FAE. Several factors contribute to the extent of fetal damage that occurs, including the level of fetal development at the time of alcohol consumption, the amount and duration of alcohol consumption, the nutritional status and overall health of the mother, and whether other substances were used during pregnancy (Jacobson, 1998).

Criteria for the diagnosis of FAS are prenatal and postnatal growth retardation, CNS abnormalities, and craniofacial malformations. While children with FAS are not typically born prematurely, nearly 80% have low birth weights. During infancy, up to 70% have severe feeding problems, often leading to failure to thrive. Children with FAS remain short and thin throughout childhood but may be of normal height and weight by adulthood (Batshaw & Conlon, 1997).

The characteristic craniofacial features of children with FAS are microcephaly; widely spaced eyes with shortened eye slits; short, upturned noses; and thin upper lips with a flattened philtrum. In addition, 20–50% of children with FAS may have some combination of ventricular septal defect, hemangiomas, and genitourinary malformations. Children with FAS may have vision problems such as nystagmus, astigmatism, strabismus, and myopia.

Developmental disabilities become evident as the infant moves through toddlerhood. Children with FAS are often hypotonic, affecting gross and fine motor development and language development. The school-aged child with FAS may demonstrate subtle fine motor incoordination and clumsiness. IQ tests of children with FAS typically fall in the mentally retarded to low average range. Most children with FAS demonstrate behavioral and emotional problems, such as poor judgment, oppositional behavior, inappropriate responses to social cues, social withdrawal, lability, and anxiety that affect their functioning in school and home environments (Alaska Health and Social Services Online, n.d.).

Children with more mild intellectual and behavioral impairments and who do not have craniofacial malformations are categorized as having FAE. These children are typically in the borderline to average range of intelligence. Children with FAE may demonstrate subtle impairments in memory, fine motor skills, and language.

Obviously, the prognosis for children with FAS and FAE depends greatly on the extent of the malformations and developmental disabilities. The occupational performance of children with FAE and FAS shows persistent delays in self-care, school-related activities, and play. The skills and abilities on which intervention typically focuses are physical, cognitive, and social-emotional. In addition, practitioners must be aware of the multiple psychosocial issues that often exist within families of children with FAS and FAE and involve the entire family in intervention programs.

Cocaine Exposure

Cocaine is a CNS stimulant that affects brain chemistry by blocking neurotransmitter uptake and thereby increasing neurotransmitter blood levels. Users of cocaine experience a short-term heightening of their body's natural responses. Each of the neurotransmitters contributes to these effects differently: Norepinephrine causes vasoconstriction, which increases heart rate, blood pressure, and feelings of euphoria; dopamine increases activity levels and sexual arousal; and serotonin decreases appetite and the need for sleep. While cocaine is not physically addictive, users develop a strong psychological dependence.

The effects of maternal cocaine use on fetal and infant development have been difficult to measure, and there is controversy about the quality of the research that has been done (Hyde & Trautman, 1989; Lindesmith Center, 2001). Experts agree, however, that the use of cocaine during pregnancy has the potential to interfere with fetal and child development (Batshaw & Conlon, 1997; Lindesmith Center, 2001).

For the fetus, increased maternal levels of norepinephrine may have serious consequences for development. Vasoconstriction decreases the placental blood supply, which can compromise fetal nutrition and/or lead to fetal hypoxemia. These fetal problems put the newborn at risk. Often neonates demonstrate withdrawal symptoms for several days after birth. Symptoms include irritability, restlessness, lethargy, poor feeding, abnormal sleep patterns, tremors, and increased muscle tone (Doberczak, Shanzer, Senie, & Kandall, 1988).

Some studies suggested that infants may continue to have neurobehavioral irregularities for several months, including mood and sleep disturbances, feeding problems, decreased attention, and interactive responsiveness (Arendt, Minnes, & Singer, 1996; Batshaw & Conlon, 1997; Howard & Beckwith , 1989). Infants who have been exposed to cocaine during fetal development may have a low threshold for overstimulation and be irritable. Even when these irregularities are temporary, they may be markers for later learning disabilities or attention problems.

The prognosis for children exposed to cocaine in utero depends greatly on the extent of the CNS involvement and developmental disabilities. The occupational performance of these children demonstrates variable performance in self-care, school-related activities, and play (Lane, 1992, 1996; Rose-Jacobs, Rank, & Brown, 1996). Intervention typically focuses on sensory motor, process, and communication/interaction skills. Effective intervention programs address the needs of the child, the mother, and the high-risk family as a unit. Often these mothers and families lack the necessary skills to meet the needs of children who have poor state control, irritability, and inconsistent social responsiveness.

NEURAL TUBE DEFECTS AND SPINA BIFIDA

Neural tube defects (NTD) are serious birth defects that involve incomplete development of the brain, spinal cord, and/or protective coverings for these organs. There are three types of NTD: anencephaly, encephalocele, and **spina bifida.** Infants born with anencephaly have no neural development above the brainstem and do not survive more than a few hours. Encephalocele is characterized by a hole in the skull through which brain tissue protrudes. Children with encephalocele who survive infancy have severe deficits, including mental retardation, **hydrocephalus,** motor impairments, and seizures (Liptak, 1997).

Spina bifida results from the congenital failure of the spine to close properly during the first month of pregnancy. Spina bifida affects about 1 in 1000 newborns in the United States (Spina Bifida Association of America, 2002). A range in the severity of the defect exists. In mild forms, the laminae of only a few vertebrae are affected, and there are no malformations of the spinal cord. More severe forms involve an extensive opening with a pouch made of up cerebrospinal fluid and the meninges (meningocele). In the most severe cases, cerebrospinal fluid, meninges, and nerve roots are all exposed (myelomeningocele).

While the specific cause of spina bifida is not known, hereditary, intrauterine, and environmental factors have all been associated with the condition. Research suggests that a combination of heredity and folic acid deficiency may account for up to half of all cases (Liptak, 1997). Spina bifida can be identified after the first month of pregnancy by amniocentesis.

The extent of motor and sensory impairment depends on the location and degree of the spinal cord defect (Table 33-2). The continuum of impairment ranges from no functional deficits, to mild muscle imbalances and sensory losses, to paraplegia and even death. Sensory and motor functions below the level of the spinal defect are impaired.

Hydrocephalus is the result of an accumulation of cerebrospinal fluid in the brain ventricles. This happens when there is an imbalance between the amount of cerebrospinal fluid produced and the amount absorbed. This imbalance is most often caused by malformations of the ventricles that obstruct the flow of fluid, although tumors can also cause hydrocephalus (Liptak, 1997). An enlarged head is an early sign of hydrocephalus in infants. After the skull has fused in older children, intracranial pressure increases. Clinical signs of hydrocephalus in infants include bulging fontanels, dilated scalp veins, separated sutures, eyes that appear to deviate downward (sun-setting appearance of the iris). Irritability; lethargy; and problems with reflexes, feeding, and tone are also common symptoms. Older children may have headaches, nystagmus, or strabismus and cognitive changes (Johnson, 1997).

The pressure of the cerebrospinal fluid on the brain may cause visual and perceptual deficits, cognitive disability, seizures, and even death. Surgical removal of obstructions is necessary. More typically, hydrocephalus is controlled by a surgically placed ventriculoperitoneal shunt, which relieves the fluid by redirecting it into the abdominal cavity where it can be absorbed (Liptak, 1997). These shunts are effective but must be carefully monitored for infection, clogging, and tube migration.

Children with neural tube defects may have perceptual and sensory processing problems. Dyspraxia and/or visual perceptual impairment contribute to fine motor difficulties (Rogers et al., 2001). Medical management for these children includes surgery for deformity repair or for shunt implantation and urologic management (Liptak, 1997). Orthotic adaptations such as bracing, casting, and assistive devices for ambulating are common. Family education in skin care, bowel and bladder programs, and diet are often essential.

Children with neural tube defects have difficulties with many areas of occupational performance. The challenges for participation increase as these children move toward adulthood. For example, mobility may not become an important issue until the middle and high school years when children move toward independence from family and are increasingly motivated to be in peer groups. Similarly, as children move through adolescence, independent management of time, school materials, and assignments becomes expected and, therefore, pressing issues. Occupational therapy practitioners assist with transition planning as adolescents with neural tube defects plan for and move into adult roles and responsibilities. Environmental adaptations using both low- and high-technology are often crucial to their occupational performance and full participation in their communities.

TABLE 33-2. **SPINA BIFIDA LEVELS**

Level of Spinal Lesion	Resultant Sensory Motor Impairments
Thoracic or high lumbar	Variable weakness and sensory loss from the abdomen distally
L3	Paralysis of ankles and feet; hip flexion and knee extension
L4 or L5	Weak or absent foot flexion and hip extension; hip flexion and knee and ankle extension
Sacral	Mild weakness of ankles and feet

ACQUIRED CONDITIONS

Pediatric Spinal Cord Injury

Injuries to the spinal column and spinal cord of children have received increasing attention since the 1980s (Brockmeyer, n.d.). While much has been learned over the years, information about basic differences between injuries to children and adults remains incomplete. While less frequent than spinal trauma in other age groups, pediatric spinal injuries do occur. A reasonable estimate is that 5% of all spinal traumas happen to children between birth and 16 years of age (Brockmeyer, n.d.).

There are significant biomechanical and anatomical differences between pediatric and adult spines. These differences explain the different injury patterns seen among age groups. The infant spine (0–2 years of age) is tremendously elastic and mobile because of incomplete calcification of vertebrae and underdevelopment of neck musculature. The large head size relative to the trunk and limbs increases the likelihood of injuries between the skull and first cervical vertebrae. The mobility of the infant spine explains the relatively low incidence of spinal column injuries; the young spine tends to stretch and not break. This, however, places the spinal cord at increased risk for stretch injuries (Brockmeyer, n.d.).

Between 2 and 10 years, tremendous changes occur in the spinal column. Muscles and ligaments strengthen, bones grow and reach a mature shape and size, and soft bone and cartilage are replaced by calcified bone. The proportion of head size to trunk changes. Because of these changes, children in this age range are more susceptible to lower cervical injuries (C5 to C6). Age-related maturation appears to be complete for the upper cervical spine by about the age of 10; while maturation of the lower cervical spine occurs somewhere around the age of 14 years (Brockmeyer, n.d.).

Mechanisms of injury also vary by age. Spinal injury caused by birth-related trauma is probably underdiagnosed. In the youngest age group (0–10 years), falls and pedestrian and automobile accidents are the most frequent causes for injury. For children between 10 and 16 years, sports-related injuries and motor vehicle accidents are the primary causes (Brockmeyer, n.d.).

Young children tend to sustain soft tissue injuries without incurring fractures, reflecting their hypermobility and skeletal immaturity, and cervical sprain is the most common type of spinal injury. Dislocation without fracture in the cervical spine, especially between the skull and C1 result in instability at the craniocervical junction. Unfortunately, many of these injuries are fatal. Dislocations between C1 and C2 (atlantoaxial joint) are less often fatal but are commonly just as serious. Fractures involving the thoracolumbar spine in children are rare but tend to involve the junction between the thoracic and lumbar spine where the relatively rigid thoracic segments join the more mobile lumbar segments. These injuries most often involve soft tissue and ligaments, resulting in cartilage or growth plate injuries (Brockmeyer, n.d.).

The principles involved in the treatment of pediatric spinal cord injury are similar to those for adults. Spinal cord injury in children is most often accompanied by a traumatic insult and some degree of neurological deficit occurs. The deficits range from an incomplete cord injury in which partial loss of function is present to a complete cord injury in which function below the level of injury is lost. Since children often sustain injury in the cervical spine, muscles of respiration and movement and sensation of the body are affected. In complete lesions, bowel and bladder functions are affected.

The prognosis for children who have had spinal trauma depends greatly on the extent and location of injury. The occupational performance of these children may be affected in all areas of self-care, school-related activities, and play. The skills and abilities on which intervention typically focuses are sensory motor and psychosocial. Environmental adaptations using both low- and high-technology may be crucial for full integration and independence

Pediatric Brain Injury

Each year >1 million children sustain brain injuries, ranging from mild-to-severe trauma (Brain Injury Association of USA [BIA], 1999). Of these children, >30,000 have permanent disabilities as a result of traumatic brain injury (TBI), making it the most common cause of acquired disability in childhood (Kraus, Rock, & Hemyari, 1990). Even when physical complications are minimal, neuropsychological impairments can lead to chronic behavioral, academic, and interpersonal problems that are enormously challenging to children, caregivers, and teachers.

Common causes of TBI include falls, sports- and recreation-related injuries, motor vehicle accidents, and assaults (e.g., child abuse). Young children are more likely to sustain brain injuries from falls, whereas older children and adolescents are most likely to be injured in motor vehicle accidents (BIA, 1999).

The range of severity of TBI, the medical management, and the general recovery stages are similar to those described for adult TBI (Chapter 39). Contrary to some perceptions, children do not have better outcomes from severe TBI than adults; mortality and recovery rates are similar (Johnson & Krishnamurthy, 1998). The emergence of cognitive and behavioral sequelae over time can make accurate assessment more complicated. Because the brains of children are still developing, the full impact of a brain injury may not become evident for many months or even years (BIA, 1999).

For children and adults, the more severe the TBI, the greater the residual deficits. As children mature and behavioral, educational, and social expectations increase, limitations usually become more obvious and limiting. Performance deficits can include sensory motor, language and communication, eating, visual perceptual, and cognitive skills. Changes in personality and behavior also commonly occur, including inattention, increased or decreased activity, impulsivity, irritability, lability, apathy, aggression, and/or withdrawal (Michaud, Duhaime, & Lazar, 1997). Such behavioral problems affect social relationships, and even with adequate cognitive ability, they can hinder academic achievement. Impairments in attention, coping, problem solving, and information processing speed can cause difficulty for children with TBI in all occupational contexts. Assistive technology and other modifications can be critical to the child's successful integration and participation in school and social environments (Michaud et al., 1997).

CONCLUSION

Children with neurological conditions offer exciting challenges and opportunities for occupational therapy practitioners who work in a variety of educational, community-based, and hospital settings. Practitioners work closely with other professionals and parents to conduct comprehensive evaluations with this population. In addition, they provide intervention services that allow children with neurological conditions to develop skills and to compensate for deficit areas to enable them to participate successfully in their valued occupations.

References

Alaska Health and Social Services Online. (n.d.). What is fetal alcohol syndrome? Available at: www.hss.state.ak.us/fas/info/Default.htm. Accessed: August 22, 2002.

Alexander, R., Boehme, R., & Cupps, B. (1993). *Normal development of functional motor skills*. San Antonio, TX: Therapy Skill Builders.

American Psychiatric Association [APA]. (1994). *Diagnostic and statistical manual of mental disorders* (4th ed.). Washington, DC: Author.

Anson, D. (1997). *Alternative computer access. A guide to selection*. Philadelphia: Davis.

Arendt, R., Minnes, S., & Singer, L. (1996). Fetal cocaine exposure: Neurological effects and sensory-motor delays. *Physical and Occupational Therapy in Pediatrics*, *16*(1–2), 129–144.

Ayres, A. J. (1981). *Clinical observations of sensory integration*. Unpublished manuscript.

Ayres, A. J. (1989). *Sensory integration and praxis tests*. Los Angeles: Western Psychological Services.

Ayres, A. J., & Tickle, L. (1980). Hyperresponsivity to touch and vestibular stimuli as a predictor of positive response to sensory integration procedures in autistic children. *American Journal of Occupational Therapy*, *34*, 375–380.

Bailey, D. B., & Nelson, D. (1995). The nature and consequences of fragile X syndrome. *Mental Retardation and Developmental Disabilities Research Reviews*, *1*, 238–244.

Barkley, R. A. (1997). Behavioral inhibition, sustained attention, and executive functions: Constructing a unifying theory of ADHD. *Psychological Bulletin*, *121*(1), 65–94.

Barkley, R. A (1998). *Attention deficit hyperactivity disorder: A handbook for diagnosis and treatment*. New York: Guilford

Baron-Cohen, S., Cox, A., Baird, G., Swettenham, J., Nightingale, N., Morgan, K., Drew, A., & Charman, T. (1996). Psychological markers in the detection of autism in infancy in a large population. *British Journal of Psychiatry*, *168*, 1–6.

Bartlett, D. (1997). Primitive reflexes and early motor development. *Developmental and Behavioral Pediatrics*, *18*(1), 151–156.

Batshaw, M. L. (1997). Fragile X syndrome. In M. L. Batshaw (Ed.). *Children with disabilities* (4th ed., pp. 377–388). Baltimore: Brookes.

Batshaw, M. L., & Conlon, C. J. (1997). Substance abuse: A preventable threat to development. In M. L. Batshaw (Ed.). *Children with disabilities* (4th ed., pp. 143–162). Baltimore: Brookes.

Batshaw, M. L., & Shapiro, B. K. (1997). Mental retardation. In M. L. Batshaw (Ed.). *Children with disabilities* (4th ed., pp. 335–360). Baltimore: Brookes.

Bayley, N. (1993). Bayley scales of infant development (2nd ed.). San Antonio, TX: Psychological Corporation.

Beery, K, (1997). *Beery-Buktenica developmental test of visual-motor integration (VMI)* (4th rev. ed.). Parsippany, NJ: Modern Curriculum.

Bobath, K. (1980). A neurophysiological basis for the treatment of cerebral palsy. *Clinics in Developmental Medicine*, *75*, 77–87.

Brain Injury Association of USA [BIA]. (1999). Brain Injury Source Pediatric Issue volume 3(3). Pediatric brain injury. Available at: www.biausa.org. Accessed: 9/19/02.

Brasic-Royeen, C., & Lane, S. (1991). Tactile processing and sensory defensiveness. In A. Fisher, E. Murray, & A. Bundy (Eds.). *Sensory integration theory and practice* (pp. 108–133). Philadelphia: Davis.

Brockmeyer, D. (n.d.). Pediatric spinal cord injury and spinal column trauma [NeuroSurgery://On-Call]. Available at: www.neurosurgery.org/pediatric/ped_spine.html. Accessed: August 22, 2002.

Brown, F. R. III, & Elksnin, N. (1994). An introduction to developmental disabilities. San Diego: Singular.

Brown, M., & Gordon, W. A. (1987). Impact of impairment on activity patterns of children. *Archives of Physical Medicine and Rehabilitation*, *68*, 828–832.

Bruininks, R. H. (1978). *Bruininks-Oseretsky test of motor proficiency*. Circle Pines, MN: American Guidance Service.

Bundy, A. (1991). Play theory and sensory integration. In A. Fisher, E. Murray, & A. Bundy (Eds.). *Sensory integration theory and practice* (pp. 46–67). Philadelphia: Davis.

Bundy, A. (1997). Play and playfulness: What to look for. In L. D. Parham & L. S. Fazio (Eds.). *Play in occupational therapy for children* (pp. 52–66). St. Louis: Mosby.

Caldwell, B., & Bradley, R. (1979). *Home observation for measurement of the environment (HOME)*. Little Rock: University of Arkansas.

Campbell, S. K., & I. J. Wilhelm (1985). Development from birth to 3 years of age of 15 children at high risk for central nervous system dysfunction. *Physical Therapy*, *65*(4), 463–469.

Case-Smith, J. (1995). The relationships among sensorimotor components, fine motor skill, and functional performance in preschool children. *American Journal of Occupational Therapy*, *49*(7), 645–652.

Castellanos, F. (1997). Toward a pathophysiology of attention deficit/hyperactivity disorder. *Clinical Pediatrics*, *36*(7), 381–393.

Chandler, L., Andrews, M., & Swanson, M. (1980). *Movement assessment of infants*. Rolling Bay, WA: Authors.

Church, M. W., Lewis, M. E. B., & Batshaw, M. L. (1997). Learning disabilities. In M. L. Batshaw (Ed.). *Children with disabilities* (4th ed., pp. 471–498). Baltimore: Brookes.

Colarusso, R., & Hammill, D. (1995). *The Motor Free Visual Perception Test—Revised*. Novato CA: Academic Therapy.

Cook, D. G. (1991). The assessment process. In W. Dunn (Ed.). *Pediatric occupational therapy: Facilitating effective service provision* (pp. 34–73). Thorofare, NJ: Slack.

Coster, W., Deeney, T., Haltiwanger, J., & Haley, S. (1998). *School function assessment (SFA)*. San Antonio, TX: Psychological Corporation.

Dawson, G., & Osterling, J. (1997). Early intervention in autism. In M. J. Guralnick (Ed.). *The effectiveness of early intervention* (pp. 307–326). Baltimore: Brookes.

Doberczak, T. M., Shanzer, S., Senie, R. T., Kandall, S. R. (1988). Neonatal neurologic and electroencephalographic effects of intrauterine cocaine exposure. *Journal of Pediatrics*, *113*, 354–358.

Dunn, W. (1999). *Sensory profile: User's manual*. San Antonio, TX: Psychological Corporation.

Dudgeon, B. (2001). Pediatric rehabilitation. In J. Case-Smith (Ed.). *Occupational therapy for children* (4th ed., pp. 843–863). St. Louis: Mosby.

Erhardt, R. P. (1990). *Developmental visual dysfunction: Models for assessment and management*. San Antonio TX: Therapy Skill Builders.

Erhardt, R. P. (1994). *Developmental prehension assessment—Revised*. San Antonio, TX: Psychological Corporation.

Fiore, T. A., Becker, E. A., & Nero, R. C. (1993). Education intervention for students with attention deficit hyperactivity disorder. *Exceptional Children*, *60*(2), 163–173.

Fisher, A. G. (1991). Vestibular-proprioceptive processing and bilateral integration and sequencing deficits. In A. Fisher, E. Murray, & A. Bundy (Eds.). *Sensory integration theory and practice* (pp. 71–104). Philadelphia: Davis.

Folio, R., & Fewell, R. (2000). *Peabody developmental motor scales—2* (2nd ed.). Austin, TX: Pro-Ed.

FraXa Research Foundation [FraXa]. (n.d.). About fragile X syndrome [Questions & Answers]. Available at: www.fraxa.org/html.about.htm. Accessed August 22, 2002.

Furuno, S., O'Reilly, K. A., Hosaka, C. M., Inatsuka, T. T., Allman, T. A., & Zeisloft, B. (1984). *Hawaii early learning profile (HELP)*. Palo Alto, CA: Vort.

Gardner, M. (1995a). *Test of visual-motor skills—Revised*. Hydesville, CA: Psychological and Educational Publications.

Gardner, M. (1995b). *Test of visual-perceptual skills (non-motor)—Revised*. Hydesville, CA: Psychological and Educational Publications.

Gersh, E. S. (1991). Medical concerns and treatment. In E. Geralis (Ed). *Children with cerebral palsy: A parents' guide* (pp. 57–90). Rockville, MD: Woodbine.

Gharai, J., & Hariri, J. (1992). Management of pediatric head injury. *Pediatric Clinics of North America, 39*, 1093–1125.

Granet, K. M., Balaghi, M. & Jaeger, J. (1997). Adults with cerebralpalsy. *New Jersey Medicine: The Purnal of the Medical Society of New Jersey, February 94*(2), 51–54.

Greenspan, S. I., & Weider, S. (1998). *The child with special needs*. Reading, MA: Addison-Wesley.

Gresham, F., & Elliot, S. (1990). *Social skills rating system*. Circle Pines, MN: American Guidance Service.

Gilfoyle, E., Grady, A., & Moore, J. (1990). *Children adapt* (2nd ed.). New York: Slack.

Haley, S. , Coster, W., Ludlow, L., Haltiwanger, J., & Andrellos, P. (1992). *Pediatric evaluation of disability inventory*. San Antonio, TX: Psychological Corporation.

Howard, J., & Beckwith, L. (1989). The development of young children of substance-abusing parents: Insights from seven years of intervention and research. *Zero to Three, 9*(5), 8–11.

Huber, C. J., & King-Thomas, L. (1987). The assessment process. In L. King-Thomas & B. Hacker (Eds.). *A therapist's guide to pediatric assessment* (pp. 3–10). Boston: Little, Brown.

Humphrey, R, (1991). The impact of feeding problems on the parent-infant relationship. *Infants and Young Children, 3*(3), 30–38.

Hyde, A. S., & Trautman, S. E. (1989). Drug-exposed infants and sensory integration: Is there a connection? *AOTA Sensory Integration Special Interest Newsletter, 12*(4), 1–3.

Jacobson, S. W. (1998). Specificity of neurobehavioral outcomes associated with prenatal alcohol exposure. *Alcoholism: Clinical and Experimental Research, 22*(2), 313–320.

Johnson, D. L. (1997). Hydrocephalus. In R. A. Hockelman, B. S. B. Froedam, N. M. Nelson, & H. M. Seidel (Eds.). *Primary pediatric care* (3rd ed., pp. 1347–1350). St. Louis: Mosby.

Johnson, D. L., & Krishnamurthy, S. (1998). Severe pediatric head injury: Myth, magic and actual fact. *Pediatric Neurosurgery, 28*, 167–172.

Kientz, M., & Dunn, W. (1997). A comparison of the performance of children with and without autism on the sensory profile. *American Journal of Occupational Therapy, 51*(7), 530–537.

Koman, L. A., Mooney, J. F., Smith, B. P. (1996). Neuromuscular blockade in the management of cerebral palsy. *Journal of Child Neurology, 11*(1), S23–S28.

Kraus, J. F., Rock, A., & Hemyari, P. (1990). Brain injuries among infants, children and adolescents. *American Journal of Diseases of Children, 144*, 684–691.

Lane, S. (1992). Prenatal cocaine exposure: A role for occupational therapy. *AOTA Developmental Disabilities Special Interest Newsletter, 15*(2), 1–2.

Lane, S. (1996). Cocaine: An overview of use, action and effects. *Physical and Occupational Therapy in Pediatrics, 16*(1–2), 15–33.

Lindesmith Center (2001). Cocaine and pregnancy. Available at: www.lindesmith.org/lib/women_index.htm. Accessed: 9/19/02.

Liptak, G. S. (1997). Neural-tube defects. In M. L. Batshaw (Ed.). *Children with disabilities* (4th ed., pp. 529–552). Baltimore: Brookes.

Logemann, J. A. (1983). *Evaluation and treatment of swallowing disorders*. San Diego, CA: College Hill.

March of Dimes. (2001). Down syndrome. Available at: www.modimes.org/HealthLibrary/334_602.htm. Accessed: August 22, 2002.

Mathiowetz, V., & Haugen, J. B. (1995). Evaluation of motor behavior: Traditional and contemporary views. In C. A. Trombly (Ed.). *Occupational therapy for physical dysfunction* (4th ed., pp. 157–185). Philadelphia: Williams & Wilkins.

Matthews, P. B. (1988). Proprioceptors and their contribution to somatosensory mapping: Complex messages require complex mapping. *Canadian Journal of Physiology and Pharmacology, 66*, 430–438.

Mauk, E. J., Reber, M., & Batshaw, M. L. (1997). Autism: And other pervasive developmental disorders. In M. L. Batshaw (Ed.). *Children with disabilities* (4th ed., pp. 425–448). Baltimore: Brookes.

Michaud, L., Duhaime, A., & Lazar, M. F. (1997). Traumatic brain injury. In M. L. Batshaw (Ed.). *Children with disabilities* (4th ed., pp. 595–617). Baltimore: Brookes.

Miller, G. A. (1981). *Language and speech*. San Francisco: Freeman.

Miller, G., & Clark, G. D. (1998). *The cerebral palsies: Causes, consequences and management*. Boston: Butterworth-Heinemann.

Miller, L. J. (1988). *Miller assessment for preschoolers*. San Antonio, TX: Psychological Corporation.

Miller, L. J., & Roid, G. H. (1994). *The T.I.M.E. toddler and infant motor evaluation: A standardized assessment*. Tucson, AZ: Therapy Skill Builders.

Morrison, C. & Metzger, P. (2001). Play. In J. Case-Smith (Ed.). *Occupational therapy for children* (4th ed., pp. 528–544). St. Louis: Mosby.

Mulligan, S. (1996). Patterns of scores of children with attention disorders on the Sensory Integration and Praxis Tests. *American Journal of Occupational Therapy, 50*(8), 647–654.

Mulligan, S. (1998). Patterns of sensory integration dysfunction: A confirmatory factor analysis. *American Journal of Occupational Therapy, 52*, 819–828.

Mulligan, S, (2001). Classroom strategies used by teachers of students with attention deficit hyperactivity disorder. *Physical and Occupational Therapy in Pediatrics, 20*(4), 25–36.

MTA Cooperative Group. (1999). A 14th month randomized clinical trial of treatment strategies for attention-deficit/hyperactivity disorder. *Archives of General Psychiatry, 56*(12), 1073–1086.

National Institute of Mental Health [NIMH]. (1999). Learning disabilities brochure. Available at: www.nimh.nih.gov/publicat/ldmenu.cfm. Accessed: 9/19/02.

National Institute of Neurological Disorders and Stroke [NINDS]. (2001). Cerebral palsy: Hope through research. Available at: www.ninds.nih.gov. Accessed: August 22, 2002.

Nichols, D. (2000). Postural control. In J. Case-Smith (Ed.). *Occupational therapy for children* (4th ed., pp. 266–288). St. Louis: Mosby.

O'Neill, M., & Jones, R. (1997). Sensory perceptual abnormalities in autism: A case for more research? *Journal of Autism and Developmental Disorders, 27*(3), 283–293.

Parham, D., & Mailloux, Z. (2001). Sensory integration. In J. Case-Smith (Ed.). *Occupational therapy for children* (4th ed., pp. 329–381). St. Louis: Mosby.

Pelligrino, L. (1997). Cerebral palsy. In M. L. Batshaw (Ed.). *Children with disabilities* (4th ed., pp. 499–528). Baltimore: Brookes.

Pierce, D. (2000). Maternal management of the home as a developmental play space for infants and toddlers. *American Journal of Occupational Therapy, 54*, 290–299.

Piper, M., & Darrah, J. (1994). *Motor assessment of the developing infant*. Philadelphia: Saunders.

Pranzatelli, M. R. (1996). Oral pharmacotherapy for the movement disorders. *Journal of Child Neurology, 11*(1), S13–S22.

Reilly, M. (1974). *Play as exploratory learning; Studies in curiosity behavior*. Beverly Hills, CA: Sage.

Reynolds, C. R., & Kamphaus, R. W. (1992). *Behavior assessment system for children*. Circle Pines, MN: American Guidance Service.

Rogers, S. J., & D'Eugenio, D. B. (1981). *Early intervention developmental profile*. Ann Arbor: University of Michigan Press.

Rogers, S. L., Gordon, C. Y., Schanzenbacher, K. E., & Case-Smith, J. (2001). Common diagnosis in pediatric occupational therapy practice. In J. Case-Smith (Ed.). *Occupational therapy for children* (4th ed., pp. 136–187). St. Louis: Mosby.

Roizen, N. J. (1997). Down syndrome. In M. L. Batshaw (Ed.). *Children with disabilities* (4th ed., pp. 361–375). Baltimore: Brookes.

Rose-Jacobs, R., Frank, D., & Brown, E. (1996) Issues of developmental measurement in clinical research and practice settings with children who were prenatally exposed to drugs. *Physical and Occupational Therapy in Pediatrics, 16*(1–2) 73–87.

Smelt, H. R. (1989). Effects of an inhibitive weight-bearing mitt on tone reduction and functional performance in a child with cerebral palsy. *Physical and Occupational Therapy in Pediatrics, 9*, 53–80.

Sparrow, S., Balla, D., & Cicchetti, D. (1984). *The Vineland Adaptive behavior scales. Interview edition: Survey form manual.* Circle Pines, MN: American Guidance Service.

Spina Bifida Association of America. (2002). Facts about spina bifida. Available at: www.sbaa.org/html/sbaa_facts.html. Accessed: August 22, 2002.

Sroufe, L. A., Cooper, R. G., & DeHart, G. B. (1992). Child development: Its nature and course (2nd ed.). Columbus, OH: McGraw-Hill.

Stewart, K. B. (2001). Purposes, processes and methods of evaluation. In J. Case-Smith (Ed.). *Occupational therapy for children* (4th ed., pp. 190–216). St. Louis: Mosby.

Swinth, Y., & Case-Smith, J. (1993). Assistive technology in early intervention: Theory and practice. In J. Case-Smith (Ed.). *Pediatric occupational therapy and early intervention* (pp. 342–368). Boston: Andover Medical.

Takata, N. (1974). Play as prescription. In M. Reilly (Ed.). *Play as exploratory learning: Studies of curiosity behavior* (pp. 209–246), Beverly Hills, CA: Sage.

Teasdale, G., & Jennett, B. (1974). Assessment of coma and impaired consciousness: Practical scale. *Lancet, 2*: 81–84.

Vaughn, B. E., Contreras, J., & Seifer, R. (1994). Short-term longitudinal study of maternal ratings of temperament in samples of children with Down syndrome and children who are developing normally. *American Journal of Mental Retardation*, 98, 607–618.

Watling, R., Deitz, J., Kanny, E., & McLaughlin, J. (1999). Current practice of occupational therapy for children with autism. *American Journal of Occupational Therapy*, 53(5), 498–505.

Williams, M., & Shellenberger, S. (1994). *How does your engine run?* Albuquerque, NM: Therapy Works.

Yasukawa, A. (1990). Upper extremity casting: Adjunct treatment for a child with hemiplegic cerebral palsy. *American Journal of Occupational Therapy, 44*, 840–846.

Zeitlin, S., Williamson, G., & Szczepanski, M. (1998). *Early coping inventory*. Bensenville, IL: Scholastic Testing Service.

CHAPTER 34

CARDIOPULMONARY DYSFUNCTION IN CHILDREN

OLGA BALOUEFF

Conditions affecting children's cardiac and respiratory systems are either congenital or acquired. They can be a child's primary condition or they can be associated with other conditions, such as in Down syndrome. Impairments exist in different degrees in children's health and occupational performance according to the severity and chronicity of the condition. This chapter addresses the implications of heart disease and respiratory conditions on occupational performance and interventions to help children with these conditions participate in life's occupations.

CARDIAC CONDITIONS

Congenital Heart Disease

All **congenital heart defects** (CHDs) originate before the end of the first trimester of gestation, because the heart develops early in embryonic life and is completely formed and functioning by 10 weeks (Damjanov, 1996). Congenital heart defects affect approximately 0.8% of all live births (Lewin, 2000). Causes of CHDs include environmental factors, such as maternal infections, drug and alcohol use during pregnancy, chromosomal abnormalities, and genetic syndromes (Damjanov, 1996). The symptoms of CHDs become evident at birth, during infancy, or even later in life (Howell, 2000). Without intervention, some heart defects are severe enough to cause death, especially in infancy.

There are two major types of CHDs: acyanotic and cyanotic. In acyanotic defects, the oxygen saturation is normal and the blood shunts from the left side of the heart to the right side. Thus oxygenated blood flows to the lungs as well as to the body (Howell, 2000). Common conditions include aortic stenosis, atrial and ventricular septal defects, coarctation of the aorta, patent ductus arteriosis, and endocardial cushion defect (Petry & Rainville, 1999).

In cyanotic defects, the blood is shunted from the right side of the heart to the left side, and unoxygenated blood is returned to the body. As a result, arterial oxygen saturation levels fall below normal values (Howell, 2000). Symptoms of CHDs are manifested in respiratory difficulties, fatigue, lack of tolerance for the prone position, poor weight gain, and feeding difficulties. Medical and surgical treatments depend on the type of defect and the child's age (Walters, 2000).

Acquired Heart Disease

The heart is vulnerable to a variety of infections (bacterial, fungal, parasitic, and viral), which may result in either endocarditis, myocarditis, pericarditis, or even in pancarditis (Damjanov, 1996). Recently, an increasing prevalence of obesity in children in the United States has been reported; these children are at risk for premature cardiovascular disease. Some of the causes for this worrisome trend can be attributed to increased portions of high-fat and high-calorie meals and snacks and a decline in physical activity. Such practices result in hyperlipidemia, a predominant risk factor for atherosclerosis and type II diabetes (McCrindle, 2000).

PULMONARY CONDITIONS

Pulmonary dysfunction can generally be divided into two types: obstructive (e.g., cystic fibrosis, asthma) and restrictive (e.g., bronchopulmonary dysplasia).

Cystic Fibrosis

Cystic fibrosis (CF) is a chronic, life-threatening disease, typically diagnosed in early childhood. It is the most common autosomal recessive disease, affecting 1 in 3300 live births in the United States (Cystic Fibrosis Foundation, n.d.). This disease is characterized by a generalized dysfunction of the exocrine glands, affecting several systems, such as respiratory, gastrointestinal, pancreatic, hepatic, and reproductive.

The predominant complication of CF pertains to the hyperviscosity of bronchial mucus, which transforms itself into viscous plugs that prevent normal respiration. The mucus accumulation is a fertile ground for bacterial growth and predisposes the child to frequent respiratory infections (Ashwell & Agnew-Coughlin, 2000). An analysis of chloride levels of the child's perspiration is used to confirm a CF diagnosis (positive sweat test). Once chloride has entered a sweat gland's lumina, that gland cannot reabsorb it, and the sweat contains an increased amount of salt (Damjanov, 1996). Parents often say that their infant tastes salty. Pancreatic dysfunction resulting in poor digestion and malabsorption of nutrients is another major problem for individuals with CF. Food malabsorption is reflected in large and foul-smelling stools, abdominal distention, and poor weight gain.

Although CF is still an incurable chronic illness, the mean life expectancy has increased owing to improved therapies. Most people with this disease die as the result of pulmonary infection before they reach adulthood. However, promising gene therapy research for treating lung abnormalities has begun, and lung transplantation for those with end-stage disease has also been successful for some individuals (Welsh & Smith, 1995).

Medical management of CF is largely supportive. It consists of prevention and treatment of upper respiratory infections, maintaining adequate nutrition, and preventing intestinal obstruction. Antibiotics (to prevent and clear infections), pancreatic enzymes, and multivitamin supplements are commonly prescribed. Respiratory therapy involving techniques such as postural drainage, percussion and vibration of the chest walls, mist tent, and aerosol therapy are employed for clearing mucus from the airways (Ashwell & Agnew-Coughlin, 2000). Proper intake of fluids and calories are important considerations in the child's daily nutrition (Cintas, 1995).

Asthma

Asthma is a chronic inflammatory disorder characterized by increased responsiveness of the bronchial tree to various types of stimuli. These stimuli are classified in two groups: intrinsic or nonallergic (e.g., viral infections, exercise, emotional factors, climatic changes) and extrinsic or allergic (e.g., pollen, mold, dust, cigarette smoke) (Magee, 2000). This condition affects 10% of children and 5% of adults in the United States, and in 50% of cases the disease begins in childhood (Damjanov, 1996).

Typical asthmatic attacks are characterized by wheezing during expiration, coughing, breathlessness, and chest tightness. These episodes may be associated with airflow obstruction that is reversible either spontaneously or with medication. Treatment is symptomatic and generated at preventing or reducing bronchospasms and bronchial inflammation to maintain pulmonary function and physical activity. Assisting children in controlling their asthmatic attacks and helping them engage in normal childhood occupations are major aspects of management for this disorder.

Bronchopulmonary Dysplasia

Bronchopulmonary dysplasia (BPD) is a chronic lung problem secondary to prolonged use of mechanical ventilation and oxygen administration to the prematurely born infant who experienced respiratory distress at birth. As a result of these interventions, a series of complications occur, such as destruction of the respiratory tract cilia, epithelium interstitial fibrosis, and alveolar growth retardation (Cintas, 1995; Kahn-D'Angelo & Unanue, 2000). The overall incidence for BPD varies from 13 to 69% for infants who weigh <1500 g. (Kahn-D'Angelo & Unanue, 2000).

A child with mild BPD may exhibit occasional increased respiratory rate and cyanosis when crying or during feeding. In more severe cases, the child can exhibit severe difficulty with breathing and circulation and can even be prone to developing congestive heart failure and pulmonary edema. Accordingly, respiratory support ranges from nasal oxygen supplementation to positive airway pressure and complete mechanical ventilation (Cintas, 1995). With age and growth, the majority of children are weaned from supplemental oxygen and show improvement in their BPD. Because of the risks associated with decreased blood oxygenation, these children may be at risk for central nervous system and developmental disabilities (Kahn-D'Angelo & Unanue, 2000; Petry & Rainville, 1999).

IMPACT OF CARDIOPULMONARY CONDITIONS ON CHILDREN'S OCCUPATIONAL PERFORMANCE

Occupational performance in children with cardiac or pulmonary impairments varies greatly from one child to another, depending on the type and severity of the medical condition, age, family, social, and cultural environment. In infancy, many children experience feeding difficulties that affect their growth and development (Ashwell & Agnew-Coughlin, 2000; Imms, 2001). As they engage in feeding, these infants may develop problems such as changes in cardiac rhythm and output, tachypnea, and cyanosis, resulting in poor oxygenation, reduced activity tolerance, and fatigue (Kelly & Dumas, 2000; Petry & Rainville, 1999). In addition, babies who have experienced oral intubation or thoracic surgery may display significant oral aversion and tactile hypersensitivity. A combination of these factors leads to problems such as refusal to eat, poor appetite, and poor weight gain (Imms, 2001; Svavarsdottir & McCubbin, 1996).

In childhood, the most commonly seen deficits are in the areas of play and activities of daily living, and feeding is often a persistent problem. The body functions most frequently affected are the sensorimotor, especially motor and neuromusculoskeletal. Social participation in school and community activities may be interrupted because of a susceptibility to respiratory and bacterial illnesses, hospitalization, and lack of stamina.

In adolescence, children with chronic illnesses often experience delayed physiological maturation and are also at greater risk for psychosocial problems, particularly anxiety, depression, poor self-esteem and body image, and poor social interactions (Ashwell & Agnew-Coughlin, 2000; Rolland, 1994). Adherence to medical treatment, medications, and therapy schedules often becomes an issue at that age, as the urge for independence, experimentation, and risk-taking behaviors increases.

FAMILY FUNCTIONING IN CHILDREN WITH CARDIOPULMONARY CONDITIONS

Families of children with chronic illnesses face some specific stresses, such as financial and physical burden of care, frequent hospitalizations, concerns regarding their child's mortality and uncertain future (as in CF), as well as the affected child's and other children's psychosocial adjustment (Imms, 2001; Svavarsdottir & McCubbin, 1996; Thompson, Gustafson, Hamlett, & Spock, 1992). Optimal functioning for children with cardiopulmonary conditions is rooted in a supportive and cohesive family that believes in a high, but realistic, potential for the child and that is supportive of the child's move toward independence (Thompson et al., 1992).

EVALUATION OF OCCUPATIONAL PERFORMANCE

Evaluation of health impairments, functional limitations, and individual strengths in children with cardiopulmonary dysfunction is a family-centered and multidisciplinary approach. Occupational therapy assessment must take into account the effects of medical and physiological instability, decreased mobility, and contextual situation—such as home environment; hospitalization; and disruptions in typical social, emotional, and physical life experiences. Occupation-centered and developmental assessments are particularly useful with this group of children (Coster, 1998). The assessment process should start with an exploration of the significant occupations of the child and the family, focusing on parental concerns, priorities, and aspirations for the child's involvement in personally satisfying activities (Cohn & Cermak, 1998; Coster, 1998). Understanding the family's daily routines and the child's own goals are key for ensuring adherence to therapeutic and lifestyle modifications.

INTERVENTION

The primary goal of occupational therapy is to facilitate the acquisition of contextual and developmental appropriate skills. Intervention is individualized, family focused, and graded to the child's level of tolerance to maximize best performance. Precautions have to be observed regarding the mode, intensity, and frequency of activities (Howell, 2000). In carrying out intervention, occupational therapy practitioners must be sensitive to sudden changes in the child, such as pallor or flushing, labored respiration, pulse rate, and decreased stamina. Education and support of the family regarding the child's developmental and special needs are an integral part of intervention, including environmental adaptations at home and at school to help the child conserve energy.

According to Ashwell and Agnew-Coughlin (2000), families benefit from strategies that permit some flexibility in intervention regimens, which promotes a better integration of the child's needs into the family routines. Families of medically fragile children are eager for education and practical strategies for taking care of their child, particularly in the area of feeding (Stimson & McKeever, 1995). As the children get older, it becomes important to educate them regarding precautions, energy-conservation techniques, responsibilities for following their therapeutic schedule, and for advocating with confidence about their strengths and limitations.

CONCLUSION

Cardiopulmonary dysfunction in children has the potential to delay the development of skills related to activities of daily living, play, and school performance. Occupational therapy intervention facilitates the development of occupational performance and supports children and their families as they cope with potentially life-threatening conditions.

References

Ashwell, J. A., & Agnew-Coughlin, J. L. (2000). Cystic fibrosis. In S. K. Campbell, D. W. Vanderlinden, & R. J. Palisano (Eds.). *Physical therapy for children* (pp. 734–763). Philadelphia: Saunders.

Cintas, H. L. (1995). Pediatric disorders. In T. M. Long & H. L. Cintas (Eds.) *Handbook of pediatric physical therapy* (pp. 52–99). Baltimore: Williams & Wilkins.

Cohn, E. S., & Cermak, S. A. (1998). Including the family perspective in sensory integration outcomes research. *American Journal of Occupational Therapy, 52*(7), 540–546.

Coster, W. (1998). Occupation-centered assessment of children. *American Journal of Occupational Therapy, 52*(5), 337–344.

Cystic Fibrosis Foundation. (n.d.). About cystic fibrosis. Available at: www.cff.org/about_cf/what_is_cf.cfm?CFID=206154&CFTOKEN=58058711. Accessed August 22, 2002.

Damjanov, I. (1996). *Pathology for the health-related professions*. Philadelphia: Saunders.

Howell, B. A. (2000). Thoracic surgery. In S. K. Campbell, D. W. Vanderlinden, & R. J. Palisano (Eds.). *Physical therapy for children* (pp. 786–810). Philadelphia: Saunders.

Imms, C. (2001). Feeding the infant with congenital heart disease: An occupational performance challenge. *American Journal of Occupational Therapy, 55*(3), 277–294.

Kahn-D'Angelo, L., & Unanue, R. A. (2000). The special care nursery. In S. K. Campbell, D. W. Vanderlinden, & R. J. Palisano (Eds.). *Physical therapy for children* (pp. 840–880). Philadelphia: Saunders.

Kelly, K. M., & Dumas, H. (2000). Children with ventilator dependence. In S. K. Campbell, D. W. Vanderlinden, & R. J. Palisano (Eds.). *Physical therapy for children* (pp. 711–733). Philadelphia: Saunders.

Lewin, M. B. (2000). The genetic basis of congenital heart disease. *Pediatric Annals, 29*(8), 469–480.

Magee, C. L. (2000). Asthma. In S. K. Campbell, D. W. Vanderlinden, & R. J. Palisano (Eds.). *Physical therapy for children* (pp. 764–785) Philadelphia: Saunders.

McCrindle, B. W. (2000). Screening and management of hyperlipidemia in children. *Pediatric Annals, 29*(8), 500–507.

Petry, J., & Rainville, E. B. (1999). The cardiovascular and the pulmonary systems. In S. M. Parr & E. B. Rainville (Eds.). *Pediatric therapy: A systems approach* (pp. 123–153). Philadelphia: Davis.

Rolland, J. S. (1994). Families, illness, and disability, New York: Basic Books.

Stimson, J., & McKeever, P. (1995). Mother's information needs related to caring for infants at home following cardiac surgery. *Journal of Pediatric Nursing, 10*, 48–57.

Svavarsdottir, E. K., & McCubbin, M. (1996). Parenthood transition for parents of an infant diagnosed with a congenital heart condition. *Journal of Pediatric Nursing, 11*, 207–216.

Thompson, R. J., Gustafson, K. E., Hamlett, K. W., & Spock, A. (1992). Stress, coping, and family functioning in the psychological adjustment of mothers of children and adolescents with cystic fibrosis. *Journal of Pediatric Psychology, 17*(5), 573–585.

Walters, H. L. (2000). Congenital cardiac surgical strategies and outcomes: Hearts. *Pediatric Annals, 29*(8), 489–498.

Welsh, M. J., & Smith, A. E. (1995). Cystic fibrosis. *Scientific American, 273*(6), 52–59.

CHAPTER 35

CHILDREN WITH HIV/AIDS AND THEIR FAMILIES

JIM HINOJOSA, GARY BEDELL and MARGARET KAPLAN

AIDS was first recognized in children in 1982. Most children with AIDS acquire it perinatally from their mothers (Centers for Disease Control and Prevention, Division of HIV/AIDS Prevention [CDC], 1997). Although research supports that zidovudine therapy (AZT) for HIV reduces perinatal transmission (CDC, 1997), prohibitive cost reduces its use worldwide (Rosenberg, 2001). In the United States, adolescents account for the greatest increase in the number of people diagnosed with HIV/AIDS (Cobia, Carney, & Waggoner, 1998). Adolescents may also become infected through unsafe sexual intercourse, intravenous drug use, and sexual abuse (Bartlett, Keller, Eckholdt, & Schleifer, 1995).

Children with HIV/AIDS are at high risk for developing cognitive, behavioral, and neurological deficits, such as progressive encephalopathy, acquired microcephaly, myelopathy, peripheral neuropathy, and pyramidal tract dysfunction (Wolters, Brouwers, & Moss, 1995). Their health may be compromised by decreased access to health care, adverse living situations (e.g., poverty, drug use), and **opportunistic infections** (e.g., *Pneumocystis carinii* pneumonia, candidiasis, *Mycobacterium avium* intracellulare, lymphocytic interstitial pneumonia) (Peckham & Gibb, 1995). The clinical picture ranges from mild impairment to severe global deficits (Wolters et al., 1995). Medical advances have improved the interventions available and the quality of life for children living with HIV/AIDS in the Western world. As children live longer, the focus of occupational therapy services may need to shift from medical to educational and community settings.

CLIENT FACTORS AND AREAS OF OCCUPATIONS

Children with HIV/AIDS commonly have difficulties caused by the virus itself, by the effects of other common risk factors (e.g., premature birth, multiple drug exposure in utero, poor prenatal care, deficient nutrition), and the effects of medication (Pizzo & Wilfert, 1998). Neurological symptoms stemming from the virus include muscle tone abnormalities and progressive loss of sensorimotor, cognitive, and language abilities. The condition of children with HIV/AIDS abilities can vary on a day-to-day basis owing to the effects of opportunistic infections, direct effects of the virus, side effects of medications and medical treatments, and multiple psychosocial issues. Pain and discomfort can cause further psychosocial issues for children. Young children have difficulty expressing pain and discomfort but may manifest it through an apparent loss of abilities, for example, a refusal to walk.

Children with HIV/AIDS often experience extensive loss of primary caregivers, siblings, other family members, or may live in foster homes. Extensive medical procedures and repeated hospitalizations contribute to isolation from peers and the community, as well as possible separation from familiar caregivers. Consequently, they may develop separation anxiety, withdrawal, anger, depression, or physical symptoms. These reactions vary among children, depending on their age, temperament, and personal situation.

As children grow older, awareness of being different and of society's reaction to HIV/AIDS can increase. The stigma attached to HIV/AIDS and related discrimination can foster patterns of secrecy within families. Families may need support in talking to each other, their children, and close friends about their own HIV status and that of their children. Children may need help in coping with the reactions of peers, teachers, and others, especially if they are able to remain in school and participate in community activities.

A **family-centered approach** to services and an attitude of **unconditional positive regard** (Rogers, 1961) are essential when working with children with HIV/AIDS and their caregivers. Practitioners may need to develop strategies to cope with their own grieving and anxiety when working with children with HIV/AIDS and their families.

EVALUATION OF CHILDREN WITH HIV/AIDS

Evaluation is typically guided by interviews with caregivers about their concerns, priorities, schedules, and other responsibilities as they affect children. Practitioners also need information about the children's developmental history, experiences with medical procedures, hospitalizations, other separations and losses, and behavior in different contexts. Observation of children engaged in school activities or play with peers or family members can contribute useful information. The areas of feeding, mobility, and self-care are often concerns of caregivers and can be assessed through observation or with functional assessments, such as the Pediatric Evaluation of Disability Index (Haley, Coster, Ludlow, Haltiwanger, & Andrellos, 1992). Information about children's school performance can be obtained by interviews with teachers and other related service providers and by administration of the School Function Assessment (Coster, Deeney, Haltiwanger & Haley, 1998).

Criterion-referenced assessments and standardized tests in specific developmental areas can be used in the same manner as they are for other children. For children with HIV/AIDS, factors such as fatigue, pain, frustration, irritability, depression, and separation anxiety must be considered during the evaluation process. Practitioners need to be sensitive to the effects of opportunistic infections or other medical conditions, such as decreased respiratory capacity, fever, nausea, diarrhea, and dehydration.

INTERVENTION FOR CHILDREN WITH HIV/AIDS

Providing a safe and supportive environment is essential for all occupational therapy intervention. The unpredictable nature of HIV/AIDS, medication side effects, and prior experiences with noxious medical procedures often create situations in which children and their caregivers have limited control and may feel socially isolated. Therapeutic relationships with children and caregivers often must be reestablished or strengthened because of the increased fear, distrust, and apathy that frequently occur from prolonged illness, hospitalization, and convalescence at home. Provision of environments in which children and caregivers can express themselves openly and explore and participate in meaningful activities safely often becomes a primary focus of intervention. Some children may have decreased feelings of self-efficacy and have difficulty initiating actions required for gratification, play, social interaction, activities of daily living (ADL), functional communication, and mobility. Encouraging children's self-directed actions, choices, and problem solving fosters a heightened sense of control.

Service delivery that is coordinated, flexible, and interdisciplinary increases the likelihood that the children's and their caregivers' needs are being met in an efficient manner. For example, rescheduling appointments during nonschool hours and developing alternative service delivery models may be necessary to minimize missing school days or to accommodate children and caregiver medical and socioeconomic needs.

Intervention to address areas of occupation is similar to that used for other children with disabilities. Some areas, however, may require special attention. For example, oral thrush, decreased respiratory capacity, sinusitis, malnutrition, and HIV wasting may complicate interventions that address oral motor abilities and feeding skills. Food may have to be softer and blander to lesson the discomfort caused by oral thrush. More in-depth neurodevelopmental and sensory or physiological state regulation interventions may be required to improve safe and efficient coordination of oral motor abilities with respiration.

Because of frequent absences related to medical illnesses and appointments, older school-aged children may need assistance with managing daily life routines, such as scheduling time needed for taking medications, making medical appointments, studying and doing homework, and pursuing leisure pursuits. Practitioners may collaborate with the children's teachers and caregivers to develop strategies, environmental modifications, and realistic plans to assist children with managing an often-chaotic daily life.

Practitioners also address particular issues with adolescents, such as identity formation, identification with a peer group, grooming and hygiene skills, dating, sexual expression, experimentation with social skills and roles, learning prevocational skills, and exploring vocational or career goals. Health promotion and illness management can be reinforced by addressing topics such as proper nutrition, stress management, balancing ADL, management of symptoms and medication side-effects, and methods to prevent transmission of HIV/AIDS to others.

Frequently, children with HIV/AIDS exhibit forgetfulness or more pronounced memory and orientation problems, disorganization in task performance, and decreased task persistence. These problems may be the result of psychosocial issues, stress, or chaotic living situations. They may also indicate central nervous system (CNS) damage. To address these problems, materials, instructions, the physical environment, and the teaching and learning process may need to be modified according to the children's abilities, requirements, and learning styles. Smaller groups may be needed for children to attend to important task performance requirements. Classrooms or living spaces may have to be organized in a way that orients and guides the children to specific activity areas and the types of behaviors that are expected in various settings (e.g., academics, free play, snack time). Providing environmental cues, feedback, reinforcement, and encouraging practice in a variety of contexts may assist children with learning daily routines and skills needed to function at home, in school, and in the community.

Children with HIV/AIDS may also exhibit problems related to postural tone, balance, motor control, and sensory modulation. These sensorimotor problems may be related to:

- The progressive encephalopathy that occurs when HIV or other HIV infections or cancers enter or develop in the CNS.
- Static encephalopathy that occurs from perinatal factors that are frequently associated with cerebral palsy.
- Opportunistic infections that do not have a progressive effect on the CNS.
- Lack of sensory and motor experiences owing to hospitalizations, extensive convalescence, or overprotective care-giving practices.
- Prior experiences with noxious medical procedures.

Practitioners can address these issues by employing interventions that use sensory integration techniques (Kimball, 1999), desensitization procedures (DuHamel, Redd, & Vickberg, 1999), methods of sensory affective regulation (DeGangi, Craft, & Castellan, 1991; Wilbarger & Wilbarger, 1991; Williams & Shellenberger, 1992), neurodevelopmental treatment (Schoen & Anderson, 1999), or motor control and learning strategies (Kaplan & Bedell, 1999).

RESEARCH NOTE 35–1

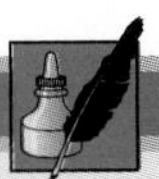

Including the Family

Intervention programs for children and families at risk for developmental problems and children with documented handicaps are a prominent proportion of occupational therapy practice. Current pediatric practice in occupational therapy is influenced by legislation that defines who will provide services, where services are provided, what specific services are delivered, and how services and outcomes are evaluated. The focus of pediatric intervention is not just on the child with a disability but also includes the family, teacher, and peers. Family-centered intervention programs are now the standard models of pediatric practice for occupational therapists. These research areas are inherently collaborative, interdisciplinary, and student centered.

Dunbar (1999) provided an instructive example using a case report of a child with a sensory processing disorder. The case report illustrates how sensory processing problems can affect all aspects of a child's life and affects his or her family and peers. To be effective, intervention must address all components of the child's environment, including home and school. Dunbar provided an illustration of a therapeutic program that includes family involvement in treatment, goal setting, and outcome evaluation.

Dunbar, S. B. (1999). A child's occupational performance: Considerations of sensory processing and family context. *American Journal of Occupational Therapy*, 53, 231–235.

Biomechanical interventions are used to improve the children's strength and endurance and to provide body and body part positioning (splints, seating, and other adaptive equipment) (Colangelo, 1999). Energy conservation, work simplification, time management principles, environmental modification, and other adaptive strategies and equipment can be discussed with and used by teachers and primary caregivers to compensate for the children's decreased strength, endurance, and mobility. Approaches that incorporate principles of teaching and learning can be used for functional skill acquisition (Kaplan & Bedell, 1999; Royeen & Duncan, 1999; Todd, 1999). Many of the aforementioned approaches can address the fine, gross, or perceptual motor abilities needed for ADL, educational activities, play, and leisure.

One of the most challenging aspects of intervention is knowing how to balance the amount of encouragement and support needed to "push" individuals to "do" and "allow" them to "just be," given their current circumstances. This is especially salient when working with children with HIV/AIDS and their caregivers. Because of the chronic and sporadic nature of the disease, it is often challenging to predict what interventions will be necessary or effective to achieve desired outcomes at a given time.

CASE STUDY 35-1

Joseph: A Boy with HIV

Joseph is a 12-year-old Hispanic-American boy who acquired HIV perinatally. He was relatively asymptomatic until 5 years ago when he was diagnosed with AIDS. Joseph lives with his mother (Lydia), maternal grandmother (Magdalena), aunt (Louisa) and uncle (John), and two cousins (Elba and Anthony) in a two-bedroom apartment in a housing project in East Harlem. Joseph's father and older sister died from complications from AIDS 10 and 12 years ago, respectively. Lydia has been periodically hospitalized and unable to be Joseph's primary caregiver for the last 3 years. However, when able, she participates in Joseph's care by preparing his meals, reading him stories, watching television with him, and visiting a neighborhood park. Magdalena is Joseph's primary caregiver and legal guardian, but Louisa and John also participate in Joseph's care.

Joseph is in the fifth grade in a regular education program in a public school and receives resource room support for reading and math. Occupational therapy services have been added to his individualized education plan (IEP) to address fine and gross motor skills needed for handwriting, using the computer, and fully participating in physical education and other social activities with peers.

Additional information about Joseph's client factors and occupations was obtained by observing Joseph in academic and nonacademic activities in his classroom, physical education class, resource rooms, and in the school cafeteria. The School Function Assessment (Coster, Deeney, Haltiwanger, & Haley, 1998) was administered by interviewing Joseph's teachers and a telephone interview was conducted with Magdalena.

Confidentiality laws makes it unlawful to disclose a child's diagnosis of AIDS on the IEP or school records to protect the child and his or her family from possible stigma and discrimination and physical harm (McFarland, 1999). Magdalena disclosed Joseph's AIDS diagnosis to his teacher in the beginning of the year because, as she reported, "He will probably have to miss a number of days of school and may need to come late or leave early due to doctors appointments . . . and I didn't want you to get the wrong idea."

Joseph is taking new HIV medications that cause serious bouts of diarrhea, nausea, and fatigue at home and in school. Magdalena reports that Joseph is self-conscious about his looks, because he lost a lot of weight and his friends are beginning to notice. He has difficulty keeping up physically with his friends during physical education and recess. Joseph's emotional status reportedly changed drastically in the last few months from being a "friendly child with a gleam in his eyes" to becoming a passive and serious child who sometimes "looks like he has the weight of the world on his shoulders."

Observations of and discussions with Joseph confirm these difficulties. Joseph is becoming increasingly frustrated and saddened by his HIV/AIDS symptoms, medication side effects, multiple medical appointments, and the impact they have on his school performance and overall daily life.

Intervention goals are discussed and agreed on with Joseph, his primary teacher, and his grandmother. The focus of occupational therapy is to develop adaptive strategies based on work simplification, energy conservation, and time management principles to assist Joseph with performing the school activities that are most important for him academically and socially. Accommodations are made to allow Joseph to leave his classroom earlier to avoid rushing to the cafeteria and physical education class. Occupational therapy focuses directly on handwriting and computer skills in the resource rooms and motor skills and activity tolerance in physical education classes. Joseph wants his primary classroom to be a place where he feels like "a regular kid," so the team agrees that the practitioner will make only periodic visits to his classroom to monitor his progress and make additional recommendations, if needed.

One of the more difficult decisions for Joseph is to replace recess time with quiet time spent resting or catching up on his academics after taking his lunchtime dosage of medications. Continued collaboration with the school nurse, counselor, and Joseph's primary health-care provider is needed to further assist him with managing his medications, side effects, and other HIV/AIDS symptoms and to provide him with a safe and supportive environment to cope emotionally and physically with living with HIV/AIDS.

Coster, W., Deeney, T., Haltiwanger, J. & Haley, S. (1998). *School function assessment (user's manual)*. San Antonio, TX: Psychological Corporation.

McFarland, W. P. (1999). Empowering professional counselors in the war against AIDS. *Professional School Counseling, 2,* 267–273.

In general, children with HIV/AIDS should be encouraged to be as active as possible. If children are verbal, practitioners and caregivers should enable them to ask for what they want or need. Nonverbal communication should be used for children who do not speak. Practitioners should wait and give children time to do something themselves before they rush in to help. Practitioners may have to assist or do more for children who are losing abilities because of illness or not feeling well because of the direct effects of the disease or medication side effects. It may be difficult to balance children's realistic need for help and children's often attempted strategy of getting others to do for them.

CONCLUSION

Practitioners' judgments and actions when working with children with HIV/AIDS and their caregivers are more likely be effective if they are sensitive to the children's physical conditions, personalities, typical coping styles, and family life circumstances. Practitioners should make a conscious effort to be open and willing to deal with issues by discussing them with the children, family caregivers, other practitioners, and supervisors and by reflecting on their own practice. In addition, practitioners need continually to update their knowledge related to the basic and applied science of HIV/AIDS and the related health and social issues.

Guidelines for the use of antiretroviral medications are regularly updated to reflect current research and can be found on the Internet (e.g., www.hivatis.org/guidelines/pediatric). Current information about incidence, research studies, and a range of interventions is available from the CDC (www.cdc.gov; 800-342-AIDS) and from the National Pediatric AIDS Network (www.npan.org; 800-646-1001). Prevention efforts are highlighted at the CDC National Prevention Information Network (www.cdcnpin.org; 800-458-5231). These organizations may be useful sources of information and support groups for parents and older children.

References

Bartlett, J. A., Keller, S. E., Eckholdt, H., & Schleifer, S. J. (1995). HIV relevant issues in adolescents. In N. Boyd-Franklin, G. L. Steiner, & M. G. Boland (Eds.). *Children, families, and HIV/AIDS: Psychosocial and therapeutic issues* (pp. 78–89). New York: Guilford.

Centers for Disease Control and Prevention, Division of HIV/AIDS Prevention. (1997). AIDS among children: United States, 1996. *Journal of School Health, 67,* 175–177.

Cobia, D. C., Carney, J. S., & Waggoner, I. M. (1998). Children and adolescents with HIV disease: Implications for school counselors. *Professional School Counseling, 1,* 41–45.

Colangelo, C. A. (1999). Biomechanical frame of reference. In P. Kramer & J. Hinojosa (Eds.). *Frames of reference for pediatric occupational therapy* (2nd ed., pp. 257–322). Baltimore: Lippincott Williams & Wilkins.

Coster, W., Deeney, T., Haltiwanger, J., & Haley, S. (1998). *School Function Assessment (user's manual).* San Antonio, TX: Psychological Corporation.

DeGangi, G. A., Craft, P., & Castellan, J. (1991). Treatment of sensory, emotional, and attentional problems in regulatory disordered infants: Part 2. *Infants and Young Children, 3,* 9–19.

DuHamel, K. N., Redd, W. H., & Vickberg, S. M. (1999). Behavioral interventions in the diagnosis, treatment and rehabilitation of children with cancer. *Acta Oncologica, 38,* 719–734.

Haley, S. M., Coster, W. J., Ludlow, L. H., Haltiwanger, J. T., & Andrellos, P. J. (1992). *Pediatric Evaluation of Disability Inventory: Development, standardization and administration manual.* Boston: New England Medical Center Hospitals and PEDI Research Group.

Kaplan, M. T., & Bedell, G. (1999). Motor skill acquisition frame of reference. In P. Kramer & J. Hinojosa (Eds.). *Frames of reference for pediatric occupational therapy* (2nd ed., pp. 401–430). Baltimore: Lippincott Williams & Wilkins.

Kimball, J. G. (1999). Sensory integrative frame of reference: Postulates regarding change and application to practice. In P. Kramer & J. Hinojosa (Eds.). *Frames of reference for pediatric occupational therapy* (2nd ed., pp. 169–204). Baltimore: Lippincott Williams & Wilkins.

Peckham, C., & Gibb, D. (1995). Mother-to-child transmission of the human immunodeficiency virus. *New England Journal of Medicine, 333,* 298–302.

Pizzo, P. A., & Wilfert, C. M. (1998). *Pediatric AIDS: The challenge of HIV infection in infants, children, and adolescents.* Baltimore: Williams & Wilkins.

Rogers, C. R. (1961). *On becoming a person.* Boston. MA: Houghton Mifflin.

Rosenberg, T. (2001, January 28). Look at Brazil. *New York Times Magazine,* sec. 6, 26–31, 52, 58–60.

Royeen, C. B., & Duncan, M. (1999). Acquisition frame of reference. In P. Kramer & J. Hinojosa (Eds.). *Frames of reference for pediatric occupational therapy* (2nd ed., pp. 337–400). Baltimore: Lippincott Williams & Wilkins.

Schoen, S. A., & Anderson, J. (1999). Neurodevelopmental treatment frame of reference. In P. Kramer & J. Hinojosa (Eds.). *Frames of reference for pediatric occupational therapy* (2nd ed., pp. 83–118). Baltimore: Lippincott Williams & Wilkins.

Todd, V. R. (1999). Visual information analysis: Frame of reference for visual perception. In P. Kramer & J. Hinojosa (Eds.). *Frames of reference for pediatric occupational therapy* (2nd ed., pp. 205–256). Baltimore: Lippincott Williams & Wilkins.

Wilbarger, P., & Wilbarger, J. L. (1991). Sensory defensiveness in children aged 2–12. Santa Barbara, CA: Avant Educational Programs.

Williams, M. S., & Shellenberger, S. (1992). *An introduction to "How does your engine run?" The alert program for self-regulation.* Albuquerque, NM: TherapyWorks.

Wolters, P. L., Brouwers, P., & Moss, H. A. (1995). Pediatric HIV disease: Effect on cognition, learning, and behavior. *School Psychology Quarterly, 10,* 305–228.

CHAPTER 36

PSYCHOSOCIAL DYSFUNCTION IN CHILDHOOD AND ADOLESCENCE

LINDA FLOREY

In 1999, the U.S. surgeon general issued the first report ever on the mental health of Americans. A primary message in the report is that mental health is fundamental to health and that mental disorders are real health conditions. Overall, 9–13% of all children have serious emotional disturbances (U.S. Department of Health and Human Services [DHHS], 1999).

Children and adolescents with notable psychopathology are identified within five distinct types of public service sectors: schools, juvenile justice, child welfare, general health, and mental health agencies. There is an underutilization of mental health services by the caregivers of children and adolescents with psychosocial dysfunction owing to stigma associated with mental health services and perceptions that intervention is not relevant or too demanding. Consequently, many youth are identified at a later age when problems are more serious. Primary care and the schools are the major settings for the potential recognition of youth with psychosocial disorders (DHHS, 1999).

Occupational therapy practitioners working in general hospitals and rehabilitation centers may work with children and adolescents who have suffered bruises, fractures, or head trauma as a result of impulsive or aggressive behavior caused by an underlying psychiatric disorder. Practitioners working in the school system encounter youngsters with significant emotional and behavioral disorders. The intent of this chapter is to review the typical deficits in performance associated with psychosocial dysfunction, the features of attention deficit hyperactivity disorder, conduct and oppositional defiant disorder, mood disorder, and autism and Asperger disorder and the types of assessments and intervention programs that may be used with this population.

TYPICAL DEFICITS IN PERFORMANCE AREAS AND SKILLS FOR CHILDREN AND ADOLESCENTS WITH PSYCHOSOCIAL DYSFUNCTION

Evaluation Methods

Typical deficits in performance of children and adolescents with psychosocial dysfunction are often invisible to practitioners. Problems in behavior or emotion are not present all of the time but may be triggered by internal or external events. Symptoms of psychiatric disorders are often exaggerations of normal behavior so affected individuals seem like youth with regular problems. It is the immaturity of the behavior or the persistence of the behavior that is troublesome. A problem in the area of behavior is often not visually obvious at first and less predictable than physical problems.

Children and adolescents with psychiatric disorders typically have problems in social and task behavior. They may be aggressive, intrusive, disruptive, argumentative, unpredictable, inattentive, bossy, or withdrawn. Some children have difficulty attending to activities and completing steps, and some may demonstrate a complete lack of interest in or satisfaction with activities. They may develop isolative or restricted patterns of interests or activities, such as watching television or playing computer games.

Many children lack social skills required for team and group activities. They may also lack executive skills such as sequencing steps to perform activities and physical skills to participate, as many are awkward and clumsy. Many youth have trouble controlling their temper, sustaining social interactions, and recognizing and interpreting social cues. Children and adolescents with psychosocial disorders often have no friends and are generally not liked by their peers. In addition to not being liked by their peers, they may not have support from adults in the environment. Teachers and coaches tend to dislike children and adolescents who are disruptive or oppositional or who have difficulty following classroom rules (Hocutt, 1966).

Children and adolescents with psychosocial disorders have usually experienced failure in task and social situations or have been teased or rejected. They have little self-confidence and are often resistant to trying. Their deficits pervade all occupational performance areas, although they may do better in some areas than others. The deficits they have in common are Cub Scout deficits; not invited to birthday party deficits; not on the team or liked by the team deficits; no one to eat lunch, play, or hang out with deficits; and no best friend deficits.

Occupational Behavior: A Focus for Intervention

The **Occupational Behavior** frame of reference targets the broad parameters of play, student role, and socialization as the primary concern of occupational therapy. The purpose of this subsection is to present a conceptual map for assessments and intervention.

Developmental Progression in Occupational Behavior

Occupational behavior focuses on the developmental continuum of play and work and how these phenomena are incorporated into occupational roles throughout the life cycle (Reilly, 1966). There is a developmental progression in the manner in which work and play phenomena are incorporated into occupational role. The progression is from player to student to worker, homemaker, or volunteer to retiree (Moorhead, 1969). The occupational role of preschool children is that of player, as play is the major activity during this period. Work activities are emerging as preschoolers learn the basics of dressing and other self-care behaviors and preschool expectations. In middle childhood and adolescence, the major daily activity is attending school; thus the occupational role during this period is student. The dominant theme is productive activity in school and displaying self-reliant behavior and completing chores at home. Play activity takes up less time than in early childhood but is critical for mastering cooperation, teamwork, and competition.

Occupational role behavior involves learning social expectations and specific ground rules for social behavior within different and expanding contexts. For example, children have to recognize and learn the social rules appropriate to the schoolroom, the playground, the soccer team, the sand lot, the religious setting, the camp, and other people's homes (Fig. 36-1). The roles of student and worker emanate largely from the social institutions of school and work, and many expectations are formally taught through these vehicles.

Developmental Focus in Play, Student Role, and Socialization

Occupational therapy focuses on determining the extent to which injury or illness has disrupted or impoverished occupational behavior and on identifying steps to ameliorate dysfunction and to foster development. Children and adolescents with psychosocial dysfunction experience difficulty in the social aspects of play and the role of student.

The Occupational Role of Player

The occupational role of player changes throughout development, but it remains as the primary arena in which social relatedness is learned, rehearsed, and mastered. Social play

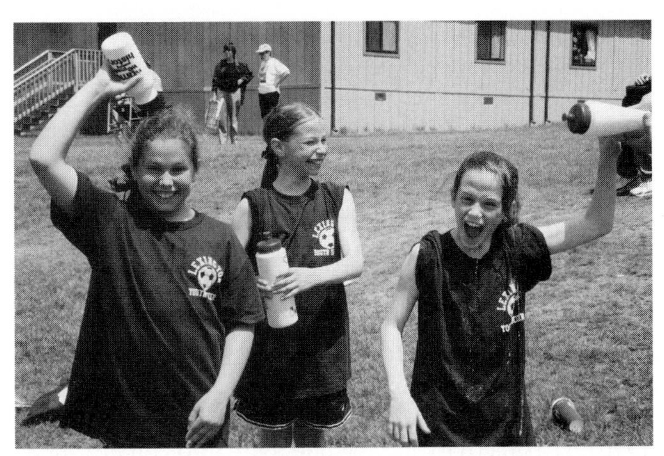

FIGURE 36–1. During middle childhood, games with rules, such as soccer, are common occupations. (Courtesy of L. Berkowitz, Lexington, MA)

during infancy and toddler years consists of exploring social influence through playful interactions, intentionally eliciting social responses, and engaging in symbolic social play. Between the ages of 2 and 5, social interactions become more frequent, more sustained, and more complex (Mussen, Conger, Kagan, & Huston, 1990). In these preschool years, sociodramatic play is prominent, as is constructive play. Sociodramatic play permits children to frame play in terms of role expectations, to coordinate these roles, and to communicate in and out of the roles. Simple group and board games allow children to practice rules of reciprocity and turn taking.

Play in middle childhood, ages 6–12, is characterized by increasing complexity in peer relationships. During this period, the structure of social groups changes from informal gangs with few formal rules and rapid turnover in membership to more structured, formal, and cohesive groups with more elaborate membership requirements. Friendships move from being easily established and terminated to being stable over longer and longer periods (Mussen et al., 1990).

Games with rules are dominant. Children go through different stages in their understanding of rules during this period. In the beginning of middle childhood, rules are vague and children are often unable to put the rules of the game above the need to win. Games such as baseball are conceived of typically as action: as *hitting* the ball and *running* around the bases. Toward the end of this period, children become more aware that they can negotiate rules among themselves and determine them by consensus. Games are characterized by competition and often take the form of sports.

In adolescence and adulthood, it is believed that the qualities that children exhibit in play are the ones adults continue to seek. In adolescence, sports and special-interest clubs continue to be prominent as does hanging out. Social relationships continue to be very much in evidence.

The Occupational Role of Student

The social institutions of the school and the laws regulating schooling largely define the role of student. In school and after-school contexts, children must master both academic and social curricula. Within the school setting, the academic curriculum is formally taught: The social curriculum is often not taught and must be learned informally. Children must be able to recognize and modulate their actions based the particular norms and cues of each setting. They must learn appropriate actions for different classroom, lunchroom, hallway, and recess behavior within the school itself. This includes how to enter discussions, when to raise hands, how to join a game in progress, how to share the attention of the teacher and classmates, how loud to talk, and when and how silly they can be. Academically, they must learn how to read, write, spell, and calculate and generally master information about the world they live in. They must be able to listen, pay attention, and focus on tasks.

Typical Performance Deficits in Play, Student Role, and Socialization

Typical performance deficits of children and adolescents with psychosocial dysfunction are in the player and student roles, because social and task behavior are embedded within them. Most children designated as **emotionally disturbed**—formerly designated as seriously emotionally disturbed (SED)—in the school system are failing academically, are socially rejected, and have poor evaluations of themselves and their potential contributions to society (Combrinck-Graham, 1996). Data from the National Longitudinal Transition Study of Special Education Students (NLTS) indicate that more than three quarters of students with SED had failed one or more courses, which was the highest failure rate of any category of students with disabilities. High school students who are SED demonstrated a pattern of disconnectedness from school activity. They were the least likely to belong to clubs or social groups at school and had high rates of absenteeism (Wagner, 1995).

The combination of maladaptive behaviors, poor social skills, and poor coping strategies place children and adolescents with psychosocial dysfunction on the margins of the classroom, playground, lunchroom, and gymnasium. They have difficulty fitting in, and they are at extreme risk for being disconnected from the major institution that prepares them for adulthood and from the social fabric of the community.

The major focus of occupational therapy intervention with these youths is to identify high-risk areas and to teach skills in the task and social components of player and student roles to reconnect them to school, community, and productive patterns of living.

PROMINENT PSYCHIATRIC DISORDERS IN CHILDHOOD AND ADOLESCENCE

Risk factors that make youths vulnerable to psychiatric disorders include chronic medical conditions that limit typical childhood activities, brain damage, intrauterine exposure to toxins (e.g., lead and alcohol), severe parental discord, exposure to acts of violence, parental psychiatric disorders or deviance, poor parenting, and family dysfunction (DHHS, 1999; Offord & Fleming, 1996). Social and environmental risk factors, including prolonged separation between parent and child, physical or sexual abuse, poverty, and instability in the family environment also contribute to mental dysfunction (Zigler & Finn-Stevenson, 1996). The causes of disorders are often difficult to determine but are increasingly conceptualized from a biopsychosocial perspective that encompasses the traditional environmental, interpersonal and psychological models, and the biological–medical model (Garfinkel, Carlson, & Weller, 1990). One factor may play a lead role in a specific disorder, but generally a multiplicity of biopsychosocial vulnerabilities or stressors are implicated.

Six disorders are discussed here: **attention deficit hyperactivity disorder** (ADHD), **oppositional defiant disorder** (ODD) and **conduct disorder** (CD), mood disorders, and **autism** and **Asperger disorder.**

Attention Deficit Hyperactivity Disorder

ADHD is one of the most common psychiatric disorders of childhood and adolescence (American Academy of Child and Adolescent Psychiatry [AACAP], 1997a). There are three types of ADHD: predominantly inattentive, predominantly hyperactive–impulsive, and combined. Symptoms of inattention include failing to give close attention to details or making careless mistakes, difficulty sustaining attention or listening, difficulty organizing, and avoidance of sustained mental effort. Symptoms of hyperactivity include fidgeting, being out of seat, and running or talking excessively. Symptoms of impulsivity include blurting out answers, difficulty waiting turns, and interrupting or intruding on others. These behaviors are inconsistent with the child or adolescent's developmental level and intellectual ability. Functional impairment is present in two or more settings and causes significant impairment in social, academic, and occupational functioning (AACAP, 1997a; Danckaerts & Taylor; 1995; Weiss, 1996).

Children with ADHD often have difficulty inhibiting impulses in social behavior and in cognitive tasks. They are often unpopular with age mates because of aggression and impulsivity and are underachievers in school (AACAP, 1997a; Weiss, 1996). Signs of ADHD may not be observable when the child or adolescent is in highly structured situations, is receiving one-on-one attention, or is engaged in interesting activity (AACAP, 1997a.) Prominent features of ADHD vary with age. In preschool children, gross motor overactivity, oppositional and aggressive behavior, and difficulty playing quietly are common complaints of parents (DHHS, 1999). In older children, impairments in functioning in school, home, and with peers is common. Adolescents with this disorder tend to present as restless rather than hyperactive, although fidgeting is common. Inattention, poor impulse control, poor peer relations, and poor problem solving are common (AACAP, 1997a).

ADHD is more prevalent in boys than girls. Prevalence is estimated to be 3–5% (American Psychiatric Association [APA], 1994). The cause of ADHD is unknown, although neurotransmitter deficits, genetics, and perinatal complications have been implicated (DHHS, 1999). Intervention focuses on support and education of parents, appropriate school placement, and pharmacology with psychostimulants (AACAP, 1997a).

There is a high co-occurrence or co-morbidity of ADHD with oppositional defiant and conduct disorders (AACAP, 1997a; Danckaerts & Taylor; 1995; Taylor; 1994; Weiss, 1996). Hyperactivity may be one route into conduct disorder, and it is a risk factor for the outcome of aggressive and antisocial behavior and delinquency (Taylor, 1994).

Oppositional Defiant Disorder and Conduct Disorder

ODD and CD are the predominant disorders seen in mental health and community clinics (Loeber, Burke, Lahey, Winters, & Zera, 2000). These disorders and ADHD are collectively referred to as *disruptive disorders*. The essential features of ODD are a recurrent pattern of negativistic, defiant, disobedient, and hostile behavior toward authority figures. ODD typically includes problem behaviors such as persistent fighting and arguing, deliberately annoying or being spiteful to others, refusal to comply with requests or rules, and blaming others for one's own mistakes.

The essential features of CD are a repetitive and persistent pattern of behavior in which the basic rights of others or societal norms or rules are violated. Children or adolescents with CD behave aggressively by fighting, bullying, physically assaulting, or being cruel to people or animals. These patterns of behavior cause significant impairment in social, academic, or occupational functioning (APA, 1994). A pattern of antisocial behavior usually involving physical aggression is common, and this behavior is typically regarded as unmanageable by significant others (Earls, 1994). Diagnostically, there is controversy about whether aggressive symptoms should be part of ODD or CD (Loeber et al., 2000).

Conduct disorder is the more serious of the two disorders, and ODD is sometimes a precursor of conduct disorder (DHHS, 1999). Both are of great concern because of their high degree of impairment and antisocial behavior. A proportion of children with ODD develop CD and a proportion of those with CD meet criteria for antisocial personality disorder (Loeber et al., 2000).

Children and adolescents with conduct disorder and oppositional defiant disorder typically have low self-esteem and, to hide this, they may portray themselves as tough and uncaring. Adolescents with conduct disorder are likely to show academic deficiencies, high rates of truancy, high rates of injury and school expulsion, and diminished social skills in relationship to peers and adults (DHHS, 1999).

There is no single cause of ODD or CD. High motor activity, marital discord, and disrupted childcare are risk factors for ODD. Prominent risk factors for CD include parental dysfunction and deviance (e.g., alcoholism and criminal behavior of the father), family characteristics (e.g., inconsistent or lax childrearing practices), and contextual conditions associated with a variety of untoward living conditions (e.g., low socioeconomic status and familial aggregation) (AACAP, 1997b; Earls, 1994; Kazdin, 1995). Intervention focuses on long-term management of symptoms.

ODD and CD frequently co-occur with other psychiatric disorders. There is a high co-morbidity of conduct disorder with ADHD, anxiety disorders, mood disorders, and substance use. Children with symptoms of ADHD and conduct disorder are at greater risk for poor outcomes than those with either disorder alone. Children with conduct and anxiety symptoms are less likely to have police contacts or be perceived by peers as bullies, as it is believed that the presence of anxiety serves as a braking system on the seriousness of antisocial behavior (Earls, 1994; Kazdin, 1995).

Mood Disorders

Mood disorders in children and adolescents are classified into two major types: unipolar depressive disorder and **bipolar disorder.** In bipolar disorder, combinations of manic and depressive symptoms are found (Weller, Weller, & Svadjian, 1996). Bipolar disorder was once believed to occur rarely in children and adolescents, although developmental variation in presentation, symptom overlap with other disorders, and lack of clinician awareness have led to underdiagnosis or misdiagnosis (AACAP, 1997c). In this section, attention is directed to depression in children. Brief descriptions of manic episodes are given to differentiate them from symptoms found in children with ADHD.

Depressive Disorder

Major depressive disorder (MDD) and **dysthymic disorder** (DD) are common and recurrent disorders in both children and adolescents (AACAP, 1998). The primary features of a depressive episode are at least a 2-week period of pervasive change in mood characterized by either depressed or irritable mood and/or loss of interest and pleasure. Symptoms must represent a change from previous functioning and produce impairment in relationships or in performance of activities. In children and adolescents, mood may be cranky rather than sad. Somatic complaints, irritability, and social withdrawal are common in children (APA, 1994). Adolescents experience hopelessness and feelings that things will never change for the better. The most serious complication is suicidal thoughts, including recurrent thoughts of death or actual attempts at suicide (Weller et al., 1996). Suicide is the third leading cause of death for the adolescent population (DHHS, 1999).

Dysthymic disorder has fewer symptoms than MDD and is more chronic. DD involves a persistent, long-term change in mood. Depressed youths withdraw, view minor issues as overwhelming, interact less with others, develop behavioral problems, and have poor school performance (AACAP, 1998). Two thirds of children and adolescents with MDD have another psychiatric disorder. The most commonly associated disorders are DD, anxiety disorder, disruptive or antisocial disorders, and substance abuse disorders (AACAP, 1998; DHHS, 1999).

The prevalence of depression increases with age. The prevalence of MDD in children is approximately 2%, and in adolescents, 4–8% (AACAP, 1998). Among depressed children, the sex ratio is nearly equal, but by adolescence, female preponderance is manifest (Harrington, 1994). Numerous causes may lead to the expression of depressive symptoms. Genetic, biologic, psychosocial, and environmental factors have been implicated (Harrington, 1994; Weller et al., 1996). Children and adolescents are at high risk for recurrence of the illness. Intervention focuses on psychotherapy and pharmacology.

Manic Symptoms

Symptom patterns of mania vary by age. Children younger than 9 years of age, present with irritability and emotional lability; whereas older children typically demonstrate euphoria, elation, paranoia, hypersexual behavior, and grandiose delusions. Hyperactivity, push of speech, and distractibility may be present in both age groups (Weller et al., 1996). Manic children usually display more affect than do children with ADHD and are more euphoric or irritable. They also display a more pronounced shift in mood than do children with ADHD, and their activity tends to be more goal directed (Harrington, 1994). Adolescents with mania often feel energetic, confident, and special. They may complain that their thoughts are racing, and they do schoolwork in a disorganized, chaotic fashion. They may become overconfident and engage in reckless or risky behavior, such as fast driving or unsafe sex (DHHS, 1999).

Autism and Asperger Disorder

Autism and Asperger disorder are two of the **pervasive developmental disorders** (PDDs; see Chapter 33). The central defining feature of all the PDDs is a serious problem in socialization. These disorders are characterized by patterns of delay and deviance in the development of social, communicative, and cognitive skills. There is a wide range of syndrome expression in that symptoms change over the course of development (AACAP, 1999). Autism is characterized by a distinctive pattern of deficits in social dysfunction, communicative deviance, and restrictive and repetitive behaviors and interests (APA, 1994; Lord & Rutter, 1994; Volkmar, 1996). Social dysfunction is manifest primarily in difficulties in reciprocal social interaction and the ability to form relationships. In infancy, there is often lack of eye contact, poor attachments to key individuals, and difficulty with the give-and-take of social relatedness. In preschool years, children with autism typically demonstrate a lack of interest in other children, a limited range of facial expression, and rare eye contact. They may be distressed by separation from their parents but often do not greet parents in positive ways when rejoined (Lord & Rutter, 1994; Volkmar, 1996).

Communicative deviance is evident in the failure to develop expressive language. Those individuals who develop speech demonstrate a lack of or an unusual social quality. Speech may be characterized by echolalia, pronoun reversal, and failure to use language for social interaction. Restricted and repetitive interests and behaviors may include preoccupation with a specific part of a toy (e.g., spinning wheels on a toy truck) or stereotypic movements (e.g., hand flapping, toe walking). Most children with autism show some abnormalities or delays in these areas before the age of 3.

Children with Asperger syndrome have qualitative impairments in social interaction of the same kind observed in autism; but there is lack of delay in language, cognitive, or adaptive behavior early in life. Motor milestones are described as being delayed and motor clumsiness and awkwardness are commonly reported by parents (AACAP, 1999). Approaches to peers and novel adults may be unusual or idiosyncratic, but attachment to family members is established. Children often lack knowledge of how to approach others. Social deficits become more apparent as children enter school and are exposed to peers. Individuals with Asperger syndrome may become intensely interested in one or two subjects or interests, which may interfere with their acquisition of other skills. However, these children may be able to successfully earn a living, despite having inept social skills (Tanguay, 2000).

The prevalence of autism is approximately 1 in 2000, and the prevalence of autism and Asperger syndrome together is 1 in 1000 (Tanguay, 2000). These disorders occur more frequently in males than females. Mental retardation frequently co-occurs with autism but not with Asperger syndrome. Individuals with these disorders may exhibit many behavioral difficulties, including hyperactivity, attentional problems, obsessive–compulsive behaviors, stereotypies, and affective symptoms (AACAP, 1999).

Autism is believed to have a neurobiological base, although the identification of specific pathology remains elusive (Lord & Rutter, 1994). Intervention planning is lifelong, particularly for individuals with autism. Intervention focuses on symptom management; behavioral adjustment; adaptive, academic, social, and communicative skills; and educational or vocational preparation (AACAP, 1999).

EVALUATION OF CHILDREN AND ADOLESCENTS WITH PSYCHOSOCIAL DYSFUNCTION

The purpose of the occupational therapy evaluation is to identify strengths and weaknesses from which goals and intervention strategies may be developed. Behavioral, affective, and communication/interaction areas should be evaluated first, relative to individual and interpersonal aspects of play, school, and daily living routines. Children are screened routinely for visual motor and motor problems, because children with psychosocial disorders frequently demonstrate deficits in these areas. Additional assessments of visual motor, sensory motor, and motor function follow only when screening indicates that problems are evident and further understanding of the child is necessary. The evaluation process is ongoing throughout the practitioners' total contact with a child or adolescent. Children with psychosocial disorders may have more than one psychiatric disorder, and they may also have other disabilities that contribute to their overall level of functional performance. They frequently have learning disabilities, speech disorders, and cognitive disabilities or limitations. The occupational therapy practitioner can observe and target areas of vulnerability and refer to other professionals.

Evaluation Methods

Observation underlies all forms of evaluation. Structured observations involve either setting up a particular event or activity to be observed or observing in natural settings and recording, as objectively as possible, the specific behaviors exhibited. An observation guide or checklist facilitates the recording of a specific behavior, such as task behavior.

The interview is an important source of information about how children and adolescents communicate information and how they view their own experiences. How they choose to report activities and events should be recorded, even though the accuracy of the report may be questionable. For example, some children report having "millions" of friends, but are unable to name any friends or any activities or games they play with other children. The occupational therapy practitioner must probe areas in which children and adolescents give vague or general responses. For example, many children say they play with toys, and adolescents respond that they hang out with their friends. The practitioner needs to explore areas that are not clear or verify information by reading the medical chart or by interviewing the parents or primary caregivers.

Standardized tests provide information regarding performance, with reference to a normal standard. Interest checklists and inventories can be self-administered and can provide information related to the child or adolescent's preferences.

Evaluation of Preschool and School-Age Children

The purpose of evaluation with preschool- and school-age children is to determine the level of function in play and social behaviors and in visual motor skills. Developmental assessment is done when immaturity in skills is suspected.

Play and Social Behavior

With preschool children, two evaluative situations are used: one structured and one unstructured (Fig. 36-2). In structured

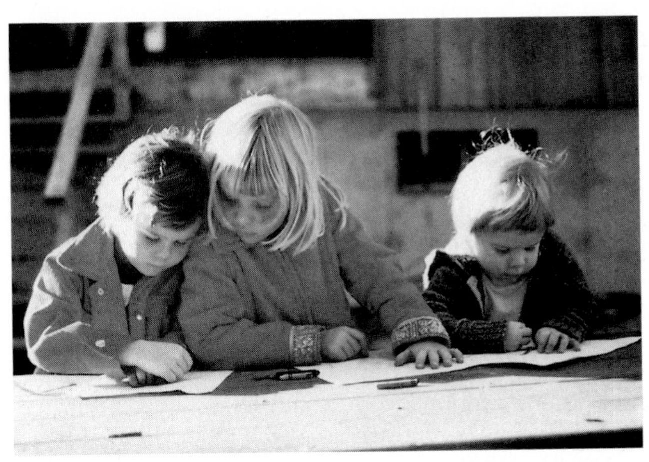

FIGURE 36–2. Preschool children engaged in parallel play.

play, the child is seen alone and is given a sample of a simple project, such as an animal macaroni collage and materials to construct one. Attention span, process–product orientation, attention to detail, manipulation, and construction are assessed. In unstructured play, the child is provided with a range of toys and materials suitable for sensorimotor, dramatic, and constructive play. The child is observed alone and with a peer. What the child does with the materials and how he or she engages with the practitioner and peer are evaluated. The Knox Preschool Play Scale—Revised (Knox, 1997) or the developmental play classification developed by Florey (1971) are useful guides for interpreting observational data.

With children who are functioning younger than a developmental age of 3, only the unstructured play situation is used, because collage construction is too advanced. Interviewing parents using Takata's (1974) play history is useful for understanding immediate and past play experiences. This yields a perspective on the longitudinal nature of the child's play repertoire and can be helpful in determining a starting point for intervention.

School-age children are interviewed individually with respect to their play activities and friends. The purpose of the interview is to gain the children's perspective of daily living, school, chores, social relationships, and overall time use in addition to specific play activities. Interview questions target play preferences, interests, friends and playmates, types of activities in which the family may engage, and after-school activities. Children are asked to describe a typical day and typical weekend day in their living setting. Whenever possible, information should be validated by the parents or caretaker. Children are given a simple craft project, such as copper tooling using a template, in which a successful outcome is key. Children with psychosocial dysfunction have frequently experienced failures because of impulsivity, inattentiveness, or inability to organize and focus tasks; thus it is important that their experience in occupational therapy be successful.

The practitioner observes the child's attention span, ability to make decisions, follow directions, use tools and materials correctly, and solve problems. Children are observed with peers in a game or activity situation to evaluate the quality and quantity of their social interactions with peers.

The behavior observation guide given in Box 36-1 is useful for observing and recording behavior in different settings. Although the categories of task, social, and general behavior are all interrelated, they are used to help practitioners focus on different aspects of the child's performance in many situations. For example children with ADHD may be able to focus on simple steps in an activity on a one-to-one basis with an adult. Yet in the presence of others, they may have difficulty focusing and sharing materials and space with others, may interrupt others, or may have difficulty waiting their turn.

Other assessments to guide observations in context are the Early Coping Inventory (Zeitlin, Williamson, & Szczepanski, 1988) designed for children aged 4–36 months, the Coping Inventory (Zeitlin, 1991) designed for children aged 3–16 years, and the School Function Assessment designed for use in the school setting (Coster, Deeney, Haltiwanger, & Haley 1998).

Developmental Assessments

Developmental assessments provide an indicator of functional level, regardless of chronological age. The Denver Developmental Screening Test (Revised) is a standardized screening test for children aged 1 month to 6 years. The domains assessed include personal–social, fine motor adaptive, language, and gross motor functions. The Miller Assessment for Preschoolers is a standardized screening tool used to identify children aged 2 years, 9 months to 5 years, 8 months who are at risk for school-related problems (Richardson, 2001).

In working with school-age children and with adolescents, if there is a question of maturity in communication, daily living skills, socialization, or motor skills, the Vineland Adaptive Behavior Scales can be used. This assessment is useful for documenting immaturity in performance of an individual with average intelligence and may help establish qualifications for eligibility for special services in the school system. The Vineland scale is used with children from birth to 18 years, 11 months and employs a semistructured interview administered to the parent or caretaker of the child (King-Thomas & Hacker, 1987).

Visual Motor Assessments

The Beery-Buktenica Developmental Test of Visual-Motor Integration is a developmental test of visual motor integration that provides age norms and describes the developmental sequence for copying geometric forms. It is used with children 2–15 years of age (King-Thomas & Hacker, 1987). There are separate motor and visual subtests of this assessment to further evaluate any problems. If children score below the norm for their chronological age in this area and if they demonstrate motor problems in developmental testing, the Motor-Free Visual Perception Test (MVPT) may be administered if the child is 4 years or older. The MVPT focuses on

BOX 36–1 BEHAVIOR OBSERVATION GUIDE

TASK BEHAVIOR

- How long can the child attend to an activity? Does the child become easily distracted or have difficulty concentrating?
- Is the child able to follow instructions and use materials and tools correctly? What type of instruction works best? Verbal? Visual? Demonstration? How many steps can the child follow at one time?
- Does the child take time with the task or rush through it?
- Is the child disorganized in performing steps in a task or is he or she preoccupied?
- Is the child able to handle a mistake?
- Can the child stay seated throughout the task? Can he or she sit without moving around in the chair or playing with desktop objects?
- Is the child proud of his or her efforts?

SOCIAL BEHAVIOR

- Does the child establish eye contact when in the company of others?
- Is the child able to maintain appropriate personal space with others?
- Does the child isolate himself or herself from others or from an ongoing activity?
- Does the child approach others of the same age? Younger? Older?
- Does the child approach adults more often than peers?
- Can the child share materials, space, and attention of adults with peers?
- Can the child wait turns in games or activities? In conversations?
- Does the child engage in negative behavior for attention from others?
- Is the child disruptive to others (e.g., excessive talking, interrupting, clowning)?
- Is the child able to abide by the rules of the group, activity, or situation?
- Does the child pick up social cues or learn from feedback from others?

GENERAL BEHAVIOR

- Is the child in a heightened mood most of the time (e.g. sad, angry, giddy, and irritable)?
- Does mood change frequently from one extreme to another?
- Does the child engage in unsafe or impulsive behavior?
- Does the child's affect match the situation in which he or she is engaged?
- Does the child become easily angry or aggressive? Deliberately provoke others?
- Does the child make sexual remarks frequently? Engage in masturbation?
- Does the child make any odd noises, have peculiar movements or behavior, engage in any rituals?
- Does the child have difficulty with transitions or changes in routine?

visual perception not requiring a motor response (King-Thomas & Hacker, 1987). The Bruininks-Oseretsky Test of Motor Proficiency (BOTMP) may be administered to assess gross and fine motor skills for children ranging in age from 4½ to 14½ years (King-Thomas & Hacker, 1987).

Evaluation of Adolescents

The purpose of evaluations with adolescents is to assess socialization, task performance, daily living skills, and time management behaviors. Cognitive skills are also assessed as an adjunct to determining underlying abilities and limitations in task performance and daily living skills. Visual motor functioning is routinely assessed, and additional motor and developmental skills are assessed when there is a question of function in these areas.

Time Management, Daily Living Skills, Task Performance, and Socialization

Adolescents are interviewed with respect to their interests, activity patterns, and friends (Fig. 36-3). This is done using

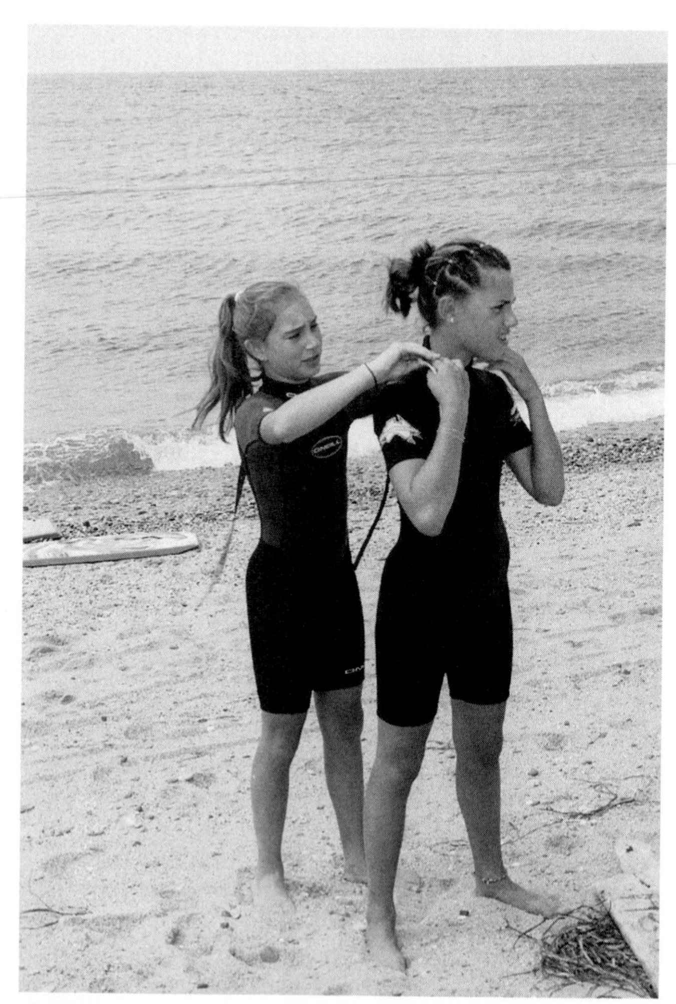

FIGURE 36–3. Adolescent girls giving support to each other while enjoying a day at the beach. (Courtesy of L. Berkowitz, Lexington, MA)

the typical weekday and typical weekend day semistructured interview format. The interview provides a snapshot of the organization of role behavior with respect to daily living skills, chores and responsibilities, school and after-school activities, and peer and friendship patterns. The adolescents are given a choice of simple craft projects and are asked to complete one project. Task behavior is also assessed using the Allen cognitive level (ACL) test to provide a quick estimate of the adolescent's current ability to learn. This test, with implications for daily performance activities, provides valuable information regarding the kinds of cues the adolescent may need to perform role activities (Allen, Earhart, & Blue, 1992). The frequency and content of social interactions with peers and adults are assessed by observations made in various settings. The behavior observation guide give in Box 36-1 may be used to direct observation and interpretation.

INTERVENTION GOALS AND PRINCIPLES

This section focuses on developing goals and identifying broad principles of intervention that may be used in a variety of service contexts, such as health-care settings and the school system, for children and adolescents with psychosocial dysfunction.

Goals and Teamwork

Findings from assessments used in the occupational therapy evaluation are summarized to reflect strengths and problem areas. The problem areas become the focus for goals, whereas the strengths may be used to facilitate goal achievement. For example, if an adolescent has problems in socialization with peers, and strengths in task skills, establishing a goal of teaching a step in a task to a peer incorporates both elements. Goals should be drawn from the problem areas, prioritized, and stated in measurable terms. Goals such as "increasing peer socialization" and "increasing self-esteem" are too broad and unmeasurable and have no beginning or end. Measurable goals should address the what, when, and how of expected behavior in occupational therapy (Brands, 1977). The *what* describes the behavior in which the child or adolescent is expected to engage, *when* specifies how frequently or how long the behavior is expected to occur in any treatment setting or session, and the *how* indicates under what circumstances the behavior is to take place. For example, a measurable goal for a child might be to attend to task or group (the what) for 45 min (the when) with prompts and redirection to task if inattention occurs (the how). Goals are modified throughout the intervention process and are paced to encourage increasing levels of difficulty, responsibility, and behavioral control.

An interdisciplinary team approach is typical in psychosocial programs for children and adolescents. The number of members and composition of the interdisciplinary team varies from setting to setting. Each member of the team contributes a unique focus, with the goal of formulating a broad perspective of the child and of providing an integrated intervention approach. The occupational therapy practitioner needs to report information in a concise, descriptive manner, free from occupational therapy or psychiatric jargon. It is more relevant to know how and under what circumstances a particular behavior is evident than simply to report that the child is angry, depressed, happy, anxious, or needs moderate assistance to complete a task.

Another shared focus of the team is to develop a system to manage behavior in group settings. Behavior management systems range from expectations for behavior within the setting, such as school, to formal approaches based on principles of behavior modification, such as token economy. The occupational therapy practitioner must incorporate elements of the behavioral management system into each person's occupational therapy program.

Characteristics of the Occupational Therapy Intervention

Intervention for children and adolescents consists of creating play and task environments in which there are opportunities for association with peers and adults. Social behavior and learning should be embedded within both the play and task environments. Intervention suggestions for children and adolescents with psychosocial dysfunction are discussed below.

- *Use natural childhood and adolescent activities*. The overall process of the activity should be emphasized and not the product. The goal of play with toys, crafts, or games focuses on sharing materials, engaging in social banter, not fighting with others, and achieving a sense of pride in task accomplishments rather than simply making a coin purse or playing a game (Fig. 36-4).

Florey and Greene (1997) suggested analyzing and structuring the cognitive, motor, and social complexity of activities

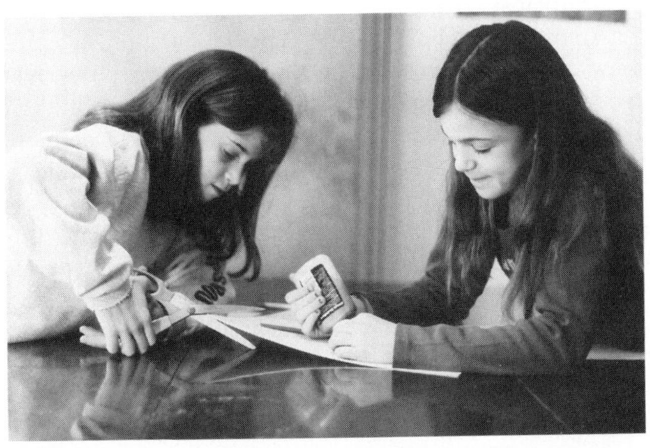

FIGURE 36–4. School-age children sharing materials in an occupational therapy group.

to optimize an individual's success. Cognitive complexity refers to the problem-solving processes involved in mastering steps and controls necessary to complete the activity sequence. Activities should be examined with respect to the number of steps required, the sequence and complexity of steps, and the degree of patience and persistence required. Motor complexity refers to the range of fine motor or visual motor skill required. Social complexity refers to the opportunities the situation affords for social exchange, such as sharing and cooperating in the use of space, materials, and adult and peer attention and interaction.

Often social goals cannot be realized because the activity itself is too complex or frustrating, and this triggers poor social coping strategies. The cognitive and motor complexity of activities may be initially simplified to facilitate and model social learning. For example, children often talk with one another and share more frequently when engaged in simple repetitive activities such as stringing with medium-size beads, because they easily master the task requirements.

• *Vary activities to support child and adolescent's developmental skills*. Many children and adolescents with psychosocial disorders engage in isolative and solitary activities, such as video games and TV watching. Variety in activities offers a chance to sample and learn skills under the guidance of adults. The occupational therapy practitioner may work with other members of the team to engage children in a variety of activities throughout a day or week.

The functional level of an activity for a child or adolescent is one of the most difficult areas to determine. Children with psychosocial disorders may have learning, speech, and cognitive disabilities or previous failures that result in a hesitancy and resistance to try new activities. The starting point for any activity should have simple steps and use materials that are easy to control. For example, when finishing wood projects, painting is more difficult to control than staining. Simple crafts, such as copper tooling, tile boxes or trivets, wood projects, clay slip projects, candle making, leather lacing, staining frames, coloring within designs, and bead stringing are favorites of both children and adolescents. A sample of a completed craft project helps youngsters anticipate steps.

An example of how to handle a social situation, or a preview of a social situation by the practitioner, provides a model for what is expected. Starting simply helps children build a feeling of success. Any activity can be made more complex and challenging, but it is difficult to simplify a complex task, once engaged.

For younger children, simple group games facilitate turn taking and reciprocity, and imaginative play permits children to frame play so that coordination and communication within and outside of roles can occur. Such games often provide a common ground for interaction among unfamiliar peers (Bergen, 1987).

In middle childhood, intervention should emphasize clubs or small groups that have a distinctive identity. Children of this age seek to belong and to be part of a larger social environment. Rituals or distinctive ways of proceeding, such as special beginnings or endings and special handshakes and ways of greeting or dressing serve to bind children to the social groups. Social skills can be emphasized, modeled, and taught within organized groups such as scouts or informally constructed clubs. A club format may also be used for social and task skill instruction in which children name the club (e.g., Problem Solvers not Problem Makers) and they decide on any special features (secret handshakes, code words, or the wearing of special symbols, such as a hat or T-shirt). Models for working in the school system may include academic skills, such as a handwriting club in which part of the agenda can be friendship or activity partnership.

In adolescence, emphasis is on constructing game, sport, and hobby models as well as on activities promoting more independence (e.g., cooking, occupational exploration, and work skills groups). Rituals are also important with this age group, although they may be subtler and take the form of code words and distinct manner of dress. These groups focus on learning specific skills with more explicit and abstract standards for behavior and outcome. For example, in working on a social goal, treating others with respect is emphasized rather than a concrete behavior, such as waiting one's turn, as might be emphasized with younger children.

• *Populate play and task situations with peers*. One-on-one intervention with an adult may be desirable and necessary at first, as children and adolescents benefit from positive social interactions with adults and may need an opportunity to learn the specifics of a craft or game. As soon as feasible, peers should be included. It is within the peer group that the learning and practicing of sharing materials, equipment, space, and the attention of others including the practitioner occurs. Being able to function in a peer group is critical for children with psychosocial dysfunction, and grading the learning and practice of social skills within naturalistic play and task domains is critical.

One strategy for incorporating peers of different developmental levels within a play or task group is using more mature or older children and adolescents as helpers for less mature children. The younger children benefit from learning a task or skill within a sibling model and the older children have an opportunity to practice their skills with a less intimidating age group.

• *Use task and play environments for teaching social skills*. Numerous social skills checklists and training guides are available, but the best interventions occur in daily interactions with others in a variety of settings. Occupational therapy practitioners help model and frame interactions by giving praise for positive interactions—"I like the way everyone is working together"—or by correcting negative interactions when they occur—"How else could you have done or said that?"

There are developmental considerations in teaching social skills, as certain capacities evolve with age, including the child's ability to take the perspective of another person,

CASE STUDY 36-1

Tim: A Boy Admitted to a Psychiatric Hospital's Inpatient Service

Tim, 8 years, 2 months old, is admitted to the inpatient service of a psychiatric hospital for impulsivity, rages, and aggression toward peers and adults, including throwing furniture at school. He lives with his adoptive mother and 5-year-old adoptive sister. He was admitted with a diagnosis of ADHD, rule out mood disorder, and rule out oppositional defiant disorder. The stimulant he was placed on by his primary pediatrician was discontinued to assess his baseline behavior without medication.

HISTORY

Tim was removed from his biological mother at age 2 because of neglect. He was placed in a foster home, and 1 year later, adopted by his foster mother. Tim's adoptive mother reports that he was always an active and aggressive child. She was called to his preschool several times because of repeated instances of fighting with others. He had problems in the first grade, but they had moved to a new location, and the mother attributed his problems to the move. Tim had difficulty with schoolwork in the second grade. He frequently fought with peers and could not focus on classroom work. His pediatrician prescribed a stimulant to help Tim focus on schoolwork. Recently, Tim started fighting and becoming aggressive with his adoptive sister.

OCCUPATIONAL THERAPY EVALUATION AND TREATMENT

Tim was interviewed regarding his play interests and friends, instructed in a copper-tooling project, and given the Beery-Buktenica Developmental Test of Visual-Motor Integration. Tim was difficult to interview because he was in and out of his chair repeatedly and answered questions with one-word responses. He liked sports, and that was it. He had difficulty naming sports in which he engaged. He said everyone at school was his friend, but when asked if it was hard or easy to make friends, he said hard, because "they're mean to me." When asked how they were mean, he said they will not play with him, but he did not specify why. On the copper-tooling task, he needed refocusing to work on the details of the template and to slow down. He was delighted with his end product.

Tim's performance on the developmental test was the equivalent of 6 years, 1 month, and he required prompts to slow down. It was unclear whether his poor score on the test was the result of impulsivity or a deficit in visual motor integration. Additional testing using the visual and motor subsections of the test might be useful closer to discharge. Tim was observed in informal groups and in a craft group to assess his interaction with others. The other children initially liked Tim, because he was friendly and outgoing; but he soon angered them because he was bossy and took play materials from them. He tried to win card games by cheating and tried to win in everything.

Tim participated in multiple occupational therapy groups throughout his 10-day hospitalization. He was in craft skill groups, cooking groups, a scout group, a social skills group called the Problem Solvers and in outing groups. The focus of occupational therapy was to help him with both task and social skills with children of his age. He worked best and followed directions when in a small group with an adult. He had major problems in attention to tasks and became overly physically active in unstructured situations such as on the open sport deck. In those situations, he jumped on furniture and was unsafe with sport equipment. He became argumentative and aggressive with peers. With staff intervention, he was able to take 2-min time-outs, calm himself, and re engage in an activity.

No one on the team had observed any changes in mood, any extreme irritability or giddiness, or hypersexual behavior—as might be typical of a child with a mood disorder. The team also concurred that he was able to respond positively to situations with structure and firm limits, suggesting that his aggression and limit-testing behavior were probably related to ADHD and not ODD. He was placed on a different stimulant from the one he had been on previously to help him focus on tasks and activities.

During his hospitalization, nursing personnel taught Tim's mother behavior management techniques. His mother attended different intervention sessions, including those led by the occupational therapy practitioner, to assist her in applying behavioral techniques in an activity context. The occupational therapy practitioner gave Tim the visual and motor subtests of the developmental test to determine any underlying visual motor integration problem. He received an age equivalent score of 8 years, 1 month in the visual component and a score of 5 years, 6 months in the motor component, suggesting problems in fine motor skills.

Continues

OUTCOMES

The 10-day hospitalization was only the beginning of the intervention process for Tim. The team concurred that Tim had probably missed learning numerous skills because of ADHD. He tried to succeed any way he could, often engaging in behavior that alienated school personnel, peers, and his family. Upon discharge, the occupational therapy practitioner recommended engagement in small social skills or supervised skill groups to help Tim learn positive peer negotiation and interaction. They also suggested occupational therapy in the school system to address fine motor problems and social skills deficits.

the conceptualization of friendship, problem-solving ability, and communication skills. Differences in gender and cultural context should be considered as well (Cartledge & Milburn, 1995).

For preschool children and children functioning at lower social levels, being able to work in the same environment with others, regarding and responding to others, eye contact, simple cause-and-effect sequences, and reciprocal turn taking are appropriate goals. Being able to express positive social behaviors (e.g., laughing and/or smiling) and generally giving positive attention, sharing, and/or compromising; showing affection and/or acceptance; and entering ongoing peer activities may also be reinforced (Cox & Schopler, 1996).

HISTORICAL NOTE 36–1

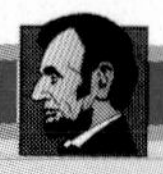

Ruggles's Work with Children: The Care Required by Children

SUZANNE M. PELOQUIN

Ora Ruggles's work with an 11-year-old boy named Ramon exemplifies her practice among children. Ramon had little voluntary control, and he twitched and jerked constantly. Painfully shy, he hid himself in dark corners so as not to be noticed. One day, when the rest of her charges complained that their clay was so lumpy that they were wasting time pressing it through a screen, Ruggles walked Ramon from a corner into the workroom.

As soon as he saw the other children making clay figures, he reproached Ruggles. She countered by showing him how to press clay through the screen. His uncontrolled shaking worked to his advantage, and the other children soon thanked him for producing clay with such a fine texture. Ramon felt useful and appreciated. The task gave him a chance to connect with others in a venture that highlighted his capacity for fellowship rather than his disability.

Although in her biography, the word *diagnosis* is never used, Ruggles's practice took the patient's symptoms and needs into deep consideration.

Carlova, J., & Ruggles, O. (1946). *The healing heart.* New York: Messner.

Higher-level social behaviors for older children and adolescents include changing behavior in response to the needs of friends and acquaintances. These are subtle and sophisticated skills that include joining groups, being accepted by others, being tactful, giving support, offering attention, and helping peers. Good eye contact and the ability to communicate are critical. Examples of targeted skills are successfully joining a group, sharing and playing cooperatively, and giving compliments (Cox & Schopler, 1996).

Social skills training per se is not the complete answer to the performance deficits of children and adolescents with psychosocial dysfunction. Cox and Schopler (1996) caution that there is a big difference between training in controlled settings and generalizing skills to the typically spontaneous, fluid, and unstructured aspects of the real world.

- *Make expectations for behavior explicit and known*. Behavioral expectations may be part of a larger behavior management system or they may be specific to the occupational therapy program. Rule behavior is a major focus in childhood, and expectations for behavior can be phrased as specific rules. Rules for safety and the general manner of proceeding should be established by the practitioner, and the consequences of rule following and rule violation should be clearly communicated. Children enjoy constructing rules and can be given an opportunity to contribute to the rules of the group or the use of the play or game space or materials. Adherence to rules may be promoted by verbal praise or concrete symbols for good effort, such as earning stickers or special privileges (e.g., a visit to the vending machines). Children and adolescents with behavior or emotional problems often have trouble identifying when they have done something right, and social feedback or concrete rewards serve this purpose. The children should identify their positive behaviors and those they may need to work on so that behavioral regulation is under their control.

The intervention principles serve as guidelines for the development of programs for children and adolescents. Program examples include arts and crafts, social skills, cooking and baking, indoor and outdoor games, open houses for parents, and talent shows. Functional skills such as food shopping, money handling, crossing the street, riding the bus, and cleaning up after activities may be incorporated in these programs. Programs may be individually or group focused; and if group focused, individualized goals are addressed within the group. For example, having one child wait his or her turn and follow directions in a game situation and having another child initiate positive social interaction with a peer can both be accomplished within an existing play group. The content of the activities, tasks, and situation in the groups are selected and paced to encourage increasing levels of skill, responsibility, interpersonal responsiveness, and emotional control.

CONCLUSION

Children and adolescents with psychosocial dysfunction are likely to have difficulties in social and task behaviors. Intervention is based on the occupational behavior frame of reference that emphasizes an understanding of normal development and the parameters of play, socialization, and school roles to strengthen social behaviors.

References

Allen, C., Earhart, C., & Blue, T. (1992). *Occupational therapy treatment goals for the physically and cognitively disabled*. Bethesda, MD: American Occupational Therapy Association.

American Academy of Child and Adolescent Psychiatry [AACAP]. (1997a). Practice parameters for the assessment and treatment of children, adolescents, and adults with attention-deficit/hyperactivity disorder. *Journal of the American Academy of Child and Adolescent Psychiatry, 36*(10 Suppl.), 85S–121S.

American Academy of Child and Adolescent Psychiatry [AACAP]. (1997b). Practice parameters for the assessment and treatment of children and adolescents with conduct disorder. *Journal of the American Academy of Child and Adolescent Psychiatry, 36*(10 Suppl.), 122S–139S.

American Academy of Child and Adolescent Psychiatry [AACAP]. (1997c). Practice parameters for the assessment and treatment of children and adolescents with bipolar disorder. *Journal of the American Academy of Child and Adolescent Psychiatry, 36*(10 Suppl.), 157S–176S.

American Academy of Child and Adolescent Psychiatry [AACAP]. (1998). Practice parameters for the assessment and treatment of children and adolescents with depressive disorders. *Journal of the American Academy of Child and Adolescent Psychiatry, 37*(10 Suppl.), 63S–83S.

American Academy of Child and Adolescent Psychiatry [AACAP]. (1999). Practice parameters for the assessment and treatment of children, adolescents, and adults with autism and other pervasive developmental disorders. *Journal of the American Academy of Child and Adolescent Psychiatry, 38*(12 Suppl.), 32S–54S.

American Psychiatric Association [APA]. (1994). *Diagnostic and statistical manual of mental disorders* (4th ed.). Washington, DC: Author.

Bergen, D. (1987). Stages of play development. In D. Bergen (Ed.). *Play as a medium for learning and development* (pp. 49–66). Portsmouth, NH: Heinemann.

Brands, A. (Ed.). (1977). *Individualized treatment planning for psychiatric patients*. Rockville, MD: U.S. Department of Health and Human Services.

Cartledge, G., & Milburn, J. (1995). *Teaching social skills to children and youth* (3rd ed.). Boston: Allyn & Bacon.

Combrinck-Graham, L. (1996). The development of school-age children. In M. Lewis (Ed.). *Child and adolescent psychiatry, a comprehensive textbook* (2nd ed., pp. 271–278). Baltimore: Williams & Wilkins.

Coster, W., Deeney, T., Haltiwanger, J., & Haley, S. (1998). *School Function Assessment*. San Antonio, TX: Psychological Corporation.

Cox, R., & Schopler, E. (1996). Social skills training for children. In M. Lewis (Ed.). *Child and adolescent psychiatry: A comprehensive textbook* (2nd ed., pp. 902–908). Baltimore: Williams & Wilkins.

Danckaerts, M., & Taylor, E. (1995). The epidemiology of childhood hyperactivity. In F. Verhulst & H. Koot (Eds.). *The epidemiology of child and adolescent psychopathology* (pp. 179–209). Oxford, UK: Oxford University Press.

Earls, F. (1994). Oppositional-defiant and conduct disorders. In M. Rutter, E. Taylor, & L. Hersov (Eds.). *Child and adolescent psychiatry modern pproaches* (3rd ed., pp. 308–329). Oxford, UK: Blackwell Scientific.

Florey, L. (1971). An approach to play and play development. *American Journal of Occupational Therapy, 25*, 275–280.

Florey, L., & Greene, S. (1997). Play in middle childhood: A focus on children with behavior and emotional disorders. In L. D. Parham & L. Fazio (Eds.). *Play in occupational therapy for children* (pp. 126–143). St. Louis: Mosby.

Garfinkel, B., Carlson, G., & Weller, E. (1990). Preface. In B. Garfinkel, G. Carlson, & E. Weller (Eds.). *Psychiatric disorders in children and adolescents* (pp. xv–xvi). Philadelphia: Saunders.

Harrington, R. (1994). Affective disorders. In M. Rutter, E. Taylor, & L. Hersov (Eds.). *Child and adolescent psychiatry modern approaches* (3rd ed., pp. 330–350). Oxford, UK: Blackwell Scientific.

Hocutt, A. (1996). Effectiveness of special education: Is placement the critical factor? *Future of Children, 6*(1), 77–102.

Kazdin, A. (1995). Conduct disorder. In F. Verhulst & H. Koot (Eds.). *The epidemiology of child and adolescent psychopathology* (pp. 259–290). Oxford, UK: Oxford University Press.

King-Thomas, L. & Hacker, B. (1987). *A therapist's guide to pediatric assessment*. Boston: Little, Brown.

Knox, S. (1997). Development and current use of the Knox preschool play scale. In L. D. Parham & L. Fazio (Eds.). *Play in occupational therapy for children* (pp. 35–51). St. Louis: Mosby.

Loeber, R., Burke, J., Lahey, B., Winters, A., & Zera, M. (2000). Oppositional defiant and conduct disorder: A review of the past 10 years, Part I. *Journal of the American Academy of Child and Adolescent Psychiatry, 39*(12), 1468–1484.

Lord, C., & Rutter, M. (1994). Autism and pervasive developmental disorders. In M. Rutter, E. Taylor, & L. Hersov (Eds.). *Child and adolescent psychiatry modern approaches* (3rd ed., pp. 569–593). Oxford, UK: Blackwell Scientific.

Moorhead, L. (1969). The occupational history. *American Journal of Occupational Therapy, 23*, 329–334.

Mussen, P., Conger, J. Kagan, J., & Huston, A. (1990). *Child development and personality* (7th ed.). New York: Harper & Row.

Offord, D., & Fleming, J. (1996). Epidemiology. In M. Lewis (Ed.). *Child and adolescent psychiatry: A comprehensive textbook* (2nd. ed., pp. 1166–1178). Baltimore: Williams & Wilkins.

Reilly, M. (1966). The educational process. *American Journal of Occupational Therapy, 23*, 299–307.

Richardson, P. (2001). Use of standardized tests in pediatric practice. In J. Case-Smith (Ed.). *Occupational therapy for children* (4th ed., pp. 217–245). St. Louis: Mosby.

Takata, N. (1974). Play as a prescription. In M. Reilly (Ed.). *Play as exploratory learning* (pp. 209–246). Beverly Hills, CA: Sage.

Tanguay, P. (2000). Pervasive developmental disorders: a 10-year review. *Journal of the American Academy of Child and Adolescent Psychiatry, 39*(9), 1079–1095.

Taylor, E. (1994). Syndromes of attention deficit and overactivity. In M. Rutter, E. Taylor, & L. Hersov (Eds.). *Child and adolescent psychiatry modern approaches* (3rd ed., pp. 285–307). Oxford, UK: Blackwell Scientific.

U.S. Department of Health and Human Services [DHHS]. (1999). *Mental health: A report of the surgeon general*. Rockville, MD: Author

Volkmar, F. (1996). Autism and the pervasive developmental disorders. In M. Lewis (Ed.). *Child and adolescent psychiatry: A comprehensive textbook* (2nd. ed., pp. 489–497). Baltimore: Williams & Wilkins.

Wagner, M. (1995). Outcomes for youths with serious emotional disturbance in secondary school and early adulthood. *The Future of Children*, 5, 90–112.

Weiss, G. (1996). Attention deficit hyperactive disorder. In M. Lewis (Ed.). *Child and adolescent psychiatry: A comprehensive textbook* (2nd. ed., pp. 544–563). Baltimore: Williams & Wilkins.

Weller, E. Weller, R., & Svadjian, H. (1996). Mood disorders. In M. Lewis (Ed.). *Child and adolescent psychiatry: A comprehensive textbook* (2nd. ed., pp. 650–665). Baltimore: Williams & Wilkins.

Zeitlin, S. (1991). *Coping inventory*. Bensenville, IL: Scholastic Testing Service.

Zeitlin, S., Williamson, G., & Szczepanski, M. (1988). *Early coping inventory*. Bensenville, IL: Scholastic Testing Service.

Zigler, E., & Finn-Stevenson, M. (1996). National policies for children, adolescents and families. In M. Lewis (Ed.). *Child and adolescent psychiatry: A comprehensive textbook* (2nd. ed., pp. 1186–1195). Baltimore: Williams & Wilkins.

CHAPTER 37

CHILD ABUSE AND NEGLECT

DEBORA A. DAVIDSON

Families who enact patterns of maltreatment toward their children are experiencing dysfunction that causes victims immediate distress and possibly lifelong occupational performance problems (Bagley & Mallick, 2000; Jasinski, Williams, & Siegel, 2000; Libow, 1995). Practitioners who work in schools, pediatric rehabilitation centers, and early intervention facilities address the needs of parents and families as a part of their responsibility toward the children who have been referred for service. Occupational therapists often work with children and families on a regular basis and over substantial periods of time; this positions practitioners to prevent and ameliorate problems related abuse or neglect.

Delayed development is both a risk factor for and an effect of child maltreatment. Research indicates that the incidence of abuse and neglect may be as high as 3.4 times greater for children with disabilities than for those without (Sullivan & Knutson, 2000). Disabilities associated with an increased risk of maltreatment include communication disorders, mental retardation, behavior disorders, physical impairments, and craniofacial anomalies (Jaudes & Diamond, 1985; Sullivan & Knutson, 2000; Verdugo, Bermejo, & Fuertes, 1995; Wald & Knutson, 2000). Conversely, chronic episodes of abuse place children at increased risk of acquiring delayed social, language, and emotional skills (Egeland, Sroufe, & Erickson, 1983; Haskett & Kistner, 1991; Hoffman-Plotkin & Twentyman, 1984; Jaudes & Diamond, 1985). Most of the pediatric clients seen by occupational therapy practitioners have delayed development in one or more areas and are, as a group, at increased risk of abuse and neglect. By developing an awareness of the risk factors for and signs of child abuse, occupational therapists can use their knowledge and skills to take an important role in preventing, identifying, and ameliorating this major public health problem.

IDENTIFICATION AND PREVENTION

Epidemiology

An understanding of the nature and dynamics of a problem is prerequisite to its prevention. In 1998, approximately 903,000 American children (or 1.3%) were diagnosed as victims of abuse or neglect (U.S. Department of Health and Human Services [DHHS], 2002). Some experts assert that this figure underrepresents the number of true cases, because many children do not receive assistance (Sedlak & Broadhurst, 1996; Starr, Dubowitz, & Bush, 1990). Child abuse may be categorized as neglect, physical abuse, sexual abuse, or emotional maltreatment. In many cases, children experience multiple types of maltreatment.

Definitions of Terms

Neglect makes up about 60% of cases and is defined as the withholding of nutrition, shelter, clothing, and medical care such that the child's health is endangered. Undersupervision and abandonment are included in this category. **Physical abuse** affects about 23% of victims and includes punching, shaking, kicking, biting, throwing, burning, and other forms of injurious punishment. **Sexual abuse** is estimated at about 12% and includes any seduction, coercion, or forcing of a child to observe or participate in sexual activity for the sexual gratification of a more powerful individual.

Emotional maltreatment has been established in about 6% of cases and includes the withholding of affection as well as chronic humiliation, threatening, or criticism. This type of maltreatment is the most difficult to measure, and figures are likely to be underrepresentative of incidence (DHHS, 2000).

CAUSES OF CHILD MALTREATMENT

The causes of child maltreatment are multiple, and no single feature or condition has been found to be causal. Research has repeatedly demonstrated that characteristics of the child, the parents, and the social environment interact dynamically to affect the level of risk for abuse.

Children are at greater risk for abuse and neglect if they have increased dependency needs because of medical or developmental problems, have a difficult temperament, are the product of an unwanted pregnancy, or are considered by the mother to be of an undesirable gender (Frodi, 1981; Steele, 1987). Younger children are at higher risk for serious injuries than older children and adolescents (Sedlak & Broadhurst, 1996). Qualities of the parents (particularly the mother, who is usually the primary caretaker) have also been identified as risk factors. These include having a history of being malparented; having a personality that is characterized by immaturity, egocentrism, and impulsivity; and engaging in alcohol or drug abuse (Main & Goldwyn, 1984; Ogata, Silk, Goodrich, Lohr, Westen, & Hill, 1990; Steele, 1987; Wolfner & Gelles, 1993).

Characteristics of the larger community make up the third level of factors that affect the risk of malparenting. Poverty has been shown to correlate positively with increased rates of child abuse and neglect (DHHS, 2000; Coulton, Korbin, Su, & Chow, 1995; Sedlak & Broadhurst, 1996). Although poverty is linked to increased levels of child abuse, high levels of social integration and community morale appear to be mediating factors that can reduce levels of child abuse even in low-income neighborhoods (Gabarino & Kostelny, 1992). Social isolation and conflict represent risk factors for abuse and neglect. Single-parent families are at significantly higher risk of abuse than two-parent families (Sedlak & Broadhurst, 1996).

Successful intervention and prevention programs address family and community needs for positive leadership and safe places to gather (Steele, 1987; Vondra, 1990). A meta-analysis of abuse prevention and family wellness programs indicated that the most effective programs involved a strengths-based, empowerment approach that lasted over 6 months and provided at least two sessions per month (MacLeod & Nelson, 2000). Occupational therapists have opportunities to intervene with individuals and families through direct service and with community agencies and policy-making bodies via program development, consultation, and administrative roles.

REFERRAL TO PROTECTIVE AGENCIES: MEETING LEGAL MANDATES

All states mandate that health-care and educational professionals report suspected cases of child abuse and neglect to state protective agencies (DHHS, 2002). Most reports to child protective services agencies are generated by the public schools (Sedlak & Broadhurst, 1996). In many cases, a decision to refer a family to child protective services is made by a team, and the team's leader actually makes the report. However, in the absence of a team decision, if an individual therapist has reason to suspect maltreatment, he or she is legally and ethically responsible to make a referral independently (DHHS, 2002).

All reports made in good faith are acceptable, even if it becomes apparent that maltreatment has not occurred. The identity of the referring party is confidential. Referrals involve making a telephone call, followed by a letter that outlines the client's name, age, and address and a summary of the reasons for concern. Reports are categorized by severity and type, and investigations are scheduled accordingly.

Ideally, a referral to child protective services should be made with the parents' knowledge, but this may not be possible if the child's or another's safety might be jeopardized. Repeated reports should be made if continued observations of the problem behaviors occur; multiple referrals are sometimes needed before a case qualifies for an in-depth child protective services evaluation or a legal intervention. The average time period between referral and the initiation of intervention services is 29 days (DHHS, 2000).

Approximately 21% of reported child abuse and neglect cases reach the courts (DHHS, 2000). For documentation to serve as credible evidence in court it must be completed in a reliable and valid manner (Barth & Sullivan, 1985; Kreitzer, 1984). Reliable evidence is documented close to the event's occurrence and, when possible, by more than one observer. Repeated observations or measures taken over a period of time strengthen the report. Valid evidence employs a variety of direct measures, involves standardized tests as much as possible, and is based on objective information, rather than the therapist's interpretation.

Involving child protective services in a case adds another facet to the treatment team. The role of child protective services is to screen families who have been referred for possible abuse or neglect, evaluate those whose problems meet intake criteria, and intervene in identified cases of child abuse. In addition, many child protective services agencies offer an array of services to families who are admitted to the caseload. Services typically include case management, mental health counseling, in-home support, and respite care (DHHS, 2000).

Child protective services agencies are frequently recipients of criticism by the media and the community at large. They are traditionally overburdened and underfunded (Faller, 1985; Roche, 2000). Child protective services caseworkers are typically paraprofessionals who carry large, emotionally stressful caseloads and find limited resources to meet clients' complex needs. They earn relatively low wages for long and sometimes dangerous work. Occupational therapists whose clients are involved with child protective services should strive to initiate and maintain regular contact with their clients' caseworkers to share information and form a positive working relationship. Child protective services workers can, in turn, support therapeutic efforts by encouraging parents to attend appointments and work with the therapist.

OCCUPATIONAL THERAPY EVALUATION

The goals of an occupational therapy evaluation in cases of known or suspected child abuse and neglect are as follows:

- To help determine the child's developmental and functional status and ways to enhance it.
- To help the child and his or her family by supportively, but objectively, contributing to assessment of the parents' current ability to adequately care for the child.
- To evaluate the social and physical environments to identify needs and resources.

Evaluation of the Child

A comprehensive developmental assessment provides an excellent opportunity for observing and documenting the problems common to abused and neglected children. Norm-referenced evaluation tools should be employed as much as possible to maximize the credibility of the information (Helberg, 1983). Developmental assessment of children suspected or identified as being abused can help with securing needed services and designing intervention programs. It may also be of assistance in evaluating the extent to which environmental factors have contributed to delayed development. Standardized developmental assessment before and after therapeutic intervention or foster home placement may indicate rapid developmental spurts that coincide with the intervention. Such findings support a hypothesis for significant environmental contribution to the child's problems (Martin, 1972).

Throughout the evaluation process, the child's physical appearance and affective and social behavior should be observed and noted, as well as hygiene, appropriateness of dress, and the presence of bruises or scars. Problematic behaviors that may reflect maltreatment include rejection of social contact, clinging, aggression, overactivity, underactivity, and noncompliance (Hoffman-Plotkin & Twentyman, 1984; Vondra, 1990). Some children from abusive environments develop adultlike skills secondary to assuming caretaking responsibilities in an effort to gain parental approval or to meet family needs (Martin, 1972). A case example illustrates these points.

When 7-year-old Thomas came to his first occupational therapy session, his hair was dirty and he was wearing overalls that were too small. Thomas was solemn of expression and spoke only when directly questioned. When asked about his daily routine he reported that he always got up early to prepare his mother's breakfast and to care for his infant sister before catching the bus to school. By the end of the session, Thomas had climbed up onto the therapist's lap, uninvited, and presented her with a picture he had drawn for her. When asked who his best friend was, Thomas replied, "You are."

Parenting Assessment

Qualities of the parent may be deduced from interviews at intake, while interviewing for developmental history, and from observations of parent–child interaction. The development of rapport and subsequent progress in treatment requires the therapist to enter the relationship with an attitude of support and a belief that the parents are invested in their children's well-being (Pollack & Steele, 1972). The requirement for confidentiality is counterbalanced by the necessity to ensure client safety and follow legal mandates; this becomes a major issue in situations of possible abuse. Parents should be informed early in the evaluation process that the practitioner will maintain information in confidence but is legally mandated to report cases of possible maltreatment to the appropriate state agency. Some facilities have a brief document for new clients that includes this statement along with other introductory information about the services. If a child is in the custody of child protective services, the legally appointed guardian must grant permission to share information with other individuals or agencies.

An evaluation of parenting skills and practices should include an initial interview and observation of parent–child interactions in structured and unstructured situations. The initial interview is a time to set the tone of the therapeutic relationship and to observe spontaneous behaviors of the parent and child. Advice and recommendations are generally inappropriate at this stage.

Although interviews can quickly provide concentrated information, family relationships are complex and often difficult to characterize adequately in words. Asking the parent to interact with the child through developmentally appropriate activities allows the therapist to observe spontaneous, natural behavior that provides clues regarding problems and assets in occupational performance. A case example illustrates these points.

During an initial interview, Joyce reported that her daughter, 3-year-old Hannah, had "an evil temper, just like her dad." Joyce was especially distressed because Hannah's day care was in jeopardy since Hannah had bitten other toddlers. The therapist asked Joyce to teach Hannah to play with a toy box with multiple buttons and levers that released pop-up toy figures. Joyce showed the box to Hannah, who became excited and reached for the toy. Joyce quickly became frustrated by Hannah's inability to immediately use the levers and buttons and so pulled the toy out of Hannah's reach to play with the box herself. Hannah then hit her mother and collapsed in anguish, as Joyce rolled her eyes and said, "See what I mean? She's violent!"

OCCUPATIONAL THERAPY INTERVENTION

Effective treatment of abused children and their families requires an interdisciplinary team approach that addresses the needs of the family as a system as well as the needs of individual family members. In many settings, the team includes social workers, teachers, psychologists, physicians, nurses, speech therapists, and/or physical therapists.

Intervention for the Parents

The occupational therapist can assist parents by helping them identify and build on their family's strengths, by teaching concepts and skills that may be lacking, and by assisting with building a natural social support system. The development of a support system begins with the parent–therapist relationship, which is facilitated via communication of caring and respect. When the parent views the therapist as someone in whom to trust and confide and as someone who will try to help, a milestone has been reached. Parent groups may facilitate the formation of helpful social relationships, as participants learn that they are not uniquely troubled and may discover mutually helpful solutions. More enduring forms of support can be developed by helping parents develop mutual relationships with reliable friends, family, and community resources.

Parent education should include behavior management techniques, such as praising approximations of desirable behaviors, sticker charting, and gentle time-outs. Information related to normal child development of social, daily living, and safety skills can reduce frustration and danger caused by parents' unrealistic expectations. Role-playing and practice of new skills in parent–child activity-based sessions help consolidate new knowledge and skills. Assertiveness training may help parents develop child management skills, improve general communication abilities, and facilitate empowerment. Education and practice of crisis prevention techniques (e.g., list making; financial budgeting; planning work, leisure, and health-care obligations around child care and transportation resource availability) is often useful. Carefully timed and tactful referral for further help, such as that afforded by psychotherapists, child-care programs, and adult educational or vocational training programs can also significantly affect family functioning.

Intervention for the Child

Emotional bonding with a caring adult has been postulated to be a prerequisite to healthy personality development (Bowlby, 1988; Jernberg, 1979; Martin, 1972). Ideally, this type of relationship should be developed with a caregiver who is a permanent member of the child's world. Sometimes the therapist must assist the child in establishing initial trust in therapy and then transferring this new ability to a caregiver in the larger world. The therapist may facilitate a child's ability to form relationships through activities found in healthy parent–child interactions, including cuddling and holding, feeding, grooming, and teaching developmentally appropriate skills. Reliability, gentleness, and communication of caring are essential features in this kind of therapy. Approaches for addressing the abused child's psychosocial needs may be combined with occupational therapy techniques used in treating other developmental needs, such as motor skills, dressing, and eating. Therapeutic activities based on sensory integration theory, neurodevelopmental treatment, and behavioral approaches are easily performed with attention to the nature and quality of the therapeutic relationship.

Intervention for the Parent–Child Relationship

As the parent and child become better able to receive and respond to support from the therapist, the likelihood of facilitating their own positive interactions increases. The occupational therapist can select activities to elicit appropriate caregiving behaviors by grading the amount of interaction and external structure required. Activities should be selected for appropriateness in terms of the parent's and the child's developmental levels and presented in a supportive, nonevaluative mode. The therapist may need to demonstrate and teach some of the activities initially. In all activities, gentle physical contact, pleasant conversation, and mutual enjoyment are the main goals. The occupational therapist can also use parent–child sessions to teach concepts of child development. Parent–child sessions can also allow parents to observe and practice behavior management skills, such as praising and correcting behaviors.

CONCLUSION

Unlike most of the causes of developmental disabilities, such as prenatal distress and genetic error, child abuse is a common problem that occupational therapists can help prevent. Occupational therapists who work in school- and community-based settings are in a strategic position to screen children routinely for abuse, to provide preventive intervention and referral, and to help ameliorate the consequences of abuse.

The negative effects of physical abuse have been documented as early as infancy and have been shown to persist through adulthood. Chronic child abuse in families tends to perpetuate an intergenerational cycle of troubled interpersonal relationships, emotional distress, and malparenting (Main & Goldwyn, 1984; Ogata et al., 1990; Prodgers, 1984). Effective intervention with families who engage in violence toward their children is an investment in the occupational performance and well-being of this and future generations.

References

Bagley, C., & Mallick, K. (2000). Prediction of sexual, emotional and physical maltreatment and mental health outcomes in a longitudinal cohort of 290 adolescent women. *Child Maltreatment*, *5*, 218–226.

Barth, R., & Sullivan, R. (1985). Collecting competent evidence in behalf of children. *Social Work, March-April*, 130–136.

Bowlby, J. (1988). *A secure base: Parent-child attachment and health*. New York: Basic.

Coulton, C., Korbin, J., Su, M., & Chow, J. (1995). Community level factors and child maltreatment rates. *Child Development*, *66*, 1262–1276.

Egeland, B., Sroufe, A., & Erickson, M. (1983). The developmental consequences of different patterns of maltreatment. *Child Abuse and Neglect*, *7*, 459–469.

Faller, K. C. (1985). Unanticipated problems in the United States child protection system. *Child Abuse and Neglect*, *9*, 63–69.

Frodi, A. (1981). Contribution of child characteristics to child abuse. *American Journal of Mental Deficiency*, *85*, 341–345.

Gabarino, J., & Kostelny, K. (1992). Child maltreatment as a community problem. *Child Abuse and Neglect*, *16*, 455–464.

Haskett, M., & Kistner, J. (1991). Social interactions and peer perceptions of young physically abused children. *Child Development*, *62*, 979–990.

Helberg, J. (1983). Documentation in child abuse. *American Journal of Nursing*, *2*, 236–239.

Hoffman-Plotkin, D., & Twentyman, C. (1984). A multimodal assessment of behavioral and cognitive deficits in abused and neglected preschoolers. *Child Development*, *55*, 794–802.

Jasinski, J. L., Williams, L. M., & Siegel, J. (2000). Childhood physical and sexual abuse as a risk factor for heavy drinking among African-American women: A prospective study. *Child Abuse and Neglect*, *24*, 1061–1071.

Jaudes, P. K., & Diamond, L. J. (1985). The handicapped child and child abuse. *Child Abuse and Neglect*, *9*, 341–347.

Jernberg, A. (1979). *Theraplay*. Washington, DC: Jossey-Bass.

Kreitzer, M. (1984). Legal aspects of child abuse: Guidelines for the nurse. *Nursing Clinics of North America*, *16*, 149–160.

Libow, J. (1995). Munchausen by proxy victims in adulthood: A first look. *Child Abuse and Neglect*, *19*, 1131–1142.

MacLeod, J., & Nelson, G. (2000). Programs for the promotion of family wellness and the prevention of child maltreatment: A meta-analytic review. *Child Abuse and Neglect*, *24*, 1127–1149.

Main, M., & Goldwyn, R. (1984). Predicting rejection of her infant from mother's representation of her own experience: Implications for the abused-abusing intergenerational cycle. *Child Abuse and Neglect*, *8*, 203–217.

Martin, H. (1972). The child and his development. In C. Kempe & R. Helfer (Eds.). *Helping the battered child and his family*. (pp. 93–114). Philadelphia: J.B. Lippincott.

Ogata, S., Silk, K., Goodrich, S. Lohr, N., Westen, D., & Hill, E. (1990). Childhood sexual and physical abuse in adult patients with borderline personality disorder. *American Journal of Psychiatry*, *147*, 1008–1013.

Pollack, C., & Steele, B. (1972). A therapeutic approach to parents. In C. Kempe & R. Helfer (Eds.). *Helping the battered child and his family* (pp. 3–21). Philadelphia: J.B. Lippincott.

Prodgers, A. (1984). Psychopathology of the physically abusing parent: A comparison with the borderline syndrome. *Child Abuse and Neglect*, *8*, 411–424.

Roche, T., August, M., Grace, J., Harrington, M., Hylton, H., Monroe, S., & Willwerth, J. (2000, November). The crises of foster care. *Time Canada*, 156(20), 52.

Sedlak, A. J., & Broadhurst, D. D. (1996). *Executive summary of the third national incidence study of child abuse and neglect*. Washington, D.C.: U.S. Department of Health and Human Services, National Center on Child Abuse and Neglect.

Starr, R. H. Jr., Dubowitz, H., & Bush, B. A. (1990). The epidemiology of child maltreatment. In R. T. Ammerman & M. Hersen (Eds.). *Children at risk: An evaluation of factors contributing to child abuse and neglect* (pp. 149–165). New York: Plenum.

Steele, B. (1987). Psychodynamic factors in child abuse. In R. E. Helfer & R. S. Kempe (Eds.). *The battered child* (4th ed., pp. 81–114) Chicago: University of Chicago Press.

Sullivan, P. M., & Knutson, J. F. (2000). Maltreatment and disabilities: A population-based epidemiological study. *Child Abuse and Neglect*, *24*, 1257–1273.

U.S. Department of Health and Human Services [DHHS]. (2000). *Child maltreatment 1998: Reports from the states to the National Child Abuse and Neglect Data System*. Washington, DC: U.S. Government Printing Office.

U.S. Department of Health and Human Services [DHHS]. (2002). National Clearinghouse: Child abuse and neglect information. Available at: www.calib.com/nccanch/. Accessed: August 22, 2002.

Verdugo, M. A., Bermejo, B. G., & Fuertes, J. (1995). The maltreatment of intellectually handicapped children and adolescents. *Child Abuse and Neglect*, *19*, 205–215.

Vondra, J. I. (1990). Sociological and ecological factors. In R. T. Ammerman & M. Hersen (Eds.). *Children at risk: An evaluation of factors contributing to child abuse and neglect* (pp. 149–165). New York: Plenum.

Wald, R. L., & Knutson, J. F. (2000). Childhood disciplinary experiences reported by adults with craniofacial anomalies. *Child Abuse and Neglect*, *24*, 1623–1627.

Wolfner, G., & Gelles, R. (1993). A profile of violence toward children: A national study. *Child Abuse and Neglect*, *17*, 197–212.

CASE STUDY ANALYSIS: UNIT IX

OLGA BALOUEFF

This analysis addresses the clinical reasoning process for assessment and intervention planning in a public school setting, for 9-year-old Patrice Douce who sustained a traumatic brain injury (TBI).

PREPARING THE OCCUPATIONAL PROFILE: INITIAL DATA GATHERING

Both Susan and Mary have worked in the Pierce Elementary School, Patrice's school, for some time. Over the years, they have built a strong rapport with the school principal, the teachers, and the director of special education. They all value these occupational therapy practitioners' expertise and understand the many roles the therapists fill at the school, ranging from consultant to the classroom teacher to providing direct services to the children with special needs.

Susan and Mary are well aware that Patrice's return to reengage and participate in everyday classroom activities is not only difficult but also daunting at times. Before formally evaluating Patrice's needs, Susan arranged for time to talk with his classroom teacher and his parents to understand their perspective on his school reentry. Meanwhile, Mary observes Patrice in the playground and in the classroom, recording her observations on a checklist she and Susan have developed for all initial data gathering and evaluation at the school.

On the playground, Mary sees Patrice playing basketball with his peers. He has trouble making baskets, stumbles, and drops the ball. On several occasions, he lashes out at his friends, shouting out at them and threatening to hit them. Later in the day, in the classroom during a math lesson, Patrice yawns repeatedly and finally puts his head on the desk. In the reading circle, he fidgets more than the other children and needs help to find his place in the book. Mary notes that Patrice is more alert early in the day but that toward the end of the day he becomes tired and irritable. His behavior is often distracting to the teacher and his classmates.

When talking to his teacher, Susan finds out that on his return to school Patrice has been well received by his classmates. They are generally supportive and helpful, particularly two of the girls who take it on themselves to redirect him in classroom assignments when he loses his place in the book or in transcribing letters and numbers from the blackboard into his notebook. The teacher feels that Patrice's attention and his performance are generally better in the early part of the morning, but that he becomes easily distracted, short-tempered, and even tired by noon. She knows that he was a good student before his injury; but now, although he seems to understand most of the new materials presented in class, he needs help starting and finishing tasks and has trouble concentrating and getting organized. She adds that she didn't know much about TBI before Patrice's coming to her class, but that she has begun reading about it and found out that he presents many of the behaviors commonly seen in children with this injury.

The teacher also believes that Patrice sometimes does not seem to fit in with friends and classmates, particularly at recess or when the class gets animated. She feels sorry for him and is looking forward to collaborating with the occupational therapy practitioners, the speech therapist, the other team members, and his parents to create strategies and an educational plan suitable to his needs.

When meeting with Mr. and Mrs. Douce, Susan explains to them that her role as an occupational therapist is to help Patrice develop skills and strategies to assist his learning in school. She asks for their input about their goals for their son and what they think Patrice's present needs are. At first, they are surprised by the question and are reluctant to speak up. Trying to put them more at ease, Susan finds out that generally in Haiti professionals are considered to be in charge and thus tell parents what to do and not the reverse. After a while, the parents become more comfortable and talkative, they express their joy about their son's recovery but also bewilderment and sadness about his changed behavior, although the hospital staff had prepared them for that.

When asked about their immediate concerns, they lament that Patrice, who before his injury had been a good student, is now lazy, stubborn, and unwilling to do his homework. He also frequently interrupts conversations and speaks out of turn. Furthermore, Patrice often fights with his younger brother and appears to act younger than his age. He sleeps a lot, particularly when he comes home from school and often seems disoriented when he wakes up. They add that their goal for their son is for an improvement in his behavior at home and at school. They want him to be a good and well-disciplined student and to be polite and respectful to adults.

Finally, Susan meets with Patrice. She wants to understand his perspective on the school reentry and on his strengths and needs. By engaging him in a conversation, she hopes to get a window into his thinking processes, his feelings, and his speech patterns. She puts the young boy at ease by talking about favorite basketball players and TV shows and about having been herself out of school for a while, because of an illness, when she was a child.

When asked if he is happy to be back in school, he says, "Oh yes! But it is hard!" When questioned about what is hard, he tells her that he gets tired at school and that he is unable to play basketball with his friends like he used to. "I must also be very dumb now because I forget things, and I often get confused," Patrice adds. Finally, Susan asks him to tell her three things he wants to do better in the future. To that, he answers, "Playing basketball, not fighting with my friends, and making my parents proud of me." Susan tells him that together with him, his teacher, and his parents, they will work at finding ways for him to get stronger and meet his goals.

CONCEPTUAL BASES GUIDING THE EVALUATION PROCESS

After reflecting on frames of reference to guide Patrice's evaluation, Susan chooses the Model of Human Occupation (MOHO; Kielhofner, 1995), which considers the child's total functioning within the environment. To address the movement patterns and sensorimotor characteristics underlining Patrice's skilled behavior, she uses also the Neurodevelopmental Treatment (NDT) approach (Schoen & Anderson, 1999).

Patrice's occupational therapy evaluation is summarized in Table IX-A. The table identifies concepts from the MOHO and NDT frames of reference and the occupational therapy practice framework.

PATRICE'S OCCUPATIONAL THERAPY INTERVENTION

At the individualized education program (IEP) meeting with Mr. and Mrs. Douce, team members present their evaluation results and discuss an education plan for Patrice. The IEP addresses both academic and personal modifications, specific instructional needs, measurements to determine success, and Patrice's present levels of performance.

Patrice will receive direct and consultative occupational services twice a week. Mary, the certified occupational therapist assistant, will provide the direct service, which will involve working with Patrice during recess, gym, and in his classroom. She will assist the teacher in the classroom in meeting the educational goals for Patrice. She will consult regularly with Susan, the occupational therapist. Susan will also observe in the classroom and consult with the teacher about modifications to the learning environment that will enhance Patrice's learning.

Mr. and Mrs. Douce approve the IEP. To promote communication between school and home, the team and the Douces decide to use a notebook to record observations and strategies regarding Patrice's needs. The Douces agree to contribute to the notebook, so that school personnel can gain an understanding of Patrice's performance at home. The notebook is to be sent home daily at the beginning of the school year, changing to weekly when his performance improves and stabilizes. Although Patrice is not present at the meeting, Susan, reviews the information shared at the meeting with Patrice. The team identified the following goals and strategies for Patrice.

1. Patrice will improve his social skills so that he remains calm in frustrating situations and follows the rules in the classroom, lunchroom, and playground. To increase Patrice's social skills and promote appropriate classroom behavior, the teacher and the special education team will
   - Present clear rules of conduct and repeat them frequently.
   - Post classroom rules and review them daily.
   - Recognize and reward appropriate behavior immediately.
   - Be sensitive to Patrice's cues of confusion and tiredness.
   - Prepare Patrice for changes and transitions.
   - Model calm, friendly behavior and negotiating skills.
   - Create opportunities for success each day.
2. Patrice will increase his attention and concentration so that he can remain on task for longer periods of time and with fewer modifications in the classroom.
   a. To increase Patrice's attention and concentration in the classroom the teacher will
      - Place Patrice's desk close to hers and that of a well-organized classmate.
      - Place Patrice's desk away from door and other high-activity areas.
      - Keep instructions short and concise.
      - Keep the environment organized and without excessive distraction.
      - Monitor and refocus Patrice as needed.

   b. The occupational therapist will observe Patrice periodically; given these observations, the teacher and occupational therapist will develop additional strategies to meet Patrice's needs more effectively.
3. Patrice will improve his gross motor coordination and endurance so that he can sit comfortably for

TABLE IX–A. **PATRICE'S OCCUPATIONAL THERAPY EVALUATION**

Areas of Occupation	Assessment Tools	Principal Findings
Factors Within School Context		
Activities of daily living	School Function Assessment[a]	Independent in most activities of daily living but needs a few modifications for full participation in activities (e.g., transitions from one area of school to another, carrying a meal tray, carrying books)
Educational activities	School Function Assessment[a] and interview and questionnaire for teacher, parents, and Patrice	Participates in most activities in regular classroom with some assistance (e.g., short breaks, slower pace, redirection, supervision of arithmetic and spelling)
Play and leisure activities	School Function Assessment[a] and interview and questionnaire for teacher, parents, and Patrice	Participates in half the activities he did before; has difficulty with running at recess and team sports; tires easily
Self-concept	Self-Perception Profile for Children[b]	Feels less worthy than peers in athletic and behavioral conduct
Interests and values	Interview for teacher, parents, and Patrice	Wants to be a good student, play ball, and have friends
Social	Social Skills Rating System (three versions for child, parents, teacher)	Aggressive and acts out when frustrated; impulsive
Factors that Influence Occupational Performance		
Visual motor integration	Developmental Test of Visual Motor Integration[c]	Difficulties with reproduction of diagnosis and eye–hand coordination
Gross and fine motor skills	Bruininks-Oseretsky Test of Motor Proficiency[d]	Poor balance and coordination; difficulty with jumping; slow moving; poor eye–hand and bilateral coordination
Neuromusculoskeletal (muscle tone, strength, endurance, postural control, postural alignment)	Observations from an NDT perspective	Weak postural muscles, leading to increased fatigue; diminished equilibrium reactions in standing; diminished overall strength (e.g., slides off chair easily)
Process skills (attention span, initiation and termination of activity, sequencing, inquiries, adaptation)	Teacher's report and School Function Assessment[a]	Attention span is poor when tired; easily distracted; needs help in starting and ending activities; irregular performance in class with homework
Mental functions (spatial relationship, visual discrimination, figure–ground, visual closure, visual memory)	Motor-Free Visual Perception[e]	Difficulties with visual memory, certain aspects of spatial relationships, and visual discrimination; complains of test being hard and eyes getting fatigued

[a]Coster, Deeney, Haltiwanger, & Haley (1995).
[b]Harter (1985).
[c]Beery (1997).
[d]Bruininks (1978).
[e]Colarusso and Hammill (1995).

longer periods in class and be successful in physical education class and in the playground.

a. To enable Patrice to sit comfortably in class, the occupational therapist will
   - Modify Patrice's usual chair in the classroom to include a platform to support his feet, a raised chair back, and armrests for lateral supports.
   - Modify Patrice's desk at school to include raising the desktop and tilting it to 45° to promote upper body stability and wrist extension and to decrease energy requirements.

b. To develop Patrice's gross motor coordination (postural and truck control, equilibrium reactions, overall muscle strength) the certified occupational therapy assistant will
   - Provide gross motor activities for Patrice and a small group of children with a large ball, scooter board, and mat equipment.
   - Practice basketball-related skills (e.g., catching, dribbling, throwing the ball into the basket).

4. Patrice will improve his fine motor coordination so that he can engage more successful in writing and art activities.
   a. To develop Patrice's fine motor coordination, the certified occupational therapy assistant will work with him on bilateral arm and hand activities during art and writing classes.
   b. The occupational therapist will observe Patrice performing fine motor activities and suggest additional approaches to the certified occupational therapy assistant as Patrice improves.
5. Patrice will increase his visual-processing skills so that he can read more easily, participate in mathematics activities, and use the computer with less strain.
   a. To increase Patrice's visual-processing skills, the teacher and the special education team will
      - Allow extra time for Patrice to examine visual input; repeat auditory instructions; and, when expected, to give written and oral responses.
      - Teach Patrice to follow written text by using his finger, by underlining, or by covering part of the page to create a window while reading.
      - Teach Patrice to use of color cues on the sides of page for left-to-right cuing.
      - Use large-print calculator and large-print books when appropriate.
      - Teach strategies for resting he eyes.
   b. To increase Patrice's visual-processing skills, the certified occupational therapy assistant will provide activities for Patrice and a small group of classmates that include visual discrimination, spatial relations, and visual figure-ground perception skills.
   c. The occupational therapist will observe Patrice and suggest modified approaches to the certified occupational therapy assistant as Patrice improves.

During periodic meetings with the Douces, the team will address Patrice's progress and make suggestions to them for improving his functional performance at home. These suggestions will reinforce the following goals:

- Develop Patrice's gross and fine motor coordination: (1) enroll Patrice in a karate class or other activity that encourages gross motor development and (2) modify Patrice's usual chair at home to include a platform to support his feet, a raised chair back, and armrests for lateral supports.
- Increase Patrice's attention and cooperation: (1) discuss strategies for keeping Patrice focused on task completion and his ability to comply with directions and (2) help the Douces understand that Patrice's behavior is not always intentional and that he is not purposively distracting others or daydreaming.

The strategies cited in Patrice's IEP were derived from the following resources: Begali (1992); Bell, (1994); Drummond (1996); Savage and Wolcott (1994); and Wolcott, Lash, and Pearson (1995).

SUMMARY

Together with Patrice, Mr. and Mrs. Douce, the classroom teacher, and the rest of the team, Susan and Mary formulated an evaluation and an IEP to meet the boy's educational needs. Because Patrice's needs will change as his brain recovers, the IEP has to remain flexible and must be revised regularly. Communication among the family, the classroom teacher, and the team members is crucial. Patrice's motivation and involvement are central to the implementation of the plan.

American Occupational Therapy Association. (In press). Occupational therapy practice framework: Domain and process. American Journal of Occupational Therapy.

Beery, K. (1997). Beery-Buktenica developmental test of visual-motor integration (VMF) (4th rev. ed.). Parsippany, NJ: Modern Curriculum.

Begali, V. (1992). *Head injury in children and adolescents: Resources and review for school and allied professionals*. Brandon, VT: Clinical Psychology.

Bell, T. A. (1994). Understanding students with traumatic brain injury: A guide for teachers and therapists. *AOTA School System Special Interest Section Quarterly*, *1*(2), 1–4.

Bruininks, R. H. (1978). Bruininks-Oseretsky test of motor proficiency. Circle Pines, MN: American Guidance Service.

Coster, W., Deeney, T., Haltiwanger, J., & Haley, S., (1998). School function assessment (SFA). San Antonio, TX: Psychological Corporation.

Colarusso, R., & Hammill, D. (1995). The Motor Free Visual Perception Test-Revised. Novato, CA: Academic Therapy.

Drummond, C. W. (1996). Inclusion and school-based occupational therapy. AOTA *School System Special Interest Section Quarterly*, 3(3), 1–3.

Harter, S. (1985). The self perception profile for children. Denver, CO: University of Denver.

Kielhofner, G. (Ed.). (1995). *A model of human occupation: Theory and application* (2nd ed.). Baltimore: Williams & Wilkins.

An education-based reasoning model to support best practices for school-based OT under IDEA 97. AOTA *School System Special Interest Section Quarterly*, 8(2), 1–4.

Savage, R. C., & Wolcott, G. F. (Eds.). (1994). *Educational dimensions of acquired brain injury*. Austin, TX: Pro-Ed.

Schoen, S. A., & Anderson, J. (1999). Neurodevelopmental treatment frame of reference. In P. Kramer & J. Hinojosa (Eds.). *Frames of reference for pediatric occupational therapy* (2nd ed., pp. 83–118).

Wolcott, G., Lash, M., & Pearson, S. (1995). *Signs and strategies for educating students with brain injuries: A practical guide for teachers and schools*. Houston, TX: HDI.

UNIT *ten*

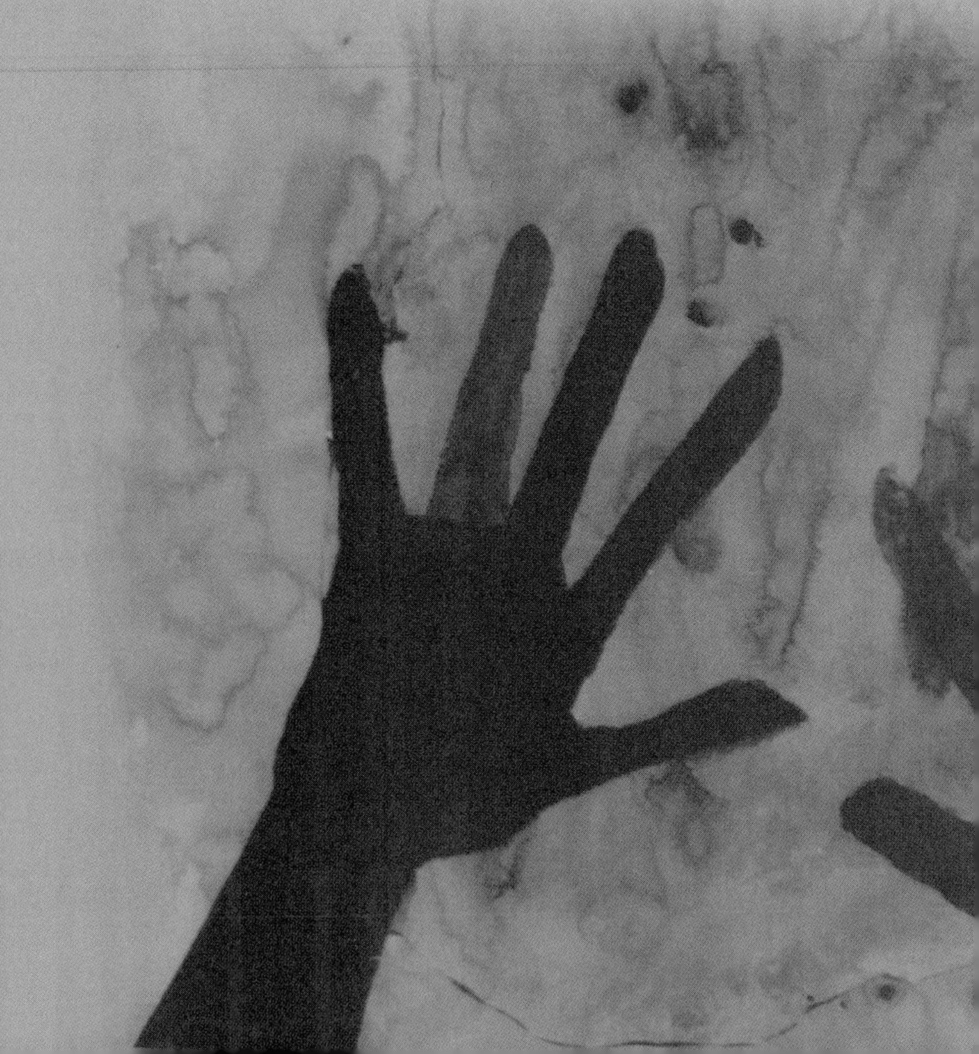

Diagnostic Considerations in Adult and Older Adult Practice

Learning Objectives

After completing this unit, readers will be able to:

- Describe the population served by occupational therapy practitioners working with adults and older adults.
- Explain core approaches to understanding life-span development in adults and older adults and relate these to occupational performance.
- Describe common diagnoses and health-care interventions for adults and older adults receiving occupational therapy, including the following:
  - *Neurological dysfunction:* Cerebral vascular accident, traumatic brain injury, Parkinson disease, amyotrophic lateral sclerosis, multiple sclerosis, spinal cord injury, and Guillain-Barré syndrome.
  - *Orthopedic and musculoskeletal dysfunction:* Hand injuries; fractures of the hip, back, pelvis, and lower extremities; upper and lower extremity amputations; and arthritis.
  - *Cardiopulmonary dysfunction:* myocardial infarction, chronic obstructive pulmonary disease, congestive heart failure, and tuberculosis.
  - *Immune system dysfunction:* HIV, infection, and cancer.
  - *Psychosocial dysfunction:* Dementias, mood disorders, substance abuse, eating disorders, borderline personality disorder, and schizophrenia.
  - *Skin system dysfunctions:* Burns.
- Explain the effects of illness and disability associated with common diagnoses on occupational performance in adulthood and old age.
- Identify and support selections of occupational therapy evaluation and intervention strategies for adults and older adults who are experiencing one or more of the common diagnostic conditions.

This unit looks at the way common medical and psychiatric diagnoses in adults influence occupational therapy evaluation and intervention. Diagnostic conditions are often associated with particular patterns of occupational performance difficulties, environmental stressors, and body system-body function impairments. For example, a person with a fractured hip will likely have initial difficulty with functional mobility for sitting, toileting, and bathing. Alternatively, someone with a persistent mental illness may be able to move with little difficulty but be challenged by distorted thinking processes and the social stigma still common to mental illness. Practitioners who are aware of some of the common problems associated with given diagnoses will be skillfully able to elicit client concerns, target evaluations, and tailor interventions to accommodate diagnostically related factors.

All diagnostic conditions pose certain precautions related to occupational therapy intervention. Fractured bones require sufficient healing time before too much pressure is placed on them, and fragile psyches require sensitivity in grading performance demands. To keep clients safe, practitioners need to be aware of precautions associated with diagnoses along a continuum from acute to chronic stages or as phases of recovery. These precautions require an understanding of specialized medically and psychologically related medications, equipment, and procedures. Practitioners who are not aware of these precautions can seriously harm clients.

Diagnostic conditions, then, can influence therapists' choice of evaluation methods and intervention approaches and methods. Practitioners are also influenced by the client's occupational profile and concerns (see Units VII and VIII), conceptual models guiding practice (see Unit VI), and professional and service factors (see Units XI and XII). (Note: Words in **bold** type are defined in the Glossary.)

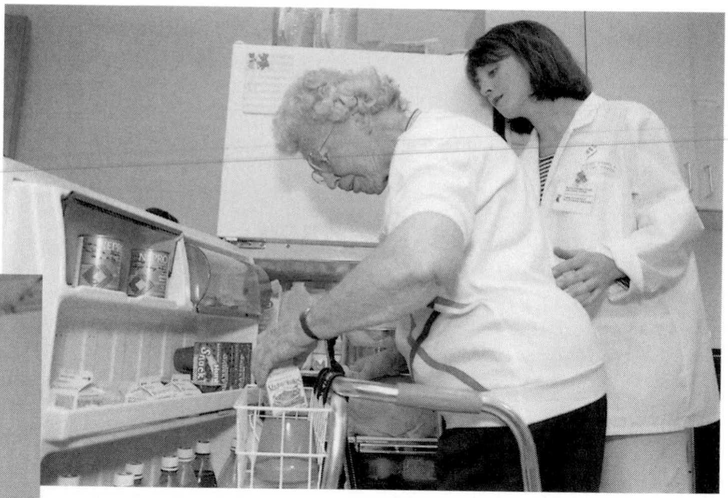

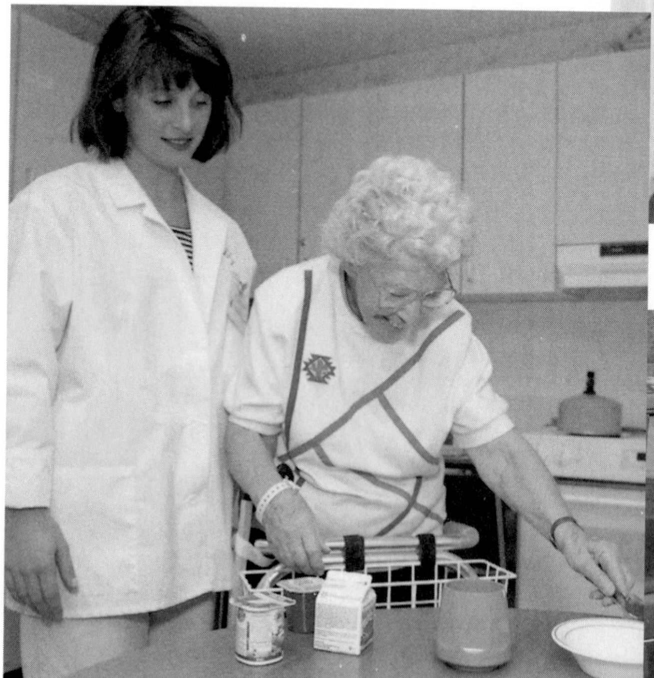

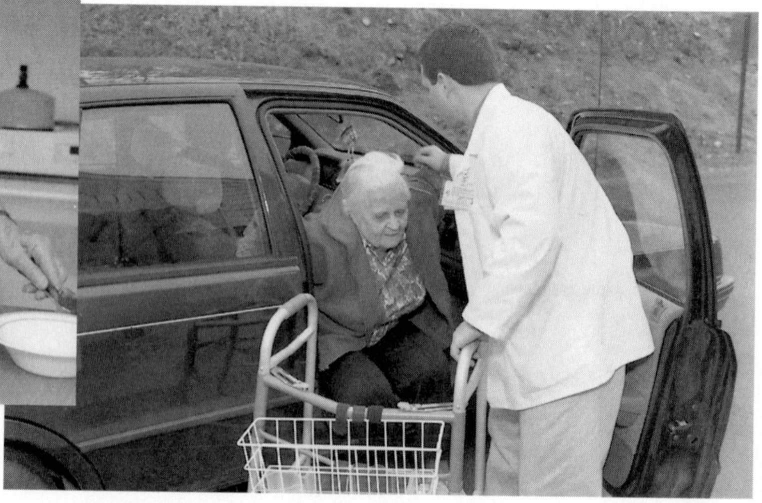

Preparing to go home after a stroke or hip fracture requires thinking about how to do familiar tasks in new ways, (*left & right*) such as making a meal safely. (Courtesy of G. Samson, UNH Photographic Services, Dimond Library, University of New Hampshire, Durham.) (*bottom*) The practitioner coaches a woman on how to get out of a car while using a walker. (Courtesy of G. Samson, UNH Photographic Services, Dimond Library, University of New Hampshire, Durham.)

CHAPTER 38

INTRODUCTION TO ADULT AND OLDER ADULT POPULATIONS

BETTY R. HASSELKUS

In recent decades, adulthood and old age have been recognized as complex, dynamic stages of life that offer tremendous challenges and rich contexts of practice for health care professionals. The American Occupational Therapy Association (AOTA) membership invoice questionnaire for 2000 revealed that >60% of all occupational therapy personnel in the United States work primarily with adults and older people, and 37% of all personnel work primarily with people who are 65 years of age or older (AOTA, 2000). As the demographics of the world shift to a larger and larger proportion of elderly, increasing numbers of occupational therapists are drawn to geriatrics and its various subspecialties as areas of practice.

In this chapter, I will briefly review the many ways that life-span developmentalists have characterized adult life and old age. Next, I examine human occupation during adulthood and aging, focusing on self-care, work, and leisure. Finally, I discuss adult development and aging within the context of health and illness, focusing on caregiving processes and the relationship of adult development to mental retardation, mental illness, and physical disability.

THE CONCEPT OF LIFE-SPAN DEVELOPMENT

The term *human development* typically refers to a patterned sequence of changes in the human being that occurs over a considerable length of time (Kaluger & Kaluger, 1984; Newman & Newman, 1984). Until the second half of the twentieth century, the primary focus of the field of human development was clearly on early life developmental changes. In the last half of that century, however, the emphasis broadened to a decidedly life-span view (Erikson, 1959; Hatch, 2000; Reese & Overton, 1970; Vaillant, 1977); adulthood and old age are now firmly ensconced in the concept of human development, extending the study of development throughout maturity to very old age and death.

Human development in adulthood and old age encompasses physiological, psychological, and sociological aspects of change (Dannefer & Perlmutter, 1990). These aspects of development provide a way to organize the study of life-span changes and have led to the use of several different **metaphors** to portray development in adulthood and aging. A number of these metaphorical images are discussed here.

Passages

In 1976, Sheehy introduced the term *passages* to describe critical transitions that define development in adult life. "Life after adolescence is not one long plateau. Changes are not only possible and predictable, but to deny them is to be an accomplice to one's own unnecessary vegetation" (p. 12). Passages are shifts in one's internal self. "Pulling Up Roots," for example, is a passage that takes place when young adults gradually shift themselves emotionally and physically away from a self that is centered within the parental home to a new separate self with its own authenticity within its own peer group. The "Urge to Merge" is the passage that leads to coupling and thoughts of marriage.

Passages occur across the life span. In a later book, Sheehy (1995) extended the concept of passages beyond mid-life and into older age, including passages such as the "Flaming Fifties." She described the fifties as a time that requires courage and rebelliousness as individuals forge ahead into the second half of life.

Marker Events

Neugarten (1977) discussed the idea of marker events across the life span and their relationship to personality development and adaptation. Marker events are social occasions, such as graduating, marrying, starting a job, or getting a driver's license. Such events have been shown to trigger periods of change and development in people's lives (Lowenthal, Thurnher, & Chiriboga, 1975). Neugarten (1977) proposed that the occurrence of a marker event itself does not promote development; rather it is when such events occur "off time" rather than "on time" that major changes occur. For example, retirement earlier in life than normally expected would be off time, and, because of this, the event would generate significant developmental change within the individual. Retirement at the usual time in life would not lead to such a major adjustment.

More recently, Settersten and Hagestad (1996a, 1996b) investigated what they called "cultural age deadlines" and their meanings in contemporary American society. In their research on transitions, they found that the men and women in their study did, by and large, have the perception that cultural age deadlines exist for family, work, and educational spheres of life (with some differences by gender); but a considerable flexibility is also perceived to be present. Little or no consequences were perceived to exist for missed deadlines related to family, work, or education, for example. The authors concluded from these findings that "cultural thinking about age timetables . . . seems relatively loose and flexible" (1996a, p. 612).

Seasons

In his book on adult development, Levinson (1978) used yet another image of development, the image of seasons. Levinson used the term *life cycle* rather than *life span*, to convey a sense of a process or journey that has an underlying universal pattern and shape. The pattern is made up of periods or stages of life; these are the seasons of life, and each has its own distinctive character and quality. To Levinson, each season in the cycle of life has its own time and needs to be understood in its own terms. "No season is better or more important than any other" (p. 7). A transition is required for a shift from one season to the next.

Life as a Composition

Bateson (1989) introduced the themes of composition and improvisation into **life-span development** theory. Adults have the capacity to manipulate and recombine familiar and unfamiliar components of their lives, thus creating new directions for themselves, moving into previously unknown territory. Bateson stated that adults need to "recognize the value of lifetimes in continual redefinition" (p. 7). Life is like a work in progress; individuals need to improvise constantly. Life is a composition that people refocus and redefine throughout their lifetimes.

Life as a Narrative

Closely related to the concept of life as a composition is the metaphor of life as a narrative. A narrative is an account of something that contains more than a mere sequence of events; a narrative has a coherence and wholeness (a plot) that binds its components together (Polkinghorne, 1988). According to Bruner (1986), people seek to create a wholeness of their lives from beginning to end by building a coherent narrative across the life span. Within this metaphor of the life span, adulthood and aging become the middle and ending of the life narrative. Mattingly (1991, 1998) introduced the concept of narrative to occupational therapy, suggesting that therapists use the structure of narrative to make meaning out of clinical situations. Therapists create stories with their clients—stories with specific beginnings, middles, and endings—and they seek to fit these stories into the larger narrative of each client's life as well as into their own life narratives.

These, then, are major images of human development from a life-span perspective. Other important frameworks do, of course, exist (Atchley, 1989; Gilligan, 1982; Hatch, 2000; Kaufman, 1986). Adulthood and aging are, indeed, rich and varied periods of life.

OCCUPATION AND LIFE-SPAN DEVELOPMENT

Embedded in occupational therapy's professional values and practices are beliefs that occupation—the everyday purposeful activity of human beings—is related to human development (Moyers, 1999). Occupation, then, offers another framework within which to organize and study development in adulthood and aging.

Work, play, and self-care are the everyday occupations of life (American Occupational Therapy Association, 1995). The activities that make up these occupations and the routines and patterns of these occupations change across the life span. These shifting characteristics and patterns of occupation are linked to human development in two ways: They contribute directly to developmental change, and they provide a mirror in which therapists can see developmental change reflected.

For example, a 40-year-old woman who returns to graduate school after years of being at home with two children is experiencing a major shift in the patterns of her daily occupations. The shift in occupations contributes directly to the woman's development; she will be changed during the graduate school experience—intellectually, socially, and psychologically. This shift is also a reflection of much developmental change that has already occurred in this woman's life—the shift from a focus on at-home parenting to a focus on out-of-the-home activities. This leads to a newly defined sense of purpose and self-image that were not present 5 years earlier, such as a heightened level of confidence.

The relationship of occupation to life-span development has been examined from a number of perspectives (Townsend, 1997; Wilcock, 1998; Wood, 1998). The traditional concepts of occupation as work, play, and self-care are used here in the discussion of occupation within this developmental context.

Work

Havighurst (1953, 1964) developed a theory of developmental tasks to describe the lifelong process of vocational development. To Havighurst (1953), a developmental task is one "which arises at or about a certain period in the life of the individual, successful achievement of which leads to his happiness and to success with later tasks, while failure leads to unhappiness in the individual, disapproval by the society, and difficulty with later tasks" (p. 2). Starting with identification with a worker in childhood (mother, father, other significant person), human beings proceed through five other stages of vocational development, ending with the older retired person who "contemplates a productive and responsible life" (1964, p. 216). Along the way, the individual develops work habits and skills and roles, all of which both contribute to the individual's development and reflect his or her growing mastery and productivity in society.

Palmer (2000) offered a different view of work in his book *Let Your Life Speak: Listening to the Voice of Vocation*. Palmer's portrayal of vocational development in life is akin to one of spiritual development. Instead of focusing on the acquisition of skills and the completion of tasks as did Havighurst, Palmer described a gradual lifelong unfolding of a person's innate inner vocational resources. It is to the voice of these inner resources that Palmer encouraged us to listen.

Benner (1984) proposed another work-related model of development in her study of the acquisition of skills in nursing. Based on a model proposed by Dreyfus and Dreyfus (1980), Benner described the changes in proficiency that occur from novice to expert across time in nursing practice. The changes include development within the individual from fragmentary thinking to holistic thinking (see Chapter 13).

A focus on end-of-career retirement as a developmental transition has emerged in recent years, as researchers have approached retirement from an experiential perspective (Jonsson, Josephsson, & Kielhofner, 2000; Savishinsky, 2000). Findings from this research, in sharp contrast to Havighurst's contemplative image, reveal the dynamic and flexible nature of the retirement experience and the continuing importance of purpose, relationships, and a sense of community.

Leisure

Leisure, too, may be conceptualized both as an occupation that contributes to development and one that reflects developmental changes throughout adulthood and aging. Kleiber and Kelly (1980) presented a persuasive discussion of the strong links between leisure activities and psychosocial development across the life span. For example, in young adulthood, shared leisure contributes to the development of intimacy; in middle age, a parent who has been home centered for several years may find new friendships through involvement in community sports. Focusing more on the link between leisure and inner development, Lydon (1997) wrote about the contribution that the ordinary hobby of knitting makes to her own inner growth: "After all, the important thing is not so much what you knit as what happens to you while you knit it. Where the interior journey takes you. . . . How you are transformed" (p. 11).

In recent years, gender-specific issues have been imbedded in the study of leisure (Henderson, 1990; Henderson,

Bialeschki, Shaw, & Freysinger, 1996). Henderson (1990) argued that the long-time definition of leisure as nonwork was derived from the male-oriented model of work as an activity that was separated from the home. Henderson suggested that a redefinition of leisure as a subjective experience is a better fit in the complex world of women today. Perhaps this redefinition is a better fit for men as well.

In addition to gender, the study of leisure and aging has received increasing attention since the 1990s (Kelly, 1993). Specific aging concerns include the relationship between leisure and well-being in old age, leisure and friendships among older adults, and leisure opportunities in assisted living settings. Findings from a large prospective study in Denmark demonstrated a strong relationship between moderate leisure-time physical activity and reduced risk of mortality in men and women aged 20–93 (Andersen, Schnohr, Schroll, & Hein, 2000); this interest in the relationship between an active lifestyle, well-being, and life expectancy is evidenced by a large body of research.

In an ethnic research focus, Allen and Chin-Sang (1990) studied the meaning of leisure for aging black women. Many of the women in the study said that they had had no leisure in the past and any leisure that they experienced after retirement was imbedded in the contexts of work and service, such as volunteer activities in churches or in senior centers. It can be seen that the leisure of these retired black women reflected their lifelong patterns of work while also contributing to their continuing socialization in old age.

Self-Care

Activities that individuals engage in on their own behalf to maintain their health and well-being are activities of self-care (Orem, 1980). Orem stated, "Normally, adults voluntarily care for themselves. Infants, children, the aged, the ill, and the disabled require complete care or assistance with self-care activities" (p. 35). While Orem's statement overgeneralizes people's situations, most people know intuitively that self-care capabilities do gradually develop in the child and adolescent; that they continue to shift and change in adulthood; and that, for many people, self-care needs and capabilities change in old age.

To occupational therapists, self-care has come to refer collectively to basic personal care tasks, including bowel and bladder management, bathing, dressing, eating, grooming and hygiene, and mobility (Christiansen, 1994). Just as these basic skills develop and change across the life span, so, too, do the more complex instrumental activities of daily living, such as meal preparation, medication monitoring, and financial management. The new college student living away from home for the first time dramatically illustrates change through his or her increasing capabilities and independence in cooking, budgeting, and laundering clothes. The new parent experiences continuing development and change as he or she gradually learns to care for the needs of a newborn infant while providing continued care of the self.

Self-care may have a different meaning to elderly people than it does to young adults. Scott-Maxwell (1968), in describing her everyday experiences as a woman in her eighth decade of life, wrote, "I have a duty to all who care for me—not to be a problem, not to be a burden. I must carry my age lightly for all our sakes, and thank God I still can. Oh that I may to the end" (p. 31). The fierce desire not to be a burden imbues self-care with a new and different meaning in old age.

Much of the emphasis in self-care literature has been on activities that are related to illness and people's responses to illness. Using a sample of adults from age 20 to 79, Segall (1987) studied the relationship of age to the way people respond to illness symptoms. Segall found age differences in subjects' responses to certain symptoms. For example, when experiencing a loss of appetite, young adults tended to self-treat and older adults tended to consult a doctor. People of all ages in the study sought physician help for some symptoms such as shortness of breath and frequent headaches.

The meaning of the changes in self-care that occur with illness can be powerful. In Albom's (1997) sensitively written chronicle of his visits with a former professor during the last month's of the professor's life, the markers of Morrie's progression toward death are clearly in the realm of self-care. After his seventh visit, Albom wrote, "Morrie lost his battle. Someone was now wiping his behind. . . . With the exception of breathing and swallowing his food, he was dependent on others for nearly everything" (p. 115). For Morrie, this final defeat led to a shift in his inner self from an initial desire to "fight all this" to eventually figuring, "Forget what the culture says. . . . I am not going to be ashamed. What's the big deal?" (pp. 115–116). To Morrie, his self-care was a complex activity that both reflected his prior life experiences and contributed to further developmental change.

In summary, the everyday occupations of adults and older people can be used as a framework for understanding the developmental changes of adulthood and old age. Work, play, and self-care are multidimensional categories of activity that reflect aspects of life, including age and developmental stage. The foundations of occupation learned in childhood are expanded and adapted throughout life, providing support for changes across the life span in human beings. In his delightful short essay on what he learned in kindergarten, Fulghum (1986) summarized his philosophy for daily life as follows: "Learn some and think some and draw and paint and sing and dance and play and work every day some" (pp. 6–7). These are the occupations of life. Occupational therapists use these occupations to guide their therapeutic activities and to enhance life-span development in clients.

IN SICKNESS AND IN HEALTH

I turn now to examining the meaning of occupation in the life-span development of people with chronic illnesses and of their caregivers. Individuals who are born with a disability or who live for years with a long-term illness experience their everyday occupations, and thus their development, in ways that are influenced by the disability.

Life-Span Development and Developmental Disabilities

People with developmental disabilities may have as part of their life experiences recurrent hospitalizations, periods of institutionalization, and frequent contacts with health professionals and service agencies in their homes and in the community. The goal of all this health care and service is to enhance the person's well-being and ability to have quality of life; however, paradoxically, the disruptions in daily life imposed by this ongoing interaction with special services "can dramatically interfere with the acquisition of adult life skills" (Neistadt, 1987, p. 433). Furthermore, living with a chronic disability means living in an environment that is often physically inaccessible and with societal attitudes that are largely patronizing and embedded in negative stereotypes. The disruptions that occur in education, social relationships, and family life are apt to be of such magnitude that Becker (1997) referred to the life of a person with disabilities as "a chaotic world".

Kielhofner (1981), in his research on adults with mental retardation (one type of developmental disability), described the altered everyday world of the participants in his study:

> *For retarded persons, it is a matter of living in a world that pays a tremendous amount of negative, curious, patronizing, or humorous attention to them and that directs extraordinary social action toward them. . . . In this way, everything about the retarded person's everyday world was altered from that experienced by normal persons. (p. 140)*

In this altered world of people who have mental retardation, the typical passages, markers, and seasons of life may be not typical at all or may be totally absent. Individuals with mental retardation may never get a driver's license, cast their ballots, pull up their roots, or establish their own households. Kielhofner's study (1981) focused on the everyday life of residents in a group home. The lack of opportunity for occupation presented by this environment was obvious:

> *Only a few [of the residents] had any control over their immediate living environment. Almost none of them performed such basic functions as cooking, shopping, traveling, cleaning, laundering, and so forth. . . . Almost all of them had little or nothing to do with their time.(p. 138)*

Without occupational opportunities, the developmental changes that occupation helps bring about will not occur or will be markedly curtailed.

Another focus of attention related to persons who have mental retardation is on the aging sector of this population (Segal, 1990; Seltzer & Krauss, 1987). The provision of residential facilities for older mentally retarded people is a key concern, since many aging adults with mental retardation have lived all their lives with their now aging and dying parents (Seltzer, Begun, Seltzer, & Krauss, 1991; Seltzer, Krauss, & Tsunematsu, 1993). Long-held patterns of dependency and relative isolation may need to be overcome to facilitate new competencies in social skills and activities of daily living (Heller, 2000; Nochaski, 2000).

Life-Span Development and Long-Term Illness and Disability

The deinstitutionalization movement of the 1960s and 1970s led to the discharge of many adults with chronic disabilities and older people from long-term care facilities to community living. Gradually, community-based programs and living facilities have developed to support people with chronic illness as they engage in the occupational tasks of independent living.

For individuals with persistent mental illness, a new type of supported living setting emerged called the halfway house (Friedlob, Janis, & Deets-Aron, 1986). The mission of a halfway house is to provide "a bridge between the hospital and the community via a therapeutic milieu designed to prepare residents for resuming their roles in society" (p. 272). Enabling the residents to learn skills in daily occupations—such as health and hygiene, nutrition, household management, interpersonal relationships, and leisure activities—was a prominent component of the concept as well as vocational training, employment, and eventually moving to more independent settings.

Recognition of the importance of successful engagement in everyday occupations to people with persistent mental illness now permeates mental health practice in most settings. Research in occupational therapy is being carried out on the occupational behavior of clients with depression (Neville-Jan, 1994) and schizophrenia (Laliberte-Rudman, Yu, Scott, & Pajouhandeh, 2000) and on models of practice used by therapists as they seek to enhance the occupational functioning of clients with psychiatric illness (Legault & Rebeiro, 2000; Muñoz, Lawlor, & Kielhofner, 1993). The role of work in the lives of people with mental illness has also been the focus of research, as difficulty in maintaining steady employment is viewed as one of the defining features of the illness (Scheid & Anderson, 1995; Sullivan, 1993). Successful vocational activity is often described as central to community living and a significant sign of being well.

LIFE ISSUES TO CONSIDER IN PRACTICE 38-1

Mr. R: A Man with Rheumatoid Arthritis

Mr. R was an older man who had lived his entire life in the Midwestern state of Wisconsin. He and his wife lived in a one-bedroom apartment in Madison, having sold their home when Mr. R was 78 years old. Both a married son and a married daughter lived in the same city.

Mr. R retired at age 66, after holding a variety of work positions, including those of tavern keeper and telephone lineman. All his life, he had enjoyed participating in sports activities such as golfing, fishing, hunting, and bowling; and, for several years after retirement, his involvement in these activities continued and even increased. He was especially proud of his championship bowling record.

I came to know Mr. R when I was the occupational therapist with an interdisciplinary geriatric home-care program affiliated with the Veterans Administration Hospital in Madison. He was referred to the program when he was 81 years old. The primary medical reason for referral was for management of rheumatoid arthritis (RA) which had been diagnosed when Mr. R was 77 years old. Mr. R had experienced persistent inflammation associated with the RA, leading to a daily life of pain, fatigue, and gradually increasing difficulty in carrying out his everyday activities. At the time of referral to home care, he had totally abandoned his previous sports activities, including his much loved bowling. Mr. R stated that he had not stepped inside a bowling alley for 2 years.

On our early team visits to Mr. R, we learned that he spent his time primarily within the confines of his apartment, taking care of his personal needs, handling the financial aspects of the household, and assisting with some light housekeeping tasks. For leisure, he watched television, did some reading, and worked crossword puzzles. Socialization was limited largely to family visits (which were frequent) and home visits by the home-care team. Mr. R was the driver for himself and his wife for appointments and grocery shopping in the community, thus maintaining a role he had filled throughout their marriage.

DISEASE PROGRESSION

Over the course of the 2 years after the referral to home care, Mr. R's rheumatoid arthritis continued to be active. Management efforts included medication trials and adjustments, adapted equipment, splinting, assistive mobility devices, training in joint protection principles, and activity modification. In spite of these carefully planned and monitored health-care strategies, Mr. R's joint inflammation proliferated, involving his hand joints, wrists, shoulders, cervical vertebrae, knees, ankles, and feet. The persistent swelling from the inflammation began to weaken the periarticular structures of many of his joints. For example, the joint stress from simply using his thumb to push down the heat control lever in his car one winter day ruptured the tendon of his flexor pollicis longus muscle. The metacarpophalangeal joints of his right hand showed increasing ulnar deviation, aggravated by the pressure exerted during use of a cane for walking.

At some point in those 2 years, it became evident that Mr. R was clinically depressed. His affect became increasingly flat; his interest in activities that were still within his capability waned; and he seemed mentally sluggish, giving slow and sometimes confused answers to questions. His wife reported having to prod him repeatedly to get up in the morning. Mr. R, himself, stated that he felt like he was "under a big blanket" for much of the day.

The long-term use of prednisone (a synthetic steroid and anti-inflammatory agent) led to a number of side effects, including cataracts and general susceptibility to infection. The cataracts affected Mr. R's vision to the extent that it was difficult for him to read or do crossword puzzles. The sudden appearance of an infection in his left great toe proved to be a significant turning point for Mr. R (this situation is described in some detail below).

IMPACT ON LIFE

The change in Mr. R's daily life and activity patterns during these 2 years was marked. His life space became almost totally limited to his apartment, except when persuaded and assisted by his wife or children to go on an outing. His daily routine became more and more sedentary, with long periods of time spent just sitting without engagement in any accompanying activity such as TV watching or reading. He gave up driving during this period, a decision that seemed necessary but that obviously contributed to his diminished activity beyond the apartment.

Mrs. R gradually began to assume responsibility for the financial aspects of their life, feeling defeated in her efforts to persuade "Dad" to continue to take care of these tasks and feeling somewhat concerned about his level of capability, having witnessed the episodes of confusion. His participation in chores around the apartment decreased to the single activity of helping with the dishes. When first referred to the home-care team,

Continues

Mr. R had been independent in all basic self-care tasks; after 2 years, he needed assistance with tub bathing, dressing, cutting up food, and going up and down stairs. He was still independent in shaving, toileting, transferring onto and off of furniture such as the bed and his easy chair, and generally moving about the apartment.

OCCUPATIONAL THERAPY

As the occupational therapist on the home-care team, I was extensively involved with Mr. R in his ongoing care. One of my primary responsibilities was to provide support for him as he tried to carry out his usual activities of daily living. In cooperation with the other members of the interdisciplinary team, I monitored Mr. R's functional level, documenting changes in function and planning therapeutic interventions with him and his wife to try to maximize his capabilities in everyday activities. This approach included regular systematic assessments of his functional performance combined with planning and carrying out interventions to maintain or increase Mr. R's independence.

Over the course of the 2 years, a number of pieces of adaptive equipment were provided to assist Mr. R with his daily activities. These included bathing equipment (a bath bench, grab bar, and hand-held shower hose), a long-handled shoehorn and a shoelace adapter, a car door opener and car key holder, a large-handled knife to assist with cutting food, magnifiers for reading, and a medication dispenser to help Mr. R keep track of his medication schedule. In addition, Mr. R was measured for and trained in the use of a cane to assist with walking; subsequently the cane handle was padded to reduce the stress to his hand as he used it.

Time was spent helping both Mr. and Mrs. R gain understanding about the RA disease process and principles of joint protection. This included teaching ways to adapt activity to minimize stress to the joints, such as learning how to get in and out of an easy chair with minimal twisting of the knees. A commercially available resting splint for the right wrist was fitted to Mr. R to support and reduce stress in those joints during activity. In addition, a small splint was constructed to support the interphalangeal joint of the right thumb, enabling Mr. R to continue to use the thumb in activities requiring light opposition, in spite of the tendon rupture.

I made an effort to reintroduce some type of leisure sports activity into Mr. R's life since it had held such importance to him before the onset of rheumatoid arthritis. Initially, I tried to think of different ways that Mr. R could continue involvement in bowling, such as being a score keeper or even just watching. These ideas were firmly rejected. Ultimately, I talked with him about a swimming program that was available and designed especially for people with arthritis. This idea appealed to him, and I made arrangements for him to attend. Several members of the home-care team took turns accompanying him to the swim program once a week for a period of a few months. Finally, I made a point to encourage Mr. R to reminisce about his past achievements and experiences in his sporting activities. I had developed a monthly newsletter for the home-care program, and each issue featured a story about one of our patients. It was easy and delightful to develop a feature story about Mr. R and his bowling accomplishments. He and his wife searched and found the newspaper clippings, pictures, and trophies that documented Mr. R's achievements. They both contributed anecdotes about especially exciting tournaments and scores. I was able to write such details as "High score for a single game was 289 when Donald got nine strikes in a row, then pulled a spare and ended with a strike. He remembers that occasion well as the spectators gathered around in the tenth frame." A sense of accomplishment was strong for Mr. R during the planning and preparation of the newsletter article; we were all pleased with the end result.

THE TURNING POINT

During the third year of our involvement with Mr. R, a problem arose that seemed initially to be readily manageable but that proved, instead, to be the trigger for a rapid deterioration in his health status. On one of our home visits, Mr. R complained of a sore toe. Upon examination, the great toe on his left foot was indeed red and swollen around the toenail. After an unsuccessful trial with oral antibiotics, Mr. R was hospitalized for 6 days for more vigorous treatment of the infection.

During the hospitalization, Mr. R displayed significant and persistent confusion; I was taken aback one day when I visited him on the ward and found that he didn't know who I was. His functional abilities and mobility had declined further, so that he needed assistance with all self-care activities and primarily used a wheelchair to get around. After his return home, our efforts to help him regain his prehospitalization level of endurance and mobility were not successful, and his cognitive status remained marginal. We introduced a wheeled walker for moving about the apartment and attempted to instruct Mr. R in its safe use. We arranged for a home health aide to come twice a week to help with bathing. Mr. R's days consisted of being helped with his personal care needs, resting, and watching a little television.

Continues

Within 3 weeks, it became obvious that the daily care that Mr. R required was exhausting to both him and his wife. Mrs. R and the family expressed deep concern about being able to continue to care for Dad at home. A meeting was arranged for the family and key members of the home-care team to discuss the situation. The family tearfully proposed, and the health team members agreed, that nursing home placement was needed. Mr. R moved to a nursing home 5 days after the meeting; he died just 2 months later.

From the standpoint of occupation and occupational health, Mr. R had adapted his lifestyle on retirement, substituting engagement in outdoor sports and home management activities for previous involvement in work. A few years after retirement, a health problem, in the form of rheumatoid arthritis, emerged and became a major disrupting factor in his occupational life. During his last few years, Mr. R experienced a gradual shift from a daily balance of work, leisure, self-care, and rest to an everyday existence consisting almost entirely of assisted self-care and rest. Through the use of adaptive equipment, modified activity, and new substitute activities, the health-care team strove to help Mr. R maintain a balance of occupation in his life for as long as possible during the years of decline. (The theoretical approaches used for Mr. R's intervention are discussed in Case Analysis: Unit X, at the end of this unit.)

QUESTIONS AND EXERCISES

1. What are some of the developmental challenges that Mr. R faced?
2. If he had not had occupational therapy, how would Mr. R's occupational life have been different?

Serving a broader population, Neistadt and Marques (1984) described an independent living skills training program that offered training for adults with multiple disabilities in tasks such as banking, attendant care management, and personal health care for adults with diagnoses such as cerebral palsy, multiple sclerosis, and spina bifida. The program participants gained competencies and confidence in their abilities.

With a focus on physical dysfunction and adult development, Quigley (1995) studied the role experiences of five women who had sustained traumatic spinal cord injuries in adulthood. The women in the study consistently used strategies of adaptation and negotiation to resume their occupations—redefining their roles and adapting their surroundings, daily routines, and relationships. Each of the women had developed a new role of self-advocate as she dealt with the barriers in the community imposed by societal attitudes and architectural features. Quigley referred to the adaptation by the women as a process of "recomposing their lives"; the women "accomplished this feat by combining, amending, and contrasting their past lifestyles into their present and anticipatory roles" (p. 784). Quigley concluded that occupational therapists can assist people with disabilities to reconstruct their lives and facilitate continuing life-span development.

Finally, Gillen (2000) described an occupational therapy program aimed at increasing activities of daily living abilities in a 31-year-old man with ataxia syndrome secondary to multiple sclerosis. Therapy included adapted positioning, orthotic prescription, adapted movement patterns, and use of the environment for trunk and limb stability. In addition to improved independence in activities of daily living, the client was able to return to his previous living situation and was able to resume part-time work with his previous employer. The disruption of this man's daily occupations, imposed by the ataxia, was markedly modified by the therapy program, enabling him to once again engage in developmentally appropriate activities.

CONCLUSION

Illness and disability are viewed as disruptions in a person's healthful life patterns and development across the life span. The most recent language of the World Health Organization (2001) related to disability includes body functions-body structures, activities, and participation. This new language represents a shift away from the prior emphasis on pathology to an emphasis on health as engagement in occupation and participation in society. In occupational therapy and other health-care disciplines, too, the emphasis has shifted to a focus on life skills and the provision of a safe environment in which to gradually regain prior occupations and develop new competencies and roles in society.

References

Albom, M. (1997). *Tuesdays with Morrie*. New York: Doubleday.

Allen, K. R., & Chin-Sang, V. (1990). A lifetime of work: The context and meanings of leisure for aging black women. *Gerontologist, 30*, 737–740.

American Occupational Therapy Association. (1995). Occupation. *American Journal of Occupational Therapy, 49*, 10151018.

American Occupational Therapy Association (2000). *"2000" Membership Invoice Questionnaire*. Bethesda, MD: Author.

Andersen, L. B., Schnohr, P., Schroll, M., & Hein, H. O. (2000). All-cause mortality associated with physical activity during leisure time, work, sports, and cycling to work. *Archives of Internal Medicine, 160*, 1621–1628.

Atchley, R. C. (1989). A continuity theory of normal aging. *Gerontologist, 29*, 183–190.

Bateson, M. C. (1989). *Composing a life*. New York: Plume.

Becker, G. (1997). *Disrupted lives: How people create meaning in a chaotic world*. Los Angeles: University of California Press.

Benner, P. (1984). *From novice to expert: Excellence and power in clinical nursing practice*. Menlo Park, CA: Addison-Wesley.

Bruner, J. (1986). *Actual minds, possible worlds*. Cambridge, MA: Harvard University Press.

Christiansen, C. (1994). A social framework for understanding self-care interventions. In C. Christiansen (Ed). *Ways of living: Self-care strategies for special needs* (pp. 3–26). Bethesda, MD: American Occupational Therapy Association.

Dannefer, D., & Perlmutter, M. (1990). Development as a multidimensional process: Individual and social constituents. *Human Development, 33*, 108–137.

Dreyfus, S. E., & Dreyfus, H. L. (1980). *A five-stage model of the mental activities involved in directed skill acquisition*. Unpublished manuscript, U.S. Air Force Office of Scientific Research [contract F49620-79-C-0063], University of California at Berkeley.

Erikson, E. H. (1959). Identity and the life cycle. *Psychological Issues, 1*, 1–171.

Friedlob, S. A., Janis, G. A., & Deets-Aron, C. (1986). A hospital-connected halfway house program for individuals with long-term neuropsychiatric disabilities. *American Journal of Occupational Therapy, 40*, 271–277.

Fulghum, R. (1986). *All I really need to know I learned in kindergarten: Uncommon thoughts on common things*. New York: Fawcett Columbine.

Gillen, G. (2000). Improving activities of daily living performance in an adult with ataxia. *American Journal of Occupational Therapy, 54*, 89–96.

Gilligan, C. (1982). *In a different voice*. Boston: Harvard Press.

Hatch, L. R. (2000). *Beyond gender differences: Adaptation to aging in life course perspective*. Amityville, NY: Baywood.

Havighurst, R. J. (1953). *Human development and education*. New York: McKay.

Havighurst, R. J. (1964). Youth in exploration and man emergent. In H. Borow (Ed.). *Man in a world of work* (pp. 215–236). Boston: Houghton Mifflin.

Heller, T. (2000). Supporting adults with intellectual disabilities and their families in planning and advocacy: A literature review. *Physical and Occupational Therapy in Geriatrics, 18*(1), 59–73.

Henderson, K. A. (1990). The meaning of leisure for women: An integrative review of literature. *Journal of Leisure Research, 22*, 228–243.

Henderson, K. A., Bialeschki, M., Shaw, S., & Freysinger, V. (1996). *Both gains and gaps: Feminist perspectives on women's leisure*. State College, PA: Venture.

Jonsson, H., Josephsson, S., & Kielhofner, G. (2000). Evolving narratives in the course of retirement: A longitudinal study. *American Journal of Occupational Therapy, 54*, 463–470.

Kaluger, G., & Kaluger, M .F. (1984). *Human development: The span of life*. St. Louis: Times Mirror/Mosby.

Kaufman, S. R. (1986). *The ageless self: Sources of meaning in late life*. Madison: University of Wisconsin Press.

Kelly, J. R. (Ed.). (1993). *Activity and aging*. Newbury Park, CA: Sage.

Kielhofner, G. (1981). An ethnographic study of deinstitutionalized adults: Their community settings and daily life experiences. *Occupational Therapy Journal of Research, 1*, 125–142.

Kleiber, D. A., & Kelly, J. R. (1980). Leisure, socialization, and the life cycle. In J. E. Iso-Ahola (Ed.) *Social psychological perspectives on leisure and recreation* (pp. 91–137). Springfield, IL: Thomas.

Laliberte-Rudman, D., Yu, B., Scott, E., & Pajouhandeh, P. (2000). Exploration of the perspectives of persons with schizophrenia regarding quality of life. *American Journal of Occupational Therapy, 54*, 137–147.

Legault, E., & Rebeiro, K. L. (2000). Occupation as means to mental health: A single case study. *American Journal of Occupational Therapy, 55*, 90–96.

Levinson, D. J. (1978). *The seasons of a man's life*. New York: Knopf.

Lowenthal, M. F., Thurnher, M., & Chiriboga, D. (1975). *Four stages of life: A psychosocial study of women and men facing transition*. San Francisco: Jossey-Bass.

Lydon, S. G. (1997). *The knitting sutra: Craft as a spiritual practice*. New York: HarperCollins.

Mattingly, C. (1991). The narrative nature of clinical reasoning. *American Journal of Occupational Therapy, 45*, 998–1005.

Mattingly, C. (1998). *Healing dramas and clinical plots: The narrative structure of experience*. Cambridge, UK: Cambridge University Press.

Moyers, P. A. (1999). The guide to occupational therapy practice. *American Journal of Occupational Therapy, 53*, 247–322.

Muñoz, J. P., Lawlor, M., & Kielhofner, G. (1993). Use of the model of human occupation: A survey of therapists in psychiatric practice. *Occupational Therapy Journal of Research, 13*, 117–139.

Neistadt, M. (1987). An occupational therapy program for adults with developmental disabilities. *American Journal of Occupational Therapy, 41*, 433–438.

Neistadt, M. E., & Marques, K. (1984). An independent living skills training program. *American Journal of Occupational Therapy, 38*, 671–676.

Neugarten, B. L. (1977). Personality and aging. In J. E. Birren & K. W. Schaie (Eds.). *Handbook of the psychology of aging* (pp. 626–649). New York: Van Nostrand Reinhold.

Neville-Jan, A. (1994). The relationship of volition to adaptive occupational behavior among individuals with varying degrees of depression. *Occupational Therapy in Mental Health, 12*(4), 1–18.

Newman, B. M., & Newman, P. R. (1984). *Development through life: A psychosocial approach*. Homewood, IL: Dorsey.

Nochaski, S. M. (2000). The impact of age-related changes on the functioning of older adults with developmental disabilities. *Physical and Occupational Therapy in Geriatrics, 18*(1), 5–21.

Orem, D. E. (1980). *Nursing concepts of practice* (2nd ed.). New York: McGraw-Hill.

Palmer, P. J. (2000). *Let your life speak: Listening for the voice of vocation*. San Francisco: Jossey-Bass.

Polkinghorne, D. E. (1988). *Narrative knowing and the human sciences*. Albany: State University of New York Press.

Quigley, M. C. (1995). Impact of spinal cord injury on the life roles of women. *American Journal of Occupational Therapy, 49*, 780–786.

Reese, H. W., & Overton, W. F. (1970). Models of development and theories of development. In L .R. Goulet & P. B. Baltes (Eds.). *Lifespan developmental psychology: Research and theory* (pp. 115–145). New York: Academic.

Savishinsky, J. (2000). *Breaking the watch: The meanings of retirement in America*. Ithaca, NY: Cornell University Press.

Scheid, T. L., & Anderson, C. (1995). Living with chronic mental illness: Understanding the role of work. *Community Mental Health Journal, 31*, 163–176.

Scott-Maxwell, F. (1968). *The measure of my days*. New York: Penguin.

Segal, R. (1990). Helping older mentally retarded persons expand their socialization skills through the use of expressive therapies. *Activities, Adaptation, and Aging, 15*, 99–109.

Segall, A. (1987). Age differences in lay conceptions of health and self-care responses to illness. *Canadian Journal on Aging, 6*, 47–65.

Seltzer, G. B., Begun, A., Seltzer, M. M., & Krauss, M. W. (1991). Adults with mental retardation and their aging mothers: Impacts of siblings. *Family Relations, 40*, 310–317.

Seltzer, M. M., Krauss, M. W., & Tsunematsu, N. (1993). Adults with Down syndrome and their aging mothers: Diagnostic group differences. *American Journal on Mental Retardation, 97*, 464–508.

Settersten, R. A. Jr., & Hagestad, G. O. (1996a). What's the latest? Cultural age deadlines for family transitions. *Gerontologist, 36*, 178–188.

Settersten, R. A. Jr., & Hagestad, G. O. (1996b). What's the latest? II. Cultural age deadlines for educational and work transitions. *Gerontologist, 36*, 602–613.

Sheehy, G. (1976). *Passages: Predictable crises of adult life*. New York: Dutton.

Sheehy, G. (1995). *New passages: Mapping your life across time*. New York: Random House.

Stancliff, B. (1996). OT practitioners work with more elderly patients. *OT Practice*, 17.

Sullivan, W. P. (1993). "It helps me to be a whole person": The role of spirituality among the mentally challenged. *Psychosocial Rehabilitation Journal, 16*, 125–134.

Townsend, E. (1997). Occupation: Potential for personal and social transformation. *Journal of Occupational Science: Australia*, 4(1), 18–26.

Vaillant, G. E. (1977). *Adaptation to life*. Boston: Little, Brown.

Wilcock, A. A. (1998). Reflections on doing, being and becoming. *Canadian Journal of Occupational Therapy*, *65*, 248–256.

Wood, W. (1998). The genius within. *American Journal of Occupational Therapy*, *52*, 320–325.

World Health Organization. (2001). International classification of functioning, disability and health [ICIDH-2, final draft, full version]. Geneva: Author. Available at: www.who.int/icidh. Accessed: August 27, 2001.

CHAPTER 39

ADULT NEUROLOGICAL DYSFUNCTION

KAREN HALLIDAY PULASKI

Occupational therapists working with adults with neurological problems must understand clients' neurological dysfunction before beginning evaluation and intervention. The abilities to evaluate accurately clients who have neurological deficits, to define functional outcomes, and to provide efficacious intervention are largely based on the therapist's understanding of how neuroanatomy and neuropathology relate to impairment and disability in functional activity. If the therapist does not understand the functional impact of a neurological deficit, as well as potential secondary problems that might arise, he or she will not be able either to individualize a clients' intervention or to help clients set realistic short- and long-term goals that are achievable within a set time frame. With health-care reforms affecting the total amount of intervention time insurance companies will allow, it is imperative for therapists to be able to evaluate clients effectively and efficiently and to help them achieve their highest level of functioning in the least restrictive environment.

A complete review of neuroanatomy and neurophysiology is beyond the scope of this chapter, but a brief review is provided. The main focus of this chapter is to provide a general overview of neuroanatomy as it relates to function, a description of several adult neurological diagnoses, and a description of typical deficits associated with those diagnoses. Prognosis and secondary complications are also discussed. The occupational therapy interventions within specific settings are described. Finally, some case examples are provided to illustrate how specific neurological insults can affect function.

This chapter does not cover every neurological diagnosis that an occupational therapist may encounter; indeed, there are hundreds of neurological diseases that are so little known they do not even have a name. It is important for the occupational therapist working with clients who have neurological disorders to be able to categorize like information together and to generalize from known neurological disorders the relevant information about likely deficits, secondary complications, evaluation, and intervention.

CATEGORIZATION OF ADULT NEUROLOGICAL DYSFUNCTION

There are several ways to categorize or organize specific neurological dysfunction for the adult population: type of onset, upper motor neuron versus lower motor neuron, and hemisphere of lesion are just a few.

Onset

The onset of neurological events can be categorized as sudden and traumatic versus chronic or progressive. Sudden-onset or traumatic events are viewed as those insults to the central nervous system (CNS) that occur suddenly or traumatically. Examples of this type include **cerebrovascular accident** (CVA), **traumatic brain injury** (TBI), **Guillain-Barré syndrome,** and **spinal cord injury** (SCI). Chronic or progressive neurological events are generally viewed as those insults that have a gradual onset during the adult phase (i.e., they are not congenital) and may cause a progressive decline in the client's functional ability over time. Examples of this include **Parkinson disease** (PD), **amyotrophic lateral sclerosis** (ALS), and **multiple sclerosis** (MS). The sudden versus chronic category of neurological diagnosis affects current and future occupational therapy intervention. For example, short-term intervention for a client with a sudden CVA might be focused on muscle reeducation and strengthening during self-care tasks to help the client become more self-sufficient. In contrast, intervention for a client with chronic and advanced MS might be focused on energy conservation and preparing for future wheelchair adaptations to allow the client to remain active in the community as his or her mobility declines.

Upper Versus Lower Motor Neuron

Another way to delineate neurological insults is to categorize them based on the location of the **lesion** (injured tissue) in terms of upper motor neuron lesions versus lower motor neuron lesions. Upper motor neuron lesions occur within the brain or spinal cord motor tracts. Clients with lesions in upper motor neurons experience a loss of voluntary muscle control and a loss of inhibition on reflexive movement, causing hyperreflexia. This causes spasticity or excess muscle tone in the affected muscle. Lower motor neuron lesions occur within the cell bodies or axons of the peripheral nerves that innervate or synapse with the muscle fibers. The cell bodies of lower motor neurons are located in nuclei of the brainstem (cranial nerves) or anterior horn cells of the spinal cord (spinal nerves); the axons are in the peripheral nerves. Clients with lower motor neuron lesions also experience a loss of voluntary muscle control but experience loss of the reflex arc with a consequent decrease in muscle tone. The upper versus lower motor neuron categorization is useful for motor neuron diseases (Lundy-Elkman, 1998).

Localization of Lesion

A third way to organize information about neurological dysfunction is to understand how the location of the lesions within the CNS (brain and spinal cord) relates to impairments. It is important to realize that the function of the brain as a whole is greater than the sum of its parts. Examining various areas of the brain is valuable for better understanding of how brain functions affect behavior, but it yields an incomplete picture of how the brain works. Little is known about how the brain functions as a whole. Categorization by lesion site is, therefore, not perfect by any means; but it can, at least, provide some direction to practitioners about the impairments they may see when observing functional activity. Table 39-1 organizes diagnoses by site of lesion, type of onset, demographic information, cause, and functional implications.

TABLE 39–1. **NEUROLOGICAL CONDITIONS, RELATED FACTORS AND INTERVENTION IMPLICATIONS**

Condition	Site of Lesion	Onset	Age Range (years)	Causes	Implications
Cerebrovascular accident	Brain	Sudden, traumatic	Any; more common >60	Embolic thrombosis; hemorrhage	All occupational areas and all client factors can be affected, depending on specific location of lesion
Traumatic brain injury	Brain	Sudden, traumatic	Any; more common 18–24 and 70+	Motor vehicle accident; fall from greater than one's height; sports injury; work-related injury; gunshot wound	All occupational areas and client factors can be affected, depending on location of lesion and type of injury
Parkinson disease	Brain	Chronic, progressive	Usually 50–69	Unknown; possible toxin exposure; sequelae to specific form of encephalitis	All occupational areas, neuromusculoskeletal and some mental functions, and motor skills can be affected
Amyotrophic lateral sclerosis	Brain and spinal cord	Chronic, progressive	50–70	Unknown; possible toxin exposure; hormonal imbalance; autoimmune problems	All occupational areas, neuromusculoskeletal, and especially motor skills can be affected
Multiple sclerosis	Brain and spinal cord	Chronic, progressive	20–40	Unknown	All occupational areas and client factors can be affected, depending on location of lesion
Spinal cord injury	Spinal cord	Sudden, traumatic	Any; more common 16–30	Motor vehicle accident; fall; act of violence; sports injury	All occupational areas; neuromusculoskeletal, sensory, genitourinary, and especially motor skills can be affected
Guillain-Barré syndrome	Peripheral nerves	Sudden, traumatic	Any	Unknown; possible toxin exposure; viral infection	All occupational areas, neuromusculoskeletal, motor skills, and especially sensory can be affected

Various areas of the brain are involved in controlling different factors that allow a client to function in different occupational areas. When observing a client engaged in an occupational activity, such as activities of daily living (ADL), the therapist should form hypotheses about why that client is unable to perform independently. Understanding what areas of the brain and what functions have been affected by the neurological event helps the therapist form these hypotheses. One way to understand this better is to break the brain down into localized areas and to delineate the functions of those areas (Arnadottir, 1990).

Frontal Lobes

The frontal lobes are primarily responsible for executive cognitive functions (e.g., ideation and concept formation, judgment, abstract thought, intellectual functions), personality, intention and execution of voluntary motor function contralaterally (in the area of the precentral gyrus), voluntary eye movements, and programming of the motor component of speech. The frontal lobes are also related to the sequencing, timing, and organizing of action and behavior as well as initiation and planning of action. These lobes also play a role in emotions.

Parietal Lobes

The parietal lobes are primarily involved in reception of somatic sensation (e.g., fine touch, pain and temperature, proprioception, kinesthesia) and perception and interpretation of sensory information. These lobes are also involved in tactile localization and discrimination as well as stereognosis. The parietal lobes assist with the recognition of tactile, visual, and auditory input. The parietal lobes store motor programs (praxis) as well as an appropriate body scheme and its relationship to the environment. This area of the brain is also responsible for the comprehension of language and pragmatics, which refers to the skills associated with communication (e.g., turn taking, eye contact, and nonverbal expression).

Occipital Lobes

The occipital lobes are primarily responsible for visual reception, and integration of visual information. They assist with the perception of visual spatial relationships and the formation of visual memory.

Temporal Lobes

The temporal lobes are primarily involved in auditory reception and comprehension. They assist with the perception of sound and music. The temporal lobes are also responsible for memory and the learning of visual and auditory patterns. In addition, they are related to emotions, motivation, and personality.

Limbic Lobes

The limbic lobes are intimately involved in emotion and memory through their connections to the medial aspects of the frontal and temporal lobes. The exact function of the limbic lobes is not well understood.

Brainstem

The brainstem (midbrain, pons, and medulla) is responsible for controlling eye movements, facial movements, and spontaneous respiration. The brainstem also has input into the auditory nerve and thus can affect balance and equilibrium.

Cerebellum

The cerebellum is the center for controlled coordinated movements. It controls coordination by modulating the synaptic activity that produces movement. The cerebellum makes sure the muscles contract at the right time, with the right amount of force for the activity, to produce the right amount of movement. The cerebellum also is the storehouse for remembering motor programs. It has direct connections to the vestibular nucleus (through the vestibulocerebellar pathways) and thus influences balance as well.

Spinal Cord

The spinal cord begins at the foramen magnum at the base of the skull and continues to the lower border of the first lumbar vertebrae. Muscle movement (contraction) and sensation are controlled by mixed nerves: efferent fibers control muscle movement and afferent fibers control sensation. These mixed nerves carry the messages from the brain to the muscles and carry sensory information back up to the brain. Efferent myelinated axons synapse with skeletal muscle fibers to produce movement. Axons located medially in the spinal cord control axial muscles, and axons located laterally in the spinal cord control appendicular movement. Afferent sensory axons are both ascending and descending and allow information to flow from the brain to the muscles as well as from the muscles back up to the brain to permit refinement in movement. There are also several spinal reflexes that can be inhibited or facilitated in a mature human to permit purposeful movement. Movement is controlled ipsilaterally in the spinal cord (Arnadottir, 1990; Lundy-Elkman, 1998).

Hemisphere of Lesion

Brain functions can also be categorized by hemisphere. The left hemisphere of the brain is generally responsible for movement of the right side, processing of sensory information from the right side, perception of the right visual fields, visual and verbal processing, bilateral motor planning or programs (praxis), verbal memory, auditory reception, speech, and processing of verbal auditory information. The right hemisphere is generally responsible for movement of the left side, processing of sensory information from predominantly the left side, left visual fields, visual spatial processing, contralateral motor planning (praxis), nonverbal memory, bilateral auditory reception, processing of pragmatics (nonverbal language), and attention to incoming stimulation and emotion (Adams, Victor, & Roper, 1997; Arnadottir, 1990; Lundy-Elkman, 1998).

A spinal cord injury is one example of how a therapist might use neuroanatomy functionally to understand the lesions by location. An SCI causes sensory or motor impairments but does not cause cognitive or perceptual impairments. Another example is a left hemisphere CVA. This lesion causes right, not left, hemiplegia. Further use of this classification for improved understanding of impairments is discussed as it relates to specific neurological diagnoses. Additional review of neuroanatomy and neurophysiology is recommended for understanding specific client cases; some useful sources are included in the references to this chapter.

RECOVERY OF FUNCTION

It is possible for many clients with neurological dysfunction to improve their abilities to perform functional activities either through recovery of uninjured neurological tissue or through learning how to compensate for lost neurological function. The amount of recovery depends on several factors: site of the lesion, size of the lesion, the client's age, and the client's general health.

Relative to the site of the lesion, some recovery of neurological function is possible after brain and peripheral nerve lesions, but not with spinal cord lesions. With brain lesions, recovery of neurological function may be secondary to the brain's ability to use uninjured areas to assume function of injured areas, the ability of uninjured brain neurons to grow new axonal branches and form new synapses with other intact neurons, or activity-related changes in neurotransmitter release (Held & Pay, 1999; Lundy-Elkman, 1998; Neistadt, 1994). With peripheral nerve injuries, recovery of function is linked to the capacity of peripheral axons to regenerate (Adams et al., 1997; Lundy-Elkman, 1998).

Relative to size of lesion, larger lesions may cause more damage and have worse prognoses for recovery than smaller lesions. Older adults and those with poor overall health generally have a poorer prognosis for recovery than younger adults and those in good health (Neistadt, 1994). Gender and life experiences and pharmacological intervention at the time of insult may also be factors in the prognosis (Held & Pay, 1999). When conducting an evaluation and planning an intervention, occupational therapists need to be aware of the recovery potential of adults with neurological injuries.

OCCUPATIONAL THERAPY EVALUATION AND INTERVENTION

Record Review

A complete review of available medical and psychosocial records is a good starting place for an evaluation. Therapists must be careful not to form a fixed picture of clients' functioning based on records, however. Therapists should remain neutral in their clinical impressions of clients until they have the opportunity to complete a thorough evaluation. The medical records can provide therapists with:

- A history of the client's premorbid health problems.
- A neurological diagnosis.
- Information on the location(s) of the lesion(s).
- Information on any secondary complications.
- Information on medical precautions and contraindications.
- A review of the course of the most recent neurological event.
- A list of medications the client is taking.
- Psychosocial information.
- A summary of the client's current life roles and ability to function within those roles.

Any information obtained from a client record should always be verified with the client, or a significant other if the client cannot communicate or has severe cognitive deficits. No information about the client's ability to function should be simply transferred from the medical record onto an evaluation form, except to reflect reported history. A therapist is always responsible for assessing the client's current level of functioning and recording the assessment results.

Client Interview and Goal Setting

The next step in the evaluation is a client interview. It is essential for therapists to form therapeutic relationships with clients and to allow clients to relate, in their own words, what their medical experiences have been like for them. The client interview should focus on the clients' understanding of their neurological diagnosis, the clients' description of their strengths and weaknesses, and the clients' goals for rehabilitation. It is important to keep in mind that goal setting may depend on the type of setting in which the client is receiving intervention. A client who is in the acute care or inpatient rehabilitation phase after a CVA may be unable to provide specific goals and may need assistance from the therapist to determine these goals. This same client may be quite self-directed by the time he or she reaches outpatient rehabilitation. It is also appropriate and important to involve a client's family or significant other (with the permission of the client, if possible) as soon as possible. The family and/or significant other can be a great resource for further information and may be the primary source if the client is unable to speak for himself or herself.

Practitioners must remember that they are not doing therapy *to* clients but are attempting to form a partnership *with* clients to help them reach their goals. For example, if a client needed assistance with dressing before the recent neurological event and chooses to continue to receive assistance, then goals for independence in dressing are not appropriate. It is important that the goals are established *with* the client, not *for* the client.

Evaluation of Occupational Areas

The evaluation should then proceed to assessment of occupational areas, such as ADL, work, leisure, and other valued activities (see Chapter 24). The areas a therapist assesses are often determined by the client's ability to perform valued activities, the level of recovery a client has reached, and the type of setting in which the therapist practices. An inpatient rehabilitation therapist working with a client who was undergone a new **exacerbation** of MS may focus on bathing, dressing, transfers, and some light homemaking. The therapist working in an outpatient or home-health setting with this same client 4 weeks later may be focusing on instrumental activities of daily living (IADL), such as full homemaking, banking, adapted driving, and leisure activities.

In some cases third-party payers will not reimburse for therapy in occupational areas that a client and therapist may feel are important. For instance, leisure activities may not be covered because the payers do not see leisure as a necessity; may not understand that motor, process, and social skills training can be accomplished with these activities; and may not understand the health maintenance benefit of

TABLE 39-2. **FOCUS OF CARE THROUGHOUT THE CONTINUUM**

Acute

- Clients are generally not medically stable
- Major focus of occupational therapy intervention is on evaluation and recommendations for the next most appropriate venue of care (i.e. inpatient rehabilitation, home with follow-up services, extended care)
- Clients who will be going directly home from acute care are priority clients
- Intervention for those patients going home often focuses on client and family education as well as improving performance of activities that client must be able to do (usually with assistance) to go home, such as self-care and basic mobility.
- Intervention for patients not going home generally focuses on addressing those occupational areas and client factors that affect functioning in anticipated discharge context

Inpatient Rehabilitation

- Clients are generally transferred as soon as they are medically stable and can tolerate intensive rehabilitaiton (usually 3 hr minimum per day)
- Focus is to evaluate and assist the client with occupational areas necessary to move on to the next level of care (home) as soon as possible
- Good evaluation of the home environment and supports is crucial
- Intervention is focused on ADL and critical IADL.
- Clients are discharged when they are able to manage safely at home, with supports in place
- Clients generally require some assistance at home for the above activities

Outpatient and Home Health

- Clients and therapists must work closely together to establish the specific goals of what activities the client wishes to resume and the purpose of therapy
- Intervention may still be focused on both basic ADL and IADL, as many clients who are discharged home require assistance for these activities
- Intervention should also focus on social participation and valued occupational areas, including education, work, and leisure
- Home programs should be extremely functionally oriented, and the client and/or family must assume a great deal of responsibility for carrying out the home program and for incorporating what is gained from therapy into everyday life

Extended

- Clients are often referred from the acute care to an extended care if they are not able to tolerate an intensive rehabilitation program but have the end goal of returning home
- Clients may go directly home from this setting or may gain enough strength to be admitted to an inpatient rehabilitation program with eventual discharge home
- Focus of intervention is often the same as inpatient rehabilitaiton but is provided at a less-intensive level
- Intervention may also be provided to long-term residents who have a change in medical status resulting in a decline in ability to function more independently
- Intervention focuses on areas that have been affected by the decline

helping people remain engaged in active lifestyles. Therefore, with leisure activities in particular, occupational therapists need to emphasize the skills training and time-management issues to educate third-party payers about the benefits of those activities.

It is crucial for practitioners to have a clear understanding of their role within a particular setting to maximize a client's benefit from an inpatient rehabilitation stay or a certain number of visits to an outpatient clinic. The overall goal of all therapeutic intervention should be to assist the client to function as independently as the client desires in the least restrictive environment (LRE). An inpatient practitioner should focus on those occupational areas, such as functional mobility and self-care, that are critical to permitting discharge from an inpatient setting. An outpatient or group home practitioner should focus on those occupational areas, such as homemaking and budgeting, that the client needs to live independently in the community.

Table 39-2 highlights the focus of intervention based on the setting in which occupational therapy is provided. Failure of therapists to recognize their role within the continuum of care may result in situations in which clients fail to be able to move from more restrictive environments (extended-care facilities) to less restrictive situations (home).

Therapists should have documentation forms for the evaluation that are sensitive to the type of setting. For example, a home-health form is typically different from an acute care one. Occupational therapy evaluations should always focus on occupational areas. When occupational performance problems are identified, additional areas on the form should permit documentation of which client factors, skills, and contextual features appear to be affecting performance. When clients are acutely ill or able to participate only minimally, it may be necessary to prioritize or defer assessments of occupational performance until clients can more actively participate.

Evaluation of Client Factors

During the evaluation of occupational areas, the therapist should begin to observe what a client can and cannot complete. The therapist should also begin to observe which client factors and skills may be preventing a client from completing occupational tasks. The therapist should then evaluate specific client factors and skills to determine if his or her observations are correct (see Chapter 25). The therapist should also use information about the location of the lesion to understand the observations. It may be difficult to determine exactly why a client is having difficulties completing a task until an evaluation of client factors is made. By completing an evaluation in this manner, the therapist is also able to observe which strengths and strategies a client may use to compensate for impairments in other client factors.

For example, a 19-year-old woman, whose diagnosis is Guillain-Barré syndrome, is seen by an occupational therapist to evaluate homemaking in the client's house. The client chooses to make a simple meal consisting of baked chicken, baked potato, and peas. The therapist observes that the client is able to organize the activity and plan the menu. The therapist also notes that the client has difficulty carrying objects within the kitchen, lifting heavy pans, using both upper extremities at the same time (e.g., when washing the potato at the sink or opening the package of peas), and maintaining her balance throughout the activity. The therapist may hypothesize that this client has decreased strength in her upper extremities, decreased balance caused by poor trunk control, decreased lower extremity strength, and possible sensory impairments. The therapist then decides to specifically evaluate range of motion (ROM), strength, coordination, and sensation to determine if the hypotheses are correct. The therapist also notices which performance routines and contextual factors are affecting the client. For instance, the woman may habitually choose a heavy iron skillet over a lighter-weight one, making the task harder. Thus the intervention plan evolves from determining which specific client factors are impaired and which contextual features are affecting performance. Interventions then reflect strategies to restore skills as well as to modify the context so that the woman is able to function optimally.

Special Considerations

Many factors may impede therapists' ability to assess occupational areas or client factors for neurologically involved clients. Examples are medical complications, such as uncontrolled blood pressure or seizures; premorbid conditions, such as myocardial infarcts or other disease processes; and current restrictions placed on the client, such as weight-bearing restrictions for a fractured extremity. Clients may also demonstrate behavioral manifestations of the neurological event that interfere with assessment, such as lethargy, agitation, inattention, or **perseveration.** There may be language deficits, such as **aphasia,** that make it impossible for clients to provide information or understand the therapist's requests for activities. There may also be perceptual or motor complications (e.g., a left neglect, a **hemianopsia,** or a premorbid amputation) that make evaluation more difficult. Therapists must find a way to modify their assessments to

RESEARCH NOTE 39–1

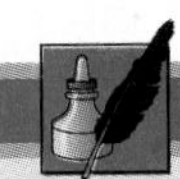

What Are the Most Effective Occupational Therapy Interventions?

KENNETH J. OTTENBACHER

The development of an appropriate occupational therapy intervention program requires that the therapist has a clear understanding of the distinctions among body systems, impairment, activity, and participation as defined by the World Health Organization (2001). In the past, intervention and research activities for adults have focused on impairments and body systems—that is, on the physical and organic structures associated with pathology or on the ability to perform specific physical activities.

One challenge of occupational therapy research in the twenty-first century is to establish a connection across assessment and intervention at the levels of body systems, activity, and participation. Trombly and Wu (1999) provide an excellent example of this type of research in a their study comparing the effect of a goal-directed action and rote exercise in the organization of reaching behavior in individuals who have experienced a stroke. In their study, patients with stroke performed either a rote exercise (reaching to a location in space) or a goal-directed reaching exercise (reaching for food). In a second experiment, individuals with stroke either reached to pick up either the receiver of a telephone that was ringing or a wooden dowel. A detailed kinematic analysis was performed for all movements. Goal-directed action produced significantly smoother, faster, more forceful, and more preplanned movements than did the rote exercise.

Trombly, C. A., & Wu, C. (1999). Effect of rehabilitation tasks on organization of movement after stroke. *American Journal of Occupational Therapy,* 53, 333–344.

World Health Organization (2001). *International classification of functioning, disability and health (ICF).* Geneva, Switzerland: Author.

gain an accurate picture of what the client can and cannot do. Therapist may need to use gestures and the context of a task to assess accurately clients with aphasia. Therapists may need to schedule their sessions in the morning, when clients are more alert or less agitated or see such clients in frequent, short intervention sessions, rather than one long session. Any modification made to standardized assessment processes used for the evaluation should be clearly documented.

Intervention should evolve out of the therapist's evaluation of occupational areas, client factors, and performance context as well as the client's input in terms of goals, future performance contexts, and intervention activities. Specific occupational therapy interventions are discussed within the context of specific diagnoses.

CEREBROVASCULAR ACCIDENT

Definition, Cause, and Demographics

CVA or cerebral vascular disease (CVD) can be defined as a vascular insult that causes a lesion to the brain resulting in neurological deficits. It is commonly referred to as a stroke because of its sudden onset. A CVA is characterized by an interruption of blood flow to a specific area of the brain, resulting in brain damage owing to lack of oxygen. There are many causes of this interruption but the most common ones are thrombosis, embolism, and hemorrhage.

A *thrombosis* is a blood clot that forms somewhere in the vascular system and causes a block in the blood supply. In a CVA, the thrombosis occurs somewhere in a cerebral vessel. An *embolism* occurs when a blood clot that is formed somewhere else in the vascular system (often the heart) breaks free and travels to a cerebral vessel, where it becomes lodged and interrupts blood flow. In either case, the resulting interruption of blood flow causes *ischemia*, or lack of nutrients and oxygen essential to maintaining viable brain tissue. A *hemorrhage* is a rupturing in the vessel wall, causing the vessel to bleed out intracerebrally or into the subarachnoid space. This causes pressure on the surrounding tissue and interruption of the blood supply to the brain tissue. All three causes result in brain damage.

Some clients may experience a **transient ischemic attack** (TIA), which causes neurological disturbances similar to a CVA. These disturbances resolve within a short period of time, usually 24–48 hr. A TIA is often a warning or precursor to a CVA.

There are numerous factors that can contribute to a CVA. Some of the most common ones are hypertension, obesity, age, diet, sedentary lifestyle, diabetes, and history of vascular disorders and myocardial infarcts. Clients who have experienced a CVA once are often at higher risk for another one. CVAs are more common in older adults who often exhibit several risk factors; however, they may occur at any age from infanthood through all of adulthood.

In addition to being categorized by origin, CVAs can be categorized by the major cerebral vessel that is occluded. There are six major vessels that may be used as descriptors for diagnosis: the internal carotid artery (ICA), the anterior cerebral artery (ACA), the middle cerebral artery (MCA), the posterior cerebral artery (PCA), the basilar artery, and the cerebellar branch. Each of these arteries, along with numerous ancillary arteries, feed different parts of the brain. Table 39-3 lists common impairments that occur with damage to these arteries.

Deficits

Lesions from CVAs are focal—that is, they are localized in the specific area supplied by the affected blood vessel. The resulting impairments are directly related to that area of the brain. Common impairments include hemiplegia (on the contralateral side of the lesion), sensory impairment, cognitive disturbances, motor impairments, language impairments, and visual perceptual impairments. Sensory deficits may include tactile, pain, temperature, proprioception, and kinesthesia impairments. Cognitive disturbances may include

TABLE 39-3. **COMMON EFFECTS OF OCCLUSIONS OR HEMORRHAGES OF CEREBRAL VESSELS**[a]

Artery	Common Effects
Internal carotid	Contralateral hemiplegia, sensory problems, aphasia (usually left hemisphere), and hemianopsia
Anterior cerebral	Contralateral hemiplegia, cognitive deficits, sensory deficits, and aphasia (usually left hemisphere)
Middle cerebral	Contralateral hemiplegia (primarily the upper extremity), contralateral hemianopsia, sensory deficits, and language deficits
Posterior cerebral	Contralateral hemiplegia, ataxia, visual deficits (e.g., field cuts, cortical blindness, and normal pursuit eye movements)
Basilar	Double vision, facial paralysis, visual deficits, and balance or vestibular disturbances
Cerebellar	Vertigo, difficulties in swallowing, ipsilateral ataxia, and changes in sensation

[a]Data from Arnadotiir (1990), Bartels (1998), and Gresham and Stason (1998).

deficits in attention, organization, sequencing, concentration, problem solving, judgment, and safety. Motor impairments may include changes in tone, disruption of active movement, and apraxia.

Some clients experience language deficits, called aphasias, that may interfere with receptive or expressive language, understanding of pragmatic or nonverbal language, and written expression. Common visual deficits are visual field cuts, visual field neglects, double vision, problems in scanning or difficulty with depth perception, and figure-ground perception problems. Clients may also display changes in behavior or personality as well as changes in their affect. These deficits may limit clients' abilities to perform some or all of their occupational activities, basic ADL and IADL, education, work and leisure activities, and social participation (Arnadottir, 1990; Bartels, 1998; Gresham & Stason, 1998).

Prognosis

There are many indicators neurologists use to suggest the prognosis for a client with a CVA, including the location of the lesion, the size of the lesion, and the age of the client. The neurologist also takes into account the client's prior health history and the course of initial recovery the client exhibits within the first 72 hr as well as within the first 2 weeks (Macciocchi, Diamond, Alves, & Mertz, 1998; South African Medical Association, 2000; U.S. Department of Health and Human Services, 1995).

Secondary Complications

The course of recovery varies from client to client, depending on the location of the CVA and the severity. Secondary factors can also affect prognosis. Secondary factors include edema or swelling within the brain, extensions of the original CVA, and vasospasms that can occur in the vessels surrounding the initial CVA. Clients may also have other medical complications, including pneumonia, uncontrolled diabetes, and cardiac disturbances.

Some initial symptoms of oncoming CVA are incoordination in an extremity, changes in sensation or tingling in an extremity or the face, slurred speech, difficulty swallowing, balance disturbances, visual or cognitive disturbances, or severe headache (Bartels, 1998; Fisher, 1995). A CVA may take as long as 48 hours to fully evolve, and clients may eventually become unconscious or unresponsive if the CVA is severe enough.

Stages of Recovery and Occupational Therapy Evaluation and Intervention

Evaluation should begin with assessment of occupational areas if possible. If a client has experienced a more severe CVA, the acute care therapist may need to start the evaluation with a focus on client factors that may eventually affect occupational areas. Evaluation at this stage may concentrate on sensory processing, ROM (both passive and active), tone, and cognitive and perceptual skills. If a client is able to engage in activity, the evaluation should start with assessment of basic occupational areas, including self-care activities and basic mobility within functional tasks, such as getting out of bed. Many clients also experience difficulties with swallowing or dysphagia, and this should be evaluated as soon as possible to prevent possible aspiration. Dysphagia or swallowing evaluations are often done by both the speech therapist and the occupational therapist.

Clients are generally transferred from acute care to inpatient rehabilitation once they are medically stable and able to participate in intensive rehabilitation. Evaluation at this point should always start with assessment of occupational areas that directly affect the client's ability to return to his or her desired living situation. These areas often include the following:

- Self-care activities such as bathing and dressing, toileting, grooming, and eating.
- Mobility within the context of activity such as bed, toilet, and tub transfers.
- Homemaking activities such as meal preparation, laundry, and light housekeeping.

The therapist should hypothesize about why a client is unable to complete a task (e.g., hemiplegia; poor trunk control; impaired balance; difficulties with attention, organization, and sequencing; disturbances in visual perception). The hypotheses should be based on observation and understanding of the neurological basis of impairment. These hypotheses should then be substantiated by specific assessment of client factors. Intervention should focus on improving performance in desired activities and reduction of impairment using activities selected for their therapeutic potential. Often both can be addressed by engaging the client in the activities he or she must be able to do more independently for a transition into the community.

Once a client is able to transition to the community, the outpatient or home-health practitioner continues to expand the focus on occupational activities, including ADL and IADL; education, work and leisure activities, and social participation within the home and community. Practitioners should attend to the role that the client plays within his or her family context and social network. Evaluation should focus on assessing the activities the client values and is unable to complete, with further evaluation of the impairments or contextual factors that prevent function. Intervention should focus on assisting the client in being able to perform those valued activities within his or her social network, home, and community.

Client education is an integral part of the rehabilitation process from the beginning. It is crucial that families, caregivers, and clients understand the changes that have occurred and what the process of rehabilitation can offer. Clients and families may need to receive the same information repeatedly so they can make sense of all the changes

CASE STUDY 39-1

Sarah James: A Client with a Stroke

CLIENT HISTORY

Sarah James is a 72-year-old retired piano teacher who has been married for 52 years to Leonard, a retired postman. They have one adult son living nearby. Sarah loves to garden, listen to jazz, and play cards. She and her husband lead an active social life and have a wide circle of friends. They live in a one-story ranch house. Sarah fell one morning getting out of bed. Her husband brought her to the emergency room. She complained of weakness in her right arm and leg, disturbances in her balance, and problems with her vision. A CT scan showed a lesion in the left posterior cerebral artery. Sarah was admitted to the acute hospital but was transferred 36 hr later to an inpatient rehabilitation center.

OCCUPATIONAL THERAPY EVALUATION AND INTERVENTION

On evaluation in the rehabilitation center, Sarah required assistance for all ADL, including bathing and dressing, transfers, and simple homemaking tasks. The therapist observed that she had difficulty maintaining her balance, using her right upper extremity, and locating objects. The therapist hypothesized that Sarah was experiencing contralateral hemiplegia and ataxia, which were affecting her balance and ability to use the right upper extremity, and a right hemianopsia, which was affecting her visual abilities in locating items during functional activity. The therapist tested this hypothesis by further evaluating the client's active ROM, muscle strength, coordination, and visual fields.

Intervention focused on improving strength and ROM, improving coordination, and teaching Sarah compensatory strategies for the hemianopsia. Intervention was provided through functional activities, including bathing and dressing, grooming, homemaking, and leisure activities.

QUESTIONS AND EXERCISES

1. What was the practitioner's implicit frame of reference for his or her work with this client?
2. What alternative frame(s) of reference might be useful for organizing evaluation and intervention for this client?
3. How would this frame of reference change your evaluation and intervention for this client?
4. In thinking through revisions to occupational therapy evaluation and intervention for this client, what types of clinical reasoning are you using?

they are experiencing. The earlier families can become involved with the care of a loved one, the easier it is for them to comprehend and become a part of the process. Practitioners can facilitate this by educating families about the causes and sequelae of CVA as well as about specific interventions families may be able to provide to a loved one. These include helping the client to reengage in valued activities by offering physical and emotional support as well as assisting in restorative or preventative routines, such as ROM, interaction with clients who have language deficits, and stimulation for clients with left neglect. Education should be ongoing in all rehabilitation settings, and families and clients should be made aware of outside opportunities for education and support (e.g., stroke clubs).

TRAUMATIC BRAIN INJURY

Definition, Cause, and Demographics

TBI can be defined as any injury resulting from a traumatic event that causes direct or indirect damage to the brain. The most common causes of TBI are high-speed motor vehicle accidents (often involving alcohol, drugs, or both) and falls from heights greater than that of the person's height. Other common causes include sports injuries and injuries from violence, gunshot wounds, and work-related injuries (National Institutes of Health Consensus Panel [NIH], 1999).

TBI is generally categorized into two different types, based primarily on the cause. A focal contusion is a bruising of the brain as a result of a direct blow to the head. This can occur, for example, from a fight or a sports injury. Diffuse axonal damage results from twisting, tearing, or stretching of the axons of the nerve fibers throughout the brain. This primarily occurs because of velocity, when the brain and body are moving forward at a certain speed and are suddenly stopped short. This causes the brain to bounce back and forth within the skull, leading to diffuse damage. This may also be called a shearing injury. This type of injury can occur in a motor vehicle accident or a fall greater than the person's own height. Some clients may experience both focal contusions and diffuse axonal damage; for example when, in a motor vehicle accident, the individual hits the head on the windshield (focal) and sustains damage from the impact of velocity (diffuse).

Focal contusions are visible on specialized imaging studies (MRI and CT scans), once the bruising or lesion has formed. Diffuse axonal damage is not visible on imaging studies and is generally diagnosed through medical history and assessment of the client's behavior. Factors that suggest diffuse axonal damage are causes of injury that involve velocity, loss of consciousness, and cortical posturing (specific body tonal postures that occur as a direct result of severe injury).

The most common profile of a person with a head injury is a generally young (aged 15–24) male with a history of high-risk behaviors (NIH, 1999; Winkler, 1995). The second most common profile is an older adult (aged 70+) with either balance or cognitive difficulties, whose injury results from a fall within the home. The third largest group is children under the age of 5 (NIH, 1999). Obviously, there are many survivors of TBI who do not fit any of these profiles, but knowledge of these patterns can provide practitioners with possible clues relevant to assessment and intervention.

Deficits

TBI affects all occupational areas, including ADL and IADL, education, work, leisure activities, and social participation. Clients can experience difficulty in a broad range of body functions and performance skills because of the nature of the TBI. Clients often have motor disturbances with abnormal tone, resulting in hemiplegia, paraplegia, triplegia, or quadriplegia. They may have restricted ROM, poor postural control, and poor motor control. Often, clients experience sensory disturbances. They may also have cognitive impairments in level of arousal, orientation, attention, memory, sequencing, and organizing. They may be unable to problem solve effectively or to learn new information. Clients often display visual perceptual deficits and may have problems with spatial relations, position in space, and figure-ground and depth perception. Many clients have language deficits that interfere with their abilities for self-expression and socialization. Often, clients have a great deal of difficulty controlling their emotions and can easily become overwhelmed (Winkler, 1995).

Specific impairments in client factors are directly related to the location of the lesion(s). Clients who have unilateral or bilateral frontal contusions may not experience any motor or sensory deficits at all but may have significant problems in cognitive, psychological, and social performance skills. Clients who endure significant diffuse axonal damage may have deficits in occupational areas caused by impairments in all of their abilities and skills. It is the therapist's job to determine which occupational areas are affected, develop hypotheses based on the neurological diagnosis and observation about which client factors are affected, and then substantiate the hypotheses with a thorough evaluation. Intervention should consist of using purposeful activities to address both occupational areas and client factors that may be affected by the traumatic brain injury. As always, contextual factors are also addressed to support performance.

Prognosis

The prognosis for individuals who have experienced a TBI depends on several things. Neurologists usually assess the patient's age, the size and location of the injury, the type of injury, the level of consciousness at the time of injury, and the length of coma if loss of consciousness occurs. Prognostic indicators that support a favorable outcome include a young age, a small lesion in a noncritical part of the brain, focal rather than diffuse injury, and a short episode of loss of consciousness (<1 day) (Katz, 1992).

Secondary Complications

Secondary complications also affect prognosis. These include edema or swelling of the brain (which can increase the pressure on the brain and thus cause more damage), hygromas (collections of cerebrospinal fluid that pool because of a tearing of the membranes that surround the brain), hematomas (a collection or pooling of blood that can increase intracranial pressure), and infections of the brain or of the membranes that surround the brain. Intracranial pressure caused by any of these can be monitored and controlled by medications and by pumping mechanisms or surgery to remove the fluid and reduce the pressure. Another secondary complication that can occur is anoxia, or loss of oxygen, to the brain. This may be caused from bleeding, a severe drop in blood pressure, or respiratory failure. All of these secondary complications can cause further damage to the brain; therefore, they have a direct effect on prognosis.

Stages of Recovery and Occupational Therapy Evaluation and Intervention

There are many different descriptions about the stages of recovery through which clients with TBI may pass. Most descriptions use the client's cognitive status as an indicator for recovery. It is important to remember that not all clients experience all stages and that clients can become fixed in any stage along the road to complete recovery. It is also important to remember that any set of stages is merely a description and that clients at any point in their recovery may exhibit characteristics of more than one stage (Dobkins, 1996).

In general, clients initially suffer a loss of consciousness, during which they may not respond to any stimulus at all. Often clients at this stage require a **tracheostomy** as well as a ventilator to assist them in respiration. Clients at this stage of recovery receive their nutrition through a feeding tube (either a nasal gastric or gastric tube) and, obviously, are dependent for all care. Clients may experience changes in their muscle tone (either hypotonic or hypertonic), which may limit their ROM.

Occupational therapists who work with clients in the acute stage of recovery must rely on family and significant others to provide information about these clients' occupational history. Therapists evaluate client factors, such as observing passive and active movement, that may affect future occupational areas. Therapists also provide controlled stimulation and an opportunity for purposeful response to stimuli, such as deep touch, pain, light touch, gustatory, olfactory, visual, and kinesthetic stimulation. The purpose of sensory stimulation is not to speed up a client's recovery but rather to determine when a client transitions from coma level to a low arousal level.

Intervention at this stage often focuses on family education; preventative strategies designed to preserve ROM, skin integrity, and respiratory function and to manage tone; and providing opportunities for purposeful response.

The next, low-arousal level, is generally characterized by spontaneous eye movement, visual tracking of objects or people in the room for brief periods (2–3 sec), and some type of purposeful response to stimulation, such as eye opening to auditory stimulation or withdrawal from painful stimulation.

Practitioners who provide evaluation and intervention at this stage of recovery (acute or inpatient rehabilitation) continue to monitor musculoskeletal, cognitive, and sensory factors but also begin to try to elicit even more purposeful responses, especially in terms of following one-step commands or spontaneously attempting basic occupational areas; for example, washing one's face or combing one's hair, within a structured context. Practitioners provide intervention in a quiet environment and keep verbalizations to a minimum. Tasks can be introduced through objects, such as handing the client a washcloth or comb and pairing it with a simple one-step command. Evaluation and intervention can be graded up, depending on the client's ability to arouse, attend, and participate. The client who begins to follow one-step commands with any consistency is usually transitioning to a posttraumatic amnesia (PTA) state.

Clients in the PTA stage usually experience a state of confusion or disorientation, with no awareness of time or place. Clients at this stage have extremely impaired attentional skills and an inability to form memories secondary to severe inattention. Clients may be agitated and restless or lethargic. They may exhibit uninhibited behaviors, such as using inappropriate language. Therapists working with clients in this stage (usually inpatient rehabilitation) want to begin to evaluate which occupational areas clients can perform, how much assistance they need, and why they require assistance. The occupational area assessed may be determined by how confused the client is, and the occupational routines may need to be broken down into smaller tasks, such as combing one's hair instead of full bathing and dressing.

Although clients in this stage have significant memory deficits, they are often able to relearn commonly performed tasks, like bathing and dressing, through processes known as procedural learning or procedural memory (Giles & Shore, 1989; Miller, 1980). Therapy focuses on basic occupational areas and skills, such as activities encouraging attention and controlled motor skills. Intervention also focuses on evaluating and improving client factors, such as decreased ROM, that may prevent a client from being able to complete the tasks.

The length of this stage is often directly related to the length of the client's coma stage—that is, the longer the coma the longer the period of PTA. As clients become less confused, they move into a postconfusional state.

Clients in a postconfusional state may demonstrate impairments in higher-level attention and concentration as well as impairments in memory. Clients at this stage may still be agitated or disinhibited, with an inability to control frustration or anger. Some clients have the opposite problem, displaying difficulty initiating activity or interaction, and showing little or no affect. Most higher-level cognitive skills, such as reasoning, concentration, problem solving, safety, and judgment, are also usually impaired.

Practitioners who provide intervention at this stage of recovery (inpatient or outpatient rehabilitation or home health) focus on more complex ADL, both in the home and in the community, as well as helping the client to return to or identify new occupational activities to meet their goals for education, work, leisure, and social participation. Clients make the transition to outpatient or home-health therapies when they can safely return to community living with existing supports: family, sitters, or group homes.

Many clients experience depression and isolation because of the change in their abilities to manage occupational areas independently and to function in prior life roles as family members, workers, and friends. TBI severely interrupts a person's place in his or her life phases, whether that be a senior in high school getting ready for college or an adult who has two young children and an active career.

PARKINSON'S DISEASE

Definition, Cause, and Demographics

Parkinson disease is a progressive degenerative disease, characterized by the degeneration of dopaminergic neurons in the substantia nigra, deep in the brain (Fox & Alder, 1999). Dopamine is an inhibitory neurotransmitter that greatly affects motor control. Clients with Parkinson disease experience a reduction of dopamine available within their CNS, which causes an imbalance between the inhibitory and the excitatory effects of the neurotransmitters used for motor control. The exact cause of Parkinson disease is unknown in most cases, although it can be caused in a few cases by toxic poisons or as sequelae to a specific form of encephalitis.

Deficits

As with the previously discussed conditions, all occupational areas can be affected by Parkinson disease. Clients often experience impairments in neuromusculoskeletal factors, such

CASE STUDY 39-2

Tim Rouse: A Client with a Head Injury

CLIENT HISTORY

Tim Rouse is a 17-year-old senior in high school who lives with his mother. Tim's parents are divorced, but his father remains active in his life. His mother is a nurse who works the night shift at a local hospital. Tim was involved in a high-speed motor vehicle accident. He was the driver and collided head-on with another vehicle. The passenger in his car was killed instantly.

At the scene, Tim was found unconscious and unresponsive, even to painful stimulation. His respiration was labored, and his blood pressure was dropping. He was intubated at the scene and rushed to the hospital emergency room. A CT scan showed multiple contusions in both frontal lobes as well as in the right fronto-parietal-temporal region. The physician concluded that Tim had endured diffuse axonal brain damage owing to the nature of the accident and loss of consciousness. Tim was placed on a ventilator to assist his breathing.

During his intensive care stay, Tim had intracranial pressure, secondary to edema and multiple infections. He first showed signs of arousal—spontaneous eye opening and tracking people in his room—27 days after the accident and followed his first command 35 days after injury.

OCCUPATIONAL THERAPY EVALUATION AND INTERVENTION/OUTCOME

Tim was transferred to inpatient rehabilitation, where he presented with poor attention, agitated behavior, and left hemiplegia. He required assistance with both ADL and IADL (e.g., mobility and morning self-care routines) and with leisure activities (e.g., operating his CD player). His skills gradually improved during his inpatient stay, so that he could complete basic self-care and was able to participate in some educational and leisure activities.

When he made the transition to outpatient therapy, he was independent in basic ADL and was able to initiate and participate in other activities with minimal assistance. He continued to experience difficulties with higher-level cognitive functions, such as concentration, judgment, and problem solving, and had diminished use of his left upper extremity.

Currently, Tim is in outpatient therapy. He becomes easily frustrated and says he feels as if "life had gone on without him." Many of his friends have gone to college or are working. The outpatient therapist is helping Tim set realistic goals in terms of education and work as well as IADL at home and within the community, such as cooking, shopping, and banking. The therapist is also working with Tim to improve the functional use of his left upper extremity. Tim is involved in many groups at outpatient therapy aimed at helping his social participation by reestablishing his leisure interests and helping him develop a social network.

QUESTIONS AND EXERCISES

1. What was the practitioner's implicit frame of reference for his or her work with this client?
2. What alternative frame(s) of reference might effectively organize evaluation and intervention for this client?
3. How would this frame of reference change your evaluation and intervention for this client?
4. In thinking through revisions to occupational therapy evaluation and intervention for this client, what types of clinical reasoning are you using?

as ROM, reflexes, muscle tone, strength, and soft tissue integrity; motor skills, such as gross and fine coordination, motor control, endurance, postural control, and alignment oral motor control; and eventually, mental processes such as short-term memory and perception. It is unclear exactly how Parkinson disease affects a client's cognitive skills, but these changes are thought to be related to the connections of the substantia nigra to other areas of the cortex (Fox & Alder, 1999; Schultz-Krohn, Foti, & Glogoski, 2001).

Prognosis

Parkinson disease is progressive, and there is no cure for it. Numerous medications can be used to slow the progression of the disease. These medications are generally dopamine agonists used to increase the amount of available dopamine within the CNS. Surgery may also used to reduce some of the motor manifestations, including tremor and rigidity. The average life span after diagnosis is 13 years; death is usually the result of heart disease or infection (Lundy-Elkman, 1998).

Initially, clients with a diagnosis of Parkinson disease often experience a tremor of the hand or foot that may be present only with intentional movement. As the disease progresses, the tremor may spread to include all extremities, as well as the trunk and head, and be present at all times or absent only during sleep. Clients experience increases in muscle tone, rigidity that may lead to *cogwheeling* (intermittent resistance to passive movement), decreased ability to initiate movement, disturbances in postural control and alignment, alterations in gait, fatigue, and decreased control of motor output. The onset of the disease is usually gradual and generally occurs between the ages of 50 and 69 (Lundy-Elkman, 1998; Schultz-Krohn et al., 2001).

Secondary Complications

Secondary complications arising from Parkinson disease include changes in soft tissue integrity, reduced passive and active ROM leading to contractures, reduced muscle strength, skin and respiratory problems, infections, dysphagia, and disruptions in speech production. Clients may also experience masking, or an inability to produce facial expression, secondary to the weakness of facial muscles. Eventually in the late stages of Parkinson disease, clients may experience changes in cognition and perceptual skills. Depression is often part of the clinical presentation, although it is difficult to know if this is a clinical manifestation of the disease itself or simply an understandable psychological reaction to issues of loss and change.

Occupational Therapy Evaluation and Intervention

Clients with Parkinson disease may be provided with occupational therapy on either an inpatient rehabilitation or outpatient basis, depending on the progression of the disease. Practitioners working with clients with Parkinson disease must keep in mind that this disease is progressive and that extreme fatigue can exacerbate the symptoms. Evaluation should be focused on specific activities that have become difficult for the client to accomplish. Intervention should include remediation of neuromusculoskeletal functions and motor skills, as well as assisting the client with adapting his or her current lifestyle. Practitioners must be sure to focus on remediation of only those client factors that can be changed—such as strength, active and passive ROM, soft tissue dysfunction, and endurance. In part, this may also consist of vigilant observation on how medications are affecting performance, to help physicians monitor dosages. Use of adaptive equipment and environmental modifications may allow clients to remain more independent for a longer time. Practitioners can also help clients learn energy-conservation techniques.

A further focus of intervention should be on education for clients and their families to facilitate understanding and acceptance of the disease process. As the disease progresses and clients lose their ability to communicate or express emotions facially, the ability to connect with loved ones may be greatly strained. By assisting clients with remaining in their own environment for as long as possible and as independently as possible, a practitioner can have a great influence on their quality of life as well as that of the family.

AMYOTROPHIC LATERAL SCLEROSIS

Definition, Cause, and Demographics

ALS (also called motor neuron disease and Lou Gehrig's disease) is a degenerative process that destroys motor neurons in the cortex, brainstem, and spinal cord. It affects both upper motor neurons and lower motor neurons. This disease causes massive loss of anterior horn cells in the spinal cord as well as in the lower brainstem, leading to weakness and muscle atrophy (hence the term *amyotrophic*) (Francis, Bach, & DeLisa, 1999; Hallum, 1995). It also causes demyelinization of corticospinal and corticobulbar tracts, secondary to the degeneration of the motor cortex, resulting in upper motor neuron lesions (thus the term *lateral sclerosis*) (Hallum, 1995). The cause of this disease is unknown, although research has investigated several possible factors, including exposure to toxins, exposure to viruses, hormonal imbalances, and autoimmunity problems (Hallum, 1995; Schultz-Krohn et al., 2001).

Most clients who have a diagnosis of ALS are between 40 and 70 years of age and more men are affected than women (Hallum, 1995; Schultz-Krohn et al., 2001). There is no specific medical test for ALS; a diagnosis is based on clinical manifestations. Onset is gradual, and often the client has adapted to the slow loss of muscle strength long before noticing significant changes and seeking medical assistance.

Deficits

Initial symptoms often include complaints of an inability to perform functional tasks, such as buttoning buttons or climbing stairs. Another symptom may be cramping or muscle twitching in the muscle groups that are weakened. These are often described as *fasciculations*. Upper motor neuron problems may include hyperreflexia and spasticity. Weakness can occur anywhere in the body. At first it is slightly more common in the lower extremities, rather than the upper extremities, and is more distal rather than proximal. Onset of weakness is also usually asymmetrical. Clients may experience involvement of the cranial nerves, resulting in poor oral motor and facial control, with eventual dysphagia and speech disturbances (Francis et al., 1999; Hallum, 1995; Schultz-Krohn et al., 2001).

Prognosis

ALS is fatal, and death is usually the result of respiratory failure, secondary to weak musculature and eventual paralysis. The average life span following diagnosis is approximately 3 years (Lundy-Elkman, 1998). There is no medical intervention for ALS itself, but many interventions can allow the client to remain as active as possible and, eventually, as comfortable as possible. These include rehabilitation therapies, pain medications, alternative nutritional sources (including diet alteration and feeding tubes if the client wishes) and use of mechanical ventilation (again, if the client so wishes).

Secondary Complications

Secondary complications can include infections, changes in soft tissue integrity, skin breakdown, and respiratory complications, such as dyspnea. Clients may also understandably experience depression and fear. Depression and fear may lead to a less active lifestyle that can result in further muscle atrophy (Francis et al. 1999; Hallum, 1995).

Occupational Therapy Evaluation and Intervention

Occupational therapy practitioners are most likely to see clients with ALS in outpatient or home settings, although they may also be seen in inpatient rehabilitation settings. It is crucial for the therapist to have a clear understanding of the course of the disease and the prognosis to assist the client in setting realistic goals and to develop an appropriate intervention plan. Practitioners must be careful not to allow clients to overexert themselves and thereby cause an overuse syndrome. Should clients engage in activities that cause an overuse syndrome, they may actually lose muscle strength.

Evaluation should begin with a thorough assessment of what clients are able to do in terms of desired activities within the context of their home, work, and other occupational environments. Thorough assessment of the clients' occupational performance concerns, coupled with performance observations, illuminates the difficulties these clients may be experiencing. Therapists have a generalized idea of what impairment is contributing to any disability, such as decreased muscle strength, but should further evaluate specific impairments in neuromusculoskeletal functions and motor skills. This may include evaluation of ROM, muscle tone, strength, endurance, and soft tissue integrity. Therapists also evaluate gross and fine motor coordination, motor control, and oral motor control in cases in which clients have difficulty with eating and basic communication.

Intervention should be focused on countering declines in function through use of functional activities, such as maintaining upper extremity strength through performance of self-care activities. As the disease progresses, clients may benefit from adaptive equipment to maintain independence for as long as possible, as well as to minimize the work of caregivers. This may include equipment for bathing and dressing, eating, and mobility. It may also include adaptation of the home and work environments as well as adaptations to leisure activities.

Client and family education is essential, from the time of diagnosis, to assist clients and families in making decisions, especially about quality-of-life issues, such as tube feedings, and use of mechanical ventilation. As a client becomes more dependent for ADL, education should focus on teaching the family how to assist the client and on helping the client learn to direct his or her caregivers. Teaching caregivers how to perform ROM and how to position the client may also help with pain management and avoidance of pressure sores on the skin in the later stages of ALS.

As with any progressive degenerative disease that is eventually fatal, clients may experience depression and feelings of loss of control over their lives. Many clients also experience anger, denial, and apathy. It is important for the practitioner to recognize that these emotions are an anticipated part of adjusting to living with ALS. Support groups and one-on-one counseling may be helpful, as well as informal networking with other clients and families dealing with ALS. Educating clients and families and assisting clients to remain in control of valued occupational activities as long as possible can help reduce the feelings of helplessness. It is also essential to support clients to make their own end-of-life decisions with dignity.

MULTIPLE SCLEROSIS

Definition, Cause, and Demographics

Multiple sclerosis is a progressive disease with a gradual onset that is characterized by a demyelinization or destruction of the myelin sheaths that cover the nerve fibers within the CNS. The myelin sheath allows nerve impulses to be carried from the brain to various parts of the body. As the myelin sheath is destroyed, so is the body's ability to send messages via the nervous system. The destroyed myelin sheath is eventually replaced by plaques or sclerotic (hard) patches within the white matter of both the brain and the spinal cord; hence the term *multiple sclerosis*.

The cause of MS is unknown. This disease is characterized by a series of exacerbations and **remissions,** with each exacerbation potentially resulting in some residual loss of function. Many factors are thought to contribute to an exacerbation, including fatigue, increased physical demand, stress, poor nutrition, and cold weather. The average age for diagnosis of this disease is usually between the ages of 20 and 40 and it affects three times as many women as men (Lundy-Elkman, 1998; Schultz-Krohn et al., 2001).

Deficits

Clients with MS may experience difficulty in all of the occupational areas of their lives. Clients' abilities to engage actively in these tasks often fluctuate, depending on whether they are in acute exacerbation. Ongoing evaluation of clients' ability to perform various activities is required as they pass through an acute exacerbation into remission. Therapists must be able to evaluate and help clients understand and adapt to any residual disability that may exist after an exacerbation.

Impairments in client factors are directly related to where in the CNS the disease strikes. Clients may experience impairments in sensory processing (any sensation or vestibular changes), neuromusculoskeletal factors (ROM, muscle tone, strength, endurance, postural control, postural alignment, and soft tissue integrity), and motor functions and skills (gross and fine coordination, motor control, praxis, and oral motor control). Mental functions and processing skills may also be affected (memory, organization, sequencing, problem solving, insight, judgment, new learning, potential psychotic episodes, mood swings, and depression). MS has the potential to affect every client factor, because it can attack any part of the CNS.

Initially, clients may experience only incoordination of a limb; **paresthesias** of the limbs, trunk, or face; and fatigue. Exacerbations may resolve in as little as 1–2 weeks. Exacerbations generally leave behind some residual impairment. Over time, with multiple exacerbations, clients are less and less able to recover from each exacerbation and return to their baseline functioning abilities (Lundy-Elkman, 1998; Schultz-Krohn et al., 2001).

As with any progressive disease, clients often experience feelings of hopelessness, anger, denial, and depression. Many clients describe feelings of losing control over their lives as well.

Prognosis

MS is rarely fatal. The life span for an individual diagnosed with MS varies tremendously, depending on how frequent and severe the exacerbations are; however most clients with MS live a normal life span (Lundy-Elkman, 1998; Schultz-Krohn et al., 2001).

Secondary Complications

Secondary complications can be extremely varied, often depending on what part of the CNS is affected. They may include contractures, compromised respiratory system, infections, and skin breakdown.

Occupational Therapy Evaluation and Intervention

A large part of intervention focuses on providing the client with education about the disease process and assisting clients in adjusting to the ongoing, degenerative nature of the disease. Intervention must include a way for clients to learn to grade activities, based on their current level of functioning. Intervention should also focus on teaching energy conservation, work simplification, and safety awareness. Clients must learn to identify for themselves when they are becoming too fatigued, because the fatigue itself can trigger an exacerbation. By providing clients with avenues to adjust activities, the practitioner also helps them retain control over their daily life. As the disease progresses, the practitioner may need to introduce adaptive equipment and environmental adaptation to allow clients to continue to function as independently as possible.

Clients diagnosed with MS may be seen in any type of setting, depending on how significant their exacerbations are. Some clients may be able to remain at home and continue to work, perhaps with a modified schedule, if their exacerbations are not severe. Other clients may experience exacerbations so severe or so debilitating that they require inpatient rehabilitation. Practitioners who provide intervention in the acute or inpatient rehabilitation phase should be focused on evaluating which functional activities clients are able or unable to perform that are important to them and that will influence discharge to the home environment. Practitioners must be careful not to overexert clients or cause undue fatigue during evaluation and intervention.

Intervention in an inpatient rehabilitation phase may include focusing on ADL, such as bathing, dressing, grooming, and eating. Functional mobility is also a focus, including toilet transfers, bed transfers, and tub transfers. If the exacerbation is severe enough, the practitioner may need to introduce an alternative method of mobility, such as a wheelchair. When ordering equipment for clients with MS, practitioners must attend to the potential for the equipment to meet the clients' changing needs. For instance, a wheelchair should be one that can be easily adapted and modified to allow for further decline (e.g., manual to power conversion, addition of head support, lateral supports, and tilt-in-space mechanisms). Further adaptation of the home environment may be needed to assist with transfers, safety, and other mobility concerns.

Once clients can safely manage at home, they will transfer to outpatient or home-health therapies. The practitioner in these settings should focus on clients' ability to manage occupational activities within the home and the community. This may include home management, child care, banking, and adaptation of the workplace.

Because the average age of diagnosis is between 20 and 40 years of age, many clients are in a highly productive phase of their lives. They may be engaged in various roles in life, including that of spouse, worker, and parent. Practitioners must work to help clients remain active in these important life roles in whatever capacities are possible. Evaluation of functional activity should be completed as it relates to the individual client's life roles, and intervention should focus on the same activities.

Ongoing client and family education is absolutely necessary to help clients and the families understand the disease process and adapt as the disease progresses. A good understanding of the possible consequences of the disease process allows clients and their families to plan for future activities that they may no longer be able to do because of physical or mental decline. This planning can significantly affect the quality of life for both clients and families as the disease progresses. Referral to support groups, such as those sponsored by the Multiple Sclerosis Society, may also be of great benefit.

SPINAL CORD INJURY

Definition, Cause, and Demographics

SCI can be defined as any traumatic event that results in damage to the spinal cord. SCI can be caused by laceration, puncture, or compression of the cord. This injury is often caused by a fracture in the vertebral column. Common causes of spinal cord injury include motor vehicle accidents (44.5%), falls (18.1%), acts of violence (16.6%), and sports injuries (12.7%), such as diving accidents (Staas, Formal, Freedman, Fried, & Read, 1998). Almost one fourth of all spinal cord injuries are related to drug and alcohol use (Marion & Pryzbylski, 2000). The most common profile of a person with spinal cord injury is a male (80%) between the ages of 16 and 30 who is either a student or employed (Staas et al., 1998; Zejdlik, 1992).

SCI may result in damage that is permanent or temporary. Damage may further be defined as complete, incomplete, or transient. A complete lesion is characterized by complete loss of function below the level of the lesion. Incomplete lesions are those that result in partial loss of function below the level of the lesion. Transient injuries are usually caused by compression from a fracture or edema; as the pressure is removed, function eventually returns. Transection or partial transection of the spinal cord causes spinal shock, loss of motor control and sensation, and alterations in muscle tone (initially flaccid and then spastic).

Deficits

Deficits resulting from SCI are directly related to the site of the lesion. Function is impaired below the level of the lesion. Clients can experience impairments in sensory and neuromusculoskeletal functions and related motor skills. Clients commonly experience problems with many occupational performance areas, particularly ADL, work, leisure, and social participation. It is important for the clinician to understand that sensory motor impairments and related skill deficits are based on the level of the lesion. The impairments are more difficult to predict if a lesion is incomplete. Clients with lesions below C8 or T1 will have full use of their upper extremities and will be considered to have paraplegia. Clients with lesions above this level will have impairment in their upper extremities and will be considered to have quadriplegia. Table 39-4 shows what movements can be expected after injury at different levels, how each injury can affect function, and what the intervention goals might be for a client with that injury.

Practitioners who provide intervention for clients with SCI must also be fully aware of the emotional, social, and self-management problems a client may experience. Common stages of adjustment may include denial, anger, bargaining, depression, and acceptance. Clients may also experience feelings of isolation, despair, frustration, and hopelessness. It is often extremely beneficial for clients to receive therapy in a rehabilitation center that offers a dedicated SCI program so that the client is able to interact and gain psychological and social support from other people with similar experiences (Marion & Pryzbylski, 2000). Other clients may be able to offer encouragement and motivation in a way that a healthcare professional cannot. The ability for clients who are in the early phases of rehabilitation to interact with a client who is more independent can often have a major impact on the total rehabilitation process. Individual and group counseling may also be beneficial.

Prognosis

In the 1950s, most people with spinal cord injuries died either immediately or within 1 year of injury. Owing to the tremendous advances in the medical management for persons with SCI, individuals now experience close to full life expectancies after injury. There are still numerous secondary complications that can cause disruption in a client's life, and a great deal of responsibility lies with the client to safeguard against these complications (Staas et al., 1998; Zejdlik, 1992).

Secondary Complications

Because of the way in which SCIs occur, co-existing problems may include head injury and fractures. Further damage may be caused at the scene of the injury by failure to stabilize the vertebral column while moving the injured person. Secondary complications may also include respiratory distress or arrest, problems with skin maintenance, urinary tract infections, and problems with blood pressure such as **autonomic dysreflexia** (Marion & Pryzbylski, 2000; Zejdlik, 1992).

Stages of Recovery and Occupational Therapy Evaluation and Intervention

Evaluation of occupational performance concerns needs to proceed with an understanding of which functional movement and sensation a client has. This can be achieved through consideration of diagnosis as well as specific manual muscle testing and sensory testing. This testing may need to be done in an ongoing fashion for incomplete or transient lesions, because as the swelling and edema subsides more function returns.

The role of the practitioner in acute and inpatient settings is to help the client begin to develop strategies necessary to regain desired occupational performance skills. Therapeutic interventions focus on maintaining passive and active ROM, improving motor skills and functions, providing appropriate wheelchair and bed positioning to preserve respiratory and skin functions, and evaluating the need for adaptive equipment and methods to allow a client to function as independently as possible. Fabrication of adaptive equipment and splinting may be used to meet these goals. Some examples of equipment are universal cuffs, self-care

TABLE 39–4. **SPINAL CORD INNERVATION LEVELS AND IMPLICATIONS FOR INTERVENTION**[a]

Last Innervated Level	Key Muscles	Active Movement	Affected Occupational Areas	Possible Intervention
C1–C3	Sternocleidomastoid; possibly partial trapezius and diaphragm	Can assist with respiration; neck movement; partial scapular elevation	• Dependent in basic ADL and most IADL • Mobility augmented through use of power wheelchair • Communication and leisure activities may be met through adapted equipment • Work and productive activities may be met through some adaptive equipment • Able to engage in educational and vocational tasks within limits, using adaptive equipment	• Use of power wheelchair controlled by head or chin control units • Client to use portable respirator • Mouthstick for use of computers; tape recorders; and for educational, leisure, and vocational activities • Use of environmental control units for managing things in the environment and for leisure activities • Able to direct caregiver
C4	Full innervation of diaphragm; trapezius	Full respiration; neck movements; scapula movement; scapula retraction	• Dependent in self-care • Client may be able to use adaptive equipment for drinking • Dependent in home management tasks • Functional and community mobility augmented through use of power wheelchair • Social participation, work, and leisure activities may be possible through use of adapted equipment • Able to engage in educational and vocational tasks within limits	• Use of power wheelchair controlled by head, chin, or sip-and-puff control units • Client not reliant on portable respirator • Long straw for drinking • May use externally powered arm supports for upper extremity use in activities • Continued use of adapted equipment as stated for C1-C3 • Client generally with better endurance and more options for educational, leisure, and vocation
C5	Partial deltoid; partial biceps; rhomboids; partial rotator cuff	Shoulder flexion and abduction to 90°; partial elbow flexion; supination	• Can participate in basic ADL such as bathing, dressing, grooming, and eating with adapted equipment • Mobility most practical with power wheelchair • May assist with transfers • Continued participation in education, vocational, and leisure activities with adapted equipment • Client may be able to engage in wider range of activities	• Use of secure shower seat, washcloth mitt, and adapted shower head for ADL • Dynamic tenodesis splint and long opponens splint with mobile arm support for eating and typing • More options for wheelchair and environmental control units • More options for educational, vocational, and leisure activities as well as more options in how to engage
C6	Partial serratus anterior; partial pectoralis; partial latissimus dorsi; deltoid; biceps; carpi radialis	Scapula adduction; shoulder flexion and extension; weak trunk control; elbow flexion; wrist extension (tenodesis for grasp)	• Able to complete basic ADL independently with adapted equipment (bathing, dressing, grooming, eating) • Can assist in sliding board transfers • Can use manual chair with adaptations for mobility • Able to use communication devices without adaptation • Can engage in light IADL • Increased variety for educational, work, and leisure activities • Can drive with adaptations	• Tenodesis splints for activities requiring hand grasp • Adaptive ADL equipment (razor holders, eating utensils, dressing loops and friction pads, adapted long handled sponge and wash mitt, adapted leg bag for continence) • Knobs on wheelchair rims and on steering wheel with hand controls • Return to work environment that is wheelchair accessible
C7	Triceps; extrinsic finger flexors and extensors; partial wrist flexors	Moderate trunk control; elbow extension; functional grasp and release	• Independent in all basic ADL, requires less use of adapted equipment • Can use manual wheelchair and transfer independently to most surfaces • Light home management tasks in wheelchair accessible home • Return to many educational, leisure, work, and social participation activities without requiring as much adapted equipment • Environment must be wheelchair accessible	• Equipment may still be needed (button hook or pant loops) but less adaptation/effort required • May still require bathing equipment • Less adaptation for eating required • May still require adaptive equipment for toileting • No longer require splinting for upper extremity use
C8–T1	Intrinsics of the hand, including thumb	Full use of upper extremities	• Independent in all ADL • Can participate in numerous educational, leisure, and work activities in wheelchair-accessible environment	• Use of manual wheelchair that should be adapted to client's lifestyle • May still use some adapted equipment for self-care (long-handled sponge, suction holder for soap) • Client often can engage in numerous activities without further adaptation

[a] Data from Pulaski (1998), Spencer (1988), and University Hospital, Physical Therapy Section (1998).

CASE STUDY 39-3

Mark Jonis: A Client with a Spinal Cord Injury

CLIENT HISTORY

Mark Jonis is a 32-year-old computer analyst. He is married and has one child. He and his wife have no family in the immediate living area but have a wide circle of friends. Mark was involved in a motor vehicle accident that resulted in an SCI at the C-6 level. X-ray examination showed that the injury was a complete transection and was caused by severe displaced fractures of the vertebral column. Initially, Mark experienced a great deal of swelling in the spinal cord owing to the traumatic nature of the injury.

OCCUPATIONAL THERAPY EVALUATION AND INTERVENTION/OUTCOME

When the therapist in the acute care setting initially evaluated Mark, he found that Mark was breathing on his own (C1-C3), and demonstrated some shoulder flexion and abduction and elbow flexion; however, Mark had no sensation below the level of the lesion. Therapy focused initially on improving ADL and leisure options, by introducing adaptive equipment and encouraging Mark's participation. The practitioner also helped Mark improve his motor skills by maintaining ROM, increasing Mark's ability to be more upright in bed and eventually in a wheelchair, and attending to bed and wheelchair positioning to preserve respiratory status and prevent decubitus.

When Mark was medically stable and able to tolerate a more intensive rehabilitation setting, he was transferred to an inpatient rehabilitation center with a dedicated SCI program. The new therapist interviewed Mark about his occupational goals and assessed Mark's active and passive ROM. Mark could demonstrate shoulder extension, forward reach, internal rotation, adduction, and wrist extension. This active movement was consistent with the initial diagnosis of complete transection at the C-6 level and indicated that Mark's initial edema had resolved.

Mark and his practitioners focused on activities such as use of the computer with adapted equipment to improve upper extremity strength and endurance. They helped Mark become more independent in mobility (bed mobility, transfers, wheelchair mobility), self-care activities (eating, bathing, dressing, grooming), and leisure and work activities.

The therapist determined that Mark could use tenodesis for functional activities and so provided him with a universal cuff for eating, writing, bathing, and grooming. The practitioner also worked with him on learning to use a sliding board for transfers, using compensatory techniques and adapted equipment for dressing and bathing, resuming use of a computer, and incorporating adaptations to his activities related to child care. The therapist provided education and referral to a specialist when Mark and his wife began to seek information about sexuality. The therapist also provided a home evaluation before discharge to assist Mark, his wife, and their 2-year-old child in adapting the house for a wheelchair.

When Mark reached the level at which he and his wife could manage safely at home, he was discharged from the inpatient setting and began therapy at a local outpatient center. The outpatient practitioner focused on assisting Mark in reintegrating into the community and back into the life roles that he had previously enjoyed, including computer analyst, husband, and father. The practitioner assisted him in community mobility, community accessibility, adapting his work environment to allow for a wheelchair, and adapted driving. The practitioner also focused on adaptations to allow him to participate in child care. The practitioner encouraged Mark to participate in a number of groups with other clients to help him in his adjustment. Mark and his wife also received personal counseling.

QUESTIONS AND EXERCISES

1. What was each practitioner's implicit frame of reference for his or her work with this client?
2. What alternative frame(s) of reference might effectively organize evaluation and intervention for this client?
3. How would this frame of reference change your evaluation and intervention for this client?
4. In thinking through revisions to occupational therapy evaluation and intervention for this client, what types of clinical reasoning are you using?

adaptive equipment, and long opponens splints that allow the client to perform bathing, dressing, eating, and work activities independently.

The outpatient or home-health practitioner should assist the client in focusing on occupational activities occurring within the home and community. Every practitioner who interacts with the client needs to have a clear understanding of what that client's goals are as well as the life roles the client was engaged in before injury and what life roles the client wishes to engage in after injury. Environmental adaptations in the home and workplace may allow a client to function independently in both of these arenas.

Again, client and family education are essential throughout the entire rehabilitation process. A major focus of education includes teaching the client how to direct a caregiver in assisting him or her in daily activities, if the client requires this help. Family involvement at an early stage helps both the client and the family cope with the numerous changes that are occurring as a result of the spinal cord injury.

GUILLAIN-BARRÉ SYNDROME

Definition, Cause, and Demographics

Guillain-Barré syndrome is generally characterized by an acute inflammation of multiple nerves leading to rapid progressive muscular weakness, potential paralysis, and sensory disturbances or loss. The inflammation causes damage to the myelin sheath that covers the nerve fibers within the CNS; it may, in more severe cases, cause axonal damage within the nerve fiber. In some cases, the onset of inflammation may be more gradual, although this is rare.

The exact cause of Guillain-Barré syndrome is unknown; however, it often occurs after recovery from or exposure to an infectious viral disease, surgery, or immunization. Diagnosis is made based on the client's clinical presentation of the foregoing characteristics as well as an elevated protein level in the cerebrospinal fluid, determined by spinal tap. Guillain-Barré syndrome may result in death from respiratory failure because of paralysis or secondary complications from paralysis, but it is usually a transient motor unit disease that generally ends in full recovery. Some clients may experience residual weakness, which may be a result of prolonged hypoxia in the acute phase.

This syndrome can occur in a mild form, causing some paresis in only the lower extremities, or in a severe form, causing quadriplegia and respiratory failure. The extent of the disease directly depends on which nerves are involved and how many nerves are involved. The disease process generally occurs in three stages: the acute phase, which begins with the onset of symptoms and lasts until no further new symptoms are present; the plateau phase, which is characterized primarily by no significant changes; and the recovery phase, which is when remyelination and axonal regeneration occur and the client begins to show improvement. The acute phase generally lasts 1–3 weeks, the plateau phase can last several days to 2 weeks, and recovery can span 6 months to 2 years. Guillain-Barré syndrome can attack all people at all stages of life (Reed, 2001).

Deficits

Clients may experience impairments in sensory processing, neuromusculoskeletal, and motor skills. Clients may have no sensation or may be hypersensitive. They may experience paresthesias that can be particularly painful. Clients may have disturbances in ROM, muscle tone, strength, endurance, postural control, or soft tissue integrity. They often present with poor coordination and motor control from both proximal and distal motor weakness as well as sensory changes. They may also have impairments with their oral motor control, resulting in swallowing deficits and placing them at risk for aspiration. These impairments have a tremendous influence on the client's ability to participate in ADL and valued occupations (Reed, 2001).

Prognosis

Clients are often treated with steroids to reduce the inflammation. As the inflammation recedes, muscle activity and sensation gradually return. Complete recovery may take as little as 2 months or as long as 2 years. More acute onset generally results in a more rapid recovery, whereas a slower onset may take longer to resolve or may leave the client with permanent residual weakness. Aggressive exercise programs or interventions that place a great physical demand on the client are contraindicated, as this may cause an increase in muscle weakness or even cause a relapse (Reed, 2001).

Secondary Complications

Secondary complications include respiratory failure, unstable blood pressure, skin breakdown, urinary tract infections, muscle atrophy, soft tissue shortening, and extremely poor endurance. Clients may also be depressed, angry, apathetic, or frustrated. Clients often also experience a great deal of pain, caused by the inflammation of the sensory axons in the nerves. This pain can be medically controlled to a certain point and improves over time (Reed, 2001).

Stages of Recovery and Occupational Therapy Evaluation and Intervention

The role of the acute-stage therapist is to determine at what level the client is able to participate. Often, therapists may intervene while clients are still being maintained on a ventilator, which limits the client's ability to participate. Evaluation would then focus on assessment of passive and active ROM, strength, bed positioning for skin and respiratory maintenance, soft tissue integrity, muscle tone, coordination, and sensation. Practitioners may need to provide splinting and specialized positioning to prevent loss of ROM and changes in soft tissue integrity as well as to help decrease the amount of pain the client is experiencing. Practitioners also work with the client and care staff to maximize client control of the context. For example, special adaptations may be needed to control bed position, use call lights, and control the television.

For clients who are no longer ventilator dependent, the therapist may be able to complete a bedside evaluation for swallowing and oral motor impairments that affect clients' ability to eat. When clients are able to tolerate a diet by mouth, the practitioner can begin to assist them to self-feed. Acute-stage practitioners may need to provide adaptive equipment for this. Clients may be transferred to an inpatient setting before being able to tolerate a diet by mouth; in these cases, self-feeding is a focus for the inpatient practitioner.

Clients are transferred to an inpatient rehabilitation setting once they are medically stable and can tolerate more intensive rehabilitation. The inpatient rehabilitation therapist focuses evaluation on desired ADL, such as bathing, dressing, grooming, eating, and toileting; motor skills, including bed mobility, transfers, wheelchair mobility, and functional ambulation during task performance; and other valued occupational activities associated with education, work, leisure, and social participation. Further evaluation is based on developing hypotheses about which specific deficits are causing each client's difficulty with these tasks. Possible deficits include sensory and neuromusculoskeletal impairments, with resulting limitations in motor skills. Practitioners may need to provide specialized splinting or adaptive equipment to facilitate independence during this transitional stage. It is important to remember, however, that most clients with Guillain-Barré syndrome make a complete recovery. This affects which equipment the therapist recommends for these clients. Therapists would not, for example, recommend a power chair for clients in the earlier stages of the disease, even for clients who are presenting with quadriplegia. Therapists should consider the cost of equipment and how long a client may use that equipment before recommending purchase. Sometimes practitioners are able to loan a piece of adaptive equipment to a client or to fabricate an inexpensive piece of equipment if the client will not be using it over an extended period of time. Once these clients have reached a level at which they can be safely managed at home, they make the transition to outpatient or home-health services.

Practitioners working with clients at the outpatient or home-health stage of recovery focus on identifying which occupational challenges are important for the client to overcome, whether they relate to IADL, work, education, leisure, or social participation. Again, hypotheses should be developed to determine why such a client needs assistance, and intervention is focused on restoring function, developing skills, and/or providing compensatory strategies so the client can become fully functional again.

Throughout the rehabilitation process of providing intervention for clients recovering from Guillain-Barré syndrome, practitioners must have an excellent ability to grade activities as well as to teach clients to grade activities to prevent too great a demand on the client. Overexertion can cause further muscle weakness or a relapse. Client and family education should be ongoing throughout the rehabilitation process.

CONCLUSION

Occupational therapy practitioners who provide rehabilitation services to adult clients with neurological impairments are faced with great challenges in helping their clients overcome a wide variety of occupational performance problems. It is crucial for practitioners to have a working knowledge of neuroanatomy and neurophysiology as it relates to neurological insult if clients are to receive the maximum benefit from therapeutic intervention. Practitioners must always remember that the focus needs to be on goals that clients value, which may not always be the same goals that practitioners value. Therapists must be able to observe clients performing valued activities, develop hypotheses quickly about why clients may have difficulty performing these tasks, and develop intervention plans based on assessments. For conditions for which improvement in body functions and structures is likely, interventions involve a combination of reengaging the client in occupational activities that are designed to restore skills and of developing social and environmental supports. For conditions that are degenerative in nature, intervention centers on adaptive strategies, including task modification, energy-saving methods, adapted devices, and environmental modifications.

Practitioners must be extremely focused in their intervention and make sure they have a specific goal for every interaction that occurs with clients. Practitioners must also be constantly reevaluating the interventions they are providing to make sure they are truly assisting clients in reaching their goals in the most efficacious way.

References

Adams, R., Victor, M., & Roper, A. (1997). *Principles of neurology*. New York: McGraw-Hill.

Arnadottir, G. (1990). *The brain and behavior*. St. Louis: Mosby.

Bartels, M. (1998). Pathophysiology and medical management of stroke. In G. Gillen & A. Burkhardt (Eds.). *Stroke rehabilitation: A function-based approach* (pp. 1–30). St. Louis: Mosby.

Dobkins, B. H. (1996). *Neurologic rehabilitation*. Philadelphia: Davis.

Fisher, M. (1995). *Stroke therapy*. Boston: Butterworth & Heinemann.

Fox, C. M., & Alder, R. N. (1999). Neural mechanisms of aging. In H. Cohen. (Ed.). *Neuroscience for rehabilitation* (2nd ed., pp. 401–418). Philadelphia: Lippincott, Williams & Wilkins.

Francis, K., Bach, J. R., & DeLisa, J. A. (1999). Evaluation and rehabilitation of patients with adult motor neuron disease. *Archives of Physical Medicine and Rehabilitation*, 80(8), 951–963.

Giles, G., & Shore, M. (1989). A rapid method for teaching severe brain injured adults how to wash and dress. *Archives of Physical Medicine and Rehabilitation*, *70*, 156–158.

Gresham, G. E., & Stason, W. B. (1998). Rehabilitation of the stroke survivor. In H. Barnett, J. Mohr, B. Stein, & F. Yatsu (Eds.). *Stroke pathophysiology, diagnosis and management* (pp. 1389–1401). New York: Churchill Livingston.

Hallum, A. (1995). Neuromuscular diseases. In D. A. Umphred (Ed.). *Neurological rehabilitation* (pp. 375–393). St. Louis: Mosby-Year Book.

Held, J. M., & Pay, T. (1999). Recovery of function after brain damage. In H. Cohen.(Ed.). *Neuroscience for rehabilitation* (2nd ed., pp. 419–439). Philadelphia: Lippincott, Williams & Wilkins.

Katz, D. J. (1992). Neuropathology and neurobehavioral recovery from closed head injury. *Journal of Head Trauma Rehabilitation, 7,* 1–15.

Lundy-Elkman, L. (1998). *Neuroscience fundamentals for rehabilitation.* Philadelphia: Saunders.

Macciocchi, S. N., Diamond, P. T., Alves, W. M., & Mertz, T. (1998). Ischemic stroke-relation of age, lesion location and initial neurologic deficit to functional outcomes. *Archives of Physical Medicine and Rehabilitation,79*(10), 1255–1257.

Marion, D. W., & Pryzbylski, G. J. (2000). Injury to the vertebrae and spinal cord. In K. Mattex, D. Feliciano, & E. Moore (Eds.). *Trauma* (pp. 451–472). New York: McGraw-Hill.

Miller, E. (1980).The training characteristics of severely head injured patients: A preliminary study. *Journal of Neurology, Neurosurgery and Psychiatry, 43,* 525–528.

National Institutes of Health Consensus Panel [NIH]. (1999). National Institutes of Health Consensus Panel on rehabilitation of persons with traumatic brain injury. *Journal of American Medicine, 282*(10), 974–983.

Neistadt, M. E. (1994). The neurobiology of learning: Implications for treatment of adults with brain injury. *American Journal of Occupational Therapy, 48,* 421–430.

Pulaski, K. H. (1998). Adult neurological dysfunction. In M. E. Neistadt & E. B. Crepeau (Eds.). *Willard and Spackman's occupational therapy* (9th ed., pp. 660–680). Philadelphia: Lippincott.

Reed, K. L. (2001). *Quick reference to occupational therapy* (2nd ed.). Gathersburg, MD: Aspen.

Schultz-Krohn, W., Foti, D., & Glogoski, C. (2001). Degenerative diseases of the central nervous system. In L. W. Pedretti & M. B. Early. (Eds.). *Occupational therapy practice skills for physical dysfunction* (5th ed., pp. 702–730). St. Louis: Mosby.

South African Medical Association. (2000). Stroke therapy clinical guideline. *South African Medical Journal, 90,* 276–278, 280–289, 292–306.

Spencer, E. (1988). Functional restoration: Neurological, orthopedic, and arthritic conditions. In H. Hopkins & H. Smith (Eds.). *Willard and Spackman's occupational therapy* (pp. 483–502). Philadelphia: Lippincott.

Staas, W. E., Formal, C. S., Freedman, M. K., Fried, G. W., & Read, M. E. (1998). Spinal cord injury. In J. A. DeLisa & B. M. Gans. (Eds.). *Rehabilitation medicine: Principles and practice* (3rd ed., pp. 1259–1291). Philadelphia: Lippincott-Raven.

U.S. Department of Health and Human Services. (1995). *Clinical practice guideline: Post stroke rehabilitation.* Rockville, MD: Agency for Health Care Policy and Research.

University Hospital, Physical Therapy Section. (1988). *Functional significance of spinal cord levels.* Unpublished manuscript, Boston, Massachusetts.

Winkler, P. (1995). Head injury. In D. A. Umphred (Ed.). *Neurological rehabilitation* (pp. 421–453). St. Louis: Mosby-Year Book.

Zejdlik, C. P. (1992). *Management of spinal cord injuries* (2nd ed.). Boston: Jones & Barlett.

CHAPTER 40

OCCUPATIONAL THERAPY: DIAGNOSTIC CONSIDERATIONS IN ADULT AND OLDER ADULT PRACTICE

SECTION I

Adult Orthopedic Dysfunction

CATHY DOLHI

MARY LOU LEIBOLD

JODI SCHREIBER

Consider the following scenario in which an occupational therapist is meeting a client for his first treatment session:

> THERAPIST: *Good morning, Mr. Smith! I'm Mary, your occupational therapist. What would you like to work on today?*
> MR. SMITH: *I want to walk.*
> THERAPIST: *That's physical therapy's job. My job is to help you take care of yourself when you go home.*
> MR. SMITH: *My wife will take care of me. All I want to do is walk.*
> THERAPIST: *Okay. I'll start you on an exercise program right away to build up your arm strength so that you can walk with a walker, or I will have you discontinued from occupational therapy so that you can concentrate on your physical therapy.*

In this situation, the therapist and client have missed an opportunity to identify performance concerns other than walking. The practitioner has also overlooked a chance to help the client promptly resume participating in meaningful occupations. Observe the difference when the therapist responds to the client's desire to walk in the following way:

> MR. SMITH: *I want to walk.*
> THERAPIST: *Great! Where do you want to go and what do you want to do when you get there? What is a typical day like for you?*
> MR. SMITH: *I get up, get showered, dress, and then I walk my dog. When I get back, I make cream of wheat in the microwave and turn on the coffee pot. Next I read the newspaper while I eat and then I run my errands to the grocery store, post office, and pick up the things we need at the pharmacy.*

Look at the difference! By listening to the client and by asking appropriate occupationally centered questions, the occupational therapist has elicited critical information about the client's premorbid routine and habit patterns. In doing so, she has helped him think about the activities that are important to him and consider performance concerns.

These are not uncommon interactions between occupational therapy practitioners and clients who are experiencing orthopedic disorders affecting the back and lower extremities. Since mobility is the most obvious functional deficit in these conditions many occupational therapy practitioners incorrectly assume that their clients require only physical therapy services. Although physical therapists do focus on the remediation of the motor skill deficits and mobility impairments, occupational therapy can make significant contributions to the client's recovery. First, the occupational therapist must help the client identify important areas of occupation and performance deficits that restrict the client's participation. Next, the occupational therapy practitioner collaborates with the client to identify strategies that will facilitate the client's reengagement in meaningful occupations.

Orthopedic conditions involve the bones, joints, and related structures (muscles, tendons, ligaments, and nerves). This section focuses on helping clients who have conditions that affect the lower extremities and back; the next section addresses conditions of the upper extremities. Orthopedic conditions may result from a variety of causes, including trauma, cumulative stress, falls, and degenerative joint disease, or they may be related to congenital or chronic conditions experienced by the individual.

ORTHOPEDIC IMPAIRMENTS AND MOTOR SKILL LIMITATIONS

Occupational therapy practitioners working with clients who have orthopedic impairments and motor limitations must be knowledgeable about these conditions and their effects on occupational performance. These impairments may be directly related to the injury or disorder (e.g., lower extremity amputation secondary to diabetes) or may be imposed on the client during a recovery phase (e.g., hip precautions following a total hip replacement). Limitations or restrictions differ by diagnosis and even among physicians for the same diagnosis. Thus the practitioner must confirm the specific facility and physician protocols.

Three common types of acute-care restrictions encountered by clients who have orthopedic problems in the lower extremities and back are *weight bearing, hip precautions,* and *incision management*. The occupational therapy practitioner must understand the clinical and functional relevance of these restrictions before engaging the client in occupational activities.

Weight Bearing

Individuals who have sustained injuries to the back, pelvis, or lower extremities may be restricted in standing and bearing weight through the legs by the physician. The duration of these restrictions depends on whether the client has had a surgical procedure, the type of fixation device used, and the physician's protocol for managing the condition. Table 40-1 provides descriptions of commonly used weight-bearing restrictions (Goldstein, 1999).

Hip Precautions

Hip precautions are restrictions typically associated with clients who have had a total hip replacement or a hip fracture with a closed reduction. These restrictions are designed to protect the hip joint and avoid further injury, such as dislocation (Lawrence, DiLima, & Evans, 1992; Platt, 1996). Restrictions include, but are not limited to, the avoidance of the following:

- Hip flexion beyond 90°.
- Hip internal rotation and trunk rotation that may result in hip internal rotation.
- Crossing the legs at the ankles or knees.
- Lying or rolling onto the uninvolved side.

Most surgeons permit clients to lie in supine or on the affected side. Lying on the unaffected side is avoided because it promotes internal rotation of the affected hip.

Incision Management

If the client has a surgical incision, the practitioner must help the client manage its care. Keeping the incision clean and dry is critical, and the client should be reminded to dry the area carefully after bathing. Practitioners should check with the physician to determine when the incision is sufficiently healed to permit showering. Nurses typically apply and change dressings, but practitioners should help ensure that clients are compliant with wound care instructions. Practitioners should also help clients identify activities and position changes that may result in strain on the incision site and offer alternatives.

TABLE 40-1. **WEIGHT-BEARING LEVELS FOR THE LOWER EXTREMITIES**[a]

Status	Description
Non-weight bearing (NWB)	• Unable to put any weight on lower extremity(ies) • If restriction involves both extremities, activity is limited to those completed while sitting or in bed • May complete transfers using a sliding board
Touch-down weight bearing (TDWB)	• Majority of weight bearing is through both arms on the ambulation device[a] and the unaffected extremity for functional mobility • Weight bearing on involved extremity is limited to using toes to make contact with floor, primarily to maintain balance
Partial weight bearing (PWB)	• Typically refers to bearing 50% of body weight on involved extremity • Restriction can be measured objectively with commercially available devices but is frequently estimated by client and/or practitioner and requires sustained effort and attention
Weight bearing as tolerated (WBAT)	• Amount of weight put on extremity is left to discretion of client based on level of comfort
Full weight bearing (FWB)	• No restrictions on amount of weight put on the extremity

[a]Physical therapists typically recommend strategies for safe ambulation and prescribe a mobility device to help clients adhere to weight-bearing precautions. Close collaboration between the physical therapy and occupational therapy practitioners is essential so that the client is able to engage in areas of occupation safely and effectively while using the device.

COMMON CONDITIONS AND AREAS OF OCCUPATIONAL THERAPY INTERVENTION

Eight orthopedic conditions that affect the back, pelvis, and lower extremities and that are commonly seen by occupational therapy practitioners are presented in Table 40-2. In most cases, clients experiencing these conditions with no co-morbidities can complete feeding, grooming, or upper body dressing and bathing with only minor assistance. Because of mobility problems, these activities may be accomplished in a different manner than they were premorbidly and may require some setup by another person. For example, a caregiver may need to bring water and toiletries to the client who is long sitting in bed so that upper body bathing may be completed. Similarly, a caregiver can assist the client to transfer out of bed to a wheelchair so that he may get dressed more independently after retrieving his clothes from the closet.

The occupational performance deficits most commonly encountered include those that involve bending, lifting, functional mobility, transfers, and lower body activities of daily living (ADL). Many areas of occupation have the potential to be problematic for clients with these types of conditions and may be overlooked if the client focuses on ambulation as the primary goal. Areas of occupation that should be thoroughly addressed by the practitioner include bed mobility, toileting, lower body bathing and dressing, transfers, home management, care of others or pets, child rearing, community mobility, meal preparation and cleanup, safety procedures and emergency responses, sexual activity, shopping, work or school, play, leisure, and social participation.

Table 40-2 presents a brief description of each condition, an overview of related precautions, targeted intervention strategies, and equipment options associated with each condition. Boxes 40-1 to 40-5 present selected client examples that highlight the concepts presented in the table. Although these cases focus on the orthopedic deficit experienced by the

BOX 40-1 MARITA: A CLIENT WITH A TOTAL HIP REPLACEMENT

Occupational therapy referral: The occupational therapy consult is "status post left total hip replacement as a result of degenerative joint disease."

Occupational profile: Marita is a divorced 63-year-old who resides alone in a two-story home. Premorbidly, she completed all housekeeping independently, including cooking, cleaning, and shopping. She attends weekly group activities at the senior citizens' center and engages in church activities.

Treatment setting: Inpatient rehabilitation hospital.

Disposition setting: Home.

Occupational therapy goals: While observing hip precautions and weight bearing as tolerated, Marita will, in 1 week, be able to:

- Prepare a frozen food entrée in the microwave with minimal assistance while ambulatory using a standard walker and walker basket.
- Independently don and doff shoes and socks using adaptive equipment while seated in an armchair.
- Develop a plan with minimal assistance for securing temporary help from others for obtaining groceries and mail.

BOX 40–2 SOPHIA: A CLIENT WITH A HIP FRACTURE WITH ORIF

Occupational therapy referral: The occupational therapy consult is "status post right hip open reduction with internal fixation (ORIF) because of a hip fracture."
Occupational profile: Sophia is a single 83-year-old who resides in a nursing home. She participates in facility recreation programs. Before her fall, she completed basic ADL with minimal assistance and ambulated within the facility with supervision (no device).
Treatment setting: Long-term care facility.
Disposition setting: Long-term care facility.
Occupational therapy goals: Sophia will, in 1 week, be able to:

- Transfer to and from toilet, bed, and chair with supervision using prescribed ambulatory device.
- Complete lower body dressing and grooming with minimal assistance and using adaptive devices as appropriate while seated in an armchair.
- Independently complete facial and oral care while standing at the sink for 10 min, to build endurance so she can resume a restorative walk-to-dine program.

client, in practice, clients often experience several conditions simultaneously. The therapist must consider the effect of all of those conditions during intervention. For example, a client who experienced a stroke may fall and fracture a hip several years later. In this case, the therapist must be mindful of the residual deficits from the stroke as well as the implications and precautions associated with the hip fracture.

BOX 40–3 JEAN: A CLIENT WITH A KNEE REPLACEMENT

Occupational therapy referral: The occupational therapy consult is "status post right knee replacement."
Occupational profile: Jean is a married 72-year-old who resides with her husband in a retirement community townhouse. She is responsible for light homemaking and laundry and participates in community leisure activities, including bocce ball, Bingo, and the garden club.
Treatment setting: Acute care hospital.
Disposition setting: Home.
Occupational therapy goals: Jean will, in three sessions, be able to:

- Transfer in and out of the family automobile with minimal assistance from her husband.
- Complete toileting with supervision by husband for clothing management.
- Retrieve clothing and dress independently while ambulating with a standard walker.

BOX 40–4 ANTONIO: A CLIENT WITH A LOWER EXTREMITY AMPUTATION

Occupational therapy referral: The occupational therapy consult is "status post right above the knee amputation as a result of a motor vehicle accident." The client is in the preprosthetic training phase.
Occupational profile: Antonio is a married 58-year-old who resides with his wife in a one-story home. He is a self-employed exterminator and the father of three adult sons. Premorbidly, he completed all home management tasks involving the lawn, car, and home maintenance. He played golf weekly and attended movies regularly.
Treatment setting: Acute care hospital.
Disposition setting: Outpatient rehabilitation facility to complete preprosthetic training
Occupational therapy goals: Antonio, in 1 week, will be able to:

- Transfer to the bed and toilet with minimal assistance while using a prescribed ambulatory device.
- Demonstrate understanding of and independently incorporate the desensitization regime to the residual limb during his morning ADL routine.
- Increase bilateral upper extremity strength to good in all major muscle groups so he can safely engage in his ADL routine using the prescribed ambulatory device.

BOX 40–5 JOY: A CLIENT WITH A LOWER EXTREMITY AMPUTATION

Occupational therapy referral: The occupational therapy consult is "status post left below the knee amputation because of diabetes." The client is in the prosthetic training phase.
Occupational profile: Joy is a widowed 78-year-old who lives alone in a third-floor apartment; she receives Meals-on-Wheels. She is a retired high school teacher who enjoys TV game shows and reading the Bible. Her two adult daughters reside out of state.
Treatment setting: Skilled nursing facility (while endurance is low).
Disposition setting: Inpatient rehabilitation center (when she is able to tolerate 3 hr of treatment per day).
Occupational therapy goals: Joy, in 1 week, wearing the prosthesis will be able to:

- Complete her morning grooming activities while standing at the bathroom sink with moderate assistance for maintaining standing balance.
- Complete lower body dressing while seated in an armchair at bedside with moderate assistance using adapted methods.
- Inspect her left lower extremity residual limb with a mirror and correctly identify areas of potential skin breakdown to the therapist with minimal assistance.

TABLE 40–2. **OCCUPATIONAL THERAPY CONSIDERATIONS FOR CLIENTS WITH ORTHOPEDIC CONDITIONS OF THE BACK AND LOWER EXTREMITIES**[a]

Condition	Description	Precautions	Intervention Considerations and Equipment
Hip fracture with closed reduction Total hip replacement or total hip arthroplasty	Break in any portion of femur that can be manipulated into its natural position without major surgery Surgical removal of a diseased or injured hip joint, which is replaced with a prosthetic appliance	Weight bearing established by physician; hip precautions	• Eating, grooming, and upper body dressing typically require assistance from another person for gathering, setting up, and putting away needed supplies; client can then complete tasks either long sitting in bed with over-the-bed table or seated on edge of bed, seated in wheelchair, or seated in armchair at table or sink • Lower body dressing can be accomplished with equipment or adaptations as needed (e.g., reacher, dressing stick, sock aid, long shoehorn, elastic shoelaces, and/or hook-and-loop tape shoe closures); oversize clothing may ease dressing; standing should be encouraged during dressing (client can alternate sitting and standing during activities) • Toileting equipment must enable client to maintain hip precautions; options include standard elevated toilet seat (or model designed for hip injuries) with bilateral arm supports or bedside commode with adjustable legs for use alone or positioned over toilet • Bathing may be completed using transfer tub bench, hand-held shower, nonskid mat, and long-handled sponge; client may choose to sponge bathe at sink or bedside instead • Abduction wedge pillow used to prevent internal rotation of affected hip while in bed or seated • Walker bag or basket and/or wheeled cart may be used to retrieve and transport items safely
Hip fracture with open reduction and internal fixation	Surgical procedure that uses wires, screws, or pins applied directly to fractured bone segments to keep them in place	Weight bearing established by physician	• Clients often do not require strict hip precautions, treatment considerations as described above may be implemented to enhance performance and minimize pain; this may be especially beneficial immediately post surgery, and equipment can be loaned to client
Knee replacement	Implantation of device to substitute for damaged joint surfaces	Weight bearing established by physician	• Typically, active movement of knee is encouraged during *all* activities; client's ability or willingness to flex knee may initially be limited because of fear or pain; twisting motions that put undue stress on joint should be avoided • All ADL and IADL can be completed in a manner selected by client once safety is demonstrated and knee flexion is promoted; completion without use of adaptive equipment is encouraged to promote normal movement; however, it may be used initially in some instances to enhance performance, encourage participation, and minimize pain • Walker bag or basket and/or wheeled cart may be used to retrieve and transport items safely while client uses ambulation device • If needed, equipment may be used on long-term basis for independence

Continues

TABLE 40–2. **OCCUPATIONAL THERAPY CONSIDERATIONS FOR CLIENTS WITH ORTHOPEDIC CONDITIONS OF THE BACK AND LOWER EXTREMITIES**[a] *(Continued)*

Condition	Description	Precautions	Intervention Considerations and Equipment
Vertebral compression fracture (without CNS involvement)	Fracture of vertebral body, often associated with osteoporosis	Rolling in bed restricted to log rolling technique; orthotic device may be used to restrict vertebral mobility (e.g., corset type or rigid body jacket); wearing schedule determined by physician	• Eating, grooming, and upper body dressing typically require assistance from another person for gathering, setting up, and putting away needed supplies; client can then complete tasks either long sitting in bed with over-the-bed table or seated on edge of bed, in wheelchair, or in armchair at table or sink • If orthotic device is worn only when out of bed, the following sequence is recommended: client lies in bed without device; completes upper body bathing while semireclined; dons thin T-shirt or undershirt; resumes supine position, log rolls and dons orthotic device; returns to supine and fastens orthotic device—client is now ready to assume seated position on edge of bed • Lower body dressing can be accomplished with equipment or adaptations as needed (e.g., reacher, dressing stick, sock aid, long shoehorn, elastic shoelaces, and/or hook-and-loop tape shoe closures); oversize clothing may help accommodate orthotic device • Standing should be encouraged during dressing; client can alternate sitting and standing during activities • Use of elevated toilet seat and bilateral arm supports for toileting may enhance performance by increasing safety, decreasing anxiety, and increasing confidence • Bathing restricted to long sitting in bed without brace or sitting in chair with orthotic device in place • Walker bag or basket and/or wheeled cart may be used to retrieve and transport items safely
Pelvic fracture	Break in any part of pelvic ring or acetabulum	Hip flexion limited to 60°; non-weight bearing for both lower extremities	• Eating, grooming, and upper body dressing typically require assistance from another person for gathering, setting up, and putting away needed supplies; client can then complete tasks long sitting in bed with bed inclined to 60° to adhere to precautions • Lower body dressing and bathing can be accomplished long sitting in bed with bed inclined to 60° and with equipment and adaptations as needed (e.g., reacher, dressing stick, sock aid, long shoehorn, elastic shoelaces, hook and loop tape shoe closures, and/or long-handled sponge); client typically requires assistance with lower extremity dressing and bathing in conjunction with long-handled equipment • Toileting is managed either in bed with bedpan or using bedside commode with drop arms and backrest that allows client to maintain hip flexion at 60° • Bed mobility may be enhanced by use of trapeze bar placed on hospital bed • Reclining wheelchair is necessary for mobility to adhere to precautions; choice of proper wheelchair cushion is necessary to maintain skin integrity due to non-weight-bearing status • Completing functional transfers usually requires another person to assist with lower extremities during transfer; sliding board may also be necessary to secure safe, confident transfers

TABLE 40–2. **OCCUPATIONAL THERAPY CONSIDERATIONS FOR CLIENTS WITH ORTHOPEDIC CONDITIONS OF THE BACK AND LOWER EXTREMITIES**[a] *(Continued)*

Condition	Description	Precautions	Intervention Considerations and Equipment
Lower extremity amputation: preprosthetic training phase	Loss of any part of legs or feet (before artificial limb replacement)	Balance precautions owing to change in center of gravity; fall risk owing to phantom limb sensation and balance deficits	• Addition of antitipper bars and/or counterbalancing to wheelchair to avoid tipping should be considered to accommodate for change in center of gravity • All ADL and IADL can be completed in a manner selected by client once safety is demonstrated; client completes tasks either from wheelchair or ambulatory level, depending on variety of factors (e.g., medical condition, balance, activity tolerance, cognition, and environmental accessibility) • Use of elevated toilet seat and bilateral arm supports for toileting may enhance performance by increasing safety, decreasing anxiety, and increasing confidence • Bathing may be completed with use of tub transfer bench, tub seat, or sponge bathing
Lower extremity amputation: prosthetic training phase	Period in which client learns to use lower extremity prosthesis	Preprosthetic precautions as applicable; maintenance of skin integrity, especially during prosthetic use	• All ADL and IADL can be completed in a manner selected by client once safety is demonstrated; client completes task either from wheelchair or ambulatory level, depending on variety of factors (e.g., medical condition, balance, activity tolerance, cognition, and environmental accessibility) • The following dressing procedures are recommended: client with one prosthesis sits on edge of the bed or in armchair, dresses prosthesis first, then dons device and dresses other leg; client with bilateral prostheses sits in armchair or in bed, dresses both prosthetic devices, and then dons them; socks and shoes on prosthesis should be inspected, cleaned, and changed as needed • Use of elevated toilet seat and bilateral arm supports for toileting may enhance performance by increasing safety, decreasing anxiety, and increasing confidence • Bathing may be completed with use of tub transfer bench, tub seat, or sponge bathing; cleaning of prosthesis is done on regular basis as instructed by prosthetist; residual limb should be kept dry to maintain skin integrity and avoid skin breakdown; client's bathing schedule should be arranged to allow a maximum amount of time so residual limb and prosthesis may dry thoroughly

[a]Data from Bear-Lehman (2002); Goldstein (1999); Jacobs (1999); Lawrence et al. (1992); Nicholas (1996); Petty (1991); Platt, (1996); Rockwood, Green, Bucholz, and Heckman (1996); Venes (2001); and the authors' clinical experience.

In addition to orthopedic precautions, practitioners can expect clients to experience pain, which may vary daily. Practitioners must respect the client's pain and caution against engaging in movements or activities that intensify it. At the same time, clients should be encouraged not to unduly limit participation in activities because of anticipation of pain and fear of injury. By helping the client identify and overcome any cause of participation limitations, practitioners may expedite recovery.

Phantom pain is a condition unique to clients who have had an amputation. Therapists should reassure clients who describe pain in the amputated limb that it is not an outlandish perception and that many individuals with amputations experience similar symptoms. Clients should be encouraged to try a variety of techniques for pain management, which may include physical agent modalities, relaxation exercises, guided imagery, massage, and repositioning.

CONCLUSION

As in all of occupational therapy practice, each case is unique and intervention must be tailored specifically to the client and his or her specific health condition. In addition, physicians manage cases differently in regard to weight bearing, activity level and the use of precautions; therefore, practitioners should consult with individual physicians in each case.

SECTION II

Upper Extremity Musculoskeletal Impairments

ELINOR ANNE SPENCER

This section presents a brief introduction to musculoskeletal impairments of the upper extremities experienced by adults who are referred for occupational therapy intervention.

TYPICAL EFFECTS OF UPPER EXTREMITY INJURIES

Trauma and disease of the musculoskeletal system ranges from sudden, acute, and catastrophic injuries to gradual changes in function owing to impairments of joints, nerves, and connective tissue. Secondary effects such as muscle contractures or atrophy, limitations in joint mobility, deformity in alignment, weakness, sensory dysfunction, and chronic pain can occur (Goldstein, 1999).

Performance Areas

Because the use of the arms and hands is critical to many of the activities humans perform, upper extremity dysfunction can result in limitation or loss of independence in all performance areas. This loss affects self-esteem and motivation and may impose changes in family roles. An adult may need to adjust to accepting assistance with personal tasks from a child, family member, or stranger. Dependence on others may extend to household tasks, driving, shopping, care giving, and other significant duties. Upper extremity dysfunction can also lead to disruption of work and social participation. These disruptions can tax the psychological coping skills of the injured worker and others around him or her. The family may or may not be capable of adjusting to the daily effects of disability on the client. Loss of work time and the possible need for vocational redirection also have economic implications.

Upper extremity dysfunction can limit leisure activities, resulting in loss of ability to engage in previously enjoyed activities. Time away from work may not transfer to enjoyment in forced or extended leisure time. Choices of activity now depend on the nature of the disability and adaptive options available. The work and leisure activity balance is affected. Changes in the daily pattern become necessary. Exploration of methods to provide motivation and satisfying activity for recuperation becomes important (Cooper, 2002).

Impairments

Sensory and neuromusculoskeletal functions and structures are the primary factors affected by injury or illnesses of the upper extremity. These can lead to a variety of deficits in skills and performance areas, which in turn can adversely impinge on mental health. For instance, laceration, penetration, or compression of tissue can cause discontinuity of nerve pathways, resulting in temporary or permanent change in sensory awareness and sensory functions. The loss of pain and touch sensations is a safety hazard; without this sensory feedback clients may burn or scrape themselves without knowing it. Persistent pain contributes to fear and reluctance to move the extremity or part, hindering return of mobilization and function. There may be specific deficits in tactile discrimination, localization, and stereognosis that affect the motor functions of grasp, release, coordination, and reach.

Disruption of nerve pathways interferes with the nervous system's control of movement. Impairments in range of motion (ROM), strength, and endurance result from a disruption of essential neuromuscular integration processes. This loss of neuromuscular integration also hinders postural control, body alignment, and motor control of isolated muscles and joint movements. The person with an injured extremity may lack motor power for gross and fine coordination tasks that require strength or manipulation of resistive materials. Limitations may affect bilateral capabilities by necessitating compensatory strength and coordination from the unaffected extremity (Cooper, 2002; Praemer, 1992).

The psychological effect of disease or injury on the client will vary. In some situations, long-term functional potentials may not initially be recognized or accepted by the client and family, because of feelings of confusion, fear, insecurity, anger, inadequacy, and disequilibrium. These clients and families see the illness or injury changing previous levels of life adjustment and activity to unfamiliar, unknown, and unacceptable conditions or situations. Other clients and families are able to recognize potential functional gain and work toward recuperation and positive outcomes.

Injury and disease interfere with the developmental process. Age, gender, education, work experience, lifestyle, and family involvements affect the client's attitude toward dysfunction. The adolescent or adult who has experienced life as an able-bodied person, with few or no physical limitations, may meet sudden debilitating trauma with shock, disbelief, anger, and denial. Perceptions of illness and disability vary within cultures and socioeconomic groups. As in all occupational therapy interventions, programming provided to the client must be geared toward the individual's personal and social context to be acceptable and appropriate to his or her particular motivations, interest, abilities, and goals.

EVALUATION FOR PEOPLE WITH UPPER EXTREMITY INJURIES

Evaluation procedures must be understood and tolerated by the client to ensure participation in the occupational therapy program. The more the client understands and becomes involved in the procedures, the better the rapport between therapist and client and the more complete the progress. Evaluation methods include interview, standardized assessments and situational testing such as observation of task performance. The evaluation provides objective feedback to the client on his or her present functional levels and encourages a discussion of treatment priorities and potentials. Unit VII includes information on specific evaluation methods.

Performance Areas

Assessment of performance of both basic ADL and instrumental activities of daily living (IADL) identifies self-care potentials, the need and potential for use of adaptive methods and assistive devices, the level of dependence in self-care and daily activity responsibilities, and the pretrauma daily activity pattern. Methods of assessment may include checklists for self-evaluation, interviews with the client concerning the home environment, observation of ADL functions, and discussion of feasible alternatives to present task approaches.

Assessments of work include discussion of the daily work context and schedule, work demands and pretrauma performance capabilities, imposed changes in daily routine relative to family relationships and responsibilities, options for temporary adjustment in work patterns, and alternative work readiness options for those who may not be able to return to their previous employment. Interviews with the client elicit general occupational history; the effect of the injury or condition on daily work activity; the financial burden; and the client's expectations, needs, and priorities. Performance tests indicate work readiness, endurance, and functional capacity related to job requirements. Evaluation of safety and the client's awareness of precautions and limitations are important aspects of assessing the client's ability to perform work activities as well as home tasks, child care, and general daily activities.

Early in the intervention process, therapists should also identify leisure activities that the client habitually engages in for individual enjoyment and social interaction. Checklists or the development of an activity schedule of the client's daily or weekly pattern can be helpful when planning home programs to gain functional ability through these types of activities during recuperation and time off from work.

Impairments

Evaluation of client factors begins with assessment of the client's sensory awareness of the extremity, positioning of the extremity at rest and with movement, functional ability, and subjective feelings regarding the injured extremity. Visual attention to and verbal discussion of the extremity may be diminished owing to limitations in sensation or hypersensitivity to the injury or disability. Specific levels of sensory disturbances in tactile localization, static and moving stimulus perception, one- and two-point discrimination, sensory discrimination, and stereognosis are determined. The cause, location, and extent of pain are also evaluated to learn precautions and limitations.

Assessments of neuromusculoskeletal factors and functions include tests of ROM of both upper extremities, strength of both upper extremities, endurance in general movement and activity, pain, postural control and alignment, and the effect of the injury on the soft tissue. During assessments, the therapist should ensure that, as much as possible, the extremity is positioned in the optimum alignment and in a pain-free position.

Assessments of motor skills include standardized tests for gross and fine motor movements and observation of these movements in ADL and in work or leisure activities. Performance is assessed against normative data, when available, as well as against the noninjured extremity, which can serve as a guide for normal function of the individual. Bilateral limitations are also evaluated, with particular attention to the hand dominance of the client.

Assessment of psychological aspects begins with developing rapport with the client and identifying the client's behavior and feelings about the injury. Feelings might include anxiety, impatience, anger, fatigue, distractibility, or sadness. Personal concepts of functional and cosmetic damage can positively or negatively affect the client's motivation for recuperation. Personal contextual variables must also be considered. The client's interpretation of the injury may be influenced by his or her cultural and social background. In addition, the client's developmental experiences influence attitudes toward injury and illness and the ability to cope with adverse conditions. It is essential that adult clients be recognized as having a developmental history. Disability brings dependence, which is often a difficult reminder of the dependency of childhood. The dependent adult must be treated as an adult in all aspects of therapeutic intervention. Collaborating in setting treatment objectives based on evaluation results enables the adult client to take an adult role. During the evaluation process, practitioners must maintain flexible and open attitudes for meeting the variety of cultural variables that are found in individual clients and families. Changes from the premorbid pattern of behavior are noted as early as possible.

INTERVENTION FOR PEOPLE WITH UPPER EXTREMITY INJURIES

Functional restoration is the primary objective of rehabilitation. Assisting a person to build or restore his or her life to its fullest use and satisfaction is a philosophical mandate of occupational therapy. Therapeutic intervention can reverse disability, improve ability, and prevent further disability.

Performance Areas

The client learns to minimize the disruption of established routines of self-sufficiency by setting priorities for basic ADL functions and problem solving. Examples of common priorities are the following:

- Application and removal of splints and prostheses.
- Performing tasks with adaptive devices.
- Developing adaptive techniques for temporary use.
- Working toward maximal functional independence.
- Understanding precautions relevant to deficits.
- Using therapy techniques at home in between therapy visits.

Intervention programs related to IADL and work include training in such areas as:

- Adaptive techniques for homemaking and other daily activities.
- Energy conservation and work simplification procedures.
- Use of adaptive equipment to improve skill levels.
- Increasing work capacity and endurance.
- Use of long-term splints and prostheses.

In addition, occupational therapy practitioners provide assistance in helping the client to explore alternative work options when the nature of the injury necessitates job changes.

Leisure activities are used to foster positive involvement, enjoyment, and family and community participation. The client may discover new economic benefits from recreational interests.

Impairments

Treatment of sensory deficits includes the following goals:

- Reduction of and adaptation to pain.
- Training in sensory awareness and discrimination.
- Desensitization.

- Sensory stimulation.
- Facilitation of body image adjustment and acceptance.
- Training regarding the safety hazards of decreased sensation.
- Facilitation of positive social interaction.

Treatment of neuromusculoskeletal impairments focuses on several areas:

- Passive and active ROM.
- Movement and function in activities to encourage extremity control and trunk alignment.
- Activities to improve general endurance.
- Methods to adjust to pain and limitations.
- Strengthening of affected areas and extremities.
- Involvement in overall body movement.

Interventions to improve motor skills include motor exercises and activities, use of activities requiring bilateral functions of extremities, and involvement in task performance to develop gross and fine motor coordination and dexterity. The occupational therapist must make every effort to involve the client in planning and executing appropriate progressive exercises and activities both in the clinic and at home.

The psychological aspect of the treatment program involves client education about current limitations and treatment objectives as well as likely limitations on active participation and the benefits of adaptations. Practitioners also address psychological issues by collaborating with clients to determine treatment priorities, focusing treatment on the client's goals.

Successful intervention also helps clients regain pretrauma skills, develop newly needed skills, and accept functional limitations for a temporary or permanent period. Changes in activity competency or method require adjustment and adaptation. Participation in a functional activity program individually and with others contributes to this adjustment and helps clients view themselves as valuable functioning members of adult society.

Before the injury, the person may have been a high-functioning member of a family and neighborhood, known to have certain interests, skills, and roles within a unique culture. Following injury, disability, and recuperation, the person must be equipped to reenter that familiar community and lifestyle, perhaps with a brace, a splint, prosthesis, assistive device, or significant scar. The client will then need to educate the community about his or her personal challenges, limitations, and potentials.

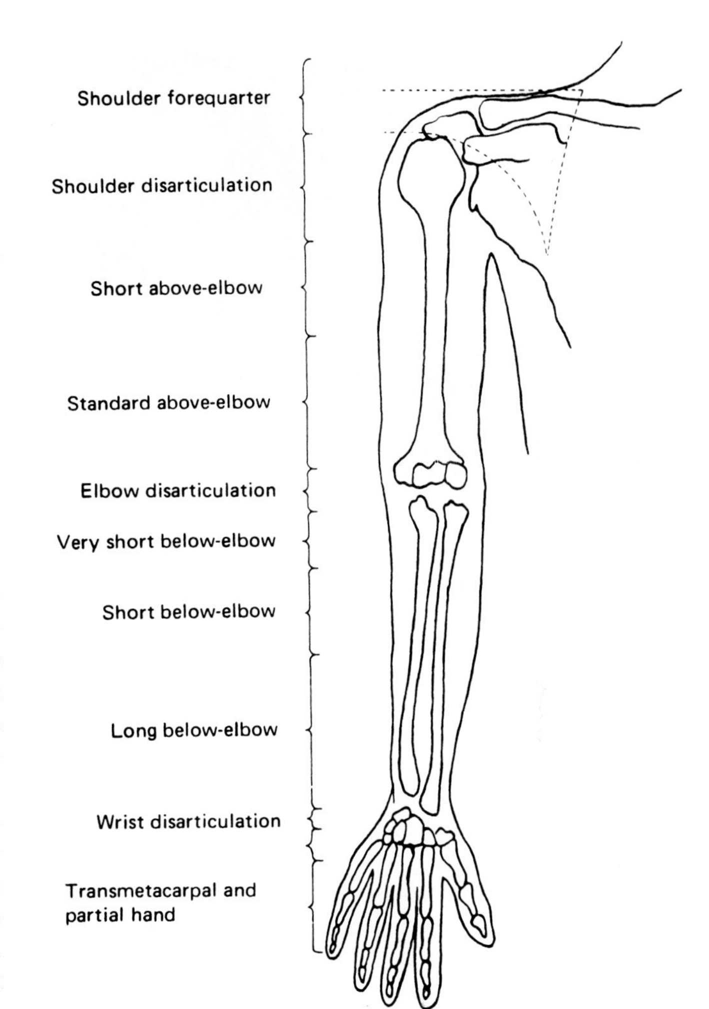

FIGURE 40–1. Amputation levels of the upper extremity.

UPPER EXTREMITY AMPUTATION

To have an amputation is to be without a limb or part because of congenital anomaly, injury, or disease. Common causes of amputation in the upper extremities are external trauma, prolonged infection, severe neuromuscular impairment, and tumors. Typical signs and symptoms include loss or impairment of bone, neurovascular tissue, muscle tissue, functions of the extremity, distal sensations, and cosmesis. The higher the level of the amputation, the greater these losses will be (Fig. 40-1). In many cases, a **prosthesis** or artificial limb is recommended to help substitute for some of the lost functions.

Early fitting of a prosthesis hastens psychological adjustment, reduces pain and edema, and can facilitate tissue and psychological healing by introducing an adaptive response to the patient and his or her family. Early fitting also limits phantom limb sensations by early prosthetic contact and function. The prosthesis is prescribed by the medical team and fabricated by a certified prosthesis. The occupational therapist performs a check of the fit and function and educates the client in the wear, operation, precautions, and functions of the prosthesis in daily activity.

Performance Areas

Independent functions in basic ADL are affected by partial or complete lack of hand and perhaps arm function and the

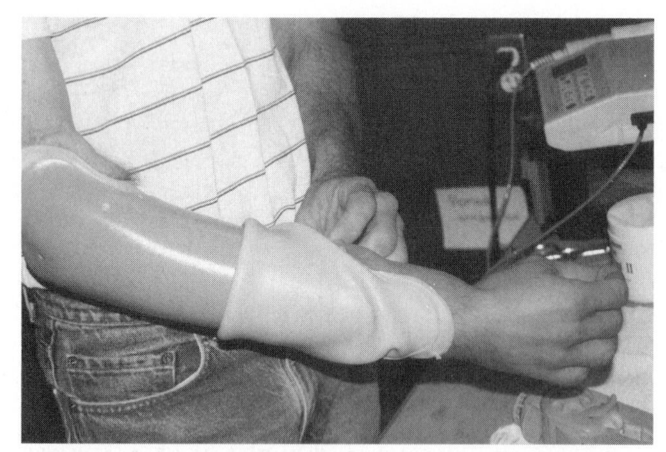

FIGURE 40–2. Clients must learn to put on and take off the prosthesis. Some clients own two terminal devices: One that is more cosmetically attractive for social occasions and another that is hardier for work. (Courtesy of Barbara Schell, Gainesville Hand Clinic, Gainesville, GA.)

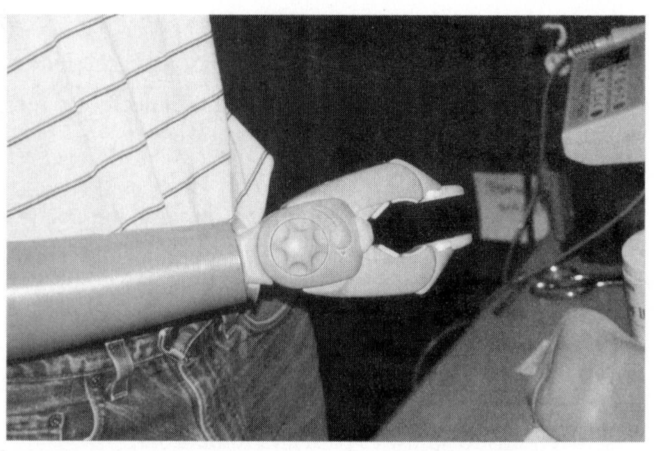

FIGURE 40–3. Clients must learn to control the terminal device for appropriate tension during grasp and release. (Courtesy of Barbara Schell, Gainesville Hand Clinic, Gainesville, GA.)

loss of bilateral functions. The client must also contend with the effects of the amputation on body image, cosmesis, personal care, and functional lifestyle. The client must adjust to the care of the residual limb and the prosthesis, as well as to the appearance and use of the prosthesis in the environment (Fig. 40-2). Assistive devices enhance early preprosthetic use of the residual limb in bathing and hygiene as well as other self-care tasks. Use of the extremity enhances integration of the limb and prosthesis into the body image for independent daily activity.

The loss or change in upper extremity unilateral and bilateral functions and related changes in postural control affect performance in IADL and work performance. These changes, in turn, result in loss in work time and, typically, in changes in the daily activity routine, job capability, and future planning. To respond to these limitations, interventions focus on helping the person learn preprosthetic and prosthetic use of the affected area in coordination and grasping activities (Fig. 40-3).

A return to work assessment assists clients in recognizing their capabilities as related to the feasibility of either a safe return to their former occupation or undertaking a vocational redirection. Specific tasks, such as safe and efficient tool, equipment, and material handling, are used to determine work-related skills (Fig. 40-4). Assessment of attitudes, aptitudes, work habits, work tolerance, and skills using standardized tests and work-simulated tasks are included, as well as observation of household tasks, driving, and child care. Chapter 24 includes information on assessing work skills and related performance areas.

Participation in previously enjoyed individual and social leisure activities may require adapted equipment or techniques. Resumption of these activities during treatment assists in general body conditioning, integration of the prosthesis into the client's lifestyle, and the development of a positive image. Hobbies and sports activities provide motivation and social interaction, while promoting coordination and strength development.

Impairments

Amputation results in pathological changes in body image and awareness. Sudden trauma results in localized pain from the injury or surgery. Because sensory representation of the limb remains in the brain after the limb has been removed, sensation of the missing part (phantom sensation) can be triggered or reinforced by sensory input from elsewhere in the body (Celikyol, 2002; Cummings, Alexander, & Gans, 1984). The client may experience painful sensations (phantom pain), such as tingling, gripping, clenching, burning, or cramping. Pain can also result from edema, infection, or neuroma in or around the amputation site. Postsurgical scar tissue, fragile skin areas, and bony prominences can hinder

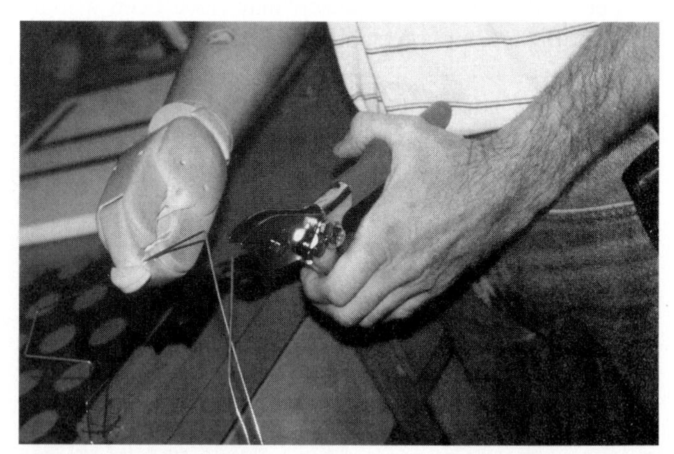

FIGURE 40–4. The client practices a two-handed activity that is similar to one that he is required to do at work. (Courtesy of Barbara Schell, Gainesville Hand Clinic, Gainesville, GA.)

sensory tolerance of socket contact and the prosthetic control system. The therapist teaches clients to monitor the skin on the stump to prevent secondary sensory deficits caused by pressure from ill-fitting prostheses.

Loss of neuromusculoskeletal tissue results in limitations in passive and active ROM relative to the site and type of amputation, strength of the extremity, general functional endurance, and postural alignment. After the amputation, changes in weight, sensation, and use of the missing part cause a shift in the client's center of gravity. Atrophy of the musculature on the side of the amputation, scoliosis, and compensatory curves may occur if the client does not engage in appropriate overall body exercise in both isolated and integrated movement patterns.

With loss of body tissue, there is loss of sensory, motor, and coordination functions in both the directly affected and surrounding tissue of the limb. The higher the amputation, the more the client must depend on the prosthesis for replacement of bodily function. The shorter the stump, the greater the coverage of the stump socket, which adds weight, limits proximal joint functions, and limits sensory contact of the extremity. Before the client receives a prosthesis, he or she must develop strength and tolerance in the stump for prosthetic operations. The training goals are preventing faulty body mechanics, developing sufficient ROM and strength for prosthetic operation, and maintaining optimum body alignment. Motor control of the prosthesis involves learning the control motions for the hook or the hand (terminal device) for grasp and release combined with reach.

The cognitive challenge of accepting and functioning with a changed physical body requires productive sensory and motor activity with and without the prosthesis. To be functionally useful, the prosthesis must be integrated into the functional body schema and become a viable part of the client's functional perspective. If the trauma was caused by an electrical accident or crush injury, the client may show signs of cognitive dysfunction, The occupational therapist assists the client in understanding and accepting the functions and limitations of the prosthesis.

Becoming familiar with the prime psychological concerns of the client is an essential part of the initial contact. The client may express guilt, shame, depression, anger, or impatience about the amputation. The client may have lost a dominant hand. It is essential for the practitioner to provide opportunities for working through emotional and physical adjustment via activity, individually and in groups. Involvement of family members in the training program can be beneficial. Participation of the client in the choice of the prosthesis is also important; each client puts a different value and stress on the functional (hook, gripper) versus cosmetic (prosthetic hand) aspects of a prosthesis.

Adjustment to potential changes in ability and performance is affected by premorbid developmental factors. A child born with a congenital anomaly usually develops body functions and a body image incorporating that anomaly during the growth process. The adult, having passed this developmental period in physical performance, suffers the traumatic amputation as a loss that disrupts both the body image and the integration of previously developed and habituated functions and skills. The prosthesis is an addition to the natural developmental process and must be incorporated into a meaningful relationship with the body to become an acceptable functional part of it. People with either traumatic or congenital amputations must adapt to the mechanical or electronic replacement of natural functions.

Adjustment to prosthetic wear and use can be enhanced or hindered by cultural views and expectations. When preparing clients for prosthetic wear, therapists begin with orienting clients to the functional and cosmetic options of prostheses relative to their needs and expectations. The need for and potential value of the prosthetic replacement depend partly on each client's limitations as a result of the amputation, his or her avocational and vocational needs and interests, and personal attitude toward prosthetic potential. The latter begins with the client's attitude toward the loss of the limb, the meaning of the loss, and the perspectives and influence of family and friends. The priorities of the client's personal habits, home life, work, hobbies, social life, and aspirations affect the choice of prosthetic components and the success of prosthetic wear and operation.

ARTHRITIS

Arthritis is a common chronic condition of the joints that results in pain, loss of motion, deformity, and associated functional deficits. Arthritis is caused by joint disease or direct trauma to bone and soft tissue. *Rheumatoid arthritis* (RA) is a progressive systemic disease characterized by remissions and exacerbations of destructive inflammation of connective tissue, particularly synovial membranes in synovial joints. RA results in limitations in ROM and causes deformity. Connective tissue changes may cause sensory impairments in the hands and feet. The disease can occur at any age and is manifested by swollen, reddened, and painful joints during and after excessive use. Rheumatoid arthritis affects the client's functional ability, physical appearance, and mental and physical tolerance (Kelley, 1993; Springhouse Corporation [Springhouse], 1995).

Osteoarthritis (OA), or degenerative joint disease (DJD), is a slowly progressive joint disease that commonly affects the joints of the fingers, elbows, hips, knees, and ankles. OA is characterized by degeneration of the articular cartilage and swelling in the joints. It generally accompanies the aging process, affecting the weight-bearing joints. It is also experienced by people who have been active in sports and by those whose jobs have caused strain in their fingers and legs. Traumatic injury to bone or joints may result in chronic intermittent joint pain exacerbated by heavy use of the extremity or changes in temperature or humidity (Maher, 1993; Springhouse, 1995).

Performance Areas

The person with arthritis pain and deformity develops difficulties in basic ADL owing to changes in sensation, ROM, and strength in the upper and lower extremities and trunk. Decreased comfort, speed of movement, and endurance in daily task completion result in physical dependence and loss of self-esteem. Adaptations are available to simplify physical challenges, decrease pain in grip, and extend grip and reach. For example, a college student with arthritis can continue to write in school by using custom-made hand, wrist, or finger splints and large rough or rubber-textured pencils and pens for easy traction grip, even with hand deformities and pain. Client education and practice in activity analysis, work simplification, and energy conservation aid the client in daily pacing of tasks to prolong activity.

The problems of arthritis affect the IADL and work activities of the client by limiting the timely independent accomplishment of specific job tasks and responsibilities, often requiring job sharing, if available, in the home or in the workplace. Certain tasks may exacerbate the painful condition by requiring repetitive motions or prolonged resistive force of movement without rest. With decreases in sensitivity, grip strength, and ROM, tolerance for the physical forces in tool and material handling is lowered, rendering the person vulnerable to further joint damage and inability to meet work demands. Change in work capability may lead to wage loss.

A change in leisure activities may result from decreased facility in activities requiring strength and coordination, along with the social loss from decreased participation in activities with family and friends. This can affect self-esteem, relaxation, and general enjoyment. Change of position or methods of performing activities of interest can facilitate continued participation. The balance of work, play, rest, and leisure is vitally important within the daily activity pattern, particularly when disability interferes with past or future independent activity.

Impairments

A major problem for individuals with arthritis is intermittent or chronic pain, which can temporarily or permanently limit physical functions needed for task accomplishment. Perception and tolerance of pain vary with individuals. When joint inflammation is active, the client may complain of severe pain, and there may be visible inflammation of the joints. During this time, joint protection is essential. Restricting mobility during inflammation promotes function after this period. Improper use of joints and lack of attention to therapeutic positioning of the body can cause or increase pain. Denial, frustration, or tension may result in improper use of joints, which puts undue stress on them. When there is a reduction of swelling and inflammation, rehabilitation procedures can begin. In addition to pain, people with arthritis, especially RA, may have decreased sensory perception in the hands and feet. Numbness, tingling, or decreased coordination in object handling may indicate the possibility of sensory deficits.

Neuromusculoskeletal deficits in arthritis include limitations or loss in ROM, strength, and endurance, leading to abnormal postural alignment and joint deformities. Misalignment or deformities in positions of hyperflexion, hyperextension, abduction, adduction, and ulnar deviation may be present. Improper fit of wheelchairs and crutches, walkers, splints, and other tools and utensils exacerbates misalignment of joints and overuse of muscles in resistive activity. Deformities may prevent functional use of muscles. Functional hand splints can assist in alignment of muscles, tendons, and bones. Activities requiring strength are used carefully in the therapeutic program; too much resistance can cause joint pain and fatigue. In the presence of subluxation or dislocation, it is important to avoid overactivity of the affected joints and excessive resistive exercise and activity of the muscles controlling these joints. Passive and active joint ROM can prevent muscle atrophy (Sobel & Klein, 1995).

Motor skill limitations are often observed in gross and fine motor coordination, awkward dexterity, decreased movements in hands and arms, decreased speed of movement, and limitations in task completion and endurance. Functional problems may be caused by internal joint damage, fear of pain, actual pain, decreased strength and sensation, and deformity. When presenting functional challenges, the practitioner must remain alert for signs of mental, psychological, and physical fatigue, as well as the client's subjective responses to the intervention process. The most effective way to prevent deformity is to incorporate therapeutic positioning and movement into ADL. Clients need education in the following:

- Joint protection.
- Use of adaptive equipment.
- Conservation of energy.
- Therapeutic use of joints through balance of activity and rest.
- Pacing of daily activities and exercises.

Assistive devices should be used only to increase function or to protect impaired joints. They should be lightweight, comfortable, and simple to use. If the client cannot use or accept the device easily, he or she will soon discard it. Splinting may be used with arthritis to provide support to diseased joints, alleviate pain, prevent deformity, maintain and promote function, and establish functional alignment of bones.

Psychological adjustment to progressive disability and augmentation of natural ability with splints and assistive devices challenge both the individual and his or her family. Because the disease is progressive, the client experiences a gradual decrease in functional ease and capacity owing to decreasing strength, mobility, coordination, and pain-free movement. Because of pain and instability, some clients with arthritis fear further damage to the joints; therefore, they avoid using them. On the other hand, other clients deny the disability and avoid preventive precautions, causing joint destruction and deformity.

Intervention must be geared toward assisting clients to combat the debilitating effects of the disease and to maintain maximal independent functions. Occupational therapy practitioners aid clients in developing a self-directed program of joint protection and function that can continue at home. Alternating the degree of physical and mental stress in a daily plan of scheduled activities enables clients to engage in work and rest activities, gross and fine motor functions, and in sitting and standing positions. Daily plans similar to these help adults maintain activity tolerance, and realistic productivity according to their needs, desires, and abilities (Fries, 1999).

Developmentally progressive limitations in independent functions in self-care, work, and play activities hinder the self-esteem of young and older adults. Arthritis may cause lifestyle changes.

The social and cultural contexts of the client's home environment and general routine influence his or her willingness to adapt to change. For example, concern about appearance may keep a client from accepting home adaptations, such as entrance ramps. Perceptions of illness and disability may vary between the client and family; each may have different ideas about how much assistance is needed. The family may err in giving too much assistance to the client, building dependence, and depriving the client of the needed exercise of independent daily choices of functions through exercise and activities.

HAND INJURIES

The degree of dysfunction related to a hand injury depends on the type of trauma, location of trauma, and the extent of the injury. Direct trauma may result in sprains, strains, fractures, and dislocations of bone. Repeated trauma may result in inflammation of muscles, tendons, or nerves. Severe lacerations and bone injuries may result in structural and functional damage to skin, nerves, muscles, tendons, and other soft tissue. The course of the injury may be limited to the immediate and residual effects of direct trauma, or it may result in progressive symptoms of dysfunction from cumulative trauma related to occupational illness or injury (Pascarelli, 1994).

A common environment for hand injuries is in the workplace where injuries occur from overexertion of the body, blows from an object, or a fall. Tools, machinery, or tasks in the home, as well as during sports activities also may cause hand injuries. Typical signs and symptoms of hand injury include these:

- Disruption of skin integrity.
- Localized pain.
- Decreased ROM.
- Possible sensory loss.
- Decreased functional use.

Hand injury is typically followed by a period of immobilization or limited use of the extremity. The client may experience fear and denial of the functional prognosis.

Performance Areas

As with other upper extremity impairments, injury to the hand affects independence in most performance areas because of the following:

- Temporary or permanent disruption of hand dominance (if that is the affected hand).
- Dependence in bimanual hand use.
- Presence of splints or other devices to promote healing.
- Decreased comfort, function, and endurance in task performance.

Individuals injured at work may be excused from work with compensatory financial assistance; but if disability from the injury is permanent, the client may be unable to return to the former job. The financial loss for both the client and the family can be significant. Loss of ability to participate in leisure activities occurs with forced change in physical functions. The client may experience imposed leisure time without the ability to perform activities habitually enjoyed. If participation in effective individual and social leisure activity is not available, the client's psychological health may suffer.

Impairments

Impairments in sensory functions of the hand include changes in overall sensory awareness of the body part, changes in sensation, and increases in pain levels. Changes in sensory functions can significantly affect the neuromuscular functions of movement and coordination (Cailliet, 1994). Chapter 25, Section 1 includes information about how to conduct assessments related to sensation. Because pain is a subjective response, the therapist evaluates the presence of pain through the client's ability to tolerate palpation, movement, force, and object manipulation. Edema and swelling affect the sensory response of the client because the edema chemically irritates and compresses nerve endings. A volumeter is commonly used to measure changes in hand mass caused by edema in comparison to the uninjured hand. Circumference measurements are also obtained by using a tape measure or calipers. After identification of sensory deficits, the occupational therapist works out a functional program to limit pain, increase the client's pain tolerance and increase sensory awareness (see Chapter 30, Section 1).

Impairments in neuromuscular functions include effects of sensory and motor disturbances on postural alignment and control, limitation or loss in ROM, limitation in extremity strength and endurance, and development of positive or negative compensatory positions. Neuromuscular functions are generally limited by restrictions of surgery, pain, and the client's fear of moving the hand or arm.

Static splints are used to position the hand or arm in optimum alignment for tissue healing and to prepare the client for passive and active programs. The physician may also prescribe them for therapeutic exercise after the casting and healing periods. Ideally, splints should be put on and removed by the client, according to the therapist's instructions. Dynamic or functional splinting allows and encourages joint movement against progressive resistance and may be used in light and graded activities. A splint can help or hinder motion or function. It must be augmented by exercise and activity, as medically and functionally appropriate (Boscheinen-Morrin, Davey, & Conolly, 1995). Chapter 31, Section 3 provides information on using splints.

Motor skills limitations affect gross motor and fine motor coordination, limitations in dexterity, decreased functional ability in the extremity, limitation in endurance and strength, and dependence on adaptive functioning and assists.

Psychological issues that must be addressed when dealing with individuals with hand injuries include the following:

- Emotional response to trauma.
- Ability to adapt to restrictions in function.
- Adjustment to the disability and prognosis.
- Changes in relationship to family roles.
- Concerns regarding work expectations and potentials.

Attention to the priorities of the client is crucial in developing the intervention program and assisting the client to accept long-term limitations of cosmesis and function, if necessary. Assistance in vocational redirection, referral to other needed health personnel, and therapeutic involvement in work-simulated tasks, as appropriate, allow the client to progress with a positive outlook.

In the developmental continuum, hand injuries most often occur to the working-age male or female from direct or cumulative trauma. The effect of a hand injury on the daily lifestyle and future planning of the client varies with the seriousness of the injury. The working adult who has lost economic security at the beginning or prime of occupational accomplishment and advancement may or may not have the tolerance, interest, or ingenuity to redirect either work or other important life activities. Once again, these responses are mediated by cultural and personal perceptions of illness and disability. The family's attitudes and behaviors also positively or negatively influence the client's progress. It is important to consider the treatment program of the client within the context of his or her lifestyle to ensure maximum participation.

HISTORICAL NOTE 40–1

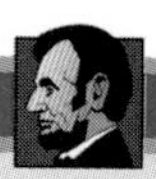

Dunton's Reflections about Adults: Collaborative Care

SUZANNE M. PELOQUIN

William Rush Dunton Jr. described an early encounter with adult patients when he was an assistant physician at Sheppard and Enoch Pratt Hospital in Towson, Maryland. At the time, Dunton organized dramatic plays for the patients. He remembered:

> ***We had a scene painter as a patient and I was able by much bossing to make him paint some attractive sets. Each morning, he would say: "Won't you let me off today?" And I would harden my heart and refuse. . . . It is probable that in later years I would not have been so brutal in my treatment of my scene-painter patient and I would have drawn him back to his vocation by easy stages, but experientia docet and I wanted new scenery. (Dunton, 1943, p. 245)***

Dunton's reflection that experience teaches (*experientia docet*) reminds us that we can welcome the opportunities for learning—about occupation, about illness, and about people—that present themselves in practice. Dunton's story also seems to be a plea that we treat adults as such, engaging with them in the collaborations and personal reflections that turn mistakes into the wisdom of maturity.

Dunton, W. R. (1943). How I got that way. *Occupational Therapy and Rehabilitation, 22,* 244–246.

CONCLUSION

This section reviewed the effects of orthopedic conditions, amputation, arthritis, and hand injury on adult occupational functioning. All of these conditions are common in adults. Each condition requires practitioners to become familiar with variations, which often must be explored further in relevant technical material. Each client is unique, presenting a personal situational context. Although prognoses may be generally assessed, success in recuperation depends on the attitude and effort of the client. Occupational therapy practitioners provide essential services by progressively reengaging the client in valued occupational activities both to restore function and to help the client learn required adaptive responses.

ACKNOWLEDGMENTS

With heartfelt thanks I acknowledge the encouraging contributions of Florene Black, Jane Horton, Mary Katsiaficas-Libby, Kathy A. Long, Gigi Leonard, Peg MacDonald, Barbara Ramsey, Lois Rosage, Blue Hill Memorial Hospital, and the spirit of Patricia Curran to these pages.

References

Apley, A. G., & Solomon L. (1994). *Concise system of orthopaedics and fractures*. Cambridge, UK: Butterworth.

Bear-Lehman, J. (2002). Orthopaedic conditions. In C. A. Trombly & M. V. Radomski (Eds.). *Occupational therapy for physical dysfunction* (5th ed., pp. 909–925). Philadelphia: Lippincott Williams & Wilkins.

Boscheinen-Morrin, J., Davey, V., & Conolly, W. B. (1995). *The hand: Fundamentals of therapy* (2nd ed.). Boston: Butterworth-Heinemann.

Cailliet, R. (1994). *Hand pain and impairment* (4th ed.). Philadelphia: Davis.

Celikyol, F. G. (2002). Amputations and prosthetics. In C. A. Trombly & M. V. Radomski (Eds.). *Occupational therapy for physical dysfunction* (5th ed., pp. 1045–1070). Philadelphia: Lippincott, Williams, & Wilkins.

Cooper, C. (2002). Hand impairments. In C. A. Trombly & M. V. Radomski (Eds.). *Occupational therapy for physical dysfunction* (5th ed., pp. 927–963). Philadelphia: Lippincott, Williams, & Wilkins.

Cummings, V., Alexander J., & Gans, S. O. (1984). Management of the amputee. In A. P. Ruskin (Ed.). *Current therapy in psychiatry* (pp. 212–219). Philadelphia: Saunders.

Fries, J. F. (1999). *Arthritis: A take care of yourself health guide for understanding your arthritis*. Cambridge, MA: Perseus.

Goldstein, T. S. (1999). *Geriatric orthopaedics: Rehabilitative management of common problems* (2nd ed.). Gaithersburg, MD: Aspen.

Jacobs, K. (Ed.). (1999). *Quick reference dictionary for occupational therapy* (2nd ed.). Thorofare, NJ: Slack.

Kelley, W. N. (1993). *Textbook of rheumatology*. Philadelphia: Saunders.

Lawrence, K. E., DiLima, S. N., & Evans, D. M. (Eds.). (1992). *Geriatric patient education resource manual: Vol. 1, 1991–1998*. Gaithersburg, MD: Aspen.

Maher, A. B. (1993). *Orthopedic nursing*. Philadelphia: Saunders.

Nicholas, J. J. (1996). Rehabilitation of patients with rheumatic disorders. In R. M. Buschbacher, D. Dumitru, E. W. Johnson, D. J. Matthews, & M. Sinaki (Assoc. Eds.). *Physical medicine and rehabilitation* (pp. 711–727). Philadelphia: Saunders.

Pascarelli, E. F. (1994). *Repetitive strain injury: A computer user's guide*. New York: Wiley.

Petty, W. (1991). *Total joint replacement*. Philadelphia: Saunders.

Platt, J. V. (1996). *Occupational therapy practice guidelines for adults with hip fracture/replacement*. Bethesda, MD: American Occupational Therapy Association.

Praemer, A. (1992). *Musculoskeletal conditions in the U. S.* Park Ridge, IL: American Academy of Orthopaedic Surgeons.

Rockwood, C. A., Green, D. P., Bucholz, R. W., & Heckman, J. D. (1996). *Rockwood and Green's fractures in adults*. Philadelphia: Lippincott-Raven.

Sobel, D., & Klein, A. C. (1995). *Arthritis: What exercises work*. New York: St. Martins.

Springhouse Corporation. (1995). *Professional guide to diseases* (5th ed.). Springhouse, PA: Author.

Venes, D. (Ed.). (2001). *Taber's cyclopedic medical dictionary* (19th ed.). Philadelphia: Davis.

CHAPTER 41

CARDIOPULMONARY DYSFUNCTION IN ADULTS

REGINA FERRARO DOHERTY

The purpose of this chapter is to help occupational therapy practitioners understand basic cardiopulmonary diagnoses and their implications for occupational therapy intervention. This information is important even for practitioners who do not specialize in cardiopulmonary rehabilitation. Many clients have cardiopulmonary disease either in their past medical history or secondary to multiple trauma, multisystem failure, or neurological injury. Consequently, all occupational therapy practitioners working in settings serving people with physical disabilities should be knowledgeable in the medical and surgical interventions used in the care of clients with cardiopulmonary dysfunction.

ACTIVITY LIMITATIONS AND PERFORMANCE AREAS

There are many functional limitations experienced by clients with cardiopulmonary dysfunction. These clients may be impaired by disease for prolonged periods, as are clients with chronic obstructive pulmonary disease (COPD), or may be impaired by sudden onset, as are clients with acute myocardial infarction (MI). In both of these scenarios, the client with cardiopulmonary dysfunction must undergo lifestyle and role changes that, in turn, affect occupational performance.

Activities of daily living (both basic and instrumental), work, play, education, and leisure activities are the occupational performance areas that can be affected by cardiopulmonary dysfunction. Impairments in endurance, strength, coordination, emotional coping skills and, at times, mental functions may also contribute to limitations in activity and occupational engagement. Cardiopulmonary disease is a somewhat unique disorder in that it imposes multiple lifestyle changes on clients and their families. Noncompliance with cardiopulmonary activity limitations, medications, and diet can lead to worsening of disease processes, severe medical complications, and sometimes death. Occupational therapy practitioners, because of their education in the psychosocial as well as the physical frames of reference, play a key role in the treatment of this client population. Occupational therapy's foundation in activity analysis and activity adaptation allows practitioners to be vital and integral parts of the cardiopulmonary rehabilitation team.

EVALUATION

Evaluation of clients with cardiopulmonary dysfunction can be broken into four essential components: medical chart review and history taking, client interview, functional evaluation, and physiological evaluation.

History Taking

It is critical to do a detailed medical chart review before beginning an evaluation with a client. The occupational therapy practitioner should look for the following information: the client's presenting primary diagnosis, the secondary diagnosis, past medical history, surgical procedures, medications, and results of laboratory or other diagnostic tests. In addition, information about the client's work history and social support system should be noted. Physician recommendations relative to activity levels are also important. The occupational therapy practitioner is responsible for understanding the medical information in the chart. Any terminology that is unfamiliar should be looked up in a medical dictionary or discussed with the client's medical team before evaluation.

The primary precaution for clients with cardiopulmonary disease is the risk of fatal cardiac or respiratory arrest. Activity levels that overtax clients' diseased cardiac or pulmonary systems can trigger those arrests. The chart review should give the occupational therapy practitioner an idea of what activities are safe for particular clients.

Client Interview

The initial interview for clients with cardiopulmonary disease begins with a discussion about their functional performance levels. The occupational therapist also needs to engage clients in a discussion regarding their preadmission roles and coping skills. During this time, therapists should particularly focus on identifying activity routines that are likely to present challenges for the client. For instance, because stair climbing requires a lot of cardiopulmonary work, it is important to ask clients about the number of stairs in their work and home environments. During the interview, the occupational therapist should observe the clients' breathing pattern, level of comfort or discomfort, posture, and information-processing skills (see Chapter 22).

Functional Evaluation

An initial occupational therapy evaluation for this population includes assessment of clients' current level of functioning in activities of daily living (ADL), with particular attention to their physiological response to functional activity. These physiological responses indicate clients' activity tolerance or endurance. Psychological coping skills also need to be assessed. Chapters 24 and 25 contain more information on assessment approaches.

Clients with cardiopulmonary dysfunction should also be screened for upper extremity range of motion (ROM), strength, gross and fine motor coordination, and sensation (see Chapter 25). Therapists need to check with the medical staff about any special precautions before performing these evaluations.

Physiologic Evaluation

Vital Signs Monitoring

Clinicians working with clients with cardiopulmonary disease need to be competent in monitoring **vital signs,** because these indicate a client's physiological status. Vital signs require monitoring during evaluation and intervention, both at rest and in response to therapeutic activities. Therapists need to keep a watchful eye on their clients and monitor how they are responding to given activities. Therapists also need to identify cardiopulmonary distress quickly. Cardiopulmonary distress is defined by Krider (1995) as labored, rapid, irregular, or shallow breathing that may be accompanied by coughing, choking, wheezing, dyspnea, anxiety, chest pain, or cyanosis of the oral mucosa, lips and fingers.

Vital signs are often the first and most important indicator that a client's clinical condition is changing (Krider, 1995). The vital signs most commonly monitored in the cardiopulmonary population are pulse or heart rate (HR), respiratory rate (RR), blood pressure (BP), and oxygenation.

Pulse

Pulse is the rhythmical dilation of the arteries, produced by the blood being pumped into the arteries by the contractions of the heart. Therefore, the pulse indicates heart rate—the number of times the heart contracts, or beats, per minute. The normal pulse, or HR, for adults is 60–100 beats per minute (bpm), with an average of 72–78 bpm. A pulse rate >100 bpm is termed tachycardia (abnormally fast HR). A pulse rate <60 bpm is termed bradycardia (abnormally slow HR). Pulse is evaluated for rate, rhythm, and strength.

The most common location to palpate the pulse is at the site of the radial artery in the wrist. Once palpated, the number of beats per minute is counted and recorded. If a client is suffering from a low BP, pulse is more easily palpated from a carotid artery in the neck, because the carotid artery is closer to the heart than the radial artery.

Respiratory Rate

Respiratory rate is counted by watching the abdomen or chest wall move in and out with breathing, a motion caused by the expansion and deflation of the lungs. Each full cycle of chest or abdominal movement (in and out) counts as one breath. The normal range for the adult RR is 12–22 breaths per minute. Tachypnea refers to a RR above normal. This elevated rate can be the result of exercise, fever, pain, or anxiety. Bradypnea refers to a slow RR. This rate is the less common of the two, yet may occur as a side effect of medication or in a client with central nervous system damage. It is important for the practitioner to count the RR without letting the client know that this is being done. When clients are aware that they are being monitored, they can alter the rate of their breathing. Movement of the supraclavicular fossae, at the union of the neck and shoulders, may be used in cardiopulmonary clients whose chest or abdominal wall movement is difficult to see.

Blood Pressure

Blood pressure is the force exerted against the walls of the arteries as the blood moves through the arterial vessels. BP is measured with a sphygmomanometer, and is recorded in millimeters of mercury (mm Hg). The BP cuff of the sphygmomanometer is wrapped around the client's brachial artery and inflated to a pressure 30 mm Hg higher than the client's average, which results in temporary obliteration of the pulse. If the client's average BP is unknown, the cuff should be inflated to 200 mm Hg. This obliteration creates turbulence in the brachial artery. The turbulence creates sounds (Korotkoff sounds) that can be heard with a stethoscope held over the brachial artery as the cuff is deflated.

Systolic blood pressure (SBP) is the peak force that occurs when blood is circulated through the systemic and pulmonary systems during contraction of the heart. It corresponds to the first sound heard in the brachial artery as the BP cuff deflates. The normal adult range for SBP is 90–150 mm Hg, with the average being 120 mm Hg. Diastolic blood pressure (DBP) is the force that occurs in the blood vessels when the heart is relaxing. It is during this period that the heart is filing with blood. The adult range for DBP is 60–90 mm Hg, with the average being 80 mm Hg. This corresponds to the last sound heart in the brachial artery as the BP cuff deflates. BP consistently greater than 140/90 is referred to as hypertension (high blood pressure). BP consistently lower than 90/60 is referred to as hypotension (low blood pressure).

Other Assessments

Additional diagnostic tests are used to assess physiological and cardiopulmonary function. One of the most commonly used laboratory tests to assess respiratory function is arterial blood gases (ABGs). The ABGs are measured from the arterial blood supply, which contains oxygen and carbon dioxide levels indicative of lung function. Measurements of ABGs provide information on the oxygenation status of the blood and the acid–base balance in the blood (Wilkins, 1995). Three relevant measurements of oxygenation provided by ABGs are PaO_2, SaO_2, and CaO_2.

PaO_2 is the partial pressure of oxygen in plasma and reflects the ability of the lungs to transfer oxygen from the environment into the circulating blood. The normal adult range for PaO_2 is 75–95 mm Hg on room air. A PaO_2 of less than the predicted range indicates hypoxemia (abnormally low oxygen levels in the blood). PaO_2 has a clinical significance because clients who sustain a low PaO_2 are at risk for cognitive compromise because the brain is not receiving adequate oxygen. These clients are generally in need of oxygen therapy (discussed later in this chapter).

SaO_2 is the amount of oxygen bound to hemoglobin. The normal value of SaO_2 is >95%. CaO_2 is the total content of oxygen in arterial blood and is one of the most important blood gas determinations because it influences tissue oxygenation. The normal range for CaO_2 is 16–20 mL/dL blood. CaO_2 levels need to be stable before intervention so that exercise does not further compromise tissue oxygenation.

Equipment

There are many different types of medical equipment used to monitor a client's physiological status in cardiopulmonary dysfunction settings. Equipment used with this population extends from the inpatient setting to the outpatient arena and is vast and ever developing. Practitioners who wish to specialize in this area should be thoroughly oriented in the purpose, operation, and precautions for the equipment housed on their particular unit. Some frequently used equipment is described here.

Arterial Pressure Line

An arterial pressure line (A-line or art-line) is a catheter that is inserted into an artery, most commonly the radial artery in adults, to monitor blood pressure and provide a port by which to obtain arterial blood gas measurements. Usually, the reading is projected onto a monitor at or above the client's bedside. Therapists should use caution not to confuse an A-line with an intravenous line, because the two entail different precautions for movement and activity.

Oximeter

An oximeter is a noninvasive instrument that measures the percentage of hemoglobin saturated with oxygen. As noted above, the normal adult value for oxygen saturation is >95%. Oximetry is often used during occupational therapy intervention sessions to monitor a client's physiological response to activity. When clients are unable to maintain adequate oxygenation with activity, they are said to be in desaturation.

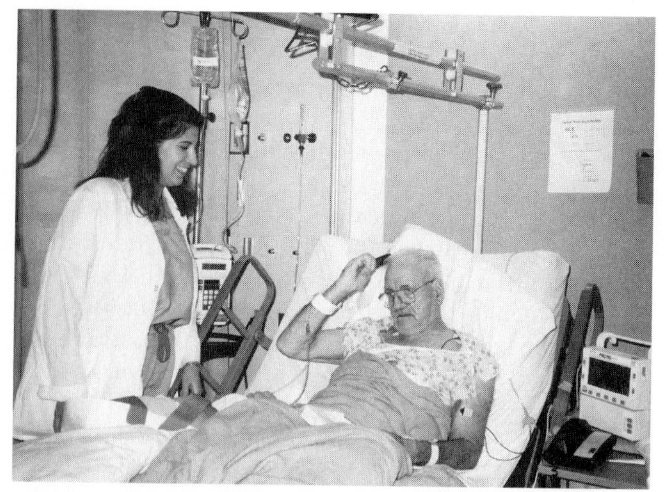

FIGURE 41-1. The client performs an ADL task while the therapist monitors his cardiopulmonary status via ECG and oximetry. Photo courtesy of R. F. Dougherty, Boston, MA.

Electrocardiogram

An electrocardiograph (ECG) is a machine that graphically records the heart's electrical activity through electrodes, or leads, placed over the chest. ECG monitoring can be performed on a continuous basis in the intensive care unit (ICU), or by a portable 12-lead ECG. The purpose of performing a 12-lead ECG is to obtain 12 different views of the electrical activity in the heart. These electrical currents are then recorded, or traced, by the ECG on special graph paper. The ECG tracings are clinically evaluated for abnormalities in several different variables. Abnormalities in ECG tracings are termed dysrhythmias. Dysrhythmias, or arrhythmias, are any abnormality in the rate, regularity, or sequence of cardiac electrical activity. Occupational therapists working with clients who require 12-lead ECG monitoring with activity should pursue continuing education in this area.

Holter Monitor

A Holter monitor is a small recording unit that stores a client's ECG tracings from surface electrodes for a preprogrammed time period. It is, in essence, a portable ECG unit. Clients wear the unit and electrodes while keeping a diary of activities. Later, a cardiologist can interpret the tracings to see if arrhythmias occur over time and if particular activities cause abnormalities in the electrical activity of the heart. The ability to link specific activities to heart function helps determine safe activity levels for clients with cardiopulmonary dysfunction. Holter monitors are also sometimes used with clients who do not have a primary diagnosis of cardiac dysfunction. For example, many clients who are admitted to acute care hospitals for cerebrovascular accidents are placed on Holter monitors. The monitors identify the presence of an arrhythmia, which assists in the confirmation of an embolism as a stroke's cause. In total, cardioembolic phenomena cause 15–20% of all strokes (Roth, 1993).

Other Monitors

Many medical devices that can monitor HR, oxygen saturation, BP, and ECG concurrently are commercially available. Use of this type of equipment is helpful during the early phases of activity progression (Fig. 41-1). It is critical that, in the initial evaluation of the client with cardiopulmonary dysfunction, the occupational therapist pays close attention to the physician-directed activity level and vital signs limitations. Contrary to previous beliefs, there is no longer a role for rest therapy, or prolonged bedrest, in the management of the client with cardiovascular disease (Kottke, Haney, & Doucette, 1990). Early mobilization has become common practice during acute hospitalization and has been deemed beneficial to the client's recovery process (Ishii, 1995; Wegner 1984).

INTERVENTION

The ultimate goal of occupational therapy intervention for adults with cardiopulmonary disease is to help them resume their valued life activities and reduce their disease-related risk factors, such as cigarette smoking. To accomplish these goals, occupational therapy practitioners use activity grading and monitoring, energy conservation and work simplification, relaxation and stress management, and prevention and home programs. Occupational therapy practitioners work closely with other members of the cardiac rehabilitation team—such as nursing, physical therapy, and exercise physiology—to customize a client's rehabilitation program. Occupational therapy practitioners in traditional and consultative roles often co-lead groups with their rehabilitation colleagues and help clients understand the connection between exercise, functional activity, risk modification, and role performance.

Activity Grading

Treatment of clients with cardiopulmonary disease begins in the acute care setting and extends to rehabilitation hospitals, skilled nursing facilities, outpatient clinics, and the home. Once a client's functional and physiological status is evaluated and documented, intervention begins. Clients with cardiopulmonary dysfunction require regulated activity during the rehabilitative process. The main reason for regulating activity is to reduce or control the stress or workload placed on the heart. The greater the cardiac workload, the greater the oxygen demand on the myocardium.

Because of the need for regulated activity, an essential component of intervention for the client with cardiopulmonary disease is the use of graded activity. Clients who have experienced prolonged hospitalizations because of cardiopulmonary instability are, for the most part, largely deconditioned and significantly impaired in ADL performance. For these clients, a simple bathing activity, such as face washing, may cause desaturation. It is essential that activity implementation with this population be modified and graded according to client progress. Progression through graded activities enables the client with cardiopulmonary disease to regain or enhance activity tolerance.

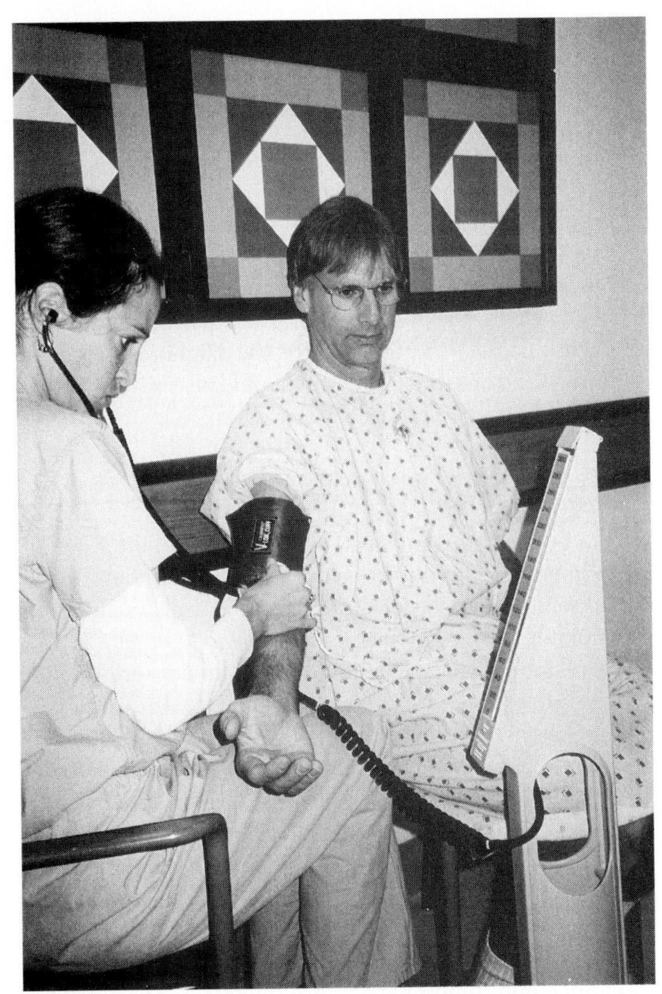

FIGURE 41-2. The practitioner uses a sphygmomanometer to obtain a client's blood pressure during a therapy session. Photo courtesy of R. F. Dougherty, Boston, MA.

Activity Monitoring

As an ADL task or exercise program is graded, the client's physiological tolerance of those activities must be monitored and documented (Fig. 41-2). At the beginning of each therapy session, the occupational therapy practitioner should take the client's vital signs at rest. Pulse, blood pressure, respiration rate, and oxygen saturation should be measured and recorded. If the client's resting vital signs are not within the ranges considered medically safe for him or her, the session should be discontinued. If the client's resting vital signs are within a medically safe range, then intervention can continue. Vital signs should be measured again 5–10 min into the session. The meaning of changes in vital signs is different for each client: For some, a small change indicates physiological instability; for others, this is not true. Therefore, a careful review of the client's history, medical status, medications, and physician-guided vital sign limitations is helpful.

In general, oxygen saturation should be maintained at ≥90% during functional activity, and HR should be limited to an increase no more than 20–30 bpm above the resting rate. A HR of <50 bpm is considered an inappropriate response, and the activity being performed should be terminated. Afterward, the client should be monitored and the physician notified (Shanfield & Hammond, 1984). BP responses can be variable even in healthy individuals, so medical guidance relative to safe parameters for individual clients is advisable. As a general rule, BP should be limited to an increase or decrease of no more than 15–20 mm Hg (Kottke et al., 1990; Krider, 1995; Ogden, 1979; Shanfield & Hammond, 1984).

If the cardiovascular response to activity is deemed appropriate by the monitoring clinician, the activity is continued and the vital signs are recorded again 5 min after completion of activity. The practitioner should record the client's vital signs in graph form on the initial evaluation and intervention notes. Doing so will assist the client and the practitioner in recognizing progress. Elevated HR and BP may present as one of the initial cardiopulmonary response to activity because of the increased work required by the heart. As the conditioning effect occurs, the resting and working HR and BP should decrease to more appropriate levels.

Clients with cardiopulmonary dysfunction require education about the symptoms of increased cardiac work before activity progression. This teaching is needed in advance so that the client may adequately provide feedback to the practitioner in the event of a nonadaptive physiological response. Physiological signs and symptoms of cardiopulmonary distress include dizziness, fatigue, chest pain, palpitations, headache, nausea, shortness of breath, diaphoresis (profuse sweating), and anxiety. Clinicians should also be alert to the nonverbal signs of client discomfort.

Cardiac Rehabilitation

The most substantial benefits of cardiac rehabilitation include improvements in activity tolerance, symptoms, blood lipid levels, and psychosocial well-being as well as reductions in smoking, stress, and mortality (Wegner et al., 1995). These all in turn lead to improved occupational performance and enhanced quality of life for the client with cardiopulmonary dysfunction. There are four phases of cardiac rehabilitation. Phase 1 is the acute hospitalization period. Activity during this stage is limited to bed to chair transfers, basic ADL, and slow walking. Orthostatic intolerance and sinus tachycardia are often present during activity progression in phase 1.

Phase 2 begins at the time of discharge and extends 12 weeks after the cardiac event. Phase 2 focuses on regaining endurance and improving activity tolerance. Reconditioning and risk modification programs are implemented. No isometric exercise is permitted at this time. Mild endurance exercise training is begun to increase aerobic capacity.

In phase 3, rigorous risk factor modification is begun, strength training is performed to induce physiological adaptations to exercise, and the client is prepared for return to work. Exercise training is aimed at lowering BP and HR to decrease myocardial workload. Phase 4 is considered the maintenance phase. During this phase, exercise habits are established, and risk factor modification is ongoing.

As clients proceed through the phases of cardiac rehabilitation, activity levels are increased, based on the client's physiological responses to activities. All purposeful tasks place an energy demand on the cardiopulmonary system. The metabolic equivalent (MET) is considered the unit of choice to measure energy expenditure in the cardiopulmonary population (Ogden, 1979). The MET is the energy expended in a resting state: 1 MET is equal to 3.5 mL oxygen per kilogram of body weight per minute. The energy cost of activities is then rated based on the resting MET. For example, if an activity is rated as 5 METs, that means that it requires five times the oxygen expended at rest. Minimal or very light cardiac activity is considered to require 1–2 METs; light cardiac activity requires 2–3 METs; moderate cardiac activity requires 3–4 METs; and heavy cardiac activity requires 4–5 METs. Table 25-18 provides examples of appropriate functional activities for distinct levels of cardiac activity. The MET levels appropriate for a given client in a given phase of cardiac rehabilitation should be determined in conjunction with the client's physician.

Energy Conservation and Work Simplification

The principles of **work simplification** for energy conservation are fundamental to the treatment of clients with cardiopulmonary dysfunction. Work simplification is the performance of a task in an organized, planned, and orderly way, such that body motions, workload, and fatigue are reduced to a minimum. Energy conservation is essential for clients with cardiopulmonary dysfunction because it enables them to save their energy for fundamental tasks or for times during the day when more energy is needed. The following work simplification and energy conservation techniques are recommended:

- Balance work and rest (e.g., if a client has a social function to attend in the evening, recommend resting in the afternoon); avoid rushing, and take frequent rest breaks to prevent fatigue.
- Whenever possible perform a task while sitting instead of a standing position.
- Avoid reaching and bending by prearranging work at comfortable levels.
- Maintain good posture; be especially cautious of a prolonged stooped posture.
- Avoid lifting and holding; use a rolling cart or slide items when possible.
- Rest for at least 60 min after meals so that the blood needed for digestion will not be interrupted by exercise.
- Work in a properly lit and well-ventilated environment.
- Prioritize tasks, practice delegation, and eliminate steps that are unnecessary to task completion.

Clients with cardiopulmonary disease may need assistance in deciding how to conserve energy. They should be guided in their decision-making process about how they wish to use their energy. An interest checklist may be helpful for these clients. For example, a client with limited activity tolerance may choose to employ a homemaker for house-cleaning tasks to save energy to perform an alternative task. A different client may take great pride in his or her role as a homemaker and, hence, employ work simplification techniques for the successful performance of this task. Adaptive equipment plays a role for clients with cardiopulmonary dysfunction, especially in the home environment. Tub seats and long-handled sponges increase bathing independence for clients with limited activity tolerance.

Relaxation and Stress Management

Principles of stress management and relaxation are appropriate for integration into occupational therapy intervention protocols for clients with cardiopulmonary dysfunction. Physicians often instruct clients with cardiopulmonary dysfunction to make lifestyle changes. Learning to reduce and better cope with stress is one of these changes. These clients require education in the physiological effect that stress has on their body, the warning signs of stress, and methods to reduce stress. The stress-induced flight-or-fight response stimulates the release of a variety of hormones, including norepinephrine. These hormones can increase BP and cholesterol levels. Epinephrine may cause constriction of the coronary arteries, reducing blood flow to the heart (Stuart, Deckro, DeSilva, & Benson, 1993). Instruction in the relaxation response and cognitive behavioral stress management techniques serves to lower rates of coronary disease and increase coping skills (see Chapter 30, Section 8). The carryover of these techniques is essential to lifestyle modification in the client with cardiopulmonary dysfunction.

Prevention and Home Programs

Prevention education and home program implementation for the promotion of healthy lifestyle changes in clients with cardiopulmonary dysfunction are essential. Risk factor modification needs to begin in the rehabilitative program and be carried out in the home. Clients must be educated in the coronary and pulmonary risk factors that they can control. Coronary disease factors that clients can control are smoking, high BP, sedentary lifestyle, overweight, high cholesterol, and stress. Pulmonary risk factors that clients can control are smoking and environmental conditions. Clients may be at a point at which role performance is rapidly altered by physical limitations or physiological impairments. Because of this, the client's ability to gain a sense of control is key to successful disease management.

During acute hospitalization, clients retain little information concerning their conditions. Education must include written handout materials and demonstrative learning when possible. Education of cardiac clients cannot be considered complete without the inclusion of their partner and family members, owing to the high anxiety they experience and the important role they play in caring for the cardiac client (Tooth & McKenna, 1995). Clients with COPD who suffer from anxiety coupled with dyspnea (shortness of breath) also benefit from being given written procedures. Education should bridge the gap between hospital and home.

Pederson (1993) stated that "a successful home care plan depends on careful assessment and planning before discharge" (p. 24). Compliance with home programs can be fostered by suggesting the client keep a journal and by partner and family encouragement. The positive effects of exercise and diet change, such as feeling better and having more energy, should be emphasized to the client during this difficult lifestyle change.

The preceding information is of general relevance to evaluation and interventions for this population. The following sections deal with specific cardiopulmonary diagnoses and include information about medical aspects of these conditions as well as specific occupational therapy interventions.

MYOCARDIAL INFARCTION

Demographics

All occupational therapy practitioners who work with adults will encounter clients who suffer from coronary artery disease (CAD). One of the most frequently seen clinical manifestations of CAD is myocardial infarction. Nearly 1.5 million Americans sustain an MI or heart attack each year. Of these, 50,000 episodes are fatal (Wegner et al., 1995). MI is not an affliction of the elderly population alone; 45% of MIs occur in individuals <65 years of age. MI occurs more frequently in men than in women.

Definition

The heart is a muscle that receives its vascular blood supply from the coronary arteries and their respective branches. Inadequate blood supply or sudden interruption of blood flow to the myocardium leads to ischemia (tissue damage). If the blood supply does not resume, then infarction (tissue death) develops. The most common cause of inadequate blood flow is narrowing of the coronary arteries by atherosclerotic disease or by thrombotic or embolic occlusion. Acute ischemic syndromes include acute MI, angina, and sudden ischemic death.

Signs and Symptoms

The primary presenting symptom for the diagnosis of MI is usually a pressure like chest pain that is unrelenting and severe. The pain is located substernally, and can radiate to the arms, back, or upper jaws. Secondary symptoms are dyspnea (shortness of breath), nausea and vomiting, and confusion, particularly in the elderly. Some people present with only these secondary symptoms.

MIs are classified according to which coronary artery is occluded and which ventricle is involved. Most frequently, they affect the left ventricle. The different types of left ventricular MIs are classified according to which wall of the left ventricle has been affected— anterior, inferior, septal, posterior, or anterolateral (Miracle, 1988). There are differences in the medical management of the different types of MI, which are beyond the scope of this chapter. In general, after a left ventricular MI, a client is more likely to develop dysrhythmias; whereas, after a right ventricular MI, a client is more likely to develop decreased cardiac output.

Angina is sometimes associated with MI. Angina is a transitory syndrome characterized by episodic pain when the oxygen supply to the heart is insufficient to meet the heart's needs. It can occur as a result of an increased oxygen need in high-cardiac-output conditions (Klein, 1988).

Medical interventions

Medications

During the acute hospitalization period, pharmacological treatment of acute MI is used to relieve pain and anxiety, limit the extent of heart muscle necrosis, and prevent complications. The following are some of the common medications used for the acute MI population:

- *Nitrates:* To improve myocardial oxygen supply by dilating the coronary arteries and collateral vessels (e.g., nitroglycerin),
- *P-adrenergic blockers:* To decrease heart rate, blood pressure, and the force of contraction, thereby decreasing the myocardial oxygen demand and preventing ischemia (e.g., metoprolol/Lopressor)
- *Calcium channel blockers:* To inhibit calcium entry into smooth muscle and myocardial cells; they decrease BP by peripheral vasodilatation and relieve coronary vasospasm by dilating the coronary arteries (e.g., verapamil and nifedipine).
- *Inotropic agents:* To increase cardiac output and increase blood flow (e.g., dopamine).
- *Anticoagulants/antiplatelet agents:* To decrease the clotting ability of the blood to prevent clots and blockages in blood flow from forming (e.g., Coumadin and aspirin).

Surgery

There are different types of surgical procedures used with individuals who have sustained MIs. The goal of these procedures is to restore myocardial profusion.

Thrombolytic Therapy

Thrombolytic therapy is an early treatment used to improve the survival rate of MI clients. It is started, within the critical time frame of 0–6 hr after symptomatic onset, by direct infusion of a thrombolytic agent into an occluded or infarct-related artery. Examples of thrombolytic agents are tissue plasminogen activator (tPA), urokinase, and streptokinase. This procedure can dissolve some or all of the blockage in the infarct-related artery, which limits the infarct size and improves outcome. The smaller the area of myocardial damage, the better the heart's overall functioning will be.

Percutaneous Transluminal Coronary Angioplasty

Percutaneous transluminal coronary angioplasty (PTCA) involves dilation of the affected, or acutely occluded, coronary artery by balloon angioplasty to open the vessel for myocardial profusion. PTCA has the advantage of not requiring clients to undergo open-heart surgery. It is most often indicated for clients with proximal, single-vessel CAD (Halperin & Levine, 1985; Tommaso, Lesch, & Sonnenblick, 1984).

Intra-Aortic Balloon Pump

The intra-aortic balloon pump (IABP) is a mechanical support device used for acute myocardial reperfusion. The balloon device is inserted into the femoral artery and passed to the ascending aorta. While using ECG or hemodynamic monitoring, the balloon is inflated with helium during diastole and deflated during systole. This serves to increase cardiac output and decrease myocardial oxygen consumption. IABP is often used as a temporary support of systemic or coronary profusion in conjunction with other procedures, such as thrombolysis and PTCA (Webb & Hochman, 1997).

Coronary Artery Bypass Graft

Coronary artery bypass graft (CABG) is a surgical procedure that was devised in the late 1960s for the treatment of CAD. It is currently one of the most commonly performed major surgical operations and holds only a 1–2% risk of mortality (Tommaso et al., 1984). During this procedure, a vein from another part of the body, usually the saphenous vein in the lower extremity, is grafted onto the heart surface to bypass or detour the atherosclerotic or narrowed coronary artery. This creates a patent (open) artery, thereby permitting improved blood flow to the myocardium. Clients who have undergone this procedure are advised to use caution in reaching, bending, and lifting as well as getting in and out of bed so that the sternum (breastbone), which is cut during surgery, is given time to heal.

Occupational Therapy Intervention

The principles of cardiac rehabilitation are used in the occupational therapy treatment of clients after an acute MI or cardiac reperfusion surgery. The client is gradually progressed through the appropriate activity level, as described earlier. These clients are seen in a variety of intervention settings, ranging from acute care hospitals to outpatient clinics. The role of the occupational therapy practitioner in the treatment of the client with cardiac dysfunction is to maximize independence, increase activity tolerance, and support adaptive emotional responses while promoting reintegration into all desired performance areas within established activity limitations.

CONGESTIVE HEART FAILURE

Demographics and Definition

The National Heart, Lung, and Blood Institute (NHLBI) estimates that >4 million Americans have heart failure and that about 400,000 new cases are diagnosed each year

(Konstam et al., 1994). It is the most common diagnosis in hospitalized clients age 65 and older (NHLBI, 1996). Congestive heart failure (CHF) is a clinical syndrome in which the heart fails to maintain an adequate output, resulting in decreased blood flow to the tissues and congestion in the pulmonary or the systemic circulation, or both. A client who is experiencing heart failure has a weak heart with reduced pumping power.

Signs and Symptoms

For most clients, heart failure is a chronic condition, which means that it can be treated and managed but not cured. The most common causes of heart failure are CAD (usually with previous MI), cardiomyopathy, hypertension, and heart valve disease. The signs and symptoms of CHF are difficulty breathing, especially on exertion or when lying flat in bed (nocturnal dyspnea); waking up breathless at night; frequent dry, hacking cough, especially when lying down; fatigue and weakness; dizziness or fainting; edematous (swollen) feet, ankles, and legs; and nausea with abdominal swelling, pain, or tenderness. These signs and symptoms occur because the heart is pumping with less power and force than normal. The echocardiogram is considered one of the most useful diagnostic test in the medical evaluation of clients with heart failure (Advisory Council to Improve Outcomes Nationwide in Heart Failure, 1999). This test provides the medical team with the measurement of a client's left ventricular ejection fraction (EF). Clients with a left ventricular EF of ≤40% are generally considered to have systolic dysfunction.

Medical Interventions

Medications

Initial medical management of congestive heart failure includes rest to decrease cardiac work and initiation of pharmacological agents. The following are some of the common medications used for the CHF population:

- *Diuretics:* Started immediately when the client presents with symptoms of volume overload; often referred to as "water pills" because they help remove excess fluid and salt from the blood (e.g., furosemide/Lasix).
- *Angiotensin-converting enzyme (ACE) inhibitors:* Relax the blood vessels, making it easier for the heart to pump (e.g., captopril).
- *Digitalis glycosides:* Increase the contractile state of the heart, strengthening each heart beat so more blood can be pumped (e.g., digoxin).
- *β-Adrenergic receptor blockers (β-blockers):* Used to inhibit the affects of the sympathetic nervous system on the heart and prevent the progression of heart failure in clients with left ventricular dysfunction; generally used together with diuretics and ACE inhibitors (e.g., carvedilol).

Surgery

Some clients with CHF benefit from surgical revascularization. Clients with CHF are generally candidates for revascularization if they have viable myocardium fed by stenotic arteries (Konstam et al., 1994). Two types of surgical revascularization procedures considered for clients with CHF are CABG and balloon angioplasty. Use of CABG prolongs life in clients with worsening heart failure. Valve replacement or valve repair is undertaken if the cause of CHF is valvular dysfunction.

Recent technological advances have resulted in the use of mechanical assist devices for clients with end-stage heart failure and cardiomyopathy who are awaiting transplantation. The surgical implantation of a left ventricular assist device (LVAD) allows clients to maintain hemodynamic stability, while beginning the process of rehabilitation and reconditioning for enhanced pretransplant status and operative recovery. These devices serve as a bridge to transplantation.

Heart transplantation is also considered for those clients who continue to have repeated hospitalizations despite aggressive medical therapy. Cardiac transplantation recipients must meet specific selection criteria. Clients with end-stage coronary disease or idiopathic cardiomyopathy (a condition that affects the muscular function one or both ventricles) and who have a potential of survival of <6–12 months are appropriate candidates for transplantation (Myerowitz, 1987; Schroeder 2000).

Practitioners working with the heart transplant population must be aware of precautions for clients with compromised immune systems. To prevent a transplant recipient from rejecting the tissue transplant or graft, the client is treated with immunosuppressive therapy. This therapy includes antirejection drugs, such as azathioprine and cyclosporine. These drugs inhibit the immune response and prevent tissue rejection but also increase the client's risk of contracting infection. The immunocompromised client cannot fight off a simple cold. Practitioners working with this population are required to follow institution-guided precautions, including treatment in isolation rooms during early stages and gowning, gloving, and masking.

Clients who have undergone cardiac transplantation are appropriate for cardiac rehabilitation with slight modifications. Therapists must remember that clients undergoing cardiac transplantation have been debilitated for prolonged periods. They may have presurgical functional and MET capacity limitations influencing the initial phases of cardiac rehabilitation.

Client Education

Heart failure is one of the most common causes for hospital readmission. Proper discharge planning and client education are essential for preventing unnecessary readmissions. Education of this client population includes general counseling about the disease process, symptoms of worsening heart failure, risk factor modification, prognosis, activity restrictions, and medication management. Clients with CHF are advised to keep a diary of their daily weight and to inform their physician if a weight gain of 3–5 lb or more occurs within 1 week. This weight gain means that the client is retaining fluids and medication regiments may need to be altered.

Occupational Therapy Intervention

Occupational therapy treatment of the client with CHF uses principles of cardiac rehabilitation, with a focus on ADL training and maximizing activity tolerance. Energy conservation and work simplification techniques need to be integrated into the client's daily occupational routines to facilitate psychosocial adaptation in the face of physiological impairments and altered performance in occupational roles.

CHRONIC OBSTRUCTIVE PULMONARY DISORDER

Demographics and Definition

Chronic obstructive pulmonary disorder affects >13.5 million Americans. It is the fourth leading cause of death in the United States and is 1.8 times more prevalent in men than in women (Johannesen, 1994; NIH, 1995; National Institutes of Health [NIH], 2000). COPD is the term used to describe a variety of pulmonary disorders, including chronic bronchitis, asthma, emphysema, and bronchiectasis. It is, however, generally restricted chronic bronchitis and emphysema, because unlike asthma, COPD implies irreversible and generally progressive airway damage (Celli 1998; Fishman, 1988). COPD is characterized by progressive limitation in the flow of air into and out of the lungs.

Emphysema is the destruction of the walls of the bronchioles and alveoli, resulting in abnormally enlarged air spaces. The most common cause of emphysema is the inhalation of tobacco smoke, which induces an imbalance between protease and antiprotease activity in the lung, resulting in a destruction of the elastic fibers in the alveolar walls.

Chronic bronchitis is characterized by excessive mucus secretion in the bronchial tree, which leads to obstruction of airflow and mucus plugging. It is manifested by persistent productive cough. Chronic bronchitis is diagnosed when cough and symptoms are present on most days for a minimum of 3 months for at least 2 successive years or 6 months during 1 year.

In COPD, the walls of the small airways and alveoli lose their elasticity. The alveolar walls become thickened and the air passageway becomes plugged with mucus. Air enters the alveoli during inhalation but may not be able to escape during exhalation because the air passages collapse, trapping stale air. This leads to decreased gas exchange, tiring of respiratory muscles, increased carbon dioxide accumulation, and hypoventilation.

As COPD progresses, the disease process places a large burden on the heart. The right side of the heart needs to produce high pressures to force blood through the narrow blood vessels to the lungs. This causes the right chambers of the heart to enlarge and thicken. Cor pulmonale is a condition in which the right ventricle of the heart is hypertrophied secondary to lung disease.

Signs and Symptoms

The client with COPD usually presents with the following symptoms: dyspnea (difficulty breathing), morning cough, and expiratory wheeze; in the later stages of the disease, the clients displays breathlessness that prevents him or her from lying down. Dyspnea is the hallmark of COPD and is often viewed as the single greatest contributor to functional difficulties (Leidy, 1995).

Medical Interventions

There is presently no cure for COPD; however, positive lifestyle changes can result in a longer, more comfortable life (Johanneson, 1994). In many instances, some irreversible damage has already occurred by the time COPD is diagnosed. Management of COPD is through health-care education, smoking cessation, pharmacological therapy, supplemental oxygen, infection protection, nutritional therapy, and pulmonary rehabilitation.

Health Education

Individuals with COPD need general health education to promote healthy lifestyles. In addition, these individuals are advised to avoid exposure to dust and fumes, curtail physical activities during air pollution alerts, and to avoid extremes in temperature and humidity, because these conditions trigger hyperreactivity in their irritated airways (Johanneson, 1994). Smoking cessation is essential to prevent the progression of COPD. Cigarette smoking results in destruction of lung tissue. Practitioners should refer these clients to smoking cessation programs for assistance with this lifestyle change.

Medications

Pharmacological therapy for the client with COPD includes the use of bronchodilators, steroids, antibiotics, diuretics, and mucolytics. Bronchodilators, such as ipratropium bromide, act as anticholinergic agents. Once inhaled, they block the muscarinic cholinergic receptors, decrease vagal tone, increase smooth muscle contraction, and decrease mucus secretion. Corticosteroids (such as prednisone) are used in the treatment of COPD to decrease airway inflammation. Antibiotics (e.g., tetracycline and amoxicillin) are used in clients with COPD, usually during acute exacerbation, to decrease the duration of the episode and improve expiratory flow rates. Antibiotic prophylaxis (given in anticipation of infection) is also used with this population. Diuretics, such as furosemide (Lasix), are used to prevent water retention. Mucolytics (guaifenesin) are used to decrease the viscosity of the mucus and to facilitate mucociliary clearance. Clients with COPD are also encouraged to keep their airways clean by mobilizing secretions with aerosol treatments, chest percussion, and postural bronchial drainage.

Surgery

Lung transplantation is a surgical option for some clients with advanced COPD. Lung transplant selection criteria vary among transplant centers. In general, transplant is considered when the client's life expectancy is 1–3 years and maximal medical therapy has failed (Celli, 1998; Smith, 1998). Contraindications include organ failure, active infections (other than in the lung), obesity, CAD, smoking or drug abuse, and age >60.

Other Medical Treatments

Oxygen

Supplemental oxygen reduces mortality in clients with COPD. It can also improve a client's exercise tolerance and cognitive abilities. Oxygen therapy is generally recommended for clients with a sustained PaO_2 <55 mm Hg or an oxygen saturation <88% and evidence of cor pulmonale.

Infection Protections

The excess thickened mucus in the lungs of clients with COPD is an excellent growth medium for bacteria. Infection protection in the COPD population includes prophylactic vaccination against influenza and pneumococcal pneumonia, avoidance of exposure to persons (especially children) with respiratory infection, and maintaining adequate hydration to thin mucous secretions.

Nutritional Therapy

Nutritional therapy in the COPD population is essential because weight loss and nutritional deficiencies decrease respiratory muscle strength. A high-fat, low-carbohydrate diet is recommended.

Occupational Therapy Intervention

Education

Clients with COPD require considerable education in proper breathing techniques to facilitate improved oxygenation, increase ventilatory muscle endurance, and promote relaxation. Clients with COPD are often taught how to use the pursed-lip breathing technique. In this technique the client breathes in slowly through the nose, purses lips as if to whistle or kiss, and breathes out very slowly through the pursed lips. The pursed lips serve to control the flow of air with exhalation. Rehearsal of this technique can lead to better-breathing patterns in clients with cardiopulmonary dysfunction.

Pulmonary Rehabilitation

Pulmonary rehabilitation is implemented for clients with stable COPD. Its goal is to return the client to the highest level of functional capacity through education, exercise training, and psychosocial support. The demonstrated benefits of pulmonary rehabilitation are reduction of respiratory symptoms, reversal of anxiety and depression, improved self-esteem, enhanced ability to carry out ADL, increased exercise tolerance, and improved quality of life (Johannsen, 1994; Shanfield & Hammond, 1984).

Occupational therapy interventions in pulmonary rehabilitation programs should include the use of the following:

- Graded activities.
- ADL and instrumental ADL training.
- Exercise training programs to increase activity tolerance.
- Client and family education in principles of energy conservation, work simplification, stress management, and relaxation techniques.
- Pursed-lip breathing.
- Establishment of home programs.

During the rehabilitation process, clients with COPD need to learn problem-solving skills that they can use in the home environment.

TUBERCULOSIS

Demographics and Definition

Tuberculosis (TB) is a major world health problem. It is estimated that there are 1 billion individuals infected with TB worldwide, making it one of the most prevalent infections in the world (Enarson & Rouillon, 1998; Fishman, 1988). TB is more prevalent in urban areas. It is also more common among Hispanics, African Americans, Asians, Native Americans, drug-dependent individuals, the homeless, people in residential-care facilities and other closed institutions, alcoholics, prison inmates, and individuals with HIV (Advisory Council for the Elimination of Tuberculosis, 1999; Rieder, Kelly, Bloch, Cauthen, & Snider, 1991). Tuberculosis is an infectious disease that is caused by *Mycobacterium tuberculosis* or, rarely in the United States, *M. bovis*. This infectious bacterium is airborne, acid fast, and slow growing.

The TB infection is transmitted primarily by inhalation of contaminated droplets of respiratory secretions dispersed through the air by coughing, sneezing, or talking. There are three types of TB: primary, reactivation or postprimary, and extrapulmonary. In primary TB, the client is infected with the TB bacteria but may not have any clinical manifestation. The body's immune system fights the infection, rendering the bacteria inactive. In other clients, especially those with weakened immune systems owing to aging, malnutrition, or infections such as HIV, the TB bacteria become active and cause disease.

In adults, reactivation TB is the most common form of TB disease. It is the active presentation of the disease. On average, people infected with M. *tuberculosis* have a 10% chance of developing active TB sometime in their life (NIOSH, 1999). Extrapulmonary TB is the infection's involvement in any organ outside the lung. Extrapulmonary TB involvement occurs in two thirds of clients infected with HIV. Low CD4 cell counts, the white blood cells that play a central role in the immune response, are associated with greater probability of extrapulmonary TB in clients with HIV (Friedman, 1994).

Signs and Symptoms

The classic symptoms of TB are cough, hemoptysis (spitting up blood), fever, night sweats, and weight loss. TB is typically diagnosed by a smear-positive acid-fast bacilli (AFB) culture of mucus, blood, bone, or tissue.

Medical Interventions

Hospitalization

Medical management of TB is centered on eradicating the infecting organism and preventing the emergence of drug-resistant strains. Clients with active TB are hospitalized and kept in respiratory isolation during the initial phase of treatment. Just 2 weeks of medical therapy greatly decreases the infectiousness of clients with pulmonary TB. However, occupational therapy practitioners working with this population should adhere to respiratory precautions, as dictated by the institution in which they practice. Generally these clients are bedded in private reverse air pressure rooms with antechambers. In the United States, clinicians involved in direct contact with these clients are required to wear specialized masks to comply with the National Institute for Occupational Safety and Health (1999) requirements for prevention of disease transmission.

Medications

The pharmacological management of TB involves the administration of multiple medications. The current acceptable minimal duration of therapy is 6 months; this is greatly shortened from the 1970s when 18 months was the norm. HIV-infected clients with TB should be treated for a minimum of 9 months. A typical medication regimen for the treatment of TB includes medication with chemotherapeutic agents such as isoniazid, rifampin, and pyrazinamide.

There has been an increase in the number of people with multidrug-resistant TB (MDR-TB), which is caused by strains resistant to two or more drugs. These clients require the use of second-line TB drugs, and drug therapy for 13–24 months may be necessary. Lung resection surgery may also be used in the advanced treatment of drug-resistant TB.

Occupational Therapy Intervention

Occupational therapy has historically maintained a place in the treatment of clients with TB. Occupational therapy was one of the first programs instituted in TB sanitariums, where reading, entertainment, and the development of craft activities were used therapeutically to make the prolonged hospital stay of the client more tolerable (Northrop, 1978). The concept of graded activity may have originated in German tuberculosis sanatoria in the late 1300s (Creighton, 1993). At present, the effectiveness of medications has made it possible for shortened lengths of stay in the hospital and earlier return to work for clients with tuberculosis. However, occupational therapy treatment continues to be an essential service to clients who experience functional limitations secondary to infection with M. *tuberculosis*. The elderly and immunocompromised with TB are appropriate for occupational therapy intervention focused on education concerning energy conservation, work simplification, and graded activity to maximize endurance.

CONCLUSION

Occupational therapy practitioners play a vital role in the rehabilitation of the client with cardiopulmonary dysfunction. This is a growing client population, and occupational therapy practitioners are involved with these clients in a variety of settings. To be effective, occupational therapy practitioners need to have a comprehensive understanding of the cardiopulmonary disease process and its wide-reaching implications. The use of activity gradation and adaptation, which remains unique to the occupational therapy profession, significantly enhances the quality of life for individuals who have these illnesses. Occupational therapy practitioners bring together function and physiology to complement the cardiopulmonary rehabilitation team.

References

Advisory Council for the Elimination of Tuberculosis. (1999). Tuberculosis elimination revisited: Obstacles, opportunities and a renewed commitment. *Morbidity and Mortality Weekly Report, 48*,(RR09), 1–13.

Advisory Council to Improve Outcomes Nationwide in Heart Failure. (1999). Part 1: evaluation of heart failure—Clinical features. *American Journal of Cardiology, 83*, 2A–8A.

Celli, B. R. (1998). Standards for the optimal management of COPD: A summary. *Chest, 113*(4), 283S–287S.

Creighton, C. (1993). Graded activity: Legacy of the sanatorium. *American Journal of Occupational Therapy, 47*, 745–748.

Enarson, D. A., & Rouillon, A. (1998). The epidemiological basis of tuberculosis control. In P. D. O. Davies (Ed.). *Clinical tuberculosis* (2nd ed., pp. 35–52). New York: Chapman & Hall.

Fishman, A. P. (Ed.). (1988). *Pulmonary diseases and disorders* (2nd ed.). New York: McGraw-Hill.

Friedman, L. N. (Ed.). (1994). *Tuberculosis current concepts and treatment*. Ann Arbor, MI: CRC Press.

Halperin, J. L., & Levine, R. (1985). *Bypass*. New York: Times Books.

Ishii, K. (1995). Physical capacity assessment of the acute cardiovascular patient. *Journal of Cardiac Nursing*, 9(4), 53–63.

Johannsen, J. M. (1994). Chronic obstructive pulmonary disorder: Current comprehensive care for emphysema and bronchitis. *Nurse Practitioner, 19*(1), 59–67.

Klein, D. (1988). Angina. *Nursing, 18*(7), 44–46.

Konstam, M., Dracup, K., Baker, D., Brooks, N., Dacey, R., Dunbar, S., et al. (1994). *Heart failure: Management of clients with left ventricular systolic dysfunction* [Quick Reference Guide for Clinicians, No. 11; AHCPR Publication No. 94-0613]. Rockville, MD: U.S. Department of Health and Human Services.

Kottke, T. E., Haney, T. H., & Doucette, M. M. (1990). Rehabilitation of the patient with heart disease. In F. J. Kotte & J. F. Lehmann (Eds.). *Krusen's handbook of physical medicine and rehabilitation* (4th ed., pp. 874–903): Philadelphia: Saunders.

Krider, S. J. (1995). Vital signs. In R. L. Wilkins, S. J. Krider, & R. L. Sheldon (Eds.). *Clinical assessment in respiratory care* (3rd ed., pp. 35–46). Boston: Mosby.

Leidy, N. K. (1995). Functional performance in people with chronic obstructive pulmonary disease. *IMAGE: Journal of Nursing Scholarship, 27*, 23–34.

Miracle, V. (1988). Understanding the different types of MI. *Nursing, 18*(1), 53–56.

Myerowitz, P. D. (1987). Selection and management of the heart transplant recipient. In P. D. Myerowitz (Ed.). *Heart transplantation* (pp. 73–88). Mount Kisco, NY: Futura.

National Heart, Lung, and Blood Institute [NHLBI]. (1996). *Congestive heart failure in the United States: A new epidemic* [NIH Data Fact Sheet]. Bethesda, MD: U.S. Department of Health and Human Services.

National Institutes of Health [NIH] National Heart, Lung, and Blood Institute (1995). *Chronic obstructive pulmonary disease* [NIH Publication No. 95-2020]. Bethesda, MD: U.S. Department of Health and Human Services.

National Institutes of Health [NIH]. (2000). *Morbidity and mortality: 2000 chart book on cardiovascular, lung and blood diseases*. Bethesda, MD: U.S. Department of Health and Human Services.

National Institution for Occupational Safety and Health. (1999). *TB respiratory protection in health care facilities: Administrators guide* [NIOSH Publication No. 99-143]. Atlanta: Centers for Disease Control and Prevention.

Northrop, C. (1978). Pulmonary disease: Tuberculosis. In R. Goldenson (Ed.). *Disability and rehabilitation handbook* (pp. 525–540). New York: McGraw-Hill.

Ogden, L. D. (1979). Activity guidelines for early, subacute and high risk cardiac patients. *American Journal of Occupational Therapy, 33*, 291–298.

Pederson, B. (1993). Home care management of the chronic obstructive pulmonary disease patient increases patient control and prevents rehospitalization. *Home Healthcare Nurse, 10*, 24–30.

Rieder, H. L., Kelly, G. D., Bloch, A. B., Cauthen, G. M., & Snider, D. E. (1991). Tuberculosis diagnosed at death in the United States. *Chest, 100*, 678–681.

Roth, E. (1993). Heart disease in patient with stroke: Incidence, impact and implications for rehabilitation part I: classification and prevalence. *Archives of Physical Medicine and Rehabilitation, 74*, 752–757.

Schroeder, J. S. (2000). Cardiac transplantation. In E. Braunwald, A. S. Fauci, K. J. Isselbacher, D. L. Kasper, S. L. Hauser, D. L. Longo, & J. L. Jameson (Eds.). *Harrison's Online*. New York: McGraw-Hill.

Shanfield, K., & Hammond, M. A. (1984). Activities of daily living. In E. Hodgkin, J. E. Zorn, & G. Long Connors (Eds.). *Pulmonary rehabilitation: Guidelines to success* (pp. 171–193). Philadelphia: Lippincott.

Smith, C. M. (1998). Lung transplantation. In W. Kelley (Ed.). *Textbook of internal medicine* [Primary care online]. (2nd ed.). Philadelphia: Lippincott, Williams & Wilkins.

Stuart, E. M., Deckro, J. P., DeSilva, R. A., & Benson, H. (1993). Cardiovascular disease: The heart of the matter. In H. Benson, & E. M. Stuart (Eds.). *The wellness book* (pp. 363–398). New York: Simon & Schuster.

Tommaso, C. L., Lesch, M., & Sonnenblick, E. H. (1984). Alterations in coronary function in coronary artery disease, myocardial infarction, and coronary bypass surgery. In N. K. Wenger & H. K. Hellerstein (Eds.). *Rehabilitation of the coronary patient* (2nd ed., pp. 41–65). New York: Wiley.

Tooth, L., & McKenna, K. (1995). Cardiac patient teaching: Application to patients undergoing coronary angioplasty and their partners. *Patient Education and Counseling, 25*, 1–8.

Webb J., & Hochman, J. S. (1997). Pathophysiology and management of cardiogenic shock due to primary pump failure. In B. J. Gersh & S. H. Rahimtolla (Eds.). *Acute myocardial infarction* (2nd ed., pp. 308–337). New York: Chapman & Hall.

Wegner, N. K. (1984). Early ambulation after myocardial infarction: Rationale, program components, and results. In N. K. Wegner & H. K. Hellerstein (Eds.). *Rehabilitation of the coronary patient* (2nd ed., pp. 97–110). New York: Wiley.

Wegner, N. K., Froelicher, E. S., Smith, L., Ades, P., Berra, K., Blumenthal, J., et al. (1995). *Cardiac rehabilitation as secondary prevention* [Clinical Practice Guideline No. 17, AHCPR Publication No. 96-0673]. Rockville, MD: U.S. Department of Health and Human Services.

Wilkins, R. L. (1995). Interpretation of blood gases. In R. L. Wilkins, S. J. Krider, & R. L. Sheldon (Eds.). *Clinical assessment in respiratory care* (3rd ed., pp. 103–124). Boston: Mosby.

CHAPTER 42

OCCUPATIONAL THERAPY FOR ADULTS WITH IMMUNOLOGICAL DISEASES: AIDS AND CANCER

MICHAEL PIZZI and ANN BURKHARDT

The immune system defends the body against microorganisms, such as bacteria and viruses, and destroys abnormal cells produced by dysfunctions in cellular DNA. When the immune system is impaired, the body is especially susceptible to infection from microorganisms and the unchecked proliferation of abnormal cells. Two common adult immunological diseases are **human immunodeficiency virus** (HIV) infection, which leads to **acquired immunodeficiency syndrome** (AIDS), and cancer. In HIV infection, a virus directly attacks the immune system, rendering it ineffective in fighting off infections from microorganisms. In cancer, the immune system is ineffective in controlling the growth of abnormal cells. This chapter describes occupational therapy evaluations and interventions specific to adults with these two diseases.

HIV INFECTION AND AIDS

Causes and Demographics

HIV infection is caused by a retrovirus, Retroviruses contain RNA but not DNA; they use their RNA to produce DNA once they have gained entry to a host cell—a reversal of the usual sequence during which DNA directs the production of RNA. HIV specifically targets cells in the body that have CD4 receptors on their surface membranes: the

T-4 helper lymphocytes (also known as CD4+ cells) and some cells in the central nervous system (CNS), gastrointestinal tract (GI), and uterine cervix. HIV ultimately destroys its target cells, causing immune, CNS, GI, and uterine dysfunctions. The damage to the immune system makes people vulnerable to a wide range of opportunistic infections (microorganisms that take advantage of the opportunity afforded by a compromised immune system). Death from HIV infection is usually the result of these opportunistic infections (Kassler, 1993; Springhouse Corporation [Springhouse], 1995).

HIV is transmitted by exposure to blood or body secretions of individuals who are infected with the virus. This can occur through sexual transmission, blood transfusion, sharing of needles, and gestation (mother to child). AIDS was first described in the homosexual populations in New York and California in 1981. Soon thereafter, it was found among children, intravenous drug users, and hemophiliacs and other individuals who had received blood transfusions. The disease is now becoming especially prevalent in heterosexual women and young adults who have no known risk factors other than their sexual behavior (Kassler, 1993; Springhouse, 1995).

Stages of HIV Infection: Signs and Symptoms

There are four stages of HIV infection

- *Acute infection:* The body's initial short-lived flulike response to the virus.
- *Asymptomatic disease:* HIV continues to replicate in the body and affect the immune system, but not enough to cause signs and symptoms.
- *Symptomatic:* HIV has done enough damage to the immune system to cause signs and symptoms.
- *Advanced disease or AIDS:* The immune system is severely compromised.

Beginning in the asymptomatic stage, the CD4+ cell count begins to drop from its normal level of $>1000/mm^3$ of blood; in AIDS, CD4+ counts are $<200/mm^3$. Diagnosis of any stage depends on both laboratory and clinical findings (Kassler, 1993; Springhouse, 1995).

HIV transforms itself rapidly, thus creating difficulty for researchers to develop a vaccine or cure. However, the drug treatments to improve life quality have dramatically altered the life spans of people with HIV. Currently, there are drugs that are made to alter the attachment of the HIV to the T-cell or interfere with reverse transcriptase action within the cell. The most profound discovery is the use of protease inhibitors, which inhibit HIV's final assembly before leaving the cell, and the drug cocktails, which combine three or more drugs that interact with one another and interfere with HIV at many levels. These have proven to be the most effective defense against HIV infection. On the horizon are drugs that work outside of the cell membrane and that have no side effects thus far in clinical trials (Park, 2001).

Occupational therapists working with people who have HIV should have knowledge of the infection's pharmacology and side effects as they affect occupational performance. Drugs that are extending the lives of people with HIV and AIDS provide occupational therapists more opportunities to explore wellness and health promotion in community-based interventions.

Occupational Therapy Diagnostic Considerations

There are a variety of sequelae associated with the symptomatic and advanced stages of HIV infection. One common sign is generalized lymphadenopathy, or enlargement of the lymph nodes. Other signs include fever and diarrhea. These problems can deplete the client's energy and tolerance for activity. Neurological disorders often accompany advanced stage disease (AIDS). Cognitive impairment, affective and sensory changes owing to dementia, myelopathy (pathology of the spinal cord), and peripheral neuropathies can occur as a direct result of the disease itself or as side effects of pharmaceutical treatments.

Cognitive impairment that leads to poor safety may limit the choices for home care. Affective changes interfere with communication and expression. Personality is often altered and interpersonal relationships are often changed. Sensory changes can interfere with the simplest of basic activities of daily living (ADL), especially if an individual cannot hold on to tools and implements they use daily: feeding utensils, combs, tissues, money, and the telephone.

If hyperesthesia (unusual sensibility to stimuli) is part of the sensory change, touch can be painful and aversive. Visual changes can occur because of some opportunistic infections. For example, cytomegalovirus infection can cause retinopathy and result in low vision or blindness. When both vision and somatic sensation are impaired, engaging in and successfully completing simple daily tasks become problematic. Life roles are adversely changed.

Wellness and HIV

Occupational therapists, through occupation and client-centered care, foster the promotion of health and wellness, including healthy attitudes and habits and routines for living (Finn, 1972; Johnson, 1993; Pizzi, 1990a; Reitz, 1992; White, 1986; Wiemer & West, 1970). Given the vastly improved drug regimen afforded people with HIV and AIDS, people are living longer than when the epidemic began in the 1980s. Examples of the drugs being used are the following (Park, 2001):

- *Zidovudine therapy (AZT):* This drug keeps HIV from converting its viral genome into one that is compatible with human DNA.
- *Protease inhibitors:* These hinder HIV's final assembly before leaving the cell.
- *New drugs:* Fusion or entry inhibitors (e.g., T-20 and T-1249) that potentially keep HIV from penetrating

the cells are currently being tested in clinical trials; if they are effective they have the advantage of keeping the immune system intact.

- *Molecular decoys:* Research is being conducted on the development of decoy, or fake, CD4 cells, which could lure HIV away from the human cell.

Approximately 30% of people taking drugs have the dual problems of toxicity and resistance. Either the body wears out or the individuals cannot or will not keep up with their drug schedules. Occupational therapy can help people gain the new habits required to maintain these demanding drug regimens. In addition, practitioners can help people adapt activities as needed to accommodate the drugs' side effects that impact occupational performance.

Factors Affecting Occupational Performance

Physical Functions

Fatigue, shortness of breath, visual impairments, peripheral and central neuropathies, various forms of cancer, opportunistic infections, cardiac problems, and the wasting syndrome may all develop over the course of infection with HIV. Physical pain may occur from a variety of causes, including peripheral nervous system (PNS) damage. Postural changes, with or without a formal underlying neurological diagnosis, may occur in association with extreme weight loss. These postural changes can also result in pain (Galantino, Mukand, & Freed, 1991). Damage to the central nervous system (CNS) results in dementia, spinal cord dysfunction, and stroke. Both PNS and CNS dysfunctions may be accompanied by gait disturbances, balance impairment, and restricted mobility, as well as changes in muscle tone. Range of motion (ROM), strength, coordination, and sensation can be affected, resulting in mild to severe changes in function. Physical problems must be fully assessed for their effect on occupational roles (Galantino & Pizzi, 1991).

Mental Functions

The disease caused by HIV is often viewed only in terms of its progressive course. The psychosocial effect of hearing the diagnosis may result in depression, anxiety, and guilt. People infected with the disease may become preoccupied with death and the process of dying. Anger accompanies the adjustment process—anger at the disease, at the prospect of a lonely and painful death, at the lack of available medical treatment, at the medical staff, and at oneself.

Anxiety, manifested as tension, stress, tachycardia, agitation, insomnia, anorexia, and panic attacks, serves to perpetuate an already maladaptive cycle of behavior. Neuropsychiatric symptoms, such as forgetfulness, lack of concentration, apathy, withdrawal, and decreased alertness, can occur. In the later stages of disease, confusion and disorientation may become evident.

Physical disfigurement caused by AIDS often leads to problems with self-image. This coupled with neuropsychiatric dysfunction may result in limited social and occupational activity. Feelings of lost control over their life and loss of mastery of the self may lead clients with AIDS to state that the disease seems to be controlling their life. Such ideas, in turn, contribute to the development of feelings of helplessness and hopelessness, and thus to clinical depression. Occupational therapy practitioners need to help clients rediscover meaning in the presence of such life-altering change (Pizzi, 1991). Adaptation of life roles is needed. Grief and bereavement issues related to the loss of prior life roles should be considered by the occupational therapy practitioner in conjunction with other team members.

Contextual Factors

The inability of family members and significant others to cope with revelations concerning disease-related risk behaviors of a loved one can lead to alienation of clients with HIV infection. Partners may leave the relationship because of fear, guilt, illness, or perceived inability to care for a person with a chronic condition. Occupational therapy practitioners must be aware of how these possibilities can affect the occupational therapy process and the client's functioning.

The physical environment may become too challenging for people who experience fatigue, shortness of breath, and visual or somatic sensory losses. Their restricted mobility at home, work, or in the community may make it difficult for them to balance the activity demands of self-care, work, and leisure. Visual and somatic sensory problems may also make it difficult to negotiate physical environments.

Physical and social environments may be affected by a change in job status and income. Individuals who do not have adequate disability coverage can lose their homes, families, and friends. The threat of homelessness may be quite real. Once-pleasurable avocational activities, such as going to the movies or out to dinner, may be beyond their current economic resources. The occupational therapist must consider the economic situation of clients before making intervention recommendations, particularly if clients must purchase equipment and materials to maintain productivity (Pizzi, 1991).

Occupational Therapy Evaluation

Clients with HIV must prioritize their goals. Long-term goals may become short-term ones, necessitating shifts in habits, time management, and engagement in productive pursuits. Personal values become more meaningful, and they often shift from concrete materialism to a more spiritual arena. Symbolism, control, temporal rhythms, occupation, and occupational role and environment are themes that guide occupational therapy practice for clients with HIV and AIDS (Clark & Jackson, 1990).

Before an assessment, therapists must determine the need to observe any special infection precautions. When therapists have a cold or the flu, they should wear a mask to avoid infecting their clients with compromised immune systems. Therapists should follow infection control precautions (**universal precautions**) with all clients, regardless of their HIV status. In addition, special infection control precautions should be followed when these are posted outside a client's room.

Relative to universal infection precautions, all practitioners should be familiar with the infection control procedures at the facilities and agencies in which they work. Generally, occupational therapy practitioners need to wash their hands before and after seeing each client. Gloves are worn when assisting with ADL, if it is likely that the occupational therapy practitioner is coming into contact with body fluids or blood. Gowns, masks, and goggles are worn if there is risk of body fluid splashes (e.g., a client who is spitting up sputum or experiencing diarrhea).

Because people with HIV infection have specialized problems and needs, it is advisable to use specific assessment batteries created for this population. Pizzi developed two assessments for use with this population: The first focuses on wellness and the second is designed for timely assessment of clients with less endurance.

The Pizzi Holistic Wellness Assessment (PHWA) was developed to capture subjectively the narrative of clients' lives; clients assess their level of well-being in eight categories of health (Pizzi, 2001). People with HIV who have been given the assessment found it helpful for discovering their self-perceptions of well-being; for learning how to take action in different areas to create healthier living; and, with the coaching of an occupational therapist, for developing meaningful ways to engage or reengage in health-promoting occupations. The positive attitude of the occupational therapist—an attitude in which HIV is viewed as a chronic but life-altering challenge—is quintessential in occupational therapy assessment and intervention. It is one that promotes well-being across the HIV continuum.

The second assessment is the Pizzi Assessment of Productive Living (PAPL) for adults with HIV infection and AIDS (Pizzi, 1993). This assessment was developed to assess holistically, in a short time, all domains of function and occupational behaviors of a client (Box 42-1). The time variable is important, because many people with HIV and/or AIDS have limited endurance. In addition, because managed care limits therapists' ability to provide more than a pre-fixed amount of care, time management is essential.

For ADL, work, and leisure, therapists must weigh the importance of activity participation for the person involved. If basic ADL consume too much time and energy, the therapist may recommend that the client allow a caregiver to do at least one such activity, so that he or she has the energy and time to participate in an activity of greater meaning. It is also important to assess if there are particular times of day when the client feels more energetic, so activities can be planned to make use of the enhanced tolerance at those times. Consideration of stress triggers is also important for evaluation, case management, and intervention planning, because stress contributes to immunosuppression.

As people live longer via improved drug regimens and improved education about strategies for survival, occupational therapy practitioners have the opportunity to engage clients in occupation-based activities that support continued wellness through a balance of engagement in spiritually meaningful self-care, work, play/leisure and restful tasks. The following observations and strategies listed in the intervention section will help optimize the clients ability to live with greater quality and dignity.

Occupational Therapy Intervention

The purpose of occupational therapy intervention for adults with HIV infection is to enhance competent performance of self-chosen occupations that contribute to valued roles. Data from assessments, such as the PAPL, outline problem areas to be addressed during intervention.

There are several special considerations for therapists when developing intervention plans and goals for the person with HIV infection. Medical conditions that may accompany HIV infection are infectious processes and require special isolation procedures. In a hospital setting, the isolation procedure is often posted at the door of the room or is available at the nursing station. If there are no special precautions, the practitioner should use universal precautions with all clients, regardless of their HIV status. Subtle cognitive and physical changes can occur rapidly, so frequent informal reevaluation of these areas is important.

Discrimination against and negative social judgments of people with HIV infection are inappropriate. All clients are entitled to nonjudgmental care and acceptance as people. Many clients with this disease have dealt with a number of personal losses during their illness. Mourning is a natural reaction to this loss.

The lack of a cure for HIV infection, at the time of this writing, affects the hope of and the reality that will be faced in the future. Alternatives and modifications to allow a client to continue working are valuable. Fatigue and weakness limit activity tolerance and the client's ability to participate. Thus energy conservation, work simplification, and occupational adaptations can enhance productivity.

Although adaptive equipment and positioning may enhance activity participation and preserve skill, clients who are in denial may not be able psychologically to accept these alternatives when they are needed. This denial must be respected until clients can deal with the underlying issue.

Self-esteem can be enhanced when clients are given some control over their schedule and routine. As skill competence is challenged with disease progression, control through choices facilitates positive feelings of self-worth and empowerment. Complementary and alternative medical techniques may enhance the quality of life and decrease pain and dependency on drugs. Some of the techniques used include progressive relaxation, biofeedback, prayer, therapeutic touch, Chinese traditional medicine, energy work, myofascial release, craniosacral therapy, imagery, and visualization.

BOX 42–1 PAPL[a]

DEMOGRAPHICS

Name ______ Age ______ Sex ______
Lives with (relationship) ______
Identified caregiver ______
Race ______ Culture ______ Religion (practicing?) ______
Primary occupational roles ______
Primary diagnosis ______
Secondary diagnosis ______
Stage of HIV ______
Past medical history ______
Medications ______

ADL (USE ADL PERFORMANCE ASSESSMENT)

Are you doing these now? ______
Do you perform homemaking tasks? ______

For Areas of Difficulty

Would you like to be able to do these again like you did before? ______
Which ones? ______

Work

Job ______
When last worked ______
Describe type of activity ______
Work environment ______
If not working, would you like to be able to? ______
Do you miss being productive? ______

Play/Leisure

Types of activity engaged in ______
If not, would you like to? Which ones? ______
Would you like to try other things as well? ______
Is it important to be independent in daily living activities? ______

PHYSICAL FUNCTION

Active and passive ROM ______
Strength ______
Sensation ______
Coordination (gross and fine motor or dexterity) ______

Visual–Perceptual

Hearing ______
Balance (sit and stand) ______
Ambulation, transfers, and mobility ______
Activity tolerance and endurance ______

Pain

Location ______
Does it interfere with doing important activities? ______

Other

Sexual function ______

Continues

BOX 42–1 PAPL[a] *(Continued)*

Cognition (attention span, problem solving, memory, orientation, judgment, reasoning, decision making, safety awareness) ______

______

TIME ORGANIZATION

Former daily routine (before diagnosis) ______
Has this changed since diagnosis? ______
If so, how? ______
Are there certain times of day that are better for you to carry out daily tasks? ______
Do you consider yourself regimented in organizing time and activity or pretty flexible? ______
What would you change, if anything, in how your day is set up? ______

BODY IMAGE AND SELF-IMAGE

In the last 6 months, has there been a change in your physical body and how it looks? ______
How do you feel about this? ______

SOCIAL ENVIRONMENT

Describe support available and used by patient ______

PHYSICAL ENVIRONMENT

Describe environments in which the patient performs daily tasks and the level of support or impediment for function ______

STRESSORS

What are some things, people, or situations that are/were stressful? ______
What are some current ways you manage stress? ______

SITUATIONAL COPING

How do you feel you are dealing with:
Your diagnosis ______
Changes in the ability to do things important to you ______
Other psychosocial observations ______

OCCUPATIONAL QUESTIONS

What do you feel to be important to you right now? ______
Do you feel you can do things important to you now? ______
In the future? ______
Do you deal well with change? ______
What are your hopes, dreams, aspirations? ______
What are some of your goals? ______
Have these changed since you were diagnosed? How? ______
Do you feel in control of your life at this time? ______
What do you wish to accomplish with the rest of your life? ______

OCCUPATIONAL THERAPY

Plan ______
Short-term goals ______
Long-term goals ______
Frequency ______
Duration ______
Therapist ______

[a]Adapted from Pizzi, M. (1991). HIV infection and occupational therapy. In J. Mukand (Ed.). *Rehabilitation for patients with HIV disease* (pp. 283–326). New York: McGraw-Hill.

Wellness is inextricably connected with nutrition. Occupational therapy practitioners can collaborate with nutritionists to develop strategies clients can use to follow a sound nutritional program. Sometimes after assessing the safety of oral feeding, therapists may recommend alternative nutritional methods. For example, feeding tubes can assist clients in obtaining the calories needed to feel stronger, if eating by mouth becomes too energy-consuming or painful. Oral candidiasis (yeast infection) can cause dysphagia. Neurological manifestations of AIDS can also contribute to dysphagia. Sometimes a feeding tube gives a client a new lease on life. If the client regains the ability to swallow, oral feeding can be resumed. For people with loss of appetite, the tube can be used to supplement caloric intake. If they recover from the dysphagia or loss of appetite, the tube can be pulled.

The intervention focus must change and be modified throughout the course of a client's HIV infection. For clients who are symptomatic, the treatment is tailored to the sequelae exhibited. People with neurological sequelae may benefit from compensatory training, caregiver education, and adaptive equipment. In general, energy conservation, health promotion, and wellness strategies can enhance immunocompetence and physical and psychosocial well-being. As the disease progresses, adaptive strategies, environmental modification, and modification of ADL techniques can be added to preserve a sense of mastery and self-control (Denton, 1987; Gutterman, 1990; Pizzi, 1988, 1989, 1990a, 1991; Weinstein, 1990).

Pain management becomes increasingly important over time. Myofascial release, craniosacral therapy, acupressure, biofeedback, imagery, and visualization may be useful (Galantino et al., 1991). As the disease progresses, the strategies used should be adapted to the level of participation and understanding of the recipient.

In the later stages of the disease process, adjustment to dying, grief, loss, and bereavement become central issues of daily life. The theme of therapy may then shift to focus on projects with inherent symbolism for the client. For example, a project such as making a memory book or a time capsule to leave behind for friends and loved ones is often valuable. Spiritual needs must be expressed. A sense of accomplishment with one's life is key to issues of self-esteem and feelings of self-worth. Assistance with the achievement of comfort during all occupations, including sleep, supports the quality of life.

At later stages in the disease, the therapeutic use of self is individualized and depends on the level of comfort of the practitioner given the situation. Some practitioners want to support the family through the death experience. For others, this is too intense or too draining. Therapists who are less comfortable with spirituality and the concept of death may withdraw or take a respite from the case at this time. Teaching and training caregivers may be the most effective use of treatment time as the disease progresses (Pizzi, 1990b).

CANCER

Causes

Cancer is a malignant neoplasm. Neoplasms are proliferations of abnormal cells that arise from organs within the body. These abnormal cells usually form a solid mass, or tumor, as in breast cancer. Sometimes neoplasms do not form solid tumors, as in leukemia in which the abnormal cells are lymphocytes. Neoplasms are characterized as *malignant* when they invade surrounding cells, disrupting the function of those cells. Malignant tumors can also metastasize, or send abnormal cells to other parts of the body through the blood or lymph systems. The branch of medicine that deals with cancer is called oncology.

Cancers may be low grade or high grade. Low-grade tumors tend to be slower growing, and their cell structures are more uniform and consistent. They often respond well to surgery, chemotherapy, hormone treatment, and radiation. One example of a low-grade tumor is prostate cancer. Adenocarcinoma (malignancy of epithelial tissue of a gland) of the prostate is quite slow growing and not highly metastatic. In contrast, high-grade tumors are rapidly growing and tend to metastasize to other organs. They are generally more resistive to conventional oncological treatment. One example of a high-grade tumor is inflammatory breast cancer. It is aggressive, resistive to chemotherapy and radiation treatment, and metastasizes readily to other areas of the body (e.g., lung, brain, liver, and bone).

Cancers are staged from the time of the diagnosis through progression of the disease. There are many staging systems in use. Perhaps the easiest to understand is the tumor, metastasis, node system (TMN). The presence of tumor(s) and the number of primary tumors is designated by the "T" number. The number of metastases is represented by the "M," and the "N" signifies the number of positive lymph nodes. For example, a client who presents with T1, M0, and N0 has a detectable tumor that has not spread. The general prognosis still depends on the virulence of the tumor type itself, but the staging tells the therapists that the cancer was detected before any perceivable spread of the disease. In contrast, a client who is staged at T1, M2, and N12 has more advanced disease (Burkhardt & Joachim, 1996).

Demographics and Sequelae

People of all ages, from infancy through old age, can develop cancer. When people develop cancer, they often lose or gain a significant amount of body weight for no logical reason. Tumors have a higher metabolic rate than normal tissues. Many cancers grow extensive circulatory networks around themselves and withdraw nutrients from the bloodstream, which leads to weight loss. This increased metabolism of tumors allows them to grow and replace themselves more rapidly than normal tissue. It is also what makes the tumor cells more vulnerable to cell death from chemotherapy and radiation treatment.

Other sequelae experienced by clients with a diagnosis of cancer are caused by the effect of the primary cancer itself on normal tissues; the extent and location of the surgery performed to resect or bypass the tumor; and the side effects of chemotherapy, hormone therapy, immunotherapy, or radiation therapy.

Direct Effects of Cancer

Primary tumors can develop in virtually any organ of the human body. The sequelae from a primary tumor may be related to the function of the primary organ. For example, in liver cancer the liver enzymes may become elevated, and the client may become jaundiced. The increase in liver enzymes makes the person fatigue easily, complain of arthralgias (joint pains), and have a low tolerance for activity.

Effects of Surgery

Many tumors can be completely resected from the body. That is, the tumor is removed en bloc, in a whole piece. With limb tumors, if the tumor has not entangled itself with the nerves or blood vessels (the neurovascular bundle), amputation can be avoided. These surgeries are referred to as limb sparing. If the tumor involves the neurovascular bundle, an amputation may be the only recourse. If internal organs, such as the pancreas or the liver, are involved, it may be necessary to remove part or all of the organ and replace its function with supplemental medication. If tumor resection is not possible, sometimes bypass surgery is done to bypass a tumor-related obstruction and allow the affected organ to continue functioning as the disease advances.

Chemotherapy

There are several classes of drugs used in chemotherapy: alkylating agents, antibiotics, antimetabolites, mitotic inhibitors, and miscellaneous drugs. The majority of these agents are synthetic chemicals, although some of the antibiotics and mitotic inhibitors are derived from natural, organic constituents. These drugs are considered to be hazardous substances (Briggs, Freeman, & Yaffe, 1990). The high metabolism of tumors makes them susceptible to controlling with chemotherapy, because tumors absorb the chemotoxins before the normal tissues do. Consequently, the concentration of chemotoxins in the blood used by tumors is higher than the concentration in freely circulating blood.

The sequelae associated with chemotherapy depend on the type of chemotherapy used and its effect on normal tissues of the body. Some chemotherapy drugs are mild, with side effects often imperceptible or identifiable only by minor changes in constitutional symptoms, such as changes in bowel activity. Other chemotherapy agents cause highly perceptible changes, such as hair loss, paresthesias (sensory changes characterized by tingling and numbness of the distal extremities), muscle weakness, or vascular changes in the limbs and may result in increased incidence of orthostatic hypotension or permanent nerve damage.

It is important for health-care workers who work around chemotherapy agents to be careful of their own exposure to the drugs. These can induce cancer in the caregiver over time. Standard precautions, such as the use of gloves, is indicated to protect health-care workers and others from exposure to the chemotoxins (National Institute for Occupational Safety and Health, 1998)

Hormones

Use of hormones in treatment can produce premature menopause or accentuation of secondary sexual characteristics. For example, diethylstilbestrol (DES), a synthetic estrogen used in the treatment of prostate cancer, can cause enlargement of the breasts in the men being treated with the hormone. Some hormones used to treat prostate cancer produce a chemical orchiectomy (render the testes inactive). In women, hormone-blocking agents are used to prevent the bonding of estrogen to estrogen-dependent breast tumors or progesterone to progesterone-receptor-positive tumors. These drugs can cause premature menopause and weight gain and can lead to the development of primary cancer of the ovaries or uterus.

Radiation

Radiation kills tumor cells by raising their temperature above the their tolerance level. Radiation, however, also affects normal tissues. Near the end of several weeks of radiation treatment, soft tissues become erythematous (red); the skin may be painful, often sustaining the equivalent of a superficial second-degree burn; and local edema is present. While the client is actively undergoing radiation treatment, the use of lotions and topical ointments may be restricted, because lotions and creams change the surface tension of the skin and, in doing so, can enhance the action of the radiation, rather than soothing the sequelae.

Once the radiation treatment is completed and the skin heals, the soft tissues in the path of the radiation continue to change. This process, known as radiation fibrosis, can last for several years. During this time, clients report feeling tightness of soft tissues with movement. This sensation is associated with a loss of elasticity and resultant tightening of the tissues. People with this problem are at risk for losing movement, particularly when the radiation was given over or adjacent to a joint. For instance, clients with head and neck cancer or breast cancer may have radiation involving their glenohumeral joint. Their shoulder may progressively stiffen, and they can develop adhesive capsulitis as part of the fibrosis.

ROM and soft tissue mobilization techniques, such as myofascial release, may preserve or restore normal movement. These techniques may be needed for the 3-year window of time in which the fibrosis is active. Once the fibrosis settles down, clients can generally keep the motion they have without further exercise. Therefore, ROM and mobilization techniques are strategic during and after radiation therapy treatment while radiation fibrosis is occurring. Scar management, especially using silicone gel pads, can assist by softening the irradiated tissues and preserving the elasticity of the soft tissues during the postradiation phase of recovery (Burkhardt & Weitz, 1990).

Another unfortunate side effect of radiation treatment is the loss of myelin from nerves, resulting in decreased sensory and motor nerve function of the demyelinated nerves. One common example is brachial plexopathy (demyelinization of the nerves branching off from the brachial plexus). Clients who receive radiation for breast or lung cancer may develop brachial plexopathy. Radiation-induced plexopathy is a permanent loss of nerve function. It is often progressive and results in significant functional loss in the client's affected upper extremity. The associated sensory changes may or may not result in pain. If the individual experiences burning hyperesthesias that interfere with sleep and significantly impair quality of life, the affected nerve may be blocked to remove the sensation of pain (e.g., phenol block or electrical stimulation blocks), or the client may be placed on specific drugs to diminish the neuropathic pain. Transcutaneous electrical nerve stimulation (TENS) may be used near the origin of the point of pain to block pain messages. TENS should never be used on a limb in which lymph nodes have been removed or irradiated. Sometimes use of superficial vibration can positively influence the hyperesthesia.

When sensation is impaired, safety is an issue that must be addressed in therapy. Functional changes are managed with positioning and use of adapted ADL devices or treatment techniques to compensate for lost function (Cook & Burkhardt, 1994).

Occupational Therapy Evaluation

Occupational therapy evaluations should encompass physical, psychological, and social aspects of living, because all of these areas affect the client's life occupations. Evaluations should be done to assess both client factors and contextual factors affecting occupational performance. The therapist should evaluate the following:

- Mobility, including all of the usual subsets of movement (ROM, muscle strength, dexterity, coordination, speed of movement, and purpose of movement).
- Sensation (protective and discriminative).
- Cognition.
- Vision (acuity and visual perception).
- Basic and instrumental ADL.
- Work activities.
- Leisure activities.
- Social participation.
- Ability to plan and obtain adequate rest.

Occupational Therapy Intervention

The type of occupational therapy intervention depends on the course of the disease and treatment and the client's medical status at the time of referral. In a hospital setting, immediately after surgery, or during chemotherapy or radiation treatment, the purpose of an occupational therapy referral may be to improve general mobility and basic self-care ability. Swallowing may also be an issue if the client develops dysphagia from neurological damage, surgical resection involving the oral or oral pharyngeal cavity, or fungal infections of the oral pharyngeal cavity (fungal infections commonly occur in all immunosuppressed people).

After the initial staging and treatment of the disease, referrals are often made to treat limitations in joint mobility (e.g., early onset of adhesive capsulitis); lymphedema (edema caused by obstruction of the lymphatics); difficulty eating or swallowing; instability involving the trunk or a limb(s); loss or impairment of hand or upper extremity function; scar management, splinting, and positioning; fabrication of cosmetic devices (in the event of soft tissue compromise); alterations in body image; depression; an adjustment disorder; or somatosensory pain syndromes.

With progression of the disease, or in the event of progressive conditions associated with treatment, such as radiation-induced brachial plexopathy, the emphasis of treatment shifts to supportive care: positioning to optimize functioning or to reduce pain, or rehabilitative approaches to substitute for lost function (Dietz, 1974). Counseling concerning changes in life roles is important at this point. Some practitioners fail to recognize the value of counseling at this juncture. Developing support for self-esteem and engendering hope can make the difference between a feeling of well-being and the assumption of the sick role. Also, other health-care professionals may not be aware that occupational therapy practitioners address these issues.

With advancing disease, palliative or comfort care becomes the focus of intervention (Dietz, 1974). The occupational therapy practitioner's role in palliative care is to help the client maintain some degree of mastery over the environment and to meet emotional needs. Sometimes clients need only low-technology equipment, such as a long-handled reacher, to control their environments. When the cancer has caused severe disability, technologically advanced equipment, such as computerized communication and environmental control systems may be needed. For emotional needs, occupational therapy practitioners can empower individuals by helping them successfully complete activities of importance to them. Practitioners can also interact in ways that tell clients they are valued. For instance, accepting compliments from clients with advancing disease allows them to realize that their opinion still matters. Sharing something they love, such as a piece of literature, a poem, or music, communicates respect and appreciation. Allowing reminiscence and formulating tapes or writings of things remembered can also be helpful. The use of techniques such as massage or guided imagery may promote a sense of well-being or pleasure.

Preventative care is also an important aspect of any rehabilitation program (Dietz, 1974). In reference to cancer, providing wellness strategies while intervening with a population at risk for cancer is important. For instance, smoking tobacco leads to lung cancer, breast cancer, head and neck cancer, and cardiovascular disease. Working on smoking cessation, in all occupational therapy settings, is a viable form of preventative care (Williams, Burkhardt, & Royce, 1995). Another example of prevention is teaching stress reduction techniques with all populations of clients, because stress can lead to other risk behaviors that can contribute to cancer, such as poor diet and abuse of drugs or alcohol.

Factors Influencing Treatment

There are several precautions that are important to consider when treating clients with cancer. When someone has had surgery, initial precautions include protection of the incision or resection site and mobility limitations. Practitioners need to be careful not to pull skin incision open during procedures such as ROM. Once the incision is healed, full movement should resume, unless there was reconstruction to the site.

Reconstructive procedures have highly specific mobility allowances that should be obtained directly from the surgeon(s). For example, if a tendon transfer or a flap has been done, the surgeon may wish to ensure the reconstruction is stable before movement training is begun. Although similar to reconstructive procedures done with hand injuries, the orders for these cases may need to be individualized, because there is greater tissue compromise associated with a tumor resection. Radiation may have had an additional influence on the site as well.

Chemotherapy can cause several conditions that warrant treatment precautions. The first and foremost of these is thrombocytopenia, a diminished platelet level. Platelets assist the blood to clot and are important in terms of recovery from trauma. When the universal platelet level dips to low levels, such as <45,000–50,000 units, resistive activity should be avoided (Burkhardt & Joachim, 1996). Care should be taken to avoid cuts and bruises when platelets are low, because bleeding can readily result and may require extensive time to be controlled.

Myelosuppression is also a concern for clients who are receiving chemotherapy or undergoing bone marrow transplantation. Myelosuppression predisposes individuals to infections. Sometimes common infections can be fatal for a person with myelosuppression because the immune response is severely suppressed. Anemia, another side effect of chemotherapy, lowers tolerance for activity, because often even basic ADL may result in shortness of breath and fatigue. Pacing and conservation of energy are important with all of the aforementioned complications. Arrhythmias may also occur in response to chemotherapy; in these clients, occupational therapy treatment should be avoided until the arrhythmia is stabilized with medication.

Orthopedic precautions are a concern if the individual is at risk for a pathological fracture owing to bony metastases or if there has been bony resection of a limb. There is a drug now being used for people who have bony lesions from breast cancer or multiple myeloma (Berenson, Lichtenstein, Porter, Dimopoulos, Bordonie, & George et al, 1998). This drug Aredia (Novartis Pharmaceuticals Corporation, 1999) helps reduce the chance of bone complications from fractures, surgery, and radiation. Aredia can be effective in treating bone complications, whether or not the client has already experienced evidence of bone metastases. Aredia can decrease bone pain in some breast cancer and multiple myeloma patients. Studies have demonstrated that some clients needed fewer doses or a lower strength of pain medication; others were able to switch from narcotics to over-the-counter pain relievers.

Often, clients are encouraged to use their limbs for light ADL activities, despite the risk of a pathological fracture, because disuse leads to significant decreases in limb function. The presence of metastases to bone may limit tolerance for activities with inherent torsion and torque, because these activities may result in a fracture. When a client has had resection of a bony lesion, the precautions depend on the presence of a joint replacement, bone graft, or fusion. Limb-sparing procedures may have a different outcome than noncancer arthroplasty surgeries, as resection of soft tissue may be necessary, depending on the infiltration of the tumor. Specific postoperative protocols should be obtained from or developed in collaboration with the surgical team.

Swelling of a limb(s), may occur as a result of compression of the lymphatics, lymphatic invasion by tumor, decreased functioning of the lymphatics associated with lymph node resection or irradiation, or cellulitis (inflammation of the involved limb) (Burkhardt & Joachim, 1992). With lymphedema, the person may have pain and decreased use of the arm or leg. Energy conservation and work simplification may be important aspects to consider in developing a treatment plan.

LIFE ISSUES TO CONSIDER IN PRACTICE 42-1

Dying and End-of-Life Care

QUESTIONS AND EXERCISES

1. What do you personally, and as a health-care professional, believe about death and the process of dying?
2. Do you think you would have the objective insight and honest communication skills needed to help individuals work toward end-of-life goals?

ETHICS NOTE 42–1

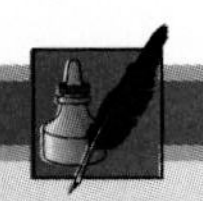

Cultural Issues in Client Education

Christine is a devout Muslim, born and raised in the United States. Sam recently immigrated to the United States from Agra, India. After being on a waiting list, both are in the interdisciplinary patient education program for individuals with neurofibromatosis. The occupational therapy department donates its time to do a cooking group to demonstrate safety techniques. The menu for the evening group is roast pork, mash potatoes, peas, and a salad.

The therapist begins her discussion, and immediately Christine voices concerns about the menu since it is against her religion to eat pork. Sam objects to any kitchen activities. He angrily states he has never been in a kitchen, does not cook, and does not want any part of this activity since no respectable Indian man would do any cooking. The therapist is taken aback by these objections.

QUESTIONS AND EXERCISES

1. **What, if any, are the therapist's responsibilities to be aware and sensitive to cultural issues regarding foods?**
2. **What are her obligations to the hospital's patient education program?**
3. **Does it make any difference that the activity is a volunteer service rather than a reimbursed form of intervention?**

Issues of Death and Dying

Clients' concepts of death and their spiritual beliefs influence their abilities to cope with the diagnosis of cancer, especially if the disease is likely to be progressive. Adults may find spirituality for the first time when they are dealing with a diagnosis of cancer. Some people tell of renewed faith and strong beliefs in the power of prayer. Guilt may be expressed concerning the suspected influence of past behaviors that may have contributed to the development of a diagnosis of cancer (such as smoking for a person with lung cancer).

Many people do not reach a level of acceptance concerning death. The greatest challenge is for the individual to remain hopeful, despite the progressive nature of the disease. Other clients, who actually have a good prognosis, need education and reassurance to accept the reality that many people today who have such a diagnosis are treated and continue to survive, without any life span shortening.

Consistently doing what you promise to do, making repeat visits, listening, and generally demonstrating a caring attitude engender trust and a sense of well-being between practitioner and cancer survivor. Accountability is the underlying issue supporting the development of trust (Burkhardt & Joachim, 1996). Some practitioners wax and wane in their ability to work with people facing life decisions. In your own practice, you may find this to be something about which you are introspective and acutely aware. Attempting to treat a client may also unexpectedly awaken

CASE STUDY 42–1

Valerie: A Woman Dying of Breast Cancer

EVALUATION

Valerie, a 42-year-old woman with a diagnosis of breast cancer, was referred to occupational therapy for management of her left arm lymphedema. She had recently had a recurrence of her breast cancer. The initial diagnosis of breast cancer was made 3 years earlier. At the time of diagnosis, Valerie had a modified radical mastectomy. Then, 5 months before the recurrence, she underwent reconstructive surgery: a transrectus abdominis mammoplasty (TRAM). She was last seen by the plastic surgeon 2 weeks before the referral for an episode of cellulitis in the involved arm. At that time she was treated with a broad-spectrum antibiotic and was started on a diuretic regimen. She continued to have swelling and also complained of reflex muscle spasm in her shoulder and upper back.

On evaluation, it was noted that Valerie had erythema of her breast and chest wall. Her sensory evaluation was significant for intermittent tingling, in a glovelike distribution, in her left arm. Her shoulder ROM was severely limited in a capsular pattern of mobility. Her strength was diminished in a pattern consistent with upper brachial plexopathy involvement. On palpation, an enlarged, hardened cervical lymph node was felt. Valerie stated that she refused chemotherapy with this exacerbation, because she had doubts that the chemotherapy had helped the first time. She had been seeing a homeopathic physician and practiced chelation therapy.

Valerie was fitted with a tubular support bandage and a wrist support. She was provided with several items of adapted equipment, including Dycem, a bath

Continues

sponge, a buttonhook, and a dressing stick. She was given resources and recommendations for additional items she might find useful. A referral was made back to her primary oncologist for a further workup relative to the erythema and the neurological findings.

Valerie's primary oncologist diagnosed metastases to the skin and brachial plexopathy and referred her for emergent radiation therapy. She complained of discomfort positioning her arm. The paresthesias worsened and disrupted her sleep. The doctor placed Valerie on a regimen of amitriptyline (Elavil) to decrease the neuropathic pain, decrease the edema, and enhance relaxation for sleep (the medication was taken at night).

INTERVENTION

Valerie purchased a reclining lounge chair to sleep in at night. She continued to complain of pain in her arm. A program of TENS was begun to control the discomfort. Also, Valerie was fitted with a swathe and sling of foam construction to support the arm during ambulation. She was advised to stop taking the diuretic, because her lymphedema had hardened owing to the drug's dehydration effect. Valerie was instructed in the positioning of her arm during ADL for maximum comfort and function. She was advised not to massage her arm until her medical treatment was completed (because of the degree of lymphadenopathy). Valerie reported that her sleep pattern improved.

Valerie is the mother of three children. She verbalized her concerns over the progression of the cancer and the effect it would have on her boys and her husband. She was concerned how her husband would manage when she was gone. Valerie noted that she wanted to continue her sexual relationship and sought advice on positions that would allow maximum comfort and relief of pain during the activity. She was grateful for the recommendations made and reported that they helped her maintain her physical relationship with her husband, which she still valued.

She was encouraged to begin memory books for her family and to write a series of letters to her family and friends, to gain some control and closure over her fear of leaving everyone behind. She did not want her children to think she had not fought her disease hard enough. The oldest was 14 years old and the youngest was 3. Her husband and parents were supportive of her throughout the advancement of the disease. She wanted so much to be able to give back something to each of them.

Spirituality was extremely important to her. She joked, "My sister-in-law took me off the prayer list because I was doing so well. I called and asked her to put me back on and never to take me off of it again." Valerie stated that prayers others said for her were important to her. She said it made her feel less alone, facing metastatic cancer. It was important to her to have her caregivers understand these feelings and values. She asked everyone she met to keep her in their prayers. It gave her hope. That hope spurred her on to do her best to live as normal a life as her progressing disease allowed.

Valerie was admitted to the hospital one more time, 4 months before her death. She was able to manage her edema and position her arm for maximal comfort. She continued to be able to participate in her basic ADL and homemaking with one person's assistance. She arranged to have hospice care at home so she could be with her family throughout the remainder of her life. Occasionally, she would call her occupational therapist for advice concerning positioning or her lymphedema or with questions that arose concerning daily activities. When she had a doctor's appointment at the medical center, she would schedule a therapy appointment to upgrade her home program as well.

The family, in particular her father and husband, always accompanied her and listened to or were trained to assist with the advice and home program prescribed or upgraded. Valerie freely expressed her concerns over the effect her death would have on her family. Despite her concerns, she almost systematically continued to develop reminiscence strategies to communicate her feelings to her family and to put them at ease about her death. She had a calm perspective concerning her own short yet meaningful life. Valerie was grateful for her family, and she was able to use each moment to the fullest to show her appreciation to them.

Although the practice of the occupational therapist was hospital-based, the approach to case management (balancing visits in person with phone communication) was more of a community-based model. The occupational therapist served as a consultant on lifestyle adjustment and modifications in activities defining Valerie's roles as homemaker, wife, mother, and independent person, always in charge of her own personal care. The choices she made were somewhat unorthodox, from an allopathic medical perspective, but they were her own choices—for better or worse.

CASE ANALYSIS

Valerie was a young woman who had advancing disease. She had made particular choices, against her physician's advice, to opt out of chemotherapy and into alternative medicine solutions. When she was referred to occupational therapy, she was presenting with lymphedema and pain. These complications alone were not enough to indicate a change or worsening of her disease process, but they were limiting relative to her ability to engage successfully in her daily occupations.

Valerie also had developed brachial plexopathy. In view of her lack of other contributing risk factors associated with cancer treatment, the plexopathy indicated an advancement of the cancer condition in her body. Valerie's physicians referred her to a therapist for supportive care. After the discovery of her advancing cancer, her goals became palliative in nature. The intervention had to deal with the emergent issues of edema, pain, and lost function. It also required the therapist to be realistic in assisting Valerie to set new goals that were focused on planning how she wanted to use the rest of her time and energy to prepare her family and herself for her diminishing functional capacity and her eventual death. The focus of the care was occupation-based, despite the reliance on management of critical aspects of her condition that were impairment related. The steps of the treatment that managed impairments were done to allow greater daily activity and social participation.

QUESTIONS AND EXERCISES

1. What is the practitioner's implicit frame of reference in this case?
2. What are some alternative frames of reference that might have effectively organized evaluation and intervention for Valerie?
3. Describe the changes in the frame of reference needed when shifting perspective from prevention focused to restorative-focused to supportive focused and, finally, to palliative focused care.
4. When do you think it is appropriate to switch the focus of treatment from supportive to palliative care?
5. How would you handle a situation in which a terminally ill client wanted to have his or her occupational therapy program focused on restorative goals? For example, suppose a client who has brain lesions and permanent loss of his or her dominant upper extremity wants to regain use of the arm. However, you know that sensory and motor function return will never occur, because of the severity of their condition. What is an appropriate response to that client?

the therapist's own fears and pain of past or recent loss. Using supervision to manage a case, and the therapist's own issues, is important under these circumstances.

Each client that therapists interact with throughout their careers adds new dimensions to their observations and understanding. As therapists grow and experience life, their coping abilities change, as well. Sharing in a client's fears can be threatening to the unprepared or spiritually challenged practitioner. The strength of practitioners to confront their own issues head-on is crucial and the core of the therapeutic use of self.

CONCLUSION

HIV and cancer need to be approached from a holistic perspective, one that integrates both updated medical knowledge and spiritual meaning. Using occupation-based activity supports wellness and nourishes spirit. This chapter illustrates that intervention can be most effective for people experiencing life threatening illnesses when they are treated from wellness models of care. Daily life occupations can be carried out to their fullest, and productive living can be facilitated for any person with HIV or cancer with the right mixture of knowledge, education, and human kindness.

References

Berenson, J. R., Lichtenstein, A., Porter, L., Dimopoulos, M. A., Bordonie, R., George's et al. (1998). Long-term pamidronate treatment of advanced multiple myeloma patients reduces skeletal events. *Journal of Clinical Oncology, 16*, 593–602.

Briggs, G. G., Freeman, R. K., & Yaffe, S. J. (1990). *Drugs in pregnancy and lactation* (3rd ed.). Baltimore: Williams & Wilkins.

Burkhardt, A., & Joachim, L. (1992). Occupational therapy techniques used in the treatment of the edemas. *Occupational Therapy Practice, 4*(1), 8–21.

Burkhardt, A., & Joachim, L. (1996). *A therapist's guide to oncology: Medical issues affecting management*. San Antonio, TX: Therapy Skill Builders.

Burkhardt, A., & Weitz, J. (1990). Oncological applications for silicone gel sheets in soft-tissue contractures. *American Journal of Occupational Therapy, 45*, 460–462.

Clark, F., & Jackson, J. (1990). The application of the occupational science negative heuristic in the treatment of persons with the human immunodeficiency infection. *Occupational Therapy in Health Care, 6*(4), 69–91.

Cook, A., & Burkhardt, A. (1994). The effect of cancer diagnosis and treatment on hand function. *American Journal of Occupational Therapy, 48*, 836–839.

Denton, R. (1987). AIDS: Guidelines for occupational therapy intervention. *American Journal of Occupational Therapy, 41*, 427–432.

Dietz, J. H. Jr. (1974). Rehabilitation of the cancer patient: Its role in the scheme of comprehensive care. *Clinical Bulletin*, 4, 104–107.

Finn, G. (1972). The occupational therapist in prevention programs. *American Journal of Occupational Therapy, 26*, 59–66.

Galantino, M. L., Mukand, J., & Freed, M. M. (1991). Physical therapy management of patients with HIV infection. In J. Mukand (Ed.). *Rehabilitation for patients with HIV disease* (pp. 257–282). New York: McGraw-Hill.

Galantino, M. L., & Pizzi, M. (1991). Occupational and physical therapy for persons with HIV disease and their caregivers. *Journal of Home Health Care Practice, 3*(3), 46–57.

Gutterman, L. (1990). A day treatment program for persons with AIDS. *American Journal of Occupational Therapy, 44*, 234–237.

Johnson, J. (1993). Wellness. In H. Smith & H. Hopkins (Eds.). *Willard and Spackman's occupational therapy* (8th ed., pp. 843–852). Philadelphia: Lippincott.

Kassler, W. (1993). *An introduction to HIV*. Redwood City, CA: Cummings.

National Institute for Occupational Safety and Health. (1988). *Guidelines for the protection and health of health care workers* [DHHS (NIOSH) Publication No. 88-119]. Washington, DC: U.S. Government Printing Office.

Novartis Pharmaceuticals Corporation. (1999). What is Aredia? Available at: www.aredia.net/patients/about_aredia/. Accessed October 22, 2001.

Park, A. (2001, January 15). The hunt for cures. *Time*, pp. 70–72.

Pizzi, M. (1988). Challenge of treating AIDS patients includes helping them lead functional lives. *OT Week*, *31*, 6–7.

Pizzi, M. (1989). Occupational therapy: Creating possibilities for adults with HIV infection, ARC and AIDS. *AIDS Patient Care*, *3*, 18–23.

Pizzi, M. (1990a). The transformation of HIV infection and AIDS in occupational therapy: Beginning the conversation. *American Journal of Occupational Therapy*, *44*(3), 199–203.

Pizzi, M.(1990b) The model of human occupation and adults with HIV infection and AIDS. *American Journal of Occupational Therapy*, *44*, 257–264.

Pizzi, M. (1991). HIV infection and occupational therapy. In J. Mukand (Ed.). *Rehabilitation for patients with HIV disease* (pp. 283–326). New York: McGraw-Hill.

Pizzi, M. (1993). HIV infection and AIDS. In H. L. Hopkins & H. D. Smith (Eds.). *Willard and Spackman's Occupational Therapy* (8th ed., pp. 716–729). Philadelphia: Lippincott.

Pizzi, M. (2001). The Pizzi Holistic Wellness Assessment. In Velde, B. and Wittman, P. (Eds.) *Occupational Therapy in Health Care* (Special issue on community based practice), *13*, 51–66. Binghamton, NY: Haworth Press.

Reitz, S. M. (1992). A historical review of occupational therapy's role in preventive health and wellness. *American Journal of Occupational Therapy*, *46*(1), 50–55

Springhouse Corporation [Springhouse]. (1995). *Professional guide to diseases*. Springhouse, PA: Author.

Weinstein, B. (1990). Assessing the impact of HIV disease. *American Journal of Occupational Therapy*, *44*, 220–226.

White, V. K. (1986). Promoting health and wellness: A theme for the eighties. *American Journal of Occupational Therapy*, *40*, 743–748.

Wiemer, R., & West, W. (1970). Occupational therapy in community health care. *American Journal of Occupational Therapy*, *24*, 323–328.

Williams, V., Burkhardt, A., & Royce, J. (1995). Helping you call it quits: O.T. practitioners are in a unique position to help clients quit smoking successfully. *OT Week*, 9(9), 18–20.

CHAPTER 43

ADULTS WITH MENTAL ILLNESS

SECTION I

Psychiatric Diagnoses and Related Intervention Issues

JUDITH D. WARD

The following psychiatric diagnoses were selected for discussion because occupational therapy practitioners encounter them in their work in mental health settings, in physical rehabilitation, and in long-term care and community-based practice. Although many diagnoses were left out, the ones that are included exemplify cognitive, behavioral, and psychosocial problems associated with most mental and many physical disorders seen by occupational therapy practitioners. Depression is everywhere. Substance abuse is the cause of problems occupational therapy practitioners see in nursing homes, trauma centers, and in physical and cognitive rehabilitation settings. The people occupational therapy practitioners treat in these settings may also display the effects of dementia. Finally, people with severe and persistent mental illness share many of the problems discussed in the sections on borderline personality disorder and schizophrenia.

Although people with these mental impairments are seen in a variety of settings they are discussed in this section primarily from the point of view of practice in mental health settings. Each disorder is examined in terms of the American Psychiatric Association (APA) diagnostic criteria. However, enough information is given to show the implications for occupational therapy in a variety of practice situations.

BOX 43-1 THE DSM'S MULTIAXIAL SYSTEM FOR ASSESSMENT[a]

The DSM provides a multiaxial system for assessment. Each axis provides domains of information that guide the gathering of data on a patient so that a comprehensive picture can be obtained. The five axes are as follows:

- *Axis I:* Clinical disorders; other conditions that may be a focus of clinical attention; includes all mental disorders except personality disorders and mental retardation.
- *Axis II:* Personality disorders; mental retardation.
- *Axis III:* General medical conditions; includes any medical conditions, such as diabetes or heart disease, that may be relevant in managing a client's mental disorder.
- *Axis IV:* Psychosocial and environmental problems; includes any life events or familial, economic, or environmental circumstances that are relevant to the client's mental illness or recovery.
- *Axis V:* Global assessment of functioning (GAF); includes scale that rates the client's current functioning in social, occupational, and psychological functioning.

[a]Data from APA (2000).

THE DIAGNOSTIC AND STATISTICAL MANUAL OF MENTAL DISORDERS

The Diagnostic and Statistical Manual of Mental Disorders (DSM) is the APA's guide to the diagnosis of mental disorders (Box 43-1). It provides the criteria for diagnosis, description of symptoms, information on familial patterns, and the prevalence and course of the disorders. The manual provides International Classification of Diseases (ICD) codes for most diagnoses (APA, 2000). The DSM is descriptive and does not discuss theories about causation unless specific biological factors are known. The purpose of the manual "is to provide clear descriptions of diagnostic categories in order to enable clinicians and investigators to diagnose, communicate about, study, and treat people with various mental disorders" (APA, 1994, p. xxvii). Since the manual is used to provide a means of communication among a diverse population of mental health and legal professionals, work on it included liaison with organizations interested in its construction. Among them was the American Occupational Therapy Association.

THE MENTAL STATUS EXAMINATION

The *mental status examination* is a formal procedure used to examine and diagnose the mental functioning of a client. It serves the same function in psychiatry as the physical examination does in medicine. A psychiatrist or psychologist conducts the mental status examination, and occupational therapy practitioners may contribute information about their observations of the client to enable a diagnosis to be made.

The mental status examination is conducted through an interview in which the examiner considers the client's verbal responses and observes related psychomotor behaviors and appearance to evaluate the individual and diagnose the condition. A general description of the client is recorded, including his or her appearance, motor behavior, speech, and attitude.

The emotional expression is noted and, equally important, the context in which the emotions are expressed are observed. For example, if a client laughs while describing the death of a close family member, the examiner attempts to determine the significance of this inappropriate response. Perceptual disturbances such as hallucinations, illusions, and depersonalization are identified. Thought processes and thought content are explored.

During the interview, the examiner explores the client's intelligence by noting vocabulary and level of education. If problems are suspected, the patient is given a standardized intelligence test. Orientation and memory are also assessed. Orientation to person, place, and time refers to the client's ability to know who he or she is, where he or she is located, and the current date and time. Remote, recent-past, and short-term memory functions are also assessed (Scheiber, 1988).

Knowledge of the client's social history as well as information from the mental status interview help the examiner assess the impulse control and judgment of the client. Finally, the individual's insight into and understanding of the extent and origination of the problem is explored (Scheiber, 1988). Many of the functions noted in the mental status examination are interrelated. For example, perceptual disturbances can interfere with thought process and content. Memory loss results in disorientation. In the following discussions of diagnoses, note how problems with different mental functions are displayed.

DEMENTIA OF THE ALZHEIMER'S TYPE AND OTHER DEMENTIAS

The term **dementia** is used to designate cognitive disorders that are caused by a general medical condition, head trauma, or the persistent effects of a substance (APA, 2000). The APA classifies Alzheimer's disease as a dementia. When the symptoms of dementia are present and all identifiable causes are ruled out, a diagnosis of Alzheimer's is made. Dementias include the following (APA, 2000):

- Dementia of the Alzheimer's type.
- Vascular dementia.
- Substance-induced persisting dementia.
- Dementia owing to multiple causes.
- Dementia caused by HIV disease.
- Dementia caused by head trauma.
- Dementia caused by Pick disease.
- Dementia caused by Parkinson disease.
- Dementia caused by Huntington disease.
- Dementia caused by Creutzfeldt-Jakob disease.

Symptoms

Regardless of cause, the dementias present common symptoms. These always include impairment of memory and may include the inability to think abstractly or plan and carry out complex actions. Apraxia, aphasia, or agnosia may also be present. These symptoms are severe enough to impair social or occupational functioning in a person who, earlier in life, was unimpaired (APA, 2000). Symptoms associated with dementia are as follows (APA, 2000):

- *Memory impairment:* Affects the ability to learn new information (registration) and affects remote memory, or remembering old information (retention and recall).
- *Disturbed executive functioning:* Includes impairment of abstract thought and an inability to plan, sequence, and carry out complex activities.
- *Confabulation:* Reciting imaginary events to fill in for gaps in memory.
- *Aphasia:* Impairment of language, including receptive aphasia (inability to understand spoken or written language) and expressive aphasia (impaired use of verbal and written language).
- *Apraxia:* Inability to perform motor activities, although sensory motor function is intact and the client understands the requirements of the task.
- *Agnosia:* Inability to recognize familiar objects, although sensory capacities are intact.

Dementia of the Alzheimer's Type

Alzheimer's disease is the most prevalent dementia (Kaplan & Sadock, 1998). Its onset is insidious, and there is progressive deterioration of cognitive functioning. It occurs mainly in the aged but can have an early onset. The initial signs of Alzheimer's dementia are memory impairments, social withdrawal, apathy, and sleep disturbance. The individual may be unable to concentrate and may have hypochondriacal complaints. Early signs of dementia can be difficult to distinguish from depression. In dementia and depression, thinking is slowed and recall difficult (Kaplan & Sadock, 1998). To complicate matters, people with dementia may also be depressed about their condition.

Short-term memory is commonly the first to be lost in Alzheimer's. This loss may not be noticeable in individuals who live in familiar surroundings and do the same jobs or activities they have done for years. Sometimes, the first symptoms, noticed by the family, are emotional. People with dementia may be frustrated and depressed about their failing abilities and become irritable and withdrawn. One man who was upset about his trouble with work, was testy at home. When his wife engaged him in marital counseling, things got worse because the Alzheimer's wasn't identified. He said:

> *I knew something was wrong. I could feel myself getting uptight over little things. People thought I knew things about the plant that I—I couldn't remember. The counselor said it was stress. I though it was something else, something terrible. I was scared. (Mace & Rabins, 1991, p. 9)*

The emotional reactivity may not be only in response to the condition. It may be a function of the brain changes that occur with Alzheimer's. In these cases, the behavior cannot be controlled.

Initially, people with Alzheimer's disease can accommodate their impairment by creating systems for remembering; but as deterioration progresses, the adaptations no longer work. Even in the early stages, symptoms become more pronounced if there is extreme stress or a change in the usual environment. For example, a woman who functions well in her own home may become disoriented during a weekend stay with relatives. When the familiar landmarks and routines are absent the dementia is revealed. She is unable to become accustomed to (learn) the new environment and her ingrained habits do not serve her in new routines.

In more advanced stages, the person with Alzheimer's is unable to hold a job that demands organization of thought and recent memory. The inability to remember recent events can cause disorientation and paranoia. For example, the man who forgets that he just paid for groceries may accuse a family member of stealing the money from his wallet. Memory loss can be dangerous when clients forget they have lit a burner on the stove or if they take a walk and get lost. Memory impairment also sabotages one's sense of time:

> *The other day I walked out of the room and returned in less than a minute. She looked at me accusingly and said, "Where have you been? I've been waiting hours for you to come back." Don't argue because her sense of time is gone. For her to understand how much time has passed means she must also remember what she did in the immediate past. She can't do that because she can't recall the immediate past and has no concept of time. (Murphey, 1988, p. 39)*

It can be frustrating and exhausting to live with a person who has Alzheimer's. As memory deteriorates, long-term memory is affected and the individual may not recognize family members. Bennett (1995) noted the magnitude of memory loss in his mother when he visited her in a nursing home:

> *Mam's memory has almost gone, leaving her suffused with a general benevolence. It is a beautiful day and we walk on the sands. "Has Gordon been to see you?" I ask. "Oh yes," she says, happily. "Though I'm saying he has, I don't know who he is." "Do you know who I am?" She peers at me. "Oh yes, you're . . . you're my son, aren't you?" "And what's my name?" "Ah, now then." And she laughs, as if this is not information any reasonable person could expect her to have. (pp. 76–77).*

Bennett's mother is cheerful and easygoing. Not everyone is. Alzheimer's affects the individual's personality as well. People who were kind and gentle souls all their lives may turn surly and aggressive. A person who had been fastidious may become sloppy and disheveled. An individual who was always self-reliant and independent may now follow a caretaker around like a shadow. Confusion can result in socially inappropriate behavior: "One teenage boy came home to find his father sitting on the back porch reading the newspaper. He was naked except for his hat" (Mace & Rabins, 1991, p. 130). This man stripped because he was hot, unaware of his public display.

Psychotic symptoms can also accompany Alzheimer's. The delusional thinking can be a function of memory impairment or can arise unrelated to forgetfulness. The behaviors stimulated by the delusions can be difficult to manage, as Bennett (1995) described in his diary:

> *This evening Mam is convinced that there are people outside the house and that they are waiting to take me away. I get her off to bed but she keeps coming down, anxious to be taken away in my place. At one point she gets outside in the bitter cold, and eventually I go to bed in order to stop her coming downstairs. I drift off to sleep three or four times, but each time she wakes me, wanting to know if I am all right. (p. 70).*

Some individuals get worse in the evening or they may awake in the night and become disoriented. This is called *sundowning*. It is not known what causes this phenomenon. Some researchers have attributed the confusion to waking in the dark and being unable to get one's bearings. A night light sometimes helps these clients. For others, sundowning may be a sign of fatigue and lowered stress tolerance at the end of the day (Mace & Rabins, 1991) or a sign of overmedication (Kaplan & Sadock, 1998).

People with Alzheimer's may become agitated and anxious for no apparent reason and sometimes overreact to seemingly inconsequential things. This is known as catastrophic reaction, and occasionally the individual will strike out at others. Sometimes it is possible to identify a reason for the reaction:

> *Mother hit me. She isn't strong enough to hurt me physically. But, along with the verbal tirade, I reacted badly. I yelled back and she got worse. . . . Mother wasn't angry at me even though she shouted when she struck me. She gets that way when the TV gets loud, a lot of action takes place, or when several people come into the room. Even if she used to know them, they are strangers now and their presence confuses her. (Murphey, 1988, p. 128)*

Family members need to understand the limits Alzheimer's dementia places on the client. Health-care professionals need to understand the stress families endure as they live with someone whose brain is slowly dying. Both the affected individual and his or her caregivers are considered clients in need of intervention.

Communication becomes more and more difficult with time. Problems with verbal expression can start with getting words mixed up. For example one woman said "You know I don't like to eat carburetors." when discussing cauliflower with her daughter (Murphey, 1988, p. 10). It is often the names of things that go first. Bennett's (1995) mother stood before the mantelpiece staring at the clock, trying to name it: "It's one of those things," she said, "with things that go round, and then when they get there they've had it for a bit" (p. 75). Some people ramble on, talk and talk without making sense; others revert to silence.

Motor abilities are affected as the disease progresses. Sometimes motor planning is impaired, so the person might lie the wrong way, across the bed or try to sleep standing up. One woman said of her husband: "He's had trouble opening his eyes lately. He will complain, 'Fern, I can't see,' but when I explain to him that he has his eyes closed, he counters with, 'I can't open my eyes.' And later, he opens his eyes without effort" (Konek, 1991, p. 88). Experienced carpenters who have Alzheimer's may lose the ability to work with tools. The simple task of dressing may be impossible. This is not because people lose the ability to move their arms or fingers, but they don't know how to accomplish these tasks (apraxia).

Alzheimer's disease ultimately ends in death after an average duration of 8–10 years (APA, 2000). Some people die of other diseases of aging. Those who don't may progress to a vegetative state and require constant care.

General Goals in the Management of Dementias

Dead brain cells cannot be revived, and there is currently no cure for Alzheimer's disease. It is important, however, to differentiate Alzheimer's from dementias that have a treatable cause. For example, if the dementia is caused by cerebrovascular disease, it is possible to intervene in the progress of dementia by treating the vascular disease.

Medical treatment of Alzheimer's disease includes treatment of physical problems, provision of nutrition, and maintenance of health. The symptoms of dementia are managed by creating an environment that supports function and facilitates social interaction. Psychotic symptoms, agitation, and depression can be treated by medication. But care must be taken, as older people are more likely to have unusual responses to these drugs than younger clients (Kaplan & Sadock, 1998).

Occupational Therapy

Occupational therapy practitioners in many areas of practice work with people exhibiting the symptoms of dementia. Cerebrovascular accidents (CVA), Parkinson disease, meningitis, and HIV infection can all result in temporary or permanent dementia. The therapist must assess the cognitive abilities of clients for whom dementia may be a complication of their condition. Instruction in treatment activities must be geared to cognitive abilities with consideration of impairments. If the problem is irreversible and progressive, treatment plans must take this into account.

Structure and predictability are important aspects of the milieu in which people with dementia live. The performance skills of the person with dementia depend not only on cognitive abilities but also on the individual's motivation and the nature of the environment. People with Alzheimer's may be unable to learn new skills; but old skills and habits remain deeply ingrained, and these can be used long into the disease (Borell, Sandman, & Kielhofner, 1991).

People with Alzheimer's are likely to live with their families during some of their illness. Education and support of the family are critical. Families need to understand the disease and learn what they can expect in terms of confusion and apparent inconsistencies of behavior. There are a number of excellent books about living with and caring for individuals with Alzheimer's that give examples of the variety of problems that can be encountered and how to manage them (Mace & Rabins, 1991; Murphey, 1988). Families can be helped to find resources, such as support groups for caregivers and respite care services.

Occupational therapy practitioners can help families identify the environmental factors that facilitate maximum function and support peace of mind. The individual's capacities, including functional communication skills, are assessed to determine current strengths and limitations. Whether the client is living with family or in an institution, he or she requires appropriate sensory and social stimulation in an environment that supports function and minimizes disabilities. Because sensory abilities become impaired, environmental stimulation needs to be intensified (Levy, 1987a). Care must be taken, however, because overstimulation can cause agitation, confusion, and catastrophic reaction.

Daily routines that are predictable and reflect the rhythm of the larger society, with the opportunity for activity and a chance to rest, help keep the person in touch with the world. Familiar objects and lifestyle also help keep the client grounded in reality. A sense of autonomy can be maintained if people are given the freedom to choose their activities from a variety of options (Levy, 1987a). Occupational behavioral approaches can help practitioners identify ways to address these issues systematically (see Chapter 18).

Allen's cognitive disability approach is useful for managing Alzheimer's disease (see Chapter 21, Section 4). This approach measures the cognitive level of the individual and identifies the sensory cues to which the client, at a particular level, is able to attend. When caregivers and practitioners understand the cognitive level of the client, they are able to understand how to provide the correct stimulation to engage that person in activity. They will also understand the cognitive limitations of the client and provide stimulation for only those responses that are possible.

The therapist can help fashion the environment to the client's abilities, interest, and comfort level and help maintain their dignity (Levy, 1987b). Because in Alzheimer's and other degenerative dementias, cognitive abilities decrease over time, the environment must be adapted accordingly. Even when abilities are simple, it is possible to provide occupation:

> *Grandpa's fascination with paper helped him to pass the time. We now put colorful advertising supplements from the newspaper, old catalogs, and junk mail on the table in the family room for him. These were his playthings for hours because he could no longer do more complex things. (Honel, 1988, p. 187)*

MOOD DISORDERS

The mood disorders are classified in two major categories: depressive disorders and bipolar disorders (Box 43-2). Depressive disorders are those in which there is a prolonged emotional state of sadness. Bipolar disorders have periods of mania and periods of depression, the two poles. All the mood disorders have the following characteristics:

- Disturbance of mood.
- Psychomotor symptoms that affect thought processes, attention, activity level, sleep patterns, and appetite.

See Box 43-3 for additional kinds of depression.

Depressive Disorders

Depression is pervasive in our society. The lifetime prevalence of *major depressive disorder* is 13% for males and 21% for females (Carson, Butcher, & Mineka, 2000). All the depressive disorders share similar symptoms, but the degree of severity varies. A depressed mood has many faces. The person may feel tired, sick, heavy, hopeless, or sad. The depression can also manifest itself as irritability and anger. This condition depresses function as well as mood. To the depressed person everything seems harder to do. Or, such an individual may feel life is not worth the effort. In her autobiographical novel, *The Bell Jar*, Plath (1971) describes the depression of her main character, Esther, who hasn't slept for a week. She hadn't washed her hair and has worn the same clothes, without washing them, for three weeks because it seemed so silly:

> *I saw the days of the year stretching ahead like a series of bright white boxes, and separating one box from another was sleep. It seemed silly to wash one day when I would only have to wash again the next. It made me tired just to think of it (pp. 104–105).*

Esther, like many depressed people can't find meaning in life and this attitude colors her perceptions. Why should she care for her grooming when life is an "infinitely desolate avenue" (p. 104)? She is not even able to escape this desolation through sleep, a common problem in depression. Depression kills the ability to experience pleasure (anhedonia) and even those things that were enjoyed in the past no longer hold meaning.

The APA (2000) describes two types of depressive disorders: major depressive disorder and dysthymia. These disorders have many of the same symptoms, but the onset, duration, and severity of the depressions differ.

Major Depressive Disorder

Major depressive disorder is severe depression that is present almost all of every day for at least 2 weeks. There is a noticeable change in the person's usual mood, which is evident through sadness, and a loss of pleasure in almost everything. People with major depression lose their appetite and often cannot get a full night's sleep. Some people experience hypersomnia. There is frequently an overwhelming fatigue that immobilizes the individual. This inertia is so paralyzing that it is impossible to pull oneself together to do the simplest activities. Knauth (1975) remembered how he felt as he heard his visiting son's footsteps:

> *It was my son returning unannounced from Vietnam. . . . If ever there was a situation in which a man would do everything possible to pull himself together, this was it. But although I felt this overwhelmingly, there was absolutely nothing I could do. I sat rooted in my chair and waited, trembling like a man condemned. I heard the footsteps stop outside the door; I saw the handle turn. I shrieked inwardly at myself: "Get up! Get up!" Then he was there.*
>
> *To me he looked seven feet tall. The brass on his uniform glittered, the ribbons were flashes of color on his chest, his boots shone like twin mirrors. He was everything I was not—strong, healthy, alive. . . . I don't believe I will forget that moment, or my own dreadful sense of helplessness, until the day I die. (p. 93)*

BOX 43–2 APA CLASSIFICATION OF MOOD DISORDERS[a]

DEPRESSIVE DISORDERS

- Major depressive disorder
- Dysthymic disorder
- Depressive disorder not otherwise specified

BIPOLAR DISORDERS

- Bipolar I disorder
- Bipolar II disorder
- Cyclothymic disorder
- Bipolar disorder not otherwise specified

[a]From APA (2000).

BOX 43–3 DEPRESSION IS UBIQUITOUS[a]

In addition to depression classified under mood disorders, the APA recognizes other types of depression:

- Adjustment disorder with depressed mood.
- Alzheimer's and other dementias with associated depression.
- Depression associated with a medical condition.
- General anxiety disorder with major depressive disorder.
- Posttraumatic stress disorder with major depressive disorder.
- Schizoaffective disorder—depressive type.
- Substance-induced depression.

[a]From APA (2000).

Knauth was not physically paralyzed but he was unable to respond. This inertia is called psychomotor retardation. Everything slows. It is hard to concentrate; thoughts and actions are sluggish. Making decisions becomes an impossible hurdle and self-esteem plunges. Irrational thoughts of worthlessness and guilt may become obsessive. Knauth explained:

> *In my own eyes I became worthless. . . . I reviewed my life and saw everything that I had done wrong. Not even the most trivial detail escaped this deadly scrutiny. . . , I realized what a poor excuse for a father I had been. I recalled the details of my divorce, and I understood precisely why my first wife had left me for another man. Viewed in the merciless gloom of this early-morning self-analysis, even my work appeared to me to have been a fraud. At last I was being shown up for the hapless faker that I was and this was my punishment. (pp. 35–36).*

In some people, the feelings of guilt and worthlessness may take on the severity of psychotic delusions or other psychotic features. A major depressive episode can develop in a day or over weeks. It may last for months. If untreated, it can last longer than 4 months. In most cases, with remission, the individual returns to premorbid functioning (APA, 2000) but recurrences are common (Kaplan & Sadock, 1998).

Dysthymia

Dysthymia has a slower onset than major depression, and it tends to be chronic rather than episodic (Kaplan & Sadock,1998). Its symptoms are not as pronounced as those of major depressive illness, and the individual is usually able to work and does not need to be hospitalized. It is a serious disease, however, and 75% of people with dysthymia who are seen clinically go on to develop major depression (APA, 2000).

To be diagnosed with this condition, the individual must be depressed "for most of the day, for more days than not" (APA, 2000, p. 380) for at least 2 years. This depression takes the form of fatigue, listlessness, blunted pleasure, or irritability. The individual may carry out essential activities but with great effort and without enjoyment. Self-esteem is low, and function may be impaired by poor concentration or the inability to make decisions. Appetite and sleep are affected. People with dysthymia may be so accustomed to being depressed that they take it for granted (APA, 2000). It took Love, a psychologist, years to recognize her own depression. She said:

> *The way it affects me is that I have a gloomy outlook on life. Life doesn't excite me. it puts a negative slant on life for me. . . . It's difficult to think positively. This is like having a really bad hangover. It feels almost like a physical residue of a drug in my tissues. . . . It's in your cells. . . . My body feels gloomy. (Cited in Cronkite, 1994, p. 49)*

Bipolar Disorder

Bipolar disorder is sometimes called manic-depression because people with the disorder go through cycles of both moods. The depression associated with bipolar disorders is like the depression described earlier in this section. Mania is the polar opposite of depression. Mania is characterized by excessive energy with flight of ideas associated with an elevated, expansive, or irritable mood. This mood must persist for at least 1 week or be severe enough to require hospitalization for the diagnosis to be applied (APA, 2000).

Additional symptoms of mania include sleeplessness and grandiose thinking with inflated self-esteem. The person may dress flamboyantly, behave in a dramatic manner, may spend money lavishly (running up huge credit card or phone bills). Speech is often pressured, loud, and nonstop. Individuals with mania seem to talk to hear themselves talk, punning and singing without listening to others. Judgment is impaired, and people with mania may be sexually overactive and promiscuous (APA, 2000). During manic episodes, patients may have, "excessive involvement in pleasurable activities that have a high potential for painful consequences" (APA, 2000, p. 363). These behaviors are calamitous to families and the cause of humiliation and regret when the individual is in remission.

There are degrees of mania. Fieve (1975) described the extreme delirious mania of one of his patients:

> *On the psychiatric ward she developed a great excitement and overactivity. She said she had so much to do that she no longer had time to eat. After five days of starvation she required tube feeding. . . . She entered a phase of great physical activity. She paced the floor, and went into patients' rooms, causing considerable disturbance. She was distractible, mis-identified people, and was disoriented in time and place. Her condition seemed to approach a state of ecstasy when she sang religious hymns and unabashedly stripped in front of everyone. Once she became violent and struck another patient. On another occasion she broke the window in her room. (p. 23)*

This is an extreme case of mania. In other individuals the mania is milder and less destructive, but such states are considered mania if they are intense enough to impair social and/or occupational functioning (APA, 2000).

Bipolar I and Bipolar II Disorders

The DSM distinguishes two bipolar disorders. Both have episodes of major depression, but bipolar I disorder has occurrences of full-blown mania or mixed symptoms, whereas bipolar II disorder has recurrent depressive episodes with hypomania. Hypomania is a persistent state of inflated or irritable mood that is distinctly different from the individual's usual nondepressed behavior. During the hypomanic episode, the client may have any of the symptoms described for mania, but these symptoms are milder and do not impair social and occupational functioning and do not require hospitalization (APA, 2000).

Mixed Episodes

Associated with bipolar I disorder are mixed episodes that present concurrent symptoms of mania and depression. The individual may have flight of ideas and grandiose thinking while breaking into sobs or feeling despairing anxiety, all at the same time (Duke & Hochman, 1992). These mixed episodes are severe enough to interfere with social and occupational functioning or to require hospitalization.

Cyclothymic Disorder

Cyclothymia is a chronic mood disturbance in which there are periods of hypomania and periods of depressive symptoms. The symptoms are less severe than, or do not meet all the criteria for, a manic episode or major depressive episode, and they last for at least 2 years. Cyclothymia has a slow, gradual onset in adolescence or early adulthood, and it appears to predispose the individual to other mood disorders (APA, 2000).

Causal Factors and the Course of Mood Disorders

The causes of unipolar depressive disorders are both biological and psychosocial. External stress, such as job loss, death of a loved one, or illness can lead to depression. However, it appears that these stressors are more important in the first episode of depression than in subsequent ones. This has led to the theory that the original stressors produce changes in the brain cells, which create long-term susceptibility to depression ("Update on Mood," 1995). Women who have a family history of depression have a greater risk for experiencing depression themselves than the general population (Kaplan & Saddock, 1998). Genetic factors play a stronger role in bipolar disorders than in any other major psychiatric disorder (Carson et al., 2000). Approximately 50% of people with bipolar I disorder have a parent with a history of a mood disorder (Kaplan & Saddock, 1998).

A National Institute of Mental Health (NIMH) study found that 89% of people with bipolar disorder had further manic or depressive episodes after their first hospitalization ("Bipolar Disorder," 1994). Mood disorders may become chronic and worsen over time (Box 43-4). More than 50% of people who undergo one major depressive episode will have another. And those who have two episodes have an 80% chance of a third. On average, a treated episode of major depression will last 3 months (Kaplan & Saddock, 1998).

BOX 43–4 MOOD DISORDER SPECIFIERS

SPECIFIERS FOR THE SEVERITY OF THE CURRENT EPISODE

- Severe with psychotic features.
- Severe without psychotic features.
- Moderate.
- Mild.
- Partial remission.
- Full remission.

SPECIFIERS FOR THE NATURE OF THE CURRENT OR MOST RECENT EPISODE

- *Chronic:* Applied to the depressive episodes of major depression and bipolar disorders; major depressive episode must be present for at least 2 years.
- *Catatonic features:* Psychomotor disturbance in which the individual is motorically immobile or excessively overactive for no apparent purpose.
- *Melancholic features:* Applied to the most recent major depressive episodes; loss of pleasure or lack of reaction to pleasurable stimuli; depression is often worse in the morning, and sleep disturbance is characterized by early morning awakening; excessive or inappropriate guilt, loss of appetite, and psychomotor retardation or agitation may be present.
- *Atypical features:* Mood lightens in response to pleasurable stimuli (mood reactivity); may include increase of appetite, excessive sleeping, and a feeling of heaviness in the arms or legs; may have social sensitivity, which impairs social or occupational functioning.

SPECIFIERS FOR THE COURSE OF RECURRENT EPISODES

- *With or without full inter-episode recovery:* The most recent period between episodes of recurrent major depression or the bipolar disorders; prominent symptoms are sometimes present between episodes (classed as "without inter-episode recovery"); may show full remission between episodes.
- *Seasonal pattern:* The most common pattern begins in fall or winter and ceases in spring (sometimes known as seasonal affective disorder).
- *Rapid cycling:* Applied to an individual with bipolar disorder who has had at least four episodes of major depression, mania, mixed, or hypomanic moods within 1 year.

[a]From APA (2000).

Treatment

Treatment for depression depends on the severity, persistence, and cause. If the depression is associated with a medical disorder or is substance induced, these factors must be addressed. Psychotherapy is effective for some people, but there needs to be more research to identify the more effective methods. Researchers at the NIMH found that interpersonal therapy, which examines the social context of the depression, was slightly more effective than cognitive behavioral therapy for patients with major depression. However, cognitive therapy is effective for people with depression who are not excessively guilty or pessimistic ("Update on Mood," 1995). If mood changes are seasonal, the systematic, controlled use of bright light is effective. ("Seasonal Affective Disorder," 1993). The NIMH study found that medication worked better and faster than other treatments.

Psychotherapy and medication are frequently used together; the medication lightens the mood, and the therapy provides support and stress management.

Electroconvulsive therapy (ECT) is helpful for at least half of depressed patients who don't respond to medication. It is most valuable for cutting short a depressive episode. ("Update on Mood," 1995).

Antidepressant medications, which affect the biochemistry of the brain, fall into three major categories: the tricyclic antidepressants (TCAs), which block norepinephrine reuptake; the selective serotonin reuptake inhibitors (SSRIs); and the monoamine oxidase inhibitors (MAOIs), which prevent norepinephrine and dopamine from being broken down. All three types of drugs are effective treatments for depression. The SSRIs have the fewest side effects, and Prozac, one of them, is the most widely prescribed psychoactive drug in the United States ("Update on Mood," 1995).

The antimanic medications include lithium carbonate, antipsychotic medications, and anticonvulsants. Lithium carbonate is the most commonly used, but it has many side effects; the anticonvulsants are considered as useful. Antipsychotic medications are used for psychotic symptoms of depression and mania, sometimes in combination with other medications (Kaplan & Saddock, 1998).

Implications for Occupational Therapy

Depression and Depressive Episodes of Bipolar Disorders

Depending on the degree of severity, depression affects all areas of performance. The individual with dysthymia can often carry on necessary activities but without enjoyment. The severely depressed client may actually be in a state of catatonia (APA, 2000), in which they do nothing for themselves or are occupied with purposeless excessive motor activity.

When working with a client who has depression, it is important to consider the psychomotor retardation that slows motor and cognitive functioning. The therapist may need to give directions in a simple, one-step fashion and allow the client plenty of time to respond. During conversations, the therapist must be able to tolerate the time required for the client's cognitive integration of information received and his or her verbal response. The psychomotor retardation alters social functioning. Clients who are depressed become isolated and may even be unable to ask for help or convey the magnitude of their depression.

There is always a risk of suicide with depression. Ironically, it is more likely to occur after a deep depression has somewhat lifted, and the individual gains the energy to carry out the act.

Therapists walk a fine line when working with clients who have depression. Care must be taken not to insult their intellects when grading activity for psychomotor retardation. Therapists may feel the need to provide the energy for the interaction, but that may engender what Styron (1990) described as "humiliated rage" when his art therapist conducted sessions, which Styron called "organized infantilism" (p. 74). He wrote:

> *Our class was run by a delirious young woman with a fixed, indefatigable smile, who was plainly trained at a school offering courses in Teaching Art to the Mentally Ill; not even a teacher of very young retarded children could have been compelled to bestow, without deliberate instruction, such orchestrated chuckles and coos. (p. 74).*

On the other hand it is also important to help these clients mobilize themselves. When Knauth (1975) reflected on his depressive illness he realized that the most elementary actions helped him survive. Each morning he forced himself to get out of bed, make coffee, and make his bed:

> *If this sounds too trivial to mention, it is not. It proved to me, day after day, that I was still able to accomplish something, even though my mind was telling me I was a total loss. By the act of getting out of bed I proved that I could still command my body and had at least a semblance of free will. By the act of making coffee I proved that I could still do something to preserve myself and thus deny my growing wish for death. By the act of making my bed I proved that I had not fallen completely into the state of sloth and disarray that my disorganized mind constantly told me I was in: I still cared (pp. 87–88).*

Since stress can precipitate depression, it is valuable to address stress management. There is a link among stress, depression, and physical illness and between mood disorders and alcohol and **substance abuse.** If the occupational therapy practitioner is aware of the client's medical and social history these factors can be addressed.

Mania

Individuals with mania or hypomania may be exceptionally productive or creative (Richards, 1992). This does not mean that all people with mania are creative. Nor does it mean that it is easy to work with a manic or hypomanic client. The description of Frieve's deliriously manic patient illustrates how these individuals can lose control and present danger to others. It may be impossible for them to engage in purposeful activity.

During a manic episode, these clients are likely to be disruptive of groups because of their verbal or motor overactivity. They can take over a group, intimidating other clients and subverting the therapist. People with mania can be dangerous to themselves (e.g., careless with tools, without regard for self-injury). It is unwise to foster excessive activity in people who are manic, because they may be unable to recognize their own physical exhaustion.

When the manic symptoms fade, the occupational therapy practitioner and client can address daily living patterns to assess routines and habits for stressors that might precipitate future relapses. People who have had chronic mood disorder for most of their adult lives may not have developed mature occupational skills and may need help learning time management, parenting skills, and other adult roles. This instruction is more effective when the disease has responded to medication, and the manic symptoms are modified enough for the individual to attend and be able to concentrate.

When a person is suffering from a mood disorder, judgment is impaired. The person with depression has an exaggerated gloomy outlook, and the person with mania may not feel that anything is wrong. Thus it is helpful to assist the client and family members to recognize precursors of the manic or depressive episodes to arrange for prompt intervention. Even when clients respond well to medication, it is important for them to know how to maintain a balanced life to prevent relapse. The actress Patty Duke, who has learned to live with her bipolar illness, which is well controlled by lithium, said:

> *You still have to deal with reality. And reality is hard. . . . It takes practice to do it differently than you used to, and to recognize your norm for tolerance of aggravation, or of stress, or of sleep deprivation, or hunger. (Duke & Hochman, 1992, p. 248)*

> *I'd be less than honest if I said that manic depression is not part of my life today. . . . I am who I am, with behavior patterns that have been going on for years. Just taking a pill doesn't mean I'm going to become a different person. The whole world doesn't immediately turn rosy. So I keep working really hard to break behaviors I don't like in myself. I practice. . . . It is a question of relearning—or maybe learning for the first time—how to behave the way you want to behave. (pp. 239–240)*

SUBSTANCE ABUSE

When people use drugs in a compulsive or self-destructive way they are said to abuse substances. In this discussion of substance abuse the terms *drug* and *substance* will be used interchangeably to refer to any psychoactive chemical, including alcohol and inhalants, illicit and prescribed drugs and medications.

Substance Dependence and Abuse

When describing the effects of the misuse of psychoactive drugs the DSM (APA, 2000) distinguishes between *substance dependence* and *substance abuse*. Substance dependence, often called drug addiction, refers to repeated self-administration of drugs that leads to significant cognitive, behavioral, and physiological problems. Included among the problems of dependence may be the development of drug tolerance and unpleasant withdrawal symptoms. Those who are addicted to substances spend a great deal of time obtaining the drugs or recovering from the effects. Thus social and occupational function is impaired. Often addicted individuals want to control their use of drugs but are unable to regulate the amount used or they use the substance over a longer period of time than intended. People who are substance dependent continue maladaptive patterns of use even when they know that they have physical or psychological problems associated with abuse (APA, 2000).

In substance abuse, individuals do not develop tolerance or withdrawal symptoms but experience social consequences of drug use, which leads to failures in fulfillment of role responsibilities and poor school or work performance. Abusers use in spite of engaging in activities, such as driving, which are hazardous when impaired by drugs. When abuse results in legal complications, these individuals may continue to use despite these problems (APA, 2000). The distinction between substance abuse and dependence "is neither precise nor fixed for any given person" ("Treatment of Drug Abuse," 1995a, p. 1).

Drug abuse and dependence are not simple problems. In the American population, 39% of alcohol abusers and 50% of people who have other drug problems have a second psychiatric disorder. Antisocial personality, borderline personality, anxiety, and mood disorders are the most common secondary diagnoses. Although it is unclear which problem comes first, the consensus among experts is that the drug abuse must be treated before other psychiatric problems can be addressed ("Treatment of Drug Abuse," 1995b).

Additional complications in the treatment of drug addiction are that many users are involved with more than one drug, and there is a high incidence of AIDS among intravenous drug users. Approximately 30% of new cases of HIV infection in the United States are the result, directly or indirectly, of intravenous drug use ("Treatment of Drug Abuse," 1995b).

Drug Tolerance and Withdrawal

Tolerance occurs when individuals require increasingly more of a drug to obtain the desired effect or experience a diminishment of effect when continuing to use the same amount of the substance (APA, 2000). Withdrawal symptoms are behavioral, cognitive, and physiological changes that occur in an individual who has used a substance regularly, over a prolonged period and then ceases to use the drug. These symptoms abate when drug intake is resumed. The degree of tolerance and the seventy of withdrawal symptoms vary with the substance (APA, 2000).

Causes of Substance Abuse and Dependence

There is no single cause that can be attributed to all substance abuse. Even when considering a single substance, it is impossible to isolate a single cause.

Biological Factors

There is some evidence of a genetic predisposition to **alcoholism.** Studies have reported that one third of alcoholics have an alcoholic parent and greater than 40% of males who have two alcoholic parents develop alcoholism. However, these studies did not rule out the environmental factors, such as the modeling that could take place in alcoholic families (Carson et al., 2000). Other substances, too, are thought to have biological and/or genetic factors in their use. However, Goldstein (1994) cautions against misunderstanding the genetic vulnerability to drug addiction. He wrote, "Drug addiction differs from clear cut genetic diseases, which do not depend on external factors. The position may be closer to that of diseases with strong hereditary influences, like the common kinds of heart disease or like colon and rectal cancers, in which environmental factors play a major role" (p. 87).

Psychosocial and Environmental Factors

The three most commonly cited reasons for beginning to use heroin are curiosity, pleasure, and peer pressure. However, the family is an important influence on substance abuse in adolescence. Children who are not closely supervised or who are brought up in unstable families in which at least one parents abuses drugs or alcohol are more likely to develop problems with substances (Carson et al., 2000).

There can be a vicious cycle in substance abuse, by which people who enter the drug culture become so immersed in it that they are isolated from the larger world. This often happens at a young age, and the youth develops a sense of inadequacy at dealing with the adult world. This can be a self-perpetuating dilemma in which the addict then uses drugs and alcohol to escape personal anxieties (Carson & Butcher, 1992). Some people get hooked on drugs when they are prescribed for pain during illness or after surgery. This is more common in middle-aged and older people who use alcohol and pills for sleeping as well as pain.

Treatment

Whatever the cause of substance abuse, it is agreed that the first step in treatment is to stop using the substances. This begins with the acknowledgment that there is a problem. There is much denial associated with substance abuse. Betty Ford, in her book, *Betty: A Glad Awakening,* described her denial:

> *My makeup wasn't smeared, I wasn't disheveled, I behaved politely, and I never finished off a bottle, so how could I be alcoholic? And I wasn't on heroin or cocaine, the medicines I took—the sleeping pills, the pain pills, the relaxer pills, the pills to counteract the side effects of other pills—had been prescribed by doctors, so how could I be a drug addict?* (Ford & Chase, 1987 p. 7)

Sometimes problems with the law, such as drunk driving charges, will awaken clients to the seriousness of their use. In Ford's case, the family held an intervention, in which they carefully confronted her with the effect her abuse had on them. This was done in the company of professionals who could offer help.

Detoxification and the Use of Drugs for Treatment

Addiction to opiates, alcohol, and other sedatives may require supervised withdrawal from the drug. In the case of severe withdrawal symptoms—delirium and seizures—hospitalization may be required. Detoxification is the beginning, not the end, of treatment. Ironically, drugs with similar effects to the abused drug are sometimes used to ease the detoxification process. And, in the case of opiate addiction, the drug methadone, a synthetic opioid is prescribed for long-term use. This replaces addiction to an illegal, self-administered drug with a supervised, orally administered addictive drug. Methadone maintenance programs are controversial and regulated by law and health agencies. But for people who were living in crime and completely involved in obtaining drugs for the next fix, methadone gives their lives stability and enables these individuals to maintain a job ("Treatment of Drug Abuse," 1995a).

The drug disulfiram (Antabuse) was the first medication used in the intervention of alcoholism. If alcohol is ingested while taking disulfiram, the individual becomes nauseous, creating a kind of negative reinforcement. Newer medication (naltrexone and nalmefene), opioid antagonists that reduce cravings for alcohol, are now being used. These drugs appear to be safer than disulfiram ("Treatment of Alcoholism," 2000).

Group Treatment

Individual therapy is part of many treatment programs but is seldom used alone. Most drug treatment programs employ various forms of group treatment. Substance abusers tend to isolate themselves and feel they are alone with their problem, and groups help them find those who have been through the same experiences.

Residential Therapeutic Community

Residential therapeutic communities are for individuals whose lives have been consumed by their addiction. Former drug addicts staff them. The life of the community is highly structured, and all members engage in household and other responsibilities required to maintain the environment. The community is monitored closely, and residents have little contact with outsiders. Standards of behavior are clearly defined and regimented.

Through regular individual and group therapy sessions, residents continuously confront their drug use and the concomitant problems. An important element in such a program is the learning gained from formerly addicted staff members. The philosophy behind the therapeutic community is that "drug abuse is regarded as a disease of the emotions that requires a transformation in thinking, feeling, and behavior leading to the development of self-reliance, a sense of responsibility, and a work ethic" ("Treatment of Drug Abuse," 1995a, p. 3).

Chemical Dependency Programs

Chemical dependency programs usually take place in a special unit of psychiatric or general hospitals and are run by professionals and some individuals who were once drug abusers themselves ("Treatment of Drug Abuse," 1995a). Length of stay can vary from a matter of days to a month, and private insurers usually reimburse intervention costs. Various aftercare follow-up programs are included, and clients are encouraged to join a twelve-step program, such as Alcoholics Anonymous (AA) or Narcotics Anonymous.

Twelve-Step Programs

Twelve-step programs are self-help programs fashioned after AA and have abstinence as the goal. In all these programs, members acknowledge their inability to control their addiction and refer to themselves as recover*ing* rather than recover*ed*. AA and Narcotics Anonymous emphasize seeking help from a higher power. Newer 12-step groups have a more secular approach, while acknowledging the need for help from others.

Occupational Therapy

Occupational therapy practitioners who work in programs to help clients who abuse substances usually work in psychiatric and specialized drug treatment centers. However, in other settings, occupational therapy practitioners work with people whose problems result from substance abuse. Dementia and amnestic disorder are psychiatric disorders that may be caused by prolonged use of substances, and 68% of disabilities caused by trauma are a result of risk-taking behavior under the influence of drugs and alcohol (Heinemann, 1993).

Occupational therapy practitioners who work in substance abuse programs do so as part of a team that may consist of psychiatric social workers, nurses, physicians, drug counselors who may be recovering drug abusers, and recreation therapists. The problems occupational therapy addresses are those having to do with life management (Raymond, 1990). Skills in daily living are likely to be impaired in anyone who abuses substances. The following description of the effect of abstinence on a recovering alcoholic aptly describes the difficulties encountered by any individual who abuses drugs.

> *Alcoholics in the first few years of abstinence have been compared with returning prisoners of war. Their world is unfamiliar, because they have been living in an environment created by alcohol. Feelings that have been blunted or suppressed come back to trouble them. They have lost a great deal of time and must start where they left off. Being sober, like being free after imprisonment, entails new responsibilities. Thus alcoholics in the early stages of abstinence often suffer from anxiety and depression and may find it difficult to hold a job or preserve a marriage. The resolution of these problems comes when they establish new personal relationships, rebuild old ones, and begin to develop confidence in their power to control their lives ("Treatment of Alcoholism," 1987b, p. 2).*

Perhaps the greatest contribution occupational therapy can make to the lives of recovering substance abusers is the refinement or acquisition of practical skills of life management that will meet their immediate and long-term needs and develop a sense of control over their lives (Ramond, 1990). In doing so, the problems discussed in the following subsections are addressed:

Social Isolation

Substance abusers often feel alienated from the outer world. Their lives are lonely and consumed by getting drugs and getting high (Robak, 1991). Callahan (1990) described this situation:

> *All that winter and into the spring I lost ground to booze. I was now drinking a maintenance fifth, usually of tequila, plus "social" drinks amounting to another fifth. Gradually I stopped going out and just drank my two fifths at home. I avoided situations where being drunk would seem inappropriate and I avoided people who weren't also drunks—99 percent of the real world. (p. 106)*

Group activities help recovering abusers cut through their loneliness, and occupational therapy programs in drug treatment units usually consist of groups in which recovering clients help each other. They promote drug-free socialization and create a climate of mutual understanding, which may ease the transition to self-help programs in the larger community. Some abusers benefit from groups that are directly related to the development of social competence. Many of these clients lack the very foundation of social competence, that of trusting others.

> *I feel I need to mention the importance of relationships—friendships as well as intimate relationships. As I began my recovery, for a long time I couldn't allow someone to love me. If somebody wanted to do something for me, I would instantly ask myself, "What do they want?" It felt like a set-up. You see, the street is a place where everybody takes advantage of everybody else. If I help you on the street and you accept that help, you instantly owe me. And every time we look at each other we both know it. I had to come to terms with the fact that everyone needs help. (Gorman, 1993, p. 16)*

Social skill development includes assertiveness training, learning communication skills, and working on interpersonal and social responsiveness training. All of these are done in a reflective manner in which the recovering client learns to think before acting. Psychoeducation techniques are often used in these groups in which life skills are learned through information sharing, practicing skills, role playing, and homework assignments (Raymond, 1990).

Basic Life Skills

Raymond (1990) found that money management was the topic most requested for occupational therapy groups when she surveyed clients in an inpatient drug and alcohol abuse unit. Users are often surprised to discover how much money they spent on their drugs and/or they never learned to manage money because it was consumed by their drug use. One cannot assume that clients possess the most ordinary habits of daily living. The administration of an activities configuration to identify use of time may reveal other basic skills that have fallen into disuse or were never acquired.

Time, Leisure, and Stress Management

Substance abuse leads to a narrowing of life and time. With abstinence, time takes on new dimensions. The individual needs to find satisfying ways to fill leisure time, which in the past was spent using a substance. A new, clean-and-sober, social network is needed. Recovering clients need to identify times they are likely to use, and develop ways of coping with stress and boredom without resorting to psychoactive substances. Occupational therapy groups that can address these needs include those in stress management, relaxation training, social recreation, and leisure planning.

Work

Vocational planning and the assessment of work skills are not issues that can be addressed in short-term, inpatient treatment environments. But employment issues cannot be ignored, and plans to engage in or return to work are a critical part of aftercare programs. Referral to vocational services and local employment and training agencies such as junior colleges or technical schools can assist the client in making necessary connections and developing work skills.

Problem Solving and Goal Setting

Problem-solving and goal-setting skills are needed to address the larger issues that clients in recovery face. These clients need to learn to approach problems in a thoughtful, structured way. Often individuals who abuse have very low self-confidence and do not believe they will be successful. They avoid problems for fear of failing to overcome them (Robak, 1991). By learning to formulate attainable goals and to approach problems proactively, clients gain psychological strength while learning practical approaches. Problem solving and goal setting can be offered as separate groups dealing with these concepts, or they can be structured into all functional groups as part of their goals (Raymond, 1990).

Dual Diagnosis

Special consideration may need to be given to clients who have a dual diagnosis of substance abuse and another psychiatric disorder or mental retardation. Raymond (1990) reported on a team approach she found successful in her work with inpatient clients who experienced both psychiatric disorders and substance abuse. She preferred to co-lead her occupational therapy groups with another staff member who was familiar with the person's psychiatric symptoms. She also found that these individuals needed more specific skill training and practice than her clients whose sole problem was substance abuse. The psychiatric clients had a more difficult time conceptualizing their life outside of the hospital and would want to focus on current problems and events on the inpatient unit.

Substance Abuse and Physical Disability

Drug or alcohol abuse often contributes to accidents that cause brain or spinal cord injuries, but substance abuse treatment for this population is inadequate because of communication and architectural barriers (Callahan, 1990; "CSAT Offers," 1999). Heineman (1993) claimed that professionals in physical rehabilitation medicine often avoid confronting the substance abuse of their patients, yet it is likely that those who abused substances before their injuries will abuse them after rehabilitation. Gorman (1993), who is paraplegic as a result of an injury sustained while driving under the influence, said:

> *The loss of both my legs was not even enough to make me give up my drugs and alcohol. My friends smuggled booze to me in the intensive care unit at the hospital. I watched the clock waiting for my morphine shot every three hours. I didn't have much pain, but I liked the morphine high. Pain was an excuse to get high and I used it. A doctor at the rehabilitation hospital asked if I liked beer. I told him, "No, but I like hard liquor every once in a while." So he wrote in my chart that I could drink while in rehabilitation. (I remember how he wrote it . . . "Let Ken have his spirits.")* (pp. 12–13)

EATING DISORDERS

Anorexia nervosa and *bulimia nervosa* are eating disorders found primarily in women of modern industrialized societies. The onset for both disorders is in adolescence and early adulthood (APA, 2000).

Anorexia Nervosa

Anorexia nervosa is a chronic condition with medical and psychological components that affects 0.5–1% of female adolescents (Kaplan & Sadock, 1998). It is self-induced starvation caused by severe restriction of food intake, purging, and excessive exercise or binging and purging (APA, 2000). The APA (2000) diagnostic criteria for anorexia nervosa are as follows:

- Because of purposeful restriction of food intake, the individual weighs <85% of what is considered normal for height and age.
- The client has an obsessive concern with weight and a fear of becoming fat; self-esteem is tied to thinness, and weight loss is considered an achievement.
- The client has a distorted body image and denies that there is a problem.
- Postmenarcheal women have amenorrhea for at least three menstrual cycles.

Although people with anorexia may hide their shape under baggy clothes, they are severely emaciated. They often have yellowish dry skin and fine downy hair (lanugo) over their bodies. (Luder & Schebendach, 1993). Bruch (1979) described Alma, a 20-year-old patient with anorexia:

> *When she came for consultation she looked like a walking skeleton, scantily dressed in shorts and a halter, with her legs sticking out like broomsticks, every rib showing, and her shoulder blades standing up like little wings. . . . Alma's arms and legs were covered with soft hair, her complexion had a yellowish tint, and her dry hair hung down in strings. Most striking was the face—hollow like that of a shriveled-up old woman with a wasting disease, sunken eyes, a sharply pointed nose on which the juncture between bone and cartilage was visible. When she spoke or smiled—and she was quite cheerful—one could see every movement of the muscles around her mouth and eyes, like an animated anatomical representation of the skull. Alma insisted that she looked fine and that there was nothing wrong with her being so skinny. "I enjoy having this disease and I want it. I cannot convince myself that I am sick and that there is anything from which I have to recover." (pp. 2–3).*

Anorexia nervosa is a paradox. People with this disease starve themselves, and although they are skeletal they claim to feel fat. They become obsessed with their weight and profess not to be hungry, although those who recover say that they thought about food all the time while anorexic. In their effort to control food intake, people with eating disorders develop rituals around eating, cutting food into tiny pieces, or eating very slowly (Kaplan & Sadock, 1998).

There are two types of approaches that people with anorexia use: those who achieve their excessive thinness through severe restriction of eating and excessive exercise, and those who binge and purge or starve and purge to achieve weight loss. About 50% of people with anorexia induce vomiting and use laxatives (Brotman, 1994).

People with anorexia often resist treatment and deny that they have a problem even as they suffer medical consequences. Menstruation ceases, and in 25% of cases it does not resume when normal eating is reinstituted. This results in sterility and osteoporosis. These clients may develop cardiac arrhythmia, and the death rate is as high as 20%. (Brotman, 1994).

Along with the physical problems of anorexia nervosa are the cognitive and emotional problems associated with starvation. Thinking becomes distorted and may exacerbate the person's irrational fears of getting fat. Luder and Schebendach (1993) described this distorted thinking:

> *Personal encounters with patients who would not converse over the phone, fearing caloric transmission if the other party was eating while conversing; would not watch television commercials, fearing transmission of calories through the television screen; and would not eat off of glass dinnerware, convinced that it retained calories from previously eaten foods, all illustrate just how bizarre these fears can be. (p. 55)*

After recovery, one woman noted:

> *Instead of feeding my brain, I was starving it. This is where the distorted thinking took over. When I saw I was twenty pounds underweight, I was so frightened, I became thirty pounds underweight. The thought of gaining twenty pounds was overwhelming. I felt locked in with no options, and unable to change. (Meyers, 1989, p. 36)*

Another woman described her state of mind: "I had begun to feel that there was some sort of glass partition between me and the rest of the world" (MacLeod, 1981, p. 106). In fact, people with both anorexia and bulimia do become isolated from the rest of the world (APA, 1993). Their eating disorders can take over their lives, leaving little time for fun and social activities.

Bulimia Nervosa

Bulimia nervosa consists of binge eating followed by self-induced vomiting or the use of laxatives, excessive exercising, or fasting to compensate for the binge. Unlike those with anorexia nervosa, people with bulimia have normal weight and irregular menstruation. The APA (2000) diagnostic criteria for bulimia nervosa are as follows:

- Binging is characterized by a lack of control over eating that lasts for a discrete period of time; during that period, the client eats more than most people would, and he or she cannot stop eating or control what is eaten.
- To compensate for overeating, the client engages in excessive exercise; induces vomiting; and/or overuses laxatives, enemas, or diuretics to prevent weight gain.

This binge-and-purge behavior occurs at least twice a week for 3 months. The self-esteem of the individual with bulimia nervosa is unreasonably tied up in weight and body shape (APA, 2000).

The prevalence of bulimia among females is 1–3% (APA, 2000). Therapists cannot identify a client with bulimia by appearance, as weight is usually normal. But, as with anorexia, people with bulimia are preoccupied with their weight and exercise excessively. They can become socially isolated, as they are secretive in their episodes of overeating and vomiting.

Medical complications of bulimia are a result of the vomiting and laxative abuse. These include fluid and electrolyte imbalances, sore throat, abdominal pain, and esophageal or gastric rupture caused by frequent vomiting. People who engage in vomiting also have dental enamel erosion and may exhibit Russell's sign, skin changes on the dorsum of the hand from rubbing against the teeth when inducing vomiting. Laxative abuse causes dehydration and electrolyte depletion. And there may be irregular menstruation (Kaplan & Sadock, 1998).

Approximately 40% of people with severe bulimia have a history of anorexia ("Eating Disorders," 1997). Bruch (1973) described Celia who, when hospitalized for anorexia, began to binge and purge:

> *Celia said that the hospitalization took away her anorexic behavior, which was her only source of feeling strong and independent. She began to have eating binges, eating out of a sense of panic, or out of emptiness; she denied that they ever occurred out of feelings of hunger, "I don't eat when I feel an inner strength derived from being independent, but when this independence is destroyed my defenses against eating also are." Sometimes she would throw up after such eating binges; usually she refused meals for several days. Though she never had been heavy, she was preoccupied with the fear of getting fat and fear of being rejected. Paradoxically, she also felt that food gave her a sense of security. "I feel always more secure when I have eaten a lot, when I have a full stomach. It is just as I would be gratified from getting attention, socializing successfully. Quantity is an important element; the more I can get into my stomach the safer I feel." . . . But when she ate she felt exceedingly guilty, full of self-contempt and disrespect for herself which contributed to her sense of worthlessness, "because food has become my only source of satisfaction; because I can't control my eating or my feelings." . . . When she could control her eating and would lose weight, she felt strong and cheerful. When she gave in to the urge for food she became depressed and suicidal.* (pp. 268–269)

Causal Factors, Onset, and Course

People with eating disorders can sometimes pinpoint the event that triggered their problem. For some, it may have been incidental weight loss that elicited praise and compliments. Some feel pressure from those around them to lose weight. They may have been brought up in families who are excessively weight conscious and gradually develop an eating disorder. For example, Celia, like most people who develop anorexia nervosa, was not obese before beginning to diet. But when her 130-lb boyfriend remarked that she weighed almost as much as he did, she started to diet (Bruch, 1973). What starts as "normal" dieting becomes an obsession in people with eating disorders.

Biological Factors

Eating disorders run in families, and there is some suggestion, based on twin studies, that heredity is partly implicated. There are abnormalities in hormone and neurotransmitter regulation in people with eating disorders, and they also have trouble interpreting internal sensations of hunger and fullness (APA, 1993). However, when examining biological factors, cause and effect are hard to determine. ("Eating Disorders," 1992).

Psychological Factors

Psychological theories about causation include the idea that people with eating disorders use dieting and weight control measures to compensate for feelings of personal ineffectiveness and low self-esteem (APA, 1993). The personality of women with anorexia are depicted as "shy, serious, neat, quiet, conscientious, perfectionistic, hypersensitive to rejection, and inclined to irrational guilt and obsessive worrying" ("Eating Disorders," 1992, p. 3). They have a desire for control and a need to feel special. The eating disorder is viewed as a means of gaining control when the individual feels that he or she lacks autonomy.

Some researchers feel that anorexia is the response of young women to the pressures of sexuality and adult independence. Women with anorexia feel that they don't know their own desires and live to please others. The obsessive control of eating is an area in which they express their independence (Kaplan & Sadock, 1998).

People with bulimia are more outgoing than people who are anorexic. They are also more emotional and impulsive. Some experts have theorized that, as children, people with bulimia were fed to soothe them or to put them to sleep and that they were encouraged to eat when they were not hungry. Other researchers propose that food takes the place of love ("Eating Disorders," 1992).

Family Factors

The APA (1993) suggested that families of people with eating disorders are pathological. The family member with the eating disorder is viewed as exhibiting a pathology that is really family dysfunction. However, it may be the stress of having a child with an eating disorder that creates family problems ("Eating Disorders," 1992).

Sociocultural Factors

Foods eaten, patterns of food consumed, and body image are influenced by culture. Approximately 90% of individuals with anorexia are women (Brotman, 1994), and there is a great deal of social pressure on women to be slender.

The more intense the social pressure for slimness, the more likely it is that a troubled girl or young woman will develop an eating disorder rather than some other psychiatric symptom—especially if she also regards self-control in eating as a sign of the discipline needed for high achievement and social success. In our society, richer and better-educated women tend to be thinner than average, and they may also be at higher risk for eating disorders.

Anorexia and bulimia are especially common among women athletes and ballet dancers. One survey found that 15% of female medical students have had an eating disorder at some time; another study found bulimia to be five times more common in college women than in working women of the same age ("Eating Disorders," 1993, p. 1).

Other Factors

Depression is associated with eating disorders, and some theorists conceive of eating disorders as a variant of depression. Serious depression is found in 40% of anorexic patients. Women who suffer from severe depression have double the rate of bulimia and eight times the rate of anorexia than the general population. It is not clear if the depression is the effect of dieting or if people who are depressed develop eating disorders ("Eating Disorders," 1992).

Treatment

Treatment Goals

The treatment goals for people with anorexia are to restore weight to within 10–15% of ideal (Brotman, 1994) and to restore menstruation. In addition, for both clients with anorexia and those with bulimia, the following are common goals (Brotman, 1994; APA, 1993):

- Address physiological factors associated with the eating disorder (e.g., effects of starvation, emotional and cognitive, personality changes).
- Restore normal eating patterns.
- Address the psychological, social, and behavioral factors that may underlie the problem.
- Treat associated mood disorders.
- Challenge distorted cultural values.

Treatment of Malnutrition and Other Biological Problems

Hospitalization is not required for uncomplicated bulimia (APA, 1993). However, hospitalization is required for people with anorexia if weight is less than 30% of minimal healthy weight or if medical complications (e.g., slow pulse, low blood pressure causing dizziness, loss of potassium, cardiac arrhythmias) are present (Brotman, 1994). Although longer stays are more beneficial, insurance currently does not pay for more than a few days in the hospital (Brotman, 1994). Since starvation brings about distorted thinking, it is difficult to address the psychological factors when the individual is not thinking well. The goal of hospitalization is weight gain and medical stabilization. Weight gain is not the cure, but it is necessary to clarify thinking, which is distorted by starvation, so that underlying factors can then be addressed.

Medication

Medication is used for these clients if there are accompanying problems: Antidepressants for depression and/or obsessive-compulsive behavior, and antianxiety medication for anxiety. Medication for clients who are anorexic helps with depression and anxiety but it does not address the eating disorder (Brotman, 1994). For clients with bulimia, even when depressive symptoms are not evident, antidepressant medication may reduce binge eating and purging (APA, 1993).

Treatment of Psychological, Behavioral, and Social Problems

Anorexia is a complex, life-threatening illness and requires ongoing attention. Currently, the best, immediate results come from a combination of weight restoration followed by individual and family psychotherapy (APA, 1993). The goal of psychotherapy is to address the psychological issues that are at the foundation of the eating disorder. Psychodynamic therapies help facilitate insight and sometimes the subject of food and weight is avoided ("Comparing Treatments," 1994). In this noncoercive approach, patients with anorexia do not feel that their need for control is being threatened (APA, 1993). It has been found that bulimia also "can be treated without direct attention to eating habits and weight, simply by relieving depression and improving the patient's social life" ("Comparing Treatments," 1994).

Often the onset of anorexia occurs in girls young enough to be living with their family of origin, and family therapy is included in the treatment regime. Whether families have a major role in the cause of the eating disorder or are suffering the effects, the family is involved. Family therapy practitioners view the family as a system in which the roles, rituals, and rules are addressed ("Eating Disorders," 1992).

Cognitive behavioral treatment is effective for both anorexia and bulimia (Brotman, 1994; "Comparing Treatments," 1994). This treatment addresses the clients' attitudes and is especially effective in helping people with bulimia change eating habits and body image, reduce perfectionism, and enhance self-esteem. In one study, cognitive therapy was found to be most effective at changing attitudes of people with bulimia toward food and weight and 36% effective in addressing binging and purging ("Comparing Treatments," 1994). Other facets of treatment may include nutritional counseling (Brotman, 1994) and expressive therapies for people who have trouble with verbal communication (APA, 1993). Group interpersonal therapy has been found to be 44% effective for the binging-and-purging symptoms of bulimia ("Comparing Treatments," 1994).

Outcome

Most people with bulimia respond to individual and group therapy ("Eating Disorders," 1993). Anorexia tends to be a chronic problem, requiring years of treatment. "The anxiety and frustration of care givers and family members is extraordinary. It is painful to watch helplessly as a young woman starves herself to death" (Brotman, 1994, p. 8).

Occupational Therapy Intervention Considerations

People with eating disorders are usually able to function in work or school (Shimp, 1989), unless they are suffering from starvation effects. At first glance, these women appear to be competent and functional, because they are often perfectionistic high achievers. However, Bridgett (1993) suggested a number of areas that can be addressed by occupational therapy practitioners (Box 43-5).

One of the first goals of treatment articulated by Bridgett (1993) is to gain physical, cognitive, and social awareness. A step toward identifying internal cues of hunger and satiation and gaining a more realistic body image can include activities that involve multisensory stimulation of visual, tactile, and proprioceptive receptors. This may include the appropriate use of exercise (Bridgett, 1993).

BOX 43–5 OCCUPATIONAL THERAPY ASSESSMENTS FOR CLIENTS WITH EATING DISORDERS[a]

- Occupational history.
- Activity configuration.
- Self-image (self portrait, string test, estimation of body size).
- Interest inventory.
- Locus of control.
- Physical assessment (muscle strength, balance, endurance).

[a]From Bridgett (1993).

People with eating disorders are not only out of touch with their bodies but also are out of touch with their own psychological and social needs and desires. Particularly clients with anorexia may not be in touch with what they want for themselves because they are so eager to please others. Bruch (1979) described a girl who was always trying to second-guess what her parents wanted of her so she could satisfy them. This included trying to find out what they had gotten her for Christmas, so she could express an interest in it. Assertiveness training may be a good addition to the treatment regime for these women and girls to help them identify their own needs and how to fulfill them.

Because many clients with anorexia have trouble talking about their problems (APA, 1993), expressive activities such as art, dance, crafts, and music may help with self-expression. The occupational therapy practitioner must recognize the multiple benefits of expressive activities: They are forms of multisensory input and can address self-assertion. Furthermore, they promote self-awareness through emotional expression and sensory stimulation (Bailey, 1986). The practitioner can implement expressive activities in ways that address all of these elements.

Time management to include leisure activities and social contact is another occupational therapy goal (Bridgett, 1993). People with eating disorders often become so preoccupied by exercise, food rituals, and work or school performance that they do not include leisure in their lives. If they do engage in recreation it takes on a pressured feeling from which they derive little enjoyment. Bridgett (1993) described the activity configuration of one of her patients who had anorexia. This 17-year-old girl's typical day consisted of 8 hours of school or school work, 6 hours on the job, 6 hours of sleep, and 2 hours of exercise. She neglected meals, spent little time with her family, and increasingly avoided involvement with peers.

Psychoeducational groups to develop stress management skills are helpful. The goals of such groups are to seek ways to broaden leisure and social activities by examining current activities and interests, exploring community resources and developing a plan of action to broaden and balance life activities (Bridgett, 1993).

There remains the question of food, nutrition, cooking, and eating: Should these be occupational therapy activities? Shimp (1989) reported on an occupational therapy program in a short-term treatment program for people with eating disorders that consisted of a family-style meal group. In these groups, patients planned, shopped for, prepared, and ate a meal. The purpose of these groups was to channel the need for control of eating into healthy functional control rather than the unhealthy behaviors associated with eating disorders. Each individual formulated personal goals for the meal: " 'To eat without panicking,' 'not to worry about amounts so much,' to eat without anger,' and 'to be cooperative in preparing the meal instead of just doing things my own way' "(p. 2). Shimp noted:

> *Eating the meal is hard, but the patients learn to take their own adequate portions and complete their meals in 30 min. without negative statements (although initially seldom without tears). In this high-stress area, the patients also find it difficult to get the "right" amount of food without measuring portions, to eat with others (especially for those who are new to the unit), and to deal with the temptation to binge with the extra food on the table while they are waiting for the others to finish. Some patients even have trouble sitting down with others and then not getting up to clean the kitchen without eating as they have done in the past (especially those with families). (pp. 2–3)*

Occupational therapy practitioners who engage in cooking and nutrition groups should heed the following caution from Luder and Schebendach (1993), who work with people who have eating disorders:

> *Nutrition plays an important role in eating disorders, for it is as much a part of the symptom as the cure. The patient's obsession about nutrition issues often makes the nutritionist a popular member of the treatment team. However, care must be taken to avoid a proselytizing attitude about "good" versus "bad" nutrition. Indeed, the concept of nutrition as a process that transcends a specific food, food group, or daily intake must be clearly conveyed and continually reinforced. (p. 61)*

It is also important to remember that studies have found that people with eating disorders can be treated without direct attention to eating habits (APA, 1993; "Comparing Treatments," 1994).

BORDERLINE PERSONALITY DISORDER

Borderline personality disorder is classified on Axis II of the DSM. It is among the most ambiguous of the personality disorders in the spectrum of mental illness. Personality traits are the characteristic ways in which people think, feel, and act. They are enduring qualities that persist over time. People who have personality disorders suffer from long-standing, maladaptive personality traits. Borderline personality was not classified by the APA until 1980 and is not considered a highly reliable diagnosis. The term *borderline* refers to the characteristics that border on psychosis and neurosis. Sometimes it is difficult to distinguish personality disorders from depression, anxiety disorders, schizophrenia, or adjustment disorders ("Borderline Personality," 1994a).

Characteristics

People with borderline personality disorders share one or more of the following characteristics (APA, 2000):

- Instability of thought, mood, and behavior.
- Unstable interpersonal relationships.
- Problems with self-image.

Instability of Thought, Mood, and Behavior

People diagnosed with borderline personality tend to be impulsive. They are quick to anger and likely to abuse drugs and alcohol. There is a 60% rate of major depression in people with borderline personality. Their depression is qualitatively different from others who suffer from chronic depression. In borderline personality disorder, there is less guilt, lethargy, and appetite loss than in mood disorders. Instead, these clients complain of loneliness, boredom, and a feeling of emptiness ("Borderline Personality," 1994a).

Self-mutilation and suicide attempts are serious problems in people with borderline personality. Some people engage in cutting themselves, claiming that it "makes me feel real." Others have chronic suicidal tendencies, which are sometimes viewed by their therapists as bids for attention. However, suicidal gestures cannot be dismissed, since people with borderline personality are impulsive and have the same rate of suicide as people with schizophrenia and bipolar disorder ("Borderline Personality," 1994c).

Unstable Interpersonal Relationships

People with borderline personality disorder can be a challenge for those who work and live with them. Their instability of thought and mood results in unpredictable behavior. They appear to overreact to events that others find unremarkable. They invest a great deal of importance and intensity in relationships but inexplicably reject the individual they once idolized. It is thought that this occurs because people with borderline personalities have such an intense need for others that it is impossible for others to live up to those expectations. These clients eventually feel betrayed and angry when their unreasonable demands of others are not met.

For example, Mary, a 30-year-old woman with borderline personality disorder felt rejected and angry when her friend canceled a lunch date because of a death in the family. Kernberg (1984), a psychotherapist, reported that a patient with borderline personality disorder "let me know that she wanted me to say only perfect and precise things that would immediately and clearly reflect how she was feeling and would reassure her that I was really with her. Otherwise I should say nothing but listen patiently to her attacks on me" (p. 129).

Another factor in the relationships of people with borderline personality is their use of splitting. Splitting is a primitive defense mechanism in which individuals view themselves and others as all good or all bad (Carson et al.,

2000). Cognitive therapists call splitting dichotomous thinking, which is thinking that places everything in discrete categories, black or white, rather than conceptualizing that there are continuous dimensions to reality (Beck & Freeman, 1990). This kind of all-or-nothing thinking may explain why a person with borderline personality seems quite suddenly to turn against a friend or a therapist. It may be that the client's perfect image of the friend was marred in some way and, instead of being able to acknowledge that no one is perfect, the client now thinks of the friend as completely bad.

In therapeutic situations, the consequences of dichotomous thinking are that the client might classify staff as either good or bad; if care is not taken, staff and other patients may be drawn into this splitting. This produces division among staff as well as among staff and patients, damaging the therapeutic environment. It is important to recognize this phenomenon and maintain good communication.

Problems with Self-Image

People with borderline personality disorder have not achieved an integrated sense of self or they have a sense of impaired self (Miller, 1994). They may express their feelings of inadequacy:

> *It has always been there, for as long as I can remember, even back in school, even in middle school . . . it is like a rating scale. . . . I don't give people numbers. I just rate them against me and I never met anyone that I was equal to or better than, no matter what. Even if it is a bum on the street, there is something that makes him better than me. (Miller, 1994, p. 1217).*

Feeling inadequate leads to estrangement and despair. One person with borderline personality disorder said she feels "separated in a way, not quite in there with the rest. . . . I think it is because I already feel I'm different, so I feel I should separate myself from everyone else in some way" (Miller, 1994, p. 1217). A study in which people with borderline personality disorder were interviewed found that "each person revealed an ever-present wish not to be alive" (Miller, 1994, p. 1217).

People with borderline personality disorder are not always in turmoil (Beck & Freeman, 1990). They go through periods of holding jobs and maintaining relationships. In social situations, they do best in settings such as work, where the structure permits them to maintain control. Mental health workers see borderline patients when they are feeling out of control and decompensated, but, for some, there are periods of high functioning.

Cause

The cause is unknown, but many people with borderline personality disorder have a history of persistent abuse in childhood. Other theories about cause include a biological deficit in the regulation of affect/mood and inconsistent parenting. It is primarily a diagnosis of women, who make up 70–77% of all those diagnosed (Linehan, Tutek, Heard, & Armstrong, 1994), and it is found in 2% of the general population (APA, 2000).

Biological Theories

There is a hereditary component to personality, and some studies propose that borderline personality disorder may be caused by an inherited brain malfunction, since there is a higher rate of borderline personality in certain families. Limited research has found brain damage and/or injury to the limbic system or frontal lobes in some people. These areas of the brain modulate impulses and emotions ("Borderline Personality," 1994a).

Psychodynamic Theories

Kernberg attributes borderline personality disorder to the use of immature defense mechanisms: "splitting, poor reality testing, a weak ego, and inadequate integration of identity—inability to make sense of the contradictory aspects of oneself and others" ("Borderline Personality," 1994a, p. 3). These attributes are caused by the unstable early childhood interactions with the caretaker, which have been characterized as unpredictable, alternately smothering and rejecting. Psychodynamic theories consider the first 2 years of life significant in the development of people with borderline personalities. It is thought that during these years, parenting practices that foster aggression and frustration interfere with the child's development of a stable ego identity. Later in life, the person with borderline personality disorder may re-enact this childhood relationship, resulting in reinforcement of maladaptive interactions ("Borderline Personality," 1994b).

Associated Factors

There is a high rate of substance abuse among individuals diagnosed with borderline personality disorder, and other forms of self-destructive behaviors are common. About 25% of people with borderline personality disorder are also diagnosed with posttraumatic stress disorder, which is the result of persistent abuse as a child (Herman, 1992).

Posttraumatic stress disorder is a condition of anxiety, flashbacks, and problems with interpersonal relationships as a result of a highly traumatic experience in which one's life or well-being was threatened. It can also occur in an individual who witnessed the traumatic experiences of another. The symptoms usually have their onset after the trauma and can cause severe debilitation of social and occupational function (APA, 2000).

Treatment

Treatment of borderline personality disorder follows the frame of reference of the clinician and the setting. Sometimes people with borderline personality require hospitalization when there is danger of suicide or severe regression. It is advised that hospitalization be kept brief and that these individuals understand that the purpose of the protective environment is not to foster the sick role but to help them regain control of their life.

Psychotherapy

A variety of psychotherapies, from psychoanalytic to supportive psychotherapy, have been used for borderline personality disorder. Evaluations of treatment approaches are inconclusive, because there has been little systematic research done. Researchers believe that it is difficult to change personality, which is, by definition, ingrained, enduring patterns of thought and behavior ("Borderline Personality," 1994b).

Dialectical Behavior Therapy

Dialectical behavior therapy is a cognitive behavioral technique that has been helpful in treating important symptoms of borderline personality disorder. It combines individual and group therapy, using methods to help individuals control impulses and soothe themselves. The theory behind this treatment is that people with borderline personality disorder have problems with regulation of impulses and emotions. They lack skills in stress tolerance and self-regulation, which in turn interferes with interpersonal relationships. This maladaptive behavior is believed to be caused by a combination of personal factors and an environment that fosters and reinforces these characteristics (Linehan et al., 1994).

Dialectical behavior therapy methods include "psychoeducation, problem solving, social skills training, modeling, homework assignments, and behavioral rehearsal" ("Borderline Personality," 1994c, p. 1). These methods address problems with impulsive responding and the inability to modulate feelings, anger, and self-destructive behavior. The goals of dialectical behavior therapy are to (Linehan et al., 1994):

- Reduce suicidal and other life-threatening or self mutilating behaviors.
- Lessen noncompliant behaviors that interfere with treatment.
- Change behavior patterns that lead to inpatient psychiatric care and interfere with quality of life.
- Enhance coping skills.

Medication

In the past, drug therapy was avoided but now medication is used for the symptoms the individual exhibits. Thus medication can be used for anxiety, depression, mania, and psychotic symptoms. Antipsychotic medication appears to be effective for many of these symptoms when found in people with borderline personality disorder ("Borderline Personality," 1994c).

Implications for Occupational Therapy

It is important for all who work with people with borderline personality disorder to be consistent and trustworthy. This can be a challenge, because these clients have such difficulty trusting others and seem to sabotage relationships (Beck & Freeman, 1990). On one hand, they have great dependency needs. They feel empty and inadequate and wish that others could help them. On the other hand, these clients are terrified of intimacy for fear of rejection and abandonment.

Kernberg (1984) suggested that the treatment setting provide a homelike environment in which work and leisure routines can be maintained. Task groups are important as a means to gain leadership and collaborative skills and to test ego function, but they are not the place to explore feelings and intrapsychic conflict. In inpatient settings or day treatment, "bridges between hospital life and the external social environment" (p. 344) are created while individual and group therapy is carried out. Kernberg stressed the importance of the personal as well as professional attributes of the staff, since they use their interpersonal interactions with the clients to work through borderline issues. It is important that the analysis of client–staff interaction sticks to here-and-now events. Members of the health-care team are cautioned to "consistently preserve socially appropriate behavior toward patients and clearly delimit their personal boundaries from their professional functions. To be spontaneous and open in their interactions with patients does not mean that members of staff should talk about their personal lives" (p. 345). Communication among staff is critical to support the therapeutic community and to prevent splitting.

Because people with borderline personality disorder who are in crisis are so difficult, there is the danger that staff will despair of satisfactory recovery. One woman with the disorder articulated the effect this had on her:

> *I know that things are getting better about borderlines and stuff. Having that diagnosis resulted in my getting treated exactly the way I was treated at home. The minute I got that diagnosis people stopped treating me as though what I was doing had a reason. All that psychiatric treatment was just as destructive as what happened before.*
>
> *Denying the reality of my experience—that was the most harmful. Not being able to trust anyone was the most serious effect. . . . I know I acted in ways that were despicable. But I wasn't crazy. Some people go around acting like that because they feel hopeless. Finally I found*

a few people along the way who have been able to feel OK about me even though I had severe problems. Good therapists were those who really validated my experience. (Herman, 1992, p. 56)

Outcome

Borderline personality disorder appears to be a chronic problem that may require long-term, intermittent therapy during periods of crisis. Therapy is supportive to help the individual regain some equilibrium and to intervene in self-destructive behavior. The *Harvard Mental Health Letter* summed up the outcome of the disorder:

If they live through their 20's without disaster, persons diagnosed as borderline often reach a kind of equilibrium. Their extremes of mood and impulsive behavior are moderated and suicide attempts almost cease. Several studies of long-term outcome in formerly hospitalized borderline patients have come to the same conclusion: Little change over a 5-year period, but much improvement after 15 years and more. . . . Most had freed themselves of their worst addictions, married, become parents, and kept jobs. They were doing about as well as patients committed to the same hospital at the same time for depression. . . . In middle age most patients in the outcome studies no longer qualify for a diagnosis of borderline personality. ("Borderline Personality," 1994c, p. 3)

The people who fared best in the outcome studies were those who were more intelligent, who found satisfaction in work, and who had special talents ("Borderline Personality," 1994c).

BOX 43-6 SCHIZOPHRENIA AND OTHER PSYCHOTIC DISORDERS[a]

SCHIZOPHRENIA SUBTYPES

- *Paranoid type:* Persecutory or grandiose delusions and/or hallucinations; speech and behavior is more organized than other types; affect and cognition relatively well preserved.
- *Disorganized type:* Flat or inappropriate (silly) affect; marked disorganization of speech and behavior.
- *Catatonic type:* Disturbed psychomotor behavior, either excessive purposeless activity or immobility.
- *Undifferentiated:* Symptoms meet the general criteria described in the text.
- *Residual type:* A history of at least one episode of schizophrenia and continuing evidence of negative symptoms, atypical beliefs, and odd perceptions; no prominent hallucinations or delusions.

OTHER PSYCHOTIC DISORDERS

The following disorders share most of the characteristics of schizophrenia with differences in duration, cause, or concurrent symptoms. The treatment and management of the psychotic symptoms are similar, and occupational therapy considerations are often the same if functional impairment accompanies the disorder.

- Schizophreniform disorder.
- Brief psychotic disorder.
- Schizoaffective disorder.
- Substance-induced psychotic disorder.
- Delusional disorder.
- Shared psychotic disorder (folie a deux).
- Psychotic disorder due to general medical condition.

[a]From APA (2000).

SCHIZOPHRENIA

Schizophrenia is probably a group of related psychotic disorders, rather than a single entity (Box 43-6). The disturbed thought processes and psychotic symptoms associated with schizophrenia lead to difficulties with communication, interpersonal relationships, and reality testing. Schizophrenia is found in 1% of the population and is slightly more common in males than in females. The age of onset is between late adolescence and the mid-30s. For the diagnosis to be made, the symptoms must be significantly severe enough to impair social or occupational function and must be present for at least 6 months (APA, 2000).

Characteristic Symptoms

Characteristic symptoms of schizophrenia include disturbances of thought content, affect, process of thought, volition, perception, and sense of self. There may also be social withdrawal and disturbed psychomotor behavior. No single feature is always present, but the APA (2000) diagnosis of schizophrenia specifies that at least two of the following symptoms must be noted: delusions, hallucinations, disorganized speech and/or behavior, and negative symptoms.

Positive and Negative Symptoms of Schizophrenia

Positive symptoms are those that are conspicuously disturbing to others. Symptoms are active, florid, and characterized by excessive or peculiar activity. The individual experiences bizarre delusions and insulting or commanding auditory hallucinations. They may go into sudden, unexplained rages, and their speech and thinking are incoherent.

Negative symptoms are less conspicuous than positive symptoms. Individuals are passive, speak with a toneless voice, and exhibit little facial expression (flat affect). They avoid eye contact and rarely smile or return greetings. They do not initiate activity and make few spontaneous movements. Speech is empty, and thoughts are obscure. These clients have trouble concentrating and seem to take little pleasure in anything. Negative symptoms can be confused with depression and can look like the side effects of antipsychotic medication. Often, negative symptoms are the prevailing condition, with positive symptoms emerging periodically (APA, 1994).

Disturbance of Content of Thought

Delusions are false ideas, which may be fragmented and bizarre or organized and systematic. Common schizophrenic delusions are thought broadcasting, by which individuals believe that they are able to send out their thoughts to others. Sometimes clients believe someone is putting thoughts into their heads. This thought insertion can consist of unpleasant and disturbing delusions. Thought withdrawal occurs when it seems as if thoughts had been removed. This may be an expression of the impoverished thought process associated with schizophrenia. Sometimes individuals have delusions of being controlled and they believe they are being given instructions that they feel impelled to follow.

Thought Process: Disorganized Thinking

Disorganized thinking has been referred to as the most important symptom of schizophrenia (APA, 2000). The disturbances of thought patterns take many forms and can be observed through the clients' speech or writing. People with schizophrenia may have vague, overly abstract or overly concrete thinking. Some speak in repetitive stereotyped phrases. Some people are so incoherent that their speech has been described as a "word salad" (APA, 2000). North (1989) described her thought processes during a psychotic episode. Note how her incoherent associations are related to her delusional thinking, in her description of the result of her attempt to keep her thoughts from being broadcast to others:

> *Most of all, I wanted to keep my mother from hearing my thoughts. Whenever it seemed she was tuning in on my thought waves, I purposely substituted nonsense words for my true thoughts, or intentionally scrambled the words as they came to me. But in the process, my thoughts sometimes got so hopelessly jumbled that I needed to write them down to straighten them out for my own comprehension. To keep anyone from being able to read the thoughts I was writing, I invented a private code of original characters symbolizing letters, words, phrases, and tenses all mixed up in such a way that no one could possibly read it. On paper it looked like endless columns of nonsensical symbols. (p. 37)*

Perceptual Disturbances

People with schizophrenia experience all kinds of hallucinations, but the most common type are auditory, in the form of voices or sounds. Tactile hallucinations can take the form of burning, tingling, and electrical sensations. Some feel their body mysteriously change and may actually envision the changes. Others may have exceptional sensitivity to sound, sight or smell.

North (1989) described her visual hallucinations:

> *My thoughts weren't the only thing giving me trouble. My perceptions had changed. I had become vaguely aware of colored patterns decorating the air. When I first noticed them, I realized I had actually been seeing them for a long time, yet never paid attention to them before. I thought that everyone saw them, that they were a visual equivalent of background noise, like a fan's hum that goes unnoticed. These patterns, composed of tiny spicules and multicolored squiggly lines, wiggled and wormed their way around and through each other like people milling in a crowd. The patterns looked like what I imagined the visual equivalent of radio static to be, so I called them Interference Patterns. (p. 37)*

North's term *interference pattern* is wonderfully descriptive and apt. Hallucinations, of every kind, interfere with people's perceptions of the world. Whether they hear voices or see or feel these sensory misperceptions, they are distracted and impaired by the phenomena. It is difficult to think straight, to organize and carry-out purposeful action, and to relate to people.

Disturbances of Affect

Affect refers to the emotional tone of individuals demonstrated by their facial expression and voice inflection. When the affect lacks intensity it is called blunt. If there is no emotional expression, the person is said to have a flat affect. Sometimes people with schizophrenia have an inappropriate affect; for example, they laugh or smile when talking about sad events. Or they look terrified when there is nothing obviously frightening.

All of the symptoms of schizophrenia are interrelated. Hallucinations pull people with schizophrenia away from reality. Their affect reflects their perceptions rather than those of the observer. When patients are preoccupied with their inner reality, their cognitive and motor responses to the external environment are slow or are bizarrely irrelevant. To the observer, these individuals' thought processes, affect, and behavior seem inappropriate. North (1989) wrote:

> *Dr. Hemingway had no idea of the high activity level of the voices as we talked, and he didn't know that the*

voices were heavily influencing me. To him I looked flat, vacant, catatonic. I moved slowly, and left giant gaps between my words. I talked very little as far as he could tell, but I felt I was talking a lot. After all, I was carrying on simultaneous conversations with him and the voices. (p. 187)

Disturbed Sense of Self

It seems reasonable that if one is hallucinating and delusional one might be perplexed about one's identity. One woman said that her son, who was schizophrenic, kept asking her if he was Jesus. He'd say: "I'm not Jesus. I'm not Jesus, am I Mom?" The person might know that the delusion doesn't make sense but cannot get rid of it. Some have no doubts about their delusional thinking and hallucinations.

A disturbed sense of self can also become evident when the individual becomes obsessed by the meaning of life or feels controlled by outsiders. There may be a loss of ego boundaries, and the patient does not have a sense of self. Vonnegut (1975) described how his delusional thinking led him to question how he could negotiate his way within his new view of the world:

When I looked at someone they were everything. They were beautiful, breathtakingly so. They were all things to me. The waitress was Eve, Helen of Troy, all women of all times, the eternal female principle, heroic, beautiful, my mother, my sisters, every woman I had ever loved. Everything good I had ever loved. Simon was Adam, Jesus, Bob Dylan, my father, every man I had ever loved. They were whatever I needed and more. I loved them utterly.

I worried about how complicated this could make my life. Maybe it was enlightenment but it brought up not inconsequential problems of engineering. Who sleeps with whom was one, but there were lots of others. Like what if two people I loved wanted me to do different things? Who would I spend time with, who would I talk with, who would I dedicate my life to? If I loved everyone there was no way to focus any more, no reason to spend time with anyone in particular (p. 117).

Decreased Volition and Disorganized Behavior

People with schizophrenia have trouble initiating action and engaging in goal-directed activity. Their interest in the world is muted, and they often lack the drive to follow up a course of action to its conclusion. This makes it difficult to live independently, because they have trouble with the most mundane tasks. To the outsider this appears as "laziness" but as Vonnegut (1975) said, he sometimes "had trouble walking and remembering to breathe" (p. 112). Here is how Maxine, a woman who had schizophrenia all her adult life, is described:

Maxine had never been able to survive on her own, even in a room at the Y. She was careless and lazy. The neighbors came over one day after Maxine had put all the dirty dishes in the kitchen sink and turned the water on—"so the dishes would wash themselves"—and found water all over the floor. (Sheehan, 1995, p. 205)

Maxine was not a stupid woman, but her schizophrenia impaired her judgment. Vonnegut (1975) described some of the psychotic perceptions and thoughts that interfere with completing a task:

Small tasks became incredibly intricate and complex. It started with pruning the fruit trees. One saw cut would take forever. I was completely absorbed in the sawdust floating gently to the ground, the feel of the saw in my hand, the incredible patterns in the bark, the muscles in my arm pulling back and then pushing forward. Everything stretched infinitely in all directions. Suddenly it seemed as if everything was slowing down and I would never finish sawing the limb. Then by some miracle that branch would be done and I'd have to rest, completely blown out. Then I found myself being unable to stick with any one tree. . . . I began to wonder if I was hurting the trees and found myself apologizing. Each tree began to take on a personality. I began to wonder if any of them liked me. I became completely absorbed in looking at each tree. (p. 99)

Withdrawal

Because people with schizophrenia are preoccupied with delusions and hallucinations, they seem to have withdrawn from the world. If their delusions are paranoid they do not trust others and avoid the dangers interaction would foster. For some, the withdrawal seems emotional, they appear detached and unconcerned.

Disturbance in Psychomotor Behavior

Disturbance in psychomotor behavior can take many forms. When Vonnegut described pruning the trees, he probably appeared as slow moving and preoccupied as he felt. He worked slowly, resting between the cutting of each branch as he closely examined each tree. Some people with schizophrenia engage in bizarre posturing or excessive motor activity, pacing, rocking, and other excited actions that seem unrelated to environmental stimuli.

Other Features

People with schizophrenia may be disheveled or eccentrically groomed. They are not socially adept, rather, withdrawn and isolative; some are obnoxious. Depression, anxiety, and anger sometimes accompany the disorder. Sylvia Frumpkin, a woman with schizophrenia, was angry a lot of the time, and people found her aggressive and difficult. Her attire was interesting (Sheehan, 1983):

> *Miss Frumpkin seemed unaware of the [hot and humid] weather that morning, she was wearing a blouse, a vest, a pair of blue jeans, and a quilted jacket. She had tied another pair of blue jeans around her neck. She also wore around her neck a chain with a pop top from a soda can on it. On her feet were a pair of socks and the high heeled gold sandals. On her head was a bandanna. Knotted into the bandanna was a spoon. (p. 104)*

BOX 43–7 OUTCOME OF SCHIZOPHRENIA[a]

- 30% recover and remain symptom free for 5 years.
- 60% respond to medication and other treatments and live in the community with outpatient treatment; they have varying degrees of social and occupational impairment and personality impoverishment and may need brief hospitalization for psychotic behavior, often because of failure to comply with the medication regime.
- 10% remain profoundly disabled.

[a]Data from Carson and Butcher (1992).

Causal Factors

The cause of schizophrenia is unknown. Twin and adoption studies suggest a genetic basis for schizophrenia, but there is also an environmental connection ("How Schizophrenia Develops," 2001). A disproportionate number of people with schizophrenia are born in the late winter or early spring, which fosters the theory that infectious diseases may have a prenatal effect ("Schizophrenia," 1999). Birth complications have been noted in the medical histories of people with schizophrenia ("Birth Complications," 1999). Also, schizophrenic symptoms that are not treated by drugs become worse over time, suggesting that the psychotic process, itself, might damage the brain ("How Schizophrenia Develops," 2001).

Brain-imaging technology enables researchers to view the structure and activity of the living brain. People with schizophrenia show pathology in a number of brain functions, but there is no single pathology common to all. Some have enlarged lateral ventricles (APA, 2000). Antipsychotic medications, used to treat the symptoms of schizophrenia, successfully reduce hallucinations and delusions in a variety of diagnoses. These drugs affect the activity of a number of neurotransmitters, including dopamine and glutamate. The newer medications affect the interplay of those neurotransmitters and norepinephrine and serotonin and have been successful in improving both positive and negative symptoms. The action of these drugs supports the theory that there are irregularities in brain chemistry associated with schizophrenia ("How Schizophrenia Develops," 2001).

Treatment and Implications for Occupational Therapy

The first-line treatment of schizophrenia is medication. The examples just given to illustrate the symptoms of schizophrenia are of people who were not being treated by medication at the time. Antipsychotic medication reduces most of the psychotic symptoms for many people. However, medication alone is not enough to ensure a good quality of life for most clients. Even with successful response to medication, individuals with schizophrenia are still left with little experience dealing with the world (Box 43-7). The disease strikes so early in adulthood, that clients may not have ever experienced normal adult life.

An important role of occupational therapy is to assess these clients in terms of adult occupational roles. Instruction in everyday activity may be required to help clients organize their lives and alleviate stress. Relapse can be caused by stress, and people with schizophrenia are less resilient than others.

Stress

When thinking about schizophrenia and stress it helps to keep in mind Vonnegut's claim that he had trouble walking and remembering to breathe. The claims of everyday life are magnified by the impairments of schizophrenia. For people with schizophrenia, stress may be having to smile at the customer while handing out change at a fast-food restaurant or sorting laundry and remembering to put the soap in the washing machine.

The verbal skills of some people with schizophrenia may mislead therapists into believing these clients can hold jobs and maintain multiple life roles. This is not true for all. They may need to work in an environment that is quiet and not socially demanding. Occupational therapy practitioners work with the 60% of people with schizophrenia who have only partial recovery and live marginal lives.

Stress management includes staying healthy, clean, and sober. Street drugs and alcohol can bring relapse. In Vonnegut's case, drugs triggered his psychosis. Therefore, it is important to teach people with schizophrenia to recognize early symptoms of relapse and how to respond by getting help.

Often the occupational therapy practitioner, more than any other mental health professional, is aware of the discrepancy between verbal proficiency and functional performance skills of the mentally ill. Even clients who have good verbal skills cannot be assumed to be capable of organizing thought and action. Studies have shown that people with schizophrenia have trouble with tasks that require problem solving and novel thinking ("Schizophrenia," 1992). The implications for occupational therapy are that people with schizophrenia must be carefully taught strategies for solving everyday "problems." They need to learn to anticipate predictable difficulties so that they will be prepared, for example, to phone the doctor and arrange for transportation. Practice of skills and rehearsal of social behaviors are critical for learning. Liberman (1988) recommended periodic "booster sessions" of instruction to maintain skills successfully.

Studies also show that people with schizophrenia have trouble with the coordination and integration of multisensory information. They have difficulty grouping objects and ideas by form and meaning or emotional relevance ("Schizophrenia," 1992). Thus, when introducing new learning, occupational therapy practitioners must break down activities to manageable components and give concrete instruction. Even social skills need to be specifically taught and rehearsed. Some clients need explicit instruction on affiliative skills, holding a conversation, being a friend, or dating. Behavioral approaches to learning are effective when the therapist acts as teacher, prompter, coach, and reinforcer (Liberman, 1988).

Activity

A study of 35 people with schizophrenia examined what quality of life meant to them. The results suggested that it was important to feel socially connected, which led to a sense of belonging and of being supported. Engagement in activity was related to being connected to others and to feeling normal, both important aspects of quality of life. Being active was also viewed as a means of gaining skills in time management and acquisition of vocational skills, which then led to a feeling of having control of their life (Laliberte-Rudman, Yu, Scott, & Pajouhandeh, 2000). Occupational therapy practitioners, who are concerned with quality of life must consider these aspects when working with people with schizophrenia.

Structured group activity programs, in any treatment setting, have been found to improve bizarre behaviors and obsessive ruminations (Hayes, 1989). In spite of the difficulty people with schizophrenia have with multisensory integration, one study of activity and verbal groups found more verbal interaction among people with schizophrenia engaged in a group construction task than in a verbal group (Odhner, cited in Hayes, 1989). In some activity groups, the occupational therapy practitioner acts as a facilitator of social interaction and problem solving, while the clients work cooperatively or in parallel (Hayes, 1989). Other groups can be geared to learning specific skills, and in those groups, the therapist acts as teacher and coach.

Family Education and Support

People with chronic schizophrenia need supportive living environments and may live with their families. Family members benefit from learning management skills that help reduce the stress of living with a person with schizophrenia. They need education about the disease and its management; how to communicate, verbally and nonverbally, with the client; and how to deal with problems (Liberman, 1988).

Creating a Functional Sense of Self

Psychiatrist Davidson engaged in phenomenological research in which he examined interviews of 74 people with schizophrenia who had been hospitalized for severe psychotic symptoms. Davidson (1994) noted: "We have come to understand that reconstructing a functional sense of self in the midst of persisting psychotic symptoms and dysfunction is an important aspect of the improvement process in schizophrenia" (p. 113). Here is how one of the people in his study talked about her improvement:

> *It is being active, and I take pride and I'm independent to a certain extent . . . like in my jazz music, like I'll turn on my jazz radio, and I'll love it . . . it's my interest. I turn the radio on myself, no one had it going to nourish themselves, to entertain themselves, like parents would at a house. I turn it on, I'm responsible, I enjoy the music, I make notes and draw while I'm hearing it . . . then I turn it off, then I have some evidence, I've got something done, I've been productive, I have the drawings to look at. Maybe they're damn fine drawings. . . it was for me and by me. My own nurturing. So I'm proud of this effort, but I do need that active state of mind to be steady, to be constant. (p. 109)*

CONCLUSION

In this section, mental illness was discussed according to diagnosis. The diagnosis helps therapists communicate by naming the condition. Diagnostic categories give healthcare professionals consistent terminology and criteria with which to discuss particular disorders, and they lend baseline information for research. An understanding of the typical symptoms and prognoses is an important aspect of the clinical reasoning process. Therapists can expect to use specific assessments and precautions based on diagnoses. Even when practitioners do not know the diagnosis, they make assumptions as they interact with each client and get clues that might point to a diagnosis.

The use of diagnosis can enhance communication and facilitate the intervention process, but it can also stereotype people. It is important to remember that the assumptions therapists make about a diagnosis may not hold true for the particular individual they are seeing. And, although practitioners cannot work without the shared language that a diagnosis provides, it is ultimately the individual who is the concern. The individual transcends the diagnosis.

SECTION II

Interventions for People with Serious Mental Illness

CATANA BROWN

DEFINITION OF SERIOUS MENTAL ILLNESS

Serious mental illness as a term is generally used to describe conditions in which the illness has a major impact on the person's function (Rothbard, Schinnar, & Goldman, 1996). This impact in function may be reflected in repeated hospitalizations, difficulty maintaining employment, or a lack of social relationships. Diagnoses that are most often associated with serious mental illness include schizophrenia, severe forms of bipolar disorder, and major depression. One of the reasons it became important to distinguish serious mental illness from "less serious" mental illness is to the general disregard for the needs of this population in our society. When the community mental health movement began, after a period of time it became clear that the people who had the most serious illnesses were receiving the least services. By specifying serious mental illness, greater attention was drawn to the population.

There is a down side to this terminology. The term *serious mental illness* places the emphasis on deficits. Unfortunately, the prevailing approaches for people with serious mental illness have too often centered on managing the psychosis, providing custodial care, and protecting the public rather than supporting full community inclusion and participation. Occupational therapists' knowledge of occupational performance can contribute to change in intervention approaches both through services provided at the individual level as well as through advocacy for system change. This section discusses intervention approaches that appreciate individuals for their uniqueness and differences, accentuate strengths and empowerment, and support people to participate in daily life.

PROMOTING EMPOWERMENT

Consumer *empowerment* involves reducing reliance on professionals and helping clients take action and control over their own lives (Dickerson, 1998). It is a political movement involving consciousness raising and social change. This can be unsettling for the occupational therapist. Empowered consumers are more likely to question and critique professionals. In addition, it can be difficult for professionals to listen and come to terms with their own roles in dehumanizing and repressive systems. On the other hand, when professionals embrace consumer empowerment, the experience can be liberating for both parties. A cooperative and collaborative working relationship can be established in which the consumer is the expert in terms of the experience of living with a mental illness and the occupational therapy practitioner is the expert in supporting participation in daily life. Promoting empowerment and a client- and consumer-centered approach to practice go hand in hand. Box 43-8 lists attributes of this approach.

There are many benefits to the use of consumer-centered approaches. Law (1998) reviewed the research evidence and found that consumer-centered approaches:

- Increased adherence to intervention recommendations.
- Improved client satisfaction with services.
- Resulted in better functional outcomes.

RECOVERY MODEL

The *recovery model* encompasses empowerment but is a larger construct. Emerging from the consumer movement,

BOX 43-8 CHARACTERISTICS OF CONSUMER-CENTERED PRACTICE[a]

- Services are directed toward what the consumer wants and needs in his or her life.
- The occupational therapist provides information on all of the available options and the pros and cons of the options.
- The consumer is the ultimate decision maker.
- The consumer's experience as the one living with the mental illness is valued.
- The consumer is involved in all aspects of the occupational therapy process.
- The consumer is "allowed" to make mistakes or exercise poor judgment, and these are viewed as typical life experiences.
- Consumers are encouraged to voice opinions, give feedback, and provide evaluations; consumer input is regarded as beneficial and essential.

[a]From Deegan (1996), Dickerson (1998), and Law (1998).

the model speaks to a process that includes recovery from mental illness and, more important, the effects of mental illness (e.g., poverty, loss of dignity) (Deegan, 1996). Based on a qualitative study of individuals experiencing recovery, Young and Ensing (1999) identified five components of the recovery process: overcoming stuckness, discovering and fostering empowerment, learning and self-redefinition, returning to basic functioning, and improving quality of life. Spirituality is important in all steps of the process and essential to the last stage. Spiritual practices employed as part of the recovery process can inspire change, support positive views of self, provide rituals and habits, and give meaning to life.

Use of Narrative

Creating a *self-narrative* is an intervention approach that can be used to support self-redefinition (Ridgway, 2001). People who have experienced serious mental illness often must grapple with identifying who they are. This includes an analysis of what parts of their identity reflect who they've been all along and what parts are new. The intervention process can include helping clients develop their story. Many methods for storytelling may be used. Journaling, letter writing, poetry, collage, or drama are some media that are amenable to narrative work. The occupational therapy practitioner may help initiate the process by posing questions or themes or creating a timeline to fill in. The occupational therapy practitioner may also be involved in identifying or creating venues in which the story can be told (e.g., publication sources, audiences).

Advocacy

Advocacy includes standing up for individual rights as well as addressing public policy. One component of advocacy intervention is education. Consumers should be provided with knowledge of the American's with Disabilities Act of 1990 as well as other policies and laws that guarantee rights to individuals with serious mental illness. In addition, intervention includes the development of skills needed for the act of advocacy. Advocacy skills include the ability to communicate, negotiate, and organize a group into action. For example, an occupational therapy practitioner may educate consumers regarding issues of mental health insurance parity in their state, discuss methods of contacting state representatives regarding the issue, and actually conduct a visit to the state legislature. On a smaller scale, intervention may involve supporting consumers to self-advocate with their landlord for needed apartment repairs.

Self-Management

Self-management involves developing strategies that support recovery both in basic functioning and in enhanced quality of life. The general public is becoming more aware of the role that lifestyle can play in an individual's overall satisfaction with life. The need for health-promoting practices can be even more important to people with vulnerabilities related to mental illness. Self-management includes topics such as nutrition, exercise, stress management, smoking cessation, development of support systems, and engagement in meaningful occupation. Occupational therapy intervention can incorporate information about and techniques for supporting self-management practices. The Wellness/Recovery Action Plan, a framework for creating a personalized self-management plan developed by Copeland (1997), provides an outline for individualizing self management practices during all phases of recovery from stabilization to crisis.

Supporting Dream Building and Future Planning

Fundamental to recovery is fostering hope, identifying dreams, and making plans for the future. Interpersonal strategies can foster hope when the therapist expresses a belief in the consumer's potential and strength and accepts setbacks as a normal part of the recovery process (Russinova, 1998). Intervention also includes helping the consumer identify dreams and find meaning in life. Interest inventories can be useful in this process (see Chapter 22, Section 2). Once dreams are recognized, intervention can focus on creating and implementing a plan and identifying external and internal supports to help realize the dream.

FACILITATING PERSONAL CHANGE

Occupational therapy interventions are often directed at making a personal change; however, rarely is the change

TABLE 43-1. **MOTIVATIONAL STRATEGIES FOR STAGES OF CHANGE**

Stage of Change	Characteristics	Motivational Strategies
Precontemplation	Not yet considering change, not even thinking about the problem	Establish rapport; express empathy; reflective listening; help client express own concern about behavior
Contemplation	Willing to consider the problem and possibility of change but still highly ambivalent	Elicit pros and cons of change; provide information and incentives to change; accentuate the positives of change
Preparation	Deciding to take steps to change; making plans; committed	Offer options, expertise, and advise; help consumer enlist social support; clarify goals and strategies for change; anticipate pitfalls and problem solve
Action	Having a plan and taking steps to change	Affirm self-efficacy; offer information on variety of action options; acknowledge difficulties
Maintenance	Behaviors becoming firmly established	Help practice new coping strategies; support lifestyle changes; feedback regarding length of time for sustained change
Recurrence	Problem behaviors have returned	Help reenter the change cycle; frame recurrence as a learning experience

[a]Data from DiClemente (1991).

process itself considered as an intervention goal. Understanding the stages of change and techniques for facilitating change can result in more successful outcomes.

Stages of Change Model

Prochaska and DiClemente (1982) developed a transtheoretical model to conceptualize the stages of change by examining how people change without professional intervention. The stages are presented in Table 43-1. It is important to recognize that the stages are not linear but cyclical, and people move back and forth through them. Therapy generally operates at the action stage; however, people receiving services are frequently at an earlier stage of change. Recognizing the stage of change allows therapists to design intervention strategies to match clients' readiness.

Motivational Interviewing

Motivational interviewing is an intervention approach used to help people recognize a problem and do something about it. It is particularly designed to resolve the ambivalence associated with change. Motivational interviewing was initially developed for treating alcohol abuse but has since been applied across many intervention situations (Miller, 1983). The goal of motivational interviewing is to increase the consumer's intrinsic motivation. The five general principles of motivational interviewing are the following:

- *Express empathy:* Understand the consumer's perspective without criticizing.
- *Develop discrepancy:* Help the consumer recognize the dissonance between current behavior and broader goals.
- *Avoid argumentation:* If resistance is detected, take this as a signal to change strategies.
- *Roll with resistance:* Involve the consumer in problem solving; acknowledge that ambivalence is normal.
- *Support self-efficacy:* Recognize the possibility for change and the range of alternative approaches the consumer can use.

Examples of motivational interviewing strategies for each stage of change are listed in Table 43-1.

COGNITIVE BEHAVIORAL APPROACHES

Cognitive behavioral approaches were developed to address distorted thinking in depression (Beck, 1997) but have since been extensively applied across concerns that involve distorted thinking processes. For example, common cognitive distortions in depression include viewing the self as unlovable or inadequate and the future as hopeless. Anorexia nervosa typically involves overreliance on body image for a sense of self worth. And in generalized anxiety disorder, thinking is excessively pessimistic. Delusional thinking and resistance to medication adherence have also been addressed through cognitive behavioral approaches. The practitioner and consumer work collaboratively in cognitive behavioral therapy to create experiments that test distortions in thought. The process involves the following steps:

1. *Eliciting automatic thoughts:* The practitioner can ask the consumer to describe certain events and what he or she was thinking at the time

2. *Identifying themes or schemas:* Collaboratively, the practitioner and consumer reflect on the automatic thoughts and look for consistent patterns of thinking.
3. *Challenging automatic thoughts:* The practitioner encourages the consumer to identify evidence that refutes the automatic thoughts.

For example, a student may express concerns about an upcoming test. The student makes comments like, "I am so stupid. Everyone else in the class is going to do better than me. I'm going to fail this test and the entire course." The student's comments along with previous discussions suggest themes related to inadequacy and incompetence. To challenge this thinking the practitioner might ask questions such as, "How have you made it so far? What did you get on the last test? Have you been to class? Have you read the material? Have you studied?" As the student provides answers indicating past achievement and current abilities, this evidence is pointed out. After spending time discussing the situation, the student is asked to reflect again on the upcoming test with the expectation that thinking will be more positive.

Cognitive therapy is not limited to a verbal interchange but is most effective when supported by taking action. A component of cognitive therapy is the development of a sense of competence and mastery. Therefore, the consumer is encouraged to engage and reflect on activities that support more accurate or positive ways of thinking.

SKILLS TRAINING

Many people with serious mental illness developed their illness during late adolescence or early adulthood, which often interferes with typical opportunities to acquire independent living skills. Therefore, training in skills such as cooking, money management, use of public transportation, and conversation skills can improve occupational performance outcomes. Skills training typically uses an educational approach that incorporates presentation of the skill followed by repeated practice and feedback.

For example, consumers learning how to ride the bus may receive information about bus schedules and routes, cost, and social etiquette. This would be followed by practice of actually taking the bus on routes that the consumer intends to use. Initially, the occupational therapy practitioner may accompany the consumer. Eventually, the consumer practices the skill on his or her own, perhaps with the use of a cue card provided by the practitioner. Ideally, at least some of the practice is done in the consumer's natural environment. The research on skills training indicates that people with serious mental illness can acquire and maintain new skills (Penn & Mueser, 1996). Skills training approaches use social learning principles to foster skill acquisition. When teaching new skills to people with serious mental illness it is important to compensate for cognitive impairments. Important strategies to incorporate in skills training are outlined in Box 43-9.

BOX 43-9 STRATEGIES FOR SKILLS TRAINING

- Incorporate motivators that match content of the program.
- Provide opportunities for application in real life.
- Repeated practice.
- Provide feedback about performance.
- Evaluate knowledge and/or skill acquisition to determine learning needs.
- Match instruction to environmental and individual needs.

ENVIRONMENTAL MODIFICATIONS

Often times the most efficient and effective interventions to support occupational performance are environmental modifications. In analyzing a task to determine potential modifications, it is important to identify what environmental features act as barriers to performance. Given the cognitive impairments and sensory processing needs of people with serious mental illness, environmental modifications that simplify the executive processing and attentional demands of a task, reduce the sensory overload of an environment, and accentuate salient cues can be beneficial. The following list provides examples of simple-to-implement environmental modifications.

- Make sure necessary equipment and supplies are available.
- Simplify and write out steps of a task.
- Place materials in sequential order.
- Create a quiet place for cognitively demanding work.
- Use checklists, calendar, labels, timers, etc. as cues.
- Organize drawers, closets, etc.
- Underline, bold, or use color to highlight salient information.
- Enlist naturally occurring supports (e.g., family, friends, store clerks, bus drivers).

COMMUNITY-BASED SERVICE MODELS

Most of the psychosocial services for people with serious mental illness are provided in community-based settings with hospitalization reserved primarily for crisis and stabilization. There are several different models of community-based service delivery in current practice. Some state systems rely primarily on one model, whereas others use a combination of models.

Clubhouse

The original clubhouse, Fountain House, was established in 1948 by a group of former patients. The primary mission of Fountain House, which continues today in clubhouses around the world, is to provide a place for people with serious mental illness to belong, where participation is voluntary and membership is lifelong (Macias, Jackson, Schroeder & Wang, 1999). The work-ordered day forms the core of the clubhouse program. Clubhouse activities are organized in work units such as maintenance, clerical, and food service to maintain the clubhouse. Clubhouses also provide transitional and independent employment. Through contracts with community employers, the clubhouse places members in temporary, transitional employment positions to learn the skills of work. When ready, members move on to independent employment positions.

Intensive Case Management

In intensive case management, the case manager acts not only as a coordinator of services but also as a clinician, providing direct service across multiple areas of need. There are two prominent models of intensive case management: the *Program for Assertive Community Treatment* (PACT) and the *strengths model* (Mueser, Bond, Drake, & Resnick, 1998). Both models provide highly individualized services to individuals with serious mental illness in their natural environment. The PACT model uses a multidisciplinary team with a shared caseload, and the strengths model uses one-on-one case management. Another difference lies in the emphasis of each approach as addressed in their titles. The PACT model stresses assertiveness, meaning that case managers seek out consumers; the strengths model stresses capitalizing on assets of the consumer.

Supportive Housing, Employment, and Education

Consumer choice is a major feature of supportive housing, employment, and education (Carling, 1993; Drake & Becker, 1996). The consumer selects the preferred setting, whether it be an apartment complex, job site, or school, Then services are provided that will foster success in that setting. Identifying and implementing reasonable accommodations becomes the dominant intervention.

In supported employment, prevocational training is minimized and rapid placement is the goal. Supports are provided during the job search and employment for as long as needed. Job coaches are often used to assist with the process. In supported housing, the consumer receives support when looking for housing as well as for maintaining a particular housing situation. This could include training or assistance in home management. Supports for education are tutors, note takers, and other academic accommodations.

DECIDING WHICH MODELS TO USE

The models discussed in this section are applicable to all people with serious mental illness. The models are primarily designed for application in community settings, since they place a strong emphasis on natural environments. However, many of the principles and techniques are applicable to hospital-based practice. For example, supporting dream building and future planning from the recovery model may be particularly important for someone transitioning from a hospital setting. The models are not diagnosis specific; instead, the choice of model depends on the focus of the intervention. In addition, the models are compatible, meaning that more than one model can and generally is used for an individual person or within a program. For example, principles from the recovery model may be used to help an individual develop a self-management plan related to improved nutrition. Motivational interviewing approaches are used to determine where the individual is in terms of making a change in self management, and cognitive behavioral approaches are implemented to change distorted views about the person's self image. Skills training approaches provide education in nutrition, and the person's kitchen is modified to support cooking more nutritious meals. The client currently receives these needed services through a combination of staff and consumers at the clubhouse, case management team, and supported housing program.

CONCLUSION

People with serious mental illness often have needs related to multiple areas of successful and satisfying community living. Community-based settings providing services to people with serious mental illness use philosophies and intervention approaches that focus on supporting community participation. Occupational therapy's focus on occupational performance can contribute both to the needs of the population and to the service settings.

References

American Psychiatric Association [APA]. (1993). Practice guidelines for eating disorders. *American Journal of Psychiatry, 150*(2), 212–223.

American Psychiatric Association [APA]. (1994). *Diagnostic and statistical manual of mental disorders* (4th ed.). Washington, DC: Author.

American Psychiatric Association [APA]. (2000). *Diagnostic and statistical manual of mental disorders* (4th ed., tr). Washington, DC: Author.

Americans with Disabilities Act [ADA]. (1990). Pub. L. 101-336, 42 U.S.C. §12101.

Bailey, M. K. (1986). Occupational therapy for patients with eating disorders. *Occupational Therapy in Mental Health* 6(1), 89–116.

Beck, A. T. (1997). The past and future of cognitive therapy. *Journal of Psychotherapy Practice and Research*, 6, 276–284.

Beck, A. T., & Freeman, A. (1990). *Cognitive therapy of personality disorders*. New York: Guilford.

Bennett, A. (1995, May). Notes from offstage. *The New Yorker*, pp. 68–78.

Bipolar disorder: Outcome and treatment effects. (1994, Oct.). *Harvard Mental Health Letter, 11*, 7.

Birth complications and schizophrenia. (1999, November). *Harvard Mental Health, 16*, 7.

Borderline personality disorder. Part 1. (1994a, May). *Harvard Mental Health Letter, 10*, 1–3.

Borderline personality disorder. Part 2. (1994b, June). *Harvard Mental Health Letter, 10*, 1–4.

Borderline personality disorder. Part 3. (1994c, July). *Harvard Mental Health Letter, 10*, 1–3.

Borell, L., Sandman, P. O., & Kielhofner, G. (1991). Clinical decision making in Alzheimer's disease. *Occupational Therapy in Mental Health, 11*(4), 111–124.

Bridgett, B. (1993). Occupational therapy evaluation for patients with eating disorders. *Occupational Therapy in Mental Health, 12*, 79–89.

Brotman, A. W. (1994, January). What works in the treatment of anorexia nervosa. *Harvard Mental Health Letter, 10*, 8.

Bruch, H. (1973). *Eating disorders: Obesity, anorexia nervosa, and the person within*. New York: Basic.

Bruch, H. (1979). *The golden cage: The enigma of anorexia nervosa*. New York: Vintage.

Callahan, J. (1990). *Don't worry, he won't get far on foot*. New York: Vintage.

Carling, P. J. (1993). Housing and supports for persons with mental illness: Emerging approaches to research and practice. *Hospital and Community Psychiatry, 44*, 439–449.

Carson, R. C., & Butcher, J. N. (1992). *Abnormal psychology and modern life* (9th ed.). New York: HarperCollins.

Carson, R. C., Butcher, J. N. & Mineka, S. (2000). *Abnormal psychology and modern life* (11th ed.). Boston: Allyn & Bacon.

Comparing treatments for bulimia. (1994, May). *Harvard Mental Health Letter, 10*, 8.

Copeland, M. E. (1997). *Wellness recovery action plan*. Brattleboro, VT: Peach.

Cronkite, K. (1994). *On the edge of darkness: Conversations about conquering depression*. New York: Doubleday.

CSAT offers practical advice in guide for treating disabled. (1999, February). *Brown University Digest of Addiction Theory and Application, 18*(2), 9.

Davidson, L. (1994). Phenomenological research in schizophrenia: From philosophical anthropology to empirical science. *Journal of Phenomenological psychology, 25*(1), 104–130.

Deegan, P. E. (1996). Recovery as a journey of the heart. *Psychiatric Rehabilitation Journal, 19*, 91–97.

Dickerson, F. B. (1998). Strategies that foster empowerment. *Cognitive and Behavioral Practice, 5*, 255–275.

DiClemente, C. C. (1991). Motivational interviewing and stages of change. In W. R. Miller & S. Rollnick (Eds.). *Motivational interviewing: Preparing people to change addictive behavior* (pp. 191–202). New York: Guilford.

Drake, R. E. & Becker, D. R. (1996). The individual placement and support model of supported employment. *Psychiatric Services, 47*, 473–475.

Duke, P., & Hochman, G. (1992). *A brilliant madness: Living with manic-depressive illness*. New York: Bantam.

Eating disorders. Part 1. (1992, December). *Harvard Mental Health Letter*, 8, 1–4.

Eating disorders. Part 2. (1993, January). *Harvard Mental Health Letter, 9*, 1–4.

Eating disorders. Part 3. (1997, October). *Harvard Mental Health Letter, 14*, 1–5.

Fieve, R. R. (1975). *Moodswing*. New York: Bantam.

Ford, B., & Chase, C. (1987). *Betty: A glad awakening*. New York: Doubleday.

Goldstein, A. (1994). *Addiction: From biology to drug policy*. New York: Freeman.

Gorman, K. K. (1993). Addicted and disabled: One man's journey from helplessness to hope. In A. W. Heinemann (Ed.). *Substance abuse and physical disability* (pp. 11–20). New York: Haworth.

Hayes, R. (1989). Occupational therapy in the treatment of schizophrenia. *Occupational Therapy in Mental Health*, 9(3), 51–68.

Heinemann, A. W. (1993). An introduction to substance abuse and physical disability. In A. W. Heinemann (Ed.). *Substance abuse and physical disability* (pp. 3–9). New York: Haworth.

Herman, J. L. (1992). *Trauma and recovery*. New York: Basic Books

Honel, R. W. (1988). *Journey with grandpa*. Baltimore: Johns Hopkins University Press.

How schizophrenia develops: New evidence and new ideas. (2001, February). *Harvard Mental Heath Letter, 17*, 1–4.

Kaplan, H. I. & Sadock, B. J, (1998). *Kaplan and Sadock's synopsis of psychiatry* (8th ed.). Baltimore: Williams & Wilkins.

Kernberg, O. (1984). *Severe personality disorders: Psychotherapeutic strategies*. New Haven, CT: Yale University Press.

Knauth, P. (1975). *A season in hell*. New York: Harper & Row.

Konek, C. W. (1991). *Daddyboy: A memoir*. St. Paul, MN: Graywolf.

Laliberte-Rudman, D., Yu, B., Scott, E., & Pajouhandeh, P. (2000). Exploration of the perspectives of persons with schizophrenia regarding quality of life. *American Journal of Occupational Therapy, 54*, 37–147.

Law, M. (1998). Does client-centred practice make a difference. In M. Law (Ed.). *Client-centered occupational therapy* (pp. 19–28). Thorofare, NJ: Slack.

Levy, L. L. (1987a). Psychosocial intervention and dementia. Part 1: State of the art, future directions. *Occupational Therapy in Mental Health, 7*(1), 69–107.

Levy, L. L. (1987b). Psychosocial intervention and dementia. Part 2: The cognitive disability perspective. *Occupational Therapy in Mental Health, 7*(4), 13–36.

Liberman, R. P. (1988). Psychosocial management of schizophrenia: Overcoming disability and handicap. *Harvard Mental Health Letter, 5*(5), 4–6.

Linehan, M. M., Tutek, D. A., Heard, H. L., & Armstrong, H. E. (1994). Interpersonal outcome of cognitive behavioral treatment for chronically suicidal borderline patients. *American Journal of Psychiatry, 151*, 1771–1775.

Luder, E., & Schebendach, J. (1993). Nutrition management of eating disorders. *Topics in Clinical Nutrition*, 8, 48–63.

Mace, N. L., & Rabins, P. V. (1991). *The 36-hour day* (rev. ed.). Baltimore: Johns Hopkins University Press.

Macias, C., Jackson, R., Schroeder, C., & Wang, Q. (1999). What is a clubhouse? Report on the ICCD 1996 survey of USA clubhouses. *Community Mental Health Journal, 16*, 9–23.

MacLeod, S. (1981). *The art of starvation*. London: Virago.

Meyers, S. K. (1989). Occupational therapy treatment of an adult with an eating disorder: One woman's experience. *Occupational Therapy in Mental Health*, 9(1), 33–47.

Miller, S. G. (1994). Borderline personality disorder from the patient's perspective. *Hospital and Community Psychiatry, 45*, 1215–1219.

Miller, W. R. (1983). Motivational interviewing with problem drinkers. *Behavioural Psychotherapy, 11*, 147–172.

Mueser, K. T., Bond, G. R., Drake, R. E., & Resnick, S. G. (1998). Models of community care for sever mental illness: A review of research on case management. *Schizophrenia Bulletin, 24*, 37–74.

Murphey, C. (1988). *Day to day: Spiritual help when someone you love has Alzheimer's*. Philadelphia: Westminster.

North, C. S. (1989). *Welcome silence: My triumph over schizophrenia*. New York: Avon.

Penn, D. L., & Mueser, K. T. (1996). Research update on the psychosocial treatment of schizophrenia. *American Journal of Psychiatry, 153*, 607–617.

Plath, S. (1971). *The bell jar*. New York: Harper & Row.

Prochaska, J. O., & DiClemente, C. C. (1982). Transtheoretical therapy: Toward a more integrative model of change. *Psychotherapy: Theory, Research and Practice, 19*, 276–288.

Raymond, M. (1990, September). Life skills and substance abuse. AOTA *Mental Health Special Interest Section Newsletter, 13*(3), 1–2.

Richards, R. (1992, April). Mood swings and everyday creativity. *Harvard Mental Health Letter, 8*, 4–6.

Ridgway, P. (2001). Re-storying psychiatric disability: Learning from first person accounts of recovery. *Psychiatric Rehabilitation Journal, 24*(4), 20–32.

Robak, R. (1991). *A primer for today's substance abuse counselor*. New York: Lexington.

Rothbard, A .B., Schinnar, A. P., & Goldman, H. (1996). The pursuit of a definition for severe and persistent mental illness. In S. M. Soreff (Ed.). *Handbook for the treatment of the seriously mentally ill* (pp. 9–26). Kirkland, WA: Hogrefe & Huber.

Russinova, Z. (1998). Promoting recovery from serious mental illness through hope-inspiring strategies. *Community Support Network News, 13*(1), 1, 4–6.

Scheiber, S. C. (1988). Psychiatric interview, psychiatric history, and mental status examination. In R. E. H. J. A. Talbott & S. C. Yudofsky (Eds.). *Textbook of psychiatry* (pp. 163–194). Washington, DC: American Psychiatric Press.

Schizophrenia and the brain. Part 2. (1999, June). *Harvard Mental Health Letter, 15*(12), 1–3.

Schizophrenia: The present state of understanding. Part 1 (1992, May). *Harvard Mental Health Letter, 8*, 1–4.

Seasonal affective disorder. (1993, February). *Harvard Mental Health Letter, 9*, 1–4.

Sheehan, S. (1983). *Is there no place on earth for me?* New York: Vintage

Sheehan, S. (1995, February 20). The last days of Sylvia Frumkin. *The New Yorker*, pp. 200–211.

Shimp, S. L. (1989). A family-style meal group—Short-term treatment for eating disorder patients with a high level of functioning. *Mental Health Special Interest Section Newsletter, 12*, 1–3.

Styron, W. (1990). *Darkness visible: A memoir of madness*. New York: Random House.

Treatment of alcoholism. Part 2. (1987). *Harvard Mental Health Letter, 4*, 1–3.

Treatment of alcoholism. Part 1 (2000, May). *Harvard Mental Health Letter, 16*, 1–4.

Treatment of drug abuse and addiction. Part I (1995a, August). *Harvard Mental Health Letter, 11*, 1–4.

Treatment of drug abuse and addiction. Part 2. (1995b, September). *Harvard Mental Health Letter, 11*, 1–3.

Update on mood disorders. Part 2 (1995, January). *Harvard Mental Health Letter, 11*, 1–4.

Vonnegut, M. (1975). *The Eden express*. New York: Bantam.

Young, S. L., & Ensing, D. S. (1999). Exploring recovery from the perspective of people with psychiatric disabilities. *Psychiatric Rehabilitation Journal, 22*, 219–231.

CHAPTER 44

SKIN SYSTEM DYSFUNCTIONS: BURNS

ELIZABETH A. RIVERS

The skin injuries most frequently seen by occupational therapists are burns. Burns affect people of all ages. The annual incidence of burn-related injuries in the United States is estimated at 1.25 million, of which greater than 45,000 require hospitalization and 4,500 die (American Burn Association [ABA], 1999).

REVIEW OF SKIN ANATOMY AND FUNCTIONS

The skin is the largest organ in the body. Its structure and appendages provide an extensive, complex, flexible, physical barrier for protection from environmental stresses (Harris & Harris, 1999). Skin functions include thermoregulation; sensation; prevention of water loss; protection from chemical, bacterial, and other foreign body invasion; protection from ultraviolet rays and mechanical trauma; and provision of form, shape, and color to body areas. Skin damage results in myriad and complex systemic, physiologic, and functional problems (Falkel, 1994). The compound systemic effects of burn trauma noted in the cardiovascular, respiratory, endocrine, central nervous, gastrointestinal-digestive, genitourinary, and metabolic systems are beyond the scope of this chapter. The reader is referred to burn or wound texts, since therapy assessment and treatments are based on knowledge of the total extent of anticipated burn responses.

Skin has two distinct layers: epidermis and dermis. The epidermal cells originate in the basal layer and undergo a process of keratinization as they migrate to the surface to form a protective barrier of keratin. Other cells in the epidermis are Langerhans cells, Merkel cells, and melanocytes. Researchers do not yet understand the full role of Langerhans and Merkel cells. Melanocytes found at the dermoepidermal junction produce melanin to provide protection from the ultraviolet rays of the sun (Falkel, 1994). Epidermal cells lining the hair follicles and sweat glands (epidermal appendages embedded in the dermis) serve as a source of epithelium for healing wounds. Sebaceous glands, other epidermal appendages embedded in the dermis, are found in most areas, except where there is no hair. Secretion from sebaceous glands, sebum, moves toward the surface and probably enhances barrier properties by moisturizing and lubricating the skin (Johnson, 1994).

The dermis is made up of vascular connective tissue. Interlacing collagen fibers interspersed with elastic fibers in this layer give the skin strength and elasticity. Dermis does not regenerate. It heals by scar formation.

BURN CLASSIFICATION

The signs and symptoms of burns relate to the classification of the burn. Burn centers classify the seriousness of injury by the cause of injury, depth of injury, percentage of total body surface area (TBSA) involved, location of the burn on the body, and age of the client.

Depth

Burn depth is estimated from clinical observation of the appearance, sensitivity, and pliability of the wound (Wachtel, 1985). Superficial (historically called first-degree) burns involve only the outer layers of the epidermis. The skin is red but is not blistered. These burns are painful briefly but heal uneventfully in 4–8 days. A mild sunburn is a good example of a superficial burn.

Partial-thickness (historically called second-degree) burns can be superficial or deep. Superficial partial-thickness wounds involve only the epidermis and generally blister. When the blister is removed, the wound is erythematous (red), weeping, and quite painful. Superficial partial-thickness wounds generally heal in 10–14 days, with minimal permanent changes. Deep partial-thickness burns involve the epidermis and varying depths of the reticular dermis. Hair follicles, sweat glands, and sebaceous glands are spared to some extent. These wounds are either hemorrhagic or waxy white in appearance. They are generally soft, dry, edematous, and occasionally insensate, with pain increasing as wound healing progresses. A deep partial-thickness wound can convert to a full-thickness injury. Deep partial-thickness wounds require greater than 3 weeks to heal and nearly always result in some amount of scar as well as poor skin quality. A surgeon generally applies skin grafts early in areas that affect function.

Full-thickness (historically called third-degree) burns involve the epidermis, dermis, and the epidermal appendages. Full-thickness burns are dry, tan, or deep red in color, with thrombosed vessels visible. The skin is cold, hard, and insensate. Edema is present owing to capillary damage causing fluid shifts from the intravascular to extravascular space. Edema, eschar (burned tissue) tightness, and wound inelasticity restrict movement and circulation. The surgeon may cut through the eschar (escharotomy) to improve circulation. Surgical treatment with skin grafts speeds wound closure. Scars and disfigurement are frequently the outcome (Johnson, 1994).

Body Surface Area Involved

The extent of the burn is classified as a percentage of the TBSA. Two methods for estimating burn size are the rule of nines and the Lund and Browder (1944) chart. The rule of nines is simple and quick but relatively inaccurate. It divides body surface into areas made up of 9%, or multiples of 9%, with the perineum making of the final 1%. The head and neck are 9%, each upper extremity is 9%, each leg is 18%, and the front and back of the trunk are each 18%. This method is modified for children up to 1 year of age, with the head and neck being 18% and each lower extremity 14% (Harris & Harris, 1999). The percentages for the head and neck and lower extremities are gradually modified from ages 1 to 10 years.

The Lund and Browder chart provides a more accurate estimation of the TBSA. This chart assigns a percentage of surface area for more specific body segments by equating proportions of each segment to the TBSA. An example of body segments is the division of the arm into the upper arm, forearm, and hand. (Details are available in Lund and Browder [1944].) A client's palm print, excluding the fingers, is about 0.5% of the TBSA and may be used as a quick estimate of burn surface area involvement (Sheridan et al., 1995).

Severity of Burn

In 1999 the American Burn Association (ABA) listed 140 burn centers in the United States, about 15 of which have successfully met the ABA burn care standards. Sheridan, Weber, Prelack, and Petras, Lydon & Tompkins (1999) confirmed decreased complications when children are transferred to a burn center early. Patients with the following burns should be treated in a specialized burn facility after initial assessment and treatment at an emergency department:

- Partial- and full-thickness burns greater than 10% TBSA in clients younger than 10 or older than 50 years old.
- Partial- and full-thickness burns greater than 20% TBSA in other age groups.
- Partial- and full-thickness burns with serious threat of functional or cosmetic impairment that involve face, hands, feet, genitalia, perineum, and major joints.
- Full-thickness burns greater than 5% TBSA in any age group.
- Electrical burns.
- Chemical burns with serious threat of functional or cosmetic impairment.
- Inhalation injury with burn injury.
- Circumferential burns of the extremity and chest.

All of these conditions are considered major or severe injuries.

In addition to the area exposed, the severity of a burn injury depends on the duration and intensity of thermal exposure. Therefore, ambulance emergency medical technologists and hospital staff immediately identify the mechanism of the burn injury. Superficial partial-thickness burns typically occur after a brief contact with hot liquids or flames. Deep partial-thickness burns are caused by longer exposure to intense heat, such as with hot water immersion scalds or contact of flaming materials with the skin. Full-thickness burns result from longer exposure to flames; prolonged immersion scalds; contact with hot oil, tar, or chemical agents; and electrical contact.

Age of Client

Age is an important variable in hospital course and prognosis after a burn. Babies and older adults generally are more fragile physiologically. Thin skin and slow circulation allow them to absorb more heat than they can dissipate. Complications associated with the burn arise from massive fluid shifts, infections, and treatments (e.g., surgical procedures). Donor areas heal poorly. Acceptable pain management is difficult for these frail individuals, their families, and the burn care staff (Sorenson, Fisher, & Rivers, 2002). Age, burn size, severity of injury, and severity of associated problems—such as an inhalation injury and head injury—are all considered in predicting prognosis.

FLUID RESUSCITATION

A burn injury causes translocation of body fluids. With large burn injuries, burn shock can occur owing to extensive intravascular fluid loss that causes decreased plasma volume, blood volume, and cardiac output. If fluid resuscitation is inadequate or the client does not respond to the resuscitative efforts, acute renal failure and death ensue (Wachtel, 1985). Several formulas are available for calculating fluid requirements for burn patients; however, the specifics regarding the type of fluid, hourly rate, and amount used are determined by the individual physician's philosophy.

WOUND CARE

Various topical agents are available for treating people with burn injuries. Their purpose is to delay colonization and reduce bacterial counts on or in the wounds. Silver sulfadiazine, silver nitrate soaks, and Sulfamylon are just a few examples (Richard & Staley, 1994; Weber & Thompkins, 1993). Although all burn wounds are generally treated with some type of topical antibacterial agent, these drugs do not substitute for surgical treatment if the need is indicated. When the depth and extent of the wound are known to require 3 weeks or more for healing, surgery is generally needed to decrease burn morbidity and mortality (Heimbach & Engrav, 1984).

Surgical treatment for burn wounds consists of excision (removal) of the burned tissue and placement of skin grafts. Transplantation of the person's own skin from one site to another is referred to as an *autograft*. *Split-thickness skin grafts* (STSGs) are either meshed to expand the coverage, assist drainage, and help wound adherence or applied in sheets. Meshed grafts leave a permanent mesh pattern on the mature wound. Microvascular skin flaps *(full-thickness skin grafts)* are used when the wound is limited in size but the defect is so deep that tendon survival or graft adherence is doubtful. When adequate autograft is not available because of the extent of body surface area involvement or when wound depth is such that graft take is questionable, a temporary biologic dressing is frequently used.

Biologic dressings, either viable or nonviable, can be used as a temporary wound covering (Heimbach & Engrav, 1984). The proposed benefits of biologic dressings are that they reduce fluid loss, decrease pain, inhibit bacterial growth, and protect the wound until autografting is possible. The unfavorable potential is that biologic dressings usually become inelastic. Examples of biologic dressings homografts, which are made from processed cadaver skin; xenografts, which are made from processed skin of another species such as pigs; synthetic products such as Biobrane, which is a nylon–silicone mesh coated with collagen; or other artificial skin substitute (Saffle & Schnebly, 1994).

HYPERTROPHIC SCARS

Burn scar and contracture are common sequelae after a deep burn injury; collagen is the primary structural component of scars. The quality of burn wound maturation is affected by numerous factors, some of which occur during the early phases of burn care. A significant determinant in potential for scar development is the number of days required to achieve wound closure.

Infection in a burn wound can increase the inflammatory response and delay healing. Spontaneous healing of full-thickness burns is a prolonged, painful process, resulting in thick scars. Strict adherence to infection control procedures, the use of topical antibiotics, scrupulous cleansing of the burn wound, and early surgical burn wound repair minimize the potential for burn scar contracture (Johnson, 1994). Despite these procedures and surgical interventions, scarring continues to be a major deterrent in recovering full function after a major burn injury.

Race, age, anatomic location, and depth of the burn wound can influence scar formation. Hypertrophic scars rise above the skin surface anytime from 4 to 12 weeks after wound closure. Initially, the hypertrophic areas appear thick, rigid, and hyperemic (congested with blood). Their functional or cosmetic significance varies with the anatomic location of the wound. Hypertrophic scars that cross joints can limit range of motion (ROM) and function. Collagen contraction or skin shortening over the joint also limits ROM. If contractures are left untreated, shortening of the muscle and fibrous contraction of the joint capsule eventually occur. Scars on the face distort facial features and limit jaw, lip and eyelid function.

Numerous anecdotal reports of successful scar treatments are available; but few randomized, prospective, controlled studies have been published. With maturation, the hypertrophic scar softens, thins, and flattens, and collagen synthesis and degradation become balanced. Surgeons generally agree that hypertrophic scars will not develop in wounds that epithelialize and become lighter in color 2–3 weeks after the injury. The process of collagen degradation in hypertrophic scar is still not fully understood (Chang, Laubenthal, Lewis, Rosenquist, Lindley-Smith, & Kealey, 1996).

EVALUATION

Occupational therapy practitioners specializing in burn care evaluate, treat, and reassess clients of all ages, as ordered by the physiatrist or surgeon, from the time of the burn injury until all wounds are mature and the client has returned to preburn family, home, work, school, and community life. Wounds are mature when they are durable, soft, mobile, of proper color, and as flexible as possible. All phases of burn healing overlap because an injury is rarely of a single depth and different parts of the body heal at different speeds (Rivers & Fisher, 1991).

A client with a severe burn injury who is admitted to the hospital undergoes a multitude of emergency procedures conducted by many personnel. Doctors place endotracheal airways; intravenous fluid lines; do escharotomies; estimate burn size; and order medications, activity, diet, x-rays, and analgesics. Nurses cleanse the wounds, apply topical antimicrobial agents and dressings, place tubes to decompress the stomach and bladder, and weigh the client.

At this acute phase, an important role of the occupational therapist is to prevent likely deformities that could impede function. Therefore, when possible, the occupational therapist views the client's wounds during these initial procedures and determines areas of involvement that may require positioning or splints or both. Therapists do this initial therapy evaluation in hydrotherapy if possible. If the client is alert and willing, therapists also evaluate functional motions. Although it is easier for some clients to move without their dressings, with adequate analgesia, it is possible to assess active ROM when dressings are in place. Goniometer measurements over dressings are possible by making allowances for the bandage thickness. Active ROM of uninvolved areas is also documented. Although it is difficult to assess strength objectively at this time because of edema and pain, therapists should note whether the client can move each joint through a full ROM against gravity. They also obtain hand dynamometer and pinch gauge measurements if the hand is not involved, or if the burn is only a superficial partial-thickness burn with minimal surface area involvement and no edema is present.

Once immediate positioning needs are handled, it may be possible to obtain the client's preinjury level of function through interview with the client. When this is not possible or when the client is intubated (using an oral or nasal airway for breathing), a close family member may be able to provide this information. Communication about earlier occupational roles and habits as well as any prior impairments is important. These may include client factors, such as previous musculoskeletal injuries, sensory deficits, hand dominance, personality traits, activity of daily living (ADL) and instrumental activity of daily living (IADL) function, job title and a basic description of work skills, educational level achieved, cultural requisites, and recreational activities.

Maximizing client choice and control in the care plan increases client motivation (Law, Baptiste, & Mills, 1995). However, Caplan (1988) noted that the capacity for voluntary autonomy must be re-created in clients who experience sudden, severe, and incurable impairments. Spiritual beliefs (Egan & DeLaat, 1992) and cultural influences (Leslie, Blakeney, Moore, Desai, & Herndon, 1996) also sway client participation. For example, some Southeast Asians may refuse grafts, because they fear the spirit escapes during surgery. This results in prolonged, poor healing and increased scars. During the interview, the occupational therapist must indicate respect for any unique characteristics of the client. All of this information becomes the basis for an individualized intervention plan. The practitioner's attitude, approach, general maturity, experience, and creativity also become facets of the strengths and resources available to a burned client and his or her family.

When interviewing or working with the client, all staff observe universal infection control precautions according to the hospital's procedures. The following are included in most universal precaution protocols. Wash hands before and after each client contact; don protective garb, aprons, caps, or gloves before client contact and discard immediately after leaving the bedside or room; change gloves whenever contaminated with secretions or excretions from one site before contact with another site; and decontaminate all equipment, materials, and surfaces between client contacts (Weber & Thompkins, 1993).

Burn occupational therapists evaluate wound condition, scar density, ROM, strength, endurance, and function at frequent intervals during hospitalization and after hospital discharge to identify specific problem areas and decreases in function that commonly occur. Although changes in function are generally attributed to the scarring associated with burn wound healing, hospitalization and the metabolic effects of a burn injury also contribute to decreases in strength, endurance, and ADL and IADL performance. Consequently, it is important to monitor skin and scar status, sensation, emotional responses, and coping skills (Leman & Ricks, 1994). The client's collaboration, understanding, memory, posttraumatic stress situation, and ability to assume responsibility for long-term care are important considerations. Although basic splint designs, specific resting positions for burned body areas, and exercise techniques are frequently taught as the standard for burn rehabilitation, every intervention plan reflects the specific needs for each particular client. Unfortunately, clients often substitute use of uninjured extremities during ADL and IADL performance. Therefore, therapist and family supervision are necessary to assist recovery of the original fluidity of motion.

PHASES OF RECOVERY

The focus of the burn team and related intervention techniques change with the phase of recovery. In 1997, the ABA defined three phases of burn recovery: the burn shock phase (acute care), the wound surgery phase (including postoperative care), and the rehabilitation phase (wound maturation). Whether the client goes through all three phases depends on the depth and extent of the burn injury. Because of the mixed nature of the burn injuries, these stages usually overlap.

The burn shock, or acute care, phase consists of fluid resuscitation, client stabilization, and initial wound care procedures. With superficial or partial-thickness wounds that heal without surgery, the acute care phase is also considered the period from the date of injury until epithelial healing. When the wounds are superficial, this is the only phase the client experiences, and occupational therapy is generally not indicated. However, very young infants and very old clients may require occupational therapy when the wounds are partial thickness in depth, do not require surgery, but take more than 2–3 weeks to heal because slow wound healing with concomitant pain impairs function. The expenditure of energy for wound healing may foster withdrawal, decreased activity, and—without therapy—healing with permanent impairment.

After acute resuscitation and stabilization of major burn injuries, the second phase of healing for deep partial- or full thickness wounds is the wound surgery and postoperative phase. During this phase, the client undergoes multiple surgical procedures and immobilization periods. This is also the period when infections and other medical complications can sometimes occur.

The third phase is the rehabilitation phase. This phase starts with wound closure and continues through wound maturation. For individuals with severe burn injuries, therapy assumes the primary role during the rehabilitation phase.

TREATMENT GOALS FOR RECOVERY PHASES

The occupational therapy practitioner working with burned individuals must constantly integrate and use physical, environmental, and psychosocial intervention skills. The physical and cosmetic disabilities, often the sequelae of a burn injury, challenge the family, client, and therapist. Although specific rehabilitation goals may be the primary responsibility of certain burn team members, depending on individual burn center policies, everyone focuses on restoring or maximizing the client's functional capacity. Therefore, the burn rehabilitation goals discussed next are also goals of the occupational therapist. In the following sections, there may be overlap of other disciplines with occupational therapy, and the goals are referred to as rehabilitation goals (Richard & Staley, 1994).

Burn Shock (Acute Care)

During the acute care phase, resuscitation and wound care are the foci of the burn team. When the wounds are superficial, the goal of rehabilitation therapy is to prevent loss of strength and endurance by promoting normal function. Limb elevation decreases the risk of edema and alleviates pain. Skin care education includes moisturization to combat the itching and dryness frequently experienced with epithelial healing. With adequate analgesia and burn team coaching, independent ADL and IADL are continued.

When burn wounds are deep partial thickness or full thickness, the acute care rehabilitation goals are to control edema; prevent loss of joint mobility, functional strength, and endurance; promote self-care; provide orientation activities and stimulation; and begin client and family education about wound healing and rehabilitation.

Wound Surgery (Postoperative Care)

During the surgical phase of care, immobilizing the grafted area in prescribed positions for prescribed amounts of time enhances graft adherence. Immobilization is necessary to prevent displacement of skin grafts during their vascularization. The position and length of time of immobilization vary with the body area treated, the depth of the excision, the type of surgical procedure performed, and the physician's preference. Postoperative immobilization is 3–7 days. Joints are generally immobilized one joint proximal and one joint distal to the grafted joint.

During this phase, occupational therapy goals are to

- Design splints and implement positioning techniques for immobilization in consultation with the surgeon.
- Teach the family to provide appropriate sensory stimulation to decrease frustration with client disorientation.
- Provide adaptive devices to increase self-care skills when appropriate.

Other rehabilitation interventions at this time are designed to:

- Continue client and family education.
- Prevent thrombophlebitis, skin tightness, and disuse atrophy of areas not immobilized by implementing a controlled exercise plan for areas proximal and distal to the grafted site.

Rehabilitation

The rehabilitation phase starts during wound closure. A client with a severe burn can enter this phase before all wounds are healed. Many times, a client with a severe burn injury needs one or two more surgical procedures or has certain small areas still requiring topical antibiotics upon entering the rehabilitation phase.

The rehabilitation phase is the most challenging of all for burn clients and their families. It is the period when burn scar and contracture can be recognized and the client, usually in a state of depleted energy, must assume responsibility for self-care. This includes initiation and independent performance of ADL, IADL, work, and leisure activities. The need for care does not end with hospital discharge when wounds are often still flat and mobile; it continues until wound maturation is complete. This is particularly difficult for clients who view hospital discharge as the end of the discomfort, pain, and burn care.

Although burn wound maturation may take several years after injury, each client is unique. The time needed for wound maturation varies from 9 months in a light-pigmented adult up to 5 years in a growing or darkly pigmented child. Client perseverance, patience, and a sense of humor can defuse anger during this rigorous, prolonged phase.

INTERVENTION

Client and Family Education

Education about burn care is crucial to help the client, family, and community contacts cope with the multiple facets of burn care. Education starts at the beginning of the recovery process to ensure the client and family's understanding of the long-term needs associated with burn recovery. Pain, immobilization, medications, shock, exhaustion, sleeplessness, and lengthy hospitalization often alter the client's thinking and memory. The appearance of his or her wounds during the stages of recovery is disconcerting. It can be depressing for a client to hear a burn team member saying that the wound looks good if the client does not understand that this is only one phase in the healing process. Experience shows that clients cope more easily with constant changes when they learn what to expect.

Family education and understanding occur at a slower pace than that of the client (Jordan, Allely, & Gallagher, 1994). The client speaks to the burn team constantly, whereas the family may see a burn team member for a few minutes during visiting hours. Convening family groups to discuss nutrition, exercise, pain, wound changes, and other common topics augments learning and maximizes staff time. Talking about the frustration of watching a family member struggle to function independently may comfort relatives, and life-long friendships and support systems often develop in waiting rooms. The recovery process is shorter when staff, clients, and family share outcome goals and clearly record progress. Discharge should never be a surprise.

Functional recovery after a burn injury is a dynamic process. Scarring and deconditioning occur during hospitalization and bedrest. Since burn recovery is a painful process, it is important that clients become actively involved with their rehabilitation program at the beginning. A client who learns and uses management techniques for pain and stress early, often carries out a successful outcome. Advances in patient-centered pain management continue with improved understanding of drugs and physiology (Ehde, Patterson, & Wiechman, 2000; Fauerbach, Lawrence, Schmidt, Munster, & Costa, 2000; "Pain management," 1995). Successful clients allow the accident to become a part of their unchangeable past and assume responsibility for their long-term recovery. They understand the purpose of specific treatments, potential outcomes if they avoid or discontinue treatment, the prolonged burn recovery time, pain management techniques, and methods for independently assessing scar maturation. They also develop support and encouragement resources from family, community, or counselors. In addition, they empower themselves to resume leisure, work, and other occupations as soon as they are able.

Exercise and Activities to Promote Movement

The goal of exercise is to improve physical function through increased muscle strength, endurance, flexibility, and power. Physical and occupational therapists collaborate in implementing plans to restore physical function. A thorough history helps determine the type of ROM that will safely meet the mutual goals of the client, physician, and therapist. Although clients tend to avoid movement in general, when they do move, it is painful, slow, and labored. As the burn wound closes, a number of factors often limit a burn client's willingness or ability to exercise. These include scar tightness, hypersensitivity, pain and discomfort from stretching scars, the client's emotional adjustment, and a generalized feeling of fatigue. During this period, motions often appear robot-like, with no fluidity of movement; spontaneity is absent, normal motions are limited, and joint ROM is limited. If these movement patterns are allowed to persist, functional limitations develop.

Clients develop painful joints if they do not regain full active ROM quickly after the burn. Pain can be the result of tight contractures of soft tissue, tendons, ligaments, blood vessels, and nerves surrounding the involved joint. It can be from skin contractures or hypertrophic scar bands. Pain also develops from cartilage deterioration owing to poor nutrition caused by lack of complete joint gliding. If joints remain stiff, clients may have difficulty with self-care activities or returning to work. Clients may also experience postural strain from substitution when they are not able to move their extremity in a full arc of motion.

Although activity and active exercise are needed for muscle strength and endurance, continuous passive motion (CPM) devices can be used as an adjunct to the exercise regime (Covey, Dutcher, Marvin, & Heimbach, 1988). Covey et al. (1988) demonstrated increased recovery and no tissue damage with controlled passive motion machines. CPM devices are beneficial when the client's active motion is limited secondary to pain, edema, or anxiety. Although the therapist must monitor the client's response when initially using the device, a CPM device is an extension of treatment when the therapist is not available. With adequate analgesia, it is especially appropriate for use when the client is resting or sleeping.

Free weights using the Delorem method or electronically controlled dynamometers are examples of strengthening techniques (see Chapter 30, Section 2). Using a bicycle ergometer for endurance is also appropriate in burn rehabilitation. Although exercise tolerance in the hypermetabolic client is a concern, monitoring pulse rate, blood pressure, and respiration assist in safely grading exercises.

An important role of rehabilitation activities is to stretch burn scars to prevent or reduce contractures. All members of the burn care team are involved in helping the client in this process. Preexercise stretching prevents injury, as does massaging a lubricating cream into the maturing tissues to prevent skin rupture from dryness and scar rigidity. This also helps decrease itching (Field, Peck, Hernandez-Reif, Krugman, Burman, & Qzment-Schenck, 2000). Complex motions and resistive exercises are added as tolerated. Flexibility exercises (combined joint movements) are complex motions. A burn scar limits motion of the joint it crosses and the joints proximal and distal to it. Therefore, it is important to provide exercises and activities that require concurrent joint motions. For example, an exercise program for a person with an upper extremity burn may emphasize elbow function but should also incorporate coordinated movements of the shoulder, elbow, and hand.

A unique role of the occupational therapy practitioner is the careful analysis of the total effect of scarring on the client's occupational performance. Occupational therapy practitioners identify ADL, IADL, work, and leisure activities that stretch contractures as a natural part of performance. Working with clients and their families, customized activity routines are designed. Since burn contractures are dynamic, fluidity of full motion is more pivotal to recovery than regaining early function with adapted equipment or substitution of motions. Frequently, updated home worksheets such as those produced by Glass and Bruns (2000) encourage active patient and family commitment.

Positioning

Positioning techniques were first developed for the acute phase of burn care. To understand and effectively use positioning techniques, the therapist must understand the problem. In response to fear of pain, the burn client frequently assumes a protective childlike posture of adduction and flexion of the upper extremities, flexion of the hips and knees, and planar flexion of the ankles. Hand burn pain causes clients to hold their hands in a dysfunctional thumb-adducted, wrist-flexed position. Using a pillow when there are neck burns and resting with the head of the bed in an upright position when there are trunk burns contribute to inappropriate posturing. If the burn client remains in a flexed, fetal, withdrawal position as wound healing progresses, contractures develop and limit function. In general, therapeutic burn positioning entails encouraging some degree of extension of all involved areas when resting. Therapeutic positioning of a cooperative client with burns aids in edema control and reduction, maintains normal muscle length when resting, ensures wound coverage immediately after placement of skin grafts, limits the degree of scar contracture, and teaches the client methods for combating the skin tightness that affects function.

During the acute phase of care, the main purpose for positioning is to limit edema formation. Although there is an initial diffuse capillary leak with a severe burn, the severity or impact of distal extremity edema formation can be limited with elevation of the limb at or slightly above heart level. Foam wedges or pillows are used to elevate hand and arm burns. In these cases, extension of the elbows is important to prevent restriction of venous return. Raising the foot of the bed reduces foot or leg edema. Clients should avoid flexing the hips more than 30° when the legs and hips are burned and should keep their knees extended. For people with face and neck burns, raising the head of the bed at least 30° or using a foam elevation wedge helps reduce edema.

As wound closure begins and progresses, practitioners address more proximal positioning concerns. When the axillae and anterior trunk are involved, abduct the arms to 90° using armboards attached to the side of the bed or overhead suspension. Blanket rolls placed along the upper trunk also promote shoulder abduction. If any portion of the neck is involved, the client should not use a pillow for head support. Use a small towel roll behind the neck instead.

Postoperative immobilization positions may entail many of the techniques already described but may also be specific for the type of procedure used or area treated. When a skin graft is used for wound coverage, the body area or joint treated is usually held in some degree of extension or abduction. When a skin flap is performed, positioning specifics change to prevent stress on the suture lines and blood supply. Knowledge of the surgical procedure performed and determination of potential postoperative complications, such as suture-line stresses or graft shifting, enable the therapist to institute effective, safe positioning techniques. If functionally limiting contractures develop from poor positioning at home, practitioners should have clients use splints for positioning.

Activities of Daily Living

Once medically stable, the client begins independent eating, although dressings and edema may alter performance. Adapting utensils to increase grasp may be needed temporarily. Avoid extending utensils and straws because using the elbow at the habit level promotes more normal ROM. Remember that ADL independence without adaptations is one of the least painful methods to achieve full active ROM. Therefore, remove adaptive devices as soon as possible to avoid dependence on them.

Clients usually receive hydrotherapy on a daily basis as part of wound care. Nurses cleanse the wounds, but patient participation in bathing and grooming should be encouraged. Although it is difficult for patients to reach all body areas, getting involved in bathing is a beginning point for wound healing education while fostering independence in self-care. Overall, ADL practice during this early phase of care focuses the client toward recovery, emphasizes abilities, and provides a means for discharge education.

As wound closure is achieved and the client nears discharge from the hospital, normal independent self-care proceeds. Independence in bathing, grooming, eating, toileting, and dressing skills should be evaluated. The client should perform bathing and grooming in a bathroom with appliances similar to those used at home. The therapist should help the client practice dressing skills with clothes from home so the client and family realize that adapted clothing is rarely necessary. With major burn injuries, adaptations may be needed to encourage self-care independence. Clients can be encouraged to use a mirror to assess self-care skills. Clients who can see their scar stretching may understand the benefit of improved function.

Experience has shown that many clients fear hot water, especially if they were injured in the shower or bathtub. These clients are eager to learn how to safely test water temperatures and to set the thermostat of their hot water heater less than 120°F. Cooking is another activity that many clients avoid at home because they fear heat or they were injured while cooking. Cooking activities in the clinic decrease fears and permit teaching about safe cooking procedures to be used at home.

The therapist can teach the client to don vascular support or compression garments. Performance with a therapist brings an awareness and understanding of the time and benefits of ADL and IADL tasks, developing patience, and planning time to perform tasks independently.

The therapist should also teach the client to avoid sun exposure injuries. Unprotected sun exposure to a healed wound results in blotchy, unpredictable tanning. If pigment is absent in the healed wound, severe tissue damage can result from sun exposure. Wearing a wide-brimmed hat is recommended for anyone with maturing face and neck burns. Clients exposed to sun and heat learn to work in shaded areas; wear light-colored, lightweight, nonrestrictive clothing; don a cool flap hat or wide-brimmed hat; use a battery fan or spray bottle; wear sunglasses; drink enough fluids; and avoid vasoconstricting drugs such as cigarettes (Rivers & Fisher, 1991). Skin protection using a block with a sun protection factor (SPF) of 30 should be recommended. Sunscreens should be applied anytime a client is in the sun, even if simply riding in a car.

Because circulation is permanently changed in scarred areas and sweat glands may be absent, heat exposure is a problem. Injured skin is sensitive to temperature extremes. Severely injured patients may need to remain in air-conditioned areas if the temperature is greater than 70°F. Often a fan and spray bottle of water are adequate coolants. The clients also must learn to prevent frostbite and cold injuries in a cold outdoor environment. Therapist should teach them to keep their vehicles well maintained; carry a cell phone, stay with the vehicle in difficulties; and keep blankets, extra mittens, warm clothing, boots, candles, and snacks in the car. At work, the client should be encouraged to wear insulated, waterproof boots; safety shoes with fiberglass toes and shanks, if approved by the employer; flap hats or insulated hood; and multiple layer, nonrestrictive clothing of wind-resistant fabric. Clients recovering from burns should avoid vasodilating drugs (alcohol) and vasoconstricting drugs (cigarettes) (Rivers & Fisher, 1991).

Splints

The use of splints in burn care varies with the phase of wound healing but, more important, with the philosophy of the burn center. Traditionally, splints were taken off for meals, dressing changes, and exercise. Today, analgesia for background and breakthrough pain makes activity possible during acute care. When used, acute care splints are generally static in design and used at night or for short periods.

The primary splint still used in acute burn care is the burn hand splint. The time of application may be only when ROM becomes limited to only postoperatively. Miles and Grigsby (1990) recommended waiting 48–72 hr after injury to apply the hand splint. This is because the extreme fluid shifts that occur during acute resuscitation can greatly affect splint fit. The purposes of the burn hand splint are to prevent ligamentous stress at the interphalangeal joints, to assist in edema reduction, and to allow flow to the intrinsic muscles of the hands by emphasizing the distal transverse arch of the hand. This splint prevents the burn claw deformity, which is flexion of the wrist, hyperextension of the metacarpophalangeal joints, and flexion of the interphalangeal joints.

The burn hand splint differs from other hand splints by the position of its components. Usually made out of a low-temperature thermoplastic material, the splint positions the wrist in 30–35° of extension, the metacarpophalangeal joints in 50–70° flexion, the interphalangeal joints in extension, and the thumb in abduction (Fig. 44-1). The splint positions

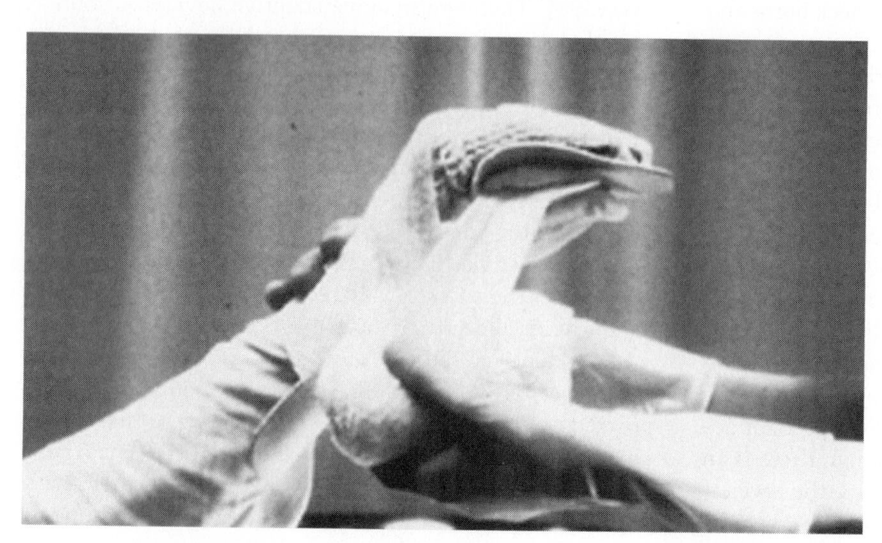

FIGURE 44–1. Gauze wraps are used to maintain the hand position with a burn hand splint.

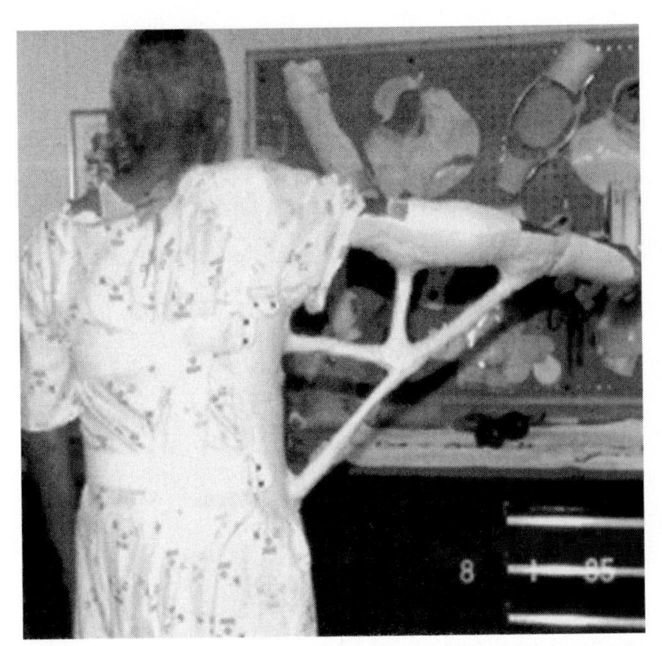

FIGURE 44–2. An airplane splint allows mobility while maintaining the shoulder in 90° of abduction.

described are used for dorsal hand burns; the specific positions for a given client depend on the surface area burned. When there are circumferential hand burns, the positions can be modified.

These splints are usually secured with gauze. Straps are not used because of infection control concerns and the possibility of distal edema. When an acute splint is used, it is usually a conformer splint that has total contact with the surface area being treated and generally places the body area in an extended position. Frequent splint readjustments accommodate fluid volume changes in the extremity and variations in dressing bulk.

A conforming positioning splint may be needed after skin grafts are applied. Owing to the bulk of the postoperative dressing, plaster strips are frequently used for splinting during operations. Most postoperative splints hold the joint or limb in extension, with the exception of a foot splint, which positions the ankle in dorsiflexion, and the airplane splint, which positions the shoulder in about 90° of abduction (Fig. 44-2).

Although static splints may be needed during burn wound maturation, the therapist should not restrict activity, if possible. Low-temperature thermoplastic dynamic splints may be appropriate when scar contracture is present. The purpose of a dynamic splint is to assist or regain function or to provide slow dynamic stretch to contracting tissues. When fabricating and fitting a dynamic splint, use caution to prevent the splint components from exerting ligamentous stress, friction, or joint compressive forces. There are a few commercially available dynamic splints for elbows, knees, and ankles; but these should be used with caution.

Plaster casts maintain correct positions or stretch and soften contractures. The advantages of plaster casting are the low cost of materials and the characteristics of accurately conforming, nonremovable circumferential contact. Plaster, as with all circumferential wrappings, should be applied distal to proximal on the limb to assist venous return. In some cases, parts of the cast are cut out, permitting desired movement, such as elbow extension, while blocking flexion. Adding this type of "drop-out" feature increases patient control to stretch gently. Serial casting and a dynamic plaster casting technique have both been described for treatment of scar contractures of the hand, wrist, elbow, knee, and ankle (Staley & Serghiou, 1998).

In many instances, it is difficult to discuss burn splinting as a separate treatment entity without including scar management principles (Daugherty & Carr-Colllins, 1994). Splints such as the total-contact transparent face mask and neck splints are more appropriately presented as methods of scar management, with positioning techniques used acutely. Splint design should be specific for the particular wound-healing problem. Knowledge of basic splinting principles; frequent assessment of client function, needs, skin condition, and splint fit; and design creativity are necessary for any successful splint program. (see Chapter 31, Section 3).

Scar Management

Mechanical pressure has long been advocated as a way to influence scarring and has been used as treatment for or prevention of hypertrophic scars (Carr-Collins, 1992). As a scar develops, it becomes hyperemic (red), raised, and rigid (Johnson, 1994). Effective scar management is often the long-term goal of the entire burn team. Long-term scar care includes the use of splints and compression or external vascular support garments (Fig. 44-3).

The purpose of using elastic compression garments and splints on maturing burn wounds is to apply perpendicular pressure that approximates capillary pressure, because it has

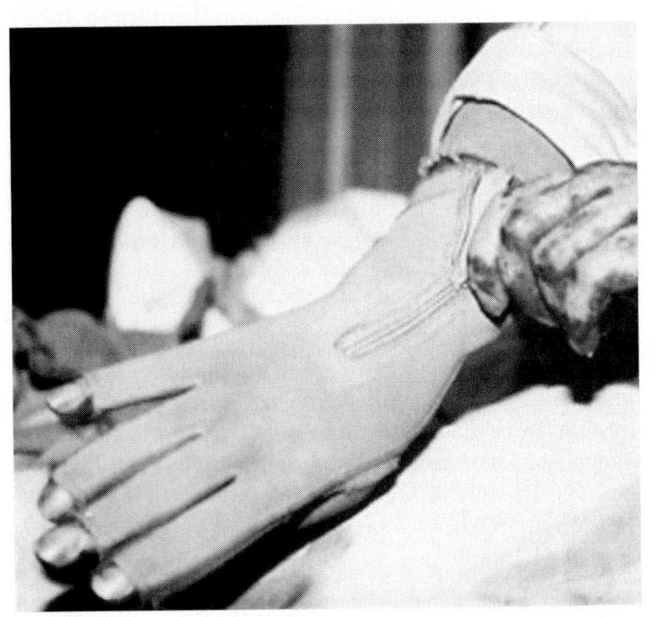

FIGURE 44–3. A custom-fitted external compression and vascular support glove is worn 23 hours a day to minimize scarring, edema, and vascular pooling. Open fingertips in the gloves can improve fingertip prehension and sensation.

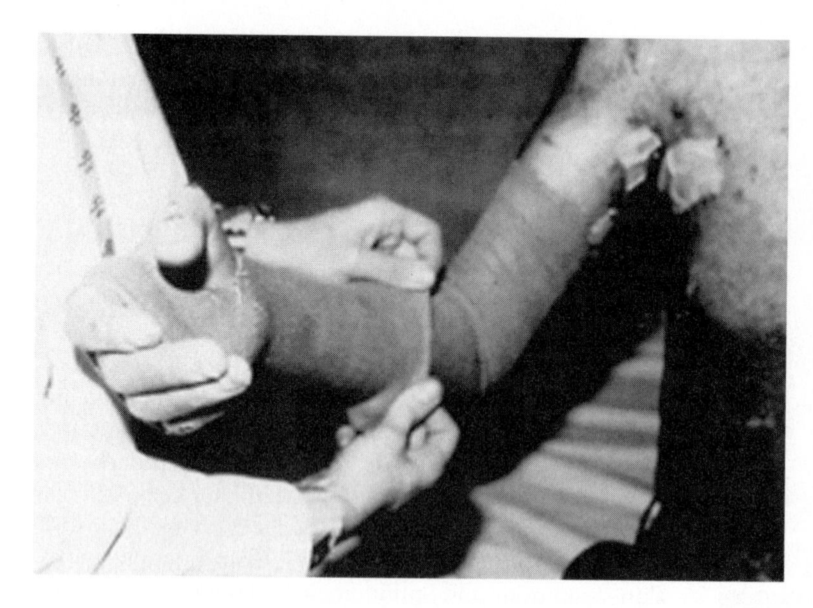

FIGURE 44–4. Tubular elastic dressings are used for skin conditioning on the extremities. The hand or foot must be included in the dressing to prevent distal swelling.

been postulated that wounds mature more rapidly with fewer scars when deprived of excessive circulation and oxygen. Elastic wrap supports prevent dependent edema under grafts on dependent extremities. Scar hypertrophy and collagen contraction generally are not noted until after wound closure. When the healed wound tolerates the shear of donning a sleeve, the wraps can be replaced with cotton and rubber tubes or custom-measured garments. Providing for normal motions while maintaining adequate scar control and coverage is difficult. Occupational therapy practitioners must have creativity, skill, and perseverance while always questioning what else can be done to assist the client. No pressure appliance or garment is perfect, and frequent reassessment is needed to ensure appropriate pressure and fit.

Numerous pressure dressings and techniques are available for use early during wound healing (Ward, 1991, 1993). Traditionally, vascular support and compression techniques are applied early. Vascular supports control edema, minimize vascular and lymphatic pooling in the extremities, and condition the new skin for the shear force demands of commercial garments. Elastic wraps applied over gauze dressings in a figure-eight, gradient fashion is the initial treatment choice in most burn centers. They are also considered the first stage of graded pressure therapy.

As the wounds heal and bandage needs diminish, compression therapy can be progressed to using tubular elastic dressings that are pulled on. Interim pressure garments begin skin desensitization and sensory reeducation, teach independent dressing or garment-donning skills, and provide timely compression therapy education. Elastinet™ and Tubigrip™, available in rolls of various circumferences, are frequently used for intermediate compression therapy on the extremities (Fig. 44-4). Interim pressure on the hand can be accomplished by progressing to an intermediate spandex glove that is made by the therapist, by using manufactured presized gloves, such as Isotoner, or by applying a total-contact Coban™ wrap (Fig. 44-5). The therapist must consider the cost and purposes for using interim pressure when choosing a method. Skin condition, the need to decrease edema, and the client's functional abilities and understanding are a few of the significant points.

Although custom garments are made from sequential measurements of the client, actual garment fit is not perfect. To be effective, the elastic garment must exert equal pressure over the entire area. This is not always possible because of body contours, bony prominences, and postural adjustments by the client. When the garment does not fit consistently, a therapist adds inserts or overlays to distribute pressure uniformly. Areas frequently needing inserts are the superior anterior chest, breast areas on women, web spaces on the hand, anterior surface of the toes, the upper and lower lip areas, and nasolabial folds on the face. Inserts are also needed to prevent garment overlap and folding in the antecubital areas of the elbows, posterior aspect of the knees, axillary folds, and anterior aspect of the ankle.

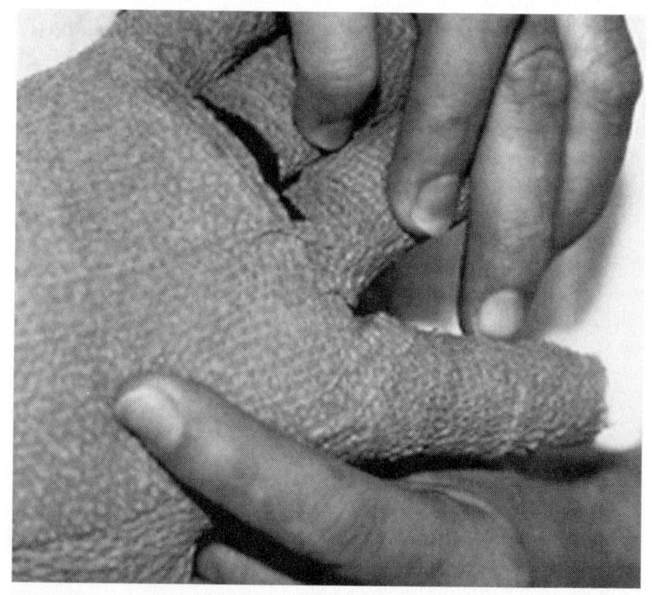

FIGURE 44–5. Coban™ wraps are used to minimize edema and to prepare the hand for a custom-fitted glove. A strip placed dorsal to volar provides web-space control.

Pressure inserts were originally made from thermoplastics, but problems of skin maceration under the inserts were common. Today, thermoplastics are used only for fairly large surface areas when positioning is also needed. Today, most inserts are made from more flexible materials, such as orthopedic felt, silicone, or closed-cell foam. Friction and skin maceration are not common with these flexible materials. Therapists should frequently assess and replace torn or flattened pressure inserts. Skin reaction, cost, safety, wound changes, and the client's ability to keep the insert in the correct position under the garment influence insert use.

Despite advances in scar control using garments and inserts, splints may still be needed for certain body areas. There are also areas where effective pressure distribution is not possible with elastic garments. The neck, face, and mouth are good examples of areas where an alternate method for pressure therapy is needed. Neck mobility, ineffectiveness of elastic garments, and dysfunctional postural adjustments that the client may make in response to scar tightness and discomfort contribute to neck contractures. Scar involvement of the neck region can extend from the face to the superior aspect of the chest, causing distortion of the lower face and lip commissures, eversion of the lower lip, limited neck rotation and extension, and shoulder protraction (Fig. 44-6). Fricke et al. (1999) recommend consultation with an orthodontist as the best way to maintain dental and facial relationships during burn scar management.

Early splint designs for neck contracture prevention consisted of a total-contact neck conformer made from a thermoplastic material (Willis, 1970). Problems encountered with this neck conformer are mandibular retraction, minimal to no neck rotation allowed, and decreased surface contact with neck motion. An advancement of this splint design is a rigid, total-contact, transparent chin and neck orthosis (Rivers, Strate, & Solem, 1979) (Fig. 44-7). Fabricating a transparent plastic splint is an involved process but allows more precise alterations and assessment of fit compared to opaque thermoplastic materials. An alternate splint design is the triple-component neck splint, which consists of a chin cup, chin strap, and modified neck conformer (Leman & Lowery, 1986) (Fig. 44-8).

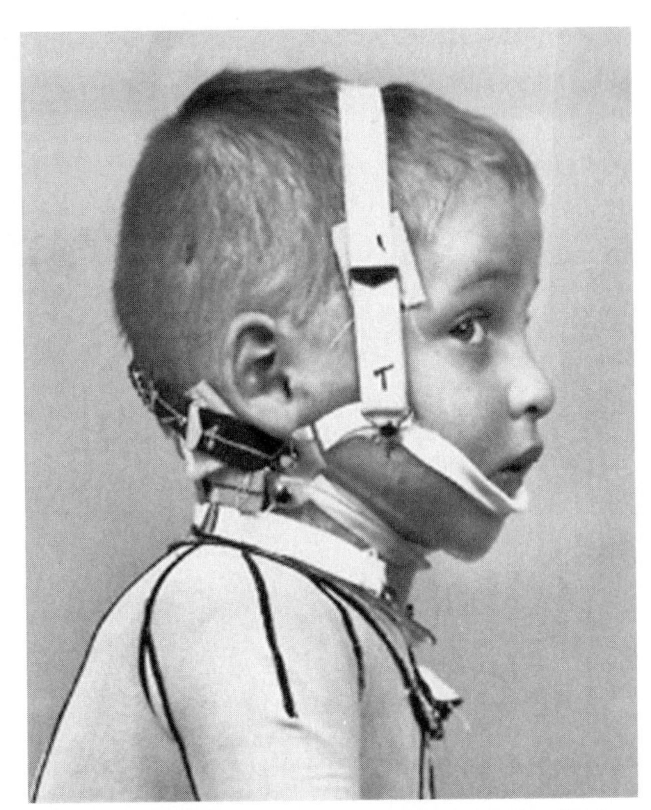

FIGURE 44–7. Profile of a transparent chin and neck orthosis worn with a custom external vascular support garment. Similar devices are used with adults.

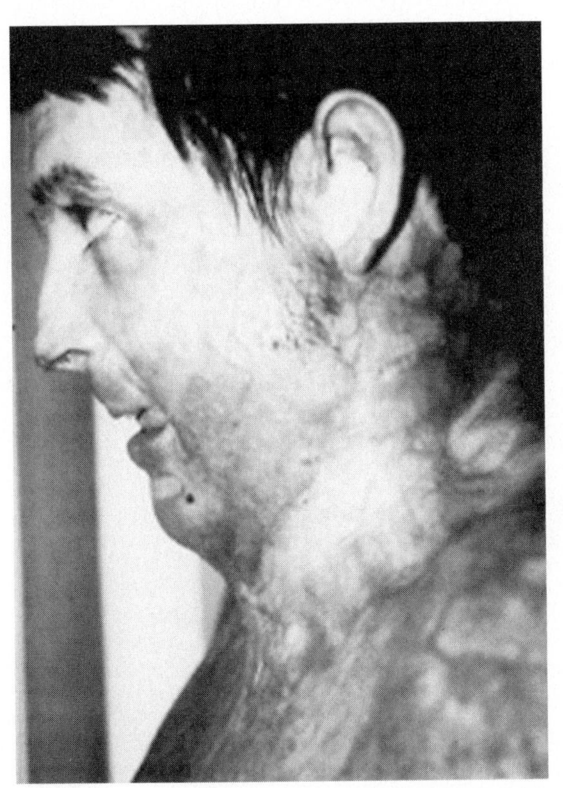

FIGURE 44–6. When a neck scar shortens by contraction, the chin shelf and cervicomental angle are lost, and ROM is restricted.

Burn scar contracture of the perioral facial region may lead to cosmetic and functional impairment. Microstomia, or contracture of the oral commissures, affects intubation for surgery, eating skills, oral hygiene, dental care, facial expression, and sometimes speech. Due to the structure of the perioral region and the need for stretching pressure when scar is developing, an elastic hood without an insert increases circumoral contractures. A microstomia-prevention appliance is commercially available for preventing or decreasing microstomia during wound healing (Carlow, Conine, & Stevenson-Moore, 1987). The commercial appliance is effective in preserving the horizontal width and can be adapted to increase vertical stretching by molding a piece of thermoplastic to its acrylic sections. Problems with this approach are distortion of the tissues surrounding the oral commissures and potential pressure sores of the oral mucosa. Some therapists construct a modified microstomia-prevention splint. (Fig. 44-9). The advantage of

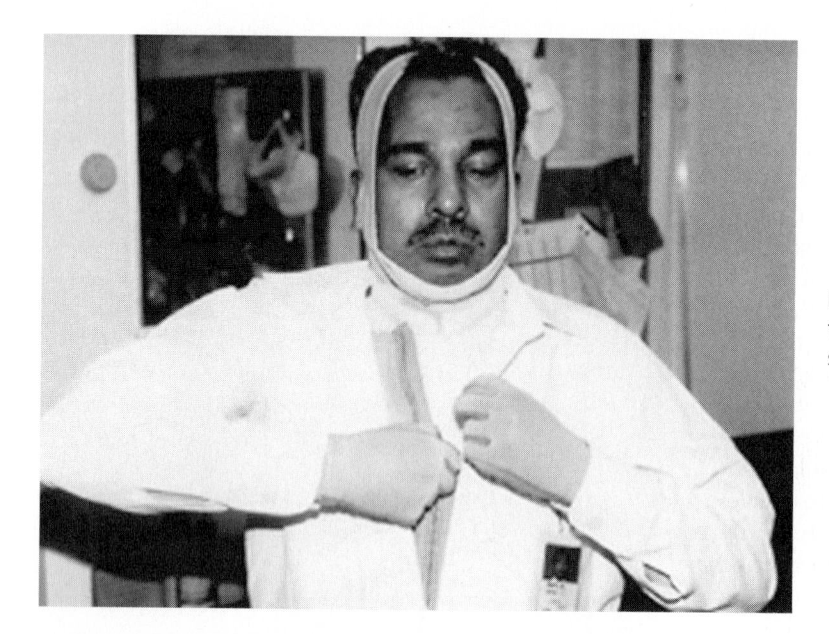

FIGURE 44–8. A patient independently donning a triple-component neck splint and external compression and vascular support garment.

this design is its flexibility in allowing modification of the splint's commissures without adding additional material.

Facial pressure devices include elastomer inserts under elastic garments, low-temperature thermoplastic masks, and total-contact, transparent face orthoses (Figs. 44-10 and 44-11). The advantages of a transparent mask are that more precise alterations are possible, the amount of scar contact can be easily assessed, and facial contours can be emphasized. Many clients prefer the transparent mask because it is simple to don and doff, is less obtrusive, and the hair is uncovered, allowing some identity.

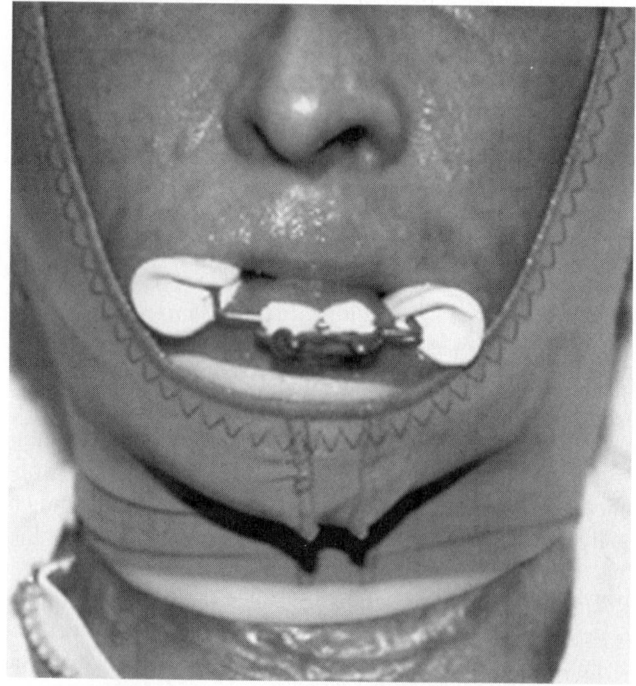

FIGURE 44–9. A therapist-made microstomia splint and a thermoplastic chin cup, worn under the elastic chin strap, which was molded to the patient to preserve the cervicomental angle and chin shelf.

Scar management is a long-term process that requires frequent assessment and adjustment of garment and splint fit. Increasing the person's ability to don and doff garments and splints is an important objective in design selection (Fig. 44-8). In most cases, success depends on the person's creativity, persistence, and ability to assume responsibility for self-care.

Skin Care

Whether or not scar contracture develops during burn wound maturation, the new skin (epithelium) will never look or react to exposure or contact like the skin did before injury. Common problems include edematous, insensate or hypersensitive, dry, and unusually fragile skin (Fig. 44-12).

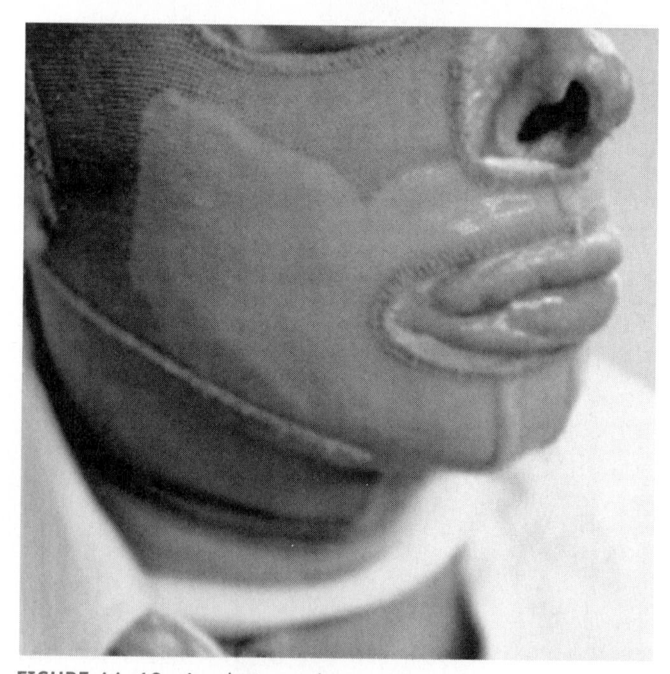

FIGURE 44–10. An elastomer insert worn under a custom-measured mask distributes pressure more uniformly.

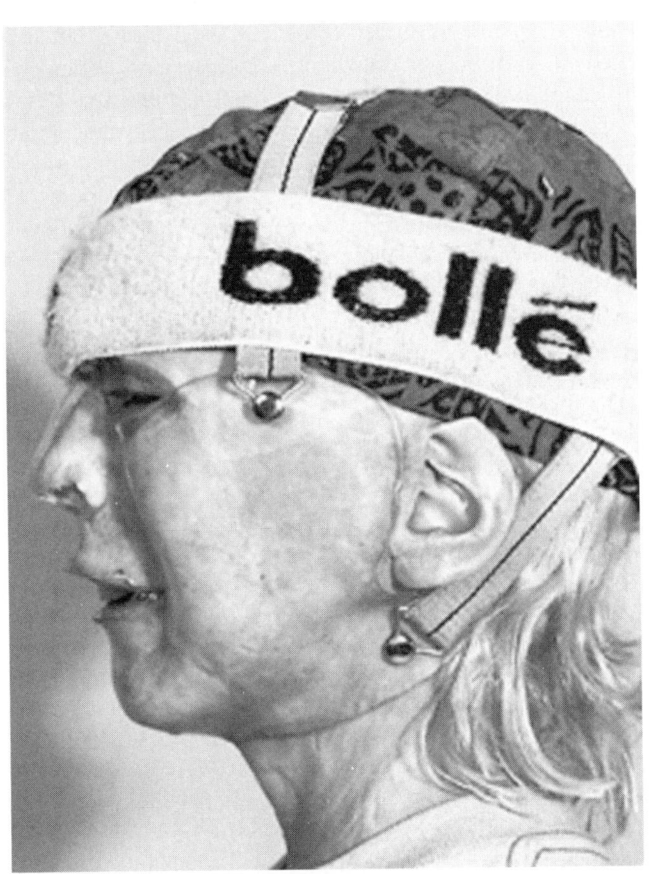

FIGURE 44–11. A transparent facial orthosis. Headbands are frequently used for forehead scar control.

Newly healed skin is also vulnerable to exposure to ultraviolet light, extremes of temperature, and chemical irritation (Rivers & Fisher, 1991). Because of changes in elasticity, shear tolerance, sensation, and pigmentation, skin care and conditioning should be part of self-care education in every burn intervention plan for these clients.

Before hospital discharge, the client should learn how and when to lubricate the skin. This is necessary because most deep partial-thickness and full-thickness burns damage epidermal appendages that contribute to the skin's moisture balance. Lubrication should be done every day after bathing and at intervals during the day when the skin feels exceptionally dry, tight, or itchy (Field et al, 2000).

Improving skin tolerance and sensitivity to friction or trauma is also part of skin care. Scratching, rubbing, bumping into something, and the shearing forces of custom-made, external vascular support garments can cause blisters. Clients should be taught not to be alarmed when blisters occur and to leave small blisters intact. If the blister is large, it should be drained, and mercurochrome and dry gauze should be applied. A disposable contact layer of gauze, cloth, or paper towel under the pad decreases perspiration and contact dermatitis. Interim pressure dressings and presized garments; massage, exercise, and activity while wearing interim garments; and desensitization activities are also effective in increasing skin tolerance and decreasing sensitivity. Vibration or tapping with a cool pack decreases itching.

It is important for the therapist to be aware of possible complications of contractures and scar control devices. Deformities such as delayed skeletal growth from the scar management devices have been reported (Fricke, Omnell, Dutcher, Hollender, & Engrav, 1999; Leung, Cheng, Ma, Clark, & Leung, 1983). Robertson, Zuker, Dabrowski and Levinson (1985) reported that sleep apnea as a complication of burns to the head and neck of children, especially children who wore chin straps at night. More recently, Nahieli, Kelly, Baruchin, Ben-Meir, and Shapira (1995), reported oromaxillofacial skeletal deformities resulting from burn scar contractures of the face and neck in a client who did not wear support or compression garments or splints. Frequent follow-up in a burn clinic with both physician and therapist assessment is important for safety.

RETURN TO OCCUPATIONAL ACTIVITIES

The physical demands of jobs and other life tasks include many motor skills, such as reaching, stooping, pulling, lifting, and manipulating. Because the emphasis of burn

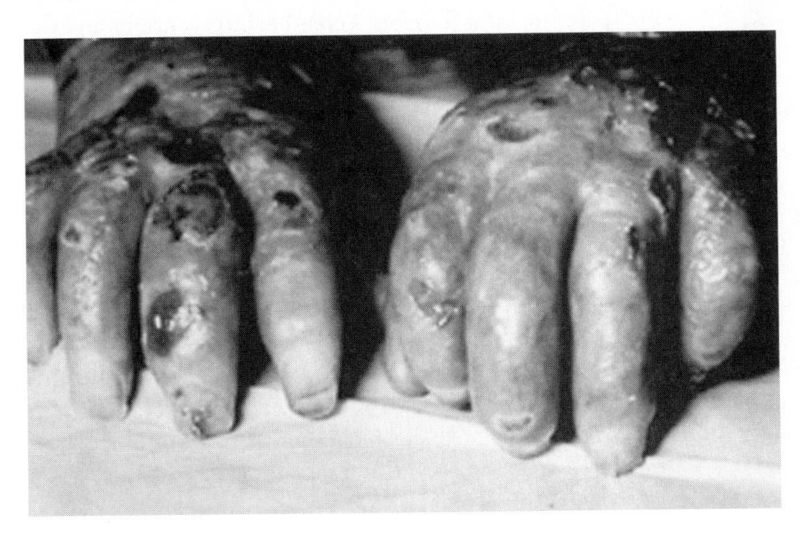

FIGURE 44–12. Burn wounds that heal without surgery are frequently edematous, fragile, and prone to blistering. Skin conditioning and intermediate garments are used to prevent these problems.

rehabilitation is on functional recovery, a resourceful occupational therapist uses activities that incorporate desired motions and also are occupationally relevant, such as the Valpar Small Tools Work Sample (Fig. 44-13). Return to leisure activities may occur before return to job responsibilities. Sports with friends, such as casting for and catching a fish gives clients opportunities for sun or cold protection, improving gross motor and fine motor skills, inner satisfaction, and socialization.

Identifying and integrating job skills in the acute care treatment plan decreases the potential for loss of skills and fosters the client's realization that he or she is going to be okay. Returning to work before final scar maturation preserves function and improves the client's self-concept. This is possible, however, only after reintegration into the family and resolution of socialization concerns. Mutual expectations from the employer or teachers with surgeons, nurses, social workers, and therapists encourage early return to productive activity.

Preparing a burn client for return to work is a shorter process when intervention plans incorporate both job demands and basic functional needs. Therefore, the job description can provide a basis for identifying and analyzing intervention activities that promote restored function. If the client was injured on the job or is lacking confidence in his or her abilities, many psychosocial issues may emerge when discussing return to work. Fear, anger, appropriate boundaries, and pain need to be addressed early and when needed, with a psychologist (Watkins, Cook, May, & Ehleben, 1988; Robert, Meyer, Villarreal, Blakeney, Desai, & Herndon, 1999). The person may not feel capable of performing the job again, may be anxious about being injured again, or may be self-conscious about appearance. Job desensitization can take place when the client goes to the workplace, observes the job, and discusses concerns with coworkers and a supervisor and later with the therapist. Group sessions that include both inpatients and outpatients have also had positive results in resolving return to work issues. Work provides distraction, control, and independence often desired by clients recovering from burns.

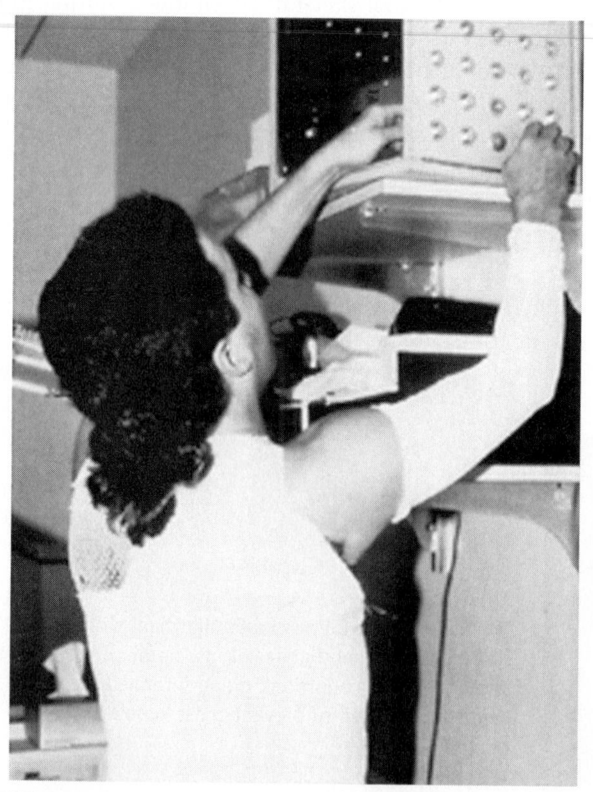

FIGURE 44-13. Work samples, such as the Valpar Small Tools Work Sample, can be used to simulate both functional motions and work skills during acute or outpatient care.

CONCLUSION

People who have burn injuries have improved outcomes, owing to advances in burn care. Today, most clients recovering from a burn injury can expect to return to a near-normal life, including return to school or work early during the recovery process. To achieve this goal, a team approach to client-centered care is necessary (Gorga et al., 1999; Sheridan et al., 2000). Despite advances in burn care, challenges loom ahead. According to the U.S. Department of Health and Human Services (Administration on Aging, 2001), by 2030, there will be about 70 million older persons, more than twice the number in 1999. Most older persons have at least one chronic condition and many have multiple conditions. Senior clients with burns often also have arthritis, hypertension, hearing impairments, heart disease, cataracts, orthopedic impairments, sinusitis, and diabetes (Still, Law, Belcher, & Thiruvaiyaru, 1999). Conscientious therapists include burn prevention and first aid in all types of intervention programs.

As technology grows, new communication media expedite computer interaction for distant clients. Therapists need licenses in each state where they provide telemedicine consultation. Whenever possible, burn center therapists guide, encourage, direct, counsel, coach, and protect distant therapists, clients, and families during video evaluation. Praise for the local therapist's creative interventions and the client's exertion is motivating. Hoffman, Doctor, Patterson, Carrougher, and Furness (2000) recently explored virtual reality as an adjunctive pain control during burn wound care in adolescent patients. Future developments for electronic client self-documentation, evaluation, and treatments seem unlimited.

Practitioners refer clients to numerous burn-related programs. School reentry programs (Blakeney et al., 1995, Doctor, 1995), burn camps (Rosenstein, 1986), groups for recovered burn clients, and local and national organizations are just a few of the programs for these clients. For health-care professionals, the ABA, a national organization, is an important resource, dedicated to burn rehabilitation, education, research, and prevention.

References

Administration on Aging. (2001). A Profile of Older Americans: 2000 [U.S. Department of Health and Human Services]. Available at: www.aoa.dhhs.gov/aoa/stats/profile/. Accessed: June 21, 2001.

American Burn Association [ABA]. (1999). *Burn care resources in North America, 1999–2000*. Available at http://www.ameriburn.org/pub/resourcedir.php3: Author.

Blakeney, P., Moore, M. A., Meyer, W. III, Bishop, B., Murphy, L., Robson, M., & Herndon, D. (1995). Efficacy of school reentry programs. *Journal of Burn Care and Rehabilitation, 16*, 469–472.

Caplan, A. L. (1988). Informed consent and provider-patient relationships in rehabilitation medicine. *Archives of Physical Medicine and Rehabilitation, 69*, 312–317.

Carlow, D. L., Conine, T. A., & Stevenson-Moore, P. (1987). Static orthoses for the management of microstomia. *Journal of Rehabilitation Research and Development, 24*(3), 35–42.

Carr-Collins, J. A. (1992). Pressure techniques for the prevention of hypertrophic scar. In R. E. Salisbury (Ed.). *Clinics in plastic surgery* (vol. 19, pp. 733–743). Philadelphia: Saunders.

Chang, P., Laubenthal, K. N., Lewis II, R. W., Rosenquist, D., Lindley-Smith, P. & Kealey, G. P. (1996, March). Prospective randomized study of the effect of pressure garment therapy on the rate of wound maturation in burn patients. Abstract of paper presented at the *Proceedings of the American Burn Association Annual Meeting, USA*, Vol. 28, p. 83, Nashville, TN.

Covey, M., Dutcher, K., Marvin, J. & Heimbach, D. (1988). Efficacy of continuous passive motion (CPM) devices with hand burns. *Journal of Burn Care and Rehabilitation, 9*, 397–400.

Daugherty, M. B., & Carr-Colllins, J. A. (1994). Splinting techniques for the burn patient. In R. L. Richard & M. J. Staley. (Eds.). Burn care and rehabilitation: Principles and practice (pp. 242–323). Philadelphia: Davis.

Doctor, M. E. (1995). Commentary. *Journal of Burn Care and Rehabilitation, 16*(4), 466–468.

Egan, M., & DeLaat, M. D. (1992). Considering spirituality in occupational therapy practice. *Canadian Journal of Occupational Therapy, 61*, 95–101.

Ehde, D. M., Patterson, D. R., Wiechman, S. A., & Wilson L. G. (2000). Post-traumatic stress symptoms and distress 1 year after burn injury. *Journal of Burn Care and Rehabilitation, 21*(2), 105–111.

Falkel, J. E. (1994). Anatomy and physiology of the skin. In R. L. Richard & M. J. Staley. (Eds.). Burn care and rehabilitation: Principles and practice (pp. 10–28). Philadelphia: Davis.

Fauerbach, J. A., Lawrence, J. W., Schmidt, C. W., Munster, A. M., & Costa, P. T. (2000). Personality predictors of injury-related posttraumatic stress disorder. *Journal of Nervous and Mental Disease, 188*(8), 510–517.

Field, T., Peck, M., Hernandez-Reif, M., Krugman, S., Burman, I., & Ozment-Schenck, L. (2000). Postburn itching, pain, and psychological symptoms are reduced with massage therapy. *Journal of Burn Care and Rehabilitation, 21*(3), 189–193.

Fricke, N., Omnell, M., Dutcher, K., Hollender, L., & Engrav, L. (1999). Skeletal and dental disturbances in children after facial burns and pressure garment use: A 4-year follow-up. *Journal of Burn Care and Rehabilitation, 20*, 239–249.

Gorga, D., Johnson, J., Bentley, A., Silverberg, R., Glassman, M., Madden, M., Yurt, R., Nagler W. (1999). The physical, functional, and developmental outcome of pediatric burn survivors from 1 to 12 months postinjury. *Journal of Burn Care and Rehabilitation,. 20*(2), 171–178.

Glass, T. M., & Bruns, M. M. (2000). *Exercises for pediatric burn therapy*. San Antonio, TX: Therapy Skill Builders.

Harris, S., & Harris, J. (1999) *The skin* [Permachart Quick Reference Guide]. Concord, Ontario, Canada: Papertech.

Heimbach, D. M., & Engrav, L. H. (1984). *Surgical management of the burn wound*. New York: Raven.

Hoffman, H. G., Doctor, J. N., Patterson, D. R., Carrougher, G. J., & Furness, T. A. (2000). Virtual reality as an adjunctive pain control during burn wound care in adolescent patients. *Pain, 85*(1–2), 305–309.

Johnson, C. (1994). Pathologic manifestations of burn injury. In R. L. Richard & M. J. Staley (Eds.). Burn care and rehabilitation: Principles and practice (pp. 29–48). Philadelphia: Davis.

Jordan, C. L., Allely, R., & Gallagher J. (1994). Self-care strategies following severe burns. In C. Christiansen (Ed.). *Ways of living* (pp. 305–332). Bethesda, MD: American Occupational Therapy Association.

Law, M., Baptiste, S., & Mills, J. (1995). Client-centered practice: What does it mean and does it make a difference? *Canadian Journal of Occupational Therapy, 62*, 250–257.

Leman, C., & Lowery, C. (1986). The triple-component neck splint. *Journal of Burn Care and Rehabilitation, 7*, 357–361.

Leman, C. J., & Ricks, N. (1994). Discharge planning and follow-up burn care. In R. L. Richard & M. J. Staley. (Eds.). *Burn care and rehabilitation: Principles and practice* (pp. 447–472). Philadelphia: Davis.

Leslie, G., Blakeney, P., Moore, P., Desai, M. H., & Herndon, D. N. (1996, March). *Native Americans: A challenge for the pediatric burn team*. Poster presented at the American Burn Association annual meeting, Nashville, TN.

Leung, K. S., Cheng, J. C. Y., Ma, G. F. Y., Clark, J. A., & Leung, P. C. (1983). Complications of pressure therapy for post-burn hypertrophic scars: Biochemical analysis based on 5 patients. *Burns, Including Thermal Injury, 10*, 434–438.

Lund, C., & Browder, N. (1944). The estimation of area of burns. *Surgical Gynecology and Obstetrics, 79*, 352–355.

Miles, W., & Grigsby, L. (1990). Remodeling of scar tissue in the burned hand. In J. Hunter, L. Schneider, E. Mackin, & A. Callahan (Eds.). *Rehabilitation of the hand: Surgery and therapy* (3rd ed., pp. 841–857). St. Louis: Mosby.

Nahieli, O., Kelly, J. P., Baruchin, A. M., Ben-Meir, P., & Shapira, Y. (1995). Oro-maxillofacial skeletal deformities resulting from burn scar contractures of the face and neck. *Burns, Including Thermal Injury, 21*(1), 65–69.

Pain management of the burn patient. (1995). *Journal of Burn Care and Rehabilitation, 16*(3), 343–376.

Richard, R. L., & Staley, M. J. (Eds.). (1994). *Burn care and rehabilitation: Principles and practice*. Philadelphia: Davis.

Rivers, E. A., & Fisher, S. V. (1991). Advances in burn rehabilitation. In F. J. Kottke & E. A. Amate (Eds.). *Clinical advances in physical medicine and rehabilitation* (pp. 334–357). Washington, DC: Pan American Health Organization.

Rivers, E., Strate, R., & Solem, L. (1979). The transparent face mask. *American Journal of Occupational Therapy, 33*, 108–113.

Robert, R., Meyer, W., Villarreal, C. K., Blakeney, P., Desai, M., & Herndon, D. (1999). An approach to the timely treatment for acute stress disorder. *Journal of Burn Care and Rehabilitation, 20*, 250–258.

Robertson, C. F., Zuker, R., Dabrowski, B., & Levinson, H. (1985). Obstructive sleep apnea: A complication of burns to the head and neck in children. *Journal of Burn Care and Rehabilitation, 6*, 353–357.

Rosenstein, D. (1986). Camp celebrate: A therapeutic weekend camping program for pediatric burn patients. *Journal of Burn Care and Rehabilitation, 7*(5), 434–436.

Saffle, K. R., & Schnebly, W. A. (1994) Burn wound care. In R. L. Richard & M. J. Staley (Eds.). *Burn care and rehabilitation: Principles and practice* (pp. 119–176). Philadelphia: Davis.

Sheridan, R., Hinson, M. I., Liang, M. H., Nackel, A. F., Schoenfeld, D. A., Ryan, C. M., Mulligan, J. L., & Tompkins R. G. (2000). Long-term outcome of children surviving massive burns. *Journal of the American Medical Association, 283*(1), 69–73.

Sheridan, R., Petras, L., Basha, G., Salvo, P., Cifrino, C., Hinson, M., McCabe, M., Fallon, J., & Thompkins, R. G. (1995, April). *Should irregular burns be sized with the hand or the palm: A planimetry study*. Paper presented at the American Burn Association annual meeting, Albuquerque, NM.

Sheridan, R., Weber, J., Prelack, K., Petras, L., Lydon, M., & Tompkins. R. (1999). Early burn center transfer shortens the length of hospitalization and reduces complications in children with serious burn injuries. *Journal of Burn Care and Rehabilitation, 20*(5), 347–350.

Sorenson, W., Fisher, S., & Rivers, E. (2001). Burn rehabilitation. In B. O'Young & M. A. Young (Eds.). *Physical medicine and rehabilitation secrets* (pp. 352–361). Philadelphia: Hanley & Belfus.

Staley, M., & Serghiou, M. (1998). Casting guidelines, tips, and techniques. *Journal of Burn Care and Rehabilitation, 19*(3):254–260.

Still, J. M., Law, E. J., Belcher, K., & Thiruvaiyaru, D. (1999). A regional medical center's experience with burns of the elderly. *Journal of Burn Care and Rehabilitation. 20*(3), 218–223.

Wachtel, T. (1985). Epidemiology, classification, initial care, and administrative considerations for critically burned patients. In T. Wachtel (Ed.). *Critical care clinics* (pp. 3–26). Philadelphia: Saunders.

Ward, R. S. (1991) Pressure therapy for the control of hypertrophic scar formation after burn injury: A history and review. *Journal of Burn Care and Rehabilitation, 12*(3), 257–262.

Ward, R. S. (1993). Reasons for the selection of burn-scar-support suppliers by burn centers in the United States: A survey. *Journal of Burn Care and Rehabilitation, 14*(3), 360–367.

Watkins, P. N., Cook, E., May S. R., & Ehleben, C. M. (1988). Psychological stages in adaptation following burn injury: A method for facilitating psychological recovery of burn victims. *Journal of Burn Care and Rehabilitation*, 9(4), 376–384.

Weber, J. M., & Thompkins, D. M. (1993). Improving survival: Infection control and burns. *American Association Critical Nursing*, *4*(3), 414–423.

Willis, B. (1970). The use of Orthoplast isoprene splints in the treatment of the acutely burned child. *American Journal of Occupational Therapy*, *24*(3), 187–191.

CASE ANALYSIS: UNIT X
EVALUATION AND INTERVENTION WITH MR. R. USING TWO THEORETICAL PERSPECTIVES

BETTY R. HASSELKUS

EVALUATION AND TREATMENT USING TWO THEORETICAL PERSPECTIVES: THE NARRATIVE

Mr. R., the man with rheumatoid arthritis who was described in the Case Study 38-1 on page 762 was referred to the home care team when he was 81-years-old.

THE MODEL OF HUMAN OCCUPATION

In the Model of Human Occupation, it is a general therapeutic principle that therapy is an event that comes into a life that has both a history and a future that extend beyond the therapeutic experience. In Mr. R.'s situation, we, as team members, would be described as coming "into a life in progress" (Kielhofner, 1995, p. 253). In this Model, appreciation of the life that has been lived before and that will be lived in the future should always be a part of the therapeutic process. This principle is imbedded in the concept of life as a narrative or story.

In the Model of Human Occupation, disease or injury are viewed as disruptions in a person's life story; when such disruptions occur, it is necessary to *reorganize* one's life into a new or modified story. The reorganization represents the healing process that is needed after illness or injury, enabling the individual to re-create meaningful new directions for the life that lies ahead. Therapy represents a process that facilitates the reorganization of the life story into a new plot (Kielhofner, 1995).

In the narrative above, I tried to enter Mr. R.'s life with an appreciation for his history and for the life that lay ahead of him. To enter a life that is in old age is, of course, very different from entering at other life stages. Mr. R.'s history was long and rich with many life roles, experiences, and personal accomplishments. At 81 years old, Mr. R.'s future was likely to be short by comparison. With that in mind, the challenge for me, when working with this older person, was to fit occupational therapy into that long and rich life in a way that would facilitate a reorganization and meaningful continuation of his life narrative, for as long as that narrative lasted.

Perhaps the therapeutic activity that fit most powerfully with Mr. R.'s personal narrative was the development of the feature story for the monthly home care newsletter. In creating the story, Mr. R. reconnected with his past and brought selected experiences from that past story into the present; in the process, he also connected with many other people through the sharing of that part of his history. Ideally, then, engagement in the newsletter story served to help restore a sense of wholeness to Mr. R.'s life narrative, a wholeness that had been disrupted by the rheumatoid arthritis. The newsletter activity provided a way to link the present with the past, and vice versa. The rheumatoid arthritis, in fact, served as a vehicle that brought Mr. R. access to the newsletter because of his need for home health care. Up until that point in time, the disease had been linked only to giving up important parts of his life — the hunting, fishing, and bowling. Alternatively, in the development of the newsletter article, the disease provided the entreé to an occupation that helped reorganize his life in such a way that the past was not discarded; rather, it continued to offer meaning to the present.

Another principle of the Model of Human Occupation is the following: "The only tool which therapists have at their disposal is to change the relevant environment to support or precipitate a change in the human system" (Kielhofner, 1995, p. 261). Much of the occupational therapy focus with Mr. R. was on modifying his environment. Examples are the assistive devices that became a part of his life space such as the bathing equipment, magnifiers, medication dispenser, car door opener, and cane. In tandem with these environmental changes, the emphasis in therapy was on Mr. R.'s skills and functional performance, that is, his ability to get in and out of the bathtub, to take his medication independently, to continue to drive, to be able to do crossword puzzles and read. This is in contrast to other theoretical frameworks which focus on bringing about change in the underlying neurophysiological capacities of the mind-brain-body performance subsystem.

"The loss of roles and habits requires swift replacement" (Kielhofner, 1995, p. 264). This is a third principle in the Model of Human Occupation. Kielhofner likens a person's loss of roles and habits to the collapse of the scaffolding which holds up much of everyday life. Such losses can lead to strong emotional reactions and disorganization of a person's way of life. Mr. R.'s role losses were numerous, including the roles of hunter, fisherman, champion bowler, driver, and keeper of the financial records to name only a few. He also experienced losses in his daily routines and habits as the arthritis gradually necessitated modifications and changes in the way he carried out his self-care and household activities. It is probable that Mr. R.'s depression was a reaction to these losses of roles and habits.

The assistive devices described above served to help support Mr. R.'s continuation of familiar daily activities and routines. Participation in the arthritis swim program provided Mr. R. with a new role and new routines as partial replacement for the losses. As the occupational therapist, I negotiated with Mr. R. to help bring about this opportunity for a new social role. In this process of negotiation, I respected Mr. R.'s choice not to take part in former activities such as bowling, even in a modified way; he was clearly telling me that this previous highly valued activity was no longer desirable under the new conditions of his life. It was my challenge to provide the opportunity for replacements, ones that fit into the narrative of Mr. R.'s life — past, present, and future.

THE REHABILITATION FRAME OF REFERENCE

The occupational therapy engaged in with Mr. R. might also be described within the Rehabilitation Frame of Reference. The strong emphasis in therapy with Mr. R. on the maintenance of independent function in daily activities and the use of compensatory techniques and equipment to facilitate function are part of the philosophy and goals of rehabilitation. Within this framework, the changes in functional performance secondary to the rheumatoid arthritis are viewed as occupational dysfunction for which compensatory methods are needed.

In my occupational therapy evaluation of Mr. R., I focused on monitoring his function in work, self-care, and leisure over time. I administered the Barthel Index at 6-month intervals to monitor Mr. R.'s functional performance in daily self-care activities (Hasselkus, 1982; Mahoney & Barthel, 1965). The Barthel Index is an evaluation of basic self-care and includes the following ten items: eating, transferring, toileting, ambulation, personal hygiene, bathing, dressing, going up and down stairs, and continence of bowel and bladder. Mr. R.'s score upon referral to the home care team was 90, meaning he was independent in all self-care items except eating and bathing for which he needed minimum assistance. At the time he was discharged from home care to nursing home care, his score had dropped to 45; Mr. R. was wholely or partially dependent in all but toileting and bowel and bladder continence. The Barthel Index provided a systematic method of monitoring for changes in function; when changes were detected, compensatory techniques and equipment were introduced in an effort to restore previous levels of competence and independence or increase safety during the activity.

The Rehabilitation Frame of Reference is strongly associated with the biomedical view of health and illness. In the biomedical view, the human being is viewed as an organism made up of organ subsystems and physiological processes. One understands illness by understanding the pathologies represented in these subsystems and processes. Rheumatoid arthritis represents pathology in the musculoskeletal subsystem. As the occupational therapist, in addition to monitoring function as described above, I watched carefully for signs of periarticular changes in Mr. R.'s involved joints. I was especially attentive to his hands and wrists, examining him regularly for signs of active inflammation such as swelling, redness, fever, tendon or ligament damage, early deformities. I questioned him about the duration of his morning stiffness and about his level of pain. I taught him joint protection techniques to "protect" his joints from undue stress that might exacerbate the disease activity and put his joints in further jeopardy. I constructed a small splint to support the damaged IP joint of his thumb; I fitted Mr. R. with a commercially available splint to put his right wrist at rest, thus helping to control the inflammation in the carpal joints.

All of this therapy was carried out within the context of medical management of the rheumatoid arthritis. I was part of Mr. R.'s medical management, along with the physician and pharmacist who also monitored the disease activity and regulated his medications, the nurse who monitored his general health, the physical therapist who evaluated and treated his gait and mobility problems, and the social worker who attended closely to the family needs. While this was a very interdisciplinary team, and we all tried to be holistic in our approach to the home care patients, nevertheless, much of our activity was governed by the rehabilitation model, emphasizing the body systems and their pathologies. With Mr. R., the team focused strongly on the pathology of rheumatoid arthritis and the need for compensation in his daily life.

Occupational therapy with Mr. R., thus, represented more than one theoretical frame of reference. The Model of Human Occupation and the Rehabilitation Frame of Reference area both represented in the occupational therapy process that evolved with this older person. The two frameworks overlap and complement each other in several ways. Both emphasize function in activities of daily living. The Rehabilitation Framework also emphasizes the capacities that underly that function, those that are more at the level of the body organ subsystems and physiological processes. Both emphasize the importance of the environment as a modality that can be modified to enhance function; the Rehabilitation Framework refers to the environment as a source of compensation and the Model of Human Occupation refers to it more as a resource to support the reorganization of the person's narrative of life. Different forms of clinical reasoning seem to be emphasized in each framework. Procedural reasoning is evident in the rehabilitation framework, especially in the therapy that focused on the pathology of rheumatoid arthritis and in the therapeutic skills such as splint-making and teaching joint protection. Narrative reasoning fits well with the therapy that was guided by the principles of the Model of Human Occupation; conceptualizing Mr. R.'s life as a narrative and searching for ways to fit into that narrative and help with its reorganization led to the idea for the feature story in the newsletter. The swim program was the result of more narrative reasoning, but also conditional reasoning and interactive reasoning — as the therapist, I was able to imagine Mr. R. in the new role of a swimmer and I reasoned together with him to create a shared view of him in that role.

Near the end of the story of Mr. R., conditional and interactive reasoning were strongly emphasized as the team worked together — with other community health workers, with Mrs. R., and with the rest of the family — to imagine what his future would be and then to agree on the appropriate plans to bring that future about. The move to a nursing home was another major disruption in Mr. R.'s life narrative. Perhaps his death two months later is testimony to the magnitude of the shattering effects of the move. For a person's life story must somehow maintain a wholeness and integrity to the end. Occupational therapists must continue to seek ways to make that possible.

Hasselkus, B.R. (1982). Barthel self-care index and geriatric home care patients. *Physical & Occupational Therapy in Geriatrics, 1* (4), 11–22.

Kielhofner, G. (1995). Change making: Principles of therapeutic intervention. In G. Kielhofner (Ed.), *A model of human occupation: Theory and application*, 2nd edition (pp. 251–270). Philadelphia: Williams & Wilkins.

Mahoney, F., & Barthel, D. (1965). Functional evaluations: The Barthel index. *Maryland State Medical Journal, 14*, 61–65.

UNIT *eleven*

Issues in Service Provision

Learning Objectives

After completing this unit, readers will be able to:

- Explain how public policy, legislation, regulatory factors, and funding mechanisms influence occupational therapy practice.
- Describe key factors that will influence the shape of occupational therapy practice in the future.
- Discuss occupational therapy management issues relative to planning, marketing, quality assurance, and documentation of services.
- Define and discuss communication relative to interdisciplinary teams, supervision of occupational therapy personnel, and fieldwork supervision.
- Discuss the ethical and legal responsibilities of occupational therapy personnel in regard to issues of abuse and neglect and their role in the prevention and protection of clients from abuse and neglect.
- Describe occupational therapy services in institutional-based care in physical dysfunction and mental health settings.
- Describe the differences between community-based settings in relation to goals, staff, clients, and occupational therapy roles.
- Describe the roles of occupational therapy personnel in consultation and program development.

The day-to-day practice of occupational therapy is influenced by administrative, reimbursement, and legislative issues, and occupational therapy practitioners can, in turn, influence this process through collective and individual action. Occupational therapy personnel must be proactive in a rapidly changing health-care environment to ensure the delivery of services in established settings and to expand services to new practice arenas. This unit provides an overview of the legislative and reimbursement issues for occupational therapy services and the management and supervision issues inherent in the delivery of occupational therapy services. It examines current practice in institutional and community settings and describes ways that occupational therapy personnel can develop services to meet the emerging needs of new populations. (Note: Words in **bold** type are defined in the Glossary.)

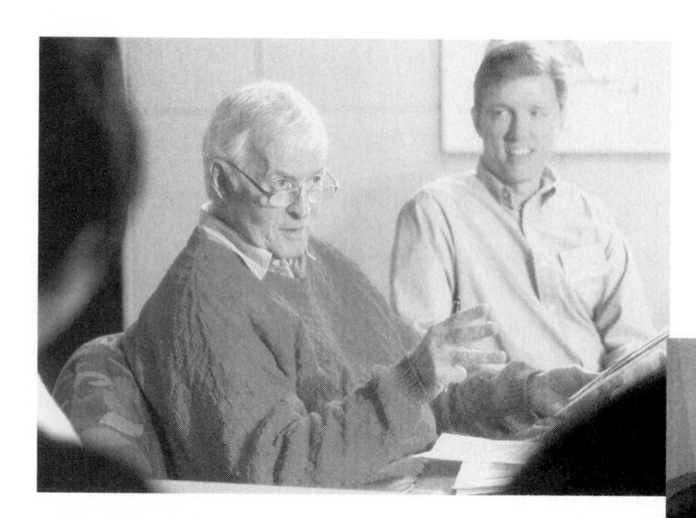

Occupational therapy practice involves cooperation and communication among colleagues and team members. Team meetings foster interdisciplinary collaboration and sharing. ((*top*) Courtesy of K. Clineff, Winchester, MA (©KINDRACLINEFF 2001); (*middle*) Courtesy of G. Samson, Photographic Services, University of New Hampshire, Durham, NH) (*bottom*) Supervision and collaboration are important aspects of the role of occupational therapy practitioners. (Courtesy of G. Samson, Photographic Services, University of New Hampshire, Durham, NH.)

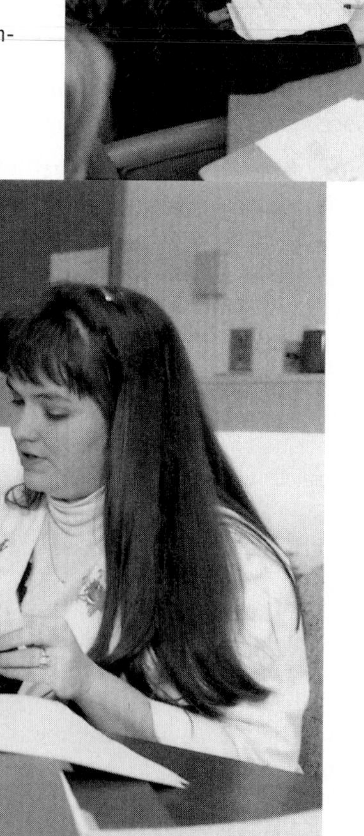

CHAPTER 45

OCCUPATIONAL THERAPY REIMBURSEMENT, REGULATION, AND THE EVOLVING SCOPE OF PRACTICE

MARY EVANOFSKI

The provision of health-care services in the United States, including occupational therapy, is a highly regulated industry accounting for 13.6% of all spending in the country, making it the most costly in the world. In 2000, per capita health expenditures in the United States totaled $4187. The nearest expenditure by any other country was France at $2369 per capita (Landers, 2001). Health policy in the United States grew out of our history. In the early years, independence from the monarchy and from government interference was a deep-seated value (Adams, 1931, Kraus, 1959). Federal responsibility related to health care throughout the 1800s was limited to the protection and medical care of the active military (Gritzler & Arluke, 1985). Since that time, a proliferation of legislative actions and events has shaped U.S. health care.

In this chapter, I first focus on major U.S. health-care policy trends in the twentieth century and their influence on occupational therapy practice. I briefly contrast current

U.S. health-care funding with health-care funding worldwide to demonstrate the differences in the organization and provision of health services. Next, I review the regulations and accreditation standards that have influenced the practice of occupational therapy. Finally, I address the scope of practice including opportunities and challenges that occupational therapy practitioners will face in the future.

AN ORIENTATION TO HEALTH-CARE POLICY IN THE UNITED STATES: 1930–2001

A comprehensive national health-care policy has eluded U.S. legislative approval for more than two centuries. Table 45-1 shows the complicated array of laws, regulations, business, and charitable enterprises that have prevailed in the absence of a comprehensive federal approach to health policy. Advocates for private enterprise and capitalism drove the evolution of a huge and profitable insurance industry, which continues to provide employer-based medical benefits. Meanwhile, major changes in health-care funding occurred in 1965, when federal mandates led to the introduction of both Medicare and Medicaid. Four major health-care reimbursement systems emerged during this time: indemnity insurance, health maintenance and managed care organizations, Medicaid, and Medicare.

TABLE 45-1. **LAWS, REGULATIONS, AND ORGANIZATIONS THAT PERTAIN TO HEALTH-CARE REIMBURSEMENT**

1777	President Washington orders inoculation of troops
1798	U.S. Public Health Service provides insurance for seamen
1847	American Medical Association sets up against quackery
1910	New York sets up workman's compensation, and American Medical Association lobbies for national health insurance
1920	American Medical Association leadership changes, restricting number of medical schools and no longer favoring national health insurance
1930	American Medical Association and American Hospital Association endorse privatized health insurance with medical controls
1935	Social Security Act of 1935
1942	Blue Cross/Blue Shield set up in each state
1943	International Ladies Garment Workers Union gets medical benefits
1945	Kaiser Permanente, the first HMO established
1960	Medicare and Medicaid established
1970	Cost control through Medicare-sponsored Professional Standards Review Organizations (PSRO)
1983	Medicare reform: prospective payment and diagnosis-related groups
1987	Omnibus Act of 1987 ensuring Medicare coverage for nursing home patients
1992	Market-driven health care versus health-care reform debate
1997	Balanced Budget Act of 1997
2000	Balanced Budget Act Reform
2001	Patient Bill of Rights

Indemnity Insurance, Third-Party Payers, and Cost Containment

In the 1930s, the American Medical Association (AMA) and American Hospital Association promoted indemnity plans as an alternative to national health insurance (Corning, 1969). The insurance industry grew as a direct result of federal tax incentives provided for employers who provided medical benefits to workers (Herzlinger, 1997). Indemnity insurance was the form of insurance coverage provided by most employers who purchased health benefits for their employees from the 1930s to the 1970s (Tufts Health Plan, 1995). It is closely identified with fee-for-service forms of reimbursement. With an indemnity plan, employees are able to access health care from any health-care provider at any point—at the emergency room, at the hospital, at the physician's office.

Beginning in the 1970s, insurance companies, which served as third-party payers to employers, began to introduce strategies to contain costs. These efforts continue today. Contractual agreements with providers (hospitals, physician offices, clinics, and outpatient settings) stipulate discounts in exchange for guaranteed volume. Other strategies used by third-party payers include deductibles, per diem rates, case rates, and exclusion of services. Table 45-2 provides definitions for some of these terms.

However, health-care costs rose faster than employers anticipated (Herzlinger, 1997). Some employers could no longer afford to pay health benefits. One cost-saving response was to reduce the number of employees who received health-care coverage by hiring more part-time and contractual workers. As a result, from 1995 to 1998, the percentage of uninsured Americans grew from 15.1% to over 16.5%, leaving more than 44.3 million Americans uninsured (Gardner, 2001).

Several stopgap measures were taken, and by 2000, the numbers of uninsured Americans dropped to 14.3% (38.7 million people) (Gardner, 2001). With a waning economy, few health-care experts were optimistic about sustaining the downward trend (Gardner, 2001). Another approach to containing health-care costs was the development of managed care plans designed on principles established by health maintenance organizations.

TABLE 45-2. DEFINITIONS OF REIMBURSEMENT TERMINOLOGY

Balanced Budget Act of 1997 (BBA of 1997): Congress authorized many Medicare cuts in attempt to balance the U.S. budget.

Balanced Budget Refinement Act of 2000 (BBA of 2000): In response to public pressure, Congress passed legislation to restore some of the benefits eliminated in 1997.

Case rate: A fee negotiated for a specific case, based on the diagnosis and anticipated needs of the patient.

Deductible: A percentage of the bill that is most often passed on to the claimant.

Fee for service: A fee paid for every service provided.

Health maintenance organization (HMO): Services are delivered on a prepaid budgeted basis; patients must use HMO providers and usually pay a fee at the time of the visit.

Managed care organization (MCO): Any type of health coverage by which the member's care is managed through a series of cost-containment components and oversight.

Medicaid: A federal program, run and partially funded by individual states, to provide medical benefits to certain low-income people.

Medicare: A federal health insurance program for people 65 years and older and for certain younger people with disability.

Per diem rate: A negotiated per-day rate for a hospital stay that includes all services.

Prospective payment: Reimbursement based on a predetermined formula rather than on services actually provided to the patient.

Retrospective payment: A fee-for-service system in which the provider charges Medicare after the service occurs.

Health Maintenance and Managed Care Organizations

The first health maintenance organization (HMO), Kaiser Permanente, was founded in the 1940s. At its inception, Kaiser provided medical care to all of the workers of a company for a monthly fee. Many of these employees were immigrants who worked on the railroads and western expansion projects in remote areas, where risks were high and medical care scarce. For practical reasons, Kaiser insisted on prevention and education as a strategy for health maintenance (Kongstevdt, 1997). By the 1970s, the traditional indemnity insurance providers who were beginning to investigate ways to contain costs modified the Kaiser model to meet their needs. The new term *managed care* emerged to describe programs that sought to control the use of health-care services (Tufts Health Plan, 1995).

The new HMOs had an emphasis on education, prevention, and screening and used pricing strategy similar to the Kaiser model in which per-member-per-month fees are paid to the HMO regardless of service provided. The passage of the HMO Act of 1973 marked a new era for HMOs (Herzlinger, 1997). The law provided financial incentives that allowed employers to shift from traditional indemnity plans to HMO and other managed-care plans to provide health-care coverage for their employees. Soon, groups of physicians, large providers, and newly formed physician-hospital organizations (PHOs) entered the marketplace, each with their own version of a managed care organization (MCO) (Kongstevdt, 1997).

Like insurance companies, HMOs, and MCOs negotiate contracts with providers. A major cost-containment strategy is to control the use of services by controlling physician behavior. Indeed, through practice guidelines, peer review, incentives, and sanctions related to payment, MCOs have been able to change the way doctors practice medicine (Kongstevdt, 1997). In a common model, primary-care physicians serve as gatekeepers for all medical care that a patient receives. Patients must have authorization from their primary-care physician and the managed-care provider before seeing a specialist or receiving hospital care. These managed-care strategies are not limited to physician interactions; the same limitations apply to other providers, including occupational therapy practitioners (Kongstevdt, 1997).

By the 1990s, managed care promised to be the health-care solution for U.S. citizens, who were reluctant to allow full federal control of their health care and who have consistently favored competition as a means to ensure high quality and cost control. Again, private enterprise eliminated the need to define a comprehensive federal health-care-funding policy. However, the limits on choice and treatments and the need for authorizations have frustrated people as they seek health care (Kaiser/Harvard School of Public Health, 2001). Doctors and other health-care practitioners, including occupational therapy practitioners, are also frustrated as they respond to stricter controls on their practice through approval requirements, limitation of visits, and fee schedules (Hall & Berenson, 1998).

Occupational therapists report that they have had to respond to managed-care impositions and to use different assessment procedures, to be more efficient, as a result of these changes. Furthermore, they have had to learn how to delegate care to family members, occupational therapy assistants, or aides (Walker, 2001). Therapists also express concern about the amount of time devoted to documentation, delays in treatment while waiting for authorization, and the general feeling that they have to fight constantly for funding (Walker, 2001). Yet many occupational therapy practitioners and leaders see opportunities for professional growth and have optimism for the future (Abreu, 1996; Christiansen, 1996; Walker, 2001). Occupational therapy practitioners have been involved in developing critical pathways (Abreu, Seal, Podlesak, & Hartley, 1996; Harkleroad, Schirf, Volpe, & Holm., 2000; Novalis, Messenger-Fricke, & Morris, 2000), have found a natural role as case managers (Fisher, 1996) and have developed and expanded measurement methods to demonstrate cost effectiveness and occupational therapy value (Ellenberg, 1996).

Medicaid

Because indemnity insurance, HMOs, and MCOs are closely connected to benefits provided by employers, people who are unemployed and those who are unable to work are not covered by these plans. Medicaid, a federally legislated program that began in 1965, was created to provide medical assistance for people with limited income who meet other eligibility requirements. Originally, Medicaid provided health care only to medically indigent women and children. It now includes people who are blind or otherwise disabled and the poor elderly.

Although this is a federal program, states design and administer the program to meet the particular needs of their citizens. Consequently, Medicaid has a high degree of variation from state to state. The federal government pays a share of the expenditures based on a matching formula that is different for each state. By law, the matched funds cannot be lower than 50% or higher than 83%. For example, for a state with 50% matched funds, the federal government matches every $200,000 of state expenditures with $100,000 of federal money. For health-care providers, including occupational therapy practitioners, each state has developed unique methods of referral, authorization, and documentation. States also differ in the number of visits allowed and the reimbursement rates (Hoffman, Klees, & Curtis, 2001).

Medicare

In 1944, Merril G. Murray, social security administrator, proposed government health insurance coverage for social security beneficiaries (Corning, 1969). Between 1950 and 1963, the elderly population grew from 12 to 17.5 million. Hospital costs doubled (Hoffman et al., 2001). From the 1940s to the early 1960s, Congress deliberated many health insurance bills, but it was not until 1964 that public support for Medicare was widespread (Corning, 1969). On July 9, 1965, President Johnson, with former President Truman in attendance, signed Title XVIII of the Social Security Act designated as Health Insurance for the Aged and Disabled into law. This law is commonly known as Medicare (Hoffman et al., 2001). Medicare continues to provide health-care coverage for persons 65 years and older and for those who receive Social Security for disability.

This historic bill defined a new policy by creating an obligation of the U.S. government to pay for the health-care needs of the elderly (Corning, 1969). Part A of Medicare covers care in hospitals, skilled nursing facilities (SNFs), home-health services, and hospice. Part B covers outpatient services, long-term care in nursing facilities, and assistive devices. At the time of its inception, Medicare was based on a retrospective payment system and reimbursed reasonable cost. Medicare soon accounted for the largest single health-care expenditure in the United States (Hoffman et al., 2001).

When Congress passed Medicare, occupational therapy practitioners and their professional organization, the American Occupational Therapy Association (AOTA), had little political power, as exemplified by the restrictions placed on occupational therapy for Medicare beneficiaries. AOTA and occupational therapy practitioners worked successfully over the following two decades to ensure inclusion of occupational therapy services in Medicare reimbursement (Gritzler & Arluke, 1985). By the mid-1980s, Medicare recipients had become the largest group of clients seen by occupational therapy practitioners (Scott, 1985).

In 1984, in the face of the rising health-care costs, Congress enacted a major reform of Medicare. This reform transformed Medicare from a retrospective payment system to a prospective payment system (PPS). Hospitals were reimbursed for each admission according to preestablished rates for each of 471 diagnosis-related groups (DRGs). Hospitals began to use a formula to develop an average length of stay (ALOS) for each diagnostic group and attempted to limit the length of stay to that average. The result was a significant reduction to length of stay and fewer hospital admissions (Leiter, 1985).

Because hospitals were discharging patients more quickly, they were referred to occupational therapy during more acute stages of their illness (Abreu, 1996). Outpatient and home-based care increased to provide ongoing treatment after discharge from the hospital. SNFs began to take more critically ill patients. Subacute care emerged as a new category of service offered in hospitals, in rehabilitation hospitals, SNFs, and nursing homes (Kongstevdt, 1997). Occupational therapy practitioners were in high demand (Baum, 1985). In 1982, approximately 2.5% of occupational therapy practitioners worked in outpatient care, 3.8% in home-health care, and 6% in long-term care. By 1999, about 40.3% of practitioners worked in long-term care, 23% in outpatient care, and 13% in home health (Baum, 1985; Health Policy Alternative, 1996).

DRG exemptions were granted to psychiatric hospitals, children's hospitals, freestanding rehabilitation hospitals, and rehabilitation units within hospitals. An exemption meant that the PPS was not applied and that these specific services would continue to be paid based on reasonable cost. Despite the implementation of the prospective payment system, these exemptions and other loopholes led health-care providers to embark on a proliferation of new business ventures that took advantage of niche markets in specialized care. Medicare spending, despite the PPS, remained out of control.

Because of the continued increase in Medicare expenditures, Congress approved managed care components for Medicare in the early 1990s. The MCOs eagerly moved into the Medicare market. Unfortunately, owing to the complex needs and high variation of use within the growing over-65 age group, it proved difficult to care for this population in a managed care environment. Within 5 years, most MCOs retreated from the Medicare market (Johannsson, 1998).

Balanced Budget Acts of 1997 and 2000

The 1997 Balanced Budget Act (BBA) and the corresponding changes in Medicare reimbursement had a major impact on occupational therapy in every practice setting (AOTA, 2000). Using complicated formulas and anecdotal evidence of Medicare fraud and waste, Congress was convinced that it could balance the budget by making drastic cuts in reimbursement for Medicare beneficiaries. Provisions of the BBA of 1997 mandated a full prospective payment system in SNFs, using resource utilization groups (RUGs). Because of this change, over $2.1 billion in payments to SNFs were withdrawn. Those Medicare patients deemed medically complex, many of whom required rehabilitation services, saw their services drastically reduced (AOTA, 2000).

In the outpatient arena, the BBA of 1997 established a $1500 cap for occupational therapy services under Medicare Part B. The limit affected recipients of occupational therapy services in private practice, in clinics, at rehabilitation agencies, SNFs, and outpatient settings. Again, it was the medically complex patients who were most affected (AOTA, 2000).

Perhaps the most significant provisions of the BBA of 1997 were those that sought to control home-health costs. Again, a PPS was mandated, this time for Medicare patients seen in the home. The Congressional Budget Office estimated a reduction in Medicare expenditures for home care of over $16.2 billion over 5 years; however, these estimates proved to be grossly miscalculated (AOTA, 2000). SNFs, nursing homes, and home-care providers needed to make choices between food, nutrition, and medications at the expense of rehabilitation and activities. Patients and their families were shocked and dismayed; thousands wrote their representatives, saying that they felt betrayed by their government (AOTA, 2000).

Many occupational therapy practitioners were laid off, moved to part-time positions, or were subjected to salary cuts. New graduates were unable to find jobs in their chosen field (AWP Research, 1999). In a 1999 AOTA-sponsored study, 21% of the occupational therapy practitioners reported a decrease in their income, and 18% reported across-the-board salary cuts at their place of work. In this same survey, 38.5% of occupational therapy practitioners reported an increase in caseload (AWP Research, 1999). Mergers of departments and health-care organizations became common. Furthermore, pressure to use occupational therapy aides rather than occupational therapists and occupational therapy assistants, where possible, increased (AWP Research, 1999).

This time, AOTA had a well-developed Federal Affairs Department and grass-roots organization and were able to play a significant leadership role in bringing about amendments favorable to occupational therapy clients and the practitioners who served them. By the summer of 2000—in response to patient, family, and provider pressure—Congress passed legislation to restore some of the eliminated benefits. The Balanced Budget Refinement Act of 2000 secured a 2-year suspension on the $1500 cap on occupational therapy services. It also increased the RUG rate payments to SNFs by 20% and made new provisions for medically complex patients, specifically ensuring increases in rehabilitation categories.

Comparison of U.S. Health-Care Funding with Other Industrialized Countries

Health care in the United States is consumer driven, with people demanding high-quality, innovative technological care, convenience, and choice. The United States is the only country in the industrialized world to rely primarily on an optional employer-based health insurance. Access to care is not a legal right in this country as it is in European countries, Canada, and most other industrialized countries. Every country has a unique approach to funding and providing health care to its citizens, but it is possible to generalize the approaches into five categories (Table 45-3) (Morrison, 2000).

Yet, citizens of other countries have their own complaints about health care. Although other industrialized countries guarantee access to care, long waits are common, and there is little choice in care (Morrison, 2000). Most of these systems offer private medical insurance that enable subscribers to opt out of the state-sponsored plan or to provide additional services beyond those of state-sponsored plans (PricewaterhouseCoopers, 1999).

A close examination of the development of the different systems, makes it clear that health care is culturally defined—a product of politics, economy, and policies that reflect basic societal values (Morrison, 2000). No country has the perfect compromise. Each health system is challenged in its attempt to balance cost, access, quality of care, universality, and responsiveness to the public. It is apparent that the kinds of health-care systems are converging, each country looking to improve their systems through adoption of programs and funding schemes practiced by others (PricewaterhouseCoopers, 1999).

TABLE 45-3. **CATEGORIES OF HEALTH CARE ACROSS THE WORLD**

Category	Characteristics	Example Countries
Socialized medicine	The state owns, funds, and controls virtually all facets of the health-care system	United Kingdom, Sweden, Denmark
Socialized insurance	The government provides basic insurance to its citizens, covering medically necessary services	Canada, France, Australia
Mandatory health insurance	Organized around large employers, unions, or work-based associations, health insurance is through sickness funds or government-sponsored programs	Japan, Germany, Belgium, Netherlands, Luxembourg
Voluntary insurance	There is no guarantee of universality	United States, South Africa
Three-tiered system	(1) clinics for the very poor, (2) insurance coverage to working people and their families, and (3) insurance for the private sector, catering to the elite	Mexico, Brazil, Argentina

REGULATION AND ACCREDITATION OF OCCUPATIONAL THERAPY PRACTICE

While it is the ethical obligation of occupational therapy practitioners to practice competently, various forms of certification, licensure, and regulations provide protection to the people seeking occupational therapy services. These include certification and licensure of occupational therapy practitioners and regulation of those agencies and institutions providing occupational therapy services.

Certification and Licensure to Practice Occupational Therapy

The National Board of Certification of Occupational Therapy (NBCOT) certifies occupational therapy practitioners. This ensures that anyone practicing occupational therapy has met the standards established by NBCOT. Currently, these standards include graduation from an accredited occupational therapy or occupational therapy assistant program, completion of fieldwork experience, and passing the certification examination administered by the NBCOT. NBCOT is independent of the AOTA, which is typical for other professional certification boards (Grossman & Cleary, 1997).

To ensure ongoing professional competence of certified occupational therapy practitioners, NBCOT is developing a program for recertification (AOTA and NBCOT, 2001). It has proposed a plan for certification renewal, which includes a self-assessment, a professional development plan, and a portfolio of ongoing professional activities. In the program design, NBCOT intends to award points for various types of professional development. If this plan is approved, to maintain their certification, practitioners will need to obtain a total of 50 points over the 5-year renewal cycle. NBCOT will conduct random audits at the end of the 5th year (NBCOT, 2002).

In addition to certification by NBCOT, occupational therapy practitioners in 42 states must also maintain licenses to practice. State licensure laws, or practice acts, are the most common form of regulation of a profession (Grossman & Cleary, 1997). A practice act defines a profession's scope of practice and authorizes the specific services provided by the profession covered by that law. Licensure laws and their regulations protect the citizens of the state from quackery and fraud. Each state has regulatory bodies that oversee occupational licensing.

Because occupational licensing occurs at the state level, specific regulation of professional practice varies from state to state (Benemerito, 2000). For example, states licensing laws may differ on the scope of practice of occupational therapy. This means that there may be variation from state to state on specific interventions included in the occupational therapy practice act and interventions excluded from occupational therapy practice by the practice acts of other professions. For instance, some occupational therapy licensure laws include the use physical agent modalities (PAMs) within the scope of practice, while others do not. Exclusion clauses contained in the practice acts of other professions prohibit occupational therapy practitioners from using certain techniques or interventions. For example, psychologists may include an exclusion clause in their practice act that would preclude other professions, such as occupational therapy, from using behavior modification or cognitive therapy techniques. If an occupational therapy practitioner used behavioral modification or cognitive behavioral therapy in that state, this action would be interpreted as practicing psychology without a license.

Health-Care Organization Accreditation and Accountability

While professional certification and licensure ensure the competence of individual occupational therapy practitioners, there is still variation in the quality of health care provided from setting to setting (Herzlinger, 1997). The quality of the institutions and agencies providing health care influences the quality of care provided within these institutions and agencies. As a result, independent, nonprofit organizations, interested in protecting the public interest relative to health-care quality have evolved to oversee the provision of health-care services. These organizations, called accreditation agencies, assign and set standards and monitor activities through surveys and site visits. Accreditation provides a high level of control over occupational therapy practice. Occupational therapy practitioners must know and comply with the standards set by the accrediting agencies. These criteria include standards related to the delivery of services, documentation, quality improvement, and patient satisfaction.

Three agencies that define standards that are important to occupational therapy providers are the Joint Commission on Accreditation of Health Care Organizations (JCAHO), the National Commission for Quality Assurance (NCQA), and the Commission on Accreditation of Rehabilitation Facilities (CARF) (Table 45-4).

Joint Commission on Accreditation of Health Care Organizations

Since 1951, JCAHO has developed standards for hospitals and health-care organizations and evaluated their compliance against these criteria. It accredits many of the places in which occupational therapy practitioners work. Hospitals and other health-care providers must demonstrate compliance to JCAHO standards to receive Medicare funds (JCAHO, 2001).

National Commission for Quality Assurance

NCQA, established in 1991, assesses and reports on the quality of the nation's managed-care plans (NCQA, 2001). Although this program is voluntary, about 90% of the HMOs in the nation are currently involved in the NCQA accreditation. NCQA standards are especially concerned with member satisfaction, quality of care, access, and services. Ultimately, only those agencies that can meet the rigorous quality review of NCQA are successful in procuring contracts for HMO and MCO patients.

Commission on Accreditation of Rehabilitation Facilities

Finally, CARF, founded in 1966, also promotes, oversees, and measures health-care quality. With its focus on programs that cater to people with disabilities and others in need of medical and vocational rehabilitation, CARF is the preeminent accrediting agency for rehabilitation providers. CARF accreditation is voluntary for rehabilitation providers, but again the incentive to participate is increased by standards set by payers, who are more likely to offer contracts to accredited rehabilitation programs (CARF, 2001).

Summary

Formerly, medicine focused on curing and controlling infectious disease, but today chronic disease and social problems are the leading causes of death (Grossman & Cleary, 1997). Health habits, lifestyle, and social factors (e.g., violence, drug abuse, and poverty) have become the domain of health professionals (Grossman & Cleary, 1997). These types of health problems require multiple interventions by a variety

TABLE 45-4. **HEALTH-CARE REGULATORY AGENCIES**

Agency	Authority	Performance Measurement Standard
Joint Commission on Accreditation of Health Care Organizations	• Hospitals • Health-care networks • Home-care organizations • Long-term care facilities • Assisted-living facilities • Behavioral health organizations • Ambulatory care • Clinical laboratories	ORYX©
National Commission for Quality Assurance	• Managed-care organizations • Managed behavioral health-care organizations • Credentials verification organizations • Physician organizations	HEDIS© (Health Plan Employer Data and Information Set)
Commission on Accreditation of Rehabilitation Facilities	• Adult day care • Assisted living • Behavioral health • Employment and community services • Medical rehabilitation • Vocational rehabilitation	Not applicable

of professionals. As society changes and becomes more complex, the work roles of the health-care professionals become more complex and varied (Grossman & Cleary, 1997). As occupational therapy practice changes and grows, it must do so within the boundaries of established regulation (Arnold, Hill, & Shepherd, 2001; Smith, 2000). While occupational therapy practitioners have an ethical obligation to provide competent care, the checks and balances of regulation, licensure, and certification provide additional safeguards for the public.

THE SCOPE OF PRACTICE EVOLVES

Today, occupational therapy practitioners continue their roles within traditional health-care settings but also venture into broader health and wellness arenas (Waldman, Petralia, & Moskow, 2001). In hospital, rehabilitation, mental health, long-term care, home-care, and outpatient settings, occupational therapy practitioners of the future will continue to work as part of a multidisciplinary team to address occupational performance related to self-care and independence. They will continue to work in schools and other community agencies to provide occupational therapy services to children, youth, adults, and the elderly. However, the broader health and wellness arenas present new opportunities for occupational therapy practitioners. Next, I examine some of the trends and technological advances that will influence the future of occupational therapy practice.

Computers and Consumers

Consumers of health care are seeking more and more information and communication from their health-care providers. By recent estimates, 52 million Americans with Internet access have used the World Wide Web to obtain health or medical information (Dyer, 2001). The Baby Boomers have become the key purchasers of health care for themselves and for their aging parents. With easily searchable health information, consumers are sensitive to value and are willing to spend their funds for convenient and high-quality services. Telecommunication will lead to telemedicine, as these educated consumers seek communication, information, consultation, and treatment via the Internet (PricewaterhouseCoopers, 1999).

Occupational therapy practitioners will need a high degree of computer expertise so that they can create and use new Web-based tools with their clients. E-mail reminders and queries will keep them in touch with clients and their families (Wooten, 2000). Virtual environments and telerehabilitation will provide occupational therapy recipients with virtual treatment regimes, providing immediate feedback and practice that goes beyond half-hour treatment sessions (Zeigmann, Cole, Lichtenberg, & Brooks, 2001).

Assistive devices and compensatory tools will include technologically advanced gadgets, robots, home and automobile automation, and palm devices that do the work of reminding and coaching (Mazer, Sofer, Korner-Bitensky, & Gelinas, 2001). Palm devices will transform documentation of intervention and evaluation (Waldman et al., 2001). Practitioners will communicate with other team members and with payers via electronic, digital, or cellular means (Wooten, 2000). Consequently, practitioners will need to keep pace with the hardware and software that will permeate both delivery and administration of their services.

Genomics and Biotechnological Advances

Perhaps the most significant event that will affect health and health care is the completion of the Human Genome Project. This project, a $3 billion international endeavor, provides a map of the entire human genome, a blueprint for the human being, which consists of 140,000 genes and 4 billion units of DNA. The very concept of illness will change with the ability to predict health risk based on inexpensive and readily available testing. By 2010, experts anticipate major diagnostic advances for genomic variations of infectious disease, cardiovascular disease, and cancer. In the future, scientists will be able to map disease-linked genes to specific chromosomes. A person's genetic profile will be used to design custom drugs. Clinical trials will be more focused to specific populations, improving speed and results. Through these activities, scientists hope that the need for surgery and treatments for chronic illness will decrease (PricewaterhouseCoopers, 1999).

In venues that emerge from improvements in genetic diagnostics, occupational therapy practitioners will find consultative niches that they are uniquely able to fulfill. Life care planning is an emerging field for occupational therapy practitioners. These practitioners consult with families and third-party payers to identify the future costs, the services, and the equipment that people with catastrophic illness or injuries will require for the remainder of their lives (Hobart, 1998). Individuals who have specific disease or health risks, identified through their personal genetics map, will seek the help of occupational therapy practitioner, because of their skills and expertise in occupation and in new arenas such as lifestyle counseling and lifestyle training (Yousey, 2001).

Emerging genetic knowledge will also influence existing practice areas such as pediatrics. Practitioners frequently visit families in their homes and become a trusted source of information. Consequently, practitioners are in a position to help families find answers to questions about genetics. When a child has a developmental delay without a definite diagnosis, or when questions about siblings or parents arise, occupational therapy practitioners may find themselves giving advice about when genetic testing and/or genetic counseling may be appropriate (Adams, 2000). These practitioners will need to have a good understanding of genetic abnormalities. They will need to keep abreast of the most current genetic testing available. They will also need to understand the complex issues surrounding genetics advances, in terms of medical, legal, social, and ethical issues.

The potential changes in health care and health as a result of the Human Genome Project are just beginning to emerge, but there is no doubt that the very way we think about illness will change and that this change will have corresponding changes for the delivery of occupational therapy services.

Delivery of Services Related to Mental Health and Illness

With the reduction in the prevalence of infectious disease, heart disease, and cancer, we may predict that some of the most difficult health challenges will fall within the realms of mental illness and psychosocial impairment. According to a report of the U.S. surgeon general, 44 million Americans suffer from a mental illness or addiction (U.S. Public Health Services, 2000). In addition, antisocial behaviors leading to the growth of violence and risky sexual behaviors are on the rise globally (Institute for Alternative Futures, 1998).

Despite great strides in diagnosis, pharmaceuticals, and other treatments, mental illness continues to lack parity with other health concerns. Although Medicare and some third-party plans cover acute episodes of mental illness, manifested by physical symptoms, there are usually strict limits to benefits, and benefits are likely to be inadequate to meet most of the needs of people who experience the recurring symptoms of chronic mental illness. While occupational therapy can trace its roots to mental health treatment (Gritzer & Arluke, 1985), the number of occupational therapy practitioners working in the field of mental health has dramatically declined since the 1980s owing to deinstitutionalization and changes in funding.

Yet, occupational therapy focused on mental health, behavioral health, and psychosocial adaptation is increasingly found in unlikely places. For example, Follis and Nolen (2001) described their community development program in transitional housing facilities in Memphis, Tennessee. In another example, Goodman and Shapiro (2000) linked occupational therapy with adventure programming for high-risk adolescents. In more traditional settings, other occupational therapy practitioners are expanding services to include psychosocial treatment, breaking down the artificial barrier between physical and mental health services that exists in many health-care settings. Leslie (2001) described the expansion of psychiatric occupational therapy at the Cleveland Clinic (Cleveland, Ohio). Working with the consultation liaison section that manages psychopharmacology, Leslie has introduced psychiatric occupational therapy services for patients who are depressed and terminally ill or who are severely injured. In another example, Hahn (2000) introduced mental health interventions as an adjunct to sensory and fine and gross motor intervention in two public schools.

Implications for Occupational Therapy Practice

Currently, the scope of practice delineated in the guide to occupational therapy practice indicates "occupational therapy practitioners are concerned with the engagement by persons in meaningful and purposeful occupations in the performance areas of ADL, work and productive activities, and play/leisure" (Moyers, 1999, p. 8). This scope of occupational therapy practice will evolve as the result of changes in societal needs, research, outcome studies, and theoretical developments.

As explained earlier in this chapter, the scope of practice is also determined at the state level by occupational therapy practice acts. These acts vary from state-to-state and may prohibit practice in an emerging role or may require specific advanced training (Arnold, Hill, & Shephard, 2001; Benemerito, 2000; Smith, 2000). As occupational therapy practitioners pursue new opportunities, it is their ethical and legal responsibility to guarantee that they are working within the scope of practice articulated by the profession, their training, and their state licensure laws (Youngstrom, 2000).

CONCLUSION

In 1999, U.S. health-care costs exceeded $1 trillion. Public spending by federal, state, and local government accounted for over 45%, or $524 billion, and while corporate and private payers spent $600 billion. Cost containment and cost controls, advances in medicine and technology, and incremental changes in health-care policy will continue to form the backdrop for health care and occupational therapy in the future.

How will we frame occupational therapy practice? Baum (2000) urged us to return to the fundamentals of the profession to guide us in shaping the future. In presentations around the country, she repeatedly advocated for occupational therapy practitioners to bring an occupational performance perspective to rehabilitation programs, hospitals, schools, and community practice. Baum repeated this refrain, chiding us to "to stick to our knitting"—reminding us that it is through the understanding of occupation that occupational therapy practitioners will help our clients to succeed.

References

Abreu, B. C. (1996). Occupational therapy in a managed care environment. *American Journal of Occupational Therapy, 50*(6), 407–408.

Abreu, B. C., Seal, G., Podlesak, J., & Hartley, L. (1996). Development of critical paths for postacute brain injury rehabilitation: Lessons learned. *American Journal of Occupational Therapy, 50*(2), 417–427.

Adams, J .T. (1931). *The epic of America*. New York: Atlantic Monthly.

Adams, L. K. (2000). Genetic breakthroughs shape occupational therapy intervention. *OT Practice, 5*(19), 17–20.

American Occupational Therapy Association. (2000, April). National policy forum. Forum at the American Occupational Therapy Association annual conference and business meeting, Seattle.

AOTA and NBCOT renew partnership. (2001). *OT Practice, 6*(11), 20.

Arnold, M., Hill, D., & Shephard, J. (2001) State licensure, the law and ethics. *OT Practice*, 6(11), 16.

AWP Research. (1999). *OT Week employment survey, top-line report*. Herndon, VA: Author.

Baum, C. M. (1985). The Evolution of the US Health Care System. In J. Bair (Ed.). *The occupational therapy manager* (pp. 3–25). Bethesda, MD: American Occupational Therapy Association.

Baum, C. M. (2000). Reinventing ourselves for the new millennium. *OT Practice*, 5(1), 2–15.

Benemerito, T. (2000). Why you need to know your practice act. *OT Practice*, 5(9), 10.

Christiansen, C. (1996). Managed care: Opportunities and challenges for occupational therapy in the emerging systems of the 21st century. *American Journal Occupational Therapy*, 50(6), 409–412.

Commission on Accreditation of Rehabilitation Facilities [CARF]. (2001). About CARF. Available at: www.carf.org. Accessed December 17, 2001.

Corning, P. A. (1969). The evolution of Medicare . . . From idea to law. Available at: www.socialsecurity.gov/history/corning.html. Accessed November 20, 2001.

Dyer, K. A. (2001). Ethical challenges of medicine and health on the Internet. *Journal of Medical Internet Resources*, 3(2), 1–27.

Ellenberg, D. B. (1996). Outcomes research: The history, debate, and implications for the field of occupational therapy. *American Journal of Occupational Therapy*, 50(6), 435–442.

Fisher, T. (1996). Roles and functions of a case manager. *American Journal Occupational Therapy*, 50(6), 452–454.

Follis, D., & Nolen, A. (2001). Our journey into the community. *OT Practice*, 6(9), 12–16.

Gardner, J. (2001). Numbers don't tell the whole story. *Modern Healthcare*, 33(41), 16–17.

Goodman, J., & Shapiro, M. (2000). OTs in the trees. *OT Practice*, 5(23), 17–20.

Gritzler, G. M., & Arluke, A. (1985). *The making of rehabilitation: A political economy of medical specialization, 1890–1980*. Berkeley: University of California Press.

Grossman, J., & Cleary, W. (1997) *A study of professions: Progress report to the American Occupational Therapy Association*. New York: MAGI Educational Services.

Hahn, C. (2000). Building mental health roles into school system practice. *OT Practice*, 5(21), 14–16.

Hall, M., & Berenson, R .A. (1998). Ethical practice in managed care: A dose of realism. *Annals of Internal Medicine*, 128, 395–402.

Harkleroad, A., Schirf, D., Volpe, J., & Holm, M. (2000) Critical pathway development: An integrative literature review. *American Journal Occupational Therapy*, 54(2), 148–158.

Health Policy Alternative, Inc. (1996) *Health care and market reform: Workforce implications for occupational therapy: Report prepared for the American Occupational Therapy Association*. Washington, DC: Author.

Herzlinger, R. (1997). *Market driven health care*. Reading, MA: Addison Wesley.

Hobart, K. (1998). The occupational therapist as a life care planner. *OT Practice*, 3(6), 45–47.

Hoffman, E., Klees, B. S., & Curtis, C. (2001) *Brief summaries of Medicare and Medicaid: Title XVIII and Title XIX of the Social Security Act*. Available at: www.hcfa.gov/pubforms/actuary/ormedmed/default4.htm. Accessed November 30, 2001.

Institute for Alternative Futures. (1998). Trends and forecasts: Health care 2010. Available at: www.altfutures.com. Accessed December 1, 2001.

Johannsson, C. (1998). Why HMOs pull out of medicare, *OT Practice*, 3(10), 5.

Joint Commission on Accreditation of Healthcare Organizations [JCAHO]. (2001). About us. Available at: www.jcaho.org. Accessed February 18, 2001.

Kaiser/Harvard School of Public Health Program on the Public and Health Privacy. (2001). *Consumers report problems with their health plans*. Boston: Kaiser Family Foundation.

Kongstevdt, P. R. (1997). *The managed care handbook* (3rd ed.). Gaithersburg, MD: Aspen.

Kraus, M. (1959). *The United States to 1865*. Binghamton, NY: Val-Balou.

Landers, S. (2000, August 28). The world's healthcare: How do we rank? *American Medical News* [On-line]. Available at: www.ama-assn.org/sci-pubs/amnews/pick_00/gvsa0828.htm. Accessed December 17, 2001.

Leiter, P. (1985). Facility planning. In J. Bair (Ed.). *The occupational therapy manager* (pp. 65–82). Bethesda, MD: American Occupational Therapy Association.

Leslie, C. A. (2001). Psychiatric occupational therapy: Finding a place in the medical/surgical arena. *OT Practice*, 6(7), 10–14.

Mazer, B. L., Sofer, S., Korner-Bitensky, N., & Gelinas, I. (2001). Use of the UFOV to evaluate and retrain visual attention skills to clients with stroke: A pilot study. *American Journal of Occupational Therapy*, 55(5), 552–557.

Morrison, I. (2000). *Health care and the new millennium*. San Francisco, CA: Jossey Bass.

Moyers, P. A. (1999). The guide to occupational therapy practice. *American Journal of Occupational Therapy*, 53(3).

National Board of Certification for Occupational Therapy [NBCOT]. (2002). Proposed plan for certification renewal. Available at: www.nbcot.org/programs/executive_summary.htm. Accessed March 18, 2002.

National Committee for Quality Assurance [NCQA] (2001). Overview. Available at: www.ncqa.org/Pages/about/overview3.htm. Accessed February 18, 2001.

Novalis, S. D., Messenger-Fricke, M., & Morris, L. (2000). Occupational therapy benchmarks within orthopedic (hip) critical pathways. *American Journal of Occupational Therapy*, 54(2), 155–158.

PricewaterhouseCoopers. (1999). HealthCast 2010: Smaller world, bigger expectations. Available at: www.pwchealth.com/healthcast_future3.html. Accessed December 17, 2001.

Scott, S. J. (1985). Payment for occupational therapy services. In J. Bair (Ed.). *The occupational therapy manager* (pp. 325–341). Bethesda, MD: American Occupational Therapy Association.

Smith, K. (2000). Refining regulation to enhance public protection. *OT Practice*, 5(18), 10.

Tufts Health Plan. (1995). *Managed care 101: Employee handbook*. Boston, MA: Author.

U.S. Public Health Services. (2000) Mental health: A report of the surgeon general. Available at: www.surgeongeneral.gov/library/mental-heatlh/chapter6/sec1.html. Accessed November 21, 2001.

Waldman, K. F., Petralia P. B., & Moskow, A. R. (2001). Keep PDA users functioning. *OT Practice*, 5(20), 20.

Walker, J. (2001) Adjustments to managed care: Pushing against it, going with it, making the best of it. *American Journal of Occupational Therapy*, 55(6), 621–628.

Wooten, J. O. (2000). Health care 2025: A patient's encounter. *The Futurist*, 34(4), 18–22.

Youngstrom, M. J. (2000). Considerations for effectively translating occupational therapy into new arenas. *OT Practice*, 5(8), 7–9.

Yousey, J. (2001). Life coaching: A one-on-one approach to changing lives. *OT Practice*, 6(1), 11–14.

Zeigmann, M., Cole, E. Lichtenberg, A., & Brooks, R. (2001) Tele-rehabilitation: New tools for providing in-home brain injury rehabilitation. *OT Practice*, 6(20), 12–15.

CHAPTER 46

DOCUMENTATION AND MANAGEMENT OF OCCUPATIONAL THERAPY SERVICES

JUDITH M. PERINCHIEF

Practitioners at any level should have knowledge of management functions within an organization, including the role of the manager. A manager is any person whose role is to ensure, monitor, and regulate work, organizations, production, and operations (American Occupational Therapy Association [AOTA], 1993). This knowledge is important to the smooth functioning of the organization, the program, and the delivery of an individual service (e.g., occupational therapy.) The use of this knowledge also assists in alleviating potential problems within the workplace. The purpose of this chapter is to define and describe management functions in occupational therapy, including marketing, quality assurance, and documentation.

MANAGING

Managerial Competencies

Historically, managers have had designated functions: primarily organizing and planning, directing, controlling, and evaluating. It is imperative that the manager and those being managed understand these functions and the effect these functions have on the day-to-day performance of duties within the practice setting (Christie, Mansfield, Rausch, & Townsend, 1988a, 1988b)

Organizing and Planning

The manager's role of organizing involves activities aimed at maintaining the formal structure for the accomplishment of tasks within a system. The key to effective management is understanding organizational behavior and styles and philosophies of management and selecting those with which the manager feels most comfortable. Studies of organizations and managers have identified that no one theory or style is the definitive or correct way to manage and that different environments and situations call for different approaches on the part of the manager. It is also commonly accepted that management styles can be modified or changed through formal education or self-training in response to environmental change. Managers today must be willing to take risks and have a vision for the future as they participate on the focused management teams now prevalent in health care.

Planning takes many forms within an organization. It is the process of making decisions in the present to bring about an outcome in the future. It is one of the more complex and frustrating aspects of managing in the health-care industry because this system is, by nature, nonsystematic. Health-care managers employ planning processes in an attempt to promote order in what is frequently viewed as a disorganized system.

Directing

Directing continues to be a basic responsibility of a manager. This involves shaping and modifying employee behavior through directing, so that an employee can acquire the necessary knowledge and skills to perform assignments in compliance with policies and procedures. Directing includes being an effective leader in the issuing of orders and in the appropriate use of discipline to improve employee behavior. The objectives of a good leader are to raise the level of member motivation, improve the quality of all decisions, develop teamwork and morale, further individual development of members, and increase readiness to accept change. These are important skills that should be developed by the practitioner so that he or she is prepared to function in the health-care arena of today.

Controlling

Within any organization, there are inherent features that control the behaviors and processes of its individuals. These may be emphasized to a greater or lesser degree in a given work setting. They include tables of organization, job descriptions, policies, and procedures. Because the job description enumerates all aspects of a job, the employee is assured that all parties know significant elements of the job. Job descriptions must be written to include essential job functions as a result of the Americans with Disabilities Act of 1990 (ADA, 1991).

The roles of the occupational therapist and the occupational therapy assistant have evolved into a collaborative partnership in the delivery of occupational therapy services. Though each has separate roles and responsibilities in practice, they work closely together (AOTA, 1990). The occupational therapist is commonly the supervisor of the occupational therapy assistant and, therefore, must be aware of the subtleties of their roles and responsibilities. With the changes taking place in practice, occupational therapists might very well be supervising a number of occupational therapy assistants. Therapists do not necessarily have a comprehensive knowledge of assistant practice and are, perhaps, uncomfortable in the supervisory role (Johnson, Lamere-Wallace, & Gardner, 2000). Thus there is a need for practitioners to understand the delineation of their roles as identified in job descriptions and professional organization standards.

Policies and procedures are necessary to control effectively administrative management of a service, department, and organization and to provide structure to daily operations. The extent of the policies or procedures is dictated by the size and complexity of the organization, and they exist to greater or lesser degrees, depending on the level of bureaucracy within the organization. Policies are controlling in that they set forth regulations regarding why something is to be done. Procedures should state precisely how and in what specific order an activity is to be carried out. These are organized into manuals that are required by accrediting bodies, such as the Joint Commission of Health Care Organizations (JCAHO, 2000) and the Commission on the Accreditation of Rehabilitation Facilities (CARF, 1999). These policies and procedures should be readily available to staff in hard copy and electronic form.

Evaluating

For the manager, evaluation may assume many names, but essentially it is the managerial function that ensures quality of service. The manager must evaluate every aspect of the program, the outcomes of service providers, and the ethical responsibility to provide optimal care. However, consumers also demand excellent health care, making the evaluation process an essential component of ensuring consumer satisfaction.

A discussion of the evaluating function of a manager would be incomplete without including issues of performance appraisal and credentialing. The evaluation of job performance relates specifically to an individual and the assurance that the individual is qualified and performing duties at a determined level of quality. Performance appraisals are formal mechanisms used by managers to provide positive and constructive feedback regarding the individual's performance, compared to prescribed expectations. The criteria are described in job descriptions and in policies and procedures. It is generally assumed that in using these measures a level of objectivity can be ensured in the process. As a result of performance appraisals, training needs can be identified and areas of noncompliance can be used more effectively to build on the practitioner's areas of competence.

Credentialing through certification and licensure ensures the public that the personnel who provide care are qualified to do so. It is the responsibility of a manager to verify credentials on employment and to guarantee that employees maintain appropriate credentials on an ongoing basis. Therefore, it becomes imperative that the manager be current in the requirements of the credentialing agencies for occupational therapy and local licensing regulations. It is also mandatory that practitioners be cognizant of the regulations and maintain their credentials as prescribed on a national and local level.

Impact of Environment on Management Skills

What has changed for the manager is the environment in which these activities take place, and this necessitates additional competencies beyond those mentioned above (Schell & Slater, 1998). In response to the changing health-care environment, service delivery has been restructured. This restructuring includes major shifts from a single-system to a multisystem model of management, from a direct-service to a multiple-service model, from department to program management, and from individual professional standards to market-driven standards. These shifts require the manager to implement new strategies for flexible staffing and service delivery, new communication practices and procedures, and new methods of staff support within decentralized models of management. These decentralized models have established a compressed, nonhierarchical management structure that has complicated administrative relationships and roles. The models support the program manager concept rather than discipline-specific management. The program manager may be from a different professional background than those being supervised and may not have daily contact with staff in each of the sites managed. As a result, new strategies for communication, collaboration, and supervision must be developed. The program manager is also responsible for other program resources, such as equipment.

The role of leadership has also changed. Leadership, rather than being identified with the designated administrator, resides in a number of individuals and is the responsibility of everyone on the team, regardless of the level of his or her expertise. The required skills have been expanded and now include the abilities to accept change readily, to be sensitive to issues of timing, to maintain composure, to learn to make an impact with influence, to use power effectively, and to cultivate a long-term perspective (Abreu, 1997).

Practitioners need to remain competitive in today's health-care market. To compete successfully they must have the confidence to explain occupational therapy; document their services; and communicate effectively with payers, referral sources, and utilization reviewers. Practitioners must be able to adjust their pace in providing services in a timely manner. Last, but far from the least of new skills, practitioners must have business and finance acumen, which is necessary to respond to reimbursement issues to understand the development of product lines and cost-efficiency methods and to implement the strategies crucial to adapting to changes in managed health care (Walker, 2001).

Planning as a Component of Program Development

Planning may be formulated around a program, such as in a new service or an extension of an existing service, or in the physical arrangement of either new or renovated space. In any event, planning is based on the mission, philosophy, and goals of the organization. Regardless of the program to be developed and the setting, certain principles are involved in devising the plan of action.

There are three major elements that must be considered in approaching organizational planning: surveys, interviews, and evaluation. Surveys are used to identify a need for the program. This includes the population to be served, the source of referrals, the needs of staff, the treatment methods, and the potential for reimbursement. Interviews are conducted with top-level management within the organization to determine their perception of the program being proposed. Fiscal considerations and administrative restrictions must be accommodated. Potential consumers must also be interviewed, and community leaders should be consulted. Evaluation translates the information gathered into a workable plan that matches facilities and personnel with the needs of the organization, the program, and the community.

At the end of the twentieth century, as health-care organizations intensified their competitive strategies and moved into new markets, planning became more important. This trend continues with an emphasis on community-based programs in outpatient services, specialized services, work-related programming, and new technology sectors. Careful, cost-effective planning is essential to meet the needs of the health-care consumer. The use of staff planners or planning consultants to initiate planning within a health-care service has become more or less obsolete; therefore, the practitioner of today needs to be prepared to participate actively in all phases of planning for occupational therapy services.

Planning tests managers. All planning, regardless of the system used, involves the expenditure of effort to collect data, to identify trends, and to project into the future. Countless meetings are required among those involved in the planning process. Good planning mandates close interrelations between the planners and executive, but also requires participation from all levels in the organization. A participatory management style that values the input of all personnel facilitates commitment to the planning process.

Strategic Planning

Regardless of the purpose of planning, a systematic approach is strongly recommended. Strategic planning deals with three basic questions:

- Where are we?
- Where do we want to be?
- How do we get there?

These questions are asked throughout the planning process. The use of the strategic planning process is well

BOX 46–1 STEPS IN STRATEGIC PLANNING

ASSESSMENT

Assessment involves the construction of a thorough evaluation of the current and future state of the organization. At this stage, there is the opportunity to involve many managers and employees who have special expertise. By involving groups of employees in the development of assessments, they will feel a sense of ownership of the strategic plan. Through the assessment phase, issues are identified and are then ranked in order of priority.

ANALYSIS

To develop focus, issues are selected from the assessment that could influence the organization's response. A literature review is essential at this point in the process. Trends should be analyzed, and brainstorming of implications for the future should take place.

DECISION MAKING

Next, the advantages and disadvantages are discussed concerning each of the issues that were analyzed. At the decision-making stage, preferred options are determined and ranked; these become the actual objectives of the strategic plan.

IMPLEMENTATION

Methods to implement the plan must be developed. Because this is the stage at which failure commonly occurs, it is advantageous to determine action steps, set time tables, and allocate resources for each step.

EVALUATION

In the evaluation step, the outcome of the planning process is reviewed. The usual way to do this is to measure the actual outcome against a standard. Questions should be asked to determine when an issue is resolved and how this can be measured. If the plan is not working within a particular parameter, then the individuals involved in planning should return to the decision-making stage to consider ways of improving or eliminating the action plans or to develop new ones.

documented in health care, and there are numerous published resources available for reference. It entails a five-step process: assessment, analysis, decision making, implementation, and evaluation (Box 46-1). This process is commonly used in approaching health-care planning across the spectrum of service.

Successful strategic planning results in values and themes that guide and strengthen the organization's ability to succeed in changing environments. There are, however, potential pitfalls of the process. The process has been criticized in the past for requiring too much time and losing the original focus of the process (Hayes, 1989). Problems develop if inadequate time is allocated to the process, if planners are hired (which minimizes staff involvement and commitment), or if goals are not tested adequately to be sure that they are the appropriate ones to pursue (Steiner, 1979). Despite these findings, strategic planning continues to be used in the health-care industry as well as in other industrial businesses.

Program managers are continuously involved in planning both within a specific unit and across program lines. At the program level, managers need to be intimately aware of the resources necessary for various programs and the financial implications of providing these resources. Cost–benefit analysis must be done, including projected revenues. The manager must also identify the probability of securing the staff necessary for expanding or new programs. Staffing projections should be based on productivity estimates grounded in treatment standards within the specific discipline or specialty area. There are no national standards for staffing ratios, owing to variations imposed by practice setting, client diagnosis, complexity of problems, referral rates, and length of stay. To identify and provide appropriate levels of resources in a cost-effective manner, the manager must conduct an analysis of space and equipment needs. Safety features and accessibility standards must be included in planning the physical space needs for the program. The provision of communication systems is dictated by the specific needs of the specialties to be treated.

MARKETING

Marketing Functions

A discussion of planning would be incomplete without inclusion of an overview of marketing issues and strategies. Strategic planning identifies the organization's mission and goals and considers economic alternatives in planning services. In contrast, marketing identifies the needs and desires of the consumer and is concerned with public relations and sale methods. Marketing is not just advertising a product; it is identifying and serving the evolving needs of the consumers and the public. Both marketing and strategic planning are inextricably linked, because there must be a match between goals and mission of the institution and the needs of the consumer in the development of any new service.

Marketing experts suggest that health-care professionals have neglected market research and have overlooked the development of market strategies in their pursuit of methods to produce quick results. Marketing in health care is a growing discipline that combines knowledge of health care, its environment, and its analytic design, with a study of their interactions. Analysis of consumer behavior, attitudes, knowledge, and beliefs are changing the way health-care systems are now planning for service expansion. The number of programs being offered that emphasize lifestyle change, disease prevention, and alternatives to hospital care reflects this consumer orientation.

Managers of occupational therapy services can successfully incorporate marketing into their administrative practices by combining proven marketing strategies with practice methods. This technique maintains professionalism, delivers high-quality care, and satisfies the needs of potential clients, while ensuring the viability of the program. Marketing concepts can be used effectively to demonstrate occupational therapy services to others within the organization. Methods of internal marketing strategies might include an open house, in-services for other team members (e.g., nurses, nutritionists, teachers), or feature articles in employee newsletters. Progress notes and service reports as well as participation in case conferences are other methods that demonstrate the benefits of occupational therapy and, therefore, can be construed as marketing tools. Marketing can also be used externally to educate consumers to the need and availability of occupational therapy services, such as community newsletters, workshops for special disability groups, and participation in health fairs within the community.

The occupational therapy service manager must educate personnel about the merits of marketing to the well-being of the organization. Many staff members do not perceive themselves as having a role in marketing of services. Staff can be reminded that the impression they create with clients or visitors in a practice setting is, in fact, a marketing measure. Staff can also be informed that marketing is necessary to create public awareness of the value of occupational therapy services and to differentiate occupational therapy practitioners from competing health-care practitioners.

Marketing Through Service Delivery

One mechanism of capitalizing on the unpredictable is to embed marketing into aspects of daily practice (e.g., describing the value of occupational therapy while providing direct service, speaking to parents about the benefits of occupational therapy while waiting to pick up one's child from an after-school program, or presenting on health and wellness at a local senior center). Marketing the value of occupational therapy is the collective responsibility of all practitioners. It takes an ongoing commitment from practitioners to innovate, evolve, redefine, and reinvent themselves. It requires that practitioners instantly respond to new demands and seize the new opportunities, designing new products and services for changing, smaller markets.

Because marketing is an important part of service delivery, it is vital that all practitioners understand it. One might argue that as a professional service, occupational therapy has historically not been well marketed. Practitioners assumed that individuals who referred patients to therapy for service understood what it was occupational therapy could deliver—that is, that the physicians knew what the product was. Today, occupational therapy practitioners realize that is not true and probably never has been.

Unfortunately, occupational therapy practitioners have not done a good job of marketing to potential consumers. The potential consumer has no idea what the product is, except perhaps parents of children with developmental disabilities, but they are already consumers of the services. Practitioners need to focus on the value of occupational therapy—its benefits rather than its features. Traditionally, occupational therapy practitioners and health-care organizations have developed their products on the basis of what they thought the consumer wanted relative to the plans of the practitioners and organizations. Marketing reverses this process.

Marketing Strategies for Service Managers

Marketing can be described as a business philosophy aimed at improving profits by identifying the needs of key consumer groups and offering a product package that serves their needs more fully and effectively than does the competition. Marketing, therefore, aims at profit improvement, focuses on consumer requirements, targets certain market segments or consumer groups, and develops a product and service package that offers value to consumers in the served markets. There are four key dimensions to marketing.

- Identifying consumer requirements and expectations.
- Targeting consumer groups or segments to serve.
- Developing the service package to satisfy the consumer.
- Improving profit performance.

The once protected market segments are now open to truly competitive enterprise. There is a wide range of services in the health-care market for which quality, productivity, and technological advances outdistance the competition for the market share. The key strategy is for regaining and building market share and profitability by concentrating on developing market plans, identifying consumer requirements and expectations for each market segment, developing service packages for each segment, and organizing and managing around the needs of the consumers who ultimately make the buying decisions.

As with the planning function of management, marketing requires some strategies, too. These are the result of market research, competitive analysis, and benchmarking. Benchmarking is the identification of best practices in related and unrelated settings to emulate as processes or use as performance targets within the current planning setting.

Marketing Through Consumer Satisfaction

One of the bottom-line issues in marketing is customer satisfaction; thus the focus of marketing should be to satisfy the consumer and create new markets. The total quality of the service must meet the consumers' requirements and exceed their expectations. While it may be difficult to satisfy each consumer fully all the time, it is certainly a worthy objective. Potential consumers refers to internal as well as external consumers. Other departments depend on the services, information, interventions, reports, and instructions that occupational therapy practitioners supply in the normal course of transacting business. If the internal line breaks down in delivering important requirements, then the satisfaction of the external consumer is put at risk.

To become consumer focused and market driven, people throughout the organization must develop an orientation and sensitivity to people who are their customers. Listening to the market is now everyone's job. Listening for and understanding consumer expectations are key features for marketing.

The assessment of consumer satisfaction is closely tied to quality assurance (QA) and continuous quality improvement (CQI). Postservice satisfaction is classically derived by the relationship between the consumers' expectations and the services' perceived performance. Future use of health care is derived from people returning for additional services and new consumers. While there is a direct link between patient satisfaction and repeat use, the influences imposed by intermediaries on compliance and provider change are important to the evaluation of repetition in health-care behaviors of the consumer. Loyalty and word-of-mouth satisfaction are more closely related to reputation than to actual measures of overall consumer satisfaction.

ENSURING QUALITY

Quality Assurance and Outcome Management

Quality assurance is the continuous measurement of outcomes against criteria and then taking corrective action when problems are identified. For instance, a problem may be caused by structural difficulties, such as inadequate equipment, or by procedures that do not meet client needs. New equipment purchases can be justified because a problem has been identified related to the quality of service. Likewise, identification of procedural problems directs occupational therapy personnel to examine the procedure and revise it to alleviate the problem. The problem may be related to the competence of occupational therapy practitioners. Training programs can address this process need. New programs may also evolve from the process. There are five stages in quality assurance outcome monitoring. Monitoring may be measured concurrently with the delivered care and retrospectively after discharge (Box 46-2).

BOX 46–2 STAGES OF QUALITY ASSURANCE MONITORING

STAGE 1

The indicators of quality care are identified; indicators are the aspects of care that have high priority, high risk, and high volume and are perceived as solvable should a problem occur.

STAGE 2

Measurable data are collected; for example, standardized performance measures that reflect the indicators.

STAGE 3

Cause is determined; if a problem is found, remedial action is indicated.

STAGE 4

The remedy is implemented; an important step and sometimes overlooked step; the remedy should be short and simple and should not be too costly to implement.

STAGE 5

The measurement process is repeated to determine if the problem has been solved; if not, the process reverts to stage 3 and the cause is reinvestigated; if so, the situation is monitored periodically, with lengthened measurement intervals, to determine that no further complications have occurred.

Links to Evidence-Based Practice

Evidence-based practice is supported through QA outcome studies conducted in the occupational therapy clinical setting (see Chapter 53). Within the health-care system, quality assurance is mandated by federal legislation and accreditation standards (Chapter 45). Since 1988, the JCAHO (2000) has included QA, utilization review, and program evaluation within its standards. In addition, AOTA has produced several excellent resources on quality assurance (AOTA 1990; Forer, 1996). These sources are updated regularly to reflect the requirements of the accrediting bodies.

Program Evaluation

Program evaluation is an outcome-monitoring system that reflects the results of services on consumers by defining and reviewing the outcomes of care (CARF, 1999). It is obvious that this process lends itself readily to the application of evidence-based practice. CQI is a frequently used system in the rehabilitation setting (Slater, Evans, & Small, 1993). The actual method of evaluation varies from one program to another and from one department to another. Accrediting agencies, such as JCAHO and CARF, require that a system for evaluating programs of care be in place in accredited institutions.

Diagnosis or service generally guides the methods for program evaluation. The studies involve the identification of goals, purpose, indication for intervention, recommended services, discharge status of the client, and the need for follow-up or community-level services. Examples of occupational therapy program evaluation studies include achievement of functional goals for clients with head trauma, evaluation of levels of self-care skills as determined by the Functional Independence Measure (FIM™) for clients with left hemiplegia, examination of parallel group participation in individuals performing on an Allen cognitive level 4, and client and family satisfaction with training programs in occupational therapy. Data on outcomes are related to those consumers who achieved the goals or who demonstrated change as a result of receipt of service. A committee consisting of management-level staff or designees determines strengths, weaknesses, and shortcomings of the program being evaluated. The results of the study are shared with those involved with the program, and plans are made for implementing any changes to improve the program or service.

DOCUMENTATION

Documentation is one of the most important functions performed by occupational therapy practitioners. Next to assessment and intervention, documentation accounts for a major portion of time in the daily schedule of practitioners. It is the key to communicating service provision to other providers on the professional team and to third-party payers. The relation of documentation in professional practice to reimbursement issues cannot be stressed enough. Because documentation is a form of communication, issues of language and the correct use of terminology are paramount. It is crucial to use the terminology appropriate to the setting (i.e., medical terminology in a medical setting and educational language in a public school). Efforts to standardize terminology increased in the 1990s, and as a result, two systems have been universally accepted as documentation standards for occupational therapy.

Occupational Therapy Practice Framework

The Occupational Therapy Practice Framework (AOTA, in press) is the fourth in a series of documents intended to standardize occupational therapy terminology. The newest edition is designed to frame occupational therapy's unique perspective clearly and to define the constructs and terms that guide practice. This document supports the *Guide to Occupational Therapy Practice* (Moyers, 1999). Both the framework and the guide have been identified as the definitive references for occupational therapy terminology.

International Classification of Functioning, Disability, and Health

The International Classification of Functioning, Disability, and Health (ICF) reflects the trend away from terms like *disability* and *handicap* and to a focus on social participation. The code classifies human functioning at the level of the body, the whole person, and the person within the complete social and physical environmental context (World Health Organization, 2001). AOTA currently recommends that the ICF be used in documentation of occupational therapy outcomes. The classification system provides a uniform language for documentation of services and assists in tracking outcomes.

Purposes of Documentation

The documentation of assessment and intervention is the only evidence of professional decision making and clinical reasoning. It is the only method that ensures that something has actually taken place in the eyes of reimbursement agencies and accrediting bodies.

There are four principal purposes for documentation (AOTA, 1995):

- Facilitate effective intervention.
- Justify reimbursement.
- Stands as a legal document.
- Provides communication among practitioners, client, and family.

Therefore, documentation has legal, ethical, and financial ramifications.

Documentation is not a simple skill that can be acquired in one setting and transferred to another. Knowledge must be continually updated in terms of standards set forth by reimbursement agencies, regulators, and accreditors. AOTA has published numerous documents that serve as reference material for the documentation process, including *Practice Guidelines* (AOTA, 1996), *Managed Care: An Occupational Therapy Sourcebook* (American Occupational Therapy Association—Managed Care Project Team, 1996), *Elements of Clinical Documentation* (AOTA 1995), and *Occupational Therapy Practice Framework* (AOTA, in press).

Documentation Systems

Problem-Oriented Medical Record

Weed (1971) developed the problem-oriented medical record (POMR) as a means of providing structure for progress note writing. This documentation system has become a standard method of client-care documentation in many medical settings today. The system is based on a list of problems that is generated by assessing the client's abilities and limitations. This is a master list developed by the treatment team collectively. The problems are numbered, and each subsequent progress note, called a SOAP note, is written with reference to the problem list. The decision to use the POMR is generally an institutional one. The structure of a SOAP note is as follows:

- S = *subjective:* Where the practitioner records information as reported by the client, the family, or significant other; might include what a client says that cannot be measured.
- O = *objective:* Where the practitioner records measurable, observable data, usually obtained through formal evaluation or assessment tools; includes specific medical information and history.
- A = *assessment:* Where the practitioner records his or her professional judgment or opinion on occupational performance expectations or limitations, given the objective data noted in the previous section.
- P = *plan:* Where the practitioner records a specific plan of action to be followed to resolve identified problems; may include short- or long-term goals and how long and how often the intervention should be provided.

BOX 46-3 SAMPLE SOAP NOTE

- Patient name: James Jones
- Date: 12/20/01
- Time: 2:40 P.M.
- Problem 3: Lower extremity dressing
- *S*: "Ever since my surgery to replace this left hip, I need help putting on my pants and shoes. They won't let me bend to reach my feet cause it will damage the hip."
- *O*: Mr. Jones is 48 hr postsurgery for left THR. He is limited in active and passive hip flexion to 90° and left hip abduction at neutral by postsurgical precautions. Right hip ROM is WNL. He has normal UE strength and ROM bilaterally. Sitting balance and posture in wheelchair are good. He is able to sit at the side of the bed unsupported with good balance. Patient can transfer from wheelchair to bed independently, NWB on left LE. Mr. Jones can dress his UEs independently. He requires assistance to place underwear and trousers over his feet, but can pull the clothing up from his knees. He is unable to put on shoes and socks.
- *A*: Mr. Jones will be independent in all LE dressing, observing postoperative hip precautions, within 2 days.
- *P*: Secure long-handled dressing stick, sock donner, long shoehorn, and stretch laces for Mr. Jones. Train Mr. Jones with adapted equipment during two intervention sessions. Educate Mrs. Jones in the use of equipment so that she can support her husband's level of independence.

NWB, non weight bearing; *LE*, lower extremity; *ROM*, range of motion; *THR*, total hip replacement; *UE*, upper extremity; *WNL*, with no limitations.

The POMR and SOAP notes are commonly used in acute care medical and rehabilitation settings. The SOAP format may be used for initial notes, treatment notes, progress notes, and discharge notes. These notes are written in an integrated section of the record to which all disciplines contribute, rather than in discipline-specific sections. Each provider writes SOAP notes to the problems that are appropriate to his or her intervention (Box 46-3).

In some settings, outcome criteria or goals are added to the SOAP format. The use of G (for goals) is becoming a common practice. The goal section should contain long- and short-term goals of the particular health-care practitioner writing the note. In some instances, the system has been adapted to a particular setting. DAP notes are a variation of the SOAP format. In this system, D (for data) is used rather than the S and O of the SOAP format. BIRP notes are sometimes used in practice settings to replace the SOAP format. In this system, the letters are identified as follows:

- B = behavior of the client.
- I = intervention provided.
- R = response to intervention.
- P = plan for continued intervention.

The BIRP format might be found in specialized treatment settings, such as partial hospitalization programs or substance-abuse programs.

Documentation Practices

Documentation practices vary from setting to setting. Sometimes these differences are dictated by public policy (such as educational settings that use individualized education plans), sometimes by accrediting bodies (such as CARF), and sometimes by the preference of the individual practice setting.

In mental health settings, the problems, goals, and interventions are often multidisciplinary and may be written in a different format and in a less-specific language. Occupational therapy services are frequently included as adjunctive therapy, where roles overlap and identities are blurred. Reimbursement is usually not discipline specific, and therapy services are included in a room or per diem rate for the facility. Treatment plans in mental health are usually multidisciplinary. In this setting, the individualized treatment plan (ITP) is the accepted method of documentation. It becomes a contract between the client and the members of the treatment team. ITPs can be long because of the multidisciplinary nature of the documentation. Geropsychiatric services are an exception to mental health documentation standards, because the patients are insured through Medicare. The documentation in these settings must adhere to Medicare requirements.

In school-based practice, occupational therapists develop individualized education plans (IEPs) and write problems, goals, and interventions focused on behaviors and skills the child needs to be successful in school. The IEP is multidisciplinary and is based on the assessment from each discipline. Problem statements focus exclusively on occupational performance in the educational setting. The timeline for goal statements is based on the academic year, and interventions must relate to the educational setting, regardless of whether the individual may require intervention for other areas of occupational performance.

Medicare or Medicaid covers most clients who receive therapy services in long-term care settings, and documentation methods in these sites are federally mandated. The Minimum Data Set (MDS) is the comprehensive, multidisciplinary assessment used for all long-term care residents. Often the MDS is divided so that each discipline has its own part to complete.

Nelson and Glass (1999) demonstrated that the occupational therapists' involvement in the completion of MDS has been limited to only self-care areas of the assessment. Clients are then divided into resource utilization groups (RUGs), according to how much care they need. Inappropriate assessment for RUGs may result in denials of coverage. Practitioners working in these settings must learn to be concise in providing the necessary information in the fewest words possible. Full participation in the MDS process is a professional responsibility to the client.

Practitioners should keep in mind that documentation requirements vary substantially from one setting to another. These variations stem from the differences in the mission of the practice setting, the needs of the consumer, and reimbursement and regulatory requirements.

CONCLUSION

Just as the delivery of services is every practitioner's responsibility, so too are the practice issues of documentation, marketing, and assurance of quality services. Each time occupational therapy practitioners encounter clients and their families, they are in a position to market their profession. Through daily contact with consumers in clinical, educational, and consultation capacities, others become more informed and knowledgeable about occupational therapy services. Each time the practitioner documents intervention plans and assessments, it is a reflection of the profession. These are responsibilities of each practitioner, whether or not he or she bears a managerial title.

References

Abreu, B. C. (1997) Interdisciplinary leadership: the future is now. *OT Practice*, 2(3), 21–25.

American Occupational Therapy Association. (1990). Role delineation for OTRs and COTAs. *American Journal of Occupational Therapy, 44*, 1091–1102.

American Occupational Therapy Association. (1993). Occupational therapy roles. *American Journal of Occupational Therapy, 47*, 1087–1099.

American Occupational Therapy Association. (1995). Elements of clinical documentation (revision). *American Journal of Occupational Therapy, 49*, 1032–1035.

American Occupational Therapy Association. (1996). *Practice guidelines*. Bethesda, MD: Author.

American Occupational Therapy Association. (In press). Occupational therapy practice framework: Domain and Process. *American Journal of Occupational Therapy*.

American Occupational Therapy Association—Managed Care Project Team. (1996). *Managed care: An occupational therapy sourcebook*. Bethesda, MD: AOTA.

Americans with Disabilities Act of 1990 [ADA]. P. L. 101-336, 104 Statute 327-378, (1991).

Christie, B., Mansfield, M., Rausch, G., & Townsend, B. (1988a). Managerial competencies. *Administration and Management Special Interest Section Newsletter*, 4(1), 3–4.

Christie, B., Mansfield, M., Rausch, G., & Townsend, B. (1988b). Managerial Competencies. *Administration and Management Special Interest Section Newsletter*, 4(2), 3–4.

Commission on Accreditation of Rehabilitation Facilities [CARF]. (1999). *Standards manual for organizations serving people with disabilities*. Tucson, AZ: Author.

Forer, S. (1996). *Outcome management and program evaluation made easy: A tool kit for occupational therapy practitioners*. Bethesda, MD: American Occupational Therapy Association.

Hayes, R. (1989). Strategic planning—Forward in reverse? *Harvard Business Review*, 67(6), 111–120.

Johnson, D. G., Lamere-Wallace, D., & Gardner, E. A. (2000). Brief or new: Supervisory preparedness of occupational therapists. *American Journal of Occupational Therapy, 54*, 97–98.

Joint Commission of Accreditation of Healthcare Organizations [JCAHO]. (2000). *The quality assurance guide*. Chicago: Author.

Moyers, P. (1999). Guide to occupational therapy practice. *American Journal of Occupational Therapy, 53*, 247–322.

Nelson, D. L., & Glass, L. M. (1999). Occupational therapists' involvement with the minimum data set in skilled nursing and intermediate care facilities. *American Journal of Occupational Therapy, 53*, 348–352.

Schell, B. A., & Slater, D. Y. (1998). Management competencies required of administrative and clinical practitioners in the new millennium. *American Journal of Occupational Therapy, 53*, 744–750.

Slater, C. A., Evans, R. W., & Small, L. (1993, October). *Clinical program evaluation: An example of continuous quality*. Paper presented at the American Speech and Hearing Association annual symposium, Anaheim, CA.

Steiner, G. A. (1979). *Strategic planning: What every manager must know*. New York: Free Press.

Walker, K. F. (2001). Adjustments to managed health care: pushing against it, going with it and making the best of it. *American Journal of Occupational Therapy, 55*, 129–137.

Weed, L. L. (1971). *Medical records, medical evaluation and patient care*. Chicago: Yearbook Medical.

World Health Organization. (2001). International classification of functioning, disability, and health (ICF). Available at: www.who.int/icidh/. Accessed April 12, 2001.

CHAPTER 47

INTERDISCIPLINARY COMMUNICATION AND SUPERVISION OF PERSONNEL

ELLEN S. COHN

TEAMS AND TEAMWORK

In the often-cited poem about Hinduism, "The Blind Men and the Elephant," John Godfrey Saxe described the plight of six men, all blind, who happened on an elephant. The first man, feeling the elephant's side, reported it was like a wall. The second, feeling the tusk, interpreted the creature to be like a spear. The third, finding its trunk, declared it to be like a snake, and so on. Thus when each observer stated his opinion of the elephant, "each was partly in the right, and all were in the wrong!" (Saxe, 1871, p. 260). Herein lies the concept underlying the use of the interdisciplinary team communication. Although each member, representing a different perspective, is hardly blind, a single way of observing limits the ability to comprehend the whole. It is the combined vision, evaluation, and coordinated intervention plan that provides a complete picture of the whole client receiving intervention.

For most areas of practice, interdisciplinary team interactions are the norm. Successful intervention involves a collaborative and mutual process during which practitioners and clients develop the care plan together (Golin & Duncanis, 1981; Humphry, Gonzalez, & Taylor, 1993; Leff & Walizer, 1992). According to Parham (1987), occupational therapists are "concerned with understanding the occupations of human beings, the ways in which people organize the activities that fill their lives and give their lives meaning" (p. 555). To understand how a particular client experiences illness or disability within the context of his or her occupations and daily life, the occupational therapy practitioner needs to collaborate with other members of the team involved in providing care for that client.

The team is made of a variety of different specialists who have different backgrounds, training, values, worldviews, and sometimes different goals. These specialists work together in different configurations, depending on the needs of the client. Each team member addresses the client's concerns from a unique perspective, and all perspectives are then coordinated to structure the client care plan. It is assumed that this coordinated perspective will make a difference in the ultimate outcome for the recipient of the care plan (Crepeau, 1994a, 1994b; Unsworth, Thomas, & Greenwood, 1995).

Ideally, interdisciplinary team members share a common concept of the client's concerns and a common philosophy of care management, synthesize the diverse information gathered from their own evaluations and those of outside consultants, and work together to formulate and implement a comprehensive care plan based on the available data. Most important, the team should act as a functional unit whose members are willing to learn from each other and modify, when appropriate, their own opinions, based on the combined observations and expertise of the entire group (Perlmutter, Bailey, & Netting, 2001). The advantages of a team approach are a more holistic approach to client care, integrated interventions, the reduction or elimination of duplicated services and fragmentation or gaps in care, and quicker and more informed decisions for client plans (Stancliff, 1995).

Historically, health-care teams have generated a client's care plan behind closed doors, without the client's input, and then shared their plans with the client. In current practice, however, additional voices are influencing the team process. Incorporation of the client as a member of the team is now espoused by health professionals and is viewed as crucial to the eventual success of the care plan (Baum,1998; Crepeau, 1994a, 1994b). In the managed-care environment, which focuses on both cost containment and quality of care, the third-party payer's perspective is increasingly considered another crucial factor in the team's decision-making process.

An understanding of the potential contributions of the various people and professionals involved in the client's life enables the practitioner to develop a more meaningful plan for each client. The members of the team have interrelated functions. Depending on the practice environment, the occupational therapy practitioner's interactions with other professionals and with the important people in the client's life vary. In a medical setting, such as an acute care hospital or a rehabilitation unit, the team members may operate under a physician's order, and practitioners might interact with team members numerous times a day. Alternatively, a practitioner in private practice or employed by a home-care agency might not have frequent contact with other specialists but may have more repeated contact with family members or other significant people in the client's life.

Regardless of the environment, occupational therapy practitioners need to be aware of the roles of the other members of the team, so practitioners may be clear about the contributions occupational therapy can make and how everyone can work together for the client's benefit. Therefore, occupational therapy practitioners need to interpret their role and contribution to the intervention team, for it is never safe to assume that other members of any particular team have a full understanding of the potential contributions of occupational therapy. Consider, for example, Rose's story.

Rose is a 72-year-old who recently underwent a total hip replacement and is now receiving occupational therapy services in her home. Although her husband is devoted to her, he is unable to help her maintain the home. A social worker is available to consult with the intervention team. Together, the occupational therapist, the client, her husband, and the social worker determined that seeking the services of a Meals-on-Wheels program would alleviate the pressure of preparing meals. This team decision-making process helped the occupational therapist determine the focus of occupational therapy intervention. With Rose's homemaking duties alleviated, the occupational therapist was able to focus on helping Rose regain and monitor her strength and endurance so that she had the resources to again join her husband at their weekly singing group. With the assistance of the intervention team, occupational therapy focused on a meaningful activity for Rose and her husband.

Although practically every medical and allied health professional may be called on to provide services to address the range of client conditions seen by occupational therapy practitioners, the professionals listed in Box 47-1 may be especially relevant (Wachtel & Compart, 1996).

Team Interaction Models

Each client usually has an identified case manager or team leader. The case manager is the designated person on whom clients and their family can consistently rely to explain, clarify, or acquire necessary information. This case manager may also serve the role of the client ombudsman. The leadership of the team or the case management may change over time, according to the identified concerns of a particular client, the members of the team, the nature of the task, and the structure of the organization. In a traditional medical model, the physician is often the leader of the team. Today, especially in community-based or educational settings, a therapist, special service coordinator, or teacher may lead or coordinate the team and simultaneously serve as the case manager.

BOX 47–1 MEDICAL, REHABILITATION, AND EDUCATIONAL PROFESSIONALS

- *Adapted physical educator:* Adapts sporting equipment and games for individuals with special needs.
- *Administrator:* Applies and enforces federal, state, and local laws that regulate finances, standards, and environments for most health and educational programs; has valuable expertise in management of personnel, space, and finances.
- *Audiologist:* Specializes in diagnosis and treatment of hearing impairments; administers a variety of tests to determine hearing level and site of damage to the auditory system; recommends hearing aids and other assistive devices to enhance residual hearing loss or the need for special training.
- *Biomedical engineer:* Specializes in the application of scientific theory and technology to the development of devices and techniques for medical treatment, rehabilitation, and research; provides technical expertise in recommendation of commercial products and the modifications of existing devices or the design and fabrication of custom equipment or adjusted environments.
- *Chaplain:* Focuses on religious and spiritual needs of clients; provides nondenominational individual and family counseling; offers special services.
- *Orthotist and prosthetist:* Orthotist makes and fits braces to support or correct body parts weakened by disease, injury, or congenital deformity or to help prevent deformities; prosthetist designs and fabricates artificial limbs, with special attention to enhancing fit, function, and appearance.
- *Physical therapist:* Evaluates physical capacities and limitations; administers treatment designed to alleviate pain, correct or minimize deformity, increase strength and mobility, and improve general health.
- *Physicians (specialists):* Usually specialists to whom a client has been referred by the primary-care physician (e.g., orthopedists, ophthalmologists, neurologists, cardiologists, physiatrists, psychiatrists).
- *Psychologist:* Provides psychological, projective, and behavioral assessments; provides individual, couple, family, and group psychotherapy related to behavioral or adjustment issues.
- *Rehabilitation counselor:* Assists individuals with physical, mental, cognitive, or sensory disabilities to become or remain self-sufficient, productive citizens; helps clients cope with societal and personal problems, plan careers, and find and keep satisfying jobs.
- *Rehabilitation nurse:* provides goal-directed, personalized care that encompasses preventive, maintenance, and restorative aspects of nursing; administers medication and instructs client and significant others in care management and health maintenance programs.
- *Respiratory therapist (inhalation therapist):* administers oxygen and mists for medical purposes, provides oxygen-assessment programs and client education.
- *Social worker:* Assists client, family, or other important people in the client's life to achieve a maximal level of social and emotional functioning; provides client and family counseling, discharge planning, and education on entitlements and other available resources; assists in identifying transportation and attendant care resources.
- *Special educator:* Serves as a teacher of children with either unusually high intellectual potential or children who are handicapped by mental illness, learning disabilities, or developmental deviations; may have advanced skills in teaching children who are blind, deaf, emotionally disturbed, mentally retarded, or physically handicapped.
- *Speech and language pathologist:* Specializes in speech disorders, the development of language and speech production, the physiology of speech, theories, and measurement of hearing and phonetics.
- *Teacher:* Certified to provide education at the early childhood, kindergarten, elementary, secondary, or high school level.
- *Therapeutic recreation specialist (recreation therapist):* Facilitates the enjoyable use of leisure time to promote mental and physical well-being; uses social and recreational activities to aid in adjustment to disability and participation in community activities.
- *Vocational counselor:* Provides diagnostic evaluation of transferable skills, achievement levels, aptitudes, and interests to determine employability and job placement potential; works with employers to facilitate successful work placements.

Teams may be organized into multidisciplinary, interdisciplinary, or transdisciplinary models. Often, however, a team moves from one model to another and functions in its own unique variation of the classic models. In the multidisciplinary approach, team members work side by side, and each member has a clearly defined role with specific areas of responsibility. Evaluation, planning, and therapy take place independently. Generally, families and clients meet with the team members of each discipline separately.

In an interdisciplinary approach, team members share responsibility for providing services, often sharing roles. Team members conduct separate evaluations, but share the results to develop an integrated and coordinated care plan. Clients and families or other significant people in clients' lives meet with the team or a representative of the team, such as the team leader or case manager.

In a transdisciplinary team, members commit to teaching, learning, and working across disciplinary boundaries to plan and provide integrated services. The team assimilates the perspectives of the various team members to make joint decisions. Traditional role boundaries are crossed, and the skills of other disciplines are integrated into a total care plan.

Creating Shared Meaning and a Common Language

Professionals and clients may have different viewpoints or priorities for intervention, or they may have the same goals, yet differ in the meaning of the goals or the approach for reaching goals. Therefore, it is essential for the team members to develop shared meaning about the client's entire condition. For the intervention to be effective, the team must understand each client's (Crepeau, 1994a; Salisbury, 1992):

- Beliefs
- Attitudes
- Ways of making meaning of his or her life world
- Knowledge of his or her condition
- Expectancies for the future
- Expectancies about treatment

The constructionist process, as described by Buckholdt and Gubrium (1979) and Crepeau (1994a, 1994b), involves the individual clinical reasoning of the team members and the collective reasoning of the group. Formal lines of communication and methods for sharing these interpretations often develop through team meetings, collaborative intervention sessions, written evaluations, and progress notes. Each team member makes his or her own interpretation of the client's lived experience and then articulates this interpretation to the other team members. The team collectively reconstructs the interpretation to create a unified image from the diversity of their individual perspectives. Through this constructionist process, team members discover, interpret, and negotiate their understanding of the client by "sorting out conflicting data to arrive at a common definition of the problems faced by the patient" (Crepeau, 1994b, p. 161).

To develop a cohesive treatment team that uses a constructionist process, the team must focus its energy and creativity to establish a shared mission. Only in a climate of mutual trust and respect can a group of people with diverse perspectives develop into a cohesive team (Zenger, Musselwhite, Hurson, & Perrin, 1994). Thus it is important to acknowledge that team building is a developmental process; it takes time and energy to learn about each member's values, goals, and communication style (Blechert, Christiansen, & Kari, 1987).

Although teams may have different needs at different times, Blechert et al. (1987) found that team development can be described in terms of life stages. In the first stage, team members explore and define their roles within the context of the team and work setting. Each team member identifies his or her area of expertise and interest, thereby defining each member's unique contribution. Once the team has worked together, adjustment and rearrangement of roles may be necessary to progress to the next stage. Finally, as team members redefine their roles and learn to value each other, they begin to think about issues from multiple points of view. When functioning well, the team members are able to see the issues as a whole. Similar to the blind men with the elephant, the image developed by the team is broader and richer when multiple perspectives are shared to construct a unified image.

SUPERVISION

Supervision Story

Barbara, an occupational therapist with 3 years of experience, has just started working in a day school program for children with developmental disabilities. Within 4 weeks of her involvement in the program, Barbara is required to complete annual evaluations for five children. Barbara is unfamiliar with the assessment tools used by the occupational therapy department in the day school program, yet believes she should know how to administer them. Initially, Barbara is reluctant to reveal to her supervisor that she is unfamiliar with the assessments, because she perceives the lack of this knowledge as incompetence and fears her supervisor's disapproval. Nonetheless, she understands the purpose of **supervision** and challenges herself to seek the guidance she needs. Barbara's supervisor is pleased that Barbara was able to identify her learning needs, and together they develop a learning plan for Barbara.

This situation highlights the complexity of the supervisory process. Tasks include ensuring quality while teaching and developing skills, all within the context of an interpersonal relationship. This occurs among all levels of occupational therapy personnel, from aides, students, and staff therapists to all occupational therapy practitioners. The following sections address definitions, the supervisory relationship, functions, goals, and components of the supervisory process as well as staff development.

Definition

Supervision is a dynamic, interactive process in which the supervisor has been assigned or designated to assist in and direct the work and growth of the supervisees. The word *supervisor* is derived from the Latin words *super*, "over," and *videre*, "to watch, to see" (Mish, 1997). Therefore, the supervisor is assigned or designated by the organization administration to oversee or watch over the work of another, and the supervisee is expected to be accountable to the supervisor. The supervisory process, as defined by the American Occupational Therapy Association (AOTA; 1999), is "a process in which two or more people participate in a joint effort to promote, establish, maintain, and/or elevate a level of performance and service" (p. 592). Supervision is viewed as a mutual process that "fosters growth and development; assures appropriate utilization of training and potential; encourages creativity and innovation; and provides guidance, support, encouragement, and respect while working toward a goal" (p. 592).

These definitions of supervision all identify the supervisor as a person who has some official responsibility to direct, guide, and monitor the supervisee's practice. These authority, evaluation, and accountability functions distinguish supervision from consultation or mentorship. In the mentorship or consultative role, the more experienced practitioner guides or coaches the apprentice, without the authority function of evaluating performance and maintaining the standards and viability of the organization.

Supervisory Relationship

The importance of the relationship between supervisors and supervisees is inherent within the supervisory context. Each member in the relationship enters with his or her own assumptions and expectations. These expectations are based on the supervisee's past experiences with other supervisors, parents, and authority figures. These experiences, together with supervisee's emerging images of occupational therapy and professional goals, provide the foundation for the supervisory relationship. Supervisors, in turn, have a notion of the behaviors, skills, and attitudes necessary for effective practice in their settings. Initially, the delineation of expectations of both supervisors and supervisees is a primary focus of supervision. Later, the focus shifts to providing feedback related to the stated expectations.

The feedback provided by supervisors is critical to supervisees' development. Feedback is defined as sharing knowledge of the results of an individual's performance with the intent of changing that individual's behavior in a desirable direction. It refers to a particular aspect of behavior, to a total behavioral sequence or performance, or to the nature of the message itself. For example, the message may convey information about supervisees' attitudes toward clients. This definition connotes an expectation that "some change will occur in the supervisee's understanding, attitude, or behavior in response to feedback" (Freeman, 1985, p. 5).

Feedback can help identify the next step in the change process, clarify steps that have taken place, evaluate whether a particular step meets performance criteria for a specific task and whether it relates to or achieves the overall goals, and clarify or modify those goals or expectations as needed. One of the key sources for feedback is the supervisor. It is important for supervisees to recognize that supervisors are not judging their worth or goodness but are assessing how well they are performing. "Feedback, given honestly and sincerely is often the most valuable change agent" (Freeman, 1985, p. 109).

Functions

Supervisors assume multiple roles as they promote the growth of their supervisees. The educational role focuses on learning and performing. In this role, the supervisor acknowledges that the supervisee is an adult learner and assumes the supervisee will take an active role in the supervisory process. Drawing on the principle of adult learning that learners should be empowered to share responsibility for planning and evaluating their learning experiences, the supervisor works with the supervisee to plan and achieve acceptable goals (Knowles, 1980). The learning may begin with the direct transmission of information essential to perform one's job responsibilities, such as orientation to the organization of the facility and department, including structure, function, policies, and procedures. The supervisor then teaches or coaches the supervisee to explore the range of possibilities to promote quality delivery of services. As in Barbara's situation, the supervisor may negotiate a learning contract that outlines specific skills and theories to be mastered and delineates a plan to meet specific objectives.

In the administrative function, the performance of the supervisee is observed to ensure the maintenance of job requirements and professional standards. The supervisor evaluates and documents the supervisee's ability to meet these requirements and standards. If the job requirements and standards that are consistent with professional, state, and department guidelines have not been achieved, the supervisor assumes the teaching role to promote successful performance.

Both the administrative and educational roles require the supervisor to be a supportive role model. The role model is widely recognized as central to assisting others in the traditions and standards of practice (Rogers, 1982). Many clinical situations provoke reflection on complex, intense issues of life and death, personal loss, disease, and disability. Given the potential for personal responses to these issues, the supervisor must attend to the supervisee's reactions to these issues and to his or her ability to cope with the situations present. The supervisor can help the supervisee identify behavior and feelings that may affect his or her interactions with clients or the ability to provide quality care. However, it is beyond the role of the supervisor to provide psychotherapy to a supervisee. When psychotherapy is indicated, supervisors should make the necessary recommendation.

Components of the Supervisory Process

Anderson's (1988) analysis of the supervisory process identified several components, discussed in the following sections.

Understanding the Supervisory Process

For the supervisory process to be effective, both the supervisor and supervisee need to be prepared for their roles. Thus the supervisory process should include ongoing discussions relative to expectations, concerns, needs, learning styles, and perceptions of the supervisory experience. Through these ongoing discussions, expectations, goals, and approaches may be modified in response to the evolving process.

Planning

Planning begins as soon as the supervisory process begins. It is a joint process in which the supervisor and supervisee identify the supervisee's ability to problem solve, the degree of involvement each participant desires, the ability of the supervisee to observe and analyze his or her behavior, and the supervisor's flexibility in adapting his or her style to the supervisee's needs. Together, the supervisor and supervisee determine the objectives and methods for accomplishing the given objectives.

Observing

The observational component of the supervisory process involves data collection and recording by both supervisor and supervisee for further analysis and interpretation, which can then lead to performance evaluation. The most traditional form of observation is for the supervisor to watch the supervisee perform a given task and simply to write evaluative statements reflecting his or her perceptions of the appropriateness of the supervisee's performance. Other forms of observation include tallies of specific behaviors, use of specific rating scales, verbatim recording, selective recordings, observing nonverbal behavior, and audiotaping or videotaping the therapy sessions.

Goals

The goal of supervision "is the professional growth and development of the supervisee and the supervisor, which it is assumed will result ultimately in optimal service to clients" (Anderson, 1988, p. 12). Subsumed in this broad goal emphasizing learning and service are the following subgoals:

- Develop a sense of professional identity.
- Increase theoretical knowledge and apply this knowledge to the complexities inherent in practice.
- Develop reflection on practice.
- Name, frame, and solve problems in an organized, thorough, and analytical fashion.
- Make thoughtful decisions in a reasonable time period.
- Be objective, flexible, and independent in thought and action.
- Develop self-awareness and make changes in behavior on the basis of such awareness.
- Cultivate individual abilities.

To achieve these goals, the supervisor must establish a safe and trusting relationship with his or her supervisee. This type of relationship fosters a mutual sharing of questions, concerns, observations, and speculations and allows identification of alternative or multiple approaches to solving the complexities of practice. Some of the goals of supervision are similar to those of staff development. Indeed, as the following section shows, supervision is an essential component in any comprehensive staff development program.

ETHICS NOTE 47–1

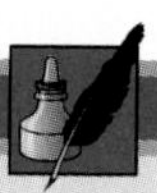

Who Should Be Responsible for Ensuring Competence?

PENNY KYLER and RUTH A. HANSEN

Tom, who is a registered occupational therapist, worked in acute physical rehabilitation for the last 12 years. During a recent reorganization of the hospital, many staffing changes were made. Tom now is working half-time in adolescent psychiatry. He has no previous experience working with adolescents who have a primary psychiatric diagnosis. He is now working alone on the unit.

QUESTIONS AND EXERCISES

1. **Does Tom have the credentials and the competencies to provide services in adolescent psychiatry?**
2. **Does Tom have the right to refuse to work in adolescent psychiatry?**
3. **Does the employer have the right to expect that Tom can provide occupational therapy services on the unit?**
4. **What actions should the employer and Tom take to ensure that he can deliver competent services for patients?**

Staff Development

Staff development is critical to achieving and maintaining quality delivery of services in any organization. Although the components of a staff development program depend highly on the nature and resources of that particular facility, most organizations take a performance-oriented approach. When viewed from this perspective, the purpose of staff development is to facilitate the growth of employees so they can achieve the highest performance possible. An effective staff development program should focus on the integration of the organization's and the employee's goals (Lieberman & Miller, 1979). However, the increasingly complex climate of managed health care, which emphasizes productivity and meaningful outcomes, may leave managers with less time to establish clinical competence in their employees. The health-care environment of today demands that practitioners be competent and ready to provide quality services as soon as possible.

Traditional staff development programs generally consist of formal courses, workshops, conferences, or a series of in-service training units that teach specific skills and procedures. Orientation programs to introduce new staff members to policies, procedures, evaluation tools, and documentation requirements are common in many settings. A more highly developed program for new staff members may include lectures on topics specific to the clinical population receiving services. These programs focus on immediate skill development and establish facility standards.

To address employee personal and professional goals from a developmental perspective, Smith and Elbert (1986) recommended using a self-appraisal approach—that is, employees complete an assessment of their competence and then write objectives for future learning. Self-appraisals include content relative to clinical knowledge and skills as well as content relative to professional development, such as time and stress management, communication skills, interdisciplinary communication, and professional standards and ethics. Once employees identify their goals, they can develop an individualized development program by drawing on the resources of the facility, their supervisors, and the educational opportunities in their community and the broader professional communities.

Lieberman and Miller (1979) recommended using the work itself to stimulate and reinforce professional growth and development. Drawing on Schön's (1983) notion of reflection in action, in which practitioners critically examine or reflect on the reasoning processes used in everyday practice, Slater and Cohn (1991) advocated videotaping and analyzing therapy sessions in either peer-learning or small-group situations. While examining the videotapes, learners and supervisors can stop the action and discuss the various approaches used and explore new interpretations to address therapy from a broader perspective.

SUPERVISION OF OCCUPATIONAL THERAPY PERSONNEL

Guidelines and Standards

The amount and nature of supervision in a particular setting are closely determined by the structure of the setting, the role functions of the practitioner, and the practitioner's expertise in his or her various roles. AOTA (1999a) provided guidelines for supervision that indicate patterns and types of supervision. The guidelines describe supervision along a continuum that includes close, routine, general, and minimal levels of supervision. Close supervision requires daily, direct contact at the site of work. Routine supervision requires direct contact at least every 2 weeks at the site of work. Interim supervision occurs through indirect methods, such as telephone or written communication. General supervision requires at least monthly direct contact, with supervision available as needed by other methods. Minimal supervision is provided only as needed and may be less than monthly (AOTA, 1999a).

Referring to the supervision story earlier in the chapter, Barbara requires functional supervision to assist her in learning needed skills. A functional supervisor provides information and feedback relative to a particular function, such as implementing a particular intervention technique or learning a particular assessment.

AOTA (1999a) maintained the principle that "overall clinical supervision specific to the application of occupational therapy principles must be overseen by an OT" (p. 592). Administrative supervision can be provided by others, such as special education directors, principals, facility administrators, or other health-care providers (AOTA, 1999a). It is recommended that entry-level practitioners receive close supervision of their occupational therapy practice by intermediate- or advanced-level practitioners for service delivery aspects. Although not required, it is recommended that intermediate-level practitioners who have mastery of basic role functions receive routine to general supervision from advanced practitioners, and it is recommended that advanced practitioners obtain minimal supervision within their area of expertise and general supervision for the administrative aspects of their work (AOTA, 1999a).

Although professional guidelines recommend minimal levels of supervision, the consumers of occupational therapy and occupational therapy practitioners have a certain amount of faith in the occupational therapy process, without much empirical evidence to document the efficacy of a given intervention. As a profession, occupational therapy is are just beginning to measure therapy outcomes. In this context, supervision becomes a critical mechanism to encourage occupational therapy practitioners to examine the underlying assumptions and postulates for changes that guide the intervention process. Supervision then becomes a vehicle to examine the reasoning behind the daily actions of practice. Thus supervision is a valuable and often overlooked process for even the most experienced practitioner.

Occupational Therapy Students

The consensus within the occupational therapy profession is that the fieldwork experience plays an integral role in professional development. In 1923, the first standards requiring fieldwork experiences were approved by AOTA (Pressler, 1983). Fieldwork continues to function as the critical link between the academic world of theory and the clinical world of practice (Cohn & Crist, 1995). This component of education functions as the gateway into the profession, because all students must complete fieldwork requirements to become eligible to take the certification examinations for occupational therapists and occupational therapy assistants.

The process and content of fieldwork experiences have been debated over the years. Yet the value of having an opportunity to integrate academic knowledge with application skills at progressively higher levels of performance and responsibility has always been acknowledged as important (Pressler, 1983). Christie, Joyce, and Moeller (1985) highlighted that value by documenting the fieldwork experience as having the greatest influence on the development of a therapist's preference for a specific area of clinical practice. Of the 131 therapists surveyed, 55% indicated that clinical practice preferences were either formed or changed during the fieldwork experience, and another 24% noted that fieldwork experience expanded their interests to other areas of practice. Thus the fieldwork experience can be rich and rewarding, and as such, it is likely to have a tremendous bearing on a student's career choices.

Purpose and Levels of Fieldwork

The AOTA Standards and Accredited Educational Program for Occupational Therapist and Occupational Therapy Assistants (AOTA, 1999c, 1999d) outline the general fieldwork requirements for all students. The requirements are divided into two classifications: level I and level II fieldwork. Level I fieldwork offers students practical experiences that are integrated throughout the academic program. The AOTA standards describe level I fieldwork as "experiences designed to enrich didactic course work through directed observation and participation in selected aspects of the occupational therapy process" (1999c, p. 581; 1999d, p. 588). The ultimate goal of level I fieldwork is for students to "develop a basic comfort level with and understanding of the needs of clients" (AOTA, 1999c, p. 581). Through level I fieldwork experiences, students are exposed to the values and traditions of occupational therapy practice and have the opportunity to examine their reactions to clients, systems of service delivery, related personnel, and potential role(s) within the profession. Because the academic level performance expectations and specific purposes of the level I fieldwork experience vary in each occupational therapy curriculum, the timing, length, requirements, and specific focus of the experience are negotiated with each academic program on an individual basis (AOTA, 2000a).

The purpose of level II fieldwork for the occupational therapy student is to "promote clinical reasoning and reflective practice; to transmit the values, beliefs, that enable ethical practice, and to develop professionalism and competence as career responsibilities" (AOTA, 1999c, p. 582). For occupational therapy assistant students the purpose of level II fieldwork is "promote clinical reasoning, appropriate to the occupational therapy assistant role" as well as to achieve professionalism and competence (AOTA, 1999d, p. 589). Under close supervision, students test firsthand the theories and facts learned in academic study and have a chance to refine skills through interaction with clients.

The requirements established by AOTA include a minimum of the equivalent of 24 weeks full-time of level II fieldwork for occupational therapy students (AOTA, 1999c) and a minimum of the equivalent of 16 weeks full-time for occupational therapy assistant students (AOTA, 1999d). To offer occupational therapy students experience with a wide range of client ages and a variety of occupational performance conditions, the 6 months are usually divided into two 3-month experiences in different settings. Alternatives to full-time fieldwork, such as part-time models or 12-month experiences, are becoming more common (Adelstein, Cohn, Baker, & Barnes, 1990; Phillips & Legaspi, 1995). Successful completion of level II fieldwork is a requirement for certification as a registered occupational therapist (OTR) or certified occupational therapy assistant (COTA). Fieldwork provides students with situations in which to practice interpersonal skills with clients and staff and to develop characteristics essential to productive working relationships (AOTA, 2000a).

For students, the overall purpose of the fieldwork experience is to gain mastery of occupational therapy clinical reasoning and techniques to develop entry-level competence. Effective oral and written communication of ideas and objectives relevant to the roles and duties of an occupational therapist or occupational therapy assistant, including professional interaction with clients and staff, is expected of all students. Students are responsible for demonstrating a sensitivity to and respect for client confidentiality, establishing and sustaining therapeutic relationships, and working collaboratively with others. Another expectation—more internal to the students' development of positive professional self-images—includes taking responsibility for maintaining, assessing, and improving self-competence. Students are responsible for articulating their understanding of theoretical information and identifying their abilities to implement evaluation or intervention techniques. Moreover, the ability to benefit from supervision as a resource for self-directed learning is critical to professional development. Thus understanding and articulating one's individual learning style becomes essential to the supervisory process.

Transition from Student to Professional

The shift from the academic setting to the fieldwork setting is an obvious, yet often underestimated, life change. Occupational therapy students are making the environmental transition from the classroom to the fieldwork setting while simultaneously emerging from the role of student to the role of occupational therapy practitioner. As with any transition, occupational therapy students leaving academia face a process of change from one structure, role, or sense of self to another. The struggle to assimilate into a new environment and to develop a new role may jolt students into disequilibrium, and some may have trouble adjusting to the new role. As is true of all life changes, this disequilibrium can be an opportunity for growth, especially in the context of a supportive supervisory relationship.

This time of transition for students results in changes in assumptions about themselves and the world and requires a corresponding change in behaviors, relationships, learning styles, and self-perceptions. As they move into fieldwork settings, students may begin to reassess their suppositions about occupational therapy, the theories they learned in school, and their views of themselves as practitioners, learners, and individuals. Because individuals differ in their ability to adapt to change and because each student is placed in a different fieldwork setting, the transition has a different effect on each student.

The nature of the fieldwork environment is fundamentally different from that of the academic environment. Knowing

TABLE 47-1. **DISTINCTIONS BETWEEN ACADEMIC AND FIELDWORK SETTINGS**

Characteristic	Academic Setting	Fieldwork Setting
Purpose	Dissemination of knowledge, development of creative thought and student growth	Provide high-quality client care
Faculty/supervisor accountability	To student; to university/college	To client and significant others; to fieldwork center; to student
Student accountability	To self	To clients and significant others; to supervisor; to fieldwork center
Pace	Depends on curriculum; adaptable to student and faculty needs	Depends on clients' needs; less adaptable
Student:educator ratio	Many students to one faculty member	One student to one supervisor; small group of students to one supervisor; one student to two supervisors
Source of feedback	Summative at midterm or end of term; provided by faculty	Provided by clients and significant others, supervisor, and other staff; formative
Degree of faculty/supervisor control of educational experience	Able to plan; controlled	Limited control; various diagnoses and length of client stay
Primary learning tools	Books, lectures, audiovisual aids, case studies, simulations	Situation of practice; clients, families, significant others, and staff
Conceptual learning	Abstract, theoretical	Pragmatic, applied in interpersonal context
Learning process	Teacher directed	Client, self, peer; supervisor directed
Tolerance for ambiguity	High	Low
Lifestyle	Flexible; able to plan time around class schedule	Structured; flexible time limited to evenings and weekends

and acknowledging some of the distinctions between the two settings may ease the transition and provide students with support to accept the challenges of fieldwork experiences (Table 47-1). Within the fieldwork environment, the learning focus shifts to the application or implementation of therapy techniques in an applied interpersonal context. Techniques that were introduced in a simulated context now must be mastered and applied with attention to the client's emotional needs.

Abstract questions appropriate in the academic environment shift to pragmatic questions to reduce the possibility of error in one's thinking. For example, rather than thinking about a client's function in the kitchen from an abstract perspective, the student has to think about the client's function in the context of a specific kitchen in a certain small apartment and to attend to the client's concerns about his or her family. Because the student recognizes that his or her actions have an influence on the client's life, tolerance for ambiguity or uncertainty declines during fieldwork.

In the academic setting, students are accountable to themselves, and performance is evaluated on a summative basis through tests, assignments, and grades. Students choose whether to disclose their grades to family or peers, and their performance does not affect others. In the fieldwork center, a student's performance is evaluated on a formative basis and may be observed by the entire health-care team, especially at team meetings. Performance is no longer the private matter it was at school but is publicly observed, because it has direct and critical consequences for clients. Colleagues, clients, and their families then may offer meaningful feedback. Although all these opportunities may create disequilibrium or tension, they likewise constitute new ways in which students learn about themselves and their profession. The broad and diverse experience within the fieldwork setting challenges students to redefine their sense of self.

Fieldwork takes place in a situation over which fieldwork educators have little control. The organizational factors of the health-care setting, combined with client-care factors, such as the nature and complexity of the client's problem, the length of stay, and fluctuation in client load, make planning difficult, especially in acute care settings. In settings that provide extended care for clients, however, the fieldwork educators are able to plan ahead, because the client population is more constant and the fieldwork educator knows which clients will be available during student placements.

Fieldwork educators' primary responsibility is client care; they have an ethical imperative to ensure the welfare of clients. This appropriate professional ethic may constrain activities that may be desirable from the standpoint of education. However, the supervisory relationship allows fieldwork educators to adapt to the constraints of the setting.

This unique relationship is a positive aspect of the fieldwork environment, because fieldwork educators can adapt the fieldwork experiences to meet the needs of the learner.

Roles and Responsibilities

After completion of the prerequisite academic coursework, occupational therapy and occupational therapy assistant students are eligible to begin their fieldwork experiences. Clearly defined objectives and guidelines help students organize their efforts toward achieving clinical competence. Working toward mastery of the entry-level skills required for high-quality client care is a mutual undertaking between the fieldwork educators and the students. Both are responsible for the process of evaluating student progress and modifying the learning experience within the environment.

Students are responsible for fulfilling all duties identified by the fieldwork educators and academic fieldwork coordinators within the designated times and complying with the professional standards identified by the fieldwork facility, the education program, and the Occupational Therapy Code of Ethics (AOTA, 2000b; see Appendix C). The people responsible for the fieldwork education program and direct supervision of occupational therapy students must be occupational therapists who meet state practice acts and regulations and have a minimum of 1 year of practice experience, subsequent to the requisite initial certification. For occupational therapy assistant students, supervision can be provided by a registered occupational therapist or a certified occupational therapy assistant, also with a minimum of 1 year of experience.

Although the minimum requirement is 1 year of experience, fieldwork educators should be competent clinicians who can serve as good role models or mentors for future practitioners. The people responsible for supervising students are formally titled fieldwork educators, although the terms *clinical educators*, *fieldwork supervisors*, and *student supervisors* are also used (AOTA, 2000a). Two areas of responsibility of fieldwork educators are administrative functions and direct day-to-day supervision. The administrative responsibilities of the fieldwork educator include, but are not limited to, collaborating with the academic fieldwork coordinator to develop a program that provides the best opportunity for the implementation of theoretical concepts offered as part of the academic educational program and creating an environment that facilitates learning, clinical inquiry, and reflection on one's practice.

Each education program has an academic fieldwork coordinator who functions as a liaison between the academic setting, the fieldwork educators, and the students. The academic fieldwork coordinators assign eligible students to fieldwork experience and are available for consultation with both students and fieldwork educators.

Fieldwork Evaluation

Frequently, students receive informal feedback during supervision meetings; however, formal mechanisms for providing feedback and evaluation of a student's performance, judgments, and attitudes are built into the fieldwork experience. There are two distinct purposes in fieldwork evaluation. One is the formative, ongoing process of directing student learning throughout the fieldwork experience; the other is summative, documenting the level of skills attained at the completion of the fieldwork experience. Although these two processes are different, they are not mutually exclusive. The formative process occurs throughout the fieldwork experience so that students and fieldwork educators can compare perceptions, assess which student activities are important and which are less so, review objectives, plan new learning opportunities, and make necessary modifications in behaviors. The second process, which is cumulative, requires documentation of a student's performance after completion of the fieldwork experience.

The Fieldwork Evaluation (FWE) is the instrument adopted by AOTA for evaluating the performance of professional-level occupational therapy students in all fieldwork education centers (Commission on Education [COE], 1986). The FWE consists of two sections. The first section has 51 behavioral statements depicting competent performance in five areas: evaluation, planning, treatment, problem solving, and administrative or professionalism. The student is evaluated in each area on the basis of performance, judgment, and attitude on a rating scale ranging from excellent to poor. The second section is a written summary of performance, indicating particular strengths and weaknesses and any other information useful in documenting professional growth and learning. This form should serve as a summary of what students already know of their performance. Completion, administration, and subsequent use of the FWE should be conducted with consideration of all legal and ethical implications for each student assessed. Such consideration includes the right to nonprejudicial evaluation, the right to privacy of information, and the right for students to appeal (COE, 1986).

The Fieldwork Evaluation Form for the Occupational Therapy Assistant Student (FWE/OTA) is the instrument adopted by AOTA for evaluating the performance of occupational therapy assistant students in all fieldwork centers. Developed in 1983, this instrument contains 24 competency items, divided into four sections: evaluation, treatment, communication, and professional behavior. Each of the 24 items on the FWE/OTA is rated on a scale of 1 to 5, with criteria stated for each level. The FWE/OTA is used in a formative manner at midterm to provide students with feedback and to develop strategies for improving performance. It is used in a summative manner after completion of the fieldwork experience, because the AOTA states that the FWE/OTA final scores be based on the last 2 weeks of the fieldwork experience (COE, 1983).

Finally, the intent of the fieldwork evaluation is not to differentiate between students, but to measure their achievement of specific competencies. Future employers want assurance that students satisfy the entry-level requirements. The

FWE data may be synthesized to provide the foundation for employment references.

Students also have the opportunity to provide the fieldwork educators and fieldwork facility with feedback. AOTA (2000c) recommends the Student Evaluation of Fieldwork Experiences (SEFWE) form. This form allows students to provide feedback about the orientation process, supervisor interaction, and the entire learning experience. The fieldwork sites use this information to improve fieldwork programs, and the academic programs share the information with future students who are interested in training at those sites.

A profession usually defines its boundaries by setting up criteria for entry. In occupational therapy, the fieldwork experience is an essential component of the entry criteria. Fieldwork is the beginning of a lifelong process of connecting theory with practice. The depth of the experience depends greatly on the degree to which students and fieldwork educators share the responsibility for teaching and learning.

Occupational Therapy Aides

To provide efficient and cost-effective occupational therapy services, many occupational therapy departments are employing occupational therapy aides. An occupational therapy aide is an individual assigned by an occupational therapist to perform delegated, selected, client- and non-client-related tasks for which the aide has demonstrated competency. Ultimately, the occupational therapist or assistant is responsible and accountable for the overall use of aides in implementing services. The use of occupational therapy aides must be conducted in accordance with state laws and regulations, and practitioners must use professional judgment to determine which tasks to delegate to an occupational therapy aide in each particular situation. Finally, site-specific training must be provided along with appropriate supervisory mechanisms to continuously monitor competency (AOTA, 1999b).

Certified Occupational Therapy Assistants

AOTA (1999a) states that a certified occupational therapy assistant must receive supervision from a registered occupational therapist for direct service and that all occupational therapy practitioners must practice and manage occupational therapy programs in accordance with applicable federal and state laws and regulations. These regulatory mandates often identity specific standards for supervision. Most of the state regulatory boards include provisions for the regulation of occupational therapy assistants. Therefore, the registered occupational therapist has a legal and ethical responsibility to provide supervision of the certified occupational therapy assistant.

Supervision must be an interactive process to establish service competence—that is, whenever an occupational therapist delegates a task to an occupational therapy assistant, he or she must ensure that the assistant can perform the same or equivalent procedures with the same results. The supervisor needs to consider the setting and the client population. For example, the certified occupational therapy assistant who is working with a person whose condition is rapidly changing will require more supervision because of the need for frequent evaluation, reevaluation, potential therapy modifications, and the amount of potential risk involved. Regardless of the setting and formal qualifications, the supervisor and supervisee have mutual responsibility to understand each other's educational backgrounds, role competencies, and responsibilities to work as a team (see Chapter 13).

Entry-Level Registered Occupational Therapists

The AOTA (1999a) recommends that entry-level therapists receive close supervision by an intermediate-level or advanced-level registered occupational therapist. It is essential for individuals with limited clinical experience to obtain appropriate supervision and to negotiate for this level of supervision during the initial job interview. Valuing and directly requesting appropriate levels of supervision help ensure quality care.

CONCLUSION

Today's health-care environments are becoming more and more complex. To be successful in these complex situations, practitioners must be able to make judgments based on thoughtful inquiry, analysis, and reflection on practice. All occupational therapy practitioners, regardless of their job title or years of experience, deserve and can benefit from the opportunity to reflect on and analyze their practice. It is through the telling of their experience to others that practitioners can become aware of their unshared biases and presuppositions that affect every interaction with clients. Indeed, clinical supervision is a precious gift that therapists must give to each other and to themselves.

References

Adelstein, L. A., Cohn, E. S., Baker, R. C., & Barnes, M. A. (1990). A part-time level II fieldwork program. *American Journal of Occupational Therapy, 44,* 60–65.

American Occupational Therapy Association. (1999a). Guide for the supervision of occupational therapy personnel in the delivery of occupational therapy services. *American Journal of Occupational Therapy, 53,* 592–594.

American Occupational Therapy Association. (1999b). Guidelines for the use of aides in occupational therapy practice. *American Journal of Occupational Therapy, 53,* 595–598.

American Occupational Therapy Association. (1999c). Standards for an accredited educational program for the occupational therapist. *American Journal of Occupational Therapy, 53,* 575–582.

American Occupational Therapy Association. (1999d). Standards for an accredited educational program for the occupational therapy assistant. *American Journal of Occupational Therapy, 53,* 583–589.

American Occupational Therapy Association. (2000a). Guidelines for an occupational therapy fieldwork experience Level I & II. Bethesda, MD: Author.

American Occupational Therapy Association. (2000b). Occupational therapy code of ethics. *American Journal of Occupational Therapy, 54*, 617–616.

American Occupational Therapy Association. (2000c). Student evaluation of fieldwork experience. Bethesda, MD: Author.

Anderson, J. L. (1988). *The supervisory process in speech-language pathology and audiology*. Boston: Little, Brown

Baum, C. (1998). Client-centered practice in a changing health care system. In M. Law (Ed.). *Client-centered occupational therapy* (pp. 29–45). Thorofare, NJ: Slack.

Blechert, T. F., Christiansen, M. F., & Kari, N. (1987). Intraprofessional team building. *American Journal of Occupational Therapy, 41*, 576–582.

Buckholdt, D. R., & Gubrium, J. F. (1979). Doing staffing. *Human Organization, 38*, 255–264.

Christie, B. A., Joyce, P. C., & Moeller, P. L. (1985). Fieldwork experience 1: Impact on practice preference. *American Journal of Occupational Therapy, 39*, 671–674.

Cohn, E. S., & Crist, P. (1995). Back to the future: New approaches to fieldwork education. *American Journal of Occupational Therapy*, 49, 103–106.

Commission on Education [COE]. (1983). *Fieldwork evaluation for the occupational therapy assistant*. Rockville, MD: American Occupational Therapy Association.

Commission on Education [COE]. (1986). *Fieldwork evaluation for the occupational therapists*. Rockville, MD: American Occupational Therapy Association.

Crepeau, E. B. (1994a). Three images of interdisciplinary team meetings. *American Journal of Occupational Therapy, 48*, 717–722.

Crepeau, E. B. (1994b). Uneasy alliances: Belief and action on a geropsychiatric team. (Doctoral dissertation, University of New Hampshire, 1994). *Dissertation Abstracts International*, 9506410.

Freeman, E. (1985). The importance of feedback in clinical supervision: Implications for direct practice. *Clinical Supervisor, 3*, 5–26.

Golin, A. K., & Duncanis, A. J. (1981). *The interdisciplinary team*. Bethesda, MD: Aspen.

Humphry, R., Gonzalez, S., & Taylor, E. (1993). Family involvement in practice: Issues and attitudes. *American Journal of Occupational Therapy*, 47, 587–593.

Knowles, M. (1980). *The modern practice of adult education*. New York: Association Press.

Leff, P. T., & Walizer, E. H. (1992). *Building the healing partnership: Parents, professionals, and children with chronic illnesses and disabilities*. Cambridge, MA.: Brookline.

Lieberman, A., & Miller, L. (1979). *Staff development: New demands, new realities, new perspectives*. New York: Columbia University Press.

Mish, F. (Ed.). (1997). *The Merriam-Webster dictionary*. Springfield, MA: Merriam-Webster.

Parham, D. (1987). Toward professionalism: The reflective therapist. *American Journal of Occupational Therapy, 41*, 555–561.

Perlmutter, F. D., Bailey, D., & Netting, F. E. (2001). *Managing human resources in the human service*. New York: Oxford University Press.

Phillips, E. C., & Legaspi, W. S. (1995). A 12-month internship model of level II fieldwork. *American Journal of Occupational Therapy*, 49, 146–149.

Pressler, S. (1983). Fieldwork education: The proving ground of the profession. *American Journal of Occupational Therapy, 3*, 163–165.

Rogers, J. C. (1982). Sponsorship: Developing leaders for occupational therapy. *American Journal of Occupational Therapy, 36*, 309–313.

Salisbury, C. (1992). Parents as team members—Inclusive teams, collaborative outcomes. In B. Rainforth, J. York, & C. MacDonald (Eds.). *Collaborative teams for students with severe disabilities* (pp. 43–68). Baltimore: Brookes.

Saxe, J. G. (1871). *The poems of John Godfrey Saxe*. Boston: Fields, Osgood.

Schön, D. (1983). *The reflective practitioner: How professionals think in action*. New York: Basic.

Slater, D. Y., & Cohn, E. S. (1991). Staff development through analysis of practice. *American Journal of Occupational Therapy, 45*, 1038–1044.

Smith, H. L., & Elbert, N. F. (1986). *The health care supervisor's guide to staff development*. Rockville, MD: Aspen Systems.

Stancliff, B. L. (1995, November). Rehabilitation teams versus individual departments. *OT Practice*, 21–22.

Unsworth, C. A., Thomas, S. A., & Greenwood, K. M. (1995). Rehabilitation team decisions on discharge housing for stroke patients. *Archives of Physical Medicine and Rehabilitation, 76*, 331–340.

Wachtel, R. C., & Compart, P. J. (1996). Preparing pediatricians. In D. Bricker & A. Widerstorm (Eds.). *Preparing personnel to work with infants and young children and their families: A team approach* (pp. 181–198). Baltimore: Brookes.

Zenger, J. H., Musselwhite, E., Hurson, K., & Perrin, C. (1994). *Leading teams: Mastering the new role*. Homewood, IL: Business One Irwin.

CHAPTER 48

PROTECTING VULNERABLE CLIENTS

DEBORA A. DAVIDSON

Occupational therapy practitioners define their role as the promotion of safe, socially acceptable occupational performance that is valued by the client and involves healthy interaction with the environment (Moyers, 1999). The Occupational Therapy Code of Ethics cites beneficence, or the demonstration of concern for the well-being of clients, as its first principle (American Occupational Therapy Association, 2000). This clearly includes preventing the abuse and exploitation of occupational therapy clients. Fortunately, occupational therapy practitioners are well positioned to provide this service, as they often establish helping relationships in the settings where clients live, work, and recreate. Furthermore, occupational therapists working with others can initiate and guide systemic improvements that are essential to preventing and ameliorating victimization.

ABUSE, NEGLECT, AND EXPLOITATION

The term **neglect** refers to the withholding of shelter, food, safety, medical care, or positive social and emotional interaction—all of which are necessary for mental and physical health. Abuse is deliberate harm toward a person who is dependent and includes physical actions such as striking or shaking, sexual actions such as fondling or raping, and social actions such as belittling or intimidating (Child Abuse Prevention and Treatment Act, 1996). Exploitation is the unethical use of another, including taking his or her money or belongings (Sampson, 1996).

People with a variety of disabilities are at significantly increased risk of neglect, abuse, and exploitation throughout their life spans (McAllister, 2000). The National Clearinghouse on Child Abuse and Neglect (1995) sponsored a study of 35 representative child protective service agencies that indicated an incidence of maltreatment that was 1.7 times higher for children with disabilities than for those without. In 47% of the cases, the child's disability was thought to have been a causative factor in the abuse. In a survey of agencies serving survivors of sexual abuse and assault, Sobsey (1988) found that 54% of the clients had mental retardation. Another study of women with mild mental retardation found that 71% of the sample had experienced forced or coerced sexual contact (Stromsness, 1993). At least 0.5 million elderly Americans experienced abuse or neglect in 1996 (National Center on Elder Abuse at the American Public Human Services Association, 1998).

Abuse occurs in every setting frequented by persons with disabilities, including homes, schools, work settings, group homes, and residential care facilities (Lumley & Miltenberger, 1997; Marchetti & McCartney, 1990).

CAUSES OF ABUSE AND NEGLECT

Abuse and neglect are the outcomes of dynamic problems that involve the victim, the perpetrator, and their environment (Hoffman-Plotkin, & Twentyman, 1984; McAllister, 2000). A trait shared by most people who become victims of domestic or institutional abuse or neglect is prolonged dependency on others for basic needs, such as shelter, food, clothing, medical care, and belonging. This group includes many people who seek occupational therapy. In addition to dependency, these people may have inherent and learned traits or behaviors that increase their risk of harm by a caregiver. Examples of this include having a high level of activity, being unable to communicate effectively, and responding aggressively.

Those who are unable to report or resist mistreatment are at increased risk of abuse and neglect (Lumley & Miltenberger, 1997; Vondra, 1990). People with cognitive disabilities are often acculturated to be passive and compliant (Tharinger, Horton, & Millea, 1990). They are expected to trust and obey a wide array of caregivers and are often rewarded for being "good" (Lumley & Miltenberger, 1997). Assertive disagreement or resistance to following directives may be construed as problematic or even symptomatic and treated accordingly. Many individuals with limited independence have reduced social lives and are eager to please potential friends, increasing their vulnerability to all types of abuse and exploitation.

People who perpetrate abuse range from the overwhelmed caregiver who occasionally reacts harshly out of exhaustion and despair to the calculating sociopath who deliberately seeks and systematically hurts victims (MacNamara, 1992). Caregivers who are neglectful may lack resources or knowledge of the medical or daily care needs of the individual in their care. Sometimes caregivers have health or life complications of their own and are unable to manage the demands of juggling a complex array of responsibilities (McAllister, 2000). A caregiver's alcohol and drug use increases the risk of abuse, as do mental and personality disorders (Windham, 2000).

Further increasing the risk of abuse is the isolation experienced by family and paid caregivers (Steele, 1980). The community's prevailing attitudes about how to resolve conflict and the value of individuals with disabilities influence individuals' behaviors. Some communities are cohesive and interactive, resulting in available positive support and social scrutiny, a combination that tends to reduce antisocial behavior (Sampson & Groves, 1989). In communities where people commonly verbally and/or physically batter one another, or where neighbors rarely interact at all, vulnerable people are at higher risk of victimization (Vondra, 1990).

THE ROLE OF OCCUPATIONAL THERAPY IN THE PROTECTION OF VULNERABLE CLIENTS

MacNamara (1992) stated, "One reason for the persistence of the problem [of abuse] is that it tends to be treated episodically and not systematically" (p. 4). Occupational therapy practitioners can influence the individual, the caregivers, and the wider environment. Helping clients develop skills that reduce dependency in activities of daily living reduces caregivers' stress and necessary intrusion. The routine involvement of people with disabilities in community functions is another way of reducing the risk of victimization. Not only is social isolation reduced but also the disabled individual has opportunities to develop social and decision-making skills that are antithetical to acting like a victim.

Assertiveness training that specifically teaches individuals to recognize and respond to dangerous or exploitative situations may help clients avoid victimization (Khemka & Hickson, 2000; Lumley & Miltenberger, 1997). Because it is impossible for clients to make good choices without adequate information, sexuality education is especially important (Lumley & Miltenberger, 1997; Tharinger et al., 1990). Occupational therapy practitioners who have completed appropriate educational preparation can make important contributions here, either independently or in conjunction with other professionals on the intervention team.

Most abuse is caused by someone who knows and has access to the victim (Sobsey & Doe, 1991). Caregivers can benefit from a supportive educational approach that includes hands-on training and performance evaluation, which facilitates a sense of empowerment along with needed skills. Helping family caregivers develop a network of family or community members who can regularly provide physical and emotional assistance eases some of the risk of abuse at home. Connecting families with consumer-support groups and social service agencies that provide professional respite, day programs, supervised group living, transportation, or other services to disabled individuals also reduces the risk of abuse and neglect.

When clients enter institutional care, their likelihood of experiencing sexual abuse significantly increases (Lumley & Miltenberger, 1997). Occupational therapy practitioners can provide needed support and information to institutional workers via consultation and during direct intervention (Marchetti & McCartney, 1990). An even more sustaining approach is to advise management on ways to maximize the quality of staffing. Establishing shifts that are predictable and of reasonable duration, providing supervision that is regular and frequent, and requiring staff development and

WHAT'S A PRACTITIONER TO DO? 48-1

Possible Sexual Harassment

Iris is a 23-year-old with Down syndrome who has started to work in a discount retail store, where she stocks shelves and sweeps the floor. Iris receives weekly job coaching by an occupational therapy practitioner, who has been impressed by Iris's developing work habits and social skills. One week, the practitioner noticed that Iris appeared subdued and preoccupied. When she asked Iris how things were going, Iris characteristically answered, "Fine." The practitioner mentioned the changes in Iris to the shift manager, who said that Iris had missed 2 days of work the previous week.

The practitioner then observed Iris and a male coworker, Bob, as they stocked shelves. Bob teased Iris by "accidentally" knocking items off the shelves so that she would then bend over to pick them up as he watched. He called her "hot stuff," which made Iris blush and look uncomfortable. When the practitioner privately asked Iris how she felt about working with Bob, Iris replied, "He bugs me!" Further questioning revealed that Bob had touched Iris inappropriately on occasion.

QUESTION AND EXERCISES

1. Are there indications of harassment or abuse?
2. What ethical considerations are raised?
3. What should be done?

SUMMARY

This situation involves both the client and another employee, and confidentiality is an issue. Iris may feel uncomfortable discussing her concerns in front of others, so the practitioner should sit down with her privately to explore what has happened with Bob. Then Iris, with the practitioner present, should inform the store manager of the concerns. This presents an opportunity for Iris to practice self-reliance. Iris should be praised for her good judgment and courage in doing this. A plan of action that is satisfactory to Iris and the practitioner is then worked out with the manager; this might include the manager's giving Bob a formal warning and reassigning him to another area. The practitioner then agrees to stop by on a daily basis until it is evident that the situation has stabilized.

training help reduce the risk of abuse in institutional settings (MacNamara, 1992).

Another level of preventive intervention lies in the community. Occupational therapy practitioners are positioned to help facilities develop programs that bring community members into the facility and that take residents out into the world. Institutions that encourage volunteer opportunities and open social events and that establish a high profile in the community, provide a healthier environment for both staff members and residents.

RESPONDING TO SITUATIONS OF ABUSE AND NEGLECT

Unfortunately, it is not always possible to prevent abuse from occurring. Occupational therapy practitioners can play an effective role in identifying and altering existing cases of abuse. Often the signs of ongoing physical or sexual abuse are subtle and indirect, especially if the client has limited language, is intimidated, or is habitually compliant. Practitioners must be sensitive to changes in demeanor and nonverbal communication to evaluate the possibility of abuse (Tharinger et al., 1990). Behaviors that may indicate abuse include a client who acts anxious or out of character in the presence of a particular individual, interactions that reflect a pattern of domination or intimidation by one person over another or physical evidence of neglect or abuse.

Practitioners are legally mandated to know their state's regulations and procedures for reporting suspected abuse and to refer cases of suspected abuse or neglect to the appropriate state agency (Schauer, 1995; Tharinger et al., 1990). Individuals who report reasonable concerns to protective services are legally protected from prosecution, even if the situation is determined to be benign. The identities of those making reports remain confidential.

CONCLUSION

Occupational therapy practitioners are strategically positioned, have the knowledge and skills, and are ethically and legally mandated to address the public health concerns of abuse, neglect, and exploitation. Creating and maintaining environments that are free of abuse and exploitation is essential if our society is to reach the goal of full inclusion. All occupational therapy practitioners should be proficient in preventing, identifying, and intervening in cases of suspected or actual abuse.

References

American Occupational Therapy Association. (2000). Occupational therapy code of ethics 2000. Available at: www.aota.org. Accessed 10/7/02.

Child Abuse Prevention and Treatment Act. (1996). P.L. 104-235. 42 U.S.C. 5101, et seq.

Hoffman-Plotkin, D., & Twentyman, C. (1984). A multi-modal assessment of behavioral and cognitive deficits in abused and neglected preschoolers. *Child Development, 55*, 794–802.

Khemka, I., & Hickson, L. (2000). Decision-making by adults with mental retardation in simulated situations of abuse. *Mental Retardation, 38*, 15–26.

Lumley, V., & Miltenberger, R. (1997). Sexual abuse prevention for persons with mental retardation. *American Journal on Mental Retardation, 101*, 459–472.

MacNamara, R. D. (1992). *Creating abuse-free caregiving environments for children, the disabled, and the elderly: Preparing, supervising, and managing caregivers for the emotional impact of their responsibilities*. Springfield, IL: Thomas.

Marchetti, A., & McCartney, J. (1990). Abuse of persons with mental retardation: Characteristics of the abused, the abusers, and the informers. *Mental Retardation, 28*, 367–371.

McAllister, M. (2000). Domestic violence: A life-span approach to assessment and intervention. *Lippincott's Primary Care Practice, 4*, 174–189.

Moyers, P. (1999). The guide to occupational therapy practice. [Special issue]. *American Journal of Occupational Therapy, 53*, 251–322.

National Center on Elder Abuse at the American Public Human Services Association. (1998). The national elder abuse incidence study: Final report. Available at: www.aoa.dhhs.gov/abuse/report. Accessed 10/4/02.

National Clearinghouse on Child Abuse and Neglect. (1995). Abuse and Neglect of Children with Disabilities: Report and Recommendations. Available at: www.calib.com/nccanch/. Accessed 10/4/02.

Sampson, D. (1996). KELN annotated bibliography: Elder abuse: Financial exploitation by a conservator. Available at: www.keln.org/bibs/sampson.html. Accessed 10-4-02.

Sampson, R. J., & Groves, W. B. (1989). Community structure and crime: Testing social-disorganization theory. *American Journal of Sociology, 94*, 775–802.

Schauer, C. (1995). Protection and advocacy: What nurses need to know. *Archives of Psychiatric Nursing, 9*, 233–239.

Sobsey, D. (1988, December). *Sexual abuse and exploitation of people with severe handicaps*. Paper presented at the annual conference of the Association for Persons with Severe Handicaps, Washington, DC.

Sobsey, D., & Doe, T. (1991). Patterns of sexual abuse and assault. *Sexuality and Disability, 9*, 243–259.

Steele, B. (1980). Psychodynamic factors in child abuse. In R. E. Helfer & R. S. Kempe (Eds.). *The battered child* (3rd ed., pp. 49–85). Chicago: University of Chicago Press.

Stromsness, M. M. (1993). Sexually abused women with mental retardation: Hidden victims, absent resources. *Women and Therapy, 14*, 139–152.

Tharinger, D., Horton, C. B., & Millea, S. (1990). Sexual abuse and exploitation of children and adults with mental retardation and other handicaps. *Child Abuse and Neglect, 14*, 301–312.

Vondra, J. (1990). Sociological and ecological factors. In R. E. Helfer & R. S. Kempe (Eds.). *The battered child* (3rd ed., pp. 49–85). Chicago: University of Chicago Press.

Windham, D. (2000). The millennial challenge: Elder abuse. *Journal of Emergency Nursing, 26*, 444–447.

CHAPTER 49

FACILITY-BASED PRACTICE SETTINGS

PAM ROBERTS and MARY EVENSON

Occupational therapy practitioners work in facilities that provide services to children and adults in need of institutional care. They may also provide services to community-based programs such as adult day services or residential programs such as group homes or assisted living. The reasons that individuals require institutional care are often a result of a diagnosis or condition that requires medical, surgical, psychiatric, rehabilitative intervention, and/or social circumstances. As a consequence, individuals experience difficulty performing daily life activities and may be at risk for safely and independently participating in social roles within their communities (World Health Organization, 1998). In these circumstances, occupational therapy assessments and interventions may offer services to help these individuals resume participation in meaningful and productive roles in their daily lives.

TYPES OF FACILITIES

According to the American Hospital Association survey in 1998, there are approximately 5000 hospitals in the United States, 57% not for profit, 15% for profit, and 28% governmental (local, state, and federal). Teaching hospitals account for approximately 20% of facilities and almost 66% of hospital employees work in facilities with more than 1000 workers (U.S. Department of Commerce, 1997).

Facility-based health-care services include skilled care for medical, surgical, rehabilitation, and psychiatric or mental health needs and nonskilled custodial care (meals, housekeeping, etc.) that are provided within the context of an inpatient care setting. Facility-based health-care is a labor-intensive industry operating on a 24-hr-per-day, seven-day-per-week basis (Sultz & Young, 2001). The market trend is to limit facility-based interventions because of the high operating costs of maintaining the physical plant, overhead (e.g., electricity and gas), supplies, and use of personnel over 24 hours per day.

Typically, personnel make up one of the highest percentages of cost expenditures. Personnel needs of licensed versus unlicensed staff are based on patient acuity. Because of the medical instability of intensive care patients. There is usually a higher nursing to patient ratio (1:1 ratio) in intensive care units compared to inpatient rehabilitation. For community-based residential settings such as group homes and assisted living, staffing ratios vary based on state regulations and/or the organizational structure of personnel management.

REIMBURSEMENT ISSUES

According to the Health Care Financing Administration (HCFA)—now called the Centers for Medicare and Medicaid

Services (CMS)—private insurance funds approximately 33% of the total health-care services. Public funds, including Medicare and Medicaid, contribute approximately 45%, out-of-pocket costs account for approximately 18%, and the remaining 4% is from other private funds such as foundations (Health Care Financing Administration Office of the Actuary, 1998). Children and adults under the age of 65 who are not disabled may be covered by a managed care organization or private insurance. Adults who are injured on the job are often covered under worker's compensation, depending on state law. If individuals are uninsured, they may be eligible to apply for state assistance under the Medicaid system or may need to pay privately for health-care services. Individuals who are under the age of 65 and are disabled may be eligible to apply for state or federal assistance. Veterans of the United States military service are eligible to receive health care via the Veterans Administration. In 1966, Medicare was enacted as a means of providing health coverage for the elderly (age 65 and older) and the disabled. Older adults may opt to subscribe to Medicare for health benefits or to receive coverage from a managed care organization, or a combination of benefits.

In an effort to contain costs and standardize care, Congress implemented the Medicare **Prospective Payment System (PPS)** for acute hospitals in 1983. PPS is a means to pay for Medicare services based on criteria set by the government. Since the PPS enactment, a temporary exemption has been in effect for rehabilitation hospitals and units, children's hospitals and units, alcohol and drug programs, long-term care, cancer specialty hospitals, and psychiatric hospitals and units. The acute care PPS is based on over 490 diagnostic related groups (DRGs).

The effect of DRGs has been significant. For many acute diagnoses, the length of stay is usually 1–2 weeks, depending on co-morbidities and complications. Hospital lengths of stay have become shorter, and discharges to all types of postacute care providers, such as inpatient rehabilitation, skilled nursing, and long-term care providers, has risen. In an effort to control costs in the post-acute care arena, the Balanced Budget Act (BBA) of 1997 was enacted. The BBA mandated PPS for nursing facilities in 1998, home-health agencies in 2000, and inpatient rehabilitation in 2001. In the future, PPS requirements will be developed for other exempt units.

CONTINUUM OF CARE AND HEALTH-CARE REGULATIONS

For all facility-based practice, regulatory and legal requirements are the basis of each site's policies and procedures for operation, service delivery, and quality. The purpose of the health-care system must be to reduce the impact and burden of illness, injury, and disability and to improve the health and functioning of the people of the United States (President's Advisory Commission on Consumer Protection and Quality in the Health Care Industry, 1997).

The **continuum of care** is an array of health-care services that are available to individuals based on acuity, level of disability, and resultant level of social participation in the community. These continuum of care services are provided through emergency room care, intensive care, acute care, transitional care, inpatient rehabilitation, inpatient psychiatric, long-term care, adult day services, and residential care. All levels of care are regulated to ensure quality and safety. Standards are intended to reflect current practice or best practice and are administered through such regulatory agencies as the Joint Commission for the Accreditation of Health Care Organizations (JCAHO), the Department of Health and Human Services (DHHS), the Rehabilitation Accreditation Commission (CARF), and individual state departments of public health. Each of these agencies set standards for care, which are revised annually. Standards serve as guidelines to continuously improve the value and responsiveness of quality programs and services. Some examples of standards address safety and security, ethics, patient rights, and staff competencies.

In keeping with a client-centered perspective, it is important for occupational therapy practitioners to take responsibility for facilitating communication in support of the client's transition between the various levels of care. This communication may occur formally or informally with the client, caregivers, and practitioners at each level within the continuum of care. A practitioner's **clinical reasoning** is affected by his or her knowledge and experience and is further shaped by the interactions with the client and team, the severity of the client's condition, the setting, and the level of the continuum of care.

CLIENT-CENTERED CLINICAL REASONING IN FACILITY-BASED PRACTICE

Rehabilitation is a multifaceted process that may involve prevention, evaluation, and intervention for medical conditions; restoration of functional capabilities; facilitation of reintegration; and enhancement of quality of life. Other aspects of rehabilitation include commitment to the continuity of care, interdisciplinary team process, goal-directed interventions, skill development, functional enhancement, and discharge planning. Essential to this process is the direct involvement of clients and/or their caregivers to identify needs, wants, priorities, and desired outcomes.

Occupational therapy practitioners in institutional settings assess how an individual's roles may be affected by illness or injury. An important element of the evaluation process is the occupational therapist's striving to understand the client in terms of his or her life roles, expectations, abilities, and environments. This philosophical approach is in keeping with a top-down model (Mathiowetz & Haugen,

1994; Trombly, 1995a, 1995b), in which occupational therapy practitioners determine what clients perceive to be the important occupational performance issues that are causing them difficulty in carrying out their daily activities in work, self-maintenance, leisure, and rest (Baum & Law, 1997).

A key insight to understanding the client is collaborating with him or her to identify and use intervention activities that are personally meaningful and culturally and developmentally relevant (Christiansen, 1994; Clark et al., 1991; Gray, 1997, 1998). For example, occupational therapy intervention for a man with a traumatic brain injury who wants to return home and resume cooking may involve activities such as making breakfast. This cooking activity also addresses the development of motor skills, such as coordination and mobility, and process skills, such as organization and sequencing (American Occupational Therapy Association, in press; Moyers, 1999).

Clinical reasoning is defined as a dynamic process of inquiry into action that takes place in the context of occupational therapy evaluation and treatment. This process consists of several elements: recalling information and theory, reflecting on one's own observations; analyzing and interpreting the results of the constantly changing problem–decision–action process; and revising the perceived goals, strategies, and procedures. The clinical reasoning process includes a consideration of client's prior level of function, living situation, and medical history. The client's current status, the severity of condition, his or her perception of the disability, and the resources available must also be considered.

The emphasis of occupational therapy needs to focus on the client's abilities to perform his or her occupational roles and activities within the anticipated environmental context. Here, occupational therapy practitioners use their conditional reasoning to imagine what possibilities may lie ahead in the future for a given client (Mattingly & Fleming, 1994). A storytelling, or narrative reasoning, approach may be useful for the practitioner and client to construct an image of the client's future (Mattingly & Fleming, 1994). Priorities may include prevention of secondary complications, remediation to reduce deficits, compensation to limit or adapt to residual limitations, and the maintenance of long-term function. For facility-based care, the ultimate goal of occupational therapy is to return the client to full participation in daily life within the individual's capabilities.

Within many acute care facility-based systems, the occupational therapist's role has shifted from one of providing acute medical or psychiatric intervention to one of performing screenings and assessments to facilitate discharge recommendations and identify needs for continued care. As part of the evaluation process, it is essential for the therapist to use interactive reasoning skills in talking with clients and/or their caregivers and social supports about their daily routines and occupational performance problems. Interviewing may be accomplished informally or formally. Factors that may prohibit occupational therapists' ability to gather necessary information include the acuity or severity of the client's condition and limited or no access to family or caregivers (Neistadt, 1995).

Use of formal assessment measures has been found to optimize **client collaboration** in goal setting and maximizing goal achievement (Neistadt, 1995). Client collaboration is defined as an approach to treatment that uses a philosophy of respect for, and partnership with, the individual receiving the service. Specifically, formal measures such as the Occupational Performance History Interview (Kielhofner et al., 1998), the Canadian Occupational Performance Measure (COPM) (Law et al., 1994), and use of goal attainment scaling (Ottenbacher & Cusick, 1990) may assist occupational therapists in identifying clients' priorities when shaping the intervention plan. Using a comprehensive occupational performance approach, such as the COPM, occupational therapists are able to obtain information about the individual client's perception of his or her abilities and satisfaction with performance in the areas of self-care, work, productivity, and leisure performance.

Neistadt's (1995) survey of adult physical disabilities settings suggested that therapists inconsistently use formal assessment measures and procedures. Many clients' underlying problems are identified, and occupational therapy

HISTORICAL NOTE 49–1 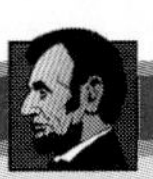

Johnnie on the SPOT: The Profession's View of Environments

SUZANNE M. PELOQUIN

Although the founders of the Society for the Promotion of Occupational Therapy (SPOT) held singular views, they shared the common perspective that occupation could help individuals in a variety of circumstances. The letters that abbeviated the Society's name pleased George Edward Barton:

> ***I am strongly in favor of the National Society for the Promotion of Occupational Therapy as a title. I know that it is long but it does tell the story and the S. P. O. T. suggests the ever alert "Johnnie." (quoted in Licht, 1967, p. 272)***

Some among us may not recall that the early-twentieth-century phrase Johnny-on-the-spot, which designated a person in the right place with the just-right timing and ever-handy tool. Many current therapists enjoy a similar reputation.

Barton's reference to the "spot" in question reveals the long-standing interest that occupational therapists have had in the environments, or spots, within which individuals find and occupy themselves. The continuity of the profession, embedded within the larger issue of its relevance, hinges on the degree to which therapists stay alert to the environments within which they practice.

Licht, S. (1967). The founding and founders of the American Occupational Therapy Association. *American Journal of Occupational Therapy, 21,* 269–277.

TABLE 49–1. **CHARACTERISTICS OF FACILITY-BASED PRACTICE SETTINGS**

Type of Care	Who Benefits?	Typical Settings	Special Services Provided	Role of Occupational Therapy	Typical Length of Stay	Requirements
Acute medical or surgical care	Need for medical or surgical stabilization; 24-hour physician and nursing care; *typical diagnoses:* cerebral palsy, stroke, brain injury, spinal cord injury, congestive heart failure, pulmonary disease, hip fracture, cancer	Private, community, or Veteran's, Administration, or specialty hospital	Trauma services; ICU; medical services; surgical services; consultations by allied health-care providers	Positioning, ROM, and sensory stimulation; assessment of client's abilities, roles, habits, and routines; safety assessment; functional survival skills such as eating, dysphagia, grooming, hygiene, and toileting; discharge planning; recommendations for continued services at the next level of care	Depends on diagnosis (DRG), usually 1–2 weeks	Need for medical or surgical diagnosis or intervention; admitted from the emergency room, direct admit, or transfer from another facility
Skilled nursing	People who require special, 24-hour care for either a short or extended period of time; *diagnoses:* acute care	Unit in a hospital; freestanding nursing home	Physician; nursing; physical therapy; occupational therapy; speech therapy; social services; activity therapy; other services by consultation	Short-term care is more intensive with specified frequency; long-term care is by consultation; self-care skills such as eating, dysphagia, grooming, upper and lower body dressing, hygiene, and toileting; mobility skills during ADL such as transfers and locomotion activities; home management and community skills such as car transfers, kitchen activities, public dining, care of pets	Short term: not to exceed 100 days; long term: indefinite or as needed	Bridge the gap with another level of care; admitted from acute care hospital; skilled intervention such as intravenous medication, wound care; disability with a new functional deficit
Inpatient rehabilitation	People who require a comprehensive rehabilitation program; 75% of clients must have a diagnosis within the HCFA 10 diagnostic groups (Stroke, spinal cord injury, congenital deformity, amputation, major multiple trauma, lower extremity fracture, brain injury, polyarthritis including rheumatoid arthritis, neurological disorders, burns)	Freestanding rehabilitation center; unit within a hospital; Veteran's Administration	Rehabilitation physician; rehabilitation nursing; physical therapy; occupational therapy; speech therapy; recreational therapy; neuropsychology or psychology; social services; other services by consultation	Comprehensive evaluation; participation in functional outcome such as FIM™; self-care skills; functional mobility, communication, and social cognition during ADL; home management skills; community reintegration; discharge planning; recommendations for continued services at the next level of care	Usually 2–4 weeks; target length of stays by diagnostic categories, usually from national benchmarks	Transfer from a hospital, nursing home, or home; must be able to tolerate intensive therapy for a minimum of 3 hours per day 5–6 days per week; must require care from two disciplines

Inpatient psychiatry	People who require special, 24-hour care for either a short or extended period of time; *typical diagnoses (DSM IV-TR):* depression, schizoaffective disorders, mood disorders, obsessive compulsive disorders, anxiety, phobic disorders	Community or private hospital; unit within a hospital; Veteran's Administration	Psychiatry; nursing; occupational therapy; therapeutic recreation; psychology; social services; mental health workers; art, expressive or music therapy; behavior management; other consultations as needed	Assessment of client's abilities, roles, habits, and routines; safety assessment; functional skills such as self-care, home and community function; may administer the Allen Cognitive Level Screen; individual and/or group treatment; discharge planning; recommendations for continued services at the next level of care	Usually 1–3 weeks	Need for psychiatric diagnosis or intervention; admitted from the emergency room, direct admit, or transfer from another facility; client who requires 24-hour monitoring for safety; may be court ordered as with forensic cases in which clients require secured (locked) units because of safety risk to self or others
Partial hospitalization	People who require episodic focused psychiatric intervention; *diagnoses:* inpatient psychiatry	Community or private hospital; unit within a hospital; Veteran's Administration	Psychiatry; occupational therapy; therapeutic recreation; psychology; mental health workers; social services	Assessment of client's abilities, roles, habits, and routines; continuity of care for self-management goals with emphasis on productive living for home and community; individual and/or group treatment; recommendations for continued services at the next level of care	Usually 1–3 months	Transition from inpatient or as an alternative to acute psychiatric hospitalization; structured program
Long-term care (physical and mental)	People who need constant 24-hour care for an indefinite period of time and for whom a functional recovery may be not be possible or who lack the resources to be safe at home; *diagnoses:* mental retardation and see acute care and inpatient psychiatry	Community, private, or state hospital; freestanding or private nursing home; Veteran's Administration	Physicians or psychiatrists; nursing; mental health workers; therapy consultation as indicated for positioning, functional mobility during ADL, adaptations, and caregiver training; behavioral management; custodial care such as eating, dysphagia, grooming, and bathing	Individual assessment and interventions as indicated; consultant to program for ADL, environmental adaptations, and behavior management	Variable; indefinite	Transfer from a hospital, nursing home, or home; bridge gap between inpatient setting and home versus determine need for permanent placement; person needs assistance with ADL
Adult day services	Attend on a planned basis; people who are older than 18 with any type of functional impairment; elderly; physical disabilities; mental disabilities; developmental disabilities	Community-based program (usually freestanding); associated with a senior	Physician order; nursing; therapy; social services; art; music; movement; games; current events; computer; meals;	Consultation; individual assessment and interventions as indicated; wellness programs; activities programs; directors of adult day services	Average 18–26 months for elderly populations; maybe long term for	Varies by individual programs

Continues

TABLE 49–1. **CHARACTERISTICS OF FACILITY-BASED PRACTICE SETTINGS** *(Continued)*

Type of Care	Who Benefits?	Typical Settings	Special Services Provided	Role of Occupational Therapy	Typical Length of Stay	Requirements
		center, community-based mental health center, assisted-living organization; hospital; or skilled nursing facility	transportation; community outings		individuals with neurological and/or degenerative diagnoses	
Group homes	People who need 24-hour residential care; *diagnoses:* developmental disabilities, brain injury, spinal cord injury, mental health/behavioral diagnoses	Congregate living in a house	Physician order; mental health workers; therapy consultation as indicated for positioning, functional mobility during ADL, adaptations, and caregiver training; behavioral management; custodial care such as eating, dysphagia, grooming, and bathing	Consultation; individual assessment and interventions as indicated	May be transitional or long term	Vary by state regulations
Assisted living	Need for residential care to some degree; *diagnoses:* Alzheimer disease, frail elderly, neurologically impaired, developmentally disabled, HIV/AIDS, general aging population	Congregate living; home-like building; apartment	Physician order; nursing; therapy consultation as indicated for positioning, functional mobility during ADL, adaptations, and caregiver training; social services; art; music; movement services; dance; games; current events computers; library; transportation; chaplaincy; pharmacy; beauty salons; health spas; custodial care such as eating, dysphagia, grooming, and bathing	Individual assessment and interventions as indicated; wellness programs; swim programs; activity programs	Average 18–27 months	Usually people who no longer want to care for their own homes, lost spouse, losing memory, falling at home; children feel parents are unsafe

ADL, activities of daily living; *DRG,* diagnosis-related group; *FIM™,* Functional Independence Measure; *HCFA,* Health Care Financing Administration; *ICU,* intensive care unit; *ROM,* range of motion.

practitioners select interventions geared toward improving the performance components without active involvement of the client and caregivers. Changes realized in performance components do not necessarily create changes in occupational performance. Whereas use of an adaptive approach, using occupationally based activities, has been shown to enhance achievement of occupational outcomes (Gray, Kennedy, & Zemke, 1996; Trombly, 1995a).

Based on the information from the evaluation process, ideally, the client, caregivers, occupational therapy practitioner, and the team collaborate to finalize the intervention plan, which is influenced by the context of the setting and the needs and goals of the client. Furthermore, the occupational therapy practitioner may assume the role of an advocate, representing the client's goals to the team of health-care providers. The format of intervention depends on the specific client's needs and may include individual and/or group intervention sessions. Some institutions may have protocols, clinical pathways, or care maps that constitute a standardized course of care for a given diagnosis or condition. Regardless of intervention method, outcomes are the true test of the client's ability to function successfully after discharge from the facility.

The insurance industry, state and federal governments, employers, and consumer groups also focus on using outcomes research to assist in making better and more informed decisions about health care. In general, these measures often include the client's functional status, well-being, and satisfaction with services and care (Sultz & Young, 2001).

FACILITY-BASED PRACTICE SETTINGS

According to regulations by JCHAO, facilities must provide age-appropriate services for infants, toddlers, children, adolescents, adults, and older adults. Discrete physical areas are required for pediatrics and adult populations. In most instances, facilities provide general care for a variety of individual needs; however, specialized programs may be offered within a facility or as a separate freestanding program. In physical medicine and rehabilitation settings, specialized services include, but are not limited to, congenital problems such as cerebral palsy, stroke, spinal cord injury, brain injury, and orthopedic, arthritis, cardiac, and pulmonary conditions. For psychiatric settings, specialized programs include services that address, but are not limited to, failure to thrive, substance abuse, depression, eating disorders, mood disturbances, schizoaffective, schizophrenia, anxiety, and phobic conditions.

Long-term care settings, such as nursing homes or state hospital and community-based residential settings provide skilled and nonskilled services to assist individuals with chronic conditions who require extended or permanent placement. Examples of chronic conditions are developmental delay, mental retardation, autism, psychosis, dementia, and neurological or degenerative diagnoses (e.g., muscular dystrophy, cystic fibrosis, multiple sclerosis).

For acute or short-term care, planning for discharge from the hospital should begin on the day of admission and involve a systematic process, resulting in a collaborative decision made by the client, physician, family members, and hospital personnel. The level of assistance required by the individual to manage self-care, bladder and bowel, and mobility must be considered. Furthermore, medical and/or disability insurance coverage and psychosocial resources are also important factors in discharge planning. Collaborative discharge planning goals often focus on identifying a safe place of residence, providing training for family and/or caregivers, and making arrangements for continued medical, psychiatric, therapeutic, and/or residential services. When possible, preferable discharges are to home or community settings.

Table 49-1 describes the continuum of care in a variety of settings. Community-based discharges include returning an individual to their prior living situation, relocation to live with family or friends, or relocation to alternative community settings such as group homes or assisted living. Adults living at home may be entitled to adult day services, which are sometimes associated with a facility such as a hospital or community-based mental health center. Other examples of residential programs are group homes and assisted living. These programs provide congregate living in a variety of settings from a house to an apartment. Populations served by these settings include individuals who are at risk for independent living in the community.

In each of these settings, a physician's order is required to initiate occupational therapy evaluation and intervention. Within these settings, occupational therapy practitioners work with other health-care providers. The composition of the team depends on the needs of the client. Usually, the facility-based team includes a physician, nurse, and allied health professionals. The community-based team includes a combination of skilled and unskilled care providers.

CONCLUSION

Today's health-care environment is ever changing and complex. Facility-based occupational therapy practice needs to be focused on the clients based on where they are receiving services within the continuum of care. Other factors that may affect the client's transition through the continuum, and ultimate outcome, are the severity of the disability, comorbidities, and personal resources such as social and financial support systems. Facility-based care requires teamwork, which can be informal or formal. Occupational therapy practitioners have the opportunity to advocate for clients to identify necessary transitions and resources at the next level within the continuum of care. Examples of such referrals are to home care, outpatient, and community-based settings.

Occupational therapy practitioners must keep in mind clients' priorities as related to satisfaction and participation in everyday life. The role of occupational therapy is to support the clients' successful reintegration into the home and community.

References

American Hospital Association. Resource Center fact sheet: Fast fax on U.S. hospitals from hospital statistics. http://www.ana.org/resource. Accessed August 14, 2000.

American Occupational Therapy Association. (in press). Occupational therapy practice framework: Domain and process. *American Journal of Occupational Therapy*.

Baum, C. M., & Law, M. (1997). Occupational therapy practice: Focusing on occupational performance. *American Journal of Occupational Therapy, 51*, 277–288.

Christiansen, C. (1994). Classification and study in occupation: A review and discussion of taxonomies. *Journal of Occupational Science (Australia), 1*(3), 3–21.

Clark, F. A., Parham, D., Carlson, M. E., Frank, G., Jackson, J., Pierce, D., Wolfe, R. J., & Zemke, R. (1991). Occupational science: Academic innovation in the service of occupational therapy's future. *American Journal of Occupational Therapy, 45*, 300–310.

Gray, J. M. (1997). Application of the phenomenological method to the concept of occupation. *Journal of Occupational Science (Australia), 4*(1), 5–17.

Gray, J. M. (1998). Putting occupation into practice: Occupation as ends, occupation as means. *American Journal of Occupational Therapy, 52*, 354–364.

Gray, J. M., Kennedy, B. L., & Zemke, R. (1996). Application of dynamic systems theory to occupation. In R. Zemke & F. Clark (Eds.). *Occupational science: The evolving discipline* (pp. 309–324). Philadelphia: Davis.

Health Care Financing Administration, Office of the Actuary. (1998). The nation's healthcare dollar: 1998, Where the healthcare dollar went. Available at: www.hcfa.gov/stats/nhe-oact/tables/chart.html. Accessed July 1, 2000.

Kielhofner, G., Mallinson, T., Crawford, C., Nowak, M., Rigby, M., Henry, A., & Walens, D. (1998). *A user's manual for the Occupational Performance History Interview* (version 2.0). Chicago: University of Illinois.

Law, M., Baptiste, S., Carswell, A., McColl, M., Polatajko, H., & Pollock, N. (1994). *The Canadian Occupational Performance Measure* (2nd ed.). Toronto: Canadian Association of Occupational Therapists.

Mathiowetz, V., & Haugen, J. B. (1994). Motor behavior research: implications for therapeutic approaches to central nervous system dysfunction. *American Journal of Occupational Therapy, 48*, 733–745.

Mattingly, C., & Fleming, M. H. (1994). *Clinical reasoning: Forms of inquiry in a therapeutic practice*. Philadelphia: Davis.

Moyers, P. A. (1999). Guide to occupational therapy practice. *American Journal of Occupation Therapy, 53*, 247–322.

Neistadt, M. E. (1995). Methods of assessing client's priorities: A survey of adult physical dysfunction settings. *American Journal of Occupational Therapy, 49*, 428–436.

Ottenbacher, K. J., & Cusick, A. (1990). Goal attainment scaling as a method of clinical service evaluation. *American Journal of Occupational Therapy, 44*, 519–526.

President's Advisory Commission on Consumer Protection and Quality in the Health Care Industry. (1997). *Quality first: Better health care for all Americans: Final report to president of the United States*. [DHHS Publication No. HE 20.6502: Q 2/2]. Washington, DC: U.S. Government Printing Office.

Sultz, H. A., & Young, K. M. (2001). *Healthcare USA: Understanding its organization and delivery*. Gaithersburg, MD: Aspen.

Trombly, C. A. (1995a). Occupation: Purposefulness and meaningfulness as therapeutic mechanisms. *American Journal of Occupational Therapy, 49*, 960–972.

Trombly, C. A. (1995b). Theoretical foundations for practice. In C.A. Trombly (Ed.). *Occupational therapy for physical dysfunction* (4th ed., pp. 15–27). Baltimore: Williams & Wilkins.

U.S. Department of Commerce. (1997). *County business patterns* [Economics and Statistics Administration, U.S. Census Bureau, CBP/97-6]. Washington, DC: U.S. Government Printing Office.

World Health Organization. (1998). ICIDH-2: *International classification of impairments, disabilities, handicaps: A manual of classification relating to the consequences of disease*. Geneva: Author.

CHAPTER 50

COMMUNITY-BASED PRACTICE ARENAS

LOU ANN GRISWOLD

Community-based occupational therapy practitioners support people in the context of their daily lives. Their goal is to enable people to function within their natural environments to play, work, and experience a sense of belonging (Grady, 1995). Through community-based interventions practitioners help people acquire skills to address their immediate occupational needs and to learn strategies for greater long-term life satisfaction (Baum, 1998). Beyond providing services to individuals, community-based practitioners may provide services to community agencies, taking on the role of consultant, program planner, evaluator, or staff trainer (Scaffa, 2001).

Each community setting has a particular mission with its own goals and priorities, often quite different from medical-model settings. For example, public schools are organized within an educational model, whereas early intervention and home-health care use a family-centered model for service delivery. Community-based practitioners draw on their full range of occupational therapy knowledge, skills, and values to provide services, individuals, and community agencies. Practitioners must be flexible and use a variety of intervention approaches in the community: establishing or restoring skills, selecting a setting or task to ensure a better match between skills and expectations, modifying the task demands, preventing additional problems, and creating circumstances that enhance task performance (Dunn, Brown, & McGuigan, 1994). Furthermore, strong communication skills are essential when practitioners collaborate with clients, family members, and other team members.

This chapter describes occupational therapy practice in community settings where occupational therapy services are well established. Beyond the public school setting, these include agencies that provide early intervention, work hardening, home health care, community mental health services, and adult day care. Scenarios are given for each setting, using pseudonyms for the client examples. The chapter closes with a brief discussion of emerging opportunities for occupational therapy practitioners to serve their communities.

EARLY INTERVENTION

Early intervention programs use a family-centered model to meet the developmental, educational, and social needs of children under 3-years of age who have a disability, have a developmental delay, or are at risk for delay (Case-Smith, 1998a). These services build on the strengths of families and provide resources and expertise to meet the needs of all family members (Case-Smith, 1998a; Rosenbaum, King, Law, King, & Evans, 1998). An early intervention team typically includes an early childhood educator, speech-and-language pathologist, occupational therapy practitioner, physical therapist, social worker, and family members. In family-centered models, family members are equal members of the team and participate in all aspects of planning the child's care (Case-Smith, 1998b).

Occupational therapy practitioners in early intervention often work in a transdisciplinary manner, sharing their expertise with other team members and implementing therapeutic activities from other professionals. In this setting, occupational therapy focuses on enhancing a child's ability to play and interact with family members and participate in age-appropriate eating and dressing tasks. The practitioner works toward these goals by promoting the child's ability to move with purpose and develop gross and fine motor skills while enhancing social and cognitive abilities. Occupational therapy practitioners also help parents understand their child's behavior, enable the child and family to compensate for the disability, and support family members (Case-Smith, 1998b).

A Day in Early Intervention

Joan has a car full of toys, as she travels from house to house to provide services to children and their families. Joan usually visits five to six children in a day. Her first stop is Sam's house, where she helps Sam's mother give him a bath. Sam has recently been diagnosed with cerebral palsy, so Joan focuses both on Sam's needs and on his parent's concerns. First, Joan makes suggestions to decrease the stiffness in Sam's body for easier bathing and dressing. Then she spends about 20 minutes talking with Sam's mother about their adjustment.

The other children Joan sees are a 15-month-old little boy who is blind, two children with Down syndrome, one little girl who had neurological damage after falling into a lake, and two children who have general developmental delays. For each child, Joan provides play activities that focus on developing his or her movement patterns and cognitive skills. Joan includes parents and older brothers and sisters in the these activities—and even a family dog who retrieves a ball kicked by a 2-year-old as Joan facilitates balance reactions. Joan also talks with the parents to be sure that the interventions fit with the feelings, needs, and goals of each family.

SCHOOL SYSTEMS

Schools teach children how to read, write, and understand and use mathematical concepts. They also socialize students to collaborate with others and to become aware of the world in which they live to prepare the children for their future roles as community members. Children who have a disability that prevents or inhibits them from learning often receive special education. These students may have difficulty moving within their environment; using their hands to write; taking in, processing, and using information; or getting along with others. Teachers (classroom, physical education, and special education), the student's parents, a speech-and-language pathologist, an occupational therapy practitioner, a psychologist, and a guidance counselor form the school placement team. The team determines if the student has a disability that interferes with learning. If so, the team members develop an **individual education program** (IEP) to meet the student's educational needs and goals.

An IEP addresses the child's learning needs in an environment that is most typical for students at that age (Giangreco, 1995; Hanft & Place, 1996). Practitioners support the child's successful participation in regular classroom activities by modifying the environment, adapting tasks, or introducing learning activities to promote skill development. Practitioners consult with teachers and school personnel to support the student's performance, to work with a group of children in a classroom, or sometimes to see the child individually (Dunn & Campbell, 1991).

A Day in a School Setting

Mike begins his workday at 7:45 with a team meeting to discuss Rachel, a 10-year-old with learning disabilities. Together, the team of eight members discusses modification of classroom activities that will enhance Rachel's learning but are similar to those of her classmates. Mike then provides four children with 20 minutes of sensory motor activities to improve their ability to organize and sequence their work in the classroom. Mike observes a student's performance in class and during recess. He also leads class activities to help children with their coordination and manipulation skills and attends two gym classes, adapting the activities for children with disabilities, so that all of the children may participate. Mike is pleased to note that his adaptations result in greater peer interaction for the children with disabilities.

During lunch, Mike meets with a teacher about the child he observed to develop strategies to help the student stay on task. He spends 1 hour after lunch evaluating a student's motor abilities and the next 30 minutes working on a report that he will finish at home in the evening. He ends his day in an after-school meeting with the school's kindergarten teachers to discuss prerequisite skills for handwriting and introduces them to activities that enhance manipulative skills.

WORK REHABILITATION PROGRAMS

Work programs are designed for people who have a work-related injury to enable them return to the workforce. Clients may have a wide range of problems, the most common being lumbar spine injuries, carpal tunnel syndrome, cervical spine injuries, shoulder injuries, and hand/wrist tendonitis (King, 1993). Because active, physical jobs are more likely to result in injury, the majority of work program clients are males between 26 and 46 years of age (King, 1993). The team in work programs generally consists of occupational therapy practitioners and physical therapists working with employment supervisors to modify work sites and production lines.

Goals for an injured employee relate specifically to each person's job and diagnosis. Typical goals are reconditioning, controlling symptoms, and managing stress. Occupational therapy services include evaluating physical capacity and functional limitations and developing skills by providing graded work simulation. Work site modifications or assistive devices may also improve performance and prevent future injuries. As people are forced to recognize physical limitations they may experience a change in self-esteem. Occupational therapy practitioners also address this and other disability-related psychosocial issues (Biernacki, 1993) and help people examine the variety of roles and abilities they have to modify their self-perceptions.

Beyond its rehabilitative focus, occupational therapy emphasizes prevention of injury and cumulative trauma in work settings. This involves an understanding of ergonomics, the study and design of work sites and methods to enable safe and productive performance (Isernhagen, Hart, & Matheson, 1998; Jundt & King, 1999). Work-site assessment and education to prevent injury is a crucial part of the practitioner's concern (King, 1993).

A Day in a Work Rehabilitation Program

Catherine begins her day by providing an early morning educational program to the employees at a manufacturing company. She shares information about body mechanics and provides general recommendations regarding sitting posture and work-space adjustments to prevent shoulder and neck pain. She sets up appointments with individual employees to assess their specific work site.

Catherine then goes to the outpatient unit of a hospital where she assesses a new client for his strength and work capacity, using job-related functions. She continues her day working with clients in job simulations, using work simulators of physical demands of their jobs and aerobic training equipment (Wyrick, Niemeyer, Ellexson, Jacobs, & Taylor, 1991).

Catherine meets with a young man to discuss how he can use leisure activities to reduce the stress, anxiety, and depression he is experiencing because of his disability. She ends her day with a job-site analysis for a client who had been injured on the job. Her analysis includes assessing the work environment; the physical demands of the job; the machines, tools, and equipment used, and the worker traits required for the job (McCormack, 1990; Niemeyer, 1989). Catherine's job analysis has a dual purpose: adapting the job tasks for the client referred for therapy and preventing future injuries for him and his colleagues. She will report her recommendations to the factory supervisor next week.

HOME HEALTH CARE

Home health care promotes independent functioning to enable people to live at home. It blends the medical model and family-centered model, as services are medically determined, yet provided with greater awareness of the home environment and family dynamics. Home health practitioners support people who have an injury or illness, promoting their ability to perform self-care, home-making, or leisure tasks independently and safely. Although any age group can receive home health care, most clients are elderly. The most common diagnoses include neurological, orthopedic, and general medical conditions (Gifford, Wooster, Gray, & Chromiak, 2001).

Some clients have rehabilitation goals designed to increase their skills, while others need modification of daily tasks to compensate for functional losses. In addition, because the caregivers may have multiple demands on their time and energy, home-health providers also address the caregivers' physical and emotional needs (Brittingham & Dempster, 1990; Clark, Corcoran, & Gitlin, 1995; Toth-Cohen, 2000). Team members include nursing personnel, physician, physical therapist, speech therapist, and home-health aide.

Occupational therapy supports clients in reaching the highest level of competence and satisfaction in daily life. A practitioner might modify a task or an aspect of the environment to enable greater independence or train the client in techniques for energy conservation and task simplification or train caregivers to provide assistance for functional mobility and transfers (Gifford et al., 2001).

A Day in Home Health

Renee has learned to be flexible in her role as a home-health occupational therapist. As she travels around the city to clients' homes, she never knows the issues that might arise and the professional and personal skills she will need to use. Her days begin at various times, depending on the clients she will visit that day. Today, Renee begins at 9:00 to assist Mr. Tully in daily living skills. Mr. Tully has **Parkinson disease** and is experiencing rigid movements and decreased mobility; he wants to improve his ability to care for himself in the morning to reduce the help his wife must give him. Renee observes Mr. Tully as he showers and dresses himself. She recommends modifications to the bathroom and shows Mr. and Mrs. Tully some safety hazards they need to consider relative to Mr. Tully's shuffling gait. They discuss these hazards and potential solutions. Mr. and Mrs. Tully report that he is most unsafe as he walks down the long hallway in their home. Renee suggests better lighting and a handrail for Mr. Tully to hold onto as he walks.

Next, Renee assesses Mrs. George, who has just been discharged from the hospital after having hip surgery. Mrs. George is concerned about her leisure activities, especially gardening. She wants to continue to tend her rose bed. Rene and Mrs. George discuss various stools and seats that would enable Mrs. George to continue gardening within the limits of her range of motion. Mrs. George's son agreed to go to the garden center to try several of these options and bring home the gardening stool that works the best.

On her third visit for the day, Renee works with Mr. and Mrs. Watters. Mr. Watters is recovering from a stroke that has left him with severe right-sided hemiplegia and little speech. Consequently, he depends on his wife for his care. Renee helps Mrs. Watters devise a new routine so that she can tend to her husband's needs and have the time to pursue her quilting hobby. They discuss the possibility of a home-health aide to reduce some of Mrs. Watters's responsibilities. Renee calls the nursing supervisor to request these services before she leaves. Renee dictates notes in her car about each of the therapy sessions, which a secretary will transcribe for her. Her day ends with another home evaluation and hour in the office to order equipment and call the clients whom she will see tomorrow.

COMMUNITY MENTAL HEALTH

Community mental health programs have emerged because of federal legislation that deinstitutionalized care for people with pervasive mental illness such as **schizophrenia** and **bipolar disorder** (Scheinholz, 2001). Because many people with chronic psychiatric illness have difficulty living independently, these programs focus on providing support to foster greater community integration and prevent decompensation and hospitalization (Richert & Merryman, 1987).

Community mental health teams include psychiatrists, psychiatric nurses, rehabilitation workers, social workers, occupational therapy practitioners, and other therapists who provide art, music, or movement therapy. Occupational therapy services focus on teaching and promoting basic living skills for work, self-care, and leisure using a home and community environment (Wilberding, 1991). Occupational therapy promotes personal hygiene, home management, interpersonal skills, coping strategies, job readiness, money management, transportation, and participation in leisure activities. (Azok & Tomlinson, 1994; Brown, Shiels, & Hall, 2001; Earle-Grimes, 1994; Richert & Merryman, 1987; Wilberding, 1991).

A Day in Community Mental Health

Karen works in a community mental health center that uses the clubhouse model (Royeen & Ramsay, 2000; Scheinholz, 2001). Clients who participate in the program are considered members of the club. All members participate in decision making, clerical work, meal preparation, and maintenance of the clubhouse. About 20 members participate daily from 9:00 A.M. until about 4:00 P.M.

The day begins with a club meeting during which the community makes decisions about activities and behavioral expectations. Karen frequently co-leads this meeting with the nurse. At 10:00, members join an activity group. These groups reflect member interest and vary substantially from one week to the next. Karen rotates among the groups, but

RESEARCH NOTE 50–1

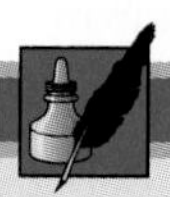

Community-Based Services: A Rich Opportunity for Occupational Therapy Research

In a health policy report sponsored by the Institute of Medicine, Iglehart (1995) predicted that by the year 2005 the majority of all health-care services in the United States will be provided outside traditional hospital and rehabilitation facilities. This migration to home- and community-based service delivery represents an unprecedented research opportunity for occupational therapists.

Occupational therapy interventions, when properly planned, implemented, and evaluated, have their greatest impact in the clients' natural (home or community) environment. Helewa et al. (1991) reported an example of the effectiveness of a home-based program of occupational therapy intervention for individuals with rheumatoid arthritis. A total of 105 clients between 18 and 70 years of age were randomly assigned to receive a 6-week comprehensive program of occupational therapy (experimental group) or to receive no occupational therapy treatment (control group). At the end of the 6 weeks, the control subjects began to receive occupational therapy and the subjects in the experimental group continued to receive intervention as needed. Outcomes were measured at baseline, 6 weeks and 12 weeks. At 6 weeks, individuals in the experimental group receiving occupational therapy scored significantly higher on global measures of functional assessment. Helewa et al. concluded "occupational therapy leads to a statistically significant and clinically important improvement in function in patients with rheumatoid arthritis (p. 1453)".

Helewa, A., Goldsmith, C. H., Lee, P. Bombardier, C., Hanes, B. Smythe, A., & Tugwell, P. (1991). Effects of occupational therapy home service on patients with rheumatoid arthritis. *Lancet*, 337, 1453–1456.

Iglehart, J. K. (1995). Health policy report: Rapid changes for academic health centers. *New England Journal of Medicine*, 332, 407–411.

spends most of her time in the kitchen where a group prepares lunch for all club members. Karen incorporates nutrition, time management, and basic cooking information into the morning activities. Karen and the other staff eat lunch with all club members, modeling social interactions and communication skills.

After lunch, Karen goes to the greenhouse. As members tend to the plants, Karen supports the development of their attention to task and their ability to collaborate with others in a respectful manner. The development of these skills will contribute to their goal of returning to work.

In the late afternoon, Karen accompanies Joe, a young adult, to a fast-food restaurant where he is just beginning a job as a cook. She observes Joe working to assess his ability to meet job demands, most especially his ability to follow the steps necessary to cook hamburgers and french fries, maintain consistent focus on the task, and collaborate with other staff members. After the observation, they discuss his performance and ways to improve his ability to follow instructions and to communicate with other staff members.

ADULT DAY CARE

Adult day-care services provide meaningful, structured activities designed to provide a safe environment so that people with severe disabilities or chronic illness can continue to live at home. Adult day care enables caregivers to continue working or to have a respite from the day-to-day responsibilities involved in caring for a family member who may have diagnoses such as cerebrovascular accident, rheumatoid arthritis, Parkinson disease, multiple sclerosis, and dementia. In addition, these programs provide the opportunity for social interaction and engagement for people who otherwise would be alone at home.

Adult day-care programs vary but often provide health, social, and recreational services for the clients and supportive services for family members (Van Slyke, 2001). Adult day care programs are typically interdisciplinary with nursing personnel, occupational therapy practitioners, social workers, and recreational therapists collaborating to develop individual client programs (Van Slyke, 2001).

Occupational therapy focuses on a person's ability to engage in self-care and leisure activities while maintaining or enhancing cognitive abilities and communication skills (American Occupational Therapy Association, 1986a). Practitioners may work with individuals on specific goals or may provide consultation to the program to promote general activities to meet the clients' needs (Van Slyke, 2001) or foster overall health or retard decline (Clark et al., 1997).

A Day in Adult Day Care

Susan consults 2 days a week at an urban adult day-care center. She begins her day in a meeting with administrative and day-care staff to identify client needs. Susan greets participants and their caregivers as they arrive at the center in the morning, spending time talking with a family member of one of the clients who has requested her advice regarding memory techniques to aide her mother-in-law's self-care routine. Susan then co-leads an exercise group to improve mobility and coordination. After the exercise session, Susan leads a craft group that is making Valentine's Day decorations for the day program's party that the group decided to have for the kindergarten class in the school next door.

Next, she goes into the kitchen where a group of people is preparing a mid-morning snack for everyone. She shows one woman how to use joint protection techniques while she cuts up apples for the snack.

In the afternoon, Susan provides staff education on strategies for improving clients' opportunities to have control over the daily schedule at the center. She ends her day with a team meeting to review participants' progress and activity level. Before leaving, she makes some calls to locate information on bathroom adaptations needed by a caregiver (American Occupational Therapy Association, 1986b, Hasselkus, 1992).

CONCLUSION

Many opportunities exist for occupational therapy practitioners to develop community-based programs that influence the health and well-being of people of all ages (Baum & Law, 1998) through direct services and consultation. Fazio (2001) suggested that events and trends in the community provide the catalyst for innovative community-based occupational therapy programs. For example, an after-school program would benefit from occupational therapy involvement in the design and pacing of the activities for the children to consulting with staff about behavior management techniques. Fazio described occupational therapy programs in the community as a "clearly focused effort and activity [to meet] the needs of an identified group" (p. 62). Goals of the program depend on the members of the particular community group but could include intervening with an identified problem, preventing future problems, and ultimately helping community members feel that they belong and are productive members of the group.

The role of the occupational therapy practitioner may be as direct service provider, consultant, or program administrator. Examples of programs are providing constructive activities in boys and girls clubs, consulting and providing education to staff and families at a health clinic, and implementing a violence-prevention program in elementary schools (Quirk, 2001).

Work in community settings is extremely rewarding as occupational therapy practitioners work closely with clients and family members while addressing a wide range of immediate and long-term needs. Practitioners working in these settings must have a strong sense of what they have to offer, because they usually work without contact with other occupational therapy personnel. Working in these settings requires practitioners to collaborate with other team members and know when and how to seek support and supervision from colleagues in the setting and occupational therapy practitioners working outside the setting but who are familiar with the particular community-based practice area.

References

American Occupational Therapy Association. (1986a). Occupational therapy in adult day-care [Position paper]. *American Journal of Occupational Therapy, 40*, 814–816.

American Occupational Therapy Association. (1986b). Roles and functions of occupational therapy in adult day-care. *American Journal of Occupational Therapy, 40*, 817–821.

Azok, S. D., & Tomlinson, J. (1994). Occupational therapy in a multidisciplinary psychiatric home health care service. *Mental Health Special Interest Section Newsletter, 17*(2), 1–3.

Baum, C. (1998). Client-centred practice in a changing health care system. In M. Law, (Ed.). *Client-centered occupational therapy* (pp. 29–45). Thorofare, NJ: Slack.

Baum, C., & Law, M. (1998). Community health: A responsibility, an opportunity, and a fit for occupational therapy. *American Journal of Occupational Therapy, 52*, 7–10.

Biernacki, S. D. (1993). Reliability of the worker role interview. *American Journal of Occupational Therapy, 47*, 979–803.

Brittingham, K. M., & Dempster, M. (1990). Occupational therapists in home health care: Ensuring positive outcomes through collaboration. *Occupational Therapy Practice, 2*(1), 32–44.

Brown, F., Shiels, M., & Hall, C. (2001). A pilot community living skills group: An evaluation. *British Journal of Occupational Therapy, 64*, 144–150.

Case-Smith, J. (1998a). Defining the early intervention process. In J. Case Smith (Ed.). *Pediatric occupational therapy and early intervention* (2nd ed., pp. 27–48). Boston: Butterworth-Heinemann.

Case-Smith, J. (1998b). Foundations and principles. In J. Case Smith (Ed.). *Pediatric occupational therapy and early intervention* (2nd ed., pp. 3–25). Boston: Butterworth-Heinemann.

Clark, C. A., Corcoran, M., & Gitlin, L. (1995). An exploratory study of how occupational therapists develop therapeutic relationships with family caregivers. *American Journal of Occupational Therapy, 49*, 587–594.

Clark, F., Azen, S., Zemke, R., Jackson, J., Carlson, M., Mandel, D., Hay, J., Josephson, K., Cherry, B., Hessel, C., Palmer, J., & Lipson, L. (1997). Occupational therapy for independent-living older adults. *Journal of the American Medical Association, 278*, 1321–1326.

Dunn, W., Brown, C., & McGuigan, A. (1994). The ecology of human performance: A framework for considering the effect of context. *American Journal of Occupational Therapy, 48*, 595–607.

Dunn, W., & Campbell, P. H. (1991). Designing pediatric service provision. In W. Dunn (Ed.). *Pediatric occupational therapy: Facilitating effective service provision* (pp. 139–160). Thorofare, NJ: Slack.

Earle-Grimes, G. (1994). Psychiatric home health care: New horizons for occupational therapy. *Mental Health Special Interest Section Newsletter, 17*(2) 3–4.

Fazio, L. S. (2001). *Developing occupation-centered programs for the community: A workbook for students and professionals*. Upper Saddle River, NJ: Prentice-Hall.

Giangreco, M. F. (1995). Related services decision-making: A foundational component of effective education for students with disabilities. *Physical and Occupational Therapy in Pediatrics, 15*(2), 47–68.

Gifford, K. E., Wooster, D. A., Gray, L., & Chromiak, S. B. (2001). Home health. In M. Scaffa, (Ed.). *Occupational therapy in community-based practice settings* (pp. 188–222) Philadelphia: Davis.

Grady, A. P. (1995). Building inclusive community: A challenge for occupational therapy. [Eleanor Clarke Slagle Lecture]. *American Journal of Occupational Therapy, 49*, 300–310.

Hanft, B., & Place, P. A. (1996). *The consulting therapist*. San Antonio, TX: Therapy Skill Builders.

Hasselkus, B. R. (1992). The meaning of activity: Day care for persons with Alzheimer disease. *American Journal of Occupational Therapy, 46*, 199–206.

Isernhagen, S., Hart, D., & Matheson, L. (1998). Rehabilitation ergonomics: Ergonomics and education: Fad, failure or fraction of back injury prevention? *Work: A Journal of Prevention, Assessment and Rehabilitation, 10*, 293–297.

Jundt, J., & King, P. M. (1999). Work rehabilitation programs: A 1997 survey. *Work: A Journal of Prevention, Assessment and Rehabilitation, 12*, 139–144.

King, G., Tucker, M. A., Alambets, P., Gritzan, J., McDougall, J., Ogilvie, A., Husted, K., O'Grady, S., Brine, M., & Malloy-Miller, T. (1998). The evaluation of functional, school-based therapy services for children with special needs: A feasibility study. *Physical and Occupational Therapy in Pediatrics, 18*(2) 1–27.

King, P. M. (1993). Outcome analysis of work-hardening programs. *American Journal of Occupational Therapy, 47*, 595–603.

McCormack, K. F. (1990). Job site analysis. *Occupational Therapy Practice, 1*(2), 35–43.

Niemeyer, L. (1989). Program models for work hardening. In L. O. Niemeyer and K. Jacobs (Eds.). *Work hardening: State of the art* (pp. 13–66). Thorofare, NJ: Slack.

Quirk, F. M. (2001). *Walking a fine line: Occupational therapists in emerging areas of pediatric practice*. Unpublished master's thesis, University of New Hampshire, Durham.

Richert, G. Z., & Merryman, M. B. (1987). The vocational continuum: A model for providing vocational services in a partial hospitalization program. *Occupational Therapy in Mental Health, 7*(3), 6–19.

Rosenbaum, P., King, S., Law, M., King, G., & Evans, J. (1998). Family-centred service: A conceptual framework and research review. *Physical and Occupational Therapy in Pediatrics, 18*(1), 1–20.

Royeen, M., & Ramsay, D. (2001). Way station: A model of excellence in community mental health programs. *Occupational Therapy in Health Care, 12*(4), 65–78.

Scaffa, M. (2001). Community-based practice: Occupation in context. In M. Scaffa (Ed.). *Occupational therapy in community-based practice settings* (pp. 3–18). Philadelphia: Davis.

Scheinholz, M. K. (2001). Community-based mental health services. In M. Scaffa (Ed.). *Occupational therapy in community-based practice settings* (pp. 291–317). Philadelphia: Davis.

Toth-Cohen, S. (2000). Role perceptions of occupational therapists providing support and education for caregivers of persons with dementia. *American Journal of Occupational Therapy, 54*, 509–515.

Van Slyke, N. (2001). Adult day-care programs. In M. Scaffa (Ed.). *Occupational therapy in community-based practice settings* (pp. 163–172). Philadelphia: Davis.

Wilberding, D. (1991). The quarterway house: More than an alternative of care. *Occupational Therapy in Mental Health, 11*(1), 65–91.

Wyrick, J. M., Niemeyer, L. O., Ellexson, M., Jacobs, K., & Taylor, S. (1991). Occupational therapy work-hardening programs: A demographic study. *American Journal of Occupational Therapy, 45*, 109–112.

CHAPTER 51

A CONSULTATIVE APPROACH TO OCCUPATIONAL THERAPY PRACTICE

EVELYN G. JAFFE and CYNTHIA F. EPSTEIN

SECTION I: Overview of Consultation
SECTION II: Prevention
SECTION III: Community-Based Practice

Consultation is the process of helping others identify issues and analyze the environment to address concerns. It is an indirect service, working with the client rather than directly with the problem, and involves mutual decision making, advice, and recommendations, within the client's perspective. This is compared to direct service, which provides more prescriptive, active intervention to solve the problem (Jaffe & Epstein, 1992). Almost all occupational therapy practitioners, whether or not it is readily apparent, provide some form of consultation during the implementation of direct intervention activities (American Occupational Therapy Association—[AOTA], in press). Meeting with families of a client, discussing cases with another colleague, planning discharge and/or community activities, or educating client caregivers and community personnel, all have a consultative component. Consultation also may be a discreet practice activity. Many occupational therapy practitioners have established consultation practices in the community as their primary role (American Occupational Therapy Association [AOTA], 1993).

The ultimate goal of consultation is to help the client or client system develop skills to prevent future problems. Consultation enables the client to assume a proactive stance and to anticipate and forestall problems, thus preventing further problems within the context of client-centered occupational performance (Epstein & Jaffe, 1996; Jaffe & Epstein, 1992). The consultation concepts presented in this chapter help practitioners enhance their practice in this rapidly changing world (Epstein & Jaffe, 1996).

This chapter provides an overview of consultation concepts, the process of consultation, and the important skills and knowledge needed to perform the role of consultant. Consultation practice is considered from two perspectives: first, as an integral component of a practitioner's clinical practice and, second, as a discrete practice activity. Inherent in consultation concepts are the basic principles of **prevention** and a systems approach. Therefore, this chapter includes an overview of a systems approach through an **environment and systems analysis** and a discussion of prevention programs. In addition, recent entrepreneurial trends in occupational therapy **community-based practice** are discussed.

Consultation is not a new role for occupational therapy practitioners. As a model of service delivery, it expanded in the mid-1960s as health-care legislation, personnel shortages, economic concerns, scientific discoveries, and biotechnology increased (Jaffe & Epstein, 1992). In the early 1970s, many occupational therapists became consultants in school systems (Education of the Handicapped Act of 1975). In fact, their role incorporated both direct service, as educationally related therapy for children with special needs, and indirect service, via consultation with teachers, related services personnel, and others in the school system (Gilfoyle, 1980).

In the late 1970s, greater numbers of occupational therapy practitioners were engaged to work in contractual arrangements in hospitals, rehabilitation centers, long-term care facilities, and home-care agencies. While often called consultants, their services were essentially the same as those practitioners employed by the facility (Jaffe, 1996). Many of these practitioners had varied assignments and wereexposed to multiple systems and organizational designs. They learned techniques and approaches that were shared at new assignments. While their main role continued to be direct service to clients, a consultative approach to service evolved. These collegial and collaborative activities helped develop the practitioner's role in such settings (Epstein, 1991; Lerner, 1992).

As the need for occupational therapy services continued to expand in the late 1980s and into the 1990s, occupational therapy practitioners established private practices. These practitioners found increasing opportunities for providing consultative services as part of their service delivery model (Dorando-Unkle & Weiss, 1993). Morris, Madachy, and Cawley (1996) identified important consultative activities and approaches provided by occupational therapy practitioners working with the elderly in both traditional and nontraditional settings. An explosion of community-based, innovative programs marked occupational therapy's entrance into the twenty-first century. Many of these programs resulted from collaborative efforts between occupational therapy students, working with guidance from their academic programs, and practitioners in community programs (Dudgeon & Greenberg, 1998). **Entrepreneurship** in the community became a focal point for many practitioners as they sought new avenues for service delivery. Use of consultation perspectives was inherent in all of these activities.

SECTION I

Overview of Consultation

Consultation is the interactive process of helping others solve existing or potential problems by identifying and analyzing issues, developing strategies to address problems, identifying resources, and preventing future problems from occurring (Jaffe & Epstein, 1992). Consultation activities include counseling; giving advice; and offering opinions, recommendations, alternatives, suggestions, support, and, above all, help. Inherent in any definition of consultation is the concept of an interactive process between consultant and client that is characterized by sharing, problem solving, mutual respect, equality, and collaboration. Helping the client develop problem-solving strategies is basic to any consultation experience.

The models of consultation and levels of consultation determine the setting, target, status, and outcome of the consultation. Basic concepts of a systems approach and the principles of prevention are an integral component of consultation activities (Jaffe & Epstein, 1992).

TABLE 51–1. **THEORETICAL MODELS OF CONSULTATION**[a]

- *Clinical or intervention model:* Specific-case or client-focused model based on diagnosis and recommendations for remediation
- *Collegial or professional model:* Peer-centered model based on egalitarian, collaborative problem solving
- *Behavioral model:* Behavior-focused model based on control, adaptation, modification, or change of learned behavior
- *Educational model:* Information-centered model involving staff development, in-service training, and workshops led by the consultant or trainer
- *Organizational development model:* Management-focused model based on organizational structure, leadership styles, and administrative or employee relationships
- *Process management model:* Group-based model focused on dynamics and process of client system, involving staff development and team building
- *Program development model:* Service-centered model focused on development or modification of programs to improve services.
- *Social action model:* Social reform model focused on social values and policies to facilitate social change
- *Systems model:* Systems-centered model based on the specific values, mission, goals, and culture of the client system

[a]Epstein & Jaffe (1996) and Jaffe & Epstein (1992). Adapted with permission from Mosby.

THEORETICAL MODELS OF OCCUPATIONAL THERAPY CONSULTATION

Understanding the foundations of consultation and the various approaches drawn from the theoretical models provide the consultant with a frame of reference, much like planning an intervention program. The approach depends entirely on the given situation, the client system, the specific needs, and the degree of change required. Just as with occupational therapy direct service intervention, in which practitioners may draw from one or more frames of reference, models of consultation may be derived from different theory bases. These models may be used separately, in conjunction with another or progressively in the consultation process (Epstein & Jaffe, 1996; Jaffe & Epstein, 1992) (Table 51-1).

A thorough understanding of the models and the theoretical concepts supporting them allows the consultant to choose the model from which to develop the appropriate approach for each specific situation and client system.

LEVELS OF OCCUPATIONAL THERAPY CONSULTATION

Beyond the theoretical models, consultation typically involves one or more levels of consultation activity (Table 51-2).

TABLE 51–2. **LEVELS OF CONSULTATION**[a]

Level I: Case-Centered Consultation

- *Target:* Specific patient or individual
- *Goal:* To produce appropriate behavioral or physical change

Level II: Educational/Collegial Consultation

- *Target:* Specific client group (staff, clinicians, teachers, administrators, caretakers)
- *Goal:* To improve functional efficiency through skill development

Level III: Program and/or Administrative Consultation

- *Target:* Specific system (school, agency, corporation, health facility, etc.)
- *Goal:* To promote institutional change through program planning and administrative consultation

[a]Epstein & Jaffe (1996), and Jaffe & Epstein (1992). Adapted with permission from Mosby.

Level I: Case Centered

Case-centered consultation is the traditional clinical or intervention model and usually involves specialized assessments or collaborative discussions to help resolve the individual case or client problem. Occupational therapy clinical expertise is essential in addressing a particular client's problem. The goal is to produce appropriate behavioral or physical change. For example, an occupational therapy practitioner working in a public school might consult with a third-grade teacher regarding a specific child's distractible behavior. The goal is to assist the teacher to structure the classroom environment for this child so that he or she can attend to schoolwork more successfully. The consultant may suggest having the child work in a cubby or sheltered area, away from the noise and distractions of other children.

Level II: Educational and Collegial

Educational and collegial consultation addresses the consultant's role as trainer, educator, mentor, information specialist, or process facilitator. Problem identification and problem solving are central to this process. The client group may consist of staff, other clinicians or professional colleagues, teachers, supervisors, managers, or administrators who have sought the assistance of a consultant to help their group improve its function, efficiency, and ability to address issues critical to the system. This is a collegial or professional peer-centered consultation based on an egalitarian, collaborative problem-solving relationship with professional colleagues. At this level, consultation focuses on both group process and information using behavioral and educational models, and may involve staff development and in-service training, with the consultant acting as educator and trainer.

Using the same setting as the previous example, the occupational therapy school consultant may be invited by the

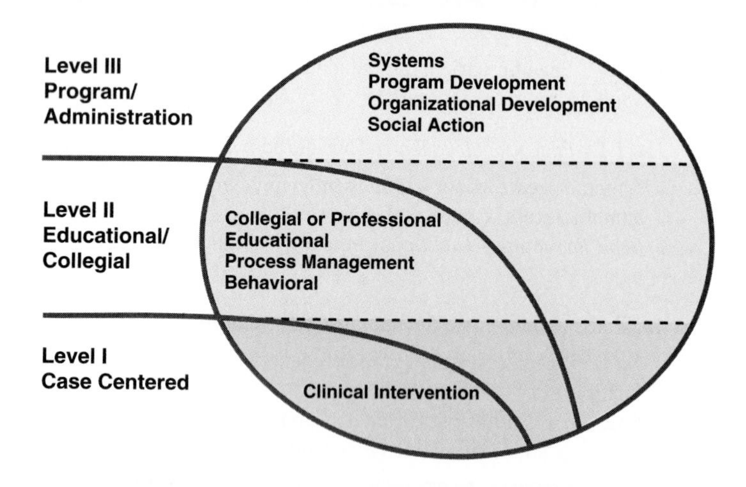

FIGURE 51–1. The interrelationship among the theoretical levels and the models of consultation. Jaffe & Epstein (1992). Adapted with permission from Mosby.

teacher to discuss the unsettled behavior of the class after recess, which the teacher believes is the result of some disruptive children on the playground. The consultant collaborates with the teacher to brainstorm and problem solve. They mutually develop ideas to improve the situation, which include having the consultant provide some in-service training to all the third-grade teachers and aides regarding strategies for diffusing the negative behavior that resulted and the subsequent inability of the whole class to attend to schoolwork after recess.

Level III: Program and Administration

The program and administration level requires a systemwide collaboration with a more global perspective and addresses the needs of a specific system (school, agency, corporation, health facility, etc.), with the goal of promoting institutional change. This approach involves program planning, enhancing management skills, strategic planning, and administrative consultation. At this level, the consultant focuses on the broader organization and may incorporate approaches derived from one or more of the following models: program development, organizational development, social action, and/or systems.

Continuing the previous example to this level, the school principal asks the occupational therapy consultant to review the problems of all the children on the playground at recess time. Other classes have experienced similar problems, and the teachers are feeling overwhelmed and at a loss to handle all the disruptive behavior. The occupational therapy consultant investigates the issues by observing the children at recess and interviewing many of the teachers. The consultant prepares a proposal for a schoolwide activity program during recess and after-school hours. This plan is adopted by the school system after discussions with the entire teaching and administrative staff. Drawing from program development and organizational development models, the consultant focuses on adaptation and modification of the school system recess program, which results in global changes in this school and nearby neighboring schools, culminating in a total system approach.

Figure 51-1 shows the relationship among the levels of consultation and the models a consultant may apply at each level. The consultant attains a rich palette from which to draw the most suitable approaches for the particular client system and setting by moving from one level to another, using different theoretical models and possible roles. Although the case example describes a school setting, the concept of theoretical models and levels of consultation applies to all consultative settings. For example, after the terrorist attacks of September 11, 2001, Pascarelli (2001) became an active, visible consultant helping individuals and groups cope at Ground Zero. He used his clinical consultative skills at Level I to help schoolchildren overcome their fear of a repeat attack at their school, which was located close to the World Trade Center. Concurrently, working at Level II, he used educational and process management models to help workers overcome stress and exhaustion. At the same time, he worked at Level III to help a group of psychiatrists further expand their work on behalf of victims of terrorism at the site and throughout the nation and world (Pascarelli, 2001).

In addition to the models and levels, the consultant must understand the various roles he or she will assume in the consultation process. Figure 51-2 shows the relationship between the levels of consultation and these roles.

CONSULTATION ROLES

The nature of a consultant's role is an outcome of the many issues and concerns addressed in each experience. During the course of consultation, the consultant invariably assumes

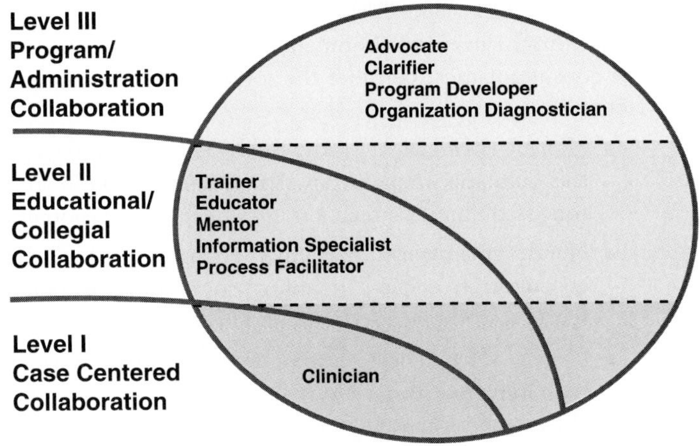

FIGURE 51–2. The collaborative relationships among the consultation levels and the roles of occupational therapists.

multiple roles. Role choice is determined by the degree of directiveness the consultant assumes, the extent to which the consultant is internal or external to the organization, and the type of collaborative roles required.

Directive and Nondirective Roles

Role choices may be viewed along a continuum of the degree of directiveness (Lippitt & Lippitt, 1986). In a nondirective role, the consultant serves as a clarifier, raising questions for client reflection and consideration. In this capacity, the consultant also provides information to help the client initiate problem solving. A directive role is that of trainer or educator. Active leadership is necessary to teach specific skills and/or procedures.

Role choice becomes an integral part of the intervention strategy for a given consultation situation. It is based on the values and sensitivities of the consultant and the needs of the client. Many times, role blurring occurs with the ebb and flow of the consultation experience. It is the consultant's responsibility to monitor the client's response and to shift roles and styles when required (Epstein & Jaffe, 1996; Jaffe & Epstein, 1992).

Internal and External Roles

Internal consultants are usually employees of the system with which they are asked to consult, whereas external consultants are brought into the organization from outside the system. The client chooses an internal or external consultant based on the particular client system and the issues, concerns, and desired outcomes of that system. Role expectations are usually different for the internal and external consultant. Each functions quite differently, even if working in similar consulting settings, and adapts personal behaviors and consulting style to be appropriate for the specific system. The consultant's effectiveness depends on awareness of situational differences. For example, the external consultant, who is an independent agent, is less constrained and can be more aggressive than the internal consultant, who "lives with" the client and, therefore, must be more cautious (Epstein & Jaffe, 1996; Jaffe & Epstein, 1992).

Internal Consultant

The internal consultant may be asked to provide consultation services within the organization to another department or program. The internal consultant usually understands the history and policies of the entire system and may have inside knowledge of its power and politics.

External Consultant

The external consultant is often an independent agent, engaged by the client system as a private contractor or a member of a consulting firm. The external consultant has minimal, if any, organizational or political relationship with the client system and, therefore, may be considered an outsider to the organization. Frequently, the external consultant can bring a more global, fresh approach to the issues and concerns of the system.

Opportunities for consultation arise in varied practice environments. In most cases, occupational therapy expertise initially is sought at a clinical level. As the practitioner's service delivery evolves, opportunities may occur that require a shift from clinician role to a consultant role. A knowledgeable practitioner assesses the need for consultation and, when indicated, takes on a consultative perspective that involves understanding the system, its values, culture, mission, and goals. It is through this understanding that the consultant can effect change in the system.

UNDERSTANDING THE CONSULTATION CONTEXT THROUGH ENVIRONMENTAL AND SYSTEMS ANALYSIS

A major element of consultation, in addition to occupational therapy expertise, is an understanding of systems and the client environment. A review of all aspects of the client system, including the internal and external environmental factors that influence the system, is basic to all consultation activities. Using a systems approach to the study of the problems, concerns, or issues, an occupational therapy consultant can help the client consider new or enhanced information, values, attitudes, and skills. In traditional medical-based, direct-service settings, the concerns of the practitioner have a more narrow approach, directed to the specific injury, disease, or disability. The move to community-based programs requires greater understanding of systems and environments from a broad, client-centered perspective.

The specific context of each client system is an integral part of the consultation process. The first step in assessment of the client system is to develop an occupational profile of the client, viewing the client from an occupational performance perspective (AOTA, 1995, in press; Dunn, Brown, & McGuigan, 1994; Jaffe & Epstein, 1992). This is achieved by conducting an environment and systems analysis.

Environment and Systems Analysis

An analysis of environmental factors, including social, economic, and political trends or issues that affect the system, help the consultant determine the frame of reference for the consultative activities. Successful consultants are knowledgeable and skilled in understanding the many environments in which their services are requested. Consultants may be called in to help a system respond quickly to changes. Therefore, the consultant must understand and address the many factors influencing the organizational process and even personal, social problems of the system.

The environment consists of a complex of internal and external conditions or factors that surround an individual or community and influence behavior and organizational structure on both macroenvironmental and microenvironmental levels. An environment and systems analysis involves the study of several forces.

- *Macroenvironment:* Forces in the external environment of the client system that influence the organization; for example, local or national legislative acts and regulatory policies; local or national economic concerns; the political climate; and the social climate, cultural mores, customs, attitudes, and values that shape the system's occupational life.
- *Microenvironment:* Forces close to the client system; for example, administrative policies and procedures of the organization; internal resources of funds, staff, and supplies; the corporate culture; and the mission and goals of the organization.

Within the macroenvironments and microenvironments, the consultant must consider the following environmental factors:

- *Human environment:* Individuals who may influence the outcome, including patients, clients, administrators, staff, families, teachers, and health professionals.
- *Natural environment:* Particular setting(s) in which the consultation occurs, including community agencies, schools, workplace settings, and health-care facilities.
- *Physical environment:* External factors or conditions that influence the consultation, including space, architecture, accessibility, and physical structure.

Reviewing all facets of the environment prepares the occupational therapy consultant for the development of the consultative activities. Performing an environment and systems analysis, as described above, provides the consultant with the stepping-stones from which all consultation strategies follow (Baum, 1991; Holm, Rogers, & Stone 1998; Jaffe & Epstein, 1992; Spencer, 1998).

CONSULTATION PROCESS

The consultation process begins with the initiation of entry into the system. It involves eight basic steps (Table 51-3) (Epstein & Jaffe 1996; Jaffe & Epstein 1992; Lippitt & Lippitt, 1986).

Entry into the System

Entry into the system or organization is the first step in the process. Entry is based on exploration of the potential for

TABLE 51-3. **BASIC STEPS OF CONSULTATION**[a]

- *Entry into the system:* Opportunity for entrance into a consultation experience
- *Negotiation of contract:* Delineation of the general terms and focus of the consultation
- *Diagnostic analysis:* Trends and system analysis and problem identification
- *Goal setting and planning:* Development of mutual understanding, respect, and trust
- *Maintenance:* Ongoing intervention, strategies, implementation, and feedback
- *Evaluation:* Analysis of the outcomes, assessment and feedback of consultation strategies
- *Termination:* Conclusion of the consultation activities
- *Renegotiation:* Extension or revision of contract for further consultation, if appropriate

[a]Epstein & Jaffe (1996), Jaffe & Epstein (1992), and Lippitt & Lippitt (1986).

TABLE 51-4. **ENTRY INTO THE SYSTEM**[a]

- *Planned entry:* Consultant develops a strategy and presents a proposal
- *Opportunistic entry:* A situation arises spontaneously and the consultant seizes the moment
- *Uninvited entry:* Consultant perceives a need and attempts to enter the system
- *Invited entry:* Consultant is invited because of his or her specific skills

[a]Epstein & Jaffe, (1996) and Jaffe & Epstein (1992). Adapted with permission from Mosby.

consultation in the system. An opportunity to develop a consulting relationship may evolve in several ways (Table 51-4).

- *Planned entry:* Requires the development of specific tactics to enter the system, including deliberate, systematic strategies chosen for a particular client system, developed in phased or sequential steps.
- *Opportunistic entry:* Usually occurs without prior planning, as a result of hearsay, media announcements, or articles about the organization.
- *Uninvited entry:* Usually is initiated by a third-party recommendation, based on the potential consultant's expertise; requires preplanning and initiative to determine the value of the consultation. *Note:* No matter how the entry is initiated, the final entry must be by client invitation.
- *Invited entry:* Occurs when the client system recognizes that it will benefit from the specific expertise and skills of the consultant.

Negotiation of Contract

Negotiation of the contract involves delineation of the general terms and focus of the consultation. Clear communication and understanding are essential when establishing a collaborative relationship. This formal document defines the purpose of the consultation and the qualifications of the consultant; identifies the obligations and expectations of both parties; and delineates procedures, time constraints, and the method and amount of compensation (Beich 1999; Shenson, 1990).

Diagnostic Analysis: Trends and Systems Analysis and Problem Identification

The consultant must understand the nature of the client environment as a whole, and its component parts through an ongoing data-gathering process. Frequently, the consultant performs a needs assessment of the client environment to review issues related to the organization that help identify problems. This assessment helps the consultant understand the client's desired occupational performance or outcome. In addition, the systems analysis forms the basis from which consultation strategies are developed (see Chapter 18, Section 2).

Goal Setting and Planning

Establishing collegial, collaborative client relationships is an essential component of consultation. The development of mutual understanding, trust, and respect with the client must occur before collaborative planning is initiated.

Maintenance

The maintenance phase is the ongoing intervention or strategy of the consultation. Communication and feedback between the client and the consultant are necessary for a successful consultation.

Evaluation

Evaluation procedures and reports should be specified at the beginning of the consultation. Frequently, they are included

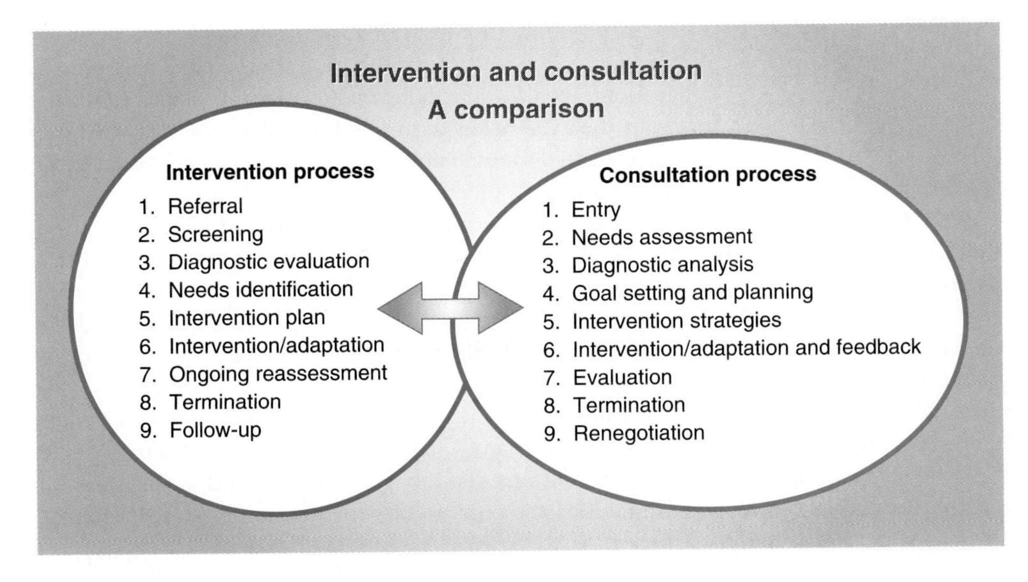

FIGURE 51–3. A comparison of intervention and consultation. Jaffe & Epstein (1992). Adapted with permission from Mosby.

in the initial contract. Evaluation reports may include an analysis of the outcomes and assessment and feedback of consultation strategies.

Termination

Termination occurs at the conclusion of the consultation activities. The client usually has achieved a sufficient degree of skill in addressing the current and future issues and problems of the organization. Therefore, the services of the consultant are no longer needed.

Renegotiation

The client may request an extension or revision of the initial contract for further consultation. New issues may have arisen as a result of changes in the client system environment, including changes in organizational structure, changes in environmental impacts, new or expanded programs, and changes in personnel (Epstein & Jaffe, 1996; Jaffe & Epstein, 1992; Lippitt & Lippitt, 1986).

Practitioners use various strategies in direct intervention for planning programs for their clients. The process is similar to that of consultation (Fig. 51-3). In both processes, there is an emphasis on the need for continual feedback, monitoring, and evaluation, which lead to modification and refinement of the intervention, whether direct service intervention plans or consultation intervention strategies (Epstein & Jaffe, 1996; Jaffe & Epstein, 1992).

CONCLUSION

Occupational therapy practice focuses on improving the ability of individuals to engage in their daily routines to take charge of their lives (Yerxa, 1983). The individual and the practitioner work collaboratively to design and implement required services (AOTA, 1995). Similarly, occupational therapy consultation requires collaboration between the client and the consultant. The goal of consultation also is to enable the client to achieve valued goals. The consultant's task is to develop an environment in which positive change can take place, thereby leading to improved client performance.

SECTION II

Prevention

CONSULTATION PRACTICE SETTINGS

Occupational therapy consultants may practice in many of the same settings as clinical practitioners. Many perform clinical activities for a majority of their time and use consultative approaches for specific situations. Therefore, their primary role may still be that of providing direct intervention. However, there are increasing opportunities for practitioners to assume primary roles as consultants in community-based programs. A prominent area for consultation is in educational and advocacy activities. Collaborative educational consultation and advocacy are particularly important in school settings, where parents often struggle to obtain appropriate services for their children with special needs. In addition to the more traditional case consultation regarding specific intervention or program plans, the occupational therapy consultant can provide education to teachers and parents regarding resources, support groups, and information sources. The consultant, in an advocacy role, may help parents obtain essential services.

In addition to educational and advocacy consultation, another major area for consultation is program development in home health and industry. Accessibility issues resulting from the Americans with Disabilities Act of 1990 (ADA) have created innumerable opportunities. Occupational therapy consultants practice in industries, in private and public businesses and corporations, and with individuals in their private homes. Legislative support for people with disabilities has increased, causing more employers and lawyers to seek guidance regarding employment of disabled individuals (Sampson, 1992; Shamberg, 1993). Ergonomic concerns in the workplace, home, and community offer additional opportunities for occupational therapy consultation. Consultants are in demand to assist with development of reasonable accommodations for job performance and work capacity evaluations for employees with disabilities. (Hoelscher & Taylor, 2000).

TABLE 51-5. **PREVENTION PRINCIPLES**[a]

- *Primary prevention:* Activities undertaken before the onset of a problem to avoid occurrence of malfunction or disability in a population potentially at risk
- *Secondary prevention:* Early diagnosis identification and detection of populations at risk to prevent dysfunction or permanent disability
- *Tertiary prevention:* Rehabilitation and remediation of a problem or illness to prevent further problems, loss, or disability

[a]Jaffe & Epstein (1992).

The continual development of technological devices has resulted in more public demand for the most recent assistive devices, expanding the need for occupational therapy consultation to professional colleagues and to individual clients and families.

PREVENTION PRINCIPLES

Prevention of disease or dysfunction and facilitation of health in clinical settings, organization, or communities is an accepted occupational therapy goal. The practitioner must assist clients to develop self-help skills that promote healthy lifestyles and environments. The generation of knowledge, responsibility, and positive attitudes are major objectives in the quest for client health and **wellness.**

Prevention activities are proactive. Prevention is action that reduces the probability or exacerbation of the incident (disease, illness or disability). Prevention may empower people and encourage self-responsibility. The principles of prevention have a direct relation to consultation activities (Table 51-5) (Jaffe & Epstein, 1992).

The occupational therapy consultant must understand basic prevention principles and use them to achieve positive outcomes. Using the concepts of prevention, the occupational therapy consultant helps the client focus on a proactive approach to the issues, which results in improved occupational performance for the client and client system. Changes in health-care delivery models, combined with both younger and older populations, which are growing rapidly because of life-sustaining technology and pharmacology, have brought prevention techniques to the forefront of practice. Increasingly, the need for intervention at both ends of the developmental spectrum has opened the door for consultation with children, adults, and the elderly.

WELLNESS AND HEALTH PROMOTION

Health promotion usually refers to programs and activities that enhance health and foster wellness. Opatz (1985) described health promotion as systematic efforts by an organization to enhance the wellness of its members through educational activities, behavioral changes, and cultural support to enhance and foster social well-being. Health promotion programs are primarily educational, rather than clinical, and may involve lifestyle changes. The aim of health promotion is to transform the concept of wellness into action.

Therefore, wellness is both a goal and a process, rather than a state or condition. It is the process of adapting patterns of behavior that lead to improved health and heightened life satisfaction (Opatz, 1985). Wellness involves an integration of the many dimensions of human life that represent the wholeness of mind and body from physical, mental, spiritual, social, and environmental perspectives. Occupational therapy consultants can provide assistance to health and wellness curricula at all grade levels in schools. They also can provide wellness programs in the community, at recreational and sports facilities, day-care centers, and workplace settings.

There are increasing opportunities for consultation to health and fitness programs in the adult population at the workplace and community health centers. People 65 years old or older are a growing constituency of the population, making greater use of community-based services, including day-care activities programs, water aerobics, and other sport and recreational activities geared for this age group (Jaffe, 1986, 1989a, 1989b).

The expertise of the occupational therapy practitioner in developing age-appropriate prevention and health promotion activities for community-based programs provides a fertile ground for consultation. The focus in the well community is at a secondary and even primary level of prevention, rather than the tertiary level of prevention used in most long-term care or rehabilitation settings. As more lives are saved and the population lives longer, the need for prevention-focused, community-based occupational therapy consultation will increase.

The increased interest in health and wellness programs has resulted in a proliferation of modes and methods of community activities, from tai chi to Pilates, from yoga to aerobics, from coaching to visioning. As the demand for professionals trained in these and other alternative health and wellness programs increases, the opportunities for collegial and program development consultation will continue to grow.

CONCLUSION

Governmental leaders and health care practitioners nationwide finally have accepted prevention and health promotion concepts. National health policymakers, insurance company officials, corporation administrators, community leaders, and health professionals have embraced proactive prevention principles and the development of effective programs. Occupational therapy practitioners can seize this opportunity to be among those leading the development of prevention and wellness programs.

SECTION III

Community-Based Practice

Entrepreneurship
Risks
Rewards
Requirements
Marketing
Conclusion

Community consultation practice environments have expanded greatly since the early 1990s. Continual changes in the health-care industry, including reduction of traditional medical model facilities, has led many occupational therapy practitioners to consider developing community-based services. New and exciting opportunities exist for knowledgeable and creative practitioners. Establishing a community-based consultation practice offers these individuals an opportunity to open new doors for occupational therapy services.

ENTREPRENEURSHIP

As the occupational therapy practitioner explores the need for consultation in the community, opportunities may arise to initiate services independently, in partnership with others, or by establishing a corporation. Challenges associated with establishing a consultation practice, therefore, require broadening the focus to consider entrepreneurship. The establishment of a business requires extensive preparation. An in-depth analysis must occur. A prospective entrepreneurial consultant must consider an environment and systems analysis. Many resources are available to help in this analysis, including information from the American Occupational Therapy Association, the Small Business Administration, business literature, World Wide Web search engines, business schools, and colleagues who have entered the business world (Beich, 1999; Hertfelder & Crispen, 1990; Koomar, 1996).

Vision and mission statements are developed to provide information to prospective clients regarding the nature of the consultation services. The vision statement is the consultant's ultimate goal, providing the focus for the direction and organization of the consultation practice. It is the framework for best practice and guides the organization's future development. The following is the vision statement for a hypothetical practice called Therapy Consultants:

The vision of Therapy Consultants is to be recognized as the premier therapy-consulting group in the state.

The mission statement reflects the purpose of an organization and expresses the basic philosophy or identity of the organization. Therapy Consultants' mission statement looks like this:

The mission of Therapy Consultants is to provide comprehensive, quality, cost-effective consultation services to consumers in health care, educational, and community environments in the state and to maintain a supportive, enriched professional environment for employees of the organization.

Vision and mission statements help focus the consultation practice and facilitate recognition of services to potential target markets. The new entrepreneur must consider key issues, such as the three R's: the risks, rewards and requirements of establishing a business.

Risks

Financial issues, time commitments, and work responsibilities are primary concerns of an entrepreneurial practice. Consultation is a service, which in an entrepreneurial consultation practice is regarded as the business product. New and developing service organizations cannot expect a consistent flow of income. Therefore, funding sources must be identified to help support the initial period. Long hours, extensive research requirements, networking demands, and the heavy responsibilities inherent in the establishment of a new business, radically skew the balance of work and play.

Consultants and entrepreneurs must be able to shift gears at a minute's notice. They must stay constantly alert for possible business opportunities, ready to respond quickly and effectively. A new venture may mean playing all supporting roles, including receptionist, secretary, janitor, and maintenance engineer, along with that of business owner, marketing representative, and most important, expert consultant.

Rewards

Establishing a consulting business can be exciting, challenging, fulfilling, and when successful, personally and financially rewarding. It can offer autonomy, flexibility, and opportunities to practice in both traditional and nontraditional environments. Often at the forefront of practice, the consultant has an opportunity to support individuals and groups seeking important aspects of change (Biech, 1999; Epstein & Jaffe,

TABLE 51-6. **BUSINESS PLAN**[a]

- *Business concept:* Defines where (geographic location), what (specialized aspects of occupational therapy consultation), when, and how the practice will be established
- *Vision and mission statements:* Define the nature of the consultation services (the business's product); identifies the target market(s) or clientele
- *Organizational plan:* Delineates the structure of the business, personnel, and financial management, including fee structure
- *Market assessment:* Analyzes potential occupational therapy consultation needs in the targeted geographic area; identifies a possible client pool
- *Marketing:* A system for organizational planning developed from an information base

[a]Biech (1999) and Epstein (1992a).

TABLE 51-7. **MARKETING MIX: THE FOUR P'S**[a]

- *Product:* Tangible or intangible attributes to satisfy a need or want
- *Price:* Financial, physical, and psychological costs to people of doing business
- *Place:* How a product will be distributed to a market or how a market gets access to a product
- *Promotion:* Development of tools and strategies to market the product

[a]Epstein (1992b) and Epstein & Jaffe (1996).

1996; Dorando-Unkle & Weiss, 1993). The consultant-entrepreneur is challenged to expand his or her skill and knowledge regarding the specific consultation environment as professional growth and development opportunities arise. Concurrently, the consultant provides important information and analysis to the client. With each new consulting experience, the consultant builds greater expertise, resources, and information, which become assets for use in future consultative activities.

Requirements

Creation of a thoroughly researched and well-analyzed business plan forms the basis for decision making. Table 51-6 outlines the major components of a business plan. The plan is an organizational tool to guide business decisions. A business plan should include a description of the business, the business's vision and mission statements, an organizational plan that acknowledges management needs and anticipates necessary initial expenditures, and a market assessment.

The money necessary to support the consultant during the initial phase is always a consideration. An occupational therapy practitioner interested in establishing a new consultation practice might consider starting up a part-time consulting practice while maintaining his or her primary job of direct intervention services. The new consultant is prudent to engage others in providing professional support, including an attorney, accountant, banker, and/or other specialists.

Marketing is another important consideration. The consultant-entrepreneur must identify a target market. A critical assessment should be performed to determine the best geographic location and type of potential clientele. An accurate analysis brings prospective clients to the consultant's door, rather than to a competitor. Stepping into the world of business by considering these three R's helps the new consultant-entrepreneur develop an effective, detailed, and well-laid-out plan.

MARKETING

A consultation practice grows and flourishes in direct relationship to the marketing approach used by the entrepreneur. "Marketing is a system for organizational planning that is developed from an information base. . . . A market is a group of individuals who have an actual or potential interest in purchasing the consultant's services" (Epstein, 1992b, p. 651). Understanding marketing variables help the consultant establish a successful business. These variables are known as the marketing mix and are commonly called the four P's of marketing. Table 51-7 summarizes these concepts. Marketing is an inherent part of the consultant-entrepreneurs business.

Effective marketing occurs when prospective clients receive a proposal that effectively incorporates the four P's. The consultation proposal is an essential component of effective marketing. A proposal that is well written clearly describes the process of the consultation and the product (i.e., the consultation service). In addition, the proposal includes a fee that is at fair market value. The proposal, therefore, becomes the consultant's best promotional tool (Epstein, 1992a, 1992b; Epstein & Jaffe, 1996).

Indirect marketing, using various forms of personal selling, increases the potential for referral and request of services. There are a variety of indirect strategies, including attending business meetings (Chamber of Commerce, Rotary, and Lions, etc.), speaking at conferences, writing articles, networking with colleagues, and sending out free newsletters. The best referrals are those from satisfied clients. The consultant can successfully expand visibility and business opportunities through networking approaches.

Stepping into the entrepreneurial world, the occupational therapist experiences professional demands from new and challenging perspectives. The demands of starting and marketing such a business require determination, dedication of time and energy, allocation of funds, and a salable consultation product. The consultant must bring excellent skills and knowledge to the task and a high degree of self-confidence. Many opportunities exist for those interested in taking on this challenge to open new professional vistas and to advocate for and support change.

CONCLUSION

Consultation offers the occupational therapy practitioner the opportunity to expand current roles and assume new, exciting, and innovative approaches to practice, especially in community-based programs. The occupational therapy consultation model described in this chapter emphasizes the interactive, dynamic, and ongoing nature of the process, which must involve evaluation and understanding of all aspects of the client environment. The consultation process includes concepts of prevention, a systems approach, and occupational performance, all within a human perspective that focuses on the needs of the client. Consultative services that include program development, evaluation, educational services, and advocacy offer the occupational therapy practitioners an opportunity to address the changing environment of health-care delivery.

A consultative approach in a variety of practice settings help ensure that health-care consumers receive occupational therapy services that are expedient and efficacious and that provide quality care in a cost-effective manner. Consultation approaches may be incorporated in all areas of occupational therapy services, either as a separate entrepreneurial practice or as an indirect service as a component of direct service intervention.

Marketing these occupational therapy services occurs after an assessment of potential clients and consultation needs. Attractive, well-defined proposals and effective networking in the community promote occupational therapy consultation services. The development of vision and mission statements and a comprehensive business plan guides the entrepreneurial practice and helps focus the services. The creative occupational therapy practitioner can meet the challenges of an entrepreneurial consultation practice.

Health-care consumers are demanding efficient and cost-effective responses to their varied health needs. Changes in the health-care environment require occupational therapy practitioners to adapt their practice to meet new challenges. Consultation assumes greater importance as practitioners become more involved in community-based programs. Incorporating consultative practice approaches enhance services and ensure that occupational therapy is a viable and essential component of the health-care delivery system.

References

American Occupational Therapy Association. (1993). *1993 Member data survey*. Bethesda, MD: Author.

American Occupational Therapy Association. (1995) Concept paper: Service delivery in occupational therapy. *American Journal of Occupational Therapy, 49*, 1029–1031.

American Occupational Therapy Association (in press). Occupational therapy practice framework: Domain and process. *American Journal of Occupational Therapy*.

Baum, C. (1991). Professional issues in a changing environment. In C. Christiansen & C. Baum (Eds.). *Occupational therapy: Overcoming human performance deficits* (pp. 807–817). Thorofare, NJ: Slack.

Beich, E. (1999). *The business of consulting: The basics and beyond*. San Francisco: Jossey-Bass/Pfieffer.

Dorando-Unkle, M., & Weiss, D. (Eds.). (1993). Occupational therapists as consultants. [Special issue]. *Occupational Therapy Practice, 4*(4).

Dudgeon, B. J., & Greenberg, S. L. (1998). Preparing students for consultation roles and systems. *American Journal of Occupational Therapy, 52*, 801–809.

Dunn, W. W., Brown, C., & McGuigan, A. (1994). The ecology of human performance: A framework for thought and action. *American Journal of Occupational Therapy, 48*, 595–607.

Education of the Handicapped Act of 1975. P. L. 94-142, 20 U.S.C. 31401.

Epstein, C. F. (1991) Specialized restorative programs. In J. M. Kiernat (Ed.). *Occupational therapy and the older adult* (pp. 285–300). Gaithersburg, MD: Aspen.

Epstein, C. F. (1992a). Developing a consultation practice. In E. G. Jaffe & C. F. Epstein (Eds.). *Occupational therapy consultation: Theory, principles, and practice* (pp. 634–649). St. Louis: Mosby Year Book.

Epstein, C. F. (1992b). Marketing: A continuous process. In E. G. Jaffe & C. F. Epstein (Eds.). *Occupational therapy consultation: Theory, principles, and practice* (pp. 650–674). St. Louis: Mosby Year Book.

Epstein, C. F., & Jaffe, E. G. (1996). Consultation: A collaborative approach to change. In M. Johnson (Ed.). *The occupational therapy manager* (pp. 533–574). Bethesda, MD: American Occupational Therapy Association.

Gilfoyle, E. M. (Ed.). (1980). *Training: Occupational therapy educational management in schools*. Rockville, MD: American Occupational Therapy Association.

Hertfelder, S. D., & Crispen, C. (Eds.). (1990). *Private practice: Strategies for success*. Rockville, MD: American Occupational Therapy Association.

Hoelscher D., & Taylor S. (2000). Ergonomics consultation: An opportunity for occupational therapists. *OT Practice, 5*(1), 16–19.

Holm, M. B., Rogers, J. C., & Stone, R. G. (1998). Person-task-environment interventions: Decision-making guide. In M. E. Neistadt & E. B. Crepeau (Eds.). *Willard & Spackman's occupational therapy* (9th ed., pp. 471–498). Philadelphia: Lippincott.

Jaffe, E.G. (1986). Prevention: "An idea whose time has come": The role of occupational therapy in disease prevention and health promotion. *American Journal of Occupational Therapy, 39*, 499–503.

Jaffe, E. G. (1989a). From the editors. In J. A. Johnson & E. G. Jaffe (Eds.). *Health promotion and preventive programs: Models of occupational therapy practice* (pp. 1–4). Binghampton, NY: Haworth.

Jaffe, E. G. (1989b). Medical consumer education: health promotion in the workplace. In J. A. Johnson & E. G. Jaffe (Eds.). *Occupational therapy: Program development for health promotion and preventive services* (pp. 5–24). Binghampton, NY: Haworth.

Jaffe, E. G. (1996). Occupational therapy consultation in a managed care environment. *OT Practice, 1*(3), 26–31.

Jaffe, E. G., & Epstein, C. F. (Eds.). (1992). *Occupational therapy consultation: Theory, principles, and practice*. St. Louis: Mosby Year Book.

Koomar, J. (1996). *Plan for success*. San Antonio TX: Therapy Skill Builders.

Lerner, S. L. (1992). Hospital based consultation. In E. G. Jaffe & C. F. Epstein (Eds.). *Occupational therapy consultation: Theory, principles, and practice* (pp. 311–323). St. Louis: Mosby Year Book.

Lippitt. G., & Lippitt. R. (1986). *The consulting process in action* (2nd ed.). San Diego: University Associates.

Morris, A. L., Madachy, P. B., & Cawley, C., (1996). Consultation amplifies the impact of occupational therapy in the community. In K. O. Larson,

R. G. Stevens-Ratchford., L. W. Pedretti, & J. L. Crabtree (Eds.). *The role of occupational therapy with the elderly* (pp. 415–450). Bethesda MD: American Occupational Therapy Association.

Opatz, J. P. (1985). *A primer of health promotion: Creating healthy organizational cultures*. Washington, DC: Oryon.

Pascarelli, F. R. (2001, November 4). Ground zero: An OT and former firefighter's perspective on the recent terrorist attacks. *Atlanta Journal—Constitution Pulse Magazine*, pp. 3, 8.

Sampson, L. (1992). Consultancy issues concerning accessibility. In E. G. Jaffe & C. F. Epstein (Eds.). *Occupational therapy consultation: Theory, principles, and practice* (pp. 385–394). St. Louis: Mosby Year Book.

Shamberg, S. (1993). The accessibility consultant: A new role for occupational therapists under the Americans with Disabilities Act. *Occupational Therapy Practice*, 4(4), 14–23.

Shenson, H. L. (1990). *Shenson on consulting*. New York: Wiley.

Spencer, J. C. (1998). Evaluation of performance contexts. In M. E. Neistadt & E. B. Crepeau (Eds.). *Willard & Spackman's occupational therapy* (9th ed., pp. 291–309). Philadelphia: Lippincott.

Yerxa, E. J. (1983). Audacious values: The energy source for occupational therapy practice. In G. Kielhofner (Ed.). *Health through occupation: Theory and practice in occupational therapy* (pp. 149–162). Philadelphia: Davis.

UNIT *twelve*

Professional Issues

Learning Objectives

After completing this unit, readers will be able to:

- Define ethics and research and explain their importance to occupational therapy practice.
- Identify utilitarian or teleological reasoning and deontological reasoning and distinguish between them.
- Explain the uses and purposes of a professional code.
- Discuss each principle of the Occupational Therapy Code of Ethics, including the core ethical concepts described in each.
- Examine current ethical dilemmas in occupational therapy, discuss the issues and conflicts involved, and generate possible solutions to the dilemmas.
- Explain the research process, including the difference between qualitative and quantitative research.
- Critically analyze a research article.
- Define and explain evidence-based practice and its importance to the profession.
- Identify crucial professional decisions that influence occupational therapy's potential contribution to society in the changing environmental context of a new millennium.

Central to the practice of occupational therapy are three interrelated topics: ethics, research, and the future of occupational therapy. Occupational therapy's professional ethics articulate the core values and beliefs that direct practitioners' actions as they provide intervention for the people who seek their services. These ethics and values also undergird occupational therapy research priorities and efforts. Consequently, practice must be based on the current research evidence that demonstrates the effectiveness of the interventions to promote full participation of clients in society. Finally, practitioners must look to the future to anticipate the challenges they will encounter and to embrace them with creativity and focused action. (Note: Words in **bold** type are defined in the Glossary.)

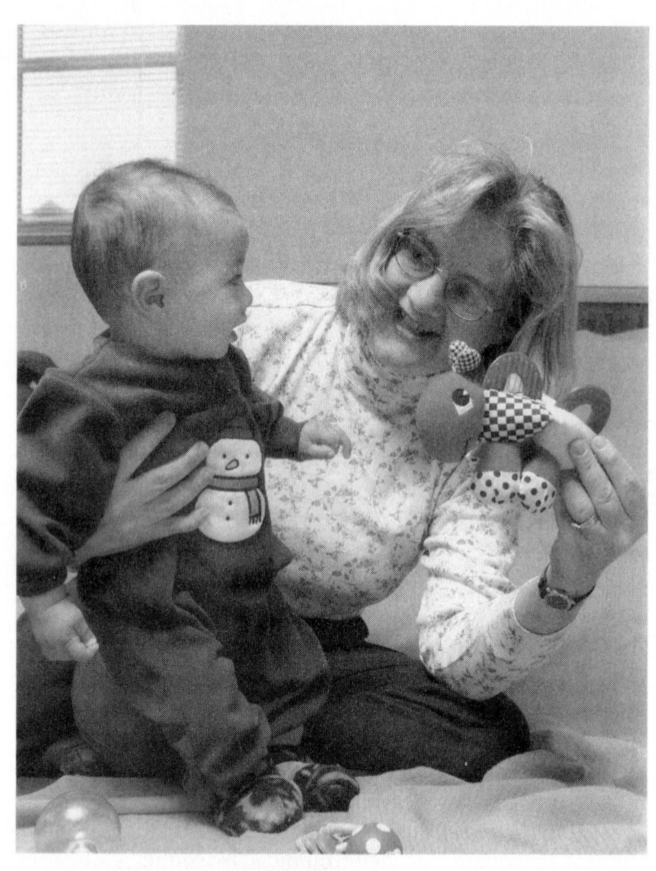

Research involves collecting data, often by observing behavior, reviewing data, and planning poster sessions for conference presentations or writing papers. It is essential that all aspects of research be conducted with the highest ethical standards. This occupational therapy researcher is studying the development of infants and toddlers. (*top*) (Courtesy of D. Prince, Photographic Services, University of New Hampshire, Durham, NH.) Collaborative research entails both individual and collective efforts. These scholars are studying data they have collected for a joint research project. (*middle*) (Courtesy of L. G. Littlefield, GKM Instructional Resource Center, Sargent College, Boston University, Boston, MA.) Poster sessions are one form of professional communications. These doctoral students and their mentor are preparing a poster for a scientific conference. (*bottom*) (Courtesy of E. Chu, Occupational Therapy Department, Sargent College, Boston University, Boston, MA.)

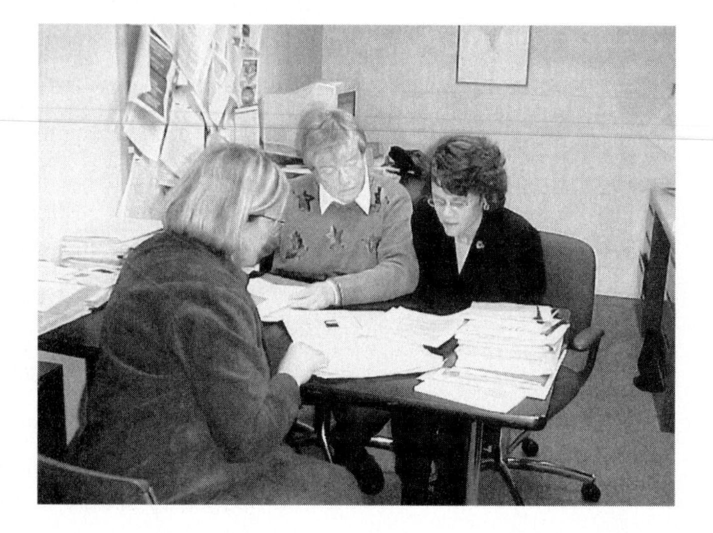

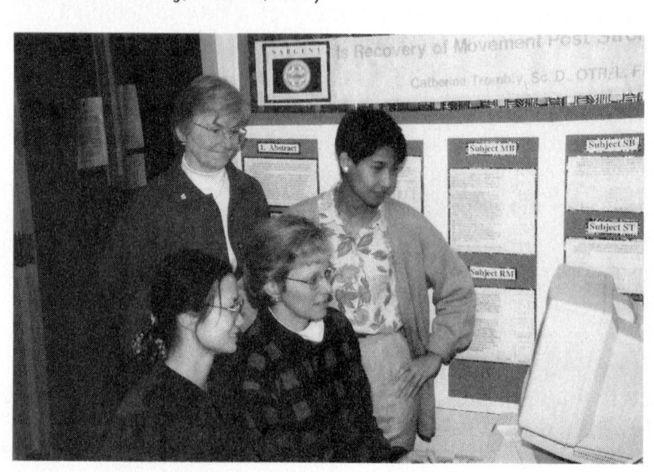

CHAPTER 52

ETHICS IN OCCUPATIONAL THERAPY

RUTH ANN HANSEN

Making ethical decisions is part of our daily lives. You may have noticed that *ethics* is a word that is being used more and more frequently by individuals in discussions of their personal lives and of public issues. The public media—television, radio, newspapers, and magazines—have made us all aware of the unethical conduct of public figures.

Struggling with decisions about what is the right thing to do can cause both intrapersonal and interpersonal tensions and create stress. We decide what is right based on personal, professional, and societal values. Ethical dilemmas occur when we face situations in which the right or correct action is not clear. This may mean there is more than one right answer or that you are struggling to select from several less-than-desirable options. Ethical conflicts occur when our values clash with those of others—friends, relatives, and professional colleagues. These situations cause us to feel uneasy, upset, and perplexed.

What follows is a summary of some of the concepts that are critical when discussing ethical issues within the occupational therapy profession. First we need to understand some basic terminology. Keeping these basic ideas in mind, I then discuss several theoretical perspectives we might use when deliberating ethical issues (Box 52-1). There are associations and relationships among many of these terms.

In discussions of ethical issues, people will talk about both beneficence and nonmaleficence. Beneficence conveys the idea of doing good or what is best for an individual or group of people, whereas nonmaleficence infers an effort to avoid doing harm of a physical, financial, psychological, or social nature. To examine the difference between these two terms, let's think about a practitioner (occupational therapist or occupational therapy assistant) who is working with someone with severe burns. From one perspective, the treatment is beneficent, since the ultimate goal is to enable the person to regain as much movement as possible. Treatment, on the other hand, is often quite painful. Some individuals may consider that serious harm (pain and psychological distress) is being inflicted on the person over the short term. Conversely, practitioners are likely to consider that withholding treatment (avoiding pain) would cause long-term harm. The individual would have contractures and serious limitations in range of motion and mobility. As you can see, the people involved (practitioner, person, family)

BOX 52-1 KEY TERMS

- *Autonomy.* The right of an individual to be self-determining; the right to make independent decisions about one's life.
- *Beneficence.* The act or attitude of doing good or causing good to happen for others; the duty to try to do what is best for another person.
- *Compensatory justice.* Provision of resources to a wronged or injured individual.
- *Competence.* Having the cognitive and psychological ability to make decisions that others judge to be rational; it is necessary to be able to communicate these decisions to others.
- *Distributive justice.* A method of determining how to dispense or allocate resources (e.g., equal shares to all; first come first served).
- *Equity.* The belief that all individuals are equal and that being treated equally is a right; this is particularly at issue when scarce resources are being distributed.
- *Ethics.* The values and beliefs that are part of a particular group (social, cultural, professional); they are a guide for the members of the group when determining right from wrong.
- *Fidelity.* The duty to be faithful to another person and to that individual's best interests; included is the idea of holding information about that person in confidence.
- *Informed consent.* The right to be make decisions about health care that occurs after the person has a complete understanding of the options available and the possible consequences of various alternative forms of care.
- *Justice.* Rules for determining how to allocate resources (materials, goods, supplies, money, personnel).
- *Metaethics.* The branch of philosophy that examines the commonalties in the ways that humans make decisions about what is right or moral.
- *Nonmaleficence.* The obligation to avoid doing harm to another or to avoid creating a circumstance in which harm could occur to another.
- *Normative ethics.* The study of individuals' deliberations about what is right.
- *Paternalism.* Acting or making decisions for another; there is usually a presumption that the decision maker is acting in the best interest of the other person and is doing so without that person's consent.

may describe this treatment in different ways, depending on their view of the situation.

Autonomy, or self-determination, competency and informed consent are interdependent concepts. In our society, as well as in many others, we place a high value on an individual's being able to make an independent decision. This right is predicated on the person's ability to make competent decisions and having the necessary facts on which to make an informed decision. Not everyone is able to make autonomous decisions. Individuals may have a temporary or permanent loss of cognitive or psychological functioning that interferes with their ability to reason and make sound judgments. Those who cannot speak are frequently assumed to be unable to make decisions for themselves.

Determining whether individuals are competent to make decisions about their lives is crucial. Making these determinations is not easy. Often, legal judgments are what determines if individuals are competent and whether they need a guardian. Those who are competent must have the necessary information to choose a course of action. As helping professionals, we must remind ourselves that all individuals have the right to make autonomous decisions. People who have physical, psychological, or cognitive disabilities and the young and old have the right (and should be encouraged) to remain as autonomous as possible in their daily lives. We have an obligation in all cases to inform those we serve of the nature of the therapy being provided, the goals of treatment, the expected outcomes, and the availability of other treatment options.

Justice is also an important principle. Most people agree that all individuals have the right to fair and equal treatment, but whether that equity extends to equal access to health, education, and social services is a thorny question. Do all people have the right to receive all services (resources) that they need or want? Obviously, there are limits to the money, time, personnel, equipment, and other resources that are available. Do the current reimbursement mechanisms ensure fair and equal access to treatment? In this era of managed care, third-party payers are making decisions about the types and amount of resources that are provided. Payment mechanisms determine if people receive specific services.

Understanding this terminology is necessary, but we also must have some knowledge of the basic theoretical foundations of ethics.

THEORETICAL PERSPECTIVES

Philosophical

Graber (1988) organized the basic philosophical theories used in medical ethics into two groupings: teleological and deontological. Graber made three key comparisons between these two theories of moral obligation. First, when deciding how to determine right from wrong, the teleologist looks at the consequences of the act, whereas the deontologist weighs the duties that an individual has in the situation. Second, the goal in teleology is to do good and avoid harm. In deontology the emphasis is on being respectful of others' rights. Finally, there is a principle within each perspective to help in the resolution of conflict. In the teleological approach, producing the greatest good for the greatest number is the guide. From a deontological perspective, the way to resolve conflict is to weigh the conflicting duties in the situation and determine which duty is primary.

When reading and talking about ethics, we need to determine the orientation of the author or speaker. Individuals make different choices about right action, depending on whether they consider the consequences or the obligation to carry out duties to have the higher priority. Knowing how people set these priorities aid in understanding why they make certain choices.

Let's go back to the example of the person who has severe burns. The teleologist examines the consequences of treatment and makes a decision about ethical practice by deciding what would cause the greatest good for the greatest number of people involved—the person, the person's family and significant others, and society. The deontologist decides the right thing to do by balancing the duties that the practitioner has against the various individuals and groups of concern. If you are thinking that this still does not give you the answer, you are correct. What it does is help you understand the thinking process that might be used in coming to a decision.

I hope that this example helps you realize that even though discussions of philosophical theory may seem far removed from everyday decisions, they are not. Conflicts with colleagues about right choices may have at their roots a disagreement about how to prioritize duties. In another situation, conflicts may arise because of a disagreement about what is the greatest good or whether that good should take priority over a specific duty.

Modern Perspectives

A logical extension of these philosophical foundations is the work of some modern philosophers and educators in the United States. Morrill (1980) organized this information into four categories, and I added the feminist perspective to this list.

Values clarification helps individuals identify and clarify their personal values and identify the values that are most important. The goal is for people to be able to establish a personal system of values. This occurs through the active process of choosing and prizing personal beliefs and being able to act on those beliefs (Raths, Harmin, & Simon, 1966).

Values inquiry provides individuals with the opportunity to examine and try to understand the values that others hold. In this process, people become more aware of the general values that motivate human choice and decision making. The goals are a commitment to a reasonably stable set of values and an understanding of that value system within society (McGrath, 1977).

Moral education and moral development propose that moral reasoning changes and matures in a predictable sequence. Kohlberg (1984) proposed six stages of cognitive-moral development that are grounded in the concepts of fairness and justice. Each stage describes a unique pattern of reasoning that the person uses to determine right from wrong. The emphasis from this perspective is on the cognitive structures used to process moral issues rather than on a personal awareness of specific values. The highest or sixth stage of moral reasoning is the Golden Rule—Do unto others as you would have them do unto you. Kohlberg maintained that the person first makes moral judgments and then acts on them. The person has a commitment to act on moral judgments (Kohlberg & Candee, 1984).

Numerous individuals have criticized Kohlberg's theory and research. Critics have faulted Kohlberg for interviewing male subjects exclusively when arriving at his original construction of stages. Other critics voice a concern that his theory has a bias toward the Western culture. They maintain that the dominant themes of moral decision making in this culture are the principals of justice, contract keeping, and rights. Gilligan (1982) found that women used the ideas of responsibility, caring, and mutuality when deliberating about certain ethical dilemmas (Haste & Baddeley, 1991).

Feminist perspectives of moral reasoning have emerged since the 1980s. In their chapter on moral theory and feminist culture, Haste and Baddeley (1991) discussed their own research and the more current writings of Gilligan. They found a clear association between being female and having a predominant moral orientation of responsibility and caring. They also found that males were more likely to make moral decisions using a rights-and-justice orientation. However, Haste and Baddeley make the important point that both men and women can reason from the alternate perspective under appropriate conditions.

"While the moral orientations are gender linked, it is clear that both sexes are aware of each orientation and can use both. Such evidence undermines the notion that impermeable boundaries and peculiar experience are the sine que non for the development of particular orientations or ways of knowing, but it does not undermine the concept of separate culture per se" (Haste & Baddeley, 1991, pp. 234–235).

"Feminist ethics is best characterized as a special challenge to traditional ethical theory" (Ladd, 1996, p. 30). The more traditional ethical perspectives develop rules to guide and gauge public behavior. Women have, typically, been involved in a domestic role that requires intensely personal relationships with particular, unique individuals (Ladd, 1996; Sichel, 1992). Feminist theory shifts the focus to that which is private and personal in peoples' lives. It favors partiality rather than detachment. As Ladd stated, "It is a natural human tendency to favor 'our own.' The question is when, if ever, it is justified to do so. Can partiality be a part of morality" (p. 30)?

Normative and applied ethics enable individuals to explore and justify right action in a specific and familiar situation. This method is particularly useful for exploring issues of professional ethics, professional codes of ethics, and professional responsibility (Morrill, 1980).

OCCUPATIONAL THERAPY ETHICS

Within our profession there are two key American Occupational Therapy Association (AOTA) documents that describe aspects of the moral stance of occupational therapy. These documents are the *Core Values and Attitudes of Occupational Therapy Practice* (AOTA, 1993) and the *Occupational Therapy Code of Ethics* (AOTA, 2000b) (see Appendix B and C).

Core Values and Attitudes of Occupational Therapy Practice

AOTA's core values document is a statement of the values and attitudes that are evident in the official documents of the association. The documents used to write this paper were *Dictionary Definition of Occupational Therapy* (AOTA, 1986), *The Philosophical Base of Occupational Therapy* (AOTA, 1979), *Essentials and Guidelines for an Accredited Educational Program for the Occupational Therapist* (AOTA, 1991a), *Essentials and Guidelines for an Accredited Education Program for the Occupational Therapy Assistant* (AOTA, 1991b), and the *Occupational Therapy Code of Ethics*. These documents directly state or infer the values and beliefs undergirding the occupational therapy profession in the United States. Kanny (1993) identified seven core values and attitudes: altruism, equality, freedom, justice, dignity, truth, and prudence (Box 52-2).

BOX 52–2 CORE VALUES AND ATTITUDES OF OCCUPATIONAL THERAPY

- *Altruism* is the unselfish concern for the welfare of others. This concept is reflected in actions and attitudes of commitment, caring, dedication, responsiveness, and understanding.
- *Dignity* emphasizes the importance of valuing the inherent worth and uniqueness of each person. This value is demonstrated by an attitude of empathy and respect for self and others.
- *Equality* requires that all individuals be perceived as having the same fundamental human rights and opportunities. This value is demonstrated by an attitude of fairness and impartiality.
- *Freedom* allows the individual to exercise choice and to demonstrate independence, initiative, and self-direction.
- *Justice* places value on the upholding of such moral and legal principles as fairness, equity, truthfulness, and objectivity.
- *Prudence* is the ability to govern and discipline oneself through the use of reason. To be prudent is to value judiciousness, discretion, vigilance, moderation, care, and circumspection in the management of one's affairs, to temper extremes, make judgments, and respond on the basis of intelligent reflection and rational thought.
- *Truth* requires that we be faithful to facts and reality. Truthfulness or veracity is demonstrated by being accountable, honest, forthright, accurate, and authentic in our attitudes and actions.

Occupational Therapy Code of Ethics

The second AOTA document is the *Occupational Therapy Code of Ethics* (AOTA, 2000b). Before examining the contents of this document, we need to understand why professions develop codes of ethics. What is the purpose of a professional code of ethics? Members of many professions, particularly health-care and service-providing professions, have privileges that are not granted to the nonprofessional. In turn, professions develop principles of conduct or codes of ethics that hold members of that profession to a higher standard of behavior.

For example, as occupational therapists, we have access to personal information about the people we serve. We are also allowed to touch and physically manipulate their bodies to administer therapy. Under most other circumstances, this type of access is illegal. Having personal information about another individual is an invasion of privacy and physical contact can be deemed an assault. Because occupational therapists have these extraordinary rights, we also have the duty to hold information in confidence, to avoid doing harm, and to respect the client's privacy and integrity.

The *Occupational Therapy Code of Ethics* (AOTA, 2000b) describes the correct professional conduct for occupational therapy practitioners. The Code also provides guidance for occupational therapy students as future practitioners and for all people, other than occupational therapists and occupational therapy assistants, who may be providing occupational therapy services (aides, technicians, etc.). The Code consists of seven principles of conduct, which provide general guidance. They are not specific and do not give the solution for a particular ethical dilemma.

Principle 1 states, "Occupational therapy personnel shall demonstrate a concern for the well-being of the recipients of their services (beneficence)" (AOTA, 2000b, p. 614). This statement reminds us that our services must be provided equitably. We must not exploit the individuals that we serve in any way. We must take precautions to avoid causing harm to them or to their property. This principle also covers the duty to charge fees that are fair and reasonable and to act as an advocate for individuals to obtain services.

Principle 2 covers the concepts of not causing harm to recipients of services and reminds us that we need to avoid any associations that could compromise professional judgment and objectivity (AOTA, 2000b).

Principle 3 emphasizes respect for the rights of our clients (autonomy, informed consent, privacy, right to refuse treatment) (AOTA, 2000b). This means that we need to collaborate with service recipients in setting treatment goals. Ideally, the recipients are the ones who select the goals of treatment, and the practitioner helps them to find ways of reaching those goals. We must ensure that recipients are fully informed about the type of treatment, any risks involved in treatment, and the expected outcomes of therapy. We must respect their right to refuse treatment and maintain confidentiality about privileged information. The code provides guidance to professionals in a variety of roles: practitioner, educator, researcher, and manager. Thus this principle also covers the rights of research subjects to be fully informed when giving consent before participation in any study. Subjects must understand the potential risks as well as the possible outcomes of the study.

Principle 4 describes the duty that we have to remain professionally competent (AOTA, 2000b). We have an obligation to maintain appropriate national and state credentials. First, practitioners must acquire the appropriate entry-level credentials (registered occupational therapist, certified occupational therapy assistant). Beyond entry level, the practitioner must maintain competency. One way to do this is by obtaining recognized advanced credentialing in areas like sensory integration and hand therapy. In addition, the practitioner must seek the necessary supervision and training when learning new skills. We must also comply with "the standards of practice and other appropriate AOTA documents relevant to practice" (AOTA, 2000b, p. 615), participate in professional development activities, and base our professional activities on accurate and up-to-date information.

Also, we are responsible for the competence of all those we supervise. This means that we must carefully assign tasks to make sure that the person assuming the duties has the qualifications, experience, and training necessary to carry them out safely and responsibly. The supervisor must decide how much and what type of supervision is necessary for the designated individual to carry out the assigned duties. We must always provide adequate supervision in these situations. Finally, if we feel that the services being requested are outside our area of competence we should refer clients to other providers or consult with those providers.

Principle 5 is a reminder of our duty to comply with all local, state, federal, and institutional laws governing our professional activities (AOTA, 2000b). This includes the responsibility to follow the AOTA policies and guidelines for the profession. Not only must we abide by and comply with these rules but also we must be sure that our employers are aware of them and that our professional colleagues are aware of and follow the *Occupational Therapy Code of Ethics*. This principle also covers documentation. All professional documentation must be accurate and complete. This means, of course, keeping accurate and complete patient records and billing correctly. It also requires accuracy in our professional résumés, professional presentations, and scholarly writing.

Principle 6 covers the concepts of veracity or truthfulness. It states, "Occupational therapy personnel shall provide accurate information about occupational therapy services" (AOTA, 2000b, p. 615). We must accurately represent our qualifications, education, and level of competence. We must be aware of and report any potential conflict of interest, and we must represent our qualifications, credentials, and capabilities accurately. We must accurately present the scope and limits of our personal expertise and refrain from making exaggerated or unfounded promises or guarantees about the outcomes of the professional services provided.

Principle 7 emphasizes the need for fidelity and veracity. We need to safeguard all confidential information about colleagues and staff as well as acknowledging the contributions and findings of colleagues (AOTA, 2000b). Included is the obligation to report the illegal or unethical conduct of professional colleagues to appropriate authorities. *Whistle blowing* is the term used to describe this obligation.

The members of AOTA write and maintain the Occupational Therapy Code of Ethics. The AOTA reviews this document every 5 years to make sure that the content is current and relevant to member concerns. The members of AOTA have designated that the AOTA Commission on Standards and Ethics (SEC) has the responsibility to maintain, revise, and enforce this code. The Representative Assembly must approve all revisions of the code before the document becomes official.

The Occupational Therapy Code of Ethics and the "Core Values and Attitudes of Occupational Therapy Practice" are two AOTA documents. They are *key* because they describe the values, attitudes, and moral beliefs that guide occupational therapy practice in the United States.

Ethical Jurisdiction

Three specific agencies have jurisdiction and concerns about the ethical conduct of occupational therapy personnel. These three groups are AOTA, the National Certification Board for Occupational Therapy (NBCOT), and state regulatory boards (licensure, registration, or trademark).

AOTA

AOTA is a voluntary membership organization that represents and promotes the interests of individuals who choose to become members. Because membership is voluntary, AOTA has no direct authority over practitioners and students who are not members. AOTA has no direct legal mechanism for preventing nonmembers who are incompetent, unethical, or unqualified from practicing. The SEC is the volunteer-sector component of AOTA that is responsible for writing, revising, and enforcing the *Occupational Therapy Code*. SEC is also responsible for informing and educating members about current ethical issues and for reviewing allegations of unethical conduct by AOTA members.

When the SEC receives a complaint about a member, the chairperson requests that a designated individual conduct a confidential, preliminary investigation. Currently, that individual is the ethics program manager, who is a member of the AOTA national office staff. This investigation provides the members of SEC with necessary information to determine if the allegation warrants deliberation by the commission. If they decide that the allegation is a violation of the Occupational Therapy Code of Ethics, they can impose one of four types of disciplinary action (AOTA, 2000a):

- Reprimand is a formal expression of disapproval of conduct communicated privately by letter from the chairperson of the SEC.
- Censure is a formal expression of disapproval that is public.
- Suspension requires removal of membership for a specified period of time.
- Revocation prohibits a person from being a member of AOTA indefinitely.

NBCOT

NBCOT is the national credentialing agency that certifies qualified individuals as registered occupational therapists and certified occupational therapy assistants. This is accomplished by successfully passing a written certification examination. This organization, because of it purpose, has jurisdiction over all NBCOT-certified practitioners as well as those currently eligible to sit for the next examination.

The three main categories of violations that warrant disciplinary action are incompetence, unethical behavior, and impairment. When NBCOT receives a complaint, they initiate an intensive, confidential review process to determine whether the allegations are warranted. If so, the Disciplinary Action Committee (DAC) may select one of several sanctions, depending on the seriousness of the misconduct. Below is a listing of the available options, starting with the least severe action and progressing to most severe. All sanctions are made public except for reprimand and ineligibility (NBCOT, 2002).

- Reprimand is a formal, written expression of disapproval of conduct communicated privately and retained in the individual's certification file.
- Censure is a formal expression of disapproval that is publicly proclaimed.
- Ineligibility to take the certification exam may be determined indefinitely or for a specific period of time.
- Probation requires that the individual fulfill certain conditions such as education, supervision, or counseling for a specified time. The individual must meet these conditions to remain certified.
- Suspension is the loss of certification for a specified period of time. The DAC uses suspension when they determine that the person must complete specific amounts of public service or participate in a rehabilitation program.
- Revocation means that the individual loses certification permanently.

State Regulatory Boards

State regulatory boards (SRBs) are public bodies created by state legislatures to ensure the health and safety of the citizens of that state. Their specific responsibility is to protect the public from potential harm that incompetent or unqualified practitioners may cause. State regulation may be in the form of licensure or registration. The legal guidelines of each state usually specify the scope of practice for the profession and the qualifications that professionals must meet to practice. In addition, the board usually provides a description of ethical behavior. In most cases, the SRBs have adopted the AOTA Occupational Therapy Code of Ethics for this purpose.

Each state regulatory board has direct jurisdiction over therapists practicing in that state. By the very nature of this limited jurisdiction, each state can monitor the practitioners in that state more closely than can national organizations, such as AOTA and NBCOT. They have the authority by state law to discipline members of a profession practicing in that state if they have caused harm to citizens of that state. SRBs can also intervene in situations in which the individual has been convicted of an illegal act that directly affects professional practice (e.g., the misappropriation of funds through false billing practices).

The primary concern of each state is to protect the people living in that state. It, therefore, limits its review of complaints to those involving such a threat. When an SRB determines that an individual has violated the law, it can elect several different sanctions as a disciplinary measure. Examples of disciplinary actions are public censure, temporary suspension of practice privileges, and permanent prohibition from practice in that state.

Where to Go First

As you can see the AOTA, NBCOT, and SRBs have specific jurisdictions over occupational therapy. Among the three groups, some areas of concern overlap. Others are separate and distinct. If you need information or want to file a complaint, it is helpful to know which of the three is the most appropriate to contact. To do so you should ask yourself the following three questions (Hansen, 2000b, p. 23):

- Did the alleged violation take place in a state that regulates occupational therapy practice?
- Is the individual a member of AOTA?
- What consequences do I consider appropriate if the complaint is determined to be justified?

Certainly in some instances, you would have a choice of any of the three agencies. For example, all three have concerns if there has been harm or potential harm to a consumer. On the other hand, ethical violations of professional values that have no potential to cause harm would likely be of interest to AOTA alone. For example, AOTA is not concerned with a violation of a verbal contract to provide a continuing education workshop, but NBCOT and SRBs would.

WHAT'S A PRACTITIONER TO DO? 52-1
Ms. Garcia

Ms. Garcia is an occupational therapist and an employee of a for-profit health-care agency. In her current position, she provides home-health services. Mr. Alexander is 68 years old and had a stroke 6 weeks ago. Under the managed care plan, Ms. Garcia is allowed six home visits. The main goal of therapy is to help Mr. Alexander regain as much self-care independence as possible so that he can remain in his home. Of course, safety is a primary concern, taking into consideration not only his physical abilities but also his judgment. His partner is employed full-time. Once the funding runs out for a home-health aide, Mr. Alexander will be home alone from 7:30 A.M. to 5:30 P.M.

At the end of six visits, Mr. Alexander is able to bath, dress, and groom himself with standby verbal cuing and some physical assistance. He must be able to perform these activities with minimal verbal cuing and no physical assistance to stay at home with his partner.

Ms. Garcia has ten years of experience as an occupational therapist and has primarily worked in home health. Her professional judgment is that with three more visits, Mr. Alexander will be able to reach the goal safely performing his self-care activities with minimal assistance. The case manager is reluctant to allow more visits and wants Ms. Garcia to discontinue her intervention.

QUESTIONS AND EXERCISES

1. What should the practitioner do in this situation?
2. What is the likelihood that the case manager will allow more visits? [In the current environment, containment of costs is a primary concern. What sort of track record does Ms. Garcia have for getting good outcomes within the specified number of visits? If she has a record of good outcomes the case manager is more likely to allow the extension. There is also the legal concern that the home-health agency may be liable if Mr. Alexander is discharged before he can perform his daily living activities safely.]
3. What if the case manager refuses? [Mr. Alexander does not have the resources to have someone in the home at all times, nor do he and his partner have sufficient financial reserves or insurance coverage to pay for an assisted living facility. Can Ms. Garcia find another way to cover the cost of the three additional visits? What if Ms. Garcia decides to provide the additional visits for free (otherwise, known as pro bono, i.e., "for the good")?]
4. What is the best way to provide the greatest good for the greatest number? To whom does Ms. Garcia have a primary duty? Does she decide what to do by relying on the rules of justice or based on her feelings of partiality for Mr. Alexander and his partner? If she decides to provide free services, does that obligate her to provide similar services to other clients, now and in the future? Can you provide a justification for not providing free occupational therapy services to all others but, rather, to only a few.
5. Does the sexual orientation of Mr. Alexander and his partner make a difference in how you decide to resolve this dilemma? Should sexual orientation be an influential factor? Give a rationale for your response.

You should also consider what disciplinary action you would consider appropriate for a particular violation. Do you want to revoke or restrict the person's state licensure? Do you want the organization to either suspend or revoke the individual's certification? Would it be more appropriate in your mind to restrict or prohibit the person's ability to be a member of AOTA? You need to seek advice before filing a complaint to be sure that you have selected the agency with the jurisdiction to achieve the consequences you consider commensurate to the violation (Hansen, 2000a, 2000c).

Several years ago, AOTA, NBCOT, and the SRBs established a network for communicating and publishing the disciplinary actions of the respective groups. The Disciplinary Action Information Exchange Network (DAIEN) provides a mechanism for notifying the public and other organizations when any disciplinary action is taken against an occupational therapy practitioner. The DAIEN list is usually published each quarter on NBCOT's Web site (www.nbcot.org) and in AOTA's *OT Practice*. This is a master list of individuals who have been subject to disciplinary action since the previous publication of the list.

ETHICAL DILEMMAS FOR DISCUSSION

It is never easy trying to make the transition from abstract ideas to practical solutions. In this section, I help you see how you can use the ethical concepts (terms and principles) and translate them into action plans when ethical dilemmas arise. I present two problems for you to try out an analytic process that you might find useful. One describes a practice dilemma and the other describes a management and supervisory predicament. First, you should read the details of the dilemma and be sure that you understand the situation. Then you should consider a series of questions. By answering

WHAT'S A PRACTITIONER TO DO? 52-2
Jeremy

Jeremy is the director of a rehabilitation services department in a large metropolitan hospital. There are eight occupational therapists, two occupational therapy assistants, and one occupational therapy aide on the rehabilitation team right now. The corporation that owns the hospital has recently merged with several other health-care businesses in the area. They are initiating a plan to right-size the organization. They have issued a mandate to all departments to establish measures that will reduce costs. Jeremy must also eliminate unnecessary services while providing services of increasingly higher quality. Jeremy has been told to reduce the number of occupational therapists to two and, in their place, to hire more occupational therapy assistants and aides to deliver treatment.

Jeremy believes that some changes in the distribution of levels of occupational therapy personnel are possible. However, his main concern is that the quality of the services provided would be seriously compromised if he initiates such a dramatic change. His main concern is for those patients who are seriously and acutely ill. They need high levels of sophisticated expertise to ensure that they receive safe and competent treatment. An example is the neurology unit where there are currently two occupational therapists and one occupational therapy assistant. The patients on this unit are primarily individuals who have had recent spinal cord injuries and traumatic brain injuries.

QUESTIONS AND EXERCISES

1. What steps should Jeremy take to make sure that there is a proper balance between providing competent treatment and being cost effective?
2. What are the legal and ethical guidelines that describe the practice of occupational therapists and occupational therapy assistants? What if any differences are there between the roles of each? What type of supervisor is needed? What credentials must the supervisor have? How much time must the supervisor spend to make sure that the aide or assistant is providing safe and competent services?
3. Would a change in staffing allow the department to maintain all services currently provided, including those in such areas such as the neonatal intensive care unit and the neurology unit? If not, how should Jeremy make decisions about what services to discontinue?
4. Are all the occupational therapists now on staff capable of providing the type of supervision necessary? Are they willing to reduce their direct patient contact and take on these supervisory responsibilities? How can Jeremy help them acquire the skills needed to take on new roles? Should he be doing this?
5. Is it realistic to expect that there are certified occupational therapy assistants and aides available in the community who want to apply for these new positions?
6. If the department is successful in making this transition, does it set a precedent for further shifts in staffing in the future?

those questions you should be able to come to some a conclusion about what you think should happen.

Read What's a Practitioner to Do? 52-1 about Ms. Garcia. You could take several approaches in this situation. One is to examine the conflict among Ms. Garcia's duties to her employer, the third-party payer, and Mr. Alexander. You, of course, may need more information to develop a solution. Many times a dilemma exists because we do not have all the information that we need to make an educated decision. For the present, take this case at face value. What are some of the options that you might consider in bringing this issue to a satisfactory resolution?

Naturally, you will come up with other questions that you want to take into account. Develop different scenarios and options and discuss them with your colleagues. Try to reach a consensus on a plan of action that all, or most of you, can agree on. After doing this, role play the situation of explaining your decision to Mr. Alexander, his partner, the case manager, the employer, and yourself, as Ms. Garcia.

Now read What's a Practitioner to Do? 52-2 about Jeremy. Obviously, there are no clear answers to these questions. Discuss this dilemma with your peers. Explore the resources that are available to you that would help you come up with a solution. Try to look at this situation not only from Jeremy's perspective but also from that of the president of the hospital, the present and future occupational therapy staff, and the patients in the hospital. Again, you can test possible solutions by role playing that you must explain your solution to each of the parties involved in this scenario.

CONCLUSION

Struggling with right and wrong in given situations is part of everyday life. We find ethical dilemmas throughout our profession—in clinical practice, supervision, management, teaching, research, and consultation. The conflicts that are described in the two cases are current versions of common ethical dilemmas. The current health-care environment demands cost-effective care and requires major changes in the nature and delivery of services. The conflicts that arise between provision of quality services and cost-effectiveness create serious tensions for all of us—provider and recipient, alike.

I hope that these cases provide a springboard for the discussion and clarification of other ethical dilemmas that you encounter. I urge you to explore the literature on health care and human services ethics more deeply. My hope is that you can remain well versed about the issues involved in the emerging ethical challenges facing us in our professional lives. I also hope that you acquire the understanding and reasoning ability necessary to analyze and confront these challenges.

References

American Occupational Therapy Association. (1979). The philosophical base of occupational therapy. *American Journal of Occupational Therapy, 33*, 785.

American Occupational Therapy Association. (1986, April). *Dictionary definition of occupational therapy*. Bethesda, MD: Author.

American Occupational Therapy Association. (1988). Occupational therapy code of ethics. *American Journal of Occupational Therapy, 42*, 795–796.

American Occupational Therapy Association. (1991a). Essentials and guidelines for an accredited educational program for the occupational therapist. *American Journal of Occupational Therapy, 45*, 1077–1084.

American Occupational Therapy Association. (1991b). Essentials and guidelines for an accredited educational program for the occupational therapy assistant. *American Journal of Occupational Therapy, 45*, 1085–1092.

American Occupational Therapy Association. (1993). Core values and attitudes of occupational therapy practice. *American Journal of Occupational Therapy, 47*, 1085–1086.

American Occupational Therapy Association. (2000a). Enforcement procedure for occupational therapy code of ethics. *American Journal of Occupational Therapy, 54*, 617–621.

American Occupational Therapy Association. (2000b). Occupational therapy code of ethics. *American Journal of Occupational Therapy, 54*, 614–616.

Gilligan, C. (1982). *In a different voice: Psychological theory and women's development*. Cambridge, MA: Harvard University.

Graber, G. C. (1988). Basic theories in medical ethics. In J. F. Monagle & D. C. Thomasma (Eds.). *Medical ethics: A guide for health professionals* (pp. 462–475). Rockville, MD: Aspen.

Hansen, R. A. (2000a). Disciplinary action: Whose responsibility? In P. Kyler (Ed.). *Reference guide to the occupational therapy code of ethics* (p. 21). Bethesda, MD: American Occupational Therapy Association.

Hansen, R. A. (2000b). Ethical jurisdiction of occupational therapy: The role of AOTA, AOTCB and state regulatory boards. In P. Kyler (Ed.). *Reference guide to the occupational therapy code of ethics* (pp. 22–24). Bethesda, MD: American Occupational Therapy Association.

Hansen, R. A. (2000c). Guidelines for responding to questions about ethical dilemmas. In P. Kyler (Ed.). *Reference guide to the occupational therapy code of ethics* (p. 20). Bethesda, MD: American Occupational Therapy Association.

Haste, H., & Baddeley, J. (1991). Moral theory and culture: The case of gender. In W. M. Kurtines & J. L. Gewirtz (Eds.). *Handbook of moral behavior and development. Vol. I: Theory* (pp. 223–249). Hillsdale, NJ: Lawrence Erlbaum.

Kanny, E. (1993). Core values and attitudes of occupational therapy practice. *American Journal of Occupational Therapy, 47*, 1085–1086.

Kohlberg, L. (1984). *Essays on moral development. Vol. II. The psychology of moral development: The nature and validity of moral stages*. San Francisco: Harper & Row.

Kohlberg, L., & Candee, D. (1984). The relationship of moral judgment to moral action. In W. Kurtines & J. Gerwitz (Eds.). *Morality, moral behavior and moral development* (pp. 52–73). New York: Wiley Interscience.

Ladd, R. E. (1996). Partiality and the pediatrician. *Journal of Clinical Ethics, 7*, 29–34.

McGrath, E. (1977). Institutional alternative for an education in values. *Counseling and Values, 22*, 5–19.

Morrill, R. (1980). *Teaching values in education*. San Francisco: Jossey-Bass.

National Certification Board for Occupational Therapy. (2002). Procedures for disciplinary action. Available at: http://nbcot.org/nbcot/scripts/programs/disciplinary-action-procedures.asp. Accessed 10/7/02.

Raths, L., Harmin, M., & Simon, S. (1966). *Values and teaching*. Columbus. OH: Merrill.

Sichel, B. (1992). Ethics of caring and the institutional ethics committee. In H. B. Holmes & L. M. Purdy (Eds.). *Feminist perspectives in medical ethics* (pp. 113–123). Bloomington: Indiana University Press.

CHAPTER 53

RESEARCH: DISCOVERING KNOWLEDGE THROUGH SYSTEMATIC INVESTIGATION

DIANA M. BAILEY

SECTION I

Introduction to Research

Throughout your educational program for occupational therapy, you will be asked to read and critically assess research found in occupational therapy and other professional journals. Your instructors may use research studies to help you gain a greater understanding of the effectiveness of specific interventions, to analyze the context of intervention, to put course material in a clinical context, and to instill the habit of reading professional literature with a critical eye. Consequently, you will have the skills to base your practice on research evidence and your clinical reasoning rather than relying on the traditional, but untested, approaches to intervention (Portney & Watkins, 2000).

As you read research articles you will ask yourself, "Is this an intervention I would want to use with my clients?" Some ideas to help you critically appraise research are presented in this chapter, along with a brief discussion of **qualitative research** and **quantitative research** and evidence-based practice.

THE PROCESS OF RESEARCH

Most of the research you will read will be in peer-reviewed journals such as the *American Journal of Occupational Therapy* and other journals in occupational therapy and related fields. These journals publish only those articles that meet

RESEARCH NOTE 53–1

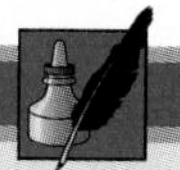

Research Priorities for the Profession

KENNETH J. OTTENBACHER

Since the 1980s, occupational therapy has addressed the challenge of research and emerged as a viable and respected health-care discipline. Research, however, represents a dynamic challenge that must continue to be a professional priority. The changes in our health-care system have generated a new set of research questions and issues. Determining the answers to these questions and raising new ones ensure that occupational therapy remains a viable health-care specialty in the twenty-first century.

The American Occupational Therapy Foundation (n.d.) identified the following as research priorities for the profession:

- Development and standardization of instruments for clinical practice and research.
- Studies that examine the effect of occupational therapy services, relative to some aspect of the occupational therapy knowledge base.
- Studies that examine and/or compare various strategies of intervention and the reasoning and decision-making process required by practice.
- Theory development, refinement, and testing.
- Studies regarding occupation in so far as it relates to wellness and adaptation in society; such studies may focus on healthy or disabled persons of any age group.
- Efforts to develop, modify, or apply innovative research methods to determine their relevance to the research needs of the profession.

The foundation also provides information on research priorities and research competencies for occupational therapists.

American Occupational Therapy Foundation (n.d.). Practice parameters and research priorities for occupational therapy. Retrieved October 10, 2002, from www.aotf.org/html/priorities.html

the standards of a panel of peer reviewers, typically drawn from its editorial board. People recruited for editorial boards are recognized for their expertise in the field. Their review of submitted papers ensures high quality research publications. Journal articles are of several types, including reviews of the literature, opinion articles, and empirical research. Empirical research involves posing a research question and collecting and analyzing data to answer this question.

Empirical research tends to be a cyclical process. Although this is not always the case, researchers usually start with a question in mind, go through the investigative stages, and end up with not just an answer to the original question but also further questions that arise during the analysis and interpretation of the data. These questions often lead to additional research. The steps required to complete a research project follow a logical sequence (Bailey, 1997):

1. Identify a problem that needs to be solved or a question that needs to be answered.
2. Review the existing research on that issue.
3. Formulate a question or **hypothesis** about the problem based on the reading.
4. Design a research method that will address the question or hypothesis.
5. Carry out the research design.
6. Collect data and interpret the findings.
7. Publish the answer to the question so that others may benefit from the identified knowledge.

QUALITATIVE AND QUANTITATIVE RESEARCH

Researchers ask a wide variety of questions and it is these questions that shape the methods researchers use in conducting their work. Tseng and Chow (2000) were interested in "identifying factors associated with slow handwriting" (p. 84) in school-age children. This question called for a correlational research design that involved comparing a sample of slow- and normal-speed handwriters. In contrast, qualitative researchers are interested in understanding how people experience the world around them. Primeau (1998) examined "the nature of parent-child play and its orchestration within the daily occupations of families" (p. 189). The data generated by these two studies differ dramatically. Tseng and Chow assessed children with a variety of instruments and compared the children's performance on these tests by using statistical analysis. In contrast, Primeau used extensive observations and interviews to understand how parents and children play. She generated themes from the data based on her observations and interviews. These themes contained rich descriptions and interpretations of the patterns observed.

Quantitative research answers questions that require standardized measures, generate numerical data, and impose controls (e.g., sampling procedures to decrease variability) (Portney & Watkins, 2000). An assumption that underlies quantitative research is that there is an objective reality

TABLE 53-1. **DIFFERENCES BETWEEN QUANTITATIVE AND QUALITATIVE RESEARCH**

Characteristic	Quantitative	Qualitative
Purpose	Theory testing; to establish facts, show causal relationships among variables; goal to generalize	Theory development; to describe multiple realities and interpretations; to understand perspective of participants in a setting
Design	Predetermined and structured; does not change during study; formal and specific to a study; used as a plan of operation	General and flexible; evolves during study; used as a hunch for how to proceed
Data	Quantifiable and statistical, using counts and measures; variables are defined ahead of time and managed in predetermined manner using statistical procedures	Descriptive data deal with qualities that are not measurable; may be field notes, artifacts, people's own words, personal or official documents
Participants	Often large samples requiring random selection; in experimental design use of control groups for extraneous variables	Small sample chosen according to the goals of the study
Investigator's relationship with participants	Roles of researcher and participant are distinct and short term; objective; no personal involvement lest data be influenced	Intense contact with participants over long periods; emphasis on trust and empathy; egalitarian relationship
Methods and techniques	Experiments, structured surveys, interviews, or observations, variable manipulation, control, statistical analysis	Observation, participant observation, reviewing documents and artifacts, open-ended interviewing, coding, searching for patterns, narrative and displays for portrayal of data
Instruments and tools	Tests and scales, inventories, questionnaires, hardware	Researcher is tool for data collection; observations and interviews aided by audiotape or videotape recordings
Data analysis	Occurs at end of data collection; deductive; use of statistical manipulation; seeks evidence to prove or disprove predetermined hypotheses	Ongoing throughout study; recursive; inductive, leading to models, themes, concepts; use of coding, note taking, event listing, pattern matching, charting, matrices, and triangulation; theory emerges as data are analyzed
Outcome	Study answers specific research question by producing statistical evidence to prove a point; brief statistical outcomes followed by discussion of findings	Lengthy, descriptive text presenting data as words; text is rich, anecdotal, full of description in narrative form; provides verification of existing theory or new grounded theory and resulting research questions to be investigated
Problems	Difficulty controlling variables that will affect the study; validity may be questioned; controlled experimental studies may have little relevance to daily life; researcher and data collection methods my affect participants	Procedures are not standardized and cannot be replicated; difficulty of managing large quantities of data; extremely time-consuming nature of data collection and data analysis

that can be observed and measured. From this perspective, concern for bias on the part of the researcher or in any aspect of the research process is paramount, because this threatens the objectivity of the findings.

In contrast, qualitative research is highly contextualized because of its grounding in understanding the experience of research participants from their own perspective. Qualitative research is emergent—that is, questions may change during the course of the research, often because the researcher has a better understanding of the people being studied (Lincoln & Guba, 1985).

Answering qualitative and quantitative research questions requires different approaches to the research process. The quantitative investigation begins with a theory and specific hypotheses that address one defined issue, whereas a qualitative investigation begins with research questions that may be multifaceted and broad. The questions may evolve throughout the qualitative study process. Some qualitative studies end by posing specific hypotheses and theoretical constructs (Glaser & Strauss, 1967), whereas others strive solely for an understanding of the phenomena being studied (Denzin & Lincoln, 2000).

The phenomena that can appropriately be studied using these two styles of research are quite different. For example, in a study using qualitative methods, understanding and the discovery of meaning are the goals rather than measurement of variables (Denzin & Lincoln, 2000). Qualitative methods lend themselves to the study of individuals or small groups of participants, and issues are typically judged from an emic, or insider's, point of view (Agar, 1986). With quantitative methods, on the other hand, measurement of variables in controlled conditions, sampling to ensure representation of the population, and determining the appropriate sample size are critical (DePoy & Gitlin, 1994). Issues are viewed from an etic, or outsider's, point of view.

Research questions may require the use of both methods (DePoy & Gitlin, 1994). Some of the reasons researchers may use multiple methods in their studies are to add power to the findings, to gain a comprehensive understanding of a phenomenon by uncovering different aspects with different techniques, and to compensate for the flaws of one design with the strengths of another. Perhaps the most common reason for a researcher to use both qualitative and quantitative designs is to achieve triangulation of methods. The purpose of triangulation of methods is to confirm information about a phenomenon by measuring it in several ways (DePoy & Gitlin, 1994). Table 53-1 presents the differences between quantitative and qualitative research designs.

CONCLUSION

The thought process and procedures that researchers engage in has been described. It is important that you have a grasp of the process of research so you not only can engage in research as beginning investigators, but also so you can read an article analytically and critically. The next section of the chapter will describe how to read a research article.

SECTION II

How to Read a Research Article

Well-informed practitioners know the literature and are familiar with the leading researchers in their particular areas of practice. They keep current with the issues and advances in their specialty in order to offer their clients the best possible care. Reading professional literature, specifically research studies, is one method of updating knowledge. Knowing when research studies are sufficiently well-designed to trust the results requires a solid grasp of the principles of research design. This section guides you through the process of reading empirical research reports, enabling you to critique the research and to know when the results are sufficiently trustworthy to be incorporated into your own practice.

THE COMPONENTS OF A RESEARCH ARTICLE

The general format for quantitative research reports tends to be similar in most journals. Articles from quantitative research are usually divided into the following sections: front material, problem, background, purpose, hypotheses or questions, method, results, discussion, and references. Qualitative research papers may follow a similar organization or may use different organizational strategies. Despite the variation in organization, qualitative research papers contain similar categories of information.

Front Material

The front material is found at the beginning of the article and usually consists of the title of the piece, the authors and their affiliations, key words that describe the research, and an abstract. Titles indicate the focus of the article. Titles that do not address the content, however eye catching, are not helpful to the potential reader, or to those performing a literature search. It is useful to know the author's affiliation because this can inform you about the environment for the study (such as a hospital or a school), possibly the school of thought from which the author comes, and if the author works in a facility known for the topic under discussion. There is usually sufficient information to contact the author should you wish to discuss the article.

Key terms, selected by the author, allow the article to be indexed appropriately in electronic databases so that it may be retrieved efficiently by those conducting literature searches. Key terms also give you further information about the important content in the article. The abstract provides a complete summary of the problem, questions, procedures, and results and allows you to decide if you wish to continue reading.

Problem

The problem is the major issue the researcher wishes to address in the study. It may not be clearly labeled as such but should be obvious in the first paragraph or two when the researcher writes about why the issue poses a problem, why it needs a solution, and what will be better as a result. Perhaps there are clients who will benefit, programs that will be improved, practitioners who will have more knowledge or skill, or client–practitioner relationships that will be enhanced. Look for an explanation of how the research question and design relate to the identified issue for an indication of whether or not this particular study actually addresses the larger problem. You should be able to tell what is likely to be improved as a result of the study. This is often referred to as the significance of the study.

For instance, Tseng and Chow (2000) noted that "proficiency in handwriting is essential if students are to accomplish an acceptable amount of work in the classroom" (p. 83) and that many school tasks are performed under time constraints. This poses a problem for children who write slowly and is the larger problem being addressed in the study. The investigators examined factors they thought might contribute to slow handwriting. The significance of the study is that contributing factors might be able to be ameliorated, ultimately helping children with slow handwriting increase their output.

Background

Most of the background material is a review of literature relevant to the problem under study. Authors summarize findings from previous studies that have addressed the issue and locate their study in relation to those findings. For example, Tseng and Chow (2000) investigated differences in perceptual-motor measures and sustained attention between children with slow and normal handwriting speeds. First, they described why proficiency in handwriting is essential, pointing out that remedying handwriting difficulties is one of the most important areas of school-based occupational therapy. Second, they cited research describing the constellation of skills necessary for efficient writing, culminating in sustained attention and perceptual motor skills. Next, they pointed out that most studies have focused primarily on illegibility, visual perception skills, fine motor skills, and visual motor integration. Finally, they summarized the findings of the few studies that do address handwriting speed.

You must judge if the author has treated controversial issues fairly by presenting various points of view and if all the important research about the issue has been included. It is usually possible to make such judgments only if you are familiar with the topic. Authors should end their review of the literature by making clear if their study will fill a gap in previous studies or replicate a study with which they were dissatisfied, possibly improving the design or examining a different population.

Purpose

Early in the article, authors explain the purpose of the study; what they hope to accomplish and why the study is worth doing. Tseng and Chow (2000) stated, "we attempt to identify more clearly the factors associated with slow handwriting in the hope that this may help to elucidate the underlying mechanisms" (p. 84). Once you understand the researchers' aims for the study, you will be able to assess if those aims were met.

Hypotheses or Research Questions

Look for a formal statement of the hypotheses or research questions being addressed. If you find hypotheses, you can be fairly sure that you are reading an experimental, quantitative study that is looking for a cause and effect between variables (one variable caused something to happen to another) or a correlation (relationship) among variables. If you see one or more research questions, the study is likely to be

ETHICS NOTE 53–1 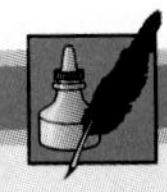

Who Owns Intellectual Property

PENNY KYLER AND RUTH A. HANSEN

Doug is a newly hired instructor in a well-established occupational therapy program. He needs to begin to do research. He has spent long hours, when he was not on a teaching contract, working on a grant proposal. He asks his department chairperson to review and evaluate his proposal. The chair tells him that the proposal needs more work. Then 6 months later, Doug finds out that, without his knowledge, the chair submitted Doug's proposal for funding and that if funded the chair will be the project director.

QUESTIONS AND EXERCISES

1. **Who owns the ideas for this grant proposal?**
2. **Does the department chairperson have the authority and the right to submit this grant without Doug's knowledge or agreement?**
3. **What options does Doug have in this situation? What are the benefits and risks with each potential course of action?**

qualitative. For example, Primeau (1998) listed four questions for her study beginning with, "What does parent-child play look like" (p. 188)?

In the study on handwriting, Tseng and Chow (2000) stated, "We hypothesized that children with slow handwriting would obtain lower scores on a series of standard visual-perception, motor, visual-motor integration, and attention tests than did children with normal handwriting speeds" (p. 84). In contrast to Primeau's participant observation study, this study was correlational in nature.

Method

The methods section describes in detail how the study was conducted. It should contain sufficient detail to allow you to assess the appropriateness of the method to the purpose of the study. To continue with the handwriting investigation, if the aims of the study were to investigate "differences in perceptual-motor measures and sustained attention between children with slow and normal handwriting speed" and to examine "the relationship between these factors" (p. 83), you would expect to see in the method section that the authors located groups of children known to have slow and normal handwriting speeds and that they tested them on perceptual motor skills and attention. In fact, Tseng and Chow located 34 slow handwriters and 35 normal speed handwriters in elementary schools in Taiwan and administered three perceptual motor tests and a vigilance task to assess their attention. They compared the test scores of the slow- and normal-speed handwriters to identify the best set of predictors for handwriting speed.

The description of the method also allows you to determine what is done similarly to or differently from other studies described in the literature review. If you are knowledgeable about the study topic you will be aware of issues that could influence the outcome of the study. For the handwriting study, issues might include the lack of norms for Chinese children, coupled with all the usual problems associated with testing young children, such as anxiety, motivation, interest, and attention span. You should look to see if these issues have been addressed.

The method section contains several subsections that will further describe the study.

Sources of Data

The people or items (such as clinical records) from whom information has been gathered are the sources of data. It is customary for researchers to say what criteria they used to determine which individuals were eligible to be in the study (population) and the methods they used to select those actually included in the study (sample). You must assess if the criteria suit the purpose of the study. The demographics of the participants help you judge if the findings are likely to be relevant to your clients.

Participant Selection

Generally for an experimental research study, it is desirable to have random selection of participants from the targeted population to ensure control for external variables, such as age or race and ethnicity (Polit & Hungler, 1999). Items such as these might have an effect on the outcome, and you should question the appropriateness of the results of an experimental study that does not make some attempt at random selection.

In contrast, qualitative researchers chose participants because they hold a distinct position in a group, have a particular relationship with other members in the group, or have certain characteristics that the researcher plans to investigate. Key informants are chosen because they hold exactly the qualifications or characteristics the researcher wishes to study (Goetz & LeCompte, 1993).

Sample Size

The research design guides the size of the sample. For studies using statistical analysis, the sample must be large enough to establish statistical power (DePoy & Gitlin, 1994). The choice of how many participants depends entirely on the type of research and the statistical analysis selected. A large survey may have several hundred participants who were selected by a random method to increase the probability that the sample represents the population. In contrast, qualitative research such as an ethnographic study may need only three for four key informants, while a case study is limited to a single case.

The author should clearly state how many people were solicited to participate in the study, how many accepted, and how many dropped out during the study. You can then make an informed decision regarding the number and characteristics of the remaining participants and whether the data will be sufficient to answer the research question, given the type of research study.

Tseng and Chow (2000) solicited nominations from teachers at two elementary schools for children evaluated as slow-speed ($n = 70$) and normal-speed ($n = 35$) handwriters. These 110 children were potential participants in the study and made up the study population. The investigators tested these children and selected those who fell one standard deviation below the norm for the slow handwriting group ($n = 34$); those who tested above the cutoff were assigned to the normal-speed handwriting group ($n = 35$). These 69 children made up the study sample. Children whose teachers' evaluations and test scores were inconsistent were eliminated from the study ($n = 41$).

Instruments

The methods section should also include a description of all tools and hardware used (Currier, 1990). You do not need details about common instruments such as goniometers and pinch grips, but will want information about a survey that the authors designed themselves or an unusual paper-and-pencil test or psychological instrument. Look for data on **reliability** and **validity** if a standardized tool was used, so that you can judge the credibility of the results. If the instrument has not been standardized, you should ask yourself what that means for the results and if you trust the authors' conclusions.

To help you assess the **trustworthiness** of the results, look for details about pretests and posttests, frequency of test administration, test administrators, and the test conditions. Qualitative studies based on interviews should include a description of the interview process and list some of the questions asked.

Procedures

The procedures to collect data should be described, including the instructions to the participants, what tasks were performed during the study by the researcher and by the participants, and how the data were collected. It is expected that procedures will be described in sufficient detail that the study could be replicated. It is just as important for procedures to be clarified in qualitative research.

Results

The results section in a quantitative study briefly describes the statistical analysis used, tells you if the hypothesis was supported, and then reports the data in detail, often using tables or graphs. This is usually the part of the article that new consumers of research are tempted to skip. If you keep in mind what the investigators are trying to find out and how they are going about that task, it will be easier to make sense of the statistical presentation. If the researchers have conducted a survey, they often report the results in a table showing what percentage of respondents answered questions in a particular way.

Many other types of research designs besides surveys use descriptive statistics to describe, organize, and summarize the findings. Authors might use frequencies, percentages, descriptions of central tendency (mean, median, mode), and descriptions of relative position (range, standard deviation). Tseng and Chow (2000) used tables to present demographic data on their participants as well as results from the perceptual motor and vigilance tests. Remember, they were trying to identify factors contributing to children's slow handwriting and were testing to see if perceptual motor difficulties and lack of sustained attention might be among the contributing factors.

Sometimes correlation analysis is used to see if two variables are related to one another. An inferential test, such as the Pearson product moment correlation analysis used by Tseng and Chow (2000), is appropriate for this purpose. Tseng and Chow wanted to see if there was a relationship between handwriting speed and the perceptual motor subtests and the vigilance test. They found a significant correlation among handwriting speed, age, and several of the test results.

Researchers will also tell you the significance level of any relationships they find, represented as a p value. In simple terms, if the authors report $p < .05$, this means the probability that the finding occurred by chance was less than 5 times in 100, or < 5%. There will almost always be a p value mentioned when statistical data are reported, and more often than not it will be given at the .05 level, although sometimes .01 or .02 are used. Just remember that these numbers indicate the chances (1%, 2%, or 5%) that the findings were the result of an error in the study procedures.

Other ways researchers may analyze numerical data are by looking for differences, perhaps between the same participants' pretest and posttest, or between outcomes after treatment for two groups (an experimental group and a control group), or between several variables related to a group of participants to see how they vary among each other. Tseng and Chow (2000) used an inferential test called multivariate analysis of variance to look for differences between the scores of slow writers and normal-speed writers on perceptual motor tests and the vigilance task. They found significant differences at the $p < .05$ level on all but two of the subtests.

The hypotheses and methods section should make clear what the investigators are trying to find out when using statistical procedures, and a careful reading of the titles of tables and figures will let you know if the authors are simply describing data about their participants or if they are looking for relationships and/or differences between participants' performances.

Discussion

Papers reporting qualitative research may be organized in separate results and discussion sections. However, more typically these are presented in an integrated way in which research findings and interpretation are merged, because in the actual research process data collection and data analysis are not separated into two different stages. Rather, analysis of data begins soon after data collection starts. This merging enables the qualitative researcher to adapt the research approach as an understanding of the topic emerges.

This section is generally the longest portion of the qualitative article and uses narrative, rather than statistical analysis, to report the results. Extended quotations of participants or descriptions of the setting, often organized thematically, are hallmarks of qualitative research (Miles & Huberman, 1994; Strauss & Corbin, 1998).

You should ask if the qualitative researchers are justified in their conclusions by careful scrutiny of the data. Did they ensure trustworthiness by using multiple sources to be sure their interpretation is an accurate reflection of the setting (triangulation)? Did they discuss their conclusions with the participants to see that they conveyed the

Questions to guide reading and critiquing a quantitative research study		
Topic:		
Title:		
Author(s)		
Source:		
Year:	Volume:	Pages:
1. What was the purpose of the study?		
What questions were asked and were they precisely and clearly stated?		
What hypotheses were stated or implied? Write them in either research or null form.		
2. To what extent did the researcher give evidence of having reviewed literature relevant to the study?		
Were any areas of literature that may have been relevant to the study not reviewed?		
3. From what population was the sample selected?		
How was the sample selected and how large was it? What was the rationale for how the sample was selected, for sample size and such?		
Was subject attrition reported? Explain.		
Could the results of the study be generalized to a larger group? Specify.		
(Answer 4.a. for descriptive and correlational studies and 4.b. for pre-experimental, experimental, and quasi-experimental studies.)		
4.a. What variables were studied and were they consistent with the stated purpose of the study?		
What evidence of instrument reliability and validity was provided?		
4.b. What intervention (independent variable) was studied? Was the described intervention consistent with the stated purpose of the study?		
What outcome measures (dependent variable) were used in the study? Were these measures appropriate operational definitions of the variables studied?		
What evidence of instrument reliability and validity was provided?		
5. What was the design of the study and what are its inherent limitations?		
6. All aspects of a research project should be controlled except the ones being studied by the researcher. List all factors controlled in the study and how they were controlled.		
Controlled Factors Method of Control		
A.		
B.		
C.		
D.		
E.		
List all factors not controlled in the research study that you believe could have affected the results of the study. Briefly explain how each factor could have influenced the research results.		
Uncontrolled Factors Potential influence		
A.		
B.		
C.		
D.		
E.		
7. How were the data analyzed and what were the results? Were the data analysis procedures appropriate for the design of the study, the sample size, and so on.		
8. What were the strengths of the study?		
9. Did the researcher(s) describe the limitations of the study? Are there any other limitations to the study that were not described by the researcher(s)?		
10. Does the study have implications for practice? What are they?		

FIGURE 53–1. Questions to guide the reading and critiquing of a quantitative research study. From Dietz, J. C., & Crepeau, E. B. (1998). Qualitative and quantitative research: Joint countributors to the knowledge base of occupational therapy. In M. E. Neistadt & E. B. Crepeau (Eds.), *Willard and Spackman's occupational therapy* (9th ed., p. 849). Philadelphia: Lippincott. Reprinted with permission.

viewpoint of the participants (member checking)? Did they discuss the data with peers to be sure their perspective did not skew the findings (peer examination) (Lincoln & Guba, 1985)?

In the discussion section of quantitative research, investigators should compare their findings with those reported in the literature review and comment on points of agreement and departure. Look for suggestions as to why the authors' findings might be different and see if you agree.

Researchers should also comment on any findings that do not support the hypotheses and offer thoughts on why they might have occurred. Do the authors suggest how these

Questions to guide reading and critiquing a qualitative research study		
Topic:		
Title:		
Author(s)		
Source:		
Year:	Volume:	Pages:
1. What was the purpose of the study? Were research questions asked? If so, what were they and were they clearly stated?		
2. To what extent did the researcher give evidence of having reviewed literature relevant to the study? Were any areas of literature not reviewed that may have been relevant to the study?		
3. Who were the participants and what was the rationale behind their selection? Did the researcher provide you with adequate information about the participants and the context of the phenomenon studied?		
4. What sources of data were used and what were the methods for data collection and analysis? What were the coding categories and what was the reasoning process for thematic analysis? Did they make sense to you?		
5. Was there congruence between the chosen research tradition and the methods for data collection and analysis?		
6. How did the researcher establish the trustworthiness of the data? What is your evaluation of the researcher's process and findings?		
7. How did the researcher report his or her involvement in the process and how did the researcher explain the effect of this involvement on the reported results of the study? Do you agree with the researcher's assessment?		
8. What were the reported results of the study? Did they make sense to you? Are there other plausible interpretations of the data? Did you find the study to be trustworthy? Why? Why not? Be specific.		
9. How do findings from this study link to research findings from other studies? What further research questions did the study inspire?		
10. Does the study have implications for clinical practice or for theory refinement or development? Explain.		

FIGURE 53–2. Questions to guide the reading and critiquing of a qualitative research study. From Dietz, J. C., & Crepeau, E. B. (1998). Qualitative and quantitative research: Joint contributors to the knowledge base of occupational therapy. In M. E. Neistadt & E. B. Crepeau (Eds.), Willard and Spackman's occupational therapy (9th ed., p. 850). Philadelphia: Lippincott, reprinted with permission.

problems might be avoided in future studies or how participants who did not find the treatment beneficial may be approached in future studies? It is important that authors remark on the shortcomings of the study so that others may repeat the study (replication) and make improvements.

The discussion section for both qualitative and quantitative research is simply the authors' speculation about what the results mean. You are entitled to draw your own conclusions based on a careful reading of the entire article. Part of the critique of the article should be if the authors gave you sufficient information to allow you to make your own decisions about its quality and utility. Ultimately, you are deciding if this is a study whose findings you wish to incorporate into your own practice. To make this decision, you ask yourselves these types of questions: What has been contributed? How has the study helped solve the original problem? What conclusions and theoretical implications can be drawn from this study?

References

The final portion of the paper presents all publications and other materials that were cited in the text. Enough information is provided to allow you to identify and find the material.

CONCLUSION

Figures 53-1 and 53-2 present worksheets to assist your reading and critiquing of qualitative and quantitative research articles. Ultimately, the goal for research is to enable practitioners to change their practice based on their own clinical reasoning and the findings of research studies. Those who do so systematically are using evidence-based practice, which is discussed in the next section.

SECTION III

Evidence-Based Practice: The Link between Research and Practice

When you use the results of research studies to shape your practice, you are using evidence-based practice (EBP). EBP helps you select the most clinically effective and cost-efficient interventions. EBP is much more than simply reading articles and using some components in practice. It is a way to aid and enhance the clinical reasoning skills you have developed from education and experience. It is a way to integrate research study findings—evidence—into practice by helping you select the best evaluation methods and tools as well as the best intervention techniques and approaches for each client.

Sackett, Richardson, Rosenberg, and Haynes (1997) defined EBP as "the conscientious, explicit and judicious use of current best evidence in making decisions about the care of individual patients" (p. 2). While Greenhalgh (1997) wrote that "the science of finding, evaluating, and implementing the results of medical [occupational therapy] research can, and often does, make patient care more objective, more logical, and more cost effective" (p. xv).

WHY SHOULD OCCUPATIONAL THERAPY PRACTITIONERS USE EVIDENCE-BASED PRACTICE?

In the daily hubbub of practice, it is difficult to systematically gather evidence from clients and their families, peers, and consultants. It is part of human nature to gravitate to ideas and solutions that fit with our own beliefs and experiences. In contrast, we tend to be less attentive to ideas about assessment and intervention that do not fit with our beliefs and experience. EBP was developed partly in response to this tendency and encourages us to consider new and different evidence that may be better suited to each particular client (Holm, 2000).

However, evidence gathered from published studies that were not carried out with similar clients and settings may not apply to your particular situation. Although it is possible to generalize from the research to your setting, you must also gather evidence from your clients, their families, and colleagues. Thus the most effective assessment and interventions for clients is generated from evidence gathered from published studies and experience.

EBP will enhance your clinical reasoning to achieve the collaborative goals you set with clients. EBP provides the tools for organizing evidence to guide assessment and intervention planning. It involves evaluating evidence for its currency and validity and using the best evidence to achieve the occupational outcomes (Holm, 2000; Tickle-Degnen, 1999).

THE PROCESS OF EVIDENCE-BASED PRACTICE

Sackett and Haynes (1995) suggested the following steps to introduce EBP into your practice:

1. Formulate the problem by converting information needs into answerable questions.
2. Track down the best evidence with which to answer these questions.
3. Critically appraise the evidence, assessing its validity and usefulness for your own practice.
4. Implement the most valid and applicable findings in one's own practice.
5. Evaluate your performance in light of new introductions.

Each of these points is examined in some detail.

Formulate the Problem as an Answerable Question

You will be faced with many types of problems that can be resolved by gaining evidence from the research literature and other practitioners. These problems include instances concerning the choice of the best assessment procedure or intervention to use. EBP may also be used to examine strategies to improve communication with clients, such as ways of increasing the collaborative process.

To formulate one of these problems as an answerable question, you should identify clients similar to the one whose intervention is being reconsidered, identify one or two occupation-based intervention strategies that would be appropriate, and describe the occupational performance outcomes you hope the client will achieve. You might ask questions that inform you regarding the context of the intervention, such as, "Are comprehensive psychometric assessments and simulator tests more effective than one session of behind-the-wheel performance, for an elderly person showing early signs of dementia who is referred for a driving evaluation?" or "Which would be the best way to help a person with schizophrenia begin to learn grocery shopping, working on pricing and food selection in a clinical setting or shopping in a supermarket?" or "Is group intervention or individual intervention more effective in enabling persons with traumatic head injury relearn how to negotiate their home environment?" Also, you can ask questions about your interactions with clients that might affect the outcome of an intervention: "When treating clients from a very different culture than my own, would encouraging them to discuss their culture with me or learning about their culture ahead of time be more likely to engage them in intervention?"

Identify the Evidence by Conducting a Literature Search

Once a clinical question has been developed, you begin your search for evidence in the literature. There are many ways to gather evidence regarding clients, such as attending conferences and workshops, obtaining bibliographies and other resources, belonging to an AOTA special-interest section (SIS), joining an electronic mailing list related to your specialty area, or joining professional associations and other groups concerned with the client group they are serving.

But perhaps the most productive way to gain the evidence to answer particular questions is by conducting a search of the literature. You may do this by searching your own collection of journals and resources. However, a systematic review of the literature via electronic databases such as OT SEARCH, MEDLINE, or CINAHL provides a wide sweep of the research literature. Librarians, especially reference librarians, can be helpful in this process.

Tickle-Degnen (2000a) asserted that "evidence be gathered in a passionately dispassionate manner. What this means is that all the evidence, most importantly that which disconfirms the practitioner's previous preconceptions and biases, must be gathered" (p. 104). You must be aware of your natural tendency to lean toward ideas and actions that confirm what you already believe and do, while avoiding ideas and actions that are outside your usual realm.

Critically Appraise the Evidence

When evaluating evidence, it is important to remember that the goal of EBP is to gather evidence that is current and will be most effective with the particular client under consideration. It is unlikely that the evidence found regarding a specific problem, be it from articles, workshop participation or discussion with peers, will yield a clear-cut answer. However, don't be discouraged. The goal is to find the best possible answer to the problem by sifting through the evidence. This can be achieved by selecting the most recent studies, because they will address the latest ideas, attitudes, and techniques regarding the topic, and by looking for review articles that critique studies related to your question (Tickle-Degnen, 2000b).

Here are ways studies can be assessed for their usefulness as evidence for treating a particular client. Assess the similarity between your client and the participants in the study in terms of diagnosis or condition, sex, age, culture, and any other condition that is deemed relevant to the intervention. Also, assess the study for its match to the client's occupational performance goals and outcomes. More often than not, the study group will not resemble the client in all aspects, in which case, you must decide if the assessment or intervention strategies should be used given the differences you have identified. Examine the study carefully to see if the author relates the individual characteristics of people in the study group and shows the different intervention outcomes for each person. This will enable you to find those study participants who most resemble your client, and to judge the effectiveness of the intervention.

As a further check on the usefulness of the study as evidence, the therapist looks to see if the researcher controlled for outside influences—that is, can the results be attributed to the intervention rather than to some other factor? Random assignment to experimental and control groups enhance the validity of a study, as does equivalent (but different) interventions with both groups.

You should also examine the study for reliability. Reliability means that the results are likely to be found again and again if the same conditions are repeated in the same manner. Reliability also addresses the consistency of results when interventions are offered by different practitioners. If you are looking for evidence concerning the best assessment tool to use, you should be sure that the author discusses the validity and reliability of the instruments in the study.

Studies with a large number of participants (60 or more) provide stronger evidence for an intervention program for your client. However, it is extremely difficult for occupational therapy researchers to obtain large numbers of participants. Sometimes you must judge the outcomes found in studies with fewer participants making decisions based on the best evidence available.

Ultimately, like practitioners in other fields, you will be making judgments about the evidence from less-than-perfect studies. The strongest evidence will come from studies in which client characteristics are similar to those of your client and in which the occupational needs and outcomes are the same as your client's needs and soals. Failing this, the best evidence possible must be gleaned from the available literature.

Implement the Most Valid and Applicable Findings

The next step is to explain the research that supports your recommended intervention or assessment to the client and family. This explanation must be clear and concise so that the client and family will understand. It is a challenge to effectively communicate the often ambiguous and confusing information to clients and their families while keeping the client's desired occupational goals in the forefront of the discussion. Once all the decision makers have agreed on the intervention, you and the client implement the intervention program. When you have been true to EBP principles and examined all the evidence equally, it is possible that you will select and implement an intervention approach that is not in your usual mode of practice. This broadening of your intervention and assessment strategies makes you a more well-rounded and effective practitioner.

Evaluate Performance in Light of New Introductions

The final step of introducing EBP is to evaluate the effectiveness of the intervention. Did the client achieve his or her goals? Were the client and his or her family pleased with the outcome? Was it cost effective? Was it a slow process or a quick process? Did it involve many resources? Were the resources at hand or difficult to acquire? Clients should be involved in the evaluation of the intervention to determine their level of satisfaction. The evaluation of a client intervention contributes to your knowledge base and provides evidence for future actions. It is crucial to maintain systematic and thorough records regarding the effectiveness of particular interventions for specific clients.

CONCLUSION

The ultimate goal of occupational therapy is to improve occupational therapy practice so that the services practitioner's provide help clients achieve the best possible outcomes. This goal can be achieved, in part, by your familiarity with the research process that will enable you to engage in EBP with clients. Doing so allows you to feel confident that you are offering the best interventions to clients, interventions that are based on relevant, valid, and reliable evidence.

ACKNOWLEDGMENT

Portions of this chapter that concern research draw heavily from Bailey (1997).

References

Agar, M. H. (1986). *Speaking of ethnography*. [Sage university paper series on qualitative research methods, Vol. 2]. Beverly Hills, CA: Sage.

Bailey, D. M. (1997). *Research for the health professional: A practical guide* (2nd ed.). Philadelphia: Davis.

Currier, D. P. (1990). *Elements of research in physical therapy* (3rd ed.). Baltimore: Williams & Wilkins.

Denzin, N. K., & Lincoln, Y. S. (2000). Introduction: Entering the field of qualitative research. In N. K. Denzin & Y. S. Lincoln (Eds.). *Handbook of qualitative research* (2nd ed., pp. 1–17). Thousand Oaks, CA: Sage.

DePoy, E., & Gitlin, L. N. (1994). *Introduction to research: Multiple strategies for health and human services*. St. Louis: Mosby.

Dietz, J. C., & Crepeau, E. B. (1998). Qualitative and quantitative research: Joint contributors to the knowledge base of occupational therapy. In M. E. Neistadt & E. B. Crepeau (Eds.). *Willard and Spackman's occupational therapy* (9th ed., pp. 847–853). Philadelphia: Lippincott.

Glaser, B. G., & Strauss, A. L. (1967). *The discovery of grounded theory: Strategies for qualitative research*. New York: De Gruyter.

Goetz, J. P., & LeCompte, M. D. (1993). *Ethnography and qualitative design in educational research* (2nd ed.). San Diego, CA: Academic Press.

Greenhalgh, T. (1997). *How to read a paper: The basics of evidence based medicine*. London: BMJ.

Holm, M. B. (2000). Our mandate for the new millennium: Evidence-based practice. [Eleanor Clark Slagle Lecture]. *American Journal of Occupational Therapy, 54*, 575–585.

Lincoln, Y. S., & Guba, E. G. (1985). *Naturalistic inquiry*. Thousand Oaks, CA: Sage.

Miles, M. B., & Huberman, A. M. (1994). *Qualitative data analysis: An expanded sourcebook* (2nd ed.). Thousand Oaks, CA: Sage.

Polit, D. F., & Hungler, B. P. (1999). *Nursing research: Principles and methods* (6th ed.). Philadelphia: Lippincott.

Portney, L. G., & Watkins, M. P. (2000). *Foundations of clinical research: Applications to practice* (2nd ed.). Upper Saddle River, NJ: Prentice Hall Health.

Primeau, L. A. (1998). Orchestration of work and play within families. *American Journal of Occupational Therapy, 52*, 188–195.

Sackett, D. L., & Haynes, R. B. (1995). On the need for evidence-based medicine. *Evidence-Based Medicine, 1*, 4–5.

Sackett, D. L., Richardson, W. S., Rosenberg, W., & Haynes, R. B. (1997). *Evidence-based medicine: How to practice and teach EBM*. New York: Churchill Livingstone.

Strauss, A., & Corbin, J. (1998). *Basics of qualitative research: Techniques and procedures for developing grounded theory* (2nd ed.). Thousand Oaks, CA: Sage.

Tickle-Degnen, L. (1999). Organizing, evaluating, and using evidence in occupational therapy practice. *American Journal of Occupational Therapy, 53*, 537–539.

Tickle-Degnen, L. (2000a). Gathering current research evidence to enhance clinical reasoning. *American Journal of Occupational Therapy, 54*, 102–105.

Tickle-Degnen, L. (2000b). What is the best evidence to use in practice? *American Journal of Occupational Therapy, 54*, 218–221.

Tseng, M. H., & Chow, S. M. (2000). Perceptual-motor function of school-age children with slow handwriting speed. *American Journal of Occupational Therapy, 54*, 83–88.

CHAPTER 54

DREAMS, DECISIONS, AND DIRECTIONS FOR OCCUPATIONAL THERAPY IN THE MILLENNIUM OF OCCUPATION

ELIZABETH J. YERXA

I explore the exciting future of occupational therapy by identifying a probable environmental context for the profession, adopting a particular set of assumptions, examining crucial decisions the profession needs to make, projecting some potential contributions of occupational therapy, and raising challenges for students.

CONTEXT OF THE FUTURE

The twenty-first century will certainly usher in an "era of chronicity" (Robinson, 1988, p. 339). As a result of the triumphs of medicine in preserving life, the population with chronic impairments will increase worldwide.

Society will become more technologically sophisticated, complex, and information driven (Postman, 1992). Organizing daily life activities, managing time, finding satisfying work (Rifkin, 1995), and achieving valued goals will require even more advanced skills than do today's activities of surfing the net or balancing the social roles of worker and mother. Such a context will create both opportunities and special challenges to people who are aging, living with disabling conditions, or trying to stay healthy. Many people will need to develop new skills and habits. For example, they might decry their lack of preparation by saying, "I don't know how to deal with my aging body. After all, I've never gotten old before."

But new knowledge of the individual human who interacts with specific environments throughout the life span will reveal unforeseen resources of adaptation (Montgomery, 1984). For example, we will know more about how humans construct their nervous systems, psyches, and culture through their own purposeful actions in adapting to environmental challenges (Goldfield, 1995). Scientists will increasingly emphasize human individuality, contextual embeddedness, and the human need for mastery (Kagan, 1996). Health, rather than being defined as the absence of pathology, will be assessed by one's capability to achieve vital goals in specific environments through the use of a repertoire of skills (Pörn, 1993). Prevention of disease and injury and promotion of health as a qualitative, positive attribute will be a high priority.

Emphasis will be placed on the significance of the context of action to successful performance, for example, by studying people's occupations in the environments in which they actually use their skills in practical endeavors (Lave, 1988). Health-care systems will provide needed services in the home, workplace, and communities in which people live and work.

Globalization will result in instantaneous exchanges of ideas and increased opportunities for communication across a variety of cultures. New knowledge will need to achieve a goodness of fit with cultural diversity to have the widest possible relevance.

The spread of capitalism with its emphasis on global markets will raise new issues of ethics and values. These will be particularly significant to health care and to the life opportunities for those deemed different or nonproductive (Nussbaum, 2001). Conflicts will arise between those who value competition and those who strive for community as well as between those who value making a lot of money and those who want to serve humankind.

However these issues are resolved, the past provides useful lessons for the future. Change is coming, often with unintended consequences. Seeking knowledge, gaining experience, and treasuring values have always proved reliable guides through the thickets of ignorance, naïveté and nihilism.

HISTORICAL NOTE 54–1

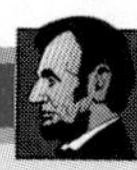

Eleanor Clark Slagle's Push for Leadership: The Call to Lead

SUZANNE M. PELOQUIN

Eleanor Clarke Slagle was a leader. Elected vice president at the first meeting of the Society for the Promotion of Occupational Therapy, Slagle eventually held every association office and for longer than anyone else. Men held many positions of authority in those early years. In medical matters, therapists deferred to male physicians; in promotional and organizational efforts, men were most often elected to high positions. Given this context, Slagle's leadership in both ideational and organizational realms is all the more remarkable.

Ora Ruggles, a reconstruction aide during World War I, remembered Slagle's leadership. During the difficult months after the death of her fiancé, Ruggles had taken a leave from occupational work. Slagle asked Ruggles to return, arguing that the occupational therapy movement needed her to "get behind it and push!" (Carlova & Ruggles, 1946, p. 113). Ruggles returned to practice and started occupational therapy programs in many locations across the United States.

Slagle's words teach this worthwhile lesson: A person can move a profession forward from a number of places. One can lead if one agrees to get behind some effort and push!

Carlova, J., & Ruggles, O. (1946). *The healing heart*. New York: Messner.

ASSUMPTIONS

First, occupational therapy consists of four essential, integrated components that need to nurture one another if it is to go forward. From practice arise the questions and puzzles that are worth pursuing because they generate new knowledge, enabling therapists to do a better job. Such questions are addressed in the realm of scholarship. Models, theories, or frames of reference that organize and synthesize new knowledge of occupation address the crucial questions from practice and suggest better interventions.

These ideas are tested and refined in the crucible of research, which enables practitioners to develop confidence in their usefulness to achieve their purposes. New ideas are transmitted back into the profession through education, as students and practitioners interact with the profession's curriculum and literature. The fruitful interaction among these four components is vital to ensure the profession's ability to progress (Yerxa, 1994).

Second, the crucial goals of occupational therapy are concerned with enduring, significant human needs for survival, challenge, contribution, mastery, and belonging. Occupational therapy is committed to improving the life opportunities, health, and capability of all people, including those with chronic impairments by employing occupation as therapy, contributing new knowledge of occupation to society, and by influencing public policy for people with impairments, disabilities, and handicaps.

Third, the profession is founded on values that have energized it for almost 100 years. These include endorsing the essential humanity and dignity of those practitioners serve by seeking higher levels of life satisfaction for patient-agents,*

* I use the term *patient-agent* for people served by occupational therapy in a medical context. It reminds me of the profession's ethical obligation to help transmute patients into agents of their own intentions.

including those with severe impairments; maintaining and enhancing health by discovering and enhancing the strengths and resources of those practitioners serve; fostering self-directedness and responsibility; maintaining a generalist, integrated, nonspecialist perspective of the human in interaction with his or her environment; using a therapeutic relationship of mutual cooperation and shared authority; viewing patient-agents as actors on the environment rather than passive reactors; possessing faith in human potential; emphasizing people's productivity and participation in society; viewing play and leisure activities along with work and rest as necessary components of a balanced life; and seeking to understand the subjective experiences or the internal world of patient-agents (Yerxa, 1983). These optimistic values need to undergird our profession's goals, science, and future decisions, so that the people who receive occupational therapy services may achieve their potential.

CRUCIAL DECISIONS

Achieving the potential of the profession depends on making thoughtful decisions in the present. These need to affirm occupational therapy's importance to society and commit practitioners to a future-oriented perspective rather than settling for what seems to be present security. False security may be purchased at the high price of reducing the profession to a set of techniques done to people or by losing its identity altogether. For example, therapists might be forced to become hybrid rehabilitation therapists (O'Neill, 1993) because corporate executives who want to maximize profits fail to see how occupational therapy is different from other professions.

What should be the appropriate knowledge base for theory, research, education and practice? Should it be centered on the natural and physical sciences, as are medicine and physical therapy? Or should it include relevant medical knowledge but also emphasize the multileveled, open human system engaged in occupation within multiple environments (**occupational science**)? Should the profession's knowledge be examined for its consistency with its philosophy and values so that practitioners can better ensure its compatibility with practice? For example, focusing unduly on pathology may be incompatible with viewing all people as potentially healthy and resourceful.

In 1934 Meyer, a psychiatrist who helped found occupational therapy, emphasized the need for a human rather than a natural science. "Our chief aim in the study of man [sic] is the determination of the range of operation of man, affecting his [sic] own course of life and that of others and of our common background, and the determination and control of the special factors making for success and failure, for health, happiness and creativity" (Meyer, 1948, p. 591). It was to be a science not of pathology but of a life where it lives, of a "he" or a "she," not a diagnosis or case.

What relation should occupational therapy seek with medicine, related professions, and other academic disciplines? Should practitioners strive to be members of an interdisciplinary medical hierarchy? Or should occupational therapy become an autonomous profession and academic discipline that communicates with many nonmedical professions and disciplines? This decision is significant in enabling occupational therapy practitioners to practice in varied environments with different groups according to their needs. Conforming to other professions' often erroneous expectations instead of defining our own scope of practice will severely limit the profession's potential to serve humankind (Yerxa, 1995).

Who should be responsible for developing the profession's knowledge and thus defining its practice: occupational scientists and occupational therapy practitioners or other disciplines? Practitioners are beginning to develop, synthesize, and transmit their own ideas (Yerxa, 2000b). These often create refreshing new models of practice that meet pressing societal needs (Jackson, Carlson, Mandel, Zemke, & Clark, 1998). For example, instead of delimiting occupational therapy practice to the use of "physical modalities" in hospitals or clinics, practitioners are helping people with chronic impairments develop independent living skills, enabling them to manage their lives in satisfying ways in the real world of home and community (Jackson, Rankin, Siefkin, & Clark, 1989). Practitioners are learning more about how to develop such skills through creating a just-right environmental challenge that helps people reclaim their resources (Montgomery, 1984).

Developing their own knowledge of occupation, in all of its complexity, will enable practitioners to practice more autonomously and to serve varied populations such as infants at risk, new mothers, frail and well elders, the homeless, people who are unemployed, troubled adolescents, prisoners, those with addictions, and other people who want to stay healthy and achieve a decent quality of life. Such knowledge will need to illuminate the special challenges to adaptation faced by those with cognitive or psychiatric impairments (Osborn, 1998). Practitioners will need to understand the biological level of people without reducing them to that level, relating their biology to their lived lives or "spontaneous total function" as Meyer (1948, p. 595) put it.

In an era of increasingly profit-driven, commercialized, managed health care, ethical decisions arise almost daily in practice and education. One dilemma is whether the profession will succumb to environmental pressures to reduce its practice to techniques that are reimbursable. Or will practitioners act as ethical professionals to meet the needs of people, advocating for them so that they may obtain needed services, including comprehensive occupational therapy, leading to mastery? The need to practice the profession competently, thoroughly, and thoughtfully is supported by studies showing that occupational therapy practitioners overuse techniques such as exercise and range of motion because they do not have time and they do not receive reimbursement for developing independent living skills (Pendleton, 1989), talking with patient-agents or family members, or following up to facilitate independence in the individual and in the community. Yet people with chronic impairments living in the community cite major unmet needs for skill development in almost every occupation of daily life (Burnett & Yerxa, 1980).

Will students learn to perceive people as complex, multileveled, whole human beings who interact with complex environments by employing occupation or will graduates adopt a specialized perspective limited to physical or mental pathology, viewing people as strokes, bipolar mood disorders, or traumatic hand injuries? The latter course not only fragments the people practitioners serve but necessarily leads to an overemphasis on sterile, repetitive technique, ignoring significant human needs related to occupation. For example, Murphy (1990), a professor of anthropology who developed a spinal cord tumor requiring rehabilitation, thought that the exercises he was supposed to do in occupational therapy were silly. Yet his vital goals of being able to manage his time, home, and transportation and continue to work apparently were not addressed by his rehabilitation program.

Osborn (1998), a young physician who sustained a traumatic head injury, provides another example of the outcome of a specialist perspective. Although she completed two stints of cognitive rehabilitation directed by psychologists, no guidance was provided so that she could accomplish the daily routines necessary for her survival in the real-life environment of New York City. As a result, she often went to bed hungry because she had botched shopping. Apparently, the program relied on a belief that since her main problem was cognitive dysfunction it could be remediated by decontextualized cognitive training. Only her family members helped her learn how to carry out the habits of daily life in her apartment and community.

One of the great strengths of occupational therapy education has been its insistence on preparing students to see people as whole and integrated and to prepare practitioners to deal with any threat to adaptation, be it in the nervous system, the culture, or the physical environment. A philosopher recently recognized the complexity of our practice by stating that it is much more difficult than rocket science. Reilly (1962) observed that the idea of occupational therapy is so vital to society that if the profession ceased to exist tomorrow, a new one based on the same idea would soon arise to take its place.

POTENTIAL CONTRIBUTIONS

The era of chronicity, in which burgeoning populations of people with impairments try to adapt to the demands of a dizzyingly complex world, could be answered by a new millennium of occupation. Through new knowledge of how people become competent and manage their environments in spite of even severe degrees of impairment and challenge, those with chronic conditions could be helped to reclaim their resources and find their place in the culture. They could learn the skills for self-direction by doing things that are satisfying, worthwhile, and of interest—thereby achieving a goodness of fit with their environments and finding their places in their culture. These occupational goals are not trivial, since engagement in occupation, self-responsibility, and autonomy have been associated in several studies with survival, longevity, health, ability to cope effectively with stress, quality of life, and happiness (Langer & Rodin, 1976; Wright, 1983).

Through occupational therapy, which develops competence, people with impairments could be connected with the mainstream of humanity. Consequently, social attitudes toward those perceived as different would change. Impairment no longer would be perceived as a barrier to full personhood or a tragedy that endlessly confers the sick role. Society would gain new appreciation of both the contributions of and the satisfactions possible for people with impairments.

Occupational therapy could promote a new concept of health. It would be perceived as possession of a repertoire of skills that enables people to achieve their valued goals in their own environments (Pörn, 1993). Thus people with chronic impairments could be seen as healthy and be assured of "equality of capability" (Bickenbach, 1993, p. 260), to have an environment and receive services that enable them to achieve their desired potential.

Occupational therapy practitioners could learn much more about how to help people develop the adaptive skills, rules, and habits that enable competence through creating a just-right challenge from the environment to enable an adaptive response. Such coaching by occupational therapy practitioners could benefit all people who need to develop skills to survive, contribute, and achieve satisfaction in their daily life activities, whether or not they have impairments.

Occupational therapy practitioners could become visible and vocal allies and advocates for people with impairments, disabilities, and handicaps. Practitioners could influence social policy to create better life opportunities for such people because their values, optimism, and knowledge demand such action as an actualization of their commitment.

The profession could search vigorously for new knowledge of people as individuals who are unique, whole, and authors of their lives through their occupations. The significance of engagement in occupation to the health and well-being of all humans could be a major area of investigation, as would the influences of varying degrees of environmental challenge on the development of competence and adaptation.

Occupational therapy practitioners who practice in medical environments would be better able to help transmute patients into agents. New knowledge would enable people to achieve higher levels of capability and skills, to achieve their goals, and manage their own lives. Such new knowledge would support the profession's autonomy in practice.

New models of practice could be developed and tested. Some of these might focus on the prevention of disability and handicap owing to impairment; development of capability across the life span; use of the play–work continuum to develop skills, rules, and habits; life organization, including management of the patient-agent's environment and resources; the development of and nurturance of intrinsic motivation for occupation via the pursuit of the patient-agent's unique interests; skill development to enable people to make necessary role transitions across the life span; restoration of healthy balances of work, rest, play, and sleep in individual lives; assessment of how to create the just-right environmental challenge necessary to enable an adaptive response; and using engagement in occupation to obtain a satisfying and healthy balance of ritual and novelty in the patient-agent's daily round of activity (Klapp, 1986). The current limited concept of activities of daily living could be broadened to include all activities that individuals need and want to do to adapt to their unique environments, obtain personal satisfaction via their own action, and contribute to their cultures.

CHALLENGES TO STUDENTS

Dyson (1995) observed that many scientists make their most creative contributions when they are new to a field but deeply immersed in its knowledge. Einstein was only 25 when he published his revolutionary relativity theory, considered the pinnacle of his creativity. Students and other newcomers could contribute revolutionary new ideas to the profession if they are deeply immersed in its concepts and values and audacious enough to perceive its issues and possibilities with fresh eyes, eschewing oversimplification and recipes.

Examples of areas that need to be better understood are environmental affordances; resources in the environment that create curiosity, act as attractors, or pose challenges that demand an adaptive response; just-right challenges, neither too difficult nor too easy, that lead to human action, skill development, and confidence in mastery; assessments of individual strengths and identification of personal and environmental resources that could be used, developed, and reclaimed to enable competence despite impairments; the significance of people's daily routines to survival, contribution, being in place in one's culture, and life satisfaction; patterns of daily living that contribute to health and happiness; how habits and repertoires relate to experiences of meaning; the relevance of the play–work continuum to the development of skills, habits, and rules and its reconstitution in the event of impairment; discovery, development, and nurturance of interests and their relationship to intrinsic motivation and capability; cultural differences and similarities in interests, skills, rules, and habits; coaching by the practitioner to elicit optimal performance and motivation; development of competence, autonomy, and self-responsibility among people with impairments or in danger of becoming social outsiders; and development of new practice environments that provide opportunities for patient-agent choice and self-direction.

Because the occupational therapy profession is founded on complex, vital ideas central to the human condition, it could contribute to society in significant ways. Students must become infected with the need to know much, much more, recognizing that understanding occupation and applying it in practice require lifelong study. My own detective work has taken two directions: reading the biographies of people with impairments, disabilities, and handicaps to discover their self-identified, unmet needs and to understand their lived lives and studying the works of great scholars from nonmedical disciplines that share the profession's values, to contribute new ideas to the science of occupation (Yerxa, 2000a).

CONCLUSION

Occupational therapy has almost limitless potential to create a significant impact on tomorrow's world. Realizing it will depend on several choices: How well will the profession integrate and nurture its four components of practice, ideas, research, and education? To what extent will today's decisions foster the profession's ethical responsibility to patient-agents, develop knowledge, further autonomy and professional self-directedness, and enhance a generalist education and outlook?

To serve humankind well will require that occupational therapy practitioners learn much more about people as agents, in their own environments, engaged in daily occupations. To learn what is needed requires that practitioners accept the challenge of becoming ardent students of life's daily activities and begin to grapple with the ambiguity and complexity of occupation, the occupational human, and the contexts in which occupation takes place. Only then will practitioners fulfill the profession's commitment to people with chronic impairments and ensure that their humanistic values are actualized in the practice of occupational therapy for a new millennium.

References

Bickenbach, J. (1993). *Physical disability and social policy*. Toronto: University of Toronto Press.

Burnett, S., & Yerxa, E. J. (1980). Community-based and college-based needs assessment of physically disabled persons. *American Journal of Occupational Therapy, 34*, 201–207.

Dyson, F. (1995). The scientist as rebel. In J. Cornwell (Ed.). *Nature's imagination: The frontiers of scientific vision* (pp. 1–11). Oxford, UK: Oxford University Press.

Goldfield, E. C. (1995). *Emergent forms: Origins and early development of human action and perception*. New York: Oxford University Press.

Jackson, J., Rankin, A., Siefkin, S., & Clark, F. (1989). "Options": An occupational therapy transition program for adolescents with developmental disabilities. In J. A. Johnson & D. A. Ethridge (Eds.). *Developmental disabilities: A handbook for occupational therapists* (pp. 197–214). New York: Haworth.

Jackson, J., Carlson, M., Mandel, D., Zemke, R., & Clark, F. (1998). Occupation in lifestyle redesign: The well elderly study occupational therapy program. *American Journal of Occupational Therapy, 52*, 326–336.

Kagan, J. (1996). Point of view: The misleading abstractions of social scientists. *Chronicle of Higher Education, 62*, A52.

Klapp, O. (1986). *Overload and boredom: Essays on the quality of life in the information society*. New York: Greenwood.

Langer, E., & Rodin, J. (1976). The effects of choice and enhanced personal responsibility for the aged: A field experiment in an institutional setting. *Journal of Personality and Social Psychology, 34*, 191–198.

Lave, J. (1988). *Cognition in practice*. New York: Cambridge University Press.

Meyer, A. (1948). The psychobiological point of view: 1934. In A. Lief (Ed.). *The commonsense psychiatry of Adolph Meyer* (pp. 590–606). New York: McGraw-Hill.

Montgomery, M. (1984). Resources of adaptation for daily living: A classification with therapeutic implications for occupational therapy. *Occupational Therapy in Health Care, 1*, 9–23.

Murphy, R. F. (1990). *The body silent*. New York: Norton.

Nussbaum, M. (2001, January). Disabled lives: Who cares? *New York Review of Books, 48*, 34–37.

O'Neill, E. H. (1993). *Health professions education for the future: Schools in service to the nation*. San Francisco: PEW Health Professions Commission.

Osborn, C. L. (1998). *Over my head: A doctor's own story of head injury from the inside looking out*. Kansas City: McMeel.

Pendleton, H. (1989). Occupational therapists' current use of independent living skills training for adult inpatients who are physically disabled. *Occupational Therapy in Health Care, 6*, 93–108.

Pörn, I. (1993). Health and adaptedness. *Theoretical Medicine, 14*, 295–303.

Postman, N. (1992). *Technopoly: The surrender of culture to technology*. New York: Knopf.

Reilly, M. (1962). Occupational therapy can be one of the great ideas of 20th century medicine. *American Journal of Occupational Therapy, 16*, 1–9.

Rifkin, J. (1995). *The end of work*. New York: Putnam.

Robinson, I. (1988). The rehabilitation of patients with long-term physical impairments: The social context of professional roles. *Clinical Rehabilitation, 2*, 339–347.

Wright, B. (1983). *Physical disability—A psychological approach* (2nd ed.). New York: Harper & Row.

Yerxa, E. J. (1983). Audacious values, the energy source for occupational therapy practice. In G. Kielhofner (Ed.). *Health through occupation: Theory and practice in occupational therapy* (pp. 149–162). New York: Davis.

Yerxa, E. J. (1994). In search of good ideas for occupational therapy. *Scandinavian Journal of Occupational Therapy, 1*, 7–15.

Yerxa, E. J. (1995). Who is the keeper of occupational therapy's practice and knowledge? *American Journal of Occupational Therapy, 49*, 295–299.

Yerxa, E. J. (2000a). Confessions of an occupational therapist who became a detective. *British Journal of Occupational Therapy, 63*, 192–198.

Yerxa, E. J. (2000b). Occupational science: A renaissance of service to humankind through knowledge. *Occupational Therapy International, 7*, 87–98.

APPENDIX A

ASSESSMENTS: LISTED ALPHABETICALLY BY TITLE

CHERYL BOOP

TABLE OF ASSESSMENTS: LISTED ALPHABETICALLY BY TITLE

Assessment Title	Author(s)	Publisher	Ages	Stated Purpose	Areas Assessed
Accessibility Checklist	Goltsman, S., Gilbert, T., and Wohlford, S.	Goltsman, S., Gilbert, T., & Wohlford, S. (1992). *The accessibility checklist: An evaluation system for buildings and outdoor settings.* Berkeley, CA: M.I.G. Communications.	Adult	Identify problems in community accessibility	Community environment
Activity Index & Meaningfulness of Activity Scale	Nystrom, E.P., and Gregory, M. D.	Gregory, M. D. (1983). Occupational behavior and life satisfaction among retirees. *American Journal of Occupational Therapy, 37,* 548–553. Nystrom, E. P. (1974). Activity patterns and leisure concepts among the elderly. *American Journal of Occupational Therapy, 28,* 337–345.	Older Adults	Examine the meaning and significance of activity and activity patterns among the elderly	Activity/leisure
Adolescent Role Assessment (ARA)	Black, M. M.	SLACK, Inc. 6900 Grove Road Thorofare, NJ 08086 800-257-8290	Adolescents	Gathers information on the adolescent's occupational role involvement over time and across domains	Childhood play; socialization with family; socialization with peers; school functioning; occupational choice; anticipated adult work
Adolescent/Adult Sensory Profile	Dunn, W.	Therapy Skill Builders 555 Academic Court San Antonio, TX 78204-2498 (800) 232-1223	10 years-up	To determine how well a subject processes sensory information in everyday situations and to profile the sensory system's effect on functional performance	Sensory processing, modulation, and behavioral and emotional responses
Adult Nowicki Strickland Internal External Control Scale (ANSIE TIM(C))	Nowicki, S., and Duke, M. P.	Educational Testing Service (ETS) Test Collection Library Rosedale and Carter Roads Princeton, NJ 08541 (609) 734-5689	Adults	Identifies a client's locus of control	Locus of control
Adult Playfulness Scale	Glynn, M. A., and Webster, J.	Glynn, M. A., & Webster, J. (1992). The adult playfulness scale: An initial assessment. *Psychological Reports, 71,* 83–103	Adults	Measures adult play behavior in the workplace.	Play/leisure
Alberta Infant Motor Scales (AIMS)	Piper, M. C., and Darrah, J.	The Psychological Corporation 555 Academic Court San Antonio, TX 78204 (800) 288-0752	Birth to 18 months	To provide a performance- based, norm-referenced measure of infant motor maturation	Progressive development and integration of antigravity muscular control in the prone, supine, sitting and standing positions
Allen Battery	Allen, C. K.	S&S Worldwide PO Box 513 Colchester, CT 06415 800-243-9232	All ages	To assess cognitive disability and suggest treatment approach	Problem-solving; following directions
Allen Cognitive Level (ACL) Screen	Allen, C. K.	S&S Worldwide PO Box 513 Colchester, CT 06415 800-243-9232	All ages	To assess cognitive disability and suggest treatment approach	Problem-solving; following directions
Allen Diagnostic Module Instruction Manual (ADMIM)	Earhart, C, Allen, C., and Blue, T.	S&S Worldwide PO Box 513 Colchester, CT 06415 800-243-9232	All ages	To assess cognitive disability and suggest treatment approach	Problem-solving; following directions

Allen Semantic Differential Scale	Allen, L.	Allen, L. (1986). Measuring attitudes toward computer assisted instruction: The development of a semantic differential tool. *Computers in Nursing, 4(4),* 144–151.	Adults	Evaluates individual's responses to webpage interventions	Comfort; creativity; function of webpage healthcare intervention
Americans with Disabilities Act Accessibility Guidelines Checklist for Buildings and Facilities	U.S. Architectural and Transportation Barriers Compliance Board	U.S. Architectural & Transportation Barriers Compliance Board. (1992). *Americans with Disabilities Act accessibility guidelines checklist for buildings and facilities.* Washington, D.C.: Author.	Adult	Identifies accessibility in the community	Community environment; workplace environment.
Arnadottir OTADL Neurobehavioral Evaluation (A-ONE)	Arnadottir, G.	Arnadottir, G. The brain and behavior: Assessing cortical dysfunction through activities of daily living. Philadelphia: Mosby. 1990.	16 years-up	Identifies neurobehavioral deficits, the impact they have on functional performance of ADL, and how they relate to the location of cortical lesions	ADL performance in dressing, grooming and hygiene, transfers and mobility, feeding, and communication
Assessment of Communication and Interaction Skills (ACIS)	Salamy, M., Simon, S., and Kielhofner, G.	AOTA Products P.O. Box 3800 Forrester Center, WV 25438 877-404-AOTA	Adults	Assess the communication/interaction skills of adults who have physical or mental illness	Communication; social interaction skills
Assessment of Living Skills and Resources (ALSAR)	Williams, J. H., Drinka, T. J. K., Greenberg, J. R., Farrell- Holtan, J., Euhardy, R., and Schram, M.	Williams, J. H., Drinka, T. J. K., Greenberg, J. R., Farrell-Holtan, J., Euhardy, R., and Schram, M. (1991). Development and Testing of the Assessment of Living Skills and Resources (ALSAR) in Elderly Community-Dwelling Veterans. *Gerontologist, 31,* 1, 84–91.	Adults	An interview that assesses a person's level of independence.	IADL
Assessment of Ludic Behaviors (ALB)	Ferland, F.	Ferland, F. (1997). Play, Children with Physical Disabilities and Occupational Therapy: The Ludic Model. Ottawa, ON: University of Ottawa Press	Children	Assess play behaviors of children with disabilities	Play/leisure
Assessment of Motor and Process Skills (AMPS)	Fisher, A. G.	Anne G. Fisher, ScD., OTR/L, FAOTA AMPS Project OT Building Colorado State U. Fort Collins, CO 80523 303-491-6253	5 years-up	Provides an objective assessment of motor and process skills in the context of performing several familiar functional tasks of the subject's choice.	Process skills, such as the ability to initiate, inquire, notice and respond, pace, sequence, organize, and terminate
Assessment of Occupational Functioning (AOF)–second revision	Watts, J. H., Brollier, C., Bauer, D., and Schmidt, W.	Watts, J. H., Brollier, C., Bauer, D., & Schmidt, W. (1989) The Assessment of Occupation Functioning: The Second Revision. In J.H. Watts & C. Brollier (Eds.), *Instrument development in occupational therapy* (pp. 61–88). New York: Haworth.	Adults	Screens overall occupational function of residents in long-term care settings	Volition; habituation; performance; values; personal causation; interests; roles; habits; skills; school and job history
Assistive Technology Evaluation	Cook, A. M., and Hussey, S. M.	Cook, A. M., & Hussey, S. M. (1996). *Assistive Technology: Principles and Practice.* St. Louis: Mosby.	Adults	To determine which, if any, assistive technology devices can allow an individual to maximize efficient performance of activities	Demographic and referral information; medical and health information; sensory and perceptual abilities; ADL; social interaction; learning and behavior; functional abilities; motor skills; mobility and positioning; and communication skills

Continues

TABLE OF ASSESSMENTS: LISTED ALPHABETICALLY BY TITLE *(Continued)*

Assessment Title	Author(s)	Publisher	Ages	Stated Purpose	Areas Assessed
Balcones Sensory Integration Screening Kit		Texas Occupational Therapy Association, Inc. P.O. Box 15576 Austin, TX 78761-5576 512-454-8682	Children in K-12	To assist in identifying special neuro-behavioral, behavioral, and/or classroom performance	Ocular-motor control; proprioception; primitive reflex-brain stem midline interaction; vestibular; tactile perception; stereognosis; visual-motor perception; lateralization
Baltimore Therapeutic Equipment (BTE) Work Simulator	Baltimore Therapeutic Equipment Company	Baltimore Therapeutic Equipment Company 7455-L New Ridge Road Hanover, MD 21076 800-331-8845	Adults	Used in work capacity evaluations to determine whether clients have the capabilities to return to work	Physical strength and endurance using a variety of attachments simulating tools
Barthel Index	Mahoney, F. I., and Barthel, D. W.	Mahoney, F. I., & Barthel, D. W. (1965). Functional Evaluation: The Barthel Index. *Maryland State Medical Journal, 14,* 61–65.	Adults	Reflects the functional status of hospital patients in activities of daily living and to assess change	Activities of daily living
Bay Area Functional Performance Evaluation (BaFPE)	Williams, S. L., and Bloomer, J.	Maddak, Inc. 6 Industrial Road Pequannock, NJ 07440 800-443-4926	Late Adolescence to Adult	To assess cognitive, affective, and performance skills in daily living tasks and social interaction skills; evaluate the effectiveness of OT	Social interaction/ behavior; ADL skills, cognitive, affective and performance skills
Bayley Scales of Infant Development	Bayley, N.	The Psychological Corporation 555 Academic Court San Antonio, TX 78204 (800) 288-0752	Birth to 4 years	To assess the current developmental functioning of infants and children	Mental, cognitive, motor and adaptive behaviors
Beery–Buktenica Developmental Test of Visual-Motor Integration–4th Edition (VMI)	Beery, K. E., and Buktenica, N. A.	PRO-ED, Inc. 8700 Shoal Creek Blvd. Austin, TX 78757 (800) 897-3202 Modern Curriculum Press 13900 Prospect Road Cleveland, OH 44136 800-321-3106	2.9 to 19.8 years	Screening instrument to assist in early identification visual motor integration abilities	Visual-motor integration skills
Behavior Assessment Rating Scale (BASC)	Reynolds, C. R., and Kamphaus, R. W.	American Guidance Service, Inc. Publisher's Building Circle Pines, MN 55014 (800) 328-2560	2.6–18.11 years	Teacher rating; parent rating; self-rating; student observation; structured developmental history	Behaviors, thoughts, and emotions of children and adolescents
Behavioral Assessment of the Dysexecutive Syndrome (BADS)	Wilson, B. A., Alderman, N., Burgess, P., Emslie, H., and Evans, J. J.	Psychological Assessment Resources, Inc. 16204 N. Florida Avenue Lutz, FL 33549 813-968-3003	16 years-up	To assess problem-solving, planning, and organizational skills over time	Temporal judgment; ability to change response patterns; problem-solving; strategizing
Behavioral Inattention Test (BIT)	Wilson, B., Cockburn, J., and Halligan, P.	National Rehabilitation Services 117 North Elm Street PO Box 1247 Gaylord, MI 49735 517-732-3866	Adults	To identify unilateral visual neglect and how it affects daily life	9 subtests reflecting daily life activities; 6 conventional pencil-and-paper tasks

Bennett Hand Tool Dexterity Test	Bennett, G. K.	The Psychological Corporation 555 Academic Court San Antonio, TX 78204 (800) 288-0752	Adults	To assess dexterity and basic hand-tool skills for manual jobs	Tool skills; safety skills
Benton Constructional Praxis Test	Benton, A. L., Hamsher, K., Varney, N. R., and Spreen, O.	Benton, A. L., Hamsher, K. deS., Varney, N. R., & Spreen, O. *Contributions to neuropsychological assessment: Clinical manual.* New York: Oxford University Press. 1983.	All ages	To assess 3-dimensional visual motor and constructional skills	Visual motor and construction skills
Berg Balance Scale	Berg, K., Wood-Dauphinee, S., Williams, J. I., and Gayton, D.	The Center for Gerentology and Health Care Research Brown University Box G-B213 171 Meeting Street Providence, Rhode Island 02912 401-863-1560 www.chcr.brown.edu/Balance.htm	Adults	To measure balance in 14 activities performed in standing	Balance
Borg Numerical Pain Scale	Borg, G.	Borg, G. *Borg's Perceived Exertion and Pain Scales,* Champaign, IL: Human Kinetics. 1998.	Adults	Self-assessment of pain	Pain
Borg Scale of Rating Perceived Exertion (RPE)	Borg, G.	Borg, G. *Borg's Perceived Exertion and Pain Scales,* Champaign, IL: Human Kinetics. 1998.	Adults	Self-assessment of exertion during activities	Perceived exertion
Boston Diagnostic Aphasia Examination	Goodglass, H., and Kaplan, E.	The Psychological Corporation 555 Academic Court San Antonio, TX 78204 (800) 288-0752	Adults	To evaluate a broad range of language impairments that often arise as a consequence of organic brain dysfunction	Perceptual modalities; processing functions; and response modalities
Box and Block Test	Mathiowetz, V., Vollard, G., Kashman, N., and Weber, K.	WisdomKing.Com, Inc. Attn. Customer Service 2410 Cades Way, Unit B Vista CA 92083 877-931-9693	7–9 years; Adults	To provide a baseline for upper extremity manual dexterity and gross motor coordination	Manual dexterity
Brief Pain Inventory	Cleeland, C. S.	Cleeland, C. S. (1991). Research in cancer pain: What we know and what we need to know. *Cancer,* 67, 823–827.	Adults	How much pain interferes with occupational performance and mood	Pain and relationship to occupational performance
Bruininks-Oseretsky Test of Motor Proficiency	Bruininks, R. H.	American Guidance Service, Inc. Publisher's Building Circle Pines, MN 55014 (800) 328-2560	4.5 to 14.5 years	To assess the motor functioning of children	Gross motor development; fine motor development
Canadian Occupational Performance Measure (COPM)	Law, M., Baptiste, S., Carswell, A., McColl, M. A., Polatajko, H., and Pollock, N.	Canadian Association of Occupational Therapists 110 Eglinton Avenue West 3rd Floor Toronto, Ontario M4R 1A3 Canada 416-487-5404	7 years-up	Measures client's perception of his/her occupational performance over time	Self-care; productivity; leisure
Caplan Indented Paragraph Test	Caplan, B.	Caplan, B. (1987). Assessment of unilateral neglect: A new reading test. *Journal of Clinical and Experimental Neuropsychology, 9,* 359–364.	Adults	Uses variable left margin to assess subtle unilateral neglect	Scanning; reading, unilateral neglect

Continues

TABLE OF ASSESSMENTS: LISTED ALPHABETICALLY BY TITLE *(Continued)*

Assessment Title	Author(s)	Publisher	Ages	Stated Purpose	Areas Assessed
Child and Adolescent Social Perception Measure (CASP)	Magill-Evans, J., Koning, C., Cameron-Sadava, A., and Manyk, K.	Magill-Evans, J., Koning, C., Cameron-Sadava, A.,& Manyk, K. (1995). The Child and Adolescent Social Perception Measure. *Journal of Nonverbal Behavior, 19,* 151–169.	6–15 years	To measure a child's sensitivity to nonverbal aspects of communication	Ability to interpret nonverbal aspects of communication
Child Behavior Checklist (CBCL)	Achenbach, T. M.	University of Vermont Psychiatry Department University Medical Education 1 South Prospect Street Burlington, VT 05401-3456	4–18 years	To record a child's competencies and problems as reported by parent or caregiver	Internalizing and externalizing psychological symptoms for children and adolescents
Child Behaviors Inventory of Playfulness (CBI)	Rogers, C. S., Impara, J. C., Frary, R. B., Harris, T., Meeks, A., Semanic-Lauth, S., and Reynolds, M. R.	Rogers, C. S., Impara, J. C., Frary, R. B., Harris, T., Meeks, A., Semanic-Lauth, S., & Reynolds, M. R. (1998). Measuring playfulness: Development of the Child Behaviors Inventory of Playfulness. In M. C. Duncan, G. Chick, & A. Aycock (Eds.), *Play & Culture Studies, Volume 1: Diversions and divergences in fields of play.* Greenwich, CT: Ablex Publishing	Children	Examines playful behaviors of children	Play/leisure
Children's Assessment of Participation and Enjoyment (CAPE)	King, G., Law, M., King, S., Harms, S., Kertoy, M., Rosenbaum, P., and Young, N.	CanChild Centre for Childhood Disability Research McMaster University, IAHS Bldg 1400 Main St W., Hamilton Ontario, Canada L8S 1C7	6 years-up	Gathers information on child's participation in everyday activities outside of mandated school activities	Social participation in non-school activities
Children's Handwriting Evaluation Scale (CHES)	Texas Scottish Rite Hospital	CHES 5530 Farquhar Dallas, TX 75209 214-366-3667	Grades 3–8	Provides a reliable measure of handwriting rate and quality	Letter size consistency; letter formation; letters on the line; spacing between letters and words
Children's Handwriting Evaluation Scale for Manuscript Writing (CHES-M)	Texas Scottish Rite Hospital	CHES 5530 Farquhar Dallas, TX 75209 214-366-3667	Grades 1–2	Provides a reliable measure of handwriting rate and quality	Copying; taking notes; presenting ideas in writing
Children's Paced Auditory Serial Addition Test (CHIPASAT)	Dyche, G., and Johnson, D.	Dyche, G. & Johnson, D. (1991). Development and evaluation of CHIPASAT, an attentional test for children: II test-retest reliability and practice effect for a normal sample. *Perceptual Motor Skills, 72,* 563–572.	Children	To detect subtle impairments in attention and speed of processing, functional observation of everyday activities	Attention and speed of processing
Choosing Outcomes and Accommodations for Children (COACH)	Giangreco, M. F., Cloninger, C. J., and Iverson, V. S.	Customer Service Department Brookes Publishing Co. P.O. Box 10624 Baltimore, MD 21285-0624 1-800-638-3775 custserv@brookespublishing.com	3–21 years	Used to develop an appropriate, individualized education program	Family interview; learning outcomes; general supports; annual goals
Classroom Observation Guide	Griswold, L.	Griswold, L. (1994). Ethnographic analysis: A study of classroom environments. *American Journal of Occupational Therapy, 48,* 397–402.	Children	Helps therapists understand classroom context	Activities of classroom settings; people in classroom settings; communication in classroom settings

Clinical Test of Sensory Integration and Balance (CTSIB)	Shumway-Cook, A., and Horak, F. B.	Shumway-Cook, A., & Horak, F. B. (1986). Assessing the influence of sensory interaction on balance: Suggestions from the field. *Physical Therapy*, 66, 1548–1550. NeuroCom 9570 SE Lawnfield Road Clackamas, OR 97015 800-767-6744	All	To assess a patient's ability to tolerate varied surfaces and sensory conditions	Balance; interaction of ocular, vestibular, and musculoskeletal systems
Cognitive Assessment of Minnesota (CAM)	Rustad, R. A., DeGroot, T. L., Jungkunz, M. L., Freeberg, K. S., Borowick, L. G., and Wanttie, A. M.	Therapy Skill Builders 555 Academic Court San Antonio, TX 78204-2498 (800) 232-1223	Adults	Screens a wide range of cognitive skills in order to identify general problem areas	Attention; memory; visual neglect; math; ability to follow directions; judgment
Cognitive Performance Test (CPT)	Burns, T.	Allen, C. K., Earhart, C. A., & Blue, T. (1992.) *Occupational therapy treatment goals for the physically and cognitively disabled*. Bethesda, MD: American Occupational Therapy Association.	Adults	Assesses how cognitive processing deficits affect performance of common activities	Cognitive processing
Community Adaptive Planning Assessment	Spencer, J., and Davidson, H.	Spencer, J. & Davidson, J. (1998). The Community Adaptive Planning Assessment: A clinical tool for documenting future planning with clients. *American Journal of Occupational Therapy, 52 (1)*, 19–30.	Adults	Examines major occupations of an individual at times of expected change	Activities involved in occupation; persons involved and their roles; physical setting; value of the occupation to self and others
Community Integration Measure	McColl, M. A., Davies, D., Carlson, P., Johnston, J., and Minnes, P.	McColl, M. A., Davies, D., Carlson, P., Johnston, J, & Minnes, P. (2001). The community integration measure: development and preliminary validation. *Archives of Physical Medicine and Rehabilitation*, 82, 429–34.	Adults	Appraise an individual's views about connecting to community	Integration into community
Community Integration Questionnaire	Willer, B., Rosenthal, M., Kreutzer, J., Gordon, W., and Rempel, R.	Centre for Research on Community Integration at the Ontario Brain Injury Association 3550 Schmon Parkway Thorold, Ontario L2V 4Y6, Canada	Adults	Helps clients examine the extent of their community participation	Household activities; shopping; errands; leisure activities; visiting friends; social events; productive activities
Competency Rating Scale	Prigatano, G.	Prigatano, G. P. *Neuropsychological rehabilitation after brain injury*. Baltimore, MD: Johns Hopkins University Press. 1986. For more information, contact: Tessa Hart, PhD. MossRehab TBI Model System Philadelphia, PA 215-456-5925.	Adult	Self-report instrument asks the client to rate his/her degree of difficulty in a variety of tasks and functions	Self-awareness following traumatic brain injury
Computer Attitude Scale	Loyd, B. H., and Gressard, C.	Loyd, B. H., & Gressard, C. (1984). The effects of sex, age, and computer experience on computer attitudes, *AEDS Journal, 18*, 67–77.	Adults	Assesses general attitudes toward computers	Computer anxiety: computer confidence; computer liking
Computer System Usability Questionnaire	Lewis, J.	Lewis, J. R. (1995) *IBM* Computer Usability Satisfaction Questionnaires: Psychometric Evaluation and Instructions for Use. *International Journal of Human-Computer Interaction, 7:1*, 57–78	All ages	Can be used to evaluate specific software programs for individuals	Usefulness; information quality; interface quality

Continues

TABLE OF ASSESSMENTS: LISTED ALPHABETICALLY BY TITLE *(Continued)*

Assessment Title	Author(s)	Publisher	Ages	Stated Purpose	Areas Assessed
Contextual Memory Test (CMT)	Toglia, J. P.	Therapy Skill Builders 555 Academic Court San Antonio, TX 78204-2498 (800) 232-1223	18 years-up	To assess awareness of memory capacity, use of strategy, and recall	Memory strategies for task completion
Coping Inventory	Zeitlin, S.	Scholastic Testing Service 480 Meyer Road Bensonville, IL 60106 (800) 642-6787	3–16 years	To assess adaptive and maladaptive coping habits, skills, and behaviors	Coping with self; coping with environment; use of personal resources; initiation of activity
Cost of Care Index	Kosberg, J., and Cairl, R.	Kosberg, J. & Cairl, R. (1986). The cost of care index: A case management tool for screening informal care providers. *The Gerentological Society of America, 26*, 273–278.	Adults	Identifies concerns of families providing care to elders	Personal and social restrictions; physical and emotional health; value placed on caregiving; characteristics of care recipient; and economic costs
Craig Handicap Assessment and Report Technique (CHART)	Whiteneck, G., Charlifue, S., Gerhart, K., Overholser, J., and Richardson, G.	Craig Hospital Research Department 3425 S. Clarkson Street Englewood, Colorado 80110 (303) 789-8202 Dave Mellick, MA	Adult	Assess behaviors related to participation	Orientation; physical independence; mobility; occupation; social integration; economic self-sufficiency
Crawford Small Parts Dexterity Test	Crawford, J.	The Psychological Corporation 555 Academic Court San Antonio, TX 78204 (800) 288-0752	Adult	Assess dexterity and fine motor skills in handling small tools and parts; Determine whether your applicant has the skills vital in positions requiring agility and strong dexterity	Eye-hand coordination; fine motor skills;
Daily Activities Checklist	Brown, C., Hamera, E., and Long, C.	Brown, C., Hamera, E., & Long, C. (1996). The Daily Activities Checklist: A functional assessment for consumers with mental illness living in the community. *Occupational Therapy in Health Care, 10 (3)*, 33–44.	Adults	Examines engagement of persons with mental illness in social settings	ADL; community living skills; socialization; quality of daily life
Daily Activity Diary	Follick, M. J., Ahern, D. K., and Laser-Wolston, N.	Follick, M. J., Ahern, D. K., & Laser-Wolston, N. (1984). Evaluation of a daily activity diary for chronic pain patients. *Pain*, 19, 373–382.	Adults	To examine time sue in relation to pain	Time spent sitting, standing, reclining and in productive activities
DeGangi-Berk Test of Sensory Integration	Berk, R. A., and DeGangi, G. A.	Western Psychological Services 12031 Wilshire Boulevard Los Angeles, CA 90025 800-648-8857	3–5 years	To measure sensory integration in preschoolers and to detect sensory integrative dysfunction	Postural control; bilateral motor integration; reflex integration
Denver Developmental Screening Test	Frankenberg, W. K., Dodds, J., Archer, P., Shapiro, H., and Bresnick, B.	Denver Developmental Materials, Inc. P.O. Box 6919 Denver, CO 80206 (800) 419-4729	Birth to 6 years	To screen for developmental delays	Personal-social; fine motor adaptive; language; gross motor, behavior during testing
Developmental Test of Visual Perception – 2nd Edition (DTVP-2)	Hammill, D. D., Pearson, N. A., and Voress, J. K.	PRO-ED, Inc. 8700 Shoal Creek Blvd. Austin, TX 78757 (800) 897-3202	4–10 years	Identifies disturbances of visual perception and visual-motor integration	Eye-hand coordination; copying; spatial relationships; position in space; figure-ground; visual closure; visual-motor speed; form constancy

Digit Span (portion of WAIS-R)	Kaplan, E., Fein, D., Morris, R., and Delis, D. C.	The Psychological Corporation 555 Academic Court San Antonio, TX 78204 (800) 288-0752	All ages	To assess short term auditory memory	Involves auditory attention, concentration, and memory tracking
Disability Rights Guide	National Council on Disability	National Council on Disability 1331 F Street, NW, Suite 1050 Washington, DC 20004 (202) 272-2004	Adults	Identifies problems in accessing community resources	Community integration
Disability Social Distance Scale	Tringo, J.	Tringo, J. L. Disability social distance scale [DSDS] (1970). In R. F. Antonak & H. Livne H. (Eds.) (1998). *Measurement of attitudes toward people with disabilities: Methods, psychometrics and scale.* pp. 153–156. Springfield, IL: Charles C Thomas.	Adults	To identify whether attitudes toward persons with disabilities are affected by the type of disability	Social interaction
Early Coping Inventory	Zeitlin, S., Williamson, G. G., and Szczepanski, M.	Scholastic Testing Service 480 Meyer Road Bensonville, IL 60106 (800) 642-6787	Birth to 3 years	To measure adaptive behavior	Sensorimotor organization; reactive behavior; self-initiated behavior
Erhardt Developmental Prehension Assessment (EDPA)	Erhardt, R. P.	Therapy Skill Builders 555 Academic Court San Antonio, TX 78204-2498 (800) 232-1223 Erhardt Developmental Products 2379 Snowshoe Court Maplewood, MN 55119 Phone: (651) 730-9004	Birth to 6 years	To measure components and skills of hand function development in children with disabilities	Arm and hand development
Erhardt Developmental Vision Assessment, Revised (EDVA)	Erhardt, R. P.	Therapy Skill Builders 555 Academic Court San Antonio, TX 78204-2498 (800) 232-1223 Erhardt Developmental Products 2379 Snowshoe Court Maplewood, MN 55119 Phone: (651) 730-9004	Birth to 6 years	To measure visual-motor development	Involuntary visual patterns; voluntary eye movements
Evaluation Tool of Children's Handwriting (ETCH)	Amundson, S. J.	O.T. KIDS 53805 East End Road P.O. Box 1118 Homer, AK 99603 907-235-0688	Grades 1–3	Evaluates a child's speed and legibility of writing in various manuscript and cursive writing tasks	Writing speed; writing legibility; sensorimotor skills
Everyday Memory Questionnaire	Sunderland, A., Harris, J. E., and Gleave, J.	Sunderland, A., Harris, J. E., Gleave, J. (1983). Everyday memory questionnaire. In D. T. Wade(Ed.), (1992). *Measurement in neurological rehabilitation.* (pp.140–141). New York: Oxford University Press.	Adults	To assess a client's general awareness of memory capabilities and knowledge about the functioning of memory and memory strategies	Memory during ADL tasks
Executive Function Route Finding Task (EFRT)	Boyd and Sautter	Boyd, T. M., & Sautter, S. W. (1993). Route-Finding: A measure of everyday executive functioning in the head-injured adult. *Applied Cognitive Psychology,* 7, 171–181.	Adults	To assess a person's ability to get from point A to point B in a familiar environment.	Understanding the task; seeking information; remembering instructions; detecting errors; correcting errors; ability to stick with the task

Continues

TABLE OF ASSESSMENTS: LISTED ALPHABETICALLY BY TITLE *(Continued)*

Assessment Title	Author(s)	Publisher	Ages	Stated Purpose	Areas Assessed
Family Assessment Device	Epstein, N. B., Baldwin, L. M., and Bishop, D. S.	Brown University/Butler Hospital Family Research Program Butler Hospital 345 Blackstone Road Providence, RI 02906	Adults	Evaluates adaptation to having a child with a head injury	General family functioning; problem-solving; communication; roles; affective responsiveness; affective involvement; behavior control
Feasibility Evaluation Checklist (FEC)	Matheson, L.	Roy Matheson and Associates 603-358-06525 or 800-4437690	Adults	To assess a person's ability to perform job functions	Productivity; safety; interpersonal behavior
Fine Dexterity Test	The Morrisby Organisation	The Morrisby Organisation, 83 High Street, Hemel Hempstead, Hertfordshire, HP1 3AH Tel: 01442 215521 - Fax: 01442 240531. Email: info@morrisby.co.uk	Ages 16 to adult	To assess candidates for small parts assembly	To measure fine motor and small tool dexterity
Fine Motor Task Assessment	McHale, K., and Cermak, S. A.	McHale, K. & Cermak, S. A. (1992). Fine motor activities in elementary school: Preliminary findings and provisional implications for children with fine motor problems. *American Journal of Occupational Therapy, 46 (10)*, 898–903.	School age	Provides a detailed picture of fine motor skills of children	Fine motor tasks; integrated fine motor tasks; other academic tasks; and nonacademic activities
FirstSTEP Developmental Screening Test	Miller, L. J.	The Psychological Corporation 555 Academic Court San Antonio, TX 78204 (800) 288-0752	Ages 2.9–6.2	Identifies preschoolers at risk for developmental delays	Cognition; communication; motor skills
Fugl-Meyer Evaluation of Physical Performance	Fugle-Meyer, A. R., Jaasko, L., Leyman, Il, Olsson, S., and Steglind, S.	Fugle-Meyer, A. R., Jaasko, L., Leyman, Il, Olsson, S., & Steglind, S. (1975). The post-stroke hemiplegic patient. I. A method for evaluation of physical performance. *Scandinavian Journal of Rehabilitation Medicine, 7,* 13–31 Fugle-Meyer, A. R., Jaasko, L., Leyman, Il, Olsson, S., & Steglind, S. (1975). Post-stroke hemiplegic patient: Assessment of physical properties. *Scandinavian Journal of Rehabilitation Medicine, 7,* 83–93.	Adults	To quantify motor recovery stages based on the Brunnstrom and Twitchell scales.	Motor recovery; balance; sensation; range of motion; pain
Functional Independence Measure (FIM)™	The Center for Functional Assessment Research at SUNY Buffalo	Uniform Data System for Medical Rehabilitation 270 Northpointe Parkway Suite 300 Amherst, NY 14228 (716) 568-0037	Adults with various physical impairments	Measures functional status; reflects the impact of disability on the individual and on human and economic resources in the community.	18 activities, 13 with a motor emphasis related to self-care; 5 with a cognitive emphasis involving communication
Functional Reach Test	Duncan, P. W., Weiner, D. K., Chandler, J., and Studenski, S.	Pamela W. Duncan Graduate Program in Physical Therapy P.O. Box 3965, Duke University Medical Center Durham, NC 27710	Adults	To assess balance impairment, detect chance in balance performance over time, and to aid in designing modified environments for impaired persons	Balance and maximum forward reach
Galveston Orientation and Amnesia Test (GOAT)	Levin, H. S., O'Donnell, V. M., and Grossman, R. G.	The University of Texas Medical Branch at Galveston 301 University Boulevard Galveston, Texas 77555-1028 409-772-9576	Adolescents and Adults	To assess orientation and memory over time to measure progress.	Orientation; memory

Glascow Coma Scale	Teasdale and Jennett	Teasdale, G., & Jennett, B. (1994). Assessment of coma and impaired consciousness: practical scale. *Lancet*, 2, 81–84.	Adult	To monitor levels of consciousness in people with traumatic brain injury	Motor, verbal and eye-opening responses
Grooved Peg Board Test	Trites, R.	Lafayette Instrument Co. 3700 Sagamore Parkway North– PO Box 5729 Lafayette, IN 47904 USA Phone 765.423.1505 Fax 765.423.4111 Toll Free 800.428.7545	Ages 5 to adult	To test manipulative dexterity. This test requires more complex visual-motor coordination than other pegboard tests	Eye-hand coordination; fine motor dexterity
Gross Motor Function Measure	Russell, D., Rosenbaum, P., Gowland, C., Hardy, S., Lane, M., Plews, N., McGavin, H., Cadman, D., and Jarvis, S.	CanChild Centre for Childhood Disability Research Institute for Applied Health Sciences McMaster University, Room 408 1400 Main Street West Hamilton, Ontario CANADA L8S 1C7 (905) 525-9140 x27850	5 months to 16 years	Evaluates change in motor function for children with cerebral palsy (has also been used for children with Down Syndrome)	Lying and rolling; sitting; crawling and kneeling; standing; walking; and running, jumping.
Hawaii Early Learning Profile (HELP)	Furuno, S., O'Reilly, K. A., Hosaka, C. M., Inatsuka, T. T., Zeistloft-Falbey, B., and Allman, T.	VORT Corporation P.O. Box 60880 Palo Alto, CA 94306 (415) 322-8282	Birth to 3 years	To assess developmental skills and behaviors	Cognitive; language; gross motor; fine motor; social; and self-help skills
Holmes-Rahe Life Change Index	Holmes, T. H., and Rahe, R. H.	Holmes, T. H., & Rahe, R. H. (1967). The social readjustment rating scale. *Journal of Psychosomatic Research, 11*, 213–218	Adults	Self-assessment to identify stressors in the client's life	Social adjustment
Home Modification Workbook	Adaptive Environments Center	Adaptive Environment Center. (1988). *Home modification workbook*. Boston: Author.	Adults	Identify architectural barriers in the home	Home environment
Home Observation and Measurement of the Environment (HOME)	Caldwell, B.	Lorraine Coulson CRTL Room 205 University of Arkansas at Little Rock 2801 S. University Little Rock, AR 72204 501-569-3423	Birth to 6 years	To assess the stimulation potential of the child's developmental environment. Used primarily as a screening instrument	Human environmental properties; Nonhuman environmental properties
Home-Based Intervention for Caregivers of Elders with Dementia	Corcoran, M. A., and Gitlin, L. N.	Corcoran, M. A., & Gitlin, L. N. (1992). Dementia Management: An Occupational Therapy Home-Based Intervention for Caregivers. *American Journal of Occupational Therapy, 46 (9)*, 801–808.	Adults	Strategy to modify household culture to support optimal occupational performance of elderly persons and caregivers	Home environment of older adults
Housing Enabler (previously known as Enabler)	Steinfeld, E., Iwarsson, S., and Isacsson, A.	Susanne Iwarsson Veten & Skapen HB Pl 2532 SE-288 93 Nävlinge Sweden Webpage =www.enabler.nu	Adults	Identifies potential problems, severe problems, or impossibility of use of assistive devices for an individual	Limitations and use of assistive devices; potential environmental barriers inside or outside the home
Individual Differences Questionairre	Paivio, A.	Paivio, A. (1971). *Imagery and Verbal Processes*. New York: Holt Rinehart & Winston.	Adults	Identifies and helps therapist create virtual contexts that are able to be used by individuals with different thinking and learning styles	Imagery and verbal thinking habits and skills

Continues

TABLE OF ASSESSMENTS: LISTED ALPHABETICALLY BY TITLE *(Continued)*

Assessment Title	Author(s)	Publisher	Ages	Stated Purpose	Areas Assessed
Infant/Toddler Sensory Profile	Dunn, W.	Therapy Skill Builders 555 Academic Court San Antonio, TX 78204-2498 (800) 232-1223	Birth–3 years	To determine how well a subject processes sensory information in everyday situations and to profile the sensory system's effect on functional performance	Sensory processing, modulation, and behavioral and emotional responses
Inpatient Rehabilitation Facility–Patient Assessment Instrument (IRFPAI)	Uniform Data System for Medical Rehabiltiation	Uniform Data System for Medical Rehabilitation 270 Northpointe Parkway Suite 300 Amherst, NY 14228 (716) 568-0037	Adults with various physical impairments	Essentially the FIM™ with quality indicators – used with PPS	18 activities, 13 with a motor emphasis related to self-care; 5 with a cognitive emphasis involving communication; quality indicators include respiratory status, pain, PUSH scale, and safety.
Interest Checklist/NPI Interest Checklist	Matsutsuyu, J. revised by Rogers, J., Weinstein J., and Firone, J.	SLACK, Inc. 6900 Grove Road Thorofare, NJ 08086 800-257-8290	Adolescents to Adult	Gathers data about a person's interest patterns and characteristics	ADL; manual skills; cultural and educational activities; physical sports; social and recreational activities
Interview-In-Place	Lifchez, R.	Lifchez, R. (1987),*Rethinking architecture: Design students and physically disabled people.* Berkeley, CA: University of California Press.	Adults	Allows a person to articulate personal environmental meanings and priorities	Meaning of personal environment
Jebsen Hand Function Test	Jebsen, R. H., Taylor, N., Trieschmann, R. B., Trotter, M. J., and Howard, L. A.	Sammons Preston, Inc. PO Box 50710 Bolingbrook, IL 60440-5071 800-323-5547	5 years-up	To assess effective use of the hands in everyday activity by performing tasks representative of functional manual activities	Writing; card turning; picking up small objects; simulated feeding; stacking checkers; picking up light and heavy objects
Klein-Bell Activities of Daily Living Scale	Klein, R. M., and Bell, B.	Educational Resources University of Washington Seattle, WA	Children & adults	Measure ADL independence to determine current status, change in status, & subactivities to focus on in rehabilitation	Dressing, mobility, elimination, bathing & hygiene, eating, & emergency communication
Knox Cube Test	Stone, M. H., and B. D. Wright	Stoetling Co. 620 Wheat Lane Wood Dale, IL 60191 630-860-9700	2–8 years 8-up years	Nonverbal mental test to measure attention span and memory	Attention span; short-term memory
Knox Preschool Play Scale	Knox, S.	Knox, S. (1997). Development and current use of the Knox Preschool Play Scale. In L. Parham & L. Fazio (eds.) *Play in occupational therapy for children.* St. Louis: Baltimore, 35–51.	Birth to 6 years	Observational assessment of play skills	Space management; material management; pretense or symbolic play; participation in play
Kohlman Evaluation of Living Skills (KELS)	McGourty, L. K., (1979, 1999)	AOTA Products P.O. Box 3800 Forrester Center, WV 25438 877-404-AOTA	Adults with cognitive impairments	Evaluate the ability to live independently & safely in the community	Self-care, safety & health, money management, transportation & telephone, work & leisure; Tends to emphasize the knowledge component of activities
Large Allen Cognitive Level (ACL) Screen	Allen, C. K.	S&S Worldwide PO Box 513 Colchester, CT 06415 800-243-9232	All ages	To assess cognitive disability and suggest treatment approach	Problem-solving; following directions

Leisure Activities Finder (LAF)	Holmberg, K., Rosen, D., and Holland, J. L.	Psychological Assessment Resources, Inc. 16204 N. Florida Avenue Lutz, FL 33549 813-968-3003	Adults	Assists clients with finding leisure activities	Play/leisure
Leisure Boredom Scale (LBS)	Iso-Ahola, S. E., and Weissinger, E.	Iso-Ahola, S. E., & Weissinger, E. (1990). Perceptions of boredom in leisure: conceptualization, reliability and validity of the leisure boredom scale. *Journal of Leisure Research, 22,* 17–25.	All ages	Measures constraints on achieving enjoyment from leisure activities	Play/leisure
Leisure Competence Measure	Kloseck, M., and Crilly, R.	Idyll Arbor 25119 SE 262nd Street PO Box 720 Ravensdale, WA 98051 425-432-3231	All ages	Measures outcomes in leisure/play activities	Leisure awareness; leisure attitude; leisure skills; cultural/ social behaviors; interpersonal skills; community integration skills; social contact; and community participation
Leisure Diagnositic Battery	Witt, P., and Ellis, G.	Venture Publishing, Inc. 1999 Cato Avenue State College, PA 16801 814-234-4561	Adolescents and Adults	Assesses an individual's "leisure functioning"	Perceived Leisure Competency Scale; Perceived Leisure Control Scale; Leisure Needs Scale; Depth of Involvement in Leisure Scale; Playfulness Scale; Perceived Freedom in Leisure - Total Score; Barriers to Leisure Involvement Scale; Knowledge of Leisure Opportunities Test; and Leisure Preference Inventory
Leisure Interest Profile for Adults	Henry, A. D.	Henry, A. D. (1997). Leisure Interest Profile for Adults (Research Version 2.0). Boston: University of Massachusetts Medical Center	Adults	To select specific play/leisure activities with which to engage an adult by assessing the client's interest and participation in play and leisure activities	Play/leisure
Leisure Interest Profile for Seniors	Henry, A. D.	Henry, A. D. (1997). Leisure Interest Profile for Seniors (Research Version 2.0). Boston: University of Massachusetts Medical Center	Older Adults	To select specific play/leisure activities with which to engage an older adult by assessing the client's interest and participation in play and leisure activities	Play/leisure
Leisure Satisfaction Scale	Beard, J. G., and Ragheb, M. G.	Beard, J. G., & Ragheb, M. G. (1980). The leisure satisfaction measure. *Journal of Leisure Research, 12*(1), 20–33	All ages	Measures a client's level of satisfaction in leisure activities	Play/leisure
Limits of Stability (LOS)	Nashner, L. M.	NeuroCom 9570 SE Lawnfield Road Clackamas, OR 97015 800-767-6744	Adult	To assess dynamic balance	Reaction time; directional control; movement velocity; movement distance; ankle range of motion
Lincoln-Oseretsky Motor Development Scale	Sloan, W.	Stoelting Company 620 Wheat Lane Wood Dale, Illinois 60191 630-860-9700	6 to 14 years	To measure unilateral and bilateral motor development	Static coordination; dynamic coordination; speed of movement; finger dexterity; eye-hand coordination; gross motor skills
Lowenstein Occupational Therapy Cognitive Assessment– Geriatric (LOTCA - G)	Elazar, B., Itzkovich, M., and Katz, N.	Maddak, Inc. 6 Industrial Road Pequannock, NJ 07440 800-443-4926	Older Adult	To identify abilities and limitations in areas of cognitive processing	Orientation; perception; visuomotor organization; thinking operations

Continues

TABLE OF ASSESSMENTS: LISTED ALPHABETICALLY BY TITLE *(Continued)*

Assessment Title	Author(s)	Publisher	Ages	Stated Purpose	Areas Assessed
Lowenstein Occupational Therapy Cognitive Assessment (LOTCA)	Itzkovich, M., Elazar, B., Averbuch, S., and Katz, N.	Maddak, Inc. 6 Industrial Road Pequannock, NJ 07440 800-443-4926	6 years-up	To identify abilities and limitations in areas of cognitive processing	Orientation; perception; visuomotor organization; thinking operations
Making Action Plans (MAPs)	Forest, M., and Lusthaus, E.	Inclusion Press/Centre for Integrated Education and Community 24 Thome Crescent, Toronto, ON., Canada, M6H 2S5 (416) 658-5363, http://www.inclusion.com	3 to 21 years	Provides a framework to more fully integrate students; to be used in conjunction with the IEP	Personal history; fears; wishes; strengths; needs; "ideal day"
Matson Evaluation of Social Skills in Individuals with Severe Retardation (MESSIER)	Matson, J. L., and LeBlanc, L. A.	Matson, J. L. (1995). *Matson Evaluation of Social Skills for Individuals with Severe Retardation*. Baton Rouge, LA: Scientific Publisher.	All ages	To measure social skills of people with severe developmental delays	Social skills
Maximum Voluntary Efforts Tests (MVE)	Hildreth, D., Breidenbach, W., Lister, G., and Hodges, A.	Hildreth, D., Breidenbach, W., Lister, G., & Hodges, A. (1989). Detection of submaximal effort by use of rapid exchange grip. *Journal of Hand Surgery, 14A*, 4. pp. 742–745.	Adult	Uses client's intra-task consistency as an indication of whether the person has exerted maximal effort	Effort in physical strength tasks
Mayo-Portland Adaptability Inventory (MPAI-3)	Malec, J. F., Moessner, A. M., Kragness, M., and Lezak, M. D.	James F. Malec, Ph.D., L. P. PM&R-3MB-SMH Mayo Medical Center Rochester, MN 55905 507-255-5199	Adolescents to Adult	To measure long-term outcomes of brain injury	Emotions; behavior; functional abilities; physical disabilities; and societal participation
McCarthy Scale of Children's Abilities	McCarthy, D.	The Psychological Corporation 555 Academic Court San Antonio, TX 78204 (800) 288-0752	2 to 9 years	To determine a child's intellectual level, strengths and weaknesses	Verbal; perceptual-performance; quantitative; general cognitive; memory; and motor skills
McGill Pain Questionnaire	Melzack, R.	Melzack, R. (1983). The McGill pain questionnaire. In Melzack, R. (Ed.) *Pain Measurement and Assessment*. New York, Raven Press, 1983. 41–48.	Adult	Self-assessment of pain	Pain
Middlesex Elderly Assessment of Mental State (MEAMS)	Golding, E.	National Rehabilitation Services 117 North Elm Street PO Box 1247 Gaylord, MI 49735 517-732-3866	Older Adults	To assess gross impairment of specific cognitive skills; designed to differentiate between organically-based cognitive impairments and functional illnesses.	12 simple cognitive tasks
Miller Assessment for Preschoolers (MAP)	Miller, L. J.	The Psychological Corporation 555 Academic Court San Antonio, TX 78204 (800) 288-0752	2 to 6 years	To identify children who exhibit moderate "preacademic problems"	Sensory, motor, and cognitive skills through verbal and nonverbal tasks
Milwaukee Evaluation of Daily Living Skills (MEDLS)	Leonardelli, C.	SLACK, Inc. 6900 Grove Road Thorofare, NJ 08086 800-257-8290	Adults with chronic mental health problems	Establish baseline behaviors to develop treatment objectives related to daily living skills	Communication, personal care, clothing care, home & community safety, money management, personal health care, medication management, telephone use, transportation usage, time awareness; subtests can be used individually or in combination

Mini Mental State Exam (MMSE)	Folstein, M. F., Folstein, S. E., and McHugh, P. R.	Folstein, M. F., Folstein, S. E., & McHugh, P. R. (1975). Minimental state: a practical method for grading the cognitive-state of patients for the clinician. *Journal of Psychiatric Research, 12*, 089–198.	Adolescents and Adults	To quantitatively measure cognitive performance	Orientation; memory; attention; calculation; recall; language
Minimum Data Set – Section G. Physical Functioning and Structural Problems Scale, Version 2.0	Health Care Financing Administration	US Government Printing Office Washington, D.C.	Residents in long term care; clients in home care	To describe baseline ADL & track changes in ADL	Bed mobility, transfer, walk in room, walk in corridor, locomotion on unit, locomotion off unit, dressing, eating, toilet use, personal hygiene & bathing
Minnesota Handwriting Assessment	Reisman, J.	Therapy Skill Builders 555 Academic Court San Antonio, TX 78204-2498 (800) 232-1223	5 to 7 years	To analyze handwriting skills and demonstrate progress resulting from intervention	Legibility; form; alignment; size; spacing
Minnesota Rate of Manipulation Tests (MRMT)	American Guidance Service	American Guidance Service, Inc. Publisher's Building Circle Pines, MN 55014 (800) 328-2560	13 year-up	To measure manual dexterity (speed of gross arm and hand movements during rapid eye-hand coordination tasks)	Placing test; turning test; displacing test; one-hand turning and placing; two handed turning and placing
Models of Media Representation of Disability	Haller, B.	Haller, B. (1995). Rethinking models of media representation of disability. *Disability Studies Quarterly, 15 (2)*, 26–30.	Adults	Identify ways in which societal beliefs and values shape an individual's views	Attitudes toward disability
Modified Dynamic Visual Processing Assessment (M-DVPA)	Toglia, J. P., and Finkelstein, N.	Toglia, J. P. & Finkelstein, N. (1991). *Manual for the Dynamic Visual Processing Assessment*, unpublished manuscript	Adults	To assess visual processing in a dynamic interaction	Visual processing
Mother-Child Interaction Checklist	Barrera, M., and Vella, D.	Barrera, M. & Vella, D. (1987). Disabled and nondisabled infants' interactions with their mothers. *American Journal of Occupational Therapy, 41*, 168–172.	Infants and Adults	Structured format to allow observation of interactions between mothers and children	Maternal behaviors; infant behaviors; reciprocal behaviors
Motor-Free Visual Perception Test- Revised (MVPT-R)	Hammill, D. D., and Colarusso, R. P.	Academic Therapy Publications 20 Commercial Blvd. Novato, CA 94949 (800) 422-7249	4 to 11 years	To test visual perception without motor involvement	Spatial relationships; visual discrimination; visual figure ground; visual closure; and visual memory
Movement Assessment Battery for Children (Movement ABC)– formerly known as Test of Motor Imprairment	Henderson, S. E., and Sugden, D. A.	The Psychological Corporation 555 Academic Court San Antonio, TX 78204-2498 (800) 232-1223	4 to 12 years	To assess children's motor skills in children with motor impairments	Static balance; dynamic balance; manual dexterity; speed of movement; eye-hand coordination; problem-solving skills
Movement Assessment for Infants (MAI)	Chandler, L., Andrews, M., Swanson, M., and Larson, A.	School of Health and Rehabilitation Sciences University of Pittsburgh 5012 Forbes Tower Pittsburgh, PA 15260 412-383-6617	Birth to 12 months	To differentiate between normal variance among developing infants versus developmental delay	Motor function; neurological function
Mulitdimensional Functional Assessment Questionnaire	Duke University Center for the Study of Aging and Human Development	Duke University Center for the Study of Aging and Human Development. (1978). *Multidimensional functional assessment: The OARS methodology*. Durham, NC: Author.	Adults	Plan optimal community living arrangements	Functional level of individual; community service use and perceived need for services

Continues

TABLE OF ASSESSMENTS: LISTED ALPHABETICALLY BY TITLE *(Continued)*

Assessment Title	Author(s)	Publisher	Ages	Stated Purpose	Areas Assessed
Multiple Errands Test	Shallice, T., and Burgess, P. W.	Shallice, T., & Burgess, P. W. (1991). Deficits in strategy application following frontal lobe damage in man. *Brain, 114,* 727–741.	Adolescents to Adults	To assess the executive function that allows an individual to act on their own initiative and to solve problems in a relatively open ended situation	Executive function, initiation and problem solving involved in activities of daily living
Neighborhood Mobility Survey	Cantor, M.	Cantor, M. (1979). Life space and social support. In Byerts, T., Jowell, S., & Pastalan, L. (Eds.), *Environmental context of aging: Lifestyles, environmental quality, and living arrangements* (pp. 33–61). New York: Garland STPM Press.	Adults	Provides a framework for evaluating how far and by what methods people travel on a regular basis to important resources in their environment	Mobility within community
Neurobehavioral Cognitive Status Screening Examination (Cognistat)	Northern California Neurobehavioral Group, Inc	The Northern California Neurobehavioral Group, Inc. P.O. Box 460 Fairfax, California 94978 (415) 457-6400	Adolescents to Adults	To screen individuals who cannot tolerate more complicated or lengthier neuropsychological tests	Language; memory; arithmetic; attention; judgment; and reasoning
NIH Activity Record	Gloria Furst OTR, MPH	National Institutes of Health Building 10, Room 6s235 10 Center Drive MSC 1604 Bethesda, MD 20892-1604	Adolescents to Adults	To identify changes in role activities	Activities of daily living
Nine Hole Peg Test	Mathiowetz, V., Weber, K., Kashman, N., and Volland, G.	North Coast Medical 18305 Sutter Boulevard Morgan Hill, CA 95037-2845 800-821-9319	Adults	To measure finger dexterity; can be more applicable to neurologically involved patients	Fine motor dexterity
Nowicki-Strickland Locus of Control Scale for Children (TIM(C))	Nowicki, S., and Strickland, B.	Educational Testing Service (ETS) Test Collection Library Rosedale and Carter Roads Princeton, NJ 08541 (609) 734-5689	Grades 3–12	Identifies a child's locus of control	Locus of control
Nursing Child Assessment Satellite Training (NCAST) feeding and teaching scales	Barnard, K. E., and Sumner, G.	University of Washington Center on Human Development and Disability Box 357920 Seattle, WA 98195-7920 206-543-7701	All ages	Measures caregiver-child interaction	Six constructs of caregiver-child interaction
Occupational Circumstances Assessment–Interview Rating Scale (OCAIRS)	Haglund, L., Henriksson, C., Crisp, M., Friedheim, L., and Kielhofner, G.	AOTA Products P.O. Box 3800 Forrester Center, WV 25438 877-404-AOTA	Adolescents to Adults	Gathers data on a client's occupational adaptation	Personal causation; values and goals; interests; roles; habits; skills; previous experiences; physical and social environments; overall occupation participation and adaptation
Occupational Performance History Interview – Second Version (OPHI-II)	Kielhofner, G., Mallinson, T., Crawford, C., Nowak, M., Rigby, M., Henry, A., Walens, D.	AOTA Products P.O. Box 3800 Forrester Center, WV 25438 877-404-AOTA	Adolescents and Adults	Gathers data on a client's occupational adaptation over time	Activity/occupational choices; critical life events; daily routines; occupational roles; occupational behavior settings

Occupational Questionnaire (OQ)	Riopel, M., and Kielhofner, G.	AOTA Products P.O. Box 3800 Forrester Center, WV 25438 877-404-AOTA	Adults	Gathers data on time use patterns and feelings about time use	Time use
Occupational Therapy Psychosocial Assessment of Learning	Townsend, S. C., Carey, P. D., Hollins, N. L., Helfrich, C., Blondis, M., Hoffman, A., Collins, L., Knudson, J., and Blackwell, A.	AOTA Products P.O. Box 3800 Forrester Center, WV 25438 877-404-AOTA	Children	Assists clinicians in identifying a child's strengths and limitations within the school environment	Student's volition (the ability to make choices); habituation (roles and routines); and environmental fit within the classroom setting
Oswestry Low Back Pain Disability Questionnaire	Fairbank, J. C. T., Couper Mbaot, J., Davies, J. B., and O'Brien, J. P.	Fairbank, J. C. T., Couper Mbaot, J., Davies, J. B., & O'Brien, J. P. (1980). The Oswestry Low Back Pain Disability Questionnaire. *Physiotherapy,* 66, 271–2.	Adults	Self-assessment of pain	Pain
OT-Quest	Schulz, E.	Schulz, E. (2000). *The OT Quest: A spirituality and quality of experience assessment tool.* Unpublished manuscript: Texas Women's University	Adults	Examines how individuals incorporate spirituality in daily life settings and occupations	Spirituality in daily life
Outcome and Assessment Information Set, B-1, M0640-M0800 (OASIS)	Center for Health Services and Policy Research	Center for Health Services and Policy Research Denver CO These forms are available for viewing, downloading, or printing from CMS' (formerly HCFA) website: http://www.hcfa.gov/medicaid/oasis/oasisdat.htm	Adults	Measures the ability to perform ADL and IADL in people in home care	Dressing; toileting; transferring; ambulation/locomotion; feeding/eating; grooming Meal preparation; transportation; laundry; housekeeping; using telephone; medication management
Paced Auditory Serial Addition Test (PASAT)	Gronwall, D. M. A.	Gronwall, D. M. A. (1977). Paced Auditory Serial Addition Task: A measure of recovery from concussion. *Perceptual and Motor Skills, 44,* 367–373.	Adults	To detect subtle impairments in attention and speed of processing	Auditory attention and processing during everyday activities
Pain Behavior Checklist	Turk, D. C., Wack, J. T., and Kerns, R. D.	Turk, D. C., Wack, J. T., & Kerns, R. D. (1985) An empirical examination of the "pain behavior" construct. *Journal of Behavioral Medicine*, 8, 119–130.	Adults	Documenting overt pain behaviors	Behavior related to pain
Peabody Developmental Motor Scales-2, revised	Folio, M. R., and Fewell, R. R.	PRO-ED, Inc. 8700 Shoal Creek Blvd. Austin, TX 78757 (800) 897-3202	Birth to 7 years	To quantitatively assess motor development of children	Gross and fine motor skills
Pediatric Evaluation of Disability Inventory (PEDI)	Haley, S. M., Coster, W. J., Ludlow, L. H., Haltiwanger, J. T., and Andrellos, P. J.	Therapy Skill Builders 555 Academic Court San Antonio, TX 78204-2498 (800) 232-1223	6 months– 7.5 years	To assess functional skills of young children, monitor progress, or evaluate the outcome of a therapeutic program	Self-care; mobility; social function
Pediatric Interest Profiles (PIP's)	Henry, A. D.	Therapy Skill Builders 555 Academic Court San Antonio, TX 78204-2498 (800) 232-1223	6–21 years	To select specific play/leisure activities with which to engage a child by assessing the child's interest and participation in play and leisure activities	Interest and participation in play and leisure activities
Pediatric Volitional Questionnaire	Geist, R., and Kielhofner, G.	AOTA Products P.O. Box 3800 Forrester Center, WV 25438 877-404-AOTA	Preschool age	Play-based observational assessment designed to evaluate a young child's volition	Motivation; personal causation; values; and interests

Continues

TABLE OF ASSESSMENTS: LISTED ALPHABETICALLY BY TITLE *(Continued)*

Assessment Title	Author(s)	Publisher	Ages	Stated Purpose	Areas Assessed
Performance Assessment of Self-Care Skills – Version 3.1 (PASS)	Holm, M. B., and Rogers, J. C.	University of Pittsburgh School of Health and Rehabilitation Sciences Pittsburgh, PA 15260	Adults with various impairments	Evaluate independent living skills in client's home and in the clinic, and to assess change	Functional mobility; personal care; home management
Planning Alternative Tomorrows with Hope (PATH)	Pearpoint, J., O'Brien, J., and Forest, M.	Inclusion Press/Centre for Integrated Education and Community 24 Thome Crescent Toronto, ON., Canada M6H 2S5 (416) 658-5363 http://www.inclusion.com	All ages	Helps clients reach their life goals, identify their strengths	Client goals
Play History	Takata, N.	Behnke, C. & Fetkovich, M. (1984). Examining the reliability and validity of the Play History, *American Journal of Occupational Therapy, 38*, 94–100.	Children and Adolescents	To identify a child's play experiences and play opportunities	Previous play experiences; actual play and opportunity for play
Playform	Ziviani, J., Rodger, S., Sturgess, J., Boyle, M., and Cooper, R.	Department of Occupational Therapy The University of Queensland QLD St. Lucia QLD 4072 Australia +61 7 3365 2652	5–7 years	Assesses a child's perception of play competence	Play
Preferences for Activities of Children (PAC)	CanChild Centre for Childhood Disability Research	CanChild Centre for Childhood Disability Research Institute for Applied Health Sciences, McMaster University, 1400 Main Street West, Room 408 Hamilton, Ontario Canada L8S 1C7 905) 525-9140 (Ext. 27850)	6 years-up	Examines a child's preferences for activities	Child's preference for activities
Preschool and Kindergarten Behavior Scales (PKBS)	Merrell, K. W.	Merrell, K. W. (1996). Social-emotional assessment in early childhood: The Preschool and Kindergarten Behavior Scales. *Journal of Early Intervention, 20*, 132–145.	3–6 years	To identify social skills and behaviors of children	Social skills
Profile of Executive Control System (PRO-EX)	Branswell, D., Hartry, A., Hoornbeek, S., Johansen, A., Johnson, L., Schultz, J., and Sohlberg, M. M.	Lash and Associates Publishing/Training, Inc. 708 Young Forest Drive Wake Forest, NC 27587 919-562-0015	Adults	To assess the executive control system in order to identify deficits in the subject's ability to plan, organize, and self-evaluate	Planning; organizing; self-evaluation
Prospective Memory Screening (PROMS)	Sohlberg, M. M. and Mateer, C.	National Rehabilitation Services 117 North Elm Street PO Box 1247 Gaylord, MI 49735 517-732-3866	Adults	To assess the ability to design and carry out planned actions appropriately	Motor and process skills in relation to activity demands
Purdue Peg Board	Tiffin, J.	Lafayette Instrument Company 3700 Sagamore Parkway North PO Box 5729 Lafayette, IN 47903 800-428-7545	5 years-up	To measure dexterity of fingertip activity and finger/hand/arm activity	Finger dexterity, fine motor coordination and speed

Quick Neurological Screening Test (QNST)	Sterling, H. M., Mutti, M., and Spalding, N. V.	Stoelting Company 620 Wheat Lane Wood Dale, Illinois 60191 630-860-9700	5 to 18 years	To assess a child's maturity and developmental skills	Large and small muscle control; motor planning; sequencing; sense of rate and rhythm; spatial organization; visual and auditory perceptual skills; balance; cerebellar-vestibular function; disorders of attention
Rabideau Kitchen Evaluation (RKE-R)	Neistadt, M. E.	Neistadt, M. E. (1994). A meal preparation treatment protocol for adults with brain injury. *American Journal of Occupational Therapy, 48 (5),* 431–438.	Adults	To evaluate the use of a meal preparation treatment protocol based on cognitive-perceptual information processing theory for adults with traumatic or anoxic acquired brain injury	Meal preparation skills
Ransford Pain Drawing	Ransford, A., Cairns, D., and Mooney, V.	Ransford, A., Cairns, D., & Mooney, V. (1979). The pain drawing as an aid to the psychological evaluation of patients with low back pain. *Spine, 1*, pp. 127–134.	Adults	Self-assessment of pain	Pain
Readily Achievable Checklist	Cronburg, J., Barnett, J., and Goldman, N.	Cronburg, J., Barnett, J., & Goldman, N. (1991). *Readily achievable checklist: A survey for accessibility.* Washington, D.C.: National Center for Access Unlimited.	Adults	To assess accessibility in the community	Community environment
Rehabilitation Institute of Chicago Functional Assessment Scale	Rehabilitation Institute of Chicago	Rehabilitation Institute of Chicago 345 East Superior St Chicago, Il 60611-4496	Adults	To evaluate client's ability to complete instrumental activities of daily living	Instrumental activities of daily living
Risk Factor Checklist	National Safety Council	National Safety Council 1121 Spring Lake Drive Itasca, IL 60143-3201 (630) 285-1121	Adults	Identifies specific workplace risks	Risks in workplace
Rivermead Behavioral Memory Test– extended version (RBMT-E)	Wilson, B., Cockburn, J., and Baddeley, A.	National Rehabilitation Services 117 North Elm Street PO Box 1247 Gaylord, MI 49735 517-732-3866	All	To detect and identify memory impairments that occur in every activity, with a broader cultural sensitivity	Memory
Rivermead Behavioral Memory Test (RBMT)	Wilson, B., Cockburn, J., and Baddeley, A.	National Rehabilitation Services 117 North Elm Street PO Box 1247 Gaylord, MI 49735 517-732-3866	Adult 16–96	Detects and identifies memory impairments daily activity	Memory
Rivermead Behavioral Memory Test for Children (RBMT-C)	Alrich, F. K., and Wilson, B.	National Rehabilitation Services 117 North Elm Street PO Box 1247 Gaylord, MI 49735 517-732-3866	Children 5–10 5 years-up	To detect and identify memory impairments that occur in every activity	Verbal recall; remembering to do a task later in the test; remember and identify pictures; remember and retell a story; retrace a route around the room Memory
Role Checklist (RC)	Oakley, F.	Frances Oakley, MS, OTR/L, FAOTA Occupational Therapy Service National Institutes of Health Building 10, Room 6S-235 10 Center Drive MSC 1604 Bethesda, MD 20892-1604	Adults	To assess productive roles in adult life	Roles significant to the client; motivation to engage in tasks necessary to those roles; perceptions of role shifting

Continues

TABLE OF ASSESSMENTS: LISTED ALPHABETICALLY BY TITLE *(Continued)*

Assessment Title	Author(s)	Publisher	Ages	Stated Purpose	Areas Assessed
Routine Task Inventory	Heimann, N. E., and Allen, C. K., and Yerxa, E. J.	Heimann, N. E. & Allen, C. K. (1989). The routine task inventory: A tool for describing the functional behavior of the cognitively disabled. *Occupational Therapy Practice* 1(1) 67–74	Adults	To assess functional behavior during typical tasks using self-report or observation	Self-awareness (eg, grooming, dressing, bathing), situational awareness (eg, housekeeping, spending money, shopping), occupational role (eg, planning/doing major role activities, pacing & timing actions), social role (eg, communicating meaning, following directions)
Safety Assessment of Function and the Environment for Rehabilitation (SAFER)	Oliver R., Blathwayt J., Brackley C., and Tamaki T.	Oliver R. Blathwayt J. Brackley C. Tamaki T. (1993). Development of the Safety Assessment of Function and the Environment for Rehabilitation (SAFER) tool. *Canadian Journal of Occupational Therapy. 60 (2).* 78–82.	Older Adults	To evaluate home safety for elders	Evaluates risks in various rooms of the home as well as general risks such as fire hazards; examines safety issues in how the individual performs various self-care and household tasks; examines the potential for wandering and the use of memory aids; and identifies how help could be summoned
Scales of Cognitive Ability for Traumatic Brain Injury (SCATBI)	Adamovich, B., and Henderson, J.	PRO-ED, Inc. 8700 Shoal Creek Blvd. Austin, TX 78757 (800) 897-3202	Adolescent and Adult	To assess cognitive and linguistic abilities in people with head injury; to gauge severity and chart progress during recovery.	Perception/Discrimination; Orientation; Organization; Recall; and Reasoning
School Function Assessment	Coster, W., Deeney, T., Haltiwanger, J., and Haley, S.	Therapy Skill Builders 555 Academic Court San Antonio, TX 78204-2498 (800) 232-1223	Kindergarten to 6th grade	To evaluate and monitor a student's performance of functional tasks and activities that support his/her participation in elementary school	Participation in elementary school setting; task supports; activity performance
School Setting Interview (SSI)	Hoffman, O. R., Hemmingsson, H., and Kielhofner, G.	AOTA Products P.O. Box 3800 Forrester Center, WV 25438 877-404-AOTA	9 years-high school	Allows children and adolescents with disabilities to describe the impact of the environment on their functioning in multiple school settings	Impact of school environment on functional performance of children and adolescents with disability
Self-Assessment of Occupational Functioning (SAOF)	Baron, K., and Curtin, C.	AOTA Products P.O. Box 3800 Forrester Center, WV 25438 877-404-AOTA	14 years-up	Self-report of client's perception of his/her occupational competence and the impact of environment on function	Volition; habituation; performance; values; personal causation; interests; roles; habits; skills
Self-Directed Search	Holland, J. L.	Psychological Assessment Resources, Inc. 16204 N. Florida Avenue Lutz, FL 33549 813-968-3003	14 years-up	Assesses career interests	Aspirations; activities; competencies; occupations
Semmes-Weinstein Monofilament Test	Weinstein, S.	Weinstein, S. (1993). Fifty years of somatosensory research: From the Semmes-Weinstein monofilaments to the Weinstein Enhanced Sensory Test. *Journal of Hand Therapy, 6,* 11–22.	All	Identifies skin pressure thresholds useful in determining degree of normal and protective sensation	Skin sensation
Sensory Integration and Praxis Tests (SIPT)	Ayres, A. J.	Western Psychological Services 12031 Wilshire Boulevard Los Angeles, CA 90025 800-648-8857	4–8.11 years	To assess praxis and sensory processing and integration of vestibular, proprioceptive, tactile, kinesthetic, and visual systems	Sensory processing; visual-spatial perception; coordination; motor planning

Sensory Organization Test (SOT)	Nashner, L. M.	NeuroCom 9570 SE Lawnfield Road Clackamas, OR 97015 800-767-6744	Adult	To objectively identify abnormalities in a patient's use of somatosensory, visual and visual systems that contribute to postural control	Postural stability in various sensory conditions/environments
Sensory Profile; Adolescent/Adult Sensory Profile; Infant/Toddler Sensory Profile	Dunn, W.	Therapy Skill Builders 555 Academic Court San Antonio, TX 78204-2498 (800) 232-1223	All Ages 3–10 years	To determine how well a subject processes sensory information in everyday situations and to profile the sensory system's effect on functional performance	Sensory processing, modulation, and behavioral and emotional responses
Skills Assessment Module (SAM)	Rosinek, M.	Rosinek, M. (1985). *Skills Assessment Module.* Athens, GA: Piney Mountain Press.	Adults	To attain a baseline of a client's ability to perform job-simulated tasks	Motor and process skills in relation to job tasks
Social Interaction Scale (SIS)	Trower, P., Bryant, B., and Argyle, M.	Trower, P., Bryant, B., & Argyle, M. (1978). *Social skills and mental health.* London: Methuen.	Adults	To rate social behavior that is exhibited during a semi-structured interview.	Social competence; voice quality; nonverbal communication; conversation
Social Skills Rating System	Gresham, F. M., and Elliot, S. N.	American Guidance Service, Inc. Publisher's Building Circle Pines, MN 55014 (800) 328-2560	3–18 years	Rates social behaviors believed to affect areas such as teacher-student relationships, peer acceptance, and academic performance	Social Skills (Cooperation, Assertion, Responsibility, Empathy, and Self-Control); Problem Behaviors; and Academic Competence (teacher ratings of reading, math performance, general cognitive functioning, motivation, and parental support).
Sociospatial Support Inventory	Rowles, G.	Rowles, G. (1983). Geographical dimensions of social support in rural Appalachia. In G. Rowles & R. Ohta (Eds.), *Aging and milieu: Environmental perspectives on growing old* (pp. 111–130). New York: Academic Press.	Adults	Catalyst for examining how an individual can evaluate alternative ways to manage community living support arrangements	Perception of support in environment
Source Book	Kelly, C., and Snell, K.	Kelly, C. & Snell, K. (1989). *The source book: Architectural guidelines for barrier free design.* Toronto, ON: Barrier-Free Design Centre.	Adults	To identify architectural barriers in the the home, work, and community	Home, work, community environments
Spinal Functions Sort	Matheson, L. N., and Matheson, M. L.	Roy Matheson and Associates 603-358-06525 or 800-4437690	Adult	To quantify the subject's perception of ability to perform work tasks that involve the spine	Perception of work tasks
Spiritual Well-Being Scale	Bufford, R., Paloutzian, R., and Ellison, C.	Ellsion, C. (1983). Spiritual Well- Being: conceptualization and measurement. *Journal of Psychology and Technology, 11 (4),* 330–340. For more information, contact Upasana Nanda, MPH at Cardinal Glennon Children's Hospital 314-268-4110	All ages	Catalyst to explore various forms of spirituality	Spirituality
Stress Management Questionnaire	Stein, F., and Nikolic, S.	Stein, F., & Nikolic, S. (1989). Teaching stress management techniques to a schizophrenic person. *American Journal of Occupational Therapy, 43,* 162–169.	Adults	Self-assessment to identify stressors in the subject's daily life	Perceptions of stress in daily life
Test of Oral and Limb Apraxia (TOLA)	Helm-Estabrooks, N.	Riverside Publishing Company 425 Spring Lake Drive Itasca, IL 60143-2079 800-323-9540	Adults	To identify, measure, and evaluate the presence of oral and limb apraxia in adults with developmental or acquired neurologic disorders	Types and severity of oral and limb apraxia

Continues

TABLE OF ASSESSMENTS: LISTED ALPHABETICALLY BY TITLE *(Continued)*

Assessment Title	Author(s)	Publisher	Ages	Stated Purpose	Areas Assessed
Test of Environmental Supportiveness	Bundy, A.	Colorado State University Department of Occupational Therapy Fort Collins, CO 80523 303-491-6253	Children	Assesses the extent to which the environment supports an individual's play	Caregivers actions, rules, and boundaries; peer, younger, and older playmates' use of cues and domination of interaction; natural and fabricated objects; amount and configuration of space; sensory environment; safety and accessibility of space
Test of Everyday Attention (TEA)	Robertson, I., Ward, T., Ridgeway, V., and Nimmo-Smith, I.	National Rehabilitation Services 117 North Elm Street PO Box 1247 Gaylord, MI 49735 517-732-3866	18 years-up	To test attention system serving different functions in everyday behavior	Selective attention; sustained attention; attentional switching; divided attention
Test of Everyday Attention for Children (TEA–Ch)	Manly, T., Robertson, I., Anderson, V., and Nimmo-Smith, I.	National Rehabilitation Services 117 North Elm Street PO Box 1247 Gaylord, MI 49735 517-732-3866	6–16 years	To test attention system serving different functions in everyday behavior	Selective attention; sustained attention; attentional switching; divided attention
Test of Gross Motor Development	Ulrich, D. A.	The Psychological Corporation 555 Academic Court San Antonio, TX 78204-2498 (800) 232-1223	3–11 years	Measures common gross motor skills	Locomotor; object Control:
Test of Handwriting Skills	Gardner, M. A.	Therapro, Inc. 225 Arlington Street Framingham, MA 01702-8723 (508) 872-9494 or (800) 257-5376	5–11 years	Standardized assessment of manuscript and cursive handwriting skills	Manuscript and cursive; writing from memory; writing from dictation; copying upper case and lower case selected letters and numbers; copying words and sentences; speed of writing; reversals; spacing, etc.
Test of Orientation for Rehabilitation Patients (TORP)	Dietz, J., Beeman, C., and Thorn, D.	Therapy Skill Builders 555 Academic Court San Antonio, TX 78204-2498 (800) 232-1223	Adolescents and Adults	To determine the existence and extent of disorientation, establish a baseline level of performance, plan intervention, monitor progress, assess effectiveness of treatment	Orientation to person and personal situation, place, time, schedule, and temporal continuity
Test of Playfulness (ToP)	Bundy, A.	Anita Bundy Department of Occupational Therapy Colorado State University Room 219, Occupational Therapy Building Fort Collins, CO 80523 970-491-6253	15 months–10 years	Assesses a child's play behavior based on playfulness rather than on motor, cognitive, or language skills	Playfulness
Test of Visual-Perceptual Skills (Non-Motor) (TVPS)	Gardner, M.	Psychological and Educational Publications, Inc. 1477 Rollins Road Burlingame, CA 94010 800-523-5775	4–12 years	To determine a child's visual-perceptual strengths and weaknesses without the use of motor responses	Visual discrimination; visual memory; visual-spatial relations; visual form constancy; visual sequential memory; visual figure-ground; visual closure

Test of Visual-Motor Skills (TVMS)	Gardner, M.	Psychological and Educational Publications, Inc. 1477 Rollins Road Burlingame, CA 94010 800-523-5775	2–13 years	To assess how a child visually perceives nonlanguage forms and translates what is perceived through hand function	Copy 26 geometric forms
Test of Visual-Motor Skills: Upper Level Adolescents and Adults (TVMS:UL)	Gardner, M.	Psychological and Educational Publications, Inc. 1477 Rollins Road Burlingame, CA 94010 800-523-5775	12–40 years	To assess how an adolescent or adult visually perceives nonlanguage forms and translates what is perceived through hand function	Copy 26 geometric forms
Test of Visual-Perceptual Skills: Upper Level (Non-Motor) (TVPS:UL)	Gardner, M.	Psychological and Educational Publications, Inc. 1477 Rollins Road Burlingame, CA 94010 800-523-5775	12–18 years	To determine an adolescent's visual-perceptual strengths and weaknesses without the use of motor responses	Visual discrimination; visual memory; visual-spatial relations; visual form constancy; visual sequential memory; visual figure-ground; visual closure
The Experience of Leisure Scale (TELS)	Bundy, A.	Bundy, A. (2000). The Experience of Leisure Scale (TELS). Fort Collins, CO: Colorado State University	Adolescents and Adults	Examines play and leisure experiences of adults and adolescents	Play/leisure
Tinetti Assessment Tool	Tinetti, M.	Dr. Mary Tinetti Yale Medical Group 300 George Street, 6th Floor New Haven, CT 06511 203-688-5238 http://www.sgim.org/TinettiTool.PDF	Adult	To measure fall-risk in adult and geriatric populations	Gait; balance
Toddler and Infant Motor Evaluation (TIME)	Miller, L. J., and Roid, G. H.	Therapy Skill Builders 555 Academic Court San Antonio, TX 78204-2498 (800) 232-1223	Birth to 4 years	To be used as a comprehensive assessment of children who are suspected to have motor delays or deviations	Mobility; stability; motor organization; social-emotional; and functional performance
Toglia Category Assessment	Toglia, J. P.	Therapy Skill Builders 555 Academic Court San Antonio, TX 78204-2498 (800) 232-1223	All ages	To assess category flexibility	Categorization; strategies; problem-solving
Valpar Component Work Samples	Valpar Corporation	Valpar Corporation 3801 East 34th Street Suite 105 Tucson, AZ 85713 800-528-7070	Adults	To generate clinical and actuarial data on universal worker characteristics	Mechanical and clerical work skills
Verbal and Nonverbal Cancellation Tasks	Mesulam, M.	Mesulam, M. (1985) Attention, confusional states and neglect. In M. Mesulam (Ed.), *Principles of Behavioral Neurology,* (pp. 125–68). Philadelphia: F.A. Davis.	All ages	To detect the presence of neglect.	Attention, visual neglect.
Vermont Interdependent Services Team Approach (VISTA)	Giangreco, M. F.	Giangreco, M. F. (1996). *VISTA: Vermont interdependent services team approach. A guide to coordinating support services.* Baltimore: Paul H. Brookes Publishing Company	Ages 3–21	To facilitate cross-disciplinary, interdependent, support service/related service decision-making and implementation for students with disabilities in schools	Support services in the school system
Vineland Adaptive Behavior Scales, Revised (VABS)	Sparrow, S. S., Balla, D. A., and Cicchetti, D. V.	American Guidance Service, Inc. Publisher's Building Circle Pines, MN 55014 (800) 328-2560	Birth to 19 years	To assess personal and social sufficiency of individuals from birth to adulthood	Communication; activities of daily living; socialization; motor skills; adaptive behavior; maladaptive behavior

Continues

TABLE OF ASSESSMENTS: LISTED ALPHABETICALLY BY TITLE *(Continued)*

Assessment Title	Author(s)	Publisher	Ages	Stated Purpose	Areas Assessed
Volitional Questionnaire	de las Heras, C. G., Geist, R., and Kielhofner, G.	AOTA Products P.O. Box 3800 Forrester Center, WV 25438 877-404-AOTA	Adults	Assesses volition by observation	Motivation; values; interests
Wadddell Signs	Waddell, G., McCulloch, J., Kummel, E., and Venner, R.	Waddell, G., McCulloch, J., Kummel, E., & Venner, R. (1980). Nonorganic physical signs in low-back pain. *Spine, 5*, pp. 117–125.	Adult	To help the therapist detect abnormal illness behavior or symptoms not consistent with typical anatomy and physiology	Back pain symptom magnification
WeeFIM™ (Guide for the Uniform Data Set for Medical Rehabilitation for Children	The Center for Functional Assessment Research at SUNY Buffalo	Uniform Data System for Medical Rehabilitation 270 Northpointe Parkway Suite 300 Amherst, NY 14228 (716) 568-0037	Children from 6 months to 7 years	Measure disability severity related to physical impairment, across health, development, educational, & community settings	18 activities, 13 with a motor emphasis related to self-care; 5 with a cognitive emphasis involving communication
West Tool Sort	Matheson, L.	Matheson L. WEST Tool Sort. Signal Hill, CA: Work Evaluation Systems Technology, 1981 Roy Matheson and Associates 603-358-06525 or 800-4437690	Adults	Self-assessment of a subject's ability to use specific tools to perform ADL and work tasks.	Motor and process skills in relation to ADL and work tasks
Work Environment Impact Scale (WEIS)	Corner, R., Kielhofner, G., and Line, F-L.	AOTA Products P.O. Box 3800 Forrester Center, WV 25438 877-404-AOTA	Adults	Examines how individuals with disabilities experience the work environment	Work environment factors and their impact on performance; satisfaction; physical, social, and emotional well-being of the worker
Work Environments Scale	Moos, R.	Consulting Psychologists Press 3803 East Bayshore Road Palo Alto, CA 94303 (800) 624-1765 or (650) 969-8901	Adults	Examines the inter-personal environment of a workplace	Workplace environment
Worker Role Interview (WRI)	Velozo, C., Kielhofner, G., and Fisher, G.	AOTA Products P.O. Box 3800 Forrester Center, WV 25438 877-404-AOTA	Adults	Gathers data on psychosocial and environmental factors related to work	Personal causation; values; interests; roles and habits related to work; influence of the environment
Workplace Workbook	Mueller, J.	Mueller, J. (1990). *The workplace workbook: An illustrated guide to job accommodation and assistive technology*. Washington, D.C.: The Dole Foundation.	Adults	To identify barriers in the workplace	Workplace environment

ADL, activity of daily living; *AOTA,* American Occupational Association; *IADL,* instrumental activity of daily living; *IEP,* individualized education program; *NIH,* National Institutes of Health.

APPENDIX B

CORE VALUES AND ATTITUDES OF OCCUPATIONAL THERAPY PRACTICE

INTRODUCTION

In 1985, the American Occupational Therapy Association (AOTA) funded the Professional and Technical Role Analysis Study (PATRA). This study had two purposes: to delineate the entry-level practice of OTRs and COTAs through a role analysis and to conduct a task inventory of what practitioners actually do. Knowledge, skills, and attitude statements were to be developed to provide a basis for the role analysis. The PATRA study completed the knowledge and skills statements. The Executive Board subsequently charged the Standards and Ethics Commission (SEC) to develop a statement that would describe the attitudes and values that undergird the profession of occupational therapy. The SEC wrote this document for use by AOTA members.

The list of terms used in this statement was originally constructed by the American Association of Colleges of Nursing (AACN) (1986). The PATRA committee analyzed the knowledge statements that the committee had written and selected those terms from the AACN list that best identified the values and attitudes of our profession. This list of terms was then forwarded to SEC by the PATRA Committee to use as the basis for the Core Values and Attitudes paper.

The development of this document is predicated on the assumption that the values of occupational therapy are evident in the official documents of the American Occupational Therapy Association. The official documents that were examined are: (a) *Dictionary Definition of Occupational Therapy* (AOTA, 1986), (b) *The Philosophical Base of Occupational Therapy* (AOTA, 1979), (c) *Essentials and Guidelines for an Accredited Educational Program for the Occupational Therapist* (AOTA, 1991a), (d) *Essentials and Guidelines for an Accredited Educational Program for the Occupational Therapy Assistant* (AOTA, 1991b), and (e) *Occupational Therapy Code of Ethics* (AOTA, 1988). It is further assumed that these documents are representative of the values and beliefs reflected in other occupational therapy literature.

A *value* is defined as a belief or an ideal to which an individual is committed. Values are an important part of the base or foundation of a profession. Ideally, these values are embraced by all members of the profession and are reflected in the members' interactions with those persons receiving services, colleagues, and the society at large. Values have a central role in a profession and are developed and reinforced throughout an individual's life as a student and as a professional.

Actions and attitudes reflect the values of the individual. An attitude is the disposition to respond positively or negatively toward an object, person concept, or situation. Thus, there is an assumption that all professional actions and interactions are rooted in certain core values and beliefs.

SEVEN CORE CONCEPTS

In this document, the *core values and attitudes* of occupational therapy are organized around seven basic concepts—altruism, equality, freedom, justice, dignity, truth, and prudence. How these core values and attitudes are expressed

From *American Journal of Occupational Therapy, 47,* 1086–1086.

and implemented by occupational therapy practitioners may vary depending upon the environments and situations in which professional activity occurs.

Altruism is the unselfish concern for the welfare of others. This concept is reflected in actions and attitudes of commitment, caring, dedication, responsiveness, and understanding.

Equality requires that all individuals be perceived as having the same fundamental human rights and opportunities. This value is demonstrated by an attitude of fairness and impartiality. We believe that we should respect all individuals, keeping in mind that they may have values, beliefs, or lifestyles that are different from our own. Equality is practiced in the broad professional arena, but is particularly important in day-to-day interactions with those individuals receiving occupational therapy services.

Freedom allows the individual to exercise choice and to demonstrate independence, initiative, and self-direction. There is a need for all individuals to find a balance between autonomy and societal membership that is reflected in the choice of various patterns of interdependence with the human and nonhuman environment. We believe that individuals are internally and externally motivated toward action in a continuous process of adaptation throughout the life span. Purposeful activity plays a major or role in developing and exercising self-direction, initiative, interdependence, and relatedness to the world. Activities verify the individual's ability to adapt, and they establish a satisfying balance between autonomy and societal membership. As professionals, we affirm the freedom of choice for each individual to pursue goals that have personal and social meaning.

Justice places value on the upholding of such moral and legal principles as fairness, equity, truthfulness, and objectivity. This means we aspire to provide occupational therapy services for all individuals who are in need of these services and that we will maintain a goal-directed and objective relationship with all those served. Practitioners must be knowledgeable about and have respect for the legal rights of individuals receiving occupational therapy services. In addition, the occupational therapy practitioner must understand and abide by the local, state, and federal laws governing professional practice.

Dignity emphasizes the importance of valuing the inherent worth and uniqueness of each person. This value is demonstrated by an attitude of empathy and respect for self and others. We believe that each individual is a unique combination of biologic endowment, sociocultural heritage, and life experiences. We view human beings holistically, respecting the unique interaction of the mind, body, and physical and social environment. We believe that dignity is nurtured and grows from the sense of competence and self-worth that is integrally linked to the person's ability to perform valued and relevant activities. In occupational therapy we emphasize the importance of dignity by helping the individual build on his or her unique attributes and resources.

Truth requires that we be faithful to facts and reality. Truthfulness or veracity is demonstrated by being accountable honest, forthright, accurate, and authentic in our attitudes and actions. There is an obligation to be truthful with ourselves, those who receive services, colleagues, and society. One way that this is exhibited is through maintaining and upgrading professional competence. This happens, in part, through an unfaltering commitment to inquiry and learning, to self-understanding, and to the development of an interpersonal competence.

Prudence is the ability to govern and discipline oneself through the use of reason. To be prudent is to value judiciousness, discretion, vigilance, moderation, care, and circumspection in the management of one's affairs, to temper extremes, make judgments, and respond on the basis of intelligent reflection and rational thought.

SUMMARY

Beliefs and values are those intrinsic concepts that underlie the core of the profession and the professional interactions of each practitioner. These values describe the profession's philosophy and provide the basis for defining purpose. The emphasis or priority that is given to each value may change as one's professional career evolves and as the unique characteristics of a situation unfold. This evolution of values is developmental in nature. Although we have basic values that cannot be violated, the degree to which certain values will take priority at a given time is influenced by the specifics of a situation and the environment in which it occurs. In one instance dignity may be a higher priority that truth; in another prudence may be chosen over freedom. As we process information and make decisions, the weight of the values that we hold may change. The practitioner faces dilemmas because of conflicting values and is required to engage in thoughtful deliberation to determine where the priority lies in a given situation.

The challenge for us all is to know our values, be able to make reasoned choices in situations of conflict, and be able to clearly articulate and defend our choices. At the same time, it is important that all members of the profession be committed to a set of common values. This mutual commitment to a set of beliefs and principles that govern our practice can provide a basis for clarifying expectations between the recipient and the provider of services. Shared values empowers the profession and, in addition, builds trust among ourselves and with others.

Prepared by Elizabeth Kanny, MA, OTR, for the Standards and Ethics Commission (Ruth A. Hansen, PHD, OTR, FAOTA, Chairperson). Approved by the Representative Assembly June 1993.

References

American Association of Colleges of Nursing. (1986). *Essentials of College and University Education for Professional Nursing. Final report.* Washington, DC: Author.

American Occupational Therapy Association. (1986, April). *Dictionary definition of occupational therapy.* Adopted and approved by the Representative Assembly to fulfill Resolution #596–83. (Available from AOTA, 1383 Piccard Drive, PO Box 1725, Rockville, MD 20849–1725.)

American Occupational Therapy Association. (1988). Occupational therapy code of ethics. *American Journal of Occupational Therapy, 42,* 795–796.

American Occupational Therapy Association (1991a). Essentials and guidelines for an accredited educational program for the occupational therapist. *American Journal of Occupational Therapy, 45,* 1077–1984.

American Occupational Therapy Association. (1991b). Essentials and guidelines for an accredited educational program for the occupational therapy assistant. *American Journal of Occupational Therapy, 45,* 1085–1092.

American Occupational Therapy Association. (1979). The philosophical base of occupational therapy. *American Journal of Occupational Therapy, 33,* 785.

APPENDIX C

OCCUPATIONAL THERAPY CODE OF ETHICS (2000)

PREAMBLE

The American Occupational Therapy Association's Code of Ethics is a public statement of the common set of values and principles used to promote and maintain high standards of behavior in occupational therapy. The American Occupational Therapy Association and its members are committed to furthering the ability of individuals, groups, and systems to function within their total environment. To this end, occupational therapy personnel (including all staff and personnel who work and assist in providing occupational therapy services (e.g., aides, orderlies, secretaries, technicians) have a responsibility to provide services to recipients in any stage of health and illness who are individuals, research participants, institutions and businesses, other professionals and colleagues, students, and to the general public.

The *Occupational Therapy Code of Ethics* is a set of principles that applies to occupational therapy personnel at all levels. These principles to which occupational therapists and occupational therapy assistants aspire are part of a lifelong effort to act in an ethical manner. The various roles of practitioner (occupational therapist and occupational therapy assistant), educator, fieldwork educator, clinical supervisor, manager, administrator, consultant, fieldwork coordinator, faculty program director, researcher/scholar, private practice owner, entrepreneur, and student are assumed.

Any action in violation of the spirit and purpose of this Code shall be considered unethical. To ensure compliance with the Code, the Commission on Standards and Ethics (SEC) establishes and maintains the enforcement procedures.

From *American Journal of Occupational Therapy, 54,* 614–616.

Acceptance of membership in the American Occupational Therapy Association commits members to adherence to the Code of Ethics and its enforcement procedures. The Code of Ethics, Core Values and Attitudes of Occupational Therapy Practice (AOTA, 1993), and the Guidelines to the Occupational Therapy Code of Ethics (AOTA, 1998) are aspirational documents designed to be used together to guide occupational therapy personnel.

Principle 1. Occupational therapy personnel shall demonstrate a concern for the well-being of the recipients of their services. (beneficence)

A. Occupational therapy personnel shall provide services in a fair and equitable manner. They shall recognize and appreciate the cultural components of economics, geography, race, ethnicity, religious and political factors, marital status, sexual orientation, and disability of all recipients of their services.
B. Occupational therapy practitioners shall strive to ensure that fees are fair and reasonable and commensurate with services performed. When occupational therapy practitioners set fees, they shall set fees considering institutional, local, state, and federal requirements, and with due regard for the service recipient's ability to pay.
C. Occupational therapy personnel shall make every effort to advocate for recipients to obtain needed services through available means.

Principle 2. Occupational therapy personnel shall take reasonable precautions to avoid imposing or inflicting harm upon the recipient of services or to his or her property. (nonmaleficence)

A. Occupational therapy personnel shall maintain relationships that do not exploit the recipient of services sexually, physically, emotionally, financially, socially, or in any other manner.

B. Occupational therapy practitioners shall avoid relationships or activities that interfere with professional judgment and objectivity.

Principle 3. Occupational therapy personnel shall respect the recipient and/or their surrogate(s) as well as the recipient's rights. (autonomy, privacy, confidentiality)

A. Occupational therapy practitioners shall collaborate with service recipients or their surrogate(s) in setting goals and priorities throughout the intervention process.

B. Occupational therapy practitioners shall fully inform the service recipients of the nature, risks, and potential outcomes of any interventions.

C. Occupational therapy practitioners shall obtain informed consent from participants involved in research activities and indicate that they have fully informed and advised the participants of potential risks and outcomes. Occupational therapy practitioners shall endeavor to ensure that the participant(s) comprehend these risks and outcomes.

D. Occupational therapy personnel shall respect the individual's right to refuse professional services or involvement in research or educational activities.

E. Occupational therapy personnel shall protect all privileged confidential forms of written, verbal, and electronic communication gained from educational, practice, research, and investigational activities unless otherwise mandated by local, state, or federal regulations.

Principle 4. Occupational therapy personnel shall achieve and continually maintain high standards of competence. (duties)

A. Occupational therapy practitioners shall hold the appropriate national and state credentials for the services they provide.

B. Occupational therapy practitioners shall use procedures that conform to the standards of practice and other appropriate AOTA documents relevant to practice.

C. Occupational therapy practitioners shall take responsibility for maintaining and documenting competence by participating in professional development and educational activities.

D. Occupational therapy practitioners shall critically examine and keep current with emerging knowledge relevant to their practice so they may perform their duties on the basis of accurate information.

E. Occupational therapy practitioners shall protect service recipients by ensuring that duties assumed by or assigned to other occupational therapy personnel match credentials, qualifications, experience, and scope of practice.

F. Occupational therapy practitioners shall provide appropriate supervision to individuals for whom the practitioners have supervisory responsibility in accordance with Association policies; local, state, and federal laws; and institutional values.

G. Occupational therapy practitioners shall refer to or consult with other service providers whenever such a referral or consultation would be helpful to the care of the recipient of service. The referral or consultation process should be done in collaboration with the recipient of service.

Principle 5. Occupational therapy personnel shall comply with laws and Association policies guiding the profession of occupational therapy. (justice)

A. Occupational therapy personnel shall familiarize themselves with and seek to understand and abide by applicable Association policies; local, state, and federal laws; and institutional rules.

B. Occupational therapy practitioners shall remain abreast of revisions in those laws and Association policies that apply to the profession of occupational therapy and shall inform employers, employees, and colleagues of those changes.

C. Occupational therapy practitioners shall require those they supervise in occupational therapy–related activities to adhere to the Code of Ethics.

D. Occupational therapy practitioners shall take reasonable steps to ensure employers are aware of occupational therapy's ethical obligations, as set forth in this Code of Ethics, and of the implications of those obligations for occupational therapy practice, education, and research.

E. Occupational therapy practitioners shall record and report in an accurate and timely manner all information related to professional activities.

Principle 6. Occupational therapy personnel shall provide accurate information about occupational therapy services. (veracity)

A. Occupational therapy personnel shall accurately represent their credentials, qualifications, education, experience, training, and competence. This is of particular importance for those to whom occupational therapy personnel provide their services or with whom occupational therapy practitioners have a professional relationship.

B. Occupational therapy personnel shall disclose any professional, personal, financial, business, or volunteer affiliations that may pose a conflict of interest to those with whom they may establish a professional, contractual, or other working relationship.

C. Occupational therapy personnel shall refrain from using or participating in the use of any form of communication that contains false, fraudulent, deceptive, or unfair statements or claims.

D. Occupational therapy practitioners shall accept the responsibility for their professional actions which reduce the public's trust in occupational therapy services and those that perform those services.

Principle 7. Occupational therapy personnel shall treat colleagues and other professionals with fairness, discretion, and integrity. (fidelity)

A. Occupational therapy personnel shall preserve, respect, and safeguard confidential information about colleagues and staff, unless otherwise mandated by national, state, or local laws.

B. Occupational therapy practitioners shall accurately represent the qualifications, views, contributions, and findings of colleagues.

C. Occupational therapy personnel shall take adequate measures to discourage, prevent, expose, and correct any breaches of the Code of Ethics and report any breaches of the Code of Ethics to the appropriate authority.

D. Occupational therapy personnel shall familiarize themselves with established policies and procedures for handling concerns about this Code of Ethics, including familiarity with national, state, local, district, and territorial procedures for handling ethics complaints. These include policies and procedures created by the American Occupational Therapy Association, licensing and regulatory bodies, employers, agencies, certification boards, and other organizations who have jurisdiction over occupational therapy practice.

References

American Occupational Therapy Association. (1993). Core values and attitudes of occupational therapy practice. *American Journal of Occupational Therapy, 47*, 1085–1086.

American Occupational Therapy Association. (1998). Guidelines to the occupational therapy code of ethics. *American Journal of Occupational Therapy, 52*, 881–884.

American Occupational Therapy Association. (2000). Occupational therapy code of ethics (2000). *American Journal of Occupational Therapy, 54*, 614–616.

Prepared by Melba Arnold, MS, OTR/L, Nancy Nashiro, PhD, OTR, FAOTA, Diane Hill, COTA/L, AP, Deborah Y. Slater, MS, OTR/L, John Morris, PhD, Linda Withers, CNHA, FACHCA, Penny Kyler, MA, OTR/L, FAOTA, Staff Liaison for The Commission on Standards and Ethics (Barbara L. Kornblau, JD, OTR, FAOTA, Chairperson).

Adopted by the Representative Assembly 2000M15

Note: This document replaces the 1994 document, *Occupational Therapy Code of Ethics* (*American Journal of Occupational Therapy*, 48, 1037–1038).

APPENDIX D

STANDARDS OF PRACTICE FOR OCCUPATIONAL THERAPY

PREFACE

The Standards of Practice for Occupational Therapy are requirements for the occupational therapy practitioner (registered occupational therapist and certified occupational therapy assistant) for the delivery of occupational therapy services that are client centered and interactive in nature (American Occupational Therapy Association [AOTA], 1995). The registered occupational therapist supervises the certified occupational therapy assistant, and both work together in a collaborative manner to meet the needs of the client. However, the registered occupational therapist is ultimately responsible and accountable for the delivery of occupational therapy services. This document identifies minimum standards for occupational therapy practice.

The minimum educational requirements for the registered occupational therapist are described in the current *Essentials and Guidelines of an Accredited Educational Program for the Occupational Therapist* (AOTA, 1991a). The minimum educational requirements for the certified occupational therapy assistant are described in the current *Essentials and Guidelines of an Accredited Educational Program for the Occupational Therapy Assistant* (AOTA, 1991b).

DEFINITIONS

Assessment. Specific tools, instruments, or interactions used during the evaluation process. An assessment is a component part of the evaluation process (Hinojosa & Kramer, 1998).

Client. A person, group, program, organization, or community for whom the occupational therapy practitioner is providing services (AOTA, 1995).

Evaluation. The process of obtaining and interpreting data necessary for understanding the individual, system, or situation. This includes planning for and documenting the evaluation process, results, and recommendations, including the need for intervention and/or potential change in the intervention plan (Hinojosa & Kramer, 1998).

Occupational therapy practitioner. Any individual initially certified to practice as an occupational therapist or occupational therapy assistant or licensed or regulated by a state, district, commonwealth, or territory of the United States to practice as an occupational therapist or occupational therapy assistant (AOTA, 1997).

Performance areas. Broad categories of human activity that are typically part of daily life. They are activities of daily living, work and productive activities, and play or leisure activities (AOTA, 1994c).

Performance components. Elements of performance required for successful engagement in performance areas, including sensorimotor, cognitive, psychosocial, and psychological aspects (AOTA, 1994c).

Performance contexts. Situations or factors that influence an individual's engagement in desired and/or required performance areas. Performance contexts consist of temporal aspects (chronological, developmental, life cycle, disability status) and environmental aspects (physical, social, political, cultural) (AOTA, 1994c).

Screening. Obtaining and reviewing data relevant to a potential client to determine the need for further evaluation and intervention.

Transition. Process involving actions coordinated to prepare for or facilitate change, such as from one functional level to another, from one life stage to another, from one program to another, or from one environment to another.

From *American Journal of Occupational Therapy*, 52, 866–869.

STANDARD I: PROFESSIONAL STANDING AND RESPONSIBILITY

1. An occupational therapy practitioner delivers occupational therapy services that reflect the philosophical base of occupational therapy (AOTA, 1979) and are consistent with the established principles and concepts of theory and practice.
2. An occupational therapy practitioner delivers occupational therapy services in accordance with AOTA's standards and policies. The nature and scope of occupational therapy services provided must be in accordance with laws and regulations.
3. An occupational therapy practitioner maintains current licensure, registration, or certification as required by laws or regulations.
4. An occupational therapy practitioner abides by AOTA's *Occupational Therapy Code of Ethics* (AOTA, 1994a).
5. An occupational therapy practitioner assures continued competency by establishing, maintaining, and updating professional performance, knowledge, and skills.
6. A registered occupational therapist provides supervision for a certified occupational therapy assistant in a collaborative manner as defined by official AOTA documents and in accordance with laws or regulations.
7. A certified occupational therapy assistant seeks and follows supervision from a registered occupational therapist in the delivery of occupational therapy services.
8. An occupational therapy practitioner is knowledgeable about AOTA's *Standards of Practice for Occupational Therapy*; the *Philosophical Base of Occupational Therapy* (AOTA, 1979); and other AOTA, state, and federal documents relevant to practice and service delivery.
9. An occupational therapy practitioner maintains current knowledge of legislative, political, social, cultural, and reimbursement issues that affect clients and the practice of occupational therapy.
10. A registered occupational therapist is knowledgeable about research in the practitioner's areas of practice. A registered occupational therapist applies timely research findings ethically and appropriately to evaluation and intervention processes and discusses applicable research findings with the certified occupational therapy assistant.
11. A registered occupational therapist systematically assesses the efficiency and effectiveness of occupational therapy services and designs and implements processes to support quality service delivery.
12. A certified occupational therapy assistant collaborates with the registered occupational therapist in assessing the efficiency and effectiveness of occupational therapy services and assists in designing and implementing processes to support quality service delivery.

STANDARD II: REFERRAL

1. A registered occupational therapist accepts and responds to referrals in accordance with AOTA's *Statement of Occupational Therapy Referral* (AOTA, 1994b) and in compliance with laws or regulations.
2. A registered occupational therapist accepts and responds to referrals for evaluation or evaluation with intervention in performance areas, performance components, or performance contexts when clients may have a functional limitation or disability or may be at risk for a disabling condition.
3. A registered occupational therapist refers clients to appropriate resources when the needs of the client can best be served by the expertise of other professionals or services.
4. An occupational therapy practitioner educates current and potential referral sources about the scope of occupational therapy services and the process of initiating occupational therapy services.

STANDARD III: SCREENING

1. A registered occupational therapist screens independently or as a member of a team in accordance with laws and regulations. A certified occupational therapy assistant may contribute to the screening process under the supervision of a registered occupational therapist.
2. A registered occupational therapist selects screening methods appropriate to the client's performance context.
3. A registered occupational therapist communicates screening results and recommendations to the appropriate person, group, or organization. A certified occupational therapy assistant may contribute to this process under the supervision of a registered occupational therapist.

STANDARD IV: EVALUATION

1. A registered occupational therapist evaluates performance areas, performance components, and performance contexts. A certified occupational therapy assistant may contribute to the evalution process under the supervision of a registered occupational therapist.
2. An occupational therapy practitioner educates clients and appropriate others about the purposes and procedures of the occupational therapy evaluation.
3. A registered occupational therapist selects assessments to evaluate the client's level of function related to performance areas, performance components, and performance contexts.

4. An occupational therapy practitioner follows defined protocols when standardized assessments are used.
5. A registered occupational therapist analyzes, interprets, and summarizes assessment data to determine the client's current functional status and to develop an appropriate intervention plan. The certified occupational therapy assistant may contribute to this process under the supervision of a registered occupational therapist.
6. A registered occupational therapist completes and documents occupational therapy evaluation results within the time frames, formats, and standards established by practice settings, government agencies, external accreditation programs, and payers. A certified occupational therapy assistant may contribute to documentation of evaluation results under the supervision of a registered occupational therapist and in accordance with laws or regulations.
7. A registered occupational therpist communicates evaluation results, within the boundaries of client confidentiality, to the appropriate person, group, or organization. A certified occupational therapy assistant may contribute to this process under the supervision of a registered occupational therapist.
8. A registered occupational therapist recommends additional consultations when the results of the evaluation indicate that intervention by other professionals would be beneficial.

STANDARD V: INTERVENTION PLAN

1. A registered occupational therapist develops and documents an intervention plan that is based on the results of the occupational therapy evaluation and the desires and expectations of the client and appropriate others about the outcome of service. A certified occupational therapy assistant may contribute to the intervention plan under the supervision of a registered occupational therapist.
2. A registered occupational therapist ensures that the intervention plan is documented within time frames, formats, and standards established by the practice settings, agencies, external accreditation programs, and payers.
3. A registered occupational therapist includes in the intervention plan client-centered goals that are clear, measurable, behavioral, functional, contextually relevant, and appropriate to the client's needs, desires, and expected outcomes. A certified occupational therapy assistant may contribute to this process.
4. A registered occupational therapist includes in the intervention plan the scope, frequency, duration of services, and the needs of the client.
5. A registered occupational therapist reviews the intervention plan with the client and appropriate others. A certified occupational therapy assistant may contribute to this process.

STANDARD VI: INTERVENTION

1. A registered occupational therapist implements the intervention plan through the use of specified purposeful activities or therapeutic methods that are meaningful to the client and are effective methods for enhancing occupational performance. A certified occupational therapy assistant may implement the intervention plan under the supervision of a registered occupational therapist.
2. An occupational therapy practitioner informs clients and appropriate others regarding the relative benefits and risks of the intervention.
3. An occupational therapy practitioner maintains or seeks current information on resources relevant to the client's needs.
4. A registered occupational therapist reevaluates during the intervention process and documents changes in the client's goals, performance, and needs. A certified occupational therapy assistant may contribute to the reevaluation process.
5. A registered occupational therapist modifies the intervention process to reflect changes in client status, desires, and response to intervention. A certified occupational therapy assistant may identify the need for modifications and may contribute to the intervention modifications under the supervision of a registered occupational therapist.
6. An occupational therapy practitioner documents the occupational therapy services provided within the time frames, formats, and standards established by the practice settings, agencies, external accreditation programs, and payers.

STANDARD VII: TRANSITION SERVICES

1. A registered occupational therapist prepares a formal transition plan that is based on identified needs. A certified occupational therapy assistant may contribute to the preparation of a formal transition plan.
2. An occupational therapy practitioner facilitates the transition process in cooperation with the client, family members, significant others, team, and community resources and individuals, when appropriate.

STANDARD VIII: DISCONTINUATION

1. A registered occupational therapist discontinues services when the client has achieved predetermined goals, has achieved maximum benefit from occupational therapy services, or does not desire to continue services. A certified occupational therapy assistant may recommend

discontinuation of occupational therapy services to the supervising registered occupational therapist.

2. A registered occupational therapist prepares and implements a discontinuation plan that addresses appropriate follow-up resources. A certified occupational therapy assistant may contribute to the implementation of a discontinuation plan under the supervision of a registered occupational therapist.
3. A registered occupational therapist documents changes in the client's status between the initial evaluation and discontinuation of services. A certified occupational therapy assistant may contribute to the process under the supervision of a registered occupational therapist.
4. A registered occupational therapist documents recommendations for follow-up or reevaluation, when applicable.

References

American Occupational Therapy Association. (1979). The philosophical base of occupational therapy. *American Journal of Occupational Therapy, 33*, 785.

American Occupational Therapy Association. (1991a). Essentials and guidelines of an accredited educational program for the occupational therapist. *American Journal of Occupational Therapy, 45*, 1077–1084.

American Occupational Therapy Association. (1991b). Essentials and guidelines of an accredited educational program for the occupational therapy assistant. *American Journal of Occupational Therapy, 45*, 1085–1092.

American Occupational Therapy Association. (1994a). Occupational therapy code of ethics. *American Journal of Occupational Therapy, 48*, 1037–1038.

American Occupational Therapy Association. (1994b). Statement of occupational therapy referral. *American Journal of Occupational Therapy, 48*, 1034.

American Occupational Therapy Association. (1994c). Uniform terminology for occupational therapy—Third edition. *American Journal of Occupational Therapy, 49*, 1047–1054.

American Occupational Therapy Association. (1995). Concept paper: Service delivery in occupational therapy. *American Journal of Occupational Therapy, 49*, 1029–1031.

American Occupational Therapy Association. (1997). *Bylaws. Article III, Section I*. Bethesda, MD: Author.

Hinojosa, J., & Kramer, P. (Eds.). (1998). *Occupational therapy evaluation of clients: Obtaining and interpreting data*. Bethesda, MD: American Occupational Therapy Association.

Prepared by the Commission on Practice (Linda Kohlman Thomson, MOT, OT(C), FAOTA, Chairperson).

Adopted by the Representative Assembly 1998M15.

Note. This document replaces the 1994 *Standards of Practice for Occupational Therapy*. These standards are intended as recommended guidelines to assist occupational therapy practitioners in the provision of occupational therapy services. These standards serve as a minimum standard for occupational therapy practice and are applicable to all individual populations and the programs in which these individuals are served.

APPENDIX E

DELINEATION OF THE AOTA STANDARDS OF PRACTICE FOR OCCUPATIONAL THERAPY

STANDARDS OF PRACTICE FOR OCCUPATIONAL THERAPY

The following table delineates the *Standards of Practice for Occupational Therapy* (AOTA, 1998) as well as the different roles of the occupational therapist and the occupational therapy assistant in ensuring delivery of services according to the standards.

STANDARDS FOR OCCUPATIONAL THERAPY

Occupational Therapy Process	Occupational Therapy	Occupational Therapy Assistant
Referral		
1. Accepts and responds to referral in compliance with laws or regulations.	X	
2. Refers clients to appropriate resources.	X	
3. Educates current and potential referral sources about the scope of services and the process of initiating services.	X	X
Screening		
1. Screens independently or as a member of a team in accordance with laws and regulations.	X	Contributes/needs supervision
2. Selects screening methods appropriate to the client's performance context.	X	
3. Communicates screening results and recommendations to the appropriate person, group, or organization.	X	Contributes/needs supervision

Continues

STANDARDS FOR OCCUPATIONAL THERAPY *(Continued)*

Occupational Therapy Process	Occupational Therapy	Occupational Therapy Assistant
Evaluation		
1. Evaluates performance area, performance components, and performance contexts.	X	Contributes/needs supervision
2. Educates clients and others about the purposes and procedures of the evaluation.	X	X
3. Selects assessments to evaluate the client's level of function related to performance areas, components, and contexts.	X	
4. Follows defined protocols when standardized assessments are used.	X	X
5. Analyzes, interprets, and summarizes assessment data to determine the client's current functional status and to develop an appropriate intervention plan.	X	Contributes/needs supervision
6. Completes and documents occupational therapy evaluation results within the time frames, formats, and standards established by practice settings, government agencies, external accreditation programs, and payers.	X	Contributes/needs supervision
7. Communicates evaluation results, within the boundaries of client confidentiality, to the appropriate person, group, or organization.	X	Contributes/needs supervision
8. Recommends additional consultations when the results of the evaluation indicate that intervention by other professionals would be beneficial.	X	
Intervention Plan		
1. Develops and documents an intervention plan that is based on the results of the occupational therapy evaluation and the desires and expectations of the client and appropriate others about the outcome of service.	X	Contributes/needs supervision
2. Prepares and documents the intervention plan within time frames, formats, and standards established by the practice settings, agencies, external accreditation programs, and payers.	X	
3. Includes in the intervention plan client-centered goals that are clear, measurable, behavioral, functional, contextually relevant, and appropriate to the client's needs, desires, and expected outcomes.	X	Contributes to process
4. Includes in the intervention plan the scope, frequency, duration of services, and the needs of the client.	X	
5. Reviews the intervention plan with the client and appropriate others.	X	Contributes to process
Intervention		
1. Implements the intervention plan through the use of specified purposeful activities or therapeutic methods that are meaningful to the client and are effective methods for enhancing occupational performance.	X	Needs supervision
2. Informs clients and appropriate others regarding the relative benefits and risks of the intervention.	X	X
3. Maintains or seeks current information on resources relevant to the client's needs.	X	X
4. Reevaluates during the intervention process and documents changes in the client's goals, performance, and needs.	X	Contributes/needs supervision
5. Modifies the intervention process to reflect changes in client status, desires, and response to intervention.	X	Identifies the need for modifications Contributes/needs supervision
6. Documents the occupational therapy services provided within the time frames, formats, and standards established by the practice settings, agencies, external accreditation programs, and payers.	X	X
Transition Services		
1. Prepares a formal transition plan that is based on identified needs.	X	Contributes to process
2. Facilitates the transition process in cooperation with the client, family members, significant others, team, and community resources and individuals, when appropriate.	X	X

STANDARDS FOR OCCUPATIONAL THERAPY *(Continued)*

Occupational Therapy Process	Occupational Therapy	Occupational Therapy Assistant
Discontinuation		
1. Discontinues services when the client has achieved predetermined goals, has achieved maximum benefit from occupational therapy services, or does not desire to continue services.	X	May recommend to occupational therapy
2. Prepares and implements a discontinuation plan that addresses appropriate follow-up resources.	X	Contributes/needs supervision
3. Documents changes in the client's status between the initial evaluation and discontinuation of services.	X	Contributes/needs supervision
4. Documents recommendations for follow-up or reevaluation, when applicable.	X	

APPENDIX F

ADDITIONAL RESOURCES

SECTION I
AGING RESEARCH AND INFORMATION WEB SITES (SELECTED)

ELIZABETH CREPEAU

Administration on Aging
www.aoa.dhhs.gov/

Alliance for Aging Research
www.agingresearch.org

American Association of Retired Persons
www.aarp.org

American Geriatric Society
www.americangeriatrics.org

Boston University Roybal Center for the Enhancement of Late-Life Function
www.bu.edu/roybal

Gerontological Society of America
www.geron.org

Guide for Caregivers
www.aoa.dhhs.gov/wecare/default.htm

International Commission on Aging and Aging Research
Dshenk@email.uncc.edu

International Network for the Prevention of Elder Abuse
Wolf4@usmhc.edu

Long Term Care Ombudsman Program
www.aoa.dhhs/ltcombudsman/default/htm

National Academy on an Aging Society
www.agingsociety.org

National Aging Information Center
www.aoa.dhhs.gov/naic/default.htm

National Council on the Aging
www.ncoa.org

National Institute on Aging
www.nih.gov/nia

Retirement Research Fund
www.rrf.org

Senior Net
www.seniornet.com

SECTION II
AIDS WEB SITES (SELECTED)

JAMES HINOJOSA, GARY BEDELL, and MARGARET KAPLAN

Centers for Disease Control and Prevention (CDC)
www.cdc.gov

Guidelines for the Use of Antiretroviral Medications
www.hivatis.org/guidelines/pediatric.

National Pediatric AIDS Network
www.npan.org

CDC National Prevention Information Network (CDC NPIN)
www.cdcnpin.org

SECTION III
ASSISTIVE TECHNOLOGY, SEATING, AND MOBILITY WEB SITES (SELECTED)[a]

TAMARA MILLS, ELIZABETH SKIDMORE, MARY ELLEN BUNING, and MARK R. SCHMELER

AbleNet
www.ablenetinc.com/

ABLEDATA on the Internet
trace.wisc.edu/tcel/abledata/index.html

AccessAbility, Inc.
4access.com

Adaptive Technology Resource Centre
www.utoronto.ca/atrc/

Adaptive Technology Links (OTPT Pages—University of Puget Sound)
otpt.ups.edu/Rehabilitation/AdapTec/html

Americans with Disabilities Act Document Center
janweb.icdi.wvu.edu/kinder

Apple Computer's Disability Connection
www.apple.com/disability

Archives of the Office of Technology Assessment (The Office of Technology Assessment closed in 1995; its archives are housed at Idaho State University)
www.ota.nap.edu

Assistive Technology, Inc.
www.assistivetech.com/

Assistive Technology On-Line
www.education-world.com

Assistive Technology Web Pages from RESNA
resna.org/taproject/at/connections.html

AZtech (A to Z Technology)
cosmos.buffalo.edu/WEB/aztech

Breaking New Ground (Adaptive Technologies for Farmers with Disabilities)
abe.www.ecn.purdue.edu/ABE/Extension/BNG/Index.html

The Canadian Seating and Mobility Conference
www.csmc.ca/

[a]An up-to-date version of this listing is available at otpt.ups.edu/Rehabilitation/Resources.html

Canine Companions (Offers trained dogs for persons with a variety of disabilities)
caninecompanions.org

Canterbury Community Internet Access Project (CCIA)
www.wbview.co.nz/ccia

Center for Universal Design
www.design.ncsu.edu:8120/cud/

Closing the Gap (Microcomputer technology for people with special needs)
www.closingthegap.com

Cornucopia of Disability Information (CODI)
http://codi.buffalo.edu

disABILITY Information & Resources (Adaptive computer products)
www.makoa.org/computers.htm

Disability and Medical Resource Mall
www.medmarket.com/index.cfm?id=disability

DO-IT (Disabilities, Opportunities, Internetworking, and Technology; program for people with disabilities to explore careers in science, engineering, and mathematics)
www.washington.edu/doit

Ease (A comprehensive software package for guiding home assessments that includes local and national database resources for prescribing environmental adaptations, individualized for each client)
lifease.com/ease300.html

Easi Project (Equal Access to Software & Information)
www.isc.rit.edu/~easi

Electronic Rehabilitation Resources (St. John's University)
www.rit.edu/~easi/itd/itdv01n1/holtzman.html

A Guide to Wheelchair Selection: How to Use the ANSI/RESNA Standards to Buy a Wheelchair (by Axelson, Minkel, and Chesney; available from the Paralyzed Veterans of America)
www.wheelchairnet.org/WCN_ProdServ/Docs/WCN_PVAguide.html

Independence Dogs, Inc. (Service dogs for the mobility-impaired)
www.independencedogs.org

Institute on Independent Living
www.independentliving.org/

International Seating Symposium
www.iss.pitt.edu/

Jim Lubin's Disability Resource List (A comprehensive compendium of disability-related links)
www.eskimo.com/~jlubin/disabled.html

Learning Independence through Computers (A resource of accessibility tools and strategies including lists of vendors throughout the United States)
www.linc.org

Manual Wheelchair Training Guide (by Axelson, Chesney, Minkel, and Perr; available at PAX Press)
www.beneficialdesigns.com/

National Center for the Dissemination of Disability Research
www.ncddr.org

National Center to Improve Practice through Technology, Media, and Materials
www2.edc.org/NCIP/

National Registry of Rehabilitation Technology Suppliers
www.nrrts.org

OT FACT (Uses dynamic questions sets, generated from a computer software program, to compile and organize large quantities of patient evaluation data so that they can be meaningfully interpreted)
www.execpc.com/~dgtldesn/otfact.htm

Quartet Technology Inc.
www.qtiusa.com/

RESNA (Rehabilitation Engineering and Assistive Technology Society of North America; an interdisciplinary association for the advancement of rehabilitation and assistive technologies)
www.resna.org/reshome.htm

RESNA Annual Conference (Offers workshops and instructional courses)
www.resna.org/

RESNA credentialing
www.resna.org/

Searchwave (A search engine for audiology and hearing-related information and resources)
www.searchwave.com

Self-Help for Hard of Hearing People, Inc. (Provides resources for persons with hearing impairment, their families, and health professionals)
www.shhh.org

TechnAbility Exchange
www.geocities.com/technability

Trace Research and Development Center (University of Wisconsin at Madison)
www.trace.wisc.edu

U.S. Architectural and Transportation Barriers Compliance Board (A federal agency committed to accessible design)
www.access-board.gov/

Yahoo online index of disability Web sites
www.yahoo.com/yahoo/Society_and_Culture/Disabilities

WheelchairNet (Information site on wheeled mobility)
www.wheelchairnet.org

Wheeled Mobility Books (Reviews of five books on wheeled mobility)
www.wheelchairnet.org/WCN_ProdServ/Docs/WCN_bookreview.html

SECTION IV
CHILDHOOD, CHILD DEVELOPMENT, AND DEVELOPMENTAL DISABILITY WEB SITES (SELECTED)

ELLEN S. COHN

American Academy of Cerebral Palsy and Developmental Medicine
www.aacpdm.org

Autism Society
www.autism-society.org

Can Child Centre for Childhood Disability Research
www.fhs.mcmaster.ca/canchild/

Family Violence Prevention Fund
www.endabuse.org

Federation for Children with Special Needs
fcsn.org

Institute for Child Health Policy
www.ichp.edu

Make a Wish Foundation
www.wish.org

Maternal and Child Health Bureau
www.mchb.hrsa.gov

Muscular Dystrophy Foundation
mdausa.org

National Institute of Child Health and Human Development
www.nichd.nih.gov

National Maternal and Child Health Clearinghouse
www.nmchc.org

National Special Needs Network Foundation, Inc.
www.nsnn.org

Office of Special Education and Rehabilitative Services (Has multiple links)
www.ed.gov/offices/OSERS/OSEP/index.html

Society for Research in Child Development
www.srcd.org

United Cerebral Palsy Association
www.ucp.org

ZERO to THREE
www.zerotothree.org

SECTION V

DISABILITY RIGHTS WEB SITES (SELECTED)

TAMARA MILLS and ELIZABETH SKIDMORE

Americans with Disabilities Act Document Center
janweb.icdi.wvu.edu/kinder/#home

Disability Legislation
www.legal.gsa.gov/legal6a.htm

Disability Rights Education & Defense Fund, Inc.
www.dredf.org/

Council for Disability Rights
www.disabilityrights.org/

Disability Rights Commission
www.drc-gb.org/drc/default.asp

Mental Disability Rights International
www.mdri.org/

Protection & Advocacy Systems: The Nation's Disability Rights Network
www.protectionandadvocacy.com/

U.S. Department of Justice, Americans with Disabilities Act Internet Home Page
www.usdoj.gov/crt/ada/adahom1.htm

U.S. Department of Justice Internet Home Page
www.usdoj.gov

U.S. Government Guide to Disability Rights Laws
www.usdoj.gov/crt/ada/cguide.htm

SECTION VI

ENVIRONMENTAL AND ASSISTIVE TECHNOLOGY SERVICE PROVIDERS AND SUPPLIERS TOLL FREE NUMBERS (SELECTED)

ELIZABETH SKIDMORE and TAMARA MILLS

Phone Number	Service Provider/Supplier
800-458-5231	Ablenet (Minneapolis, MN)
800-748-3695	Adaptive Automotive (Denver, CO)
800-225-2610	AliMed (Dedham, MA)
800-325-6233	Alternative Unlimited Inc. (Whitinsville, MA)
800-961-3273	EASE2000 Environmental Assessment and Prescription Software (New Brighton, MN)
800-323-6598	E-Z-On Product Inc. (Jupiter, FL)
800-548-7905	Electric Mobility (Sewell, NJ)
800-841-8923	Environmental Health Science Inc. (Princeton, NJ)
800-952-2248	Ford Mobility Motoring Program (Ruston, LA)
800-833-0312	TDD
800-548-4337	Guide Dog Foundation for the Blind (Smithtown, NY)
800-536-9383	Handicapped-Getaway Cruises (Saddle River, NJ)
800-622-0623	Independent Mobility Systems (Farmington, NM)
800-829-0500	Lighthouse Low Vision Products (Long Island City, NY)
800-443-4926	Maddak Inc. (Wayne NJ)
800-421-1221	National Accessible Apartment Clearinghouse (Washington, DC)
800-253-4391	Office Systems for Visually/Physically Impaired (Chicago, IL)
800-262-1984	Prentke Romich (Wooster, OH)
800-949-4232	Regional Disability and Business Technical Assistance Centers (National)
800-548-8531	Right Start Catalog (Westlake Village, CA)
800-323-5547	Sammons-Preston (Burr Ridge, IL)
800-422-7382	Wheelchair Getaway and See Go Van (Las Vegas, NV)
800-452-2085	Special Mobility Services (Portland, OR)
800-832-8697	Toys for Special Children (Hastings on Hudson, NY)
800-221-6501	Wheelchair Getaways (Lancaster, PA)

SECTION VII

EVIDENCE-BASED PRACTICE WEB SITES (SELECTED)

WENDY COSTER, SHARON CERMAK, and ELSIE VERGARA

Agency for Health Care Research and Quality
www.ahcpr.gov

American Academy for Cerebral Palsy and Developmental Medicine
www.aacpdm.org

American Academy of Pediatrics
www.aap.org

Centre for Evidence Based Mental Health
www.cebmh.com

Cochrane Library
www.cochrane.org/cochrane/edsr.htm

Dr. Fenichel's Current Topics in Psychology
www.fenichel.com

Health Web
www.healthweb.org

International Journal of Psychosocial Rehabilitation
www.psychosocial.com

McMaster OT Evidence-Based Practice Research Group
www.fhs.mcmaster.ca/rahab/ebp

National Information Center for Children and Youth with Disabilities
www.nichcy.org

Netting the Evidence
www.nettingtheevidence.org.uk

New Zealand Guideline Group: Evidence-Based Practice in Disability Support Services
www.nzgg.org.nz/disability.cfm

OT Direct
www.otdirect.co.uk

Research and Training Center on Family Support and Children's Mental Health
www.rtc.pdx.edu/

University of Michigan Health System: Evidence-Based Practice Website
www.med.umich.edu/pediatrics/ebm/index.html/

SECTION VIII

FOUNDATIONS, ASSOCIATIONS, COUNCILS, AND GOVERNMENT RESOURCE PHONE NUMBERS (SELECTED)

ELIZABETH SKIDMORE and TAMARA MILLS

Phone Number	Organization
800-555-1212	Toll-Free Directory (for updates or numbers not listed)
800-344-2666	Al-Anon Family Group Headquarters, Inc.
800-621-0379	Alzheimer's Disease Association
800-749-2257	American Association of Kidney Patients
800-424-3410	American Association of Retired Persons
800-548-2876	American Burn Association
800-424-8666	American Council of the Blind
800-527-5344	American Council on Alcoholism
800-232-3472	American Diabetes Association, Inc.
800-729-2682	American Occupational Therapy Association
800-223-2732	American Parkinson Disease Association
800-556-7890	American Trauma Society
800-782-4747	Amyotrophic Lateral Sclerosis Association
800-283-7800	Arthritis Foundation
800-727-8462	Asthma and Allergy Foundation of America
800-3au- tism	Autism Society of America
800-669-7079	Blinded Veterans Association
800-444-6443	Brain Injury Association
800-955-0906	OVID Information Technologies
800-237-6213	Captioned Films/Video for the Deaf Program
800-342-2437	Center for Disease Control and Prevention (CDC) National AIDS Hotline
800-726-9119	Center for Rehabilitation Technology
800-424-2246	Child Care Aware Hotline
800-242-4453	Children's Hospice International
800-753-2357	Cornelia deLange Syndrome Foundation
800-344-4823	Cystic Fibrosis Foundation
800-535-3323	Deafness Research Foundation
800-222-3277	Dial A Hearing Screening Test
800-572-7233	Domestic Violence Hotline
800-332-1000	Epilepsy Foundation of America
800-331-0688	Federation for Children with Special Needs
800-905-TIES	Family Together in Enhancing Support
415-252-8900	Family Violence Prevention Fund
800-548-4337	Guide Dog Foundation for the Blind, Inc.
800-676-1730	Higher Education Center for Alcohol and Other Drug Prevention
800-245-2691	HUD User
800-526-7234	Job Accommodation Network

(Continued)

Phone Number	Organization
800-558-0121	Lupus Foundation of America, Inc.
800-722-wish	Make a Wish Foundation
800-438-6233	Mothers Against Drunk Driving
800-572-1717	Muscular Dystrophy Foundation
800-541-5454	Myasthenia Gravis Foundation
800-342-2437	National AIDS Hotline
800-344-7432	National AIDS Hotline (Spanish)
800-458-5231	National AIDS Information Clearinghouse
800-424-8666	National Alliance for Blind Students
800-950-6264	National Alliance for the Mentally Ill
800-331-5362	National Association for the Dually Diagnosed
800-862-1799	National Association for Rights, Protection, and Advocacy
800-829-8289	National Alliance for Research on Schizophrenia and Depression
800-422-4453	National Child Abuse Hotline
800-729-6686	National Clearinghouse for Alcohol and Drug Information
800-622-2255	National Council on Alcoholism and Drug Dependence, Inc.
800-826-3632	National Depressive and Manic-Depressive Association
800-221-4602	National Down Syndrome Society
800-662-4357	National Drug Treatment Referral & Information Hotline
800-221-6827	National Easter Seal Society
800-POWER-2-U	National Empowerment Center
800-222-3937	National Foundation of the American Academy of Ophthalmology Public Service Programs
800-239-1265	National Foundation for Depressive Illness, Inc.
800-843-2256	National Headache Foundation
800-658-8898	National Hospice Organization
800-695-0285	National Information Center for Children and Youth with Disabilities
800-638-2045	National Institute on Drug Abuse
800-421-4211	National Institute of Mental Health
800-541-3259	National Lymphedema Network
800-969-6642	National Mental Health Association
800-553-4539	National Mental Health Consumers' Self-Help Clearinghouse
800-268-7582	National Multiple Sclerosis Society
800-323-7938	National Neurofibromatosis Foundation
800-999-6673	National Organization for Rare Disorders
800-646-1001	National Pediatric AIDS Network
800-346-2742	National Rehabilitation Information Center
800-331-2020	National Society to Prevent Blindness

(Continued)

Phone Number	Organization
800-962-9629	National Spinal Cord Injury Association
800-787-6537	National Stroke Association
800-369-7433	North American Riding for the Handicapped Association
800-422-6237	Office of Cancer Communications
800-869-6782	Parent Educational Advocacy Training Center
800-624-0100	Partnership for a Drug Free America
800-457-6676	Parkinson's Disease Foundation, Inc.
800-888-2876	Phoenix Society for Burn Survivors, Inc.
800-221-4792	Recording for the Blind and Dyslexic
800-421-8453	Sickle Cell Disease Association of America
800-772-1213	Social Security Administration
800-325-0778	TDD
800-872-5827	United Cerebral Palsy Association, Inc.
800-728-5483	United Leukodystrophy Foundation
800-426-2547	Visiting Nurse Association of America
800-899-4301	ZERO to THREE/National Center for Clinical Infant Programs

SECTION IX
MENTAL HEALTH WEB SITES (SELECTED)

ELLEN S. COHN and ALEXIS HENRY

Alcoholics Anonymous World Services
www.alcoholics-anonymous.org

American Academy of Child and Adolescent Psychiatry
www.aacap.org

American Psychiatric Association
www.psych.org

Americans with Disabilities Act
www.usdoj.gov/crt/ada/publicat.htm

Bazelon Center for Mental Health Law
www.Bazelon.org/ada.html
http://www.Bazelon.org/

Boston University Center for Psychiatric Rehabilitation
www.bu.edu/sarpsych/

Center for Mental Health Services
www.samhsa.gov/centers/cmhs/cmhs.html

Cocaine Anonymous
www.ca.org

Consumer Organization & Networking Technical Assistance Center
www.contac.org

Critical Psychology WebRing
webring.org/cgi?_bin/webring?ring=critpsy;list

Disability Rights Activist
www.disrights.org/

Electro Convulsive Therapy
www.ect.org/and http://www.banshock.org/

Hooper's Forensics Psychiatry
bama.ua.edu/~jhooper/

International Center for the Study of Psychiatry and Psychology
www.breggin.com

Job Accommodation Network
janweb.icdi.wvu.edu/

Madness
www.peoplewho.org

MadNation
www.madnation.org/

Mental and Physical Disability Law Reporter
www.abanet.org/disability/reporter/home.html

National Alliance for the Mentally Ill
www.nami.org

National Alliance for Research on Schizophrenia and Depression
narsad.org

National Depressive and Manic-Depressive Association
www.ndmda.org

National Empowerment Center
www.power2u.org National Empowerment Center

National Foundation for Depressive Illness, Inc.
www.depression.org

National Association for Rights, Protection & Advocacy
www.connix.com/~narpa

National Council on Disability—"From privileges to rights"
www.ncd.gov/newsroom/publications/privileges.html

National Consumer Supporter Technical Assistance Center
www.ncstac.org

National Institute on Drug Abuse
www.nida.nih.org

National Mental Health Association
www.nmha.org

National Mental Health Consumers' Self-Help Clearinghouse
www.mhselfhelp.org/

No Stigma
www.nostigma.org

Protection & Advocacy Agencies
www.protectionandadvocacy.com/

SAMHSA/Knowledge Exchange Network
www.mentalhealth.org/

Self-Help Sourcebook Online
www.cmhc.com/selfhelp/

Support Coalition International
www.mindfreedom.org

SECTION X
NATIONAL CIVIC ORGANIZATION PHONE NUMBERS (SELECTED)

ELIZABETH SKIDMORE and TAMARA MILLS

Phone Number	Organization
773-755-4700	Elks Organization (drug education)
317-875-8755	Kiwanis International (focus on children)
630-571-5466	Lions International (focus on sight)
215-988-1917	Masons/Shriners Lodge (may fund assistive devices, information about burn prevention and intervention)
630-859-2000	Moose International (focus on children and elderly in need)
816-333-8300	Sertoma International (focus on speech/hearing impairments)
816-756-3390	Veterans of Foreign Wars (focus on veterans)

GLOSSARY

PAT SUE SPEAR and ELIZABETH BLESEDELL CREPEAU

The following definitions are drawn from the chapters in this book and are intended as a resource for understanding. Readers are referred to the chapters in the book for reference citations relevant to these concepts and definitions, and they should cite appropriate chapter authors or original citations when referring to these constructs.

Aberrant Task Behavior Behaviors that are abnormal within the context of a task

Abstract Learning Acquisition and storage of knowledge, rules, and facts abstracted from events independently from the spatial and temporal context in which they occur

Academic Discipline A branch of knowledge, learning, and scholarly inquiry that is legitimized by university communities and that often supports the work of professions

Accreditation Council of Occupational Therapy Education of the American Occupational Therapy Association (ACOTE) Maintains standards and accredits occupational therapy education programs primarily in the United States

Active Range of Motion (AROM) The arc of motion through which the joint passes when moved by muscles acting on the joint

Activities of Daily Living (ADL) Activities involving taking care of oneself; personal and basic ADL (PADL) and (BADL) involve care of one's body, and instrumental ADL (IADL) are more oriented to self-maintenance, requiring interactions in the home and in the community

Activity Choices The activities in which clients engage during play and leisure

Activity Interests Affective responses to activities and perceptions and awareness of self and environments in relation to activities

Acute Pain Discomfort associated with tissue damage, irritation, inflammation, or a disease process that is relatively brief (hours, days, weeks), regardless of intensity

Acute Very severe or sharp, as in pain, disease, or symptoms with rapid, severe onset

Adaptation Changing in response to new expectation or demands; making tasks simpler or less demanding to promote greater success

Adaptive Response A successful response to challenge

Adaptive Seating System External stabilizer that allows people with poor trunk muscle control to sit in a chair or wheelchair

Adaptive Shortening The process whereby tissue that has been traumatized and inflamed undergoes remodeling in a shortened position because it has been immobilized in a slack position and deprived of normal stress of motion

Adequacy The efficiency of the action or process used to execute activities as well as the acceptability of the outcome or product of that action

Adjunctive Methods Intervention modalities and techniques applied to a client who is a passive recipient; usually designed to promote healing or reduce pain associated with activity

Adult Day Care Programs that provide meaningful, structured activities for people with physical and/or cognitive disabilities, provide respite for primary caregivers

Affect The emotional tone of an individual demonstrated by facial expression and voice inflection

Affective Responses Reflect the underlying affect or feeling tone that a person is communicating, serve the purpose of communicating that a person is trying to understand and is concerned about how another person feels

Agency A quality of occupational behavior that consists of being able to affect other beings or material things

Agentic Self-directed actions aimed at personal development or personally chosen goals

Agnosia Inability to recognize familiar objects in spite of intact sensory capacities

Alcoholism Chronic illness characterized by extreme dependence on alcohol and corresponding disturbances in the individual's family, social, and work life

Alter Interventions that emphasize selecting a context or task that enables the person to perform with current skills and abilities

American Occupational Therapy Association (AOTA) National professional association for occupational therapy with voluntary membership that represents and promotes member interests

American Occupational Therapy Foundation (AOTF) Nonprofit organization dedicated to expanding and refining the knowledge base of occupational therapy; provides support to research and education through grants and scholarships

Americans With Disabilities Act (ADA) Legislation that provides civil rights to all individuals with disabilities; guarantees equal access to and opportunity in employment, public accommodations, state and local government, transportation, and telecommunications

Amyotrophic Lateral Sclerosis (ALS) Progressive neurological disease in which motor neurons of the spinal cord and motor nuclei of the brain deteriorate, resulting in loss of motor control; also referred to as Lou Gehrig's disease and motor neuron disease

Anthropometrics Describes the physical dimensions and properties of the body in terms of functional arm, leg, and body movements made by a worker performing a task

Arts and Crafts Movement Social reform movement of the late nineteenth and early twentieth centuries that promoted the use of fine arts and crafts to counter the alienation of industrialism

Asperger Syndrome Pervasive developmental disorder characterized by severe and sustained impairments in social interaction and development of restricted, repetitive patterns of behaviors and interests; it is contrasted with autism by no significant delays in language

Assessment Specific tools or instruments or standardized processes used in the evaluation process

Assistive Technology Device (ATD) Items, equipment, or systems used to maintain or improve functional capacities of individuals with disabilities

Association Learning Mental linking between two events or activities so that the occurrence of one triggers initiation of the other; is mediated by subcortical or, in some cases, cerebellar structures in the brain

Asthma Condition describing difficulty breathing; characterized by sporadic narrowing of the airways

Attending Nonverbal and verbal behaviors that help communicate interest and can facilitate the development of therapeutic rapport

Attention Deficit Hyperactivity Disorder (ADHD) Neurobehavioral disorder with three hallmark features: inattention, impulsivity, and hyperactivity; alternatively defined as primarily a deficit in behavioral inhibition, linked to problems with working memory, self-regulation, internalization of speech, and reconstitution of verbal and nonverbal behaviors

Attention The cognitive ability to focus on a task, issue, or object

Autism A pervasive developmental disorder characterized by deficits in social interaction and communication, people with autism demonstrate restrictive and repetitive behavior

Autogenic Training Systematic program of verbal commands to relax body and mind

Automatic Thoughts Internal speech that involves errors in thinking and distortions

Autonomic Dysreflexia Sympathetic reflex response to adverse stimuli (e.g., distended bladder, pressure sore) that occurs in people with spinal cord injuries; can be fatal if not managed immediately

Ayres, Jean (1920–1988) Occupational therapist who developed the theory of sensory integration and standardized tests (SIPT) to evaluate sensory integration dysfunction

Bilateral Integration and Sequencing Dysfunction Problems in central vestibular processing; deficits in coordinating the two sides of the body, poor equilibrium reactions, low muscle tone, problems in communication, poor right–left discrimination

Biomechanical Having to do with the mechanics of human movement

Biomedicine Human being viewed as an organism made up of organ subsystems and physiological processes

Bipolar Disorder Mood disorder characterized by a combination of manic and depressive symptoms

Blocked Practice Rote schedule of practice that involves repetitive practice of one task before the next task is introduced

Blood Pressure (BP) Force exerted by the circulating blood against the walls of the arteries, veins, and chambers of the heart

Bronchopulmonary Dysplasia Chronic lung disease secondary to a prolonged use of mechanical oxygen administration in prematurity; effects usually outgrown by second year of life

Bulimia Nervosa Eating disorder consisting of binge eating followed by self-induced vomiting or use of laxatives; excessive exercising or fasting to compensate for the binge

Care Giving Nurturing the well-being of others

Case Manager Person who coordinates the delivery of services

Caudal Pertaining to the tail, lower, more distal

Cerebral Palsy (CP) A motor function disorder caused by a permanent, nonprogressive brain lesion or defect

Cerebrovascular Accident (CVA) An interruption of the blood supply that causes injury to the brain, resulting in neurological deficits in a specific area; also called stroke

Certified Driver Rehabilitation Specialist (CDRS) Certification credential that denotes competency in driver rehabilitation, professional ethics, and standards of practice

Childrearing Nuturing the well-being of minors

Chronic Pain Discomfort that persists for extended periods of time (e.g., months or years), accompanies a disease or associated with an injury that has not resolved within the expected period of time

Chronic Strain Stressors extended through time; may have more detrimental effects on health than intermittent stressors

Classical or Respondent Conditioning Learning in which behaviors formed by natural selection; can be elicited by new stimuli because of association

Client-Collaboration/Client-Centered Approach to treatment that demonstrates respect for and partnership with the individual or group receiving the service

Clinical Reasoning Complex multifaceted cognitive process used by practitioners to plan, direct, perform, and reflect on intervention

Clubhouse Model Rehabilitation program for people with disabilities associated with persistent mental illness; provides voluntary, lifelong membership organized around a work-ordered day in which members and staff work collaboratively with one another

Cognitive Behavioral Model Intervention approach based on the theory that individuals can make behavioral changes by changing ways of thinking, point of view, and interpretation of events

Cognitive Disability Global loss of mental ability across diagnostic categories; interferes with task behavior

Cognitive Triad Describes individuals' beliefs about themselves, the world, and the future; these cognitive appraisals affect mood and behavior

Cogwheel Tigidity Tremor superimposed on rigidity causing alternate contraction and relaxation throughout joint range of motion

Collaboration To work together in a joint effort; to cooperate reasonably

Collective Variables Fewest number of variables that completely describe a behavior

Communication and Interaction Skills Observable acts or processes that convey intentions and needs and coordinate social behavior during interactions with others

Community Mobility Being able to travel within one's own environment

Community-Based Practice Intervention strategy emphasizing delivery of services in locations within person's local places or environments of community living

Community-Centered Approach emphasizing the community as a recipient of intervention and a focus on accessibility and acceptance within physical, social, and cultural environments

Comorbidity Coexistence of two or more disease processes

Compensation The use of alternate body parts or functions to substitute for weak, painful, or missing abilities

Conduct Disorder (CD) A disruptive disorder characterized by repetitive and persistent patterns of behavior in which the basic rights of others or societal norms or rules are violated

Congenital Heart Defect Impairment of the heart and/or the large arteries and veins that is present at birth

Constant Practice Motor control concept referring to practicing the same movement task in the same way for every trial, no variations in task conditions

Consultation Relationship in which a consultant shares expertise that will assist the consultee in reaching programmatic goals

Contemporary Task-Oriented Approach Interventions based on a systems model of motor control and influenced by contemporary developmental and motor learning theories

Content Responses Verbalizations that clarify information and meaning

Context Aspects of the environment that influence performance, including cultural, physical, virtual, and social aspects, as well as individual characteristics such as spiritual and temporal factors

Contextual Interference Motor control principle about practice of multiple tasks in a random or nonsystematic but repetitive way that results in depressed performance but greater retention and transfer

Contextual Model Development viewed within a web of relations interwoven to form the fabric of meaning; mutual involvement of person in his or her social, physical, cultural, personal, spiritual, temporal, and virtual world

Continuum of Care Array of health-care services that are available to individuals based on acuity and level of disability

Contractures Tightening of muscles, tendons, ligaments, or skin that can interfere with normal joint movement

Control Parameters Motor control variables that shift a movement from one form to another movement form; act to reorganize the system

Coordination Combined activity of many muscles into smooth patterns and sequences of motion

Core Schemas Ways of understanding the world and the self that are built up over many years, not available to introspection, resistant to change

Create Interventions Approaches that focus on providing enriched contextual and task experiences; designed to enhance performance for all persons (not just persons with identified disabilities) in the natural contexts of life

Cultural Myth Unfounded or poorly founded belief about a human group, given uncritical acceptance by members of another group that operates in support of existing or traditional practices and institutions

Cultural Stereotype Mental picture based on myth that leads people to associate a characteristic or set of characteristics with a particular group of others

Cystic Fibrosis Genetic disorder of the exocrine glands resulting in hyperviscous secretions that may effect the respiratory, gastrointestinal, and reproductive systems

Declarative Memory Cognitive activity that forms the basis for conscious recollections of facts and events
Dependence Inability to perform an activity by oneself
Developmental Disability (DD) Atypical neurodevelopment that is not specific to one body system, with the onset occurring prenatally, perinatally, or in early childhood
Developmental Dyspraxia Difficulty with the planning and execution of movement patterns of a skilled or nonhabitual nature, originating in childhood
Difficulty The perceived effort required to accomplish an activity; something not easily done
Disability Activity limitation as a result of mental or physical impairment
Disease Disorder with signs and symptoms indicating abnormality of function of the organism
Distributed Models of Motor Control Descriptions where movement control is seen as a function of many working systems; can include different body systems and/or any person, task, and environmental factor
Distributed Practice Practice of task or movement interspersed with more time between the practice sessions
Down Syndrome Most common diagnosable form of developmental disability resulting from an additional chromosome 21
Duration Time needed to complete an activity
Dynamic Pattern Theory Operational approach to the study of coordinated movement used in the movement sciences
Dynamic Splint Device composed of a molded splint base, separate loops or supports, and a component that generates force such as a rubber band or that enhances or limits motion with a moving part such as a hinge
Dynamical Theory, Dynamical Action Theory (Synergetics) View of phenomenon derived from the study of how parts of systems work together; has been applied to development and motor control theories; presumes processes are nonlinear and variable, influenced by the demands, opportunities, and constraints imposed by the environment and by the capacity of the individual to respond flexibly to periods of disorganization
Dysfunction in Sensory Integration (DSI) Inability to modulate, discriminate, coordinate, or organize sensations adaptively
Dysphagia Difficulty in swallowing
Dysthymic Disorder (DD) Persistent, long-term change in mood that is less intense but more chronic than major depressive disorder and characterized by withdrawal, viewing issues as overwhelming, interacting less with others, and developing behavioral problems
Ecological Systems Analysis Integrative perspective of the individual, the interpersonal relationships, and the environment
Ecological Theory Explores the interaction between the motor (action) system and goal-directed behavior
Ecology Interaction between a person and the context or environment
Electronic Aids for Daily Living (EADL) Technological equipment used by individuals with disabilities to perform activities
Emotional Functions Relate to feelings and affective components of the mind
Emotional Maltreatment Withholding of affection as well as chronic humiliation, threatening, or criticism
Emotionally Disturbed (ED) Disability category within the Individuals with Disabilities Education Act in which students special needs are primarily of a psychosocial nature; formally called seriously emotionally disturbed (SED)
Empathy An attitude exemplified by an understanding of the feelings and perspectives of another person
Enabling Activities Therapy exercises or drills that require client involvement but are not activities typically used in the culture
Endocrine System Hormonal system
Endurance Ability to sustain a given activity over time, related to cardiopulmonary, biomechanical, and neuromuscular function
Energy and Drive Functions Psychological or physiological mechanisms that cause a person to attempt to satisfy certain needs and goals in a persistent
Enfolded Occupations Co-occur in time and/or space within the daily routine by design or default
Entry-Level Practitioner A person prepared to begin generalist practice with less than 1 year of professional experience
Ergonomics Applied science of adapting the environment and task to the worker
Essential Functions Capacities a person needs to perform job duties unaided or with reasonable accommodation
Establish and Restore Interventions Approaches to intervention that target the persons skills and abilities resulting in new or recovered functions
Ethnicity Socially constructed and potentially dynamic group membership based on subjective belief in common descent because of similarities of physical type or of customs or of both, may be self-selected or imposed from outside the group
Evaluation Ongoing process of collecting and interpreting the data necessary for intervention planning, intervention modification, and discharge planning
Evidence-Based Practice A systematic process of using research to support clinical reasoning and practice decisions
Exacerbation A woesening of a health condition or flare-up of symptoms
Experience Direct participation in an activity over time
Explanatory Models Personal accounts of illness, held by both practitioners and professionals, that describe the nature and origins of the problem and what can be done about it
Extrinsic Feedback Augmented information from an external source, can supplement intrinsic information

feedback; two forms are knowledge of results and knowledge of performance

Facilitation Enhancement or reinforcement of any action or function so that it is produced with increased efficiency and ease

Fairness in Testing Being treated in an equitable manner with respect to the context and the purpose of testing; sources of bias should be identified and eliminated

Family A group of people living together or in close contact who care for each other and their dependent members

Family-Centered Philosophy of service provision recognizing that families are the primary social context in which individuals live and receive care and that intervention is based on the family's goals and values

Fatigue Discomfort or sensation of tiredness, weariness, or exhaustion experienced during or following activity performance

Feedback Information that the learner receives about performance; critical for learning

Fetal Alcohol Syndrome (FAS) Condition characterized by significant developmental delays and physical problems resulting from the mother's excessive consumption of alcohol during pregnancy

Form of Occupation Aspects of Occupation that are directly observable

Formal Theory Explanation of observable events or relationships by stating a series of abstract propositions or principles

Fragile X Inherited, X-linked disorder affecting the production of a specific protein (FMRA) essential to early brain development, results in developmental disabilities

Frame of Reference Way of conceptualizing and carrying out practice

Free Appropriate Public Education (FAPE) Special education and related services provided at public expense that meet the standards of the state education agency

Function of Occupation Ways occupation influences development, adaptation, health, well-being, and quality of life

Functional Capacity Evaluation (FCE) Comprehensive battery of tests that yields objective measures regarding clients' current levels of function and their abilities to perform work-related tasks

Gemeinschaft Characterization of the relationships between individuals in community that are private and based on shared interests with kin or family, neighborhoods, and groups of friends

General Adaptation Response General or universal three-stage reaction to stress, alarm, adaptation, and exhaustion; involves both neurological and endocrine reactions

Generalize Ability to use skills or knowledge gained in one situation and appropriately apply them to other situations

Gesellshaft Characterization of social actions in a community that are public expressions or responses to a duty or to an organization within society

Goniometer Instrument used to measure joint range of motion

Grade Sequentially increase or decrease the demands of an activity over time to stimulate improvement in the client's function or respond to diminishing functional capacity

Group Dynamics Overt and covert patterns as well as relationships between the occupation or task, the individual, the group, and the environment

Group Phases Theoretical, predictable, periods in the life cycle of a group

Group Process Ways in which the work of small and large groups are carried out, including interactions between members, decisions, and task accomplishment

Guided Imagery Use of imagination to create relaxation or desired mental set

Guided Practice Physical guidance of the learner through the task as compared to unguided practice; may be useful to acquaint the performer with the requirements of the task

Guillain-Barré Syndrome Inflammatory disease affecting peripheral nerves

Gustation Oral activities related to taste, salivation trigger, and swallowing

Habit Training Treatment program used in by early occupational therapists that provided structured engagement in occupation for the seriously mentally ill

Habits Automatic behavior that is integrated into more complex patterns that enable people to function on a day-to-day basis; skills that are habituated are typically performed easily and with little effort

Habituation Process whereby doing is organized into patterns and routines

Health Behaviors Personal routines and behaviors that may mitigate or exacerbate the effect of stress on health

Hearing Ability to respond to, recognize, and localize auditory stimulation and the acuity of these processes

Here and Now Spontaneous action that focuses on the present

Hierarchical Model Linear model that presume a series of predictable series or steps in a process; commonly applied to motor control (the control of movement as organized hierarchically from the lowest levels in the spinal cord, to intermediate levels in the brainstem, to the highest levels in the cortex) and development in which normal development occurs in a predictable series of steps, directly related to changes in central nervous system development

Holism The view that humans are not divisible into mind and body, or form and function but rather, are agents whose activities are inexplicably linked to their own context

Home Maintainer Person who has responsibility, at least once a week, for home management tasks

Human Ecology The interaction between a person and the context

Humanistic Philosophical stance focusing on concern with human beings and their values, capacities, and achievements

Hydrocephalus Abnormal accumulation of cerebrospinal fluid in the brain ventricles; occurs when there is an imbalance between the amount of cerebrospinal fluid produced and the amount absorbed

Hypertonia Excessive muscle tone or tension resulting in slow, rigid movements and sometimes limited range of movement

Hypogonadism Underdevelopment of sexual organs and functions due to hormonal deficiency; results in failure to go through puberty naturally

Hypopituitarism A general term that refers to any under function of the pituitary gland

Hypothesis Explanation that accounts for a set of facts and that can be tested

Hypotonia Low muscle tone, floppiness, or lack of tension in muscles when a body part is moved; hyperextensibility; hyporesponsiveness to sensory stimulation

Illness Experience The meaning an individual attaches to an illness, may vary from one person to another with same diagnosis

Illness Impairment of an individual's ability to function on a day-to-day basis secondary to a disease process; also refers to the perspective of the individual versus the perspective of the physician

Impairment A deviation or loss due to problems with body structures or function (physiological or psychological)

Independence Ability to perform an activity by oneself

Independent Living Movement Organized approach by those with disability that incorporates ideas about managing personal life, participating in community life, fulfilling social roles, sustaining self-determination, and minimizing physical or psychological dependence on others

Individualized Education Program (IEP) Written plan of educationally related annual goals, objectives, strategies, and time lines to enable children with disabilities (3–21 years) to be educated in the least restrictive environment; mandated by law in the United States

Individualized Family Service Plan (IFSP) Family-centered plan written with specific outcomes and objectives outlining a family's and child's service needs in early intervention; mandated by law in the United States

Information Exchange The giving and receiving of information

Information Processing A cognitive process mediated by the brain, with the brain interpreting and relating external sensory impressions and internally stored concepts with each other and events

Intentionality A quality of behavior that consists of being oriented to or about something rather than being accidental, aimless, or random

Interviewing A shared verbal experience, jointly constructed by the interviewer and the interviewee, organized around the asking and answering of questions

Intrinsic Feedback Information gathered through the individual's available sensory avenues; the inherent sensory information from the sensory receptors during or after movement

Job Site Analysis (JSA) Assessment used to define the essential demands of a job

Knowledge of Performance (KP) Verbal postaction information feedback about the correctness of the movement pattern that the learner makes, part of motor control approaches

Knowledge of Results (KR) Verbal, terminal postaction information feedback about the movement outcome in terms of the environmental goal, part of motor control approaches

Kyphoscoliosis Abnormal convex and lateral curvature of the spinal column

Lead Pipe Rigidity Feeling of constant resistance throughout the available range of motion

Learned Helplessness A perceived loss of control, leading to dependence on others, that persists beyond the actual need for assistance

Learning A relatively permanent change in behavior or the capacity for responding resulting from practice and experience; persists with time; resists environmental changes; can be generalized in response to new tasks and situations

Learning Disabilities (LD) Describes a number of neurologically based deficits related to interpreting visual or auditory information and/or the ability to link information from different parts of the brain; typically impede academic performance in areas such as reading, writing and math

Least Restrictive Environment (LRE) The environment that provides maximum interaction with nondisabled peers consistent with the needs of the child; term associated with the Individuals with Disabilities Education Act

Lifestyle Redesign A therapeutic program that promotes people's abilities to control their lives and promote their health through the development of a customized routine of occupations

Liminal The period of time between one status and another; typically occurs during rites of passage

Major Depressive Disorder (MDD) Disorder in which there is at least a 2-week period of pervasive change in mood characterized by either depressed or irritable mood and/or loss of interest and pleasure

Major Life Events Positive or negative changes that occur in an individual's life, such as marriage, bereavement, a near fatal assault, or injury; may be stressful and result in life change

Manual Propulsion Wheelchair A wheelchair that requires the user to use muscle power to move it

Massed Practice Motor control strategy involving continuous practice with no rest periods or practice sessions; practice time is more than the time for rest between practices

Meaning of Occupation The significance of occupation within the context of real lives and the culture

Measurement Process of assigning numbers to represent quantities of a trait, attribute, or characteristic, to classify objects

Mechanistic The belief that all phenomena can be explained by analysis of parts of the whole and how parts relate to the whole

Medical Model Approach based on rational inquiry and scientific method that focuses on the identification and treatment of diseases and injuries

Memory Processes by which knowledge acquired is encoded, stored, and later retrieved

Mental Practice Performing or running through the activity in one's mind without accompanying physical practice

Mental-Hygiene Movement A social reform movement in the early 1900s promoting public health initiatives to reform care for the mentally ill

Meta-Cognitive The process of thinking or reflecting on one's own thinking

Meta-Evaluation Method of analyzing research in a topic area by grouping a variety of studies together in a meaningful way

Microtrauma Slight injury or lesion

Modify (Adapt) Approaches to interventions that revise the current context or task demands to support performance in the natural setting; also refers to ability to modulate, discriminate, coordinate, or organize sensations adaptively

Moral Treatment Nineteenth-century humanitarian approach to treatment of individuals with mental illness that centered around productive, creative, and recreational occupations

Motor Control Ability to regulate or direct the mechanisms essential to movement

Motor Cearning Set of processes associated with practice or experience leading to permanent changes in the capability for skilled acts

Motor Planning Ability to plan and execute skilled, nonhabitual motor activity

Motor Programming Models of movement control depend on a motor program, such as a central pattern generator or an abstract code in the system, that allows a movement to be carried out by any effector system

Motor Relearning Synthesis of the prevalent contemporary models of motor control and the motor learning process

Multiple Sclerosis Neurological disease in which nerves are demyelinized and axons transected by immune responses; characterized by periods of remission and exacerbation

Muscle Strength Ability to produce movement or to resist an external force

Muscle Tone Continuous mild contraction of the muscle tissue in its resting state, resistance to stretch

Narrative Account from the person's point of view expressed in the form of a story, presenting information in the form of a story

Neglect Endangering the health of another by withholding nutrition, shelter, clothing, medical care

Neural Tube Defect (NTD) Birth defects that involve incomplete development of the brain, spinal cord, and/or protective coverings for these organs, includes these three conditions: anencephaly, encephalocele, and spina bifida

Neurodevelopmental Treatment Strategies to inhibit abnormal movement patterns, normalize muscle tone, and promote more normal movement patterns in individuals with neurologically based movement problems

Nondeclarative Memory Information acquired during skill learning (motor skills, perceptual skills, and cognitive skills), habit formation, simple classical conditioning, priming, and other knowledge expressed through performance

Occupation Daily activities that reflect cultural values, provide structure to living, and meaning to individuals; these activities meet human needs for self-care, enjoyment, and participation in society

Occupational Behavior Characterization of how development over the life course, habits, and roles relate to competence in occupational performance

Occupational Choice Process through which persons select and commit themselves to occupational roles

Occupational Competence Degree to which one is able to sustain a pattern of doing that enacts one's occupational identity over time

Occupational Environment Context in which occupation occurs

Occupational Identity Cumulative sense of who one is and wishes to become as an occupational being generated from one's occupational history

Occupational Justice A critical perspective of social structures that promotes social, political, and economic changes to enable people to meet their occupational potential and experience well-being

Occupational Profile Understanding of the client's occupational history, patterns of daily living, interests, values, and needs; synthesized understanding of client's problems and concerns about engaging in occupation to identify client's priorities

Occupational Role Social expectations and behavioral enactment of activities and routines by individuals

Occupational Science Academic discipline of the social sciences aimed at producing a body of knowledge on occupation through theory generation, and systematic, disciplined methods of inquiry

Occupational Therapist A graduate of an accredited occupational therapy program who has completed fieldwork and passed the certification examination administered by the National Board for Certification of Occupation Therapy; also referred to an certified occupational therapist or registered occupational therapist (OTR)

Occupational Therapy Aide An individual assigned by a certified occupational therapist to perform delegated, selected, skilled tasks in specific situations under intense close supervision by occupational therapy practitioners

Occupational Therapy Assistant (OTA) An individual who has graduated from an accredited occupational therapy assistant program (OTA) and who has been certified by the National Board for Certification of Occupational Therapy; also referred to as a certified occupational therapy assistant (COTA)

Occupational Therapy Practitioners Occupational therapists and occupational therapy assistants

Oculomotor Control Coordination of eye movements

Olfaction Ability to detect, identify various odors, to smell

Operant Conditioning Form of learning in which behaviors increase or decrease in frequency of occurrence based on the consequences of performing them for the organism

Operational Definition Precise meaning of a term, provides guidelines for performance and measurement

Opportunistic Infection Infection that occurs in people whose resistance is lowered by other diseases or drugs

Oppositional Defiant Disorder (ODD) Disruptive disorder involving recurrent patterns of negativistic, defiant, disobedient, and hostile behavior toward authority figures

Orientation Awareness of self in relation to time, place, and identification of others

Orthotic Device Relatively permanent device worn to substitute for impaired or lost muscle function

Pain Unpleasant sensory and emotional experience associated with actual or potential tissue damage

Pain Interference The effect of pain on mood and occupational engagement

Paradigm An example or model, a way of thinking about phenomenon

Parallel-Distributed Processing (PDP) Theory of motor control describing how the nervous system as a network processes information for action

Paraphrasing Repetition of another's verbalizations using similar or related words to clarify meaning

Parkinson Disease (PD) Chronic progressive neurological disease characterized by tremor, muscle rigidity, and slowed movement patterns

Part Practice The practice of a movement that is separated into practice of the component parts and not the movement task in its entirety

Passive Range of Motion (PROM) Arc of motion through which the joint passes when moved by an outside force

Perception Mental process involving recognizing and meaningfully interpreting sensory information

Performance Capacity Underlying objective mental and physical abilities; also lived experiences that shape performance

Performance Discrepancy Performance problems that occur when performance demands exceed a person's capacities

Performance Skills People's capacities and effectiveness, related to observable elements of an action

Perseveration Persistent repetition of behaviors

Personal Causation Beliefs held by a person regarding his or her ability to influence others and the environment

Personality Set of mental characteristics that make a person unique

Personal Theory Private understandings based on experience

Pervasive Developmental Disorders (PDD) Broad classification of conditions in which serious socialization problems are the defining feature; these disorders are characterized by patterns of delay and deviance in the development of social, communicative, and cognitive skills

Physical Abuse Punching, shaking, kicking, biting, throwing, burning, and other forms of injurious punishment

Physical Capacity Evaluation (PCE) Assesses the physical and biomechanical aspects of the client's level of function, including active range of motion, muscle strength, posture, gait, sensation, and cardiopulmonary status

Physicality Using the body to communicate with others

PL 101–476 1990 Individuals with Disabilities Act (IDEA) Law reauthorizing educational services for children with disabilities from 3 to 21 years in the United States; the Individualized Education Plan may include transition and assistive technology services

PL 102–119 IDEA Amendments Reauthorization of early intervention laws; established Federal Interagency Coordinating Council in the United States

PL 94–142 1975 Education for All Handicapped Children Act (EHA) Law mandating free and appropriate education in the least restrictive environment for all children with "handicaps," ages 5 through 21 years in the United States

PL 99–457 1986 amendment to the Education for All Handicapped Children Act creating programs for preschoolers (3–5 years) with handicaps, including early intervention for infants and toddlers (birth to 2 years) in the United States

Play and Leisure Activities Intrinsically motivating activities that provide pleasure, relaxation, and expression of creativity

Play and Leisure Participation The client's engagement inactivities that provide pleasure, relaxation, and expression of creativity that are typically expected of and available to other people of the same age and culture in home, school, work, and community settings

Population Group that shares a specific set of characteristics or criteria; in research, denotes group of concern to researcher

Postural Adaptation Ability of the body to maintain balance automatically and remain upright during alterations in position and challenges to stability

Postural Symmetry Alignment of both sides of the body

Powered Wheelchair A wheelchair that is propelled by a motor

Predriving Assessment Assessing an individual's abilities related to operating a motor vehicle; determines the appropriateness of an on-the-road practicum

Preparatory Methods Intervention techniques focused on client factors and designed to help the client function more effectively in targeted activities

Present Levels of Educational Performance Information from the special education evaluation results that describe the student's school performance; includes how the student's disability affects involvement and progress in the general education curriculum

Pressure-Reducing Cushions Seating pads or systems designed to minimize pressure on bony prominences and/or to distribute body weight evenly

Prevent Interventions Approaches designed to avoid or minimize the occurrence or evolution of barriers to occupational performance; may be aimed at client, context, or activity variables

Profession Form of paid employment distinguished by its service to the public through schooled application of a specialized knowledge base and skill

Program Manager A person who coordinates, directs, and controls all aspects of an identified health service

Progressive Muscle Relaxation Systematic program of tensing and relaxing the major muscle groups

Proprioceptive Processing Interpretation of sensations generated from active movements of the muscles and joints, which provide feedback about the spatial orientation of the body, the rate and timing of movements, the amount of muscle force being exerted, and how fast and how much a muscle is being stretched

Prospective Payment System (PPS) System to pay for Medicare services based on criteria set by the government

Prosthesis Device that substitutes for a lost body part

Public Health System of services dealing with the protection and improvement of community health through organized efforts of preventive medicine, as well as environmental and social sciences

Purposeful Activity Therapeutic activity that is selected by the practitioner because it is generally congruent with the client's interests and promotes specific outcomes

Purposiveness Quality of occupational behavior that consists of being able to organize and execute multiple actions in accord with some goal or purpose

Qualitative Research Systematic investigation that seeks to understand phenomena using natural settings as sources for data gathered through observation, interviews, and examination of artifacts

Quality of Life Comparative state of well-being and functioning that includes level of comfort, enjoyment, and ability to participate in meaningful activities or occupations

Quantitative Research Use of numerical data under standardized conditions to answer research questions and hypotheses

Random Practice A schedule of practice that involves nonsystematic but repetitive practice of the same set of tasks

Range of Motion (ROM) Arc of motion through which a joint passes

Reasonable Accommodation Modification or adjustment that enables persons with disabilities to perform a job or task they are otherwise qualified to perform

Reductionistic Reduction of complex phenomenon to component parts to simple terms; oversimplification

Reflex Involuntary, stereotyped response to a particular stimulus

Reflex Model of Motor Control Theory that considers reflexes as the basis of all movements

Reinforcement An event that follows a behavior and that increases the likelihood that the behavior will be repeated; reinforcers can be either social or tangible; associated with operant conditioning

Related Services Term used in special education to refer to transportation and such developmental, corrective, and other supportive services (including speech-language, audiology, psychological, and physical and occupational therapy services) needed to help children learn in school

Relations The maintenance of appropriate relationships within an occupation

Relative Mastery A state that includes the properties of efficiency, effectiveness, and satisfaction to self and society

Reliability The degree to which errors in measurement are minimized, resulting in similar findings from repeated measures

Remission Reduction or disappearance of symptoms

Representational Learning Development of an internal image of an event or task so that an action or a series of actions can be repeated without reference to directions

Rigidity Simultaneous increase of muscle tone in agonistic and antagonistic muscles resulting in increased resistance to passive movement in any direction throughout the ROM

Risk Factors Characteristics associated with individuals that may include demographic variables, behavioral risk factors, and environmental factors that may interfere with positive growth and development or well-being

Roles Behavioral expectations that accompany a person's occupied position or status in a social system

Sample Subset of the population selected to participate in a research study

Satisfaction Experience of pleasure and contentment with one's performance

Schema (pl. Schemata) Complex cognitive representations of phenomena; a way the brain organizes information; also called chunks

Scope of Practice The domain of concern for a profession delimiting its range of interest

Screening Cursory evaluation to determine if a more thorough evaluation is needed

Sensation The transmission to the brain of nerve impulses cause by stimulation of a sensory receptor site; results in awareness of that stimulation

Sensory Discrimination Dysfunction Problem in the organization and interpretation of the temporal and spatial characteristics of sensory stimuli

Sensory Integration Organization of sensations to form perceptions, behaviors, and to learn; a neurological process and a theory of the relationship between the neural organization of sensory processing and behavior

Sensory Modulation Dysfunction (SMD) Problem in the capacity to regulate and organize the degree, intensity, and nature of response to sensory input in a graded and adaptive manner

Sensory Reeducation Techniques used to teach people with peripheral nerve injuries how to interpret and make functional use of the abnormal impulses injured nerves relay to the brain

Service Competency The process of demonstrating that comparable results are achieved by two or more people performing the same task; often used in reference to assuring appropriate delegation of tasks by occupational therapists to occupational therapy assistants

Services on Behalf of the Child Includes supports for parents and school personnel that can included specialized training that helps them to work with the child more effectively

Settlement House Movement A social reform movement in the early 1900s that established urban centers of art, music, drama, and writing for immigrants and disenfranchised persons

Sexual Abuse Any seduction, coercion, or forcing to observe or participate in sexual activity for the sexual gratification of a more powerful individual

Skills Training Practice model focusing on the acquisition of daily living skills

Social Support Presence of individuals or groups who buffer the negative effects of stress on health via emotional and practical help

Socialization Acquisition of roles, attitudes, and behaviors consistent with the norms of the social group

Societal Standards Normative expectations of a society

Socioeconomic Status Occupational, educational, and income achievements by individuals or groups

Socioemotional Factors Client factors that relate to socioemotional health, such as temperament and personality, energy and drive, and emotional functions

Spasticity Excessive tone in a muscle, typically caused by an upper motor neuron lesion

Special Education Specially designed instruction to meet the unique needs of children with disabilities

Specially Designed Instruction Individualized instruction to meet the unique needs of a student to receive free and appropriate public education in the least restrictive environment

Spina Bifida Neural tube defect in which the spine is cleft or split because the vertebrae do not enclose the spinal cord during the first month of pregnancy; ranges in severity, resulting in varying levels of paralysis and other neurodevelopmental problems

Spinal Cord Injury Impairment of the spinal cord that results in partial or complete paralysis and sensory impairment below the level of the lesion

Spirituality Fundamental orientation of a person's life, that which inspires and motivates the individual

Splint Temporary device used to facilitate recovery from an injury or to enhance function

Standardized Assessments Assessment procedures in which processes are clearly identified, along with guidelines for interpretation of results; may have established and tested normative data with which to compare results

Static Progressive Splint Removable device similar to a dynamic splint with a molded base, outrigger, finger loops and method to apply static force to a joint

Static Serial Splint Molded device worn continually or nearly continually supporting contracted tissue in a static position at the end of its available range; frequently remolded or replaced to accommodate gains in range of motion

Static Splint A molded device that has no moving parts and is designed to support tissue, usually of the upper extremity, in a desired position

Strengths Model A model of intensive case management for people with psychiatric disabilities; emphasizes personal assets and takes advantage of naturally occurring community supports

Stress Physical, emotional, or intellectual strain or tension disturbing normal equilibrium

Supervision Dynamic interactive process in which the supervisor assists in and directs the work and growth of the supervisee

Supplemental Aids and Services Aids and services, in addition to specially designed instruction or related services, provided for a student to receive free and appropriate public education in the least restrictive environment

Tactile Processing Processing of touch through the discriminatory and protective tactile systems

Target Focus of prevention or intervention

Task-Oriented Model Theory of movement that assumes that control of movement is organized around goal directed functional tasks

Task-Oriented Theories Explain motor control by identifying what problems the central nervous system has to solve to accomplish a motor task

Teleology Human capacities to foresee and plan over time for an anticipated future goal

Temperament Constitutional disposition of a person that encourages him or her to react to situations in a particular way

Therapeutic Intervention Collaboration between the person, the family, and the occupational therapy practitioner

There and Then Reflection and exploration of meanings based on past experiences, usually familial in origin

Thinking Errors Familiar but erroneous ways of interpreting events in the environment

Tone Management Therapeutic positioning and handling strategies designed to normalize muscle tone in people with spasticity

Tracheostomy Surgery to open an area in the windpipe to facilitate breathing

Training Occurs when performers are provided with the solutions to problems rather than actively solving the problem

Transactional Relationship An interaction in which both the person and environment dynamically define and transform each other over time as components of a unitary whole

Transfer of Learning The ability to use something that has been learned in a different situation; also known as generalization

Transient Ischemic Attack (TIA) Temporary loss of blood flow to an area of the brain

Traumatic Brain Injury (TBI) Damage to the brain because of a car accident, fall, gunshot wound, or other trauma

Triangulation Use of multiple methods to observe, measure, describe, or analyze phenomenon

Trustworthiness Logic of justification concerned with the truth-value, transferability, dependability, and neutrality of qualitative research

Unconditional Positive Regard Attitude of nonjudgmental acceptance toward others

Universal Design Design of environments and products to be usable by all people, to the greatest extent possible, without the need for special arrangements or adaptations

Universal Precautions Standard set of procedures used with all clients to prevent transmission of infectious diseases

Useful Field of View Measure that reflects decline in visual sensory function, slowed visual processing speed, and impaired visual attention skills

Validity Psychometric property that is concerned with the capacity of the measurement instrument to measure what it is supposed to measure

Values Beliefs and commitments that define what is good, right, and important

Varying Practice Motor control strategy that involves alteration of the conditions of the movement task across practice trials

Vestibular System Structures of the inner ear associated with balance and position sense

Vicarious Learning Learning of a behavior or of an association based on the observation of others performing the behavior

Vision Ability to see; involves light perception, conjugate movement, visual field, visual activity, visual range of motion

Visual Perception Cognitive process of obtaining and interpreting visual stimuli from the environment and includes visual discrimination, memory, spatial relations, form constancy, figure-ground, and visual closure

Visual Motor Integration The ability of the eyes & hands to work together in smoothly coordinated patterns

Volition Process by which persons are motivated toward and choose what they do

Wellness Actions that lead to a healthy lifestyle; includes nutrition, exercise, stress reduction, and other strategies

Whole Practice Practice of an entire movement and not its component parts

Work Hardening A structured, goal-oriented rehabilitation program designed to return individuals to work

Work Simplification Performance of a task in a planned and orderly way, so that body motions, workload, and fatigue are reduced to a minimum

Xenophobia An unreasonable fear or hatred of those different from oneself

INDEX

Page numbers followed by *f* indicate figures.
Those followed by *t* indicate tables.

C

Q

R

T